MAYES' MIDWIFERY

For Baillière Tindall:

Senior Commissioning Editor: Mary Seager
Project Development Manager: Mairi McCubbin
Project Manager: Derek Robertson
Designer: Judith Wright
Illustrations Manager: Bruce Hogarth

MAYES' MIDWIFERY

A TEXTBOOK FOR MIDWIVES

Thirteenth edition

Christine Henderson MA MTD DPHE DipN RN RM

Research Fellow, School of Health Sciences, University of Birmingham, Birmingham, UK;
Editor, British Journal of Midwifery

Sue Macdonald MSc PGCEA ADM RM RN ILTM FETC

Education and Research Manager, Royal College of Midwives, London, UK;
Formerly Principal Lecturer, Midwifery, Middlesex University, London, UK

Foreword by
Dame Karlene Davis DBE
General Secretary, Royal College of Midwives, London, UK

Baillière Tindall

EDINBURGH   LONDON   NEW YORK   OXFORD   PHILADELPHIA   ST LOUIS   SYDNEY   TORONTO   2004

BAILLIÈRE TINDALL
An imprint of Elsevier Limited

© Baillière Tindall 1997
© Harcourt Publishers Limited 1999
© Elsevier Science Limited 2003. All rights reserved.
© 2004, Elsevier Limited. All rights reserved.

Twelfth edition 1997
Thirteenth edition 2004

ISBN 0 7020 2616 6

British Library Cataloguing in Publication Data
A catalogue record for this book is available from the British Library

Library of Congress Cataloging in Publication Data
A catalog record for this book is available from the Library of Congress

Notice
Knowledge and best practice in this field are constantly changing. As new research and experience broaden our knowledge, changes in practice, treatment and drug therapy may become necessary or appropriate. Readers are advised to check the most current information provided (i) on procedures featured or (ii) by the manufacturer of each product to be administered, to verify the recommended dose or formula, the method and duration of administration, and contraindications. It is the responsibility of the practitioner, relying on their own experience and knowledge of the patient, to make diagnoses, to determine dosages and the best treatment for each individual patient, and to take all appropriate safety precautions. To the fullest extent of the law, neither the publisher nor the editors or authors assumes any liability for any injury and/or damage.

The Publisher

The
Publisher's
policy is to use
paper manufactured
from sustainable forests

Printed in China

Contents

Contributors vii
Foreword xi
Preface xiii
Acknowledgements xiv

PART 1
THE CONTEXT OF CHILDBIRTH 1

1. Sociological and Cultural Context 3
2. Psychological Context 14
3. Grief and Bereavement 27
4. Evidence-based Practice 48

PART 2
SEXUALITY, FERTILITY AND CONCEPTION 63

5. Anatomy of Male and Female Reproduction 65
6. Female Reproductive Physiology 89
7. Sexuality 105
8. Fertility and its Control 114
9. Infertility and Assisted Conception 129
10. Preconception Care 143

PART 3
PREGNANCY 159

11. Fertilization 161
12. Genetics 172
13. Implantation and Development of the Placenta 190
14. Embryonic and Fetal Development 205
15. The Fetal Skull 220
16. Confirming Pregnancy and Care of the Pregnant Woman 235
17. Maternal and Fetal Physiological Responses to Pregnancy 288

18. Antenatal Investigations 312
19. Maternal Nutrition 327
20. Complementary Therapies in Childbearing 338
21. Health Promotion in Midwifery 355
22. Education for Parenthood 371
23. Physical Preparation before Childbirth 383

PART 4
LABOUR AND DELIVERY 399

24. Place of Birth 401
25. Physiological Changes in Labour 410
26. Care in the First Stage of Labour 428
27. Relief of Pain During Labour 458
28. The Pelvic Floor 476
29. Care in the Second Stage of Labour 492
30. Care in the Third Stage of Labour 507

PART 5
THE NEWBORN BABY 525

31. Physiology, Assessment and Care 527
32. Thermoregulation 573
33. Infant Feeding 591
34. The Preterm Baby and the Small Baby 628
35. Respiratory and Cardiac Disorders 649
36. Congenital Anomalies, Fetal and Neonatal Surgery, and Pain 670
37. Neonatal Jaundice 684
38. Metabolic and Endocrine Disorders 696
39. Infection 703
40. Sudden Infant Death Syndrome 715

PART 6

THE PUERPERIUM 721

41. Content and Organization of Postnatal Care 723

42. Morbidity Following Childbirth 736

PART 7

CONDITIONS AND COMPLICATIONS OF CHILDBIRTH 749

43. Nausea and Vomiting 751

44. Bleeding in Pregnancy 758

45. Hypertensive Disorders of Pregnancy 780

46. Medical Disorders of Pregnancy 793

47. Sexually Transmitted Diseases 815

48. Abnormalities of the Genital Tract 829

49. Multiple Pregnancy 839

50. Preterm Labour 853

51. Induction of Labour and Post-term Pregnancy 862

52. Disordered Uterine Action 876

53. Malpositions and Malpresentations 884

54. Mental Health Problems 918

PART 8

OBSTETRIC EMERGENCIES 937

55. Shoulder Dystocia 939

56. Presentation and Prolapse of the Umbilical Cord 954

57. Disproportion, Obstructed Labour and Uterine Rupture 960

58. Procedures in Obstetrics 970

59. Complications of the Third Stage of Labour 987

PART 9

HEALTH, SOCIAL SERVICES AND PUBLIC HEALTH 1003

60. The Changing National Health Service 1005

61. Quality in Midwifery 1021

62. Epidemiology 1034

63. Children Act and Social Services 1050

PART 10

THE MIDWIFE 1069

64. A History of the Profession in the UK 1071

65. International Perspectives 1100

66. Statutory Framework for Practice 1116

67. Ethics and the Midwife 1133

68. Law and the Midwife 1142

69. Management and Leadership in Midwifery 1167

70. The Midwife as a Lifelong Learner 1185

71. Drugs and the Midwife 1209

Index 1229

Contributors

Belinda Ackerman MA PGDip PGCEA ADM HV RM RN
Consultant Midwife, Guy's and St Thomas'
NHS Trust, London,UK
33 Infant Feeding
66 Statutory Framework for Practice

Carmel Bagness MA RGN RM ADM PGCEA
Head of Midwifery, Thames Valley University,
Slough, UK
12 Genetics

Debbie Barber BSc(Hons) MSc PGDE PGCMU DipCouns RGN
RM NT MCG1
Lecturer in Specialist Clinical Practice, Oxford
Fertility Unit, Oxford; Associate Lecturer, City
University London and Oxford Brookes University,
Oxford; Chair, Royal College of Nursing – Fertility
Nurse Group, London, UK
9 Infertility and Assisted Conception

Christine A. Bewley BEd MSc RN RM ADM
Principal Lecturer in Midwifery and Academic
Group Chair, School of Health and Social Science,
Middlesex University, London, UK
45 Hypertensive Disorders
46 Medical Disorders of Pregnancy

Debra Bick BA(Hons) PhD MMedSc RM
Professor of Midwifery and Women's Health, Faculty
of Health and Human Sciences, Thames Valley
University, Slough, UK
41 Content and Organization of Postnatal Care

Jane Susan Bott MSc PGCEA RN RM ADM
Senior Lecturer in Midwifery, Faculty of Health and
Social Care Sciences, Kingston University and
St George's Hospital Medical School, London, UK
47 Sexually Transmitted Diseases

Maureen Boyle MSc PGCEA ADM RN RM
Senior Lecturer in Midwifery, Thames Valley
University, London, UK
18 Antenatal Investigations

Eileen Brayshaw MSc MSCP SRP FETC
Clinical Associate, University of Huddersfield,
Huddersfield, UK; Clinical Specialist in Women's
Health Physiotherapy
23 Physical Preparation before Childbirth

Margaret I. Brock MA RGN RM ADM PGCEA
Delivery Suite Manager, Women's Centre,
John Radcliffe Hospital, Oxford, UK
57 Disproportion, Obstructed Labour and Uterine
Rupture

Helen Bryant MSc PGCEA ADM RM RGN
Senior Lecturer in Midwifery, Thames Valley
University, Slough, UK
12 Genetics
27 Relief of Pain during Labour

Rosemary Buckley BSc RN RM
Clinical Risk Manager, Maternity Unit,
Nottingham City Hospital, Nottingham, UK
61 Quality in Midwifery

Barbara Burden MSc PGCEA RN RM ADM
Principal Lecturer in Midwifery, Education Centre,
University of Luton, Milton Keynes, UK
5 Anatomy of Male and Female Reproduction
10 Preconception Care
15 The Fetal Skull
63 Children Act and Social Services

Sarah Church MSc PGDipEd CertResearch RGN RM ENB997
Senior Lecturer, University College Northampton,
Northampton, UK
52 Disordered Uterine Action

Terri Coates MSc RN RM ADM DipEd
Freelance lecturer and writer; practising Midwife,
Salisbury, UK; Formerly Midwifery Course Director,
Distance Learning Centre, South Bank University,
London, UK
55 Shoulder Dystocia

Margie Davies RGN RM
*Midwifery Liason Officer, Multiple Births
Foundation, Queen Charlotte's and Chelsea Hospitals,
London, UK*
49 Multiple Pregnancy

Frances Day-Stirk MHM ADM DN(Lond) RM RN
*Director of Learning, Research and Practice
Development, Royal College of Midwives, London, UK*
69 Management and Leadership in Midwifery

Tandy Deane-Gray BSc MA PGCEA RN RM ADM
*Senior Lecturer in Midwifery, University of
Hertfordshire, Hatfield, UK*
22 Education for Parenthood

Jane Denton RGN RM
*Director, Multiple Births Foundation, Queen
Charlotte's and Chelsea Hospitals, London, UK*
49 Multiple Pregnancy

Bridgit Dimond MA LLB DSA AHSM
*Barrister-at-Law, Emeritus Professor of the
University of Glamorgan, Treforest, Pontypridd, UK*
68 Law and the Midwife

Jean Donnison BA(Oxon) PhD
*Formerly Senior Lecturer, Department of Social
Policy and Administration, University of East
London, London, UK*
64 A History of the Profession in the UK

Soo Downe BA(Hons) MSc PhD RM
*Professor of Midwifery Studies, Midwifery Studies
Research Unit, University of Central Lancashire,
Preston, UK*
29 Care in the Second Stage of Labour

Jacqueline Dunkley-Bent MSc PGCEA RGN RM ADM MRIPH
*Consultant Midwife in Public Health, Guy's and
St Thomas' NHS Trust, St Thomas' Hospital,
London, UK*
21 Health Promotion in Midwifery

Tina Harris BA(Hons) SRN SCM ADM
*Senior Lecturer in Midwifery, De Montfort
University, Leicester, UK*
30 Care in the Third Stage of Labour

Christine Henderson MA MTD DPHE DipN RN RM
*Research Fellow, School of Health Sciences,
University of Birmingham, Birmingham, UK;
Editor, British Journal of Midwifery*

Tina Heptinstall BSc(Hons) MSc RN RM ADM PGCEA
*Senior Lecturer, School of Health and Social Care,
University of Greenwich, London, UK*
 1 Sociological and Cultural Context
24 Place of Birth

Simon Hettle BSc(Hons) PhD AIBMS MILTHE
*Lecturer in Biological Sciences, Department
of Biological Sciences, University of Paisley,
Paisley, UK*
12 Genetics

Tracey Hodgson MSc SRN RM ADM PGCEA
*Senior Lecturer, University College Northampton,
Northampton, UK*
52 Disordered Uterine Action

Karen Jackson BSc(Hons) RGN RM
*Midwife Teacher, University of Nottingham,
Nottingham, UK*
7 Sexuality

Patricia Jones BA(Hons) RN RM ADM
*Antenatal Screening Co-ordinator, Fetal Medicine Unit,
Elizabeth Garrett Anderson Hospital, London, UK*
10 Preconception Care

Shirley R. Jones MA RGN RM ADM CertEd SoM ILT
*Professor of Midwifery, Head of School of Women's
Health Studies, Supervisor of Midwives, University of
Central England, Birmingham, UK*
67 Ethics and the Midwife

Tara Kaufmann
*Change Manager, Service Transformation Team,
Barts and the London NHS Trust
London, UK*
60 The Changing National Health Service

Chris Kettle PhD DipMid(Practitioner) CertRM SRN SCM
*Clinical Midwife Specialist, University Hospital of
North Staffordshire, Stoke on Trent, UK*
28 The Pelvic Floor

Gay Lee BA MMedSci RN RM
*Palliative Care Nurse and Freelance Writer,
London, UK*
 1 Sociological and Cultural Context
24 Place of Birth

Paul Lewis BSc MSc DipN PGCEA RM RN RMN ADM
*Professor of Midwifery Practice and Development
and Academic Head of Midwifery, Bournemouth
University, Bournemouth, Dorset, UK*
53 Malpositions and Malpresentations

Patricia Lindsay MSc PGCEA RN RM ADM
Midwife, Rosie Hospital, Cambridge, UK
43 Nausea and Vomiting
44 Bleeding in Pregnancy
48 Abnormalities of the Genital Tract
50 Preterm labour
56 Presentation and Prolapse of the Umbilical Cord
59 Complications of the Third Stage of Labour

Christine MacArthur BSc MSc PhD
*Professor of Maternal and Child Epidemiology,
Department of Public Health and Epidemiology,
University of Birmingham, Birmingham, UK*
42 Morbidity following Childbirth

Sue Macdonald MSc PGCEA ADM RM RN ILTM FETC
*Education and Research Manager, Royal College of
Midwives, London; formerly Principal Lecturer,
Midwifery, Middlesex University, London, UK*
70 The Midwife as a Lifelong Learner

Gaynor D. MacLean BA PhD RN RM MTD
*Consultant, Safe Motherhood, Maternal and
Neonatal Health, Swansea, UK*
65 International Perspectives

Pat McGeown MSc RN RM SoM
*Head of Midwifery Department, Perinatal Institute
for Maternal and Child Health, Birmingham, UK*
51 Induction of Labour and Post-term Pregnancy

Mary McNabb BA BSc MSc RN RM ADM PGCEA
*Senior Lecturer in Midwifery and Women's Health,
London South Bank University, London, UK*
 6 Female Reproductive Physiology
11 Fertilization
13 Implantation and Development of the Placenta
14 Embryonic and Fetal Development
17 Maternal and Fetal Physiological Responses to Pregnancy
25 Physiological Changes in Labour

Stephanie Meakin RN RM BA MA
*Head of Midwifery Education and Deputy Lead for
Post Qualifying Education, University of
Southampton, Southampton, UK*
58 Procedures in Obstetrics

Maggie Meeks MD MRCPCH
*Consultant Neonatologist, Department of
Neonatology, Leicester General Hospital, University
Hospitals Leicester, Leicester, UK*
37 Neonatal Jaundice

Stephanie Michaelides PGCEA ADM RM RGN
*Senior Lecturer, Midwifery and Neonatal Issues,
Middlesex University, London, UK*
31 Physiology and Care
32 Thermoregulation
37 Neonatal Jaundice

Eileen Powell BA(Hons) PGCEA ADM FPN RM RN
*Senior Midwifery Lecturer, Faculty of Health and
Human Sciences, Thames Valley University, Slough, UK*
16 Confirming pregnancy and care of the pregnant
woman

Carolyn Roth
*Lecturer in Midwifery, City University London,
London, UK*
4 Evidence-based Practice

Catherine Rowan MA RGN RM ADM PGCEA
*Senior Lecturer, Faculty of Health and Human
Sciences, Thames Valley University, Wexham Park
Hospital, Slough, UK*
16 Confirming pregnancy and care of the pregnant
woman

M. Susan Sapsed BPS BA(Hons) MPhil RN RM ADM MTD
*Senior Lecturer, Midwifery and Women's Health,
Education Centre, University of Luton, Luton, UK*
15 The Fetal Skull

Jancis M. Shepherd MA MTD RGN RM ADM PGCEA
*Senior Midwifery Lecturer, Faculty of Health and
Human Sciences, Thames Valley University, Slough, UK*
16 Confirming pregnancy and care of the pregnant woman

Mary Sidebotham MA ADM/DPSM RM RGN
*Consultant Midwife, Women's Unit, Stepping Hill
Hospital, Stockport, UK*
54 Mental Health Problems
62 Epidemiology

Joyce Sihwa MSc LLB(Hons) DipLegalPractice CertEd RN RM ADM
*Programme Leader, Continuing Professional
Development for Midwives, Department of
Midwifery, City University, St Bartholomew School
of Nursing and Midwifery, London, UK*
4 Evidence-based Practice

Maria Simons BSc RN RM
*Midwife, Maternity Department, Milton Keynes
General NHS Trust, Milton Keynes, UK*
5 Anatomy of Male and Female Reproduction

Carol Simpson RGN RM ENB405
Independent Midwife, Christchurch, New Zealand
34 The Preterm Baby and the Small Baby
35 Respiratory and Cardiac Disorders
36 Congenital Anomalies, Fetal and Neonatal Surgery,
     and Pain
38 Metabolic and Endocrine Disorders
39 Infection
40 Sudden Infant Death Syndrome

Catherine Siney RN RM
*Specialist Midwife and Substance Misuse/Bloodborne
Viruses and Infection Control Manager, Liverpool
Women's Hospital, Liverpool, UK*
71 Drugs and the Midwife

Jenni Thomas OBE
*Founder and President, The Child Bereavement
Trust; Maternity and Paediatric Bereavement
Facilitator, Buckinghamshire Hospitals NHS Trust,
High Wycombe, UK*
3 Grief and Bereavement

Denise Tiran MSc RGN RM ADM PGCEA
*Principal Lecturer, Complementary Medicine/
Midwifery, University of Greenwich, London, UK;*

*Director, Expectancy Ltd – the Expectant Parents'
Complementary Therapies Consultancy, London, UK*
2 Psychological Context
19 Maternal Nutrition
20 Complementary Therapies in Childbearing

Rosemary Towse BA(Hons) MTD RN RM
*Midwife Teacher, University of Surrey,
Guildford, UK*
8 Fertility and its Control

Margaret Yerby MSc PGCEA ADM C&G730 RN RM
*Formerly Senior Lecturer, Midwifery, Thames Valley
University, London and Slough, UK*
12 Genetics
27 Relief of Pain during Labour

Denis Walsh MA RGN RM DPSM PG DipE
*Independent Midwifery Lecturer and PhD student,
University of Central Lancashire, Preston, UK*
26 Care in the First Stage of Labour

Helen Wenman BA(Hons) PGDipAppSocSt CQSW PGDipEthics
*National Lead Adviser, Qualifying Social Work
Training, General Social Care Council, London, UK*
63 Children Act and Social Services

Foreword

I was delighted to be asked to write the Foreword for this thirteenth edition of *Mayes' Midwifery*, a text which has been revised and further developed to continue in its tradition as the key midwifery text for student and qualified midwives. The range of authors and their expertise reflects the diverse and impressive array of talent that the midwifery profession holds within it.

For those midwives working in the NHS, change is ever present and demands midwives who are unswerving in their commitment to providing care that is appropriate and effective, as well as critical and analytical about midwifery practice.

This requires a knowledgeable and confident doer able to work within a team. I believe the research and evidence-based content of this text, with its objectives, range of references and reflective activities, will bring the theory of midwifery to life and into practice in an engaging and inspiring way. It will also be of use in supporting mothers to plan their care and make decisions on the options locally available.

This is an exciting time to be a midwife. Maternity-specific initiatives, entwined with an ever-changing NHS and society itself, can sometimes make midwifery a challenging choice of profession yet many individuals still choose midwifery. It is a role in which no two days are ever the same, where as a practitioner you crave the 'normal' and where, though you may at times become frustrated, tired and challenged, you are never bored. However, it is also a time of much opportunity. Government policy across the UK is to encourage locally accessible services and in many areas these are being provided by the development of midwife-led care for a large population of women. This includes the midwife being the first point of contact for pregnant women, assisting them to understand the options available and to exercise informed choice.

Today's midwife truly needs to be committed to being a lifelong learner in order to operate within the complex realities of midwifery and with a variety of client groups and service users. I believe that this text will be an invaluable resource to student midwives to support their preparation programmes, midwives undertaking return to practice and adaptation programmes and for practising midwives as part of their ongoing updating.

London, 2004

Dame Karlene Davis, DBE
General Secretary,
Royal College of Midwives

Preface

The previous edition of *Mayes' Midwifery* began the transition to a multi-author and multi-expert resource for the midwife of today and developed an international reputation. When midwives were surveyed regarding a further revised edition the response was overwhelmingly positive. This edition continues in that style but has been extensively revised and updated, in sections that reflect the needs of the contemporary midwife, women and their babies.

There have been huge changes within midwifery in the past 10 years, many of which were new or even unanticipated when the last edition was published. These began with the House of Commons Health Committee review of maternity services chaired by Nicholas Winterton (1992) and the setting up of an Expert Maternity Group, with a remit to improve maternity services. The recommendations and action plan identified in the Changing Childbirth Report (1993) have come to fruition and new initiatives have been developed within maternity care. The publication and implementation of the NHS Plan (2000), the development of National Service Frameworks, the Modernisation agenda and Government targets are all changing the landscape within which midwives are practising, offering new perspectives, opportunities and challenges. The profile of the midwife is also changing. Educational programmes preparing students for midwifery are now at degree or diploma levels, providing an academic background for students, which can equip them with the knowledge, skills and confidence to provide a high standard of care to women and their babies. It also equips them to function autonomously within the wider healthcare team. Midwives already in the system increasingly have opportunities to access academic and practice developments and this is reflected in new and emerging roles such as the consultant midwife, professor of midwifery and practice development midwives.

We had the challenge of providing a text which reflects these changes and those yet to come, a resource which will be useful for student midwives, qualified midwives and for other practitioners who are looking for more information on maternity care, care of the newborn, and midwifery generally. We have been fortunate in working with an extremely committed group of authors who are experts and leaders in their field. They have worked incredibly hard to produce a dynamic and accessible text. Many have taken a fresh approach, introducing new thinking and new ideas.

The book has a strong physiological basis. There are chapters focusing wholly on maternal, fetal and neonatal physiology and others, such as the chapters dealing with care in labour and the care of the newborn, that weave physiology into applied practice. All chapters are fully referenced and well supported by research and evidence. We feel that different approaches and perspectives appear throughout the text, making it an interesting and challenging resource for all of those interested in women's health and childbirth – both qualified and student readers.

An important part of the text development has been to provide clear guidelines for the reader at the beginning of each chapter, with a 'summing up' at the end of the chapter. We have included a range of reflective activities within each chapter, providing opportunities for readers to consider how what they read can be implemented and applied into practice. We hope it will also encourage readers to question practice and ask women about their experiences, helping midwives and potential midwives to make the maternity services safer and more user-friendly.

This textbook will undoubtedly raise many questions, stimulate debate and hopefully encourage a spirit of enquiry. We see it as a stepping-stone for readers to explore beyond its pages to look at new evidence and the care we give as our knowledge expands; bearing in mind that evidence includes women's and midwives experiences as well as research.

We hope you enjoy using the 13th edition of *Mayes' Midwifery*. If you have any comments about the book we would be pleased to hear from you.

London and Birmingham,   Christine Henderson
March 2004   Sue Macdonald

REFERENCES

Department of Health (2000) *The NHS plan: a plan for investment, a plan for reform*. London: HMSO: 144.

Department of Health (1993) *Changing childbirth. Report of the Expert Maternity Group*. Chaired by Baroness Cumberlege. London: HMSO.

House of Commons Health Committee (1992) *Maternity services. Second report of Session 1991–1992*. Chaired by Nicholas Winterton. London: HMSO.

ACKNOWLEDGEMENTS

With this sort of text, there are many people to thank: the authors – all busy people who have worked hard on developing their chapters, and strived to deliver to deadlines; colleagues; and our Institutions – the University of Birmingham, Middlesex University and the Royal College of Midwives, who have been supportive during the gestation period of the book. However, special thanks are due to our friends and family who have supported us in many ways as the paper mountain grew, and have been patient with our commitment to the computers, proofs and library! A special thank you to Alison Macdonald, who provided expert advice on several issues.

To Chester whose walks were sometimes curtailed in the latter stages, and Timmy and Cassie who reclined on the chapters when being proofed!

Also a special mention for Mary Seager and Mairi McCubbin who worked brilliantly as a double act, supporting, and helping us develop the final product.

PART 1

THE CONTEXT OF CHILDBIRTH

1. Sociological and Cultural Context 3

2. Psychological Context 14

3. Grief and Bereavement 27

4. Evidence-based Practice 48

Sociological and Cultural Context

Tina Heptinstall and Gay Lee

LEARNING OUTCOMES

By the end of the chapter the reader will be able to:

- describe what sociology is and trace its historical developments
- understand the relevance of sociology to midwifery and how it is useful in helping midwives to understand a range of everyday situations in midwifery practice

- critically evaluate the construction of social differences between individuals and its influence on midwifery practice
- critically evaluate the ways in which stereotyping occurs and how it undermines positive midwife–mother relationships.

Sociology is the study of social interaction among people in a society over a particular time span. A sociological perspective is one that looks beyond assumptions that are made about a society and questions events as they appear at face value. Sociology involves a critical and systematic appraisal of the accepted norms in society, power structures, social inequalities and the differences between groups.

HISTORICAL DEVELOPMENTS

Western sociology had its origins in the Industrial Revolution during the late 18th and 19th centuries, a time that witnessed enormous social change. Significant changes in the organization of economic production were brought about through capitalism, and new social relationships were linked to private ownership of the means of production. This refers not only to the means of production of material goods but also to what happened to people in these new production methods (Giddens, 1997). One of these significant social changes was the move away from a population that was predominantly agrarian to one that became largely urban. New populations emerged as large conglomerations of people gathered around cities, and a new male workforce developed in the large-scale industries.

The social commentators during this time included philosophers such as Auguste Comte and political economists such as Adam Smith and Karl Marx. The sociologists Max Weber and Emile Durkheim also considered the changing world around them and tried to make sense of it by constructing theoretical explanations of different aspects of industrial life. Durkheim was concerned about moral values and social cohesion and Weber's interests lay in the bureaucratic organization of large institutions (Giddens, 1997). Their influential ideas and theories about social action, social change and social order led to new ways of thinking about society and laid the foundations for sociology as a social science. Subsequently, many other sociologists have commented upon, and accounted for, social action and social organization. Many sociologists shared two main concerns: social control and social change. The different ways of seeing things gave rise to a variety of theories that provided explanations for the structures that developed and for the events that occurred. Sociology has been informed by philosophy, social history, economics, politics, natural sciences and feminism. Yet these disciplines are not discrete schools of thought. There is an overlap, as each one draws on aspects of another's theory.

As recognition of the complexity of western societies developed, their study has been divided up into smaller parts, into categories for analysis. Such categories may include social class and the institutions of marriage, the family and childbearing. However, they are often presented as if they are naturally emerging rather than categories that are generated out of the perceptions of the authors. The philosopher Michel Foucault considers that these categories have no intrinsic meaning. He argues that reality does not exist independently of perception (Fillingham and Susser, 1994). For example, the categorization of people into groups such as social class is only significant because meaning has been ascribed to the work people do.

Since sociology has gained most of its material from western industrial societies, it has developed in a narrow European social context and therefore cannot claim to provide any universal description of human action. Joseph *et al.* (1990) criticize the dominance of European ideas and concepts in all social science disciplines. They argue that a predominant European perspective in the social sciences neglects alternative sources of knowledge and legitimizes international systems of inequality. For example, the theory of child development, expounded by Jean Piaget, is based on western rational and scientific reasoning. It has been a universally applied theoretical yardstick for cross-cultural comparisons of 'natural' cognitive development. Joseph *et al.* (1990) argue that such a notion is Eurocentric, not only because it overlooks the values and histories of non-western societies, but also because it fails to acknowledge its own social origins.

SOCIOLOGY AND MIDWIVES

For midwives, sociology is not just about observing social action and being social commentators: it is also about being part of the action itself and having an influence upon it. This chapter gives a brief overview of what sociology is and how it developed, not because midwives need to be sociologists but because midwives can use sociology as a tool for their work. This enables them to stand back and see themselves and the women they work with as actors in a social setting, with their own particular perspective and also with their own particular influential action in that setting.

In his book *Thinking Sociologically*, Bauman (1990) is enthusiastic about sociology. As he guides readers through his book he wants 'to show how the apparently familiar aspects of life can be interpreted in a novel way and seen in a different light' (Bauman, 1990: 18). For midwives, the relevance of sociology may be examined in the light of thinking, 'not to "correct" your knowledge, but to expand it; not to replace an error with an unquestionable truth, but to encourage critical scrutiny of beliefs hitherto held; to promote a

habit of self-analysis and of questioning the views that pretend to be certainties' (Bauman, 1990: 18).

'Critical scrutiny of beliefs' and 'questioning the views …' can be very useful in midwives' individual encounters with women and in the context of the midwife as a member of a maternity service undergoing change. For example, midwives need to be aware of their own views about formula and breast milk and how they may influence first-time mothers in the context of infant feeding. Women may come from backgrounds where mixed feeding is the norm or backgrounds where it is frowned upon. Into the discussion go the midwife's personal views and the professional information she has acquired (which may or may not coincide).

WAYS OF LOOKING AT THE WORLD

A sociological perspective demonstrates that the world around us is not a 'given fact' but that it is socially created and given meanings. Views of biological processes are also related to specific social settings. As Stacey comments, 'The ways in which a society copes with the major events of birth, illness and death are central to the beliefs and practices of that society and also bear a close relationship to its other major social, economic and cultural institutions' (Stacey, 1988: 1).

Sociology examines the ways in which certain assumptions about social thought and social organization are made. For example, the nature of knowledge itself is a construct. Scientific knowledge cannot be regarded as a collection of objective facts. Generally created in a masculine form, it is transmitted through culture and it legitimates the status, control and authority of those in power (Turner, 1995). For example, Ehrenreich and English (1979) described how, during the early medical developments in the late 19th to the early 20th century, ideas about women's health were based on the understanding that the female body and female functions, particularly menstruation, were inherently pathological. Leap and Hunter (1993) provide a vivid insight into women's experiences of health that include their views on contraception, abortion and birth in the first half of the last century. Women's own writing of their experiences of health, children and motherhood are examples from bodies of knowledge through which women understand and explain their lives (Finger, 1990; Gieve, 1989; Maushart, 2000).

Antenatal screening for genetically inherited conditions is a contemporary example of ways of 'looking at the world'. Women have a range of views on antenatal screening, and the concept of 'risk' for women may be very different from the views held by health professionals (Kolker and Burke, 1994; Marteau *et al.*, 1993). In addition, cultural assumptions determine the questions that scientists/doctors ask as well as how they interpret the data. A sociological perspective offers a challenge to the dominant idea that antenatal screening is a 'good thing' and that disability is something that should be prevented. Conrad and Gabe (2000) provide an overview on sociological perspectives on the new genetics and explore arguments that surround the social construction of 'genetic disorders'. Phil Hammond (1994) takes a wry and sceptical look at antenatal screening tests but poses some more serious questions about the way such tests are presented to women and how women are expected to make choices and cope with difficult test results. His short article illustrates the point that one event is perceived differently by different people.

Language is also not a 'given fact'. Spender (1985) explores the social construction of language, particularly in the context of women's subordination. The language of obstetrics and midwifery is value laden. It changes as it imparts meanings, expresses attitudes and illuminates the balance of power (Hewison, 1993). Leap (1992) suggests a reconsideration of such words as 'confinement', 'management', and 'allow' in the context of caring for pregnant women. Value is also implied by phrases such as 'the advances in perinatal medicine' and 'the fashion of waterbirth'. By becoming conscious of the language, midwives can become conscious of the practice that generated it; attempts to change words are attempts to change practice.

The assumption of the objectivity and neutrality of science has also been challenged; science is socially constructed. The dilemmas of the scientific method have been explored by Oakley (1990) and McNabb (1989) with regard to research concerning childbearing women. McNabb questions the use of the randomized controlled trial (the epitome of the objective scientific method) to investigate activity during labour, by attempting to isolate 'parts' of labour such as ambulating and positions in labour. She argues that: 'it is a completely inappropriate research method when applied to a dynamic process such as labour' (McNabb, 1989: 58). The subtle interplay between the physical, psychological and cultural dimensions of labour does not lend itself to reducing labour to discrete 'parts' for observation, manipulation and control.

Childbirth is a socially significant and universal event and the different meanings that are ascribed to it vary over periods of time and between cultures. Herein, culture does not solely refer to the practices, values and attitudes of racial groups but also to cultures within and between the occupational groups of midwives and obstetricians (Kitzinger *et al.*, 1990).

The culture of control around birth in western societies in present times may be exemplified through the institutionalization of birth. This was premised on assumptions that pregnancy and childbirth are hazardous events needing medical intervention (Campbell and Macfarlane, 1994). However, Macintyre (1977) cautions against romanticized notions of childbirth in pre-modern times and in non-western cultures where maternal and infant mortality are often high. She acknowledges that many women are dissatisfied with their experiences of modern practice but she considers that: 'The point is not what childbirth was once like … but what it could be like in our society now or in the future' (Macintyre, 1977: 22).

Technology is now a commonplace feature of pregnancy and birth. An obvious example is the 'active management of labour'. Here, the activity and progress of labour is measured according to set criteria over a given time span (O'Driscoll and Meagher, 1993). It is the obstetrician or midwife who is active, in so far as they may intervene in labour, for example by using intravenous Syntocinon infusions, in order for progress to be 'normal'. The cultural milieus of such labours are in sharp contrast to the culture of 'active birth' whereby the woman herself and not her objectified uterus is the focus of labour (Balaskas, 1992).

Another example of intervention with technology which midwives often view as a mixed blessing, is the use of the cardiotocograph (CTG). Research has shown that use of the CTG does not improve perinatal mortality and long-term outcomes for the babies who are born having had their heartbeats continuously monitored in this way, whatever the risk they are considered to be at (NICE 2001; Thacker and Stroup, 2001). Yet it is usual for 'high-risk labours' to be continuously monitored because midwives and obstetricians fear that if something subsequently goes wrong they will be blamed for not having monitored the labour closely enough, even though rational judgement tells them the research evidence should back a 'low-tech' approach. This is an example of the overuse, and sometimes misuse, of technology. The skill for midwives and obstetricians is in using intervention and technology appropriately.

Perhaps a useful concluding perspective on the matter is one from Burnett Lunan, a consultant obstetrician and gynaecologist. He believes that the health of women today is a major factor in the improvement of maternal mortality statistics. However, a more important one, both here and particularly in the developing world, is good primary care (provided in the UK by midwives) but with excellent facilities for referral to hospital-based specialists, with appropriate technology, should problems arise (Lunan, 1996). This requires good clinical and decision-making skills on the part of midwives to distinguish the normal from the abnormal. It also requires good obstetric skills on the part of doctors (or specially trained non-medical personnel in the developing world). Leap and Hunter (1993) say something similar; they found that maternal mortality at home was very low because 'handywomen' seemed to know when they needed medical help.

WOMEN, MIDWIVES AND MEDICINE

Midwives have existed in all societies. In the 16th and 17th centuries women as healers were seen as a threat, particularly to men (Donnison, 1988). Men organized themselves into the profession of medicine, which originally formally excluded women. Medicine gained ascendancy through the legitimization of 'science'. It gradually encroached into aspects of people's lives and this was characterized in the 19th century by the medicalization of madness (Showalter, 1987; Szasz, 1971) and the medicalization of 'women's conditions', especially of pregnancy and childbirth (Oakley, 1984). According to Gabe and Calnan (1989: 223), medicalization may be defined as 'the way in which the jurisdiction of modern medicine has expanded in recent years and now encompasses many problems that formerly were not defined as medical entities'. By the early 20th century the regulation and control of women, and in particular women's sexuality, had passed from Church to State to medicine (Turner, 1995). The control of pregnancy, childbirth and motherhood had passed from a primarily social domain to a primarily medical domain (Oakley, 1980, 1984). The locus of control in childbirth had also changed from the sphere of women to that of men and medicine (Stacey, 1988).

Historically, some midwives were in alliance with doctors; the power struggle was broadly middle-class midwives versus working-class midwives and women, the former wanting to bring up the status of trained midwives to that of trained nurses (Leap and Hunter, 1993). This historical background is explored in detail by Heagerty (1997) who shed new light on material from the Royal College of Midwives' archive.

The expansion of medical power and control in pregnancy and childbirth was characterized by a view of women that separated their physical and reproductive lives from their social and emotional lives. The metaphor of the body, and specifically the uterus, as machine and the doctor as mechanic helps to explain the early development of obstetrics, in which a woman's body is fragmented and reduced to component parts (Martin, 1987; Oakley, 1989). Thus, although medicine and medical men may not consciously wish to accrue it, the increasing domination of technology over natural childbirth results in increased power of doctors over childbearing women.

THE SOCIAL CONSTRUCTION OF MOTHERHOOD

The way in which women become mothers is culturally determined and socially controlled (Holdsworth, 1988). Girls are strongly socialized to become mothers, and motherhood remains the proof and hallmark of adulthood, womanhood, and femininity (Oakley, 1980).

Traditionally it has been expected that all women want children, and implicit within this norm is that women, within a particular age range and with a partner, should have a certain number of babies. Areas that have aroused interest are outside this 'norm'. These may currently include 'teenage pregnancy' (Chambers *et al.*, 2000; Murcott, 1980; Phoenix, 1991), 'older mothers' (Berryman, 1991) and fertility (Stacey, 1993). The interest in these areas obscures the view that normal reproduction is socially constructed. There has been little interest in why white, married, and middle-class women (considered to be the norm) have or want to have children. Perhaps this is because certain values are presented as 'normal' by those who have power in a society, and their definition becomes the yardstick by which everything else is measured.

In her book *Who's Fit to be a Parent?* Campion (1995) introduces the notion of 'fitness' to be a parent and explores perceptions of parents and professionals in the context of 'disabled parents', 'gay parents', 'drug-addicted mothers' and 'working mothers'. This author focuses on groups of people who have been marginalized in a society by those who have the power to define good, bad or problematic parenting. This form of social construction that examines 'parents on the edge' needs to be viewed within a particular historical, economic and social context, informed by the beliefs and values of dominant groups.

SOCIAL DIFFERENTIATION

In a similar way, society divides individuals into categories such as race, social class and gender, which tends to imply homogeneity within groups. Such an oversimplification ignores the complexities of these individual lives and does not account for differences in life events and an individual's quality of life. However, it is a practical way of examining aspects of society that are of interest and help us understand social organization and social interaction (Giddens, 1997).

Reflective Activity 1.1

Think of some of the stereotypical statements made about the following women; how do you think these views may influence the care these women receive? Discuss your views with others.

- A pregnant 16-year-old, with one child
- A refugee, pregnant for the first time
- A 48-year-old first-time mother
- A physically disabled wheelchair user seeking fertility treatment
- A pregnant woman with learning disabilities.

Race

'Race' is a social construct that has more to do with social structures and power relationships than with biology (Phillips and Rathwell, 1986). The imbalance of power in society enables the views of the powerful to dominate. It is within this context that the issues relating to minority ethnic groups are often seen in terms of individual pathology rather than as a result of inequalities in the social structure and it is in this way that racism develops (Smaje, 1995). Often the differences are seen as problematic (Douglas, 1992; Phoenix, 1990). Phoenix (1990) asserts that Asian women are socially constructed as inferior to white people; features perceived to be representations of their culture are negatively stereotyped as strange and exotic, and hence devalued.

Much of the work on race has concentrated on areas concerning health, and particular interest has been shown in diet, maternity care and diseases affecting certain racial groups (Douglas, 1992; Katbamna, 2000). Phoenix (1990) argues that the experiences of black and Asian women in the health service as both clients and health workers reflects the racial discrimination that is institutionalized in British society. She maintains that Asian women are perceived by the health services to have extraordinary needs and are thus regarded as causing a problem. She considers that some of these needs are shared by all women regardless of their cultural background. She illustrates this by considering that many women do not like hospital food and that many women find it difficult to understand what the medical staff say to them. Moreover, a lot of women dislike internal examinations, particularly by male doctors.

In a study which investigated the provision of maternity care to women of South Asian descent, Bowler (1993) describes how midwives used stereotypes of women to make judgements about them in order to provide care. She identified four main themes in the stereotype: communication; failure to comply with care and service abuse; making a fuss about nothing; a lack of normal maternal instinct. She also reported that the midwives tended to see Asian women as a homogeneous group with the same needs. Bowler (1993) suggested that service delivery can be affected, particularly in the areas of family planning, pain control and breastfeeding.

Neile (1997) argues that black and minority ethnic group women have not benefited from the organizational changes in the maternity services over the past years; inequalities in care and outcomes persist. The way forward lies in midwives becoming more aware of the experience of these women and acting in ways that address these issues. Tackling racism, promoting equality of access, improving communication and enhancing multiculturalism within midwifery education are among the strategies that need to be undertaken in order to bring about a more sensitive and appropriate maternity service for all women.

Refugees and asylum seekers are categories of minority ethnic groups; issues around this population group are poorly understood. The care of childbearing refugees and asylum seekers, who have needs unique to their difficult circumstances, is often poorly understood.

A refugee is defined under the 1951 United Nations Convention Relating to the Status of Refugees as someone who has a well-founded fear of being persecuted for reasons of race, religion, nationality, membership of a particular social group or political opinion. Such people may be 'internal' refugees in another place in their own country or may seek asylum (i.e. refugee status) in another country.

Although the current rise in immigration is a significant recent social change in this country, refugees and asylum seekers are part of a wider tradition of immigration that has been going on for hundreds of years and has always been considered a good thing, which can also be problematic (Home Office, 2004; Woollacott, 2001).

Immigrants bring specialist skills or do essential, unpopular unskilled work and are usually young, thus rectifying the skew towards an ageing population. While some people are 'economic migrants' rather than refugees, it is often impossible and unhelpful to distinguish those at risk of persecution in their own country, those trying to escape chronic and debilitating poverty and those encouraged to come because their skills are in short supply (for example midwives and computer specialists).

Asylum seekers' welfare benefits have been greatly reduced over the years. They are now being administered by the Home Office National Asylum Support Service (NASS), and are subject to stringent assessment criteria. Those who achieve refugee status have full benefit rights. It is important to realize that all asylum seekers are entitled to the same access to NHS services as most other UK residents.

Asylum seekers are usually housed in the worst accommodation. Some, considered to be in danger of absconding, are detained. As with other homeless people, hard-to-let housing or 'bed and breakfast' accommodation may be used, overcrowded and lacking in facilities as it so often is. Relatives or friends may provide accommodation but most of those without such contacts are being dispersed from London and the South East to areas probably far away from their own ethnic group and from expert help. Yet many will return to the larger cities (Robinson, 2003).

Refugee and asylum seeker mothers' needs for special health and social care can arise from:

- post-traumatic stress and other mental health problems (these are often more prevalent than physical health problems)
- malnutrition
- growth retardation of the baby
- infections, including TB, HIV, malaria and intestinal parasites
- exhaustion
- injury from torture or rape
- female genital mutilation which may be a problem during birth, as for some other ethnic groups
- communication problems for non-English speakers (Burnett and Fassil, 2002) – readily available and sensitive interpreting services are essential
- barriers to successful breastfeeding (Kennedy and Murphy-Lawless, 2001) in the form of the health

problems above, lack of social support and suitable accommodation.

The special needs of refugee and asylum-seeking, child-bearing women stem from their special experiences of loss: of home, family (often including partners and other children), social roots, customs and country, and from their experiences of suffering: abuse and the journey to escape it. Inevitably this will 'impact on their physiological, psychological and social profile during pregnancy' (Kennedy and Murphy-Lawless, 2001: 8).

Schott and Henley (1996) emphasize the importance of effective communication with all pregnant women, regardless of ethnicity. They challenge the use of stereotypes and show how these can result in simple misunderstandings, insensitivity or racist behaviour. Developing a better understanding of the nature of differences between individuals can result in improved planning and delivery of care. Moreover, cultures are not static and individuals within a groups are not all the same. And the perception of a culture may be different as seen from the outside, in contrast to the view from within it. Thus, examining ourselves is as significant as examining others.

Social class

Social class remains an enduring theme within sociology. Differences in class within capitalist society depend on a person's work, so that the basic idea behind class comes from economics. The use of class as a social category has often been accepted uncritically and taken for granted as a 'natural' category. Oakley (1992) describes how social class can be regarded as a designation introduced by statisticians to describe occupational and social differences between people.

The categorization of people into social class according to occupation by the British Registrar General is a commonly used classification (Table 1.1).

However, this classification focuses primarily on families where an employed man is the head of the household; women, retired people and the unemployed are poorly reflected. Hence, it is likely that new forms of social classification will be used in the future. Using official government categorizations, sociologists have conducted studies that have provided an array of descriptive data including lifestyle differences between occupational groups (Blaxter, 1990; Graham, 2000b).

Sociologists have used these and other government data to conduct studies which paint a picture of the

Table 1.1 Examples of occupations in their social class (Graham, 2000a)

Social class		Occupations
I	Professional	Accountant, lawyer, doctor
II	Managerial	Sales manager, teacher, journalist, nurse
IIIN	Skilled non-manual	Secretary, shop assistant, cashier
IIIM	Skilled manual	Joiner, bus driver, cook
IV	Partly skilled manual	Security guard, machine tool operator, farm worker
V	Unskilled manual	Building labourer, cleaner, laundry worker

lives of people in different occupations. Importantly for health professionals and health policy makers, data using social class differentials such as birth and death rates (including perinatal mortality) are also collected by social class. This has proved very useful in the production of evidence about social inequalities between different groups and how these are linked to health (Oppenheim, 1993; Walker and Walker, 1997).

Inequalities in health have persisted over years, even after the inception of the NHS in 1948. One of the most significant reports that revealed health inequalities was the Black Report in 1980 (DHSS, 1980) and similar findings were reiterated in *The Health Divide* by Margaret Whitehead in 1988 (Townsend *et al.*, 1988). Subsequent evidence demonstrates how such inequalities continue to prevail, as shown in the commentaries by Walker and Walker (1997) and Graham (2000b). In recent years the links between health and wealth have been recognized and this public health aspect of midwifery has been brought into sharper focus. This is exemplified by current initiatives around smoking cessation, domestic violence and young motherhood. Some of the emerging consultant midwife posts are concerned with these specific groups (Dennett, 2003).

Jean Davies (2000) has demonstrated how enhanced midwifery care can contribute to improving the lives of women in areas of socioeconomic deprivation, particularly in relation to their health, confidence and personal aspirations.

For midwives, one result of social class categorization is that it has led to the development of class stereotypes of women using the maternity services (Green *et al.*, 1990; Kirkham, 1989). Essentially, these stereotypes undermine good communication between pregnant

women and their care-givers. The stereotype portrays women in a negative light, and assumptions are made by midwives and doctors about women's understanding and their wants. Through changes in the organization of care, the assumptions upon which the stereotypes are founded may be challenged. As Green *et al.* (1990) argue, 'Systems of care which allow midwives and mothers to get to know each other (preferably before the birth) could do much to reduce the reliance on stereotypes, with beneficial results for all concerned.' In her study of midwives working with socially and economically disadvantaged women, Davies (2000) acknowledges the differences in cultures between midwives and women. Within this context she recognizes that stereotyping may occur and comments on its deleterious effect on the midwife–mother relationship: 'Where there is a lack of openness, communication is likely to come to grief' (Davies, 2000: 139).

All women are entitled to dignity and respect. For example, pregnant women in prison have been the focus of debate among user representatives, midwives and doctors (Barnard *et al.*, 1996). Sheila Kitzinger (1999) has been especially vocal in raising awareness of the needs of these women, not least for emotional support and promoting self-esteem. She and others have campaigned for the removal of chains for women attending clinics and during birth in hospital, and for new mothers not to be separated from their babies (Barnard *et al.*, 1996). In this final comment from Sheila Kitzinger, women in prisons can be seen as a metaphor for other vulnerable groups:

> It is easy to remain ignorant of conditions in prisons. I believe that any commitment to helping childbearing women must extend to speaking out for the most vulnerable and voiceless women in our society. Women in prison are often the least educated, and are the victims of violence and sexual abuse.
>
> (Kitzinger, 1999: 18)

Gender

As social roles, social activity and health status are linked to race and class, they are also inextricably bound to issues of gender. While anatomical and physiological differences between the sexes are biologically determined, gender may be described as the socially or culturally prescribed status of women and men in a society. The associated concepts of femininity and masculinity are similarly socially constructed and, as such, they are not fixed. Ideas about a person's gender roles and behaviour may be ascribed before birth. Rothman (1994) uses the phrase 'fetal sons and daughters' as she describes how women who know the sex of their child after amniocentesis describe fetal activity in a way that is gender stereotyped. The movements of the males were more often described as 'strong' and 'vigorous' and females were described as 'lively'. Gender stereotyping continues soon after birth as appearance and behaviour are gender related. For example, Rothman (1994: 129) contrasts the 'firm grip' of the boy's 'adorable little fists' to the 'tight cling' of the girl's 'delicate tiny fingers'.

As part of the ideology of motherhood, women and mothers are seen as the unique carers of young children. The ideas of maternal–infant attachment were primarily espoused by Bowlby (1953) who argued that the quality of the early relationship between a mother and her child was significant for the child's development. Despite challenges to this theory (Rutter, 1981), it remains pervasive and underpins the gendered division of labour in the home and in the workforce. In practice, this amounts to difficulties for women seeking paid employment outside the home. This is illustrated by the over-representation of women in part-time, low-skilled and low-paid jobs, the paucity of nursery provision and the uneven career development between women and men (Davies, 1990). Rossiter (1988) argues that pregnancy, lactation and early infant attachment have acted as a justification of childrearing arrangements. She considers that they have been created in response to the changing needs of the economy, not those of dependent children. Such a situation was particularly evident in Britain during the Second World War when the needs of the economy resulted in an increase in the numbers of women in the paid workforce. This significant change was a concession to women's 'proper' and 'natural' role. It was conditional upon a return to the status quo after the war. A key element of the post-war propaganda was to encourage women to return to the hearth and for men to go back to their jobs (Holdsworth, 1988).

The pattern of work in the UK has changed since the 1970s and this has had an impact on the gendered division of labour (Davies, 1990). Individuals will no longer be in conventional, lifetime, full-time careers but will work for a number of employers in small organizations that will contract with each other. With reference to health service occupations, Davies (1990) discusses how, with flexible and contractual patterns of work, part-time work could lose its low status

and become a more accepted feature of occupational organization.

As motherhood is socially prescribed, so too is fatherhood. The traditional, gendered role for a father is to provide financially for his children. Generally, his involvement with babies and children is mediated through the mother; he rarely assesses a child's needs and he ends up being a helper. Lewis (1986) comments that men are initially excluded from the magic circle and they later take on the role of playmate. Mothers are the decision-makers. Yet, Brannen and Moss (1988) believe that this is a pseudo-power. Women have control in the home by virtue of it not being very important. Although its development is unclear, the most widespread and significant change in fathers' involvement has been their attendance at the birth of their children, but this has not been matched by their involvement in the antenatal and postnatal period (Barbour, 1990). This is a statement of good intent rather than a practical plan of action.

Kitzinger (1989) suggests that men are poorly prepared for fatherhood and that they are presented with an image which they cannot match. Much of the midwifery literature on transition to fatherhood focuses on involving men in some form of antenatal group and preparing them for an inclusive and supportive role in labour and the following early weeks of their child's life (Lester and Moorsom, 1997; Smith, 1999). In their study of the experiences of new fatherhood, Barclay and Lupton (1999) found that men looked forward positively to fatherhood but found the early weeks and months more uncomfortable than rewarding. Even though they wanted to 'be there' for their partners and babies, they often felt excluded from providing care for their child because of issues related to breastfeeding, tensions within relationships and their role as economic provider.

In spite of the rhetoric surrounding the 'New Man', there is little evidence to challenge situations that render childraising inequitable since Lewis and O'Brien (1987) commented on this. This may in part be attributed to the poor level of paternity leave and benefits, particularly in comparison to other European countries. Men in paid employment are given few opportunities to engage in sharing childcare on a basis comparable to women. Once again, inequalities arise from social structures, and expectations are rooted in the processes of socialization. Lupton and Barclay (1997) suggest that if 'new fatherhood' is to be achieved, structural and social change will be required.

As Lewis (1986) concludes:

truly participant fatherhood will not become the norm until great changes are made outside the family in child-care arrangements and in the sexual division of labour in the workplace. Certainly true symmetry between spouses cannot occur without major societal organisation.

                                          Lewis (1986: 190)

CONCLUSION

In summary, for midwives to think sociologically is for them to think critically and systematically about the social context of their own lives and the lives of the women and families around them: to think about how different groups of people understand their world and the meanings it has for them. Pregnancy, childbirth and childrearing are all social events and as such they are not fixed, but changing. Traditionally, midwifery has tended to ignore sociology and it has not made a significant contribution to it. However, with greater insights into the social organizations and social structures of their world, midwives as a unique group have an important contribution to make to sociology that is quite separate from that which doctors and the medical model of childbirth can make.

KEY POINTS

- Sociology examines 'given facts' and involves a critical and systematic appraisal of the accepted norms in society, power structures, social inequalities and the differences between groups of individuals.
- Social differences between groups are commonly discussed using the categories of social class, race and gender. This is just a practical way of examining aspects of a society and helps us understand social organization and social interaction.
- The construction of motherhood and fatherhood is socially prescribed and socially controlled. 'Fitness to parent' is a current theme and demonstrates that the roles of parents are not fixed, but change alongside moral, political and economic influences.

REFERENCES

Balaskas, J. (1992) *Active Birth: The New Approach to Giving Birth Naturally*, revised edn. Harvard: Common Press.

Barbour, R.S. (1990) Fathers: the emergence of a new consumer group. In: Garcia, J., Kilpatrick, R. & Richards, M. (eds) *The Politics of Maternity Care: Services for Childbearing Women in Twentieth-century Britain*. Oxford: Clarendon Press.

Barclay, L. & Lupton, D. (1999) The experiences of new fatherhood: a socio-cultural analysis. *Journal of Advanced Nursing* 29(4): 1013–1020.

Barnard, M., Beech, B., Blake, F. *et al.* (1996) Handcuffing women prisoners. *Midwives* 109(1296): 6.

Bauman, Z. (1990) *Thinking Sociologically*. London: Blackwell.

Berryman, J.C. (1991) Perspectives on later motherhood. In: Phoenix, A., Woollett, A. & Lloyd, E. (eds) *Motherhood: Meanings, Practices and Ideologies*. London: Sage Publications.

Blaxter, M. (1990) *Health and Lifestyles*. London: Routledge.

Bowlby, J. (1953) *Child Care and the Growth of Love*. Harmondsworth: Penguin.

Bowler, I.M.W. (1993) Stereotypes of women of Asian descent in midwifery: some evidence. *Midwifery* 9(1): 7–16.

Brannen, J. & Moss, P. (1988) *New Mothers At Work*. London: Unwin Paperback.

Burnett, A. & Fassil, Y (2002) Meeting the healthcare needs of refugees and asylum seekers in the UK: an information and resources pack for health workers. Online. Available http://www.london.nhs.uk/newsmedia/publications/asylum.refugee.pdf

Campbell, R. & Macfarlane, A. (1994) *Where to be Born: The Debate and the Evidence*, 2nd edn. Oxford: National Perinatal Epidemiology Unit.

Campion, M.J. (1995) *Who's Fit to be a Parent?* London: Routledge.

Chambers, R., Wakley, G. & Chambers, S. (2000) *Tackling Teenage Pregnancy*. Oxford: Radcliffe Medical Press.

Conrad, P. & Gabe, J. (2000) Sociological perspective on the new genetics: an overview. *Sociology of Health and Illness* 21(5): 505–516.

Davies, C. (1990) *The Collapse of the Conventional Career: The Future of Work and its Relevance for Post-registration Education in Nursing, Midwifery and Health*

Visiting. London: English National Board for Nursing, Midwifery and Health Visiting.

Davies, J. (2000) Being with women who are economically without. In: Kirkham, M. (ed) *The Midwife–Mother Relationship*. Macmillan: London.

Dennett, S. (2003) Trials and tribulations. *Midwives* **6**(12): 512–513.

Department of Health and Social Security (DHSS) (1980) *Inequalities in Health: Report of a Research Working Group* (The Black Report). London: Department of Health and Social Security.

Donnison, J. (1988) *Midwives and Medical Men: A History of Interprofessional Rivalries and Women's Rights*, 2nd edn. London: Heinemann.

Douglas, J. (1992) Black women's health matters: putting black women on the research agenda. In: Roberts, H. (ed) *Women's Health Matters*. London: Routledge.

Ehrenreich, B. & English, D. (1979) *For Her Own Good: 150 Years of the Expert's Advice to Women*. London: Pluto Press.

Fillingham, L.A. & Susser, M. (1994) *Foucault for Beginners*. London: Writers and Readers Publishing.

Finger, A. (1990) *Past Due: A Story of Disability, Pregnancy and Birth*. London: The Women's Press.

Gabe, J. & Calnan, M. (1989) The limits of medicine: women's perception of medical technology. *Social Science and Medicine* **28**: 223–231.

Giddens, A. (1997) *Sociology*, 3rd edn. Oxford: Polity Press.

Gieve, K. (ed) (1989) *Balancing Acts: On Being a Mother*. London: Virago.

Graham, H. (2000a) Understanding health inequalities. *MIDIRS Midwifery Digest* **10**(2): 144–145.

Graham, H. (ed) (2000b) *Understanding Health Inequalities*. Buckingham: Open University Press.

Green, J.M., Kitzinger, J.V. & Coupland, V.A. (1990) Stereotypes of childbearing women: a look at some of the evidence. *Midwifery* **6**: 125–132.

Hammond, P. (1994) Test pest. *Nursing Times* **90**(32): 60.

Heagerty, B. (1997) Willing handmaidens of science? The struggle over the new midwife in early twentieth century England. In: Kirkham, M. & Perkins, E.R. (eds) *Reflections on Midwifery*. London: Baillière Tindall.

Hewison, A. (1993) The language of labour: an examination of the discourses on childbirth. *Midwifery* **9**: 225–234.

Holdsworth, A. (1988) *Out of the Dolls House: The Story of Women in the Twentieth Century*. London: BBC Publications.

Home Office (2004) Online. Available http://www.homeoffice.gov.uk/rds/immigration1.

Joseph, G.G., Reddy, V. & Searle-Chatterjee, M. (1990) Eurocentrism in the social sciences. *Race and Class* **31**(4): 1–26.

Katbamna, S. (2000) *'Race' and Childbirth*. Buckingham: Open University Press.

Kennedy, P. & Murphy-Lawless, J. (2001) *The Maternity Care Needs of Refugee and Asylum-seeking Women*. Dublin: Eastern Regional Health Authority.

Kirkham, M. (1989) Midwives and information-giving in labour. In: Robinson, S. & Thompson, A. (eds) *Research, Midwives and Childbirth*, Vol. 1. London: Chapman & Hall.

Kitzinger, S. (1989) *The Crying Baby*. London: Penguin.

Kitzinger, S. (1999) Birth in prison: the rights of the baby. *Practising Midwife* **2**(1): 16–18.

Kitzinger, J., Green, J. & Coupland, V. (1990) Labour relations: midwives and doctors on the labour ward. In: Garcia, J., Kilpatrick, R., & Richards, M. (eds) *The Politics of Maternity Care: Services for Childbearing Women in Twentieth-century Britain*. Oxford: Oxford University Press.

Kolker, A. & Burke, B.M. (1994) *Prenatal Testing; A Sociological Perspective*. London: Bergin and Garvey.

Leap, N. (1992) The power of words. *Nursing Times* **88**(21): 60–61.

Leap, N. & Hunter, B. (1993) *The Midwife's Tale*. London: Scarlett Press.

Lester, A. & Moorsom, S. (1997) Do men need midwives: facilitating a greater involvement in parenting. *British Journal of Midwifery* **5**(11): 678–681.

Lewis, C. (1986) *Becoming a Father*. Milton Keynes: Open University Press.

Lewis, C. & O'Brien, M. (eds) (1987) *Reassessing Fatherhood: New Observations on Fathers and the Modern Family*. London: Sage Publications.

Lunan, C.B. (1996) Obstetrics and gynaecology in the developing world. *British Journal of Obstetrics and Gynaecology* **103**: 491–493.

Lupton, D. & Barclay, L. (1997) *Constructing Fatherhood: Discourses and Experience*. Sage: London.

Macintyre, S. (1977) Childbirth: the myth of the Golden Age. *World Medicine* **12**(18): 17–22.

McNabb, M. (1989) The science of labour? *Nursing Times* **85**(9): 58–59.

Martin, E. (1987) *The Woman in the Body: A Cultural Analysis of Reproduction*. Milton Keynes: Open University Press.

Marteau, T.M., Plenicar, M. & Kidd, J. (1993) Obstetricians presenting amniocentesis to pregnant women: practice observed. *Journal of Reproductive and Infant Psychology* **11**: 3–10.

Maushart, S. (2000) *The Mask of Motherhood: How Becoming a Mother Changes Everything and why we Pretend it Doesn't*. London: Penguin Books.

Murcott, A. (1980) The social construction of teenage pregnancy: a problem in the ideologies of childhood and reproduction. *Sociology of Health and Illness* **2**(1): 1–23.

Neile, E. (1997) Control for black and ethnic minority women: a meaningless pursuit. In: Kirkham, M. & Perkins, E.R. (eds) *Reflections on Midwifery*. London: Baillière Tindall.

NICE (National Institute for Clinical Excellence) (2001) *The Use of Electronic Fetal Monitoring*. London: NICE.

O'Driscoll, K. & Meagher, D. (1993) *Active Management of Labour*, 3rd edn. London: Mosby.

Oakley, A. (1980) *Woman Confined: Towards a Sociology of Childbirth*. Oxford: Martin Robertson.

Oakley, A. (1984) *The Captured Womb: A History of the Medical Care of Pregnant Women*. Oxford: Blackwell.

Oakley, A. (1989) Who cares for women? Science versus love in midwifery today. *Midwives Chronicle* **102**(July): 214–221.

Oakley, A. (1990) Who's afraid of the randomised controlled trial? Some dilemmas of the scientific method and 'good' research practice. In: Roberts, H. (ed) *Women's Health Counts*. London: Routledge.

Oakley, A. (1992) *Social Support and Motherhood*. Oxford: Blackwell.

Oppenheim, C. (1993) *Poverty: The Facts*. London: Child Poverty Action Group.

Phillips, D. & Rathwell, S. (1986) *Health, Race & Ethnicity*. London: Croom Helm.

Phoenix, A. (1990) Black women and the maternity services. In: Garcia, J., Kilpatrick, R. & Richards, M. (eds) *The Politics of Maternity Care: Services for Childbearing Women in Twentieth-century Britain*. Oxford: Clarendon Books.

Phoenix, A. (1991) *Young Mothers?* Cambridge: Polity Press.

Robinson, V. (2003) *Spreading the Burden*. London: Polity Press.

Rossiter, A. (1988) *From Private to Public: A Feminist Exploration of Early Mothering*. Ontario: The Women's Press.

Rothman, B.K. (1994) *The Tentative Pregnancy: Amniocentesis and the Sexual Politics of Motherhood*. London: Pandora.

Rutter, M. (1981) *Maternal Deprivation Reassessed*, 2nd edn. London: Penguin.

Schott, J. & Henley, A. (1996) *Culture, Religion and Childbearing in a Multiracial Society: A Handbook for Health Professionals*. London: Butterworth Heinemann.

Showalter, E. (1987) *The Female Malady: Women, Madness and English Culture, 1830–1980*. London: Virago.

Smaje, C. (1995) *Health Race and Ethnicity: Making Sense of the Evidence*. London: Kings Fund Institute.

Smith, N. (1999) Antenatal classes and the transition to fatherhood: a study of some fathers' views. *MIDIRS Midwifery Digest* **9**(4): 463–468.

Spender, D. (1985) *Man Made Language*, 2nd edn. London: Pandora Press.

Stacey, M. (1988) *The Sociology of Health and Healing*. London: Unwin Hyman.

Stacey, M. (ed.) (1993) *Changing Human Reproduction*. London: Sage Publications.

Szasz, T. (1971) *The Manufacture of Madness*. London: Routledge & Kegan Paul.

Thacker, S.B. & Stroup, D.F. (2001) Continuous electronic heart rate monitoring for fetal assessment during labour (Cochrane Review). *The Cochrane Library*, Issue 1. Oxford: Update Software.

Townsend, P., Davidson, P. & Whitehead, M. (eds) (1988) *Inequalities in Health: The Black Report & The Health Divide*. Harmondsworth: Penguin.

Turner, B.S. (1995) *Medical Power and Social Knowledge*, 2nd edn. London: Sage Publications.

Walker, A. & Walker, C. (1997) *Britain Divided: The Growth of Social Exclusion in the, 1980s and, 1990s*. London: Child Poverty Action Group.

Woollacott, M, (2001) Migrant storm in a teacup. *The Guardian* 5.1.2001.

FURTHER READING

Phoenix, A., Woollett, A. & Lloyd, E. (1991) *Motherhood Meaning, Myths and Ideologies*. London: Sage Publications. The authors examine aspects of the social construction of motherhood, ranging from reasons for having children or not, and its meanings for women; the experiences of 'younger' and 'older' mothers; employed mothers; mothering more than one child; and mothers and their deaf children.

Hunt, S. & Symonds, A. (1995) *The Social Meaning of Midwifery*. London: Macmillan. Everyday aspects of the working lives of midwives are examined in depth. For example, in looking at aspects of the labour ward culture, the authors look at everyday rituals.

Leap, N. & Hunter, B. (1993) *The Midwife's Tale*. London: Scarlet Press. This book is not only the midwife's story but also that of the handywoman – the person within the community who preceded and paralleled the development of the trained and professional midwife in the early part of the last century.

Schott, J. & Henley, A. (1996) *Culture, Religion and Childbearing in a Multiracial Society: A Handbook for Health Professionals*. Oxford: Butterworth Heinemann. This book is a practical guide on how to work with childbearing women with cultural and racial backgrounds different from those who are working in the National Health Service – it is about professionals asking appropriate questions and really listening to the answers, whatever the problem and whatever the cultural, religious or racial context.

2

Psychological Context

Denise Tiran

LEARNING OUTCOMES

By the end of this chapter you will be able to:

- appreciate the psychological factors that may affect a mother's experience of pregnancy, childbirth and early parenthood

- understand the basics of good communication skills, which are essential in midwifery practice.

INTRODUCTION

Pregnancy, childbirth and early parenthood are periods of immense change in the lives of women, their partners and their immediate families. Quite apart from dealing with the physical symptoms and discomforts, there will be many anxieties, worries and fears which the woman will experience and which she may be unable to express unless she receives sensitive support from her midwife. The midwife needs to have a comprehensive understanding of the psychological changes which occur so that she can contribute to the holistic care required by the mother and her family and identify women who are vulnerable to psychological difficulties or, in extreme cases, to mental illness which may be triggered by the stresses of pregnancy. This knowledge also helps the midwife to provide appropriate antenatal education, either to individuals or in groups preparing for parenthood.

COMMUNICATION IN MIDWIFERY PRACTICE

Midwifery is a profession in which communication is vital – communication between midwives, mothers and their families, and between all health professionals. A safe and satisfying childbirth experience is far more likely to be achieved when there is good communication between all those involved and priorities of communication are recognized (Tennant and Butler, 1999). Poor communication, management styles and working environments can adversely affect the quality of midwifery practice, and midwifery services should endeavour to work towards women-centred care in keeping with the philosophy of the Department of Health's strategy for the 21st century (SNMAC, 1998).

Today's parents are better informed about pregnancy and childbirth than hitherto and demand not only physical safety, but also emotional fulfilment culminating in a pleasurable, meaningful experience of birth and parenthood. They expect – and deserve to receive – adequate and appropriate information which is communicated in an open, straightforward way so that they can make informed choices about their care and retain control during pregnancy, labour and the postnatal period. Midwives who appreciate the feelings and needs of parents and make every effort to form a partnership with them so that their demands and aspirations are met, make a great contribution to their emotional fulfilment and subsequent mental health.

Verbal and non-verbal processes

Communication is a two-way process and involves verbal and non-verbal processes.

Facial expression is a powerful form of non-verbal communication and may be a better indicator of true meaning than the content of speech. The midwife needs to be alert to discrepancies between what the mother says and what she actually means. The midwife must also use her own facial expression appropriately. A smiling face (however fraught the midwife may feel) is welcoming; a sympathetic expression shows the midwife's caring side, rather than merely the professional but impersonal approach. Eye-to-eye contact enables signals to be received and feedback given. The midwife needs to acquire the skill to detect cues gained from eye-to-eye contact and respond to them. For example, when the midwife is attempting to obtain sensitive and intimate details, the mother may avoid eye contact, perhaps owing to embarrassment, or because she is either omitting facts or not answering a question truthfully. There may be many reasons for this behaviour such as trying to conceal the fact of a previous termination of pregnancy, or that she has been abused. In some cultures limited eye contact is the norm, and the midwife should be aware of and respect these cultural differences.

Head nodding is used to signify reinforcement and encouragement, and to indicate that the speaker should continue. Gestures are used to add emphasis to speech, relieve tension, for example by hand wringing, or to reveal other emotional states. Body language indicates different emotions, for example leaning forwards conveys attentiveness and concern, whereas drawing back or turning away may signify disinterest. A dominant attitude is communicated by an expanded chest, a trunk which is upright or leaning back and head and shoulders held high. The submissive person has a dejected attitude, leans forward with bowed head and drooping shoulders and appears downcast and depressed. Anxiety can be seen in someone who is tense, stiff and upright.

Orientation gives an indication of interpersonal attitudes. It refers to the position of the body and the angle at which one person interacts with another. It should be considered together with physical proximity since when direct face-to-face orientation occurs there is greater distance between people than with sideways orientation. For instance, it is preferable to sit at 90 degrees to the mother when taking a history or discussing aspects of care. A face-to-face position can be considered confrontational, especially when the barrier of a desk is present. If the midwife needs access to a computer she should attempt to keep the equipment as unobtrusive as possible so that the interaction takes place between the mother and midwife – and not between the mother and the computer.

When the midwife is higher than the mother, this gives a feeling of domination which is not conducive to a partnership in care. When seeing mothers in the antenatal clinic, the mother should be invited to remain seated until it is necessary for her to lie on the couch to be examined. In the postnatal ward or at home, the midwife should sit on a chair next to the mother when talking to her, or assisting with breastfeeding.

Personal space

Personal space may differ according to cultures – the British are renowned for 'keeping their distance' while the Italians frequently indulge in physical displays of affection. Personal space extends from about 45 cm to just over a metre, while one's intimate space, normally reserved only for those with whom there is a very close relationship, is less than 45 cm. Much of the midwife's close contact with a mother may constitute an invasion of her intimate space, but the majority of our physical touch has become functional and impersonal. This may be a subconscious strategy on the part of the midwife to overcome both her own and the mother's embarrassment; it may have evolved in response to ever-increasing workloads; or it may be a means of maintaining 'professional' distance.

Midwives must be sensitive to the needs of women and learn to use touch appropriately. Sometimes, simply reaching for a mother's hand or putting an arm around her shoulders can be more effective than any spoken word. Massage and other manual complementary therapies are increasingly being used within midwifery in an attempt to return to the nurturing so necessary to pregnant and newly delivered women (Tiran, 2000). However, it must be acknowledged that not all women wish to be touched, especially in labour. Midwives will observe women who need 'mothering' with constant physical and emotional attention, whereas others would choose to retreat into an isolated corner to labour and deliver, in much the same way that many animals do. People often treat pregnant women as objects of public property, invading their intimate space to pat their abdomens. Midwives should recognize that many women dislike this and should not develop the habit as part of their repertoire of professional gestures.

Touch is also open to various interpretations and midwives will need to use it with sensitivity. Male midwives will need to exercise exceptional discretion in the ways in which they use touch, for it would be easy for either a mother or her partner to misinterpret a gesture of kindness.

Physical appearance

Physical appearance conveys much information to others. Before even talking to an individual we are beginning to make judgements on the basis of physical appearance. As soon as the mother and the midwife meet, each will be assessing the other from the information available to them at this early stage, although it must be remembered that it is easy to make assumptions. The midwife should be alert to the underlying messages obtained from a mother's appearance. For example, a woman who is overly cheerful, jovial or perhaps aggressive, may be trying to hide extreme nervousness.

Written communication

Communication may be in the form of the written word, which can be either handwritten or computerized records. It is essential that all written communications are legible, including signatures, for both effective care and legal reasons. Professional records must be comprehensive and completed as contemporaneously as possible. Any written information given to mothers must be comprehensible using plain language; it may be necessary to provide leaflets and other information in several languages depending on the local clientele. Computerized records may offer a means of recording the main medical and obstetric details but can inhibit the documentation of social and psychological information: midwives must ensure that their records are not limited by the format of the computer program, or indeed, the format of the medical records.

Need to be understood

The essence of good communication is to consider each person as an individual. Culture, education and social class are some of the factors which affect the use of language and should be considered when making an assessment of each mother. The midwife should give frequent simple, clear explanations in terms that can be easily understood, avoiding abbreviations and jargon which may lead to confusion. It is also important to remember that intonation has a marked effect on meaning and that changes in pitch and emphasis help to clarify the spoken word.

There are many families in the UK for whom English is not their first language. Non-English-speaking women are often given less information than other women, and this prevents them from making informed decisions about their care. This greatly increases the problems of communications and the midwife should know how to obtain suitable help. Sometimes there is a member of the family who can interpret; otherwise a member of staff or a volunteer may be available to help. Explanatory and health education leaflets in various languages are available. Mothers who speak little or no English can feel very lost and isolated, especially in hospital, and staff need to make a special effort to communicate their care and empathy non-verbally as well as verbally.

Verbal communication involves speaking and listening

Attentive listening and the close observation which is part of it enable the midwife to assess the woman carefully and identify her real needs and requirements. Listening attentively is an active rather than a passive skill and needs considerable effort and practice to acquire and use effectively. A good listener concentrates totally on the speaker so that she feels valued as an individual. A relaxed, attentive attitude and encouragement in the form of a nod or smile will encourage the speaker to continue, while the listener carefully notes the non-verbal cues.

Even when the midwife cannot see the mother, she may be able to detect cues in the mother's non-verbal communications. For example, sometimes the midwife can recognize the onset of the second stage of labour simply by listening to the altered sounds of a mother's breathing in a labour room.

Skilled questioning techniques, using open and probing, rather than closed or leading, questions, are essential for good communications. Questions may be asked in a variety of ways and midwives should know how to select the appropriate type of question, since this will greatly influence the information obtained in response.

Reflective Activity 2.1

How much information can you obtain from a mother without asking her direct questions? At the booking clinic try assessing a woman as she approaches you before you start taking the history. In the postnatal period, try undertaking the routine postnatal examination without touching the mother to examine her.

Observe your colleagues: can you identify which midwives have good communication skills and why? Are there episodes when a midwife fails to communicate adequately with a particular mother?

Therapeutic counselling

Generic midwifery practice involves a combination of both directive and non-directive counselling, using a range of communication skills. Mack (2000) suggests that midwives can learn to offer a 'counselling approach' in their practice, in which focused and purposeful discussion is facilitated with mothers when necessary. A 'therapeutic distance' needs to be maintained to avoid the midwife becoming too emotionally involved with the mother, but this should not be so great that it interferes with the relationship which is being developed between the midwife and the mother. Therapeutic counselling, however, requires specialized training and application, and it would not be practical or appropriate for all midwives to be fully trained counsellors. This is an area which some midwives choose to develop as their speciality within the profession. Some trusts employ midwife-counsellors who can concentrate on those families with specific needs, such as those affected by bereavement, early pregnancy loss or fetal abnormality (Inati, 1999; Moulder, 1999; Sehdev and Wilson, 1999), or specific client groups who may need specialist help, such as teenagers or women with problems of addiction. Street and Downey (1996) describe a 'medico-collaborative' model of counselling which attempts to work in partnership *with* the client rather than '*on*' her in a directive manner. The structured counselling model which most closely fits this concept is that of Egan (1982).

PSYCHOLOGICAL ASPECTS OF PREGNANCY

Women become pregnant for a number of reasons. Raphael-Leff (1991) suggests that, in part, conscious conception is due to a desire to obtain 'genetic immortality' by prolonging the parents' existence. However, becoming pregnant is also something which assists in the process of 'growing up', of becoming an adult, as well as offering women the opportunity to emulate their own parents and repay the dependence which they had. Some people may subconsciously view the childbearing experience as a 'second chance' to give to their own child everything which they may have wished for themselves. In others, a baby represents the parents' need to be loved, to be a recipient of the unconditional love which children offer. There is also an element of control, not only in the position of parental power, but also the ability in contemporary society, to make a choice about whether, when and how to become pregnant. Societal pressure also plays a part, a factor which can add to the trauma of infertility in some couples.

The way in which a couple react to the news of the woman's pregnancy will be dependent on their individual situation. Most women and their partners will be delighted, even when the pregnancy is unplanned. This joy will be heightened if there has been a history of infertility or pregnancy loss, although this in itself will bring fresh concerns for the current pregnancy (Case scenario 2.1). Many women view conception as their transition to true adulthood and a reassurance about their femininity and sexuality, while men have proved their virility. On the other hand, both partners will face the realization of impending new responsibilities, practical and financial, and begin to consider the potential effects on their independence. The process of childbearing involves profound physiological and psychological upheaval. It is a developmental or maturational crisis and involves one of the greatest transitions in a woman's life. This transition is very rapid and involves not only major social, economic and emotional changes, but also the acquisition of a new identity, a new role and new skills. Conflict between the roles of lover and mother, employee and career woman, daughter and mother, and between independence and dependence is

Case scenario 2.1

Roberta had one child, conceived by in vitro fertilization, who was now 6 years old. He had been one of twins but the second twin had died in utero at 12 weeks. Five further attempts at IVF were unsuccessful and, after prolonged counselling, Roberta began to come to terms with having just one child. She was shocked, delighted – and terrified – when she became pregnant. She was in constant fear that the baby would die or be born abnormal (especially as she had been involved in farm work at the time of conception). Everything caused her immense anxiety, from the arrival of a new puppy promised to her son, to thoughts of the birth, to fear over the responsibilities of raising a new baby.

The booking appointment took almost 2 hours while she poured out her concerns, and the midwife referred Roberta for specialist midwife counselling to try to help her come to terms with her situation. She was encouraged to look for the positive aspects of this pregnancy, including the fact that spontaneous conception made this a very different pregnancy from her last. She slowly came to realize that many of her anxieties were normal and only partly related to her previous obstetric history. Gradually she was helped to put her concerns into perspective and as the pregnancy progressed she became calmer until, at 38 weeks' gestation, she spontaneously delivered a healthy daughter.

a common experience of pregnant women which can lead to an identity crisis that may continue into the puerperium. Fundamental changes in relationships occur during pregnancy. Although normally long since independent of her own family, the pregnant woman may discover a need to re-establish close emotional ties with her parents, particularly her mother. Family relationships and childhood events are reappraised as the woman herself faces the prospect of motherhood. This may lead to a reawakening of unresolved conflicts from her own upbringing, which may impact on the way in which a mother chooses to raise her own children.

Relationships

Childbirth is a uniquely female experience which in some ways alienates women from the opposite sex. Female relationships tend to become more important in pregnancy; thus closer ties may develop between mother and daughter and with other relatives and friends who have experienced childbirth. The woman's partner may feel left out and become jealous, especially as pregnancy advances and the woman becomes increasingly involved in the relationship with her baby. The relationship between husband and wife changes from an intense, romantic affair to the complex relationship of parenthood with its new priorities and needs. For most women, pregnancy involves giving up a job, even if only temporarily, and this results in a reduction in income and social contacts outside the home; thus the woman becomes more dependent on her partner. Conversely, she may begin to meet neighbours and make new friends from amongst those people she rarely saw whilst working, and from this she may gain a sense of being part of the local community. First-time parenthood is a demanding test of the couple's personal resources and maturity and of the strength of their relationship. In the majority of cases, couples draw closer together and their relationship is strengthened. For a few couples, however, conflicts arise and the relationship deteriorates, often because of immaturity and sometimes because there are already problems, although they may not have been openly acknowledged. When pregnancy is unplanned and unwanted, especially in fragile relationships or where the mother is unsupported, the negative impact is even more profound. The woman may need to make a decision about whether or not to have the pregnancy terminated, with all the physical, emotional, moral and social implications which that may bring, and it is not uncommon for pregnancy to be the final factor which triggers a break-up of an unstable relationship.

Adapting to pregnancy

Some women view pregnancy as a 'hurdle' to get through, whereas others consider it a developmental process. The 'hurdle' concept is held by women who regard pregnancy as a means to an end, a deviation from normality and think that, once over, they will return to their former state. Others consider pregnancy as a maturation process and recognize, albeit subconsciously, that change will lead to a reorganization of their personality. Although childbirth is now physically safer than ever before, psychological problems still abound, and may, in fact, be greater than in previous decades when the main concern was whether or not the baby would survive. To some extent these worries are caused by the very developments and technological advances which make childbirth safer. The increase in investigations and tests carried out in pregnancy, the move from home to hospital births and the marked increase in intervention has led to the 'medicalization' of pregnancy and childbirth. As a result, women feel that they have lost control over their bodies and the birth, and this can cause great distress.

Raphael-Leff (1991) identifies two groups, 'facilitators' and 'regulators', with the former enjoying relinquishing themselves to the pregnancy and the latter resisting the loss of control which pregnancy and childbirth bring. The facilitator sees pregnancy as the culmination of all that is feminine in her life. She is eager to announce her pregnancy verbally and visually to the world, communicating with her baby, actively seeking to adapt her lifestyle to the demands of the fetus and, towards term, excitedly anticipating the arrival of her baby. Conversely, the regulator feels that pregnancy is an inconvenience, a means to an end, and reluctantly makes changes to her life merely because the baby requires her to do so. She does not indulge in fantasy communication with her baby, continues to work to the last possible moment and feels encumbered by the physical demands put on her body.

The mother's mood will be related to the delight or distress she feels at being pregnant, and may also be affected by the common problems of fatigue, nausea and frequency of micturition, etc. which many women experience during the early weeks of pregnancy. The changes which are occurring in the woman's emotional state are often revealed by episodes of tearfulness and irritability at this time, which are partly hormonal and partly related to all the worries and concerns which she is experiencing. For those women who have had a previous miscarriage, or if such problems arise in the present pregnancy, this may be a particularly anxious time. Such anxieties or complications lead to women feeling insecure about their pregnancies until they are well established. Hence they may refrain from telling other people and from making preparations for their baby until they are convinced that the pregnancy is going to continue.

Attending the antenatal clinic may be the woman's first experience of hospital as a 'patient'. She may find the concept that pregnancy is a normal physiological event difficult to equate with being a hospital patient, since she associates such a role with ill-health. In many areas, a large proportion of antenatal care, including the first booking appointment, is now conducted in the mother's own home or in her local GP's surgery or health centre, to place the emphasis on health rather than on illness. However, much of standard antenatal care continues to focus on the physical aspects of pregnancy, and emotional feelings experienced by the woman may be neglected, although to her they may be of paramount importance and she becomes preoccupied with making sense of them. Many women feel that their needs and feelings are disregarded at antenatal clinics, especially when the midwives appear exceptionally busy and short of staff and time. Concern has long been expressed about the 'conveyor belt' feeling which many women experience when they attend for antenatal care (Reid and Garcia, 1989). Emphasis may appear to the mother to be solely on the care of the fetus. Early in pregnancy, women may be advised to change their dietary habits, stop smoking and reduce alcohol intake, all for the benefit of the fetus. Although most women are anxious to do what is best for their baby, some may feel resentful if their own needs and feelings receive insufficient attention, and this feeling may be exacerbated in those experiencing unfavourable environmental and social conditions, or those with inadequate emotional support from those around them. A careful history and assessment by the midwife in early pregnancy should elicit the woman's individual circumstances and psychological as well as physical needs. Midwifery care, including social and emotional support, can then be tailored to meet the woman's individual needs. A holistic framework for planning of maternity care may assist in this process (Tiran, 1999).

Importance of information and involvement (Case scenario 2.2)

Some of the examinations and investigations carried out during the antenatal period can be uncomfortable and particularly stressful. It is essential that the woman

> *Case scenario 2.2*
>
> Dorothy had a history of three previous spontaneous abortions as a result of cervical incompetence. On booking for the fourth time she was offered the opportunity to participate in a randomized controlled trial on cervical cerclage but she and her partner found it an immensely difficult decision to make. Her worries centred on the risk of entering the trial and being allocated to the control group in which no cervical suture would be inserted, which is not what she actually wanted. Her partner wanted her to enter the trial in order to help others and seemed to be putting pressure on her to do so. After a prolonged period of discussion, Dorothy finally agreed to enter the trial and was delighted that she was allocated to the 'suture' group.
>
> On her next appointment with the midwife she was relieved that this issue was resolved but now felt under pressure from her partner to continue her sick leave from work as manager of a fast-food restaurant, despite the fact that she was becoming increasingly bored and frustrated. We discussed the need to work out a balance between the physical stresses of returning to work and the emotional stresses of isolation and boredom if she did not. As she was already 23 weeks' pregnant there were not too many weeks left before she could legitimately commence maternity leave and finally she decided that she would not go back to work until after the birth.
>
> Added to her distress was her concern regarding her smoking habits, for which she was under pressure from her partner; this had the reverse effect of causing Dorothy to be so stressed that she smoked more. We focused on the positive aspects of her having managed to reduce the number of cigarettes she smoked each day, and helped her partner to put into perspective the risk factors for both Dorothy and her baby. Once the 'guilt factor' of her partner's reprimands was reduced, Dorothy was able spontaneously to cut down on the number of cigarettes she smoked each day. As she had made these decisions herself she felt empowered and as the pregnancy progressed she settled into a more comfortable frame of mind.

and, where possible, her partner are given all necessary information about such examinations and tests to enable them to make an informed decision about whether or not they wish to have them performed. The mother who considers that termination of pregnancy is morally wrong may refuse tests to diagnose fetal abnormalities as she would wish to continue the pregnancy whatever the outcome. This is her right; thus her views should be respected and she should be supported in her decision. Others may be unsure about how to proceed should a fetal abnormality be diagnosed and may need considerable counselling with their doctor and midwife, and perhaps with a minister of religion. The woman who has a raised serum alpha-fetoprotein (AFP) and subsequently has an amniocentesis may go through an agonizing period of waiting until the liquor AFP result is available. If the level is raised, the couple may suffer anguish whatever decision they make about their pregnancy. Even if the liquor AFP is normal, doubts about whether the baby is really normal or not may persist throughout pregnancy until they are able to see for themselves that the baby is as normal as any other.

In general, as the pregnancy progresses the mother may feel physically fairly well, although any problems which occur may cause her to experience feelings of guilt and she may attribute these problems to her lifestyle, behaviour or emotional state.

Clement *et al.* (1998) explore the positive and negative psychological aspects of women's experiences of ultrasound scanning and highlight the dilemmas presented to some women by either knowing too much or knowing too little. They include a discussion on facilitation by midwives and doctors of the parents' need to make decisions about – in this case – ultrasound scans. However, it should be recognized that decision-making is one of the most difficult elements of antenatal care for some couples, despite the fact that being able to make decisions is, to some extent, empowering. They need to be involved in making decisions from the very moment of conception. Women should be given sufficient information to enable them to make an informed decision, although in reality this is often extremely difficult.

Planning maternity services involves an understanding of the balance between providing standards of care that are safe and those that are what women actually want. Hirst *et al.* (1998) discuss whether all women wish to receive uniform care, and explore factors such as the gender of the care-giver, the number of visits, their preferred professional care-giver (midwife, GP or obstetrician) and whether knowing the carer provides women with sufficient satisfaction. When much *obstetric* care could be described as defensive from fear of litigation, it is important to ensure that *midwifery* care is responsive to those factors that can be readily assimilated into a system which, while taking risk into account, can also engender a sense of empowerment in women by facilitating woman-centred care.

Societal pressures also play a part in increasing anxiety for some women. The Government has attempted to focus on 'family values' so that those not in a heterosexual, monogamous, two-parent family may feel that they are unconventional, despite the increase in the number of single mothers. The media produce advertisements which seem to highlight the joys of parenthood without identifying the demands. The number of consumer books and products on pregnancy and childbirth is huge. Pregnancy is a very 'fashionable pastime' with many well-known personalities displaying their pregnancies (literally) to the world. It is also a lucrative business so that the number and variety of pregnancy-related activities and goods from which women can choose is vast. Society seems to imply that women must 'live' their pregnancies for the duration and the media's portrayal of women 'blooming' with joy and anticipation does nothing to help those for whom pregnancy is uncomfortable, worrying or unwanted. Women are reluctant to admit that they are not enjoying their pregnancies almost as if this is an admission of failure, but those who do acknowledge their feelings are relieved to have shared them and surprised to hear that many other women feel similarly.

Reactions to pregnancy

Many women experience fears and fantasies about what is happening inside their bodies. They often worry about normal physical and physiological changes and, if they are multigravidae, invariably compare the present pregnancy with their past experiences. Vivid dreams are common, which may be very disturbing and may be exacerbated by tiredness and insomnia. The dreams frequently involve the baby and may be interpreted by the mother as a premonition, often of something unpleasant. With the tiredness and other discomforts, it is often difficult to distinguish between normal emotional reactions and mental illness, which may be as high as 15% in the first trimester. Some women fear punishment for previous terminations, and are very worried that such retribution may adversely affect the present baby, causing it to die or be abnormal. These women need the opportunity to express their fears and require reassurance and support.

Psychosocial support throughout pregnancy may reduce the impact or incidence of postnatal depression, which can occur in up to 10% of new mothers, and may be informal support or formal (Oakley *et al.*, 1996;

Stamp *et al.*, 1995). Psychosocial support requirements may differ between mothers and fathers. Wheatley (1998) describes a new mother's support systems as an 'inner primary source ring' and an 'outer secondary source ring', but these may differ slightly according to the problem the mother is attempting to solve.

As the pregnancy progresses, the recognition of fetal movements, the increasing abdominal growth and seeing the baby on a scan all combine to make the developing baby a reality, although some women fail to acknowledge this until the baby is actually delivered. For others it becomes a personalized being at this stage in pregnancy and many women name and talk to their baby and are concerned about his or her well-being. All women are anxious and worried to a greater or lesser extent about the well-being of their developing fetus and have to rely on professionals to keep them informed of progress. Some women find this loss of personal control difficult to accept, especially when attending a busy antenatal clinic where they may see many different doctors and midwives during the course of their pregnancy. The system gives them little opportunity to build up a relationship with and develop confidence in the professionals caring for them, despite the changes which have been made following publication of the *Changing Childbirth* report (DoH, 1993). Trust and mutual respect between the woman and midwife is important so that concerns and issues can be freely and openly discussed, enabling the mother to retain her autonomy and make well-informed choices and decisions related to her care. The woman retains the locus of control in pregnancy and childbirth, and this is extremely important to the mental and emotional health of the majority of women.

Late pregnancy is a crucial time for some women and their identity crisis may be accentuated when they stop working, even temporarily, and hence lose daily contact with friends and colleagues. This may be the first time since early childhood that the woman has been free from schooling or a job, and for many it is the time when they feel emotionally ready to relinquish the demands of their work and mentally prepare themselves for the birth and for motherhood. However, although she may appreciate the rest and time to prepare for her baby, she may also feel lonely and isolated at home. This is particularly so for the woman who starts her family after several years of professional work, especially if this has involved progressing to a senior level. A reduction in income may further reduce the social life and independence of some couples. However, the state system of maternity benefits sometimes encourages expectant mothers to work

longer than their health allows, and midwives would do well to advise women to take as much time off before the birth as their finances permit. The transition from independent working girl to a mother with additional responsibilities means that she is unlikely ever again to have the time to do what she wants with such spontaneity.

Adjustment to new roles such as housewife and mother instead of career woman, as well as being a wife and lover, becomes more of a reality and it takes time before the woman is able to resolve the ensuing conflict by integrating these roles both in her thoughts and her behaviour. The woman also becomes preoccupied by her approaching labour and another source of role conflict at this time may be the medicalization of childbirth. On the one hand, the woman may have high hopes and expectations of childbirth as a momentous life experience under her control when she fulfils her role as a woman, yet the reality may be that it is managed by professionals as if she has a medical condition which may well culminate in an obstetric operation. Such role conflict may lead to confusion, indecision and, in some cases, to depression (Kumar and Robson, 1978). If the woman is assertive enough to 'fight for' a home birth she may be made to feel guilty that she is potentially placing her unborn baby and herself in a vulnerable position.

Changing body image can have a powerful effect on a woman and her partner in pregnancy. Some women enjoy their pregnant state until perhaps the latter weeks when they feel too heavy and cumbersome, whereas others feel unattractive and fear that they will no longer be appealing to their partner. Men, too, react in different ways, some finding the bodily changes of pregnancy attractive, while others do not find it appealing.

The woman's sexual activity and enjoyment may diminish in pregnancy, especially during the first and third trimesters when physical discomforts affect her. In early pregnancy many couples are concerned about causing miscarriage, especially if there is a history of such problems. During the third trimester sexual activity tends to decrease, largely because it is physically uncomfortable. Couples need to be encouraged and advised to find other ways of expressing their feelings for each other. Towards the end of pregnancy, however, there may be a sudden increase in libido.

Adjusting to the transition

During this phase of pregnancy the woman's coping resources are diminished and most find it more difficult to manage major upheavals in life. Holmes and Rahe (1967) produced a list of 42 life events which people find particularly stressful and assigned a score to each one. Pregnancy has a score of 40 and a new family member 39. (The maximum score for one event is 100.) Many of the changes which women have to cope with in pregnancy and over which they have little or no control are included in the list, such as stopping work, changes in financial status, social activities and sleeping patterns. Additional events over which they do have some control, such as moving house, can be particularly stressful at this time despite the number of couples who choose to move house during the pregnancy. People vary in their ability to cope with stress. Lazarus (1966) describes the factors which influence the processes of coping and readjustment. These include factors that already exist such as personality and the individual's previous experience and confidence in his or her ability to cope and adjust. Other factors are the degree of stress experienced and the quality of support which is available. Although the midwife cannot change the mother's personality or her previous experience, she can make a careful assessment of the amount of stress the woman is under, assess her coping ability and offer a high level of emotional, and in some cases, practical, support.

Stressful events in pregnancy may result in physio-pathological complications such as the onset of preterm labour, but it is possible that appropriate psychosocial support from the midwife or other professional may reduce their incidence. During the last few weeks of pregnancy, antenatal classes which the woman may have attended are usually completed and for some women this is a significant cause of stress, as they miss the peer support that has developed within the group. Encouragement by the midwife and health visitor for members of the group to keep in touch and build up their own network of support can be helpful both for the latter stages of pregnancy and for the early months and, indeed, years of parenthood.

Anxieties and fears about the pregnancy begin to subside, however, especially if all seems to be progressing normally and the survival of the baby seems assured. Women now tend to become increasingly impatient with their pregnancy and long for the delivery of their baby. Physically they feel immensely uncomfortable, the pregnancy seems interminable and they are eager to greet their new baby.

Towards the end of pregnancy, women become increasingly absorbed in preparations for the baby. In the latter 2–4 weeks of pregnancy, concentration, short-term memory and new learning ability decline and there is an increase in daydreaming and preoccupation with the approaching birth. Women who work in intellectually demanding positions right up to term or who expect to pursue intellectual work soon after delivery, often find it considerably more difficult than anticipated. Serotonin levels increase in the last few weeks of pregnancy so that the mother's natural antidepressant chemicals reduce her anxiety and fear regarding the birth. Women are often regaled with numerous 'horror stories' from friends and family about their own birth experiences and can spend many months of the pregnancy feeling immensely frightened about the delivery. This will be compounded if the woman has suffered previous difficult labours. They need to come to terms with the fact that there is no alternative but to go through the experience of labour (or caesarean section) and sensitive guidance by the midwife, both individually and in parent education classes, can assist in this.

Birth experiences

Women's perceptions and experiences of childbirth are so varied that it is difficult to consider all aspects. The woman's emotional experience of having a baby is often neglected by professionals, the emphasis being placed on physical care and monitoring progress in order to detect any deviations from the normal which may require intervention. Safety, of course, is of paramount importance, and all women want to deliver a live healthy baby (Walton and Hamilton, 1995), but women also have high emotional expectations of this momentous event in their lives. When these expectations are fulfilled, and the woman can look back on her unique experience of childbirth with pride and a sense of achievement, her confidence and self-esteem are increased and she may be less likely to suffer from postnatal depression. Communication and information-giving is essential during labour and delivery (Kirkham, 1989). Simkin (1992) found that women's long-term memories of childbirth are incredibly vivid, a factor which Kitzinger (1992) translated into the potential for long-term distress in cases where the woman feels violated by the care she received during labour. Moorhead (1996) recognizes the major changes which occur in women as a result of their childbirth experience and stresses that the impact of childbirth can never be transient but is indeed a permanent factor in the lives of these women.

No matter how well prepared the woman is, the reality is usually something of a shock. The contractions are strange, uncomfortable and increasingly powerful.

At a time when the expectant mother feels particularly vulnerable, she may be in strange, often uncomfortable surroundings. This author has cared for a woman who was due to move house 1 week prior to her expected date for delivery yet she was adamant that she should deliver in the current house where everything was familiar – and perhaps this contributed to a mental initiation of labour at 37 weeks' gestation. Developing a system of care in which women are enabled to labour at home for as long as possible with visits by the midwife to assess progress may facilitate a more normal course of events than if they are forced to go to hospital as soon as labour commences. Labour may occur in the middle of the night and this adds to the sense of unreality. They may be cared for by strangers, although caseload and team midwifery systems may improve continuity of carer. All women in such circumstances will be in a high state of arousal and it is very common for them to feel depersonalized, as if it were all happening to somebody else. There is a sense of loss of control because labour is a powerful and irrevocable process and there is no turning back. This can be frightening and a cause of panic in some women. In the transitional stage the woman has the alarming sensation of wanting to evacuate her bowels and bear down and this often produces a transient episode of panic and fear of losing control. For some women the actual moments of birth are thrilling, especially if they are well prepared and in control. Facilitating a partnership in care between the mother, the midwife and the companion accompanying the woman will give her a greater feeling of being in control of her own destiny. Midwives should also be careful in their choice of words used during interactions with labouring women, as inappropriate terminology may affect negatively the adaptation of the mother and family to the new arrival (Misch, 1999; Wells, 1999), whereas positive reassuring vocabulary and ensuring a balance between terminology that is easily understood but is not condescending can be empowering to labouring women.

After delivery

When the mother receives her baby into her arms immediately after delivery the commonest reaction is one of ecstasy and relief; the difference between the woman in pain and the mother with the baby in her arms is astounding and is virtually universal. The father is often present at the birth and shares this joyful experience with his partner but will also feel relief that his partner is now out of pain and that the baby has been delivered safely. There is a culture-constant pattern of behaviour at this time which starts with the mother greeting and engaging in eye-to-eye contact with her baby. The baby is usually awake, alert and responsive during this time immediately after birth. Then the mother begins to explore her infant, peripherally at first, then all over (Klaus and Kennell, 1970). Most mothers also talk to their baby during this time of exploration. The baby may then begin to indicate a desire to suck and the mother who wishes to breastfeed responds by suckling her child. The midwife should observe these clues and be available to give the mother assistance at this first feed so that she learns how to position her baby correctly on the breast, as this is the key to successful breastfeeding. In Ball's study (1994) mothers who fed their babies within the first hour of delivery recalled more positive feelings at that time and the highest levels of satisfaction with motherhood 6 weeks later. A successful first feed also builds up the mother's confidence in her ability to breastfeed and she continues to feed for longer (Salariya et al., 1978). Mothers who do not wish to breastfeed should be offered the opportunity to bottlefeed their infant in response to his sucking movements.

The physical contact between the mother and baby during the first hour after birth has a beneficial effect on developing the maternal–child relationship. It has also been shown to have a positive influence on the mother's satisfaction with motherhood and her emotional well-being (Ball, 1994). It should be relaxed and unhurried and include the father too so that he can share with the mother in the joy of the birth and start getting to know his baby. Midwives therefore have the responsibility to ensure that all mothers have this enriching time of close contact with their baby during the hour after birth. Ball (1994) refers to it as the fourth stage of labour and stresses that it needs the same degree of attention and care as the other three stages. Although it is an important and pleasurable time for mother–infant attachment, it is thought not to be absolutely crucial for human beings since the majority of mothers deprived of this early experience form good attachments to their babies at a later stage and develop close relationships with them. Omission of this time, however, does have an adverse effect on the mother's satisfaction with the experience of motherhood and emotional fulfilment and this is still evident at 6 weeks after delivery. If this time of close contact after delivery has to be delayed because the mother is anaesthetized or ill, the midwife should ensure that the mother has the opportunity later to have a period of uninterrupted time with her baby, together with her partner. Sometimes it is not possible at birth because the baby is ill and is transferred to the neonatal unit. The mother should always be given the opportunity to see and touch her baby, even if only briefly, and then have an uninterrupted time together with her partner so that they can share their distress and support each other. As soon as possible, usually at the time of transfer from the delivery suite to the postnatal ward, she should be taken to see her baby.

Sometimes conditions, such as birth asphyxia, which require immediate treatment prevent the mother from holding her baby immediately after birth and she will be extremely distressed and anxious at her baby's failure to breathe at once. Any concern for the baby, no matter how trivial, will be extremely alarming for the mother. Her perception of time will be altered so that attention to the baby lasting only a few seconds or minutes will seem like hours to her. The mother and her partner should be kept well informed about what is happening to their baby, reassured if appropriate and given the opportunity to see and hold their infant as soon as possible.

For a minority of women, their immediate response to their babies is flat and unemotive. Some may be disappointed about the sex of their child. Others may feel real distaste, especially if the baby is very bloodstained or soiled with meconium. Sometimes an unfavourable response follows a distressing labour and delivery, or the mother may be too sedated to respond to the birth of her child. Most of these mothers gradually accept their baby during the next 24–48 hours. Only a small minority will have difficulty in establishing a relationship with their newborn child. However, the mother who does not wish to see or hold her baby immediately should not always be viewed as a potential case of puerperal depression. Some women prefer to be washed and rested before they are ready to greet their new baby.

Early days of motherhood

During the postnatal period many women have problems adapting to their new role. Adjustments also have to be made in family relationships to make room for the baby and this sometimes causes disharmony with siblings and/or the father. The demands of caring for a newborn baby far exceed most mothers' expectations. Disturbed nights lead to extreme tiredness and affect the mother's ability to cope with everyday situations. She feels guilty that she is an imperfect mother who is unable to cope and feels isolated in the home with her baby, often experiencing a loss of identity. A supportive and understanding partner and family, and the support of the midwife can do much to help the mother through the early weeks of motherhood. A network of support, usually built up during pregnancy, has proved to be very helpful to many women struggling to cope during the first few weeks after the birth of their baby.

Most mothers gradually adjust to their new role and resume an active and fulfilling life, but a significant number develop postnatal depression which, if not recognized and treated, can continue for many months and mar their enjoyment of the early months of motherhood (see Ch. 42). A few women feel so traumatized by the childbirth experience that they suffer post-traumatic stress disorder which may lead to prolonged nightmares, a fear of future pregnancies (Menage, 1993), psychosexual difficulties and inadequately developed mother–child relationships (Ballard *et al.*, 1995). Kitzinger (1992) suggests that the delivery phase may be likened to the experience of sexual assault by some women. Midwives can help in the prevention of post-traumatic stress disorder by empowering women to retain control, respecting their wishes wherever possible, providing adequate information, enabling women to cope with their pain or providing the means to reduce it and, perhaps most importantly, by offering the opportunity to 'debrief' following labour. It is also important for staff to have an opportunity to discuss critical incidents which have occurred in the delivery suite.

CONCLUSION

Conception, pregnancy, childbirth and early parenthood are periods of immense physical, psychological, social, financial and practical change. The trend of having small families, particularly when employment and financial considerations are taken into account, may mean that some women have only one pregnancy. Women (and their partners) are keen to ensure that their childbearing experience is both safe and satisfying, and as most mothers achieve a safe, normal, physiological pregnancy and labour, there is greater emphasis on psychological satisfaction and enjoyment. Women deserve to be facilitated to achieve this and the midwife is in an invaluable position to assist them. Of all health professionals providing care for pregnant and childbearing women, the midwife is best placed to provide holistic care which adequately takes into account the psychological aspects of maternity care.

KEY POINTS

- Midwives must develop, maintain and refine their communication skills, both verbal and non-verbal, in order to provide appropriate care for all women during pregnancy and childbirth.
- Psychological care during the childbearing period is equally as important as physiopathological care but is far more likely to come within the remit of the midwife's role rather than that of medical staff.

- The pregnancy and childbirth experience is likely to be the most emotionally profound event in a woman's life and midwives have a responsibility to ensure that expectant and newly delivered mothers are as empowered as possible by all professionals involved in their care.

REFERENCES

Ball, J.A. (ed) (1994) *Reactions to Motherhood*. Hale: Books for Midwives Press.

Ballard, C.G., Stanley, A.K. & Brockington, I.F. (1995) Post traumatic stress disorder (PTSD) after childbirth. *British Journal of Psychiatry* **165**(3): 525–528.

Clement, S., Wilson, J. & Sikorski, J. (1998) Women's experiences of antenatal ultrasound scans. In: Clement S (ed) *Psychological Perspectives on Pregnancy and Childbirth*, Ch. 1, pp. 7–20. London: Churchill Livingstone.

Department of Health (DoH) (1993) *Changing Childbirth. Report of the Expert Maternity Group*. London: HMSO.

Egan, G. (1982) *The Skilled Helper*. Belmont, California: Wadsworth.

Hirst, J., Hewison, J., Dowswell, T. *et al.* (1998) Antenatal care: what do women want? In: Clement, S. (ed) *Psychological Perspectives on Pregnancy and Childbirth*, Ch. 2, pp. 27–44. London: Churchill Livingstone.

Holmes, T.H. & Rahe, R.H. (1967) Social readjustment rating scale. *Journal of Psychosomatic Research* **11**: 219.

Inati, M. (1999) Counselling for fetal anomalies. *Journal of Paediatrics, Obstetrics and Gynaecology* **25**(1): 34–36.

Kirkham, M. (1989) Midwives and information giving during labour. In: Robinson, S. & Thomson, A. (eds) *Midwives, Research and Childbirth*, Vol. 1, pp. 117–138. London: Chapman and Hall.

Kitzinger, S. (1992) Birth and violence against women: generating hypotheses from women's accounts of unhappiness after childbirth. In: Roberts, H. (ed) *Women's Health Matters*, pp. 63–80. London: Routledge.

Klaus, M.H. & Kennell, J.H. (1970) Human maternal behaviour at first contact with her young. *Pediatrics* **46**(2): 187–192.

Kumar, R. & Robson, K. (1978) Neurotic disturbance during pregnancy and the puerperium. In: *Mental Illness in Pregnancy and the Puerperium*, pp. 40–51. Oxford: Oxford University Press.

Lazarus, R.S. (1966) Psychological stress and coping process. Cited in: Ball, J.A. (ed) (1994) *Reactions to Motherhood*. Hale: Books for Midwives Press.

Mack, S. (2000) Therapies for the relief of physical and emotional stress. In: Tiran, D. & Mack, S. (eds) (2000) *Complementary Therapies for Pregnancy and Childbirth*, 2nd edn, Ch. 12. London: Baillière Tindall.

Menage, J. (1993) Post-traumatic stress disorder in women who have undergone obstetric and/or gynaecological procedures. *Journal of Reproductive and Infant Psychology* **11**(2): 221–228.

Misch, C.R. (1999) Watch those words. *Mother Baby Journal* **4**(3): 21–24.

Moorhead, J. (1996) *New Generations: 40 years of Birth in Britain*. London: National Childbirth Trust.

Moulder, C. (1999) Late pregnancy loss: issues in hospital care. *British Journal of Midwifery* **7**(4): 244–247.

Oakley, A., Hickey, D., Rajan, L. *et al.* (1996) Social support in pregnancy: does it have longterm effects? *Journal of Reproductive and Infant Psychology* **14**(1): 7–22.

Raphael-Leff, J. (1991) *Psychological Processes of Childbearing*. London: Chapman & Hall.

Reid, M. & Garcia, J. (1989) Women's views of care during pregnancy and childbirth. In: Chalmers, I., Enkin, M. & Keirse, M.J.N.C. (eds) *Effective Care in Pregnancy and Childbirth*, pp. 1331–1142. Oxford: Oxford University Press.

Salariya, E.M., Easton, P.M. & Cater, J.L. (1978) Duration of breastfeeding after early initiation and frequent feeding. *Lancet* ii: 1141–1143.

Sehdev, S.S. & Wilson, A. (1999) Views of women and their partners on general practice care received during and after a miscarriage. *European Journal of General Practice* **5**(3): 105–109.

Simkin, P. (1992) Just another day in a woman's life? Part 2: nature and consistence of women's longterm memories of their first birth experiences. *Birth* **19**(2): 64–81.

Stamp, G.E., Williams, A.S. & Crowther, C.A. (1995) Evaluation of antenatal and postnatal support to overcome postnatal depression: a randomised controlled trial. *Birth* **22**(3): 138–143.

Standing Nursing and Midwifery Advisory Committee (SNMAC) (1998) *Midwifery: Delivering Our Future*. HMSO: London.

Street, E. & Downey, J. (1996) *Brief Therapeutic Consultations*. Chichester: Wiley.

Tennant, J. & Butler, M. (1999) Communication: issues for change. *British Journal of Midwifery* 7(6): 359–362.

Tiran, D. (1999) A holistic framework for maternity care. *Complementary Therapies in Nursing and Midwifery* 5(3): 127–135.

Tiran, D. (2000) Massage and aromatherapy. In: Tiran, D. & Mack, S. (eds) (2000) *Complementary Therapies for Pregnancy and Childbirth*, 2nd edn, Ch. 7. London: Baillière Tindall.

Walton, I. & Hamilton, M. (1995) *Midwives and Changing Childbirth*. Hale: Books for Midwives Press.

Wells, B. (1999) Finding the right words. *Midwifery Matters* 81(2): 7.

Wheatley, S. (1998) Psychosocial support in pregnancy. In: Clement, S. (1998) *Psychological Perspectives on Pregnancy and Childbirth*, Ch. 3, pp. 45–59. London: Churchill Livingstone.

FURTHER READING

Clement, S. (ed) (1998) *Psychological Perspectives on Pregnancy and Childbirth*. London: Churchill Livingstone. This is a multi-contributed text which explores a range of important issues on the psychological aspects related to maternity care.

3

Grief and Bereavement

Jenni Thomas

LEARNING OUTCOMES

After reading this chapter you will be able to:

- understand the complexities of the grieving process and how this may manifest in different women, their partners and families
- consider the needs of women, their partners and families who are suffering a bereavement around childbirth
- develop practice strategies which will increase the support to families and which facilitate the positive preservation of memories
- explore your own attitudes to death and bereavement and consider how these might affect the care provided to families and colleagues.

And can it be that in a world so full and busy, the loss of one weak creature makes a void in any heart, so wide and deep that nothing but the width and depth of vast eternity can fill it up!
(Charles Dickens, *Dombey and Son*)

With better antenatal care and advances in technology, childbirth is now a relatively safe procedure and the birth of a child is usually a cause for celebration and joy rather than as in Dickens' time, when childbirth itself held significant dangers for the mother and baby (see Fig. 3.1). Sadly, even now, some babies do die – there were 3469 stillbirths and 2559 neonatal deaths recorded in England, Wales and Northern Ireland in 1999 (Office for National Statistics, 1999). In addition it is estimated that 20% of confirmed pregnancies end in miscarriage before 20 weeks' gestation.

Death is a part of life and inevitable in the experience of living, but the death of a baby before, at, or shortly after birth, because of miscarriage, termination for fetal abnormality, stillbirth or neonatal death, is unexpected and against the natural order of things. It is unique, incomprehensible and unlike any other death. When an adult or a child dies, family members have a wealth of memories to draw upon and a life to remember, but when a baby dies, parents grieve the lack of memories and any future with their child. For most parents the death of a baby is a significant and painful experience,

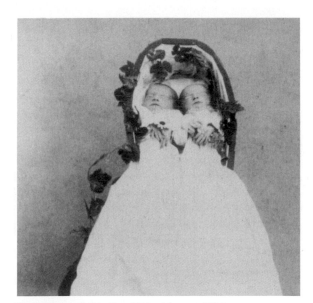

Figure 3.1 Twins in casket at home, 1890.

regardless of the cause or gestational age. These parents depend on those in the health service, including midwives, to care for them and offer relevant information to guide them in the choices they have to make in this time of crisis.

Not many years ago it was considered inappropriate for mothers to grieve over the loss of their baby. It is only in the last 15–20 years that the importance of grieving for a healthy long-term outcome has been recognized. Research at the Tavistock Clinic has shown that, following stillbirth, bereaved mothers may suffer lifelong repercussions, including hypochondria and phobias as well as disturbances in relationships (Lewis and Bourne, 1989). Appropriate professional help and support at this time and in the months ahead are essential. Recognizing and responding to the parents' very varied feelings, trying to sense what they need and helping them to make informed choices, are the particular challenges for professionals involved in caring for these parents before, during and after the birth of their baby.

There is no right way to grieve, no set way of managing these difficult situations, and the midwife needs to learn through involvement with grieving families. The insights and suggestions for practice, made in this chapter, are based on what parents have taught professionals through sharing their needs.

Reflective Activity 3.1

Tasks of mourning (see p. 31)

Review your knowledge of the stages and tasks of the grieving process. Think of a hurt or loss that you have experienced. What were some of the feelings that you experienced associated with that loss? What help did you need?

Consider the behaviour of the last person you cared for who was coping with a death or loss – perhaps a woman who had a baby with a congenital abnormality. Did the person experience any of the recognized tasks in the process of mourning? Did the person move in and out of various tasks?

Which behaviour did you find hardest to manage as a practitioner?

THERAPEUTIC USE OF OURSELVES

As individuals we naturally tend to turn away from looking at painful things, yet it is only in looking at ourselves that we can grow and ultimately help others. When a baby dies at or soon after birth, we care for parents during an immense tragedy in their lives. In touching such sadness and pain, witnessing the parents' grief and coming alongside them in their loss, we can easily be reminded of losses in our own lives.

The process of helping is an active one and assumes our willingness to become involved, by willingly putting ourselves in a place where hurt and pain are experienced. In this interaction we require the ability to share in the painful process, to be congruent, to express our concern and yet also remain separate, enabling us to offer care that is sensitive to the parents' needs.

In caring for grieving parents it is essential that we develop self-awareness and recognize our own feelings. In preparation, it can be helpful to reflect on previous life experiences that have been difficult – hurts experienced, broken relationships and other situations that have involved loss. It helps us to understand better why we react in certain ways, our own limitations and when professionally we are likely to need support. As carers, if we are able to acknowledge and appropriately express our own anger, fear, sadness and embarrassment, we are more likely to accept these emotions in other people – the way we manage our own emotions has a direct influence on how we cope when others express feelings.

When we interact with people who are profoundly distressed, it is normal to feel inadequate and helpless. In healthcare the role of the professionals is usually to make people better and to take pain away; however, in bereavement, people cannot be made better. In contrast, healing occurs when people are able to feel and express their painful feelings. When caring for bereaved families, the care-giver's feelings often mirror those of the family – anger, sadness, confusion, a sense of failure. Management that recognizes and acknowledges the value of staff's contributions in this work and their need for support helps to build individuals' self-esteem in times of stress. Having access to a professional offering support or counselling based in the hospital can be just as valuable for staff as it is for parents.

LOOKING AFTER OURSELVES AS PROFESSIONALS

Emotions are also felt physically and we carry them in different parts of our body – tension can be felt in the muscles of the shoulder, grief and sadness perhaps in the muscles around the neck, heart and stomach. Once we notice which parts of our body are affected in times of stress, we are more able to identify ways of releasing these trapped emotions. Relaxation, vigorous exercise, listening to music, counselling or perhaps watching a comedy programme on television and seeking support are therapeutic outlets.

When people feel unable to deal with their own emotions, they develop protective strategies such as distancing themselves from other people's emotions, appearing unaffected and detached or conversely becoming very busy in order to avoid their emotional pain. They may develop negative feelings about themselves and their work and see themselves as failures. This can be manifest as anger or resentment, which can colour family and professional relationships. Some of the warning signs of feeling depleted include experiencing chronic exhaustion, frequently feeling upset, having difficulty eating or sleeping or engaging with people, developing headaches or backaches, having nightmares, feeling worthless and pessimistic, avoiding contact with others, leaving work early and arriving late.

Reflective Activity 3.2

Think of your own response to stress. Do you feel that you have an effective response to stress? What do you feel would be a better way of coping?

Next time you feel that you would describe yourself as stressed, tune in to how you are physiologically responding. Notice where the emotion is in you physically. Then try out one of the strategies you have thought might be helpful, assessing the effect on your mood and body.

Support and training for midwives working in partnership with families

Caring for distressed parents is difficult and demanding. To do it well, all staff need a working environment that considers their needs and values them as individuals. Where appropriate support mechanisms are in place, midwifery teams are able to provide the best possible care to families. Bereaved parents are deeply grateful and remember the care they received throughout their lives.

Bereavement skills training and support should be an intrinsic part of maternity care, whether it is hospital or community based. Using counselling and listening skills is an essential part of the professional's role and one that requires training, enabling midwives to care effectively when managing the death of a baby.

Midwives need to know about the policies relevant to different areas of care and the choices available to parents, and to understand grief and theories related to bereavement. Ideally, student midwives should receive education and training in bereavement work in preparation for their role as midwives in managing the loss of a baby.

It is not helpful for the same members of staff to always provide the bereavement support to families as this can de-skill the other members of the team and overburdens those constantly involved in the care. There is no one person who is better equipped to care; in truth each of us has something to offer – we offer ourselves and in so doing learn from grieving families.

When closely involved with bereaved parents, midwives may feel the isolation and loneliness that the grieving family are experiencing. It is useful to be aware that these members of staff are dealing with a particularly demanding situation and may well need the opportunity to talk with colleagues about how they are managing as soon afterwards as possible. A unit policy that encompasses debriefing sessions, held after a crisis, enables staff involved to share their experience with colleagues in a supportive atmosphere. When done well, debriefing enhances team work and provides an outlet for individual members to offload and feel less alone.

Support should be available from the Supervisor of Midwives, and this may be provided on an individual or team basis. Initially the midwife may wish to talk through the experience, exploring her management of the family's care and her own feelings. The skilled supervisor can assist the practitioner in a critical reflection on the episode of care and her part in it, and, together, they can identify any educational or practice development needs, and how these can be met. It is also useful for several practitioners to meet together to reflect on the case, as this is an important way of identifying shortcomings within the system, sharing good practice and providing mutual support. Paying such attention to the needs of the staff and the parents through the episode of bereavement also highlights the organization's commitment to improving the service.

The functions of this confidential supervision fall into three categories:

- Supportive – to provide moral, psychological and emotional support for staff, enabling midwives to identify and talk about their own emotions and reactions and explore feelings of sadness, helplessness and inadequacy.
- Educational – to facilitate learning and understanding and to promote the development of skills and resources, thus integrating theory into practice. This enables midwives to identify their learning needs and develop an insight into alternative strategies of action.
- Managerial – to clarify roles, tasks and boundaries and look at ethical issues, as well as highlighting resource implications.

When staff do take the time to talk about their needs, their feelings, their reactions to situations and to understand their strengths and limitations, then work-ing with families in grief is very special.

UNDERSTANDING LOSS AND GRIEF

> If bereavement is what's happened to you, grief
> is how you feel, and mourning is what you do.
> (Dr Richard Wilson, Consultant Paediatrician)

There have been many theories advanced to explain the grieving process. Bowlby highlighted attachment theory and the tendency in human beings to make strong bonds with others and the emotional reaction that occurs when those bonds are broken. He suggested that the behavioural responses that make up part of the grieving process are geared towards re-establishing a relationship with the lost object (Bowlby, 1980). Building on Bowlby's work, Kubler-Ross (1970) and Parkes (1972) described a series of predictable grief reactions which make up stages or phases of the grief response, and Worden (1991) added to this model the concept of 'tasks of mourning'.

These tasks of mourning will be used as a guide to understanding the grieving response following the death of a baby. Worden (1991) stresses that mourning, which he defines as the emotional process that occurs after a loss, is an essential and necessarily painful heal-ing process. As with healing after physical injury, the process can be delayed or go wrong. The midwife has a significant part to play in helping parents begin to accomplish in particular the first two of the following tasks identified by Worden:

1. Accept the reality of the loss.
2. Work through to the pain of grief.
3. Adjust to an environment in which the deceased is missing.
4. Emotionally relocate the deceased and move on with life.

Accepting the reality of the loss

Initially the parents are unlikely to believe the bad news and will be in a state of shock and denial, even when a death has been anticipated. This may be mani-fest in a number of ways. Some bereaved parents cry uncontrollably, become hysterical or collapse, whereas others feel faint or numb and display little outward signs of emotion, appearing very controlled, calm and detached. The initial shock may last for hours or sev-eral days. This natural reaction is a form of emotional

protection that will disappear as parents gradually take in the full impact of what has happened. Each experience of grief is unique and previous losses may complicate the reaction to this current bereavement.

Parents may initially be unable to acknowledge what has happened and may manage by denying the reality. These parents need time and help to do what is right for them; however, it is not helpful for professionals to col-lude with denial and unreality, for example by avoiding talking about the dead baby, somehow making the child's death seem less important – not showing or fully acknowledging its significance.

Midwifery staff have an important role in enabling parents to gradually face reality. Being sensitive to par-ents' needs, discussing what other parents have valued, being offered choices such as seeing and holding their dead baby, being involved as much as possible in the preparations for the funeral, and observing rituals and traditions, all help to make what has happened real. Families from different faiths need support for the mourning rituals appropriate to their culture.

Working through to the pain of grief

As the denial and numbness gradually subside, the bereaved parents usually experience the full impact of what has happened. Intensely painful feelings may last many weeks or months. This normal reaction to an abnormal event can be overwhelming as they think about what could have been and what the future now holds. Bereaved mothers are often incapable of think-ing about anything or anybody else and are consumed with their child, themselves and how they feel. Painful reminders get in the way and are all around them. Innocent comments may get misinterpreted and cause distress and irritability. Susan Hill (1990), a writer and bereaved mother, eloquently described her extreme sensitivity after the death of her baby Imogen as 'like having one skin less'. She explained how she appreci-ated the professionals who treated her gently.

It is normal to feel extremely sad, guilty, angry and resentful. Many parents struggle with guilty feelings about some aspect of their baby's death, especially if they were initially ambivalent about becoming parents. Mothers may think about their behaviours or actions taken which they may blame for causing the death of their baby, i.e. running for a bus, or carrying heavy shopping. These punishing thoughts can intrude into all aspects of their life.

Feelings of anger are often unexpected and hard to manage. The father or mother may feel anger for the loss of control that death brings; their anger can be directed at the medical and midwifery team for not recognizing the problem sooner, for not keeping their baby alive; anger at a God who allowed it to happen; and possibly anger towards their baby for not living and leaving them. Sometimes unexpected resentment with a family member or their partner adds to this exhausting and painful time.

Grief is not a mental illness, although sleeplessness, anxiety, fear, anger and a preoccupation with self can all add up to a feeling of 'going mad'. These feelings are normal and when experienced and expressed do slowly become less intrusive and frequent. Talking about difficult experiences with someone who is interested and willing to listen is one of the healing ways to express grief, as is writing about your feelings. Attempts to cut short these emotions rarely help in the long term and may cause deep-seated problems in the years ahead. If grief is denied, or anger and guilt persist to the exclusion of other feelings over a number of months, help may be needed from someone trained in counselling.

Adjusting to an environment in which the deceased is missing

However short a time the parents had to get to know their baby, both during pregnancy and after the birth, facing a future without this child in the family is a difficult and painful process. Nothing can fill the aching void their baby has left and each day of life brings constant reminders of their baby's absence. The future seems uncertain and frightening, while a tremendous effort is required to carry on as normal. Grief is exhausting. It may take many months before the mother, particularly, is able to focus less on the sad events surrounding the death and regain some of her interest in life. Parents may also revisit the feelings of loss at what would have been significant milestones in their child's life.

Emotionally relocating the deceased and moving on with life

This involves moving on to a different and new way of life without their child, whilst remembering and holding on to precious memories. It is a process of reinvesting in life again alongside the knowledge that their baby will not be forgotten. This can often feel like a betrayal and is perhaps a more difficult task than is generally recognized.

When parents are able to move on with their lives together, there is a sense of putting the distress aside and looking to the future, whilst recalling memories of their baby and finding comfort and pleasure in these memories. It is also a way of making life meaningful

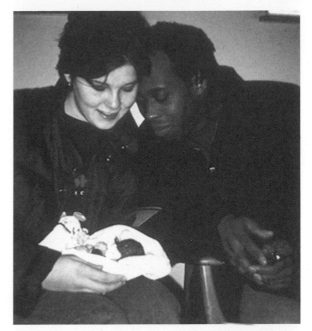

Figure 3.2 Claire and Joseph with daughter Ellie, who died at birth.

again and gaining back some control, so that the bereaved parents are not continually ambushed by memories of the death and trapped by painful feelings.

The importance of the loss

When a baby lives only a short time or dies before birth, because of miscarriage, termination for fetal anomaly or stillbirth, a common assumption is that the loss is not as significant. Pregnancy is a time of anticipation and many parents, particularly mothers, develop a strong bond with their baby long before it is born (Fig. 3.2). When a baby dies, parents grieve for all they had hoped for and the lost opportunity of getting to know their child in a future they had planned together.

This grief response is not confined to the death of a baby, as families grieve when a baby is born with a disability. These parents may experience the same feelings of loss of the healthy baby they were expecting and anger at the extinction of their hopes and plans. For some parents, the need for a caesarean section can result in a sense of failure and a reaction of grief.

A Stillbirth and Neonatal Death Society (SANDS) teardrop sticker placed on the mother's notes after a baby's death now and in future pregnancies can alert all professionals to the parents' need for sensitivity. At initial booking, it is important for the midwife to identify women who have had previous losses – whether through miscarriage, stillbirth or neonatal death, and discuss the implications for the current pregnancy. This requires opening up a potentially painful subject; however, the midwife needs to be aware that this discussion allows the dead child to be acknowledged and the baby's existence as an individual valued. In addition the midwife can also help prepare the woman for reactions and feelings that she might experience during the pregnancy and birth of this baby, which might include mixed feelings at the birth, and high levels of anxiety concerning the baby's well-being and survival (Caelli *et al.*, 1999; Hunfeld *et al.*, 1997). The healthcare team can then be alert to this mother's needs, and ensure that support systems are available during the pregnancy and puerperium. Bereaved mothers may be inclined to develop postnatal depression, particularly in cases of complicated grief.

DIFFERENT PARENTAL RESPONSES IN BEREAVEMENT

Grief is solitary – even when a couple are grieving, each parent can feel alone in his or her grief and normal patterns in relationships may become disrupted. As a father's and mother's needs are different, they may find they are unable to communicate with one another, to express the awfulness of their feelings. A mother usually finds it helpful to share her feelings of loss, while frequently the father's tendency is to repair and look to the future. The dual process model of grieving (Stroebe and Schut, 1999) illustrates the way bereaved people engage in both loss-oriented and restoration-oriented grieving behaviour and oscillate in healthy grieving between the two behaviours (Fig. 3.3).

Women naturally tend to be more loss-oriented and are more concerned with and aware of their feelings. They focus on their loss and the emotions they are experiencing. They need memories and to constantly recall, be reminded of and talk about their baby who has died.

In contrast, men are generally more restoration-oriented – they want things to return to normal and to make things better. Traditionally men are not encouraged to express feelings and so they may instinctively try to suppress them and endeavour to be strong, as society demands, and function as if nothing had happened. Although they feel the loss, it is a loss not to be acknowledged (Puddifoot and Johnson, 1997). This response may be misinterpreted by their partner, and others, as being uncaring and less interested in their baby.

These different ways of dealing with grief can put a significant strain on the parents' relationship and it is helpful for them to understand that men and women grieve differently and their partner's response to grief is natural. It is helpful to encourage parents to find ways of sharing their feelings and reaching out to one another.

When people engage in either activity to the exclusion of the other it can cause added difficulties. Women are helped when they develop some form of restorative response to enable them to move on from the intensity of the pain, and men frequently need support to explore their feelings. Relationships are more likely to survive where couples are able to help each other develop the behaviour they are less naturally inclined towards.

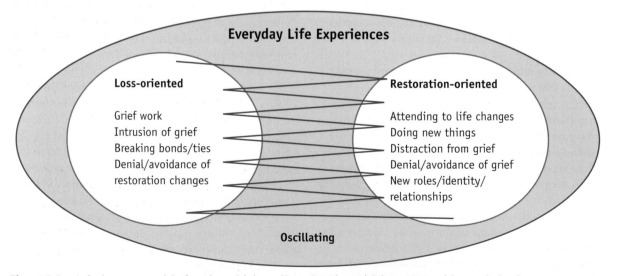

Figure 3.3   A dual process model of coping with loss. (From Stroebe and Schut, 1999, with permission.)

Supporting parents

Women and men say that the most supportive care is when professionals are able to help and encourage parents to 'parent' (CBT, 2003a), to be involved with their baby before and after death. Healthcare professionals who are sensitive and respectful of the very private emotions people experience are invaluable. There is no right way to grieve, and parents will find their own way to deal with this tragedy in their lives. Both parents need support and both need information, though it should be remembered that it is often difficult for distressed parents to absorb and understand what they are told. It is useful to ask the parents to explain to you what they have understood. They may want more information about their baby's condition or to know more about the reason for their baby's death, and so any help the midwife can provide in obtaining this information will be welcomed.

Parents appreciate staff who offer them warmth and understanding, and who are able to show they care and are not afraid to express their own emotions. In expressing feelings, professionals act as role models and tears are unlikely to be viewed negatively if genuinely felt. However, parents need support and should not have to be concerned about their midwife's feelings or experiences of grief.

Touching is the most basic form of comfort and communication. This may be a hand on the arm, or an arm around the parent's shoulder. Parents need the opportunity to talk about how they feel with someone they trust and if possible to be able to express their emotions openly. It is not helpful for parents to be told how they feel; only they can know. Parents do not want to be told the stage of grief they are seen to be at.

Often midwives spend many hours with a couple. Talking about everyday things, offering opportunities for normal conversation, can be useful, as well as being quiet and recognizing that just being there and being available to the parents is valuable. Midwives who are self-aware can be intuitive and trust their own instincts when interacting with parents; listening carefully is the key.

It is important to talk to both parents and acknowledge that both parents are grieving. It is helpful to provide information to parents who may want to do the practical things that have to be done, together.

All staff – hospital and community midwife, doctor, chaplain, counsellor and social worker, and later, GP and health visitor – need to adopt a team approach with everyone being aware of the procedures to follow when a bereavement occurs. Good team relationships are essential to provide the best possible care to bereaved parents.

Reflective Activity 3.3

Does your unit/service have a system which ensures effective communication when managing a pregnancy loss or the death of a baby? How do you personally ensure that a death has been appropriately communicated to the GP and health visitor?

BREAKING BAD NEWS

> The worst bit for me was knowing something was going wrong but no one actually told me.
> (Bereaved mother)

Parents remember the way they are told bad news and the words, actions and attitudes of the professionals involved. This places a heavy burden on the professional who has the responsibility of telling parents such sad information. Explaining bad news involves both parents together whenever possible, and should take place in a private and appropriate room. Parents appreciate honesty and a genuinely caring approach by the professional in such a situation. An interpreter will need to be present when parents do not speak or understand English. Children in the family should not be used to translate and convey information to parents.

Clear, unambiguous information needs to be sensitively given, in a way that uses language the parents understand. This may have to be repeated more than once. Questions should be answered as honestly as possible and allowances should be made for parents to respond in their own time. Offering time and actively listening to what they have to say avoids parents being left with confusing information. Parents remember when you refer to their baby by name and acknowledge the significance of their baby's death. Saying that you are sorry that their baby has died does not mean anyone did anything that requires an apology.

Reflective Activity 3.4

Think about the last time you yourself were given bad news. Can you remember finding it difficult to absorb information? What helped you at that time? Do you remember anyone who was particularly helpful to you … and what made that person helpful? Think about the words that were used, the tone of voice, the body language.

THE SCAN – THE DIAGNOSIS

The ultrasonographer may be the first person to know that something is wrong. When an appointment is made for a scan, the parents need to be clearly told and understand that the scan is being performed to detect any problem that their baby may have and that a partner or friend may accompany the mother.

When the scan reveals an abnormality or that their baby has died, the sonographer scanning the woman needs initially to explain to the parents that there is reason for concern. These situations require the presence of a doctor as soon as possible to confirm a possible diagnosis and future course of action. The mother and father should be offered an opportunity to see the scan of their baby while the doctor explains honestly and sensitively what is wrong. All staff need to be familiar with the unit policy to be followed in such a crisis. When further tests are necessary, parents need them to be carried out as soon as possible and the reliability of these tests and any risks involved carefully explained. Whether their baby's death is anticipated or occurs suddenly, the parents value the support of caring professional staff. These parents will not know what is available to them and will depend on the professional care-giver to help them through this sad and difficult time.

Parents are likely to be in shock and both the mother and father need privacy and time to absorb what they have been told and the options open to them. Keeping a scan photograph in the mother's notes for collection at a later date is helpful. It is the responsibility of the midwife looking after these parents to inform them that the community team and their GP will receive all the relevant information. This liaison between the hospital and the community is vital for parents when leaving the hospital.

MISCARRIAGE

Miscarriage is defined as a loss in pregnancy before 24 weeks' gestation. For many people the miscarriage of their baby at any gestation in pregnancy is a devastating experience (Fig. 3.4) – this may be especially so when couples have previously experienced infertility or an ectopic pregnancy. Pregnancy and the feelings associated with becoming parents are unique. Parents find phrases used by professionals such as 'blighted ovum', 'missed abortion' or 'non-viable fetus' unhelpful, meaningless and hurtful. During the second trimester, most parents-to-be acknowledge openly that they are

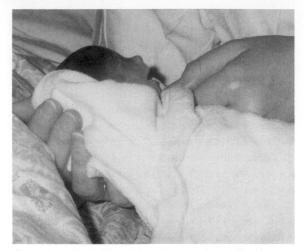

Figure 3.4   Rose Elizabeth at 21 weeks' gestation being held by her father.

expecting a baby and a miscarriage may be experienced as the stillbirth of their baby. There are no set rules to follow in caring for people at such sensitive times and staff need to recognize and respond to parents' very varied feelings, trying to sense what each individual needs. Hospitals are now being asked to offer parents a form of certificate acknowledging the birth of their baby at less than 24 weeks' gestation (SANDS Guidelines).

TERMINATION DUE TO ANOMALY

When informed about an anomaly which is detected in pregnancy, parents in distress may make decisions in haste which they later regret. It is valuable for staff to encourage parents not to hurry decisions, to acknowledge how difficult it is for them at this time and suggest they take time together, preferably at home, before making any final decisions. Parents need clear, unbiased information, in language they can understand, about their baby's condition and the options available to them, including information about the mode of delivery. Providing written information before any decisions are made is crucial. A leaflet from the organization ARC (Antenatal Results and Choices) is useful to parents. Some choose to continue with their pregnancy and need support to do what is right for them, whether their baby will have significant problems or will not live. Whatever the outcome, these parents are considering a choice that will affect the rest of their lives and their decision will involve grieving for the baby they had been expecting.

When parents have made a decision to end the pregnancy, they may not feel able to experience or express any attachment to their baby. The grief of these parents is complicated and the guilt often profound, as they have taken the responsibility for ending the life of their child; for some parents their attachment is as significant as if their baby had survived. It is important for staff not to be judgemental and to offer as much emotional support as is needed. The decision made by parents is no indication of the amount of love they have for their baby.

> ### Reflective Activity 3.5
>
> What protocols, information leaflets and booklets are available in your unit for women and their families who have lost a baby, or who are now facing perinatal bereavement? Ensure that you are aware of the range of material available, and what it includes.
>
> Have parents been asked how useful they found your unit's leaflets?

LABOUR WHEN A BABY HAS DIED OR IS NOT EXPECTED TO LIVE

A baby who has issued forth from its mother after the 24th week of pregnancy and has not at any time after being completely expelled from its mother's body breathed or shown any signs of life is a stillborn baby.

(UKCC, 1998: 37)

Hospitals can be impersonal, frightening places and the sensitive care offered by a midwife is invaluable. Providing an atmosphere in which parents are able to trust the professional caring for them is enhanced by having a suitable, comfortable and private bereavement room. The entire team needs to know when bereaved people are admitted to the unit. Professionals who are able to be human, loving and caring in their communication offer a great deal at this time. On meeting these parents, the midwife needs to immediately acknowledge the situation and say how sorry he or she is, then to spend time listening to parents, building a relationship and responding to their varied needs and feelings. Not all parents realize that the labour and delivery of their baby will need to be physically the same as giving birth to a live baby. This realization may be hard to comprehend and may cause anger and disbelief.

To find myself carrying death and, even worse, being told I had to give birth to death, was the most horrific scenario.

(Bereaved mother)

Practical considerations

The silence in the delivery room was deafening. This was the reality – this was death at birth.

(Bereaved mother)

The mother who is expecting a stillbirth or late miscarriage requires significant psychological support. However, the midwife should be aware that the principles of care during labour for this woman are similar to a woman expecting a live birth.

In situations where a baby has died in utero, the mother may request a substantial amount of pain relief, not being aware that later on, the birth of her baby may be a time she wishes she could fully remember. Experiencing the labour enables a mother to begin to face the reality of giving birth to her baby.

Discussing a birth plan and having some control in a situation where parents feel powerless is psychologically valuable. These choices provide important memories on which to focus in the process of grieving.

I didn't have any control over the situation at all and I don't think either of us really knew what was happening until well after.

(Bereaved mother)

As already discussed, the woman may be in a state of shock, and therefore it is preferable to ensure a high level of continuity of care, and the midwife providing that care should be aware of the possibility that information may not be as easily understood, and that this information needs to be simple and accessible, and may need to be repeated.

This woman may be at an increased risk of complications such as inefficient uterine action, infection, and disseminated intravascular coagulation (DIC), and therefore the care provided should include monitoring of maternal observations and well-being, and scrupulous attention to asepsis during examinations. The midwife needs to be aware that the women is often so immersed in her grief, that she will pay scant attention to what she may be physically experiencing.

Having a general anaesthetic for an emergency caesarean section creates what is a potentially complicated grief reaction. These mothers need additional help in facing the reality of what has happened: that their

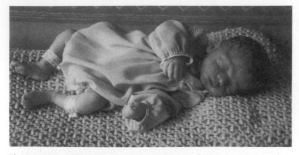

Figure 3.5 Charlie who was stillborn following an emergency caesarean section.

baby, who they will have no recollection of having, has in fact died (Fig. 3.5).

UNEXPECTED DEATH OF A BABY AT OR SOON AFTER BIRTH

When there is serious cause for concern in labour or at delivery, it is essential that the parents are informed immediately of what is suspected and that a doctor is asked to speak to the parents and provide confirmation of the prognosis. There is value in having the designated midwife present, who is then an additional support to parents' and can clarify any information should the need arise.

In this situation, practitioners themselves may experience trauma and guilt and need to be properly supported. This includes an opportunity for reflection and review, and some space to discuss the issues raised by this sad situation.

Neonatal death

Following the birth of a baby who is not expected to live, parents need to be honestly informed and given time to gradually absorb the painful information. They will need reassurance that nothing more can be done for their child and helped to be involved in any decision regarding their baby. When a decision is made to withdraw active treatment, it is vital that it is made with the parents, and that they are provided with whatever time is necessary to make these difficult choices (McHaffie, 2001). The availability of a bereavement room in the hours leading to a change from intensive to palliative care is extremely valuable, enabling parents to have the privacy, time and space they need with their child (Fig. 3.6). Some parents prefer to be alone; however they need to know when and where staff can be contacted.

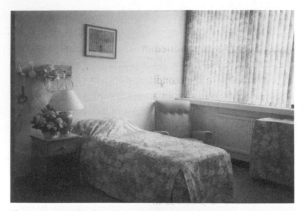

Figure 3.6 The bereavement room adjacent to the delivery suite at Wycombe General Hospital.

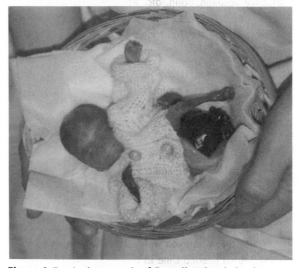

Figure 3.7 A photograph of Benedict that helped to explain why he died.

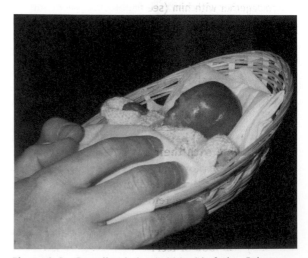

Figure 3.8 Benedict, being held by his father John.

A mother's story: Benedict – a child of mine (Warden, 1999)

Benedict had a rare condition known as 'body stalk defect', which results in a devastating set of problems in the baby (see Fig. 3.7). Clinically I had a 'termination for abnormality', but emotionally I had a baby. He died at 21 weeks' gestation.

When your baby dies, you take very little home but your memories, and if you're lucky, some tangible reminders of a precious life. Perhaps that is why it is so important what midwives and nurses do and say.

I didn't see Benedict immediately after he was born, but my husband, John, did. After Benedict was delivered I continued to bleed. John was left alone while I was in theatre. His baby was dead and he feared for me. He sat alone and wept. Those events became a recurring nightmare for him.

In hospital I had a profound sense of isolation, only reinforced by staff standing at my door asking if I was all right. Somehow it was very important that they, those who dealt with Benedict, knew how I felt about him. No one could mend my situation, but would someone sit with me and listen? Relating to me as an individual, building a relationship, made an immense difference to how I felt.

We misunderstood the words 'Just ring when you want him and ring when you want him taken back'. We assumed he needed time in the fridge. Why else would he have 'to go back'? We only had 24 hours before the post-mortem. We wanted to spend the little time we had together with him (see Fig. 3.8).

When faced with the death of your baby it's hard to know all the things you might want to do. It can also be difficult to ask. So often we rely on our midwives to talk through the possibilities and encourage us to make the choice that is right for us. There is so little time, so little opportunity and no second chance.

Our three girls continue to express their regret and resentment at not seeing Benedict. I felt too ill to see them – couldn't face them. Involving the children, being open and honest, was fundamental to us in life after Benedict. Would it have been possible to arrange for John and the girls to spend time with Benedict in a different room? As a possibility, it came to us too late and we inadvertently denied our children what we had valued most – time with Benedict.

We took a lot of photos of Benedict but have none of the three of us together. Neither do we have a photo of Benedict and those staff, special to us, who shared in what was a profound experience for us.

When I consider my record of Benedict's tiny hand and foot prints I think of the small white cardigan he wore. How I would have loved to have that too. With all these things we didn't think to ask and unfortunately no one else thought to offer.

Benedict's funeral was so important to us as a family. The funeral was an outward affirmation of Benedict's status within our family and an opportunity for everyone in the family to do something for Benedict and make their contribution. The midwife who arranged the funeral was very anxious that we would forget to attend. This rankled as it left me feeling I had failed to communicate the value we placed on our baby.

Leaving the hospital was one of the hardest things to do. I had expected a baby and now I was leaving him behind with the only people who would ever see him. We were so grateful for every kindness shown to us. It was very poignant as John and I walked alone to the main entrance. I reflected that if we had had our baby we would have been escorted. I so wanted someone to care enough to take us to the door to say goodbye and let us know when we could come back to see them later. That didn't happen, and we left with a profound sense of vulnerability and isolation.

Spending time with their baby

Initially some parents may actually fear seeing their dead baby; they may be afraid that it will make them more attached and therefore make saying goodbye even harder. For some parents, this will be their first experience of death, and they may be frightened of what their baby will look or feel like. Frequently parents are unable to accept fully what has happened and may manage by denying the reality. There is no need for parents to make any decisions in a hurry. Time and understanding are required with grieving parents, as their denial is a form of emotional protection and with time it will lessen. It is useful for the midwife to explain to the parents that other parents have also felt concerned about seeing or holding their baby, and have later valued the time they have had with their baby,

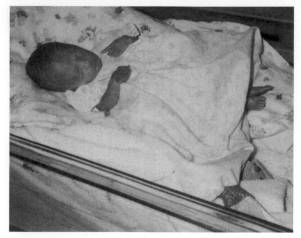

Figure 3.9   Sophie's parents appreciated being able to see her little feet and choose her dress themselves.

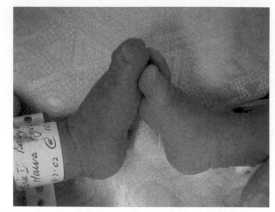

Figure 3.10   Twins, Christopher and Jessica: the photograph was sent as an email by the parents to announce the birth of the twins. (With kind permission from the Child Bereavement Trust.)

which is precious; this time will be all they have to create memories. These hours after the birth are immensely valuable. Nothing in life can prepare parents for such a tragedy and observing the staff's tenderness and interactions with their baby will remain in the parents' memories for a lifetime.

Washing and dressing the baby after death

This may be the one opportunity parents have to choose clothes for their child (Fig. 3.9). Staff can make a difference by providing information enabling parents to make choices, such as:

- Would the parents like to wash and dress their baby alone themselves?
- Would they prefer to watch their baby being washed and dressed by a member of staff?
- Do they have clothes they would like to dress their baby in?

It should be unit policy to have a selection of baby clothes from which parents can choose to dress their baby and later keep when they return home. In the months ahead parents will treasure everything that gives them a sense of their baby. Clothes their baby has worn are best left unwashed, as initially the smell of the clothes will provide parents with a tangible reminder of their baby.

The importance of memories

Midwifery and neonatal staff who help parents to get to know their baby in the brief time they have together provide a source of precious memories, which will be vitally important in the months ahead. Some units now offer parents a memory folder and memory box which can be used to store any special mementoes of

their baby. This can include photographs, their baby's name-band, foot and hand prints, a lock of hair, a page where words can be written by anyone who knew the parents and baby, a blessing or naming card, letters and perhaps the clothes their baby wore, the anniversary cards and gifts that people choose to collect and keep for the future.

The value of photographs

For many people, scan and camera photographs of their baby who has died are immensely important. These parents will be interested in what their baby looked like and will value pictures that clearly show details – their baby's profile, the tiny hands and feet, and perhaps sensitively taken pictures of their baby naked. These photographs help parents to face the reality of what has happened, to provide evidence they had a baby and that their child died. Parents may like to know they can have a photograph of themselves holding their baby, a family picture with their other children or the grandparents, or with the midwives who cared for them. When a twin dies, taking care and time to photograph the live twin and the dead twin together (Fig. 3.10) is something parents may not naturally consider and yet may so value in what can be a complicated grief process in the years ahead. Later in life the surviving twin may well be interested to know about the sibling who died and to know that his or her twin was acknowledged and mourned – parents in multiple birth and death situations have a great deal to manage and can find this information helpful. A photographic memory guide providing information and practical guidance is available for families and professionals (CBT, 2003b).

THE POSTNATAL PERIOD

Physically, the woman requires a high standard of post-natal care, and as discussed previously, this requires psychological support, as well as considering the physical aspects of involution and educational elements of ensuring the woman understands the normal physiological process of the puerperium, and what can be considered normal.

An important consideration is where the woman is cared for, and it is vital that the midwife discusses the options with the woman. The choice is usually between a rapid discharge home, a single room in the antenatal and/or postnatal ward, or on the gynaecology ward. Previous research and experience suggests that some women may wish to have contact with other mothers and babies, while some would wish to be in their home environment, and some may actually feel abandoned after being sent to the gynaecology ward (Hughes, 1987). Thinking that a woman can be 'protected' against the sounds of a crying baby may be too simplistic a view.

Wherever the woman is cared for, ideally, continuity of carer should be aimed for, and the same principles of keeping information simple and accessible should be retained. A difficulty which many women experience and find especially hard will be when a few days after the delivery, the breasts fill with milk, which is a tangible reminder that there was to be a baby to suckle. Previously bromocriptine has been prescribed to suppress lactation; however, recent concerns with women experiencing serious cardiovascular complications, including stroke and hypertension, has led to reluctance to use this. The woman needs firstly to be told that this may happen, and informed that pain relief can be prescribed, and advised to wear a supportive brassiere. For some women, homeopathic remedies may be useful: one study indicated that jasmine flowers were effective (Shrivastav *et al.*, 1988).

Reflective Activity 3.6

Consider your own unit and what policies and protocols are in place for assisting parents in gathering memories of their child. Do you feel there are sufficient resources to support the care needed, and is enough importance placed on this aspect of bereavement care?

THE HOSPITAL POST-MORTEM EXAMINATION

Parents rely on the professionals who care for them and their baby to inform them about the requirements for a post-mortem examination (autopsy). All staff should receive appropriate training in how to sensitively discuss consent for a hospital post-mortem with parents. Although a doctor may request and provide information for written post mortem consent, it is very often the midwife to whom parents turn for further information, clarification and support, and all midwives must understand the ethical, legal and emotional responsibilities involved (DoH, 2003*). Obtaining parents' consent should be seen as a continuing process, which is not limited to the signing of a form.

It is helpful to explain that a post-mortem examination may provide information as to the cause of their baby's death and that this information is important when parents are planning to have another baby in the future. Although the examination does not always ascertain the cause of death, parents can be helped by knowing what could be excluded as a potential cause. Parents need to know that the post-mortem examination will not affect their baby's face or limbs and that it will be done with the same respect and care as an operation.

When talking about the post-mortem examination all relevant aspects need to be discussed and consent obtained. It is vital to provide clear, appropriate information: that tissue blocks and slides will be kept in medical records; that consent is needed for use in medical research and education. This should be explained, as parents need to clearly understand the difference (DoH, 2003). Withholding relevant information in an effort to spare relatives' feelings is never acceptable; however, parents differ in the amount of information they need. Graphic details about the post-mortem examination may be too overwhelming for some parents. Parents need to be offered the opportunity to choose how much or how little information they would like and given time to consider their decision and ask any questions. Sensitive and caring communication is essential in this situation, to ensure consent is a process and is properly sought. It is important that parents feel in control, understand what they are consenting to and have the right to say what happens during and after the post-mortem examination.

Organ and tissue retention at post-mortem examination has become a matter of serious public and

---

* The new Human Tissue Bill will be passed as an Act in 2004, and will enshrine the Code of Practice in law.

professional concern. It is vitally important that the donation of human tissue for the purposes of medical education and research is maintained. However, this cannot take precedence over the interests and rights of bereaved families. A balance must be found between the needs of the grieving family and the desire to advance medical understanding.

What was apparent following The Royal Liverpool Children's Hospital Inquiry (RLCI, 2001) was that many parents suffered a deep sense of betrayal. These families had trusted the professionals involved after death to respect their children's bodies. It is not only difficult for parents that organs had been retained, but these parents had not been told or given a choice in any decision, and had been denied the opportunity of participating in every aspect of their child's care. The result is that, naturally, parents today need a great deal of reassurance that their child's body can only be touched with their consent. They will naturally assume that nothing is removed from their baby's body permanently. If it is a consideration that organs or tissue could be helpfully retained for the purposes of research and education, the bereaved parents must be involved in all decisions, fully aware of the reason why, and their written permission obtained (DoH, 2003).

The post-mortem procedure

Whenever possible, parents need to be told the name of the paediatric pathologist who will be doing the post-mortem examination, and at which hospital it will be carried out. In some instances, the paediatric pathologist will be available to speak to the parents. Parents need to know that their baby's body will be treated with respect and dignity and that it will be carefully restored so that, if they wish to, it will be possible for them to see and hold their baby again after the examination. The pathologist will usually make two openings, one down the front of the body and another at the back of the head. The post-mortem is usually carried out within a day or two of the death. Examination of a baby's brain requires fixing to obtain blocks and slides. This can take some weeks. If parents want their baby's brain reunited with the body, this may delay the funeral. Alternatively, parents can consent to the hospital disposing of the brain respectfully.

It is important that the consultant involved in their baby's death meets with the parents and discusses the findings of the post-mortem within 4–6 weeks of the death. Many parents value an opportunity to talk to the pathologist before or after the examination.

When a coroner's post-mortem examination is necessary

In the event of a sudden or unexplained death, a coroner's post-mortem is legally required and in this situation the parents' permission is not requested. However, parents' need for time, information and sensitive support is every bit as great as in circumstances where they are giving their consent for a hospital post-mortem. The coroner is responsible for informing parents if organs and tissue have been retained to ascertain the cause of death. The length of time an organ will be retained and when it will be returned to the body prior to burial or cremation should be discussed. It is crucial that parents are informed that, with their consent, tissue blocks and slides may be kept as part of the medical record. Parents need to understand that while enquiries into the cause of their baby's death are underway, the death cannot be registered and so final funeral arrangements cannot be made. Normally, however, when an inquest is required it is held very soon after the death and the funeral need not be delayed. Information regarding a coroner's post-mortem and whether an inquest is needed should be available for parents in written format (INQUEST, 2003).

The gift of donation

Parents will not necessarily consider asking about heart valve or other tissue or organ donation at this time of crisis. They will rely on the professionals who care for them to provide them with information to make informed choices. Most parents appreciate being offered information that enables them to make choices. Parents who are not asked may wonder why and later may even resent this lack of information. However, it is important to be aware of the circumstances when organ donation is possible and in particular that a cause of death is known.

Parents considering this possibility need to have clear information and explanations from the donor team in their particular region. They also need to be aware that heart valve donation (usually referred to as tissue donation), which can be carried out up to 48 hours after the death of a term baby, may require a large part of the heart to be retained. If a donation from their baby is to be used, blood samples will need to be taken from the mother, father and baby to test for HIV, hepatitis B and C and syphilis.

RESPECTING PARENTS

As soon as possible after their baby's death a visit from a senior doctor, accompanied by their midwives, is valuable for parents and provides acknowledgement of the importance of their baby's existence. The parents will also need time with a designated person who can help them with the practical arrangements. They need to know what steps to take next, to know about legal requirements, what the hospital can and cannot arrange and about the funeral. Providing written information, devised in consultation with families, is useful so parents can refer back to it as necessary whilst in hospital and also at home.

SPIRITUAL NEEDS

All cultures have rituals and traditions that are followed in a major life event, and these provide an opportunity to honour the importance of what has happened and help reality to be faced. When religions and cultures are different from our own, a lack of knowledge and understanding of specific spiritual needs may leave professionals feeling even more helpless, and families dissatisfied (Arshad *et al.*, 2003). Asking parents what they would like, offering them time to explore what is important for them, will be invaluable. Some parents who never go to church may find comfort in a visit from the Hospital Chaplain, a blessing or baptism for their baby, while others may like a visit arranged with their own particular religious leader. Many hospitals today keep a Book of Remembrance in which parents can later make an entry, either soon after the birth or at a later date.

Other parents who have a deep faith may choose not to have a religious ceremony. It is best to refrain from talking about your personal beliefs with bereaved families, but to be open to what may be appropriate for and a comfort to them. This illustrates the need for the midwife to be knowledgeable about different cultures and religions and their rituals, but not to make assumptions about what parents from a particular group will wish to do following a bereavement (CBT, 2003c).

INVOLVING BROTHERS AND SISTERS

It can be difficult for professionals to raise with parents that they may need to consider the involvement of their other children when a baby brother or sister has died. Children can arouse strong feelings in adults. For midwives they may evoke memories of their own childhood, their own children, or perhaps the children they had hoped to have. Professional staff increasingly recognize the importance of work with adults, but children and their emotions have often been ignored.

When a baby dies, parents may be reluctant to involve their other children. They themselves are grieving, feeling helpless and overwhelmed and may be uncertain about their own ability to regain control. It is natural for them to want to protect their children from painful situations and it can be helpful if they are told this is a normal reaction. However, this stance may leave the siblings confused, unprotected from their fantasies and unsupported in their feelings.

Communicating with siblings

The decision is not whether or not to talk to children, but who will do the talking, when and how, as it is impossible for parents not to communicate with children. They read body language, overhear conversations and notice changes in routine. Momentous situations in a family cause changes, and children quickly sense when something serious is happening. They require clear, simple, truthful and often repeated, but brief explanations about what has happened, and what may happen next. Although the children will not have known the baby and so are unlikely to be deeply grieving for their brother or sister, they will be affected by the grief of their parents.

Children do not need protecting from their feelings, but support in them. Young siblings will not grieve in the same way as older children and often express themselves through play, drawing or with friends.

Children's reactions and understanding

Children have a shorter concentration span than adults and cannot tolerate intense emotions for very long. This does not mean that they are not sometimes upset and sad. Few children under the age of 5 will understand the permanence of death. They think in literal, concrete terms and therefore metaphors or euphemisms such as 'lost' or 'gone away' are confusing. Children need adults to say the words 'has died' or 'is dead'. By 6 years of age, most children begin to understand death as permanent and that it can happen to them.

Preparation before the death

Whenever possible, it is helpful if parents prepare their other children when their baby sibling is not expected to live, giving honest information appropriate to their

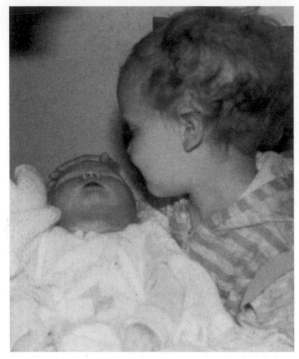

Figure 3.11 Naomi holding her baby sister Katie after she died.

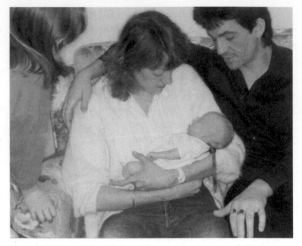

Figure 3.12 Baby Rikki with parents Jane and Adrian and sister Jaycee, who with her younger sister Donna helped to bath him after his death.

children's age. Children need to understand that most sick babies in the hospital get better and go home, but sadly sometimes babies die. It is important not to overwhelm children with information but to be guided by them and to answer their questions honestly.

Preparation after the death

Most children who have been carefully prepared and have chosen to see their dead baby brother or sister are not afraid and generally gain an understanding of death and what has happened (Fig. 3.11). What children do not know or are not told about, they often make up and their fantasies are usually worse than the reality. Sometimes they experience feelings of guilt, especially if they were not looking forward to a new sibling. They need to be reassured that the baby's death had nothing to do with their thoughts or actions, and that their parents love them and life will not always be so sad.

Parents may be concerned that frightening memories of a dead baby will leave their children with upsetting images – this is unlikely, especially when the children have been prepared for what to expect (Fig. 3.12). Children respond well to factual explanations of death and having information, such as: 'When people die it means their body doesn't work any more'. It is useful to explain that the baby may feel cold to touch and

that the skin may be mottled and the baby's lips or skin colour may be blue. It is not helpful to liken death to sleeping because people who are asleep are not dead and their bodies work very well (CBT, 2003c).

Attending the funeral

Although some parents and grandparents feel that children need to be protected from being present at the funeral, children themselves usually say that they find it helpful to be there. They need to be prepared for and included in the family's rituals of mourning. To be excluded from these events can widen the gap between the grieving parents and the child. However, a child who is frightened about attending a funeral should not be pressured or forced to do so. Some other way can be found for the child to say goodbye – such as putting a letter or flowers in the coffin, lighting a candle, saying a prayer or visiting the grave.

If children want to attend the funeral, thought needs to be given to the support that will be required. They need to know what will happen and be given the opportunity to ask questions. They may like to take an active part in the service by choosing a favourite song, poem or reading. It is often a good idea for the children to be cared for by an adult who is close to them during the service, to relieve the parents at such an emotional time.

How professionals can help

It is important for staff to make a direct offer of help to families and ensure there is time to discuss parents' worries and anxieties. However, parents are individuals and not all of them will feel able to involve their children directly or tell them about the death immediately. Different cultures will have different ways of dealing with death, and sensitivity is paramount when offering parents information so that they can make informed choices, e.g. a photograph to take home to the children of their brother or sister who has died. It is helpful for staff to explain to parents that they may meet resistance from grandparents and others, who did not receive this care years ago.

Professionals can suggest children might like to have something special for themselves – perhaps a footprint on coloured paper they have chosen or a photograph of them with their baby brother or sister. Children are helped if they are allowed to share in and create memories.

FAMILY AND FRIENDS

Grandparents too will be grieving and perhaps feeling guilty that they are still alive when their grandchild has died. They will grieve for their grandchild and for the sadness of their son or daughter. They may be a main source of comfort to the grieving parents in the months ahead and are more able to share this grief with the parents if they have been involved from the start. Other family members and friends may experience similar feelings of grief and unhappiness for the bereaved parents.

Involvement of a close family friend can also be supportive, particularly if for whatever reason a mother is having to face bereavement on her own without a partner. It is important to have someone to share the few memories of a baby's brief existence and to help when taking decisions about funeral arrangements, etc.

TAKING A BABY HOME

Parents appreciate information about taking their baby home with them before the funeral – this can usually be arranged with the local funeral director. Hospitals are large and impersonal and parents may prefer family to have the opportunity to see their baby and say goodbye in familiar surroundings (Fig. 3.13). When there is a coroner's post-mortem, permission must be sought from the coroner (CBT, 2003c).

Leaving hospital

When parents leave the hospital, where possible, a member of staff should walk with them out to their car

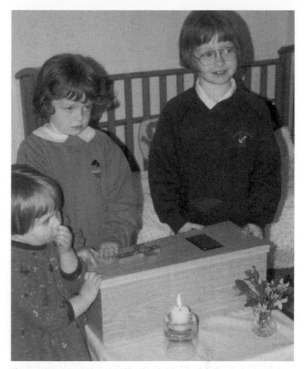

Figure 3.13   Colette, Elizabeth Ann and Eugenie with their brother Benedict's coffin at home before his funeral.

or taxi. It is crucial that community staff are aware of the baby's death and parents know who to contact once at home. Hospital policies need to be clear and enhance liaison between hospital and home in order to provide continuity of care for bereaved parents.

Making an appointment for the parents to visit the consultant again, and perhaps the midwife who cared for them, within 6 weeks for a follow-up bereavement visit is useful. They can share again what happened at their baby's death or maybe have explained anything they did not understand in crisis. This time can be a valuable way of finding out what support the parents have or may need.

REGISTRATION OF THE DEATH

Legally, when a baby is *born dead before 24 weeks' gestation* there is no birth certificate or need for registration. However, if the parents choose to have their baby buried or cremated they will need written confirmation of the birth from the doctor or midwife attending the delivery. Some units issue a form/certificate to record that the parents are taking their baby's body, and this is formally recommended as best practice.

This certificate also serves to recognize the baby's existence and can become an important memento.

After 24 weeks' gestation, when a baby is stillborn, the doctor or midwife who attended the delivery gives the parents a Medical Certificate of Stillbirth and should explain that the stillbirth of their baby must be registered by either or both parents at the registry office within 42 days.

When a baby is born alive, regardless of gestational age, and then dies within 28 days of birth, by law a doctor must confirm the death and provide a medical certificate to enable both the birth and death to be registered within 5 days of the death.

When parents are married, either or both can register, but when parents are unmarried, the registration needs to be done by the mother. The baby's father should accompany her if he wishes his name to appear on their baby's certificate.

RESPECTFUL DISPOSAL OF THE BODY

Parents of babies born dead before 24 weeks' gestation who choose to arrange a burial or cremation for their baby themselves, may need help with planning a ceremony, which can be held in the hospital chapel, in a church, or at the crematorium or cemetery (RCN, 2001). Parents do not generally know about how to manage this and may welcome the suggestion if it is made to them. Other parents may prefer not to be involved in the arrangements themselves but will want to be reassured that the hospital will treat their baby's body with respect (RCN, 2001).

All parents need information about the options available to them. An information sheet with the relevant costs and considerations is valuable, as also is plenty of time, ensuring parents are not rushed and are able to make informed choices.

THE MONTHS AHEAD

In order to begin to heal the pain of a traumatic loss, parents need to find a way to express their feelings and to communicate these feelings to a caring supportive person. Parents continue to grieve for their baby throughout their lives. They know they can never replace the baby who has died – grieving is about remembering, not forgetting. But it is the very absence of memories that makes grieving so hard when a baby dies. Parents are likely to feel a bond with the staff who cared for them and their baby. Appropriate care needs to be available in the months following the death on the unit. Parents need to know how to access support no matter how long it is since their baby died (Jennings, 2001).

In a busy unit it is not always possible for professional staff to give parents as much time as they need, both at the time of the death and on return. A designated bereavement counsellor is in a position to support the parents and the staff. Using counselling skills and working as a counsellor are two different tasks. Being a counsellor requires a professional qualification, and is a skilled task for which aptitude, training and experience are necessary. It can only happen if the client has asked for counselling.

Bereavement counselling takes time and is best offered as a home or hospital visit after the baby's death. The crucial times appear to be 3 and 6 weeks after the death and also 3, 6 and 12 months. Parents say that just knowing that as a couple, they can see a counsellor, perhaps once a month, helps them to manage their feelings and relationship. The bereavement counselling session gives them permission to talk about their feelings and their relationship and helps them to recognize that it is normal to grieve.

RETURN VISIT TO THE HOSPITAL UNIT

Some parents want to come back to the unit to see the midwife in the antenatal clinic or to see the person who cared for them and their baby. The opportunity to talk through what happened at the time of their baby's death, particularly if the mother had a general anaesthetic, can be very valuable. Ideally a time should be arranged so that when parents arrive on the unit someone expects them and they have a clear idea how long the member of staff can spend with them. Parents may want to return around the first anniversary of their baby's death, and it useful to be aware of this.

SUPPORT AGENCIES

There are a number of voluntary organizations (see Additional resources) which offer support to bereaved families in the form of helplines, parent support groups and resources for grieving families. Most parents will also welcome information about the local support groups. These agencies such as SANDS and The Child Bereavement Trust (CBT) are sources of information and support, and are also involved in developing literature and resources for bereaved parents and professionals.

Reflective Activity 3.7

Has your unit made contact with support groups locally? Has anyone in your unit been trained to facilitate bereaved parents groups?

What support agencies/groups are available to bereaved parents in your area? Do you know the contact numbers, and do you have information about what support can be offered in order to provide this information to parents? It is useful to have this information available in your diary or resource file.

CONCLUSION

The essence of working with bereaved families is to respect their wishes and feelings whatever they may be; to offer them as much time as they need to talk about what has happened; to really listen to what they have to say; to ensure they have as much information as they want and that they have understood it; to answer their questions honestly; and to make sure they have someone to contact for support in the future.

The Chief Medical Officer's recommendation that all NHS trusts should provide support and advice to families at the time of bereavement highlighted the need for the role of bereavement advisor and recognized the need for training in all aspects of dealing with grieving families (CMO, 2001). The Child Bereavement Trust has developed an audit model for the monitoring and evaluation of bereavement services (CBT, 2003d).

Midwives have to balance caring for the complex needs that the mother and her family have, which must include a consideration for physical, social, psychological and spiritual needs, at a time when she requires a high level of sensitive and skilled care. This balance requires significant self-knowledge and an ability to be truly 'with woman' through her pain and sadness, in order to support and guide her through this period. An awareness of their own needs and those of their healthcare colleagues is also imperative in ensuring a strong and supportive team.

Working with grieving parents can be difficult and emotionally draining, but knowing that the family have been helped through one of the worst periods of their lives, by what was said or done making a difference, can be immensely rewarding.

KEY POINTS

- Grief is a normal reaction to an abnormal event and the midwife's role is to identify and continually assess what parents need and help them to make informed choices.
- The way midwives manage their own emotions has a direct influence on how they manage to help others express themselves; this requires effective support systems to be in place to support them in their interactions with grieving parents.
- Seeing and spending time with their dead baby helps parents to face the reality of what has happened and creates precious memories. Most children who have been included and have chosen to see their dead sibling are not afraid and have a better understanding of what has happened.
- It is essential for staff to recognize the process of consent and always obtain written informed consent from parents for the post-mortem examination of their baby and for the retention of any tissue, blocks or slides.
- NHS trusts need to take into account the recommendations of the CMO for the role of bereavement advisor.
- Effective support needs to extend beyond the death on the unit into the community.

REFERENCES

Arshad, M., Horsfall, A. & Yasin, R. (2003) Pregnancy loss and the Holy Qu'ran. *British Journal of Midwifery*.

Bowlby, J. (1980) *Attachment and Loss: Volume 3 Loss, Sadness and Depression*. Harmondsworth: Penguin Books.

Caelli, K., Downie, J. & Knox, M. (1999) Through grief to healthy parenthood: facilitating the journey through a family pregnancy support programme. *Birth Issues* 8(3): 85–90.

Chief Medical Officer (CMO) (2001) *The Removal, Retention and Use of Human Organs and Tissue*. London: DoH.

Child Bereavement Trust (CBT) (2003a) *Information Series: The death of a baby or child; When a baby dies* (for parents); *Understanding bereaved children and young people*. High Wycombe: CBT.

Child Bereavement Trust (CBT) (2003b) *Guidance for Professionals: A Photographic Memory*. High Wycombe: CBT.

Child Bereavement Trust (CBT) (2003c) *Best Practice Guidance Series: for the care of a family when their baby dies in the maternity unit; for the care of a family when their baby or child dies in the Neonatal, Paediatric or the Accident and Emergency Units; for the taking of photographs following the death of a baby; for the care of siblings following the death of a brother or sister; for families who wish to take their baby home after death; regarding cultural and religious issues at the time of a baby or child's death*. High Wycombe: CBT. Online. Available: www.childbereavement.org.uk.

Child Bereavement Trust (CBT) (2003d) *A Bereavement Audit Model: Auditing Your Work in Bereavement Support*. High Wycombe: CBT. Online. Available: www.childbereavement.org.uk.

Department of Health (DoH) (2003) *Families and Post Mortems: A Code of Practice*. London: DoH. Online. Available: www.doh.gov.uk/tissue/families&postmortemscode.pdf.

Hill, S. (1990) *Family*. London: Penguin Books.

Hughes, P. (1987) The management of bereaved mothers: what is best? *Midwives Chronicle* 100(1195): 226–229.

Hunfeld, J.A.M., Taselaar-Kloos, A.K.G., Agterberg, G. *et al.* (1997) Trait anxiety, negative emotions, and the mothers' adaptation to an infant born subsequent to late pregnancy loss: a case-control study. *Prenatal Diagnosis* 17(9): 843–851.

INQUEST (2003) *An Information Pack for Families, Friends and Advisors*. London: INQUEST.

Jennings, P. (2001) *The First Two Years Experience of Child Bereavement Support Posts. Evaluation of the Department of Health Project*. High Wycombe: CBT.

Kohner, N. (1995) *Pregnancy Loss and the Death of a Baby. Guidelines for Professionals*. London: SANDS.

Kubler-Ross, E. (1970) *On Death and Dying*. London: Tavistock.

Lewis, E. & Bourne, S. (1989) Perinatal death. *Baillière's Clinical Obstetrics and Gynaecology*. 3(4): 935–953.

McHaffie, H.E. (2001) *Crucial Decisions at the Beginning of Life. Parents' Experiences of Treatment Withdrawal from Infants*. Oxford: Radcliffe Medical Press.

Office for National Statistics (1999) Series DH3 Mortality Statistics : Childhood, infant and perinatal. *Health Statistics Quarterly* 3: 62-69.

Parkes, C.M. (1972) *Bereavement: Studies of Grief in Adult Life*. Penguin: Harmondsworth.

Puddifoot, J.E. & Johnson, M.P. (1997) The legitimacy of grieving: the partner's experience at miscarriage. *Social Science & Medicine* 45(6): 837–845.

Retained Organs Commission (ROC) (2001) *Tissue Blocks and Slides*. London: Department of Health.

Royal College of Nursing (RCN) (2001) *Sensitive Disposal of all Fetal Remains*. London: RCN.

Royal Liverpool Children's Inquiry (RLCI) (2001) *The Royal Liverpool Children's Inquiry Summary and Recommendations*. HC12-1. London: The Stationery Office.

Shrivastav, P., George, K., Balasubramaniam, N. *et al.* (1988) Suppression of puerperal lactation using jasmine flowers (*Jasminum sambac*). *Australian and New Zealand Journal of Obstetrics and Gynaecology* 28(1): 68–71.

Stroebe, M.S. & Schut, H. (1999) The dual process model of coping with bereavement: rationale and descriptions. *Death Studies* 23(3): 197–224.

United Kingdom Central Council for Nursing, Midwifery and Health Visiting (UKCC) (1998) *Midwives Rules and Code of Practice*. London: UKCC.

Warden, A. (1999) *Benedict: a Child of Mine*. High Wycombe: CBT.

Worden, J.W. (1991) *Grief Counselling and Grief Therapy*. London: Routledge.

FURTHER READING

Burnard, P. (1992) *Effective Communication Skills for Health Professionals: Therapy in Practice 28*. London: Chapman and Hall.

Burnard, P. (1997) *Know Yourself! Self Awareness Activities for Nurses and Other Health Professionals*. London: Whurr Publishers.

Child Bereavement Trust (CBT) (1995) *Grieving After the Death of Your Baby*. High Wycombe, CBT.
In this book, parents talk about how they felt in the weeks, months and years after their baby's death, and there is a description of the many ways parents have found of expressing their feelings and remembering their baby. The parents who tell their stories in this book also talk in the video 'When Our

Baby Died', which aims to help bereaved parents and families feel less alone and understand more about how they feel.

Dent, A. & Stewart, A. (1994) *At a Loss – Bereavement Care when a Baby Dies*. London: Baillière Tindall.

Hindmarch, C. (2000) *On the Death of a Child*, 2nd edn. Oxford: Radcliffe Medical Press.
This classic text on bereavement guides the reader through the latest research on bereavement and gives prominence to the needs of grieving children and youngsters. It relates theory to practice, describes good practice guidelines and offers details of resources for further support and reading. It is illustrated with case studies and examples and is recommended reading for the many professionals who may

be involved with grieving families, including midwives, neonatal nurses, doctors, health visitors and social workers.

Houston, G. (1990) *Supervision and Counselling*. London: The Rochester Foundation.

Moulder, C. (1995) *Miscarriage: Women's Experiences and Needs*, 2nd edn. London: Pandora.

Penson, J. (1990) *Bereavement. A Guide for Nurses*. London: Harper and Row.

ADDITIONAL RESOURCES

Child Bereavement Trust (CBT) (1995) *Death at Birth* (Video). High Wycombe, CBT.
This two-part video was designed to train professionals and others who are involved in caring for parents when their baby dies, whether through miscarriage, stillbirth, neonatal death or termination for abnormality. Part One of the video looks at some of the difficulties professionals face in caring for parents when a baby dies and the needs of these parents. Part Two explores what professionals can do to improve the quality of care they offer bereaved parents. *Death at Birth: Miscarriage, Stillbirth, Neonatal Death and Termination for Abnormality* is a user's guide to the training video 'Death at Birth'.

Child Bereavement Trust (CBT) (2000) *A Baby's Death—What Policies Do We Need?* (Training video). High Wycombe, CBT.

Child Bereavement Trust (CBT) (2000) *Making Difficult Decisions: A Child of Mine* (Training video). High Wycombe, CBT.

Child Bereavement Trust (CBT) (2003) *Paediatric Post Mortem: Communicating with Grieving Families* (Training video). High Wycombe, CBT.

Child Bereavement Trust (CBT) (2004) *Supporting Parents when their Baby Dies*. High Wycombe, CBT.
A booklet written to help and guide professionals in antenatal, delivery ward, postnatal, gynaecological and neonatal teams.

Addresses

ARC (Antenatal Results and Choices)
73 Charlotte Street, London W1P 1LB
Tel: 0207 6310280

Cruse Bereavement Care
126 Sheen Road, Richmond, Surrey TW9 1UR
Tel: 0208 9404818

Ectopic Pregnancy Trust
c/o The Maternity Unit, The Hillingdon Hospital, Pield Heath Road, Uxbridge UB8 3NN
Tel: 01895 238025
Fax: 01895 259779
Website: http://www.ectopic.org.uk

Miscarriage Association
c/o Clayton Hospital, Northgate, Wakefield, West Yorkshire WF1 3JS

Tel: 01924 200799
Fax: 01924 298834
Website: http://www.miscarriageassociation.org.uk

The Compassionate Friends
53 North Street, Bristol BS3 1EN
Tel: 0117 9665202
Email: info@tcf.org.uk
Website: http://www.tcf.org.uk

The Child Bereavement Trust
Aston House, High Street, West Wycombe, High Wycombe, Bucks HP14 3AG
Tel: 01494 446648
Fax: 01491 440057
Email: enquiries@childbereavement.org.uk
Website: http://www.childbereavement.org.uk
The Child Bereavement Trust is a charity which aims to train and support professionals and believes that those who develop their learning in a supportive environment are more able to care effectively for families in grief. The charity runs a number of courses aimed at training and supporting midwives as well as providing resources for professionals and bereaved families.

The Child Bereavement Trust website contains details of training courses run by the charity and all the resources produced by CBT, which can be bought online. There is a wealth of information on bereavement, aimed at different sectors of the community. There are sections for grieving young people, for bereaved parents, for parents to help them understand how their children feel when a sibling or parent dies, for health professionals caring for bereaved families in hospital and for school teachers supporting a child who has been bereaved.

The Multiple Births Foundation
Ham House, Level 4, Queen Charlotte's and Chelsea Hospital, Du Cane Road,
London W12 0HS
Tel: 0208 7403519
Email: mbs@ic.ac.uk
Website: http://www.multiplebirths.org.uk

SANDS
28 Portland Place, London W1B 1LY
Tel: 0207 4367940
Fax : 0207 4363715
Email: support@uk-sands.org
Website: http://www.uk-sands.org

4

Evidence-based Practice

Joyce Sihwa and Carolyn Roth

LEARNING OUTCOMES

After reading this chapter you will:

- be aware of the range of sources of evidence which may inform midwifery decisions and practice, and some of their strengths and limitations
- be able to frame a question on the basis of a clinical encounter and initiate a search for relevant evidence

- be aware of the need to critically appraise research evidence prior to making use of it in practice
- have insight into the complexities of the process of translating research findings into practice
- appreciate the contexts within which midwives might apply and contribute to the development of evidence-based practice.

INTRODUCTION

There can hardly be a practitioner who has not come across the notion of 'evidence-based healthcare' (EBHC) during reading, practice and formal professional development. This chapter will examine the meaning and use of EBHC for midwifery and the skills that midwives need to incorporate it into their practice.

The idea of basing clinical practice on evidence, rather than on habit or tradition, is intended to be a means of improving the quality of healthcare interventions and establishing a rational basis for clinical decision-making. Key government policy documents incorporate the principle of evidence-based practice into the structure and management of the National Health Service and the preparation of personnel (DoH, 1997, 1999).

The first part of the chapter examines different sources of knowledge for clinical practice and their relative value in clinical decision-making. The second part will outline the process that a midwife might use for locating, appraising and applying evidence in clinical practice.

DEFINITION

At its most descriptive level, an evidence-based approach to healthcare involves basing decisions and actions on the best available evidence. Evidence-based healthcare can be viewed as a strategy and a set of tools which enable a practitioner to be aware of and locate the available evidence, judge its strength and soundness and be in a position to apply it in practice.

Central to the whole enterprise of EBHC is the concept of 'evidence'. Perhaps, not surprisingly, this is not as simple as it seems.

WHAT IS EVIDENCE?

Evidence is a familiar concept within a legal context, where it has been defined as information which may be presented to a court of law, in order for a decision to be made about the *probability* that a claim is true. In other words, it is the information on the basis of which facts are proved or disproved (Keane, 2000). In a court of law, the decision to be made on the basis of evidence results in a verdict; in healthcare, evidence is sought as the basis for clinical decision-making.

Judging what constitutes 'sound evidence' in healthcare, as in a court of law, can be problematic. Evidence can be drawn from a variety of sources: from one's own personal experience (personal testimony); from the reported experience of others (expert testimony); or from systematic research (forensic evidence). While each of these may give rise to evidence which is adequate for making decisions in practice, they also have their limitations.

The following section will consider different sources of evidence for practice and will examine their strengths and limitations.

Personal knowledge

The role of personal experience and intuition in decision-making is discussed by several authors, for example Benner and Tanner (1987). While it is indispensable to most decision-making, personal experience and what people refer to as intuition, suffer from inherent limitations. The experience of a single individual is inevitably limited in scope and quantity and may be specific to a narrow context – and hence its implications may be inapplicable to other contexts. There may be special characteristics of the people involved in the experience, their skills and resources may be exceptional, and their preferences and values may be distinct from those of the general population. Personal experience is therefore difficult to generalize.

In addition, the capacity of individuals to 'check-out' or validate the evidence generated by their experience will be constrained by their personal presuppositions and assumptions about situations.

However, personal experience is still a valuable source of evidence. The more experience one gathers, in particular if experience is critically examined and becomes the basis for learning, the greater can be its value as a source of evidence. Sharing experience with others and inviting their judgement of the evidence is another way in which experience can be strengthened as a basis for evidence.

Furthermore, personal experience frequently provides the impetus for systematic investigation of questions arising from practice and is, therefore, a powerful tool for establishing evidence for wider use.

Expert knowledge

Inherent in the idea of 'expert opinion' is the assumption that some individuals, because of their cumulative experience, are considered to have extensive knowledge or skill in a particular sphere. Conventionally within clinical practice, experts have tended to be relied upon for direction or guidance in clinical decision-making.

However, there are also problems with relying on expert opinion as a basis for clinical decision-making. While a person may have a wealth of personal experience, unless there are ways to corroborate or confirm the evidence, the validity and reliability of that person's judgement are fallible. The biases and limitations of individual experience may also apply to that of the 'expert'.

Secondly, the status of 'expert' is a socially constructed judgement and is bestowed very selectively. Thus, for example, obstetricians are more likely to be considered experts in childbirth than are midwives or women themselves (Kent, 2000; Nettleton, 1995; Oakley and Graham, 1981).

Thirdly, expertise brings with it authority and may be difficult to challenge precisely because of its authoritative status. For example, it was for a long time the expert opinion of obstetricians that elective episiotomy was preferable to spontaneous perineal tearing (Graham, 1997). This expert opinion was transmitted through textbooks and clinical teaching and was built into routine practice for a considerable time (Roth, 1998; Sleep *et al.*, 1984; Sleep and Grant, 1987).

There is a need for expert opinion to be subjected to continuing and critical scrutiny to avoid building unchallenged assumptions into clinical decision-making. Peer review, departmental reviews, audit and evaluation are some of the mechanisms that can be used to achieve this critical challenge.

Research knowledge

Knowledge derived from a research process offers the possibility of improving on the limitations of 'personal knowledge' as considered above.

All rigorous research is designed to produce evidence which gains strength because built into the research process are mechanisms that act as internal challenges to address some of the shortcomings identified above. This is true of both quantitative and qualitative research approaches, although they vary in the challenges they pose (Bryman, 1992). The research process applies systematic strategies to investigate questions, to gather and analyse data and to validate findings. This allows the knowledge to be then accepted as credible beyond the limits of the particular study.

In other words, the result of a research process is capable of presenting a 'testable' account of the situation or phenomenon under investigation.

In designing and reporting research, it is essential for the investigators to state explicitly and publicly the basis for the research design, how the study was conducted and how conclusions were drawn from their data. In quantitative studies the researcher must convince readers that the study effectively answers the question posed, that the study is valid and reliable, and that the results can be generalized to a wider population. Qualitative research must fulfil similar criteria, although the terminology used is different because of different assumptions about the nature of investigation. Researchers in this field will present support for the trustworthiness, authenticity and dependability of their results (Denzin and Lincoln, 1994; Lincoln and Guba, 1985).

Discussion of these features should be found in the methodology section of a research report in which details about the research question, sampling strategy, data collection tools and analytical processes are stated.

However, the research process, like clinical practice, takes place within a particular context and it is shaped by the values and beliefs of those carrying it out. Implicit judgements underpin all research activity. These include:

- the judgement of what is a worthwhile question to ask
- the way in which the question is posed
- decisions about what data are worth including, and
- tests applied to judge the soundness of the conclusions drawn.

The decisions at each stage of the research process are generated within, and selected by, individuals whose worldview and values have been shaped within a particular social and professional context. Thus, knowledge is shaped by its social context. In this sense, there can be no 'absolute truth'. An awareness of this can be a fruitful basis for generating new questions which reflect and incorporate wider perspectives than just those of the medical or other professions.

However, even in its own terms, research cannot offer finality in its investigation of the world. Research projects can at best offer only a partial perspective on the questions investigated – the focus of the investigation, the decisions about how to investigate it, and the process of analysing and presenting the data are all subject to a variety of constraints. Research will be shaped by the perspectives of funding bodies as well as investigators, by where the study is conducted, the personnel involved, the autonomy of research participants, the rigour of data collection and analysis, the dissemination of findings, and the debate generated by the publication of the study. Even when these factors have been well considered and addressed within the research design and interpretation of findings, the applicability of results to wider spheres may be affected by small sample size or contextual factors.

Examples of these considerations can be seen in the series of studies carried out to investigate active management of the third stage of labour, in which selection of subjects, preparation of midwives and interpretation of data have all given rise to questions affecting the translation of research findings into practice (Prendiville *et al.*, 2001).

Particular problems are encountered when a number of studies addressing the same issue present apparently conflicting results. The confusion generated may hinder implementation of results that are valid. A classic example of this is reflected in the situation relating to the use dexamethasone in preterm labour. For a period of more than 10 years, conflicting results were documented regarding the efficacy of dexamethasone in promoting maturity of the fetal lungs in the babies of women with preterm labour. A number of studies concluded that it was of value, and an equal number drew the opposite conclusion. The perinatal mortality of babies born to mothers with preterm labours continued to rise until a *systematic appraisal* of all the evidence from the research papers was conducted which confirmed the beneficial effects of dexamethasone in promoting fetal lung maturity (Crowley 1995, 2001).

Limitations can be addressed in a number of ways. For a single research report, applying a strategy for rigorous critical appraisal (CASP, 1999; Greenhalgh, 2001) can enable the practitioner to distinguish between findings that are sound and those that are not.

Systematic review Techniques such as *systematic review* attempt to address the limitations of single studies and the ambiguity of study findings. This strategy involves systematically searching for a comprehensive sample of studies on a particular issue, including a wide range of publications and the so-called 'grey literature' of unpublished studies. Studies are then selected for inclusion in the review on the basis of explicit criteria applied to research method and their evidence is evaluated.

Systematic review is a rigorous way of testing the methodology and findings of individual studies in order to overcome the limitations discussed above, for example the problems of generalizing from small local samples or evaluating conflicting results. By validating study methodology and findings, the systematic review identifies those that can be confidently applied in guiding practice (e.g. Fraser *et al.*, 1999; Prendiville *et al.*, 2000).

Meta-analysis A further development of systematic review is *meta-analysis*. This involves the 'systematic pooling of quantitative data of available evidence on a particular research question' (Li Wan Po, 1998: 101), as identified by a systematic review, and subjecting those data to further statistical analysis (e.g. Crowley, 1995, 2001; Olsen, 1997; Olsen and Jewell, 1998).

In spite of the value of the overviews provided by these two strategies, they too are not without their limitations. These include the difficulty of exhausting all possible sources of relevant studies (those published in all other languages, locating grey literature), the biases which might arise in applying inclusion and exclusion criteria, and their preoccupation with studies using a quantitative design.

However, the experience of dexamethasone demonstrates another obstacle to an evidence-based approach: 'Despite repeated randomised trials in 1987 providing incontrovertible evidence in favour of antenatal corticosteroid therapy, obstetricians all over the world have been slow to adopt this treatment. The cause of this reluctance is unclear ...' (Crowley, 2001).

Evidence derived from current literature, primary research studies, systematic reviews and meta-analyses is not the only form in which evidence is available to practitioners. Practice guidelines, issued by local standard-setting committees or by the Royal Colleges, government recommendations and WHO initiatives, when they are based on critically appraised evidence and referenced as such, present evidence in a form which is easily accessible and applicable to practitioners.

HIERARCHY OF EVIDENCE

The preceding section has considered the sources of knowledge that are drawn on to inform clinical practice and the strengths and limitations of each.

The literature promoting an evidence-based approach to healthcare (Greenhalgh, 2001; Sackett *et al.*, 2000) suggests a hierarchical order of value for different sources of evidence. This places meta-analysis at the top, followed by systematic review, a single well-conducted randomized controlled trial, cohort studies and case reports. We suggest that personal experience and knowledge are an additional source of evidence, as these should inform practice and research at every level (Fig. 4.1). Those methods at the 'top end' of the hierarchy are valued more highly because they have mechanisms built into them which are intended to counter bias.

However, it needs to be remembered that no method is free from bias and therefore all evidence must be examined in a critical way before it can be made use of.

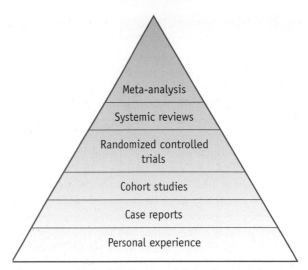

Figure 4.1 'Hierarchy' of evidence. (After Greenhalgh, 2001.)

Also, many issues requiring clinical decisions have not yet been studied in a systematic way and therefore personal experience and case reports remain important and essential in clinical decision-making.

WHAT STIMULATES THE SEARCH FOR EVIDENCE TO USE IN PRACTICE?

The search for evidence may be generated when practitioners or service users try to challenge the perpetuation of traditional practices (Romney, 1980; Romney and Gordon, 1981). This may stem from the desire to confirm and disseminate personal approaches to clinical care (McCandlish *et al.*, 1998). It may arise from an interest in investigating the nature of midwifery practice (Kirkham, 1989; Levy, 1999). It may also be stimulated by the numerous debates that surround the provision of maternity care (e.g. content of antenatal care (Sikorski *et al.*, 1996), place of birth (Macfarlane *et al.*, 2000; Olsen, 1997), nutrition in labour (Scrutton, 1999), management of the third stage of labour (Prendiville *et al.*, 1998), effectiveness, efficiency and quality of care (Green *et al.*, 1998)).

The two activities – conducting primary research to generate knowledge and critically appraising existing research findings – are closely linked. The further development of midwifery practice depends on practitioners applying both of these activities in their professional lives.

The next section of this chapter will lead the reader through the process of using evidence to answer a clinical question.

WHY SEARCH FOR EVIDENCE?

A midwife may begin a search for evidence to apply to practice for a number of reasons. The search may start with a question raised by a client, a student or another colleague, from research findings in other fields that raise questions about past practice, from media debates or because there is a tension between the practitioner's experience and the rituals and traditions in the practice context.

It may be helpful to think about the process as consisting of a series of steps that can take the individual from a clinical question or problem, to finding, appraising and applying evidence that will help to answer it.

There are basically five steps to this process. They are described below in a linear form, but in practice one might enter the process at any of the stages described.

Step 1:   This step often commences with a clinical encounter that requires a response.

Step 2:   In order to decide a response, the midwife needs to translate the situation into a question to which answers might be found.

Step 3:   This involves finding information to answer the question.

Step 4:   When the information is found, the midwife will have to make judgements about whether the information is true (valid) and reliable.

Step 5:   Having found such evidence, the last step is concerned with making use of the findings to attempt to solve the problem.

These stages, which can be summarized as shown in Box 4.1, will now be considered one by one, using a familiar clinical situation.

Reflective scenario

Consider the following situation, which midwives commonly encounter:

Kaya is in labour with her first baby. She was admitted to her local maternity unit in early labour, at 5 a.m. She is generally well, and all observations are normal. The fetus feels appropriately grown for term gestation and is lying longitudinally; the presentation is cephalic, with two-fifths of the head palpable abdominally. The fetal heart rate is 130 b.p.m. Her membranes are intact, and at initial assessment the cervix is 3 cm dilated and partially effaced; the position is left occipitoanterior.

It is now 8 a.m. and she says she is hungry and has not eaten since her tea at 6 p.m. the previous evening.

Box 4.1 Moving from clinical practice to the literature and back (after Sackett *et al.*, 2000)

1. Describing a clinical encounter
2. Posing or framing an answerable question
3. Searching for evidence
4. Critically appraising and validating the evidence
5. Implementing and evaluating the findings in practice

The midwife, Margaret, explains that the policy of the Unit is that women in established labour are kept 'nil by mouth' and only allowed sips of water or ice.

Kaya goes on to deliver at 6 p.m. the same day. She has a ventouse delivery under epidural analgesia, having experienced delay in the second stage because she was too tired to push and there were early fetal heart rate decelerations during the second stage. The baby girl is in satisfactory condition at birth, in spite of a prolonged second stage of labour.

Although it is not the first time Margaret has had to refuse a woman food in labour, she wonders all day whether Kaya's need for epidural pain relief and later delay in labour might have been related to missing her meal.

Framing an answerable question

The NHS Executive (1999) commented that defining the question is the starting point of evidence-based practice, and that once healthcare practitioners are clear about the question, this will help in locating the evidence they need to tackle the problem.

A guide for designing an evidence-based question is suggested by Sackett *et al.* (2000). A question about a healthcare intervention, like the one Margaret is considering, contains four elements. These are:

- the client population
- the intervention being considered
- the comparison or alternative intervention, and
- the outcome or outcomes the healthcare practitioner is interested in.

This format would not be suitable for *every* question generated by clinical practice, and other formats should be considered when appropriate, e.g. where the questions relate to prognosis (Laupacis *et al.*, 1994), economic evaluation (Drummond *et al.*, 1997), and guideline evaluation (Hayward *et al.*, 1995).

Kaya's situation can now be translated using the four elements outlined above.

The client population   To what client population does Kaya belong?

Kaya, who is in early labour with her first baby, is hungry and requesting food. She is anticipating a normal birth and would like to eat during the first stage of labour.

So, the definition of the client population is '*A woman in first stage of (uncomplicated) labour*'.

The intervention being considered   The midwife has carried out the existing policy, which is to refuse food to a woman in labour. The intervention therefore can be thought of as '*fasting in labour*'.

The comparison/alternative intervention   Kaya asked for food and therefore the alternative intervention can be formulated as: '*eating and drinking in labour*'.

The outcome or outcomes the healthcare practitioner is interested in   A concern that Margaret may have had might be whether Kaya's problems – delay in labour, need for pain relief, and fetal condition – might be related to fasting in labour.

The outcomes could be defined as '*prolonged labour*', '*pain relief in labour*', '*fetal distress*'.

Box 4.2 summarizes the elements recommended for constructing an answerable question and how they have been applied to the scenario.

Composing an answerable question

After identifying the key elements of the scenario, the next step is to formulate a question that can be

phrased from the above parts. This can be framed as follows:

- In women during the first stage of uncomplicated labour … (*client population*)
- does fasting … (*intervention*)
- compared to eating and drinking … (*alternative intervention*)
- lead to maternal and fetal hazards/risks, i.e. prolonged labour, increased need for pain relief and fetal distress (*outcomes of interest*).

The framed question would therefore read as follows:

In women during the first stage of uncomplicated labour, does fasting compared to eating and drinking, lead to prolonged labour, increased need for pain relief in labour or increased incidence of fetal distress?

With a question like this Margaret is likely to be in a far better position to search for the evidence on the effects of denying food to women in labour. Before moving on to consider how Margaret can search for the evidence, try formulating an answerable question for each of the scenarios presented in Reflective Activities 4.1 and 4.2.

Box 4.2 Elements recommended for constructing an answerable question (after Sackett, 2000)

Client population
Labouring women during the first stage of uncomplicated labour

The intervention being considered
Fasting in labour

Alternative intervention
Eating and drinking in labour

The outcomes of interest
Maternal and fetal hazards/risks:

- prolonged labour
- increased need for pain relief
- fetal distress

Reflective Activity 4.1

Chichi is a healthy, well-informed and well-read primigravid client. She is having a home birth. A midwife and a student midwife facilitate her care. The midwives are having an amicable conversation about perineal management during the second stage of labour.

The student states that she has worked with a number of midwives on the labour ward who have adopted varying techniques. Some have 'guarded' and massaged the perineum and flexed the fetal head as it descended whilst others have not done anything. Chichi, who was in the kitchen getting a glass of water, overhears the conversation. She asked the midwife which method would be best for her during the birth of her baby.

Can you frame a question for finding the evidence on the above scenario?

Compare your question with our suggested one at the end of the chapter (p. 62).

Searching for the evidence

> Navigating one's way through the jungle that calls itself medical literature is no easy task.
> (Greenhalgh, 2001: 13)

The process of tracking evidence in the databases is not as simple as it sounds on paper. The prerequisites for the procedure, which include keyboard skills, 'mouse' skills and search strategies, may mean that the procedure raises special challenges for some practitioners. Those who have no prior experience with information technology (IT) may be anxious and even 'phobic' about trying. This may be because of a fear of damaging expensive equipment as well as anxiety about failing to master what children seem to manage with no difficulty. It is worth remembering that no damage can be done by ordinary use, and experimentation is often part of the learning process. The situation is helped if the practitioner is in possession of a computer or can get access to one in the work or study place.

Experience of teaching evidence-based practice demonstrates that even those practitioners who are 'technophobic' and not in possession of a computer can develop the essential skills after a few sessions with a librarian or IT lecturer.

However, even those who acquire the necessary skills may have to overcome time constraints. Unfortunately, there are times when much energy and time is devoted to tracking the evidence, but the searcher may simply fail to retrieve any useful, relevant, up-to-date research articles. Whilst there are a number of areas for which evidence exists as a basis for sound decision-making, there are many clinical questions which still require evidence of good quality to be generated; this discovery in itself should be seen as a positive finding if it leads to further research.

With increased experienced, practitioners will become more efficient in their efforts. Increasingly, IT facilities are becoming part of standard clinical equipment, and searching is likely to become part of practitioners' activities at work (Littler and Weist, 1998).

Learning and developing search skills

There are an increasing number of on-line tutorials that support users through the searching process. Some of these are:

- http://www.nlm.nih.gov/bsd/pubmed_tutorial/m1001.html
- http://www.shef.ac.uk/scharr/ir/litsrch.html/
- http://www.courses.hschbklyn.edu/ebm/
- http://www.shef.ac.uk/uni/projects/wrp/index.html/.

You may wish to 'bookmark' these in your web browser (e.g. Netscape or Explorer) and add new ones as you discover them.

The searching process

The searching process requires that the practitioner define *where* the search will be made, *what words* will be used to identify relevant studies and *how* this search can be narrowed or broadened to result in a useful and relevant output which will meet the requirements.

Where to search   The searching process involves looking systematically through databases in order to locate research articles relevant to the question under investigation. (See Additional resources (pp. 61–62) for details of commonly available databases.) Searching also includes manual searching of recently published journals, because these will not yet be included in the database, for which there is usually a 6-month delay. A search may also include material located through library catalogues.

Once having located studies relevant to the question, further searching may include studies specified in the references of that study.

What words to use in the search   The words chosen for the search should be derived from the question. Care taken in defining the terms of the question will help to focus the search and, by helping to identify the key search terms, avoid wasting time locating irrelevant material.

In order to carry out an effective search, though, it may be necessary to convert the terms in the question into those recognized within the classification system in a particular database. In most databases, the references to articles are linked to *subject headings*. Where there are several alternative terms, only one of these will be used by the database. This is called 'controlled vocabulary'. Medline, CINAHL, Cochrane and DARE all use *Medical Subject Headings* (MeSH), which is a common classification system, organized in a hierarchical structure. It is possible to consult the MeSH terms, by clicking on MeSH, in order to find the ones relevant for the search. On-line searching of Medline on the PubMed site (http://www.ncbi.nlm.nih.gov) now automatically offers alternative terms if the ones used are not recognized.

There may also be related terms – for example gestation and gestational, fetal and fetus, preconceptual and preconception – several of which are relevant to your search. In such cases, you can truncate the term and add a symbol designated by the database software package as a wild card indicator. By typing gestat*, for example, the SilverPlatter database will match all words with the root indicated. The correct wildcard indicator should be checked for the software application being used.

Narrowing or broadening the search Most databases employ Boolean logic to structure the search. This means that linking terms with AND results in a narrower search, because a match will only be made if both of the named terms are found.

Using OR will result in a broader search, because matches will be made if either of the specified terms is located.

This can be tried by attempting a search for 'labour AND fasting' which should produce studies relevant to the question about Kaya's care in labour (see above). Using the Boolean connector OR can overcome the problem of language difference. One choice for searching might be: '(labour OR labor) AND fasting'.

A number of selection criteria can be built into the search strategy to refine the process so that the most relevant papers are retrieved.

The database will offer the opportunity to set *limits* regarding the references which are located. Limits can include the language, date(s) of publication and specific types of articles such as reviews or specific research methodologies. Different databases offer different options for selection of limit, and you need to consult the guidance provided with the database package.

In addition, it is possible to specify references in which the key terms appear in the title, or in the title and abstract, of articles rather than anywhere in the text.

In the event that the search yields a number of 'hits', i.e. references that are produced on the basis of the search terms, the searcher may need to eliminate those that are irrelevant or that will not help to answer the question.

Careful reading of the title and abstract of a study will help to identify those studies that will be useful to read in full.

Some helpful hints

If the search question relates to an intervention and its effects on outcomes, it is always worth starting with a search of the Cochrane Database. This will save a great deal of time and effort. Cochrane will enable location of any relevant systematic reviews of trials related to the question as well as references to trials that are listed in the Cochrane Controlled Trials Register. It may be that the answer to the question is already available in the findings of a systematic review and further searching will not be necessary.

If the term being searched has a different spelling in American English it is important to include both the English and American spellings in order not to miss studies published in the British literature e.g. (labour OR labor).

It may also be important to include a term and its opposite, in order to improve the likelihood of capturing the key term under which the research is described.

A search may work most efficiently if it is built up step by step, including new search terms one at a time (Fig. 4.2).

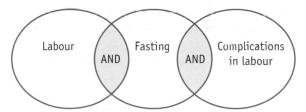

Figure 4.2 Step-by-step searching.

Judging the evidence

Practitioners may be tempted merely to look at the findings of research studies or guideline recommendations and rely on these to influence their practice. However, it is necessary to exercise critical skills, even when the source of the evidence can be expected to have applied rigorous standards in its preparation.

Again, an analogy of what happens in law might offer a useful example. In a court of law, specific criteria are used to aid the jury or judge in their decision-making when coming to a verdict. In criminal matters, the test used is that the evidence is beyond all reasonable doubt, whilst in civil matters it is judged on the balance of probabilities.

However, unlike a court, within the area of healthcare practice, there has not been the same agreed set of rules for judging evidence or determining the action to be taken once it is judged. One can view the 'evidence-based practice movement' as an attempt to establish a consensus framework both for judging evidence and for guiding practice.

Judgement can be exercised and developed by making use of the range of general and specific appraisal guides in order to validate the available research evidence (Critical Appraisal Skills Programme (CASP), 1999; Greenhalgh, 2001; Sackett *et al.*, 2000). A critical guide enables a systematic approach to appraisal, ensuring that attention is given to all elements of the research process, guarding against 'snap' decisions and ensuring that the practitioner's judgements are well grounded.

It is impossible to offer a comprehensive list of appraisal guides, as it is a rapidly developing area of literature. However, some resources that may be useful to develop a global way of appraising a research study include Rees (1997), Rose (1994), Denscombe (1998), Rudestam and Newton (2000), each of which provides a strategy for analysing and critiquing research reports.

There are also appraisal guides developed specifically to examine clinical and related studies according to the specific research problem under investigation and/or the study design. Thus, there are guides specific to examining a clinical trial, a systematic review or a qualitative study of client experience. Whatever the design of the study being appraised, it is helpful to use a tool specially designed for the purpose, which enables the important characteristics of the study to be examined. Examples of these can be found on the following websites:

CASP programme: http://www.phru.org/casp/
Wisdom Project: http://www.shef.ac.uk/uni/projects/wrp/seminar.html.

The *Journal of the American Medical Association* has produced an ongoing series 'User guides to the medical literature', each of which addresses a particular facet of searching, critiquing and making use of research evidence. A full list of this series can be found at:

http://www.shef.ac.uk/~scharr/ir/userg.html.

Once the evidence is validated, the next issue to consider is how it is put into practice.

Contexts for implementing the evidence

The 'practice' of midwifery does not happen only when the midwife is 'with woman', and the application of evidence to midwifery can be regarded as happening at several levels of practice:

- *Individual*: the decision-making that occurs at the time of giving care to an individual client.
- *Collective*: the consensus expressed in the guidelines and protocols agreed within a collaborative setting, e.g. a trust or a group midwifery practice.
- *Professional*: the body of knowledge and the implications for practice which emerge from it, as reflected for example in Royal College of Midwives' Position Papers, English National Board research and policy recommendations, Nursing and Midwifery Council (NMC) standard setting, rules and codes of practice. In addition, professional knowledge is developed, debated and published at conferences and in peer-reviewed journals.
- *Societal/public debates and consensus* as expressed in Department of Health recommendations, government policy e.g. *The new NHS: Modern and Dependable* (DoH, 1997), Clinical Governance (NHS Executive 2000), National Institute for Clinical Excellence (NICE) (NHS Executive, 1998).

It is important for midwives to contribute to and engage in debates at all these levels in order to provide rational, justifiable, equitable and good-quality care for childbearing women. The entire exercise of putting evidence into practice involves changes in practice for the benefit of clients.

At an individual level, it may seem relatively easy to implement change based on evidence. For example, individual midwives might examine and alter their usual practice in order to ensure that the women they are caring for in labour have the opportunity to hold their babies in skin-to-skin contact, which often did not happen in the past because of the usual 'hustle and bustle' of a busy labour ward. They may be scrupulous in outlining to women the evidence relating to choice of place of birth; they may facilitate women's mobility in labour.

Individual midwives will recognize, however, how difficult it is to work in a context where practice is not consistently informed by good evidence. Thus, for example many midwives face the difficulty of working in an environment where continuous electronic fetal monitoring is used in the care of most women, in spite of the absence of evidence to support this (Thacker *et al.*, 2001). The same 'evidence–practice gap' is demonstrated in the problem that Margaret, in the example above, faced, in providing food for women in normal labour (Scrutton *et al.*, 1999). So, consistent application of evidence to practice depends on more than the good intentions of individual practitioners.

Care for women and babies is delivered by more than one individual in more than one professional group. In this respect, a 'collective' approach to evidence-based practice is essential. Implementation of evidence in practice is inextricably linked to the mechanisms for quality standards and change within an organization. There are a variety of mechanisms – risk management groups, guideline development initiatives, audit activities, including meetings looking at maternal and neonatal morbidity and mortality. Midwives have to play a key role within these multidisciplinary ventures. Consultant midwives and practice development midwives are likely to make vital contributions in this sphere as their roles evolve.

However, midwives' practice is shaped by influences beyond that of their local sphere. All midwives practise within a professional framework that includes the Nursing and Midwifery Council for Nursing, Midwifery and Health Visiting *Midwives Rules* (UKCC, 1998), *Code of Professional Conduct* (NMC, 2002) and midwifery supervision.

Supervision has a special contribution to make in facilitating the development of an EBHC culture. Annual interviews can assess the needs of individual midwives for further development of required skills and encourage involvement in practice development. The use of PREP helps to identify educational and professional development and needs. Some supervisory teams (Kroll, personal communication, 2001) are encouraging midwives to engage directly in searching for and critiquing evidence in order to practise their skills, rather than merely relying on formal educational programmes as ways of keeping updated. Supervisory audits may demonstrate individual or organizational practice that is poorly supported by evidence, and action for change may be initiated.

A range of influences at the social level has relevance for creating a climate and context for evidence-based practice. In maternity care, client pressure, expressed through a range of user groups has been pivotal in compelling professionals to re-examine the evidence base for practices. Such groups include the National Childbirth Trust (NCT), Association for Improvements in Maternity Services (AIMS), Active Birth Movement, Stillbirth and Neonatal Death Society (SANDS) and many others.

The National Institute for Clinical Excellence (NICE) was set up in April 1999 with the expressed aim of providing 'patients, health professionals and the public with authoritative, robust and reliable guidance on current "best practice"', underpinned by review of the available evidence. The publication of guidelines for induction of labour and fetal heart monitoring, which are accompanied by information booklets for pregnant women and partners, are examples of their activities. The NICE guidelines are based on those published by the RCOG that had been developed by a multidisciplinary team, evidence-based and referenced, and aim to achieve consistency of practice nationally.

Another initiative, which bridges the gap between service user and professional practice, is the DISCERN instrument (http://www.discern.org.uk/background.htm), that enables consumers to evaluate the quality of the information offered to them as part of their care.

Getting research into practice

The discussion of implementation of evidence-based practice can hardly be complete without considering the complexity of the process whereby evidence is translated into practice. Individual and organizational behaviours are important elements in the translation of research into practice, and at the heart of the matter is the management of change (Broome, 1995; Enkin, 1992; Evans and Haines, 2000; Haines and Donald, 1998; Kanter *et al.*, 1992). CASP (1999) suggest that it is essential to understand the characteristics of change and its impact on organizational activity, when embarking on implementation of evidence into practice. And, not to be forgotten is the fact that evidence itself is subject to change. With further research and changing technology, the knowledge base for practice may alter very rapidly, so the search for evidence must be a continuing process.

Happily, evidence is accumulating to guide the effort to translate research into practice. A number of studies have examined the effectiveness of different strategies for disseminating and implementing research findings into practice. Bero *et al.* (1998) conducted an overview of systematic reviews on interventions for the implementation of findings. Lomas (1994) reviewed models for the dissemination of research evidence and proposes a model which illustrated the interaction between research information, appraisal, the practice environment and personnel involved in applying research findings. However, Kitson *et al.* (1998) suggest the need to go beyond these linear representations of change and offer a multidimensional model which takes into consideration three elements:

- the nature of the evidence
- the environment into which it is being introduced, and
- the process for facilitating its introduction.

Each of these elements may be more or less favourable to the change process. Kitson *et al.* (1998) propose that the model may be applied diagnostically to help in planning the implementation of change. The case studies they analyse suggest that facilitation of change is the key element to successful implementation. In the light of this suggestion, consultant or practice development midwives are strong candidates for initiating and sustaining research-based changes in practice.

Evaluating the implementation of evidence in practice

Like all change, the change process involved when evidence is translated into practice needs to be evaluated. A plan for evaluation may be part of the implementation process, or data may be collected through on-going audit activity, but there must be some thought given to measuring the impact of clinical change on client outcomes, organizational processes and staff activity.

Gray (2001) proposes an 'evidence-driven audit cycle'. This is a useful model because of the way in which it integrates the search for evidence, translation of evidence into practice and measurement of its impact using audit tools. A question is generated within clinical practice, which stimulates the search for evidence. Changes in practice can be implemented on the basis of relevant evidence and the results of such changes monitored through audit activity. Evidence is made use of by being the basis for the audit standards against which practice is measured and a means by which further questions can be generated.

HOW ARE MIDWIVES INVOLVED IN THE APPLICATION OF EVIDENCE-BASED PRACTICE?

Some midwives will be satisfied with simply applying bodies of evidence as interpreted in pre-appraised resources such as *The Cochrane Library and Evidence-Based Medicine* or in locally developed practice guidelines. Others will take a more active part by contributing to the development of evidence-based guidelines, putting into effect the skills for searching and appraising current research evidence. Some midwives will use research and appraisal strategies to challenge and change practice. A growing number of midwives will engage directly in the research process: designing and conducting primary research, participating in systematic reviews and meta-analyses. Each of these activities requires different levels of expertise in the skills for EBHC. However, all of them require a basic knowledge of the research and appraisal process.

Midwives will develop their involvement in EBHC in a variety of ways. This will be influenced to a large extent by the context in which they practice and their role within the organization in which they practice. Furthermore, the process of achieving evidence-based practice – formulating a question, searching, critically appraising and synthesizing available evidence – is time-consuming, and requires acquisition of new skills and access to resources such as electronic equipment, databases and librarians. Solutions to these constraints will develop over the long term, as the commitment to an evidence base for healthcare is disseminated more widely and provision made for its practice. However, the inclusion of the skills for evidence-based practice in the initial and on-going professional development of midwives in itself contributes to the reduction of some of these constraints (Guyatt *et al.*, 2000).

CONCLUSION

This chapter has examined ideas of evidence-based clinical practice in relation to the sources of clinical knowledge and their strengths and limitations. It has explored some ways of translating familiar clinical issues into searchable questions to enable the student to gain experience in search strategies. Tools for the critical appraisal of research papers have been introduced. Consideration is given to the processes by which validated evidence might be put into practice and the different contexts in which midwives might be involved in this process.

KEY POINTS

- Evidence may derive from personal experience, expert knowledge or systematic investigation.
- Midwives need to be discerning about strengths and limitations of different sources of evidence and

seek to strengthen the evidence base for their own practice.

- A number of tools and strategies exist, with which the practitioner should become familiar.

- A strategy for posing questions about clinical practice and searching for evidence can be a tool for challenging existing practice, revealing gaps in available evidence and developing the evidence base for practice.

- It is important that midwives gain skills in order to contribute to and engage at the individual, collective, professional and public levels in debates about the evidence for practice and the best means for using evidence to improve the care of mothers and babies.

REFERENCES

Benner, P. & Tanner, C. (1987) Clinical judgment: how expert nurses use intuition. *American Journal of Nursing* 87(1): 23–31.

Bero, L., Grilli, R., Grimshaw, J.M. *et al.* (1998) Closing the gap between research and practice: an overview of systematic reviews of interventions to promote the implementation of research findings. *British Medical Journal* 317(7156): 465–468.

Broome, A.K. (1995) *Managing change*, 2nd edn. Basingstoke: Macmillan.

Bryman, A. (1992) *Quantity and Quality in Social Research*. London: Routledge.

Critical Appraisal Skills Programme (CASP) (1999) *Evidence-based Health Care: An Open Learning Resource for Health Care Practitioners*. Luton: CASP and HCLU. Online. Available: http://www.phru.org/casp/, 23 June 2001.

Crowley, P.A. (1995) Antenatal corticosteroid therapy: a meta-analysis of the randomised trials, 1972–1994. *American Journal of Obstetrics and Gynecology* 173(1): 322–335.

Crowley, P. (2001) Prophylactic corticosteroids for preterm birth (Cochrane Review). *The Cochrane Library*, Issue 2, 2001. Oxford: Update Software.

Denscombe, M. (1998) *The Good Research Guide*. Buckingham: Open University Press (OUP).

Denzin, N.K. & Lincoln, Y.S. (eds) (1994) *Handbook of Qualitative Research*. London: Sage.

Department of Health (DoH) (1997) *The new NHS: Modern and Dependable*. London: The Stationery Office.

Department of Health (DoH) (1999) *Making a Difference*. London: DoH.

Drummond, M.F., Richardson, W.S., O'Brien, B.J. *et al.* (1997) Users' guides to the medical literature: how to use an article on economic analysis of clinical practice. *Journal of the American Medical Association* 277(19): 1552–1557.

Enkin, M. (1992) Can changes in practice be implemented? In: Chard, T. & Richards, M.P.M. (eds) *Obstetrics in the 1990s: Current Controversies*, Ch. 15. Oxford: Mackeith Press.

Evans, D. & Haines, A. (eds) (2000) *Implementing Evidence-based Changes in Healthcare*. Abingdon: Radcliffe Medical.

Fraser, W.D., Turcot, L., Krauss, I. *et al.* (1999) Amniotomy for shortening labour (Cochrane Review). *The Cochrane Library*, Issue 2, 2001. Oxford: Update Software.

Graham, I. (1997) *Episiotomy: Challenging Obstetric Interventions*. Oxford: Blackwell Science.

Gray, M. (2001) *Evidence-based Health Care*. Edinburgh: Churchill Livingstone.

Green, J., Coupland, V. & Kitzinger, J. (1998) *Great Expectations: A Prospective Study of Women's Expectations and Experiences*, 2nd edn. Hale: Books for Midwives Press.

Greenhalgh, T. (2001) *How to Read a Paper: The Basics of Evidence Based Medicine*, 2nd edn. London: BMJ Publications.

Guyatt, G.H., Meade, M., Jaeschke, R.Z. *et al.* (2000) Practitioners of evidence based care: not all clinicians need to appraise evidence from scratch but all need some skills. *British Medical Journal* 320(7240): 954–955.

Haines, A. & Donald, A. (eds) (1998) *Getting Research Findings into Practice*. London: BMJ Press.

Hayward, R.S.A., Wilson, M.C., Tunis, S.R. *et al.* 1995 Users' guides to the medical literature: how to use clinical practice guidelines. *Journal of the American Medical Association* 274(7): 570–574.

Kanter, R.M., Stein, B. & Jick, T.D. (1992) *The Challenge of Organisational Change*. New York: Free Press.

Keane, A. (2000) *The Modern Law of Evidence*, 2nd edn. London: Butterworths.

Kent, J. (2000) *Social Perspectives on Pregnancy and Childbirth for Midwives, Nurses and the Caring Professions*. Buckingham: Open University Press.

Kirkham, M. (1989) Midwives and information giving during labour. In: Robinson, S. & Thomson, A.M. (eds) *Midwives, Research and Childbirth*. London: Chapman and Hall.

Kitson, A., Harvey, G. & McCormack, B. (1998) Enabling the implementation of evidence based practice: a conceptual framework. *Quality in Health Care* 7(3): 149–158.

Laupacis, A., Wells, G., Richardson, W.S. *et al.* (1994) Users' guides to the medical literature: how to use an article about prognosis. *Journal of the American Medical Association* 272(3): 234–237.

Levy, V. (1999) Protective steering: a grounded theory study of the processes by which midwives facilitate informed choices during pregnancy. *Journal of Advanced Nursing* 29(1): 104–112.

Li Wan Po, A. (1998) *Dictionary of Evidence-based Medicine*. Abingdon: Radcliffe Medical Press.

Lincoln, Y.S. & Guba, E.G. (1985) *Naturalistic Inquiry*. London: Sage.

Littler, C. & Weist, A. (1998) Education. Front-line evidence-based midwifery. *Midwives* **1**(9): 282–284.

Lomas, J. (1994) Teaching old (and not so old) docs new tricks: effective ways to implement research findings. In: Dunn, E.V., Norton, P.G. & Stewart, M. (eds) *Disseminating Research/Changing Practice*. London: Sage.

Macfarlane, A., McCandlish, R. & Campbell, R. (2000) Choosing between home and hospital delivery. There is no evidence that hospital is safest place to give birth. *British Medical Journal* **320**(7237): 798.

McCandlish, R., Bowler, U., van Asten, H. *et al.* (1998) A randomised controlled trial of care of the perineum during second stage of normal labour. *British Journal of Obstetrics and Gynaecology* **105**(12): 1262–1272.

Nettleton, S. (1995) *The Sociology of Health & Illness*. London: Polity Press.

NHS Executive (1998) *A First Class Service*. London: DoH.

NHS Executive (2000) *Building the Information Core: Implementing the NHS Plan*. London: DoH.

Nursing and Midwifery Council (2002) *Code of Professional Conduct*. London: NMC.

Oakley, A. & Graham, H. (1981) Competing ideologies of reproduction: medical and maternal perspectives on pregnancy. In: Roberts, H. (ed) *Women, Health and Reproduction*. London: RKP.

Olsen, O. (1997) Metaanalysis of the safety of home birth. *Birth* **24**(1): 4–13, discussion 14–16.

Olsen, O. & Jewell, M.D. (1998) Home versus hospital birth (Cochrane Review). *The Cochrane Library*, Issue 2, 2001. Oxford: Update Software.

Prendiville, W.J., Elbourne, D. & McDonald, S. (2001) Active versus expectant management in the third stage of labour (Cochrane Review). *The Cochrane Library*, Issue 3, 2001. Oxford: Update Software.

Rees, C. (1997) *An Introduction to Research for Midwives*. Hale: Hochland & Hochland.

Romney, M. (1980) Predelivery shaving: an unjustified assault? *Journal of Obstetrics and Gynaecology* **1**: 33–35.

Romney, M. & Gordon, H. (1981) Is your enema really necessary? *British Medical Journal (Clinical Research Edition)* **282**(6272): 1269–1271.

Rose, G. (1994) *Deciphering Sociological Research*. Basingstoke: Macmillan.

Roth, C. (1998) *Reading Between the Lines: The Contribution of Obstetric Textbooks to Professional Authority and Power*. Occasional Paper in Sociology and Social Policy, No. 6. London: South Bank University.

Rudestam, E.K. & Newton, R.R. (2000) *Surviving Your Dissertation: A Comprehensive Guide to Content and Process*. Newbury Park, California: Sage.

Sackett, D.L., Richardson, W.S., Rosenberg, W. *et al.* (2000) *Evidence-based Medicine (Multimedia): How to Practice and Teach EBM*, 2nd edn. Edinburgh: Churchill Livingstone.

Scrutton, M.J.L., Metcalfe, G.A., Lowy, C. *et al.* (1999) Eating in labour: a randomised controlled trial assessing risks and benefits. *Anaesthesia* **54**(4): 329–334.

Sikorski, J., Wilson, J., Clement, S. *et al.* (1996) A randomised controlled trial comparing two schedules of antenatal visits: the antenatal care project. *British Medical Journal* **312**(7030): 546–553.

Sleep, J. & Grant, A. (1987) West Berkshire perineal management trial: three year follow-up. *British Medical Journal (Clinical Research Edition)* **295**(6601): 749–751.

Sleep, J., Grant, A., Garcia, J. *et al.* (1984) West Berkshire perineal management trial. *British Medical Journal (Clinical Research Edition)* **289**(6445): 587–590.

Thacker, S.B., Stroup, D.& Chang, M. (2001) Continuous electronic fetal heartrate monitoring for fetal assessment during labour (Cochrane Review). *The Cochrane Library*, Issue 3, 2001. Oxford: Update Software.

United Kingdom Council for Nursing, Midwifery and Health Visiting (UKCC) (1998) *Midwives Rules and Code of Practice*. London: UKCC.

FURTHER READING

Critical Skills Appraisal Programme and The Health Care Libraries Unit (1999) *Evidence-based Health Care*. (Distributed by Update Software: http://www.update-software.com.)
A comprehensive learning pack consisting of five units of study, each representing a key facet of the process of evidence-based healthcare. Self-directed learning with this programme is supported by a CD-ROM with interactive activities and a workbook with structured exercises.

Greenhalgh, T. (2001) *How to Read a Paper: The Basics of Evidence Based Medicine*, 2nd edn. London: BMJ Publications.
An easily understood and interesting overview of the processes of evidence-based healthcare. Guidance and

practical strategies for developing useful skills are provided. This is a useful introduction to the process but also useful for those with experience.

Sackett, D.L., Richardson, W.S., Rosenberg, W. *et al.* (2000) *Evidence-based Medicine (Multimedia): How to Practice and Teach EBM*, 2nd edn. Edinburgh: Churchill Livingstone.
This is the original formulation of a strategy for practising and teaching evidence-based healthcare. An interactive CD-ROM and pocket-sized cards are included, for help in interpreting research literature. Its particular strength is in considering a structured approach to formulating questions and suggestions about using clinical practice as a source for question development.

ADDITIONAL RESOURCES

Assia
A database for sociology, psychology, cultural anthropology, economics and politics.

Best Evidence
A huge resource available on CD-ROM. It contains abstracts of and commentaries on two major journals: *ACP Journal Club* and *Evidence-Based Medicine*. These journals (available also in hard-copy format) contain reviews from over 90 journals worldwide, and research articles that are chosen contain good study design.

BNI (British Nursing Index)
Published by the Royal College of Nursing, this lists all articles in the RCN Library. It does include some journals not listed in the American databases and is therefore especially useful for British aspects such as community care and the working of the NHS. It is available on CD and the Web.

CINAHL (Cumulative Index for Nursing and Allied Health Literature)
Contains references and abstracts from journals from all over the world but mainly in English (dates to 1982). It is available in libraries, on CD-ROM and on the Web.

Health STAR
This contains information on administration and planning of health care facilities, evaluation of patient outcomes, effectiveness of procedures and health technology.

Medline
This contains references and abstracts of 3600 medical and nursing journals throughout the world, in English and other languages. The data include literature from 1966, and thus around 12 million articles are referenced. It is American, so it is important to be aware of slight differences in spelling and terminology. It is linked to MeSH. It can be accessed at www.nlm.nih.gov, and can also be accessed in libraries, using sophisticated technology; OVID, Healthgate; WinSPIRS and SilverPlatter (CD-ROM).

MIDIRS
This includes the Midwives Information and Resource Service, and is a specialized database for midwives, focusing mainly on professional midwifery, maternity services, pregnancy, childbirth and the care of the neonate.

MIRIAD
A database of midwifery research in the UK which was established at the National Perinatal Epidemiology Unit in Oxford. This has now been integrated into the National Research Register, available on CD-ROM.

Psyclit
Contains literature and research abstracts from psychology and related disciplines, including medicine, physiology, sociology, psychiatry and anthropology.

Reviews

ACP Journal Club
This is an American source, which contains short reviews, and may be accessed through ScHARR (see below).

Bandolier
This is British and is available in print form and on the Web on http://www.jr2.ox.ac.uk:80/Bandolier/. The format is user friendly and includes evaluations of research particularly RCTs. The database has an alphabetical list which can be searched.

Cochrane Database of Systematic Reviews (CDSR)
Contains full text systematic reviews, employing a standard methodology.

Cochrane Library
Contains four databases, and is updated quarterly. It is designed to be used to answer questions on 'effectiveness', e.g. What is the effectiveness of a given intervention? What is an effective intervention for a particular situation? Is one intervention better than another in managing a situation? Available in libraries, on the Web and on CD-ROM.

Cochrane Review Methodology Database (CRMD)
Contains references to studies examining methodological issues.

Controlled Trials Register (CTR)
Contains bibliographic references and abstracts of ongoing trials.

Database of Abstracts of Reviews of Effectiveness (DARE)
Contains critical assessments of systematic reviews published in journals other than Cochrane. (DARE can also be accessed free from other websites, such as http://nhscrd.york.ac.uk/darehp.htm and ScHARR.)

Gateways

ScHARR
http://www.shef.ac.uk/~scharr/ir/netting
Based at Sheffield University, ScHARR has a rich source of information on evidence-based medicine and on health administration. Of special interest here is the Netting the Evidence gateway which links to other useful websites.

Centre for Evidence Based Medicine (in Oxford)
http://cebm.jr2.ox.ac.uk/
A gateway providing access to a variety of evidence-based medicine sources and journals. There is a link to the current issues and an index to back numbers of the journal *Evidence-Based Nursing*.

National Electronic Library for Health (NeLH)
http://www.nelh.nhs.uk/

This development from the NHS IT strategy provides clinicians with access to the best current know-how and knowledge to support healthcare-related decisions. Patients, carers and the public are also welcome to use the site, though they are referred to NHS Direct Online.

West Midlands Perinatal Institute
http://www.wmpi.net/main.htm
A useful site which has information and hotlinks around evidence-based perinatal care.

Evidence Based Midwifery Network (EBMN)
http://www.fons.org/networks/ebm/index.htm
The network started in 1998 to offer a forum for midwives in the UK to share best practice and ideas about evidence-based practice. It continues to be supported by the *British Journal of Midwifery*, which is in the process of setting up a section for the network on its website.

Journals

Journals are mostly available in print form, but some are now available electronically via the Internet, e.g. *British Medical Journal*: http://bmj.com/all.shtml allows the reader to search the *BMJ* back to 1994.
It is also possible to move from a search on CINAHL or Medline into electronic feedback, though the library will usually have to have subscribed.

SUGGESTED ANSWERS

Reflective Activity 4.1: Chichi
In women during uncomplicated second stage of labour, does guarding/massaging the perineum and flexing the fetal head compared to leaving the perineum and fetal head untouched lead to maternal/fetal risks?

Reflective Activity 4.2: Rohini
In women with a previous caesarean section, does having a vaginal birth instead of having a repeat caesarean lead to maternal and fetal risks?

PART 2

SEXUALITY, FERTILITY AND CONCEPTION

5. Anatomy of Male and Female Reproduction 65

6. Female Reproductive Physiology 89

7. Sexuality 105

8. Fertility and its Control 114

9. Infertility and Assisted Conception 129

10. Preconception Care 143

Anatomy of Male and Female Reproduction

Barbara Burden and Maria Simons

LEARNING OUTCOMES

After reading this chapter you will have:

- explored the anatomical structures of the pelvis and its corresponding joints and ligaments, and their significance for midwifery practice
- considered the dimensions, angles and axis of the pelvis and how these may influence the outcomes for birth
- examined the anatomical structures of the female reproductive system and their significance to midwifery practice
- explored how the uterus changes during pregnancy, how it functions during labour, birth and the third stage of labour, and the normal processes of involution in the postpartum period
- reviewed the structures of the male reproductive system and their significance for fertility and conception.

INTRODUCTION

An understanding of the anatomy of human reproduction enables the translation of abstract concepts of anatomy to the function and processes of conception, pregnancy, labour, birth, and postpartum and related disorders. It is envisaged that this chapter will form a foundation and reference point for application to midwifery practice, increasing the understanding of the physiological aspects of the birthing process. This approach brings together both theory and practice elements, enhancing knowledge, understanding and application to midwifery practice. This chapter includes sections on the female pelvis and the female and male reproductive systems.

A sound understanding of anatomy is essential for application to normal physiology and disease processes, and can be applied to support the midwife's role as a health promoter and practitioner. Greater understanding of the structure of the human body will increase the understanding of how it functions and why it sometimes deviates from the normal. The content of this chapter, and its supportive literature, links with other chapters and develops theory by specific examples of how anatomy and physiology may be applied to everyday practice.

THE PELVIS

The human pelvis supports the upper body and transmits its weight to the lower limbs enabling movement in an upright posture (Cruikshank and Hays, 1991). In the female, the pelvis serves as a protective bony ring encircling the reproductive organs, bladder and rectum. In pregnancy, physiological processes effect subtle changes in the composition (Sowers *et al.*, 1991), shape, plane of inclination and internal dimensions of the true pelvis. These changes enable the female skeleton to support the gravid uterus (Schneider and Deckardt, 1991) and are essential to the mechanisms involved in the process of childbirth.

The bony pelvis (Fig. 5.1)

The pelvis consists of four pelvic bones:

- two innominate
- one sacrum
- one coccyx.

Sacral foramina
Four pairs of foramina (or holes) are present in the sacrum, through which the four sacral nerves pass.

Ala
An ala projects laterally on each side of the sacral promontory and the superior surface of the first sacral vertebra. The alae extend to articulate with the ilium on both sides.
The anterior surfaces of the alae form part of the landmarks of the pelvic brim.

Acetabulum
A round cup-shaped socket on the external surface of the innominate bone with which the head of the femur articulates to form the hip joint. Two-fifths of the acetabulum is formed by the ilium, two-fifths by the ischium and one-fifth by the pubis.
Malformation, disease or injury of the hip joint can result in a reduction in abduction of the legs. This may result in hip and back pain in pregnancy, inability to abduct the hips during vaginal examination and delivery, and inability to adopt certain positions in labour such as the lithotomy or squatting position.

Symphysis pubis
A cartilaginous joint between the anterior portions of the two pubic bones. There is increased mobility and size in this cartilage during the last months of pregnancy.

Ischial tuberosity
The thickened portion of the body of the ischium providing attachment points for the sacrotuberous ligament. This is the section of the pelvis that takes the full weight of the body when sitting. Women with painful perineums can be advised to sit with their knees apart and the pelvis tilted, allowing the tuberosities to take the weight of the body, so the mother is sitting on a triangular-shaped base, relieving pressure in the perineum.
The distance between the tuberosities is estimated to be 10 cm. A reduction in this dimension may indicate a reduced pelvic outlet. Although this dimension is difficult to measure, a midwife may assess the distance by placing a closed fist on the perineum between the tuberosities. The knuckles of the fist should fit comfortably between the tuberosities in a normal gynaecoid pelvis.

Sacral promontory
The prominent upper margin of the first sacral vertebra.
The measurement between the sacral promontory and the anterior surface of the pubis is the anteroposterior diameter of the pelvic brim. A reduction in this diameter can influence the descent and engagement of the presenting part of the fetus into the pelvis.

Lumbar vertebra (5th)
Articulates with the first sacral vertebra. The position of the lumbar vertebrae influences the angle of pelvic inclination.

Ischial spine

Pubic arch
The arch created by the inferior rami of the pubes. The angle of the pubic arch is significant to the dimensions of the pelvic outlet. The optimal angle should be 90°, which is a feature of the gynaecoid pelvis.
Reduction in the pelvic outlet may result in obstructed labour, prolonged labour, persistent occipitoposterior positions and excessive fetal skull moulding.

Coccyx
A small triangular-shaped bone that articulates with the lower end of the sacrum. It is composed of four fused rudimentary vertebrae and provides attachment points for ligaments, muscle fibres of the anal sphincter and the ischiococcygeus muscle of the pelvic floor.
During the birth of the baby, the coccyx moves backwards to enlarge the pelvic outlet (see p. 69)

Ilium
Forms the upper expanded part of the innominate bone. It gives rise to the female shape of the hips.

Anterior superior iliac spine
A prominent anterior protrusion of the ilium that can be palpated through the lateral abdominal wall. The distance between the left and right anterior superior iliac spines does not necessarily indicate the capacity of the true pelvis.

Iliac crest
The curved upper border of the ilium. Women refer to this part of the pelvis as their hips.

Sacrum
Lies between the ilia, forming the rear of the pelvis. It consists of five fused vertebrae forming a wedge shape perforated by four sets of foramina through which the sacral nerves pass.
In a gynaecoid pelvis the sacrum's anterior surface is concave and a feature of the rounded cavity, allowing room for the fetal head to descend. It also plays a part in directing the baby through the pelvis around the curve of Carus (see Fig. 5.3).

Ischium
A thickened L-shaped bone that connects to the ilium posteriorly and to the pubis anteriorly. The medial surface has attachment points for the ischiococcygeus muscle of the pelvic floor.

Obturator foramen
A triangular hole created by the borders of the ischium and the pubis. It is covered by the obturator membrane, through which pass the obturator nerve and blood vessels leading to the thigh.

Pubis
Forms the anterior portion of the pelvis and has two arms called rami. The inferior ramus attaches to the ischium, and the superior ramus to the ilium at the iliopectineal eminence. It forms one-fifth of the acetabulum. The inferior ramus forms the boundary for the obturator foramen and the pubic arch, under which the baby must pass during birth.

Figure 5.1 The female pelvis. Anterior view of pelvis.

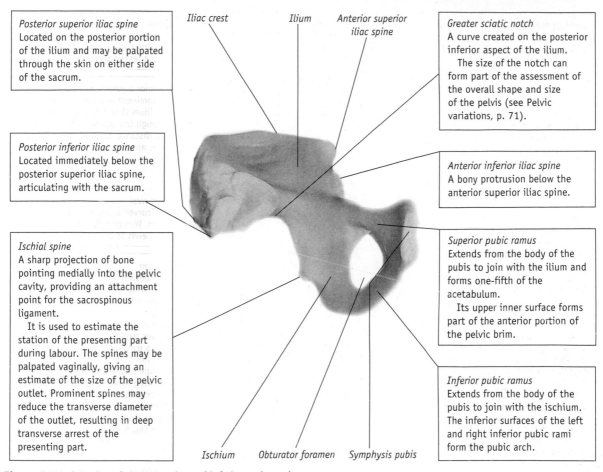

Posterior superior iliac spine
Located on the posterior portion of the ilium and may be palpated through the skin on either side of the sacrum.

Iliac crest   Ilium   Anterior superior iliac spine

Greater sciatic notch
A curve created on the posterior inferior aspect of the ilium.
   The size of the notch can form part of the assessment of the overall shape and size of the pelvis (see Pelvic variations, p. 71).

Posterior inferior iliac spine
Located immediately below the posterior superior iliac spine, articulating with the sacrum.

Anterior inferior iliac spine
A bony protrusion below the anterior superior iliac spine.

Ischial spine
A sharp projection of bone pointing medially into the pelvic cavity, providing an attachment point for the sacrospinous ligament.
   It is used to estimate the station of the presenting part during labour. The spines may be palpated vaginally, giving an estimate of the size of the pelvic outlet. Prominent spines may reduce the transverse diameter of the outlet, resulting in deep transverse arrest of the presenting part.

Superior pubic ramus
Extends from the body of the pubis to join with the ilium and forms one-fifth of the acetabulum.
   Its upper inner surface forms part of the anterior portion of the pelvic brim.

Inferior pubic ramus
Extends from the body of the pubis to join with the ischium. The inferior surfaces of the left and right inferior pubic rami form the pubic arch.

Ischium   Obturator foramen   Symphysis pubis

Figure 5.1 (*continued*) Inner surface of left innominate bone.

The innominate bones are each divided into three regions:

- ilium
- ischium
- pubis.

Joints and ligaments of the pelvis (Fig. 5.2)

The joints of the pelvis connect the innominate bones at the pubis anteriorly and to the sacrum posteriorly, and the sacrum to the coccyx. These joints are cartilaginous in type and in the pelvis consist of plates of fibrocartilage. The pelvis also provides attachment points for ligaments, which are bands of tissue connecting two structures (Guyton and Hall, 2000). In normal circumstances, ligaments do not possess the ability to stretch, and prevent excessive movements within the joints to enhance stability.

In pregnancy, joints and ligaments undergo temporary changes due to the hormones relaxin, progesterone and oestrogen, enabling some movement of the joints to facilitate birth (Miller and Hanretty, 1997). Pelvic pain can occur during pregnancy, birth or postpartum and is thought to be linked to overstretching of ligaments in the pelvis and lower spine (Mens *et al.*, 1996).

The true pelvis

The part of the pelvis significant in childbirth is known as the *true pelvis* through which the baby negotiates passage during labour and birth. This is divided into three regions known as the brim, cavity and outlet (see Fig. 5.3). It is worth considering that as the presenting part descends into the pelvis, the baby will be negotiating each aspect of the true pelvis simultaneously. For example, in a cephalic presentation, as the baby's head crowns, the presenting part negotiates

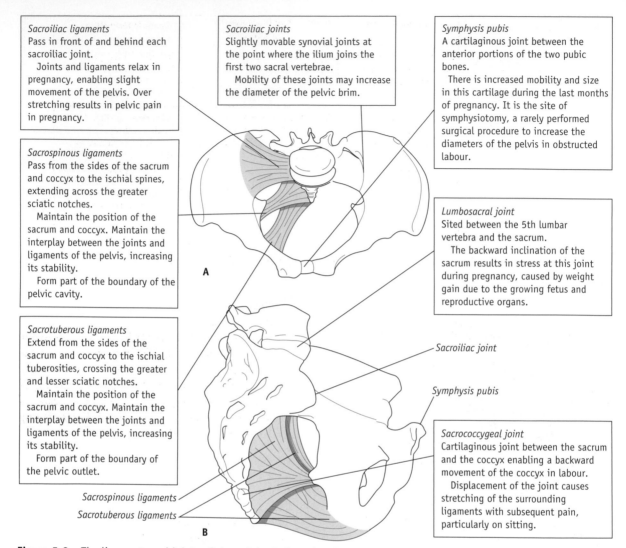

Sacroiliac ligaments
Pass in front of and behind each sacroiliac joint.
   Joints and ligaments relax in pregnancy, enabling slight movement of the pelvis. Over stretching results in pelvic pain in pregnancy.

Sacrospinous ligaments
Pass from the sides of the sacrum and coccyx to the ischial spines, extending across the greater sciatic notches.
   Maintain the position of the sacrum and coccyx. Maintain the interplay between the joints and ligaments of the pelvis, increasing its stability.
   Form part of the boundary of the pelvic cavity.

Sacrotuberous ligaments
Extend from the sides of the sacrum and coccyx to the ischial tuberosities, crossing the greater and lesser sciatic notches.
   Maintain the position of the sacrum and coccyx. Maintain the interplay between the joints and ligaments of the pelvis, increasing its stability.
   Form part of the boundary of the pelvic outlet.

Sacroiliac joints
Slightly movable synovial joints at the point where the ilium joins the first two sacral vertebrae.
   Mobility of these joints may increase the diameter of the pelvic brim.

Symphysis pubis
A cartilaginous joint between the anterior portions of the two pubic bones.
   There is increased mobility and size in this cartilage during the last months of pregnancy. It is the site of symphysiotomy, a rarely performed surgical procedure to increase the diameters of the pelvis in obstructed labour.

Lumbosacral joint
Sited between the 5th lumbar vertebra and the sacrum.
   The backward inclination of the sacrum results in stress at this joint during pregnancy, caused by weight gain due to the growing fetus and reproductive organs.

Sacroiliac joint

Symphysis pubis

Sacrococcygeal joint
Cartilaginous joint between the sacrum and the coccyx enabling a backward movement of the coccyx in labour.
   Displacement of the joint causes stretching of the surrounding ligaments with subsequent pain, particularly on sitting.

A

Sacrospinous ligaments
Sacrotuberous ligaments

B

Figure 5.2   The ligaments and joints of the pelvis. **A.** Superior view. **B.** Sagittal section.

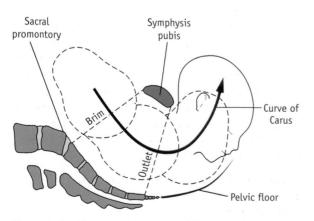

Figure 5.3   The axis of the true pelvis.

Sacral promontory
Symphysis pubis
Brim
Outlet
Curve of Carus
Pelvic floor

the outlet, most of the baby's head is in the cavity and the shoulders are at the brim.

   To assist your understanding of pelvic measurements you need to appreciate that the pelvis is three-dimensional. The pelvic measurements of the brim, cavity and outlet are abstract concepts viewed through a cross-section, whereas, measurements incorporated in the pelvic conjugates are viewed through a sagittal section. These two types of measurements inform a pelvic assessment.

Pelvic measurements (Fig. 5.4)

The pelvic brim

The landmarks of the pelvic brim are used to describe the interplay between the fetus and the pelvis as the

	Anteroposterior	Right and left oblique	Transverse
Brim	From upper inner border of the symphysis pubis To sacral promontory **11 cm**	From the sacroiliac joint To the iliopectineal eminence **12 cm**	Between widest points on the iliopectineal lines **13 cm**
Cavity	From inner border of the symphysis pubis To the curve of the sacrum **12 cm**	Right and left from the sacroiliac joint, fanning out to measure a point between the upper and lower pubic rami **12 cm**	From right inner surface of the ischium To left inner surface of the ischium **12 cm**
Outlet	From lower border of the symphysis pubis To sacrococcygeal joint **13 cm**	From the sacrospinous ligament To the obturator foramen **12 cm**	Transverse from the right to the left ischial spines **11 cm**

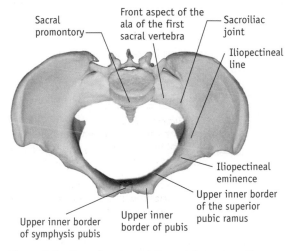

Other measurements: Sacrocotyloid diameter from sacral promontory to iliopectineal eminence – 9 cm

Figure 5.4 Pelvic measurements.

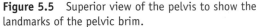

Figure 5.5 Superior view of the pelvis to show the landmarks of the pelvic brim.

presenting part descends. The landmarks are a fundamental part of the assessment of descent and engagement of the presenting part. It is not the components of the brim that are important, it is the part that the brim plays as a whole in the assessment of progress in pregnancy and labour. This is the first test that the fetus has to pass as it descends through the pelvis. The midwife assesses engagement of the presenting part during abdominal and vaginal examination (see Ch. 26).

The brim is the inlet to the true pelvis and is almost circular except posteriorly where the sacral promontory juts into the brim. The landmarks are shown in Figure 5.5.

The pelvic cavity

The cavity extends downwards from the brim to the outlet of the pelvis. In the anteroposterior view the cavity is wedge shaped; that is, shallow at the front and deep at the back. Viewed from above the cavity is circular in shape in the gynaecoid pelvis and designed to facilitate the descent and rotation of the presenting part. The boundaries of the cavity are:

1. curve of the sacrum
2. sacroiliac joints
3. sacrospinous ligaments
4. ischia
5. superior pubic ramus
6. inferior pubic ramus
7. bodies of the pubes
8. symphysis pubis.

The pelvic outlet

The outlet is diamond shaped and partly bound by ligaments. The pelvic outlet can be described in two ways: firstly, by anatomical structure and then by obstetric dimension, that is the space available through which the baby must pass during birth (see Fig. 5.6). The anatomical boundaries for the outlet of the pelvis are made up of the tip of the coccyx, the sacrotuberous ligaments, ischial tuberosities and the pubic arch. The obstetric outlet is bounded by:

1. the inner border of the base of the sacrum
2. sacrospinous ligaments
3. ischial spines
4. the lower inner border of the symphysis pubis.

Pelvic conjugates

A conjugate is a measurement taken from one point in the pelvis to another. In midwifery there are three measurements or conjugates, the anatomical, obstetrical and the internal or diagonal (Fig. 5.6). The *anatomical conjugate* is measured from the upper outer border of the symphysis pubis, measuring across the pubic bone, which adds approximately 1.25 cm to the overall measurement. This includes space not available to the baby as it enters the pelvic brim. Instead, it negotiates the smaller dimension called the *obstetric conjugate* extending from the sacral promontory to the upper inner border of the symphysis pubis.

The *internal* or *diagonal conjugate* can be estimated at vaginal examination as part of a pelvic assessment, measuring from the posterior inferior surface of the

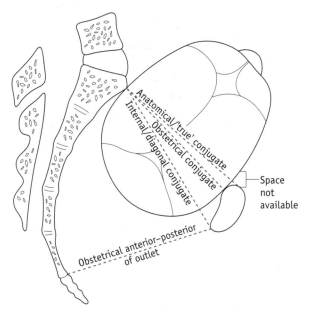

Figure 5.6   The relationship of the pelvic conjugates and the fetal negotiation of the conjugates.

symphysis pubis to the sacral promontory. This measurement varies in individual women. It is unusual to identify the sacral promontory on vaginal examination as the conjugate measures between 12–13 cm, longer than the length of most practitioner's fingers. If detected, it could indicate that the diameters of the pelvis are reduced and referral for obstetric consultation should be sought.

Angles and planes

Angles and planes are mathematical concepts applied to the pelvis. When a woman stands, the pelvis slopes into the position where the pubis is lower than the sacral promontory. This is described as an angle of 55° to the horizontal or the floor. This slope continues through the cavity reducing its angle to 15° at the outlet. The fetal head must negotiate the curve created by the changing angles within the pelvis as it enters the pelvic brim in a downward and backward direction. It emerges from the outlet in a downward and forward direction as the presenting part reaches the pelvic floor. The curve created in the pelvis is sometimes known as the *curve of Carus*.

The term *plane* is applied to the pelvis to describe its relationship to a flat surface, such as the floor. This increases the understanding of the tilt of the pelvis in a normal female skeleton. The angles are then created in relation to the degree of tilt of a particular individual and are thus hypothetical (see Figs 5.7 and 5.8). These figures show a representation of the angles in relation to the planes of the pelvis. Figure 5.8 shows the axis, or curve of Carus, an imaginary line through which the fetus rotates as it passes through the pelvis. In an abnormal pelvis the plane of the pelvis could be significantly altered and affect the axis of the birth canal and consequently the normal direction of the fetus through the pelvis. It is worth considering the axis of the birth canal when women adopt alternative positions for childbirth during labour and delivery.

1. *Sacral angle.* The angle between the plane of the brim and the anterior surface of the first sacral vertebra (Fig. 5.7). This usually measures 90° giving some indication of the size of the cavity in relation to the brim: a measurement of less than 90° suggests that the cavity is smaller than the brim; if more than 90° the cavity is larger than the brim.
2. *Angle of inclination of the pelvic brim.* The angle that the plane achieves with the horizontal when a woman is standing (Fig. 5.7) is approximately 55°. If greater than 55° there may be delay in engagement of the presenting part in the pelvis.

3. *Angle of inclination of the pelvic outlet.* This is the 15° angle the upper inner border of the obstetric outlet makes with the horizontal when the woman is in a standing position (Fig. 5.7).

Subpubic angle The angle between the two inferior pubic rami which form the pubic arch (Fig. 5.1 and Box 5.1). In a gynaecoid pelvis this should be approximately 90°, enabling two finger widths to sit in the apex of the pubic arch during vaginal pelvic assessment.

> **Reflective Activity 5.2**
>
> Rotate Figure 5.2 to represent the woman in a variety of positions, i.e. standing, 'all fours' and squatting. Note the direction of the presenting part of the fetus during descent in all positions. What is the impact of these positions on labour?

Pelvic variations

Although there are four recognized pelvic categories as identified by Caldwell *et al.* (1940) (Fig. 5.9), variations within these categories can occur (Abitbol, 1996). Some women may have mixed features, such as a gynaecoid posterior pelvis and android forepelvis. The most important factor is the true pelvic space available for the fetus to descend and emerge from the pelvis. The pelvic size and shape cannot be viewed in isolation from other factors such as position and size of fetus and the

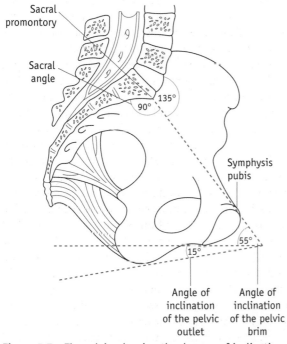

Figure 5.7 The pelvis, showing the degrees of inclination: inclination of the pelvic brim to the horizontal, 55°; inclination of pelvic outlet to the horizontal, 15°; angle of pelvic inclination, 135°; inclination of the sacrum, 90°.

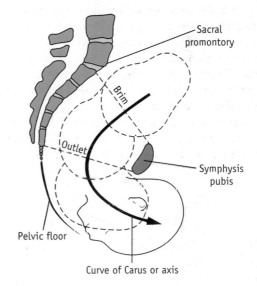

Figure 5.8 The axis of the birth canal in upright position.

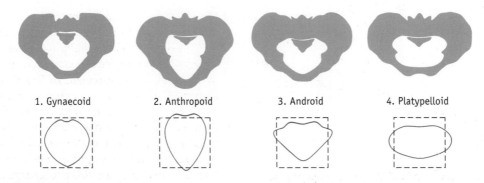

1. Gynaecoid   2. Anthropoid   3. Android   4. Platypelloid

Figure 5.9 Shapes of the pelvic brim.

Table 5.1 Pelvic categories

Characteristics	Gynaecoid/female type	Justo minor pelvis	Android/male type	Anthropoid	Platypelloid
Shape of brim	Round	Round – but small	Triangular – 'heart shaped'	Oval (widest in the anteroposterior diameter)	Bean shaped – flattened
Depth of pelvis	Shallow – straight walls	Shallow	Deep – convergent walls	Deep – straight	Shallow – divergent walls
Subpubic arch	85–90°	90°	60–75° (narrow)	More than 90°	More than 90°
Sciatic notch	Wide	Wide – but small	Narrow	Wide	Narrow
Ischial spines	Not prominent, blunt	Not prominent	Prominent and narrow interspinous diameter	Not prominent but may have narrowed interspinous diameter	Blunted, usually widely separated – not prominent
Sacrum	Deep + curved	Curved	Straight – flattened and long	Long and narrow – may be slightly curved	Broad, flat and concave
Transverse diameter of outlet	10 cm	Usually less than 10 cm May be android characteristics present which may reduced outlet	Less than 10 cm	More than 10 cm	More than 10 cm
Implications for midwifery	The gynaecoid pelvis offers the most favourable design for positive outcomes of childbirth Incidence 50%	Gynaecoid pelvis – but in miniature Outcomes depend on relationship between degree of size of pelvis and size of fetus	The fetal head may attempt to engage in the occipitoposterior position. Deep transverse arrest may result Excessive moulding and caput of fetal skull Incidence 20%	Women with this type of pelvis are said to be tall and 'well-built'. The pelvis is large and should accommodate the fetus as it descends during labour. The diameters may result in persistent occipitoposterior position leading to a face-to-pubes delivery Incidence 25%	The fetal head engages in the transverse diameter This shape of pelvis may require the fetal head to negotiate the brim using a movement called asynclitism. This movement occurs where the baby's head tilts in one direction and then the other to enable the biparietal diameter of the fetal skull to engage in the pelvic brim and for descent to occur (see Fig. 5.10). Deep transverse arrest may result, as the fetal head may be unable to rotate in the pelvic cavity Incidence less than 5%

processes of labour. Other factors that may influence the size and shape of the pelvis include injury (Olson and Pollack, 1996) and disease (Phillips *et al.*, 2000). Dietary deficiencies in young women can also have a direct influence on the growth and shape of the pelvis (Carruth and Skinner, 2000; Gallo, 1996) and therefore affect the outcome at birth; the outcome can also be affected for women who suffer pelvic fractures (Pals *et al.*, 1992).

Table 5.1 outlines the recognized characteristics of the four most common pelvic categories.

Other pelvic types identified

Any injury or disease of the pelvic bones may significantly affect the dimensions of the pelvis and subsequently impact on the outcome of labour and birth. Table 5.2 outlines the characteristics of some of the classified unusual pelves. These types may have a mixture of characteristics, as the shape will depend on the degree and timing of damage. It is important, as early as the booking visit, that the midwife consider which women may be at risk of having a damaged pelvis.

Pelvic assessment

The function of a pelvic assessment is to estimate whether the fetus will successfully pass through the pelvis during labour and delivery. The aim of this examination is to assess the pelvic size and outlet. Although this can be undertaken at any time before or during pregnancy, the relationship of the pelvis to the fetal skull can only be assessed from 37 weeks' gestation, either antenatally or during labour. The view as to whether these assessments have value has varied through time and between practitioners; however, the concepts should be understood so they may be applied to diagnostic skills and decision-making processes. Pelvic assessment is no determinant of outcome but acts as a component of an overall assessment of pelvic adequacy.

The assessment should include:

- abdominal examination to assess engagement and descent of the presenting part (Knight *et al.*, 1993)
- vaginal examination to determine the size and shape of the pelvis by assessing the following:
  - the prominence of the sacral promontory, which usually cannot be palpated on vaginal examination
  - the prominence of the ischial spines and, if identified, the distance between them
  - the angle of the pubic arch, which usually accommodates two finger widths at the apex of the arch
  - the prominence of the ischial tuberosities, which usually accommodate four knuckle widths when measured externally at the level of the perineum

It may also include:

- X-ray examination
- ultrasound scans (Gimovsky *et al.*, 1994; Thomas *et al.*, 1998)
- magnetic resonance imaging (Sporri *et al.*, 1997).

Although these activities are fundamental to diagnostic skills it is important to include a range of other factors that may enable a complete assessment to be made of the overall capacity of the true pelvis:

- assessment of the normality of the woman's gait
- height of the woman (Frame *et al.*, 1985)
- shoe size less than a 4
- previous successful vaginal delivery
- non-engagement of the fetal head at 38 weeks in primigravid women
- history of rickets or previous pelvic injury
- previous trial of labour or prolonged labour
- malpresentation such as a breech
- the extent of caput or moulding of the fetal skull present during labour.

Reflective Activity 5.3

When you are next examining a woman after the 37th week of pregnancy, consider how you assess her pelvic capacity.

Think about how you carry out a vaginal examination during labour, and its relationship to abdominal examination.

Do you carry out the following assessments:

- diagonal conjugate?
- width of pubic arch and ischial spines?
- descent and position of presenting part?
- width of sciatic notch?
- width of the ischial tuberosities?

Having considered this, construct a plan to enable you to undertake a detailed assessment of the pelvis to enable you to detect and diagnose the potential for vaginal delivery. It is understood that in clinical practice the opportunity to undertake such an assessment may only occur when a woman presents in early labour, and that it should only be conducted with her consent.

Midwifery assessment of pelvic capacity will include abdominal and vaginal assessment and may not include pelvimetry (by X-ray or ultrasound) findings. You should therefore, use this opportunity to develop your diagnostic skills.

Table 5.2 Classified unusual pelves

Characteristics	Rachitic pelvis	Asymmetrical pelvis (Naegele's type)	Robert's pelvis	Osteomalacic pelvis	Spondylolisthetic pelvis
Shape of brim	Bean shaped. Reduced anteroposterior diameter	Asymmetrical – may be absence of one sacral ala	Inlet narrow and significantly contracted	Usually grossly altered	
Depth of pelvis	Flattened	May be normal		Convergent walls	
Ischial spines		One may be prominent	Likely to be reduced interspinous diameter		
Sacrum	Lower end swings back to increase size of cavity. May be bent at the middle				May be altered – usually drastically contracted
Transverse diameter of outlet	Increased in size	May be altered	May be altered	Reduced. Bituberous diameter is less than 8 cm	
Causes	This shape may result following childhood rickets. The soft bones are distorted by the body weight. Can be caused by inadequate diet and vitamin D deficiency	Deficient development of one side of the pelvis often with bony fusion of the sacroiliac joint on the affected side, sometimes known as Naegele's pelvis. May be caused by congenital dislocation of one hip, poliomyelitis or an accident	Deficient development on both sides of the pelvis with fusion of the sacroiliac joints. A rare form of extreme pelvic contraction	A severe pelvis deformity occurring in adults as a result of vitamin D deficiency. The distortion occurring is different from that of childhood rickets as the condition occurs while walking and standing. Upward pressure on the legs and pelvis forces the sides of the pelvis inwards and the weight of the body on the spine forces the sacral promontory forwards	The fifth lumbar vertebra slips forward over the sacrum. The sacral promontory is pushed backwards and the tip of sacrum pushed forward
Implications for midwifery	This pelvic deformity may lead to obstructed labour. Fetal head may be deflexed, and usually enters the pelvis with the sagittal suture in transverse. Head – asynclitism can occur	Pelvic contraction and distortion may result in a reduced incidence of vaginal delivery	Pelvic contraction and distortion may result in a reduced incidence of vaginal delivery	In parts of the world where osteomalacia is endemic a woman may develop the condition between pregnancies, resulting in a normal vaginal delivery followed by a complicated labour or delivery.	Results in an extreme contraction of the true conjugate

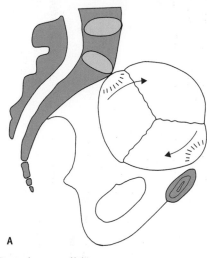
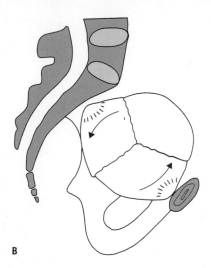

A

B

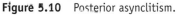

Figure 5.10 Posterior asynclitism.

FEMALE REPRODUCTIVE ANATOMY

The primary function of the female reproductive system is the production and transmission of ova and provision of a nurturing environment for the fertilized ovum and developing fetus. It has the ability to grow to accommodate the developing fetus and to expel the baby and placenta at birth, returning to its near pre-pregnant state during the puerperium. The study of the female reproductive system is fundamental to the midwife's understanding of gynaecology, pregnancy, birth and the impact birth has on the female reproductive anatomy. The structures identified with the female reproductive system include the external genitalia and the internal genitalia – the uterus, fallopian tubes and the ovaries. The female reproductive system can also be studied in relation to other organs and structures within the pelvis (Table 5.3), particularly the bladder, urethra and rectum. In addition, uterine muscular support, blood supply, nerve supply and lymphatics are identified. It is understood that the study of the pelvic floor muscles is fundamental to the understanding of the female reproductive system and they should be reviewed in conjunction with this section (see Ch. 28).

Fetal development

During the first 6 weeks following fertilization male and female gonads undergo identical forms of development. In the female fetus the ovaries descend a short distance from their position below the kidneys to sit in the pelvic cavity in close association with the fallopian tubes

Table 5.3 Anatomical relations to the vagina

View	Section of the vagina	Associated structures
Anteriorly	Upper half Lower half	Bladder Urethra
Posteriorly	Upper third Middle third Lower third	Pouch of Douglas Rectum Perineal body
Superiorly	Centrally Above lateral	Cervix Fornices Ureters and uterine arteries
Inferiorly	Vaginal orifices and vestibule	
Laterally	Upper Middle Lower	Parametrium Pubococcygeous muscles Perineal muscle Bulbocavernosus muscles

(Johnson and Everitt, 1999). Their primary function of ovum production commences under the influence of female hormones during puberty (see Ch. 6).

External genitalia

Knowledge of the anatomy of the female external genitalia (Fig. 5.11 and Box 5.1) provides a foundation for application to midwifery practice during the process of labour and birth, in relation to labial tears, perineal tears, episiotomy, tears to the urethral meatus or

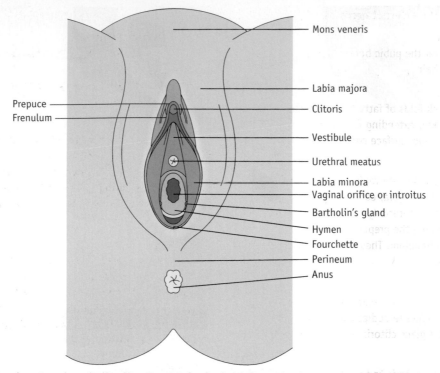

Mons veneris

Prepuce

Frenulum

Labia majora

Clitoris

Vestibule

Urethral meatus

Labia minora

Vaginal orifice or introitus

Bartholin's gland

Hymen

Fourchette

Perineum

Anus

Figure 5.11   Female external genitalia. (See Box 5.1 for further information.)

clitoris, fistulae and female circumcision (Cameron and Rawlings-Anderson, 2000).

Any of the following structures may be damaged during the birthing process and should be assessed following birth so the midwife can implement appropriate care:

- labia majora
- labia minora
- clitoris
- vestibule
- urethral meatus
- vaginal orifice
- Bartholin's glands.

Blood supply   Blood is supplied via the pudendal arteries and drainage is through corresponding veins. The external genitalia is a vascular structure that facilitates healing but which bleeds heavily when traumatized.

Lymphatic drainage   This is mainly via the inguinal glands.

Nerve supply   This is from branches of the pudendal nerve.

Reflective Activity 5.4

To facilitate your understanding of the female external genitalia, take an appropriate supervised opportunity to undertake or observe a bladder catheterization of a pregnant woman who is not in labour, such as prior to an elective caesarean section. Consider the following points:

- the appearance of the external genitalia in relation to health
- the position of the urethral meatus relative to the vaginal orifice
- the policy and practice of asepsis in relation to the technique
- the technique of catheterization
- the care and maintenance of a catheter in situ.

Internal genitalia

Knowledge of female internal reproductive anatomy (Fig. 5.12) provides a foundation on which to base an understanding of pregnancy, birth and postpartum processes. These processes include growth and development of the uterus in pregnancy (Ch. 17), uterine

---

Box 5.1 Female external genitalia

Mons veneris
A pad of fat over the pubic bone covered by skin and, after puberty, hair.

Labia majora
One of two thick folds of fatty tissue (labia majora) covered with skin, extending from the mons to the perineum. The inner surface contains sebaceous glands.

Labia minora
One of two small, smooth folds of skin (labia minora) between the labia majora, containing sweat and sebaceous glands. Anteriorly the labia minora encircle the clitoris forming the prepuce and a smaller, lower fold called the frenulum. They meet posteriorly to form the fourchette.

Clitoris
Highly sensitive erectile tissue about 2.5 cm long. Consists of two erectile bodies called the corpora cavernosa and a glans clitoris of spongy erectile tissue.

Vestibule
Extends from the clitoris to the fourchette and contains the urethral and the vaginal orifices. Contains the vestibular glands known as Skene's and Bartholin's glands.

Urethral meatus
Situated between the clitoris anteriorly and the vaginal orifice posteriorly and is the external opening of the urethra, connecting superiorly to the bladder.

Location of this structure enables the midwife to accurately undertake female catheterization, although it can be difficult to identify in women during labour and postnatally, as the structures may become distorted.

Vaginal orifice or introitus
Located posteriorly to the urethral meatus, opening into the vagina above.

Has the ability to stretch to accommodate the emerging baby at birth.

Hymen
A thin membrane partially occluding the vaginal introitus that is easily ruptured with the use of internal tampons, physical exercise and intercourse. Further rupture occurs during vaginal delivery, resulting in the remaining tissue forming tags called carunculae myrtiformes.

Bartholin's glands
The ducts of the glands emerge on either side of the vaginal orifice on the inner surface of the labia minora. They secret mucus to lubricate the vulva, and production increases during sexual arousal. They should not be palpable during vaginal examination unless obstructed or infected.

Fourchette
Created as the labia minora join posteriorly to the vaginal orifice.

It is a distinct landmark that should be identified for correct perineal alignment during perineal suturing.

Perineum
Extends from the fourchette to the anal margin, covering the pelvic floor muscles.

Prepuce
A loose fold of skin covering the clitoris.

Frenulum
A small ligament maintaining the position of the clitoris.

---

function in labour, birth and delivery of the placenta (Ch. 25), function of the muscle structures of the uterus in haemostasis and postpartum haemorrhage (see Ch. 30), involution of the uterus and return of the anatomical structures to the pre-pregnant state (see Ch. 41; Cluett *et al.*, 1997), influence of breastfeeding on involution (see Ch. 33), and infection. It is also applicable to the study of gynaecological conditions such as infection (Bartholin's abscess, postpartum infection), infertility and fertility (see Ch. 9; Forti and Krausz, 1998; Chia *et al.*, 2000), fibroids, ectopic pregnancy, uterine prolapse, carcinoma, ovarian cysts, and cervical screening.

Vagina

Description   The vagina is a fibromuscular tube directed upward and backward approximately parallel to the pelvic brim. The angle of the vagina is important to note when conducting vaginal procedures, such as vaginal examination and teaching women the correct insertion of pessaries, tampons and contraceptive diaphragms.

The vagina extends from the vulva to the cervix; the anterior wall is approximately 7.5 cm long and the posterior wall 10 cm. The walls of the vagina lie in apposition until it widens at the upper portion where

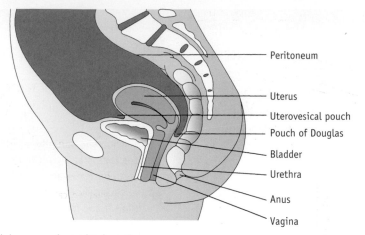

Peritoneum
Uterus
Uterovesical pouch
Pouch of Douglas
Bladder
Urethra
Anus
Vagina

Figure 5.12 Female pelvic organs in sagittal section.

the cervix projects into the vagina approximately at right angles, forming four recesses called fornices. The anterior fornix is shallow, the lateral fornices are deeper and the posterior fornix is deep. The deep posterior fornix facilitates pooling of semen during intercourse, increasing the opportunities for sperm to swim through the cervix.

There are no glands in the vagina but it remains moist because of secretions from the cervical glands and transudation of serous fluid from blood vessels. Vaginal secretions are acid and provide an unfavourable environment for spermatozoa. This is counteracted by the alkaline reaction of semen and cervical mucus. The pH of the vagina is 4.5 because it contains lactic acid produced by the action of lactobacilli (Döderlein's bacilli) on glycogen in the squamous cells of the vaginal lining. Lactobacilli normally inhabit the vagina and do not give rise to pathology. The lactic acid they produce helps to destroy pathogenic bacteria that may enter the vagina. The vagina in prepubescent girls and post-menopausal women is less acid at pH 7, which creates a favourable environment for the growth of vaginal infections, such as *Candida albicans*.

Structure The walls of the vagina have four layers:

- An interior layer composed of squamous epithelium arranged in transverse folds called rugae. This facilitates stretching of the vagina during child-birth.
- A vascular layer of elastic connective tissue.
- An involuntary muscle layer with outer longitudinal fibres and inner circular fibres.
- An outer layer of connective tissue that is part of the pelvic fascia and contains blood vessels, lymphatics and nerves.

Following childbirth the vaginal walls should be examined for damage, and assessment made to establish a plan of care.

Function The vagina is able to distend to facilitate the passage of the penis during intercourse, and the baby during childbirth.

Blood supply This is by the middle haemorrhoidal arteries, which arise from a branch of the internal iliac arteries; drainage is by the corresponding veins.

Nerve supply The vagina is supplied by sympathetic and parasympathetic nerves from the plexus of Lee–Frankenhäuser (situated in the floor of the pouch of Douglas in the region of the uterosacral ligaments) which originate from branches of the second, third and fourth sacral nerves.

Lymphatic drainage The lower third of the vagina drains into the inguinal glands and the upper two-thirds into the internal iliac glands.

Uterus

Description The uterus is a muscular, vascular, pelvic organ, often described as shaped like an upturned pear. It is situated with the bladder anteriorly and the rectum posteriorly and normally sits in a position of anteversion (i.e. leaning forward towards the bladder) and anteflexion (i.e. curved forward on itself).

The uterus is divided into the body and the cervix. The narrow end of the uterus is inserted into the vagina and the upper body communicates with the fallopian tubes at the upper lateral surfaces (Fig. 5.13 and Box 5.2).

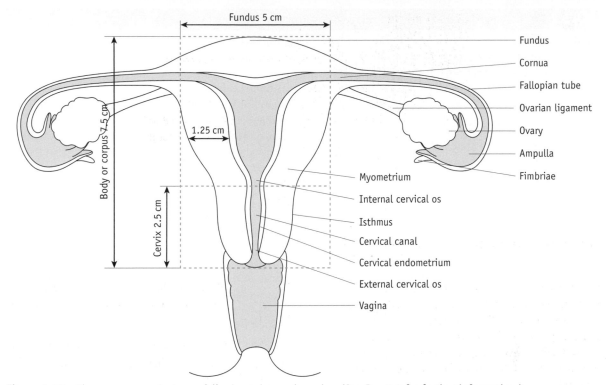

Figure 5.13   The non-pregnant uterus, fallopian tubes and ovaries. (See Box 5.2 for further information.)

Structure

Endometrium   This is the lining of the uterus and is constantly changing throughout a woman's reproductive life. It has the ability to shed during the menstrual cycle and to be maintained and thickened during pregnancy.

The endometrium is composed of vascular connective tissue, called stroma, containing tubular glands. The stroma is covered by a layer of ciliated columnar epithelium and where the stroma dips to the level of the myometrium it is covered with non-ciliated cells.

Myometrium   This is made up of plain muscle fibre and constitutes seven-eighths of the thickness of the uterine wall. In the non-pregnant state the muscle layers are not clearly defined. In pregnancy they become thicker and more defined as three layers of muscle (Fig. 5.14):

- inner circular
- middle oblique or spiral
- outer longitudinal.

The inner circular fibres are found mainly in the cornua and around the cervix, assisting cervical dilatation during labour. The middle oblique or spiral layers are thickest in the upper body of the uterus where the placenta is normally situated. These fibres contract powerfully to act as natural ligatures to blood vessels when the placenta separates from the uterine wall during the third stage of labour. The outer longitudinal fibres extend from the cervix anteriorly over the uterus to the cervix posteriorly. These fibres shorten in labour when the uterus contracts and retracts, facilitating descent and expulsion of the fetus, placenta and membranes.

Perimetrium   The perimetrium is a layer of peritoneum draped over the uterus and fallopian tubes. It is continuous with the peritoneum which covers the bladder and extends to the lateral walls of the pelvis (see Fig. 5.12). A fold in the peritoneum between the bladder and the uterus forms the uterovesical pouch, and a fold between the uterus and the rectum forms the pouch of Douglas. The latter is a recognized site for infection if the membrane is breached during surgery or trauma.

Functions   The uterus:

- provides an environment conducive to the implantation of a fertilized ovum
- is able to nurture the developing fetus
- has the ability to grow and expand to accommodate the growing fetus and placenta

Box 5.2 **The non-pregnant uterus, fallopian tubes and ovaries (see Fig. 5.13)**

Body or corpus

This includes the upper two-thirds of the uterus. The cavity of the body is triangular in shape. The structure is made up of the fundus, cornua (singular cornu) and the isthmus.

Cervix

The lowest third of the uterus. It is cylindrical in shape with its lower half projecting into the vagina at right angles.

Internal cervical os

Situated at the top of the cervical canal, its walls are in close apposition in the newly parous woman. It dilates and thins, becoming part of the lower uterine segment during the first stage of labour.

External cervical os

Situated at the bottom of the cervical canal, its walls are in close apposition in the pre-pregnant state, remaining partially dilated in parous women.

Examination of the external os forms part of the assessment of progress during labour.

Cervical endometrium or arbor vitae

The cervical endometrium is arranged in deep folds to facilitate the passage of spermatozoa through the cervical canal. The upper two-thirds is made up of columnar epithelium containing compound racemose glands secreting alkaline mucus. The cervical mucus is thin at the time of ovulation to facilitate the passage of spermatozoa. At other times it is thick in consistency, acting as a plug that assists in the prevention of infection of the uterus. The lower third is composed of stratified squamous epithelium continuous with that of the vagina.

Fundus

The upper rounded part of the body of the uterus above the insertion of the two fallopian tubes. It may be palpated:

- Antenatally:
  - to assess the growth of the fetus in relation to weeks of gestation
  - to determine the lie and presentation of the fetus
- In labour:
  - to assess uterine contractions
  - to assess contractility of the uterus following expulsion of the placenta and membranes as an assessment of potential homeostasis

- Postnatally:
  - to determine involution.

Fallopian tubes

Two tubes extending laterally from the uterus and opening into the peritoneal cavity. Each tube is approximately 10 cm long and 1 cm in diameter varying along its length. Hairs on the inner surface guide the ova towards the uterine cavity.

Scarring or obstruction caused by infection or trauma may lead to ectopic pregnancy and infertility. Tubes may be surgically ligated for sterilization purposes.

Cornu

Formed at the junction of the uterine body and the fallopian tube.

Ovarian ligament

This ligament suspends the ovary in a position close to the fimbriae of the fallopian tube to increase the probability of the ovum entering the fallopian tube.

Ovary

The female gonad that produces predetermined cells destined to become ova. Ovaries are endocrine organs producing oestrogen and progesterone and small amounts of the male hormone, androgen.

Fimbriae

Finger-like projections on the end of the fallopian tube that help to waft the ovum from the ovary to the fallopian tube.

Ampulla

Dilated distal portion of the fallopian tube where fertilization of the ovum usually occurs.

Isthmus

The junction between the body of the uterus and the cervix. During pregnancy there is growth and development of this junction, creating the lower uterine segment.

Cervical canal

This is a potential tube connecting the external os and the internal os. A plug of mucus (the operculum) forms here during pregnancy and is expelled when cervical activity and dilatation commence.

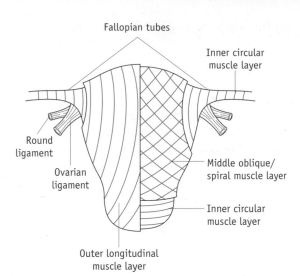

Figure 5.14   The three layers of uterine muscle.

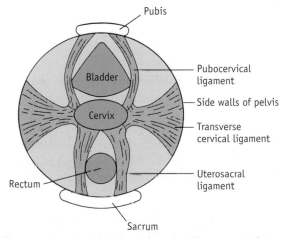

Figure 5.15   Superior view of uterine ligaments and supports.

- is able to contract, retract and expel the fetus, placenta and membranes during birth and maintain haemostasis following birth
- has the ability to return by involution to the near pre-pregnant state.

Uterine ligaments   The ligaments maintain the normal position of the uterus, which is one of anteversion and anteflexion. Damage to these ligaments may occur as a direct result of childbirth, especially prolonged labour, in chronic constipation and straining, poor lifting techniques, poor posture and obesity. The effect may not be seen until later in life at the menopause where declining levels of oestrogen cause muscle and ligament atrophy and loss of function. The result of this

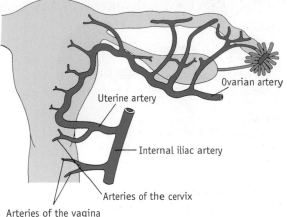

Figure 5.16   Blood supply to the uterus and its appendages.

may be uterine prolapse and associated stress incontinence and defecation difficulties (Mason *et al.*, 1999).

The uterine ligaments (Fig. 5.15) are:

- *Transverse cervical ligaments* (2): extend from the cervix laterally to the side walls of the pelvis; overstretching may cause uterine prolapse.
- *Uterosacral ligaments* (2): pass back from the cervix to the sacrum encircling the rectum, maintaining the position of anteversion.
- *Pubocervical ligaments* (2): pass forwards from the cervix to the pubic bones offering limited support to the uterus.
- *Round ligaments* (2): arise at the cornua of the uterus descending through the broad ligament and the inguinal canals to the labia majora. They help to maintain the uterus in a position of anteversion.
- *Broad ligament*: a double fold of peritoneum extending from the lateral borders of the uterus to the side walls of the pelvis.

Blood supply   Blood is supplied to the uterus via the uterine and ovarian arteries and drained by the corresponding veins (Figs 5.16 and 5.17). The uterus has a rich supply of blood vessels to facilitate the growth of the uterus and placenta during pregnancy and to support the growth and development of the fetus. The blood vessels to the uterus are twisted in the non-pregnant state, and during pregnancy they have the ability to uncoil as the uterus expands. It is important for the midwife to appreciate that this rich blood supply can give rise to massive haemorrhage if the circulatory system does not remain intact. Breaches of this system can occur during pregnancy and labour and where the normal physiology of the third stage of labour does

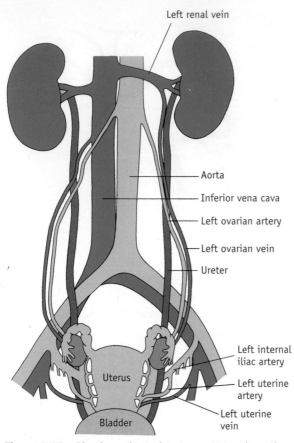

Figure 5.17   Blood supply to the uterus. Note where the ovarian vein terminates.

not take place. In addition, trauma to the genital tract may also give rise to severe haemorrhage. These events increase the incidence of mortality and morbidity for both mother and baby (DoH, 1998; Lewis, 2001; MCHRC 2000, 2001).

Uterine arteries and veins   The uterine artery arises from a branch of the internal iliac artery. It enters the uterus at the level of the internal cervical os, and then turns at right angles following a spiral course along the lateral border of the uterus, joining with the ovarian artery. It sends a branch to the cervix and vagina. The uterine veins follow the arteries and drain into the corresponding internal iliac veins.

Ovarian arteries and veins   The ovarian arteries arise from the descending aorta and cross the urethra and internal iliac arteries before passing over the pelvic brim to enter the broad ligament just below the ovary. Branches of the ovarian artery supply the fallopian tubes and connect with the uterine artery. The right

ovarian vein connects with the inferior vena cava and the left ovarian vein connects with the left renal vein.

Nerve supply   The nerve supply is both sympathetic and parasympathetic. The sympathetic nervous system to the pelvis is a continuation of the aortic plexus and is sometimes called the presacral nerve. It lies in front of the fifth lumbar vertebra and the sacral promontory. It passes downwards, joining branches of the lumbar sympathetic chain lying on the floor of the Pouch of Douglas. The parasympathetic nerve supply emerges from the sacral foramina to join the Lee–Frankenhäuser plexus. The nerves then pass to the uterus and other pelvic viscera (Waugh and Grant, 2001).

Lymphatic drainage   The lymphatic vessels and nodes drain lymph away from the pelvic organs. These vessels accompany the main arteries and veins, with nodes sited along the iliac vessels and the aorta. Drainage from the upper portion of the uterus is to the lumbar and hypogastric nodes, and drainage from the lower portion is to the hypogastric nodes.

Cervix   In women who have never been pregnant the cervix can be palpated as a firm structure similar in consistency to the tip of the nose and the cervical os is closed, whereas in a multigravid woman who is not pregnant the cervical os may remain partially dilated.

During pregnancy the cervix may appear to be blue owing to the abundant blood supply, and towards the end of pregnancy it becomes softer as it 'ripens' in preparation for labour.

Squamocolumnar junction   Carcinoma of the cervix is most likely to occur at the junction between the upper columnar epithelium and the lower stratified squamous epithelium.

Reflective Activity 5.5

Identify your local policy and procedure for undertaking cervical smears, and compare this to the current available literature.

Consider the information about the anatomy of the cervix, and how the midwife can use this in the preparation and collection of a cervical smear. You may find it useful to make notes on the instruments and techniques used throughout this procedure, and seek opportunities to discuss this procedure with a family planning practitioner at your local family planning clinic.

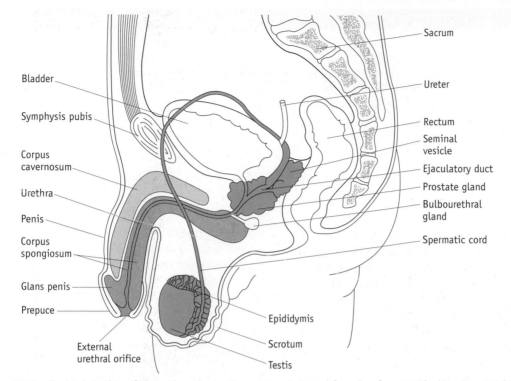

Figure 5.18 Sagittal section of the male reproductive system (adapted from Brooker, 1993). (See Box 5.3 for further information.)

MALE REPRODUCTIVE ANATOMY (FIG. 5.18 AND BOX 5.3; FIG. 5.19 AND BOX 5.4)

The function of the male reproductive system is the production of spermatozoa and their transfer to the female during sexual intercourse. The purpose of this process is the creation of new human life. It could be argued that once successful fertilization of the ovum has occurred the need for knowledge of the male reproductive system is of little importance to the midwife. However, there are a number of issues that could be considered, such as sexual intercourse in pregnancy (Oruc *et al.*, 1999), the transmission of sexually transmitted diseases (see Ch. 47) and an understanding of some of the causes of infertility (see Ch. 9).

Fetal development

As has been stated earlier, male and female gonads undergo identical forms of development during the first 6 weeks after fertilization. In the fetus the male testes are located in the abdomen just below the kidneys, in a similar position to that of the female ovary. Following this phase of organ development, the gonads form distinct structures under genetic and hormonal influences (Johnson and Everitt, 1999). In the seventh or eighth month of pregnancy the male testes descend with the spermatic cord through the right and left inguinal canals and at birth should be located in the scrotum of the term infant (Snell, 2000).

> **Reflective Activity 5.6**
>
> Seek opportunities to attend local clinics, such as genitourinary medicine, infertility and 'wellmen', to seek out health promotion information for men.
>
> Access your local policies and procedures for male health and infertility and relate them to your public health role as a midwife.

IMPLICATIONS FOR MIDWIFERY

The midwife's knowledge of anatomy of human reproduction can help identify women who might require different care, treatment and advice. In this way, the midwife can work in partnership with the woman to plan the most appropriate care for her pregnancy,

Box 5.3 The male reproductive system

Symphysis pubis
Located at the central anterior portion of the pelvis. A useful landmark when identifying other structures and positions of the male reproductive system.

Urethra
The urethra commences superiorly at the opening of the bladder, travels the length of the penis and opens onto the surface within the glans penis. The tube has the capacity to transport both urine and semen.

Penis
The root of the penis lies within the perineum, and the body or shaft surrounds the urethra and is composed of erectile tissue, fibrous tissue and involuntary muscle. The shaft ends at the glans penis. This is the organ of copulation.

Glans penis
A triangular-shaped structure covered by a mobile double fold of skin called the prepuce or foreskin.

Corpus cavernosum
One of two lateral tubes running the length of the anterior surface of the penis. It is composed of erectile tissue containing vascular spaces, connective tissue and involuntary muscle. The vascular spaces fill with blood, enabling the penis to become erect.

Corpus spongiosum
A cylinder-shaped structure surrounding the urethra. It has the same ability to facilitate erection as the corpus cavernosum.

Ureter
Duct conveying urine from the kidney to the bladder.

Prepuce
A mobile double layer of skin covering the glans penis.

Epididymis
A convoluted tube coiled on the posterior surface of each testis. Stores new spermatozoa for up to 3 weeks as they mature.

Bulbourethral gland
One of two small, pea-sized glands inferior to the prostate gland. Produces a small amount of mucus into the urethra before ejaculation.

Seminal vesicle
A tubular gland with muscular walls lined with secretory epithelium. Produces an alkaline fluid that constitutes 60% of the volume of semen produced at ejaculation.

Ejaculatory duct
An ejaculatory duct is formed on each side when the vas deferens from the testis combines with the duct from the seminal vesical. The ejaculatory ducts continue and then open into the urethra.

Prostate gland
Located at the base of, and surrounding, the urethra, the prostate gland is a capsule consisting of several glands, fibrous tissue and muscle. It produces a thin, milky fluid which makes up 30% of the total volume of semen at ejaculation.

Spermatic cord
Arises in the testis and follows a pathway within the inguinal canal into the abdominal cavity, converging with the urethra. It contains the duct known as vas deferens, blood vessels, lymphatics and nerves.

Testis
The reproductive gland of the male, situated outside the body in the scrotal sac. It is oval in shape and suspended in the sac by the spermatic cord.
   The testes are located outside the body to maintain a critical temperature 2–3°C cooler than body temperature. This is required for the production of healthy spermatozoa.

Scrotum
A bag of pigmented skin and fascia hanging between the inner thighs and the rectum that has the ability to contract and relax the enclosed muscle to maintain optimal temperature for the testes.

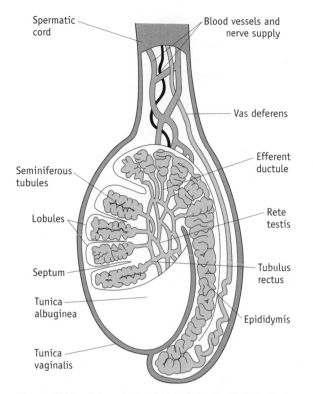

Spermatic cord · Blood vessels and nerve supply · Vas deferens · Efferent ductule · Seminiferous tubules · Rete testis · Lobules · Tubulus rectus · Septum · Tunica albuginea · Epididymis · Tunica vaginalis

Figure 5.19 Internal structures of the testis (adapted from Brooker, 1993). (See Box 5.4 for further information.)

Box 5.4 Internal structure of the testis

Tunica vaginalis
A double serous layer continuous with the pelvic peritoneum.

Tunica albuginea
Fibrous tissue surrounding the testis, dividing the testis into 200–300 lobules.

Lobules
Contain convoluted seminiferous tubules, the sites of spermatogenesis, and Leydig cells secreting androgen hormones.

Seminiferous tubules
Convoluted tubes found inside each lobule.

Epididymis
Convoluted tube coiled on the posterior surface of each testis. Stores new spermatozoa for up to 3 weeks as they mature.

Tubulus rectus
Seminiferous tubes from the lobules to the rete testis, carrying immature spermatozoa.

Rete testis
Seminiferous tubes from the tubulus rectus to the epididymis, carrying immature spermatozoa.

Efferent ductule
The tube from the rete testis into the head of the epididymis.

Vas deferens
The tube extending from the tail of the epididymis inside the spermatic cord, converging with the ejaculatory ducts.

Blood vessels and nerve supply
Testicular artery and the pampiniform plexus of veins, lymphatics and autonomic nerves.

labour and puerperium, and also identify problems which may occur in the fetus and neonate. Early contact with women can identify those women who may need further investigations, or referral to the obstetrician for specialist care.

At the booking visit the woman's medical and family history can be explored, identifying potential problems which may have been caused by nutritional issues, such as rickets and osteomalacia (Belton, 1986; Park *et al.*, 1987), or potential problems caused by conditions such as anorexia nervosa (Soyka *et al.*, 1999). The midwife can identify whether the pelvis may have changed from its original shape through trauma (Pals *et al.*, 1992), surgery (Olson and Pollack, 1996) and/or osteoporosis (DoH, 1994; Nordin, 1997; Phillips *et al.*, 2000).

Antenatally, the midwife can identify normal changes in posture (Bullock *et al.*, 1987; Gupta and Nikodem, 2000) as well as pelvic arthropathy, pelvic pain (Mens *et al.*, 1996), and symphysis pubis diastasis (Fry, 1992; Podmore and Jarrold, 1999).

During labour, an understanding of pelvic anatomy enables a midwife to assess pelvic shape and size, using the woman's history, clinical examination, abdominal palpation and vaginal examination, to provide information to help formulate a dynamic and appropriate plan of care for labour and birth (Knight *et al.*, 1993; Thomas *et al.*, 1998). The midwife may at this point be able to reduce the rate of prolonged labour, make an early identification of dystocia, and thus have a significant effect on morbidity.

During the postnatal period, the midwife assesses the uterine involution and return to its pre-pregnant state. The midwife should be able to identify deviations from normal and refer accordingly. This may include problems caused by birth trauma, male and female circumcision (Cameron and Rawlings-Anderson, 2000) stress incontinence (Glazener and Cooper, 2000; Mason *et al.*, 1999), contraceptive methods (Wu, 1996), sexually transmitted diseases (see Ch. 47) and sexual function and dysfunction (Dawson and Whitfield, 1996; Flint, 1986; Jonier *et al.*, 1995; Morgentaler, 1999; Oruc *et al.*, 1999; Riley and Athanasiadis, 1997). During neonatal examination (see Ch. 31) the midwife is establishing that the genitalia of the neonate is normal, and educating the mother accordingly.

CONCLUSION

Knowledge of human reproduction ensures that a midwife has a foundation on which to place everyday practice. An understanding of how human reproductive anatomy is constructed and functions enables a midwife to apply the concepts to both the normal physiological process of childbirth and the concepts of obstetrics. It enables midwifery practitioners to utilize a common language to discuss midwifery and obstetric practice issues with other healthcare professionals. Understanding the role of the anatomy of human reproduction in pregnancy, labour, birth and following birth enables the midwife to adopt the role of health promoter and practitioner, interpreting complex health issues and relating them accurately and in appropriate terminology to women and their families.

KEY POINTS

- A sound comprehension of the reproductive system provides a basis for an understanding of physiological and pathological conditions related to midwifery practice.
- Detailed anatomical information can be related to how the pelvis impacts on the normal and abnormal mechanisms of labour.
- Knowledge of anatomy provides a basis for understanding how pregnancy impacts on the health of the pelvis.
- Knowledge of anatomy provides a foundation for understanding of how pathological conditions and extrinsic factors impact on the pelvis during parturition.
- Knowledge of anatomy of human reproduction can be applied to the study of obstetrics, gynaecological and urogenital health and pathology to enable practitioners to offer care, treatment and advice.
- An understanding of pelvic anatomy enables a midwife to assess pelvic shape and size, providing information to help formulate a plan of care for labour and birth.

REFERENCES

Abitbol, M. (1996) The shapes of the female pelvis: contributing factors. *Journal of Reproductive Medicine* **41**(4): 242–250.

Belton, N. (1986) Rickets 'not only the English disease'. *Acta Paediatrica Scandinavica* Supplement **323**: 68–75.

Brooker, C. (1993) *Human Structure and Function*, 2nd edn. London: Mosby.

Bullock, J.E., Jull, G.A. & Bullock, M.I. (1987) The relationship of low back pain to postural changes during pregnancy. *Australian Journal of Physiotherapy* **33**(1): 10–17.

Caldwell, W., Moloy, H. & D'Espop, A. (1940) The more recent conceptions of pelvic architecture. *American Journal of Obstetrics and Gynecology* **40**(4): 558–565.

Cameron, J. & Rawlings-Anderson, K. (2000) Female genital mutilation: a global perspective. *British Journal of Midwifery* **8**(12): 754–760.

Carruth, B.R. & Skinner, J.D. (2000) Bone mineral status in adolescent girls: effects of eating disorders and exercise. *Journal of Adolescent Health* **26**(5): 322–329.

Chia, S., Lim, S., Tay, S. *et al.* 2000 Factors associated with male infertility: a case-control study of 218 infertile and 240 fertile men. *British Journal of Obstetrics and Gynaecology* **107**(1): 55–61.

Cluett, E., Alexander, J. & Pickering, R. (1997) What is the normal pattern of uterine involution? An investigation of postpartum uterine involution measured by the distance between the symphysis pubis and the uterine fundus using a paper tape measure. *Midwifery* **13**(1): 9–16.

Cruikshank, D. & Hays, P. (1991) Maternal physiology in pregnancy. In: Gabbe, S., Niebyl, J. & Simpson, P. (eds) *Obstetrics – Normal and Problem Pregnancies*, 2nd edn, Ch. 5. New York: Churchill Livingstone.

Dawson, C. & Whitfield, H. (1996) ABC of urology: subfertility and male sexual dysfunction. *British Medical Journal Clinical Research Edition* 312(7035): 902–905.

Department of Health (DoH) (1994) *Advisory group on osteoporosis report.* London: DoH.

Department of Health (DoH) (1998) *Why Mothers Die: Report on Confidential Enquiries into Maternal Deaths in the United Kingdom 1994–1996.* London: The Stationery Office.

Flint, C. (1986) *Sensitive Midwifery.* London: Heinemann Midwifery.

Forti, G. & Krausz, C. (1998) Clinical review 100: evaluation and treatment of the infertile couple. *Journal of Clinical Endocrinology and Metabolism* 83(12): 4177–1488.

Frame, S., Moore, J., Peters, A. et al. (1985) Maternal height and shoe size as predictors of pelvic disproportion: an assessment. *British Journal of Obstetrics and Gynaecology* 92(12): 1239–1245.

Fry, D. (1992) Diastasis symphysis. *Journal of the Association of Chartered Physiotherapists in Obstetrics and Gynaecology* 71: 10–13.

Gallo, A.M. (1996) Building strong bones in childhood and adolescence: reducing the risk of fractures in later life. *Pediatric Nursing* 22(5); 369–374.

Gimovsky, M., O'Grady, J. & Morris, B. (1994) Assessment of computed tomographic pelvimetry within a selective breech presentation management protocol. *Journal of Reproductive Medicine* 39(7): 489–491.

Glazener, C. & Cooper, K. (2000) Anterior vaginal repair for urinary incontinence in women. *Cochrane Database Systematic Review* (2): CD001755.

Gupta, J. & Nikodem, V. (2000) Woman's position during second stage of labour. *Cochrane Database Systematic Review* (2): CD002006.

Guyton, A. & Hall, J. (2000) *Textbook of Medical Physiology*, 10th edn. London: W.B. Saunders.

Johnson, M.H. & Everitt, B.J. (1999) *Essential Reproduction*, 5th edn. Oxford: Blackwell Scientific.

Jonier, M., Moon, T., Brannan, W. et al. (1995) The effect of age, ethnicity and geographical location on impotence and quality of life. *British Journal of Urology* 75(5): 651–655.

Knight, D., Newnham, J., McKenna, M. et al. (1993) A comparison of abdominal and vaginal examinations for the diagnosis of engagement of the fetal head. *Australian and New Zealand Journal of Obstetrics and Gynaecology* 33(2): 154–158.

Lewis, G. (ed) (2001) *Why Mothers Die 1997–99: Fifth Report of the Confidential Enquiries into Maternal Deaths in the United Kingdom.* London: CEMD: associated with NICE, RCOG.

Mason, L., Glenn, S., Walton, I. et al. (1999) The prevalence of stress incontinence during pregnancy and following delivery. *Midwifery* 15(2): 120–128.

Maternal and Child Health Research Consortium (MCHRC) (2000) *Confidential Enquiry into Stillbirths and Deaths in Infancy: 7th Annual Report.* London: MCHRC. Online. Available: www.cesdi.org.uk.

Maternal and Child Health Research Consortium (MCHRC) (2001) *Confidential Enquiry into Stillbirths and Deaths in Infancy 8th Annual Report.* London: MCHRC.

Mens, J., Vieeming, A., Stoeckart, R. et al. (1996) Understanding peripartum pelvic pain: implications of a patient survey. *Spine* 21(11): 1363–1369.

Miller, A. & Hanretty, K. (1997) *Obstetrics Illustrated*, 5th edn. Edinburgh: Churchill Livingstone.

Morgentaler, A. (1999) Male impotence. *Lancet* 354(9191): 1713–1718.

Nordin, B. (1997) Calcium and osteoporosis. *Nutrition* 13(7–8): 664–686.

Olson, S. & Pollack, A. (1996) Assessment of pelvic ring stability after injury: indications for surgical stabilization. *Clinical Orthopaedics and Related Research* 329: 15–27.

Oruc, S., Esen, A., Lacin, S. et al. (1999) Sexual behaviour during pregnancy. *Australian and New Zealand Journal of Obstetrics and Gynaecology* 39(1): 48–50.

Pals, S., Brown, C. & Friermood, T. (1992) Open reduction and internal fixation of an acetabular fracture during pregnancy. *Journal of Orthopaedic Trauma* 6(3): 379–381.

Park, W., Paust, H., Kaufmann, H. et al. (1987) Osteomalacia of the mother – rickets of the newborn. *European Journal of Pediatrics* 146(3) 292–293.

Phillips, A., Ostlere, S. & Smith, R. (2000) Pregnancy-associated osteoporosis: does the skeleton recover? *Osteoporosis International* 11(5): 449–454.

Podmore, S. & Jarrold, S. (1999) Closing the gap: diastasis symphysis pubis in childbirth. *Practising Midwife* 2(10): 20–22.

Riley, A. & Athanasiadis, L. (1997) Impotence and its non-surgical management. *British Journal of Clinical Practice* 51(2): 99–103.

Schneider, K. & Deckardt, R. (1991) The implications of upright posture on pregnancy. *Journal of Perinatal Medicine* 19(1-2): 121–131.

Snell, R.S. (2000) *Clinical Anatomy for Medical students*, 6th edn. London: Lippincott Williams & Wilkins.

Soyka, L., Grinspoon, S., Levitsky, L. et al. (1999) The effects of anorexia nervosa on bone metabolism in female adolescents. *Journal of Clinical Endocrinology and Metabolism* 84(12): 4489–4496.

Sowers, M., Crutchfield, M., Jannausch, M. et al. (1991) A prospective evaluation of bone mineral change in pregnancy. *Obstetrics and Gynecology* 77(6): 841–845.

Sporri, S., Hanggi, W., Braghetti, A. *et al.* (1997) Pelvimetry by magnetic resonance imaging as a diagnostic tool to evaluate dystocia. *Obstetrics and Gynaecology* **89**(6): 902–908.

Thomas, S., Bees, N. & Adam, E. (1998) Trends in the use of pelvimetry techniques. *Clinical Radiology* **53**(4): 293–295.

Waugh, A. & Grant, A. (2001) *Ross and Wilson Anatomy and Physiology in Health and Illness*, 9th edn. London: Churchill Livingstone.

Wu, F. (1996) Male contraception. *Baillière's Clinical Obstetrics and Gynaecology* **10**(1): 1–23.

FURTHER READING

Broome, D., Hayman, L., Herrick, R. *et al.* (1998) Postnatal maturation of the sacrum and coccyx: MR imaging helical CT and conventional radiography. *American Journal of Roentgenology* **170**(4): 1061–1066.

Podmore, S. & Jarrold, S. (1999) Closing the gap: diastasis symphysis pubis in childbirth. *Practising Midwife* **2**(10): 20–22.
This article describes the personal experience of the author who was diagnosed with diastasis symphysis pubis. The physiology of this condition and the level of pain are discussed, supported by diagrams outlining the anatomy of the pelvis in relation to vertical and horizontal displacement. The author continues by discussing the care that women should receive in labour and the puerperium.

Cluett, E., Alexander, J. & Pickering, R. (1997) What is the normal pattern of uterine involution? An investigation of postpartum uterine involution measured by the distance between the symphysis pubis and the uterine fundus using a paper tape measure. *Midwifery* **13**(1): 9–16.
This survey of 28 women aimed to measure the decline in distance between the symphysis pubis and the uterine fundus during the postnatal period as measured by the use of a paper tape measure. The authors found variability in the patterns of uterine involution with no correlation between types of infant feeding. Although this was only a small study, the authors recommend that using this type of measuring instrument should not become part of routine postpartum assessment.

Chia, S., Lim, S., Tay, S. *et al.* (2000) Factors associated with male infertility: a case-control study of 218 infertile and 240 fertile men. *British Journal of Obstetrics and Gynaecology* **107**(1): 55–61.
This case-control study aimed to determine the risk factors for infertile men with no known cause of infertility.
640 men of couples trying to conceive were recruited from an infertility clinic; 218 of these men were identified as having no known cause of their infertility. This group was compared to a control group of 240 men whose partners were pregnant. Comparisons were made for semen parameters, lifestyle activities such as smoking and drinking habits, and occupation. The findings describe the significant factors for predicting infertility as associated with smoking, occupation, and density and viability of sperm.

ADDITIONAL RESOURCES

http://www.icr.ac.uk/everyman/about/testicular.html
This site includes detailed information on testicular examination including photographs and explanations. It also outlines the symptoms of testicular cancer.

http://www.mariestopes.org.uk/
Cervical screening information.

http://www.velindre-tr.wales.nhs.uk/csw/internet/home.html
Cervical screening questions and answers.

http://synaptic.mvc.mcc.ac.uk/Pelvis/abnrml-labor.avi
Virtual museum of pelves from the turn of the century, including short case histories.

http://numedsun.ncl.ac.uk/~nds4/tutorials/index.html
'Cyberanatomy' tutorials.

6

Female Reproductive Physiology

Mary McNabb

LEARNING OUTCOMES

After reading this chapter, you will:

- be familiar with the neurohormonal aspects that regulate ovulation and menstruation
- be able to describe the menstrual cycle in relation to female health and preparation for conception
- appreciate the complex neurohormonal regulation of reproductive organs across the cycle.

INTRODUCTION

The menstrual cycle provides considerable information regarding a woman's reproductive health. All aspects of the cycle are highly sensitive to habitual dietary composition, long-term over- and undernutrition and emotional and physical stress (Ferin, 1999; Norman and Clark, 1998). Food intake and metabolism are partly regulated by neurohormonal changes during the menstrual cycle, as higher intakes of macro- and micronutrients, increased metabolic rate and increased energy expenditure have been reported during the luteal phase (Cohen *et al.*, 1987; Forman *et al.*, 1996; Solomon *et al.*, 1982; Webb, 1986).

THE MENSTRUAL CYCLE

During each menstrual cycle the lining of the uterus undergoes a cyclical process of accumulation and loss which is suspended during pregnancy and lactation. Throughout the cycle, growing ovarian follicles undergo distinct processes of development to ensure that an oocyte (immature ovum) is prepared for fertilization and implantation. Meanwhile, many organs begin to change in anticipation of pregnancy, labour and lactation. These adaptations are regulated by dynamic interactions between ovarian hormones, hypothalamic neurones and pituitary endocrine cells across the menstrual cycle. The complex interplay of these will be described later in this chapter.

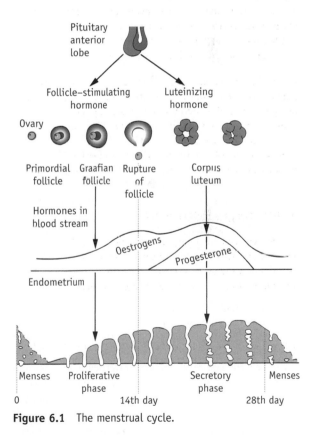

Figure 6.1 The menstrual cycle.

The menstrual cycle (Fig. 6.1) is divided into three phases which normally take place over 28 days:

1. *Proliferative phase.* This lasts about 10 days or more. Under the influence of oestrogens and local growth

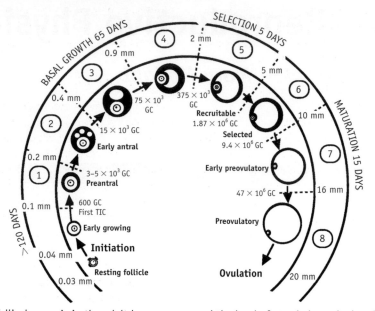

Figure 6.2 Stages of folliculogenesis in the adult human ovary and the level of atresia in each class in the process of recruiting and selecting the dominant follicle. GC, granulosa cells; TIC, theca interna cells. (From Gougeon, 1996.)

factors, blood vessels begin to proliferate the endometrium grows thicker and softer, and the tubular glands lengthen.

2. *Secretory phase*. This lasts 14 days following ovulation. Under the influence of oestrogens and progesterone, the endometrial layer becomes even thicker and the glands become tortuous as they expand with secretions.

3. *Menses*. This lasts about 4–6 days, during which the endometrial lining is shed to its basal layer. The lining is expelled with the aid of uterine contractions, and in terms of volume is around 50–100ml.

In most women the whole cycle lasts about 28 days but in some it may vary – from 21 to 42 days, or more. In a prolonged cycle, only the proliferative phase is longer. The luteal phase is always 14 days in length and is followed by the menses unless fertilization occurs. Occasionally, implantation of the ovum may cause a short implantation bleed. Therefore in obtaining information on the last menstrual period, the midwife should ascertain the duration and character of that last period.

Conception normally takes place shortly after ovulation, 14 days prior to the menstrual period. It is comparatively easy to calculate when conception occurred in women with a regular cycle, though more complex should the cycle be irregular.

A complex set of regulatory processes occurs during different phases of the menstrual cycle. Within the ovaries, a small reserve stock of growing follicles is continually drawn from the pool of mature *secondary follicles*. As illustrated in Figure 6.2, cohorts of those that have reached the *antral phase* of development are recruited in successive waves throughout the cycle, for further growth and maturation, in preparation for ovulation, fertilization and implantation (Baerwald *et al.*, 2003). At the same time, the genital tract, mammary gland, urinary, cardiovascular and fluid regulatory systems undergo a number of distinct changes in anticipation of pregnancy and lactation (Chapman *et al.*, 1998; Imagawa *et al.*, 1994; Valdes *et al.*, 2001; Vokes *et al.*, 1988). Characteristic shifts occur in a number of homeostatic systems during the luteal phase of the ovarian cycle and many of these simply accelerate following fertilization and implantation.

The *corpus luteum* is an essential endocrine organ to establish a viable pregnancy during the first 6–8 weeks (Liu *et al.*, 1995). When fertilization is followed by implantation, the life span of the corpus luteum simply extends from 2 to 42 weeks (Santoro *et al.*, 1994). To begin to understand the precise synchronization of some of the interrelated changes, this chapter will first examine the temporal regulation of ovarian activities on the menstrual cycle (Gougeon, 1996; Hodgen, 1982). It will be useful to review Chapter 5 in conjunction with this chapter.

Folliculogenesis

Fertility depends on the ability of the ovaries to produce typically one *dominant follicle* per cycle, with the capacity to *ovulate* a fertilizable oocyte. Following selection, this growing follicle regulates changes in hypothalamic–pituitary gonadotrophin activity during oocyte maturation and ovulation, and following the mid-cycle LH/FSH surge when it differentiates into a functional corpus luteum (Baker and Spears, 1999; Hodgen, 1982; Kunz *et al.*, 1998).

At mid-cycle, the dominant follicle becomes visible to the naked eye, as a large bulge under the surface epithelium of the ovary. The ovary contains thousands of highly differentiated cells, and functions as a complex neuroendocrine–autocrine–paracrine gland, synchronizing hypothalamic, pituitary, ovarian, uterine and mammary activities throughout the cycle (Armstrong and Webb, 1997; Behrens *et al.*, 1995; Hirshfield, 1991; Kunz *et al.*, 1998).

The ovarian cycle

The complete ovarian cycle takes place in the time period between successive ovulations. Current research suggests that throughout the cycle, both ovaries recruit at least two successive waves of around 10 healthy follicles that have reached 2–5 mm in diameter. The last of these enter the final stages of growth and development, which take place during the follicular phase of the next cycle (Baerwald *et al.*, 2003). These follicles leave the dynamic pool of primordial and slowly growing follicles and produce increasing amounts of steroid hormones as they embark on an exponential growth phase under the influence of pituitary gonadotrophins, while the preceding waves of growing cohorts begin to regress and undergo *atresia* or cell death (Amsterdam *et al.*, 1999; Baerwald *et al.*, 2003; Hirshfield, 1991: 47).

The *selected follicle* then demonstrates increased cell proliferation and differentiation; expansion of thecal vascularity; rapid accumulation of antral fluid and rising capacity for steroid hormone secretion (Geva and Jaffe, 2000; Gougeon, 1996). At the same time, the enclosed oocyte completes the growth phase and subsequently undergoes a profound reorganization of the nucleus and cytoplasm, in preparation for fertilization and early embryonic formation (Canipari, 2000; Moor *et al.*, 1990: 180–181).

The demise of the corpus luteum relaxes *negative feedback* and allows a slight increase in FSH/LH levels, which stimulate granulosa cell proliferation, and theca and granulosa cell compartments then begin to synthesize steroid hormones. The initial rise in oestrogens during the early follicular phase produces a negative feedback effect on circulating levels of FSH and

diminishes its stimulatory action on the non-dominant follicles of the same cohort, in both ovaries, and they subsequently undergo atresia (Amsterdam *et al.*, 1999).

Ovarian regulation

The ovarian cycle temporally modulates the secretory patterns of pituitary and hypothalamic gonadotrophins, through the changing balance of hormonal secretions, in successive cohorts of antral follicles, the dominant follicle and its successor, the corpus luteum (Baker and Spears, 1999; Hodgen, 1982). Across the cycle, ovarian steroid and peptide hormones act through negative and positive feedback mechanisms on the synthesis and pattern of release of hypothalamic gonadotrophin-releasing hormone (GnRH); pituitary gonadotrophins FSH and LH and their responsiveness to GnRH, in relation to a variety of other modulatory hormones and neurotransmitters that operate on pituitary and hypothalamic gonadotrophin cells (Smith and Jennes, 2001) (Fig. 6.3).

Selection of the dominant follicle

From the onset of the exponential growth phase, cell proliferation, fluid formation and vascularization proceed at varying speeds in the antral follicles recruited for ovulation. The most rapidly growing of these can be distinguished by rapid cell proliferation, differentiation and vascularization; upregulation in functional FSH and LH receptors and greater uptake of pituitary gonadotrophs than the remaining follicles in the cohort; and an increased sensitivity to FSH (Gougeon, 1996; Zackrisson, 2000). By day 9 of the follicular phase, the vascularity of the theca compartment in the selected follicle is double that in other follicles of the developing cohort and leads to increased delivery of LH to the *theca* and FSH to the *mural granulosa* cells (Geva and Jaffe, 2000). At the same time, selected follicles have also been shown to inhibit proliferation of granulosa cells in small follicles and to release oestrogens and progesterone, which selectively inhibit granulosa cell mitosis in mid-sized but not large antral follicles (Armstrong and Webb, 1997). These interactions enhance trophic support for the development of the selected follicle while the remainder undergo the process of atresia (Amsterdam *et al.*, 1999).

Within the dominant follicle, fibroblasts in the theca externa develop a prominent intracellular contractile system, and collagen fibres are synthesized in the theca interna (Iwahashi *et al.*, 2000). At the same time, mural granulosa cells elongate and form a pseudostratified epithelium. They express oxytocin, especially in the

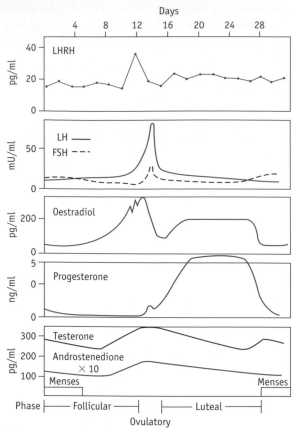

Figure 6.3 Ovarian regulation of hypothalamic–pituitary function. Note the decline in FSH during the mid-follicular phase and the rise in FSH with the demise of the corpus luteum. (Reproduced with permission from Berne and Levy, 1993: 602.)

layers nearest the antrum, while those nearest the basal lamina express oxytocin receptors. Proliferation of mural granulosa cells continues at a slower rate as they acquire LH receptors and synthesize enzymes required for steroid hormone production (Salustri *et al.*, 1993).

There is a growing ratio of fluid to tissue mass, which probably participates in temperature regulation between the dominant follicle and the surrounding stroma, resulting in a preovulatory follicle temperature of <2.3°C cooler than the surrounding ovarian stroma (Grinsted *et al.*, 1995). This suggests that although the ovaries remain in the abdominal cavity, they can provide a cooler internal environment for the preovulatory follicle, analogous to that provided for the male germ cells in the cool scrotal sac (Bujan *et al.*, 2000).

As the dominant follicle increases in size (Fig. 6.4), rising synthesis of oestrogens and progesterone lead to a parallel rise in circulating concentrations. Within the

dominant follicle, the stimulatory actions of oestrogens and FSH on LH receptors is 7–10 times greater in mural granulosa cells nearest the basal lamina compared to cumulus granulosa cells around the oocyte (Amsterdam and Linder, 1984). This gradient of LH-receptor distribution confirms the functional heterogeneity of granulosa cells and also indicates a modulatory role of the oocyte on the stimulatory actions of oestrogens and FSH on LH receptors (Eppig *et al.*, 1997).

Mid-cycle LH/FSH surges

The LH/FSH surges are temporally associated with the attainment of peak secretion of oestrogens following a rapid rise in progesterone 12 hours earlier. Just after the peak in oestrogens, mean concentration of steroids in antral fluid increases from 4829 ng/ml to 10 995 ng/ml (Gougeon, 1996: 131). This stimulates a brief positive feedback action on GnRH neurones in the hypothalamus and on FSH and LH cells in the adenohypophysis (Chappell and Levine, 2000; Smith and Jennes, 2001).

Gonadotrophin-releasing hormone neurones (GnRH)

Current evidence suggests that the frequency and amplitude of hypothalamic GnRH pulses into the hypothalamic portal circulation represent the final neuropeptide in an integrated neuronal network that generates changes in the pulsatile release of LH and FSH from the adenohypophysis across the menstrual cycle (Herbison, 1997; Smith and Jennes, 2001). Like a number of other neurotransmitters in the hypothalamus, GnRH may also act as an autocrine/paracrine regulator in several extrapituitary tissues, including ovarian follicles, at different stages of development: the uterine tubes during fertilization; the endometrium during the luteal phase of the cycle; the trophectoderm and inner cell mass of the blastocyst; and the early placenta (Casan *et al.*, 1999, 2000; Cheng *et al.*, 2000).

As illustrated in Figure 6.5, the biosynthetic and secretory activity of hypothalamic GnRH across the ovarian cycle is regulated by connections with other neurotransmitters from the hypothalamus and brainstem and by the ovarian steroid hormones, oestrogens and progesterone (Calogero *et al.*, 1996; Herbison, 1997; Herbison and Pape, 2001; Smith and Jennes, 2001). GnRH neurones in the arcuate nucleus are stimulated by ascending adrenergic neurones and inhibited by local neurones that release dopamine. The inhibitory actions of low concentrations of ovarian oestrogens are thought to act directly via membrane receptors on GnRH neurones and indirectly through adjacent dopaminergic

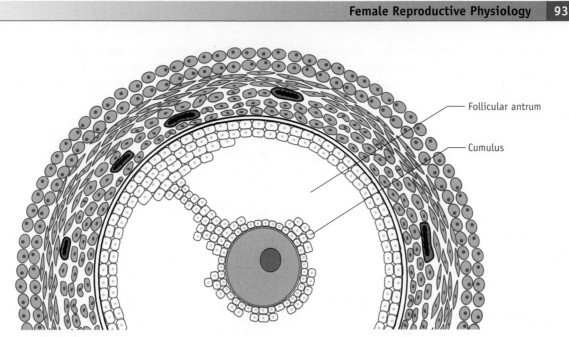

Figure 6.4 Preovulatory follicle. (Reproduced with permission from Johnson and Everitt, 1995: 65.)

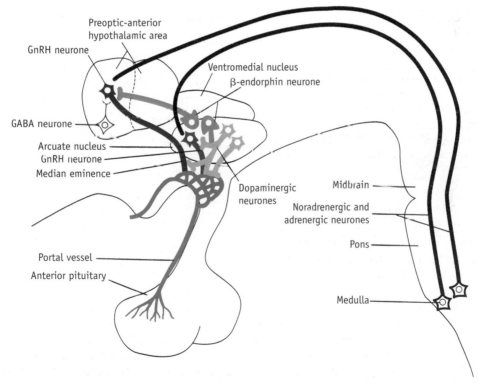

Figure 6.5 Postulated neurochemical reactions that may control GnRH secretion. (Reproduced with permission from Johnson and Everitt, 1995: 132.)

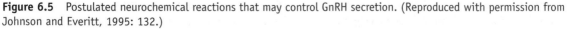

neurones (Herbison and Pape, 2001). The stimulatory effect of the preovulatory surge of oestrogens on GnRH secretion is partly mediated by noradrenaline neurones from the brainstem (Herbison, 1997).

Oestrogens may initiate the GnRH surge, by stimulating central transcription factors regulated by progesterone receptors, and may be activated by local neurotransmitters regulated by the internal circadian clock in the suprachiasmatic nucleus (Chappell and Levine, 2000; Smith and Jennes, 2001).

The adenohypophysis

The epithelial vessels of the hypothalamic–neuroendocrine system are located in the *adenohypophysis* (anterior pituitary gland) (Fig. 6.6). This is composed of at least eight interconnected groups of peptide-hormone-secreting cells regulated by the hypothalamus (Schwartz, 2000). Hormones are released in pulses from the median eminence and transported by the portal system to target cells within the anterior lobe. The rich vascular system provides the adenohypophysis with very high levels of regulatory hypothalamic peptides.

Distinct groups of cells within the adenohypophysis secrete peptide hormones with a range of homeostatic actions that are mediated by a variety of organs and tissues throughout the body. They include:

- follicle-stimulating hormone (FSH)
- luteinizing hormone (LH)
- adrenocorticotrophic hormone (ACTH), which is processed from a larger peptide, pro-opiomelanocortin (POMC), and binds to receptors in the adrenal cortex

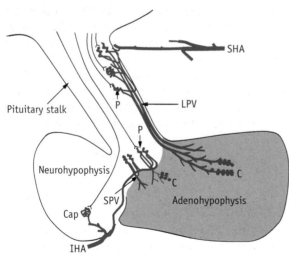

Figure 6.6   Sagittal section of the human pituitary gland to illustrate the neurovascular pathways by which nerve cells in certain hypothalamic nuclei control the output of the anterior and posterior lobes of the pituitary gland. C, epithelial cells; Cap, capillary bed in the infundibular process; IHA, inferior hypophysial artery; LPV, long portal vessels; P, capillary bed feeding the portal vessels; SHA, superior hypophysial artery; SPV, short portal vessels. (Reproduced with permission from Daniel, P. and Prichard, M.M.L. (1975) *Acta Endocrinol.* **80**: 67.)

- prolactin, a polypeptide belonging to a larger family of lactogenic hormones that includes growth hormone (GH) and human placental lactogen (hPL).

A wide variety of peptides have also been shown to interact with ovarian steroids, ions and other paracrine factors, as well as GnRH, in regulating LH and FSH secretion, particularly around ovulation. These include neuropeptide Y (NPY), nerve growth factor (NGF), β-endorphin, prolactin and oxytocin (Evans, 1999; Evans *et al.*, 2001). Plasma prolactin concentrations are lowest in the early follicular phase and progressively increase during the rest of the cycle. This pattern seems to be regulated by an indirect stimulatory influence of GnRH on prolactin-releasing cells and rising levels of ovarian steroid hormones (Brumsted and Riddick, 1992).

During the ovulatory cycle, oxytocin levels vary in the hypothalamo-hypophysial complex, medulla and cerebrospinal fluid (Evans, 1996). In the peripheral circulation, higher levels of oxytocin coincide with the mid-cycle LH surge – variations have been found in oxytocin and oxytocin receptors in granulosa and stromal cells, as well as in uterine and cervical tissue across the ovarian cycle (Behrens *et al.*, 1995; Kunz *et al.*, 1998).

Current evidence suggests that central oxytocin plays a key role in regulating the LH surge, by acting directly on pituitary gonadotrophs and by stimulating sexual behaviour around ovulation (Anderson-Hunt and Dennerstein, 1994). Uterine and cervical oxytocin cooperate in conjunction with prostaglandin E_2 and the preovulatory surge in oestrogens from the dominant follicle. These interactions promote fertilization, by softening cervical tissue and stimulating cervicofundal contractions, to rapidly transport waves of spermatozoa from the posterior vaginal fornix to the isthmic portion of the uterine tube (Behrens *et al.*, 1995; Drobnis and Overstreet, 1992; Kunz *et al.*, 1998).

The preovulatory follicle

Following the LH/FSH surges, fibroblasts within the theca externa lay down connective tissue, and theca interna and mural granulosa cells begin to differentiate from a predominantly oestrogen-secreting tissue into a highly vascularized corpus luteum with progesterone as its major steroid hormone.

Intrafollicular concentration of oestradiol decreases and progesterone sharply increases. Following the LH/FSH surges, follicular fluid oestrogen concentrations decline from 2500 ng/ml to 1000 ng/ml, while progesterone increases from 2400 ng/ml to 7700 ng/ml

(Gougeon, 1986). Under the stimulatory influence of LH/hCG, a surge in collagen type IV fibres bind to the cell surface integrin molecules on mural granulosa cells. Collagen IV has been found to *modulate* progesterone secretion, suggesting that these rapidly growing fibres play a key role in regulating the timing of ovulation to coincide with the resumption of oocyte maturation (Wasserman, 1996).

During this critical preovulatory period, the oocyte also secretes a molecule(s) that enhances oestrogen and inhibits progesterone secretion by cumulus granulosa cells. At the same time, all granulosa cells express both oxytocin and oxytocin receptors, especially the cumulus granulosa cells surrounding the oocyte, and oxytocin mRNA has also been located in the oocyte (Stock and Osterlund, 1998). Oxytocin appears to modulate progesterone secretion while stimulating progesterone receptors on granulosa cells and a variety of regulatory molecules including growth factors, integrins, prostaglandins and intracellular messengers that are involved in the process of ovulation. The presence of oxytocin and oxytocin receptors on cumulus cells and oocytes suggests that oxytocin may be involved in oocyte function and the micro-environment of fertilization (Stock and Osterlund, 1998).

A subpopulation of mural and cumulus granulosa cells demonstrates progressive accumulation and release of vascular endothelial growth factor (VEGF), which promotes endothelial cell expansion and angiogenesis, and transforming growth factor β (TGF-β), which stimulates progesterone secretion from granulosa cells following ovulation. Meanwhile, leptin and its associated gene transcription factor are expressed in polarized regions of mural and cumulus granulosa cells that co-localize with similarly polarized regions in fully grown oocytes (Antczak *et al.*, 1997).

Oocyte maturation

Throughout the growth phase of the oocyte, the progression of *meiosis* is arrested at the diplotene or germinal vesicle stage of prophase 1. Within 12 hours of the LH/FSH surge, the fully grown oocyte is reactivated to briefly resume meiosis, while complex maturational changes simultaneously occur in the cytoplasm. FSH receptors are present on the entire surface of human oocytes, suggesting that FSH has direct control of oocyte maturation (Meduri *et al.*, 2002).

In preparation for ovulation, the FSH surge may directly overcome the tonic inhibition of meiosis, while the simultaneous surge in LH may operate indirectly by inducing mRNA synthesis in the cumulus granulosa cells. Together, the LH and FSH surges initiate nuclear progression in the oocyte and expansion of the cumulus cell mass (Meinecke and Meinecke-Tillmann, 1993).

The secretion of leptin and its associated transcription factor from the cumulus granulosa cells into predetermined sites within the oocyte is thought to initiate migration of the oocyte nucleus to a polarized position prior to the breakdown of its membrane. This development allows the chromosomes to complete prophase 1, by rearranging themselves in the first meiotic spindle. The first meiotic division is then completed and 23 chromosomes are relocated to a small enclosure of cytoplasm on the periphery (Antczak *et al.*, 1997). Identified as the first polar body, this area seems to be a marker for the first polar axis in subsequent rounds of cell cleavage during early embryonic formation. This chromosomal reorganization marks the formation of a secondary oocyte containing 23 chromosomes enclosed within the larger volume of cytoplasm. These chromosomes immediately enter the second meiotic division but arrest again at second metaphase (Johnson and Everitt, 2000: 77).

During this critical period of oocyte maturation, the cumulus cell mass supplies the enclosed oocyte with a variety of intermediate molecules that are essential for maturation, sperm motility, fertilization and early embryonic formation (Seifer *et al.*, 2002). These include the regulatory protein leptin and its associated gene transcription factor which establishes the identity and fate of individual cells following fertilization, and the amino acid cystine, which is required by the oocyte until the blastocyst stage of development to synthesize the powerful antioxidant compound glutathione, which regulates the resumption of meiosis; sperm motility and lipid peroxidation; sperm–oocyte fusion and embryonic formation (Antczak *et al.*, 1997).

The cumulus cell mass also supplies:

- a brain-derived neurotrophic factor which enhances the extrusion of polar bodies
- pyruvate, which operates as both antioxidant and the glycolytic intermediate that seems to be involved in regulating the brief resumption of meiosis
- a variety of amino acids, ribonucleosides and enzymes involved in the metabolic changes that initiate the dissolution of the nuclear membrane (Motlik and Kubelka, 1990; Seifer *et al.*, 2002).

Within the main body of cytoplasm, the vesicles and tubules of the Golgi complexes also fill with dense material which coalesces to form large vacuoles that migrate to the periphery.

Mural granulosa and theca interna cells differentiate predominantly into progesterone-secreting theca-lutein and granulosa-lutein cells, which remain in the ovary following ovulation and rapidly expand to form the highly vascularized corpus luteum (Niswender *et al.*, 2000). Meanwhile, cumulus granulosa cells express an extracellular matrix of glycoproteins and type IV collagen and interact with the oocyte, to synthesize and release a well-hydrated viscous gel-like extracellular matrix composed of hyaluronic acid, a highly viscoelastic biopolymer that goes to make up the dramatically expanded oocyte–cumulus complex – there is a 20- to 30-fold increase in the oocyte–cumulus complex just before ovulation (Salustri *et al.*, 1999; Talbot *et al.*, 2003).

By 20 hours following the LH/FSH surge, extensive reorganization of microfilaments within the cumulus granulosa cells appears to initiate the synthesis of this three-dimensional matrix that seems to directly regulate both nuclear and cytoplasmic maturation of the oocyte (Chen *et al.*, 1990). Fully grown oocytes also promote matrix accumulation by modulating FSH-stimulated synthesis of plasminogen activators in surrounding granulosa cells. The quantity of follicular fluid rapidly increases and the expanded oocyte–cumulus complex becomes increasingly detached from the rest of the follicle, while mural granulosa cells remain coupled to the basal lamina (Buccione *et al.*, 1990; Salustri *et al.*, 1999).

Ovulation

As illustrated in Figure 6.7, the LH/FSH surge dramatically increases blood flow and vascular permeability in thecal capillary networks that descend to the basal lamina. The rapid increase in size and vascularization of the follicle is accompanied by the local release of the prostaglandin PGE$_2$ and of vasodilatory substances like histamine and bradykinin. PGE$_2$ initiates the breakdown of collagen fibres within the thecal compartment, and other molecules cause an inflammatory reaction from within. FSH and progesterone also initiate proteolytic enzyme activity that loosens, distends and finally erodes the follicle wall at its weakest point (Brannstrom *et al.*, 1996).

Within 12 hours of the LH/FSH surge, progesterone replaces oestrogens as the dominant steroid hormone synthesized by theca and mural granulosa cells. This shift in steroid hormone production is accompanied by

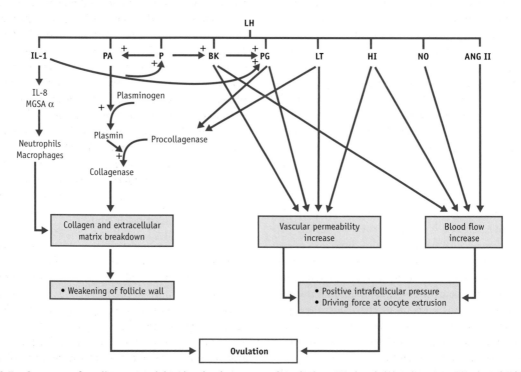

Figure 6.7 Summary of mediators participating in the events of ovulation. LH, luteinizing hormone; IL, interleukin; PA, plasminogen activator; P, progesterone; BK, bradykinin; PG, prostaglandins; LT, leukotrienes; HI, histamine; NO, nitric oxide; ANG II, angiotensin II. (From Brannstrom *et al.*, 1996.)

a rise in prostaglandin output which activates enzymes that weaken and distend the follicle wall. Between 36 and 42 hours following the surges, the apex of the follicle begins to bulge below the surface of the ovary, rupturing at its weakest point, allowing antral fluid to flow into the peritoneal cavity, carrying the expanded oocyte–cumulus complex into the fallopian tube (Brannstrom *et al.*, 1996).

At ovulation, the dominant follicle releases the hugely expanded oocyte–cumulus complex from the surface of the ovary. Immediately afterwards, the cumulus cell mass regulates the acceptance of the oocyte by the fimbriae of the fallopian tube and subsequently functions as a hormonal and metabolic unit in the lumen of the uterine cavity, optimizing conditions for the enclosed oocyte and zona pellucida to undergo final maturational changes in preparation for fertilization, implantation and embryo formation (Talbot *et al.*, 2003).

CYCLICAL CHANGES IN REPRODUCTIVE ORGANS

The uterus

During the first and second half of the menstrual cycle, changes take place within the endometrial lining, mucosal secretions of the cervix and the structure and secretions of the vagina. Successive phases of proliferation, secretion and regression of the functional zone of the endometrium occur, alongside proliferation and involution in mammary epithelial cells across the menstrual cycle (Herbison and Pape, 2001; Russo and Russo, 1987; Smith, 2001; Smith and Jennes, 2001).

The process of cyclical endometrial development that culminates with decidualization at around 8–9 days after ovulation begins towards the end of menses. During the follicular phase, rising concentration of oestrogens stimulates an intense period of proliferation of epithelial and stromal cells. This is followed by differentiation of glandular and stromal cells and continued growth and tubal formation of endometrial vascular cells, under the regulatory influence of rising levels of progesterone during the luteal phase of the cycle. Under the influence of changing concentrations of oestrogens and progesterone across the menstrual cycle, the endometrium is the site of synthesis of a wide variety of hormones, neuropeptides, growth and angiogenic factors.

During the luteal phase of the ovarian cycle, the functional zone of the endometrium is characterized by changes in cell morphology and extracellular matrix composition that transform it into a secretory, paracrine/autocrine gland.

Throughout the secretory phase, the endometrium clearly differentiates into three layers, with numerous gap junctions:

- The superficial compact zone contains decidualized stroma with attenuated non-secretory glands.
- A middle spongy zone consists of distended glands with abundant secretions.
- The basal zone has extensive development of protein synthesis and secretion (Irwin and Giudice, 1998).

Cyclic endometrial development

During the follicular and luteal phases of the ovarian cycle, a series of changes takes place in the functional layer of the endometrium and fallopian tubes, mucosal secretions of the cervix and the structure and secretions of vaginal tissue (Gipson *et al.*, 2001). As illustrated in Figure 6.8, from the mid-secretory phase of the endometrial cycle to the end of menstruation, the thickness of the functional layer of the human endometrium declines from 5–8 mm to 1–3 mm, as the superficial or functional layer of the endometrium is shed along with its connective tissue matrix, and its highly specialized arterioles are reduced to around one-third of the length they achieve by the onset of menses (Bakos *et al.*, 1993; Dockery *et al.*, 1990; Rogers, 1996; Smith, 2000; Starkey, 1993). During the premenstrual phase, endometrial cells release increasing levels of proteolytic enzymes that degrade the extracellular matrix, and highly potent and long-lasting vasoconstrictors called endothelins that act on the spiral arterioles (Ohbuchi *et al.*, 1995). From the second day after bleeding commences, the remaining stromal cells respond to the reduction in oxygen tension by synthesizing vascular endothelial growth factor (VEGF) which stimulates repair of the vascular bed and elongation of the remaining blood vessels by the fifth day of the cycle (Maas *et al.*, 2001). These blood vessels have an essential role in tissue reconstruction during the proliferative phase of the cycle (Rogers, 1996; Smith, 2001).

By around day 5 of the cycle, cell proliferation in the endometrium commences when endometrial and myometrial oestrogen receptors are stimulated by increased secretion of oestrogens from the cohort of developing ovarian follicles. During this phase, oestrogens stimulate an increase in the number of ciliated cells in the luminal epithelium and the expression of a variety of mitogenic factors including VEGF that stimulate a marked proliferation of luminal epithelial,

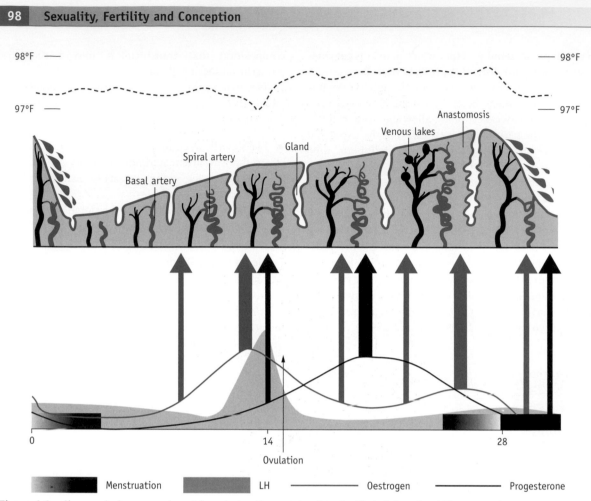

Figure 6.8   Changes in human endometrium during the menstrual cycle. Underlying steroid hormone changes are indicated below and basal temperature is indicated above. Thickness of arrows indicates strength of action. (Reproduced with permission from Johnson and Everitt, 1995: 125.)

glandular and vascular endothelial cells (Ferrara and Davis-Smith, 1997). At the same time, oestrogens directly inhibit endometrial angiogenesis, while vascular permeability rises and endometrial blood flow increases, to reach a peak just before ovulation (Ma *et al.*, 2001). Stromal fibroblasts enlarge and show signs of increased protein synthesis and association with microfibrils of collagen that become denser and thicker just before ovulation, and an insoluble pericellular matrix of collagen and fibronectin fibres forms a tight meshwork primarily around glandular and basement membranes of the luminal epithelium (Aplin, 1989; Dockery *et al.*, 1990; Fraser and Peek, 1992; Shiokawa *et al.*, 1996; Starkey, 1993).

With the surge in oestrogens that follows the selection of the dominant follicle, a three- to fivefold increase occurs in the thickness of the endometrium, and oestrogen-dependent intracellular receptors for

progesterone are synthesized. During the late proliferative phase of the cycle, the secretory glands enlarge and become thicker and more convoluted, while proliferation in epithelial and stromal cells continues until 3 days following ovulation (Irwin and Giudice, 1998; Strauss and Coutifaris, 1999). Under the influence of rising levels of progesterone following the midcycle LH/FSH surge, the cervix becomes firmer and more tightly closed and cervical secretions become scant, viscous and cellular, making it more difficult for spermatozoa to enter the uterus. In addition, relaxin and progesterone relax muscle layers in the isthmic portion of the tube, which assists the movement of the conceptus towards the uterine cavity (Downing and Hollingsworth, 1993; Johnson and Everitt, 2000: 136).

Within the uterus, endometrial glandular cells accumulate glycogen, regulatory proteins, sugars and lipids,

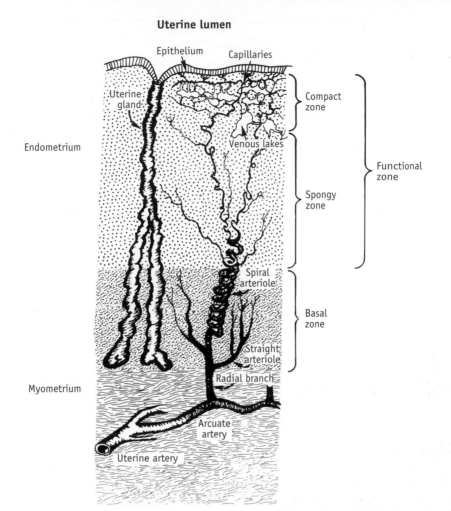

Figure 6.9 The arterial supply to the uterine endometrium. These specialized endometrial blood vessels arise within the myometrium, as the arcuate arteries. Small straight arterioles supply the basal unchanging layer of the endometrium. As they leave the basal portion and enter the spongy and compact tissue that underlies the luminal epithelium, their thick smooth muscle coat formed by circular and longitudinal layers becomes progressively thinner and by the time these blood vessels reach the subepithelial surface of the endometrium, they consist only of endothelial cells (Abberton *et al.*, 1999). (From Strauss and Coutifaris, 1999.)

and their secretory activity reaches a maximum around 6 days after ovulation. These molecules are thought to supply the conceptus with essential nutritional and regulatory molecules during and after implantation (Burton *et al.*, 2002). At the same time, progesterone stimulates increased expression of two potent angiogenic factors: angiogenin in stromal cells and VEGF in stromal cells and neutrophils associated with microvessel walls (Gargett *et al.*, 2001; Ma *et al.*, 2001). As illustrated in Figure 6.9, by the mid-secretory phase, a subepithelial capillary plexus has formed into a complex network of vessels, and the newly regrown arterioles become increasingly more spiral as they lengthen more rapidly

than the endometrium thickens (Gargett *et al.*, 2001; Strauss and Coutifaris, 1999).

Pre-decidualization

During the secretory phase, stromal cells synthesize and release a growing number of new matrix proteins together with surface expression of their receptors, including laminin, fibronectin and integrins, while the earlier cross-linking collagen fibrils are degraded. This process of matrix remodelling creates a looser and more soluble structure and, from the mid-secretory phase onwards, stromal cells also express a variety of regulatory peptides that are involved in cell replication and

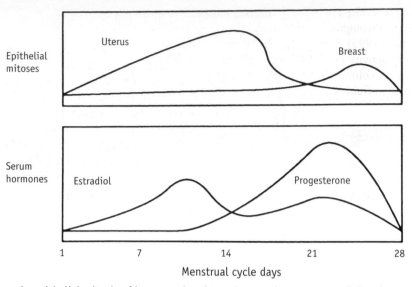

Figure 6.10 Changes in epithelial mitosis of breast and endometrium, and serum oestradiol and progesterone levels during the menstrual cycle. (From Yen, 1999.)

haemostasis. Stromal tissue undergoes further differentiation, and individual cells become larger and oedematous, which contributes to the overall thickening of the endometrium.

From the late secretory phase, further changes occur within the endometrium that are regulated by relaxin, progesterone and leptin. The endometrial stroma undergoes a process of *decidualization*, as it synthesizes a number of hormones and other molecules that provide an appropriate nutritive, regulatory and immunoprotective environment during embryo formation (Gonzalez *et al.*, 2003; Lane *et al.*, 1994; Starkey, 1993).

The cervix and vagina

There are significant changes to the cervix and vagina throughout the cycle, and these are designed to facilitate the passage of spermatozoa. During the follicular part of the cycle, under the effect of oestradiol, the muscles of the cervix relax, causing the cervical os to dilate slightly (to around 3–4 mm) at the time of ovulation. The epithelial cells begin to secret clear watery and 'stretchable' mucus, mid-cycle.

Lined with stratified squamous epithelium, the vagina is also responsive to oestrogens and progesterone. During the follicular phase, vaginal cells proliferate and begin to accumulate glycogen, which is fermented to lactic acid by the normal bacterial flora.

This provides a slightly acid environment, which acts as an anti-infective agent. During sexual excitation, the acidity of vaginal fluid is partly neutralized by the increased blood flow to the pelvic region, and this alters the pH, making it more receptive for the ejaculated sperm.

The mammary gland

The female mammary gland undergoes a surge of cell division during puberty and a cyclical pattern of proliferation and involution until the age of approximately 35 years. During this period, hormonally induced increases in cell proliferation and apoptosis do not return the glands to the starting point of the previous cycle but provide for a cumulative budding of new lobules (Vorherr, 1974: 1–18). During each cycle, episodes of increased mitosis and apoptosis follow a contrasting pattern to that of the endometrium (Fig. 6.10). Mammary epithelium shows decreased DNA synthesis and mitotic divisions during the first half of the cycle and maximal proliferation that peaks during the luteal phase of the cycle and is followed by a shorter period of increased apoptosis (Russo and Russo, 1987: 78–79). A contrasting pattern of cellular activity in uterine and mammary epithelium is reflected in cyclical differences in steroid hormone receptor concentrations in the two organs of reproduction. Mammary tissue receptors for oestrogen, like those in the endometrium, decline during the second half of the cycle; those for progesterone remain fairly constant throughout both phases of the cycle (Soderqvist *et al.*, 1993). During the second half of the cycle, secretory activity may also occur together with increases in breast volume, because of a hormonally induced increase in fluid retention.

Reflective Activity 6.1

Review the information you have gleaned from this chapter and consider how you would use this knowledge in your daily practice.

CONCLUSION

Historically, a regular menstrual flow has been viewed as a cardinal sign of female fertility, since it provides direct evidence of a regular pattern of tissue reconstruction in the endometrial lining of the uterus, in preparation for the fertile ovum. It is useful for the midwife to understand the complex mechanisms and hormonal influences that synchronize this activity with key developments within the ovaries and mammary glands across the cycle. This information will assist in calculating conception dates, and in helping the woman to understand preparatory changes for pregnancy and lactation.

KEY POINTS

- The normal menstrual cycle can indicate general health, well-being and nutritional status of the woman.
- During each cycle, the uterus facilitates reception, maturation and transport of spermatozoa from the vagina to the fallopian tube, while the inner layers of the uterus prepare to receive and directly nourish the blastocyst.
- An understanding of the complex neurohormonal relationships during the normal cycle will assist in recognizing the normal cycle and in appreciating the simultaneous changes in other organ systems.

REFERENCES

Abberton, K.M., Taylor, N.H., Healy, D.L. *et al.* (1999) Vascular smooth muscle cell proliferation in arterioles of the human endometrium. *Human Reproduction* **14**: 1072–1079.

Amsterdam, A. & Linder, H.R. (1984) Localisation of gonadotrophin receptors in the gonads. In: Motta, P.M. (ed) *Ultrastructure of Endocrine Cells and Tissues*, pp. 255–260. The Hague: Martinus Nijhoff Publishers.

Amsterdam, A., Gold, R.S., Hosokawa, K. *et al.* (1999) Cross talk among multiple signalling pathways controlling ovarian cell death. *Trends in Endocrinology and Metabolism* **10**(7): 255–262.

Anderson-Hunt, M. & Dennerstein, L. (1994) Increased female sexual response after oxytocin. *British Medical Journal* **309**: 929–910.

Antczak, M., Van Blerkom, J. & Clark, A. (1997) A novel mechanism of vascular endothelial growth factor, leptin and transforming growth factor-B2 sequestration in a subpopulation of human ovarian follicles. *Human Reproduction* **12**(10): 2226–2234.

Aplin, J.D. (1989) Cellular biochemistry of the endometrium. In: Wynn, R.M. & Jollie, W.P. (eds) *Biology of the Uterus*, pp. 89–119. New York: Plenum.

Armstrong, D.G. & Webb, R. (1997) Ovarian follicular dominance: the role of intraovarian growth factors and novel proteins. *Reviews of Reproduction* **2**: 139–146.

Baerwald, A.R., Adams, G.P. & Pierson, R.A. (2003) Characterization of ovarian follicular wave dynamics in women. *Biology of Reproduction* **69**: 1023–1031.

Baker, S.J. & Spears, N. (1999) The role of intra-ovarian interactions in the regulation of follicle dominance. *Human Reproduction Update* **5**(2): 153–165.

Bakos, O., Lundkvist, O. & Bergh, T. (1993) Transvaginal sonographic evaluation of endometrial growth and texture in spontaneous ovulatory cycles – a descriptive study. *Human Reproduction* **142**: 142–157.

Behrens, O., Mascheko, H., Kupsch. E. *et al.* (1995) Oxytocin receptors in human ovaries during the menstrual cycle. In: Ivell, R. & Russell, J. (eds) *Oxytocin*, pp. 485–486. New York: Plenum Press.

Berne, R.M. & Levy, M.N. (eds) *Principles of Physiology*. St Louis: Mosby Year Book.

Brannstrom, M., Mikuni, M. & Peterson, C.M. (1996) Ovulation-associated intraovarian events. In: Filicori, M. & Flamigni, C. (eds) *The Ovary: Regulation Dysfunction and Treatment*, pp. 113–123. Amsterdam: Elsevier Science.

Brumsted, J.R. & Riddick, D.H. (1992) Prolactin and the human menstrual cycle. *Seminars in Reproductive Endocrinology* 10(3): 220–227.

Buccione, R., Schroeder, A.C. & Eppig, J.J. (1990) Interactions between somatic cells and germ cells throughout mammalian oogenesis. *Biology of Reproduction* 43: 543–547.

Bujan, L., Daudlin, M., Charlet, J-P. *et al.* (2000) Increase in scrotal temperature in car drivers. *Human Reproduction* 15(6): 1355–1357.

Burton, G.J., Watson, A.L., Hempstock, J. *et al.* (2002) Uterine glands provide histotrophic nutrition for the human fetus during the first trimester of pregnancy. *Journal of Clinical Endocrinology and Metabolism* 87(6): 2954–2959.

Calogero, A.E., Burrello, N., Ossino, A.M. *et al.* (1996) Interaction between prolactin and catecholamines on hypothalamic GnRH release in vitro. *Journal of Endocrinology* 151: 269–275.

Canipari, R. (2000) Oocyte–granulosa cell interactions. *Human Reproduction Update* 6(3): 279–289.

Casan, E.M., Raga, F. & Polan, M.L. (1999) GnRH mRNA and protein expression in human preimplantation embryos. *Molecular Human Reproduction* 5(3): 234–239.

Casan, E.M., Raga, F., Bonilla-Musoles, F. *et al.* (2000) Human oviductal gonadotrophin-releasing hormone: possible implication in fertilization, early embryonic development, and implantation. *Journal of Clinical Endocrinology Metabolism* 85(4): 1377–1381.

Chapman, A.B., Abraham, W.T., Zamudio, S. *et al.* (1998) Temporal relationships between hormonal and hemodynamic changes in early pregnancy. *Kidney International* 54: 2056–2063.

Chappell, P.E. & Levine, J.E. (2000) Stimulation of gonadotrophin-releasing hormone surges by estrogen. I Role of hypothalamic progesterone receptors. *Endocrinology* 141(4): 1477–1485.

Chen, L., Wert, S.E., Hendrix, E.M. *et al.* (1990) Hyaluronic acid synthesis and gap junction endocytosis are necessary for normal expansion of the cumulus mass. *Molecular Reproduction and Development* 26: 236–247.

Cheng, K.W., Nathwani, P.S. & Leung, P.C.K. (2000) Regulation of human gonadotrophin-releasing hormone receptor gene expression in placental cells. *Endocrinology* 141(7): 2340–2349.

Cohen, I.T., Sherwin, B.B. & Fleming, A.S. (1987) Food cravings, mood, and the menstrual cycle. *Hormones and Behavior* 21: 457–470.

Dockery, P., Warren, M.A., Li, T.C. *et al.* (1990) A morphometric study of the human endometrial stroma during the peri-implantation period. *Human Reproduction* 5(5): 494–498.

Downing, S.J. & Hollingsworth, M. (1993) Action of relaxin on uterine contractions – a review. *Journal of Reproduction & Fertility* 99: 275–282.

Drobnis, E.Z. & Overstreet, J.W. (1992) Natural history of mammalian spermatozoa in the female reproductive tract. *Oxford Reviews of Reproductive Biology* 14: 1–45.

Eppig, J.J., Wigglesworth, K. & Pendola, F. (1997) Murine oocytes suppress expression of luteinizing hormone receptor messenger ribonucleic acid by granulosa cells. *Biology of Reproduction* 56: 976–984.

Evans, J.J. (1996) Oxytocin and the control of LH. *Journal of Endocrinology* 151: 169–174.

Evans, J.J. (1999) Modulation of gonadotrophin levels by peptides acting at the anterior pituitary gland. *Endocrine Reviews* 20: 46–67.

Evans, J.J., Pragg, F.L. & Mason, D.R. (2001) Release of luteinizing hormone from the anterior pituitary gland in vitro can be concurrently regulated by at least three peptides: gonadotrophin-releasing hormone, oxytocin and neuropeptide Y. *Neuroendocrinology* 73: 408–416.

Ferin, M. (1999) Stress and the reproductive cycle. *Journal of Clinical Endocrinology and Metabolism* 84(6): 1768–1774.

Ferrara, N. & Davis-Smith, T. (1997) The biology of vascular endothelial growth factor. *Endocrine Reviews* 18: 4–25.

Forman, M.R., Beecher, G.R., Muesing, R. *et al.* (1996) The fluctuation of plasma carotenoid concentrations by phase of the menstrual cycle: a controlled diet study. *American Journal of Clinical Nutrition* 64: 559–565.

Fraser, I.S. & Peek, M.J. (1992) Effects of exogenous hormones on endometrial capillaries. In: Alexander, N.J. & d'Arcangues, C. (eds) *Steroid Hormones and Uterine Bleeding*, pp. 67–79. Washington: AAAS Press.

Geva, E. & Jaffe, R.B. (2000) Role of vascular endothelial growth factor in ovarian physiology and pathology. *Fertility and Sterility* 74(3): 429–438.

Gipson, I.K., Moccia, R., Spurr-Michaud, S. *et al.* (2001) The Amount of MUC5B in cervical mucus peaks at midcycle. *Journal of Clinical Endocrinology and Metabolism* 86(2): 594–600.

Gougeon, A. (1986) Dynamics of follicular growth in human: a model from preliminary results. *Human Reproduction* 1(2): 81–87.

Gougeon, A. (1996) Regulation of ovarian follicular development in primates: facts and hypotheses. *Endocrine Reviews* 17(2): 121–55.

Grinsted, J., Kjer, J.J., Blendstrup, K. *et al.* (1985) Is low temperature of the follicular fluid prior to ovulation necessary for normal oocyte development. *Fertility and Sterility* 43: 34–39.

Gargett, C.E., Lederman, F., Heryonto, B. *et al.* (2001) Focal vascular endothelial growth factor correlates with angiogenesis in human endometrium. Role of intravascular neutrophils. *Human Reproduction* 16(6): 1065–1075.

Gonzalez, R.R., Leary, K., Petrozza, J.C. *et al.* (2003) Leptin regulation of interleukin-1 system in human endometrial cells. *Molecular Human Reproduction* 9(3): 151–158.

Herbison, A.E. (1997) Noradrenergic regulation of cyclic GnRH secretion. *Reviews of Reproduction* **2**: 1–6.

Herbison, A.E. & Pape, J-R. (2001) New evidence for estrogen receptors in gonadotrophin-releasing hormone neurons. *Frontiers in Neuroendocrinology* **22**: 292–308.

Hirshfield, A.N. (1991) Development of follicles in the mammalian ovary. *International Review of Cytology* **124**: 43–101.

Hodgen, G.D. (1982) The dominant ovarian follicle. *Fertility and Sterility* **38**(3): 281–300.

Imagawa, W., Yang, J., Guzman, R. *et al.* (1994) Control of mammary gland development. In: Knobil, E. & Neill, J.D. (eds) *The Physiology of Reproduction,* pp. 1033–1063. New York: Raven Press.

Irwin, J.C. & Giudice, L.C. (1998) Decidua. In: Knobin, E. & Neill, J.D. (eds) *Encyclopedia of Reproduction,* Vol. 1, pp. 823–835. Academic Press: San Diego.

Iwahashi, M., Muragaki, Y., Ooshima, A. *et al.* (2000) Type VI collagen expression during growth of human ovarian follicles. *Fertility & Sterility* **74**(2): 343–347.

Johnson, M.H. & Everitt, B.J. (1995) *Essential Reproduction,* 4th edn. Oxford: Blackwell Scientific.

Johnson, M.H. & Everitt, B.J. (2000) *Essential Reproduction,* 5th edn. Oxford: Blackwell Scientific.

Kunz, G., Noe, M., Herbertz, M. *et al.* (1998) Uterine peristalsis during the follicular phase of the menstrual cycle: effects of oestrogen, antioestrogen and oxytocin. *Human Reproduction Update* **4**(5): 647–654.

Lane, B., Oxberry, W., Mazella, J. *et al.* (1994) Decidualization of human endometrial stromal cells in vitro: effects of progestin and relaxin on the ultrastructure and production of decidual secretory proteins. *Human Reproduction* **9**(2): 259–266.

Liu, H.C., Pyrgiotis, E., Davis, O. *et al.* (1995) Active corpus luteum function at pre-, peri- and postimplantation is essential for a viable pregnancy. *Early Pregnancy: Biology and Medicine* **1**: 281–287.

Ma, W., Tan, J., Matsumoto, H. *et al.* (2001) Adult tissue angiogenesis: evidence for negative regulation by estrogen in the uterus. *Molecular Endocrinology* **15**(11): 1983–1992.

Maas, J.W., Groothuis, P.G., Dunselman, G.A. *et al.* (2001) Endometrial angiogenesis throughout the human menstrual cycle. *Human Reproduction* **16**(8): 1557–1561.

Meduri, G., Charnaux, N., Driancourt, M-A. *et al.* (2002) Follicle-stimulating hormone receptors in oocytes? *Journal of Clinical Endocrinology and Metabolism* **87**(5): 2266–2276.

Meinecke, B. & Meinecke-Tillmann, S. (1993) Effects of alpha-amanitin on nuclear maturation of porcine oocytes in vitro. *Journal of Reproduction and Fertility.* **98**: 195–201.

Moor, R.M., Nagai, T. & Gandolfi, F. (1990) Somatic cell interactions in early mammalian development. In: Evers, J.L.H. & Heineman, M.J. (eds) *From Ovulation to Implantation,* pp. 177–191. Amsterdam: Excerpta Medica.

Motlik, J. & Kubelka, M. (1990) Cell-cycle aspects of growth and maturation of mammalian oocytes. *Molecular Reproduction and Development* **27**: 366–375.

Niswender, G.D., Juengel, J.L., Silva, P.J. *et al.* (2000) Mechanisms controlling the function and life span of the corpus luteum. *Physiological Reviews* **80**(1): 1–29.

Norman, R.J. & Clark, A.M. (1998) Obesity and reproductive disorders: a review. *Reproduction, Fertility and Development* **10**: 55–63.

Ohbuchi, H., Nagai, K., Amaguchi, M. *et al.* (1995) Endothelin-1 and big endothelin-1 increase in human endometrium during menstruation. *American Journal of Obstetrics and Gynecology* **173**(5): 1483–1490.

Rogers, P.A. (1996) Structure and function of endometrial blood vessels. *Human Reproduction Update* **2**(1): 57–62.

Russo, J. & Russo, I.H. (1987) Development of the human mammary gland. In: Neville, M.C. & Daniel, C.W. (eds) *The Mammary Gland,* pp. 67–93. New York: Plenum Press.

Salustri, A., Hascall, V.C., Camaioni, A. *et al.* (1993) Oocyte–granulosa interactions. In: Adashi, E.Y. & Leung, P.C.K. (eds) *The Ovary,* pp. 209–225. New York: Raven Press.

Salustri, A., Camaioni, A., Giacomo, M.D. *et al.* (1999) Hyaluronan and proteoglycans in ovarian follicles. *Human Reproduction Update* **5**(4): 293–301.

Santoro, N.F., Goldsmith, L.T. & Weiss, G. (1994) Hormone interactions of the corpus luteum. In: Barnea, E.R., Check, J.H, Grudzinskas, J.G. *et al.* (eds) *Implantation and Early Pregnancy in Humans,* pp. 123–135. New York: Parthenon Publishing.

Schwartz, J. (2000) Intercellular communication in the anterior pituitary. *Endocrine Reviews* **21**(5): 488–513.

Seifer, D.B., Feng, B., Shelden, R.M. *et al.* (2002) Brain-derived neurotrophic factor: a novel human ovarian follicular protein. *Journal of Clinical Endocrinology and Metabolism* **87**(2): 655–659.

Shiokawa, S., Yoshimura, Y., Nagamatsu, S. *et al.* (1996) Expression of B1 integrins in human endometrial stromal and decidual cells. *Journal of Clinical Endocrinology and Metabolism* **81**(4): 1533–1440.

Smith, S.K. (2000) Angiogenesis and implantation. *Human Reproduction* **15** (Suppl. 6): 59–66.

Smith, S.K. (2001) Angiogenesis and reproduction. *British Journal of Obstetrics and Gynaecology* **108**: 777–783.

Smith, M.J. & Jennes, L. (2001) Neural signals that regulate GnRH neurones directly during the oestrus cycle. *Reproduction* **122**: 1–10.

Soderqvist, G., von Schoultz, B., Tani, E. *et al.* (1993) Estrogen and progesterone receptor content in the breast epithelial cells from healthy women during the menstrual cycle. *American Journal of Obstetrics and Gynecology* **168**(3): 847–849.

Solomon, S.J., Kurzer, M.S. & Calloway, D.H. (1982) Menstrual cycle and basal metabolic rate in women. *American Journal of Clinical Nutrition* **36**: 611–615.

Starkey, P.M. (1993) The decidua and factors controlling placentation. In: Redman, C.W.G., Sargent, I.L. & Starkey, P.M. (eds) *The Human Placenta,* pp. 362–413. Oxford: Blackwell Scientific.

Stock, S. & Osterlund, C. (1998) Expression of the oxytocin receptor and oxytocin gene in human oocytes and preimplantation embryos. In: Zingg, H., Bourque, C.W. & Bichet, D.G. (eds) *Vasopressin and Oxytocin,* pp. 323–324. New York: Plenum Press.

Strauss, J. & Coutifaris, C. (1999) The endometrium and myometrium: regulation and dysfunction. In: Yen, S.S.C., Jaffe, R.B. & Barbieri, R.L. (eds) *Reproductive Endocrinology,* pp. 218–256. Philadelphia: W.B. Saunders.

Talbot, P.D., Shur, B.D. & Myles, D.G. (2003) Cell adhesion and fertilization: steps in oocyte transport, sperm–zona pellucida interactions, and sperm–egg fusion. *Biology of Reproduction* **68**: 1–9.

Valdes, G., Germain, A.M., Corthorn, J. *et al.* (2001) Urinary vasodilator and vasoconstrictor angiotensins during menstrual cycle, pregnancy, and lactation. *Endocrine* **16**(2): 117–122.

Vokes, T.J., Weiss, N.M., Schreiber, J. *et al.* (1988) Osmoregulation of thirst and vasopressin during normal menstrual cycle. *American Journal of Physiology* **254**(23): R641–R647.

Vorherr, H. (1974) Development of the female breast. In: Vorherr, H. (ed) *The Breast,* pp. 1–18. New York: Academic Press.

Wasserman, P.M. (1996) Oogenesis: from primordial germ cells to eggs. In: Adashi, E.Y., Rock, J.A. & Rosenwaks, Z. (eds) *Reproductive Endocrinology, Surgery and Technology,* Vol. 1, pp. 341–357. Philadelphia: Lippincott-Raven.

Webb, P. (1986) 24-hour energy expenditure and the menstrual cycle. *American Journal of Clinical Nutrition* **44**: 614–619.

Yen, S.S.C. (1999) The human menstrual cycle: neuroendocrine regulation. In: Yen, S.S.C., Jaffe, R.B. & Barbieri, R.L. (eds) *Reproductive Endocrinology,* pp. 191–217. Philadelphia: W.B. Saunders.

Yen, S.S.C. & Jaffe, R.B. (eds) (1991) *Reproductive Endocrinology.* Philadelphia: W.B. Saunders.

Zackrisson, U., Mikuni, M., Peterson, M. *et al.* (2000) Evidence of the involvement of blood flow-regulated mechanisms in the ovulatory process of the rat. *Human Reproduction* **15**(2): 264–272.

FURTHER READING

Ingram, C.D., Terenzi, M.G., Housman, Q.B. *et al.* (1995) Coordination of the central actions of oxytocin in the peripartum period. In: Saito, T., Kurokawa, K. & Yoshida, S. (eds) *Neurohypophysis: Recent Progress of Vasopressin and Oxytocin Research,* pp. 339–349. Oxford: Elsevier Science.

McGee, E.A. & Hsueh, A.J. (2000) Initial and cyclic recruitment of ovarian follicles. *Endocrine Reviews* **21**(2): 200–214.

Rodway, M.R. & Rao, C.V. (1995) A novel perspective on the role of human chorionic gonadotrophin during pregnancy and in gestational trophoblastic disease. *Early Pregnancy: Biology and Medicine* **1**: 176–187.

7

Sexuality

Karen Jackson

LEARNING OUTCOMES

After reading this chapter you will be able to:

- cite a basic definition of 'sexuality'
- outline the psychological, social and physiological implications of sex and sexuality during pregnancy, childbirth and afterwards
- describe the implications of pregnancy and childbirth for women who are survivors of sexual

abuse, women who have undergone female genital mutilation and for women who are lesbians
- list some of the factors that may impact on sex and sexuality for women who are breastfeeding.

Reflective Activity 7.1

Before you start reading this chapter, think of the word 'sexuality'; what does it mean? Write down a simple definition, or words that you would associate with 'sexuality'.

Did you find the task easy? If not, why do you think 'sexuality' is difficult to define?

SEXUALITY

The word 'sexuality' is scattered liberally throughout contemporary sexual health literature, but what does sexuality actually mean. The word itself did not come into being until the modern era, and many authors are reluctant to confine it to a simple definition. This may well be because sexuality is fundamentally dynamic. It has different meanings culturally, its definition changes throughout history, and individuals' feelings and values concerning their sexuality alter as they gain more life experience.

Siectus (cited by Lion, 1982: 8) embraces sexuality as a concept which is open to transmutation as 'all those aspects of the human being that relate to being a boy or girl, woman or man, and is an entity subject to lifelong dynamic change. Sexuality reflects our human character not solely our genital nature'. This definition

encompasses the complete range of human experience, demonstrating clearly that sexuality is more than overt sexual behaviour (Pratt, 2000).

The word 'sex' is usually employed to mean the act of having sex or to distinguish between the 'sexes', i.e. male or female. Gender is the name given to socially and culturally defined characteristics of the sexes, i.e. masculinity and femininity.

PUBERTY AND TEENAGE PREGNANCY

In adolescence, humans will normally undergo puberty. The preparation of the body for puberty takes place long before any outward changes are obvious; however, it is these body changes, when the male or female is becoming sexually mature, that spark a whole range of powerful emotions. These may include fear of becoming a sexual being and/or being capable of conceiving a child, embarrassment as this change in physical appearance becomes evident, feelings of loss of childhood. Some children may welcome this 'growing-up' phase, whilst others will become confused and even rebellious.

Even when the female commences the menarche, she is likely to remain infertile for an unspecified number of cycles, but at some point she will become fertile, and it is this aspect of adolescent sexuality that is a major concern. It has been suggested that there are higher levels of complications and adverse outcomes, such as pregnancy-induced hypertension, preterm birth and perinatal mortality, associated with adolescent pregnancies (Orvos *et al.*, 1999). However, some authors report no greater risks of complications in adolescents than in older women, but state that there are many psychosocial factors specific to teenagers, such as poor social and economic standing, which must be addressed (Edwards, 2000).

The UK continues to have the highest teenage conception rate in western Europe. Evidence suggests that there are two main ways in which teenage conception rates may be tackled. The first is school-based sex education, which can be especially effective when linked to the second, the provision of accessible and confidential contraceptive services based on local need. The problem is the fallacy that such measures promote promiscuity, a dangerous myth that is not supported by studies examining the attitudes of other countries to sexuality (Chambers *et al.*, 2000).

Reflective Activity 7.2

A woman who has just had confirmation that she is 8 weeks' pregnant asks about sex during pregnancy. Which of the following statements would you agree with?

- Sex is safe for most couples throughout pregnancy
- Sex should be confined to the second trimester of pregnancy only
- All forms of sexual activity are safe throughout pregnancy
- There are certain clinical contraindications to sex in pregnancy
- Sexual activity generally decreases as pregnancy progresses

---

SEX DURING PREGNANCY

Sex during pregnancy has historically been shrouded in myth, misconceptions and old wives' tales. The advice offered during traditional British antenatal care has been one of abstention, without any evidence to substantiate this stance.

During pregnancy many couples are fearful of continuing their sexual relationship. They may feel that they may somehow provoke miscarriage, premature labour or damage the fetus; some men have expressed fear of breaking the 'bag of waters' (Kitzinger, 1985). Couples can be reassured that this is not the case.

The overriding message from most well-conducted studies is that sex during pregnancy for the vast majority of women is safe and does not lead to any increase in complications (Enkin *et al.*, 2000), although male superior position (Ekwo *et al.*, 1993) and a vagina colonized with specific microorganisms, e.g. *Trichomonas vaginalis* (Read and Klebanoff, 1993), have both been associated with preterm birth. More studies are required in this area to provide up-to-date information.

There are a few definite or relative contraindications to different sexual practices or sexual intercourse during pregnancy. Forceful blowing of air into the vagina during oral sex is an absolute contraindication as this may lead to fatal air embolism (Aston, 1997; Lumley and Astbury, 1989). The insertion of a foreign body into the vagina may cause damage to the internal structures and introduce infection (Walton, 1994). Placenta praevia, vaginal bleeding, history of premature birth and rupture of membranes are often cited as clinical reasons to avoid sex during pregnancy (Aston, 1997).

Whilst sex can be enjoyed by couples throughout the whole of pregnancy, other factors may play an important role. Change of body image, tiredness, breast changes, backache and frequency of micturition are some of the things that can affect a pregnant woman's sexuality (Aston, 1997). There are many accounts that give a very negative view of sexuality and pregnancy. Kitzinger (1985) states that some women have a distorted view of their bodies during pregnancy; they feel bigger than they really are and think that their partners must find them ugly, when in fact they often delight in pregnant women and find their physical changes exciting and beautiful.

Conversely some women have a very positive 'body image' during pregnancy. They feel incredibly attractive and womanly. It is viewed as the ultimate expression of femininity. It is an eminently powerful symbol of potency and fertility.

Physiological hormonal changes during pregnancy means that oestrogens and progesterone act together to produce marked pelvic vasocongestion, which occurs as a result of increased vascularity and venous stasis. The results can mean a heightened manifestation of all aspects of sexual intercourse including orgasm (Aston, 1997). For some, this may be the first time that they experience orgasm (Walton, 1994). For others, however, vasocongestion may predispose pregnant women to discomfort during sexual intercourse (Aston, 1997).

It is often assumed that there is a linear decrease in sexual activity as pregnancy progresses but for some women, sexual activity may well increase during the second trimester. This may be due to the disorders of pregnancy subsiding and the woman developing a sense of well-being, but it is also well recognized that sex diminishes during the third trimester (Frohlich *et al.*, 1990), most probably owing to the discomfort and mechanics of having sex with a greatly enlarged abdomen. Alternative positions to the missionary position, such as man behind woman or 'spooning', could be explored, or the woman sitting or kneeling on top of the man. Other non-penetrative options such as self or mutual masturbation, oral sex, fondling or massage or purely kissing and cuddling may also be adopted (Walton, 1994). Keeping clear channels of communication open is the most important aspect of maintaining an intimate sexual or non-sexual relationship.

SEXUALITY AND LABOUR

Labour is usually synonymous with anxiety, discomfort and pain. It is not often viewed as being a 'sexual' experience. It is clear when reading literature in this area that for some women and their partners it can be an intensely pleasurable and sexual experience. The sounds a woman makes during contractions, the organs that are used in the process of childbirth, the overwhelming energies and powers that are at work during labour, are all intimately related to sex and sexuality (Aston, 1997; Gaskin, 1990; Kitzinger, 1985; Williams, 1996). Kitzinger (1985: 210) describes it thus: 'the most intensely sexual feeling a woman ever experiences, as strong as orgasm, even more compelling than orgasm.' In her book *Spiritual Midwifery*, Gaskin (1990) quotes a number of women's and men's experiences of the sexual nature of childbirth. One woman recounts her birth experience with her husband: 'My rushes (contractions) hardly felt heavy at all, but I knew they must be because I was opening up. We just kept making out and rubbing each other. We got to places we had forgotten we could get to ... going through the birthing I felt his love very strong. It was like getting married all over again' (Gaskin, 1990: 53). Rabuzzi (1994) cites examples of other couples' erotic experiences of labour. One husband of a woman having a home birth said: 'The birth was not only painless, but very pleasurable. We had never read about this aspect ...'. He goes on to describe the noises his wife made whilst the baby's head was crowning as being 'orgasmic' and ends with: 'what a long way from the pain and agony of conventional myth'.

If labour can be such a sensual and gratifying experience, it may be a cultural or contextual aspect that makes it generally viewed negatively. It is suggested by some that the scientific and technological procedures have taken childbirth out of the hands of women and set it in the context of the powerful male-dominated institution of the hospital (Cosslett, 1994; Williams, 1996) where everything is controlled, the medical model's ultimate goal being 'safety' whatever the cost. In contrast, the natural childbirth discourse is focused on the power of the woman, which is more in evidence in home births (Cosslett, 1994; Williams, 1996). Midwives would argue that 'safety' and 'satisfaction' are both achievable.

Nipple stimulation is known to produce oxytocin, and therefore can be performed by the woman or her partner to attempt to initiate or augment labour naturally. Privacy will of course be required if she wishes to try this activity.

WOMEN REQUIRING SPECIAL CARE

There are some groups of women who may need specialized care and attention during pregnancy, labour, childbirth and afterwards.

Reflective Activity 7.3

Listed below is a group of women who you may well care for in clinical practice:

- Anne, a woman who is a survivor of sexual abuse
- Lydia, a pregnant lesbian
- Saadah, who underwent female genital mutilation as a child
- Katie, a woman who has a sexually transmitted infection
- Bernie, a woman who is breastfeeding.

What are the issues concerning sexuality for each of these woman?

It is important not to stereotype these women. All will quite probably have similar issues, but in addition, Anne may have to deal with reactivated memories of the abuse; Lydia may have to deal with homophobia and sometimes hostile behaviour; Saadah may be terrified of labour and birth; Katie may face stigma and labelling of being promiscuous; Bernie may have conflict between being a nursing mother and a sexual being.

Survivors of sexual abuse

Many authors have recognized that memories of abuse, even those which have been partially or wholly repressed, may be triggered by pregnancy and childbirth (Courtois and Riley, 1992; Kitzinger, 1990). The change in body image, the submission to physical contact, the feelings of powerlessness are all factors which are likely to make the survivor regress back to times when she encountered similar susceptibilities.

Women who have been previously sexually abused may display a range of behaviours as follows: extreme anxiety over intimate examinations; needing to be in complete control; dissociating themselves from the experience; or being quite uninhibited, engaging freely in sexual banter (Rhodes and Hutchinson, 1994). Some of the styles exhibited by sexual abuse survivors may also be adopted by women who have not been abused, but in the former group the behaviour may appear extreme.

Control has been identified as one of the key factors that is of grave importance to women who have been sexually abused (Parratt, 1994). Therefore keeping women well informed, ensuring that they are made part of the decision-making process and obtaining informed consent for all procedures are absolute requirements.

Caring for the lesbian client

It is becoming more common for lesbian couples to fulfil the desire to become parents by whatever means necessary. More and more midwives are coming into contact with lesbian couples and it is therefore imperative that the needs of these clients are recognized. Many lesbian writers and writers who have explored lesbian issues identify that lesbians as a group are largely ignored and as a consequence become invisible in texts discussing women's health (Wilton, 1996).

Midwives can do much to ensure that a lesbian's experience of pregnancy and childbirth is a positive and empowering one. They can attain this by being knowledgeable about lesbian sexuality, by using non-heterosexist language, by giving appropriate advice, by being non-judgemental and by rejecting socially constructed stereotypes (Hastie, 2000).

Female genital mutilation (FGM)

The definition of female genital mutilation 'constitutes all procedures which involve partial or total removal of the external female genitalia or other injury to the female genital organs whether for cultural or any other non-therapeutic reasons' (WHO, 1997).

In the UK it is rare for a midwife to care for a woman who has undergone FGM, apart from in certain parts of London, other large cities and some coastal areas where immigrant communities are found. The practice is deeply rooted in cultural and traditional norms, whilst it is vociferously opposed by human rights activists denouncing it as child abuse. It is not within the remit of this section to debate the political issues, but it is a health issue which has profound implications for women's short- and long-term physical, social and psychosexual well-being (Raynor and Morgan, 2000).

The impact that FGM has on a woman's sexuality and body image should not be underestimated. It also has an effect on the progress of labour and birth, e.g. it is highly likely that an episiotomy will be required. However, following delivery, repair of the genital area can only be performed for reasons connected with the labour or birth. It is illegal to repair the labia in such a way that intercourse is difficult or impossible (Raynor and Morgan, 2000). Midwives caring for these women should be knowledgeable about the practice and be able to advise and counsel women, ideally antenatally, concerning their care during labour and birth so they can ensure that they are part of the decision-making process.

Sexually transmitted infections (STIs)

There are numerous sexually transmittable infections that pregnant women may carry, for example HIV, hepatitis B, genital herpes, gonorrhoea, etc., and for this reason safe sex should be adopted and the infection treated if possible. HIV testing is now offered to all pregnant women in the UK. This means that should the result be positive, women have the choice to continue with the pregnancy or have the pregnancy terminated. If the woman chooses to continue, appropriate treatment at all stages throughout pregnancy and childbirth can dramatically reduce the number of HIV-infected infants born to these women (Lyall et al., 1998).

Quite apart from the often traumatic biophysical effects of STIs, the psychosocial effects are profound, and the repercussions on sexuality are immense. Women are often put off being screened for STIs, fundamentally because they feel that there is still a stigma attached to having an STI and they fear they may be labelled as being easy and promiscuous.

PATERNAL PRESENCE AT BIRTH

In western cultures there has been a cultural shift from men being virtually excluded from the delivery room, to men being actively encouraged to attend the birth of their child. It is not known what effect paternal presence at birth has on the process of labour or on the subsequent relationship of the couple. It does appear that the presence of a female companion such as a doula can have numerous positive effects on the outcome of labour (Kennell and Klaus, 1991). One dimension of paternal presence at birth, which is rarely discussed, is the possible adverse effects on subsequent sexual relationships. Sex therapists working with sexually dysfunctional couples have discovered that the man's experience of what was for him a traumatic labour and birth has stifled any sexual feelings for his wife/partner (O'Driscoll, 1998).

It is the responsibility of midwives to ensure that the couple realize the importance and immensity of the decision for the man 'to be there or not to be there'. The couple should be encouraged to discuss the issue openly (ideally antenatally), with the pros and cons clearly defined so that they can make an informed decision.

PERINEAL CARE

The perineum plays a major role in sex and sexuality. Perineal trauma is the main perpetrator of postnatal sexual health problems. Each year in the UK, long-term perineal pain can affect around 20% (or 120 750) of women who have sustained perineal trauma (Kettle and Johanson, 2001a). This may impact on a woman's self-image, her sexuality, her relationship with her baby and can ultimately adversely affect the couple's relationship.

There is not the scope within this chapter to discuss all the aspects of care that can improve outcomes for women in terms of preventing, minimizing and treating perineal trauma. However, midwives are well advised to become conversant with the evidence to ultimately reduce this major cause of maternal morbidity (Enkin et al., 2000; Jackson, 2000a, b; Kettle and Johanson, 2001a, b; see Ch. 28).

SEX AFTER CHILDBIRTH

As with sex during pregnancy, many social and cultural taboos surround the issue of sex after childbirth. The main issues appear to be fear of infection and trauma

but there is no evidence to support these possible complications providing that the sexual activity is considerate and gentle (Walton, 1994). The woman herself is therefore the best person to regulate when she is ready to resume sexual intercourse. In the past, there appeared to be an unwritten rule that women should abstain from sex until after the 6-week postnatal check, when the GP could give her the all clear to resume sexual relations. It was assumed that all would be well sexually after this period of time. The reality, however, is quite contrary.

From the limited research conducted in this field, all have found that childbirth causes high levels of sexual morbidity and state that this is not adequately addressed by health professionals (Barrett et al., 2000; Glazener, 1997; National Childbirth Trust et al., 1994).

There are also a number of areas related to sexuality and childbirth that appear to raise important issues for midwives and for women they care for.

It is important that family planning is discussed with the woman soon after the birth; one of the reasons for this is that a woman's fertility can return quite soon after giving birth. The fear of becoming pregnant can diminish desire for sex. A reduced libido postnatally may be an indication of underlying problems within the relationship, or it could be a symptom of postnatal depression. If this is the case, other professionals will need to be involved in giving specialized care and attention.

However, in the majority of cases, sexual problems following childbirth are directly linked to the pregnancy, the labour and birth, or the baby. Midwives and other health professionals involved in childbirth are in a prime position to counsel, guide and support parents with sexual anxieties. Here are some of the more common reasons why there may be a breakdown in sexual relations following the birth of a baby.

Body image

It has been proposed that there is a relationship between body image and sexual satisfaction (Demyttenaere et al., 1995). Many physiological changes occur during pregnancy and childbirth – weight gain, varicose veins, stretch marks and possibly perineal trauma. Whilst some women may feel that such 'landmarks of life' make them somehow more feminine and womanly, for the vast majority of women it is a time when they feel immensely unattractive and therefore undesirable.

These physical alterations in appearance are often compounded by the woman's psychological feelings about her body image. Such feelings, as with body image perceptions during pregnancy, are often distorted and amplified. As one woman explained, 'I kept looking at my disgusting jellified stomach and my huge veiny breasts and thinking how could he possibly want this (Craig, 1993). One study found that most men do still find their wives/partners desirable following the birth of the baby, their craving for sex not wavering significantly (Fischman *et al.*, 1986).

The feelings about being 'mutilated down below' or the fear of being split open with the slightest exertion can lead to sexual dysfunction (Evans, 1992). It may be useful to encourage women to examine their genitals digitally to dispel these fallacies of deformity and fragility (Evans, 1992).

The lover/mother syndrome

The woman may find herself totally infatuated with her new baby. She may immerse herself in her role of 'mother' to such an extent that the father is excluded from her physical and emotional attentions. One mother described it as 'being completely and utterly in love'; she goes on to say that 'if I am separated from my baby for more than 10 minutes, I miss him physically and my breasts start to spurt milk. There's just no room for sex' (Craig, 1993).

Adapting not only to motherhood but adapting to taking on dual roles as a mother and a lover can prove to be extremely difficult. It may be that the man has some sort of abstract fantasies about the woman being a fragile 'madonna', or the fact that his partner has now become a mother awakens memories of his own mother. Sex in these circumstances would be considered as violatory, sacrilegious or even incestuous (Raphael-Leff, 1991).

BREASTFEEDING AND SEXUALITY

The literature surrounding the effect of breastfeeding on sexuality and sexual activity is confusing and largely conflicting. Some found a positive effect on sexual activity (Masters and Johnson, 1966); some found a negative impact (Alder and Bancroft, 1983); and others still found that there was no effect on sexual interest (Reamy and White, 1987).The most up-to-date research further supports the hypothesis that breastfeeding reduces interest in sex (Barrett *et al.*, 2000; Glazener, 1997). From the evidence, no definitive conclusions can be drawn and there need to be further well-conducted studies in this area. Therefore women's sexuality may be affected in any of the ways described and each woman must be cared for, advised and counselled accordingly.

Breastfeeding, sexuality and sexual difficulties

Alder and Bancroft (1983) found that during the early postnatal period, and particularly if the baby is being breastfed, many women report a significant decrease in libido, or a complete loss of interest in sex. There may be several reasons why breastfeeding may interfere with sexual relations:

- The woman's requirements for intimacy are being met by the baby.
- She feels guilty and thrown into conflict about having sexual feelings whilst breastfeeding.
- High prolactin levels and low oestrogen levels may affect libido.
- Fatigue caused by regular feeding day and night.
- The partner's feelings of jealousy towards the baby.
- Milk ejection during intercourse.

Being sexually stimulated by a suckling baby can provoke feelings of confusion and guilt. The woman may feel that she is somehow perverted (Hulme, 1993). It is hardly surprising that breastfeeding as well as sexual intercourse brings about such pleasurable feelings; these basic actions have evolved to secure the survival of the human race (Evans, 1992). The mother should be reassured that breastfeeding is an immensely satisfying experience and one that should be relished.

Milk ejection during intercourse can be alleviated by breastfeeding the baby or expressing milk prior to coitus. Some couples incorporate this into their sexual play (Van Wert, 1996). Providing that both parties are happy with this, there is no physiological reason to discourage such an activity.

Vaginal dryness has been reported, particularly in breastfeeding mothers, possibly because of low oestrogen levels. An appropriate lubricating gel (water based if used in conjunction with condoms) may be used to alleviate the problem. This may be discussed in conjunction with family planning advice, as myths and misconceptions surrounding breastfeeding and contraception still pervade.

THE MENOPAUSE

This is a time of immense change. Initially a woman's fertility will reduce but there will come a time when she is infertile. This, together with the reduction in oestrogen and progesterone, can cause some woman to feel sexually redundant. For others, however, it is a time of sexual liberation; there is no longer the threat of pregnancy or a need for contraception. Hormone replacement therapy may be beneficial for some but not for all. All women undergoing the menopause will need time to adjust, as this will undoubtedly have an effect on their sexuality.

CONCLUSION

Just because a woman is pregnant, in labour, giving birth, or recovering from birth, she does not cease to be a sexual being. The parameters of 'normality' in terms of sexuality are wide, varied and unique to each woman. As the very essence of sexuality is embodied within childbirth, aspects of sexuality should be considered as an integral part of the care that women receive from midwives. Furthermore, midwives should have the knowledge and skills to be able to advise, support, educate and counsel women appropriately. This includes midwives acknowledging their limitations and referring to another health professional when such problems are out of their domain. For most women, the expert, sensitive care from her midwife will be all that is required.

KEY POINTS

- Sex during pregnancy is safe for the majority of women.
- Labour for some women can be an immensely satisfying, sexual experience.
- Sexuality should be an issue considered for all pregnant, labouring and postnatal women, but some women will require special care and attention: survivors of sexual abuse, lesbians, women who have undergone female genital mutilation, breastfeeding mothers.
- Sex following birth should initially be regulated by the woman, i.e. when she feels ready.
- There are wide parameters of sexual normality.

REFERENCES

Alder, E. & Bancroft, J. (1983) Sexual behaviour of lactating women: a preliminary communication. *Journal of Reproductive and Infant Psychology* 1(3): 47–52.

Aston, G. (1997) Sexuality during and after pregnancy. In: Andrews, G. (ed) *Women's Sexual Health*. London: Baillière Tindall.

Barrett, G., Pendry, E., Peacock, J. *et al*. (2000) Women's sexual health after childbirth. *British Journal of Obstetrics and Gynaecology* 107(2): 186–195.

Chambers, R., Wakley, G. & Chambers, S. (2001) *Tackling Teenage Pregnancy*. Abingdon: Radcliffe Medical Press.

Cosslett, T. (1994) *Women Writing Childbirth: Modern Discourses of Motherhood*. Manchester: Manchester University Press.

Courtois, C. & Riley, C. (1992) Pregnancy and childbirth as triggers for abuse memories: implications for care. *Birth* 19(4): 222–223.

Craig, A. (1993) Sex after stitches. Will your love life ever be the same again? *She* September: 130–132.

Demyttenaere, K., Gheldof, M. & Van Assche, F. (1995) Sexuality in the postpartum period: a review. *Current Obstetrics and Gynaecology* 5(2): 81–84.

Edwards, G. (2000) Teenage pregnancies 2. Comparative outcomes. *Practising Midwife* 3(2): 12–15.

Ekwo, E., Gosselink, C., Woolson, R. *et al*. (1993) Coitus late in pregnancy: risk of preterm rupture of amniotic sac membranes. *American Journal of Obstetrics and Gynecology* 1(1): 22–31.

Enkin, M., Keirse, M., Neilson, J. *et al*. (2000) *A Guide to Effective Care in Pregnancy and Childbirth*, 3rd edn. Oxford: Oxford University Press.

Evans, K. (1992) Getting back to nature. *Modern Midwife* 2(1): 14–17.

Fischman, S., Rankin, E., Soeken, K. *et al*. (1986) Changes in sexual relationships in postpartum couples. *Journal of Obstetric, Gynecologic and Neonatal Nursing* 15(1): 58–63.

Frohlich, E., Herz, C., van der Merwe, F. *et al*. (1990) Sexuality during pregnancy and early puerperium and its perception by the pregnant and puerperal woman. *Journal of Psychosomatic Obstetrics and Gynaecology* 11(1): 73–79.

Gaskin, I. (1990) *Spiritual Midwifery*, 3rd edn. Summertown: The Book Publishing Company.

Glazener, C. (1997) Sexual function after childbirth: women's experiences, persistent morbidity and lack of professional recognition. *British Journal of Obstetrics and Gynaecology* 104(3): 330–335.

Hastie, N. (2000) Cultural conceptions: lesbian parenting and midwifery practice. In: Fraser, D. (ed) *Professional studies for midwifery practice*. London: Churchill Livingstone.

Hulme, H. (1993) Grin and bear it. *Nursing Times* 89(6): 66.

Jackson, K.B. (2000a) The bottom line: care of the perineum must be improved. *British Journal of Midwifery* 8(10): 609–613.

Jackson, K.B. (2000b) Postnatal perineal care and the effects on sexuality. *British Journal of Midwifery* 8(12): 739–743.

Kennell, J. & Klaus, M. (1991) Continuous emotional support during labor in a US hospital. A randomised controlled trial. *JAMA* 265(17): 2197–2201.

Kettle, C. & Johanson, R. (2003a) Absorbable synthetic versus catgut suture material for perineal repair (Cochrane review). *The Cochrane Library,* Issue 2. Oxford: Update Software.

Kettle, C. & Johanson, R. (2003b) Continuous versus interrupted sutures for perineal repair (Cochrane review). *The Cochrane Library,* Issue 2. Oxford: Update Software.

Kitzinger, J. (1990) Recalling the pain. *Nursing Times* 86(3): 39–40.

Kitzinger, S. (1985) *Women's Experience of Sex.* London: Penguin.

Lion, E. (ed) (1982) *Human Sexuality in Nursing Process.* New York: John Wiley.

Lumley, J. & Astbury, J. (1989) Advice for pregnancy. In: Chalmers, I., Enkin, M. & Keirse, M. (eds) (1989) *Effective Care in Pregnancy and Childbirth*, Vol. 1. Oxford: Oxford University Press.

Lyall, E., Stainsby, C. *et al.* (1998) Review of uptake of interventions to reduce mother to child transmission of HIV by women who are aware of their HIV status. *British Medical Journal* 316(7127): 268–269.

Masters, W. & Johnson, V. (1966) *Human Sexual Response.* Boston: Little, Brown.

National Childbirth Trust, Victor, C. & Barrett, G. (1994) Is there sex after childbirth? *New Generation* 13(2): 24–25.

O'Driscoll, M. (1998) Midwives discover sex. *Practising Midwife* 1(4): 27–29.

Orvos, H., Nyirati, I. *et al.* (1999) Is adolescent pregnancy associated with adverse perinatal outcome? *Journal of Perinatal Medicine* 27(3): 199–203.

Parratt, J. (1994) The experience of childbirth for survivors of incest. *Midwifery* 10: 26–39.

Pratt, R. (2000) Introduction, sexual health and disease: an international perspective. In: Wilson, H. & McAndrew, S. (eds) *Sexual Health.* London: Baillière Tindall.

Rabuzzi, K. (1994) *Mother with Child.* Indianapolis: Indiana University Press.

Raphael-Leff, J. (1991) *Psychological Processes of Childbearing.* London: Chapman and Hall.

Raynor, M. & Morgan, R. (2000) Female genital mutilation: unveiled and deconstructed. In: Fraser, D. (ed) *Professional studies for midwifery practice.* London: Churchill Livingstone.

Read, J. & Klebanoff, M. (1993) Sexual intercourse during pregnancy and preterm delivery: effects of vaginal microorganisms. *American Journal of Obstetrics and Gynecology* 168(2): 514–519.

Reamy, K. & White, S. (1987) Sexuality in the puerperium: a review. *Archives of Sexual Behaviour* 16(2): 165–186.

Rhodes, N. & Hutchinson, S. (1994) Labour experiences of childhood sexual abuse survivors. *Birth* 21(4): 213–220.

Van Wert, W. (1996) When lovers become parents. *Mothering* 81(Winter): 58–61.

Walton, I. (1994) *Sexuality and Motherhood.* Cheshire: Books for Midwives Press.

Williams, C. (1996) Midwives and sexuality: earth mother or coy maiden? In: Frith, L. (ed) *Ethics and Midwifery. Issues in Contemporary Practice.* Oxford: Butterworth-Heinemann.

Wilton, T. (1996) Caring for the lesbian client: homophobia and midwifery. *British Journal of Midwifery* 4(2): 126–131.

WHO (World Health Organization) (1997) *Female genital mutilation: a joint WHO/UNICEF/UNPA statement.* Geneva: WHO.

FURTHER READING

Walton, I. (1994) *Sexuality and Motherhood.* Cheshire: Books for Midwives Press.
This book is an invaluable resource for midwives, as it is one of very few texts devoted entirely to the relationship between sexuality, pregnancy, childbirth and motherhood.

Andrews, G. (ed) (1997) *Women's Sexual Health.* London: Baillière Tindall.
This book takes a comprehensive look at various aspects of women's sexual health. The chapter by Gillian Aston entitled 'Sexuality during and after pregnancy' will be particularly relevant and interesting to practising midwives.

ADDITIONAL RESOURCES

FORWARD International (Foundation for Women's Health Research and Development)
40 Eastbourne Terrace, London W2 3QR
Tel: 0171 725 2606

Fax: 0171 725 2796
Email: forward@dircon.co.uk
This organization is useful for help and advice on caring for women who have undergone FGM.

National Childbirth Trust (NCT)
Alexandra House, Oldham Terrace, London W3 6NH
Tel: 0181 922 8637

Rape Crisis Foundation
7 Mansfield Road, Nottingham NG1 3GB
Tel: 0115 934 8474
Email: info@rapecrisis.co.uk

Stonewall
16 Clerkenwell Close, London EC1 ROAA
Tel: 0171 336 8860

8

Fertility and its Control

Rosemary Towse

LEARNING OUTCOMES

After reading this chapter you will be able to:

- understand the influence of the psychological effects of childbearing upon the reactions of the woman and her partner in resuming sexual intercourse and the use of contraception
- understand the importance of individual history taking from the woman prior to giving information and advice
- understand the physiological principles of each method of family planning

- evaluate the differing methods of contraception available to women and their partners including:
  - the advantages and disadvantages of the different methods available
  - the importance of accurate advice concerning the timing of resumption of the use of contraception
- know the agencies available for the woman and her partner to seek further information and advice.

Family planning involves more than just the use of contraceptive techniques. Midwives along with other health professionals have an important contribution to make in the reproductive and sexual health of women.

Worldwide there are an estimated 210 million pregnancies per year of which, within developing countries, 36% are unplanned and 20% end in abortion, whilst in the developed countries, 49% are unplanned and 36% end in abortion (Alan Guttmacher Institute, 1999). In England and Wales in 1996 the percentage of conceptions leading to a maternity was 79.3% whilst the number of legal abortions rose to 20.7%. For those under 16 years, the percentage of conceptions in 1996 terminated by abortion was 51.5% (Office for National Statistics, 1997). Britain has one of the highest rates of teenage pregnancies in Europe with 90 000 teenagers becoming pregnant every year, 8000 being under the age of 16 years (SEU, 1999). The Government has set up an action plan to try to reduce these numbers and give better support to these young people (SEU, 1999).

Having an unplanned pregnancy can be a traumatic experience for the woman and her partner and it is therefore important that both have access to information about contraception and the services available to them. This chapter will cover details of the different contraceptive methods and also the midwife's contribution to the contraceptive and sexual care of the mother. Since April 1974, both the family planning services and contraceptives have been provided free under the National Health Service. Couples or individuals requiring family planning advice and supplies may go either to their general practitioner (GP) or to a community or hospital family planning clinic. Women may register with a separate GP from their normal one for contraceptive services. In some areas there is also a domiciliary service for selected clients who for some reason do not attend the clinics. A variety of clinics may be provided, including 'drop-in' clinics for young people as well as the more traditional sessions. Some clinics may employ doctors and nurses who specialize in specific areas such as psychosexual counselling.

Reflective Activity 8.1

What services are available in your local area, both NHS and private? Do all the clinics offer a full range of services? Is there a separate clinic for young people?

If you have a woman or couple who require specialist services, such as psychosexual counselling, where or to whom would you refer? It would be useful to record these details in your resource file or diary for future use.

RESUMING RELATIONSHIPS FOLLOWING CHILDBEARING

Women vary in their approach to resuming marital relations after childbirth and also in their ability to express how they feel. It is common for newly delivered mothers to feel extremely tired and also guilty about their reluctance to have sexual intercourse. Sometimes the partner is fully occupied and does not always appreciate the whirlwind of emotions associated with the adaptation to motherhood. For many women, following childbirth it is necessary to re-establish the relationship with their partner by talking, spending time together and having non-sexual contact, and in this way they can build up towards a sexual relationship.

For the man, witnessing a delivery, particularly of a beloved partner, can be a highly emotional experience and may result in tension or guilt (Clement, 1998), and this level of emotional tension often makes it difficult for either partner to discuss the topic easily.

Mothers experiencing postnatal depression, may find their satisfaction with the relationship with their partner is reduced. This in turn may increase the man's guilt and frustration. Maternal postnatal depression is associated with a significant increase in depression in the partner (Ballard *et al.*, 1994).

Women have far better opportunities than men for obtaining advice on these intimate and delicate matters, so it is important that the midwife takes the time to provide opportunities for counselling or, where necessary, referral to specialist counsellors.

METHODS OF CONTRACEPTION

The ideal method
The ideal method should be an effective, acceptable, simple, painless method or procedure which does not rely on the user's memory. It would be:

1. 100% safe and free from side-effects
2. 100% effective
3. 100% reversible
4. easy to use
5. independent of sexual intercourse
6. used by, or obviously visible to, the woman
7. independent of the medical profession
8. able to give protection against sexually transmitted diseases
9. acceptable to both partners, all cultures and all religions
10. cheap and easy to distribute.

Reflective Activity 8.2

Using the ideals stated above, as you read, consider each of the methods of contraception. Give a rating out of 10 for each method.

Think of situations where some criteria may be considered more important to the woman/couple than others.

MALE CONTRACEPTION

Coitus interruptus
This is a method which is used by a large number of couples at some stage in their relationship. It depends on the man withdrawing his penis from the vagina before ejaculation takes place and thus requires considerable control. This may be acceptable to some couples but may cause significant frustration and stress in others.

Because of the risk of leakage of seminal fluid before withdrawal, coitus interruptus is not considered a very safe method. As there is no effective information about numbers of couples using this method regularly, it is impossible to assess its efficacy with any certainty. It may be worth providing information on other methods in case a safer method is equally acceptable. If no other alternative is acceptable, the use of a spermicide pessary or foam reduces the risk of conception by helping to destroy any sperm released into the vagina before withdrawal.

Condom or sheath
The condom or sheath is probably the most widely used contraceptive in the first few months after childbirth. As a barrier method, it not only provides protection against conception but is also effective in preventing the transmission of sexually transmitted diseases (Wootton, 1995).

For this reason many couples use this as an addition to other methods, and the regular use of condoms should be encouraged as part of the promotion of safer sex. Condoms, however, cannot protect against local infestations such as scabies and lice (Guillebaud, 1999). It is suggested that condoms may reduce the risk of cervical neoplasm (Coker *et al.*, 1992).

In the UK, condoms can be obtained free from family planning clinics, Department of Sexual Health clinics, or purchased at chemists and through many other retail outlets. A wide variety of condoms are available, including different sizes, textures and flavours, and individual preference will determine choice. Most condoms are already lubricated to make them more comfortable. The majority are made from latex. Occasionally, some men and women report sensitivity to or irritation by the latex or spermicide, and condoms containing no spermicide or those made from a hypoallergenic latex can be tried. Rarely, an allergy to the latex can occur, and the Avanti condom, which is made from polyurethane, can be used in these situations. A new condom called Ez.on is also made from polyurethane and is slightly different in shape from conventional condoms, with a tight base but looser-fitting shaft, thus theoretically making it less likely to break and allowing more sensation for the man. The midwife should never assume that either partner knows how to use condoms correctly and safely and, if necessary, she should be prepared to explain the correct method for using a condom. The golden rules for safe use of condoms include:

- only use condoms with the BSI or CE kitemark
- never use after the use-by date
- never use if the inner packaging around the condom is damaged
- condoms should only be used once
- take care with fingernails or rings, which might snag the rubber/latex
- never use with oil-based creams or fluids (including baby or bath oil, cold cream, suntan oil, vaseline, lipstick, aromatherapy oils or massage lotions) as these weaken the rubber and may cause it to break. Medicines such as nystatin or other antifungal creams and pessaries, and some oestrogen creams may have the same effect.

Following use, in the event of damage or spilling of seminal fluid, unless another contraceptive is already being used, the woman should seek advice from her GP or family planning clinic regarding the need for emergency contraception.

Effectiveness If used properly, the condom is 98% effective but effectiveness can be as low as 88%. Fewer condoms now contain spermicide as this can lead to

local dermatitis or allergy and make infections such as HIV more likely to occur (Wilkinson & Szarewski, 2003).

> ### Reflective Activity 8.3
>
> Think about the advantages and disadvantages of condoms, and how their use might best be promoted.
>
> Check the range of condoms available at your local chemist or supermarket, e.g. makes, textures, flavours, and what these cost.

Future developments

Male hormonal contraception is currently under research, and is expected to be available in about 2005. It is thought that the '*male pill*' will be based on progestagens, which inhibit follicle-stimulating hormone (FSH) and luteinizing hormone (LH) production, thus reducing sperm production. There may need to be some testosterone replacement to prevent side-effects. The aim is to prevent sperm production whilst having no effect on ejaculation. Apart from the effectiveness of this type of contraception, there is an issue of whether women would be happy to rely on their male partner for contraception of this type.

FEMALE CONTRACEPTION

Physiological methods

For some people this is the only acceptable method of contraception. The 'safe period' refers to the time during the menstrual cycle when conception is less likely to take place. It is known that ovulation occurs approximately 14 days before the onset of the next menstrual period and that fertilization is possible up to 5 days before and 2 days afterwards (Fig. 8.1). Allowing an extra day either end, intercourse should be avoided for these 10 or 11 days during the cycle. Theoretically this is very easy, but in practice to determine the exact time of ovulation takes time and patience, particularly during the postpartum period. The physiological return of ovulation following childbirth is difficult to assess and the variability of its return makes this method very unreliable in the first few months after delivery. The importance of spacing babies and of women having recovered from childbirth both physically and emotionally before starting to cope with another pregnancy is a significant factor in a mother's life. Relying

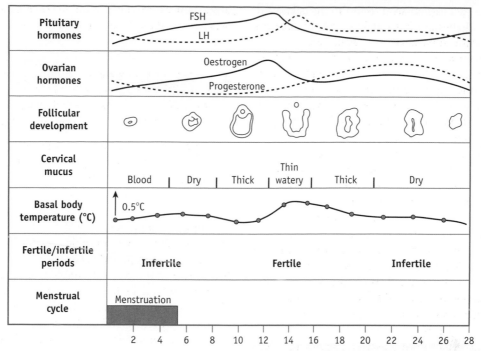

Figure 8.1 Physiological changes within the reproductive system during the menstrual cycle: FSH, follicle-stimulating hormone; LH, luteinizing hormone.

on trying to determine the 'safe period' will be difficult and may result in pregnancy. Various methods have been developed to allow the 'safe period' to be worked out. These include the standard days method; the 2 day method, lactation amenorrhoea method and the use of *Persona*.

The standard days method (SDM)

This is based on the abstinence from unprotected sexual intercourse on days 8–19 of every cycle, assuming the woman has a regular cycle of 26–32 days.

The 2 day method

This is based on the presence of cervical secretions, seen by the woman. Fertility is assumed when any secretions are present and also on the following day. Both these methods have the advantage of being simpler than the traditional calendar, temperature and Billings methods. However, any women wanting to use these physiological methods must be advised to seek expert help in order to determine their suitability to use them and ensure correct explanation of the methods.

Both the SDM and 2 day method have shown good efficacy. Multisite efficacy trials are currently being undertaken (Arevalo and Jennings, 2000).

Lactational amenorrhoea method (LAM)

This is a fairly efficient method which can be used in the fully breastfeeding mother in the first 6 months postpartum, provided certain criteria are fulfilled.

- The mother must be fully breastfeeding, day and night.
- The baby should not be receiving any feed supplements.
- The mother should be under 6 months postpartum.
- The mother should be totally amenorrhoeic. Bleeding after the birth up to 6 weeks after delivery is not included.

If any of the criteria change, the mother is potentially fertile. Provided the criteria are fulfilled, it is estimated that this method has an efficacy rate of 98% (Flynn and Kelly, 1999).

Persona

Persona combines the features of a micro-laboratory and a microcomputer and is designed to advise the woman of the potentially fertile and unfertile parts of her cycle. The device measures levels of luteinizing hormone (LH) and oestrogen breakdown products (E-3-G). The woman inserts test sticks dipped in her early morning urine into the machine, which then measures levels of the two hormones. From this, the device calculates the likely date of ovulation well in advance, and allowing for sperm survival time, the woman is then shown 'green' days when conception is unlikely and 'red' days when conception could occur. To provide the machine with sufficient information for these calculations, a minimum of 16 tests in the woman's first cycle and eight in subsequent cycles are required. Persona can only be used if the cycles are within 23–35 days in length.

Following childbirth, this is initially of limited value. It can only be used after the woman has had two successive cycles of 23–35 days. This makes it inappropriate for use in breastfeeding mothers. According to one study, with perfect use, the failure rate of Persona as a contraceptive tool is 6 per 100 woman years; however, for the typical user the rate is higher (Bonner *et al.*, 1999). Persona can be used for planning a pregnancy but there are few references to the efficacy of Persona used for this purpose.

Reflective Activity 8.4

Consider how you would explain these methods to a woman. What are the key advantages and disadvantages of each approach?

Barrier methods

Occlusive caps

These devices (Fig. 8.2) cover the cervix and mechanically obstruct the entry of spermatozoa. Caps are made in a variety of sizes and must be fitted individually by a doctor or family planning nurse. The use of occlusive caps demands a high level of motivation and confidence by the woman, since correct and conscientious use can help to reduce the failure rate of this method. The failure rate varies from 5–10 per 100 women years (Guillebaud, 1999). Cervical caps are less effective as a contraceptive in multiparous women.

The diaphragm or Dutch cap   This is one of the oldest methods of female contraception and has changed very little in design. A postnatal mother who wishes to use a diaphragm will require careful fitting and measurement. The diaphragm should not be fitted until 6–8 weeks postnatally to allow the uterus and cervix to return to a non-pregnant size and the vaginal muscles to regain their tone. The shallow rubber cap has a circular spring around the perimeter; this may be of flat metal, or a round spring allowing the cap to be compressed and

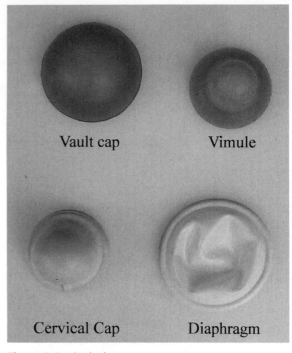

Vault cap   Vimule

Cervical Cap   Diaphragm

Figure 8.2   Occlusive caps.

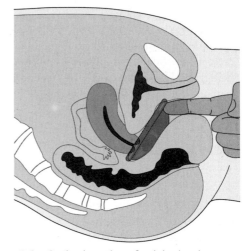

Figure 8.3   Sagittal section of pelvis showing a diaphragm in position. (From Andrews, 1997.)

inserted into the vagina rather like a tampon. Some caps have an arcing spring enabling them to be inserted under a protruding cervix. It is necessary to fit the cap so that it rests in the posterior fornix of the vagina posteriorly and on the suprapubic ridge anteriorly.

The caps come in graduated sizes and are therefore individually fitted so that the anterior wall of the vagina and cervix are covered by a diaphragm which remains comfortably and firmly in place (Fig. 8.3).

A woman who has used a cap before may require a larger size after delivery and this size may need adjustment as the vaginal muscle tone improves. A cap which is too large protrudes and causes discomfort, or may produce extra pressure, giving rise to urethritis-type discomfort. Too small a cap will move around and will not provide protection. A well-fitting cap is unobtrusive and will not be noticed during intercourse. The cap should remain in situ for 6 hours after intercourse and may then be removed at a convenient time.

Other caps   Other types of cap less commonly used may be very useful in particular cases. They all rely on suction to remain in place. The use of spermicide on both surfaces and their removal after 6 hours remain a consistent feature of use.

Vault caps   These are also graduated in several sizes and are thicker rubber than a diaphragm without a spring rim. The cap sits in the fornices of the vagina covering the cervix and remains in position by suction. The benefit of vault caps is that they can be used when vaginal muscle tone is poor and will not support a diaphragm.

The cervical cap   This is designed to fit over the cervix and it may be useful for women who have a straight-sided cervix. A disposable silicon rubber cap called the Oves cap is now available. Once the woman has been fitted for size, she can buy these herself from a chemist. The Oves cap can be kept in place for up to 48 hours.

The vimule   This combination of vault and cervical cap has a powerful suction capability and is used to cover the cervix which is small, irregular or partially amputated.

Other varieties of caps are being evaluated at present. The *Lea's Shield* is a silicone rubber cervical cap, made in one size. It is used with a spermicide and can be kept in position for up to 48 hours. With spermicide the failure rate for the Lea's Shield is 8.7% (Mauck *et al.*, 1996).

The *FemCap* is also made of silicone rubber and can be left in for up to 48 hours. One study found the FemCap had a failure rate of 13.5% (Shihata and Gollub, 1992).

Spermicidal agents

There are a variety of chemical substances that kill or inactivate spermatozoa, the most commonly used spermicide being *Nonoxynol 9*. They are incorporated into jellies, creams, pessaries, and aerosol foams.

Infrequently foams or pessaries may be used on their own where fertility is already low, to reduce the risk of pregnancy; though for women with average fertility spermicides alone would result in a high proportion of unplanned pregnancies. The use of spermicide with caps is important; the efficacy of the method is dependent on it. Spermicide is applied when the cap is introduced, and should be reapplied without removing the cap if intercourse occurs after 3 hours, by placing a spermicide pessary in the vagina. Spermicide foam is a valuable form of protection as, unlike other methods, it does not melt but remains stable at the top of the vagina for up to 4 hours.

Women complaining about 'stickiness and mess' may find the whole concept of barrier methods much more acceptable with foam.

Female condoms

The Femidom is a polyurethane tubular condom consisting of a loose-fitting polyurethane sheath with a flexible ring at either end. It is inserted so that the condom lines the vagina. A soft but firm plastic ring at the entrance covers the genitalia and needs to be steadied in position during intercourse. This condom provides protection both from pregnancy and from sexually transmitted diseases but, like all methods, it requires practice. The condoms are available from chemists and are available in limited numbers from family planning clinics.

With careful use it is up to 95% effective as a contraceptive (Guillebaud, 1999). Like caps, these can be fitted prior to sexual intercourse. The female condom contains a spermicide-free lubricant. Spermicide is not necessary but some women may choose to use one to enhance protection against some sexually transmitted diseases. Because the condom is made from polyurethane, avoidance of oil-based products is not necessary. Aesthetically some women find the Femidom less appealing than other methods.

Intrauterine contraceptive devices and intrauterine systems

The history of intrauterine contraceptive devices (IUCDs), which have been used all over the world since Biblical times, makes a fascinating study. In earlier times such devices ranged from small pebbles to vinegar-soaked sponges. Nowadays IUCDs are small plastic devices which are placed in the uterine cavity by means of a special introducer. All have copper or silver threads added, which increases the efficiency of the device.

The mode of action of IUCDs is complex and multifactorial. They act as a sterile foreign body in the uterine cavity and the resultant physiological action is potentiated by the addition of copper. The copper has a toxic effect on sperm and ova, preventing fertilization. It is rare to find viable sperm in the uterine cavity, making it very unlikely that IUCDs ever act as an abortive agent. It is also thought that the device causes some reduction in tubular contraction, thereby reducing the speed of the ovum along the fallopian tube, and there is some evidence of infrequent ovulation while the device is in situ. There may also be an increased production of prostaglandins in the uterus, which increases uterine activity and causes the expulsion of a fertilized ovum. A secondary action of inhibiting implantation is relevant when used as part of emergency contraception. In addition to inhibiting implantation, there is also a direct blastocystotoxic effect.

Contraindications to the use of an IUCD include suspected pregnancy, pelvic infection, cervicitis, menorrhagia, those taking immunosuppressant drugs, copper allergy and suspected malignancy. There is no evidence that copper IUCDs increase the risk of ectopic pregnancies, which are related to the risk of pelvic inflammatory disease (Guillebaud, 1999).

The introduction of an IUCD following delivery is generally delayed until 6–8 weeks postpartum when involution of the uterus is likely to be complete. If the device is inserted before involution is complete, it may not remain in the optimum position and is more likely to be expelled. Particular care is required after caesarean section to ensure that the wound has fully healed. In some cases a device is inserted at the time of termination of pregnancy if requested by the woman.

A variety of types are now available (Fig. 8.4). All have copper or copper and silver thread on the stem. One new variety is the GyneFIX which, unlike the other types, is frameless, consisting of six copper bands threaded onto a length of suture material. One end is provided with a knot which is inserted into the fundus and acts as an anchor.

An IUCD may be inserted at any time but commonly this is done during menstruation (except following childbearing) because it is easier to insert at this time and ensures that the woman is not pregnant before the device is introduced. Menstruation may be prolonged by a couple of days when an IUCD is in situ and the loss may be significantly increased in women who already have heavy periods, thus making this an

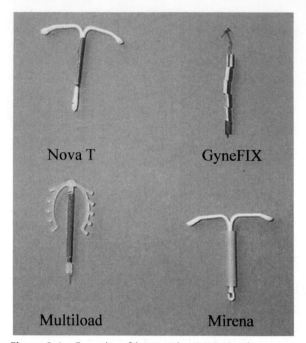

Figure 8.4   Examples of intrauterine contraceptive devices.

unsuitable method for such women. A few women with dysmenorrhoea may find the pain is worsened by the introduction of a device.

Women with recurrent infection in the reproductive tract may be advised to use another method. While the device does not introduce infection, any infection, particularly if sexually transmitted, which may occur is likely to be more difficult to treat. The devices remain in situ for 3–10 years and require only minimal supervision following insertion. They have an excellent record in preventing pregnancy with a failure rate ranging from 0.3–3 per 100 woman years (Wildemeersch et al., 1999). If pregnancy does occur when the device is in situ, removal is advised as soon as possible as there is an increased risk of mid-trimester abortion.

The *Mirena intrauterine system* (IUS) is a newer type of coil containing levonorgestrel, a progestagen, and statistically it is as effective as sterilization. The stem of this device contains a reservoir which allows a slow release of progestagen. The effects are mostly local so that ovulation frequently continues to occur. The proximity of the progestagen to the endometrium reduces its thickness, so that after an initial few weeks of erratic bleeding the blood loss diminishes, and amenorrhoea is common (Bobrow et al., 2000). The progestagen also causes a physiological mucous plug to form in the cervix, which safeguards the uterus from infection as well as impeding sperm penetration. Following removal, fertility returns rapidly to normal.

Hormonal contraception

Oral contraception

Millions of women take oral contraceptives worldwide. In 1995, in the UK, of women under 50 years using any form of contraception, 26% were using the contraceptive pill. It is the most popular method in young people with 51% of women in their early 20s using this method (Organon, 2000). The oral contraceptive pill contains either a combination of oestrogen and progestagen (the combined pill or COC), or progestagen on its own (the progestagen-only pill or POP). Over the years, the aim has been to improve the manufacture of synthetic oestrogen and progesterone and at the same time reduce the amounts of hormones needed to maintain a high efficacy of contraception. From time to time media scares concerning the COC have resulted in a panic reaction in some women, leading to unwanted pregnancies.

The main controversies have concerned the risk of venous thromboembolism (VTE) in pill takers. The background risk for VTE in women not taking hormones is 5 per 100 000. In women taking the COC the risk varies from 15–25 per 100 000 depending on the type of pill (Jick *et al.*, 2000). The risk of VTE in pregnancy is 60 per 100 000. Since 1995, the Department of Health has lifted restrictions on prescribing the newer 'third-generation' pills, allowing a much wider variety to be available to suit the individual woman's needs. Midwives should always advise any women taking the pill to seek professional advice if they have any concerns, before stopping taking the pill.

Combined pill The combined oestrogen and progestagen pill (COC) inhibits ovulation by suppressing the production of gonadotrophins from the anterior pituitary gland. It also alters the consistency of the cervical mucus, making it impenetrable to sperm, reduces the motility of the uterine tubes so that the sperm have difficulty in passing along the tube, and causes a change in the endometrium making it unsuitable for implantation. The latter three 'back-up mechanisms' are due to the action of progestagen.

The timing of administration of the combined pill is important in preventing ovulation. For complete efficiency, the course should begin on the first day of the menstrual period and continue for 21 days. This is followed by 7 days without tablets, during which time withdrawal bleeding occurs. When taken correctly the COC is virtually 100% reliable. The reported pregnancy rate is 0.18 per 100 woman years (Ryder, 1993). In cases of antibiotics being prescribed or the woman developing diarrhoea and vomiting, the COC will no longer provide reliable contraception. Other precautions, such as condoms, should be used during this time and for a further 7 days afterwards.

Major contraindications include thromboembolic disorders, breast neoplasia, liver disease and focal migraine. In diabetes mellitus, stability may be affected and it may be necessary to adjust treatment. Other relative contraindications include hypertension, heart disease, epilepsy and obesity. A family history of venous or arterial disease in close family under 45 years of age must also be considered a serious risk.

Oral contraceptives have certain side-effects which may include weight gain, nausea, breast heaviness, headaches, depression and loss of libido. Some of these may diminish in time. For women over 35 years, the COC is contraindicated if, as well as the above problems, the woman either smokes or is significantly overweight with a BMI of over 40, as there is an increased risk of thromboembolic disease, myocardial infarction and cerebral vascular accident. Other methods of contraception which do not contain oestrogen should then be employed.

After delivery, the mother who is not breastfeeding may start the combined pill 21 days postpartum. The regime of 21 days of pills followed by 7 pill-free days is followed. The oestrogen content of the pill is inclined to reduce lactation by suppressing prolactin and is also passed to the baby, albeit in small quantities, in the breast milk, so the combined contraceptive pill is not recommended for breastfeeding mothers. If started on day 21, it is effective immediately.

In 2003, the Evra patch became available. Like the COC, this transdermal patch contains oestrogen and progestagen and is changed every 7 days for 3 weeks, followed by a patch-free week.

Progestagen-only pill The progestagen-only pill (POP) is an effective method of contraception postpartum and is satisfactory for breastfeeding mothers. The progestagen does not affect lactation and any small quantity passing through the milk is not a problem for babies. The mother commences the POP at 21 days after delivery and takes the tablets continuously from packet to packet without a break. There may be some delay in menstruation, but it will be a 'proper' period when it arrives. Mothers should be advised that progestagen may cause erratic bleeding patterns, but this usually settles after a few months and the periods may gradually disappear.

Progestagen acts by causing cervical mucus to form a natural plug in the cervix and prevents the sperm entering the uterus, and also reduces the motility of the fallopian tubes. In some cases, the progestagen also causes suppression of ovulation. Women weighing over 70 kg are advised to take a double dose. The reported pregnancy rate with the progestagen-only pill is 1.2 per 100 woman years (Ryder, 1993).

The POP has to be taken within 3 hours of the same time each day, making this an unsuitable method if the woman has a bad memory or an erratic lifestyle. A new POP, called *Cerazette*, which became available in 2003, has a 12-hour leeway for missed pills, similar to the COC. In addition to the normal mode of action, it will, in many cases prevent ovulation, and frequently causes amenorrhoea.

Reflective Activity 8.5

Consider the advice that may be useful for Mrs B, who is a 24-year-old Moslem woman, and her husband. She regards menstruation as 'unclean' and any method which risks irregular (e.g. POP or progesterone injection) or prolonged bleeding (IUCD) is unacceptable. The couple also believe that touching the genital area with both hands is taboo, thus making barrier methods unsatisfactory. What sort of methods would be most appropriate to this couple?

Injectable contraceptives

These consist of a progestagen given as a deep intramuscular injection. Although only used by about 2% of women using contraception, it is becoming an increasingly popular method (Guillebaud, 1999). It has a low failure rate of about 0–1 per 100 women years for *Depo-Provera* and 0.4–2 per 100 woman years for *Noristerat*. There is no evidence that it has any detrimental long-term effect on fertility; however, by nature of its mode of action, a return to fertility may be delayed. The average time from the last injection to conception is 9 months (IMAP, 1998).

Depo-Provera   Depo-Provera (DMPA) 150 mg is most commonly used and is repeated at 3-monthly intervals. It acts by suppressing ovulation and making the cervical mucus impenetrable to sperm, causes changes in the endometrium and may lead to irregular bleeding or amenorrhoea. It is suitable for women who have been given rubella vaccination, and for those awaiting sterilization or whose partners have had a vasectomy whilst awaiting results. It is also ideal for those with a poor memory and is often used by women who are unable to take the COC, e.g. smokers over 35 years, who prefer the injection to the time limitations of the POP.

Depo-Provera can usually be commenced at 6 weeks postpartum provided the woman has not had unprotected intercourse. It is not given before 6 weeks because it may provoke bleeding and, at a time when secondary postpartum haemorrhage may occur, could make diagnosis of pathology difficult and cause unnecessary blood loss at a vulnerable time for the mother. It does not affect lactation. There is some evidence that Depo-Provera reduces the risk of pelvic inflammatory disease, endometriosis and endometrial carcinoma (Bigrigg *et al.*, 1999). Depo-Provera may cause some weight gain, acne or depression in a few women.

Noristerat   Norethisterone oenanthate 200 mg may be given intramuscularly every 8 weeks. Though it has a similar action to Depo-Provera it is used less often, and is less likely to cause irregular bleeding.

Future developments include an injectable being used in South America called *Cyclofem* consisting of a progestagen and oestrogen given monthly. It causes a monthly bleed but can be self-administered using a special injector (Muller, 1998).

Implants

Implanon is a contraceptive implant currently used in the UK. It consists of a single rod containing a progestagen on a slow-release carrier. It is about the same size as a hair grip and is inserted superficially under the skin of the upper arm using a minor surgical technique and local anaesthetic. The implant lasts for about 3 years before needing to be replaced. This regime produces highly effective care-free protection with a failure rate of 0–0.07 per 100 woman years. Like other progesterone methods, it can cause irregular bleeding, although this often reduces with time. About 25% become amenorrhoeic (Reynolds, 1999/2000). The mode of action is by inhibiting ovulation, preventing thickening of the endometrium and increasing the viscosity of the cervical mucus. The implant can be inserted from day 21 postpartum.

Care of women receiving hormonal contraceptives

Before hormonal contraceptives are prescribed, a detailed family, medical, obstetric and menstrual history is obtained. The blood pressure is checked regularly and weight is monitored if the woman is obese, though in the first few months after delivery this is of limited value as her weight is likely to change (O'Brien and Huezo, 1998). It is an ideal opportunity for health education, and discussion on issues such as safer sex, smoking, diet, breast awareness and healthy lifestyle is encouraged.

Emergency contraception

There are a variety of reasons why women are advised to seek advice concerning emergency contraception. These situations may include unprotected sexual intercourse (no contraception used, rape, failed coitus interruptus), failure of a barrier method (split condoms, dislodged caps), missed pills or injection, or expulsion of an IUCD.

Whilst some parts of the menstrual cycle may be regarded as low risk for conception, if the woman has irregular periods or is unsure of her dates, no time can be regarded as safe. In practice therefore, most women who present with such situations will be prescribed emergency contraception. There are currently two forms of emergency contraception available.

Emergency contraception (oral) The most widely used form is now a progestagen preparation called *Levonelle 2*, which has been available since 2000 (O'Brien, 2000). This consists of two tablets taken together as soon as possible after the unprotected sexual intercourse and always within 72 hours. If started within 24 hours, the percentage of pregnancies prevented is about 95%, whereas this drops to 58% if not started until 49–72 hours afterwards (Faculty of Family Planning and Reproductive Health Care, 2000). The pills will only affect the reported episode of unprotected sexual intercourse and cannot protect the rest of the cycle. Although the midwife may not need to recommend this method of contraception very often in a direct way to mothers, it is an important part of health education in the community, especially in schools and colleges.

Emergency IUCD contraception In the event of unprotected intercourse having occurred, a copper intrauterine contraceptive device may be fitted up to 5 days after the probable day of ovulation in that cycle. It can also be used later in the cycle if within 5 days of a single episode of unprotected intercourse (Guillebaud, 1999). The presence of an IUCD in the uterus will probably prevent a fertilized ovum from embedding. Although less often used, it is a highly effective method of emergency contraception with a failure rate of no more than 0.1% (Faculty of Family Planning and Reproductive Health Care, 2000).

STERILIZATION

Tubal ligation

Tubal ligation or the application of potentially removable clips to the uterine tubes are methods of sterilization which may be performed in the woman. In the male, ligation of the vas deferens is considered a permanent method of sterilization.

Before carrying out sterilization it is essential that the couple are carefully counselled. The psychosocial aspects of the decision as well as the physical factors concerned with the procedure should be considered. The emotionally stable couple usually accept sterilization without regret, but unless all eventualities have been carefully thought through, later events may lead to regret and some may use the operation to rationalize disturbances that arise later in life (IMAP, 1999a). A percentage of those who are sterilized request reversal at a later date. The commonest reasons are related to a change in marital status, sudden infant death, the death of an older child and the desire for more children. The success rate for reversal is low, so these methods should be considered permanent. The advent of contraceptive methods such as the *Mirena IUS* which is as reliable as sterilization, causes amenorrhoea in many cases and yet is removable, is an option for couples who are not totally sure about future plans.

Unless performed at the same time as a caesarean section, female sterilization is seldom carried out earlier than 6–8 weeks after delivery and by that time any problems affecting the baby which could influence the couple's decision are usually evident. The failure rate for female sterilization after 10 years is 1 in 200 and failure may occur several years after the procedure. The rate is slightly lower for older women (Peterson *et al.*, 1996; RCOG, 1999). It is worth noting that the effectiveness is less than that of the COC for women under 27 years.

Vasectomy

This is ligation of both deferent ducts (vas deferens) (Fig. 8.5). In some cases the male partner chooses to be sterilized as it is an easier and safer procedure than tubal ligation. It can be done as an outpatient procedure under local anaesthetic. Ligation of the deferent ducts prevent the sperm reaching the seminal vesicle and ejaculatory duct. As spermatozoa may survive in the ducts for some time, the couple should continue to take contraceptive precautions until two sperm-free specimens of seminal fluid are produced. This will take a minimum of 3 months. Again skilled counselling is essential before a final decision is made. The man

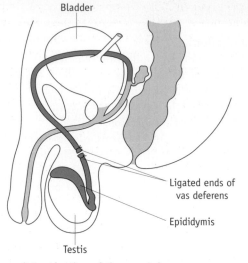

Figure 8.5   Ligation of the vas deferens.

should understand that sexual desire and activity are not affected by the operation.

There has been some concern about increased risks of testicular cancer after vasectomy, but a study by Moller *et al.* (1994) concluded that there is no increased risk.

CONTRACEPTIVE ADVICE TO WOMEN IN THE POSTNATAL PERIOD

Family planning is a specialist area and midwives, whilst knowing the principles involved, also need to be aware of limitations in their knowledge. During discussions with the mother, the midwife may detect cues which indicate a need to refer for specialist help and advice, for example in cases of medical disorders or where there are signs of psychosexual problems.

Factors to be considered

When the midwife discusses contraception with a mother and her partner, she needs to consider a variety of issues which may influence the woman's choice. It is important that the mother does not assume she carries on with her pre-pregnancy contraception without advice. The midwife should not assume that the parents have a reliable knowledge of contraception. It is useful therefore for her to confirm the woman's level of knowledge before offering advice, and this will quickly indicate if there are misunderstandings to be addressed. The midwife should appreciate that no prior contraception may have been used. By discussing the

---

Box 8.1 Factors which need to be considered in choosing contraception

- Age
- General health
- Smoking
- Obesity
- Lifestyle/employment
- Experiences of family and friends
- General views on contraception
- Cultural or religious constraints
- Previous methods used which failed
- Partner's views
- Obstetric history, e.g. parity or hypertension
- Level of intelligence/memory
- Ability or willingness to go to a family planning clinic
- Long-term plans for future pregnancies
- Stability of the relationship
- The level of efficacy demanded by the couple from their contraceptive
- The couple's feelings about each type of contraceptive
- What is available
- Any disability which could affect either partner's ability to use a particular method
- Method of feeding the baby
- History of menstrual problems, e.g. PMS
- Views about menstruation
- Periods, whether normally heavy or light
- Drugs being taken
- Risk from sexually transmitted diseases

---

factors listed in Box 8.1, the midwife will be able to give more accurate advice to the woman about choices available, as well as advising her about the best place to obtain the contraception she wants or where to get further information.

Reflective Activity 8.6

Consider your practice area, and the women to whom you provide care. What are the most popular methods of family planning in use? What are the key factors responsible for these choices?

Timing of starting contraception

The return of ovulation following delivery varies individually, but research suggests that the earliest possible ovulation occurs 30–35 days postpartum. It is therefore advisable to commence protection before this time. Mothers who breastfeed their babies on demand are likely to suppress ovulation for a long time. Exactly how long will depend on the suckling of the baby at frequent intervals and include at least two full feeds during the night. Babies who vary in their feeding requirement and occasionally sleep through the night will not stimulate enough prolactin to provide control of ovulation. The return of menstruation, when it occurs, indicates retrospective return of ovulation 14 days before. It is therefore important that the mother understands that printed information on packets of hormonal contraceptives does not relate to postpartum situations, and that the contaceptive pills need to be commenced independently of menstruation.

When oral contraception is started on day 21 postpartum, it provides full protection from the first day. If commenced later, other precautions such as condoms should be used for the first 7 days. For any sexual intercourse after day 21, some form of contraception should be used. Following a termination or spontaneous abortion, contraception can be started with immediate effect.

Special groups

Teenagers   Young people remain one of the biggest challenges for the family planning services. Accurate knowledge of sexual behaviour in young adolescents and their needs is difficult to obtain owing to the problems in getting information from this group. Sexual activity can start early, sometimes as young as 10–12 years of age, usually unbeknown to the parents. Many have unprotected sexual intercourse, partly because of their attitude towards risk-taking and partly owing to either ignorance about contraception and conception or fear of seeking advice (Burack, 1999). Young women may be at considerable pressure both from their boyfriend and from their peers to enter a sexual relationship before they themselves feel emotionally or physically ready for this. A midwife may find herself in a counselling role in assisting the young woman to make a choice not just regarding contraception, but also about entering a sexual relationship.

Many young people assume that approaching their general practitioner or attending a family planning clinic will automatically involve information being passed to their parents, and some youngsters will risk a pregnancy rather than seek contraceptive advice. There is often a difference in the attitudes of young girls and boys towards sexual activity and contraception,

with girls more likely to seek help than boys. Despite sex education at school, many young people are ignorant about basic issues such as contraception, conception and safer sex (van den Akker et al., 1999).

For young people under 16 years, no contraception can be given, even condoms, without fulfilling the Fraser (previously known as Gillick) criteria. Following the Gillick ruling in 1985, the present legal situation is that young persons under 16 years of age can independently seek medical advice and receive treatment providing they can show that they are competent to do so. In contraceptive terms, provided the doctor is assured that the young person understands the potential risks and benefits of the treatment/advice being given and if the doctor believes that the person is likely to have sexual intercourse without contraception, the doctor is not breaking the law by providing contraception if he or she believes it is in the person's best interest. The value of parental support is always emphasized and the youngsters are encouraged to talk to their parents about the consultation. All consultations are confidential regardless of age.

Reflective Activity 8.7

How would you assist a 15-year-old newly delivered mother to choose her method of contraception? You may find it useful to discuss possibilities with your local family planning clinic.

What are your own personal views of teenagers' sexual activity? How will this influence your approach to providing information and advice?

Older mothers   With an increasing number of women having babies in their 30s and 40s, contraception for this age group is an important issue. Fertility is reduced as age increases, with fertility levels at 40 years half that at 25 years (Guillebaud, 1999). This suggests that some of the methods unsuitable for the highly fertile woman may be acceptable in the older woman. The COC pill can be continued until the menopause provided the woman is not overweight, does not smoke or suffer from focal migraine. For women over 35 years with these problems, the POP is the oral contraceptive recommended.

The IUCD is another appropriate method for this age group and the Mirena IUS, in particular, is useful as it prevents menorrhagia common in older women and provides protection from endometrial hyperplasia and carcinoma.

Barriers are also popular, and for those around the menopause, *Delfen* foam may provide sufficient contraception. Many women request sterilization and the midwife should be able to refer the woman for counselling.

Medical disorders   Any woman with a long-standing or newly acquired medical disorder needs expert advice in relation to contraception. Some drugs can interfere with the effectiveness of hormonal contraception and some conditions require specialist knowledge. For women with conditions which make childbearing particularly hazardous, e.g. severe heart disease, sterilization may be requested or at least a highly effective method.

Cardiovascular disorders, haematological disorders, hypertension, diabetes, migraine and liver diseases all require individualized advice (IMAP, 1999b). Midwives should ensure that the woman knows where to seek help before deciding on any particular method of contraception.

The role of the midwife in the provision of contraceptive advice

Many women conceive their first or a subsequent child unintentionally and, while this may result in a wanted child, it is not always possible to adapt well to unplanned parenthood. The emotional toll of pregnancies which occur at inopportune times can be serious and may have long-term consequences for the whole family.

The midwife has a crucial role to play in giving information and advising women following childbirth. Many women have already decided on the method of contraception they intend to use, or use the method they have previously used. However, the midwife is in an ideal position to know of factors, either from the woman's general history or from events occurring during her pregnancy, labour or puerperium, which may require a change of plan, or methods which may suit the woman and her partner more than the original method. For teenagers in particular, the midwife may be the first health professional they have spoken to about contraception. The midwife is a prime source of information and has a key role in the government initiative relating to teenage pregnancy by supporting these young people and helping to reduce the incidence of future unwanted pregnancies (SEU, 1999).

Midwives should ensure they understand the principles of each of the main methods of contraception and be able to give appropriate advice to the women and their partners. It is also important for midwives to keep abreast of new developments in contraception, in order to provide contemporary and appropriate advice to women. In particular, they should be aware of the facilities available in their area and thus be able to refer women where necessary for more specialized advice.

KEY POINTS

- Resuming relationships following childbearing can be difficult for some couples.
- A variety of methods of contraception are available including physiological, barrier, hormonal methods and intrauterine devices.
- No one method is suitable for all couples; each couple needs to consider the best option for them.

- The role of the midwife is to give information to the woman and her partner to allow them to make an informed choice.
- The midwife should appreciate the individuality of each woman and her partner, taking into consideration age, family spacing, culture, religion and health backgrounds.

REFERENCES

Alan Guttmacher Institute (1999) Issues in brief: induced abortion worldwide. Online. Available: http://www.agi-usa.org/pubs/fb-0599.html.

Andrews, G. (1997) *Women's Sexual Health*. Edinburgh: Baillière Tindall, p 179.

Arevalo, M. & Jennings, V. (2000) Simple methods of natural family planning *IPPF Medical Bulletin* **34**(3): 3–4.

Ballard, C.G., Davis, R., Cullen, P.C. *et al.* (1994) Prevalence of postnatal psychiatric morbidity in mothers and fathers. *British Journal of Psychiatry* **164**(6): 782–788.

Bigrigg, A., Evans, M., Gbolade, B. *et al.* (1999) Depo provera. Position paper on clinical use, effectiveness and side effects. *British Journal of Family Planning* **25**(2): 69–76.

Bobrow, C., Cooling, H. & Bisson, D. (2000) Amenorrhoea despite displaced levonorgestrel intra-uterine system. *British Journal of Family Planning* **26**(2): 105–106.

Bonner, J., Flynn, A., Freundl, G. *et al.* (1999) Personal hormone monitoring for contraception. *British Journal of Family Planning* **24**(4): 128–134.

Burack, R. (1999) Teenage sexual behaviour: attitudes towards and declared sexual activity. *British Journal of Family Planning* 24(4): 145–148.

Clement, S. (1998) *Psychological Perspectives on Pregnancy and Childbirth*. London: Churchill Livingstone.

Coker, A.L., Hulka, B.S., McCann, M.F. *et al.* (1992) Barrier methods of contraception and cervical intra epithelial neoplasm. *Contraception* 45(1): 1–10.

Faculty of Family Planning and Reproductive Health Care (2000) Royal College of Obstetricians and Gynaecologists. Guidance April 2000. Emergency contraception: recommendations for clinical practice. *British Journal of Family Planning* 26(2): 93–96.

Flynn, A. & Kelly, J. (1999) The menstrual cycle, ovulation and fertility awareness. In: Kubba, A. Sanfilippo, J. & Hampton, N. (eds) *Contraception and Office Gynaecology*. London: Saunders.

Guillebaud, J. (1999) *Contraception, Your Questions Answered*, 3rd edn. London: Churchill Livingstone.

International Medical Advisory Panel (IMAP) (1998) IMAP statement on injectable contraception. *IPPF Medical Bulletin* 33(2): 1–5.

International Medical Advisory Panel (IMAP) (1999a) IMAP statement on voluntary surgical contraception. *IPPF Medical Bulletin* 33(4): 1–4.

International Medical Advisory Panel (IMAP) (1999b) Statement on contraception for women with medical disorders. *Journal of the National Association of Nurses for Contraception and Sexual Health*. Winter 1999/2000(38): 43–45.

Jick, H., Kaye, J.A., Vasilakis-Scaramozza, C. *et al.* (2000) Risk of venous thromboembolism among users of third generation oral contraceptives compared with users of oral contraceptives with levonorgestrel before and after 1995: cohort and case-control analysis. *British Medical Journal* 321(7270): 1190–1195.

Mauck, C., Glover, L.H., Miller, E. *et al.* (1996) Lea's shield: a study of the safety and efficacy of a new vaginal barrier contraceptive device used with and without spermicide. *Contraception* 53(6): 329–335.

Moller, H., Knudsen, L.B. & Lynge, E. (1994) Risk of testicular cancer after vasectomy: a cohort of 73 000 men. *British Medical Journal* 309(6950): 295–299.

Muller, N. (1998) Self injection with Cyclofem. *IPPF Medical Bulletin* 32(5): 1–3.

O'Brien, P. (2000) Emergency contraception with levonorgestrel: one hormone better than two. *British Journal of Family Planning* 26(2): 67–69.

O'Brien, P. & Huezo, C. (1998) A survey of service guidelines on the pill and blood pressure. *IPPF Medical Bulletin* 32(5): 3–4.

Office for National Statistics (1997) *Birth Statistics, England and Wales*. London: Stationary Office.

Organon Laboratories (2000) *The Economics of Implanon and other Long-term Contraceptive Options*. Cambridge: Organon Laboratories.

Peterson, H.B., Xia, Z., Hughes, J.M. *et al.* (1996) The risk of pregnancy after tubal sterilization: findings from the US collaborative review of sterilization. *American Journal Obstetrics and Gynecology* 174(4): 1161–1170.

Reynolds, A. (1999/2000) Implanon – a new contraceptive implant. *Primary Health Care* 9(10): 14–15.

Royal College of Obstetricians and Gynaecologists (RCOG) (1999) *Male and Female Sterilisation. Evidence Based Clinical Guidelines No 4*. London: RCOG Press.

Ryder, R.E.J. (1993) 'Natural family planning': effective birth control supported by the Catholic Church. *British Medical Journal* 307(6906): 723–726.

Shihata, A.A. & Gollub, E. (1992) Acceptability of a new intravaginal barrier contraceptive device (FemCap). *Contraception* 46(6): 511–519.

Social Exclusion Unit (SEU) (1999) *Teenage Pregnancy*. London: Department of Health.

van den Akker, O.B.A., Andre, S. & Murphy, T. (1999) Adolescent sexual behaviour and knowledge. *British Journal of Midwifery* 7(12): 765–769.

Wildemeersch, D., Batar, I., Webb, A. *et al.* (1999) GyneFIX the frameless intrauterine contraceptive implant – an update. For interval, emergency and postabortal contraception. *British Journal of Family Planning* January 24(4): 149–159.

Wilkinson, C., Szarewski, A. (2003) *Contraceptive Dilemmas*. St Albans: Altman.

Wootton, G. (1995) Barrier contraception: issues and trends. *Nursing Standard* 9(38): 3–8.

FURTHER READING

In the specialist area of family planning, a small number of books are available which are used as key texts for nurses practising family planning. Whilst most midwifery textbooks contain sufficient information for midwives, more detailed books can be recommended for those wishing to study in more depth.

Andrews, G. (2001) *Women's Sexual Health,* 2nd edn. London: Baillière Tindall.

An excellent book covering all aspects of sexuality and sexual health. It is easy to read and contains practical information suitable for midwives advising the women in their care, particularly in sexual health matters.

Belfield, T. (1997) *FPA Contraceptive Handbook*, 2nd edn. London: Family Planning Association.
This book is easy to read and provides clear details about each method of contraception. Some diagrams.

Guillebaud, J. (1999) *Contraception, Your Questions Answered*, 3rd edn. London: Churchill Livingstone.
A detailed book covering all aspects of contraception. Chapters are divided using the various methods of contraception. Questions are used as subheadings in order to provide appropriate information.

Social Exclusion Unit (1999) *Teenage Pregnancy*. London: Department of Health.
This is an important document for all midwives to have read. It looks at the incidence of teenage pregnancy and some of the factors relating, amongst other things, to teenage attitudes towards sex and contraception.

ADDITIONAL RESOURCES

British Pregnancy Advisory Service (BPAS)
Austy Manor, Wootton Warren, Solihull, West Midlands B95 6BX
Brook Advisory Centres
165 Gray's Inn Road, London WC1X 8UD
The Family Planning Association
27–35 Mortimer Street, London WIN 7RJ

International Planned Parenthood Federation (IPPF)
Regents College, Inner Circle, Regents Park, London NW1 4NS
The Margaret Pyke Centre
15 Batemans Buildings, Soho Square, London WIV 6JB

9

Infertility and Assisted Conception

Debbie Barber

LEARNING OUTCOMES

After reading this chapter you will:

- comprehend the biological processes of fertilization and embryology
- understand the causes of female and male infertility
- be aware of the range of investigations and treatment options

- understand the drug regimes of the treatment options available and side-effects of treatments
- appreciate the legal, ethical, socioeconomic, physical and psychological implications for health professionals and for individuals with fertility issues.

INTRODUCTION

Midwives frequently care for couples who may have received assistance in achieving their pregnancy and it is important to understand the processes couples or individuals have to go through to become pregnant. These experiences may contribute to the attitudes and anxieties they demonstrate, and could create greater challenges for the midwifery team.

Most couples will have received their fertility treatment in the private sector, and occasionally the transition into normal NHS care may itself be stressful. It is useful for midwives to establish links with their local fertility services to provide support and information on patients to ease the transition into their care. Awareness of the range of treatment options and the side-effects from treatment provides insight into both the physical and emotional condition of couples requiring midwifery care. Singleton pregnancies and the prevention of twin and triplet pregnancy are the ultimate goals of all fertility clinics – and it is essential that couples understand the risks and the care required during a multiple pregnancy. Appropriate management and monitoring of all treatments within specialist centres is the ideal way to deliver care. Many nurses and midwives have specialized in fertility and in several units provide a large proportion of care,

extending their role to perform ultrasound scanning, intrauterine insemination, embryo transfer and participating in counselling (Barber, 2002). It is important for midwives and nurses to normalize pregnancies for couples and enable them to enjoy their much-desired pregnancy.

Technological advances within the field of reproduction have increased public awareness of infertility and the demand for related services. Approximately one in six couples will experience problems conceiving a child (Hull *et al.*, 1985; Templeton *et al.*, 1990) and will seek assistance to achieve a pregnancy. It is over 25 years since the birth of Louise Brown, the world's first 'test-tube baby' and over one million babies have been born in the United Kingdom from in vitro fertilization (IVF). Research has highlighted the stigma, psychological morbidity and long-term implications caused by the experience of infertility in couples (Kerr *et al.*, 1999). These factors have an impact on couples whether treatment is successful or not. Over 95% of service provision exists within the private sector, which forms a financial hurdle that many couples must overcome prior to commencing their treatment.

The regulation of licensed clinics is governed by the Human Fertilisation and Embryology Authority (HFEA), though this only governs clinics that provide donor insemination and treatments where fertilization occurs outside of the body (in vitro). Several forms of treatment are not controlled by the HFEA, and may still potentially create problems similar to those of licensed treatments, including funding, ovarian hyperstimulation and multiple births.

HUMAN FERTILISATION AND EMBRYOLOGY AUTHORITY (HFEA)

The HFEA was created following the 1990 Human Fertilisation and Embryology Act, and was set up to license and monitor clinics providing fertility treatments (e.g. IVF, donated egg/sperm/embryo procedures, or research on embryos).

All licensed clinics must have a delegated 'person responsible' with a specific responsibility to ensure that the conditions of the licence are carried out. Annual inspections are performed by the HFEA and are a prerequisite for relicensing. Inspection includes reviewing the welfare of any potential child; clinical and laboratory standards; protocols for practice in all areas; and the safety of patients and their families.

The HFEA maintains a formal register of information regarding specific donors, donor treatments and children born from these treatments. This information could be used by offspring born as a result of donated eggs or sperm, and wishing to gather information about their genetic background. It does not permit the revelation of any identifying information whatsoever to be disclosed to applicants regarding the donors.

The HFEA produces a manual and Code of Practice (HFEA, 2001) to guide clinics on how they should carry out their licensed activities, and a patient guide containing a list of all treatments offered by each specific unit and the success rates of the respective units. Informed consent is an essential component in all licensed practices and each couple undergoing treatment must consent to all aspects of the process. The provision of independent counselling is vital to assisted reproduction treatment, and the HFEA stipulates the necessity for continuous support, information, clarification of implications and therapeutic counselling.

Reflective Activity 9.1

How do you think regulation impacts on the delivery and management of care of couples undergoing infertility treatments?

CAUSES OF INFERTILITY

Anovulation

Anovulation is a failure of the ovary to produce or release eggs. This is frequently diagnosed in primary care by the GP. In several cases the problem can be corrected by drug therapy to initiate ovulation such as the administration of clomiphene, an anti-oestrogen, which is a common treatment for polycystic ovary syndrome (PCO).

It is important to thoroughly investigate the possible cause of anovulation as this could be caused by pathology such as hyperprolactinaemia, which can be corrected, thus reducing the need for undergoing fertility treatments.

If serum prolactin is elevated (1000 mU/l) the test should be repeated. This could be caused by stress or from a prolactin-secreting pituitary adenoma or macroadenoma, diagnosed with magnetic resonance imaging (MRI). Elevated levels of prolactin inhibit the normal hormonal feedback loop that initiates ovulation. Treatment includes bromocriptine or cabergoline, which reduces the elevated levels of prolactin and restores normal endocrine activity to facilitate ovulation.

Anovulation can be divided into primary and secondary amenorrhoea; these are primarily caused by pituitary tumours, pituitary ablation, Kallmann's syndrome and cancer treatments (see Box 9.1).

Polycystic ovary syndrome (PCO)

This syndrome is often detected in women undergoing investigations for anovulation. (Kousta et al., 1999). It is characterized by cystic ovaries with more than 10 cysts, 2–8 mm in diameter distributed around and through an echodense, thickened stroma (Fig. 9.1). Endocrine features include raised serum luteinizing hormone (LH) and/or testosterone, which contribute to symptoms of acne, hirsutism (hyperandrogenism) or alopecia, oligomenorrhoea and obesity. The hypersecretion of LH is associated with menstrual irregularity and infertility. Raised body mass index (BMI – see Ch. 16)

Table 9.1   Main causes of infertility (Snick et al., 1997)

Female	Incidence (%)
Anovulation	26
Endometriosis	3
Tubal damage	13
Unexplained	30
Male factor	30

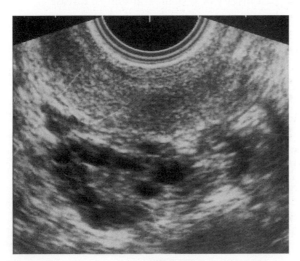

Figure 9.1 Ultrasound scan illustrating a polycystic ovary.

is associated with the increase of symptoms. Obesity leads to hypersecretion of insulin, which stimulates ovarian secretion of androgens with increased risk of the development of type II diabetes mellitus (Kousta *et al.*, 2000). Anovulation is also associated with endometrial hyperplasia due to increased oestrogen production unopposed by progesterone (Balen and Jacobs, 1997). Women with a BMI > 28 kg/m^2 and <20 kg/m^2 will have decreased fertility. There is an associated deficiency in gonadotrophin production with excessive weight loss due to diminished production of GnRH.

Acanthosis nigricans may occur – a hyperplasia and thickening of the prickle-cell layer of the epidermis characterized by grey, brown or black pigmentation in axillae and other skin folds, due to the endocrine disturbance (Balen and Jacobs, 1997).

Ovarian failure

Ovarian failure can happen at any age, but if it occurs prior to puberty is commonly associated with chromosomal abnormality such as Turner's syndrome (45X) or childhood malignancy treated by radiotherapy or chemotherapy causing sterility. Ovarian failure linked with raised gonadotrophins and cessation of periods prior to the age of 40 is linked with autoimmune failure, infection, previous surgery and cancer treatments. There is also a suggested link with familial forms of fragile X syndrome (Balen and Jacobs, 1997).

Endometriosis

Endometriosis occurs when endometrial tissue is located outside the uterus around the pelvis. It may be viewed at laparoscopy as blue/black pigmentation (old lesions), red vasculated lesions (active lesions) and white non-pigmented papules (just activating) (Gould, 2003). Retrograde menstruation is thought to be the most common cause but altered immune function is also thought to be associated with the disease. The disease causes pelvic pain, dyspareunia, dysmenorrhoea and infertility. Commonly it causes pelvic adhesions especially around the ovaries and tubes, with cystic lesions on the ovaries called *endometriomas*. Symptoms are linked with the menstrual cycle, age and hormonal therapy; treatments include drugs that interfere with the cycle. These include GnRH agonists, which cause pituitary desensitization and induce amenorrhoea. Danazol inhibits gonadotrophin secretion and also has androgenic effects that cause unpleasant side-effects such as hot flushes, acne, oily skin, hirsutism, reduced libido, weight gain, nausea and headaches. Both drugs temporarily stop menses and reduce levels of antiendometrial autoantibodies (Balen and Jacobs, 1997).

Tubal factors

Tubal damage is commonly associated with pelvic inflammatory disease (PID), ectopic pregnancies, sterilization and adhesions. Increases in sexually transmitted diseases increase the risk of PID and tubal damage. *Chlamydia* is the most frequently reported infection and is often asymptomatic, which increases the risk of cross-contamination and failure to treat (Byrd, 1993). Development of pelvic adhesions commonly results following pelvic infection. Adhesions subsequently create further problems within the pelvis, such as distortion and/or blockage of the fallopian tubes. This may lead to the development of hydrosalpinx or impaired tubal motility and movement of the oocyte. The ovary may adhere to the side wall of the pelvis, which may interfere with the movement of the oocyte into the fimbriae of the fallopian tube (Dechaud and Hedon, 2000).

Ectopic pregnancies occur in approximately 1% of the population but the risk increases with subsequent pregnancies. PID can cause damage to the lumen of the tube and subsequently increases the risk of an ectopic. Symptoms of ectopic pregnancy include bleeding, pain, shoulder tip pain and dizziness. Transvaginal ultrasound aids diagnosis, typically performed at 6 and 7 weeks' gestation. Frequently seen on ultrasound scan is a thickened endometrium with no gestation sac, free fluid and a mass in the pelvis, though not invariably. Occasionally a pseudosac may be visualized on scan but this will not contain any products of conception. Doppler blood flow assists identification of a potential pelvic mass. Serial measurements of serum human chorionic gonadotrophin (hCG) also aid diagnosis of a potential ectopic. Treatment includes surgical removal via laparoscopy or laparotomy either with a salpingostomy or salpingectomy. Medical management includes the systemic administration of methotrexate, which is injected locally into the fallopian tube.

Reflective Activity 9.2

How can health professionals help to reduce the incidence of PID?

Unexplained infertility

Unexplained infertility is classified as the inability to conceive after 1 year without any identified causative factors. It has been suggested that 40–65% of couples in this category will conceive spontaneously over the next 3 years (Balen and Jacobs, 1997). Age will have a direct effect on the duration of time to try to conceive naturally prior to commencing fertility treatment. Couples under the age of 30 years will be reassured and encouraged to try for 3 years before proceeding to treatment, as the success rates are the same as for natural conception. The older the woman the shorter the duration of waiting time. Treatment options for the unexplained category consist of improving fertility initially for the woman with drugs to enhance ovulation.

It is possible to improve sperm function by *intrauterine insemination* (IUI) – inseminating prepared sperm into the uterus.

Male factor infertility

The incidence of male factor infertility contributes to 30% of couples seeking treatment. It has been suggested that there has been a decline in semen quality over the last few decades, though research remains inconclusive with little scientific knowledge of the aetiology (Skakkebaek and Keiding, 1994). A full and comprehensive history of each case is an essential element in the assessment of male fertility and should include:

- assessment of previous fertility
- frequency of intercourse
- coital difficulties
- past history of sexually transmitted disease
- history of mumps orchitis
- history of cryptorchidism
- history of scrotal, inguinal, prostatic or bladder neck surgery
- testicular injury
- testicular cancer – exposure to gonadotoxic agents, e.g. chemotherapy/radiotherapy
- vasectomy (Thornton, 2000).

It is useful to have some idea of the quality and quantity of sperm, and these can be measured against the criteria in Table 9.2.

Endocrine assessment should include serum measurements of follicle-stimulating hormone (FSH), LH, testosterone and prolactin. Increased FSH levels could be suggestive of testicular failure. Hypogonadotrophic hypogonadism is associated with low levels of FSH and testosterone and is sometimes linked with *Kallmann's syndrome*.

Karyotyping, genetic analysis and cystic fibrosis screening should be considered in cases of azoospermia and oligospermia ($<5 \times 10^6$/ml). Cystic fibrosis gene mutations are strongly related to congenital bilateral absence of the vas deferens (CBAVD) – a defect associated with the bilateral regression of the mesonephric duct. It prevents testicular and epididymal spermatozoa from reaching the urethra and renders the patient azoospermic.

The genes responsible for spermatogenesis have been located on the long arm of the Y chromosome in a region known as the azoospermia factor (AZF). Microdeletions on the chromosome may be responsible for suboptimal spermatogenesis in certain men. There are also a host of chromosomal abnormalities that are responsible for suboptimal semen parameters, one of the best known being *Klinefelter's syndrome* (XXY), which presents a chromosomal situation that will almost inevitably result in azoospermia. Other chromosomal abnormalities have differing effects on fertility. Down's syndrome may cause hypogonadism in males, resulting in azoospermia. There are also less severe cases of trisomy 21 producing only subfertile males.

The most common congenital abnormality associated with male infertility is undescended testes which is linked with abnormal spermatogenesis. Men suffering with cryptorchidism have a sevenfold increased risk of testicular cancer (Thornton, 2000). Retrograde ejaculation may either be congenital or as a result of surgery to either the prostate or bladder neck. Sperm in these cases must be collected from alkaline urine after masturbation and then prepared for treatment. Antisperm antibodies can impair sperm motility and fertilization. A barrier exists between the blood vessels that supply the testes and the tract in which spermatozoa are produced and transported (including the testis, epididymis,

vas deferens and the urethra). A breach of this barrier exposes the spermatozoa to the immune system and consequently evokes the production of sperm antibodies. Therefore any process that threatens the integrity of the blood–testes barrier may result in the formation of sperm antibodies. The most common causes are trauma, e.g. vasectomy and vasectomy reversal, testicular torsion, testicular biopsy, varicocele, inflammatory reactions in the genital tract, infections (orchitis, prostatitis) and congenital absence of the vas deferens (seen in the majority of cystic fibrosis patients).

Various solutions to these problems exist and, indeed, micromanipulation techniques such as intracytoplasmic sperm injection (ICSI) have helped to overcome many, although not all of them. Steroids were previously administered to decrease the male immune response to improve chances of fertilization but are now rarely used. Environmental factors, toxins such as pesticides, alcohol, cigarettes and drug abuse can reduce male fertility, and a decrease in consumption of recreational toxins may sometimes improve semen parameters.

MICROMANIPULATION

Intracytoplasmic sperm injection (ICSI) (Fig. 9.2) has provided higher fertilization rates than conventional IVF. A single sperm is injected directly into the ooplasm of the oocyte, with 70% fertilization rates and pregnancy rates comparable with a conventional IVF cycle. There is concern that there seems to be an increase in the incidence of sex chromosome abnormalities in babies born after conception using ICSI.

Table 9.2 WHO criteria for a normal sperm count (WHO, 1999)

Volume	2 ml or more
pH	7.2 or more
Count	$\geq 20 \times 10^6$/ml (azoospermia is diagnosed when no sperm is found in the ejaculate and oligospermia is diagnosed when the concentration of sperm is vastly reduced)
Motility	50% or more with forward progression, or 25% or more with rapid progression (within 60 minutes of ejaculation) (abnormal = asthenozoospermia)
Morphology	The 1999 edition of the WHO manual does not define normal ranges for morphology but notes that data from IVF programmes suggest that as sperm morphology falls below 15% normal forms (teratozoospermia), the fertilization rate decreases
MAR test (antisperm antibodies)	Fewer than 50% of motile sperm with adherent particles
Immunobead test (antisperm antibodies)	Fewer than 50% of motile sperm with adherent beads

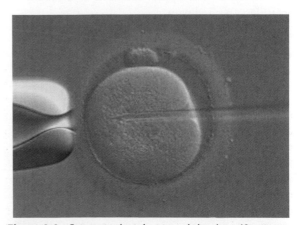

Figure 9.2 Intracytoplasmic sperm injection. (Courtesy of Dr Susan Pickering, Senior Lecturer, Division of Women's Health, Kings College, London.)

TREATMENT OPTIONS FOR FEMALE INFERTILITY PROBLEMS

Ovulation induction

There are two types of drug regime for ovulation induction, which is the most basic of fertility treatments.

Firstly clomiphene citrate, an antioestrogen, is used to treat PCO. Dosage starts at 50 mg and can increase up to 100 mg to induce ovulation. It is taken from day 2–6 of the cycle and should only be prescribed for up to six cycles where the woman has ovulated (RCOG, 2003). The drug can cause thickening of cervical mucus and can cause headaches and visual disturbances.

The other form of drug therapy involves administration of gonadotrophin, commonly subcutaneous FSH, to stimulate ovulation. Close monitoring is essential for these women as they are at risk of high-order multiple pregnancy and *ovarian hyperstimulation syndrome* (OHSS).

Ovarian hyperstimulation syndrome (OHSS)

OHSS can develop if too many follicles are stimulated during a treatment cycle of ovulation induction (OI), intrauterine insemination (IUI) and in vitro fertilization (IVF), and occurs when many follicles are stimulated especially in the case of PCO. This causes ascites, pleural and pericardial effusions, discomfort, nausea, vomiting, difficulty breathing, electrolyte imbalance leading to dehydration, and an increased risk of deep vein thrombosis.

Ultrasound examination reveals enlargement of the ovaries, which have a diameter greater than 5 cm (see Fig. 9.3). Abdominal ascites is frequently present, with fluid noted in the upper abdomen contributing to breathlessness and pain.

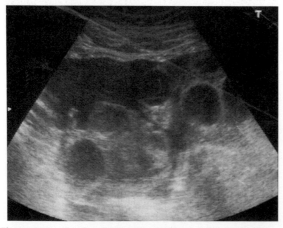

Figure 9.3   Ovarian hyperstimulation syndrome (OHSS).

Donor insemination (DI)

This treatment is appropriate for couples with azoospermia, paternal genetic abnormalities or those unable to afford IVF and ICSI. National success rates average at 9.6% per cycle (Thornton, 2000). Treatment is carried out during the woman's own natural cycle or with superovulation. Management includes monitoring with transvaginal ultrasound to identify one leading follicle prior to ovulation and insemination. When more than two leading follicles are stimulated, with superovulation, then the cycle should be cancelled to reduce the risk of multiple pregnancy.

Intrauterine insemination (IUI)

IUI involves monitored superovulation and insemination of prepared sperm 35 hours after administration of hCG to initiate ovulation. The semen may be prepared for insemination using one of a variety of techniques including sperm *swim up* and *gradient density* procedures.

The *swim up* procedure involves layering a small amount of raw semen underneath an equal amount of culture medium. The sample is left to incubate for 30–60 minutes. The motile sperm are then able to swim up and out of the seminal plasma into the medium, where they may be collected by removing the supernatant. Non-motile sperm and debris will remain in the raw semen. The sperm obtained from these procedures should then be suspended in culture medium and centrifuged to form a pellet which may then be resuspended to an appropriate volume to enable analysis.

The *density gradient* method involves layering raw semen on top of a column of sperm preparation medium (e.g. Puresperm) of varying densities, usually 40% and 80%. The sample is then centrifuged. The resulting pellet is removed, resuspended in culture medium and centrifuged. The process is repeated to ensure the removal of all of the sperm preparation medium, and the sample is then analysed for motility parameters. The density gradients select normal sperm on the basis of their density. Normal sperm should pass through the gradient and rest in the pellet at the bottom of the tube. The layers of the gradients should remove debris bacteria and abnormal sperm from the sample producing the pellet. This treatment is appropriate for slightly suboptimal sperm parameters, unexplained infertility with normal semen parameters and factors such as female age. It does not provide information on potential problems associated with fertilization and has lower success rates than in vitro fertilization (IVF).

Gamete intrafallopian tube transfer (GIFT)

GIFT has generally been superseded by IVF but there are some clinics that still offer this procedure. The process involves superovulation, removal of oocytes via laparoscopy and then deposition of a prepared sperm sample into the fallopian tube to facilitate fertilization. This process is not suitable for woman with tubal damage and yields no information on the possible problems with fertilization.

In vitro fertilization (IVF)

Louise Brown was born in 1978 following the pioneering work of Steptoe and Edwards and since that time IVF has enabled many thousands of couples to achieve a much-desired child. The technique combines superovulation, transvaginal ultrasound-guided oocyte retrieval, insemination of sperm with oocyte in the laboratory, fertilization and replacement of embryos.

Debate surrounds the number of embryos to be replaced in the uterus and many clinics in the UK routinely replace two embryos in many patients, achieving similar pregnancy rates to three-embryo replacements. Units are now using specific selection criteria stipulating replacement of one embryo to further reduce the risk of multiple, especially twin, pregnancies. Multiple pregnancies are not the desired outcome for professionals working in assisted reproduction (ART); owing to the risks encountered in fetomaternal medicine, a singleton pregnancy is the most desired outcome.

Drug management

Superovulation is achieved with the administration of FSH injections (dosages range from 50 to 350 IU), which recruits a cohort of follicles and promotes development and maturation. Purified preparations are delivered via autoinjector subcutaneously by the woman or her partner. Drugs are either developed by recombinant technology or highly purified urinary derived FSH.

To ensure maturation of the follicles and oocytes, administration of hCG is required 35 hours prior to oocyte retrieval. To establish appropriate management of superovulation and avoid premature ovulation due to the LH surge, many units incorporate GnRH agonists or antagonists to prevent ovulation. These drugs bind to GnRH receptors on the pituitary gonadotrophins and desensitize the pituitary. The agonists initiate a flare response which will cause a withdrawal bleed in the woman. The antagonists lead to immediate suppression and are used for a much shorter time. These drugs are administered by either subcutaneous injection or nasal sniffs.

Short protocol This process occurs in the first half of the cycle designed to use stored FSH, which occurs after using a GnRH agonist that is started on day 2. Then exogenous FSH is started on day 3 of the cycle. Women are monitored with transvaginal ultrasound to measure the size of the follicles, which should be approximately 18 mm in diameter, prior to administration of hCG and then oocyte retrieval. Generally lower doses of gonadotrophins are used and the time period is more patient friendly. Unfortunately management of the cycle is less flexible and most centres achieve better pregnancy rates with the long protocol.

Long protocol This process is started in the luteal phase of the cycle with the woman administrating the agonist from day 21 of her cycle. The drug can either be inhaled or injected, dependent on patient preference. Pituitary suppression is achieved within 14 days and then hormone levels are checked for desensitization via assay. Once the woman is downregulated she commences daily injections of FSH to initiate superovulation (Fig. 9.4). Once three follicles are approximately 18 mm in diameter, hCG is administrated 35 hours prior to oocyte retrieval. This regime provides maximum flexibility with cycle programming to enable scheduling of procedures during the working week.

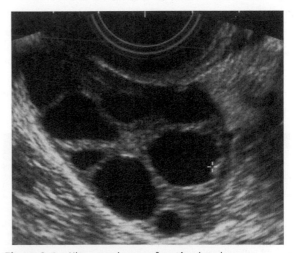

Figure 9.4 Ultrasound scan of a stimulated ovary.

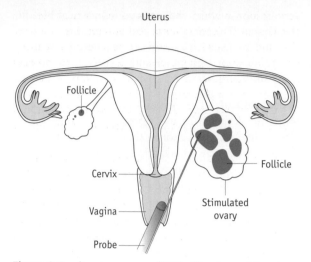

Figure 9.5 Oocyte recovery (OCR). (Courtesy of Janet Currie of the Oxford Fertility Unit.)

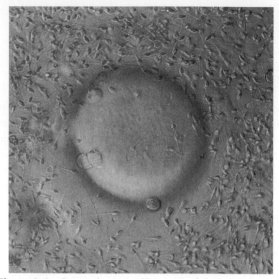

Figure 9.6 Egg and sperm. (Courtesy of Dr Susan Pickering, Senior Lecturer, Division of Women's Health, Kings College, London.)

GnRH antagonists These drugs are used to prevent the LH surge and are administered within the first half of the cycle following several days of FSH administration. Once a woman has a leading follicle of approximately 14 mm the drug is injected daily along with the gonadotrophin. This process provides a shorter treatment time and fewer injections for the woman. At this time it is the less favoured drug choice for treatment.

Oocyte collection is achieved with the use of transvaginal ultrasound undertaken as an outpatient procedure. Intravenous sedation is used to reduce levels of pain and anxiety and partners can accompany the women through the procedure if desired. Follicles are aspirated using gentle suction via a preset vacuum pump into small tubes, which are given to the embryologist for identification (Fig. 9.5). A microscope is required to identify the cumulus/oocyte mass. Follicles are frequently refilled with culture medium to encourage recovery of oocytes. Retrieved oocytes are placed in the incubator with appropriate labelling of the dishes and compartment in the incubator. All laboratory work requires double witnessing to ensure correct safety procedures.

Reflective Activity 9.3

What are the most common side-effects of fertility treatments?

Sperm preparation

Sperm samples may be collected either prior to oocyte retrieval or following the procedure but should be prepared within 30 minutes of production. Sperm preparation follows the same procedure as described in the IUI treatment. Semen samples may be frozen and subsequently defrosted for preparation prior to insemination. After insemination the spermatozoa and the oocytes (Fig. 9.6) are cultured overnight, then assessed for signs of fertilization approximately 16–18 hours later. The appearance of two pronuclei, one from the sperm and one from the oocyte, signifies normal fertilization. Occasionally more than two pronuclei are detected indicating abnormal fertilization and these embryos should not be transferred. Also noted at the fertilization check are the number and grade of the polar bodies extruded from the oocyte. These criteria can also aid in the detection of abnormal fertilization.

Embryo transfer takes place approximately 48 hours after oocyte recovery. The embryo normally contains several blastomeres at this stage, ranging from two to six in number (Fig. 9.7). Some centres culture embryos for 5 days until they have reached blastocyst stage before returning them to the uterus. There is no evidence to prove that blastocyst replacement provides better pregnancy rates than day 2 transfers, which is the routine procedure in most centres.

Fertilization

Fertilization commences when the sperm binds to the zona pellucida of the oocyte. The sperm acrosome

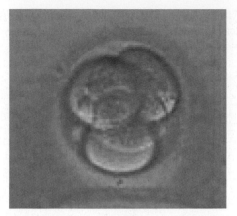

Figure 9.7   Four-cell embryo. (Courtesy of Dr Susan Pickering, Senior Lecturer, Division of Women's Health, Kings College, London.)

reacts and uses enzymes to penetrate the zona. Tail movement and enzymes ensure forward progression. The sperm enters the perivitelline space (PVS) where microvilli cover the whole surface of the human oocyte and aid sperm fusion. The post-acrosomal equatorial region of the sperm fuses with the oolemma, and the sperm nucleus and some parts of the tail and mid-piece region enter the ooplasm. This stimulates waves, or transients, of Ca^{2+} to move across the oocyte. The sperm is then propelled further into the ooplasm of the oocyte. This triggers a reaction within the oocyte that leads to the visual confirmation of fertilization, the appearance of the male and female pronuclei and the extrusion of the first polar body. Oocytes in the fetal ovary arrest during the first meiotic division and then resume division at puberty prior to ovulation. They then arrest again during the second meiotic division and only complete the process of meiosis upon fertilization when the second polar body is also extruded. After fertilization the zygote divides by mitosis into a number of smaller cells called blastomeres, in a process known as cleavage. Cleavage results in a period of intense DNA replication and cell division in the absence of growth. The blastomeres become organized in layers or groups. During cleavage each division results in blastomeres approximately half the size of the parent blastomeres.

Embryo grading

Embryos are closely monitored for quality and potential ability to implant and create a pregnancy. This visual grading process is based on morphological criteria and can neither rule out the possibility of a genetic abnormality within the embryo nor guarantee the selection of a viable embryo for replacement.

Potential genetic anomaly can be identified by using preimplantation genetic diagnosis (PGD), a process that only identifies a very small selection of genetic abnormalities including chromosomal, X-linked, autosomal recessive and dominant, and mitochondrial (ESHRE PGD Consortium Steering Committee, 2000).

The key morphological features of cleavage-stage embryos includes anucleate fragmentation, cell number (developmental speed) and cytoplasmic quality. Such gross embryo morphology is considered by many to be the most reliable indicator of embryo viability. There is a definite correlation between blastomere uniformity and a positive pregnancy test (Hardarson *et al.*, 2001). Conversely extensive zona thickening and multipronucleated blastomeres (Pelinck *et al.*, 1998) have been associated with decreased embryo quality and lower pregnancy rates. It has also been shown that those embryos that cleave (complete the first mitotic division) within 25–27 hours after insemination produce higher implantation and pregnancy rates (Lundin *et al.*, 2001). Zygote scoring has also made an impact on the way embryos are graded (Table 9.3). Combining the criteria, high cleavage morphological score, high zygote morphological score, and early cleavage timing can improve the selection process of the embryos and result in higher implantation rates.

Fragmentation   The causes of fragmentation within the embryo (Fig. 9.8) are unknown and have been linked with poor culture conditions and blastomere loss through apoptosis possibly from chromosomal abnormalities. Whatever the underlying pathology it is clearly associated with decreased implantation (Scott, 2002). The process of fragmentation has been identified as early as the two-cell stage and continues to develop throughout cleavage.

Embryo transfer (Fig. 9.9)

A speculum is inserted into the vagina and the cervix is wiped with a dry swab to remove excess mucus. The embryos are placed into a fine plastic catheter and passed through the cervix into the endometrium, sometimes under ultrasound guidance. If the cervix is convoluted or a tight internal os is encountered, the malleable outer sheath of the catheter is adapted to pass through the obstruction.

Once the embryos have been replaced the woman is placed on luteal support to circumvent the potential

Table 9.3 Embryo grading (Dale and Elder, 1997)

Embryo	Blastomeres	Fragments	Refractility	Zona
Grade 1	Even, regular, spherical	10%	Moderate	Intact
Grade 2	Uneven or irregular shape	<10% fragmentation		
Grade 3		<50% fragmentation		Intact
Grade 4		>50% fragmentation	Gross variation	
Grade 5	Embryos contain two pronuclei possibly from delayed fertilization or reinsemination on day 1			
Grade 6 classed as non-viable	Lysed, contracted or dark blastomeres			

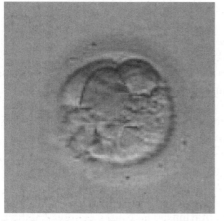

Figure 9.8 Fragmentation. (Courtesy of Dr Susan Pickering, Senior Lecturer, Division of Women's Health, Kings College, London.)

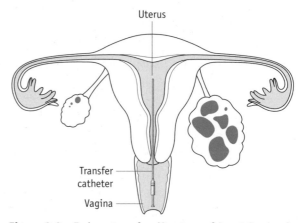

Figure 9.9 Embryo transfer. (Courtesy of Janet Currie of the Oxford Fertility Unit.)

fall in progesterone levels, as this could directly affect the function of the endometrium at this crucial time during potential implantation. Commonly progesterone pessaries are supplied and administered twice daily until the pregnancy test is performed 14 days after embryo transfer. Following IVF treatment the ovaries contain multiple corpora lutea which remain enlarged for the following few weeks. This may cause symptoms of bloating and discomfort and the woman should be advised of the symptoms.

Blastocyst transfer is another form of IVF. During normal physiological fertilization the sperm fertilizes the oocyte in the fallopian tube and the embryo moves down the tract until it eventually reaches the endometrium around day 5 after fertilization. Blastocyst development has been difficult to achieve in vitro due to inadequate culture media. As technology has developed, improved sequential media have resulted in higher rates of blastocyst development. Embryos are usually replaced on day 2 or 3, which does not correlate with implantation in vivo. As some embryos will not reach blastocyst stage but look completely normal at the day 2–3 stage, it has been suggested that blastocyst transfer enables embryologists to assess the morphological quality of the embryo at a later stage of development, thus allowing them to choose embryos with increased implantation potential (Fig. 9.10).

Cryopreservation

The cryostorage of semen is an essential service provided by the majority of assisted conception units. It is

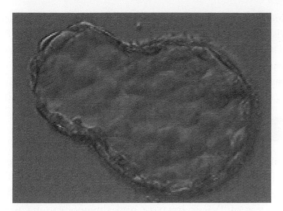

Figure 9.10 Hatching blastocyst. (Courtesy of Dr Susan Pickering, Senior Lecturer, Division of Women's Health, Kings College, London.)

offered to certain patients undergoing IVF treatment and also to patients who have been diagnosed with a malignant disease who wish to store their semen prior to chemotherapy and radiotherapy and/or potentially damaging pelvic surgery. IVF patients may request sperm storage for a variety of reasons which range from poor-quality semen following vasectomy reversal; declining sperm count; production difficulties; geographical separation of the couple at the time of oocyte retrieval; and provision of a tested, clean sample where contamination of the semen has been an issue in the past. Certain units store semen prior to a vasectomy procedure. The freeze–thaw procedure does damage the cells and may reduce the pre-freeze motility.

Embryo freezing can be performed provided enough suitable spare embryos are available after embryo transfer. Embryos may either be frozen at producer or cleavage stage (two to eight cells) and should be of a sufficient quality (grades 1, 2 and 3 or A, B and C) with less than 20% cytoplasmic fragmentation in order to attain the best chance of survival following the freeze–thaw procedure. It has been suggested that uneven blastomeres and large amounts of fragmentation could inhibit survival potential.

Cryopreservation of oocytes provides a treatment option for women about to undergo cancer treatment that may cause temporary or permanent sterility. Success rates from the use of frozen eggs is very low and only one baby has been successfully born from this technique in the UK.

Egg donation

In the UK egg donation is by anonymous donors. In some instances known donation from a family member or friend can provide the help required by a woman who may have undergone a premature menopause, has a genetic abnormality or has completed multiple failed IVF attempts. To donate eggs the donor has to undergo a full IVF cycle, which is time-consuming and not without risks. Consequently there is a national shortage of donated eggs and the National Gamete Donation Trust has been established to promote altruistic donation. Many fertility units have waiting lists as long as 2–3 years for donors, and alternative options, such as egg sharing, have been used by certain clinics. Egg sharing provides reduced cost IVF treatment to couples willing to donate half of their eggs to a recipient couple. This created ethical debate, resulting in the development of guidelines for good practice by the HFEA to further review the appropriateness of the treatment for couples. Any couple that donate eggs have to undergo thorough counselling, detailed history-taking, investigations including karyotyping, blood grouping, infection screening including hepatitis A, B and C, HIV, and syphilis, and for cystic fibrosis. Those with pre-existing disease and familial cancers are dissuaded from donation. Any uncertainty from partners will also be a cause not to go ahead with donation owing to the potential issues of existing siblings and ownership, especially in known donation between siblings.

Surrogacy

Surrogacy involves a couple commissioning a woman to act as a host for their own genetic embryo, and is a choice for women who may not have a uterus or are medically prevented from undergoing a pregnancy. It is illegal in the UK to pay a surrogate, though expenses can be paid. In English law the woman who gives birth to the baby is the legal mother of the child irrespective of the genetic origin of the child. The genetic parents therefore have to apply to adopt the child from the birth mother and this may be a problem if she changes her mind and wishes to keep the baby.

OUTCOME FROM ASSISTED REPRODUCTION TECHNIQUES

Because of the moral and ethical implications of assisted conception techniques, outcome studies have been closely monitoring the births and development of resulting children. Associated factors contributing to adverse outcome associated with ART include maternal

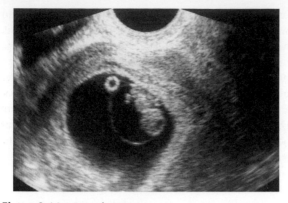

Figure 9.11   8-week pregnancy.

age, medical indications for infertility, paternal age and multiple pregnancies. The ICSI procedure has raised several issues for debate on this subject as the process can potentially use sperm carrying genetic abnormalities, and structural defects may result from mechanical or biochemical damage when introducing foreign material into the oocyte and bypassing the natural selection process of fertilization (Kurinczuk, 2003). Genetic screening is offered to couples requiring ICSI with poor sperm parameters. Mutations in the cystic fibrosis (CF) gene have been identified in men requiring ICSI; associated with these mutations is congenital bilateral absence of the vas deferens (CBAVD). Another anomaly identified with male infertility is microdeletions on the long arm of the Y chromosome that influence germ cell development and maintenance (McElreavey and Krausz, 1999). It has been established that male offspring will inherit the microdeletion and the paternal infertility (Kurinczuk, 2003).

Multiple births create further problems with morbidity and mortality of children conceived from ART (Koivurova *et al.*, 2002). Twins and triplets have increased risks of cerebral palsy; the associated risk with twins has been quoted as 13.2 per 1000 confinements, eight times more than for singletons, and 75.9 per 1000 with triplet confinements, which is 47 times higher than for singletons (Petterson *et al.*, 1993). Petterson and colleagues suggested that one in ten pregnant women with twins and one in five pregnant women with triplets, whatever the mode of conception, who reach 20 weeks' gestation will experience at least one of the following: a child with cerebral palsy, an infant death or stillbirth. One of the treatment options now offered to couples is multifetal pregnancy reduction (frequently performed in the USA). Data suggest that surviving twins from the procedure have an eightfold

increase of cerebral palsy and an eightfold increased risk of periventricular leucomalacia (Geva *et al.*, 1998). The preferred option in the UK is to replace fewer embryos, either two or one, to reduce the incidence of multiple births (Hazekamp *et al.*, 2000) (Fig. 9.11).

STRESS AND INFERTILITY

Infertility has a great impact on individuals' physical and psychological well-being (Hammarberg, 2003; Kerr *et al.*, 1999; Pfeffer and Woollet, 1983). The process of IVF is invasive and time-consuming with intimate procedures including vaginal ultrasound scanning, transvaginal ultrasound oocyte recovery, embryo transfer, administering injections and producing a sperm sample. Couples frequently feel stigmatized and embarrassed by their infertility. This contributes to a growing sense of isolation, which creates stress and anxiety in many aspects of their daily lives. Success rates are low, so many couples experience multiple episodes of grief and loss and often depression. Emotions described by couples include loss of self-esteem, mourning, threat, guilt, marital problems and also health problems (Guerra *et al.*, 1998).

The costs incurred by IVF treatment can also be a major stress for couples undergoing treatment. The Government has initiated a review of fertility treatments by the National Institute of Clinical Excellence (NICE) and the second draft for consultation has made several recommendations to increase availability of fertility treatment under the NHS.

According to the latest draft standards, three attempts of both fresh and frozen embryos provide the best chance of achieving a pregnancy. One in six couples experience problems with fertility in Britain, and there are approximately 27 000 IVF attempts every year; 80% of cycles take place in private practice. If the cycles were provided by the NHS it would cost an estimated £400m and there are concerns how the income would be generated (BBC News, 2003).

Counselling is an integral part of the process of fertility treatment at all stages. Licensed units provide independent counselling for individuals, which is an essential part of programmes, before, during and after treatment. Studies have suggested that mothers who have conceived by IVF have higher anxiety levels which relate to the survival and normality of the unborn babies, damage caused by childbirth and separation from babies after birth, compared to matched controls (McMahon *et al.*, 1997). Support from midwives during the pregnancy is crucial to these couples, who may feel more vulnerable than parents who have conceived naturally. It is important for couples to normalize the pregnancy after the intensity of the fertility treatment, which may be challenging for the team caring for the couples in primary, secondary and tertiary care.

This chapter has included the complex issues related to diagnosis, investigation and treatment of infertility. Couples who experience difficulty with conception have to deal with the stress, frustration and stigma associated with being infertile. Many undergo treatments that have a low level of success and are not available on the NHS. The whole experience may damage them and their relationships and many will not achieve a long-desired pregnancy. It is important for midwives to understand the processes that women have undergone to achieve their pregnancy. Understanding the causes of infertility and the treatment processes is important so the midwife can perceive the degree of stress and the financial burden of assisted conception.

KEY POINTS

- It is important that midwives understand the causes of infertility in men and women and are aware of their management and treatment.
- Infertility has a major impact on parents' approach to pregnancy and childbirth.
- Many women the midwife will come into contact with will have had tests or treatment for infertility, and this will impact on their experience of pregnancy and childbirth.
- Infertility and its treatment are closely regulated, and the midwife needs to be aware of the parameters of these regulations.

REFERENCES

Balen, A. & Jacobs, H. (1997) *Infertility in Practice.* London: Churchill Livingstone.

Barber, D. (2002) The extended role of the fertility nurse – practical realities. *Human Fertility* 5(1): 13–16.

BBC News (2003) 'More IVF on the NHS. Online. Available: http://news.bbc.co.uk.

Byrd, C. (1993) *Chlamydia trachomatis* genital infections. *West Virginia Medical Journal* 89(8): 331–333.

Dale, B. & Elder, K. (1997) *In Vitro Fertilisation.* Cambridge: Cambridge University Press.

Dechaud, H. & Hedon, B. (2000) What effect does hydrosalpinx have on assisted reproduction? The role of salpingectomy remains controversial. *Human Reproduction* 15(2): 234–235.

ESHRE PGD Consortium Steering Committee (2000) ESHRE Preimplantation Genetic Diagnosis (PGD) Consortium: data collection II (May 2000). *Human Reproduction* 15(12): 2673–2683.

Geva, E., Lerner-Geva, L., Stavorosky, Z. *et al.* (1998) Multifetal pregnancy reduction: a possible risk factor for periventricular leukomalacia in premature newborns. *Fertility and Sterility* 69(5): 845–850.

Gould, D. (2003) Women's health – endometriosis. *Nursing Standard* 17(27): 47–53.

Guerra, D., Llobera, A., Veiga, A. *et al.* (1998) Psychiatric morbidity in couples attending a fertility service. *Human Reproduction* 13(6): 1733–1736.

Hammarberg, K. (2003) Stress in assisted reproductive technology: implications for nursing practice. *Human Fertility* 6(1): 30–33.

Hardarson, T., Hanson, C., Sjogren, A. *et al.* (2001) Human embryos with unevenly sized blastomeres have lower pregnancy and implantation rates: indications for aneuploidy and multinucleation. *Human Reproduction* 16(12): 313–318.

Hazekamp, J., Bergh, C., Wennerholm, U. *et al.* (2000) Avoiding multiple pregnancies in ART. *Human Reproduction* 15(6): 1217–1219.

Hull, M., Glazener, C., Kelly, N. *et al.* (1985) Population study of causes, treatment and outcome of infertility. *British Medical Journal* 291(6510): 1693–1697.

Human Fertilisation and Embryology Act 1990. London: HMSO.

Human Fertilisation and Embryology Authority (HFEA) (2001) *Human Fertilisation and Embryology Authority Code of Practice,* 5th edn. London: HFEA.

Kerr, J., Brown, C., & Balen, A. (1999) The experience of couples who have infertility treatment in the United Kingdom; results of a survey performed in 1997. *Human Reproduction* 14(4): 934–938.

Koivurova, S., Hartikainen, A., Gissler, M. *et al.* (2002) Neonatal outcome and congenital malformations in children born after in-vitro fertilization. *Human Reproduction* 17(5): 1391–1398.

Kousta, E., White, D., Cela, E. *et al.* (1999) The prevalence of polycystic ovaries in women with infertility. *Human Reproduction* 14(11): 2720–2723.

Kousta, E., Cela, E., Lawrence, N. *et al.* (2000) The prevalence of polycystic ovaries in women with a history of gestational diabetes mellitus. *Clinical Endocrinology* **53**: 501–507.

Kurinczuk, J. (2003) From theory to reality – just what are the data telling us about ICSI offspring health and future fertility and should we be concerned. *Human Reproduction* **18**(5): 925–931.

Lundin, K., Bergh, C. & Hardarson, T. (2001) Early embryo cleavage is a strong indicator of embryo quality in human IVF. *Human Reproduction* **16**(12): 2652–2657.

McElreavey, K. & Krausz, C. (1999) Sex chromosome genetics '99. Male infertility and the Y chromosome. *American Journal of Human Genetics* **64**: 928–933.

McMahon, C., Ungerer, J., Beaurepaire, J. *et al.* (1997) Anxiety during pregnancy and fetal attachment after in-vitro fertilization. *Human Reproduction* **12**(1): 176–182.

Pelinck, M., De Vos, M., Derkens, M. *et al.* (1998) Embryos cultured in vitro with multinucleated blastomeres have poor implantation potential in human in vitro fertilisation and intracytoplasmic sperm injection. *Human Reproduction* **13**(4): 960–963.

Petterson, B., Nelson, K., Watson, L. *et al.* (1993) Twins, triplets, and cerebral palsy in births in Western Australia in the 1980s. *British Medical Journal* **307**(6914): 1239–1243.

Pfeffer, N. & Woollet, A. (1983) *The Experience of Infertility*. London: Virago Press.

Royal College of Obstetricians and Gynaecologists (RCOG) (2003) *Long-term Consequences of Polycystic Ovary Syndrome – Guideline No. 33*. London: RCOG.

Scott, L. (2002) Embryological strategies for overcoming recurrent assisted reproductive technology treatment failure. *Human Fertility* **5**(4): 206–214.

Skakkebaek, K. & Keiding, N. (1994) Changes in semen and the testis. *British Medical Journal* **309**(6965): 1316–1317.

Snick, H., Snick, T., Evers, J. *et al.* (1997) The spontaneous pregnancy prognosis in untreated subfertile couples: the Walcheren primary care study. *Human Reproduction* **12**(7): 1582–1588.

Templeton, A., Fraser, C. & Thompson, B. (1990) The epidemiology of infertility in Aberdeen. *British Medical Journal* **301**(6744): 148–152.

Thornton, S. (2000) *Infertility in Men*. Update Postgraduate Centre Series – Infertility. Netherlands: Excerpta Medica.

World Health Organization (WHO) (1999) *WHO Laboratory Manual for the Examination of Human Semen and Sperm–Cervical Mucus Interaction,* 4th edn. Cambridge: Cambridge University Press.

FURTHER READING

Meerabeau, L. & Denton, J. (eds) (1995) *Infertility Nursing and Caring*. London: Scutari Press.
This book presents the nurse's developing role in infertility treatments and includes a discussion of the social and political issues, and ethical and moral viewpoints.

10

Preconception Care

Barbara Burden and Trish Jones

LEARNING OUTCOMES

After reading this chapter you will:

- realize the importance of preconception care
- appreciate the concepts involved in undertaking a preconception history and screening tests

- be able to evaluate preconception care advice for parents.

INTRODUCTION

The aim of preconception care is to maximize the health of prospective parents prior to conception. This ensures they are at the peak of their health potential at the point of conception and during organogenesis (17–56 days following conception) when the possibility of fetal abnormality is highest, thus attempting to achieve maximum health potential of the developing baby. In an ideal world prospective parents would present themselves to an appropriately trained healthcare professional for health screening at least 6 months prior to a planned conception. In reality this is not usually perceived as essential by prospective parents and health professionals and it is only in retrospect when pregnancy outcome is compromised that parents seek to identify what could have prevented or reduced this outcome. Preconception care therefore needs to be aimed at any individual, male or female, with the potential for conception.

With the developing public health role of the midwife in providing total care for the family, every health promotion activity undertaken should include elements of preconception advice. Preconception care should be included in routine health screening activities offered by a variety of healthcare professionals, in health promotion literature and classes, in schools (Dickerson, 1995), during family planning or cervical screening sessions, in pregnancy testing kits, at post-abortion counselling and in any potential patient education experience. Reproductive sexual health is already discussed in schools, with the aim of reducing teenage pregnancy,

and this example could easily be applied to components of preconception care, not to advocate pregnancy but to inform adolescents of the importance of planning and preparing for pregnancy. Women who have negative pregnancy tests should also be targeted for preconception health promotion in readiness for subsequent pregnancy. Preconception advice should be offered to women during the antenatal and postnatal periods, increasing the knowledge of both pregnancy and preconception health promotion.

Preconception care varies considerably internationally, nationally and locally, reaching a small segment of the community, usually clients who are motivated, articulate and aware of their needs, or clients who have had a compromised pregnancy and are preparing for future pregnancy. It can be offered in any healthcare, educational or health promotion environment by appropriately educated individuals, targeted towards specific health needs depending on individual requirements. The type of screening available to women and their partners also varies; thus advising women on preconception care is often confusing. The difficulty with preconception care is that it is not perceived as a priority by healthcare providers and professionals and is not common knowledge in women. Only in retrospect when pregnancy outcome was not what was expected do women and their partners seek information on prevention, or advice on care for subsequent pregnancy. With appropriate preconception care the care and treatment required during pregnancy is significantly reduced. For example, providing preconception care to women with diabetes reduces hospital admissions, length of stay in hospital, intensity of care of newborn infants and subsequently shortens the infant's period of hospitalization (Herman *et al.*, 1999).

This chapter outlines some of the areas of interest to women and their partners attempting to conceive. Each area of interest is subdivided into advice a midwife could offer to women and partners and further reading or Internet addresses for additional information. It is important to remember that patterns of treatment are continually changing as new ideas and research results emerge and therefore midwives need to monitor changes and implement them into their care provision.

AIM OF PRECONCEPTION CARE

The aim of preconception care is to increase the health of prospective parents, ensuring they are at the peak of their health potential at the point where conception occurs and throughout the period of organogenesis, enhancing the health of the developing baby.

Organogenesis   This is the period of early fetal development (17–56 days following conception) where the early cell mass of conception becomes organized into three layers: ectoderm, mesoderm and endoderm; each responsible for development of different organs or body parts in the developing baby.

OBJECTIVES OF PRECONCEPTION CARE

The objectives of preconception care are to:

- maximize the health of prospective parents and hence the health of the baby during organogenesis and the duration of pregnancy, creating a constructive environment in which conception and fetal development occur
- reduce perinatal and maternal mortality and morbidity
- provide detailed information to prospective parents, enabling them to make informed choices about the care they receive and their readiness to be parents
- evaluate the genetic potential of women and their partners and the need for genetic counselling
- advise on discontinuation of contraception, enabling planning of conception and reduction of unplanned pregnancies
- inform prospective parents of elements of maternity services, enabling informed choice on the type of care required and where that care takes place.

Reflective Activity 10.1

Determine what preconception care is available to you locally. For example:

- Are preconception care clinics offered at your local health centre or hospital?
- Are there healthcare professionals willing to offer advice in areas such as HIV, genetic counselling or health promotion?

TAKING A PRECONCEPTION HISTORY

When a woman and her partner present for preconception care and advice the supporting practitioner records a personal history. The most important aspect of preconception care is the need for a full and detailed health history from both partners and others identified as being significant, such as where genetic screening is required. The aim of the session is to assess, educate and counsel prospective parents on optimum health in preparation for pregnancy. The information obtained at this interview guides the care process, providing a baseline for subsequent comparative tests.

The interview should be undertaken in an environment where clients feel at ease and confidentiality and privacy are ensured. Appropriate allocation of time for appointments should be available, enabling time to listen and advise prospective parents and undertake necessary screening tests. All tests are explained in detail, information sheets are provided and informed consent is obtained. At some point in the interview it is recommended that each partner be interviewed in private so they may disclose personal information they do not wish their partner to know.

The preconception care assessment

The process of risk assessment in preconception care presumes the potential for adverse outcome in pregnancy. The assessment focuses on identification of conditions relating to risk, assessing prospective parents' risk of complications in pregnancy and interventions required to reduce severity of those complications (Reynolds, 1998). It should contain a detailed medical, psychological and social history, physical examination and health screening of both prospective parents. The need to link risk assessment to health promotion activities ensures preconception care focuses not only on diagnosis and treatment but also on creating a healthy environment for the proposed conception through advice and guidance.

Both the woman and her partner should be involved in the discussion to provide the following information:

- health status, i.e. rubella immunity, hepatitis B status, body mass index (BMI)
- sexual history, i.e. contraceptives, sexually transmitted disease or infertility
- family history to include genetic history, even if sperm or egg donors are used
- medical/surgical history
- psychological history
- substance use, i.e. drugs, smoking, alcohol
- history of infections
- obstetric and gynaecological history
- contact with environmental hazards
- nutritional history
- occupational history.

Once a detailed history has been taken, areas of health promotion or risk are identified and screening tests performed. Dependent on individual needs and the services available, not all of the following tests will be offered or deemed necessary. However, specialist support services are available through organizations such as Foresight.

Screening tests

- Physical examination to identify any medical or surgical conditions requiring referral to members of the multiprofessional team
- Blood pressure measurement
- Cardiac function
- Thyroid function
- Respiratory function
- Review of gastrointestinal activity
- Weight
- Sexual health status, i.e. vaginal, urethral or anal swabs
- Cervical smear
- Serum screening:
  - for haemoglobinopathies
  - full blood count
  - rubella status
  - tuberculosis status
- Assessment of vitamin, zinc and lead levels
- Hair analysis:
  - nutritional state
  - exposure to toxic metals

- Karyotyping
- Urinalysis for protein, ketones, glucose and bacteriuria.

Providing information to prospective parents

Results of screening tests should be given to clients as the information becomes available, taking care not to overload the couple with details. Verbal information is supported by documents, information via the Internet and referral to others in the multiprofessional team. It is important not to assume a prior level of knowledge, particularly in relation to issues such as basic anatomy, sexual health or knowledge of support services.

NUTRITION

The importance of an adequate diet at conception and during pregnancy is identified as a key factor in adult health, with associated links to illness such as coronary heart disease (DoH, 2000). There is a direct relationship between nutritional intake, malnutrition and suboptimal nutrition in pregnancy and maternal and child health (Reifsnider and Gill, 2000). Women with conditions that require specific diets or nutritional requirements should be referred or advised to seek specialist advice from their nutritionalist or dietician (Balen and Challis, 1993). The aim is to ensure that women have a healthy body weight, sensible eating habits and suitable nutritional stores at the point of conception (Seaman, 1997). Diet in pregnancy is influenced by morning sickness, hyperemesis, pica (food cravings) and dislike of certain foods. Nutritional assessment is important because of the increase in malnutrition and the recognition that someone who is obese can also be malnourished. Current debates should be reviewed in conjunction with this section to ensure that practice is up to date; an example of this is the latest discussion on avoiding peanuts in pregnancy as this is thought to reduce the incidence of peanut allergy in children (DoH, 1998).

The body mass index (BMI) is still the recognized method of estimating nutritional status of an individual. A BMI of 20 or less is indicative that the individual is underweight whereas a BMI of 30 or over is indicative of obesity. Energy intake needs to be increased by approximately 200 calories per day during pregnancy, but no change is required while preparing to conceive.

Table 10.1 outlines the information, advice and further reading on nutrition that a midwife may find helpful when offering preconception advice on nutritional intake.

Table 10.1   Nutrition: preconception care, advice and further reading

	Information and advice	Further information
Obesity	Lack of essential nutrients in the first trimester influences organogenesis and fetal formation Advise women to achieve a BMI of 21–29 prior to conception Unsupervised dieting is not advised during pregnancy although a healthy low-fat diet may help regulate weight gain Refer to dietician	Galtier-Dereure *et al.*, 2000

Eating disorders
    Anorexia
    Bulimia
	Discussion of eating habits, although women may be reluctant to disclose information
	Advise women to achieve a BMI of 21–29 prior to conception
	Refer to general practitioner for referral to dietician, psychologist or psychiatrist
	Bulimia often improves during pregnancy with 34% no longer suffering after pregnancy
		Franko and Spurrell, 2000
		Morgan *et al.*, 1999

Vitamin deficiency and supplements	If following a healthy diet, vitamin supplements are unnecessary unless medically indicated Remember supplements are drugs Advise women that some medications contain vitamin A, which can be teratogenic, for example, treatment for acne Avoid foods high in retinoids such as liver and fish liver oil as they contain high levels of vitamin A	Smithells, 1996
Folic acid deficiency	Advise to take folic acid, remembering to take higher dose if epileptic Alcoholics, smokers and lactating women are at increased risk of folic acid deficiency. 4 mg of folic acid is taken 2–3 months prior to conception to the end of the first trimester following a previous neural tube defect or if epileptic. 0.4 mg of folic acid is taken 2–3 months prior to conception to the end of the first trimester in a first or subsequent pregnancy where there is no history of neural tube defects Increase consumption of leafy vegetables and wholemeal products	Lumley *et al.*, 2000 Elkin and Higham, 2000

Calcium deficiency
    Osteoporosis
    Rickets
    Osteomalacia
	Many women do not meet the daily recommendation of 700 mg of calcium even when not pregnant
	May influence lactation
	Advise on daily intake of calcium, milk, cheese, fish and yogurt
	Refer to dietician
		http://www.doh.gov.uk/osteop.htm

Caffeine	Reduces implantation; three cups per day reduces the rate of conception by 27%
	Advise to:
	    lower caffeine intake or cease
	    reduce intake gradually to limit side-effects, such as headaches and lethargy
		http://www.babycenter.com
		Pollard *et al.*, 1999

Anaemia	Anaemia should be diagnosed before pregnancy and the cause found and treated Advise on diet, such as bread, pulses, red meat and spinach	Seaman, 1997
GM foods	There is at present insufficient evidence on the effects of GM foods on organogenesis, pregnancy or fetal development	http://www.doh.gov.uk/gmfood.htm

INFECTION

Infection in the mother, and in some cases the father, may affect the developmental phases of the fetus. Any infections should be diagnosed and treated prior to conception and advice given on prevention of reinfection (Table 10.2). Routine serum screening can assess immunity to infections such as rubella, and where immunity is not detected, vaccination can be offered prior to conception. Infection that causes a significant rise in body temperature may result in spontaneous abortion in early pregnancy. This is particularly relevant in both measles and mumps. The impact of mumps should be considered when exploring a medical history from prospective fathers because of the link with infertility in men.

SEXUALLY TRANSMITTED DISEASE

A full and detailed sexual history must be obtained before conception to assess potential risk. This area of health is often the most difficult to discuss but needs to be explored during the interview to determine a sexual history or associated risk factors such as drug misuse. Sexually transmitted diseases, infections and infestations are on the increase and need to be routinely screened for in any health promotion encounter. Where infections are indicated, barrier methods of contraception should be used until treatment is completed. Suspected cases are referred to the genitourinary medicine clinic. Further information on sexual health is included in Chapter 47.

Reflective Activity 10.2

Access the Public Health Laboratory Service website at http://www.phls.co.uk. Review the various types of sexually transmitted diseases, evaluating them in relation to preconception care and the information required during discussion on a sexual history.

Access the following Internet sites and documents to determine the impact of the listed conditions on the prospective mother and her baby.

- Syphilis:
  - Genc and Ledger, 2000
  - Report on the National Screening Committee – Antenatal syphilis screening in the UK – http://www.phls.co.uk/publications/index.htm
- Gonorrhoea – http://www.phls.co.uk/facts/STI
- Genital warts – http://www.phls.co.uk/facts/STI
- Pubic infestations – National Guidelines for management of *Phthirus pubis* infestations – http://www.agum.org.uk
- Genital herpes – Management of herpes in pregnancy, National Guidelines for the management of genital herpes – http://www.agum.org.uk
- *Chlamydia trachomatis* – http://www.doh.gov.uk/chlamyd.htm.

MEDICAL CONDITIONS

Women and their partners who have a medical condition should attend for preconception care within a multiprofessional team, consisting of specialist practitioners, obstetricians, physician and midwives. Most medical conditions if managed effectively throughout organogenesis and the first trimester result in successful outcome for mother and baby at birth (Table 10.3). In each case early referral to the medical team is paramount.

GENETICS

One of the most important activities in preconception screening is assessment of risk of genetic anomalies in prospective children (Table 10.4). The level of risk is linked to the chance of a baby inheriting an abnormality from its family. A family pedigree is constructed as part of the preconception interview with a geneticist if indicated during the preconception history. Pregnancy is not the time for genetic screening, as ideally this should be completed before conception. Historically, genetic anomalies were linked to a given population, but now with a mobile world population it is difficult to label specific groups as being more at risk than others; therefore they should be considered in all cases and explored during discussion. At present, genetic counselling is only provided to a small sample of the community and in most cases does not reach those who are most at risk. The emphasis is currently on diagnosis and treatment during pregnancy rather than prevention before pregnancy (Harper, 1988).

ENVIRONMENT AND LIFESTYLE

The environment and our styles of life influence the development of our children, not only during childhood but also during the period of organogenesis (Table 10.5).

Table 10.2   Infections: preconception care, advice and further reading

	Information and advice	Further information
Rubella virus (German measles)	Avoid contact with infected persons for 7 days before and 5 days after rash appears Ask the GP to check immunity status and vaccinate prior to conception Avoid pregnancy for 3 months following vaccination Higher fetal risk in the first trimester Advise mothers on vaccinating children	Morgan-Capner and Crowcroft, 2000
Erythema infectiosum (slapped cheek disease)	Avoid children with the disease It is thought to be communicable 1 week before symptoms appear to 1 week after onset of symptoms	Morgan-Capner and Crowcroft, 2000
Listeriosis (*Listeria monocytogenes*)	A food-borne pathogen found in soil, water and some vegetation Wash hands when dealing with food May be present in ready-to-eat food, meat pies, pâtés, unpasteurized milk or goat's milk, soft cheeses, such as Feta, Camembert, Brie and Stilton, and can survive and multiply in refrigerators at temperatures of 6°C or above Re-heat all food to steaming point, as this kills the pathogen Avoid contact with sheep during lambing and avoid handling silage as this increases the risk of contamination Treat with antibiotics May take up to 8 weeks for the illness to emerge so advise not to become pregnant during that time	www.thebabyregistry.co.uk Silver, 1998
Toxoplasmosis	Caused by the parasite *Toxoplasma gondii* If tested prior to pregnancy and shown to carry the infection, then women are not at risk during pregnancy No risk to healthy women unless they have a compromised immune system Advise on methods to minimize chance of infection Wear gloves when dealing with cat litter boxes Wash hands thoroughly following gardening or contact with soil Ensure meat is thoroughly cooked Raw or cured meat should be avoided Wash hands after handling meat or fruit and vegetables (because of soil contamination)	Turner, 2000 www.womens-health.co.uk/toxo.htm
Tuberculosis	Treat prior to conception Vaccinate prior to travelling to areas where TB is prevalent Seek advice from GP if in contact with persons infected with the disease or individuals from areas where the disease is prevalent Advise to use barrier methods when taking antibiotics, as they reduce potential of oral contraception Contact tracing undertaken	Davidson, 1995
HIV/AIDS	Steady maintenance of low viral load and high CD4 count prior to conception reduces risks to the baby Continued unprotected sex results in an increased viral load Sperm washing and artificial insemination is available but not on the NHS. The cost is approximately £1500. This is a safer option for conception although it has a relatively low success rate Treatment with AZT Referral to sexual health team	Marina *et al.*, 1998 info@avert.org www.nam.org.uk RCPCH Reducing mother-to-child transmission of HIV infection in the UK http://www.phls.co.uk/publications/index.htm

(continued)

Table 10.2 (*continued*)

	Information and advice	Further information
Chickenpox virus (varicella zoster)	The majority of mothers who have had chickenpox develop lifelong immunity which protects their baby during pregnancy Test for VZ antibody; if not present can receive varicella zoster immune globulin 1 in 3 women suffer spontaneous abortion following infection Avoid pregnancy for 3 months following vaccination At-risk groups include schoolteachers, childcare workers and nursery nurses Avoid infected individuals. If in contact and not immune advise to use contraception until end of incubation period	Enders and Miller, 1994
Chlamydia psittaci	Transmitted from infected sheep Women should have no contact with sheep during lambing season	Blanchard and Mabey, 1994
Hepatitis B	Assess hepatitis status Vaccinate before conception if in at-risk category, for example body piercing, tattoos May recommend liver function tests to assess severity of disease Screen partners and other family members. If negative they should be offered immunization and follow-up by health services	Duff, 1998 Simms and Duff, 1993 http://www.doh.gov.uk/hepatitisb/hepatitiswomen.htm
Group B streptococcus (GBS)	May have no effect. 25% of women of childbearing age have GBS in their vaginas with no apparent symptoms Advise women they require intravenous antibiotic therapy in labour or following rupture of membranes, to reduce the incidence of transmission to their baby	www.gbss.org.uk
Cytomegalovirus	May be asymptomatic as the virus lives within the salivary glands in many 'healthy' adults Wash hands before preparing meals	Azam *et al.*, 2001
Tetanus	*Clostridium tetani* spores are found in soil, dust and gut of animals Wash hands following gardening or dusting	Fauveau *et al.*, 1993
Creutzfeldt–Jakob disease (CJD)	There is currently no known link between CJD and organogenesis; however, there is some discussion on whether the developing fetus may inherit the disease from parents	http://www.cjd.ed.ac http://www.doh.gov.uk/cjd

Stereotypical ideas of social class are now merging, making it difficult to determine the lifestyle of specific groups, as drinking, smoking and drug addiction cross all social barriers. The effect of some drugs on conception and organogenesis was first identified following the administration of thalidomide in the 1960s as a treatment for morning sickness, and as new drugs appear on the market the impact on the next generation of children has yet to be recognized (Reynolds, 1998).

The preconception history must include an assessment of risks associated with employment, exercise, drug consumption and smoking plus questions on physical abuse, use of alternative therapies and exposure to toxic substances. It is important not to make assumptions about individuals but to ask detailed questions to secure a full and detailed history.

REPRODUCTIVE SEXUAL HEALTH

Barrier methods of contraception are recommended during the preparation phase for pregnancy (Heath and Sulik, 1997). These are non-invasive methods that have no direct influence on the body and thus conception. The morning-after pill is not discussed here as its function is to terminate pregnancy rather than promote it. However, preconception care advice should be included in the packaging for distribution to women (Table 10.6).

DISABILITY

The term disability covers an extensive range of physical and mental conditions and abilities. Because the variety

Table 10.3 Medical conditions: preconception care, advice and further reading

	Information and advice	Further information
Diabetes	Involve specialist practitioners, such as diabetic liaison midwife, dieticians, physician Aim to control preconception glycaemia, reducing the incidence of fetal malformations at conception and organogenesis Measure glycosylated haemoglobin (HbA_1) as this gives information of blood glucose levels over previous 4–6 weeks	Casson et al., 1997 McElvy et al., 2000 Kirkland, 1999
Epilepsy	Seek advice on anticonvulsant therapy prior to conception as this may help reduce the incidence of fetal malformations Medication levels may be reduced Anticonvulsant drugs are teratogenic Take folic acid daily. The dose should be discussed with and prescribed by the woman's GP or physician	Hvas et al., 2000 British Epilepsy Association Helpline: 0808 800 5050 http://www.epilepsy.org.uk
Phenylketonuria	Is monogenic, autosomal recessive and affects phenylalanine metabolism Phenylalanine is present in milk, meat, fish, cheese and eggs Link with the dietician Advise woman to maintain blood phenylalanine levels between 120–360 µmol/litre through a low phenylalanine diet before conception occurs and during first trimester	Kirby, 1999
Hypertension	Review hypertensive medication as it may influence fetal development Refer to medical team to determine underlying cause (if not already aware)	Barron, 2000
Systemic lupus erythematosus (SLE)	Pregnancy is not advised in women with active nervous system involvement Control associated kidney disease for 6 months prior to conception Use barrier contraceptive methods during these 6 months Refer to physician and specialist clinics	Ramsey-Goldman, 1997 http://www.lupus-support.org.uk
Thyroid conditions	Surveillance of thyroid function required Refer to medical team	Montoro, 1997
Multiple sclerosis	Does not appear to increase obstetric complications Refer to support organizations for any individualized needs and advice	Orvieto et al., 1999
Cancer	Clients or partners receiving chemotherapy or treatments affecting spermatogenesis or oogenesis should seek advice on the advisability of storing sperm and ova because of the possible influence of treatment on fertility and conception Should have a cervical smear prior to conception Teach woman outline breast examination techniques All types of cancer have different outcomes in pregnancy so it is important to seek early advice prior to conception In some instances delay of conception may be advised to enable treatment of cancer to commence	Gottlieb, 1999 Sood et al., 2000 http://www.breastcancercare.org.uk/aware

and scope of clients' ability is so varied, it is necessary to refer women to their appropriate specialist as early as possible prior to pregnancy so that effective screening and care management can take place (see Table 10.7).

MIDWIFERY AND OBSTETRIC ASPECTS

A poor obstetric or midwifery history alerts the midwife to potential problems in a subsequent

Table 10.4 Genetics: preconception care, advice and further reading

	Information and advice	Further information
Cystic fibrosis	Lung function determines severity of maternal outcome during pregnancy Refer to dedicated cystic fibrosis team including obstetricians with experience of monitoring high-risk pregnancy	Edenborough et al., 2000 http://www.cysticfibrosis.co.uk
Sickle cell anaemia	Refer to specialist team	Cao et al., 1998 http://www.sicklecellsociety.org
Thalassaemia	Detection of carrier status Genetic counselling Referral into the healthcare system early in pregnancy to enable full exploration of options	Sickle cell and thalassaemia support project http://pages.zoom.co.uk/sctsp/index.html
Tay–Sachs disease	A fatal genetic disorder that destroys the central nervous system Autosomal recessive The child will be either a carrier or have the full disease Send woman and partner for genetic screening prior to conception Referral to genetic counsellor	http://www.ntsad.org

Table 10.5 Environment and lifestyle: preconception care, advice and further reading

	Information and advice	Further information

Employment	Advice varies with type of employment
	Review employment details to protect from occupational hazards
	Refer to health and safety representative at work for further information
	Access standards or policies at work for information on preconception and pregnancy-related issues
	Should avoid jobs which involve:
	   vibrating machines
	   toxic substances
	   excessive cold or heat
	   heavy lifting
	   long travelling times
	Advise to discuss any concerns with employer
	Remember to enquire about partner's employment
		Paul and Himmelstein, 1988
		Keleher, 1991

Stress	Avoidance of severe stress during the period of organogenesis Reduce stress by listening and advising Refer to psychologist, GP or other relevant organizations, such as employer's occupational health department	Hansen et al., 2000
Exercise	Do not take up new exercise when pregnant; take it up before pregnancy and maintain Avoid contact sports such as kickboxing Marathon running can increase the core temperature and increase spontaneous abortions Physical work increases the blood flow to the legs reducing blood flow to the uterus Avoid hot saunas, steam rooms and spas that increase core body temperature and are incompatible with conception and organogenesis Discuss with fitness instructor	Heffernan, 2000

(continued)

Table 10.5   (*continued*)

	Information and advice	Further information
Smoking	Reduces sperm count in men Both partners should stop smoking 4 months prior to conception as cigarettes produce carbon monoxide and nicotine, reducing the oxygen supply to the fetus and causing vasoconstriction of spiral arterioles in the placenta Support women and their partners to cease smoking Refer to support groups Advise to keep away from smoky atmospheres	NHS Smoking Helpline: 0800 169 0169 http://www.givingupsmoking.co.uk/home.htm
Alcohol	Alcohol readily crosses the placenta, only being metabolized by the fetus once liver enzymes mature in the second half of pregnancy and thus is toxic in early pregnancy Decreases sperm count, impairs motility of sperm and causes sperm malformations Is a direct testicular toxin resulting in poor sperm production, abnormal sperm cells and sterility and impotence Abstain from consumption of alcohol for at least 4 months prior to conception Discourage 'binge' drinking particularly during organogenesis	Jensen *et al.*, 1998
Drugs (social and prescribed)	Increased risk of structural anomalies during organogenesis, such as in the heart and great vessels, digestive system and musculoskeletal system Enquire about history, although the woman may not wish to disclose information May need to cease administration, reduce intake or supplement with less hazardous substitutes Refer to specialist practitioners such as pharmacists, and drug abuse specialists	McElhatton *et al.*, 1999 Bunford, 1997
Alternative therapies	Therapies that include administration of herbal remedies require careful monitoring of type and quantity. Treatment should be prescribed by a registered therapist, and therefore care should be taken when self-prescribing and administering Depends on the therapy, so need to consider each on an individual basis	Lee, 1999
Violence against women	Advise women on support services Refer parents to support organizations such as Relate	Bernstein *et al.*, 2000 Saunders, 2000
Pets	Special precautions should be taken when handling pets, their feeding or drinking bowls or their excrement. Direct contact is not necessary as cross-infection can occur from the handler to another person or through pet equipment such as drinking containers Toxoplasmosis is transmitted through cat faeces Advise to avoid contact with reptiles as 9 out of 10 carry *Salmonella* Salmonella from birds, insects, mammals and reptiles can result in meningitis or septicaemia, with death possible *Escherichia coli* may result in food poisoning and fetal death	Payne, 2000
Hazardous substances	Recommend organically grown foods All foods should be thoroughly washed Farmers should reduce contact with pesticides, insecticides Avoid using garden insecticides, touching pet flea collars, and anti-lice shampoos	Glenville, 1998

(*continued*)

Table 10.5 (*continued*)

	Information and advice	Further information
Solvents	Found in a variety of occupations such as printing, dry cleaning, painting, leather industries, anaesthetics, gardening, pharmaceutics and housework Limit work with solvents	Khattak *et al.*, 1999
Radiation	Avoid use of electric blankets, microwaves, sunbeds and X-rays There is debate over levels emitted by VDUs and therefore advise not to use in the 3 months prior to conception, although there is no detailed evidence available at present Advise to use safety shields when using computers Where recessive mutations occur the full effect may not be evident for several generations	Glenville, 1998 Radiation Protection Service http://www.velindre.org.uk/rps
Lead	Comes from exhaust fumes, soil, food, drinking water, lead cooking utensils Wearing of protective clothing at work if in contact Mineral analysis prior to conception Filter water and avoid lead cooking equipment High levels of lead in men linked to infertility Lead moves from maternal bones to the fetus during pregnancy	Glenville, 1998
Cadmium	Reduce contact with cigarette smoke, plumbing alloys, paint, batteries, fertilizers Filter water High levels of cadmium in men is linked to infertility Reduce smoking and alcohol intake as both activities increase cadmium levels Mineral analysis prior to conception	Glenville, 1998
Zinc	Found in red meat, cereals, cheese and nuts Levels reduced in alcohol drinkers Low levels related to infertility in men Mineral analysis prior to conception	Glenville, 1998
Aluminium	Derives from kitchen utensils, some foods cooked in aluminium pans, particularly apple and rhubarb, antacids and kitchen foil Filter water Replace kitchen ware with stainless steel, enamel or glass Advise mineral analysis prior to conception	Glenville, 1998
Mercury	Derives from tinned tuna, weed killers and dental amalgam; therefore dental treatment should be undertaken prior to conception or involve non-mercury-based amalgam Filter water Advise mineral analysis prior to conception	Glenville, 1998

Table 10.6   Reproductive sexual health: preconception care, advice and further reading

	Information and advice	Further information
Oral contraception	Cervical screening Cease administration 3 months before conception. Use alternative barrier methods, enabling the body to regulate hormones prior to conception and increase mineral stores such as copper and zinc Reduces zinc, manganese and vitamins A and B	Heath and Sulik, 1997
Intrauterine contraceptive devices	Discontinue 3 months prior to conception Use barrier methods May increase copper levels	Ashok *et al.*, 2001 Mol *et al.*, 1995

Table 10.7 Disability: preconception care, advice and further reading

	Information and advice	Further information
Disability	Refer to specialist organizations Refer to members of the multiprofessional team Vary depending on the type of disability	ParentAbility NCT: http://freespace.virgin.net/disabled.parents http://www.disabledinfo.com
Mental health	Some drugs lead to birth defects, for example diazepam causes congenital malformations if taken during first trimester Refer to psychiatry liaison team Refer to psychiatrist	O'Dwyer, 1997

Table 10.8 Midwifery and obstetric aspects: preconception care, advice and further reading

	Information and advice	Further information
Poor obstetric history	Need to know what occurred previously to manage preconception care appropriately This depends on the type of obstetric incident Refer to midwife or specialist obstetrician to review previous case(s) or advise on care in pregnancy	See relevant chapters within this book

pregnancy; therefore, it is essential to obtain a full obstetric and midwifery history when discussing preconception care (Table 10.8).

Reflective Activity 10.3

What advice would you give a woman at her 6-week postnatal examination with regard to preconception care for subsequent pregnancy?

Reflective Activity 10.4

Design a plan for use within your own area of practice identifying how you could offer preconception care advice.

CONCLUSION

The relevance of preconception care to the health of future generations still remains a minor component of health promotion, even though the impact could increase the health potential of children both in the short and long term. Improving the health of prospective parents, in turn influences the health of their children and grandchildren. What appears insignificant information in one generation may have a compounding impact in the next. By informing prospective parents of their health status, information such as sickle cell status can be documented and used to inform other family members or partners. Any healthcare activity should involve aspects of preconception care and include both partners, taking account of the diverse nature of society, human actions and the environment. In order for preconception care to be effective it must be integrated into healthcare services and health promotion opportunities. Preconception care involves a team approach and should include any health professional offering specialist advice. As preconception care involves such diverse issues it is impossible to include detailed information within this chapter. You are, therefore, reminded to access other relevant chapters within this book for more detailed advice on the implications for pregnancy, review new evidence in conjunction with this chapter, follow up the further information provided and assess your local preconception facilities, so that you can actively inform women of the local services available.

KEY POINTS

- Preconception care enhances and informs the health of prospective parents, creating the best possible environment at the point of conception.

- Opportunities exist in any healthcare encounter for healthcare professionals to offer preconception advice.

- Midwives need to have access to information on preconception care to be able to offer advice to parents, evaluate the potential outcome of pregnancy and refer to other specialists where required.

- Preconception care should have a multiprofessional approach with easy access to professionals, such as medical practitioners, diabetic liaison, psychologists, sexual health practitioners or physiotherapists.

REFERENCES

Ashok, P., Wagaarachchi, P., Flett, G. *et al.* (2001) Mifepristone as a late post-coital contraceptive. *Human Reproduction* **16**(1): 72–75.

Azam, A., Vial, Y., Fowler, C. *et al.* (2001) Prenatal diagnosis of congenital cytomegalovirus infection. *Obstetrics and Gynecology* **97**(3): 443–448.

Balen, A. & Challis, J. (1993) Dietary advice for women wishing to conceive. *British Journal of Midwifery* **1**(5): 238–241.

Barron, W. (2000) *Medical Disorders During Pregnancy*, 3rd edn. London: Mosby.

Bernstein, P., Sanghui, T. & Merkatz, I. (2000) Improving preconception care. *Journal of Reproductive Medicine* **45**(7): 546–552.

Blanchard, T. & Mabey, D. (1994) Chlamydial infections. *British Journal of Clinical Practice* **48**(4): 201–205.

Bunford, D. (1997) Cocaine and its effects on pregnancy. *British Journal of Midwifery* **5**(5): 282–286.

Cao, A., Galanello, R. & Rosatelli, M. (1998) Prenatal diagnosis and screening of the haemoglobinopathies. *Baillières Clinical Haematology* **11**(1): 215–238.

Casson, I., Clarke, C., Howard, C. *et al.* (1997) Outcomes of pregnancy in insulin dependent diabetic women: results of a five year population cohort study. *British Medical Journal* **315**(7103): 275–278.

Davidson, P. (1995) Managing tuberculosis during pregnancy. *Lancet* **346**(8969): 199–200.

Department of Health (DoH) (1998) *Peanut Allergy: the Committee on Toxicity of Chemicals in Food, Consumer Products and the Environment.* London: DoH.

Department of Health (DoH) (2000) *Coronary Heart Disease: National Service Framework for Coronary Heart Disease: Modern Standards and Service Models.* London: DoH.

Dickerson, J. (1995) Good preconception care starts in schools. *Modern Midwife* **5**: 15–18.

Duff, P. (1998) Hepatitis in pregnancy. *Seminars in Perinatology* **22**(4): 277–283.

Edenborough, F., Mackenzie, W. & Stableforth, D. (2000) The outcome of 72 pregnancies in 55 women with cystic fibrosis in the United Kingdom 1977–1996. *British Journal of Obstetrics and Gynaecology* **107**(2): 254–261.

Elkin, A. & Higham, J. (2000) Folic acid supplements are more effective than increased dietary folate intake in elevating serum folate levels. *British Journal of Obstetrics and Gynaecology* **107**(2): 285–289.

Enders, G. & Miller, E. (1994) Consequences of varicella and herpes zoster in pregnancy. *Lancet* **343**(8912): 1548–1552.

Fauveau, V., Mamdani, M., Steinglass, R. *et al.* (1993) Maternal tetanus: magnitude, epidemiology and potential control measures. *International Journal of Gynaecology and Obstetrics* **40**(1): 3–12.

Franko, D. & Spurrell, E. (2000) Detection and management of eating disorders during pregnancy. *Obstetrics and Gynecology* **95**(6): 942–946.

Galtier-Dereure, F., Boegner, C. & Bringer, J. (2000) Obesity and pregnancy: complications and cost. *American Journal of Clinical Nutrition* **71**(5 Suppl.): 1242S–1248S.

Genc, M. & Ledger, W. (2000) Syphilis in pregnancy. *Sexually Transmitted Infections* **76**(2): 73–79.

Glenville, M. (1998) Health professionals' guide to preconception care. *Foresight Research Seminars.* Online. Available: http://www.foresight preconception.org.uk.

Gottlieb, S. (1999) Pregnancy does not increase mortality from breast cancer. *British Medical Journal* **318**(7198): 1577–1591.

Hansen, D., Lou, H. & Olsen, J. (2000) Serious life events and congenital malformation: a national study with complete follow-up. *Lancet* **356**(9233): 875–881.

Harper, P.S. (1998) *Practical Genetic Counselling*, 5th edn. London: Arnold Publications.

Heath, C. & Sulik, S. (1997) Contraception and preconception counselling. *Primary Care* **24**(1): 123–133.

Heffernan, A. (2000) Exercise and pregnancy in primary care. *Nurse Practitioner* **25**(3): 42–56.

Herman, W., Janz, N. & Becker, M. (1999) Diabetes and pregnancy: preconception care, pregnancy outcomes resource utilization and costs. *Journal of Reproductive Medicine* **44**(1): 33–38.

Hvas, C., Henriksen, T. & Ostergaard, J. (2000) Epilepsy and pregnancy: effect of antiepileptic drugs and lifestyle on birthweight. *British Journal of Obstetrics and Gynaecology* **107**(7): 896–902.

Jensen, T., Hjollund, N., Henriksen, T. *et al.* (1998) Does moderate alcohol consumption affect fertility? Follow up study among couples planning first pregnancy. *British Medical Journal Clinical Research Edition* 317(7157): 505–510.

Keleher, K. (1991) Occupational health: how work environments can affect reproductive capacity and outcome. *Nurse Practitioner* 16(1): 23–37.

Khattak, S., K-Moghtader, G., McMartin, K. et al. (1999) Pregnancy outcome following gestational exposure to organic solvents: a prospective controlled study. *Journal of the American Medical Association* 281(12): 24–31, 1106–1109.

Kirby, R. (1999) Maternal phenylketonuria: a new cause of concern. *Journal of Obstetric, Gynecologic and Neonatal Nursing* 28(3): 227–234.

Kirkland, F. (1999) Preconceptual care for women with diabetes. *Journal of Diabetes Nursing* 3(4): 107–111.

Lee, L. (1999) Introducing herbal medicine in conventional health care settings. *Journal of Nurse Midwifery* 44(3): 253–266.

Lumley, J., Watson, L., Watson, M. et al. (2000) Periconceptional supplementation with folate and/or multivitamins to prevent neural tube defects. *The Cochrane Library*, Issue 1. Oxford: Update Software.

McElhatton, P., Bateman, D., Evans, C. et al. (1999) Congenital anomalies after prenatal ecstasy exposure. *Lancet* 354(9188): 1441–1442.

McElvy, S., Miodovnik, M., Rosenn, B. et al. (2000) A focused preconceptional and early pregnancy programme in women with type 1 diabetes reduces perinatal mortality and malformation rates to general population levels. *Journal of Maternal–Fetal Medicine* 9(1): 10–13.

Marina, S., Marina, F., Alcolea, R. et al. (1998) Pregnancy following intracytoplasmic sperm injection from an HIV-1-seropositive man. *Human Reproduction* 13(11): 3247–3249.

Mol, B., Ankum, W., Sossuyt, P. et al. (1995) Contraception and the risk of ectopic pregnancy: a meta-analysis. *Contraception* 52(6): 337–341.

Montoro, M. (1997) Management of hypothyroidism during pregnancy. *Clinical Obstetrics and Gynaecology* 40(1): 65–80.

Morgan, J., Lacey, J. & Sedgwick, P. (1999) Impact of pregnancy on bulimia nervosa. *British Journal of Psychiatry* 174(Feb): 135–140.

Morgan-Capner, P. & Crowcroft, N. (2000) *Guidance on the Management of, and Exposure to, Rash Illness in Pregnancy*. Report of the Public Health Laboratory Services Working Group. Online.

Available: http://www.hpa.org.uk/infections/topics_az/rashes/rash.pdf.

O'Dwyer, J.M. (1997) Schizophrenia in people with intellectual disability: the role of pregnancy and birth complications. *Journal of Intellectual Disability Research* 41(3): 238–251.

Orvieto, R., Achiron, R., Rotstein, Z. et al. (1999) Pregnancy and multiple sclerosis: a 2-year experience. *European Journal of Obstetrics, Gynecology and Reproductive Biology* 82(2): 191–194.

Paul, M. & Himmelstein, J. (1988) Reproductive hazards in the workplace: what the practitioner needs to know about chemical exposures. *Obstetrics and Gynecology* 71: 921–938.

Payne, D. (2000) Deadly risk from exotic pets. *Nursing Times* 96(24): 13.

Pollard, I., Murray, J., Hiller, R. et al. (1999) Effects of preconceptual caffeine exposure on pregnancy and progeny viability. *Journal of Maternal–Fetal Medicine* 8(5): 220–224.

Ramsey-Goldman, R. (1997) Avoiding and overcoming pregnancy-related problems of SLE. *Journal of Musculoskeletal Medicine* 14(5): 24–26.

Reifsnider, E. & Gill, S. (2000) Nutrition for the childbearing years. *Journal of Obstetric, Gynecologic and Neonatal Nursing* 29(1): 43–55.

Reynolds, H. (1998) Preconception care: an integral part of primary care for women. *Journal of Nurse-Midwifery* 43(6): 445–458.

Saunders, E. (2000) Screening for domestic violence during pregnancy. *International Journal of Trauma Nursing* 6(2): 44–47.

Seaman, C. (1997) Nutrition in pregnancy: what the papers say. *British Journal of Midwifery* 5(9): 534–537.

Silver, H. (1998) Listeriosis during pregnancy. *Obstetrical and Gynecological Survey* 53(12): 737–740.

Simms, J. & Duff, P. (1993) Viral hepatitis in pregnancy. *Seminars in Perinatology* 17(6): 384–393.

Smithells, D. (1996) Vitamins in early pregnancy: not too little, not too much. *British Medical Journal* 313(7050): 128–129.

Sood, A., Sorosky, J., Mayr, N. et al. (2000) Cervical cancer diagnosed shortly after pregnancy: prognostic variables and delivery routes. *Obstetrics and Gynecology* 95(6 Pt 1): 832–838.

Turner, A. (2000) Causes, prevention and treatment of toxoplasmosis. *British Journal of Midwifery* 8(11): 722.

FURTHER READING

Morrison, E. (2000) Periconception care. *Primary Care* 27(1): 1–12.
This review article discusses the need for counselling on folic acid and rubella plus a range of other conditions such as avoiding tobacco, substance abuse and genetic counselling. It also addresses the need for risk assessment in anticipating difficulties in pregnancy.

Perry, L. (1996) Preconception care: a health promotion opportunity, *Nurse Practitioner* **21**: 24–41.
This article outlines guidelines for preconception care and includes a table summarizing assessment, interventions and education. This paper is a comprehensive account of the principles of preconception care.

Wallace, M. & Hurwitz, B. (1998) Preconception care: who needs it, who wants it, and how should it be provided? *British Journal of General Practice* **48**(427): 963–966.
The aim of this research was to review knowledge of and attitudes to preconception care among members of primary healthcare teams and women of childbearing age. Questionnaires were used to record details from healthcare professionals and women. The article outlines the results of the project, suggesting targeting specific groups within society such as Asians, those born in other countries, primigravida and those whose education ceased at 18.

ADDITIONAL RESOURCES

Foresight: the association for the promotion of preconceptual care
28 The Paddock, Godalming, Surrey, GU7 1XD
Tel: 01483 427839

NHS Direct
Tel: 0845 4647

PART 3

PREGNANCY

11. Fertilization 161

12. Genetics 172

13. Implantation and Development of the Placenta 190

14. Embryonic and Fetal Development 205

15. The Fetal Skull 220

16. Confirming Pregnancy and Care of the Pregnant Woman 235

17. Maternal and Fetal Physiological Responses to Pregnancy 288

18. Antenatal Investigations 312

19. Maternal Nutrition 327

20. Complementary Therapies in Childbearing 338

21. Health Promotion in Midwifery 355

22. Education for Parenthood 371

23. Physical Preparation before Childbirth 383

11

Fertilization

Mary McNabb

LEARNING OUTCOMES

After reading this chapter, you will be able to:

- understand the principles of fertilization
- appreciate the different elements involved in fertilization and the journey taken by the fertilized ovum

- describe the genesis and action of hormones produced by the embryo and surrounding cells prior to implantation.

INTRODUCTION

This chapter will examine the elements of fertilization, building on previous chapters, including Chapters 5 and 6. It is important to realize that the process of fertilization includes the journey through the ampulla to the body of the uterus and critically depends on preparations that occur in reproductive organ systems across the cycle.

Spontaneous fertilization requires the coordinated maturation and transport of an oocyte–cumulus complex and thousands of spermatozoa, within a tight time span. Once the oocyte-cumulus complex has been picked up by the fimbriae of the fallopian tube, the oocyte has an estimated life span of 6–24 hours, and the spermatozoa one of 28–48 hours following their arrival in the vaginal cavity (Johnson and Everitt, 2000: 161). Both rapidly undergo a number of developmental processes, designed to ensure that only one of the 2–4 million spermatozoa that arrive in the vagina during sexual intercourse fuses with the oocyte membrane before phagocytosis (Evans, 2002; Wassarman, 1999).

Following ovulation, *the cumulus cell mass* remains metabolically coupled to the oocyte through gap junctions. These 'nurse' cells:

- protect the enclosed oocyte from oxidative stress
- undergo dynamic interactions with the surface of the infundibulum to facilitate oocyte pick-up and movement through the narrower lumen of the ampulla

- participate in regulating some of the biochemical changes in the sperm membrane and zona pellucida before *and* after fertilization
- establish a polar distribution of regulatory proteins and transcription factors within the oocyte and early embryo (Pereda and Coppo, 1984; Talbot *et al.*, 2003).

Following ovulation, the cumulus cell mass seems to release molecules that regulate final differentiation of the zona, in preparation for sperm–zona recognition and binding during fertilization (Nottola *et al.*, 1991). In relation to spermatozoa, differentiated cells in the innermost layers of the cumulus mass appear to be involved in phagocytosis, protecting the oocyte against deleterious spermatozoa, and may also be involved in maintaining a non-toxic environment around the oocyte and early embryo. The cumulus cell mass seems to participate in the induction of capacitation and acrosome reaction, initiating the cascade of events involved in fertilization that ends either in the formation of a viable zygote or degeneration of the germ cells (Wassarman, 1999).

THE FALLOPIAN TUBES (Fig. 11.1)

The fallopian tubes are a continuation of the uterus and both areas operate as a functionally integrated organ that originates from the müllerian ducts (Alexander *et al.*, 1998; Wildt *et al.*, 1998) (see Ch. 5).

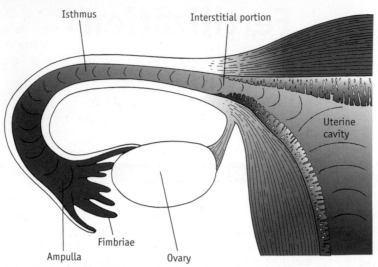

Isthmus   Interstitial portion

Uterine cavity

Fimbriae

Ampulla   Ovary

Figure 11.1   The divisions of the fallopian tube and structure of the reproductive tract.

The innermost linings are continuous with those of the uterine cavity and are made up of an internal mucosa of ciliated and secretory epithelium sensitive to changes in pituitary gonadotrophins and ovarian steroids across the menstrual cycle; and intermediate layers of smooth muscle containing blood, lymph vessels and adrenergic neurones. These nerves supply the ovaries, tubes and uterine body and are sensitive to cyclic variations in pituitary peptides and ovarian steroids (Baird, 1984; Hunter, 1988).

Around ovulation, smooth muscle fibres display characteristic movements that bring the infundibulum, or distal portion of the tube, into apposition with the ovary containing the dominant follicle, by a change in orientation of muscles surrounding the ovarian fimbriae (Hunter, 1988). One fimbria, slightly longer than the rest, reaches out to the tubal pole of the ovary and, in synchrony with ovulation, it involutes to pick up the oocyte–cumulus complex from the peritoneal cavity into the enlarged trumpet-shaped *infundibulum*, which is lined with a very dense layer of ciliated secretory epithelium.

Evidence suggests that oocyte transport to the *ampulla* is facilitated by:

- the presence of cumulus cells around the oocyte
- the sweeping movements of the cilia towards the uterine cavity
- oestrogen-induced acceleration of oocyte movement within the tube, and
- luteinizing hormone (LH)-induced relaxation of the isthmic–ampullary junction, where fertilization takes place (Johnson and Everitt, 2000: 161).

Following fertilization, the conceptus enters the *isthmus*, which is characterized by thick mucosal folds, poorly defined muscle layers, and a diameter that increases from 1–2 mm at the uterotubal junction to more than 1 cm at its distal end, with a lumen ranging from 1–100 mm. This section extends distally for 2–3 cm and contains the largest concentration of smooth muscle fibres within the tube.

The *interstitial portion* of the tube is continuous with the uterine cavity, and is characterized by a marked increase in the number of ciliated cells and by alterations in the shape of secretory cells. Muscles at the uterotubal junction are formed from four bundles characterized by hormonally sensitive interlacing spiral fibres that allow strong constriction and relaxation of the interstitial portion of the tube. Together with the high concentration of muscle in the adjacent isthmus, this is thought to regulate sperm transport and storage, and the movement of the conceptus following fertilization (Hunter, 1988; Wildt *et al.*, 1998).

There are significant variations in the muscular and epithelial tissues in their pattern of organization and degrees of thickness; and in the hormone receptor concentrations and autonomic nerve supply to different sections of the tube.

- The *isthmus* contains the greatest concentration of muscle fibres. Longitudinal and circular layers are richly innervated with high densities of adrenergic nerve terminals.
- The *ampulla* of the tube is poorly innervated and adrenergic endings are usually restricted to the walls of the blood vessels, rather than the muscle fibres.

Cyclical changes

During the menstrual cycle, the tubular mucosa under-goes cyclical alterations similar to those in the endo-metrial lining of the uterus. In the first half of the cycle, secretory and ciliated cells become larger under the influence of oestrogens. Around ovulation, ciliated cells become broader and lower while secretory cells become more distended with fluid. Following ovula-tion, microscopic holes appear in secretory cell mem-branes, which coalesce to release secretions that have accumulated during the first half of the cycle (see Ch. 6) (Hunter, 1988).

The rates of ciliary movements are also influenced by ovarian hormones. Around ovulation, beating of the dense concentration of cilia in the fimbriated por-tion is closely synchronized, which propels the oocyte–cumulus complex into the ampulla. During this period, cilia in the ampulla also beat in the direction of the isthmus, suggesting that they act to further propel the oocyte–cumulus complex towards the site of fertiliza-tion. This activity is thought to play an important role in regulating transport of the newly fertilized egg and its surrounding cells from the ampulla and subsequent movements of the zygote towards the site of implant-ation in the endometrium (Hunter, 1988).

To understand the tubular environment in relation to the changing metabolic needs of the oocyte and early embryo, research has found daily rhythms in secre-tion of growth factors and other regulatory molecules and chemical and nutritive factors present within the fallopian tubes following ovulation (de Moraes et al., 1999; Kennaway et al., 2003). The oocyte and early embryo are exposed to a rhythmic secretion of growth regulatory molecules, and precisely timed modulations occur in different parts of the tube in oxygen tension, nutrient concentrations, electrolytes and macromolecules, which complement the changing metabolic capacity of the developing oocyte and early embryo (Kennaway et al., 2003; Leese, 1995; de Moraes et al., 1999).

Findings on specific molecules indicate that during the greater part of the journey through the fallopian tube, the oocyte and early embryo are composed of non-vascularized cells that undergo a highly regulated series of cleavage divisions while they utilize exo-genous sources of nutrients and growth factors. The oocyte and early embryo shows optimal development in an alkaline environment, with low concentrations of glucose and oxygen and a plentiful supply of albu-min and growth factors (Leese, 1995; de Moraes et al.,

1999). The nutritive environment of the tubular lumen is regulated by hormonally induced secretions of the tubular mucosa and metabolic activities of the cumu-lus cell mass surrounding the oocyte (Leese, 1995).

SPERM TRANSPORT AND CHANGES IN VAGINAL AND CERVICAL TISSUE

Spermatozoa enter the genital tract in approximately 3–4 ml of seminal fluid which is thought to buffer the acidity of vaginal secretions. Over 99% are immedi-ately lost by leakage from the vagina. Those remaining spend variable times in the cervix and show differen-tial states of motility and rates of transport through the uterus. This is thought to increase the chances of fertilization, by creating a reservoir of spermatozoa in the cervix that travel in successive waves of peristalsis to a second sperm reservoir site in the isthmus, and finally to the fertilization site at the isthmic-ampullary junction (Bahat et al., 2003; Kunz et al., 1998; Wildt et al., 1998).

The structure and biological changes in the vaginal canal during the menstrual cycle provide a protected environment for the ejaculated sperm. This is mirrored by the cyclical changes seen in the cervical and vaginal tissues, which include the relaxation and widening of the cervix, and an increase in the quantity of cervical mucus, which demonstrates a characteristic 'stretchi-ness' that seems to facilitate sperm transport (Drobnis and Overstreet, 1992).

SPERM CAPACITATION

During their passage through the genital tract, sperm-atozoa undergo a final series of maturational changes before a small number are ready for fertilization. The first of these is called *capacitation*, which begins when the composition of the cell membrane undergoes a number of modifications, including the removal of cer-tain molecules added during ejaculation. This may be caused by interactions between spermatozoa and the secretions of the cervix, uterus and uterine tubes dur-ing their journey to the site of fertilization.

Capacitation seems to increase hyperactive motility, providing increased thrusting power, thought to be essential for entering the zona pellucida surround-ing the oocyte membrane (Alberts et al., 2002: 1151–1156; Drobnis and Overstreet, 1992). Sperm also acquire thermotactic responsiveness and short-lived chemotactic receptors. The former enables navigation from the isthmic reservoir to the warmer fertilization site at the isthmic–ampullary junction, while the latter are thought to be activated in sperms reaching the isthmic storage site and precisely guide the sperm towards the oocyte in the isthmic–ampullary junction (Bahat *et al.*, 2003).

FUSION OF OOCYTE AND SPERMATOZOON

The final set of transformations in spermatozoa occurs as a result of binding with the zona pellucida (see Fig. 11.2). Initially, the attachment is very loose, involving a number of spermatozoa. Firmer binding follows as an oocyte-binding protein on the sperm surface is recognized by sperm receptors on the zona pellucida. The inner plasma membrane at the apical end of the spermatozoa fuses with the outer membrane of the acrosome and forms a series of membrane-bound vesicles. Proteolytic enzymes digest sections of the zona pellucida that surround the sperm head. Subsequent movement through the zona occurs very rapidly, creating immediate access to the oocyte membrane. Only spermatozoa that have undergone this acrosomal exocytosis can fuse with the oocyte. Usually, the spermatozoon that makes first contact with the oocyte proceeds to fertilization. In the process of fusion, the plasma membrane of the sperm head is phagocytosed by the oocyte (Evans, 2002).

Immediately after the fusion of oocyte and spermatozoon, a series of ionic changes occurs in the oocyte cytoplasm, and cortical granules that were formed

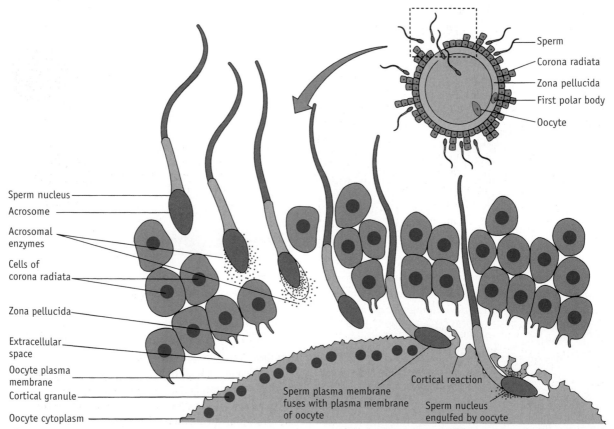

Figure 11.2 Fertilization and cortical reaction. After capacitation, the plasma membrane of the sperm and the outer membrane of the acrosome fuse and the membranes break down, releasing enzymes that allow the sperm to penetrate the corona radiata. Sperm digest their way through the zona pellucida via enzymes associated with the inner acrosomal membrane. Sperm are engulfed by the oocyte plasma membrane. Cortical granules are released when the sperm cell contacts the membrane. These granules cause other sperm in contact with the membrane to detach. (Reproduced with permission from Chiras, 1991: 471.)

following ovulation bind to the oocyte membrane, which releases their content into the space between the surface of the oocyte and the surrounding zona pellucida. This is known as the *cortical reaction*. The vesicles contain enzymes that modify the structure of the plasma membrane, providing a block to the entry of further spermatozoa.

THE ZYGOTE

The *zygote* is the newly formed cell containing maternal and paternal chromosomes and measures about 0.15 mm in diameter (FitzGerald and FitzGerald, 1994: 12). Within 2–3 hours of fertilization, the zygote proceeds with the final phase of meiosis that was halted immediately following fertilization.

Female chromosomes divide mitotically, yielding one haploid set of female chromosomes within the main body of the cytoplasm. The remaining set are discarded to a second *polar body*, on the cell periphery, which later undergoes apoptosis, along with the first polar body that was formed at ovulation (Fig. 11.3).

The cytoplasmic content of the sperm cell membrane then combines with that of the oocyte and over the next 2–3 hours the sperm nuclear membrane gradually breaks down. Between 4–7 hours following cell fusion, two sets of haploid chromosomes are formed into male and female pronuclei, as each become surrounded by distinct membranes, in opposite poles of the cell. During this period, the chromosomes synthesize DNA in preparation for the first mitotic division. As chromosomal content increases, the pronuclear membranes break down, bringing together the two sets of male and female chromosomes.

These events form the diploid complement of a new individual and the cell immediately proceeds with a first mitotic division that transforms the zygote into a two-cell conceptus (Fig. 11.4A,B). The dynamic process of cell cleavage during early embryogenesis is partly regulated by leptin and STAT3 protein secreted by the cumulus cell mass into specific predetermined sites within the oocyte cytoplasm.

Successive rounds of cleavages occur at approximately 12-hour intervals until 8–16 increasingly smaller cells have been formed within the zona pellucida and the remaining fragments of the cumulus cell mass. This process directly allocates cells to the inside and outside of the embryo; they differentiate but retain a stem cell capacity until the late blastocyst stage of development. At this point, the individual blastomeres

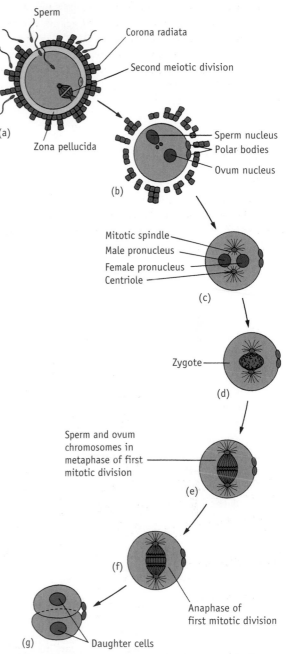

Figure 11.3 The zygote prepares for division. (a) The sperm contacts the plasma membrane of the oocyte; second meiotic division occurs. (b) Sperm and oocyte pronuclei form. (c)The pronuclei migrate towards the centre of the cell. Chromosomes condense and a mitotic spindle forms. (d) Chromosomes condense and the nuclear membranes break down. (e) Metaphase plate is formed. (f) Anaphase of the first mitotic division. (g) Two daughter cells form. (Reproduced with permission from Chiras, 1991: 472.)

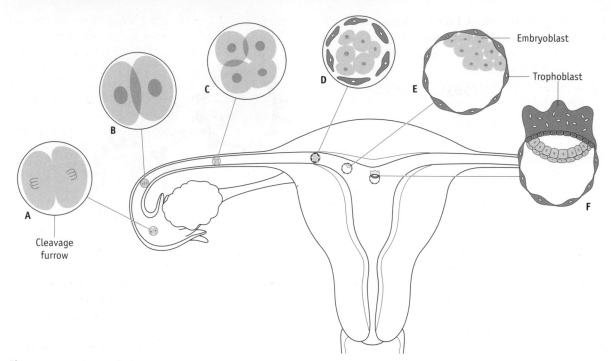

Figure 11.4 Events during the first 6 days of embryonic development. **A.** Cleavage of zygote. **B.** Two-cell conceptus. **C.** Four-cell conceptus. **D.** Morula. **E.** Blastocyst. **F.** Commencement of implantation. (From FitzGerald and FitzGerald, 1994.)

begin to nudge closer together and become visually indistinct (Schultz, 1998).

These positional changes initiate a process of morphological differentiation of the outer blastomeres from those located in the centre (Hardy *et al.*, 1996). The inner ectodermal cells develop into the embryo and germ cells, and the outer trophectoderm cells become the primitive placenta.

MORULA

When cell cleavage has produced 16 cells, the conceptus becomes known as a *morula* (resembling a mulberry) (Fig. 11.4D). Glucose is consumed in increasing quantities and the conceptus appears to require hormones and growth factors for formation. These include the leptin system that has been shown to play a key role in the development of the pre-implantation embryo (Leese, 1995). During this phase of formation, the conceptus remains within the zona pellucida. This smooth outer covering is thought to provide an overall structure for the cleaving embryo that prevents its premature adhesion to the wall of the fallopian tube and provides an immunological barrier between

maternal tissue and the genetically distinct embryo (Carlson, 1994: 45).

BLASTOCYST

Over 24 hours, the morula continues to develop until it has 16–32 cells. All inner cells express gap junctions allowing transfer of ions and small molecules directly from one cell to the next (Hardy *et al.*, 1996).

The formation of a cavity containing blastocoelic fluid begins to transform the cells of the embryo into two distinct populations. The extra-embryonic layer underlying the zona pellucida differentiates into flattened trophectoderm cells that combine with the zona to protect the inner cell mass from destruction by maternal immune cells and make contact with the endometrium to initiate implantation (Sionov *et al.*, 1993). At the same time, a cluster of smaller cells form on one side of the central cavity, giving rise to the embryo and the amniotic membrane (Carlson, 1994: 34–35). This is now the *blastocyst* (Fig. 11.4E). It is composed of 34–64 cells, and will embark on the embryonic phase of development as a free-living organism immersed in uterine secretions that are actively utilized as metabolic substrates while the exchange of oxygen and carbon dioxide occurs by diffusion (Burton *et al.*, 2002; Leese, 1995).

HUMAN CHORIONIC GONADOTROPHIN

After implantation, the embryo releases human chorionic gonadotrophin (hCG) from mitotically active cytotrophoblast cells; multinuclear syncytiotrophoblasts and possibly the extraplacental chorion, before it fuses with the amnion at around 12 weeks' gestation (Chard *et al.*, 1995). Within a week of fertilization, hCG appears in the maternal circulation and rapidly increases in the first 4 weeks following implantation, reaching peak levels of more than 100 000 mIU/ml around 60–90 days' gestation, before falling rapidly to levels under 50 000 mIU/ml from around 18–20 weeks until the end of pregnancy (Chard *et al.*, 1995; Kosaka *et al.*, 2002).

Current findings suggest that the sharp decline in hCG, at the beginning of the second trimester may be due to:

- a decidual protein – shown to inhibit hCG release by trophoblast cells in vitro
- rising levels of progesterone from 8 weeks' gestation, which inhibits the transcriptional activity of the *alpha* subunits of hCG (Yamamoto *et al.*, 2001)
- formation of the definitive placenta at around 8–10 weeks' gestation;
- the initiation of intervillous maternal blood flow, at around 12 weeks
- the development of autoregulation of hCG secretion, which is thought to maintain the low steady-state levels for the remainder of pregnancy (Ren and Braunstein, 1991).

Because of their structural similarity, hCG acts on LH/hCG receptors in theca- and granulosa-derived luteal cells of the corpus luteum and in a variety of non-gonadal tissues in maternal, placental, embryonic and fetal tissues (Alexander *et al.*, 1998; Reshef *et al.*, 1990). The luteotrophic hCG signal that initiates continued growth, relaxation of blood vessels and increased hormone production by the corpus luteum may be downregulated by the embryo and superseded by a combination of embryonic and endometrial factors that stimulate continued growth of the corpus luteum until 6 weeks and prolong its life span until the end of pregnancy (Glock *et al.*, 1995, Oon and Johnson, 2000). At the same time, increasing hCG secretion in early pregnancy, from the syncytiotrophoblast, the extraplacental

chorion and the endometrial lining of the uterus and fallopian tube regulates a wide variety of maternal adaptations; different aspects of placental and embryonic formation; and steroid hormone synthesis by the placenta, testes and fetal zone of the adrenal gland (Cronier *et al.*, 1994; Glinoer, 1997; Hermsteiner *et al.*, 2002; Jones, 1993; Seron-Ferre *et al.*, 1978).

The effects of high concentrations of hCG in early pregnancy include:

- maternal drowsiness
- nausea
- vomiting
- thirst and osmoregulatory changes
- stimulation of a transient fall in maternal TSH
- regulation of thyroid function – briefly
- modulation of the immune system
- stimulation of decidualization of the endometrial stroma in the uterus and fallopian tubes
- induction of migration and capillary sprout formation of endothelial cells
- induction of vasodilatation of endometrial and systemic blood vessels
- proliferation and differentiation of the cytotrophoblast
- stimulation of gap junctional communication during trophoblast differentiation
- modulation of trophoblast infiltration of the decidua/myometrium and spiral arteries
- relaxation of smooth muscle in the myometrium (Ambrus and Rao, 1994; Cronier *et al.*, 1994; Davison *et al.*, 1990; Glinoer, 1997, Hermsteiner *et al.*, 2002; Reinisch *et al.*, 1994; Zygmunt *et al.*, 2002).

DEVELOPMENT OF THE CORPUS LUTEUM OF PREGNANCY

When the cumulus–oocyte complex leaves the ovary, residual cells of the dominant follicle undergo rapid remodelling, including cell growth, proliferation and final differentiation, accompanied by a rapid increase in blood flow and lymphatic drainage (Alexander *et al.*, 1998; Gibori, 1993; Redmer and Reynolds, 1996). These changes allow the corpus luteum to expand rapidly to become the most active autocrine–paracrine–endocrine gland in the body (Duncan, 2000). At the peak of its activity, in the mid-luteal phase of the cycle, the corpus luteum measures up to 2 cm in diameter and produces up to 25 mg progesterone per day, although the majority of its cells are non-luteal in origin (Duncan, 2000; Niswender *et al.*, 2000; Redmer and Reynolds, 1996).

The convoluted ovarian arterial branches are enmeshed by a fine and responsive venous network surrounding the ovary, providing an effective means of adapting local blood flow to the changing state of the enclosed follicles across successive cycles (Alexander *et al.*, 1998). The close association of ovarian and utero-ovarian arterial and venous systems provides an anatomical basis for transfer of regulatory molecules from vein to artery, which allows uterine or ovarian secretions to feed back locally to regulate ovarian functions (Baird, 1984). Through this system of countercurrent transfer, hormonal secretions from the endometrium are rapidly transferred to stimulate formation of the corpus luteum (Alexander *et al.*, 1998; Redmer and Reynolds, 1996).

LUTEINIZATION

The preovulatory LH surge triggers luteinization or differentiation of theca and granulosa cells. During this complex process, theca-lutein and granulosa-lutein cells develop distinct morphological and biochemical characteristics that augment their capacity for hormonal secretion (Murphy, 2000).

Following the preovulatory LH surge, both theca and granulosa cells develop the capacity to synthesize progesterone – which subsequently becomes the primary steroid hormone produced – while also retaining the capacity to produce oestradiol (Niswender *et al.*, 2000). During the luteal phase of the cycle, small luteal cells (SLCs) are thought to synthesize oestradiol and progesterone, although large luteal cells (LLCs) produce most of the increase in progesterone during the first 10 days of the luteal phase, under the stimulatory influence of FSH, growth hormone (GH), insulin-like growth factors (IGFs), PGI_2 and PGE_2 (Apa *et al.*, 1996).

In contrast, SLCs undergo rapid cell proliferation following the LH surge and their numbers increase relative to granulosa-luteal cells as the corpus luteum matures (Hild-Petito *et al.*, 1989). Unlike granulosa-luteal cells, they respond to LH/hCG but have lower aromatase activity and low basal progesterone secretion during the first 10 days of the luteal phase of the cycle (Stouffer, 1990).

Studies on women with regular cycles and proven fertility compared ovarian steroid hormone secretion during the luteal phase of fertile and non-fertile cycles. In fertile cycles, oestrogens and progesterone concentrations were significantly higher from days 6 and 7 after the mid-cycle surge in LH/FSH (Stewart *et al.*, 1993).

The trophic hormone for enhanced steroidogenesis from the early luteal phase may be derived from both the blastocyst and the endometrium (Alexander *et al.*, 1998). From 3 days post-fertilization, the embryo expresses mRNA for hCG, and the secretory endometrium has the capacity to produce hCG, FSH and progesterone. These findings suggest that the close relationship between the uterine and ovarian arteriovenous systems may allow hCG from the endometrium and blastocyst to reach the corpus luteum quickly and stimulate increased synthesis of oestrogens and progesterone from the early luteal phase of fertile cycles.

RELAXIN

Following the LH/FSH surges, LLCs and SLCs also develop the capacity to secrete peptide and steroid hormones, in equal amounts. Relaxin, a peptide hormone of the insulin-like growth factor family is a major hormone of the corpus luteum of pregnancy. Beginning during the luteal phase of the cycle, under the stimulatory influence of LH/hCG, relaxin secretion peaks at 10 weeks' gestation, decreases by around 20% and is present in maternal plasma, at stable concentrations, for the remainder of pregnancy (Bell *et al.*, 1987).

Ovarian relaxin has a major role in stimulating endometrial stromal differentiation during the second half of the menstrual cycle and operates with hCG, to stimulate growth of the corpus luteum (Glock *et al.*, 1995; Telgmann and Gellersen, 1998). Central relaxin regulates changes in maternal thirst and osmoregulation, while central and peripheral relaxin induces renal and systemic vasodilatation, plasma volume expansion and increased adipose tissue sensitivity to insulin (Davison *et al.*, 1990; Kristiansson and Wang, 2001; Vokes *et al.*, 1988). Central relaxin also stimulates maternal pituitary GH secretion during the first half of pregnancy, while its peripheral release alters the molecular structure of ligaments, connective tissue smooth muscle and fetal membranes. This softens cervical connective tissue and pelvic ligaments, weakens fetal membranes and contributes towards a reduction in myometrial tone (Chapman *et al.*, 1997; Kristiansson *et al.*, 1996; Petersen *et al.*, 1994; Santoro *et al.*, 1994).

Current evidence from human studies suggests that peripheral relaxin has a key role in stimulating ligamental and connective tissue changes associated with the onset of labour, and raised peripheral concentration of relaxin during the second trimester is associated with preterm labour (Palejwala *et al.*, 2001; Petersen *et al.*, 1994; Vogel *et al.*, 2001).

THE LUTEAL PHASE

The luteal phase of the cycle initiates very distinct changes for mother and embryo. Hormonal secretions from the corpus luteum following the LH/FSH surge induce a whole series of maternal cardiovascular, renal, osmoregulatory and endometrial adaptations which are accelerated by embryonic and endometrial hCG just before implantation. Within the decidual endometrium, these changes create a highly specialized environment for implantation and embryonic and placental formation. At the same time, the wider systemic

changes prepare for the very different environment required to support fetal growth and development during the second and third trimesters.

CONCLUSION

An appreciation of the physiology of fertilization, implantation and early development is useful in assisting the midwife to understand the complex changes which take place at this time.

Reflective Activity 11.1

Consider this chapter in the context of information you provide to women at booking.

KEY POINTS

- Fertilization requires the fusion of a healthy oocyte–cumulus complex and one out of thousands of spermatozoa.
- This occurs during a tightly defined time span, during which the oocyte complex travels toward the uterus to implant and develop the placenta.

- During the period of embryonic formation immediately following fertilization, hormones are produced by the corpus luteum to prepare the endometrium for implantation.

REFERENCES

Alberts, B., Johnson, A., Lewis, J. *et al.* (2002) *Molecular Biology of the Cell.* New York: Garland Science, Taylor & Francis.

Alexander, H., Zimmermann, G., Wolkersdorfer, G.W. *et al.* (1998) Utero-ovarian interaction in the regulation of reproductive function. *Human Reproduction Update* 4(5): 550–559.

Ambrus, G. & Rao, C.V. (1994) Novel regulation of pregnant human myometrial smooth muscle cell gap junctions by human chorionic gonadotrophin. *Endocrinology* 135(6): 2772–2779.

Apa, R., Di Simone, N. & Ronsisvalle, E. (1996) Insulin-like growth factor (IGF)-I and IGF-II stimulate progesterone production by human luteal cells: role of IGF-I as a mediator of growth hormone action. *Fertility and Sterility* 66: 235–239.

Bahat, A. Tur-Kaspa, I. Gakamsky, A. *et al.* (2003) Thermotaxis of mammalian sperm cells: a potential navigation mechanism in the female genital tract. *Nature Medicine* 9(2): 149–151.

Baird, D.T. (1984) The ovary. In: Austin, C.R. & Short, R.V. (eds) *Reproduction in Mammals. Book 3 Hormonal Control of Reproduction.* pp. 91–114. Cambridge: Cambridge University Press.

Bell, R.J., Eddie, L.W., Lester, A.R. *et al.* (1987) Relaxin in human pregnancy serum measured with a homologous radioimmunoassay. *Obstetrics and Gynecology* 69: 585–589.

Burton, G.J., Watson, A.L., Hempstock, J. *et al.* (2002) Uterine glands provide histiotrophic nutrition for the human fetus during the first trimester. *Journal of Clinical Endocrinology and Metabolism* 87(6): 2954–2959.

Carlson, B.M. (1994) *Human Embryology and Developmental Biology*, pp. 33–50. St Louis: Mosby.

Chapman, A.B., Zamudio, S., Woodmansee, W. *et al.* (1997) Systemic and renal hemodynamic changes in the luteal phase of the menstrual cycle mimic early pregnancy. *American Journal of Physiology* 273(42): F777–F782.

Chard, T., Iles, R. & Wathen, N. (1995) Why is there a peak of human chorionic gonadotrophin (HCG) in early pregnancy? *Human Reproduction* 10(7): 1837–1840.

Chiras, D.D. (1991) *Human Biology*. St Paul: West Publishing.

Cronier, L., Bastide, B., Herve, J.C. *et al.* (1994) Gap junctional communication during human trophoblast differentiation: influence of human chorionic gonadotrophin. *Endocrinology* **135**(1): 402–408.

Davison, J.M., Shiells, E.A., Phillips, P.R. *et al.* (1990) Influence of hormonal and volume factors on altered osmoregulation of normal human pregnancy. *American Journal of Physiology* **258**(27): F900–F907.

de Moraes, A.A., Paula-Lopes, F.F., Chegini, N. *et al.* (1999) Localisation of granulocyte-macrophage colony-stimulating factor in the bovine reproductive tract. *Journal of Reproductive Immunology* **42**: 135–145.

Drobnis, E.Z. & Overstreet, J.W. (1992) Natural history of mammalian spermatozoa in the female reproductive tract. *Oxford Reviews of Reproductive Biology* **14**: 1–45.

Duncan, W.C. (2000) The human corpus luteum: remodelling during luteolysis and maternal recognition of pregnancy. *Reviews of Reproduction* **5**: 12–17.

Evans, J.P. (2002) The molecular basis of sperm–oocyte membrane interactions during mammalian fertilization. *Human Reproduction Update* **8**(4): 297–311.

FitzGerald, M.J.T. & FitzGerald, M. (1994) *Human Embryology*. London: Baillière Tindall.

Gibori, G. (1993) The corpus luteum of pregnancy. In: Adashi, E.Y. & Leung, P.C.K. (eds) *The Ovary,* pp. 261–317. New York: Raven Press.

Glinoer, D. (1997) The regulation of thyroid function in pregnancy: pathways of endocrine adaptation from physiology to pathology. *Endocrine Reviews* **18**(3): 404–433.

Glock, J.L., Nakajima, S.T., Stewart, D.R. *et al.* (1995) The relationship of corpus luteum volume to relaxin, estradiol, progesterone and human chorionic gonadotrophin levels in early normal pregnancy. *Early Pregnancy: Biology and Medicine* **1**: 206–211.

Hardy, K., Warner, A., Winston, R.M.L. *et al.* (1996) Expression of intercellular junctions during preimplantation development of the human embryo. *Molecular Human Reproduction* **2**(8): 621–632.

Hermsteiner, M., Zoltan, D.R. & Kunzel, W. (2002) Human chorionic gonadotrophin attenuates the vascular response to angiotensin II. *European Journal of Obstetrics, Gynecology and Reproductive Biology* **102**: 148–154.

Hild-Petito, S.A., Shiigi, S.M. & Stouffer, R.L. (1989) Isolation and characterisation of cell subpopulation from the monkey corpus luteum of the menstrual cycle. *Biology of Reproduction* **40**: 1075–1085.

Hunter, R.H.F. (1988) *The Fallopian Tubes*. Berlin: Springer-Verlag.

Johnson, M. & Everitt, B.J. (2000) *Essential Reproduction*. Oxford: Blackwell Scientific.

Jones, C.T. (1993) Endocrine and metabolic interaction between placenta and fetus: pathways of maternal–fetal communication. In: Redman, C.W.G., Sargent, I.L. & Starkey, P.M. (eds) *The Human Placenta*, pp. 527–557. Oxford: Blackwell Scientific Publications.

Kennaway, D.J., Varcoe, T.J. & Mau, V.J. (2003) Rhythmic expression of clock and clock-controlled genes in the rat oviduct. *Molecular Human Reproduction* **9**(9): 503–507.

Kosaka, K., Fujiwara, H., Tatsumi, K. *et al.* (2002) Human chorionic gonadotrophin (HCG) activates monocytes to produce interleukin-8 via a different pathway from luteinizing hormone/HCG receptor system. *Journal of Clinical Endocrinology and Metabolism* **87**(11): 5199–5208.

Kristiansson, P. & Wang, J.X. (2001) Reproductive hormones and blood pressure during pregnancy. *Human Reproduction* **16**(1): 13–17.

Kristiansson, P., Svardsudd, K. & von Schoultz, B. (1996) Serum relaxin, symphyseal pain, and back pain during pregnancy. *American Journal of Obstetrics and Gynecology* **175**(5): 1342–1347.

Kunz, G., Noe, M., Herbertz, M. *et al.* (1998) Uterine peristalsis during the follicular phase of the menstrual cycle: effects of oestrogen, antioestrogen and oxytocin. *Human Reproduction Update* **4**(5): 647–654.

Leese, H.J. (1995) Metabolic control during preimplantation mammalian development. *Human Reproduction* **1**(1): 63–72.

Murphy, B.D. (2000) Models of luteinization. *Biology of Reproduction* **63**: 2–11.

Niswender, G.D., Juengel, J.L., Silva, P.J. *et al.* (2000) Mechanisms controlling the function and life span of the corpus luteum. *Physiological Reviews* **80**(1): 1–29.

Nottola, S.A., Familiari, G., Micata, G. *et al.* (1991) The ultrastructure of human cumulus-corona cells at the time of fertilization and early embryogenesis. A scanning and transmission electron microscopic study in an in vitro fertilization program. *Archives of Histology and Cytology* **54**(2): 146–161.

Oon, V.J.G. & Johnson, M.R. (2000) The regulation of the human corpus luteum steroidogenesis: a hypothesis? *Human Reproduction Update* **6**(5): 519–529.

Palejwala, S., Stern, D.E., Weiss, G. *et al.* (2001) Relaxin positively regulates matrix metalloproteinase expression in human lower uterine segment fibroblasts using a tyrosine kinase signalling pathway. *Endocrinology* **142**: 3405–3413.

Pereda, J. & Coppo, M. (1984) Ultrastructure of the cumulus cell mass surrounding a human egg in the pronuclear stage. *Anatomy and Embryology* **170**: 107–112.

Petersen, L.K., Helmig, R., Oxlund, H. *et al.* (1994) Relaxin (hRLX-2)-induced weakening of human fetal membranes in vitro. *European Journal of Obstetrics, Gynecology and Reproductive Biology* **57**: 123–128.

Redmer, D.A. & Reynolds, L.P. (1996) Angiogenesis in the ovary. *Reviews of Reproduction* **1**: 182–192.

Reinisch, N., Sitte, B.A., Kahler, C.M. *et al.* (1994) Human chorionic gonadotrophin: a chemoattractant for human blood monocytes, neutrophils and lymphocytes. *Journal of Endocrinology* **142**: 167–170.

Ren, S.G. & Braunstein, G.D. (1991) Decidua produces a protein that inhibits choriogonadotrophin from human trophoblasts. *Journal of Clinical Investigation* **87**: 326–330.

Reshef, E., Lei, Z.M., Rao, C.V. *et al.* (1990) The presence of gonadotrophin receptors in nonpregnant human uterus, human placenta, fetal membranes, and decidua. *Journal of Clinical Endocrinology and Metabolism* **70**(2): 421–430.

Santoro, N.F., Goldsmith, L.T. & Weiss, G. (1994) Hormone interactions of the corpus luteum. In: Barnea, E.R., Cheek, J.H., Grudzinskas, J.G. *et al.* (eds) *Implantation and Early Pregnancy in Humans,* pp. 123–135. New York: Parthenon.

Schultz, R.M. (1998) Blastocyst. In: Knobil, E. & Neill, J.D. (eds) *Encyclopedia of Reproduction,* Vol. 1, pp. 370–374. San Diego: Academic Press.

Seron-Ferre, M., Lawrence, C.C. & Jaffe, R.B. (1978) Role of hCG in regulation of fetal zone of the human fetal adrenal gland. *Journal of Clinical Endocrinology and Metabolism* **46**: 834–838.

Sionov, R.V., Yagel, S., Har-Nir, R. *et al.* (1993) Trophoblasts protect the inner cell mass from macrophage destruction. *Biology of Reproduction* **49**: 588–595.

Stewart, D.R., Overstreet, J.W., Nakajima, S.T. *et al.* (1993) Enhanced ovarian steroid secretion before implantation in early human pregnancy. *Journal of Clinical Endocrinology and Metabolism* **76**(6): 1470–1476.

Stouffer, R.L. (1990) Corpus luteum function and dysfunction. *Clinics in Obstetrics and Gynaecology* **33**: 668–689.

Talbot, P.D., Shur, B.D. & Myles, D.G. (2003) Cell adhesion and fertilization: steps in oocyte transport, sperm-zona pellucida interactions, and sperm-egg fusion. *Biology of Reproduction* **68**: 1–9.

Telgmann, R. & Gellersen, B. (1998) Marker genes of decidualisation: activation of the decidual prolactin gene. *Human Reproduction Update* **4**: 472–479.

Vogel, I., Salvig, J.D., Secher, N.J. *et al.* (2001) Association between raised serum relaxin levels during the eighteenth gestational week and very preterm delivery. *American Journal of Obstetrics and Gynecology* **184**(3): 390–393.

Vokes, T.J., Weiss, N.M., Schreiber, J. *et al.* (1988) Osmoregulation of thirst and vasopressin during normal menstrual cycle. *American Journal of Physiology* **254**(23): R641–R647.

Wassarman, P.M. (1999) Zona pellucida glycoprotein mZP3: a versatile player during mammalian fertilization. *Journal of Reproduction and Fertility* **116**: 211–216.

Wildt, L., Kissler, S., Licht, P. *et al.* (1998) Sperm transport in the human female genital tract and its modulation by oxytocin as assessed by hysterosalpingoscintigraphy, hysterotonography, electrohysterography and Doppler sonography. *Human Reproduction Update* **4**(5): 655–666.

Yamamoto, T., Matsumoto, K., Kurachi, H. *et al.* (2001) Progesterone inhibits transcriptional activation of human chorionic gonadotrophin-a*x* gene through protein kinase A pathway in trophoblast cells. *Molecular and Cellular Endocrinology* **182**: 215–224.

Zygmunt, M., Herr, F., Keller-Schoenwetter, S. *et al.* (2002) Characterization of human chorionic gonadotrophin as a novel angiogenic factor. *Journal of Clinical Endocrinology and Metabolism* **87**(11): 5290–5296.

12

Genetics

Carmel Bagness, Margaret Yerby and Simon Hettle

LEARNING OUTCOMES

At the end of the chapter the reader will:

- have a basic understanding of genetics, including cell division, modes of inheritance and the chromosomal influences on reproduction

- be aware of methods used in diagnosing fetal genetic abnormalities
- appreciate the significance of genetic engineering for midwifery practice.

INTRODUCTION

The science of genetics would not exist were it not for man's curiosity about reproduction and inheritance, including inquisitiveness about both normal and abnormal developments. Why does one child in a family have blue eyes and blond hair when all his/her brothers and sisters have brown eyes and brown hair? Why do some babies have more than five toes on each foot? Why do certain diseases 'run in families', whilst others do not?

Genetics is the study of inheritance and variation in both individuals and populations. Much research work has been carried out in this subject over many years and it is an especially active research subject at the moment.

Virtually all pregnant women will want to know if their baby is 'normal' and advances in genetic knowledge can not only help to answer this question but can also have other great practical benefits in the field of human reproduction: e.g. the probability that a child will suffer from a particular genetic disease can be calculated, thus allowing parents to make informed choices in planning their families; it is now possible, in some cases, to replace or supplement defective genes so that the diseases they cause can be cured ('gene therapy'). Hence, it is important that practitioners in this area are aware of both fundamental principles and relevant applications of genetics.

Clearly, there are many ethical questions associated with genetic matters and it is important that these are fully addressed.

The most major recent and ongoing development in genetics research is, of course, the 'Human Genome Project' which aims to reveal the precise, detailed structure of the entire human genetic material within the next few years. The acquisition of this information is, in itself, no more than a colossal effort in data collection, but what is then done with this information may have enormous positive and negative implications for future generations.

BRIEF HISTORY OF GENETICS

Charles Darwin (1809–1882), an English naturalist who travelled widely, observed that offspring were usually both generally similar to, but also a little different from, their parents. His famous book *The Origin of the Species* (1859) summarized and synthesized his observations and conclusions from many years' work and proposed many ideas concerning inheritance and evolution. Not all his theories have subsequently proved to be correct, but his work is still of seminal importance in the whole field of the science of inheritance.

Shortly after Darwin had published *The Origin of the Species*, an Augustinian monk called Gregor Mendel (1822–1884) performed extensive breeding experiments with pea plants in the garden of the monastery in which he lived (which was in what is now the Czech Republic) that were to prove to be of fundamental and enormous significance in the science of genetics. He discovered firstly that accurate predictions of the characteristics (e.g. colour of flowers, length of stem) of subsequent generations of pea plants could be made by examining these characteristics in the parent plants. He also found that each individual plant could contain 'hidden' genetic information that was not apparent from the appearance of the plant itself, but which could reveal itself in the appearances of the offspring of that plant. He therefore suggested that each plant had two *allelomorphs* or *alleles* for each characteristic, that these different alleles resulted in different appearances in the plants that possessed them and that a particular allele could remain 'hidden' in a particular individual plant. For example, with regard to flower colour, he suggested that there were two alleles, one causing violet-coloured flowers to be produced, the other white flowers. Plants that had two copies of the 'violet' allele would clearly have violet flowers and plants that had two copies of the 'white' allele would clearly have white flowers. (Note that individual plants such as these that possess two copies of the same allele are said to be *homozygous* for that allele.) But what of plants that possessed one copy of each of the two alleles (an arrangement described as *heterozygous*)? The answer to this question was to illustrate a fundamentally important principle in genetics. By careful experimentation, Mendel was able to show that in this case, these plants had violet flowers. This showed that the 'violet' allele was 'overriding' the 'white' allele (or the 'white' allele was being 'hidden' by the 'violet' one). He described this effect as *dominance* of one allele over the other. His work on other characteristics revealed the same system operating consistently and thus he was able to classify two types of allele – *dominant* and *recessive* – for each of the characteristics he studied. In each case, the dominant allele was defined as the one whose effect was visible in the appearance of the plant that possessed one copy of each of the two alleles, i.e. the heterozygous plant. Also, he further suggested that each plant inherited one allele for each characteristic from each of its parents and thus suggested a mechanism for the transfer of hereditary information from parents to offspring. Mendel died before the significance of his work was fully appreciated and it was not until the end of the 19th/start of the 20th century that his work was rediscovered and its importance realized. It is very largely due to Mendel's persistence and accurate experimentation that the science of genetics is soundly based today (Jones, 1997).

Similar types of experiment with many other organisms, both plant and animal, have subsequently revealed the same principles of inheritance operating in them, and it is now clear that Mendel's experiments revealed universal principles of inheritance. The significance of his experiments and the conclusions drawn from them can thus hardly be overstated.

Clearly, experiments in human inheritance cannot be carried out in the same way as Mendel experimented with peas. However, evidence of inheritance within and between families can be used, and such evidence clearly shows that the principles of inheritance revealed by Mendel's experiments also apply to human genetics. For example, in 1905, one of the first findings from a human family line to be observed was that of short hands and fingers. It was noted that a parent with this trait would consistently pass it on to 50% of his/her offspring, thus showing it to be a dominant characteristic (Jones, 1994).

Early geneticists believed that the units of inheritance (the genes) were to be found somewhere in the cell, but their precise location took some years to discover. Chromosomes were first observed by Flemming in 1877: these thread-like structures in the nucleus of the cell were so named because of their affinity for certain coloured stains (Greek *chromos* – colour), but their role and significance remained obscure for several years. However, in 1903, Sutton and Boveri found that the behaviour of chromosomes during the processes of cell division provided a physical basis for the behaviour of alleles as described by Mendel. Thus, for the first time, a link was established between Mendel's principles of inheritance and a particular physical component of the cell, a crucial step in the history of genetics (Emery and Mueller, 1992).

Subsequent experiments during the early and mid 20th century (which are now rightly regarded as examples of classic work in this field) using principally bacteria and viruses investigated the chemical basis of heredity and showed conclusively that a substance known as deoxyribonucleic acid (DNA, one particular type of a class of substances called nucleic acids) was the genetic material. The molecular structure of DNA was described in detail in 1953 by Watson and Crick in another landmark in the history of genetics.

Chromosomes were known to be made up of both DNA and associated proteins (though it is only the DNA itself that is the genetic material) and thus the physical and chemical bases of inheritance were both firmly established by the middle of the 20th century. Since that period, there have been many further significant discoveries and these have led to great advances both in knowledge about the detailed mechanisms involved in different genetic processes and in the development of techniques and strategies relevant to many areas of medical (and other) practice.

For a fuller account of the history of genetics, please consult Klug and Cummings (2000) and/or Watson (1970).

CHROMOSOMES, GENES AND DNA

Please note that Klug and Cummings (2000) provide more detailed information about the material presented in this section.

Each chromosome is a long thread-like structure made up of one DNA molecule with many proteins associated with it. It has many genes arranged in a fixed manner, one after the other throughout its length (Fig. 12.1).

Deoxyribonucleic acid (DNA) is the major single component of each chromosome and it acts as an information store: it stores, in a stable and coded form, all the information necessary for all aspects of the structure, function, reproduction and development of an organism.

The DNA molecule consists of two strands wound around each other to form a double helix (Fig. 12.2): it is like a ladder in which the two uprights, whilst still remaining joined together by the rungs, are twisted round each other to form two interweaving spirals.

In the DNA molecule, the 'uprights' are made of alternating sugar residues and phosphate groups (the 'sugar–phosphate backbones') and the 'rungs' are composed of organic bases, each rung consisting of two bases. There are four different bases: two purine bases – adenine (A) and guanine (G); and two pyrimidine bases – cytosine (C) and thymine (T). Each 'rung' is made up of a pair of bases, one purine and one pyrimidine, and the pairing arrangements in these 'rungs' are very specific:

- adenine *always* pairs with thymine
- guanine *always* pairs with cytosine.

The information stored in DNA is useless unless it can be decoded and used to make cellular and organismal components. The process of decoding and using the information stored in DNA is usually referred to as the process of gene expression. Most commonly, the stored information in DNA is used to direct the production of

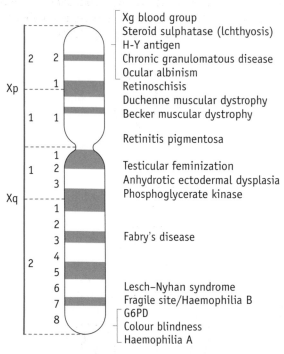

Figure 12.1   Diagrammatic representation of the human X chromosome showing some of the inherited characteristics carried.

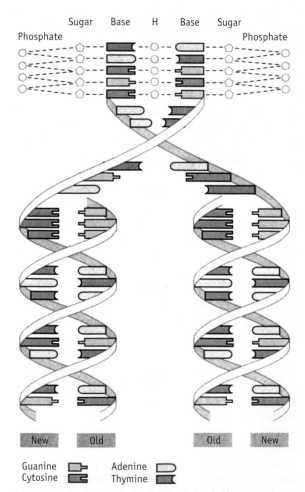

Figure 12.2   Diagram of a DNA double helix, including the process of replication.

proteins. There are literally thousands of different proteins in cells and tissues (e.g. enzymes, structural proteins such as collagen in tendons, transport proteins such as haemoglobin in red blood cells) each with its own specific role to play in the metabolism of the cell and organism. Any protein is made up of amino acids joined together in a chain and each protein has its own amino acid sequence which determines its function.

The encoding of information on a DNA molecule is achieved by specifying the precise order (sequence) of the organic bases along the molecule's length. For example, the sequence AAGCTGTCC would encode a certain piece of information; the sequence GTACTCCTA would encode another, different, piece of information. Information is stored in the form of three-base units (known as 'codons') and each codon specifies a particular amino acid in a protein. Hence, the sequence of bases in a DNA molecule directly determines the sequence of amino acids in a protein and hence the function of that protein. A gene can thus be defined as a part of a DNA molecule which contains the series of codons necessary to encode a particular protein.

The information stored in DNA is decoded using two processes: transcription and translation. In transcription (which takes place in the nucleus), part of a DNA molecule is used as a template to produce a molecule of messenger RNA (mRNA) and this mRNA then undergoes translation (on the ribosomes in the cytoplasm of the cell) to produce the protein specified ultimately by the DNA (Fig. 12.3).

Ribonucleic acid (RNA) is the other kind of nucleic acid found in the cell. Unlike DNA, it is single-stranded and it also contains the pyrimidine base uracil in place of thymine. There are three different forms of RNA found in the cell, and all of these are involved in the decoding of information from DNA. These forms are: mRNA; rRNA (ribosomal RNA – a major component of the ribosome) and tRNA (transfer RNA – crucial in translation as an 'adaptor' molecule between mRNA and protein).

Reflective Activity 12.1

Briefly review the processes involved in the expression of a gene.

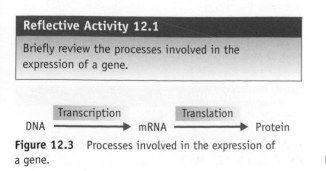

Figure 12.3 Processes involved in the expression of a gene.

THE HUMAN GENOME

The entire genetic complement of a cell or organism is referred to as its genome. Within the nucleus of all nucleated human cells (apart from developing and mature gametes) there are 46 chromosomes: thus, the human genome consists of 46 chromosomes. These chromosomes are arranged in 23 pairs (known as homologous pairs) and within each of these pairs, one member is derived from the father, the other from the mother. One of these pairs consists of the sex chromosomes: in the female, this pair consists of two X chromosomes; in the male it consists of one X and one Y chromosome. The remaining pairs are collectively known as autosomes and the chromosomes in them are numbered by length, No. 1 being the longest and No. 22 the shortest.

It now seems most probable that the human genome contains some 30 000 genes altogether, a far smaller number than had previously been suggested, e.g. 100 000–150 000 (Nicholl, 2002).

CELL DIVISION

There are two different types of cell division:

- mitosis, which leads to the production of two daughter cells identical in chromosome number to the parent cell (46 in humans; Fig. 12.4)

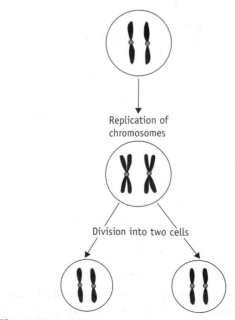

Replication of chromosomes

Division into two cells

Figure 12.4 Mitosis.

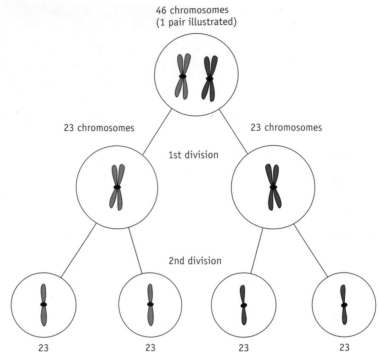

46 chromosomes
(1 pair illustrated)

23 chromosomes   23 chromosomes

1st division

2nd division

23   23   23   23

Figure 12.5 Meiosis.

- meiosis, which also leads to the production of two daughter cells, but each containing only half the number of chromosomes of the parent cell (23 in humans; Fig. 12.5).

Mitosis occurs extensively during embryonic and fetal development to increase cell numbers, and also occurs in the adult in tissues where cells are routinely lost (e.g. the skin; epithelium of the gastrointestinal tract) and in the repair processes that occur following tissue damage. Meiosis only occurs during the production of gametes in the gonads and the reduction in chromosome number that it includes is essential if sexual reproduction is to take place without doubling the amount of genetic material in each generation. Note that some rearrangement of genetic material (e.g. exchange of corresponding chromosomal segments – 'crossing-over') can occur during meiosis. This is an important part of the genetic variation that is an essential feature of sexual reproduction (Fig. 12.6).

Copying (replication) of DNA occurs during both mitosis and meiosis and it is clearly of great importance that this occurs accurately, so that errors are not introduced into the DNA, with possible consequent changes in the structure and function of an encoded protein (Nairne, 1993). One very important way in which

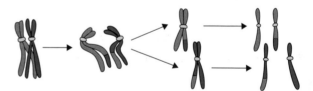

Figure 12.6 Crossover of genetic material in meiosis.

this is ensured is by the 'semi-conservative' mechanism of DNA replication: a parental DNA molecule separates into its two component strands and each of these is then used as a template for the assembly of a new strand. The strict rules of base-pairing (A always pairing with T, G always pairing with C) ensure that each new double-stranded molecule is an exact copy of the parent molecule (see Fig. 12.2).

It is also important to ensure that chromosomes move correctly into the daughter cells during cell division – if they do not, there can be very serious consequences.

Reflective Activity 12.2

Revise the processes of mitosis and meiosis.
Briefly review the semi-conservative mechanism of DNA replication.

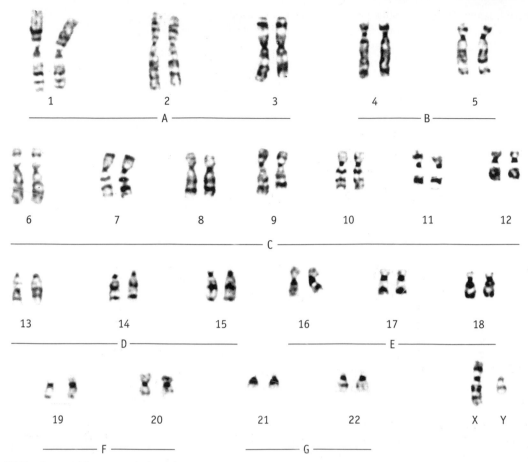

Figure 12.7 A normal human male karyotype.

CHROMOSOMAL ANALYSIS AND ANOMALIES

The study of chromosomes is called cytogenetics, and chromosomes are usually isolated from lymphocytes, cells in skin or muscle biopsies, or bone marrow cells, because of the relative accessibility of these cell types. They may also be obtained from amniotic fluid or chorionic villi when information about the chromosomes of the fetus is required.

Both mitosis and meiosis take place in a series of stages and it is only during these processes that the chromosomes of the cell are normally visible. Thus, in order to examine the chromosomes of a cell, the cell is often artificially manipulated to cause it to enter mitosis. Mitosis is halted when the chromosomes are at their most distinct, and the cell is then photographed. The pictures of individual chromosomes are cut out and the chromosomes arranged in their homologous pairs. The process of examining the chromosomes in this

way is referred to as *karyotyping* and it can provide very valuable information about them (Fig. 12.7).

Reflective Activity 12.3

Visit a cytogenetics laboratory to observe karyotyping.

If there are too many or too few chromosomes present after fertilization has taken place (usually the result of a failure of chromosomes to move correctly into the daughter cells during meiosis), or if there is some alteration in their structure, the pregnancy may result in miscarriage or an abnormal fetus. By and large, anomalies that involve whole chromosomes, or large pieces of chromosomes, are likely to have very serious effects (e.g. embryonic or fetal death) as these are very major genetic abnormalities. In fact, it has been shown that the majority of severe chromosomal abnormalities are not compatible with normal development, and thus embryos with such defects die at an early stage of development, e.g. approximately 15% of pregnancies terminate in spontaneous abortion, and about 50% of these are chromosomally abnormal (Lockwood, 2000).

Several different types of chromosomal anomaly are known:

- the presence of three chromosomes of one type (e.g. three chromosomes 18) is called *trisomy*
- the presence of just one member of a pair is called a *monosomy*
- a structural change arising from the loss of a piece of a chromosome is known as a *deletion*
- when a part of a chromosome breaks off and is added to another chromosome, it is called a *translocation*
- a *reciprocal translocation* occurs if two chromosomes exchange fragments with each other.

The commonest chromosomal birth anomaly is Down's syndrome, where there are 47 chromosomes instead of 46 (termed trisomy 21 – three copies of chromosome 21). The incidence is 1.5 per 1000 live births and this figure rises with maternal age (Harper, 1993). Most children with Down's syndrome, however, are born to women under 30 years of age, simply because more women under 30 give birth. Some children with Down's syndrome (1 in 20) have only 46 separate chromosomes, because the extra chromosome 21 is joined to another in the form of a translocation. In such cases, it is important to examine the parents genetically, because one of them may carry this translocated chromosome in a balanced fashion, having the correct amount of genetic material, but only 45 separate chromosomes. Such a parent is at high risk of having another child with Down's syndrome.

There are only two other examples of trisomies that are consistent with life – trisomy 13 and trisomy 18 – and even in these cases, the defects are many and severe, and affected individuals typically survive for only a few months after birth.

Other common chromosomal anomalies occur among the sex chromosomes, e.g. 1.3% of implanted conceptions may carry one X-chromosome without a Y or second X (monosomy X, Turner's syndrome – the only viable human monosomy). Very few of these fetuses survive – about 0.4 per 1000 live-born girls. More common at birth are other anomalies such as XXX (0.65 per 1000 girls), XYY and XXY (1.5 per 1000 boys – Klinefelter's syndrome; Harper, 1993). These sex chromosome anomalies, however, generally produce fewer ill-effects than the autosomal anomalies, though these effects can still be serious for the affected individual.

MODES OF INHERITANCE

Genetic characteristics (including genetically determined diseases) can be inherited in one of four ways:

1. autosomal dominant inheritance
2. autosomal recessive inheritance
3. sex-linked dominant inheritance
4. sex-linked recessive inheritance.

Note that the usual patterns of dominance and recessiveness do not apply in the cases of genes carried on the sex chromosomes – see below.

Common types of genetic disease include:

- enzyme deficiency states ('inborn errors of metabolism'): if due to a mutation (change) in an autosomal gene, these are very often recessive in terms of their inheritance pattern, because many metabolic processes can proceed at an adequate rate with reduced levels of enzymes
- defects in structural proteins (e.g. in connective tissue): these are, however, often inherited as dominant conditions, as reduced levels of these proteins are often insufficient to avoid the appearance of pathological effects.

Autosomal characteristics/diseases

Most human genetic diseases are due to mutations (alterations) in autosomal genes, simply because there is much more genetic material in total in the 22 pairs of autosomes than in the single pair of sex chromosomes.

Remember that a recessive allele of an autosomal gene is expressed only if its counterpart on the homologous chromosome is the same (i.e. the homozygous state), while a dominant allele of an autosomal gene will be expressed whatever the nature of its counterpart on the homologous chromosome (hetero- or homozygous state). Therefore, only one parent has to transmit the relevant allele to produce a child with a dominantly inherited autosomal characteristic/disease, whereas both parents must transmit the relevant allele to produce a child with a recessively inherited autosomal characteristic/disease.

Clearly, a homozygous person can only transmit one type of allele (normal or mutant) to any child he or she may have. A heterozygous person (sometimes referred to as a 'carrier'), however, can, equally clearly, transmit either a normal or an abnormal allele to a child. Just which allele a heterozygous parent transmits in any particular case is a random event, so there is a 1 in 2 (50%) chance of the child inheriting either allele

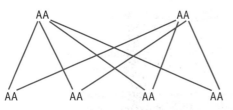

Figure 12.8 Inheritance pattern – two homozygous parents, each carrying the same allele.

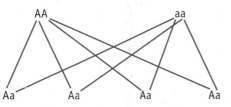

Figure 12.9 Inheritance pattern – two homozygous parents, each carrying a different allele.

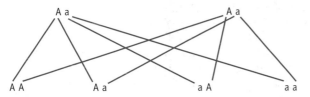

Figure 12.10 Inheritance pattern – two heterozygous parents.

from such a parent. Thus, overall, the following situations can arise:

- if both parents are homozygous for the same allele (dominant or recessive), then all their children will also be homozygous for that allele (Fig. 12.8)
- if one parent is homozygous for one allele (e.g. dominant) and the other parent homozygous for the other allele (e.g. recessive), then all their children will be heterozygous (Fig. 12.9)
- if both parents are heterozygous, then there is a 1 in 4 (25%) chance of them producing a child with a recessive characteristic/disorder (i.e. who is homozygous recessive) and a 3 in 4 (75%) chance of them producing a child with a dominant characteristic/disorder (i.e. either homozygous dominant or heterozygous) (Fig. 12.10).

These inheritance patterns have obvious consequences for the frequencies of characteristics/disorders inherited from parents of these different genetic types. Thus, whilst both autosomal dominant and recessive characteristics/diseases occur in both males and females, dominant characteristics tend to be present in each generation of an affected family, whilst recessive ones

do not typically occur in each generation. This difference arises because (unless a new mutation has occurred) a recessive characteristic can only be seen in the children of a heterozygote and either an affected individual or another heterozygote. And, if the particular recessive characteristic is rare, the probability of this happening is quite small. In practice, it is often found that parents of an individual affected by a rare recessive characteristic are related to each other (e.g. first cousins); such consanguineous matings are more likely to bring together two heterozygotes. (An exception to this general rule is the case where the relevant recessive allele is relatively common). An example is cystic fibrosis – 1 in 22 Britons carry an allele that can cause this disease.

Thus, if two parents who are themselves unaffected have a child with a recessive characteristic/disorder it indicates that both of them must carry the abnormal allele (i.e. are heterozygous). There may then be concern about whether any subsequent child they may have will also be affected. In such a case, it is important to appreciate that the risk of any one particular child suffering from the recessive condition is always 1 in 4 or 25% (see Fig. 12.10). Note too that, in the next generation, the risk of a recessive disorder being transmitted is much lower, as explained above, since the affected child would need to have a partner who is either affected or heterozygous.

Rarely, a child is born with a dominant characteristic/disorder but subsequent investigations show that neither parent carries the relevant mutant allele. In such a case, the allele must have arisen as a result of a new mutation (during the process of gamete formation in one parent) and thus the chance of a second child being born with the same disorder is very low. When the affected child comes to have children, however, the risk of him or her transmitting the mutant allele will clearly be 50% again.

(It is theoretically possible for a child to be born with a recessive characteristic/disorder and for neither parent to carry the relevant mutant allele. However, for this to happen, there must be mutations in the same gene during gamete production in both of the parents and, in practice, the chances of this happening are very low indeed. Clearly, such a child would always transmit the mutant allele to any children that he or she had.)

Further problems arise with diseases in which the disease process is either very variable in its severity (e.g. myotonic dystrophy) or does not become apparent until later in life (e.g. Huntington's disease). In the first case, it is possible for people to have and transmit the disease without suffering any serious ill-effects themselves, (although subtle signs of such diseases can often

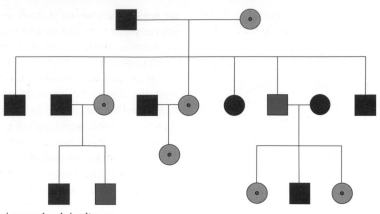

Figure 12.11   X-linked recessive inheritance.

be detected if sought). In the second, many sufferers have had their families before they realize they carry a mutant allele. In either case, parents may unknowingly pass on mutant alleles to their children and thus have several affected children.

Examples of recessively inherited autosomal conditions include phenylketonuria, galactosaemia and cystic fibrosis; examples of dominantly inherited autosomal conditions include achondroplasia, Marfan's syndrome and Huntington's disease.

Sex-linked characteristics/diseases

Sex-linked conditions are those for which the relevant genes are carried on the sex chromosomes. They are more complex in their inheritance patterns than autosomal characteristics because of the genetic difference between men and women, women having two X chromosomes in each cell, and men having one X chromosome and one Y chromosome.

Obviously, there are genes on both the X and Y chromosomes and hence both X-linked and Y-linked characteristics are known. In practice, however, there are very few genes on the Y chromosome (which is very small) and there are thus very few Y-linked characteristics. As a result of this, Y-linked characteristics are seldom considered and the terms 'X-linked' and 'sex-linked' are often used interchangeably (though this is, strictly speaking, incorrect). Note that the genes carried on the two sex chromosomes are quite different.

Only one of the two X chromosomes is active in any cell in a woman's body, the other is inactive (a 'Barr body'). Which X is inactive in any one cell is random, and differs throughout the cells of the woman's body.

A very important consequence of the difference in sex chromosome complement between men and women is that men will always exhibit a characteristic caused by a recessive allele that they carry on their X chromosome since they do not have a second X chromosome that can carry the corresponding dominant allele to 'hide' the presence of the recessive allele. With respect to women, the situation for X-linked characteristics is very similar to autosomally determined characteristics: any one woman can be homozygous dominant or recessive or heterozygous for any gene on the X chromosome. Thus a woman will only exhibit a recessive X-linked characteristic if she is homozygous recessive. In practice, since this means that such a woman must be the child of a father who exhibits that characteristic and either a 'carrier' mother or a mother who also exhibits that characteristic, and since these combinations of parents are rare, such women are, in turn, very rare.

Both X-linked dominant and recessive characteristics/diseases are known and their patterns of inheritance can be summarised as follows:

● In X-linked recessive inheritance, there is never male-to-male transmission of the characteristic, since a father must pass on his Y chromosome if the child is to be male. Also, as explained above, it is most usual to see only males affected by the condition. Thus, this type of disease is most typically carried by normal women, and affects mostly their sons. A woman who carries such a disease will transmit it (on average) to 1 in 2 of her children – thus half her sons will be affected and half her daughters will be carriers. A man who has such a condition will pass on the disease allele whenever he passes on his X chromosome: all his daughters therefore must be carriers, while his sons cannot be affected (Fig. 12.11).

● In X-linked dominant inheritance, the pattern looks very much like that for an autosomal dominant trait. However, because the mutant allele is carried on the X chromosome, an affected male cannot pass it on to his sons; however, all of his daughters will be affected. Thus, there is an excess of affected females.

Among the best-known examples of X-linked recessive diseases are Duchenne muscular dystrophy, red/green colour-blindness and the haemophilias. There are only a few X-linked dominant diseases, one example being hypophosphataemic (vitamin D-resistant) rickets.

Polygenic and multifactorial characteristics

For some traits and diseases, it is clear that individual genes are solely responsible, but much evidence is emerging that, in many cases, genes work together. It is therefore not only important to understand the particular role of individual genes, but also their location and their relationship to other genes (Judson, 1993).

Many inherited characteristics/diseases are influenced by several genes rather than just one or two. Such characteristics are said to be polygenic, and the details of their inheritance patterns are often difficult to define precisely owing to the interplay between the different alleles of the various genes involved.

(Polygenic inheritance should not be confused with situations where several genes/disorders can cause the same effect, e.g. blindness. There are many different inherited conditions that cause blindness, but most of them are simple recessive or X-linked conditions. In any one case, only one mechanism will be operating. If two blind people have children, their children will only be at risk if the parents have exactly the same condition causing the blindness, or if a dominant allele affects one of them.)

If environmental factors (e.g. diet), as well as genetic ones, are important in determining the precise nature of a physical characteristic or disease process, then the characteristic/disorder is said to be *multifactorial* in origin – examples of such disorders include neural tube defects and many cases of cleft lip and/or palate. Most characteristics (e.g. height) and diseases (e.g. atherosclerosis – a very common and serious disease of larger arteries) are, in fact, multifactorial in origin, often involving several genes and several environmental factors. It can prove very difficult to determine the precise risk status of any one individual for any particular condition in such cases owing to the large number of different contributory factors involved and the ways in which these can vary.

ORIGIN OF GENETIC DISEASES

In considering inherited disease, the problem arises as to why such conditions exist. New mutational events occur frequently, e.g. because of errors in DNA replication during cell division, or exposure to mutagenic environmental agents such as various forms of ionizing radiation (e.g. X-rays, ultraviolet light) or mutagenic chemicals (e.g. complex organic molecules in tobacco smoke).

A single new mutation can give rise to a dominant autosomal disease and sex-linked disorders. Recessive disorders, however, cannot be explained so simply because both parents must carry the same aberration for the condition to occur. Rare recessive diseases may be explained by the lack of selection against a mutation which causes the heterozygote no ill-effects, thus allowing the mutation to remain until, eventually, two people carrying the same mutation meet and produce a child who then suffers from the particular disease. There are, however, a number of relatively common recessive autosomal diseases (e.g. sickle-cell anaemia; cystic fibrosis) for which explanations of their high frequency of occurrence must be found. In general terms, such high frequencies are thought to be explained by the existence of some selective advantage that is peculiar to the carrier (heterozygote) and, in some cases, the precise nature of this advantage has been determined. For example, in the case of sickle-cell anaemia (in which the mutation occurs in the gene for one of the components of the gas transport protein haemoglobin), whilst those people who suffer from this disease (homozygous mutants) often die prematurely, those who carry one normal allele and one mutant (sickle-cell) allele show an increased resistance to malaria compared to people carrying two copies of the normal allele. Thus, in malarial areas, the heterozygous person enjoys a selective survival advantage, the mutant allele is selected for and achieves a high frequency. In other cases, the precise nature of the advantage remains to be elucidated – it could be that carriers have some advantage in sexual competition, or that gametes carrying such alleles are somehow preferred, but evidence to support these hypotheses has yet to be produced.

ASSESSMENT OF EMBRYO AND FETUS

Our increasing understanding of genetic influences on disease increases our ability to usefully assess the genetic make-up of the embryo and fetus. As we enter the 21st century, parental and social expectations of normal/perfect babies appear greater than ever before and those involved in providing care will need to be aware of these developments in order to provide adequate accurate information to women (and their partners).

The options available often seem complex and sometimes variable depending on location and economics. Consequently the Department of Health (DoH, 2000) have commissioned a report on prenatal genetic testing with a view to recommending good practice.

The process of screening and diagnosing genetic disorders has advanced significantly in recent years, making it seem easier to assess fetal normality earlier in pregnancy. Screening tests usually identify particular people or specific populations at increased risk (e.g. women over 35 years. have an increased risk of carrying a fetus affected by Down's syndrome, but not all women over 35 years will go on to have an affected fetus). Diagnostic tests are more specific and are applied to specific women who following screening are considered to be at greater risk than the general population.

GENETIC COUNSELLING/ADVICE

Women and their partners in a higher-risk category are faced with some challenging decisions early in pregnancy, or beforehand. They will need opportunities to seek accurate, relevant information and time to consider the options available. This process may be provided by specialists trained in genetic counselling, and this may be the midwife's responsibility.

Reflective Activity 12.4

Investigate where women can access genetic counselling locally, and how they may be referred.

Genetic counselling is there to facilitate effective decision-making, enabling deliberation on the internal (e.g. personal values and beliefs, previous experiences, expectations of this or subsequent pregnancy) and external factors (cultural values, religious beliefs, family and friend influences, economics, education, social circumstances) which need consideration in order for people to make a choice that is right for them. It is also important to acknowledge that where a partner is involved, it cannot be assumed that both parties will hold similar views and beliefs about the pregnancy, or abnormalities which may threaten their expectations of the child.

Counselling may be conducted before a pregnancy is begun (where there is a known or suspected family history of genetic disorders) or where a previous pregnancy was affected by a genetic disorder, in which case it may take place within months of that pregnancy or prior to planning the next pregnancy.

From the midwife's viewpoint, it should be noted that the majority of women who seek advice will be pregnant. In order to facilitate informed choices, there should be adequate explanations of the processes, risks and benefits, accuracy of the tests (including information on false positives/negatives), outcomes and alternatives for any assessments offered. This should include a focus on how far advanced the pregnancy will be before the test can be completed and how long the results may take to become available.

The key to successfully supporting women and their partners through this process lies in an awareness of the influence of effective communication skills, and of personal values and beliefs on interaction. Anderson (1999) stresses that even when information is delivered in a non-directive manner, the professional's belief system may have an effect on decision-making. Her evidence emphasizes the importance of relationship-building and knowing the women and partner's expectations and beliefs in order to facilitate autonomous decisions.

To be effective, counselling should enable couples to believe that they have made the right decision for them, which includes accepting the consequences. It should also be acknowledged that some women might not have considered the possibility of abnormality until discussed with the midwife, a circumstance which will necessitate particular sensitivity. Unfortunately, one of the difficulties with effective decision-making in pregnancy is the lack of time as gestation continues – especially for women who book later than average – which may mean that significant decisions will need to be made quickly.

For various reasons (e.g. limited family histories, variations observed in severity of a disease process), it can sometimes be difficult to provide clear guidelines as to inheritance, significance of outcomes and the effect(s) on individuals in any one particular counselling situation. Accordingly, any information given needs to clarify the gaps in knowledge as well as the advances made.

Once risk factors have been established, information should be provided on their potential impact on the fetus and neonate, including options for treatment, if any, and the nature and course of any possible resultant illnesses. Whilst advances in medicine have considerably altered the outlook for many conditions (e.g. cystic fibrosis patients now have a greatly improved life and health expectancy than previously) it is obviously important that advice is realistic, stressing the drawbacks currently experienced as well as any advances that have been made. Often, referral to specialist support groups may be useful at this time.

Case scenario 12.1

The sister of a boy with Duchenne muscular dystrophy (DMD) attends the genetic clinic with her husband. Her uncle also had the disease and died as a result. She has a 50% chance of carrying the mutant allele, because her mother must carry it. Since it is sex-linked, she would pass this allele to half her sons (and half her daughters).

There are two ways of deciding her risk of transmitting the mutant allele: firstly, her DNA could be examined directly to see if she did carry the mutant allele. This would involve using DNA probes to see if she had inherited the same, mutant, segment of X chromosome as her affected brother had. However, because the probes currently available only mark segments of chromosome close to, but not actually at the DMD locus, there is always the chance that this method may not yield results that are 100% certain, i.e. there may be a false positive result. Secondly, her blood could be tested to determine the level of a muscle enzyme, creatine kinase, found at elevated levels in the blood of affected boys: the higher this level, the greater her chance of carrying the Duchenne allele. Combining the risk figures from these two tests will provide either a very high or a very low carrier risk status.

If the final risk is more than 2–5%, she may well opt for antenatal diagnosis. At present, this usually means the termination of any male fetus. Many normal males are aborted in this way; however, it is becoming possible, in some families, to determine whether or not a male fetus will be affected, and women in these families can have sons that they know will be normal.

Case scenario 12.2

A couple attend clinic having lost a child some months before with a particular form of congenital heart disease. They wish to know what is the chance of their having another similarly affected child.

To answer this question, it would be necessary to answer these questions:

- precisely what sort of heart defect was present?
- were there any other problems with the child?
- is there any other family history of congenital heart defects?
- was there any question of rubella in early pregnancy?

The previous child had a post-mortem examination by an experienced paediatric pathologist, who identified the problem as transposition of the great vessels in a child who was otherwise normal (i.e. the pathologist was satisfied that this was an isolated defect). (This latter point is crucial, because heart defects can occur as one feature of dysmorphic syndromes that have a high risk of recurrence.)

The incidence of transposition of the great vessels in the general population is 0.4 per 1000 live births, and, given the above pathological findings and the facts that there was no family history of congenital heart defects in this case nor any rubella infection during early pregnancy, the risk of another child with congenital heart disease in this family is 1.7%, not very much higher than the 1% risk of congenital heart disease for all births.

It is equally imperative to discuss the impact of tests on the woman, and any significant other people in her life, as previously mentioned influences might be consequential to responsibility for and acceptance of any decisions made.

Women (and their partners) who have been thus counselled will then have decisions to make. The choices open to them may include:

- not becoming pregnant, and opting for fostering or adoption
- utilizing the facilities available for infertility treatments, e.g. opting for artificial insemination by donor
- continuing with the pregnancy (if appropriate) and 'hoping for the best'
- undergoing antenatal diagnostic tests, with the option to:
  - keep the pregnancy regardless of outcome
  - terminate the pregnancy if a positive diagnosis is made
- using the other alternatives that may be available in some cases, e.g. gene therapy.

The choices are nearly always complex, and consequently it is crucial that accurate knowledge is available to facilitate the best personal decisions. Case scenarios 12.1 and 12.2 illustrate situations that may arise.

SCREENING FOR RISK INDICATORS

The primary aim of screening for risk indicators/markers is to provide accurate information to facilitate fully informed decisions about proceeding with diagnostic tests to confirm or exclude a genetic disorder. There are various indicators and the utility of these in individual cases may depend on available information, previous history, the duration of gestation and parental expectations of normality.

History-taking

History-taking is a significant factor in planning care for the pregnant woman. It provides detailed information and an opportunity for relationship-building between the woman and the midwife, which although always important, may be particularly relevant for further decision-making. An accurate, detailed personal, family, medical and obstetric history is essential in identifying risk factors that expose the pregnancy to genetic disorders. This should also include personal, family and medical information about the genetic father of the fetus, where possible. Sensitivity to the fact that information is not always available is important, especially where there is no contact with the father or where infertility treatment has been used to achieve the pregnancy.

Consideration of racial and/or geographical origins may also be appropriate (e.g. Tay–Sachs disease in Ashkenazi Jews, or haemaglobinopathies in women of Mediterranean, African or Asiatic origin). Situations such as consanguinity (close relatives, e.g. cousins, achieving a pregnancy) should also be examined.

Once history-taking has been completed, the midwife and woman/couple should consider the need for further screening. Prior to any decisions, it is essential that the woman is aware that further screening may ultimately lead to a decision about keeping or terminating the pregnancy. For some women, this may be unthinkable and they should be clearly aware of this scenario, whereas for others having this choice would be essential. There may be some women who choose to continue with screening anyway, with the view that they would like to know details and prepare for the birth accordingly.

Ultrasound scanning (USS)

This is a non-invasive method of viewing the fetus. In the UK, the majority of women have access to USS, usually between 18–20 weeks' gestation. In addition to confirming the pregnancy, assessing gestational age, localizing the placenta and monitoring fetal growth, it has a significant role to play in screening for structural fetal abnormalities.

It is considered to be relatively safe, although various research studies have been somewhat inconclusively controversial about its use. Neilson (2000) reviewed nine good-quality trials up to July 1998 and confirmed that early USS enabled better assessment of gestational age, detection of multiple pregnancy and earlier diagnosis of clinically unsuspected fetal abnormalities. However, this review also concluded that the benefits of other clinical outcomes were less clear.

Many units now offer USS at 11–14 weeks' gestation, which may predict a risk of chromosomal abnormality by measuring the amount of fluid behind the neck of the fetus, specifically the nuchal fold thickness. It is measured in millimetres, computer recorded in conjunction with maternal age, and used to determine a predictive risk rate. Nicolaides *et al.* (1994) reported that this method compared favourably with screening of maternal age and serum biochemistry.

Reflective Activity 12.5

Arrange a visit to an ultrasound department, and consider both the information requested by women and their partners, and the information given to them.

What impact did this experience have on your information-giving to women?

Biochemical/serum screening

- Alpha-fetoprotein (AFP) serum screening is best carried out at 16–18 weeks' gestation. AFPs are fetal proteins present in maternal serum and amniotic fluid. It is important to have accurate information about gestational age (confirmation by USS may be necessary), as this may significantly alter results. A raised level of AFPs may indicate intrauterine death, multiple pregnancies, or, most commonly, an open neural tube defect. A lower than expected reading may imply a chromosomal abnormality, e.g. Down's syndrome. However, the work of Howe *et al.* (2000) suggested that AFP is not an effective way of screening for trisomy 21, with maternal age and mid-trimester USS detecting some 68% of cases.
- Biochemical screening tests can be combination tests used to determine risk factors. They can incorporate serum AFPs, unconjugated oestriol and human chorionic gonadatrophin, measured with maternal age and weight in relation to gestational age. There are various tests available, and some areas offer them routinely or selectively based on risk factors, whereas others only offer them privately.

Wald *et al.* (1999) suggested that using first and second trimester screening tests together, rather than in isolation, will significantly reduce (by as much as four-fifths) the number of invasive diagnostic tests necessary, with similar results and lower false positive/negatives.

DIAGNOSTIC TESTS

If an increased risk is established by any of the above procedures, the next step may be to proceed to a diagnostic test, which should, generally, provide more definite information about the fetal genetic constitution.

As stated earlier, it is essential that women are aware of the hazards attached to such procedures. These include the risks that the test may pose to the pregnancy, the risks of false positive or negative results and the danger of being faced with having to decide whether to proceed with the pregnancy or choose termination. These choices may be more difficult for some women than for others, depending on their expectations, beliefs and needs for their pregnancy, as well as multiple psychosocial influences.

The purpose of testing is to assess the status of the genome of an individual embryo or fetus. Each individual's genome is unique (with the exception of that of identical twins) and, in order to be able to recognize individual sequences of DNA, techniques have been developed to provide methods of analysis for the DNA of an individual. These techniques use genetic probes (which are labelled fragments of DNA) to determine whether a particular DNA sequence is present or absent. Embryonic/fetal genome analysis is only one application of this technology: others include forensic science and paternity disputes.

DNA can be isolated easily from any human cell that is alive and has a nucleus, including buccal cells and skin fibroblasts. The DNA probe is a copy of a relevant sequence that is identifiable and can be used as a 'probe' to hybridize a corresponding copy of the sample.

Preimplantation genetic diagnosis (PGD)

This is a recent option for diagnosing genetic disorders. It was reviewed in 1999/2000 by the Human Fertilisation and Embryology Authority (HFEA) in collaboration with the Advisory Committee on Genetic Testing (HFEA/ACGT, 1999), to consider a number of practical, ethical and legal issues associated with its viability.

This technique has to be considered before conception and involves extrauterine assessment of the embryo. It has two stages: firstly, in vitro fertilization techniques are used to create embryos, and these are then tested for particular genetic disorders or to establish their sex

(where the disorder is sex-linked) (HFEA/ACGT, 1999). Fasouliotis and Schenker (1998) reported that polar body, blastomere and blastocyst biopsies are currently performed, and the two major technologies used for single gene cell analysis involve the polymerase chain reaction (PCR – a technique to increase the amount of DNA available for analysis) and fluorescence in-situ hybridization (FISH – the use of fluorescently labelled DNA probes for the detection of single gene defects). After these tests, embryos which are considered healthy are implanted into the mother's uterus using techniques developed for infertility treatments. The success rates for this procedure remain low (16.4% live birth rate of treatments started), making this procedure risky (HFEA, 1999). Note that it is not feasible to screen the embryos for all possible genetic defects – screening is only used to establish the presence or absence of those thought to be likely to occur in a particular embryo (e.g. a defect or defects relevant to a particular genetic disease which has previously occurred in at least one of the families of the embryo's parents).

Apart from these risks, HFEA/ACGT (1999) also outlined problems with the procedure. Misdiagnosis is possible, e.g. because of technique failure or the biopsy not being typical of the fetus or because the biopsy material may become contaminated with non-embryonic material (e.g. sperm left over from the process or contaminating cells from the clinician). There are also ethical concerns, especially from those who believe in the sanctity of human life, about the numbers of embryos that may perish, either from damage during biopsy or by being destroyed following a positive diagnosis of a genetic disorder.

Currently, PGD appears to be only used for severe/life-threatening disorders. The HFEA (after public consultation in 1993) rejected the use of PGD for sex selection, on social grounds.

This technique is in its infancy, but deserves mention here because women who become aware of it may request further information. Draper and Chadwick (1999) also expressed concerns about new ethical and legal dilemmas that may be created by this, e.g. is it wrong to implant a genetically abnormal zygote? Where does the power/final decision lie in this procedure – with the woman or with the clinician?

Chorionic villus sampling (CVS)

This diagnostic test is performed in conjunction with USS. It involves placing a fine catheter/forceps intra-cervically or intra-abdominally into the chorionic tissue of the developing embryo to extract a small biopsy sample. DNA/cytogenetic analysis and some biochemical studies can be performed on the material recovered (DoH, 2000). CVS is now usually carried out no earlier than at 10 weeks' gestation, as a report from Oxford in the early 1990s suggested a high risk of fetal limb deformities when it is performed below this age. However, further research by Firth *et al.* (1994) was inconclusive about the reasons for the anomalies. Alfirevic (2000), who compared early amniocentesis with CVS, suggested an increased risk of haemangioma with CVS. Several studies also report higher associated miscarriages (1–3%; DoH, 2000), although this can be difficult to assess because of the increased risk of spontaneous miscarriage earlier in pregnancy. This may be an acceptable risk for some women who will balance this opportunity with the need to have results to allow them to make an earlier decision.

Amniocentesis

Amniocentesis involves sampling the amniotic fluid and the cells within it. The process entails guiding a fine needle into the amniotic sac, using USS to localize the placenta. The biochemical constituents of the fluid may be tested for non-specific indicators of abnormality (e.g. AFPs), for the accumulation of specific metabolites in suspected inborn errors of metabolism, or, in later pregnancy, for fetal assessment. The cells isolated from the fluid are cultured in the laboratory to determine the fetal karyotype, for more detailed DNA analyses (including fetal sexing) and/or for enzyme assays. Traditionally, amniocentesis is carried out between 16–18 weeks' gestation, when maternal age, history or screening indicate a high risk of abnormality, but this usually means that results are not available until more than 20 weeks of gestation have elapsed. Amniocentesis has thus been tried at earlier stages of pregnancy, but Alfirevic (2000) found that there appeared to be increased risks of spontaneous miscarriage and neonatal talipes associated with earlier amniocentesis, and thus these risks would need to be weighed against the possible benefits of earlier results. Results may occasionally be ambiguous, and there is also a small risk of contamination by maternal cells, or of cells failing to grow. The risk of miscarriage following amniocentesis at 16–18 weeks is commonly quoted as 0.5–1% (DoH, 2000), which is greater than the risk of spontaneous miscarriage at this stage of pregnancy.

Fetoscopy

This is the technique of observing the fetus through a fine fibreoptic telescope, during which samples of tissue may be removed, under direct vision, for analysis. It may be used to diagnose skin disease such as epidermolysis bullosa lethalis by skin biopsy. It is also possible to use it to perform therapeutic interventions, e.g. blood transfusion in rhesus incompatibility.

Cordocentesis

This technique is used to obtain a sample of fetal blood. The sample can be used to screen for chromosomal abnormalities, haemophilia and haemoglobinopathies. It is carried out using USS to guide a fine needle to the base of the umbilical cord, where a sample of fetal blood is extracted for analysis and/or karyotyping. It is usually carried out after 16 weeks' gestation and carries some risks, e.g. bleeding from the cord may compromise fetal well-being.

All screening and diagnostic tests carry some risks, psychological and/or physical; consequently the decision to proceed or not needs to be carefully measured, and the role of the midwife is in trying to ensure that couples are given the opportunity to make fully informed decisions which they are then resolved to take responsibility for.

> ### Reflective Activity 12.6
>
> Explain 'the relevance of DNA to prenatal diagnostic tests' to parents and reflect on the questions they ask you.
>
> Investigate locally to discover which methods are most favoured, focusing on the possible rationale for use, and the risks attached to each assessment.

GENETIC ENGINEERING

Research in genetics, at the molecular level in particular (described by several different terms, such as the 'new genetics', recombinant DNA technology, gene manipulation, genetic engineering), is an especially active area of scientific endeavour at the moment. It is hoped that discoveries and developments in this area will decrease the morbidity and mortality currently associated with many diseases, both those with largely genetic causes (e.g. cystic fibrosis) and those that are multifactorial in origin. In applying these technologies, as in all medicine today, the emphasis is on prevention rather than cure.

It was in the early 1970s that scientists first discovered procedures by which they could directly alter the genetic constitution of bacteria – the experimental organisms first used in this kind of work (Nicholl, 2002).

It was found that, by constructing novel DNA molecules (i.e. that were not found naturally – *recombinant DNA molecules*) in the laboratory using DNA originally isolated from different species (e.g. a bacterium and a mammal), genes from other organisms could be stably introduced into a bacterial cell. Moreover, bacterial cells containing such molecules could then produce proteins encoded by these genes that they would not normally synthesize (e.g. mammalian proteins). Since these initial experiments, recombinant DNA techniques have been very widely used in very many different fields – with microorganisms, plants, animals and human beings – and they have yielded many benefits in each of these areas (e.g. the production of human insulin by genetically modified bacteria for use by diabetic patients; Nicholl, 2002).

It is important to note that there are obvious potential problems associated with genetic manipulation, and such activities are thus closely regulated by statutory bodies (e.g. in the UK, by the Advisory Committee on Genetic Modification, a part of the Health & Safety Executive). Of particular relevance to midwifery is the fact that the manipulation of human germ cells (the gametes – spermatozoa and ova) is internationally prohibited. This is to avoid deliberately and directly changing the overall genetic constitution (the 'gene pool') of the human species, the consequences of such changes being both unpredictable and irreversible. The only human cells permitted to be genetically modified are the somatic cells (i.e. all cells other than the gametes) – see below – and modifications to these cells are tightly regulated.

One of the most obvious applications of genetic engineering in medicine is to replace or repair missing and defective alleles with normal ones – 'gene therapy'. This process involves the insertion of genetic material directly into cells to alter the functioning of those cells (e.g. to produce the normal, functional version of a protein which the defective cell cannot produce itself). This insertion of genetic material can be achieved either in vitro, prior to implantation of an embryo, or on a child or adult suffering from a genetic disorder, depending on the accessibility of the affected tissue (e.g. diseases of the bone marrow or of the respiratory tract are quite accessible to this form of therapy). The progress being made with adult, child and animal gene therapy is well reported (see in particular HFEA, GTAC and PHGU or Wellcome Trust websites (p. 189) for further information). For example, the severe and usually life-shortening disease cystic fibrosis (CF) is one disease in which various gene therapy approaches are being very actively pursued at the moment. This disease is caused by defects in a particular protein known as the cystic fibrosis transmembrane conductance regulator (CFTR) whose function is to help to regulate the flow of water across epithelial surfaces. All the different gene therapy approaches are aiming to bring about the production of normal CFTR in CF patients and thus relieve the distressing symptoms of this disease; these trials are being evaluated currently. The report of the Gene Therapy Advisory Committee (a regulatory body of the DoH) on gene therapy for cystic fibrosis (GTAC, 2000) provides more details about developments in this specific case in both the UK and US.

Since many disorders with a significant genetic component in their causation have a significant adverse impact on the health of the developing embryo/fetus, consideration has been given to the possibility of in utero gene therapy. This may be seen as the only solution to a number of degenerative genetic disorders, but may also involve considerable risk to the embryo/fetus itself. This latter point raises the question of the need for informed consent by the mother, and raises many other questions about the moral and legal status of the fetus in such situations (Bagness, 1998). Hitherto, there has been less research into in utero gene therapy performed and documented than into other applications of this therapy. A recent review (Zanjani *et al.*, 1999) examined the reality of in utero gene therapy and concluded that, although progress was promising, this form of gene therapy was unlikely to become a clinical reality in the near future.

It is a matter of simple current observation that media reports about advances in genetic technologies and their applications are both frequent and often dramatic. Consequently, parents/prospective parents may have unrealistic expectations in this area beyond the current limits of these technologies. It is therefore important to be aware of what these technologies both can and cannot achieve when dealing with parents/prospective parents.

Finally, there are resource issues to be considered in relation to these technologies, all of which are resource-intensive. Even when technology is available, consideration will have to be given to the already limited healthcare resources. It may be possible to argue in this context that the potential financial benefits of having children born free from genetic disease outweigh the cost of providing effective life care for a child/adult suffering from the condition. None the less, this will inevitably have to be balanced with the needs of the general population in allocation of funds.

CONCLUSION

The possibilities for the future are potentially vast, and the midwife will need to be aware of these technologies, as parents frequently request information following media coverage. For the midwife, this will include understanding the basis of genetics and the reality of current success in genetic engineering, including the risk : benefit ratios. The message for healthcare professionals is the need to provide appropriate and effective information to enable women and their partners to make informed decisions about the best course of action for them at present.

KEY POINTS

- A good understanding of cell division, chromosomes and diagnostic testing is important when talking to parents whose baby has an abnormality.
- An ability to apply knowledge of genetics and modes of inheritance is important in identifying women and babies who might be at risk and in selecting the appropriate screening method.

- Midwives need a sound knowledge of genetics in order to appropriately refer women and their partners for genetic counselling.
- Genetic engineering may have only a limited impact on the role of the midwife at present, but knowledge of the processes and possibilities in this field is (and will increasingly be) important in terms of effective communication with parents.

REFERENCES

Alfirevic, Z. (2000) Early amniocentesis versus transabdominal chorionic villus sampling for prenatal diagnosis (Cochrane Review). *The Cochrane Library*, Issue 2. Oxford: Update Software.

Anderson, G. (1999) Non-directiveness in prenatal genetics – patients read between the lines. *Nursing Ethics* 6(2): 126–136.

Bagness, C. (1998) *Genetics, the Foetus and the Future*. Cheshire: Books for Midwives Press.

Department of Health (DoH) (2000) *ACTG Report for Consultation on Prenatal Genetic Screening*. Online. Available http://www.doh.gov.uk/genetics/pgtintro.htm

Draper, H. & Chadwick, R. (1999) Beware! Pre implantation genetic diagnosis may solve some old problems but it also raises new ones. *Journal of Medical Ethics* 25(2): 114–120.

Emery, A.E.H. & Mueller, R.F. (1992) *Elements of Medical Genetics*, 8th edn. Edinburgh: Churchill Livingstone.

Fasouliotis, S.J. & Schenker, J.G. (1998) Pre implantation genetic diagnosis: principles and ethics. *Human Reproduction* 13(8): 2238–2245.

Firth, H.V., Boyd, P.A., Chamberlain, P.F. *et al.* (1994) Analysis of limb reduction defects in babies exposed to chorionic villus sampling. *Lancet* 343: 1069–1071.

Gene Therapy Advisory Committee (GTAC) (2000) *Gene Therapy Advisory Committee 3rd Annual Report (1996)*. London: DoH.

Harper, P.S. (1993) *Practical Genetic Counselling*, 4th edn. Oxford: Butterworth Heinemann.

Howe, D.T., Gornall, R., Wellesley, D. *et al.* (2000) Six year survey of screening for Down's syndrome by maternal age and mid-trimester ultrasound scans. *British Medical Journal* 320(7235): 606–610.

Human Fertilisation and Embryology Authority (HFEA) (1999) *Human Fertilisation and Embryology Authority Annual Report*. London: DoH.

Human Fertilisation and Embryology Authority/Advisory Committee on Genetic Therapy (HFEA/ACGT) (1999) *Human Fertilisation and Embryology Authority/ Advisory Committee on Genetic Therapy Consultation Document on Pre Implantation Genetic Diagnosis*. London: DoH.

Jones, S. (1994) *The Language of the Genes*. London: Flamingo.

Jones, S. (1997) *In the Blood: God, Genes and Destiny*. London: Flamingo.

Judson, H.F. (1993) A history of the science and technology behind gene mapping and sequencing. In: Kevles, D.J. & Hood, L. *The Code of Codes: Scientific and Social Issues in the Human Genome Project*. London: Harvard University Press.

Klug, W.S. & Cummings, M.R. (2000) *Concepts of Genetics*, 6th edn. New Jersey, USA: Prentice Hall.

Lockwood, C.J. (2000) Prediction of pregnancy loss. *Lancet* 355(9212) 1292–1293.

Nairne, Sir P. (1993) *Genetic Screening: Ethical Issues*. London: Nuffield Council on Bioethics.

Neilson, J.P. (2000) Ultrasound for fetal assessment in early pregnancy (Cochrane Review). *The Cochrane Library*, Issue 2. Update Software: Oxford.

Nicholl, D.S.T. (2002) *An Introduction to Genetic Engineering*, 2nd edn. Cambridge: Cambridge University Press.

Nicolaides, N.K., Brizot, M. & Snijers, R.M.T. (1994) Fetal nuchal translucency ultrasound for fetal trisomy in the first trimester of pregnancy. *British Journal of Obstetrics and Gynaecology* **101**(9): 782–786.

Wald, N.J., Watt, H.C. & Hackshaw, A.K. (1999) Integrated screening for Down's syndrome based on tests performed during the first and second trimesters. *New England Journal of Medicine* **341**(7): 461–469.

Watson, J.D. (1970) *The Double Helix*. London: Penguin Books.

Zanjani, E.D. & Anderson, W.W.F. Prospects for in utero human gene therapy. *Science* **285**(5436): 2084–2088.

FURTHER READING

Flanagan, G.L. (1996) *Beginning of Life*. London: Dorling Kindersley.
Fascinating content and excellent pictures, following the growth of the baby from conception to birth. The text is written for the general public, particularly for parents to be.

Keesling, A. & Watt, D. (2000) The beginning of life. In: Page, L.A. (ed) *The New Midwifery: Science and Sensitivity in Practice,* Ch. 14. Edinburgh: Churchill Livingstone.

This chapter combines the subjects of molecular biology and embryology. It is very informative and well written to encompass both subjects.

Mueller, R.F. & Young, I.D. (1998) *Emery's Elements of Medical Genetics*, 10th edn. London: Churchill Livingstone.
A comprehensive and readable textbook that covers the subject in depth.

ADDITIONAL RESOURCES

http://www.doh.gov.uk/genetics/acgt/index.htm
Advisory Committee on Genetic Testing website.

http://www.doh.gov.uk/genetics/gtac
Gene Therapy Advisory Committee website.

http://www.doh.gov.uk/genetics/pgt-ch1.htm
Provides comprehensive information about the DoH report on prenatal screening.

http://www.hfea.gov.uk
Human Fertilisation and Embryology Authority website. An informative site, focusing on the work of HFEA – also has useful link sites.

http://www.jacr.bbsrc.ac.uk
Tutorial guide to genetics and molecular biology. Some very good diagrams, outlining the chemical basis of DNA, RNA, the cell, mitosis and meiosis. Reading matter is easy to follow with many parent sites to visit. Its nickname – 'Dr Chromo's School'.

http://www.leeds.ac.uk/re/execsum.htm
Reproductive epidemiology: report on screening for cystic fibrosis.

http://www.medschl.cam.ac.uk
Public Health Genetics Unit, Cambridge, website.

http://www.ornl.gov/hgmis/project.com
The Human Genome Project website: news, history of the project, ethical issues, gene therapy. A site well worth a visit with some online connections to journals.

http://www.wellcome.ac.uk
Wellcome Trust website.

13

Implantation and Development of the Placenta

Mary McNabb

LEARNING OUTCOMES

After reading this chapter, you will be able to:

- discuss the process following fertilization during which the fertilized ovum implants and placental development takes place

- understand the process of placental formation
- describe the functions of the mature placenta.

INTRODUCTION

Hormonal variations during the menstrual cycle regulate a variety of adaptations in general and reproductive organ systems to receive the fertilized ovum (as described in Chs 6 and 11). This chapter describes implantation and placental formation.

During each cycle, the uterus facilitates reception, maturation and transport of spermatozoa from the vagina to the fallopian tube, while the inner layers of the uterus prepare to receive and directly nourish the blastocyst (Burton *et al.*, 2002). When fertilization occurs, the endometrium undergoes more extensive synchronized changes that transform it from active rejection to a brief state of receptivity for the blastocyst, during a 'window of implantation' between cycle days 20–24 (Gonzalez *et al.*, 2003; Hustin, 1992; Hustin and Franchimont, 1992; Lessey, 2000). During the first trimester the decidualized endometrium lies in direct contact with the cytotrophoblast shell, and with the placenta and fetal membranes for the remainder of pregnancy and labour (Irwin and Giudice, 1998).

In early pregnancy, distinct cells within the decidualized endometrium reduce local maternal immune responses to implantation, modulate trophoblast infiltration and provide a direct source of nutritional and regulatory molecules for the embryo after implantation, until the mature placenta begins to function and fetoplacental development begins at 11–12 weeks' gestation (Burton *et al.*, 2002; Jauniaux *et al.*, 1994; Starkey, 1993; Tseng *et al.*, 1999).

ENDOMETRIAL PREPARATION

In preparation for implantation, endometrial glandular cells accumulate glycogen, regulatory proteins, sugars and lipids and their secretory activity reaches a maximum around 6 days after ovulation. These molecules are thought to supply the conceptus with essential nutritional and regulatory molecules during and after implantation (Burton *et al.*, 2002; Hustin and Franchimont, 1992). At the same time, progesterone stimulates increased expression of two potent angiogenic factors: angiogenin in stromal cells and vascular endothelial growth factor (VEGF) in stromal cells and neutrophils associated with microvessel walls (Gargett *et al.*, 2001; Ma *et al.*, 2001). By the mid-secretory phase, a subepithelial capillary plexus has formed into a complex network of vessels (see Fig. 6.9, p. 99) and the newly regrown arterioles become increasingly more spiral as they lengthen more rapidly than the endometrium thickens (Gargett *et al.*, 2001; Starkey, 1993; Strauss and Coutifaris, 1999).

PRE-DECIDUALIZATION

During the secretory phase, stromal cells synthesize and release a growing number of new matrix proteins together with surface expression of their receptors, including laminin, fibronectin and integrins, while the earlier cross-linking collagen fibrils are degraded. This process of matrix remodelling creates a looser and more soluble structure and, from the mid-secretory phase onwards, stromal cells also express a variety of regulatory peptides that are involved in cell replication and haemostasis. Stromal tissue undergoes further differentiation and individual cells become larger and oedematous, which contributes to the overall thickening of the endometrium.

From the late secretory phase, further changes occur within the endometrium that are regulated by relaxin, progesterone and leptin. The endometrial stroma undergoes a process of *decidualization,* as it synthesizes a number of hormones and other molecules that provide an appropriate nutritive, regulatory and immuno-protective environment during embryonic formation (Gonzalez *et al.*, 2003; Starkey, 1993).

Within the myometrium, human chorionic gonadotrophin (hCG) and progesterone induce cellular enlargement and depress the excitability of uterine muscle by decreasing uptake of cellular free calcium, blocking the ability of oestrogens to stimulate α-adrenergic receptors and downregulating myometrial gap junctions (Ambrus and Rao, 1994; Niswender *et al.*, 2000). At the same time, rising levels of progesterone seem to act centrally to depress oxytocin neuronal activity, which may also contribute to a decline in uterine peristalsis during implantation (Rodway and Rao, 1995).

TROPHOBLAST-ENDOMETRIAL INTERACTIONS

Between 5 and 7 days after ovulation, the endometrium displays transient support for the attachment and implantation of the blastocyst. Growing evidence suggests that these initial processes are regulated in different ways by the inner cell mass, the outer trophectodermal layers of the blastocyst and by hormonally induced changes in the decidualized endometrium (Gonzalez *et al.*, 2000; Kumar *et al.*, 2003; Lessey, 2000). By the time of implantation, the embryo has acquired a highly differentiated trophoblast capable of attaching to the uterine epithelium, and an inner cell mass containing stem cells for germ lines and somatic cells already allocated to various tissues.

When the blastocyst hatches from the zona pellucida, trophoblast cells near the inner cell mass develop surface processes and fuse to form the syncytial trophoblast (Tabibzadeh and Babaknia, 1995). Trophoblast cells surrounding the inner cell mass make initial contact with the endometrium by close apposition of the plasma membranes of the trophoblasts with the apical plasma membranes of the surface epithelial cells, followed by proliferation and formation of junctional complexes with the surface epithelium. At the same time, the apical membranes of epithelial cells display a variety of oestrogen-induced changes that are thought to facilitate cell recognition and interaction with the trophectoderm. These include a progressive shortening of the microvilli, creating a flatter surface, and reduced thickness of the normally dense coating of glycoproteins (Hustin and Franchimont, 1992; Lessey, 2000; Tabibzadeh and Babaknia, 1995).

During the process of implantation, cell surface molecules have been characterized as a range of hormone-dependent residues known to regulate cell-adhesion (Hustin, 1992; Wegner and Carson, 1994). Infiltration follows, as low oxygen tension stimulates rapid proliferation of cytotrophoblast cells that generate specialized trophoblast cells, which displace the epithelium and enter the loose endometrial stroma. Successful implantation seems to critically depend on a progesterone-induced expression of calcitonin in glandular epithelial and stromal cells, which downregulates the expression of E-cadherin, a cell adhesion molecule at cell–cell contact sites (Kumar *et al.*, 2003; Zhu *et al.*, 1998). This relaxes lateral adhesion between cells and allows the specialized trophoblast cells to send out long, slender intercellular protrusions and establish contact with the loose network of glandular and decidual cells lying beneath the surface. During implantation, proliferating cytotrophoblast cells form a labyrinthic structure, from which the more elaborate anchoring and floating villi subsequently emerge (Hustin and Franchimont, 1992).

ENDOMETRIAL RESPONSES TO IMPLANTATION AND EARLY PLACENTAL FORMATION

The surface epithelium and underlying decidua show distinct responses to implantation. Epithelial cells around the implantation site multiply rapidly to form a complete cover for the growing blastocyst, which is enveloped in a thick layer of syncytiotrophoblast by approximately 9 days following fertilization. More extensive hormone-induced changes occur within the underlying decidua.

Decidual cells produce a range of matrix proteins, which form a loose lattice-type network that allows free passage of water, ions and large molecules between the decidua and the embryonic compartment. Following fertilization, a thickened fibrous network is formed that subsequently undergoes a degree of dissolution at the site of the implanting blastocyst. This may result from the action of trophoblast enzymes or from a progesterone-induced release of calcitonin and relaxin by the decidua (Kumar et al., 2003; Starkey, 1993).

During the first 6–8 weeks of pregnancy, the secretory pattern of epithelial gland cells extends the activity of the *luteal phase* of the cycle with a continuation of glycogen secretion and a rapid rise in the secretion of a number of glycoproteins (Burton et al., 2002; Muller-Schottle et al., 1999). These include glycodelin A, a relaxin, hCG and MUC-1, a large progesterone-dependent glycoprotein (Burton et al., 2002). Glycodelin A regulates endometrial receptivity, has potent immunosuppressive activity and may also be involved in transporting retinol to the trophoblast, yolk sac and embryo, for cell replication, differentiation and early patterning of the body axis (Johansson et al., 1999; Morriss-Kay and Ward, 1999). Recent evidence suggests that MUC-1 is taken up by the syncytiotrophoblast membrane and provides a rich and energy-free source of amino acids for its synthetic requirements (Burton et al., 2002; Seppala et al., 2002; Tseng et al., 1999).

Like the epithelial glands, decidual cells synthesize and release specific glycoproteins. One of these molecules has been identified as a growth factor binding protein that may participate in regulating the pace and extent of trophoblast implantation (Hustin and Franchimont, 1992). Decidual cells that release relaxin have also been found to contain prolactin, which is regulated by a number of factors from adjoining cells in the decidua, placenta and membranes. The physiological activity of prolactin within the decidua remains unclear but experimental findings suggest that it promotes blastocyst growth, suppresses specific aspects of the immune response and inhibits myometrial contractility, thus creating a smooth local environment for implantation (Handwerger et al., 1992; Healy, 1991).

IMMUNOSUPPRESSIVE AND ANTI-INFLAMMATORY ACTIVITIES

Trophoblast and decidual cells express modified forms of various components of the immune system. Transplantation antigens are absent from trophoblast cells,

and other antigens present are found in all human tissues and therefore tolerated by the maternal immune system. First trimester studies also indicate that the syncytiotrophoblast – situated at the maternal–embryonic interface – expresses high levels of prostaglandin E (PGE), which modulates many immune system activities. Local maternal tissue seems to be the target of PGE, as the underlying cytotrophoblast contains high concentrations of prostaglandin dehydrogenase (PGDH), an enzyme that inactivates prostaglandins and thereby protects embryonic and fetal tissues from prostaglandins produced by maternal endometrial cells (Critchley et al., 1999; Kelly, 1994). While the decidua contains all the cells necessary to produce both an immune and an inflammatory response, evidence suggests that during pregnancy many of these activities are selectively compromised by progesterone. This phenomenon has been demonstrated in T cells, natural killer cells and in small and large lymphocytes (Check, 1994; Pepe and Albrecht, 1995). Current research indicates that locally released growth factors and PGE_2 may operate in different ways to modulate immune responses to placentation (Kelly, 1994; Starkey, 1993).

DEVELOPMENT OF THE CYTOTROPHOBLAST SHELL

Early villi are composed only of cytotrophoblast cells. Once formed, they are gradually supported by ingrowth of the underlying mesoderm from cells that delaminate from the cytotrophoblast. Cytotrophoblast cells in contact with the decidua become cuboidal and contain a single nucleus with a well-defined plasma membrane. Under the influence of hCG, human placental lactogen (hPL) and growth factors, these cells act as a stem cell population. Some divide and differentiate into a continuous outer layer of multinucleated syncytiotrophoblast tissue that ceases to have distinguishable cell membranes. This forms a syncytium around the cytotrophoblast and stromal cells and is characterized by a particular requirement for reduced oxygen tension during the first trimester (Cronier et al., 1994; Ho et al., 1997; Maruo et al., 1995; Nachtigall et al., 1996). The syncytium contributes to gaseous, nutrient and waste exchange and is a key source of hormones, like hCG, growth hormone (GH), oestrogens, progesterone and hCG, that are critical for maintaining pregnancy (Kliman and Feinberg, 1992).

Other cytotrophoblast cells extend from the syncytium to form mononucleated cell columns of anchoring villi that attach the emerging placenta to the decidua (see Fig. 13.2). A final group differentiate into an invasive population of migratory extravillous cytotrophoblast cells, which completely infiltrate the decidua and the first third of the myometrium to reach the tips of the spiral arteries, where they block the flow of maternal blood into the intervillous space during the first trimester (Aplin, 2000; Caniggia and Winter, 2002). Towards the end of embryonic formation at 10–12 weeks' gestation, the intervillous space begins to open, exposing the migratory extravillous trophobast cells to a physiological increase in oxygen tension. This development seems to stimulate further differentiation of the extravillous cells to a more invasive phenotype, which allows them to enter and remodel the spiral arteries to create the low-resistance vascular system that is essential for fetal growth (Caniggia and Winter, 2002; Caniggia *et al.*, 2000; Hustin, 1992).

Chorionic villi cover the entire chorionic sac until approximately 8 weeks' gestation. Ultrasound images using a vaginal probe have been obtained for chorionic villous sampling during the first 12 weeks of pregnancy. These pictures have demonstrated that during this period of organ formation, trophoblast infiltration forms a thick undulating layer of actively growing cells called the cytotrophoblastic shell (Fig. 13.1), with primitive villi that sprout extravillous columns of differentiated cytotrophoblast cells on the maternal surface. These cells enter and plug the walls of spiral arterioles until around 10 weeks' gestation, while others remain mobile around the intervillous spaces (Hustin, 1992).

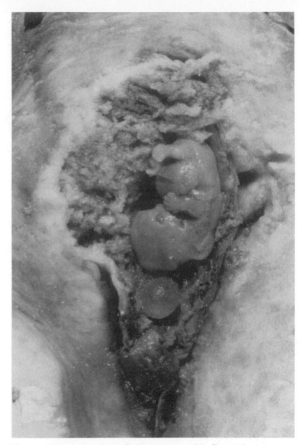

Figure 13.1 Section of the uterus with first trimester pregnancy in situ. The yolk sac appears just below the embryo. The limits of the cytotrophoblast shell appear as a thick whitish line. (Photograph courtesy of Dr J Hustin.)

FORMATION OF THE DECIDUOCHORIAL PLACENTA

During the first 12 weeks, extravillous trophoblast migration into the spiral arteries occurs primarily within the decidual segments. First the distal tips of these blood vessels are plugged with cytotrophoblast cells that are continuous with the trophoblastic shell or with the proliferating tips of the emerging villi. As illustrated in Figure 13.2, sheets of these endovascular trophoblasts migrate along the capillary walls against maternal blood flow and accumulate within the lumen when they reach the spiral arteries. During the subsequent process of vascular infiltration, cells strip away sections of the endothelium and burrow beneath this layer, to replace elastic tissue and smooth muscle with cytotrophoblast cells that appear to surround themselves with large quantities of fibrinoid material. Later, surface endothelial cells grow over the new underlying tissues. Through

this process, the convoluted walls of the spiral arteries are converted into tubes of fibrinoid material with no elastic tissue or smooth muscle fibres. As a result of these changes, segments of the spiral arteries become more dilated and lose their capacity to respond to the vasomotor influences of continued autonomic innervation (Hustin *et al.*, 1988; Pijnenborg, 1990)

During the first 10 weeks of pregnancy, ultrasound studies suggest that decidual blood vessels do not reach the intervillous space. While small amounts of plasma percolate through the plugs from these low-pressure vessels, chorionic villous sampling has rarely demonstrated the presence of maternal blood. As illustrated in Figure 13.3, this evidence suggests that during the first 10–12 weeks, the intervillous space is not immediately connected with the maternal circulation and is not yet bathed by maternal blood (Hustin and Schaaps, 1987). As illustrated in Figure 13.4, estimates of uterine blood flow also support this concept. In non-pregnant

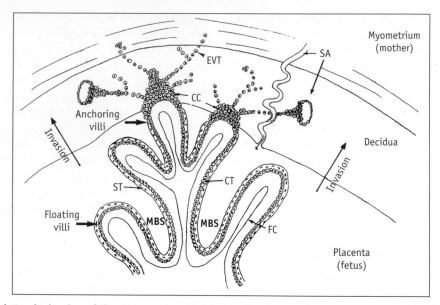

Figure 13.2   Schematic drawing of the process of trophoblast infiltration and formation of the deciduochorial placenta during the first trimester of human pregnancy. EVT, extravillous trophoblasts; CC, cytotrophoblast cell columns; CT, cytotrophoblasts; ST, syncytiotrophoblasts; FC, fetal capillaries; MBS, maternal blood space; SA, spiral arterioles. (From Jaffe, 1998.)

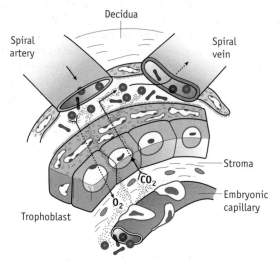

Figure 13.3   Diagram showing the uteroplacental and villous circulation and the trophoblastic barrier. (From Jauniaux and Gulbis, 1997.)

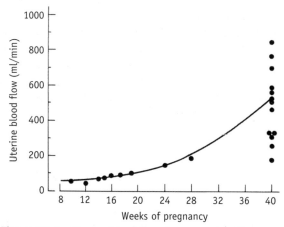

Figure 13.4   Uterine blood flow in pregnancy. (From Chamberlain and Broughton Pipkin, 1998.)

OPTIMAL ENVIRONMENT FOR ORGANOGENESIS AND EARLY PLACENTAL FORMATION

women, uterine blood flow is approximately 40 ml/min, which rises by around 10 ml/min during the first trimester. In contrast, much larger increases occur during the second and third trimesters, to reach over 800 ml/min by the end of pregnancy (de Swiet, 1991).

The first 10 weeks of pregnancy are characterized by rapid proliferation and differentiation of trophoblast cells that contrasts with much slower growth of the embryo while organogenesis occurs. Recent animal studies suggest that low oxygen tension provides the optimal conditions for embryonic and placental formation during the first trimester (Aplin, 2000; Burton *et al.*, 2002; Caniggia *et al.*, 2000; Eriksson 1999). Pre-implantation embryos exhibit increased glycogen metabolism and maximum survival rates in vitro when oxygen tension is maintained between 2.5 and 5% (Jauniaux *et al.*, 2000). This unusual environment is thought to be peculiarly suited to organ formation. Embryonic haemoglobin, which lasts for the first 8 weeks of gestation, combines with oxygen at the very low tension found in interstitial fluids. In keeping with these results, oxygen tension in the surrounding trophoblast has also been found to be lower than that in the underlying endometrium during the first 12 weeks of gestation (Jauniaux *et al.*, 2001).

These findings have led to suggestions that the embryo derives its external nutritional support from the secretory products of uterine glands (Burton *et al.*, 2002). Developments within the endometrium fully complement this notion. From the luteal phase of the cycle, glandular cells secrete rapidly increasing amounts of glycoproteins that promote cell growth and organ differentiation. At the same time the underlying decidua undergoes considerable biochemical and structural adaptations, as it forms an array of matrix proteins and differentiated secretory cells that provide growth-promoting factors for the embryo, immunoprotection for trophoblast infiltration and a variety of regulatory hormones, including prolactin, relaxin, renin, retinol-binding protein and prostaglandins (Burton *et al.*, 2002; Hustin and Franchimont, 1992; Kim *et al.*, 1999; Starkey, 1993).

FORMATION OF THE EMBRYONIC COMPARTMENT

As implantation of the blastocyst proceeds during the first 2 weeks after ovulation, the extraembryonic mesoderm progressively increases and contains isolated spaces by 12 days after fertilization. At the same time, the inner cell mass becomes a bilaminar disk, composed of high columnar cells, called the epiblast or primary ectoderm, on the dorsal surface and a layer of differentiated cuboidal cells on the ventral surface, adjacent to the blastocyst cavity, called the hypoblast or primary endoderm. Over the next few days, a wave of new endodermal cells migrate from the primary endoderm to line the blastocyst cavity and form the primary yolk sac or exocoelomic cavity during the fourth week of gestation. This cavity contains a complex fluid that is derived from the maternal circulation by transplacental diffusion, and from the secondary yolk sac, which forms at the beginning of the fourth week of gestation. Containing high concentrations of amino acids, regulatory proteins, vitamins and hormones, this fluid acts as a reservoir of molecules, prior to their use by the yolk sac and embryo during the first 8–10 weeks of pregnancy (Jauniaux and Gulbis, 2000; Jauniaux *et al.*, 1994).

As soon as the primary yolk sack forms, a thick acellular material is secreted between the exocoelomic membrane and the cytotrophoblast, called the extraembryonic mesoderm. Over the next couple of days, this tissue divides to form a second chorionic cavity, between the primary yolk sack and the cytotrophoblast. Next, an inner layer of cytotrophoblast cells delaminate to form amniogenic cells. Some of these differentiate into amnioblasts and organize into a membrane called the amnion. Formation of the primordial amniotic cavity seems to arise by cavitation of the epiblast or primary ectoderm, which opens and then reforms to create a complete membrane around the amniotic cavity containing the embryo.

Fluid formed within the amniotic cavity is secreted mainly by the embryo and contains much lower concentrations of molecules and trace elements than fluid in the exocoelomic cavity. This finding indicates that the amniotic membrane separating the two compartments is not permeable to large molecules, and most maternal and trophoblast proteins are probably absorbed by the embryo through the secondary yolk sac (Jauniaux and Gulbis, 2000; Jauniaux *et al.*, 1993, 1994). As illustrated in Figure 13.5, during the first 8 weeks of embryonic life, the amniotic cavity is dwarfed by the larger and highly dynamic exocoelomic cavity containing the free-floating yolk sac, which directly nourishes and regulates embryonic formation until around 10 weeks' gestation (Jauniaux and Gulbis, 1997; Jones, 1997).

FORMATION AND DEGENERATION OF THE SECONDARY YOLK SAC

At around 12 days following fertilization, the primary yolk sac breaks up into a number of smaller vesicles while the endoderm beneath the embryonic disk grows out to form the secondary yolk sac. As illustrated in Figure 13.6, over the next couple of weeks the secondary yolk sac grows rapidly and becomes larger than the amniotic cavity by the fifth week of gestation (Jones, 1997). With successive foldings of the embryo during the

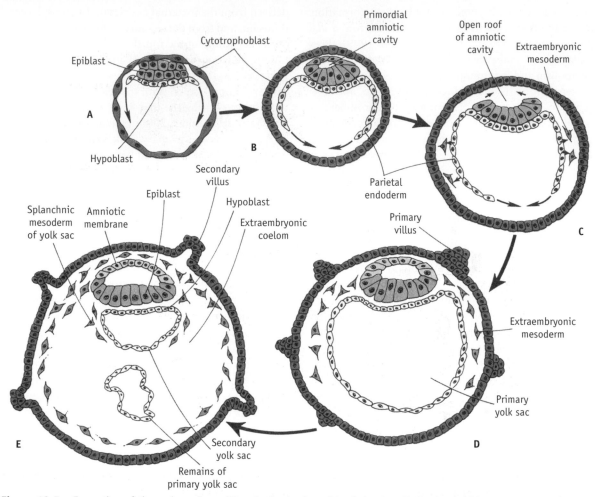

Figure 13.5   Formation of the embryonic cavities. **A.** Beginning of implantation. **B.** Implanted blastocyst at 7.5 days following fertilization. **C.** Implanted blastocyst at 8 days following fertilization. **D.** Embryo at 9 days following fertilization. **E.** Begining of third week. (From Carlson, 1994.)

dynamic process of gastrulation, which occurs between 3 and 6 weeks' gestation, the neck region of the secondary yolk sac is constricted to form the yolk stalk, which connects the definitive yolk sac to the primitive gut.

Until it begins to degenerate at around 9 weeks' gestation, the secondary yolk sac consists of three distinct layers: an outer layer of extraembryonic mesoderm that completely lines the chorionic or exocoelomic cavity; a middle splanchnic mesoderm containing blood islands; and an endodermal layer facing the yolk sac lumen (Jauniaux and Moscoso, 1992; Jones, 1997). The outer extraembryonic mesoderm has a well-developed microvillous brush border with numerous pinocytotic

vesicles within their cytoplasm which enhances its capacity for absorption of molecules from the surrounding exocoelomic fluid. The middle layer of splanchnic mesoderm contains free collagen fibrils and sinusoidal blood vessels which are induced by the innermost endodermal layer of the yolk sac. Central cells of the blood islands fuse to form primitive vascular channels that extend towards the body of the embryo where they make connections with the endothelial tubes associated with the tubular heart and major vessels (Jones, 1997). At the same time, blood cells and capillaries develop within the chorionic villi. At approximately 19 days, the two sets of vessels establish contact, thereby creating the beginnings of a vascular connection between the

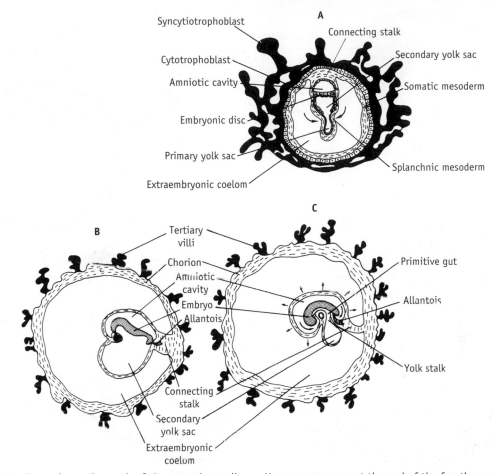

Figure 13.6 Formation and growth of the secondary yolk sac. Human pregnancy at the end of the fourth menstrual week (**A**) and during the fifth (**B**) and sixth (**C**) menstrual week. (From Jauniaux and Moscoso, 1992.)

embryonic compartment and the early placenta (Carlson, 1994: 72). Blood cell formation in the secondary yolk sac continues until haematopoiesis begins in the embryonic liver and spleen at around 8 week' gestation (Jauniaux and Moscoso, 1992).

The innermost endodermal layer of the yolk sac is made up of large columnar cells with glycogen deposits and a well-developed capacity for protein biosynthesis. These are interspersed with large microvillous-lined channels similar to bile canaliculi in hepatic parenchyma that open out into the cavity of the yolk sac and seem to be involved in the secretion of waste products. Many proteins and enzymes involved in energy metabolism and digestion are synthesized by the endodermal layer, including alpha-fetoprotein, antitrypsin, albumin and transferrin, before the embryonic liver is ready to take over this role at around 9–10 weeks' gestation (Jones,

1997). In addition, large spherical primordial sex cells appear in a restricted area of the endoderm and yolk sac stalk at the end of the fifth week of gestation and these subsequently migrate by amoeboid movement along the hind gut to the gonadal ridge where they become incorporated in the primary sex cords (Jauniaux and Moscoso, 1992; Jones, 1997).

GROWTH OF THE AMNIOTIC COMPARTMENT

Between 7 and 12 weeks' gestation, the production of amniotic fluid increases from 3 to 30 ml (Jauniaux and Gulbis, 2000). This causes the amnion to swell, until it takes over the chorionic space, bringing the amnion and chorion in contact with each other for the first time and enclosing the entire embryo, except for the umbilical

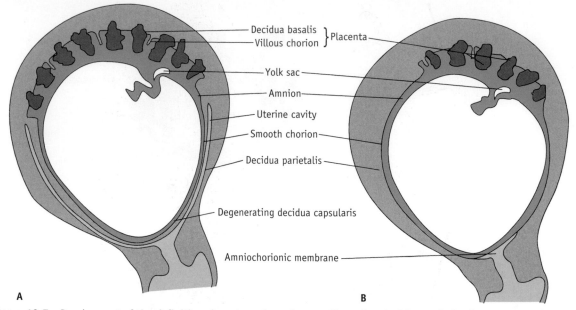

Decidua basalis
Villous chorion } Placenta
Yolk sac
Amnion
Uterine cavity
Smooth chorion
Decidua parietalis
Degenerating decidua capsularis
Amniochorionic membrane

A   B

Figure 13.7   Development of the definitive placenta and membranes. (Reproduced with permission from Moore and Persaud, 1993: 117.)

area, within a single cavity. The amnion is a specialized membrane composed of a single layer of cuboidal epithelial cells on a loose connective tissue matrix. Amniotic fluid volume increases from approximately 350–450 ml at 20 weeks, to 800–1000 ml at 36–39 weeks and then begins to decline (Moore and Persaud, 1993).

As the sac subsequently grows into the endometrial cavity, this portion of the chorion gradually becomes compressed against the decidua capsularis – the area of decidual lining that surrounds the site of implantation. With continued growth, the blood supply is reduced and these villi slowly degenerate, although the trophoblast cells between them remain viable for the remainder of pregnancy. As illustrated in Figure 13.7, this portion of the chorion, known as *chorion laeve*, forms an interface between fetal amnion and areas of maternal decidua that are not occupied by the definitive placenta.

Despite the absence of a direct blood supply, the chorion laeve has diverse layers of metabolically active tissue. It is composed of a layer of fibroblast cells that are contiguous with the amnion, a reticular layer, a type of basement membrane and 2–10 layers of trophoblast cells that are closely applied to the decidua capsularis. Taken together, these cells produce a number of enzymes that degrade locally synthesized substances including prostaglandins, oxytocin and platelet-activating factor,

all of which have a capacity to stimulate myometrial contractility (Erwich and Keirse, 1992).

SECOND PHASE OF TROPHOBLAST INFILTRATION

From 14 weeks onwards, a second wave of trophoblast infiltration extends into the myometrial segments of many spiral arteries. As in decidual segments, this activity replaces muscular and elastic tissue with unidentified fibrinoid material that converts them into widened, funnel-like tubes that have lost their capacity to respond to the vasomotor influences of continued autonomic innervation (Caniggia *et al.*, 2000). At the same time the trophoblast shell becomes thinner and more irregular as fetal growth enlarges its internal volume. An increasing number of extravillous cells become distinct from the shell surface and these gradually open up low-pressure flow of maternal blood within the intervillous space. Experimental evidence on humans and monkeys suggests that the velocity of blood flow from the spiral arterioles to the intervillous space is similar to that of an actively flowing brook entering a reed-filled marsh (see Fig. 13.8) (Ramsey *et al.*, 1976).

The onset of direct communication between maternal blood and placental villi coincides with the completion

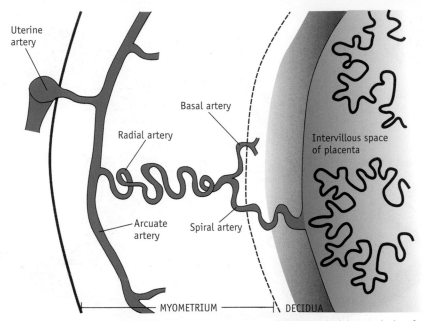

Uterine artery

Basal artery

Radial artery

Intervillous space of placenta

Arcuate artery

Spiral artery

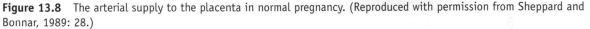

MYOMETRIUM — DECIDUA

Figure 13.8 The arterial supply to the placenta in normal pregnancy. (Reproduced with permission from Sheppard and Bonnar, 1989: 28.)

of organogenesis and the onset of fetal growth and development. During this phase, the roughly formed organs undergo progressive development and rapid growth that requires large increases in uterine size and blood volume. This suggests that the structural alterations in the decidual and myometrial segments of the uterine blood vessels allow for the emergence of an expanding low-pressure system that optimizes gas and nutritional exchange across the placental interface.

FORMATION OF THE DEFINITIVE PLACENTA

As villi of the chorion laeve disappear, those attached to the decidua basalis rapidly develop to form the mature placenta. The cytotrophoblast shell extends laterally and penetrates deeper into maternal tissue between the anchoring villi, and increasingly complex branching villi extend in the intervillous space. Each stem villus forms the centre of the villous tree. Fetal arterioles carrying poorly oxygenated blood enter the villi and break up into an extensive arteriocapillary–venous network. As illustrated in Figure 13.9, the 60–70 branching villi that make up the mature placenta provide a large surface area for gaseous and metabolic exchange between fetal blood within the villi and maternal blood circulating slowly around the external surface from the intervillous space (Sheppard and Bonnar, 1989).

> **Reflective Activity 13.1**
>
> At your next opportunity, take a small sample of placental tissue. Place this in a clear disposable container (plastic cup) and fill with water. After about 15 minutes, you can observe the chorionic villi, and the structure of the definitive placenta.

REGULATION OF AMNIOTIC FLUID VOLUME

During the first half of pregnancy, the composition of amniotic fluid is similar to that of fetal or maternal plasma and its volume increases are closely related to fetal weight. Until about 20 weeks, the dynamics of amniotic fluid volume are thought to involve a transmembrane pathway from maternal blood via the placenta and movement of fluid and other molecules across the fetal skin, which offers no impediment to the flow of fluid into the amniotic sac. From 17–25 weeks' gestation, this pattern of flow diminishes, as the fetal skin begins to keratinize. During the second half of pregnancy, the fetal kidneys and lungs make a growing contribution to amniotic fluid, while the gastrointestinal tract becomes a major pathway for its removal. Estimates of daily volumes near term suggest that fetal urine contributes 800–1200 ml, lung fluid 170 ml,

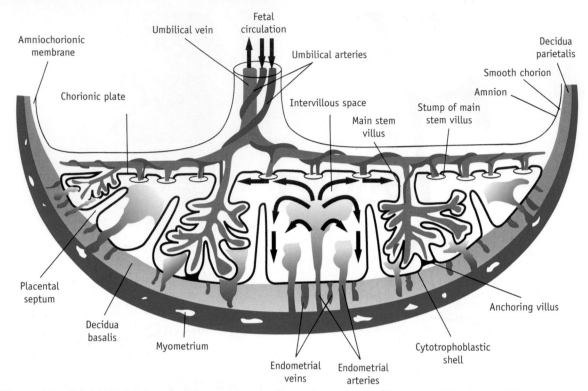

Figure 13.9 Schematic drawing of a full-term placenta illustrating one stem villous in each cotyledon with stumps indicating those that have been removed. The drawing shows: (1) the relation of the (fetal) villous chorion to the (maternal) decidua basalis; (2) uterine and fetoplacental blood flow. Maternal blood flows into the intervillous space and exchange with fetal blood occurs around the branch villi. Inflowing arterial blood pushes blood into the endometrial veins scattered over the entire surface of the decidua basalis. (Reproduced with permission from Moore and Persaud, 1993: 117.)

and 500–1000 ml is removed by fetal swallowing (Gilbert *et al.*, 1991).

At present, the mechanisms regulating amniotic fluid volume are poorly understood. During the second half of pregnancy amniotic fluid is hypo-osmolar as compared with maternal and fetal plasma. This osmotic gradient would be expected to drive water from the amniotic cavity into the maternal and fetal circulations via the umbilical cord, placenta and membranes. However, the precise volumes that move through these pathways remain to be confirmed (Brace 1995; Gilbert *et al.*, 1991).

Other evidence suggests that decidual prolactin and PGE$_2$ from the amniotic membrane and umbilical cord may be involved along with other hormones in regulating amniotic fluid volume. Concentrations of prolactin in amniotic fluid are 5–10 times higher than in the maternal circulation. Levels increase sharply in the second trimester, reaching mean values of about 3500 ng/ml around 20 weeks, before declining significantly to a second plateau of about 500 ng/ml by 34 weeks.

This pattern is thought to result from a fall in decidual production and a simultaneous rise in degradation by the fetal kidneys. Prolactin may regulate the volume of amniotic fluid, by controlling electrolyte exchange across the chorioamniotic membranes (Handwerger *et al.*, 1992; Kletsky, 1992) (Fig. 13.10).

PGE$_2$ has been found to actively regulate ion flows in a variety of epithelial-related cells. Because it is the predominant prostaglandin in the amnion, it seems possible that it may be involved in absorbing fluid across the growing amniotic membrane. The action of PGE$_2$ and other placental peptides like atrial natriuretic peptide (ANP) may regulate the removal of fluid into the maternal circulation and help to counterbalance the large inflow of fetal urine during the latter part of pregnancy (Gilbert *et al.*, 1991; Kelly, 1994).

This dynamic volume of fluid provides essential space for fetal growth and movements, particularly during the second half of pregnancy. In late pregnancy and labour, it also equalizes the pressure exerted by uterine contractions and creates a cushion for the umbilical cord,

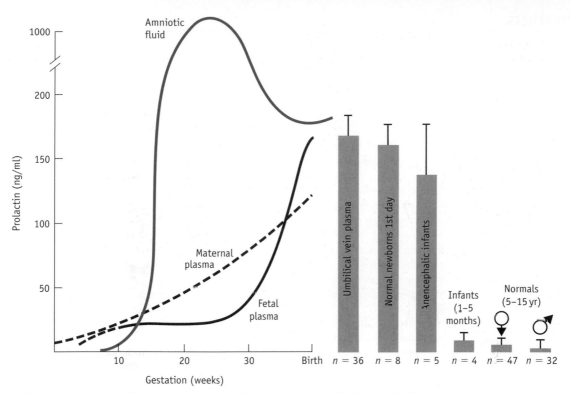

Figure 13.10 Comparison of patterns of maternal, fetal and amniotic fluid prolactin during the course of pregnancy. On the right, plasma levels of prolactin in normal and anencephalic newborns are compared with those of normal infants, children and adolescents. (Reproduced with permission from Aubert *et al.*, 1975: 159 (amended) and Schenker *et al.*, 1975: 836.)

preventing compression of the umbilical vessels between the fetus and the uterine wall during fetal movements and contractions. At the same time, liquor volume also modulates excessive overriding of the bones of the fetal skull, which protects the underlying cerebral membranes and blood vessels, as the head is moulded, during descent and rotation in the pelvic cavity.

CONCLUSION

The period of implantation and formation of the distinct biological environments for embryonic formation and early fetal growth is a time of tremendous physiological activity. This includes the implantation of the placenta, which is then prepared to fulfil all the nutritional, excretory, protective, respiratory and endocrine requirements of the fetus whilst in utero.

It is important for the midwife to appreciate the intricate processes at play from fertilization through to implantation and the development of the placenta, in order to facilitate the woman's understanding of what is happening within her body, and to support advice and information provided to the woman and her family.

KEY POINTS

- The process for successful implantation and formation of the placenta commences during the menstrual cycle.
- Optimal conditions for early embryonic development are characterized by low oxygen tension.

- An understanding of placental formation assists the midwife in providing advice and information to women about nutrition and long-term health during early pregnancy.

REFERENCES

Ambrus, G. & Rao, C.V. (1994) Novel regulation of pregnant human myometrial smooth muscle cell gap junctions by human chorionic gonadotrophin. *Endocrinology* **135**(6): 2772–2779.

Aplin, J.D. (2000) Hypoxia and human placental development. *Journal of Clinical Investigation* **105**(5): 559–560.

Aubert, M.L., Grumbach, M.M. & Kaplan, S.L. (1975) The antogenesis of human fetal hormones. *Journal of Clinical Investigation* **56**: 155.

Brace, R.A. (1995) Current topic: progress toward understanding the regulation of amniotic fluid volume: water and solute fluxes in and through the fetal membranes. *Placenta* **16**: 1–18.

Burton, G.J., Watson, A.L., Hempstock, J. *et al.* (2002) Uterine glands provide histotrophic nutrition for the human fetus during the first trimester of pregnancy. *Journal of Clinical Endocrinology and Metabolism* **87**(6): 2954–2959.

Caniggia, I. & Winter, J.L. (2002) Hypoxia inducible factor-1: oxygen regulation of trophoblast differentiation in normal and pre-eclamptic pregnancies – a review. *Placenta*: Supplement A Trophoblast Research **23**(16): S47–S57.

Caniggia, I., Mostachfi, H., Winter, J. *et al.* (2000) Hypoxia-inducible factor-1 mediates the biological effects of oxygen on human trophoblast differentiation through TGFβ3. *Journal of Clinical Investigation* **105**(5): 577–587.

Carlson, B.M. (1994) *Human Embryology and Developmental Biology*. St Louis: Mosby.

Chamberlain, G. & Broughton Pipkin, F. (1998) *Clinical Physiology in Obstetrics*. Oxford: Blackwell Scientific.

Check, J.H. (1994) The role of progesterone in supporting implantation and preventing early pregnancy loss. In: Barnea, E.R., Check, J.H., Grudzinskas, J.G. *et al.* (eds) *Implantation and Early Pregnancy in Humans*, pp. 137–160. New York: Parthenon Publishing Group.

Critchley, H.O.D., Jones, R.L., Lea, R.G. *et al.* (1999) Role of inflammatory mediators in human endometrium during progesterone withdrawal and early pregnancy. *Journal of Clinical Endocrinology and Metabolism* **84**(1): 240–248.

Cronier, L., Bastide, B., Herve, J.C. *et al.* (1994) Gap junctional communication during human trophoblast differentiation: influence of human chorionic gonadotrophin. *Endocrinology* **135**(1): 402–408.

De Swiet M. (1991) The cardiovascular system. In: Hytten, F. & Chamberlain, G. (eds) *Clinical Physiology in Obstetrics*, pp. 3–38. Oxford: Blackwell Scientific.

Eriksson, U.J. (1999) Oxidative DNA damage and embryonic development. *Nature Medicine* **5**(7): 715.

Erwich, J.J.H.M. & Keirse, M.J.N.C. (1992) Placental localisation of 15-hydroxyprostaglandin dehydrogenase in early and term pregnancy. *Placenta* **13**: 223–229.

Gargett, C.E., Lederman, F., Heryonto, B. *et al.* (2001) Focal vascular endothelial growth factor correlates with angiogenesis in human endometrium. Role of intravascular neutrophils. *Human Reproduction* **16**(6): 1065–1075.

Gilbert, W.M., Moore, T.R. & Brace, R.A. (1991) Amniotic fluid volume dynamics. *Fetal Medicine Review* **3**: 89–204.

Gonzalez, R.R., Caballero-Campo, P., Jasper, M. *et al.* (2000) Leptin and Leptin receptor are expressed in the human endometrium and endometrial leptin secretion is regulated by the human blastocyst. *Journal of Clinical Endocrinology and Metabolism* **85**(12): 4883–4888.

Gonzalez, R.R., Leary, K., Petrozza, J.C. *et al.* (2003) Leptin regulation of the interleukin-1 system in human endometrial cells. *Molecular Human Reproduction* **9**(3): 151–158.

Handwerger, S., Richards, R.G. & Markoff, E. (1992) The physiology of decidual prolactin and other decidual protein hormones. *Trends in Endocrinology and Metabolism* **3**(3): 91–95.

Healy, D.L. (1991) Endometrial prolactin and implantation. *Clinics in Obstetrics and Gynaecology* **5**(1): 95–105.

Ho, H-H., Douglas, G.C., Qiu, Q.F. *et al.* (1997) The relationship between trophoblast differentiation and the production of bioactive hCG. *Early Pregnancy: Biology and Medicine* **3**: 291–300.

Hustin, J. (1992) The maternotrophoblast interface: uteroplacental blood flow. In: Barnea, E.R., Hustin, J. & Jauniaux, E. (eds) *The First Twelve Weeks of Gestation*, pp. 97–110. Berlin: Springer-Verlag.

Hustin, J. & Franchimont, P. (1992) The endometrium and implantation. In: Barnea, E.R., Hustin, J. & Jauniaux, E. (eds) *The First Twelve Weeks of Gestation*, pp. 97–110. Berlin: Springer-Verlag.

Hustin, J. & Schaaps, J-P. (1987) Echocardiographic and anatomic studies of the maternotrophoblast border during the first trimester of pregnancy. *American Journal of Obstetrics and Gynecology* **157**(1): 162–168.

Hustin, J., Schaaps, J-P. & Lambotte, R. (1988) Anatomical studies of the utero-placental vascularization in the first trimester of pregnancy. *Trophoblast Research* **3**: 49–60.

Irwin, J.C. & Giudice, L.C. (1998) Decidua. In: Knobin, E & Neill, J.D. (eds) *Encyclopedia of Reproduction*, Vol. 1, pp. 823–835. San Diego: Academic Press.

Jaffe, R. (1998) First trimester utero-placental circulation: maternal–fetal interaction. *Journal of Perinatal Medicine* **26**: 168–174.

Jauniaux, E. & Moscoso, J.G. (1992) Morphology and significance of the human yolk sac. In: Barnea, E.R., Hustin, J. & Jauniaux, E. (eds) *The First Twelve Weeks of Pregnancy*, pp. 192–213. Berlin: Springer-Verlag.

Jauniaux, E. & Gulbis, B. (1997) Embryonic physiology. In: Jauniaux, E., Barnea, E.R. & Edwards, R.G. *Embryonic*

Medicine and Therapy, pp. 223–243. Oxford: Oxford University Press.

Jauniaux, E. & Gulbis, B. (2000) In vivo investigation of placental transfer early in human pregnancy. *European Journal of Obstetrics, Gynecology and Reproductive Biology* **92**: 45–49.

Jauniaux, E., Gulbis, B., Jurkovic, D. *et al.* (1993) Protein and steroid levels in embryonic cavities in early human pregnancy. *Human Reproduction.* **8**(5): 782–787.

Jauniaux, E., Gulbis, B., Jurkovic, D. *et al.* (1994) Relationship between protein concentrations in embryological fluids and maternal serum and yolk sac size during human early pregnancy. *Human Reproduction* **9**(1): 161–166.

Jauniaux, E., Watson, A.L., Hempstock, J. *et al.* (2000) Onset of maternal arterial blood flow and placental oxidative stress. *American Journal of Pathology* **157**(6): 2111–2122.

Jauniaux, E., Wilson, A. & Burton, G. (2001) Evaluation of respiratory gases and acid-base gradients in human fetal fluids and uteroplacental tissue between 7 and 16 weeks' gestation. *American Journal of Obstetrics and Gynecology* **184**(5): 998–1003.

Johansson, S., Gustafson, A.L., Donovan, M. *et al.* (1999) Retinoid binding proteins – expression patterns in the human placenta. *Placenta* **20**: 459–465.

Johnson, M.H. & Everitt, B.J. (1995) *Essential Reproduction.* Cambridge: Blackwell Science.

Jones, C.J. (1997) The life and death of the embryonic yolk sac. In: Jauniaux, E., Barnea, E.R. & Edwards, R.G. (eds) *Embryonic Medicine and Therapy,* pp. 180–196. Oxford: Oxford University Press.

Kelly, R.W. (1994) Pregnancy maintenance and parturition: the role of prostaglandin in manipulating the immune and inflammatory response. *Endocrine Reviews* **15**(5): 684–706.

Kim, J.J., Wang, J., Bambra, C. *et al.* (1999) Expression of cyclooxygenase-1 and -2 in the baboon endometrium during the menstrual cycle and pregnancy. *Endocrinology* **140**(6): 2672–2678.

Kletsky, O.A. (1992) Maternal and fetal prolactin. *Seminars in Reproductive Endocrinology* **10**(3): 282–286.

Kliman, H.J. & Feinberg, R.F. (1992) Differentiation of the trophoblast. In: Barnea, E.R., Hustin, J. & Jauniaux, E. (eds) *The First Twelve Weeks of Gestation,* pp. 3–25. Berlin: Springer-Verlag.

Kumar, S., Brudney, A., Cheon, Y-P. *et al.* (2003) Progesterone induces calcitonin expression in the baboon endometrium within the window of uterine receptivity. *Biology of Reproduction* **68**: 1318–1323.

Lessey, B.A. (2000) The role of the endometrium during embryo implantation. *Human Reproduction* **15**(Suppl. 6): 39–50.

Ma, W., Tan, J., Matsumoto, H. *et al.* (2001) Adult tissue angiogenesis: evidence for negative regulation by estrogen in the uterus. *Molecular Endocrinology* **15**(11): 1983–1992.

Maruo, T., Murata, K., Matsuo, H. *et al.* (1995) Insulin-like growth factor-I as a local regulator of proliferation and differentiated function of the human trophoblast in early pregnancy. *Early Pregnancy: Biology and Medicine* **1**: 54–61.

Moore, K.L. & Persaud, T.V.N. (1993) *The Developing Human.* Philadelphia: W.B. Saunders.

Morriss-Kay, G.M. & Ward, S.J. (1999) Retinoids and mammalian development. *International Review of Cytology* **188**: 73–94.

Muller-Schottle, F., Classen-Linke, I., Alfer, J. *et al.* (1999) Expression of uteroglobin in the human endometrium. *Molecular Human Reproduction* **5**(12): 1155–1161.

Nachtigall, M.J., Kliman, H.J., Feinberg, R.F. *et al.* (1996) The effect of leukemia inhibitory factor (LIF) on trophoblast differentiation: a potential role in human implantation. *Journal of Clinical Endocrinology and Metabolism* **81**(2): 801–806.

Niswender, G.D., Juengel, J.L., Silva, P.J. *et al.* (2000) Mechanisms controlling the function and life span of the corpus luteum. *Physiological Reviews* **80**(1): 1–29.

Pepe, G.J. & Albrecht, E.D. (1995) Actions of placental and fetal adrenal steroid hormones in primate pregnancy. *Endocrine Reviews* **16**(5): 608–648.

Pijnenborg, R. (1990) Trophoblast invasion and placentation in the human: morphological aspects. *Trophoblast Research* **4**: 33–47.

Ramsey, E.M., Houston, M.L. & Harris, J.W. (1976) Interaction of the trophoblast and maternal tissues in three closely related primate species. *American Journal of Obstetrics and Gynecology* **124**(6): 647–652.

Rodway, M.R. & Rao, C.V. (1995) A novel perspective on the role of human chorionic gonadotrophin during pregnancy and in gestational trophoblastic disease. *Early Pregnancy: Biology and Medicine* **1**: 176–187.

Seppala, M., Taylor, R.N., Koistinen, H. *et al.* (2002) Glycodelin: a major lipocalin protein of the reproductive axis with diverse actions in cell recognition and differentiation. *Endocrine Reviews* **23**(4): 401–430.

Schenker, J.G., Ben-David, M. & Polishuk, W.Z. (1975) Prolactin in normal pregnancy: relationship of maternal, fetal, and amniotic fluid levels. *American Journal of Obstetrics and Gynecology* **123**: 834.

Sheppard, B.I. & Bonnar, J. (1989) The maternal blood supply to the placenta. *Progress in Obstetrics and Gynaecology* **7**: 27–30.

Starkey, P.M. (1993) The decidua and factors controlling placentation. In: Redman, C.W.G., Sargent, I.L. & Starkey, P.M. (eds) *The Human Placenta,* pp. 362–413. Oxford: Blackwell Scientific.

Strauss, J. & Coutifaris, C. (1999) The endometrium and myometrium: regulation and dysfunction. In: Yen,

S.S.C., Jaffe, R.B. & Barbieri, R.L. (eds) *Reproductive Endocrinology.* pp. 218–256. Philadelphia: W.B. Saunders.

Tabibzadeh, S. & Babaknia, A. (1995) The signals and molecular pathways involved in implantation, a symbiotic interaction between blastocyst and endometrium involving adhesion and tissue invasion. *Molecular Human Reproduction* **10**(6): 1579–1602.

Tseng, L., Zhu, H.H., Mazella, J. *et al.* (1999) Relaxin stimulates glycodelin mRNA and protein concentrations in human endometrial glandular epithelial cells. *Molecular Human Reproduction* **5**(4): 372–375.

Walker, A.M. (1993) Circulatory transitions at birth and the control of the neonatal circulation. In: Hanson, M.A., Spencer, J.A.D. & Rodeck, C.H. (eds) *Fetus and Neonate: Physiology and Clinical Applications.* 1 *The Circulation,* pp. 160–196. Cambridge: Cambridge University Press.

Wegner, C.C. & Carson, D.D. (1994) Cell adhesion processes in implantation. *Oxford Reviews of Reproductive Biology* **16**: 89–137.

Zhu, L-J. Bagchi, M.K. & Bagchi, I.C. (1998) Attenuation of calcitonin gene expression in pregnant rat uterus leads to a block in embryonic implantation. *Endocrinology* **139**(1): 330–339.

14

Embryonic and Fetal Development

Mary McNabb

After reading this chapter, you will be able to:

- describe the processes involved in embryo formation
- understand the development of key organ systems during fetal life

- understand the critical importance of the fetal hypothalamic–pituitary–adrenal (HPA) axis.

INTRODUCTION

This chapter will describe the process of embryonic formation in which all major systems and structures take on a rudimentary shape during the first 8–10 weeks of gestation. By the end of this period, the nutritional and regulatory functions of the yolk sac decline and formation of the definitive placenta proceeds rapidly in preparation for fetal growth and development.

ORGANOGENESIS

During the first 3 weeks of gestation, most changes within the inner cell mass are directed towards the formation of extraembryonic structures in preparation for organogenesis. These changes begin with a differentiation of the inner cell mass into a bilaminar disc, composed of a distinct external layer called the *primary ectoderm* and an inner layer called the *primary endoderm*. A layer of ectoderm is gradually displaced by accumulating extracellular fluid. Some of these cells differentiate into amnioblasts that later form the amniotic membrane, separating the cavity from the surrounding cytotrophoblast cells (Fig. 14.1).

Having formed a surrounding cavity of extracellular fluid and the rudiments of a vascular system, the bilaminar disc embarks on a period of extensive reorganizations during the third week of gestation, that prepares the way for organogenesis. This process involves the simultaneous migration, contraction and expansion of different cell types all over the embryo. The longitudinal polar axis and bilateral symmetry of the future embryo are established as a result of these transformations.

During this critical stage of formation, a primary structure called the primitive streak is formed along the longitudinal midline of the disc. This structure seems to provide an organizing centre for all cellular activities. Following its formation, subsets of cells within the ectoderm transform into a third *mesodermal layer*. These migrate widely to form a variety of connective tissues and stromal components of individual glands (Braude and Johnson, 1990).

The formation of this trilaminar disc allows specific precursor cells for different bodily tissues to be laid down in their correct spatial positions. Over the next 6–8 weeks, each layer of the disc undergoes cell divisions, further differentiation and foldings that form basic organs and definitive body structures. Once the conceptus has entered this phase of organ formation, it becomes an embryo, as it has developed the distinct tissues that will constitute the fetus (Fig. 14.2).

Brain and central nervous system

The human nervous system begins to form at approximately 18 days after fertilization, making it the first organ system to emerge. A specific area of the ectodermal layer thickens to produce an oval-shaped portion

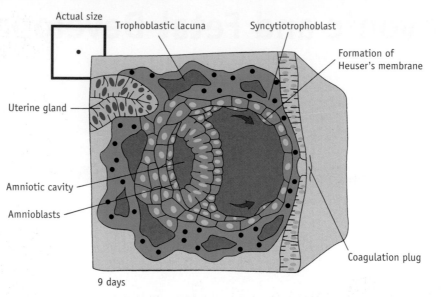

Figure 14.1 indicators:

Actual size

Trophoblastic lacuna

Syncytiotrophoblast

Formation of Heuser's membrane

Uterine gland

Amniotic cavity

Amnioblasts

Coagulation plug

9 days

Figure 14.1 By 9 days the embryo is completely implanted in the uterine endometrium. The amniotic cavity is expanding, and the hypoblast has begun to proliferate and migrate out over the cytotrophoblast to form Heuser's membrane. Trophoblastic lacunae appear in the syncytiotrophoblast, which now completely surrounds the embryo. The point of implantation is marked by a transient coagulation plug in the endometrial surface. (Reproduced with permission from Larsen, 1993: 36.)

called the *neural plate*. On either side of the midline of this plate, two longitudinal neural folds increase in size and curve towards each other, subsequently fusing to form the first outline of the neural tube. As the neural tube is formed, some neuroectodermal cells lying along the crest of each neural fold lose their attachment to neighbouring cells. These crest cells migrate and form an irregular mass on either side of the neural tube.

By 19 days' gestation, the three major divisions – forebrain, midbrain and hindbrain – are demarcated by indentations in the neural folds and a diverticulum called the infundibulum begins to grow downwards from the forebrain division, giving rise to the posterior section of the pituitary gland. At the same time an ectodermal evagination of the oropharynx begins to grow towards the infundibulum. It subsequently loses its connections with the oral cavity and forms a discrete sac known as the anterior pituitary gland.

From 4 weeks' gestation, major regions of the brain emerge and neurones start to differentiate from the epithelium of the neural tube, creating a very active phase of brain cell division. The thalamus and hypothalamus become demarcated by the end of week 5 and differentiation continues throughout embryonic development. At the end of the first 8 weeks, the head makes up almost half of the embryo and directs the first movements of the limbs.

Eyes and ears

From 5 weeks' gestation, two neuroectodermal pockets expand laterally from the hollow forebrain. These optic vesicles go through successive phases of differentiation and remodelling to form the optic cup. Mesoderm surrounding the optic cup forms the inner vascular choroid and the fibrous outer sclera, while mesenchymal tissue gives rise to the lens. At the same time the inner ear begins to form in a similar manner. Small diverticula bud from hollow otic vessels that continue to grow and reshape to gradually form the series of interconnected structures that make up the inner ear.

Cardiovascular formation and development

The cardiovascular system is essential for fetal growth and development, as it supplies nutrients and facilitates gaseous exchange in all parts of the body. Like the brain, the vascular system is largely composed of membranes that use essential fatty acids for structural formation and as precursors for a variety of prostaglandins that regulate dilatation, constriction and other thrombogenic activities. Evidence indicates that the formation of a healthy vasculature is critically dependent on low circulating concentrations of cortisol. Disruption of these conditions is associated with poor fetal growth and may be secondary to long-term problems in maternal

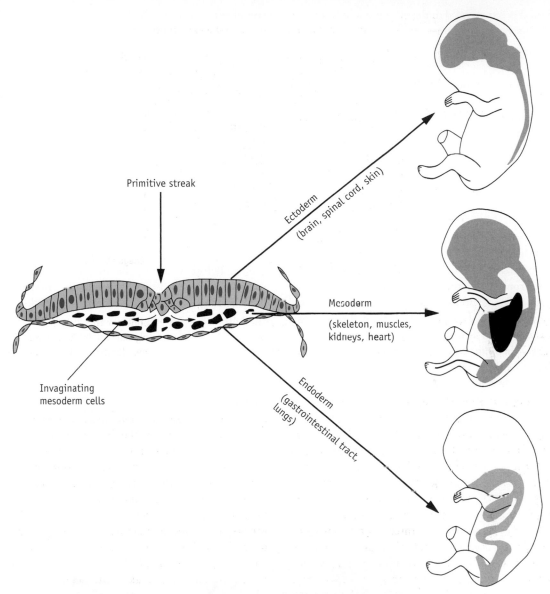

Primitive streak

Ectoderm
(brain, spinal cord, skin)

Mesoderm
(skeleton, muscles,
kidneys, heart)

Endoderm
(gastrointestinal tract,
lungs)

Invaginating
mesoderm cells

Figure 14.2 The trilaminar disk. (Reproduced with permission from Dunstan, 1990: 214.)

nutrition arising from social deprivation (Barker, 1995; Edwards *et al.*, 1993; Seckl, 1994; Wynn *et al.*, 1994).

The heart

Cells that are destined to form the primitive heart tube begin as two oval clusters of mesoderm on either side of the midline of the embryo. This precardiac mesoderm migrates towards the head and fuses in the midline, creating two parallel cords of cells. These soon enlarge and develop internal canals that become the endocardial tubes. These fold over and fuse to create the primitive cardiac tube, which is composed of one

atrium and one ventricle. Primitive blood vessels begin to form during the third week of development and pulsation of the primary cardiac tube can be detected at approximately 5 weeks' gestation. Between 5 and 8 weeks, septa are formed within the heart, which partition it into four chambers (Moore and Persaud, 2003).

Intrauterine (fetal) circulation

The fetus relies on the placenta to carry out its respiratory, nutritional and excretory functions, and fetal blood circulates throughout the placenta to meet its needs. The fetal circulation differs from the adult circulation in that blood is oxygenated in the placenta and not in the lungs. This system requires:

- larger and more numerous red cells (6–7 million/mm^3)
- higher haemoglobin content (20.7 g/dl) to pick up the maximum amount of oxygen
- a modified form of haemoglobin (HbF) which is active in the slightly more acid blood
- additional structures:
  - ductus arteriosus
  - ductus venosus
  - foramen ovale
  - two hypogastric arteries.

The basic organization of the intrauterine circulation is formed during early embryonic life: umbilical veins bring oxygenated blood to the primitive heart from the chorion frondosum; the vitelline veins return blood from the yolk sac; and the cardinal veins return blood from the rest of the body. Blood enters the heart via the sinus venous and flows through a single atrium and ventricle. When the ventricle contracts, blood is pumped through the bulbus cordis, passes into the dorsal aorta and eventually returns to deliver waste products to the chorion (Moore and Persaud, 2003) (Fig. 14.3).

During fetal life the vascular system becomes more extensive as it parallels the increasing size and complexity of individual organs and tissues. Oxygenated blood returns from a greatly enlarged placenta, via the umbilical vein. Approximately 50% of this blood enters a hepatic microcirculation and later joins the inferior vena cava via the hepatic veins. The remaining blood passes directly to the inferior vena cava, through a shunt called the ductus venosus. Blood flow through this vascular bypass is thought to be regulated by a physiological sphincter that responds to changing volume in the umbilical vein. This mechanism helps to protect the fetus from erratic fluctuations in blood pressure (Walker, 1993).

In addition to well-oxygenated blood from the placenta, the inferior vena cava also receives less-oxygenated blood from the abdomen, pelvis and lower limbs, representing more than 66% of total venous return. Before entering the heart, the inferior vena cava bifurcates into two channels: the foramen ovale links it to the left atrium and a small inlet links it to the right atrium. In the left atrium, the foramen ovale ends in a one-way valve that only permits blood flow from right to left. Flow patterns in the right atrium allow 50% of oxygenated blood returning from the placenta to be shunted to the left atrium. This right-to-left flow through the foramen ovale is maintained by the larger quantity and greater speed of blood flow from the inferior vena cava on the right, compared to that

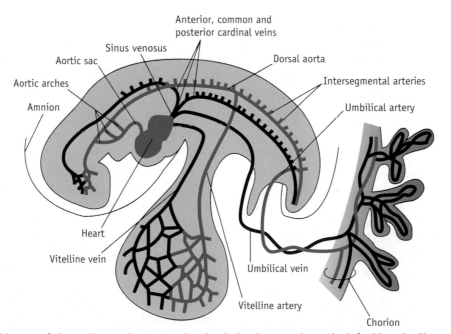

Figure 14.3   Diagram of the cardiovascular system (26 days) showing vessels on the left side only. The umbilical vein carries well-oxygenated blood and nutrients from the chorion to the embryo. The umbilical arteries carry poorly oxygenated blood and waste products to the chorion. (Reproduced with permission from Moore and Persaud, 1993: 306.)

entering the left atrium via the pulmonary veins from the lungs. During fetal life, lung tissue extracts oxygen from the low circulating blood volume that enters from the right ventricle and returns poorly oxygenated blood to the left atrium. Low venous return from the lungs is actively maintained by the exposure of pulmonary vessels to blood PO_2, which keeps them in a state of hypoxic vasoconstriction (Moore and Persaud, 1993; Walker, 1993).

A small amount of well-oxygenated blood from the inferior vena cava enters the right atrium. This is mixed with poorly oxygenated blood returning from the head via the superior vena cava, which mainly enters the right ventricle through the tricuspid valve. From the right ventricle, only 10% of blood enters the lungs via pulmonary arteries. The remaining 90% is diverted into the descending aorta via a muscular artery called the ductus arteriosus, which connects the main pulmonary artery with the aorta. Throughout fetal life, patency and therefore relaxation of this muscular artery is actively maintained by high circulating levels of PGE_2 and by the local release of PGI_2. As a result of this shunt, most blood leaving the right ventricle is responsible for perfusing the lower body and the placenta (Moore and Persaud, 1993; Walker, 1993).

In the left atrium, the pulmonary component combines with a much larger volume of more highly oxygenated blood from the inferior vena cava. From the left atrium, blood passes into the left ventricle. A small amount of this blood supplies the heart, two-thirds leaves via the ascending aorta to perfuse the upper part of the body with highly oxygenated blood, while the remaining one-third flows through the aortic isthmus to the descending aorta and then to the lower body and placenta (Walker, 1993). The two hypogastric arteries convey deoxygenated blood to the placenta.

The shunting of blood on the venous side by the foramen ovale and on the arterial side by the ductus arteriosus are structural devices designed to organize the circulation so that most blood bypasses the lungs and is directed to the placenta. This large volume of poorly oxygenated blood returning to the placenta also flows much more rapidly than the more highly oxygenated blood that supplies the upper part of the body. The rate of flow tends to be most rapid in the descending aorta. From this vessel, blood is directly pumped into the umbilical arteries and returns for gaseous exchange in the placenta (Walker, 1993) (Fig. 14.4).

During intrauterine life, the fetal–placental circulation operates as a single unit. This organization provides a low-resistance, high-capacity reservoir in the vascular bed of the placenta, which is maintained by the absence of valves in the umbilical veins. From animal experiments, total fetal–placental blood volume is estimated at 100–120 ml/kg body weight, with 80–90 ml/kg representing fetal blood volume at any given time, while the remainder is contained within the umbilical–placental circulation. This additional capacity helps to protect the fetal circulation from fluctuations in blood pressure and blood flow distribution at a time when autoregulation of regional blood flow is not fully developed. The major changes that take place in the fetal circulation at birth are described in Chapter 31.

Physiological increases in fetal cortisol during the third trimester also have a key role in stimulating a gradual increase in fetal blood pressure, in preparation for pulmonary expansion and cessation of the placental circulation. As pulmonary vascular resistance decreases to 10% of fetal values immediately after birth and pulmonary blood flow increases approximately 10-fold, cardiac output rises and myocardial contractility is stimulated by cortisol-induced maturation of the thyroid system and the labour-related surge in sympatho-adrenal activity, leading to high levels of catecholamines at birth (Nathanielsz et al., 2003; Walker, 1993).

Respiratory system

The laryngotracheal tube arises as a small protrusion from an area of the foregut, close to that which becomes the stomach. Once formed, the foregut elongates rapidly, separating the emerging stomach from the section that gives rise to the lungs. From the initial small protrusion, the lungs take shape through a series of bifurcations which begin with the emergence of right and left lobular buds that correspond in number to those in the mature organ. Between 5 and 26 weeks' gestation, these branch a further 16 times, to generate the respiratory trees. By 16 weeks, all bronchial airways have been formed and further growth proceeds by elongation and widening of existing airways. Towards the end of this phase, each terminal bronchiole divides into two or more respiratory bronchioles, while the mesodermal tissues surrounding them become highly vascularized. From 26 weeks onwards, the respiratory bronchioles continually subdivide to produce approximately 20–70 million primitive alveoli that are vascularized by a dense network of capillaries (Moore and Persaud, 2003) (Fig. 14.5).

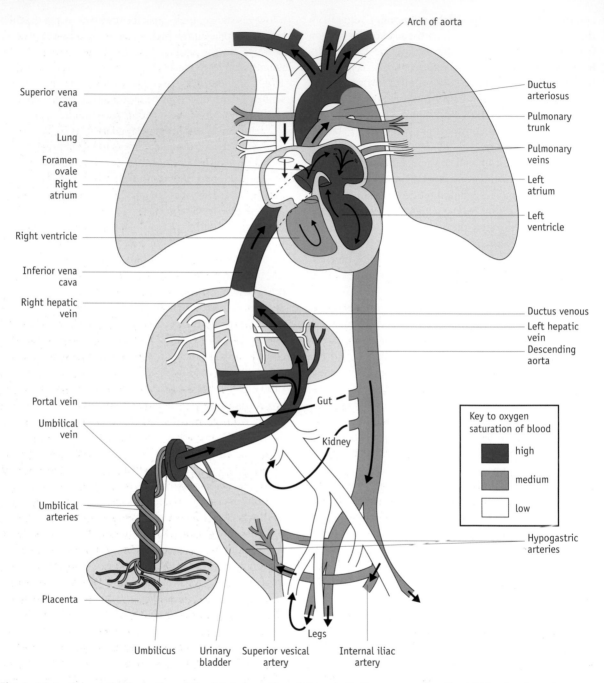

Figure 14.4 Schematic illustration of the fetal circulation. Colours indicate oxygen saturation of blood and arrows indicate the course of blood flow. Three shunts permit most blood to bypass the liver and lungs: (1) ductus venosus; (2) foramen ovale; (3) ductus arteriosus. (Reproduced with permission from Moore and Persaud, 1993: 344.)

During fetal life, these potential air spaces are filled with liquid that is actively formed by the pulmonary epithelium from the surrounding circulation. Experiments on fetal lambs have found that the volume of liquid increases from 4–6 ml/kg body weight at mid-gestation, to more than 20 ml/kg body weight near term. This liquid expansion of the potential air space maintains a small distending pressure in the lumen that approximates the functional residual capacity of the aerated lung in the newborn. In addition to this functional

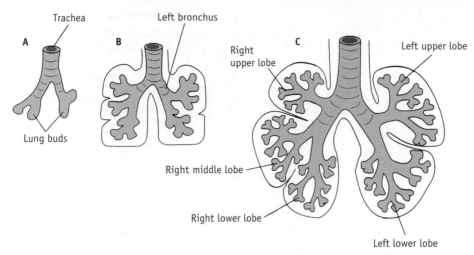

Figure 14.5   Successive stages in the development of the trachea and lungs. **A.** At 5 weeks. **B.** At 6 weeks. **C.** At 8 weeks. (Reproduced with permission from Sadler, 1990: 231.)

role in lung development, lung fluid has also been found to assist in the emergence of surfactant-producing epithelial cells that can be identified from approximately 24 weeks' gestation.

Different cellular changes occur in pulmonary tissues during successive phases of lung development. Until approximately 17 weeks, terminal and respiratory bronchioles are lined with cuboidal epithelial cells that contain abundant amounts of glycogen. These stores are thought to provide energy and precursors for the subsequent synthesis of surfactant. By 24 weeks, some cuboidal epithelial cells differentiate into thin flat cells, called type I pneumocytes, that become more closely associated with expanding networks of surrounding capillaries.

At the same time, a second type of cuboidal epithelial cell begins to differentiate within the emerging alveoli. These type II pneumocytes synthesize, store and secrete a complex substance called surfactant that is composed of a number of distinct glycerophospholipid and specialized protein molecules. As the secretion of surfactant increases, cells lining the terminal sacs also become thinner, particularly during the last 8 weeks of pregnancy. This allows the capillaries to intimately surround the alveoli, increasing the surface area potentially available for gas exchange, in preparation for the onset of respiration (Jobe, 1984; Pepe and Albrecht, 1995; Snyder *et al.*, 1985) (Figs 14.5 and 14.6).

When type II pneumocytes first appear, they contain numerous glycogen granules. From approximately 18 weeks onwards, these stores begin to decrease through a process of glycogenolysis that seems to be stimulated by increasing concentrations of a lipid molecule called platelet-activating factor (PAF). PAF is thought to trigger the enzymatic reactions involved in the synthesis of surfactant-associated phospholipids within the endoplasmic reticulum. From approximately 24 weeks onwards, increasing quantities of PAF are stored in lamellar bodies in the cytoplasm. Secretion is evident from approximately 32 weeks, and levels progressively increase with advancing gestation. Relative concentrations of the principal phospholipids also change with advancing gestation. For example, surfactant that is initially secreted contains high levels of phosphatidylinositol (PI) and very low levels of phosphatidylglycerol (PG). This ratio is gradually reversed until term when very little PI is present. As secretion rates and maturation increase, surfactant forms a lipid monolayer lining around the lumen of the alveoli. This reduces surface tension of the terminal sacs and stabilizes the membrane, which prevents them from collapsing following the onset of respiration (Jobe, 1984; Hoffman *et al.*, 1986; Pepe and Albrecht, 1995; Snyder *et al.*, 1985).

Intermittent breathing movements occur in utero from approximately 11 weeks' gestation. Results of longitudinal studies from 24 weeks suggest that the pattern of this activity is integrated with sleep cycles, fetal movements and circadian rhythms. In general, breathing movements only occur during periods of rapid eye movement sleep. Episodes of fetal movements are associated with a reduction or absence of breathing. This is particularly evident during nightly periods of gross body movements, which coincide with lowest levels of breathing. From 22 weeks onwards

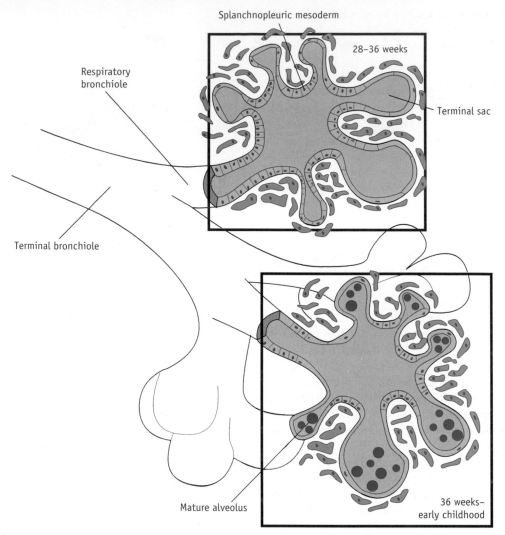

Splanchnopleuric mesoderm

28–36 weeks

Respiratory
bronchiole

Terminal sac

Terminal bronchiole

Mature alveolus

36 weeks–
early childhood

Figure 14.6 Maturation of the lung tissue. Terminal sacs (primitive alveoli) begin to form between weeks 28–36, and begin to mature between 36 weeks and birth. Only 5–20% of all terminal sacs produced by the age of 8, however, are formed prior to birth. (Reproduced with permission from Larsen, 1993: 123.)

breathing activity has been found to reach minimum levels between 1900 and 2400 hours. Episodic breathing in utero is thought to stimulate the development of lung tissue and respiratory muscles and some experimental evidence suggests that it may increase cardiac output and blood flow to vital organs including the heart, brain and placenta. The presence of breathing movements is generally taken as an indicator of fetal well-being, since periods of hypoxia have been shown to depress these movements.

Hormonal regulation

The differentiation of type II pneumocytes and the production of surfactant is closely associated with increasing levels of a number of different hormones within the fetal circulation, particularly cortisol, oestrogen, adrenaline, human placental lactogen (hPL), prolactin and thyroid hormone. In experimental studies, cortisol regulates several aspects of lung maturation. These include growth of the alveolar diameter, regulation of glycogen metabolism, enhanced synthesis and activity of enzymes involved in lipid production and stimulation of beta-adrenergic receptors. At present, prolactin and thyroid hormone are thought to act mainly by enhancing the stimulatory influences of cortisol. In recent experiments, the combined infusion of these three hormones has been found to have a greater effect on structural and secretory aspects of lung maturation compared to the effects of each hormone alone (Pepe and Albrecht, 1995; Rooney, 1992; Smith and Post, 1994; Snyder and Dekowski, 1992).

Urogenital system

Variations of mesodermal tissue give rise to the urinary and genital organs and to the outer cortex of the adrenal gland. The urinary and genital systems are very closely interwoven. They arise largely from the same type of tissue, and the excretory ducts of both systems initially enter a common cavity, the cloaca. With further development, the interconnections between the two systems remain more evident in males. During fetal life, primitive urinary ducts are transformed into the main genital duct, while in the adult, urine and semen are discharged through a common duct, the penile urethra.

In humans, formation of the definitive kidneys is preceded by a rudimentary development of a pair of nephritic vesicles and mesonephric ducts. The vesicles remain non-functional and disappear by the end of the fourth week, while the ducts produce small amounts of urine between 6 and 10 weeks' gestation. These subsequently regress in females, while in males they persist to form elements of the genital system.

Early in the fifth week a pair of ureteric buds sprout from the distal portion of the mesonephric ducts. These grow into a pouch of mesodermal tissue on either side of the sacral region – the metanephric blastema – which forms the definitive kidneys. The ureters and collecting ducts differentiate from the ureteric bud, while the nephrons or definitive urine-forming units differentiate from the metanephric blastema. Between 6 and 9 weeks' gestation, the kidneys ascend from the sacral region, to a lumbar site just below the adrenal glands (Moore and Persaud, 1993) (Figure 14.7).

From 5 to 14 weeks' gestation, the two distinct structures forming the kidneys undergo successive phases of bifurcations and extensions, as the system develops its elaborate network of calyces and tubules. When the ureteric bud first contacts the metanephric blastema, its tips extend to form an ampulla that subsequently gives rise to the renal pelvis. From 6–32 weeks' gestation, the ureteric bud undergoes numerous bifurcations that subsequently coalesce to form both major and minor calyces and collecting ducts. Meanwhile the nephrons emerge from metanephric tissue surrounding the ampulla, which differentiates to form a Bowman's capsule, the distal convoluted tubule

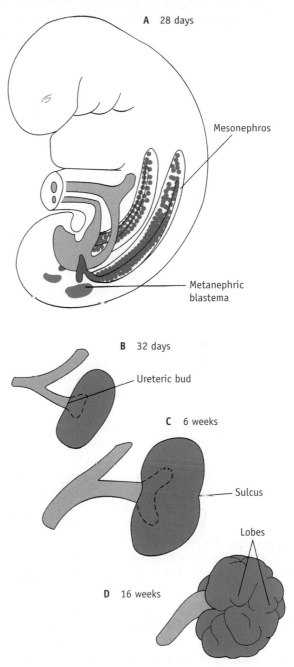

Figure 14.7 Origin of the metanephric kidneys.
A. A metanephric blastema develops from intermediate mesoderm on each side of the body's axis early in the fifth week. **B.** Simultaneously the metanephric ducts sprout ureteric buds that grow into each metanephric blastema. **C.** By the sixth week, the ureteric bud bifurcates and the two growing tips (ampullae) induce superior and inferior lobes in the metanephros. **D.** Additional lobules form during the next 10 weeks in response to further bifurcation of the ureteric buds. (Reproduced with permission from Larsen, 1993: 241.)

and the loop of Henle. At the same time a dense capillary network forms within the capsule and extends in a parallel fashion alongside the remaining sections of the tubules. During the tenth week, the distal convoluted tubules join on to the collecting ducts and the system starts to produce urine (Moore and Persaud, 1993).

Urine is formed as plasma from the glomerular capillaries and is filtered to produce a dilute filtrate which is then concentrated by the convoluted tubules and the loop of Henle. From there it passes into the bladder and out into the surrounding amniotic fluid. During fetal life the formation of urine is not used to clear waste products from the blood, as this activity is carried out by the placenta. Instead urine serves to supplement the production of amniotic fluid. During the second half of pregnancy, urine is formed at the rate of 800–1200 ml per day, making it the largest single contributor to the volume of amniotic fluid (Gilbert, 1991).

Adrenal cortex

During intrauterine life, the adrenal cortex works in conjunction with the placenta to establish interdependent hormonal interactions that cross fetal, placental and maternal compartments to provide a variety of conditions needed for fetal and neonatal development. Specific activities of this fetoplacental unit include:

- regulating placental synthesis of oestrogen, stimulating the synthesis and release of placental progesterone and maternal prolactin
- initiating a cascade of events that increases maternal plasma and red cell volume
- regulating placental metabolism of cortisol
- promoting growth of the mammary gland and stimulating its uptake of lipids during the third trimester, in preparation for lactation (Pepe and Albrecht, 1990, 1995; Winter, 1992).

Development of the adrenal glands

The central regulatory role of the adrenals is indicated by their spectacular growth and secretory capacity during intrauterine life. Cells forming the adrenal cortex appear at 3–4 weeks' gestation and enlarge rapidly to equal the size of the kidneys by the end of the first trimester. By 6–8 weeks' gestation, the cortex forms a distinct fetal zone, beneath an outer subcapsular rim of immature cells that resemble those in the outer zone of the adult gland. During the second trimester, the adrenals enlarge in direct proportion to the increase in

total body weight. At this time their relative weight is 35 times the adult value. In the third trimester, gland weights continue to increase but at a slower rate than the rest of the body. At term, the fetal adrenals are similar in size to those in the adult (Pearson Murphy and Branchaud, 1994; Seron-Ferre and Jaffe, 1981).

Most of the increased weight of the adrenals is associated with growth of an inner fetal zone that comprises approximately 80–90% of its overall volume at term. Until late in gestation, cells of the outer adult zones remain small and are less well vascularized than the larger cells of the fetal zone. The overall steroid-producing capacity of the adrenal glands also exceeds that in the adult. It is estimated that near term, the glands produce a minimum of 100–200 mg of steroids per day, compared to 20–30 mg in resting adults (Pearson Murphy and Branchaud, 1994; Seron-Ferre and Jaffe, 1981; Winter, 1992).

In the first half of pregnancy, adrenal growth seems to be largely regulated by growth factors derived from within the glands, along with those from other fetal organs, including the placenta, liver and kidneys. Until the latter part of pregnancy, the active steroid-producing fetal zone is predominantly involved in the synthesis of an androgen called dehydroepiandrosterone sulphate (DHEAS). This hormone provides placental tissue with an essential substrate for the synthesis of oestrogens (Pepe and Albrecht, 1990, 1995).

Placental hypothalamic–pituitary regulation

During the first half of pregnancy, the synthesis of DHEAS is largely stimulated by placental human chorionic gonadotrophin (hCG) and by adrenocorticotrophic hormone (ACTH)-related peptides and prolactin from the fetal pituitary gland. Since hCG first appears in the maternal circulation at the beginning of implantation and reaches highest concentrations during the first trimester, placental tissue must provide the initial stimulatory influence on the fetal adrenals. Within the fetal pituitary, cells containing ACTH-related peptides and prolactin appear between 5 and 10 weeks' gestation and are followed by the emergence of neurovascular links between the hypothalamus and the pituitary gland. By 12 weeks' gestation, corticotrophin-releasing hormone (CRH) and arginine vasopressin (AVP) are present within the hypothalamus. Together, these hormones provide essential stimulation for the development and secretory activity of ACTH-releasing cells in the pituitary (Pepe and Albrecht, 1990).

ACTH is first detectable in fetal plasma at approximately 12 weeks and shows a slight increase along with gestational age. But unlike the situation in adults, ACTH does not form the principal corticotroph during most of fetal life. Instead two other related peptides, melanocyte-stimulating hormone (MSH) and corticotrophin-like intermediate lobe peptide (CLIP), have been found in higher concentrations within the pituitary. This pattern continues until late in gestation when the proportion of ACTH increases, until it becomes the dominant hormone at term. Since ACTH has been found to stimulate growth of the adult but not the fetal zone of the adrenal gland, its low concentration throughout gestation is thought to facilitate the continued dominance of the fetal zone. At the low concentrations that characterize most of pregnancy, ACTH is centrally involved in regulating fetal zone utilization of low-density lipoprotein (LDL)-cholesterol, for the production of DHEAS. Near term, its increased concentration stimulates proliferation of the adult cortisol-producing zone of the gland (Pepe and Albrecht, 1990).

In contrast to ACTH, prolactin seems to be released in the absence of hypothalamic regulation. From approximately 14 weeks onwards, fetal serum concentrations of prolactin show a linear increase with advancing gestation. In addition to its stimulatory influence on steroid hormone production in the fetal zone of the adrenal gland, prolactin enhances the process of lung maturation during the last trimester (Thorpe-Beeston *et al.*, 1992).

Adrenal medulla

In contrast to the cortex, the chromaffin cells are formed from adjacent sympathetic ganglia that are derived from the neural crest. Unlike the cortex, this part of the gland does not become a discrete structure during fetal life. During this period, small islands of chromaffin cells are scattered throughout the cortex and larger and much more active islets form independently of the medulla, along the outside of the aorta (Mesiano and Jaffe, 1997). Immature chromaffin cells have been observed from approximately 8 weeks and significant concentrations of noradrenaline have been found from 15 weeks' gestation. No degeneration has been found to occur in these cells until the postnatal period (Phillippe, 1983).

Within the adrenal gland, small groups of cells containing measurable amounts of noradrenaline have been observed at 9 weeks but their content remains low until the third trimester. While noradrenaline remains predominant in the fetal response to stress, the rising capacity for cortisol production near term produces a sharp increase in the capacity of chromaffin

cells to produce adrenaline. The proportion of adrenaline increases progressively from approximately 28 weeks to term, when it constitutes around 50% of total catecholamine content of the gland. As measured in amniotic fluid, catecholamine metabolites increase between the second and third trimester and plasma catecholamine concentrations rise progressively during the course of labour. These changes mediate a range of cardiovascular, metabolic and respiratory responses to labour and birth (Lagercrantz and Slotkin, 1986; Lagercrantz and Marcus, 1992; Phillippe, 1983).

Following birth, involution of the fetal zone occurs rapidly during the first postnatal week, while the entire HPA axis undergoes a critical developmental period of stress hyporesponsiveness facilitated by homeostatic regulation provided by close maternal contact (Bystrova *et al.*, 2003; Hofer, 1994; Pryce *et al.*, 2002). Meanwhile the fetal zone declines more slowly over the next 2 weeks and chromaffin cells within the adrenal gland coalesce around the central vein and become innervated by autonomic fibres by 4 weeks of postnatal development (Mesiano and Jaffe, 1997).

Gastrointestinal system

Through a process of midline folding during week 4, the endodermal layer gives rise to the gastrointestinal and respiratory systems. By the fifth week of gestation, the primitive gastrointestinal tube differentiates into a foregut, midgut and hindgut. Meanwhile, hepatic, cystic and pancreatic diverticula bud from the foregut, giving rise to the liver, gall bladder and pancreas. During the sixth week, the endodermal epithelium proliferates until it fills the gut lumen. Over the next 3 weeks, the tube is recanalized and lined with definitive mucosal epithelium that differentiates from the endoderm. Soon afterwards, the gastrointestinal tract becomes involved in regulating the circulation of amniotic fluid. At 16 weeks' gestation, the fetus has been estimated to swallow 7 ml of amniotic fluid per hour, approximately 120 ml per hour by 28 weeks. This fluid has been found to accumulate in the stomach where it is absorbed into the underlying tissues (Gilbert 1991; Moore and Persaud, 1993) (Fig. 14.8).

In contrast to respiratory and cardiovascular systems, growth and maturation of the gastrointestinal and pancreatic organs extends over the period of perinatal development. The intestinal villi are well developed by 19 weeks' gestation and all cell types found in the adult intestinal lining have differentiated by the end of

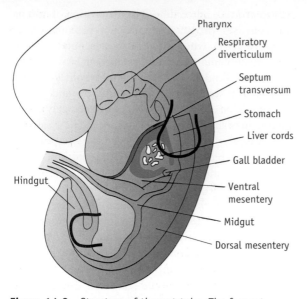

Pharynx
Respiratory diverticulum
Septum transversum
Stomach
Liver cords
Gall bladder
Ventral mesentery
Midgut
Dorsal mesentery
Hindgut

Figure 14.8 Structure of the gut tube. The foregut consists of the pharynx, located superior to the respiratory diverticulum, the thoracic oesophagus, and the abdominal foregut inferior to the diaphragm. The abdominal foregut forms the abdominal oesophagus, stomach and about half of the duodenum, and gives rise to the liver, the gall bladder, the pancreas and their associated ducts. The midgut forms half the duodenum, the jejunum and ileum, the ascending colon and about two-thirds of the transverse colon. The hindgut forms one-third of the transverse colon, the descending and sigmoid colons, and the upper two-thirds of the anorectal canal. The abdominal oesophagus, stomach and superior part of the duodenum are suspended by dorsal and ventral mesenteries; the abdominal gut tube excluding the rectum is suspended in the abdominal cavity by a dorsal mesentery only. (Reproduced with permission from Larsen, 1993: 209.)

the second trimester, but many of these cells do not acquire adult functional patterns until the onset of weaning (Carlson, 1994: 317). Intestinal motility and peristalsis begin to develop during the third trimester and intestinal growth accelerates during the final weeks of pregnancy, in preparation for the onset of enteral feeding (Menard *et al.*, 1999). At the same time, many aspects of oesophageal and gastrointestinal motility only mature during neonatal development.

At birth oesophageal motility is decreased, particularly during the first 12 hours after birth, and peristalsis is disordered, resulting in an intestinal transit time that may vary from 10–18 hours. Oesophageal reflux is common during the suckling period and true rhythmic peristalsis is not established until 3 months of age

(Blackburn, 2003; Zangen *et al.*, 2001). The enzymatic and hormonal capacities of the gut and pancreas also remain relatively underdeveloped until late pregnancy and labour when rising levels of cortisol increase hormonal and enzymatic secretions. Following birth significant maturational changes continue to occur in the functional capacity of gastrointestinal and pancreatic systems throughout the period of suckling. Maturational changes in the gut are stimulated by rising levels of neonatal cortisol and leptin, and by a wide variety of hormones and growth factors in milk, including high concentrations of insulin and leptin (Lyle *et al.*, 2001; Sangild, 1999; Shehadeh *et al.*, 2002; Wolinski *et al.*, 2003; Zangen *et al.*, 2001).

The liver

The liver is a major haematopoietic organ during embryonic and fetal life. When it initially appears, blood-forming cells have already begun to collect between hepatic cells and vessel walls. This growing activity contributes to the rapid increase in the weight of the liver, which reaches approximately 10% of body weight by 10 weeks' gestation. During the last 8 weeks of gestation, this activity declines and at birth the liver is approximately 5% of total body weight.

In contrast to the early capacity for red cell production, hepatic regulation of carbohydrate metabolism does not emerge until the latter part of gestation and shows considerably different regulatory features from those in the adult. Under basal non-stressed conditions, fetal glucose is largely supplied from the maternal circulation via the placenta. The fetal liver displays a high glucose uptake and a large capacity for glycolysis but gluconeogenic enzyme activity remains low until after birth. Glucose uptake is stimulated by raised maternal glucose concentrations and is inhibited by physiological concentrations of fatty acids, amino acids and lactate. Hepatic receptors for insulin can be demonstrated by 12–15 weeks' gestation. Although no clear association has been found between insulin receptor activity and its capacity to stimulate glucose uptake or the accumulation of glycogen, in vitro studies have shown that insulin stimulates glycogenesis in hepatocytes. Insulin has also been shown to inhibit the synthesis of gluconeogenic enzymes, thereby promoting anabolic metabolism. In keeping with this tendency, the fetal liver shows a considerably reduced sensitivity to the glucose-releasing actions of glucagon.

Substantial quantities of glycogen are deposited in the liver during the latter part of pregnancy. The onset and maintenance of this activity is largely dependent on the enhanced release of cortisol from the adult zone of the adrenal gland. When the transfer of maternal fuel is acutely interrupted at birth, these deposits are utilized, during the first 24 hours after birth, to maintain blood glucose (Jones, 1989).

Hepatic glycogen increases rapidly from approximately 36 weeks' gestation to reach 50 mg/g at 40 weeks' gestation. During late pregnancy, cortisol increases hepatic glycogen synthesis. Immediately after birth, the concomitant rise in plasma cortisol, glucagon and catecholamines and the decline in plasma insulin seem to regulate the fall in lipogenesis and stimulate the expression of enzymes required for glycogenolysis, gluconeogenesis and fatty acid oxidation that increase soon after birth (Benito *et al.*, 1982; Jones, 1989; Kalhan, 1992; Pegorier and Girard, 1998; Sadava *et al.*, 1992; Shelley *et al.*, 1975). Immediately after birth, highly oxygenated blood from the placenta is replaced by a mix of well-oxygenated blood from the hepatic artery and a larger supply of less well-oxygenated blood from the intestinal capillary bed, which enters the liver in the portal vein. During the first couple of weeks following birth, this decline in the oxygenation of hepatic blood flow plus the simultaneous decline in haematopoiesis produces a physiological enlargement of the liver which is taken up by the simultaneous increase in metabolic functions. These include the increased ability to synthesize glucose from lactate, pyruvate and amino acids and increased capacity for fatty acid oxidation from dietary lipids (Kliegman and Sparks, 1985; Pegorier and Girard, 1998).

CONCLUSION

This chapter has provided a brief overview of the formation and development of key organ systems. While increasing knowledge has been gained about the sequence of events that unfold within different layers of the inner cell mass, current understanding of human embryology remains largely descriptive in character. An understanding of the processes at play enables the midwife to give a deeper understanding to the woman regarding the changes taking place in her body, and advice around nutrition.

KEY POINTS

- The first weeks following fertilization are a time of intense activity as organogenesis takes place, and the major systems and structures of the fetus are formed.
- At the end of the fetal period of development, maturational changes have taken place in certain organs like the lungs and liver, while the HPA axis is briefly activated to regulate the onset of labour.
- Following birth the HPA axis undergoes a critical period of stress hyporesponsiveness, while the gastrointestinal and pancreatic systems mature during the oral phase of development that ends at spontaneous weaning.

REFERENCES

Barker, D.J.P. (1995) Fetal origins of coronary heart disease. *British Medical Journal* 311: 171–174.

Benito, M., Lorenzo, M. & Medina, J.M. (1982) Relationship between lipogenesis and glycogen synthesis in maternal and fetal tissues during late gestation in the rat. *Biochemical Journal* 204: 865–868.

Blackburn, S.T. (2003) *Maternal, Fetal and Neonatal Physiology*. Philadelphia: W.B. Saunders.

Braude, P.R. & Johnson, M.H. (1990) The embryo in contemporary medical science. In: Dunstan, G.R. (ed) *The Human Embryo*, pp. 208–221. Exeter: University of Exeter Press.

Bystrova, K., Widstrom, A-M., Mattheisen, A-S. *et al.* (2003) Skin-to-skin contact may reduce negative consequences of 'the stress of being born': a study on temperature in newborn infants, subjected to different ward routines in St Petersburg. *Acta Paediatrica* 92: 320–326.

Carlson, B.M. (1994) *Human Embryology and Developmental Biology*. St Louis: Mosby.

Dunstan, G.R. (ed) (1990) *The Human Embryo*. Exeter: University of Exeter Press.

Edwards, C.R., Benediktsson, R., Lindsay, R.S. *et al.* (1993) Dysfunction of placental glucocorticoid barrier: link between fetal environment and adult hypertension. *Lancet* 341: 355–357.

Gilbert, S.F. (1991) *Developmental Biology*. Massachusetts: Sinauer.

Hofer, M.A. (1994) Early relationships as regulators of infant physiology and behaviour. *Acta Paediatrica* 397: 9–18.

Hoffman, D.R., Troung, C.T. & Johnsin, J.M. (1986) The role of platelet-activating factor in human fetal lung maturation. *American Journal of Obstetrics and Gynecology* 155(1): 70–75.

Jobe, A. (1984) Fetal lung maturation and respiratory distress syndrome. In: Beard, R.W. & Nathaniel, S.Z. (eds) *Fetal Physiology and Medicine*, pp. 317–351. New York: Marcel Dekker.

Jones, C.T. (1989) Fetal maturation in late pregnancy. In: Turnbull, A. & Chamberlain, G. (eds) *Obstetrics*, pp. 119–127. Edinburgh: Churchill Livingstone.

Kalhan, S.C. (1992) Metabolism of glucose and methods of investigation in the fetus and newborn. In: Polin, R.A. & Fox, W.W. (eds) *Fetal and Neonatal Physiology*, pp. 357–372. Philadelphia: W.B. Saunders.

Kliegman, R.M. & Sparks, J.W. (1985) Perinatal galactose metabolism. *Journal of Pediatrics* 107(6): 831–841.

Lagercrantz, H. & Slotkin, T.A. (1986) The 'stress' of being born. *Scientific American* 254: 92–102.

Lagercrantz, H. & Marcus, C. (1992) Sympathoadrenal mechanisms during development. In: Polin, R.A. & Fox, W.W. (eds) *Fetal and Neonatal Physiology*, pp. 160–169. Philadelphia: W.B. Saunders.

Larsen, W.J. (1993) *Human Embryology*. New York: Churchill Livingstone.

Lyle, R.E., Kincaid, S.C., Bryant, J.C. *et al.* (2001) Human milk contains detectable levels of immunoreactive leptin. In: Newburg, D.S. (ed) *Bioactive Components of Human Milk*, pp. 87–92. New York: Plenum Publishers.

Menard, D., Corriveau, L. & Beaulieu, J-F. (1999) Insulin modulates cellular proliferation in developing human jejunum and colon. *Biology of the Neonate* 75: 143–151.

Mesiano, S. & Jaffe, R.B. (1997) Development and functional biology of the primate fetal adrenal cortex. *Endocrine Reviews* 18(3): 378–403.

Moore, K.L. & Persaud, T.V.N. (1993) *The Developing Human*, 5th edn. Philadelphia: W.B. Saunders.

Moore, K.L. & Persaud, T.V.N. (2003) *The Developing Human*, 7th edn. Philadelphia: W.B. Saunders.

Nathanielsz, P.W., Berghorn, K.A., Derks, J.B. *et al.* (2003) Life before birth: effects of cortisol on future cardiovascular and metabolic function. *Acta Paediatrica* 92: 766–772.

Pearson Murphy, B.E. & Branchaud, C.L. (1994) The fetal adrenal. In: Tulchinsky, D. & Little, B.A. (eds) *Maternal–Fetal Endocrinology*, pp. 276–286. Philadelphia: W.B. Saunders.

Pegorier, J-P. & Girard, J. (1998) Liver metabolism in fetus and neonate. In: Cowett, M. (ed) *Principles of Perinatal/Neonatal Metabolism*, pp. 610–626. New York: Springer-Verlag.

Pepe, G.J. & Albrecht, E.D. (1990) Regulation of the primate fetal adrenal cortex. *Endocrine Reviews* 11(1): 151–176.

Pepe, G.J. & Albrecht, E.D. (1995) Actions of placental and fetal adrenal steroid-hormones in primate pregnancy. *Endocrine Reviews* 16(5): 608–648.

Phillippe, M. (1983) Fetal catecholamines. *American Journal of Obstetrics and Gynecology* 146(7): 840–855.

Pryce, C.E., Palme, R. & Feldon, J. (2002) Development of pituitary–adrenal endocrine function in the marmoset monkey: infant hypercortisolism is the norm. *Journal of Clinical Endocrinology and Metabolism* 87(2): 691–699.

Rooney, S.A. (1992) Regulation of surfactant-associated phospholipid synthesis and secretion. In: Polin, R.A. *et al.* (eds) *Neonatal and Fetal Medicine*, pp. 971–985. Philadelphia: W.B. Saunders.

Sadava, D., Frykman, P., Harris, E. *et al.* (1992) Development of enzymes of glycolysis and gluconeogenesis in human fetal liver. *Biology of the Neonate* 62: 89–95.

Sadler, T.W. (1990) *Langman's Medical Embryology*. Baltimore: Williams & Wilkins.

Sangild, P.T. (1999) Biology of the pancreas before birth. In: Pierzynowski, S.G. & Zabielski, R. (eds) *Biology of the Pancreas in Growing Animals*, pp. 1–13. Amsterdam: Elsevier Science.

Seckl, J.R. (1994) Glucocorticoids and small babies. *Quarterly Journal of Medicine* 87: 259–262.

Seron-Ferre, M. & Jaffe, R.B. (1981) The fetal adrenal gland. *Annual Review of Physiology* 43: 141–162.

Shehadeh, N., Khaesh-Goldberg, E., Shamir, R. *et al.* (2002) Insulin in human milk: postpartum changes and effects of gestational age. *Archives of Disease in Childhood* 88: F214–216.

Shelley, H.J., Basset, J.M. & Milner, R.D.G. (1975) Control of carbohydrate metabolism in the fetus and newborn. *British Medical Bulletin* 31(1): 37–43.

Smith, B.T. & Post, M. (1994) The influence of hormones on fetal lung development. In: Tulchinsky, D. & Little, A.B. (eds) *Maternal–Fetal Endocrinology*, pp. 366–377. Philadelphia: W.B. Saunders.

Snyder, J.M. & Dekowski, S.A. (1992) The role of prolactin in fetal lung maturation. *Seminars in Reproductive Endocrinology* 10(3): 287–293.

Snyder, J.M., Mendelson, C.R. & Johnston, J.M. (1985) The morphology of lung development in the human fetus. In: Nelson, G.H. (ed) *Pulmonary Development Transition from Intrauterine to Extrauterine Life*, pp. 19–46. New York: Marcel Dekker.

Thorpe-Beeston, J.G., Snijders, R.J.M., Felton, C.V. *et al.* (1992) Serum prolactin concentration in normal and small for gestational age fetuses. *British Journal of Obstetrics and Gynaecology* 99: 981–984.

Walker, A.M. (1993) Circulatory transitions at birth and the control of neonatal circulation. In: Hanson, M.A., Spencer, J.A.D. & Rodeck, C.H. (eds) *Fetus and Neonate: Physiology and Clinical Applications*, Vol. 1, *The Circulation*, pp. 160–196. Cambridge: Cambridge University Press.

Winter, J.S.D. (1992) Fetal and neonatal adrenocortical physiology. In: Polin, R.A. & Fox, W.W. (eds) *Fetal and Neonatal Physiology,* pp. 1829–1841. Philadelphia: W.B. Saunders.

Wolinski, J., Biernat, M., Guilloteau, P. *et al.* (2003) Exogenous leptin controls the development of the small intestine in neonatal piglets. *Journal of Endocrinology* **177**: 215–222.

Wynn, S.W., Wyn, A.H., Doyle, W. *et al.* (1994) The association of maternal diet and the dimensions of babies in a population of London women. *Nutrition and Health* 9(4): 303–315.

Zangen, S., Lorenzo, C.D., Zangen, T. *et al.* (2001) Rapid maturation of gastric relaxation in newborn infants. *Pediatric Research* 50(5): 629–632.

FURTHER READING

Matsumara, G. & England, M. (1992) *Colouring Book of Embryology.* Edinburgh and London: Elsevier.
An interesting and creative way of increasing knowledge and understanding of embryology.

15

The Fetal Skull

Barbara Burden and M Susan Sapsed

LEARNING OUTCOMES

After reading this chapter you will be able to:

- review the process of fetal development of the structures of the skull
- assess the circumference and diameters of the fetal skull and their importance in practice
- identify the internal structures within the fetal skull and the possible complications that can occur during the birthing process

- explore the structures of the skull of the newborn baby to identify and understand the relevance of these components to midwifery practice
- describe the structures of the fetal skull and evaluate how this knowledge enables midwives to assess progress during labour, and care through the neonatal period.

INTRODUCTION

It is essential for a midwife to understand the parameters and characteristics of the fetal skull because of the role it plays during the mechanism of labour. The two key functions of the fetal skull are the protection of the brain, which is subjected to pressure as it descends through the birth canal during labour, and an ability to change shape, adapting to the process of labour in response to uterine contractions and the size and shape of the pelvis. These changes have to be achieved during labour, as the surface size of the fetal skull is large in comparison to the true pelvis; therefore some adaptation of the skull is necessary for a successful mechanism and outcome of labour. By assessing the landmarks of the fetal skull, such as sutures and fontanelles, a midwife is able to diagnose the position and attitude of the fetal head in the pelvis and determine the most likely mechanism of labour and mode of delivery.

DEVELOPMENT OF THE FETAL SKULL

As the fetus develops in utero, the mesenchyme layer surrounding the brain starts to ossify at central points, forming the various bones of the fetal skull. This process

is called intramembranous ossification and begins between 4–8 weeks of gestation. The initial development of the skull occurs from this intramembranous structure, derived from neural crest cells and mesoderm. The intramembranous structure is divided into two major components, the neurocranium, which forms the protective case of the skull and the viscerocranium, forming the bones of the face.

The neurocranium can be subdivided into the chondrocranium and the dermatocranium. The chondrocranium (cartilaginous part) is formed by the fusion of cartilages, and following ossification becomes the occipital, temporal, sphenoid and ethmoid bones. The dermatocranium (membranous part) is thought to arise from the external dermal scales developed to protect the brain. This lies under the superficial layers of the skin, covering and protecting the dorsal section of the brain, giving rise to the parietal and frontal bones.

The earliest visible signs of development can be seen on ultrasonography at about 4 weeks' gestation with calcification of the membranes and the development of the occiput. This becomes easier to determine from approximately 8 weeks when intramembranous ossification is more prominent. At 12 weeks the outlines of the individual bones become evident (Moore, 1998; Sadler, 2000) (see Fig. 15.1). Ossification of the bones

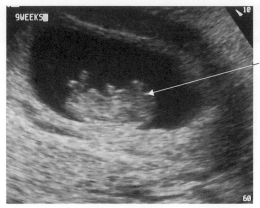

A   9 weeks side view

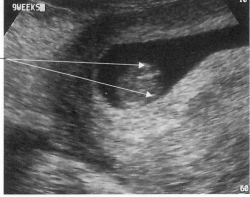

B   9 weeks top view

Initial areas of ossification – identified by white patches

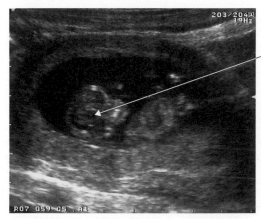

C   11 weeks side view

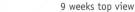

D   11 weeks top view

Developing areas of ossification of the parietal eminences and occipital protuberance – identified by the white patches

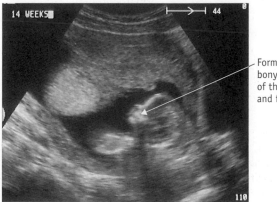

E   14 weeks side view

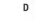

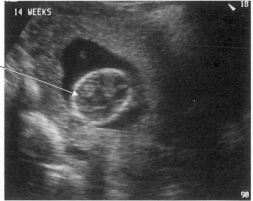

F   14 weeks top view

Formation of bony structures of the skull and face

Figure 15.1 Ultrasound images illustrating the development and ossification of the fetal skull at 9, 11 and 14 weeks' gestation. (Reproduced by kind permission of the Ultrasound Department at the Luton and Dunstable Hospital NHS Trust.)

continues throughout pregnancy with individual bones ossifying from their centre. At term the bones of the skull are thin and pliable, enabling some movement of bones to take place during labour. The two frontal bones have usually united by term.

THE EXTERNAL STRUCTURES OF THE NEWBORN SKULL (FIG. 15.2)

Following birth of the baby, the midwife examines the external structures of the newborn head, in order to

Scalp
This is the thick, soft tissue covering the pericranium. It comprises skin, hair follicles, blood vessels, connective tissue and muscle fibres.

The scalp may have puncture marks or lacerations from fetal scalp electrodes if these are used intrapartum.

The tissues of the scalp may swell during labour owing to pressure of the maternal cervix on the presenting part of the head.

Circumference – suboccipitobregmatic
Measured from the base of the head where it joins the neck, around to the centre of the anterior fontanelle and back to the neck (33 cm).

This circumference is the measurement when the fetal head is well flexed in the lower uterine segment, aiding easy entrance to the pelvic brim.

Position of anterior fontanelle under the scalp
Felt as a diamond-shaped 'cavity' under the scalp.

The fontanelle in the healthy infant is soft and spongy to touch.

A sunken fontanelle is indicative of dehydration in the newborn.

A swollen fontanelle may be indicative of raised intracranial pressure in the newborn.

Brow
Also called the sinciput, it is the area covering the frontal bone.

Vertex
This area is bordered by the anterior fontanelle, the posterior fontanelle and laterally by the parietal eminences.

This is the most common presenting part of the fetus during labour and shows that the head is well flexed.

Face
The face of the newborn baby is smaller in relation to the head than that of an adult.

It extends from the supraorbital ridges to the chin.

It cannot mould during labour.

It may sustain severe swelling or bruising in labour when the face is the presenting part.

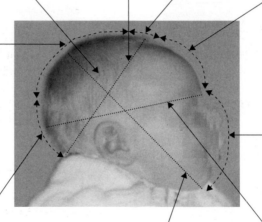

Occiput
This is the area over the occipital bone. The occiput is the denominator of the vertex used to assess and record the fetal presentation and position during the antenatal period and in labour. In a well-flexed cephalic presentation the occiput will meet the pelvic floor and produce the internal rotation of the head necessary for extension of the head under the subpubic arch of the pelvis.

Circumference – mentovertical
Measured from the point of the chin to the highest point of the vertex and back to the chin (39 cm).

This circumference presents in a brow presentation.

Circumference – occipitofrontal
Measured from the glabella (bridge of the nose) to the occipital protuberance and back to the bridge of the nose (35 cm).

This is the measurement of the skull of the newborn baby recorded at birth.

This measurement is also the presenting circumference of a deflexed head during prolonged labour associated with premature rupture of membranes.

Figure 15.2 External structures and circumferences of the newborn skull.

identify any unusual characteristics or abnormalities in the structure of the skull. Measurement of the newborn skull may also be undertaken during this procedure and documented within the child's neonatal records, although the accuracy, and therefore the relevance, of measurements at birth have been questioned (Wilshin *et al.*, 1999).

Layers of the external structures of the skull

- Skin.
- Connective tissue – containing blood vessels and hair follicles. It may become oedematous during labour resulting in a caput succedaneum.
- Aponeurosis – a fibrous sheet.
- Connective tissue – loose layer enabling movement of the scalp.
- Periosteum – a double layer of connective tissue covering and nourishing the bone. It is attached to the edges of bone.

Reflective Activity 15.1

Undertake an examination of the head of a newborn baby to familiarize yourself with the structures labelled in Figure 15.2.

Can you identify the borders of the anterior fontanelle?

Why is it important to examine the anterior fontanelle in the newborn?

THE SKULL (FIG. 15.3)

The fetal skull is a complex structure consisting of 29 irregular flat bones with 22 of these paired symmetrically: 8 bones form the cranium, 14 the face, and 7 the base. A midwife will use knowledge of the fetal skull to assess progress in labour and the health of the infant at birth, and to diagnose abnormalities during the antenatal, intrapartum and postnatal periods. Knowledge of the fetal skull in the antenatal period enables a midwife to assess the size of the fetal head in relation to the size of the pelvis (Bian *et al.*, 1997), assess engagement of the fetal skull in the pelvis (Knight *et al.*, 1993), and aid review of ultrasonography and pelvimetry reports (Altman and Chitty, 1997).

Reflective Activity 15.2

When you next examine a newborn baby, pay particular attention to the head, and the bones, sutures and fontanelles which can easily be felt under the scalp. Familiarize yourself with the importance of these structures within midwifery practice.

Sutures

The sutures of the fetal skull are soft fibrous tissues linking some bones of the skull. They enable moulding of the head to take place during labour and expansion of the brain as it develops during childhood.

The sutures of the skull are:

- frontal suture (Fig. 15.4)
- sagittal suture
- lambdoidal suture
- coronal suture.

Fontanelles

A fontanelle is a membranous, non-ossified area of the skull where three or more sutures meet.

The significant fontanelles of the skull are:

- anterior fontanelle or bregma (Fig. 15.4)
- posterior fontanelle (Fig. 15.4)
- anterolateral or temporal fontanelles
- posterolateral or mastoid fontanelles.

Sinus

A sinus is a naturally occurring cavity in the body, in this instance in the cranial bones. The sinuses associated with the frontal, ethmoidal, sphenoidal and maxillary bones change shape during puberty and are thought to be associated with voice tone. Sinuses also enable blood to circulate throughout the skull and into the membranes of the brain.

The bones and regions of the skull (Figs 15.3, 15.4)

Divisions of the skull

The skull may be divided into three main regions:

- the vault
- the base
- the face.

The vault of the skull comprises:

- two frontal bones
- two parietal bones
- two temporal bones
- one occipital bone.

Measurements of the fetal skull

The presentation and position of the fetal head, in relation to the pelvic brim, influence the degree of flexion or

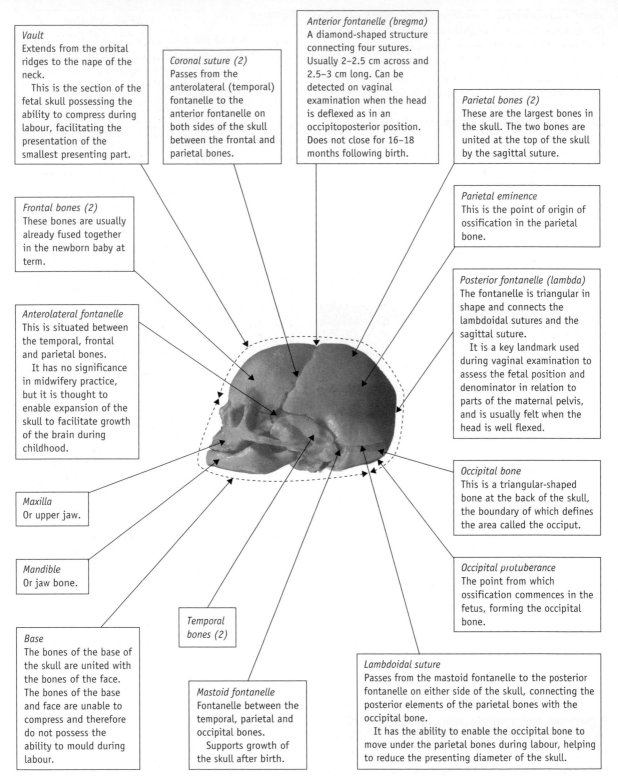

Vault
Extends from the orbital ridges to the nape of the neck.
    This is the section of the fetal skull possessing the ability to compress during labour, facilitating the presentation of the smallest presenting part.

Coronal suture (2)
Passes from the anterolateral (temporal) fontanelle to the anterior fontanelle on both sides of the skull between the frontal and parietal bones.

Anterior fontanelle (bregma)
A diamond-shaped structure connecting four sutures. Usually 2–2.5 cm across and 2.5–3 cm long. Can be detected on vaginal examination when the head is deflexed as in an occipitoposterior position. Does not close for 16–18 months following birth.

Parietal bones (2)
These are the largest bones in the skull. The two bones are united at the top of the skull by the sagittal suture.

Parietal eminence
This is the point of origin of ossification in the parietal bone.

Frontal bones (2)
These bones are usually already fused together in the newborn baby at term.

Posterior fontanelle (lambda)
The fontanelle is triangular in shape and connects the lambdoidal sutures and the sagittal suture.
    It is a key landmark used during vaginal examination to assess the fetal position and denominator in relation to parts of the maternal pelvis, and is usually felt when the head is well flexed.

Anterolateral fontanelle
This is situated between the temporal, frontal and parietal bones.
    It has no significance in midwifery practice, but it is thought to enable expansion of the skull to facilitate growth of the brain during childhood.

Occipital bone
This is a triangular-shaped bone at the back of the skull, the boundary of which defines the area called the occiput.

Maxilla
Or upper jaw.

Mandible
Or jaw bone.

Occipital protuberance
The point from which ossification commences in the fetus, forming the occipital bone.

Base
The bones of the base of the skull are united with the bones of the face. The bones of the base and face are unable to compress and therefore do not possess the ability to mould during labour.

Temporal bones (2)

Mastoid fontanelle
Fontanelle between the temporal, parietal and occipital bones.
    Supports growth of the skull after birth.

Lambdoidal suture
Passes from the mastoid fontanelle to the posterior fontanelle on either side of the skull, connecting the posterior elements of the parietal bones with the occipital bone.
    It has the ability to enable the occipital bone to move under the parietal bones during labour, helping to reduce the presenting diameter of the skull.

Figure 15.3   The characteristics of the fetal skull.

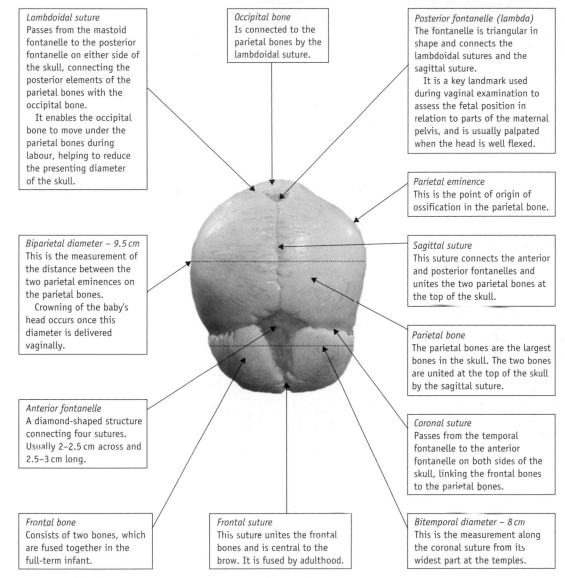

Lambdoidal suture
Passes from the mastoid fontanelle to the posterior fontanelle on either side of the skull, connecting the posterior elements of the parietal bones with the occipital bone.
   It enables the occipital bone to move under the parietal bones during labour, helping to reduce the presenting diameter of the skull.

Occipital bone
Is connected to the parietal bones by the lambdoidal suture.

Posterior fontanelle (lambda)
The fontanelle is triangular in shape and connects the lambdoidal sutures and the sagittal suture.
   It is a key landmark used during vaginal examination to assess the fetal position in relation to parts of the maternal pelvis, and is usually palpated when the head is well flexed.

Parietal eminence
This is the point of origin of ossification in the parietal bone.

Biparietal diameter – 9.5 cm
This is the measurement of the distance between the two parietal eminences on the parietal bones.
   Crowning of the baby's head occurs once this diameter is delivered vaginally.

Sagittal suture
This suture connects the anterior and posterior fontanelles and unites the two parietal bones at the top of the skull.

Parietal bone
The parietal bones are the largest bones in the skull. The two bones are united at the top of the skull by the sagittal suture.

Anterior fontanelle
A diamond-shaped structure connecting four sutures. Usually 2–2.5 cm across and 2.5–3 cm long.

Coronal suture
Passes from the temporal fontanelle to the anterior fontanelle on both sides of the skull, linking the frontal bones to the parietal bones.

Frontal bone
Consists of two bones, which are fused together in the full-term infant.

Frontal suture
This suture unites the frontal bones and is central to the brow. It is fused by adulthood.

Bitemporal diameter – 8 cm
This is the measurement along the coronal suture from its widest part at the temples.

Figure 15.4   The bones, sutures and fontanelles of the fetal skull.

extension of the fetal head and determine the precise realignment of the skull bones during labour and delivery. To assess the size of the fetal skull in relation to various diameters of the maternal pelvis, diameters of the fetal skull have been measured to correspond with common postures adopted by the fetal head as it enters the pelvic brim (Figs 15.5 and 15.6). Each of these diameters and degree of flexion and extension of the fetal head has a direct impact on the progress and possible outcome of labour. By understanding this, the midwife can suitably inform the woman so that decisions can be made on maternal positions in labour, pain relief and the subsequent care of the baby at delivery. It is important

to remember, though, that these measurements are only an estimate and will vary considerably depending on the size and weight of the baby.

INTERNAL STRUCTURES OF THE FETAL SKULL

The anatomy of the brain

It is important to understand the internal structures of the fetal skull, as although these are protected by the cranium they are vulnerable because of the ability of the

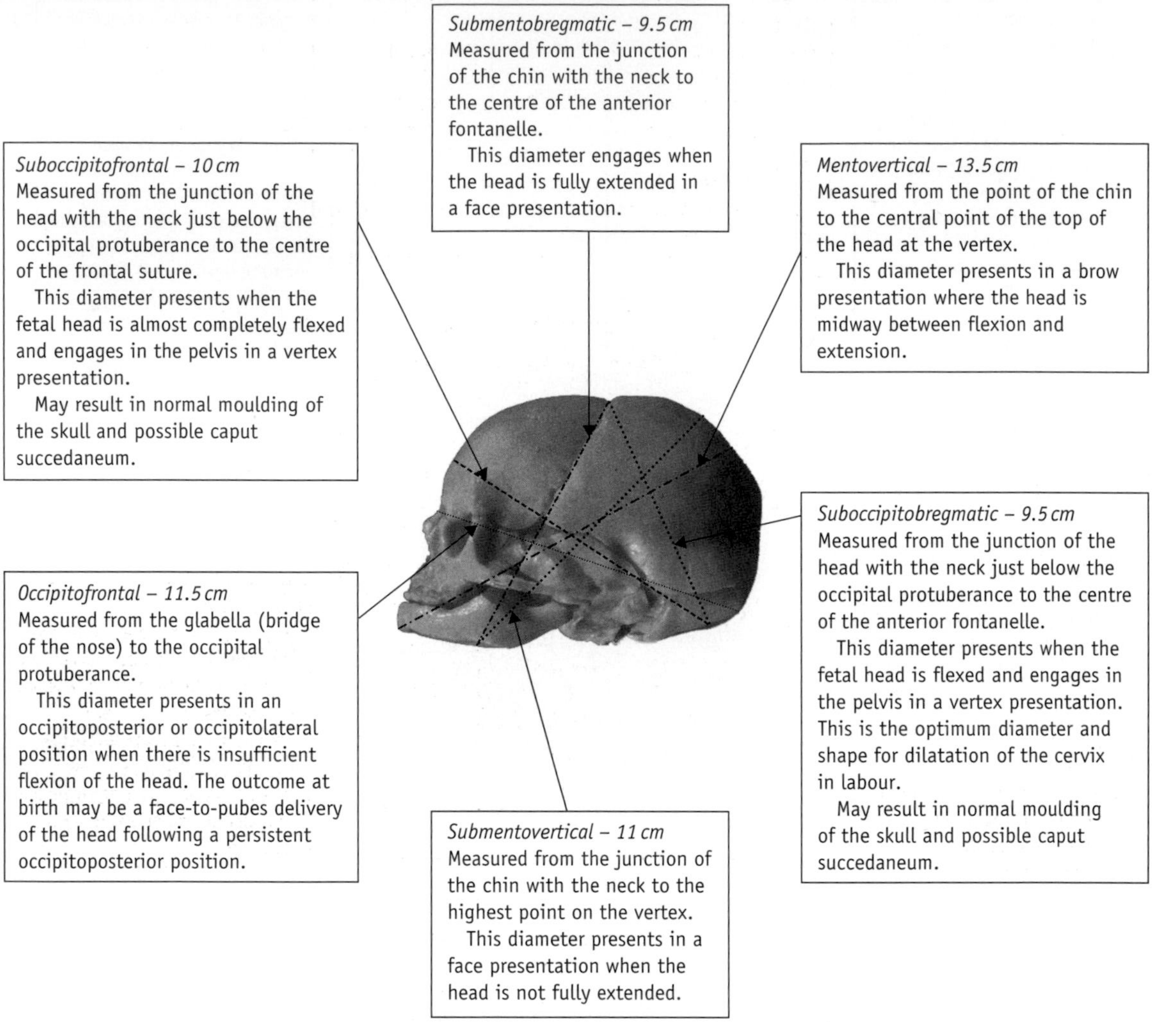

Submentobregmatic – 9.5 cm
Measured from the junction of the chin with the neck to the centre of the anterior fontanelle.
    This diameter engages when the head is fully extended in a face presentation.

Suboccipitofrontal – 10 cm
Measured from the junction of the head with the neck just below the occipital protuberance to the centre of the frontal suture.
    This diameter presents when the fetal head is almost completely flexed and engages in the pelvis in a vertex presentation.
    May result in normal moulding of the skull and possible caput succedaneum.

Mentovertical – 13.5 cm
Measured from the point of the chin to the central point of the top of the head at the vertex.
    This diameter presents in a brow presentation where the head is midway between flexion and extension.

Suboccipitobregmatic – 9.5 cm
Measured from the junction of the head with the neck just below the occipital protuberance to the centre of the anterior fontanelle.
    This diameter presents when the fetal head is flexed and engages in the pelvis in a vertex presentation. This is the optimum diameter and shape for dilatation of the cervix in labour.
    May result in normal moulding of the skull and possible caput succedaneum.

Occipitofrontal – 11.5 cm
Measured from the glabella (bridge of the nose) to the occipital protuberance.
    This diameter presents in an occipitoposterior or occipitolateral position when there is insufficient flexion of the head. The outcome at birth may be a face-to-pubes delivery of the head following a persistent occipitoposterior position.

Submentovertical – 11 cm
Measured from the junction of the chin with the neck to the highest point on the vertex.
    This diameter presents in a face presentation when the head is not fully extended.

Figure 15.5   The diameters of the fetal skull.

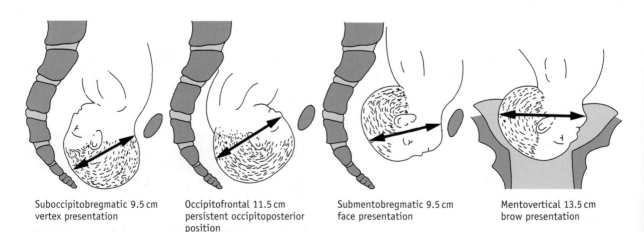

Suboccipitobregmatic 9.5 cm
vertex presentation

Occipitofrontal 11.5 cm
persistent occipitoposterior
position

Submentobregmatic 9.5 cm
face presentation

Mentovertical 13.5 cm
brow presentation

Figure 15.6   The diameters of the fetal head in relation to the maternal pelvis.

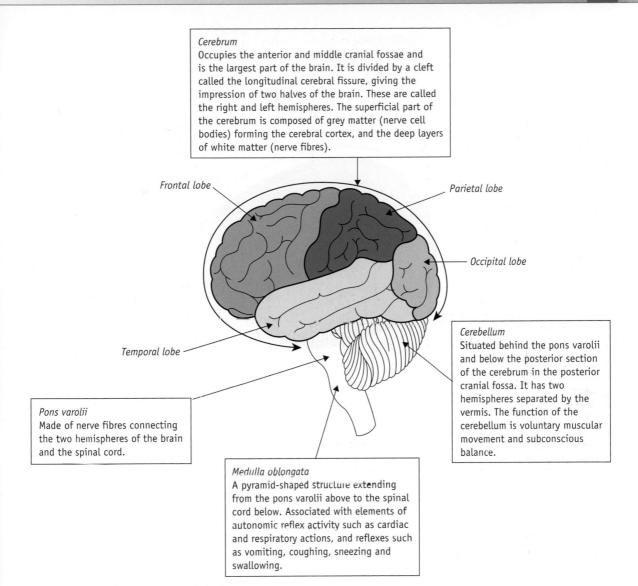

Cerebrum
Occupies the anterior and middle cranial fossae and is the largest part of the brain. It is divided by a cleft called the longitudinal cerebral fissure, giving the impression of two halves of the brain. These are called the right and left hemispheres. The superficial part of the cerebrum is composed of grey matter (nerve cell bodies) forming the cerebral cortex, and the deep layers of white matter (nerve fibres).

Frontal lobe

Parietal lobe

Occipital lobe

Temporal lobe

Cerebellum
Situated behind the pons varolii and below the posterior section of the cerebrum in the posterior cranial fossa. It has two hemispheres separated by the vermis. The function of the cerebellum is voluntary muscular movement and subconscious balance.

Pons varolii
Made of nerve fibres connecting the two hemispheres of the brain and the spinal cord.

Medulla oblongata
A pyramid-shaped structure extending from the pons varolii above to the spinal cord below. Associated with elements of autonomic reflex activity such as cardiac and respiratory actions, and reflexes such as vomiting, coughing, sneezing and swallowing.

Figure 15.7   External structures of the brain.

fetal skull to alter shape during labour and birth. Altering the shape of the skull can result in overstretching of the internal structures with subsequent tearing of tissues or rupture of blood vessels.

Regions of the cerebrum (Fig. 15.7)
The regions of the cerebrum are divided according to the bones under which they lie:

- parietal lobe
- temporal lobe
- frontal lobe
- occipital lobe.

Meninges of the brain (Figs 15.8 and 15.9)
The three membranous coverings of the brain are called:

- dura mater
- arachnoid mater
- pia mater.

MOULDING OF THE FETAL SKULL DURING LABOUR

As the measurements of the fetal head correspond closely to those of the pelvis, it is necessary to understand

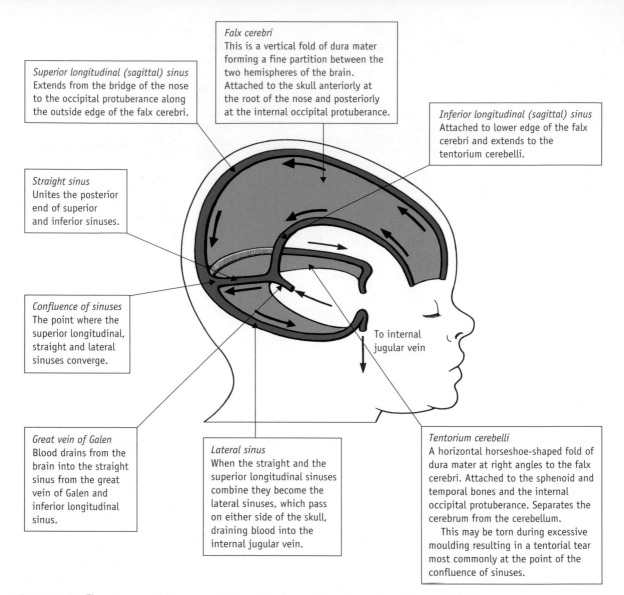

Falx cerebri
This is a vertical fold of dura mater forming a fine partition between the two hemispheres of the brain. Attached to the skull anteriorly at the root of the nose and posteriorly at the internal occipital protuberance.

Superior longitudinal (sagittal) sinus
Extends from the bridge of the nose to the occipital protuberance along the outside edge of the falx cerebri.

Inferior longitudinal (sagittal) sinus
Attached to lower edge of the falx cerebri and extends to the tentorium cerebelli.

Straight sinus
Unites the posterior end of superior and inferior sinuses.

Confluence of sinuses
The point where the superior longitudinal, straight and lateral sinuses converge.

To internal jugular vein

Great vein of Galen
Blood drains from the brain into the straight sinus from the great vein of Galen and inferior longitudinal sinus.

Lateral sinus
When the straight and the superior longitudinal sinuses combine they become the lateral sinuses, which pass on either side of the skull, draining blood into the internal jugular vein.

Tentorium cerebelli
A horizontal horseshoe-shaped fold of dura mater at right angles to the falx cerebri. Attached to the sphenoid and temporal bones and the internal occipital protuberance. Separates the cerebrum from the cerebellum.
This may be torn during excessive moulding resulting in a tentorial tear most commonly at the point of the confluence of sinuses.

Figure 15.8 The sinuses and dura mater folds of the brain. (From Bennett and Brown, 1999.)

their relationship and the effect that the pelvis has on moulding of the fetal head.

The fetal skull has a unique ability to flex during birth, and also can be adapted by prolonged compression during labour to enhance its passage through the birth canal. The skull is flexible at term although this diminishes as the gestation moves past 40 weeks. This adaptation process is termed *moulding*, a process during which the bones of the skull override each other as a result of pelvic girdle pressure. It is illustrated in Figure 15.10.

Moulding can increase or reduce the diameters of the skull by up to 1.5 cm. The usual process includes a movement of the frontal bone under the anterior aspects of the parietal bones and movement of the occiput under the parietal bones at the rear. This enables the skull to change shape but not volume. Where one diameter is decreased, another will be increased to accommodate the volume (see Table 15.1 and Figs 15.11 and 15.12). Where there is extreme or rapid moulding or abnormal compression of the fetal skull, a tear in the falx cerebri or tentorium cerebelli can occur.

The midwife present at the birth must record the degree of moulding present. During the neonatal examination the midwife reassesses moulding to ensure it is

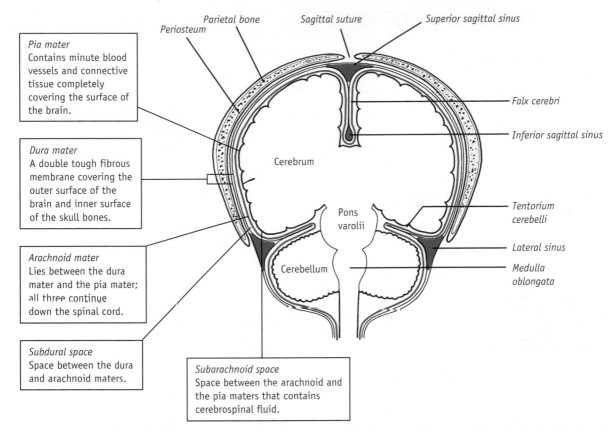

Figure 15.9   Coronal section through the fetal head to show the internal structures of the brain. (From Bennett and Brown, 1999.)

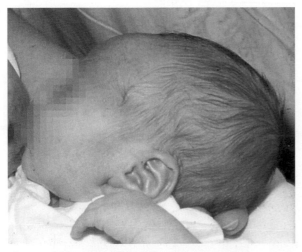

Figure 15.10   Normal moulding.

decreasing, and this may include taking measurements of the occipitofrontal circumference. Posterior moulding reduces within a few hours of birth, whereas anterior moulding is visible longer, decreasing over the first 48 hours of life.

INJURIES TO THE FETAL SKULL AND SURROUNDING TISSUES

Caput succedaneum

A caput succedaneum is an oedematous swelling within the superficial connective tissue layer of the scalp (see Figs 15.13 and 5.14). The swelling results from the pressure exerted on the fetal head by the cervix during labour. Oedema collects in the unsupported section of the fetal head, which protrudes through the hole developed by the opening cervix. The size of the swelling depends on the stage of cervical dilatation, and at full dilatation it may cover an extensive section of the presenting part. Not all babies develop a caput, as factors such as duration of labour, strength of contractions and descent of the presenting part all influence its development.

Characteristics of caput succedaneum

- Present at birth.
- May cross suture lines.
- Tends to decrease in size after delivery.

Table 15.1   Variations in the diameters of the fetal skull due to compression and moulding

Presentation	Effect on diameter
Vertex presentation with good flexion	Suboccipitobregmatic decreased Biparietal decreased Mentovertical increased
Persistent occipitoposterior position of the vertex (POP)	Occipitofrontal decreased Biparietal decreased Submentobregmatic increased
Face presentation	Submentobregmatic decreased Biparietal decreased Occipitofrontal increased
Brow presentation	Mentovertical decreased Biparietal probably decreased Suboccipitobregmatic increased

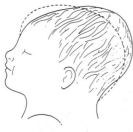 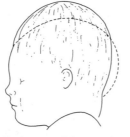 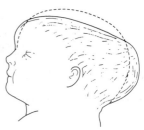

Occipitoanterior position   Persistent occipitoposterior position   Face presentation   Brow presentation

Figure 15.11   Moulding of the fetal/neonatal head.

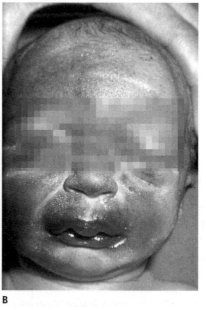

A   B

Figure 15.12   Moulding following face presentation and delivery: **A.** side view; **B.** front view.

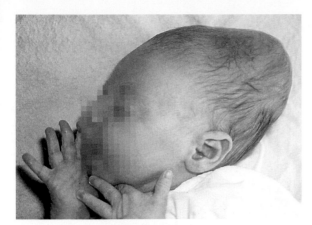

Figure 15.13   A neonate with caput succedaneum.

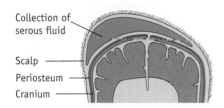

Figure 15.14   Caput succedaneum.

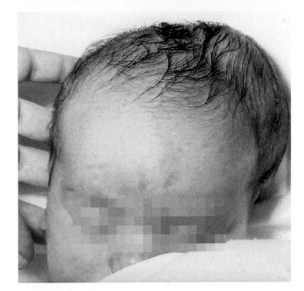

Figure 15.15   A neonate with cephalhaematoma.

- Usually a soft swelling that pits on pressure.
- No treatment is required as it generally disappears within 24–48 hours as the fluid is reabsorbed.
- Moulding of the skull will be present.

Cephalhaematoma

A cephalhaematoma is bleeding between the periosteum and the bone of the fetal skull (Figs 15.15 and 15.16). It is caused by friction of the skull against the pelvis or forceps during labour, and is associated with asynclitism of the fetal skull (the sideways rocking mechanism of the fetal head as it descends), or due to trauma following a vacuum extraction (Bofill *et al.*, 1997). The presence of a cephalhaematoma has also been linked to premature rupture of membranes (Petrikousky *et al.*, 1998). Injury to the fetal skull results in the periosteum separating from the underlying bone with subsequent bleeding between the layers. The resulting swelling is confined to the area of the affected skull bone as it is contained by the periosteum layer. A cephalhaematoma may be present in more than one bone. The most commonly affected bones are the parietal bones. The affected area is initially soft but as osmosis occurs the fluid is removed and the area becomes firm.

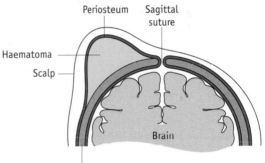

Figure 15.16   Cephalhaematoma.

Characteristics of cephalhaematoma

- Appears 12–72 hours following delivery.
- Tends to enlarge following delivery.
- Is circumscribed and does not pit on pressure.
- May be bilateral.
- Can persist for weeks and in rare cases months.
- May contribute to jaundice.

Treatment for this condition is rare, as most cephal-haematoma will disperse naturally. The neonate may be irritable, and may require gentle/minimal handling and the mother should be advised accordingly. However, as with any blood loss, the baby should be monitored for signs of anaemia, and vitamin K should be administered to increase the prothrombin level and assist with clotting. Babies are not normally perturbed by this injury but will need to be monitored for jaundice as lysis of the blood occurs.

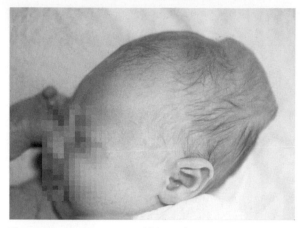

Figure 15.17   A ventouse 'chignon'.

Lacerations

Injuries may result from fetal scalp electrodes, fetal blood monitoring or forceps delivery. These involve damage to the skin of the scalp or face and result in puncture marks or lacerations usually requiring little or no treatment as they quickly heal following delivery. The aim of neonatal care in this instance involves the prevention of infection and the promotion of wound healing.

Chignon

A chignon may result following application of a vacuum extraction cup to the fetal scalp during the delivery of the baby (Fig. 15.17). The vacuum cup is applied to the scalp and suction applied, drawing the scalp into the cup. Because there is slight movement of the scalp layers, the area under the cup can become oedematous and bruised. The result is an oedematous structure the same size and shape as the vacuum cup. This condition usually disappears within a week following delivery. In rare cases vacuum extraction has been associated with *subaponeurotic haemorrhage* when bleeding occurs below the epicranial aponeurosis. The bleeding in this instance may be extensive and may be serious and so admission to a neonatal unit is necessary for observation and treatment.

INTERNAL INJURIES

Tentorial tear

The tentorium cerebelli is a fold of dura mater within which are present the venous sinuses containing blood being removed from the brain. On rare occasions the fetal head can be compromised by a difficult delivery or excessive or abnormal moulding, resulting in tearing of

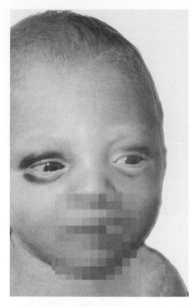

Figure 15.18   External signs of cerebral bleeding.

the membranes followed by cerebral bleeding (Fig. 15.18). This damage is often labelled as a tentorial tear.

The baby will present with signs of cerebral irritation and raised intracranial pressure, such as a tense, expanded anterior fontanelle, asphyxia (bradycardia and apnoea), and convulsions. In these instances the midwife should seek medical aid and the baby should be admitted to a neonatal intensive care unit for observation (see Ch. 36).

> **Reflective Activity 15.3**
>
> Revise the internal structures of the fetal skull.
>
> Visit your local neonatal intensive care unit to discuss the current treatment and care required by a baby with a tentorial tear.
>
> Make notes on the advice given, including signs and symptoms to enable you to detect this condition and current patterns of care available for this baby.

THE RELEVANCE OF THE FETAL SKULL TO PARENTS

It is important that midwives are able to share their knowledge with parents in order to expand the parents' understanding of the needs and care of their baby. This will commence in the antenatal period during which the midwife should discuss the nutritional needs of the fetus in development and growth, and carries through to linking the relationship between the woman and her pelvis and her baby and his skull, and the impact this has on labour.

Immediately following delivery, during examination of the neonate, the midwife can point out the key features of the skull, which include the fontanelles and sutures, and the presence of any deviations from normal, e.g. a caput, and their significance.

During the postnatal period, it is important that the midwife discusses care of the baby, which includes checking the fontanelles as a measure of the neonate's well-being. Box 15.1 provides a useful checklist for the midwife to use in educating mothers and others in the care of the baby.

Reflective Activity 15.4

Use the diagrams of the fetal skull in Figure 15.19 to revise the information outlined within this chapter. Photocopy the diagrams and revise the structures until you are confident that you know all of the components of the fetal skull and their application to midwifery practice.

CONCLUSION

Knowledge of the anatomy of the brain and the fetal skull enables practitioners to understand the role the fetal skull plays during labour and birth, helping them to assess, prevent, predict and diagnose potential and actual morbidity, while understanding the process of natural changes within the skull that help facilitate the birth of a baby.

Box 15.1 Helpful information points for parents

The following list of information will be helpful for new parents and could be used as a checklist by a midwife in the postnatal period.

- Careful handling of the head of the newborn is necessary to avoid injury.
- The newborn baby should never be shaken because of the damage that can occur to the internal structures of the skull.
- The head should be supported until about 3 months when the baby has developed some control over movement.
- The top of the head of the newborn should be washed with care because of the softness of the anterior fontanelle.
- Babies lose most of their heat through the head so in cold environments the baby's head should be covered.
- Observe the anterior fontanelle for signs of dehydration in the newborn but remember to allow time for the baby to absorb a feed once fed. The anterior fontanelle (see Fig. 15.2) is diamond shaped and feels soft and spongy to touch in the normal healthy baby.
- Injuries to the head should immediately be reported to a doctor for observation and treatment where necessary.
- A caput succedaneum should disappear within 48 hours.
- A cephalhaematoma should be absorbed within 1–4 weeks.

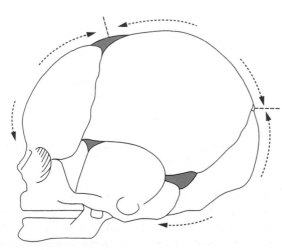 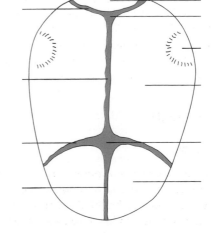

Figure 15.19 Diagrams of the fetal skull.

Following a birth the midwife uses skills of observation and diagnosis to ensure the baby's health and well-being. Knowledge of the structures outlined in this chapter enables the midwife to provide health promotion information and advice to prospective and current parents, on both the process and outcome of birth, and the subsequent care that their new baby requires.

KEY POINTS

- It is important for midwives to be conversant with the structure and development of the fetal skull.
- The impact of the fetal skull on labour influences the duration of labour, pain relief required and outcome of labour.
- The impact of labour on the fetal skull influences the amount and type of moulding and internal injuries that may occur during birth.
- The midwife should be able to anticipate and assess injuries relating to the fetal skull including the presence of caput succedaneum, cephalhaematoma, chignon, and scalp electrode injury. This assessment should include a consideration of injuries relating to the internal structures of the skull including tentorial tears.
- Midwives should use their knowledge both to inform practice and to assist families in developing their knowledge and confidence in caring for their baby.

REFERENCES

Altman, D. & Chitty, L. (1997) New charts for ultrasound dating in pregnancy. *Ultrasound in Obstetrics and Gynecology* 10(3): 174–191.

Bennett, V. & Brown, L. (eds) (1999) *Myles Textbook for Midwives*. Edinburgh: Churchill Livingstone.

Bian, X., Zhuang, J. & Cheng, X. (1997) Combination of ultrasound pelvimetry and fetal sonography in predicting cephalopelvic disproportion. *Chinese Medical Journal* 110(12): 942–945.

Bofill, J., Rust, O., Devidas, M. *et al.* (1997) Neonatal cephalhaematoma from vacuum extraction. *Journal of Reproductive Medicine* 42(9): 565–569.

Knight, D., Newnham, J., McKenna, M. *et al.* (1993) A comparison of abdominal and vaginal examinations for the diagnosis of engagement of the fetal head. *Australian and New Zealand Journal of Obstetrics and Gynaecology* 33(2): 154–158.

Moore, K. (1998) *Before we are Born: Essentials of Embryology and Birth Defects*. London: W.B. Saunders.

Petrikousky, B., Schneider, E., Smith-Levitin, M. *et al.* (1998) Cephalhaematoma and caput succedaneum do they always occur in labour? *American Journal of Obstetrics and Gynecology* 179(4): 906–908.

Sadler, T. (2000) *Langman's Medical Embryology*, 8th edn. London: Lippincott Williams & Wilkins.

Wilshin, J., Geary, M., Persaud, M. *et al.* (1999) The reliability of newborn length measurement. *British Journal of Midwifery* 7(4): 236–239.

FURTHER READING

Hankins, G., Leicht, T., Van Hook, J. *et al.* (1999) The role of forceps rotation in maternal and neonatal injury. *American Journal of Obstetrics and Gynecology* 180(1): 231–234.

Matsumura, G. & England, M. (1992) *Colouring Book of Embryology*. London: Mosby.
This book is excellent for students who have problems understanding the concepts of embryology. Colouring sections of the body enables students to explore the details of each structure of the embryo through each stage of its development, supported by detailed text of essential information.

Moore, K. (1998) *Before We Are Born: Essentials of Embryology and Birth Defects*. London: W.B. Saunders.
This book addresses all aspects of fetal development from conception to birth. The book includes photographs, scanning electron micrographs, ultrasound and MR images and drawings, all of which support learning and understanding of embryology and in particular the structures of the fetal skull and the brain.

Sadler, T. (2000) *Langman's Medical Embryology,* 8th edn. London: Lippincott Williams & Wilkins.
This detailed text outlines all aspects of clinical embryology and contains information on the genetics of birth defects. At the end of each chapter are questions relating to clinically related problems, with answers provided in an appendix.

Confirming Pregnancy and Care of the Pregnant Woman

Jancis Shepherd, Catherine Rowan and Eileen Powell

LEARNING OUTCOMES

After reading this chapter you will be able to:

- appreciate the history of antenatal care
- diagnose and confirm pregnancy by clinical and biochemical assessment, and be familiar with the tests which support this diagnosis
- obtain an antenatal history with tact and empathy, recognizing the relevance of the information given, and enable women to receive the most appropriate type of care
- identify the pregnancy changes that lead to physiological disturbance and discomfort within the various body systems; appreciate the physical and psychological effects of common disorders and discuss with women how these may be alleviated
- develop knowledge of the different maternal and fetal screening tests available
- discuss health education issues with women
- discuss with women the options for place of birth
- understand the physical skills of antenatal examination, recognize the relevance of the information obtained and evaluate the type and frequency of antenatal care required to meet individual needs
- appreciate the diversity of women's needs affected by age, socioeconomic status, race, ethnicity or disability
- identify the pregnancy changes that lead to physiological disturbance and discomfort for the woman, appreciate the physical and psychological effects of these changes and be able to discuss with women why these occur and how they may be alleviated
- recognize the signs and symptoms of symphysis pubis dysfunction (SPD) and symphysis pubis diastasis, evaluate the physical and psychological effects of SPD, and offer advice on how to reduce the symptoms antenatally, during labour and postnatally.

INTRODUCTION

This chapter will explore the care and services provided to the pregnant woman, from the point at which she believes she may be pregnant, to the onset of labour. Pregnancy is a time of enormous physical and psychological change and adaptation, as the woman and her family prepare for the addition of a baby. For most women this is an exciting and happy period of time, but may be overshadowed by fears and expectations which may have been formed by information from a variety of sources. It is important that midwives utilize the time they have in providing care to the woman, in assessing her individual needs, and in planning the most appropriate care. This should include an opportunity to increase her knowledge of her own body, the physiological effects of the pregnancy, and information on adapting to the changes which are taking place. This assists in ensuring that the woman reports anything abnormal, and in alleviating some of the minor disorders which may be experienced.

Prior to the actual pregnancy, women may have spent considerable time in planning and considering their pregnancy, and in identifying their personal fertility cycle (see Ch. 10).

HOME OVULATION PREDICTION TESTS

A home ovulation kit can identify the most fertile time of the menstrual cycle. Ovulation usually occurs within 72 hours of the peak of luteinizing hormone (LH) in the menstrual cycle; this is the most likely time for a pregnancy to occur. LH is produced by the pituitary gland and peaks at around day 14 in a 28-day menstrual cycle. The presence of LH may be detected in urine by using an ovulation detection kit, the dipstick changing colour if LH is present.

Home ovulation kits are now available with folic acid supplements. Ideally, users should be advised about preconception care and the need for folic acid supplements for the first 12 weeks of pregnancy (DoH, 1992a).

CONFIRMING PREGNANCY

Pregnancy may be suspected by the woman based on her knowledge of her menstrual cycle, sexual activity and the signs and symptoms of pregnancy. As routine pregnancy testing may not be available from the general practitioner or in many NHS trusts, women may confirm their pregnancy using a home pregnancy test. Confirmation of pregnancy may also be sought from the midwife or doctor. This is established by a detailed history and relevant clinical examination based on the signs and symptoms of pregnancy.

The signs and symptoms of pregnancy are:

- amenorrhoea
- breast changes
- nausea and vomiting
- increased frequency of micturition
- enlargement of the uterus
- skin changes
- 'quickening'

These signs will become obvious to the woman in sequential stages.

Reflective Activity 16.1

When you next undertake a 'booking' interview, discuss with the woman, and if appropriate her partner, what made her suspect that she was pregnant, how she confirmed the pregnancy – did she use a home test? What stage she discovered she was pregnant.

Signs and symptoms of pregnancy may be considered as *presumptive*, *probable* and *positive*, as illustrated in Table 16.1.

First 4 weeks

Amenorrhoea   Following implantation of the fertilized ovum, the endometrium undergoes decidual change and menstruation does not occur throughout pregnancy. Amenorrhoea almost invariably accompanies pregnancy and, in a sexually active woman who has previously menstruated regularly, should be considered to be due to pregnancy unless this is disproved.

Breast changes   Discomfort, tingling and a feeling of fullness of the breasts may be noticed as early as the third or fourth week of pregnancy, as the blood supply to the breasts increases.

Nausea and vomiting   This occurs in about 74% of pregnant women (Lacroix *et al.*, 2000). In this study 1.8% of women reported morning sickness and 80% had nausea that lasted all day.

Around 8 weeks

Nausea and vomiting usually persist in those women who are affected.

Frequency of micturition   This is due to pressure from the enlarging uterus and increased vascularity of the bladder.

Breast changes   The breasts enlarge and the superficial veins on both the chest and breasts dilate. The enlarged breasts may be painful.

Around 12 weeks

Nausea and vomiting may decrease and for some women cease altogether. Lacroix *et al.* (2000) report the mean duration of nausea to be 34.6 days with 50% of women relieved by 14 weeks' gestation.

Enlarged uterus   At 12 weeks the enlarged uterus is just palpable above the symphysis pubis.

Skin changes   Pigmentation of the skin occurs and is especially pronounced in brunettes. Areas of increased pigmentation include the nipples and areola, the linea nigra, which is the line of pigmentation from the symphysis pubis to the umbilicus and, rarely, the chloasma – 'mask of pregnancy'. The nipples become more prominent and Montgomery's tubercles are visible on the areola.

Table 16.1 Signs and symptoms of pregnancy

Timing (weeks of gestation)	Presumptive signs	Probable signs	Positive signs
4+	Amenorrhoea		
4 onwards			Positive pregnancy test, possible from the day of the expected period
4–14	Nausea and vomiting may be experienced		
3–4	Breast changes		
5–6			Fetal heart visible on ultrasound scan
6–10		*Hegar's* sign – softening of the vagina and cervix	
First 12	Frequency of micturition		
6–12	Skin changes	Softening of the cervix	
8 onwards		*Osiander's* sign – pulsation in lateral fornices *Jacquemier's* sign – lilac discoloration of the vaginal mucous membrane Changes in the uterus – size increases and shape changes	
10			Fetal heart audible with Sonicaid
14–16			Radiology, fetal skeleton visible (unlikely to be used because of danger of irradiation to the fetus)
16 onwards	Quickening – fetal movements felt by the woman		
16		Colostrum may be expressed from the breasts Uterine souffle Abdominal enlargement	
16–28		Internal ballottement	
From 20		Braxton Hicks contractions	
From 22			Fetal parts felt by examiner
24			Fetal heart audible with Pinard stethoscope

Around 16 weeks

Pressure on the bladder is relieved because the enlarging uterus has risen out of the pelvis, which reduces the frequency of micturition experienced by the woman. The fundus of the uterus is midway between the upper border of the symphysis pubis and the umbilicus.

The breasts start to secrete a little clear fluid called *colostrum*. This persists throughout pregnancy and for the first few days after delivery until milk is produced. A secondary areola may appear in brunettes.

Quickening The first fetal movements may be felt by primigravidae at 19+ weeks and by multigravidae at 17+ weeks. The time scale over which fetal movements are first felt by the mother ranges from 15–22 weeks in primigravidae and 14–22 weeks in multigravidae (O'Dowd and O'Dowd, 1985). Quickening, sometimes described as flutters, and a feeling of 'bubbles coming to the surface' rather than recognizable movements, an unreliable indicator of gestational age.

Around 20 weeks

For 90% of women, nausea and vomiting have usually diminished by 22 weeks' gestation (Lacroix *et al., 2000).

The secondary areola, if not already present, may appear.

The fundus of the uterus is just below the umbilicus.

Around 24 weeks

The fundus can be felt just above the umbilicus.

Fetal parts and movements may be felt on abdominal palpation.

Fetal heart sounds may be heard with a fetal stethoscope.

At 24 weeks the fetus is considered to be capable of an independent existence.

From 28–40 weeks

The fundus continues to rise until at 36 weeks it reaches the xiphisternum and remains at that level until the fetal head engages. *Braxton Hicks contractions*, painless irregular uterine contractions, may be palpated from about 16 weeks and these persist until the end of pregnancy.

When engagement occurs, the fundus descends slightly and together with the increased flexion of the fetus which now occurs, causes a relief of pressure experienced by the woman – *lightening*. This may not occur in multigravidae as the head often does not engage until labour is established. This lightening allows the woman to breathe with more comfort; however, the descent of the head may cause pressure on the bladder resulting in increased frequency of micturition.

Signs of pregnancy found by vaginal examination

It is now unusual practice to undertake a vaginal examination in early pregnancy, but if performed the following signs of pregnancy may be observed:

- The *softening of the vagina and cervix* is noted. This softness, together with the elongated isthmus, makes it possible to elicit *Hegar's sign* between 6 and 10 weeks. On bimanual examination, the fingers in the anterior fornix and those on the abdomen almost seem to meet because the isthmus is impalpable in contrast to the enlarged upper uterine segment and the cervix.
- *Pulsation of the uterine arteries through the lateral fornices* can be detected. This is called *Osiander's sign*.

- Increased vascularity of the vagina and cervix result in a lilac discoloration of those tissues, known as *Jacquemier's sign*.
- *Enlargement of the uterus* is noted and compared with the period of gestation.
- *Internal ballottement* may be elicited from 16 weeks. With two fingers in the anterior fornix the uterus is given a sharp tap. The fetus is pushed upwards and a slight impact on the fingers may be felt when the fetus returns to its original position.

If a vaginal examination is carried out, a cervical smear may be performed at the same time.

Positive signs of pregnancy

Although there are many physical changes experienced by the woman, which might suggest pregnancy, there are a number of positive signs which will confirm pregnancy.

The positive signs of pregnancy are:

1. *Fetal heart sounds*, which may be detected at 10 weeks using Sonicaid ultrasonic equipment. At 24 weeks' gestation these sounds can be heard with the Pinard fetal stethoscope.
2. *Fetal movements* felt by the examiner.
3. *Palpation of fetal parts*.
4. *Radiology* shows the *fetal skeleton* at 14–16 weeks. X-rays should be avoided, however, as irradiation can damage the developing fetus.
5. *Ultrasonography*. A gestational sac may be visualized at 5 weeks. At 6 weeks the fetal heart may be seen pulsating, using abdominal ultrasound. Vaginal ultrasound scanning may detect these a week earlier (Chudleigh and Pearce, 1994). A viable intrauterine pregnancy is confirmed when fetal heart pulsations can be seen in the gestational sac in the uterus.

Laboratory diagnosis of pregnancy

Chorionic tissue, which later forms the placenta, starts producing the hormone, *human chorionic gonadotrophin* (hCG), which is excreted in the urine. This hormone is usually detected in the urine from the time of the first missed period. Immunological tests depend on the detection of hCG in the urine. Pregnancy tests fall into three categories with varying sensitivities to hCG.

1. *Direct latex agglutination tests* (Fig. 16.1) where a small amount of latex particle reagent is placed on a

dark glass slide; the latex particles are coated with antibodies which will bind to hCG. The reagent is milky in appearance but when urine with hCG is added, the antibodies bind to the hCG causing the particles to agglutinate. The liquid changes to a granular consistency indicating a positive test result. Where no hCG is present, agglutination does not occur and the liquid remains milky (Wheeler, 1999).

2. *Monoclonal antibody tests/indirect agglutination tests.* Latex particles or red blood cells are coated with hCG. When the antibody solution is added, the particles or cells agglutinate. When urine containing hCG is added, the hormone binds to the antibodies, preventing them attaching to the hCG on the cells, and no agglutination occurs (Wheeler, 1999).

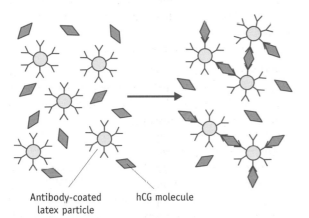

Figure 16.1 The principle of direct latex agglutination tests. (From Wheeler, 1999.)

3. *The wick or cassette method* (Fig. 16.2). This may be a simple dipstick test with an absorbent wick on a cardboard or plastic backing, or a more sophisticated wick enclosed in a case to give a cassette-type test as with home pregnancy tests; it may also contain a control window.

The absorbent wick is either passed through the urine stream, dipped into the urine, or drops of urine are placed upon the sample window. Antibodies labelled with a coloured dye placed between the application area and the result area bind to the hCG. As the urine is absorbed it travels along the wick to the result area – this appears as a coloured band. The excess urine moves further along the wick to the control panel where it is bound to another antibody and a further coloured band is displayed.

When hCG is present and the test is performed correctly, the result window and the control window will show coloured bands. If hCG is not present, no band will be visible in the result window, only in the control window. If the control window is blank, the test has not been performed correctly and should be repeated.

Up to 40 types of laboratory test kit are available in the UK (Wheeler, 1999). These have a wide range of different sensitivities from 20–1000 IU/l of hCG.

Home pregnancy tests have a more consistent range of sensitivity from 25–50 IU/l, take from 1 minute to obtain a result, appear easy to use and manufacturers claim a 99% accuracy rate. However, an American meta-analysis of the efficiency, sensitivity and specificity of tests highlighted that the diagnostic efficiency

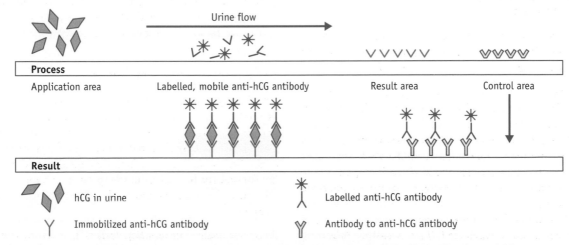

Figure 16.2 The principle of the wick test as used in dipstick and cassette devices. (From Wheeler, 1999.)

of home pregnancy tests is affected by the characteristics of the users (Bastian *et al.*, 1998). False negative results arose from testing before the recommended number of days from the last menstrual period, or from a failure to read or follow the instructions. Therefore a negative result in a woman who does not menstruate within a week should be treated with caution. The test should be repeated and laboratory confirmation sought if doubt of pregnancy exists.

The advantages of using home pregnancy tests are that they can confirm pregnancy in the privacy of the home, give the woman the information first, and provide a quick result, at an early point in the pregnancy. The average cost is £8.00 for a single test and £11–12 for a double test. However, given the varying sensitivities of home and laboratory tests it is possible that a woman may receive a positive diagnosis of pregnancy using a home pregnancy test and a negative result from a laboratory test. This may cause anxiety and confusion. If this happens, the midwife needs to ask the laboratory which test they are using and its sensitivity. A repeat test may then be requested, to confirm pregnancy. It is also possible that spontaneous miscarriage could have occurred between the two tests.

Following confirmation of pregnancy, women need to contact their midwife or doctor to commence their antenatal care.

Differential diagnosis of pregnancy

Some of the pregnancy symptoms may be found in other conditions not associated with pregnancy, and it is important that the midwife is aware of some of these symptoms, as she may need to refer the woman for further tests or specialist advice.

Secondary amenorrhoea

Where secondary amenorrhoea occurs in a woman who has previously had a normal menstrual cycle this may be due to a change of environment, emotional disturbance or general illness such as tuberculosis or thyrotoxicosis. The majority of cases are due to:

- hyperprolactinaemia, which requires investigation and management from the appropriate specialists because it may reduce the likelihood of conception
- weight loss from excessive dieting or anorexia nervosa – ovulation will not return until the woman regains her body weight
- hypothalamic insensitivity, for example following oral contraceptive use

- polycystic ovaries
- primary ovarian failure
- other hormonal imbalance (thyroid; Asherman's syndrome) (Llewellyn Jones, 1999).

Amenorrhoea also occurs around the menopause.

Vomiting

Vomiting may occur in a variety of conditions, and may be due to gastroenteritis or a prominent feature of urinary tract infection.

Enlarged abdomen

Tumours such as ovarian cysts or fibroids and ascites may be mistaken for a pregnant uterus. Obesity may also make the diagnosis of pregnancy difficult.

Fetal movements

Flatulence may be mistaken for fetal movements.

Pseudocyesis

This is a phantom or false pregnancy and may occur in women with an intense desire to become pregnant. Amenorrhoea will be present. The woman will complain of all the subjective symptoms of pregnancy, usually in a bizarre order; the abdomen may be distended and the breasts may secrete a cloudy liquid. However, she is not pregnant. The signs on which a certain diagnosis of pregnancy can be made, namely palpation of the fetus or hearing the fetal heart, are not present. Referral to a psychologist or psychiatrist may be required.

Hydatidiform mole

This occurs as a result of degeneration of the chorionic villi early in pregnancy. Severe nausea and vomiting, and severe breast tenderness may be present because of the high hCG levels. Vaginal bleeding may occur at around 12 weeks of pregnancy as the mole begins to abort (see Ch. 44).

ANTENATAL CARE

Historical review of midwifery care

To understand how current midwifery practice has developed one must refer to the historical accounts of the medical care of pregnant women (Donnison, 1988; Leap and Hunter, 1993; Oakley, 1982). Prior to the

Industrial Revolution, midwifery skills were learnt in practice with other women and passed on within families (Henderson, 1997). Knowledge about the birth process, mothering skills and baby care was learnt through observing women (Nolan and Hicks, 1997).

As discussed in Chapter 64, the development of midwifery followed a chequered course from being a community-based individualized service provided very much by women of the community through to the passing of the 1902 Midwives Act, bringing standardized education and practice to the profession. The care available to women through this time depended on factors including fashion – when engaging a doctor was considered to be more prestigious – and the wealth of the woman. Women of restricted financial means in rural locations were more likely to seek the assistance of the local midwife, and referral to a doctor was an option to be sought only in case of a deviation from normal. Midwives and families would be reluctant to seek such help because this may be costly to the family.

Antenatal care and the amount and quality of that care was reliant on the practitioner engaged, usually provided in the home and centred on the well-being of the woman. Antenatal care was mainly confined to the rich as they had the opportunity to both pay for and choose their midwife. This was usually on the recommendation of their doctor. By the time Queen Victoria came to the throne, midwives were being used mainly by the poorer sectors of society. Midwives charged less than a quarter of a doctor's fee, would deliver the woman at home and remain with the family for up to 10 days after the birth (Dowell and Price, 1998).

Provision of care for pregnant women became more structured from the start of the 20th century. Leap and Hunter (1993) relate both historical and literary accounts of 'an elite group of philanthropic women from middle, upper class and aristocratic backgrounds spearheading a campaign to regulate the training and practice' of midwifery. These reformers were also concerned with the social consequences of poverty and ill-health.

The Midwives Act 1902 resulted in the formation of the Central Midwives Board, bringing in standardized training, supervision, and a formal register of practitioners. This has been criticized as a development which made it impossible for working-class midwives to continue to practice in the long term, and by reforming midwifery practice may have altered midwives' relationship to the working class community (Heagerty, 1996; Kirkham and Perkins, 1997). However, the

alternative view is that it professionalized midwifery and contributed significantly to the reduction of morbidity and mortality of mothers and babies (Donnison, 1988).

Development of antenatal care

Formal provision of antenatal care was introduced during the First World War with the setting-up of the first clinics, though these were few and far between. The huge loss of life through the war gave an impetus to using antenatal care as a method of reducing infant and maternal mortality. The health and well-being of mothers and babies were accepted as being of prime importance to the future health of the nation.

The first hospital antenatal clinic was opened in 1915 by Doctor Ferguson in Edinburgh, and was later supervised by Ballantyne who also opened the first antenatal bed for inpatients. Until then most women had no routine antenatal care during pregnancy and were rarely seen by either a midwife or doctor until they went into labour. By that time there were often complications which may have responded to earlier diagnosis and treatment if it had been available and so improved the outcome for both mother and baby.

Antenatal care was fairly limited in the early days, with an abdominal examination, possibly urinalysis and advice or instruction on diet (Campbell, 1924, cited by Silverton, 1993).

The concept of antenatal care as a preventive measure grew slowly, and developed variably until well after the Maternal and Child Welfare Act of 1918 (Local Government Board, 1918), which encouraged local authorities to set up antenatal clinics. During the 1920s and 1930s there was little priority given to antenatal care (Leap and Hunter, 1993).

The content and intervals of antenatal visits were first specified in 1929 by the Ministry of Health (MoH, 1929). Further recommendations were added, with the inclusion of measurement of the mother's blood pressure, external assessment of the pelvis and guidelines for the minimum number of antenatal examinations to be undertaken during pregnancy (Corkhill, 1995). These were to be at 16, 24 and 28 weeks, then fortnightly until 36 weeks, followed by weekly visits until delivery. The report suggested that only the first examination and those at 32 and 36 weeks would be carried out by a doctor, with the remainder being carried out by a midwife (Silverton, 1993).

By 1935 it was estimated that 80% of women in the UK were receiving some antenatal care and the recommended intervals were similar to those of today, namely 16, 24, 28, 32, 34 and 36 weeks and then weekly until the onset of labour (Currell, 1990; Oakley, 1982). By 1946 the estimated figure for women receiving antenatal care had risen to 91% (Charles, 1992). Now, most women in the UK seek regular antenatal care and accept that it is important for their own health and that of their baby. Unfortunately those who are least likely to attend an antenatal clinic tend to be those who are most at risk of developing complications, for example women from the lower socioeconomic classes, young teenagers and women of high parity (Parsons and Perkins, 1982).

Patterns of care

From the onset of antenatal care in the UK the pattern of antenatal visits has rarely been questioned, even though when set up there was no evidence to suggest there were any benefits. The attendance ritual appeared to be generally acceptable, with neither women nor professionals questioning its rationale. There was a recommendation as long ago as 1982 that maternity providers review the number of visits for 'low-risk women' but this was never widely implemented (Hall *et al.*, 1985).

This challenge to routine practice was less likely to happen once place of birth changed and women were under further scrutiny in the hospital environment. The publication of *Changing Childbirth* (DoH, 1993) urged maternity service providers to review the system of antenatal visits, suggesting that it was not focused in the most effective way.

Reflective Activity 16.2

Discuss with your grandmother or someone from a similar age group her experiences of antenatal care. You may find it useful to discuss the same issues with your mother and make some comparisons.

Provision of antenatal care

Antenatal care is inevitably about balance. All women seek a healthy outcome to their pregnancy but not necessarily have the same antenatal care as their neighbour. Antenatal services should be acceptable to all women who use them. Wherever these are provided, there should be visible and accessible information. All staff in the team should be appropriately trained to meet the varying needs of women, particularly those who may be vulnerable and disadvantaged.

Antenatal care has several functions. It gives the health professional an ideal opportunity to share information and offer support. Earle's (2000) qualitative study exploring the relationship between women's experiences of pregnancy and the maintenance of self-identity found that the relationship between the community midwife and the woman was important to this experience and that continuity of both care *and* carer may be influential.

Aims of antenatal care

The aims of antenatal care may be summarized as:

- The establishment of open communication and a relationship of partnership between the woman and the professionals involved in her care, ensuring that she has continuity of care and carer from her lead professional.
- A source of information about all aspects of care and empowering the woman make informed choices in the knowledge that her autonomy is respected.
- The provision of appropriate support to promote psychological, emotional and social well-being in pregnancy.
- Health education to promote the maintenance and, where necessary, the improvement of health in pregnancy.
- Regular monitoring of the maternal and fetal conditions in pregnancy to ensure early detection of any deviations from normal and the instigation of appropriate referral and management.
- Preparation for labour and a safe delivery which will be a fulfilling experience for both the woman and her partner.
- The provision of education for early parenthood.
- Preparation for successful infant feeding, whether the woman chooses to breastfeed or bottlefeed.
- Preparation for the period following birth including family planning advice.

Care during pregnancy

It is important to encourage women to seek professional healthcare when they first suspect pregnancy, which is usually after one or two missed periods. The woman should be able to choose whether her first contact in pregnancy is with a midwife or her general practitioner (DoH, 1993; Health Committee, 2003; Secretary of State for Health, 2004).

She should be given clear, unbiased information and may choose whether she wishes to have a midwife, general practitioner or obstetrician as the lead professional to plan and give care during the ante-, intra- and postnatal periods. The choice of a lead professional does not prevent the woman from receiving care from other professionals if she wishes, or should it become necessary. One of the objectives of *Changing Childbirth* (DoH, 1993) is that all women should have the name of a midwife who practises locally whom they can contact for advice, even if the midwife is not the lead professional.

During the early weeks of pregnancy, many women feel exhausted, nauseated and anxious about many of the physiological changes that are occurring at that time. Early contact with their midwife or doctor provides an opportunity to express anxieties and receive the support, reassurance and advice which may be required during these early weeks.

Early booking enables women to be involved in decisions about which type of care will suit their personal, social and obstetric circumstances in the most appropriate way. Options for antenatal diagnosis for detection of fetal abnormality can be discussed and undertaken according to the decision of the woman and her partner (MIDIRS/NHSCRD, 1999a).

Where women seek care at a later stage in pregnancy it is more difficult to establish gestational age accurately by clinical examination. There may be confusion about the expected date of delivery until the gestational age is determined by ultrasound scan. After 28 weeks the assessment of gestational age by ultrasound scan is unreliable (Proud, 1997). Advice and support may be reduced, and the woman may have reduced options in terms of antenatal screening tests. Some investigations, such as the '*triple test*' for the detection of neural tube defects and Down's syndrome (see Ch. 18), are only accurate if carried out at specific times, in this case between 15–18 weeks. Early detection of these conditions enables further investigations such as ultrasound scan or amniocentesis, to be carried out at the optimum time.

The recording of the blood pressure gives an important baseline during the first trimester of pregnancy. After that time the blood pressure falls due to the physiological changes described later in this chapter and in Chapter 17. In the third trimester the blood pressure rises again and it is when this rise is greater than expected and cannot be compared with the baseline blood pressure recorded in the first trimester that problems in assessing the significance of the rise and subsequent management occur. In some cases complications have already arisen by the time the woman

books, which put both her and the fetus at risk. Such problems might be avoided with early midwifery or medical supervision.

The midwife will discuss the various options for care which are available locally for the woman. This will enable her to make an informed choice in her own time about her lead professional, arrangements for antenatal care, place of birth and postnatal care. Although many women choose their midwife or general practitioner as their lead professional, *Changing Childbirth* (DoH, 1993) recommends that all women should have the opportunity to meet an obstetrician at least once during pregnancy.

Where to give birth?

In 2002, the number of home deliveries in England and Wales was 2.9% (ONS, 2004: 38). Many professionals considered hospital birth to be safer than home birth, since the Peel Report (DHSS, 1970). However, more recently there has been increasing evidence to substantiate the view that home deliveries or *domino* schemes for women with low-risk pregnancies are safe (Chamberlain *et al.*, 1997; Lowe *et al.*, 1987; Tew, 1998).

Women need unbiased information to consider where they wish to give birth. Although a woman may request a home birth, local trusts are not obliged by law to provide this service, and the woman may have to negotiate with the trust to achieve the place of birth that she desires. Where the trust consider that they have insufficient midwives to give care to women in both the hospital and community, the hospital will be the priority for providing adequate midwifery staff levels. The woman may be asked to give birth to her baby in the hospital. Potential conflict could then arise if the woman does not wish to transfer into hospital. The midwife then faces a dilemma between her obligation to her employer and her professional responsibility to the woman. In this difficult situation both the woman and the midwife may need the support of the supervisor of midwives (UKCC, 2000).

See Chapter 24 for a detailed discussion of home birth.

Reflective Activity 16.3

Consider the discussion that you have with the woman at 'booking'. Do you think that you provide sufficient information for her to make informed decisions about patterns of antenatal care, home birth and who she would wish to see antenatally?

Alternative schemes/models of care

Wraight *et al.* (1993) indicated that numerous models of care were operating in various settings across the UK. These included domino schemes, team midwifery, and home births. The following are a selection of the differing types of schemes or provisions for antenatal care that have either been introduced in response to demands from both consumers (DoH, 1993) and midwives for an alternative type of 'care package'.

Domiciliary in and out scheme (domino scheme)

The *dom*iciliary *in* and *out* scheme (domino scheme) was considered to be an option for women who wanted community-based care (Wardle *et al.*, 1997). This model reflected the recommendations of *Changing Childbirth* (DoH, 1993), though it had been in existence for many years as a model of care in which the community midwife looked after a woman throughout pregnancy, delivered her in hospital and transferred her home within 6–24 hours to complete her postnatal care within the community.

In Scotland only 1–2% of all women receive this system of care, possibly because there is a lack of detailed information provided on the options of care, including domino. Mansion and McGuire (1998) found that the factors which influence women in their choice of using the domino scheme include dissatisfaction with various aspects of their previous births. It may also be used as an alternative option to home birth.

Other midwifery models of care, like team and caseload midwifery have replaced domino care (Wardle *et al.*, 1997). In response to the need to increase continuity of carer, many team midwifery schemes have been set up.

Team midwifery

Team midwifery involves a group of midwives in providing care to a specific number of women. The team may be based in hospital, community or a mixture of the two, and thus may be GP or geographically based or centred within the acute service. The size of the team may vary from six to over 20, though the ideal would be six to eight (RCM, 2000a; SNMAC, 1998). The model of care and the way the midwives work within the team will vary according to local agreement and issues such as whether the team are providing a total care package to low-risk women, or antenatal and postnatal care to all of the women.

Caseload/group practice midwifery

Caseload/group practice midwifery is usually accepted as a model in which care is provided to a defined number of women by a small group of midwives usually working in pairs or threes to ensure continuity of care. These models are usually based within the community, or may be 'subcontracted' by the acute trust (RCM, 2000a; SNMAC, 1998).

An evaluation of the one-to-one caseload midwifery (involving one named midwife providing care supported by a partner) found that there were high levels of continuity of carer and satisfaction achieved by both woman and midwives with a reduction in obstetric intervention in the one-to-one group (McCourt and Page (1996)).

The North Staffordshire Changing Childbirth Research Team (NSCCRT) who evaluated caseload midwifery care in comparison to traditional 'shared care' found that a caseload model could achieve very high levels of 'knowing your midwife' for pregnancy and childbirth and a significant reduction in obstetric intervention (NSCCRT, 2000).

Caseload midwifery requires effective management and support systems within the service to facilitate midwives in providing this type of care. It is also important to consider the working practices of midwives when working towards successfully implementing different service models, as additional resources may be required. A realistic analysis of what can be implemented will also assist in balancing job satisfaction and other needs of practitioners.

The changing patterns of care during the past two decades have been implemented in an attempt to improve service provision for women and their families. Increasing emphasis has been placed on improving the experience of childbirth for women, following, amongst others, publication of the *House of Commons Second Report on the Maternity Services* (DoH, 1992b) and the subsequent policy document *Changing Childbirth* (DoH, 1993). In many instances, ironically, the care provided by teams is fragmented and lacking in continuity.

One study carried out at the Royal Women's Hospital in Melbourne evaluated the effect of a new team midwife care programme on low-risk women in early pregnancy (Waldenstrom *et al.*, 2000). Satisfaction with antepartum, intrapartum and postpartum care in the standard clinic and hospital environment was measured. Doctors attended most of the women in the standard care group. Although conclusions were difficult to draw about which components of the team midwife care programme were most important, data suggest that satisfaction with intrapartum care was related to continuity of care-giver.

Antenatal day assessment units

Currently day units for minor surgery are an accepted part of healthcare delivery; however, similar units for the maternity services have been slower to develop. Scotland was one of the first places to introduce day assessment centres for women whose pregnancies were complicated by mild to moderate hypertension (Walker, 1993). Today these centres are recognized as a way to use the available resources more effectively. Audit findings in a hospital in the Midlands reported high satisfaction amongst women and a cost-effective service for the trust. It was concluded that many women with a variety of antenatal complications could be managed in the day assessment unit and that women preferred this to inpatient treatment (Knowles and Wilson, 1999). Women can either self-refer or be referred by health professionals, and this may reduce the need for antenatal admission. Recognizing that the same care can be given in a more informal environment has contributed to lowering the cost in both financial and psychological terms and for midwives the opportunity to empower women to self-refer.

Birth centres

Birth centres were first set up in the USA, and there has been a growing interest in setting up birth centres in the UK. These have evolved as a result of increasing dissatisfaction with the current provision of care.

Birth centres provide midwife-led care for women who wish to, and can safely, choose a 'low-tech' approach to birth (Rosser, 2001). They can be situated as either free-standing units or within an existing NHS site, and have clear lines of referral to a consultant-led unit when necessary. An example is the Edgeware Birth Centre (Barnet Health Authority, 2000) which is based in a community hospital in North London. Midwifery-led birth facilities show consistently better outcomes, in relation both to fewer interventions and satisfaction with care, than consultant-led delivery suites (Walsh, 2000).

Issues such as low morale, recruitment and retention difficulties, as well as difficulties in providing continuity of care and midwifery-led care may make these centres attractive to midwives. Birth centres may provide antenatal care facilities.

THE FIRST ANTENATAL VISIT

The first antenatal visit and taking of the woman's history may occur in the woman's home, health centre or general practitioner's (GP's) surgery, or at the first visit to the hospital antenatal clinic. If a combined approach is taken, this will reduce the visits that the woman may have to make.

Women may feel apprehensive at their first visit, especially if they have not met the midwives or medical staff before. Good communication skills and a non-judgemental attitude are important in enabling women to feel at ease in discussing very intimate personal details. A warm, friendly greeting and a pleasant, comfortable environment can also help to put the woman at ease. Young teenagers, women who do not speak English and those who are unhappy about their pregnancy may feel especially vulnerable. Interpreters are required for non-English-speaking clients and where possible such clients should be given written information in their own language. In many large cities where the number of teenage pregnancies is high, special 'teenagers' clinics' or clubs may be provided to meet their particular needs.

Whatever the background of the woman, or her reactions to her pregnancy, building a positive relationship with her is one of the midwife's most important aims during this first antenatal visit. This provides a foundation which will be built upon during the rest of pregnancy. The woman needs open communication with a midwife who is well-informed and committed to supporting her as an individual, encouraging the development of mutual respect, trust and partnership (Hutton, 1994). Hutton (1994) investigated users' views of the maternity services and found that there were consistent messages about the importance of the quality of the women's relationship with their midwife and how this can make or mar their experience of pregnancy, labour and the early postnatal period. One of the best memories in pregnancy about midwives was being made to 'feel special'. Thoughtless remarks casting doubt on the outcome of the pregnancy were one of the worst memories.

It is also crucial that at the beginning of the interview, the midwife discusses with the woman the purpose of the interview and issues such as confidentiality. The woman needs to understand the midwife's professional responsibilities, in terms of information which may be shared, and which may need to be discussed with other members of the team.

History-taking

When the history is taken at home or in a community clinic, the woman is likely to be more at ease. However, if the interview takes place in the hospital, the midwife should prepare the interview room to be as pleasant and non-clinical as possible in order to facilitate communication and the development of a relationship of mutual trust. The midwife should also provide privacy and sufficient time for the interview, and make this clear to the woman.

During early pregnancy the woman may be experiencing nausea and fatigue and will appreciate not having to travel to attend a busy clinic amongst strangers. Any problems can usually be discussed in private and the midwife can give information and offer advice as appropriate. Where other members of the family are present during this initial assessment this gives the midwife the opportunity to meet them, but she should also be sensitive that there may be information that the woman considers private or confidential and would prefer not to discuss in their presence.

The interview should be a two-way process of interaction between the woman and midwife. It involves assessment of the woman's social, psychological, emotional and physical condition as well as obtaining information about the present and previous pregnancies, the medical and family history. Care can then be planned in conjunction with the woman to meet her specific needs and wishes.

Methven (1982a,b) found that the antenatal booking interview merely recorded an obstetric history and that the promotion of a relationship between midwife and mother was not being achieved. Other factors which promote a more relaxed atmosphere are an informal arrangement of the room without the barrier of a desk between the mother and midwife. Sitting side by side, preferably in easy chairs at an angle of approximately 90 degrees promotes easier conversation than a face-to-face position. A few minutes spent by the midwife in introducing herself and chatting informally enable the woman to settle down and relax before personal issues are discussed. A skilled midwife can elicit most of the information required from the woman in a pleasant conversational manner without the woman realizing that she is being closely questioned. Open rather than closed questions should be employed because these encourage free responses and promote two-way interaction between the woman and midwife. Methven (1986, 1989) showed that the use of a nursing/midwifery model or framework for the

booking interview significantly increases both the quality of the communication between woman and midwife and the relevance of the information obtained for planning subsequent care. Orem's self-care model was used by Methven, but several models for midwifery have now been developed which are suitable for use at the booking interview (Hughes and Goldstone, 1989; Mayes, 1987; Midgely, 1988).

Some centres use questionnaires for obtaining the history, often sending them to women before they attend the booking clinic so that they can complete them in their own time at home and bring them to the clinic when they have their appointment. Other centres use computers which may be user friendly and midwifery oriented (Broadhurst, 1988). Lilford *et al.* (1992) conducted a randomized controlled trial to compare the effectiveness of three methods of taking an antenatal history: an unstructured paper questionnaire; a structured paper questionnaire; and an interactive computerized questionnaire. Structured questionnaires (paper or computer) were found to provide more and better information, and their use improved clinical response to risk factors. However, the focus of the questions was medically oriented and there was limited information on the social, psychological and emotional state of the woman.

Another study set out to discover if women themselves could complete part of the antenatal record at booking, instead of the midwife, and this indicated that this method is a useful alternative to the traditional way, but some women may prefer not to complete the form for a variety of reasons and their wishes should be respected (Fawdry, 1994; Galloway, 1994).

During the interview the midwife should be sensitive to the woman's attitude to her pregnancy and, if possible, to that of the father. Unusually adverse attitudes should be noted and counselling and support given as required.

Personal details

The woman's full name, marital status, address, telephone number, age, date of birth, race, religion, occupation (and that of her partner) and number of years married are clearly recorded. Her *age and duration of marriage* in a stable relationship may together be a guide to her fertility. A primigravida of 35 years may have been married only a year and be normally fertile, or she may have been married, or in a stable relationship, for 15 years and have almost given up hope of ever becoming pregnant. *Marital status* is established because some single mothers are unsupported and may need special help and understanding and referral to a social worker. Many single mothers today, however, are in a stable relationship or live an independent life and do not require any special help. In 2004, 40.6% (ONS, 2004) of infants were born outside marriage in the UK, compared with 29.8% in 1991 (CSO, 1994).

Race is ascertained because some medical and obstetric conditions are more common in certain races and thus special diagnostic tests may be carried out, where appropriate. The *religion* of the woman is recorded because of the special requirements and rituals which may be practised and affect the mother and her baby. *Occupation* gives an indication of *socioeconomic status*. Women in socioeconomic groups IV and V are more likely to have financial problems and substandard general health which may be associated with poor nutrition, smoking and inadequate housing. The outcome of pregnancy may be adversely affected and the perinatal mortality rate is increased. Extra support and health education from the midwife and referral to a social worker, if the woman wishes, may be required. Unemployment adversely affects a family's standard of living and again special support from the midwife and referral to a social worker may be required.

Present pregnancy

The date of the first day of the last menstrual period (LMP) is ascertained, care being taken to check that this was the last normal menstrual period. Some women have a slight blood loss when the fertilized ovum embeds into the decidual lining of the uterus and many mistake this for the last period. Pregnancy has been assumed to last 280 days, and to overcome the irregularity of the calendar a working rule of thumb was devised by Naegele. By counting forwards 9 months and adding 7 days from the first day of the last normal menstrual period, it is possible to arrive at an estimated date of delivery (EDD); alternatively, count back 3 months and add 7 days. This method of calculating the estimated date of delivery is known as *Naegele's rule*. However, as February is a short month

and the remaining months have 30 or 31 days, from 280–283 days may be added to the date of the LMP. Rosser (2000) states that it is unclear whether the length of pregnancy is affected by social, racial or obstetric factors. It is important to explain that it is quite normal for the actual day of delivery to be up to 2 weeks before or after this date.

Details of the woman's menstrual history should be sought: the age at which menstruation began; the duration of the periods; and the number of days in the cycle. Conception occurs shortly after ovulation. With a regular cycle of about 28 days, the standard calculation is reasonably accurate to within a few days, provided the woman knows the date of her last normal menstrual period.

In a 35-day cycle, however, ovulation would occur 21 days after the period; in a 21-day cycle, only 7 days after. Adjustments may be made, therefore, when the woman has a regular long or short cycle. If the cycle is long (e.g. 33 days), the days in excess of 28 are added when calculating the EDD (Table 16.2). With a regular short cycle such as 23 days the number of days less than 28 are subtracted from the EDD.

The calculation is difficult if the woman does not know the date of her last menstrual period, where cycles are irregular, or a normal cycle has not resumed since taking the oral contraceptive pill. If the woman has a good idea of when conception occurred, the EDD can be calculated by adding 38 weeks to this date, or subtracting 7 days from 9 months.

Women should be asked to note the date when fetal movements are first felt. Primigravidae normally become aware of fetal movements between 18–20 weeks, whereas multigravidae recognize the sensation a little earlier, between 16–18 weeks. This may be used to confirm the expected date of delivery, although with the widespread use of ultrasound in the UK, the gestational age is usually established during ultrasound examination. During the first trimester this may be by measurement of the *crown–rump length* (CRL) either by abdominal or vaginal ultrasound. From 12–24 weeks, estimation of gestational age is by measurement of the

Table 16.2 Calculation of the EDD		
Cycle 28 days	**Cycle 33 days**	**Cycle 23 days**
LMP: 12 Aug 2004	LMP: 12 August 2004	LMP: 12 August 2004
+7 days +9 months	+7 days +5 days +9 months	+7 days −5 days +9 months
EDD: 19 May 2005	EDD: 24 May 2005	EDD: 14 May 2005

biparietal diameter (BPD). The range of head shapes can influence its accuracy in the third trimester and the differences in growth and the measurements obtained may become so wide it is impossible to give an accurate estimation of gestation (Proud, 1997).

Although the use of ultrasound to estimate gestational age is very useful, some women may find it distressing if there are discrepancies between the date estimated by Naegele's rule, and that given following ultrasound examination, especially in those who are certain of the date of conception, or have a regular cycle and are certain of the date of the first day of their last menstrual period. In most cases it would be inappropriate to alter the expected date of delivery without the mother's agreement, especially when there is less than 10–14 days' discrepancy with the previously given date (Proud, 1997).

Other pregnancy symptoms such as breast changes, nausea and vomiting and increased frequency of micturition are noted. Nausea and vomiting may range from occasional slight nausea to frequent severe vomiting with ketosis, when immediate medical treatment is necessary. Any history of bleeding per vaginam since the last normal menstrual period is recorded and the woman asked to seek medical attention immediately should further bleeding occur.

In the first trimester of pregnancy a woman is quite likely to feel tired, perhaps nauseated and generally rather off-colour. A caring, approachable midwife who gives support, encourages the woman to express any worries and ask questions, and gives clear information, can be a great help to the woman at this time.

Previous pregnancies

It is necessary to ask about all previous pregnancies, including miscarriages or terminations of pregnancy. If the woman has had a miscarriage she is asked at what stage in pregnancy it occurred, whether she knows of any possible cause, if she was transferred to hospital and, if so, whether she needed either an operation to remove retained products of conception, or a blood transfusion, or both.

She is asked similar questions about terminations of pregnancy, including the reason for termination and how it was performed. Some women may not wish this information to be recorded in hand-held notes and their autonomy should be respected; however, the information should be recorded within hospital notes, and the reasons for this discussed with the woman.

Details of all pregnancies, labours and puerperia are essential:

- Was the pregnancy normal or complicated, e.g. by vomiting, hypertension or haemorrhage?
- Was the labour at term and straightforward in all three stages?
- How long did it last?
- Was the baby born in hospital or at home?
- Was the baby born normally or were any of the following required:
  - a forceps delivery?
  - ventouse extraction?
  - caesarean section?
- If so, does she know why?
- Did she have a normal healthy baby and was the baby well at birth? And now?
- If the baby died she is asked if she knows why, and what happened. This information is important to record, as the reasons for the baby's demise may indicate risks to the current pregnancy.
- The birthweight of any previous baby is important, since this gives some indication of the capacity of the woman's pelvis. A woman who has delivered without difficulty, a 3.5 kg (7 lb 8 oz) baby must have an adequately sized pelvis, while one who has had a forceps delivery of a 2.7 kg (6 lb) baby may have a small pelvis.
- Was the woman unwell after her baby's birth, or were there any problems such as haemorrhage or any other complications? The previous length of hospital stay may also be helpful, as this may reflect the normal or complicated nature of the postnatal period.
- She is asked if she breastfed her baby, if this was an enjoyable experience and for how long she was able to breastfeed. Her previous experience may influence how she intends to feed her expected baby (Foster *et al.*, 1997). If she fed artificially, the reasons for this are explored. The midwife will ensure that she is fully informed of the health benefits of breastfeeding, to both herself and her baby, to enable her to make an informed choice of feeding method, and she is asked how lactation was suppressed.

All pregnancies are dealt with in chronological order. If the history reveals any obstetric or paediatric complications and previous notes are not accessible, the information should be sought from the hospital where she delivered.

This is a useful part of the interview, as this may be the first opportunity that the woman has had for reviewing and reflecting on her previous childbirth experiences, and this provides a forum for clarifying management of problems both previously and in the future.

Medical and surgical history

This includes enquiry about any illness, operation or accident which could complicate pregnancy. It is necessary to ask by name about rheumatic fever; chorea; cardiac, respiratory and renal diseases; thyrotoxicosis; diabetes; hypertension; thromboembolic disorders; tuberculosis; epilepsy; and mental illness.

A history of psychiatric disorders, especially postnatal depression or puerperal psychosis, is of significance because such conditions may recur following a subsequent pregnancy. The woman is asked about the infectious diseases of childhood and whether she has had rubella or been vaccinated against the disease. A blood test will confirm whether or not she is immune, and if non-immune, she is warned to avoid contact with the disease, as rubella virus, if contracted in pregnancy, can cross the placenta and cause fetal abnormality.

Operations on the uterus or the pelvic floor are significant. Following caesarean section or myomectomy, there may be a weakened uterine scar, especially if the wound was infected, and there is a slight risk that it could rupture during a subsequent pregnancy or labour. Women of childbearing age sometimes have to undergo extensive pelvic floor repair operations. If a woman has had a successful operation for the relief of stress incontinence, both the woman and the obstetrician will be concerned about the mode of delivery; sometimes, another vaginal delivery is considered inadvisable and caesarean section is planned.

Relevant accidents include those involving the spine and pelvis, particularly if a fracture has occurred and deformity resulted. Deformity of the spine or pelvis following poliomyelitis or congenital dislocation of the hip would cause similar concern, since in all these instances the bony pelvis may be asymmetrical and accordingly have a smaller capacity. Enquiry may be made about back pain or symphysis pubis dysfunction and appropriate support and advice given.

Details of any blood transfusions are important, including the reason and any adverse reactions.

Drugs and medications

It is important to ask the woman whether she is taking any drugs, because many which are quite safe for her may have a teratogenic (harmful) effect on the fetus.

The woman should be informed about the risk of taking over-the-counter drugs without medical advice.

An increasing problem in pregnancy is drug addiction in women of child-bearing age. It is important that the midwife ascertain whether the woman has previously taken or currently takes prescribed drugs and/or drugs for 'social or recreational' use. It is essential that the approach and attitude of the midwife is caring, non-judgemental and constructively helpful; otherwise the woman may reject the help which the health and other specialist services can offer.

Women who are drug dependent may have increased problems during pregnancy for themselves or the fetus as they may:

- be less likely to attend for antenatal care
- be taking multiple drugs/alcohol which could increase the risk of fetal abnormality
- have unsafe injection techniques leading to infection
- have poor nutrition
- smoke tobacco
- suffer withdrawal syndrome that may lead to preterm labour
- die from accidental or intentional drug/substance overdose (DoH, 1998).

Women who misuse drugs may have a multitude of social, emotional, financial and sexual health problems that necessitate multi-agency involvement to try to minimize harm to themselves, their children and families. Practitioners need to be aware of the principles of the Children Act (DoH, 1989), which require that the appropriate authorities are informed if the baby is believed to be at serious risk of physical, psychological or sexual harm, or neglect. The midwife must explain her role and responsibilities towards child protection to the woman, with sensitivity, and discuss factors that could cause concern for the well-being of the baby. The woman may need reassurance that drug abuse alone is not a reason for removing a child and that every opportunity will be given to support her in caring for her baby. The midwife's aims of care include risk assessment of the woman and fetus/baby, referral to appropriate specialist services for consideration of detoxification, and minimization of potential harm (see Ch. 71).

Reflective Activity 16.4

Consider what protocols and guidelines are available locally to guide practice in the area of drug abuse, and whether this has a multidisciplinary approach.

Smoking in pregnancy

Midwives are ideally placed to give health education to the woman and her partner on the detrimental effects of smoking on the woman, fetus and newborn baby. The booking interview and antenatal visits are ideal times to discuss whether the woman smokes, the implications of this, and whether she would like to give up smoking (RCM, 2002). Implications of smoking include miscarriage, low birthweight, prematurity and perinatal death (Kramer, 1987), stillbirth, chest infections, asthma, glue ear, and sudden infant death syndrome (Blair et al., 1996; Haglund and Cnattingius, 1990). Smoking during pregnancy is influenced by age, socioeconomic status, and whether the partner smokes (McNeil, 1998). Psychosocial factors include depression, job strain/workload, and low levels of practical support (Borelli et al., 1996; Ryan et al., 1980; Wergeland et al., 1996).

Foster et al. (1997) reported that 85–89% of women who smoked, received advice on the effect of smoking during pregnancy, mainly from midwives. The information women are given should be unbiased and evidence based, aiming to encourage the woman to stop smoking, rather than purely frighten and stress her. Discussion with her partner and enlisting his support in reducing smoking may also be beneficial. Where interventions are introduced to help women stop smoking, e.g. provision of information on the effects of smoking, advantages of stopping, strategies to stop, particularly with individual counselling, these have shown a varied benefit in stopping smoking, increasing mean birthweight and reducing prematurity (Lumley et al., 2000).

Systematic anti-smoking programmes provided as part of routine antenatal care could significantly reduce morbidity. These strategies need to include a focus on avoiding victim blaming, social inequality and public health issues that deter women from giving up smoking (Lumley et al. 2000) (see Ch. 21).

Alcohol and pregnancy

Fetal alcohol syndrome (FAS) was recognized by Jones et al. in 1973, and defined by particular features noted in a small group of babies born to alcohol-dependent women. The assumption was made that if heavy drinking could lead to FAS, then moderate alcohol intake could lead to a milder form of harm, termed fetal alcohol effects (FAE). This led to the fear that any alcohol consumption during pregnancy has the potential for harm to the fetus.

The diagnosis of fetal alcohol syndrome requires signs in all of the three following categories (RCOG, 2000):

- fetal growth restriction
- central nervous system involvement (neurological abnormalities, developmental delay, intellectual impairment, head circumference below the 3rd centile, brain malformation)
- characteristic facial deformity (short palpebral fissures, elongated mid-face, flattened maxilla).

The RCOG (2000: 2) state: 'Other abnormalities, affecting all systems in the body, have been described and are referred to as fetal alcohol effects. Fetal alcohol syndrome is a rare event with reported incidences of 1.3, 1.7, 1.95 per 1000 live births in France, Sweden and USA respectively.'

It should be noted that heavy or moderate consumption of alcohol does not always result in FAS but it may be identified in about 30–33% of babies of mothers regularly consuming alcohol in the region of 18 units per day (RCOG, 1999: 2). Fetal response and susceptibility vary and may be affected by genetic factors (Christoffel and Salafsky, 1975); social deprivation, nutritional deficiencies, tobacco and other drug abuse, along with alcohol (Eckardt et al., 1998). This has therefore led to an understanding expressed by the RCOG Guidelines stating 'There is no conclusive evidence of adverse effects in either growth or IQ at levels below 120 grams (15 units) of alcohol per week' (RCOG, 2000: 3).

The RCOG (2000: 3), citing Mills et al. (1984) and Florey et al. (1992), note that consumption by the mother of 120 g (15 units) or more per week is associated with a reduction in birthweight of 63–66 g; more than 3 units per week in the first trimester led to an increased risk of spontaneous abortion; and in excess of 160 g (20 units) has been associated with intellectual impairment in children.

It is therefore recommended that pregnant women should limit alcohol consumption to *no more than 1 unit per day*. Even this apparently small alcohol allowance is challenged by Guerri et al. (1999), citing evidence that adverse effects of alcohol upon growth at 6 years were noted after one drink per day taken by the mother (Day et al., 1994). One or two sessions of binge drinking per week while not exceeding the weekly allowance, may be detrimental as blood alcohol levels are increased. Guerri at al. (1999) also caution against inferring that alcohol consumption below a certain level is safe, as individuals vary in their responses to alcohol. A study looking at alcohol intake, and its sequelae, in women over 30 years of age who drank during pregnancy, found the risk of intellectual impairment increased substantially for the children (Jacobson *et al.*, 1996). Currently in the UK, official guidance states 'Women who are trying to become pregnant or are at any stage of pregnancy should not drink more than 1 or 2 units of alcohol once or twice per week and should avoid episodes of intoxication' (DoH, 1995a: 34).

The midwife should use the opportunity to take a drinking history, assess the risk of alcohol dependence, or risk to the fetus from alcohol consumption, and advise and refer appropriately. The simplest way to do this may be by the use of an alcohol consumption chart (Plant, 2000). This is completed by asking the woman to recall her drinking in the last week, commencing with the preceding day and working backwards, and including all alcohol imbibed. One 'unit' of alcohol is equivalent to half a pint of ordinary strength beer, lager, stout or cider, a quarter of a pint of strong beer or lager; a small glass of table wine or sherry, or one measure of a spirit. The size of alcoholic measures may differ between a standard unit of alcohol of 8 g, and that served at home, where measures may be more generous.

Advice given to the expectant mother should be based upon the current recommended guidelines (MIDIRS/NHSCRD, 2002). The mother may appreciate her own copy of the informed choice leaflet on *Alcohol and Pregnancy* (MIDIRS/NHSCRD, 1999b).

For women with an alcohol problem, the midwife will need to offer support and referral to other agencies, e.g. alcohol dependency specialists and social services. It may be difficult to alter drinking habits and the priorities and values of the mother may differ from those of the midwife. The woman may be reluctant to attend for antenatal care, she may experience intrauterine growth restriction and will represent a challenge to the midwife in ensuring the best possible outcome for her and her fetus.

Reflective Activity 16.5

Do you consider that you provide evidence-based information with a non-judgemental approach when discussing smoking and alcohol? How would you ensure that the woman would feel 'safe' in giving you accurate information on her smoking and alcohol habits? You may find it helpful to ask a colleague to give you feedback on what he or she thinks your approach is like.

Diet in pregnancy

Inquiry is also made about the woman's diet and nutrition, and advice should be tailored to her individual circumstances, her cultural needs, whether she is vegetarian and any minor disorders that she may be experiencing. General advice to all women should include the need for a well-balanced diet that contains protein, milk, fruit, vegetables and carbohydrate. For women on low incomes, the cost of nutritious food may preclude some of these items, as women may choose to miss meals so that their children may eat (Rogers *et al.*, 1998).

Advice should be given on foods such as unpasteurized soft cheeses and mould ripened cheeses, which should be avoided in pregnancy to reduce the risk of infection with *Listeria monocytogenes*. Raw eggs and products containing raw eggs, such as mayonnaise, should be avoided because of the risk of salmonella infection, and undercooked meats and pâtés (which may be a source of *Listeria*, *Escherichia coli* and *Toxoplasma*) should also be avoided. Vegetable and salad foods should be washed prior to eating, and food should be stored at the correct temperature in the refrigerator and on the appropriate shelves to reduce the risk of infections such as listeriosis, *E. coli* and toxoplasmosis.

As high intakes (more than 10 times the recommended daily allowance) of retinol – the animal form of vitamin A – may be associated with congenital abnormality, the Department of Health (DHSS, 1990) recommend that liver and liver pâté should not be eaten. Beta carotene, the plant form of vitamin A that is found in leafy green vegetables and fruit, can be eaten safely.

The midwife should encourage women to continue with folic acid 400 μg supplements until the 12th week of pregnancy. Women who have previously had a baby with a neural tube defect should continue with 5 mg supplements until 12 weeks of pregnancy (DoH, 1992a). See Chapter 19 for a full discussion of nutrition in pregnancy.

Toxoplasmosis

Toxoplasma gondii is a microscopic single-celled organism found in raw, cured or undercooked meat, unpasteurized goats' milk products and in cat faeces. Soil that has been defecated in by infected cats may remain infectious for up to 18 months (Toxoplasmosis Trust, 2000). The organism is transmitted to humans through ingestion of food containing the organism, or by eating unwashed fruit or vegetables that have been in contact with infected soil. The effects of toxoplasmosis vary from a mild flu-like illness to a prolonged and debilitating illness similar to glandular fever (Toxoplasmosis Trust, 2000).

In Europe the incidence is between 1 and 10 in 10 000 newborn babies (Cook *et al.*, 2000) and in Scotland and England approximately 1 in 500 women acquire the infection during pregnancy (Toxoplasmosis Trust, 2000).

If a woman contracts toxoplasmosis for the first time during pregnancy, in about 40% of cases the organism may be transmitted to the fetus. This may cause miscarriage, hydrocephalus or retinochoroiditis, depending upon the trimester in which the infection is acquired.

Toxoplasmosis can be prevented, tested for, and treated during pregnancy with antibiotics and antiparasitic therapy. Unlike in some European countries, there is no national screening programme in the UK. Individuals who may have contracted toxoplasmosis are tested and treated on an individual basis.

The Toxoplasmosis Trust (2000) suggests all women should be advised how to avoid infection during pregnancy by:

- avoiding inadequately cooked meat or cured meat (Cook *et al.*, 2000)
- washing hands, food preparation surfaces and utensils thoroughly after preparing raw meat
- washing fruit and vegetables thoroughly
- avoiding unpasteurized goats' milk or goats' milk dairy products
- wearing gloves when gardening and washing hands and gloves afterwards
- covering sandpits to prevent cats defecating in them
- wearing gloves while removing cat faeces from litter trays and washing thoroughly afterwards, or asking another adult to do this.

Family history

The woman's family medical history is important. Familial diseases, such as hypertension and diabetes, are sometimes discovered during routine antenatal examinations and it is useful to know the woman's medical background. It is essential to know if any near relative has pulmonary tuberculosis, since the newborn child is very vulnerable to the infection and must be protected. Arrangements are made for the child to receive BCG vaccination before leaving hospital, as well as being segregated from the infected person.

As there is a familial tendency to produce twins, especially dizygotic twins, it is important to ask if there are

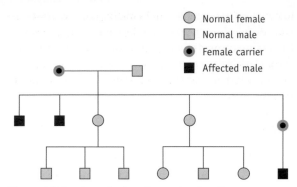

Figure 16.3   A medical pedigree showing three generations with X-linked haemophilia.

twins in the family and, if so, whether they are monozygotic (identical) or dizygotic (non-identical).

The woman should be asked if there is any history of congenital abnormality in the family (see Fig. 16.3) as she and her partner may need referral for genetic counselling (see Ch. 12). A number of diagnostic techniques are available for the diagnosis of congenital conditions in pregnancy and these may be discussed with the couple.

The midwife also carefully observes and enquires about the woman's reaction to her pregnancy, whether she is happy about it and coping with the initial minor disorders, or appears anxious, tense and unhappy. Guiding the conversation in a skilful, relaxed, unhurried manner and active listening and interpretation of both verbal and non-verbal communications help to elicit the woman's feelings and concerns. Appropriate support and help can then be offered.

It might appear that history-taking is a lengthy procedure; however, in most cases it can be completed within 30–60 minutes, as the majority of clients are healthy young women who have never been seriously ill. This personal history provides a basis on which it is possible to assess the woman's physical, psychological and emotional health and well-being and, to some extent anticipate the outcome of her pregnancy. An important aspect of this time spent taking the history is that the midwife and woman can meet and develop the relationship which has such a fundamental influence on the woman's experience of pregnancy and childbirth.

On completion the midwife can assess the woman holistically and discuss her particular needs and wishes. The midwife gives clear, accurate information about the services available to enable the woman to make informed choices, and then a care plan for pregnancy and childbirth can be discussed and agreed, tailored to the woman's individual needs. The woman should be given appropriate literature to refer to after her visit such as *The Pregnancy Book* (DoH, 2003). A future appointment may be made with the midwife and arrangements are made for any antenatal diagnostic tests to be undertaken.

HIV screening

In 1999 the UK Government drew up key national antenatal HIV targets (NHSE, 1999) to reduce the number of HIV-infected children being born by 80%, using the following time scale:

- By December 2000:
  - all women to be offered and recommended an HIV test as an integral part of their antenatal care (not including women arriving too late for antenatal care who should be offered and recommended a test after delivery)
  - an increased uptake of antenatal HIV testing to a minimum of 50%, with those health authorities already achieving 50% or more to increase uptake by a further 15%.
- By December 2002:
  - an increased uptake of antenatal HIV screening to 90% so that nationally, 80% of pregnant women with HIV are identified during their antenatal care.

The rationale for the introduction of universal screening is to reduce the vertical transmission rate and offer antiretroviral treatment during pregnancy. Midwives will need to be aware of the way in which universal HIV screening is offered to women within their own area. They may require additional training prior to a change in practice. Women require information on the implications of having the test, the test procedure, and how test results will be received. Pretest discussion and giving of information leaflets may assist women in deciding whether to give consent for the test.

or she has or has had a sexual relationship. Abuse can take many forms including physical (hitting, kicking, restraining), sexual (including assault and coercion), and psychological (verbal bullying, undermining and social isolation) (RCM, 1997).

The incidence of abuse is difficult to ascertain as it may be unrecognized or unreported through fear or shame. Estimates of abuse in pregnancy by partners vary from 1:50 (Campbell, 1986) to 1:6 (McFarlane *et al.*, 1992).

Pregnancy may act as a trigger for abuse to begin or increase (Mooney, 1993), and this may result in injury, obstetric complications such as miscarriage, intrauterine growth restriction, increased smoking or alcohol intake, or even to maternal death (Lewis, 2001).

The midwife may be the first point of contact for possible help to a woman who is abused, and the opportunity to initiate questions that may lead to disclosure of abuse can arise at the booking interview or during subsequent antenatal care. Suspicion may arise where the woman is always accompanied by her partner, especially where he constantly answers questions and undermines her. The midwife needs to have the skills to recognize potential abuse, question the woman with sensitivity, give her information of the choices available and resources to support her. Documentation of abuse should be made with the woman's consent, but not in hand-held records. Medical evidence of abuse may be needed should the case proceed to court. If the woman does not wish her disclosure to be recorded, her autonomy should be respected.

Each unit should have a multi-agency, interdisciplinary approach to the recognition, management and resources available to women who are abused. Staff training may be required prior to a new policy or guideline being introduced (DoH, 2000b).

Reflective Activity 16.6

Find out how HIV screening is offered where you work, and what information is available to women and their families.

Reflective Activity 16.7

How would you raise the issue of domestic abuse at the booking interview?

Make sure that you have a list of contact numbers for local women's aid organizations, or help groups and a copy of the local guidelines and resources in your resource file.

How may the supervisor of midwives be of use to you?

Domestic abuse

Domestic abuse is the term used to describe violence perpetrated by one adult against another with whom he

Infant feeding

Between 1980–1995 the rate of breastfeeding in the United Kingdom remained stable with 64–68% of women initiating breastfeeding. Between 1995–2000 an increase to 70% occurred (see Table 16.3), however this could be due to demographic changes in the sample. In the first 2 weeks of breastfeeding 20% of women discontinue, citing the baby's failure to suck or rejection of the breast (31%), insufficient milk (29%) and painful breasts (27%). All these are difficulties that could be overcome with skilled support. Data in the 2000 survey (Hamlyn *et al.*, 2002) does not give statistics for exclusive breastfeeding but suggests that 29% of mothers are giving breastmilk only at 5 weeks, falling to around 20% by 9 weeks. By 6 months only 10% were solely breastfeeding. This implies that, although no formula or cow's milk was given, the babies could have received water, other drinks and weaning foods. This does not meet the recommended minimum time of 4 months for exclusive breastfeeding (DOH, 1994).

Women who breastfeed are more likely to be married and having their first baby, have received full-time education beyond 16 years, be in a non-manual social class and live in the South East of the country (Foster *et al.*, 1997). Similarly, in 2000, Hamlyn *et al.* (2002) note that higher occupational groups with the highest educational levels, aged 30 or over, from ethnic minority backgrounds and having their first babies are more likely to breastfeed. Hally *et al.* (1984) found that three-quarters of mothers had already chosen their method of feeding before their booking visit. Of these women, one-third said they had made their choice before they were pregnant. This highlights some of the sociocultural factors that midwives need to be aware of when discussing breastfeeding with women. It also suggests that there is a need to start education about breastfeeding early in schools, colleges and youth clubs to enhance positive attitudes towards breastfeeding.

Many women who have chosen their feeding method in early pregnancy do not change their decision (Hally *et al.*, 1984; McIntosh, 1985), and the midwife is more likely to influence those women who are undecided about their choice of feeding method at the booking visit than those who have already decided to feed artificially. Where women have seen a friend or relative successfully breastfeed this may act as a positive influence upon their choice (Hoddinott and Pill, 1999).

Midwives need to be aware, when discussing infant feeding, that 'How do you intend to feed your baby – breast or bottle?' is a loaded question and the two choices should never be offered as if they are equal. Many women are unaware of the risks associated with artificial feeding and need appropriate and accurate information on which to make an informed choice. For women who have decided to breastfeed the values of breastfeeding should be reinforced with positive encouragement of how they can succeed. For women who express a preference for artificial feeding the reasons for their choice should be discussed and information given to them to offer the opportunity to change their mind.

During the antenatal period, women should have the opportunity to discuss with a midwife how successful breastfeeding can be facilitated. This can include information on analgesia in labour, offering the baby skin-to-skin contact and an early opportunity to suckle following delivery, correct 'latching' and positioning, the value of breast milk, baby-led feeding (both day and night), rooming in, and the benefits of continuing breastfeeding for at least 16 weeks. Dispelling myths about preparing nipples for feeding, colour of hair, and avoidance of particular foods, may enhance successful breastfeeding (MIDIRS/NHSCRD, 1999c).

Antenatal nipple preparation for inverted nipples is now known to have little bearing on the success of breastfeeding (McCandlish *et al.*, 1992), and this has led to the discontinuation of antenatal breast examination. However, this is an opportunity for the midwife to teach the woman how to examine her breasts, and increase her understanding of her own anatomy, which is a useful means of health promotion and education.

General advice should include discussion of hygiene, support of the breasts, and diet. It is advisable to avoid the use of soap on the nipples, as this may remove the natural secretions of the sebaceous and sweat glands. These secretions increase in pregnancy and not only act as a natural lubricant, but also have bactericidal properties (Newton, 1952). The application of additional creams to lubricate the nipples in pregnancy should not be required.

There is no evidence that wearing a brassière during the day and at night has any benefits; thus the woman should be advised to do what is most comfortable

Table 16.3   Incidence of breastfeeding by country

	1995 (%)	2000 (%)
	(Foster *et al.*, 1997)	(Hamlyn *et al.*, 2002)
England and Wales	68	70
Scotland	55	63
Northern Ireland	45	54
UK	66	69

for her (Alexander, 1991). As the breasts enlarge during pregnancy, a larger-sized, well-fitting brassière may be required.

Successful breastfeeding commences even before pregnancy, and that multifaceted interventions, through health intervention campaigns, health sector initiatives, peer support programmes, and media campaigns may be significant in supporting the woman in initiating and successfully breastfeeding her baby (NHSCRD, 2000).

SUBSEQUENT ANTENATAL VISITS

Hall et al. (1980, 1985) questioned the need for so many visits, particularly for those women identified as being at low risk, challenging the assumption that antenatal care is good and that more antenatal care is better. They concluded that the predictive and preventive value of routine visits was being overestimated, whilst false positive diagnosis of problems was common.

Whilst all women want to achieve a healthy outcome to their pregnancy, each woman will have particular and individual needs, so a degree of tailoring needs to be made to requirement these needs, balancing the requirement to monitor the pregnancy to prevent or detect clinical abnormalities with a supportive and educational approach.

Frequency of antenatal visits

Epidemiological and observational studies have indicated that women who receive antenatal care have lower perinatal mortality and better pregnancy outcomes. The traditional pattern of antenatal visits monthly until 28 weeks, followed by every 2 weeks until 36 weeks, then every week, has been questioned in relation to women whose pregnancies are low risk, because this schedule lacks proper scientific evaluation. Hall et al. (1985) suggested that normal multigravida should have antenatal examinations at around 12, 22, 30, 36 and 40 weeks' gestation and that primigravida should have extra blood pressure estimations and urinalysis from 34 weeks because of the increased risk of pre-eclampsia.

In 1982 the report of a working party set up by the Royal College of Obstetricians and Gynaecologists (RCOG) recommended a pattern of nine visits for primigravidae and six for multigravidae (RCOG, 1982). This recommendation was never widely implemented until it was repeated a decade later in *Changing Childbirth* (DoH, 1993), when it was suggested that providers review the pattern of antenatal care. The time saved could be used to improve the quality and effectiveness of care, providing greater support and education for those requiring it (Thorley and Rouse, 1993). It has been shown that increased social support during pregnancy may help to overcome some of the problems associated with social deprivation and to produce better outcomes for both woman and baby (Oakley et al., 1990).

Subsequent antenatal visits may be carried out by a midwife or doctor depending on whether the woman fulfils the criteria for low- or high-risk pregnancy. This may change as the pregnancy progresses. In an audit across a number of settings, the average number of visits of a multiparous woman with no pregnancy complications was 10 (Vause et al., 1996). Jewell et al. (2000) found that encouraging a more flexible approach to antenatal care conferred no significant advantage or disadvantage in terms of women's psychosocial or obstetric outcomes. This study shares similar findings to those of Sikorski et al. (1996) and Binstock and Wolde-Tsadik (1995) in that reducing the number of visits can result in women feeling that they were not being properly looked after. Discussion and debate continue in relation to the number of subsequent antenatal visits warranted for low-risk women. Professionals remain uncertain and at times unwilling to relinquish traditional patterns of delivering antenatal care, and this anxiety is transmitted to women. It is important that flexible, woman-centred care is safe, effective care. There will be a variation in the type and frequency of visits wanted by women – and this should be discussed early during the antenatal period. Some women may benefit psychologically from being seen frequently during the antenatal period (Jewell et al., 2000); others may wish to attend less frequently, to reduce time being taken off work (McDuffie et al., 1996). Most women receiving antenatal care seek reassurance, not only about their physical well-being but also their emotional state, and neither should be discounted.

International comparisons of antenatal care in developed countries have shown differences in how much antenatal care women are recommended to receive, and the professional groups who deliver that care. Blondel et al. (1985) reported that the recommended number of antenatal visits in 13 European countries ranged from three to four in Switzerland to 14 in Finland. There also appear to be differences in the models of antenatal care delivered in countries with comparable perinatal mortality outcomes.

Sikorski et al. (1996) found that women had fewer antenatal admissions and ultrasound scans with reduced visits, but some appeared more worried about the well-being of the baby antenatally and experienced more difficulties coping with the baby postnatally. Those who received fewer visits were more dissatisfied with the number of visits and felt that their expectations for care were not fulfilled. There was, however, a 30% non-response rate in this study. The dissatisfaction experienced by women could be partly related to their expectations and there is no evidence that this would persist if the new style of care became the norm.

Villar *et al.* (2001) reviewed nine trials and found that a moderate reduction in the number of antenatal care visits with increased content of the visits could be implemented without any increase in adverse biological perinatal outcomes, though women could be less satisfied with reduced visits.

There have been some concerns expressed about the reduction of visits in relation to detecting complications, especially the detection of pregnancy-induced hypertension (Redman, 1996). Another risk is of bleeding in pregnancy; however, this has many causes, none of which can be eliminated through antenatal care. Risk factors such as previous spontaneous miscarriage may be identified by history-taking, and appropriate advice given. As acute bleeding in either early or late pregnancy is likely to occur between antenatal visits, counselling and advice on what to do if this occurs is the most sensible approach (Villar and Bergsjo, 1997).

There appear to be no differences in long-term outcome between low-risk women attending the traditional 13 visits and those attending six to seven (Clement *et al.*, 1999). It has been suggested that more effective care could be provided with fewer, goal-oriented visits, particularly focused on the elements of prenatal care which are scientifically proven to be effective and have an impact on the outcomes. It is also important to ensure that the woman knows she can telephone her midwife if she has any worries or concerns which she wishes to discuss.

Medical examination

The woman usually has a medical examination generally carried out by the obstetrician once her pregnancy is confirmed, and this is focussed in content.

Examples of what might be included are:

- general appearance of the woman
- general examination of mouth and mucous membranes; palpation of glands of the neck
- height
- weight
- urinalysis
- blood pressure
- breast examination
- condition of heart and lungs
- abdominal examination
- cervical smear, if necessary
- legs, for varicose veins and oedema.

The doctor should ascertain well-being and adjustment to pregnancy and will normally ask whether she is taking folic acid supplements, and discussion should take place about their potential benefits, depending on the gestation of the pregnancy. She should also be advised to make an early appointment for a dental check-up. The gums are sensitive during pregnancy because of hormonal changes, and regular check-ups are beneficial. Dental caries are a potential source of infection.

The breasts may be examined to note pregnancy changes, a useful aid in the diagnosis of pregnancy, and to note any features such as the presence of lumps or abnormal discharge from the nipples. The breasts are likely to feel tender in the first trimester.

The heart and lungs will be checked and any deviations noted. Occasionally heart murmurs are detected at this time and referral to a specialist for further investigation may be appropriate. The abdomen is examined to ascertain whether the uterus is palpable and, if so, if its size is compatible with the estimated period of gestation. Details of the abdominal examination are given later in this chapter.

A vaginal examination is only made in pregnancy if there is a specific indication. If a routine cervical smear is due to be taken, it may be deferred until the postnatal examination. The lower limbs are examined for varicose veins. Varicosities are more likely in pregnancy because the veins become relaxed and dilated under the influence of progesterone.

Height

The woman's height and sometimes the size of her shoes are ascertained, since stature and size of feet give some indication of pelvic size (Moore *et al.*, 1983).

Weighing in pregnancy

Most women in the western world have been socialized into a society where slimness is valued (Warriner, 2000), and it is likely that most women will monitor their weight during pregnancy. It is recognized that weight gain during pregnancy is highly variable and some women even lose weight (BNF, 1994).

It is useful to record the baseline weight at the first visit but thereafter its value has been questioned (Dawes

Box 16.1 Calculation of body mass index (BMI)

$$BMI = \frac{Weight\ in\ kilograms}{(Height\ in\ metres)^2}$$

Example 1 Weight 57 kg (9 stone); height 1.68 m (5′ 6″):

$$BMI = \frac{57}{1.68^2} = 20.3$$

Example 2 Weight 64 kg (10 stone); height 1.57 m (5′ 2″):

$$BMI = \frac{64}{1.57^2} = 25.6$$

Example 3 Weight 76 kg (12 stone); height 1.57 m (5′ 2″):

$$BMI = \frac{76}{1.57^2} = 30.7$$

BMI score	Category
Less than 18.5	Underweight
18.5–24.9	Normal
25.0–29.9	Overweight
30.0–34.9	Moderately obese
35.0–39.9	Obese
40 or greater	Severely obese

Inadequate weight gain during pregnancy is associated with low birthweight (Springer *et al.*, 1992) whilst excessive weight gain may contribute to the amount retained postpartum (Rossner and Ohlin, 1995). Excessive weight gain, either preconceptually or during the pregnancy, has been recognized as a risk factor for shoulder dystocia (O'Leary, 1992; RCM, 2001), and from a long-term perspective, obesity may lead to problems such as cardiovascular disease and diabetes (DoH, 2001, 2002). It is therefore an area of health education where midwives can offer appropriate advice at a point in the woman's life when she may be more receptive to health advice. It does, however, require that midwives themselves are conversant with the principles of good nutrition, and can offer evidence-based, accurate and appropriate information.

Urinalysis

Routine testing of urine should be undertaken at every antenatal visit, for protein, glucose and ketones and is carried out using reagent strips or 'dipstick' tests. Detection of protein in the urine occurs when there are concentrations of approximately 50 mg/l. Protein concentrations depend on urine volume and specific gravity. Protein may result from contamination, particularly vaginal discharge, which may increase during pregnancy.

Asymptomatic bacteriuria   The detection of > 100 000 bacteria/ml in a single midstream urine sample is accepted as signifying an infection, and treatment with an appropriate antibiotic is essential. Up to 30% of women develop acute pyelonephritis if asymptomatic bacteriuria is untreated. Asymptomatic bacteriuria may also have a role in preterm birth or it may be a marker for low socioeconomic status and thus low birthweight (Smaill, 2001). In a prospective study evaluating the performance of reagent test strips in screening pregnant women for asymptomatic bacteriuria at their first visit to an antenatal clinic, Tincello and Richmond (1998) found that the strips were not sufficiently sensitive. They suggest that in view of the potentially serious sequelae of this condition if it is not identified, formal bacteriological investigation remains the investigation of choice.

Glycosuria is not uncommon as there is a lowering of the renal threshold in pregnancy. However, it may be due to diabetes and if there are repeated episodes, further screening will be necessary either in the form of random glucose estimates or a glucose tolerance test (GTT).

Ketones may be present if there is excessive vomiting, for example in hyperemesis gravidarum, or if the woman has not eaten for some time.

and Grudzinskas, 1991). However, Drake and Cullum (1998) suggest it is over-hasty to consider the amount of weight gained during pregnancy as unimportant. Midwives may suggest what is an average amount of weight to gain, but it is more appropriate to advise specific weight gain ranges based on pre-pregnant body mass index (BMI) – see Box 16.1 (American Institute of Medicine, 1990). Some women do find it reassuring to be weighed during pregnancy, as they perceive appropriate weight gain to be a sign of normality and a healthy pregnancy. Weight gain may vary enormously between individuals, and is affected by the cultural and social acceptance of the permissibility of gaining excess weight during pregnancy.

The growing problem of obesity in the UK will continue to impact on women and their pregnancies. The Health of the Nation's Nutrition and Physical Activities Task Forces on Obesity have highlighted pregnant women with body mass indexes over 25 as an 'at-risk group' and a focus for prevention (DoH, 1995b).

Weight gain in the past was used as an indicator of fetal growth in pregnancy along with the midwife's clinical judgement, though ultrasound is probably considered a more reliable indicator of fetal growth.

Blood pressure

Recording blood pressure in pregnancy is an integral part of the midwife's role. It is one of the screening tests taken at this and subsequent antenatal examinations and it is important that errors in interpreting blood pressure measurement are kept to a minimum, whether mercury sphygmomanometers or automated devices are used. Although mercury sphygmomanometers are in current use, they are gradually being removed from practice.

An appropriate technique must be used for taking the blood pressure. This should include positioning the woman in a sitting or left lateral position with the arm at the level of the heart. The cuff size should also be appropriately chosen and the stethoscope diaphragm applied lightly to the arm.

There has long been uncertainty about whether to record diastolic pressure at the point where the sounds muffle (Korotkoff phase IV) or when they disappear (phase V). There is now good evidence to support using the fifth Korotkoff sound when measuring diastolic blood pressure in pregnancy (Rubin, 1996) though there is a proviso that on the rare occasions in which sounds persist to zero pressure the fourth phase of muffling of sounds should be used (de Swiet, 1999; Shennan *et al.*, 1996).

Factors such as age, parity and race cause marked variability in blood pressure between individuals. Time of day, level of activity, emotions and posture may also result in variations within the same pregnant woman. The place where the antenatal visit takes place can also affect blood pressure with the 'white coat hypertension' effect being noticeable within the hospital antenatal clinic (Enkin *et al.*, 2000). This is a condition in which a normotensive subject becomes hypertensive during blood pressure measurement, but then settles to normal outside the medical environment.

Blood tests

At the first antenatal assessment visit the midwife will discuss with and obtain consent from women to undertake the following blood tests. Women and their partners must be given information regarding the reasons for and significance of undertaking these routine blood tests (RCOG, 1995). For the woman, this results in a huge amount of information and decisions to be made about her own and her baby's health, particularly in relation to screening, which can be overwhelming for her and for the midwife, especially given the time constraints of the antenatal clinic.

Full blood count   Haemoglobin levels are likely to fall because of haematological changes in pregnancy, including an increase in plasma volume. Routine administration of iron is not necessary, though local

protocols for when it should be commenced should be acknowledged.

Blood group and rhesus factor   Both have clinical significance for pregnancy and childbirth. Maternal blood is examined for the presence of antibodies and tests are repeated as required. A rhesus-negative woman will have tests carried out at regular intervals during the third trimester.

Other tests

- Rubella status
- Glucose
- Venereal Disease Research Laboratory – VDRL – test for syphilis
- Haemoglobinopathy screening
- Hepatitis B screening
- Human immunodeficiency virus (HIV).

Part of the process of choosing tests lies with the midwife and woman identifying which tests might be most appropriate. These tests are fully discussed in Chapter 18.

Risk factors

It is acknowledged that some women who appear at low risk at the outset of their pregnancy will go on to develop some problems (Tucker and Hall, 1999). The multidisciplinary team should attempt to identify such women and provide increased surveillance and care. Although it would be useful for the clinician to know which pregnancies are most likely to result in an adverse outcome, it also labels the individual woman 'high' or 'low' risk, and may also lead to a variety of interventions whose value may be questionable.

For those labelled high risk the threat of a poor outcome may create unnecessary anxiety during pregnancy and 'low risk' does not necessarily guarantee a good outcome (Enkin *et al.*, 2000). A woman labelled 'high risk' will often have normal outcomes, and a 'low-risk' woman may go on to require intervention if she develops high-risk factors. Practitioners need to appreciate that in dealing with human pregnancy and childbirth, the situation is dynamic, and therefore the label of risk should be used with caution. As with all information gathered, the midwife will share any concerns with the appropriate healthcare professional, and refer as appropriate.

ANTENATAL EXAMINATIONS

Subsequent examinations may be carried out by a midwife or doctor, depending on whether the woman is considered to be at low or high risk, and who she chooses to be her lead professional. The midwife is trained to practise normal midwifery, and thus can conduct and supervise the antenatal care of healthy women (UKCC, 1998).

Having greeted the woman in a friendly manner, the midwife asks her how she feels and whether she has any problems. It is important to ask open rather than closed questions (see Ch. 2) and to give the woman time to answer fully and discuss any matters she wishes. The midwife exercises her listening skills, noting non-verbal and verbal communications.

She can give information and advice about minor disorders and do much to dispel fears when anxieties are raised. Extra support is often required by those with social problems and with obstetric or medical complications. Referral to a social worker for additional help and support may be offered, if appropriate. The visit should provide an opportunity to discuss issues and assimilate information given by the midwife, so should not be rushed.

The following examinations are carried out at each antenatal visit after the booking interview:

- *Weighing* is still carried out in some clinics. Many women weigh themselves at home regularly because they are concerned about putting on too much weight, and it is useful for the midwife to acknowledge the woman's perspective on her weight gain.
- *Blood pressure* is measured and compared with the booking measurement and the last record, the overall trend being noted.
- *Abdominal examination* is performed to assess the height of the uterine fundus. This is usually done with a tape measure from the symphysis pubis.
  - Serial measurement of fundal height plotted on charts has been shown to increase the antenatal detection of small and large babies (Gardosi and Francis, 1999) although the value of this measurement has also been questioned (Neilson, 2000).
  - After the 28th week, examination can be undertaken to determine the lie, presentation and position of the fetus. From about 36 weeks, engagement of the head is also determined.
  - The fetal heart is auscultated.
- *Urine analysis* is undertaken to detect the presence of protein, glucose and ketones. Sometimes women are taught to test their own urine.
- Any *oedema* is noted. This may be identified in the pretibial areas, ankles and fingers. Ankle oedema may occur in pregnancy due to the increased tissue fluid in the body which tends to gravitate towards the feet and

ankles, and the increased venous pressure in the legs. Moderate ankle oedema is normal and usually settles after a night in bed. Provided the blood pressure and urine are normal, it should not be a cause for concern because it occurs in 50–80% of healthy, normotensive women. Oedema may also occur in the hands, especially in the third trimester where it may be manifested by tightness of rings. Facial oedema is difficult to recognize, unless the midwife knows the woman well. This may be recognized by friends or relatives. Generalized oedema may occur and can be observed on the abdominal wall, when the fetal stethoscope leaves a depressed ring, or as vulval or sacral oedema.

- *Varicose veins* may be noted in the legs, vulva and the anal margin and can give rise to considerable discomfort. These should be monitored for superficial inflammation, and advice provided to increase the woman's comfort.

NB: Supine hypotensive syndrome may be experienced by some women, as a feeling of faintness when they lie on their backs in the last trimester of pregnancy. This condition is caused by the gravid uterus compressing the inferior vena cava, impeding the return of the blood to the right side of the heart. The management is to turn the woman onto her left side immediately and she will rapidly recover.

Abdominal examination

An abdominal examination is carried out at every visit to the antenatal clinic. At first, only the height of the fundus is ascertained to assess fetal growth, but as pregnancy advances more information is required.

The following terms are used in relation to the fetus in utero and must be understood when learning to make an abdominal examination. It is helpful to follow a systematic process, for which the following mnemonic may be helpful:

L   Lie
A   Attitude
P   Presentation
P   Position
E   Engagement
D   Denominator

The *lie* (Fig. 16.4) is the relationship of the long axis of the fetus to the long axis of the uterus, and it may be longitudinal, oblique or transverse. In the latter weeks of pregnancy the lie should be longitudinal.

The attitude (Fig. 16.5) is the relationship of the fetal head and limbs to its body, and may be fully flexed, deflexed or partially or completely extended.

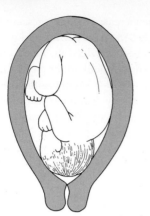
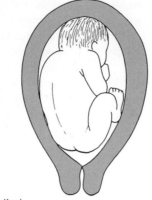
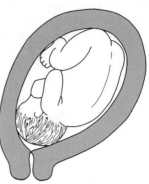

Longitudinal · Oblique

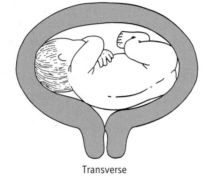

Transverse

Figure 16.4 The lie of the fetus.

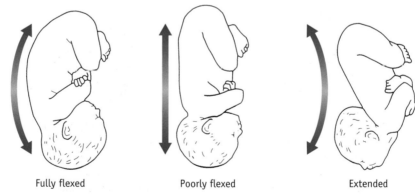

Fully flexed · Poorly flexed · Extended

Figure 16.5 The attitude of the fetus.

When fully flexed the head and spine are flexed, arms crossed over the chest, legs and thighs flexed. In this attitude the fetus forms a compact ovoid, fitting the uterus comfortably, though it can move freely.

The *presentation* (Fig. 16.6) is that part of the fetus lying in the lower pole of the uterus. A cephalic presentation is usual after about the 32nd week of pregnancy; other possible presentations are breech, face, brow and shoulder.

The *denominator* is the part of the presentation used to indicate the position:

- In a *cephalic* presentation, the denominator is the *occiput*.
- In a *breech* presentation, it is the *sacrum*.
- In a *face* presentation, it is the *mentum* (chin).

The position (Fig. 16.7) is the relationship of the denominator to six areas of the woman's pelvis.

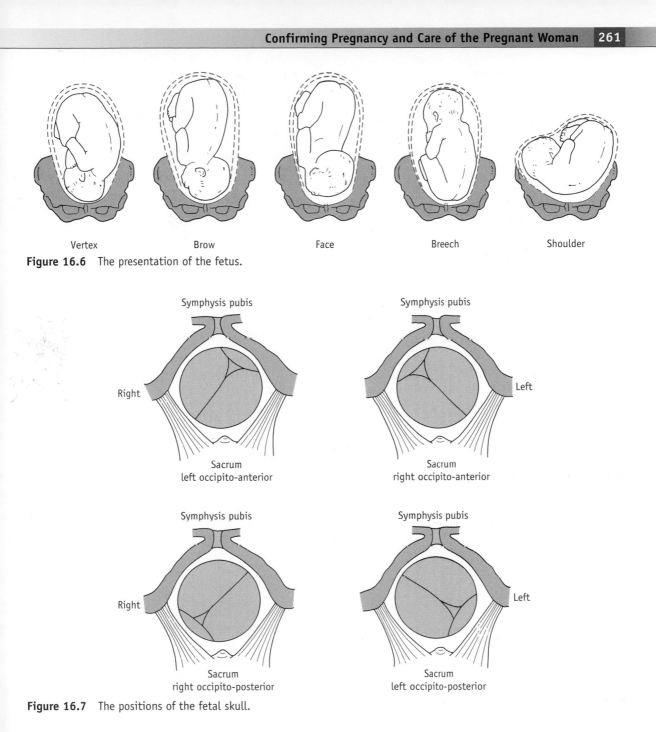

Figure 16.6 The presentation of the fetus.

Figure 16.7 The positions of the fetal skull.

These areas are:

- left and right anterior
- left and right lateral
- left and right posterior

In a cephalic presentation the occiput is the denominator, so the fetus is said to be in the:

- left or right occipitoanterior position (LOA, ROA)
- left or right occipitolateral position (LOL, ROL)
- left or right occipitoposterior position (LOP, ROP)

Anterior positions are more common than posterior positions and help to promote flexion of the fetus. In this position, the fetal back is uppermost and can flex more easily against the woman's soft abdominal wall than when it lies against her spinal column, as occurs in a posterior position. When the fetal head is well flexed, a smaller anteroposterior diameter presents to pass through the pelvis, and labour is therefore likely to be more straightforward.

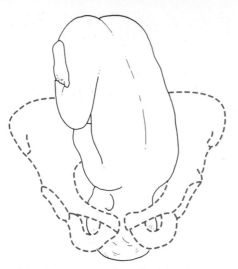

Figure 16.8 Engagement of the fetal head.

Engagement of the fetal head (Fig. 16.8) occurs when the transverse diameter (i.e. the biparietal diameter measuring 9.5 cm) has passed through the brim of the pelvis.

Engagement of the fetal head may be measured in fifths. The amount of fetal head palpable above the brim of the pelvis is assessed and described in fifths as follows (see Fig. 16.9):

- **5/5:** The fetal head is *five-fifths* palpable on abdominal examination; that is, the whole head can be palpated above the brim of the pelvis.
- **4/5:** *Four-fifths* of the fetal head are palpable above the brim of the pelvis; *one-fifth* is therefore below the pelvic brim and cannot be palpated per abdomen.
- **3/5:** *Three-fifths* of the fetal head are palpable above the brim of the pelvis; *two-fifths* are below the brim of the pelvis.

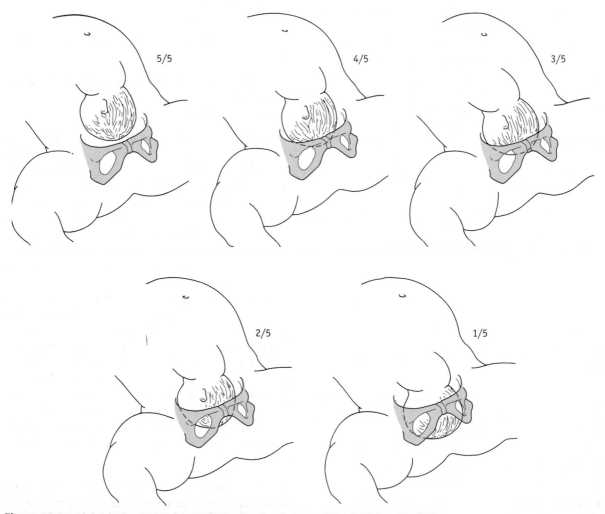

Figure 16.9 Abdominal examination to determine the descent of the fetal head in fifths.

- **2/5**: *Two-fifths* of the fetal head are palpable above the brim of the pelvis; *three-fifths* are below the brim of the pelvis. The widest transverse diameter of the fetal head has therefore passed through the brim of the pelvis and the head can be described as engaged.
- **1/5**: *One-fifth* of the fetal head is palpable above the brim of the pelvis; *four-fifths* are below the pelvic brim. The head can be described as being deeply engaged in the pelvis.

Method of abdominal examination

In addition to clinical aims, a woman-centred approach to palpation may help foster trust between a woman and her midwife, promote bonding between a woman and her baby and acknowledge a woman's expertise in her baby's health. The midwife's communication skills in explaining the examination, her attention to privacy, comfort and respect will help the woman feel reassured. The language used may also be crucial, as phrases such as 'a big baby' may frighten a women and affect her belief in her ability to give birth successfully. Technical terms may need to be explained (Olsen, 1999).

After emptying her bladder, the woman lies on a bed or couch, adopting a fairly flat position, with one pillow, unless she finds this very uncomfortable and requires a second pillow, and her knees may be flexed slightly if she wishes. Only the abdomen should be exposed. It is important that the woman should be relaxed and every effort must be made to put her at ease. Obesity, a thick, muscular abdominal wall, polyhydramnios and multiple pregnancy make the examination difficult, but provided the woman is relaxed even these difficulties may be overcome.

Three ways are used to obtain the information required:

- observation
- palpation and measurement
- auscultation

Normal findings in late pregnancy are summarized in Box 16.2.

Observation   The most important features to be noted are the size and shape of the uterus. The size should correspond with the estimated period of gestation. If there is any discrepancy, the date of the last menstrual period should be rechecked. If the dates are correct and the uterus is too large, the main possibilities are:

- large fetus
- uterine fibroids

> **Box 16.2 Normal findings on abdominal examination in late pregnancy**
>
> **Inspection**
> - Uterus a longitudinal ovoid
> - Uterus size consistent with supposed length of gestation
>
> **Palpation**
> - Cephalic presentation
> - Head engaged
> - Position left anterior
>
> **Auscultation**
> - Fetal heart sounds strong and regular
> - Fetal heart rate 140 beats per minute

- multiple pregnancy
- polyhydramnios
- hydatidiform mole.

If the dates are correct and the uterus is small, the most likely causes are:

- small fetus, probably due to placental insufficiency
- fetal death
- oligohydramnios.

If the midwife considers the girth to be excessive, she should measure it in centimetres: 95 cm at the umbilicus at 40 weeks is the average. Should a girth of 100 cm be reached or exceeded before that time, causes may be obesity, polyhydramnios, twins or a transverse lie.

The normal shape is a longitudinal ovoid, usually very clear in the primigravida, but sometimes more rounded in the multigravid woman. In late pregnancy, the unusual shape created by an oblique or transverse lie is usually unmistakable.

The dark line of pigmentation called the *linea nigra* may be seen from the umbilicus to the pubis. *Striae gravidarum* or stretch marks may be seen as red marks if new, and as silver if they date from previous pregnancy. These indicate the elasticity of the skin and the degree to which the woman has gained weight. The quality of the muscle of the abdominal wall, obliquity of the uterus, and fetal movements can also be observed. During this inspection any abdominal scars should be noted and the reason ascertained if not already recorded in the notes.

Palpation   should be carried out gently with both hands. The hands should be clean and warm and the nails short to avoid causing the woman discomfort. The

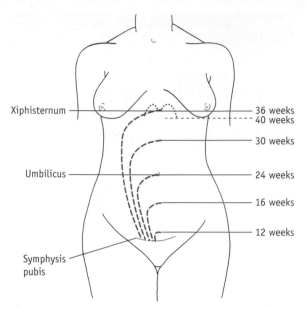

Xiphisternum ——— 36 weeks
——— 40 weeks
——— 30 weeks

Umbilicus ——— 24 weeks

——— 16 weeks

——— 12 weeks

Symphysis
pubis

Figure 16.10 The height of the fundus at different stages of pregnancy.

hands should be moved smoothly over the abdomen and the pads of the fingers used to palpate the fetal parts. A gentle, skilful touch conveys to the woman that she is being examined by a caring, competent midwife. Undue pressure produces pain and will tend to cause a tightening of the abdominal muscles, as well as stimulation of uterine contractions, and so make palpation more difficult. First the midwife places the ulnar border of the left hand on the fundus and compares the height with the size expected for the period of gestation (Fig. 16.10).

The midwife then ascertains which part of the fetus is lying at the pelvic brim and confirms the diagnosis by palpating other points of the abdomen. It should be possible to find out the lie, presentation and position and also the relationship of the fetal head to the woman's pelvis. This information is particularly important after the 32nd week of pregnancy.

There are three distinct manoeuvres (Fig. 16.11) employed in abdominal palpation:

- fundal palpation
- deep pelvic palpation
- lateral palpation.

Fundal palpation Facing the woman's head, the midwife carries out this manoeuvre to determine which part of the fetus is lying in the fundus. In most cases it will be the breech. If the head is in the fundus it can be recognized as smooth, round, hard and ballottable, separated from the trunk by a groove, the neck. This is

why it is more freely movable than the breech, which can only be moved from side to side, the back moving with it. The breech is also less hard, more irregular in outline, and lower limbs may be palpated near it.

Deep pelvic palpation This is the most important manoeuvre in abdominal palpation. The presentation is determined, and from that the lie of the fetus is deduced. If the head is presenting, the degree of flexion can be ascertained. In the latter weeks of pregnancy it is most important to determine whether the fetal head is engaged or will engage. The amount of fetal head palpable above the brim of the pelvis is assessed and described in fifths. The midwife turns to face the woman's feet and places one hand on either side of the uterus near the pelvic brim. The fingertips are allowed to sink gently into the pelvis to feel the presentation. The fetal head feels hard and round and it may be possible to ballotte it if it is not engaged. This means that, when given a gentle tap on one side by the examining fingers, it floats away and is then felt to return against the examining fingers. When the fingertips can sink into the pelvis further on one side than they do on the other, it may be because the head is flexed and the occiput is lying on the side into which the fingers sink more deeply. The position of the occiput indicates the position of the fetus. Whilst carrying out this manoeuvre the midwife should watch the woman's face for any sign of discomfort.

Pawlik's grip may occasionally be used to determine the shape, size and engagement of the fetal head. The midwife faces the woman's head, and using her right hand, grasps the fetal head through the abdominal and uterine walls. The woman is asked to breathe out through her mouth slowly while the fetal head is grasped and the mobility and engagement is assessed. The manoeuvre is now used infrequently as it may cause pain if not performed gently. Other diagnostic tests such as ultrasound scans may elicit more detailed information.

Lateral palpation This is carried out to locate the fetal back. The midwife turns to face the woman's face. One hand is placed flat on one side of the abdomen to steady it whilst the other hand gently palpates down the other side of the abdomen. The process is then reversed. The fetal back is felt as a continuous smooth resistant object, whereas the limbs are noted as small irregularities which are often felt to move. If the firm outline of the back cannot be easily palpated and fetal limbs are felt on both sides of the midline, the position is probably occipitoposterior. In this case a small depression on the abdomen just below the umbilicus may be noticed.

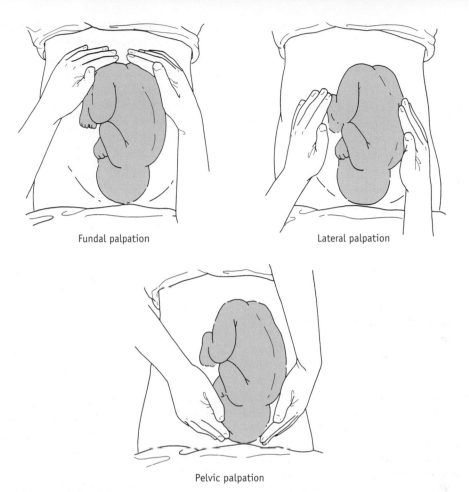

Fundal palpation

Lateral palpation

Pelvic palpation

Figure 16.11 Palpation of the abdomen.

Auscultation This can be done with the Pinard mon-aural fetal stethoscope or the binaural stethoscope, and/or with an electronic fetal heart monitor. Ideally the midwife should use the Pinard, and then the electronic monitor, as the means of monitoring the heartbeat are different, and the former is more likely to identify a true fetal heartbeat (Gibb and Arulkumaran, 1997). Having palpated the abdomen, the midwife should know where to listen for the fetal heart sounds, which are heard at their maximum at a point over the fetal shoulder. When the fetus is lying in an occipitoanterior or occipitolateral position the heart sounds are heard from the front and to the right or left according to the side on which the fetal back lies (Fig. 16.12). The fetal heart sounds like the ticking of a watch under a pillow, the rate being about double that of the woman's heartbeats observed at the wrist. The woman and her partner usually enjoy listening to their baby's heartbeat too.

A uterine souffle, caused by the flowing of blood through the uterine arteries, may be heard; this is a

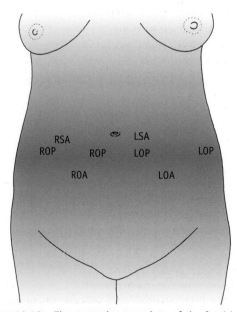

Figure 16.12 The approximate points of the fetal heart sounds in vertex and breech presentations.

soft, blowing sound, the rate of which corresponds to the woman's pulse.

Abdominal findings throughout pregnancy

At first only the height of the fundus is ascertained.

- *Week 12* (sometimes earlier): The fundus is just palpable above the symphysis.
- *Week 16*: The fundus is halfway to the umbilicus. At this stage a multigravida may have felt fetal movements.
- *Week 20*: The fundus reaches the lower border of the umbilicus and all women should be asked about movements. Fetal heart sounds may be audible.
- *Week 24*: The fundus reaches the upper border of the umbilicus, the fetus may just be palpable and the fetal heart sounds are heard.
- *Week 28*: The fundus of the uterus is one-third of the distance from the umbilicus to the xiphisternum. The fetus is now easily palpable, very mobile and may be found in any lie, presentation or position.
- *Week 32*: The uterus is two-thirds of the distance from the umbilicus to the xiphisternum. The fetus lies longitudinally and, usually, the head presents. If the midwife finds a breech presentation, she should refer the woman to a doctor. It may be decided to turn the fetus, though the doctor will probably want to wait to see whether it turns spontaneously.
- *Week 34*: The uterus extends nearly as far as the xiphisternum. Almost always the lie is longitudinal; usually the presentation is cephalic. If the breech presents then external cephalic version may be attempted or left to term.
- *Week 36*: The fundus reaches the xiphisternum. The presentation should be cephalic. In a primigravida the head may be engaged or engagement may occur a little later. If the head is engaged the fundus will be lower, at about the level of a 34-week pregnancy, and the woman will have experienced 'lightening'.
- *Weeks 37–40*: The findings will all be similar except that the fetus becomes more stable and the amount of liquor diminishes slightly.

The midwife must observe the woman carefully for signs of supine hypotensive syndrome during abdominal examinations, especially as pregnancy advances and the weight of the uterus increases.

Engagement of the fetal head

There is a popular myth that engagement of the head occurs at 36 weeks in a primigravida. In about 50% of primigravidae, engagement of the head occurs between 38 and 42 weeks (Weekes and Flynn, 1975), and in 80% of cases labour ensues within 14 days of the head engaging. In multigravidae, because of lax uterine and abdominal muscles, engagement may not take place until established labour. If the head is engaged, the pelvic brim is certainly of adequate size and the probability is that the cavity and outlet are also adequate.

Engagement is often referred to as *lightening*, because the sense of lightness women feel as the pressure is lessened on the diaphragm. In some women the head may not be engaged at term. This may be due to a full bladder or rectum or an occipitoposterior position where the presenting part tends to be deflexed. A steep angle of inclination of the pelvic brim tends to delay engagement until labour is well established. This is seen more commonly as a racial characteristic in West African and West Indian women.

If the head is high, an ultrasound scan may be performed to detect placenta praevia. It is difficult to determine cephalopelvic disproportion prior to labour because of the factors involved in labour itself.

Following this examination the findings are recorded and implications discussed with the woman.

Reflective Activity 16.8

Ask a pregnant woman what it felt like when her abdomen was palpated.

When you are present at an antenatal examination, observe the verbal and non-verbal communication that occurs between the mother and the midwife, and consider how this could be improved.

ANTENATAL RECORDS

Contemporaneous, accurate and complete records must be made of all antenatal examinations and other relevant information and should be signed and dated by the midwife. The Midwives Rules require a midwife to: 'keep as contemporaneously as is reasonable detailed records of observations, care given, and medicines or other forms of pain relief administered by her' (UKCC, 1998: 18; NMC, 2002). Records also ensure good communication between healthcare professionals and those they care for. One of the recommendations from *Changing Childbirth* (DoH, 1993) was that providers should make the necessary arrangements to ensure that all women were able to carry their own notes if they so wished. This would empower women and would increase health professionals consciousness of the language used and the content of these 'shared notes'. A recent study in New South Wales found that when women-held records were introduced into an antenatal clinic, those retaining their records were more likely to report feeling in control during their pregnancy, whereas those holding a small abbreviated card (similar to the old maternity cooperation card) were more likely to feel anxious, helpless and less likely to have information in their records explained to them (Homer *et al.*, 1999).

In some NHS trusts, antenatal notes continue to be rather cumbersome for women to carry around. A national maternity record has been devised (Harden, 1997). Standardized notes will provide continuity, convenience and safety, for women and the care team, without repetition of information for those moving home or needing care whilst on holiday. This would also provide the basis for standardizing information used for auditing, which would help in planning effective use of resources.

BIRTH/CARE PLANS

The structure of the maternity notes tends to follow a medical model; however, women should identify and discuss their own wishes for their pregnancy and birth through formulating a birth or care plan. During the 1970s, medical interventions in childbirth were growing and birth plans were seen by women as one way to regain some of the control which had been lost through birthing in hospital. These can be a useful communication tool for women and should be encouraged even though there is some evidence they do not improve control (Too, 1996; Whitford and Hillan, 1998). Too (1996) suggests women need to be educated about empowerment in order to be able to negotiate their own needs, and the midwife is well placed to initiate this. Discussion antenatally about what the woman would like to include will often avoid the wishes of the woman being ignored in labour. This can be reviewed at both antenatal visits and at parenting classes where broader discussion can take place.

Information is a fundamental part of making informed choices, and decisions must be discussed and agreed in partnership (DoH, 1993). Many trusts now recognize their relevance and birth plans are now commonly included in maternity records, and should be read and acknowledged by all practitioners involved in the woman's care. Ideally, a birth plan should incorporate the whole episode of care from antenatal to postnatal period, as this provides a useful forum for the woman and midwife to discuss the woman's total package of needs and how these can be met within the constraints of the service. This discussion is a useful educational opportunity, as for many women this may be the first opportunity to discuss issues around pregnancy and birth, and some misconceptions and 'old wives tales' can be dispelled.

WOMEN WITH SPECIAL NEEDS

Ethnic minority groups

Perinatal mortality rates are increased in infants of women from many ethnic minority groups. For example, the perinatal mortality rate in the UK in 2001 was 7.6 per 1000 births, but for babies born to mothers whose country of origin was India it was 10.7/1000, Bangladesh 9.1/1000, and for Pakistan 4.7/1000 (ONS, 2001). The antenatal care for these women therefore needs to be tailored to meet their special needs and particular problems.

Communication is one of the major problems as many women from ethnic minority groups do not speak English, or their language is very limited. These women may bring an English-speaking relative to the clinic with them, often their husband or a child, but this is not an ideal solution as sometimes the relative only interprets what he or she considers most important, misunderstandings may occur, and there is no confidentiality for the woman. One study conducted concluded that the changes Asian women considered most necessary in antenatal care were the presence of an interpreter and the need for a female doctor (Narang and Murphy, 1994). Health education and explanatory leaflets should be available in antenatal clinics in appropriate languages for non-English-speaking women. Some areas have employed link workers, or patient advocates; others have a list of healthcare workers who speak different languages. The challenges to providing appropriate and sensitive midwifery care are increasing with an increasing number of refugees and asylum seekers (McLeish, 2002).

Diet is a problem for some ethnic groups, as certain foods which are of high nutritional value may be avoided in pregnancy. Many Asian women are vegetarians and, although a good vegetarian diet can be very nutritious, not all women can access a good mixed diet. The midwife needs to discuss diet carefully and give dietary advice which is acceptable and practical for women of different cultures.

Certain health problems are more prevalent in West Indian, African, Asian or Mediterranean women and special investigations may be necessary in pregnancy. For example, *sickle cell anaemia* may be found in those who originate from Central and West Africa and parts of Asia, while *thalassaemia* may occur in those of Mediterranean origin. These inherited disorders vary in clinical severity and may have potentially crippling and serious complications. Prophylactic medication, knowledge of the condition, proper crisis intervention and expert management can help alleviate some of the complications. Screening enables potential parents to be alert to the disorders and to make informed choices. The Department of Health (2000b) have recommended that a national screening programme be introduced by 2004. Research is needed to develop information protocols that can deliver statistics on the coverage of screening and establish the incidence of haemoglobinopathies (Zeuner *et al.*, 1999).

Anaemia due to hookworm infestation or malaria may arise in some women from the African continent and other parts of the world. Infectious conditions such as tuberculosis and HIV are also more prevalent in many overseas countries.

Parent education classes tend to be poorly attended by women from ethnic minority groups, largely because of the language problem. Other women in the extended family tend to have a major influence on preparing younger members of the family for childbirth and parenthood. Some women from ethnic minority groups may be isolated because their family are still in their country of origin. Midwives therefore need to offer support and parent education on a one-to-one basis or in small groups. Women who have not been in the UK long may find this more individualized approach more acceptable and less embarrassing. Partners from some ethnic minority groups consider that support during pregnancy and childbirth is the role of women in the family and tend not to become too involved. It may be helpful for other female members of the family to be involved in preparation for childbirth and parenthood sessions too, so that they can support the pregnant woman appropriately. Although women from ethnic minorities may have particular difficulties, it is important not to make assumptions on the basis of their ethnic group, but to make an effort to establish their individual needs.

Disabled women

An increasing number of women with physical or sensory disabilities are choosing to have children; although statistics are not readily available, disabled women are more visible in the maternity system. Such women may have special problems, not only because of their disability, but also due to the negative reactions, prejudice or ignorance of some professionals, as well as members of their families. Many people are concerned about how they are going to cope with a child and underestimate the parenting abilities and determination of women with disabilities, focusing on the disability. In a report by the Maternity Alliance (1994) the chief complaint identified by disabled women was that there was insensitive, inadequate and insufficient understanding of the nature of their disability in relation to pregnancy.

Attending a busy antenatal clinic may be very difficult, if not impossible, for some women with major physical disabilities because of the problems of travel and access when they are there. Steps, small cubicles and having to move around from one area to another, climb on and off a couch and cope with a variety of different examinations and professionals may make the visit very difficult. Consideration needs to be given to the hospital environment and the accessibility of the maternity unit. Adjustable equipment will increase the independence of disabled women; therefore the right equipment and forward planning are crucial. Accessible cots, easy to use beds, baths and showers may be helpful. Some may feel disempowered by others taking over tasks for them which they are able to do with assistance (Thomas and Curtis, 1997).

Midwives should be aware of local resources and locate relevant assistance as early as possible. Help from social services may be required to provide support for the woman with the care of her baby and to make any adaptations to her home. Under the Disability Discrimination Act 1995 it is unlawful for service providers to discriminate against those with a disability by failing to make alterations to a facility, without which it may be unreasonably difficult or impossible for them to use the service.

Those with physical conditions will need care specific to their needs. Existing medication may need to be reviewed in the light of the pregnancy. Those with spinal cord injuries, or with limited mobility may be more predisposed to urinary infection and pressure sores as pregnancy advances.

Those with *hearing disabilities* may need special help (Nolan, 1994a) and there are several points to consider when caring for deaf women are as follows:

- Most deaf people lip-read, and so it is important to ensure that the speaker's mouth is clearly visible to the woman at all times and that light is sufficient.

- When talking, lip patterns may alter if the speaker speaks too loudly or softly.
- Key words should be written down, and pregnancy and birth vocabulary should be expressed in simple and clear terms.
- Written information and visual aids are particularly helpful to those who are deaf and should be used as much as possible to support verbal explanations.
- A sign language interpreter should also be available at the clinic when the woman attends for her appointments (Kelsall, 1993). The midwife addresses communications to the woman, however, and not to the interpreter.
- It is also important that the woman has her hands free for sign language. Certain procedures, e.g. blood pressure measurement, may hamper this, and the woman should be given time to communicate.
- Special equipment may be obtained such as baby alarms with flashing lights to alert the mother to the baby's cry (Kelsall, 1993).

Visually impaired women also need special help during the antenatal period, especially finding their way around a busy clinic and on and off an examination couch, and working out safe effective ways of caring for the baby. Points to consider when caring for a blind person, include (Fry, 1994; Nolan, 1994b):

- Introduce yourself, tell the woman what you are doing and where you have put things.
- Initiating interaction may be difficult – using touch and the person's name may help.
- Listening may be very tiring – be concise.
- The woman may have difficulty in assessing her need for body space as her abdomen enlarges.
- Ultrasound pictures will not be visible; the woman may be encouraged to palpate her own abdomen.
- Tactile models should be provided for parent education.
- A labour ward visit to handle equipment and become familiar with the layout of the area may be useful.
- Consider home birth.
- Skin-to-skin contact after the birth may facilitate maternal–infant interaction.
- The midwife could describe to the parents the baby's facial expression and aspects of the examination.
- A note might be placed on the door asking everyone to announce themselves on entering and leaving.
- The use of slings or backpacks enables the woman to have her hands free for dogs or canes.

One-to-one midwifery care from a very small group of midwives is most helpful for women with disabilities,

providing an opportunity to build up a relationship of trust and partnership. Like able-bodied women, they have the right to be fully informed and make choices related to their care (Nolan, 1994b), and need information and strategies for successful and responsible parenting. Options should include choice regarding place of birth, antenatal testing, delivery positions and postnatal support. Antenatal screening should be approached sensitively with awareness and understanding of inherited and non-inherited disabilities, and if an abnormality is detected the midwife should support the woman in reaching her own informed decision (RCM, 2000b).

The extent of the woman's disabilities and how she normally manages should be carefully assessed, so that appropriate strategies can be developed to cope in labour and with the care of the baby afterwards. The woman is the expert in her disability and midwives can learn from her how to adapt care to make it appropriate and as comfortable as possible for her. Providing antenatal care in the woman's own home is more relaxing for the woman, and provides the midwife with an opportunity to see how she manages in her own surroundings and assess her ability to manage with a newborn baby.

Parent education must be flexible, creative and accessible and should involve partners wherever possible. Some physically disabled women may wish to attend the usual parent education classes, but others find their disability highlighted in contrast to others and would prefer to have education provided at home. The midwife needs to assess the woman carefully and devise effective ways of helping her to develop safe and appropriate parenting skills. For the visually handicapped learning by touch is effective and models to handle can be helpful (Nolan, 1994b). Audiocassettes can also be used to support the spoken word. Those who are deaf appreciate visual aids, including demonstrations, videos, slides, films and also written information. A visit to the unit may be helpful. Care in labour will need to take account of the woman's needs, e.g. pethidine and Entonox may affect a deaf woman's powers of observation.

Postnatally, mothers may need extra support. They may feel humiliated and a nuisance by having to ask for help all the time, and fear that others may judge them to be inadequate mothers (Campion, 1997). The midwife may need to anticipate help which may be required.

Adaptations of health premises for use by disabled women may include the use of flashing lights and bells in a waiting room, ramps and more extensive use of signs in Braille. Parking spaces for disabled drivers should be clearly signposted. The Disability Discrimination Act 1995 states that every reasonable action should be taken to provide any necessary equipment, facilities or services which are needed to ensure that reasonable care can be taken of the disabled person (Dimond, 2000).

Women should enjoy care from a midwife who is knowledgeable, respectful and sensitive. Care needs to be individualized and part of a partnership that aims to maintain a high degree of dignity, privacy and independence. Midwives also need to be proactive in improving the overall physical and psychological access to maternity services for women with special needs. Meeting the needs and aspirations of those who are disabled requires extra skill, insight and imagination but is especially rewarding when the outcome is successful.

Reflective Activity 16.9

Consider your own attitudes and beliefs about women with disabilities becoming pregnant.

How would you plan care for a disabled woman in your area of practice, and what facilities are available in your unit to accommodate those with a physical disability?

Compile information from different sources in order that you could advise women, and increase your own awareness of physical, visual and auditory disabilities. Make sure that you have telephone and contact numbers.

Teenage pregnancies

In England there are nearly 90 000 conceptions a year to teenagers, with around 56 000 babies (60% of conceptions) born. Although more than two-thirds of under-16s do not have sex and most teenage girls reach their 20s without getting pregnant, the UK has teenage birth rates which are twice as high as in Germany, three times as high as in France and six times as high as in the Netherlands (SEU, 1999).

Young women experiencing an unplanned pregnancy are faced with a decision that can affect the rest of their lives. A study undertaken by the Joseph Rowntree Foundation between 1997–1999 found that decisions about continuing with, or ending an unplanned teenage pregnancy were shaped by a range of factors including the prevalence and visibility of teenage motherhood within the local area and community-wide views on the unacceptability of abortion (Tabberer et al., 1999).

Truancy, low academic achievement and poor sex education were all factors implicated in the high teenage pregnancy rates and this may also be linked to a high level of poor social, economic and health outcomes for both mother and child (NHSCRD, 1997). The midwife should avoid stereotyping teenagers, as for many, pregnancy is welcomed and a positive experience without the long-term negative outcomes.

The Government's White Paper *Health of the Nation* (DoH, 1992c) strategy identified prevention of pregnancy in girls under 16-years-old as a priority area with a target to reduce the rate of conceptions from 9.6 per 1000 in 1989 to 4.8 per 1000. Most recent figures show that the rate of conception in under-16-year-olds is 8.3 per 1000 (NHSCRD, 1997).

Sweden, Norway, Germany and the Netherlands have considerably lower teenage conception rates than those in the UK and all have an earlier and more open approach to sex education in schools (Scott et al., 1995). In the Netherlands there appears to be greater discussion between partners, more effective contraceptive use, later age at first sexual intercourse and lower levels of subsequent regret (Stammers and Ingham, 2000). The experiences of other northern European countries suggest that where teenagers are encouraged to recognize their developing sexuality at an early age and have access to contraception and sex education there are reduced rates of pregnancy, abortion and sexually transmitted diseases (Nolan, 1998).

The World Health Organization (WHO, 1989) clarified the goal that Britain amongst other countries should be aiming for:

> These young men and women are or will become the parents of the next generation and must be given every opportunity to develop to their full potential as healthy children and to avoid the dangers to themselves and to society of having children too young and too often.

One aspect of the midwife's role (UKCC, 1998) is to provide sound family planning advice, and this can be achieved by providing the necessary support, information and educational links for the adolescent (Dolby, 1998).

A number of studies have shown that good antenatal care is associated with improved pregnancy outcomes for teenagers as well as older women (McVeigh and Smith, 2000). Although most teenage mothers experience normal births, they are more likely to encounter adverse pregnancy outcomes such as low birthweight, perinatal death and pregnancy-induced hypertension

(Adelson *et al.*, 1992). They are also not as attuned to understanding behavioural cues from their babies, which can affect adaptation to motherhood.

After the birth the postpartum period is a time of rediscovery and of self-rebuilding (Hartrick, 1997). Meeting the demands of the newborn baby is challenging. There may also be social isolation, and health professionals must identify the teenager's individual needs and plan with those in mind.

This group have differing needs from traditional models: they are less likely to be in a stable relationship, are likely to be less positive about their pregnancy and lack social support (Culp *et al.*, 1988). Through appropriate and tailored parenting sessions, the midwife can offer social support, help develop a peer group network, and bring an element of realism to the pregnancy.

Midwives need knowledge of national and local organizations available to support pregnant teenagers and young parents. The Teenage Parenthood Network publishes a quarterly newsletter giving useful information about resources, groups and study opportunities. *The Really Helpful Directory* is produced in collaboration with the Trust for the Study of Adolescence, and gives information on residential and non-residential projects for pregnant teenagers and young parents across the UK.

HELPING WOMEN TO COPE WITH PREGNANCY CHANGES

Most women experience some of the so-called 'minor disorders' of pregnancy and may accept these disorders as normal 'symptoms' of pregnancy. These may be 'minor' in that they are not life-threatening, but they may be a major source of discomfort, anxiety and have *long-term morbidity*. The woman may need to cope with these disorders while continuing to work and care for her family, often having to look after other children while experiencing fatigue and discomfort. Advice on how to relieve these disorders may be sought from the midwife or doctor. Occasionally serious conditions may develop from minor disorders. The midwife needs to be alert for these and refer to medical aid where complications arise (UKCC, 1998).

Problems associated with the gastrointestinal tract

The mouth

Like all tissues with a large connective tissue component, the gums swell in pregnancy and become spongy.

Gingival oedema is not harmful but may lead to gingivitis (Hytten, 1990). As the gums may bleed, the use of a soft toothbrush is advised and the midwife should recommend regular dental care during pregnancy, which is free during pregnancy and for the year following childbirth.

Nausea and vomiting

Nausea and vomiting are common disorders affecting up to 80% of pregnant women. One study found 28% of women reported nausea and 52% reported both nausea and vomiting (Gadsby *et al.*, 1993). Lacroix *et al.* (2000) found that 74% of the pregnant population experienced nausea and vomiting from the 3rd week of pregnancy, with the median onset at 5 weeks. Nausea lasted for a mean of 34.6 days with a range of up to 114 days. Nausea had resolved by 14 weeks' gestation for 50% of the women, and for 90% of women by 22 weeks' gestation.

The aetiology is unclear; postulated theories include rising human chorionic gonadotrophin levels; and various sociocultural factors including age, parity, women with less education (Klebanoff *et al.*, 1985). It has been reported as occurring more frequently in westernized countries and rare in some African, Native American, Eskimo and Asian populations, except for Japan (Broussard and Richter, 1998).

Various remedies are available for the relief of nausea and vomiting, ranging from diet modification, rest, exercise and fresh air (O'Brien *et al.*, 1997), acupressure, treatment with pyridoxine (vitamin B_6), or antiemetics. In a review of interventions, it was highlighted that though antiemetics reduce the frequency of nausea, there are usually side-effects. Pyridoxine appears to reduce the severity of nausea, and treatment with acupressure gave 'equivocal' results (Jewell and Young, 2002). See Chapters 20 and 43.

Heartburn

Heartburn, experienced as a painful retrosternal burning sensation, commonly occurs in pregnancy. If persistent, it may be a symptom of reflux oesophagitis, resulting from the regurgitation of acidic stomach contents. This may be due to the effects of progesterone relaxing the lower oesophageal (cardiac) sphincter. Reflux may be related to a reduced 'barrier' pressure between the stomach and the lower oesophageal sphincter pressure (Ogerek and Cohen, 1989). Hytten (1990) suggests the decreased response to raised intra-abdominal pressure may allow the sphincter to become incompetent and displace into the thorax, resulting in hiatus hernia. Dodds *et al.* (1978) discount the theory that heartburn is caused by upward pressure from the uterus.

The woman should be advised to eat small, frequent meals, and avoid spicy or fatty foods and very cold liquids. Smoking, alcohol, coffee and chocolate may increase gastrointestinal irritation, as may eating before bedtime (Brucker, 1988; Larson *et al.*, 1997). An upright posture and avoiding lying down after meals may be helpful. Nocturnal heartburn may be alleviated by sleeping propped up with extra pillows.

Where simple measures are ineffective, referral to a doctor may be necessary (UKCC, 1998). In an early review, Jewell (1993) states that simple antacids can relieve heartburn, though 20–50% of the women studied by Shaw (1978) failed to gain substantial benefit from antacids. Larson *et al.* (1997) reported significant improvement of symptoms in women where conventional management was unsuccessful. In this small study, women taking ranitidine 150 mg twice daily showed improvement in symptoms compared with ranitidine 150 mg once daily or giving a placebo. This trial offers hope for the management of gastrointestinal reflux but would benefit from repetition with a larger study group. With the increased interest in alternative health therapies, the expectant woman may wish to use Shiatsu or homeopathic remedies for heartburn.

Constipation

Constipation during pregnancy is caused by the general sluggishness and decreased peristalsis of the colon due to the relaxation of plain muscle by progesterone. The problem may be compounded by increased water absorption from the colon, probably due to the increased levels of aldosterone and angiotensin (Hytten, 1990).

Constipation can be overcome by adjusting the diet, adding extra fluid, fruit, vegetables and bran cereal. Iron supplements may aggravate the problem and the supplement may need to be changed to an alternative.

If constipation persists, bran or wheat fibre supplements may be used. These absorb water and swell in the gastrointestinal tract, softening and giving bulk to the stool, and therefore the fluid intake should be increased. Though initially a bowel action may take a few days to occur, these supplements will often increase the frequency of defecation (Jewell and Young, 2001).

Liquid paraffin may interfere with the absorption of fat-soluble vitamins A and D and is rarely used, if at all. Senna preparations stimulate peristalsis and act in 8–12 hours but may cause abdominal pain and discomfort and are often badly tolerated by the pregnant woman. Lactulose is a hyperosmotic, causing an increase in fluid accumulation in the stool, distension, peristalsis and evacuation which may take up to 48 hours to act.

Laxatives should be a short-term treatment and used with information and education on dietary measures to prevent reoccurrence of constipation. The use of Shiatsu and abdominal massage for the treatment of constipation is discussed in Chapter 20.

Vaginal candidiasis (thrush)

Vaginal candidiasis (monilia or thrush) is a common yeast-like infection of the mucous membrane of the vagina caused by the organism *Candida albicans*. It occurs more frequently during pregnancy. The woman may experience a range of signs and symptoms:

- itching of the vulva and vagina
- soreness or burning of the vulva
- oedema of the vulva and vagina
- increased white non-offensive vaginal discharge
- characteristic white plaques of *Candida albicans* in the vagina or on the vulva.

The woman may be used to managing the condition for herself and be aware of the self-help measures available, which include:

- daily hygiene using simple unperfumed soap, bathing the vulva gently with lukewarm water
- avoiding wearing nylon underwear, tights or tightly fitting jeans
- wiping the vulval area from front to back after using the toilet, to minimize the opportunity of transferring the infection from the bowel
- taking Acidophilus tablets, a herbal treatment to increase the intestinal flora of *Acidophilus lactobacillus* and *Acidophilus bifidus*
- ensuring concurrent treatment of sexual partner as appropriate.

A review of topical medical treatments and trials comparing imidazole and nystatin suggested that topical imidazole seemed to be more effective than nystatin, and that 4-day courses would cure just over half the infections and a 7-day course would cure 90% of infections. Though pregnant women need longer courses of treatment than the non-pregnant, courses of over 7 days were indicated to be of no further benefit (Young and Jewell, 2001).

Skin changes in pregnancy

Skin pigmentation

Increased pigmentation of the skin is very common in pregnancy, occurring in up to 90% of pregnant women (Fitzpatrick *et al.*, 1999). The cause is uncertain, but skin changes may be due to increased oestrogen, progesterone, adrenal hormones, beta-endorphins or an increase in melanocyte-stimulating hormone (Blackburn, 2003). The face, nipples, areola, vulva, perineum and perianal region commonly darken. The tendinous middle line of the linea alba, running from the umbilicus to the symphysis pubis on the anterior abdominal wall, frequently pigments to become the linea nigra. This fades after childbirth but may never completely disappear. Freckles, naevi and scars on the abdomen may also darken. This pigmentation may be more noticeable in dark-haired, dark-complexioned women.

Striae gravidarum 'stretch marks'

Striae gravidarum may appear as red-purple linear streaks on the breasts, abdomen, thighs and buttocks, as the tension within the dermal skin layer is increased. These striae fade to silver after pregnancy. One review highlighted an RCT assessing the use of Trofolastin (a topical cream containing extract of *Centella asiatica*, alpha-tocopherol and collagen hydrolysates) in the prevention of striae gravidarum. The findings indicated that this might be useful in protecting against stretch marks developing in primigravid women, though benefit was limited to those who had previously developed striae during puberty. No significant benefit was found for multiparous women (Mallol *et al.*, 1991). Further research is needed to identify the active ingredient(s), or any potentially adverse effects (Young and Jewell, 2000a). At present this cream is only available in Spain.

Pruritus gravidarum – cholestasis of pregnancy

Pruritus gravidarum is intense itching that occurs without a rash or jaundice in late pregnancy. Itching occurs in about 17% of pregnant women (Fitzpatrick *et al.*, 1999) and may be caused by scabies, pediculosis, urticaria, atopic eczema, thrush, trichomonal infections or related to drug therapy (Jones and Black, 2002). When these causes have been excluded about 0.2–0.4% women continue to suffer from pruritus, due to an alteration in hepatic function. Black and Mayou (1995) suggested that in genetically susceptible women, normal levels of oestrogen and progesterone interfere with hepatic excretion of bile acids which then accumulate in the skin to cause pruritus. It is thought that this is a mild form of cholestasis of pregnancy. Serum alkaline phosphatase and transaminase levels may be raised, and bilirubin levels may be normal or slightly increased. Where cholestasis of pregnancy is suspected, the midwife should refer the woman for consultant care, as morbidity and mortality to woman and fetus may be increased (UKCC, 1998).

Pruritus gravidarum may be generalized or localized to the abdomen. Calamine lotion may give relief of itching in mild conditions; more severe cases may respond to antihistamine tablets, which may be prescribed by the doctor. Occasionally the condition may be so severe that the woman needs care from a consultant obstetrician as preterm delivery is indicated. The condition usually resolves spontaneously after childbirth but may recur in subsequent pregnancies, or with the use of oral contraceptive tablets (Jones and Black, 2002).

Varicose veins

Varicosities may develop in 40% of women. These are usually seen in the veins of the legs, but may also occur in the vulva and the anal area as haemorrhoids. The effects of progesterone and relaxin act on the smooth muscles of the vein walls, and the increased weight of the growing uterus also contributes to the increased risk of valvular incompetence. A family tendency is also a factor (Blackburn, 2003). Varicosities may also be associated with leg oedema, and either or both disorders may contribute to women feeling discomfort, pain, and a negative body image.

A review indicated that *rutosides* may relieve symptoms, though the safety of this during pregnancy is not known. The use of immersion in water was suggested as a means of reducing oedema, though again the long-term benefits were not clear (Young and Jewell, 2000b).

Other measures may be more helpful, such as keeping the legs elevated when at rest, increasing rest periods, exercise, such as walking and swimming, and working to avoid excessive weight gain. Some women may find support tights helpful, but constricting or tight clothing should be avoided.

The musculoskeletal system

The physiological changes of pregnancy affect the musculoskeletal system, frequently causing pain and discomfort.

Low back pain

Low back pain occurs frequently in pregnancy as progesterone and relaxin cause softening and relaxation of the ligaments of the pelvis. The weight of the pregnant uterus and the altered posture (compensatory lordosis) are likely to increase back strain, leading to pain. Sacroiliac joint relaxation may cause pain in the back, lower abdomen or radiating down the legs (Heckmann and Sassard, 1994).

Back pain may be reduced by limiting physical activity, alteration of posture, wearing low-heeled shoes and adequate rest in bed. Supportive pillows beneath the knees and abdomen and local application of heat may relieve pain. The use of an Ozzlo pillow was also found to be more helpful than the use of ordinary pillows (Young and Jewell, 2002a). Lying on the back with the feet elevated and supported approximately 60 cm above the hips for 20 minutes four times a day may relieve muscle spasm, decrease lumbar lordosis and reduce pain (Heckmann and Sassard, 1994).

Women commonly attempt to get up from a lying position by raising themselves from their back without using their arms for support. Back strain may be reduced by the midwife advising the woman to turn onto her side, and sit up as she swings her legs down from the couch/bed. A physiotherapist may teach the woman back and abdominal muscle exercises to strengthen these muscles, or apply a sacroiliac or trochanteric support (see Ch. 23). The doctor may prescribe oral analgesia, having considered the suitability of the different drugs and their effect upon the fetus. Alternative therapies to relieve back pain are discussed in Chapter 20.

Cramp

Leg cramps, usually occurring at night or in the early morning, are reported in 50% of pregnant women, and occur more frequently after 24 weeks (Blackburn, 2003). Causes are unclear, though may be linked to degree of activity, and these are more common in more sedentary women, but may be related to the changes in calcium and magnesium levels. Young and Jewell (2002b) could find no conclusive benefit in treating leg cramps with calcium, or in the use of multivitamin supplements. A single trial conducted in 1947 suggesting that sodium chloride is an effective treatment needs replication to assess whether this should be recommended; as Young and Jewell (2002b) state 'changes in dietary intake of sodium since that time may make these results less relevant'. Night cramp may be reduced by gentle leg exercises before going to bed; by

raising the foot of the bed 20–25 cm; and by dorsiflexion of the foot, and/or massage when it occurs.

Carpal tunnel syndrome

Compression of the median nerve in the wrist may lead to numbness, tingling and pain in the fingers, usually at night (Heckmann and Sassard, 1994). This usually occurs in the second and third trimesters of pregnancy. The physiotherapist may apply a lightweight splint to support the wrist, particularly at night. Heckmann and Sassard (1994), citing Wand (1990), state that the symptoms resolve completely and dramatically, often within days of delivery. Carpal tunnel syndrome may recur in subsequent pregnancies, and women who experience this may be more at risk of developing the syndrome in later life.

Reflective Activity 16.10

When you are next undertaking an antenatal clinic, make a note of which changes or disorders women seem to find most difficult to cope with. Consider the advice and information that is provided. Is it evidence based, and was the physiology discussed fully with the woman in a way she could understand?

How do you access the most information and advice for women?

Ensure that you have a personal list of local and national telephone and contact numbers of relevant helplines and self-help groups such as the SPD group.

Symphysis pubis pain

Symphysis pubis dysfunction (SPD) is the term used when the symphysis pubis joint is unable to perform its role in pelvic stabilization and impairs efficient weight bearing (Fry, 1999). This leads to pain, instability, and limitation of mobility and functioning of the pelvis. Many midwives and other health professionals are unaware of the condition or its longer-term effects, so the disabling and debilitating nature of SPD is often unrecognized. Practitioners may fail to appreciate that the woman may experience: difficulty in trying to care for her family, infant feeding problems, social isolation and depression or relationship difficulties, both during pregnancy and following childbirth.

Incidence of SPD

A diagnosis of SPD is dependent upon symptom recognition and clinical diagnosis. No national incidence has been identified but local statistics (Owens, Pearson and Mason, 2002) quoted an incidence of 1:36 in Leeds.

As midwives are the healthcare professional most likely to give continuity of care during pregnancy, labour or the puerperium (DoH, 1993) it is essential that they have the skills to recognise SPD and offer appropriate advice on its management. They need to understand how SPD affects the woman both physically and emotionally so that they may offer advice, information and moral support.

Where joint widening exceed 10 mm, this is considered abnormal and defined as symphysial separation, symphysis pubis diastasis, or symphysiolysis (Lindsey *et al.*, 1988). It is recognized that SPD occurs more frequently than diastasis, and is a cause of obstetric morbidity (Fry, 1999; Owens, Pearson and Mason, 2002; Wellock, 2002).

Pelvic pain and instability is not a new phenomenon. In 1870, Snelling described symphysis pubis relaxation thus:

> The affection appears to consist of a relaxation of the pelvic articulations, becoming apparent suddenly after parturition or gradually during pregnancy, and permitting of a degree of mobility of the pelvic bones which effectively hinders locomotion and gives rise to the most peculiar, distressing and alarming sensation. (p. 562)

It is acknowledged as an underrecognized and underdiagnosed condition (Scriven *et al.*, 1991, 1995; Taylor and Sonson, 1986). Many practitioners are unable to give optimum care as they are unaware of how SPS manifests or how disabling and debilitating the condition can be. With active treatment such as manual physiotherapy the symptoms may resolve in weeks or months; at worst, long-term morbidity may result from diastasis and necessitate surgical fixation of the symphysis pubis.

Incidence of diastasis

Where separation of the joint has been confirmed by X-ray or ultrasound the incidence ranges from one case in 300 (Kubitz and Goodlin, 1986) to one in 20 000 (Eastman and Hellman, 1966) in primigravidae and multigravidae. In the only UK study, Scriven, McKnight and Jones (1995), gave an incidence of 1:800.

Physiology of SPD

The onset of symptoms may be insidious during the second or third trimester, may be linked to a specific activity, or arise during or after delivery.

Essentially symptoms are due to instability of the symphysis pubis joint (Fig. 16.13). In the non-pregnant state, the circumferential envelope of ligaments at the joint, especially the inferior ligament, neutralizes the shearing forces on the joint allowing only minimal movement during activity. As the function of the pelvis is to transfer body weight to the legs all pelvic joints must be stable; any dysfunction in one joint will be reflected in the functioning of the others.

The literature from Gamble *et al.* (1986), Snelling (1870) through to Chamberlain (1991) and Heckman and Sassard (1994) suggests that hormonal influences are implicated in the aetiology of SPD. It has been suggested that during pregnancy the pelvic ligaments and cartilages relax in preparation for delivery under the influence of ovarian and placental hormones. Grieve (1976) noted that the normal 4–5 mm gap between the bone ends of the symphysis pubis may increase to as much as 9 mm. Gamble, Simmons and Freedman (1986) considered that enzymes, causing resorption of bone, contribute to the widening of the symphysis pubis, particularly in the third trimester. It has been suggested that high mean serum levels of relaxin are related to joint instability (Gamble, Simmons and Freedman, 1986; Chamberlain, 1991; Heckmann and Sassard, 1994), however, Peterson, Hvidman and Uldeberg (1994), Hansen *et al.* (1996) and Bjorklund *et al.* (2000) could not demonstrate this in their studies. Conversely, Kristiansson *et al.* (1996) suggested that relaxin is involved in the aetiology of symphysial, lumbar and sacral pain, and notes a positive correlation. Where hormonal influences have been implicated in the aetiology this may have led to a conservative approach to management in the belief that the condition will resolve spontaneously after delivery. More recently Damen *et al.* (2001) have demonstrated that where asymmetric laxity of the sacroiliac joints occurs, pelvic pain is increased. Where there is an underlying cause for pelvic and symphysial pain this may be relieved by treatment from a physiotherapist.

Symptoms experienced may include:

- Mild to severe groin/pubic pain that is increased by weight-bearing; pain may radiate to the medial aspect of the upper thigh(s). It may be described as a burning pain or bruised sensation in the symphysis pubis.
- A 'waddling' gait, 'dragging' of a leg.

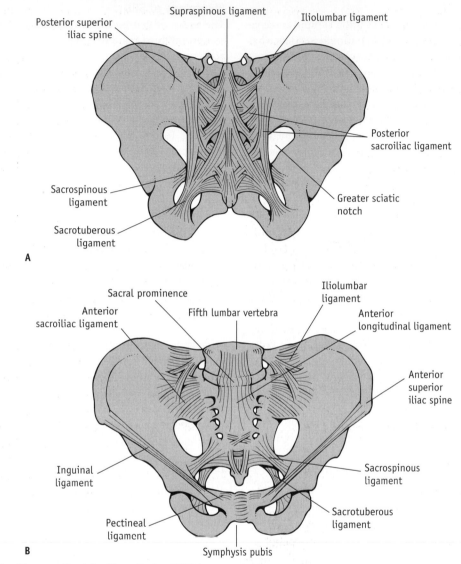

Figure 16.13 Diagram of pelvis. (From Yerby, 2000.)

- An audible or palpable 'click' and/or 'crunching' sensation felt in the joint.
- Low back pain.
- Pain on movements that involve standing on one leg such as dressing, getting in and out of the bath, climbing the stairs, or movement in bed.
- Pain on any activity that involves parting or lifting the legs such as reaching to open a window, getting in and out of the car, sexual intercourse.
- Pain on lifting and carrying any weight, e.g. baby, toddler, car seat or shopping.

It is not uncommon for explanations for these symptoms to be dismissed as 'aches and pains' of pregnancy,

round ligament strain, or urinary tract infection. Although the midwife should be alert for the two latter conditions they do not lead to the pain and limitation of function previously described.

Although it has been accepted in the literature that a separation of the symphysis pubis joint of less than 10 mm is asymptomatic but a diastasis of 10 mm or more will be symptomatic (Lindsey *et al.*, 1988), a woman can be symptomatic yet not have a demonstrable diastasis if X-rayed postnatally. Thus the term 'symphysis pubic dysfunction' denotes the symptoms experienced by the woman.

If confirmation of a diastasis is sought, ultrasound scanning using a 7.5 Mhz transducer offers a simple, relatively pain-free, procedure that does not involve ionizing radiation (Scriven *et al.*, 1995).

X-ray examination is unlikely to be performed to avoid irradiation of the gonads, however, if it is performed, a 'stork' X-ray is necessary to confirm diastasis by showing vertical shift when standing on one leg.

Traditionally diastasis has been related to traumatic or instrumental deliveries, which are still found in the literature (Kowalk, 1996; Lindsey *et al.*, 1988; Musumeci, 1994), or is associated with excessive forced hip abduction (Callaghan, 1953; Cappiello, 1995; Gherman, 1998; Kharrazi *et al.*, 1997). Cephalo-pelvic disproportion, previous or existing pelvic abnormality and multiparity are also recognized (Lindsey *et al.*, 1988). Where trauma at delivery is involved symphysial pain is usually immediately apparent. However, Driessen (1987) noted that women who have had uncomplicated, spontaneous vaginal deliveries of average weight babies have reported symptoms 12–24 hours postpartum. The reasons for this are unclear.

Driessen (1987) noted similar later onset (1–2 days) in his small study in Malawi and postulated that this was due to gradual swelling within the joint, which could account for the delay in onset. This highlights the need for the midwife to be alert for women who complain of unusually severe pain with difficulty in mobilizing postnatally that is not attributable to perineal pain.

Management of SPD

Antenatal   The aim is to limit stress on the pelvic joints, reduce pain and instigate prompt treatment. As symptoms are increased by activities such as housekeeping, walking and working (Hansen *et al.*, 1999), pain may be relieved by reducing these activities. The woman may need to rest the symphysis pubis joint. She should be encouraged to stop carrying out non-essential activities and accept offers of help with housework, childcare and shopping. Prolonged weightbearing, climbing the stairs, standing on one leg, for example, when dressing, and twisting movements of her back should all be avoided. It is also essential that she avoids abducting her hips and keeps her legs as close together as is comfortable in activities such as getting in and out of a car and turning in bed. When resting, placing a pillow between the legs and keeping the knees in apposition may be beneficial. If a shower is available this is less traumatic than a bath.

A clear explanation to both the woman and her partner of the condition and its management is vital. The explanation should avoid the use of alarming words such as 'split', 'separated' or 'broken' pelvis (ACPWH, 2000); emphasis on pelvic joint asymmetry is preferable and less frightening.

The foregoing advice and change in lifestyle can be difficult and frustrating for some women to follow but experience has shown that these strategies can noticeably reduce symptoms. However, if symptoms do not subside appreciably the woman should be referred to a specialist physiotherapist for a full pelvic and back assessment and treatment of any underlying pelvic misalignment. A pelvic support belt or a trochanteric support belt may give relief of pain but will not correct any underlying pelvic asymmetry. Where weightbearing is painful the use of elbow crutches can maintain mobility while reducing strain on the pelvis. Appropriate analgesia should be offered and prescribed.

A plan of management should be formulated for care during labour. This will require good communication between all members of the team caring for the woman both antenatally and postnatally.

Labour   The woman and her labour partner will need to be aware of the choices for pain relief and positioning during labour. Water may afford pain relief as it relieves weightbearing and allows easy changing of position. Individual assessment of the woman's mobility and safety should be evaluated, if water is her choice. Involvement and clear information may help to reduce the fear and anxiety that may be experienced. Reassurance should be given that adequate pain relief is available if needed. In severe cases elective caesarean section may be undertaken.

Where vaginal delivery is anticipated the range of hip abduction should be measured and recorded in the notes prior to labour (McIntosh, 1993). Where possible, the woman should be placed in a position within her range of pain-free hip movement. Finding a position of comfort for the labouring woman may be difficult as her mobility can be severely limited but being mobile and upright may help some women to cope with labour. A lateral position is often preferable for vaginal examination. The midwife needs to be aware that although epidural or spinal anaesthesia offers valuable pain relief, both could mask the symptoms of symphysis pubis pain and allow excessive mobilization of the joint, leading to increased postpartum pain. Where epidural/spinal anaesthesia is required the midwife should ensure that the woman's range of pain-free hip abduction is not exceeded while the anaesthesia is effective. The partner's assistance may be required to keep her legs adducted during this time. Callaghan (1953) reported that diastasis occurred when forceful and excessive hip abduction was used and Cappiello (1995) noted that diastasis occurred with epidural anaesthesia and warned against the use of excessive hip abduction because of the potential consequences. Kharazzi *et al.* (1997) report three cases where excessive hip abduction in the lithotomy position with epidural anaesthesia resulted in diastasis.

During the second stage of labour a lateral position or a supported 'all fours' position will reduce strain on the symphysis pubis. If the lithotomy position is needed for forceps delivery or Ventouse extraction, the hips should be abducted simultaneously within the pain-free range of movement and maintained for as short a time as possible. Extreme pain is likely throughout the procedure. Ideally, vaginal examination, forceps delivery and suturing would be undertaken in a lateral position. The midwife should be aware that the forced abduction of the hips that occurs when a woman pushes, while her feet are placed upon the midwives' hips, could lead to symphysis pubis diastasis so it is essential that this practice is avoided.

Postnatal period Postnatal care is very similar to antenatal management. Referral to a physiotherapist will be necessary for assessment, advice and treatment. The mother may require complete bedrest and all physical care for 24–48 hours, or until acute pain subsides.

Assessment of risk factors that predispose to deep vein thrombosis (DVT) should be undertaken, TED stockings should be worn during bedrest and thromboprophylaxis initiated if appropriate (RCOG, 2002). Ankle, calf and leg exercises may help to prevent DVT. Recently, Whitby (2003) recounted her experience of facing death through pulmonary embolism following mismanaged SPD and Barbarinsa *et al.* (1999) report two deaths of women with SPD from pulmonary embolism. Education of the mother and vigilance by the midwife throughout the postnatal period is vital.

Assistance will be needed with personal hygiene, including taking the mother to the toilet in a wheelchair and instructing her not to sit astride the bidet. The midwife will need to assist with the baby's care, handling the baby to the mother for cuddles and giving help with feeding and changing. A comfortable position will need to be found for breastfeeding and assistance given with correct positioning. Mobilization within her own capability, with the aid of elbow crutches if necessary, is then encouraged to gradually increase her activities. Pain levels will be her guide to how much weightbearing she can undertake and analgesia should be offered regularly.

Transfer home Prior to transfer, the home circumstances need careful review. Information regarding the proximity of the bathroom, number of stairs, and help available from the partner, family and friends will be required. The mother may be housebound for some days or weeks, requiring substantial help in caring for the new baby and any other children. Although the use of elbow crutches alleviates pain, their use hinders all other activities as both arms are already employed. Whether crutches are used or not, the mother may be unable to lift or carry her new baby, needing to have the baby handed to her for feeding. Carrying the baby downstairs may be impractical because of pain, and the fear of falling or dropping the baby. Changing or bathing the baby may only be possible if a surface at waist height is available. Using a pram as a changing surface may be a practical solution. Where the mother is unable to walk or to drive, her dependence upon family or friends for social activities, shopping and taking siblings to playgroup or school increases. Assistance may be needed with household tasks such as loading and unloading the washing machine or dishwasher, ironing and cleaning. Activities that involve forward flexion and rotation of the back, such as pushing a vacuum cleaner, may provoke pain.

The mother may feel inadequate in caring for her family and experience social isolation and/or relationship difficulties and these factors may increase the likelihood of depression occurring. Shepherd (2003) in a study of women's experiences of SPD noted that five of the women experienced depression and one of these was referred with a possible diagnosis of post traumatic stress disorder (PTSD). Psychological effects may adversely affect mother–infant relationships, the emotional and intellectual development of the baby and other siblings, as well as personal relationships. Health professionals need to recognize antenatal and labour factors that lead to PND and PTSD and use screening tools such as the Edinburgh Postnatal Depression Scale (Cox *et al.*, 1997, 2003) and initiate referral and treatment.

A multidisciplinary, collaborative approach to community care may be required. Social services can advise upon benefits provision and entitlement to disability living allowance if the incapacity has exceeded 3 months. A temporary 'disabled' car badge may maintain some independence, enable attendance at appointments, access to shops and reduce social isolation. An occupational therapist may be able to give advice on energy conservation and planning daily activities to limit pain. Aids such as a bath board, raised toilet seat and a 'helping hand' gadget may be supplied.

When the mother does feel able to resume her routine she can be advised that the weight of a baby in a carry sling may provoke pain and therefore should be avoided. Placing the car seat in the car and then strapping the baby into it is more practical than attempting to lift the baby in the seat. Shops and supermarkets now offer designated mother and baby car parking, assistance with shopping and packing services, however Internet or telephone shopping may be a more viable alternative. If this is available, it enables the mother to feel less dependent on friends and relatives.

Recovery Whenever the condition occurs, a very clear explanation of the condition, treatment and prognosis will be required. Albert, Godskesen and Westergaard (2001), in a study of prognosis of pregnancy-related pelvic pain report that women with symphysis pubis pain and no other pelvic joint involvement had the best prognosis. No woman in this group experienced pain beyond 6 months, postpartum. The 8.6% of women in the study who experienced pain at 2 years postpartum had all had pain in all three pelvic joints, suggesting a different aetiology. Occasionally women report that, even when symptoms have subsided, symphysial pain may be felt premenstrually. In such cases, the women should avoid activities that they know exacerbate the symptoms and initiate treatment. Rarely, with severe, chronic cases of diastasis, surgical fixation may be required to stabilize the joint.

Further research is required to determine why some women are more susceptible than others to severe pelvic instability and which form of management offers the best prognosis. The use of alternative therapies in the management of pain appears to be unevaluated. Where health professionals' knowledge of symphysial pain is increased, the postnatal incidence is markedly reduced. In women presenting with antenatal onset of symptoms, morbidity appears to be decreased where advice and active treatment is followed.

It is essential to redress the lack of awareness of SPD among some health professionals. Where the prevailing attitude is one of disbelief of the symptoms or a lack of sympathy (McIntosh, 1993) and information about this 'rare' condition is unavailable, the woman and her family may feel extremely isolated. The early recognition and management of the condition by the midwife and physiotherapist will improve the quality of life and may reduce longer-term morbidity. The midwife needs to be able to give optimum care, offering home antenatal visits where possible and visiting until 28 days postnatally if necessary before transferring care to the health visitor. During this time the midwife may need to refer the woman to the appropriate health professionals and utilize the services of voluntary agencies. Peer support and information is available for women and health professionals from www.pelvicpartnership.org.uk or by contacting the telephone helpline on 01235 820921.

> ### Reflective Activity 16.11
> Discuss with your next antenatal group how many of the women are experiencing low back pain or pelvic pain. Consider what you have read, and how you could integrate this into both antenatal care and parenting sessions.

CONCLUSION

As this chapter has demonstrated, the antenatal period is a time of tremendous physical and psychological adjustment for the woman and her family. The midwife can work in partnership to assist the process of adaptation, and aim to help increase the woman's understanding of the changes and prepare for the birth and parenting experience. A crucial part of the partnership is within the initial interview and assessment, during which the midwife can assess the woman's individual needs, plan care with her, and where there are particular needs or problems, refer accordingly so that the care and management are proactive.

Many women experience some of the so-called 'minor disorders' of pregnancy that are attributable to the physiological changes occurring within the woman's body. These disorders may range from being a minor inconvenience that the woman can cope with herself to a major source of discomfort, or even severe pain as is possible with SPD. Some women may have to contend with several of the disorders occurring simultaneously. The role of the midwife is to give information, advice and support to women to enable them to cope in the best way possible with the pregnancy, the disorder and the lifestyle changes. The midwife should always be mindful that more serious conditions can arise from the minor disorders and refer women to either a doctor or other health professional or agencies as appropriate.

The ongoing antenatal care should be provided within an environment of respect and partnership, and the midwife should aim to make every woman feel valued and every antenatal visit a positive and informative one, whether this is in the woman's home, the hospital or the community clinic.

KEY POINTS

- The midwife should be aware of the main pregnancy tests available to women, and the accuracy of these.
- The initial booking interview is an important opportunity to assess the physical, psychological, educational and social needs of the woman, and plan care accordingly.
- The antenatal period is a time of physical, psychological and social adjustment for the woman and her family, through which the midwife can guide and assist both.
- The significance of the woman's social, family, medical, and obstetric histories should be carefully assessed in order to identify any potential problems, and highlight her individual needs through the antenatal period.

- The physiological changes which are wrought by pregnancy may have effects that are uncomfortable or of concern to the woman, and an important part of the midwife's role lies in assessing the normality of the changes, ensuring the woman understands why they are occurring and suggesting strategies for increasing the comfort and well-being of the woman and her growing fetus.
- The midwife should be conversant with the physiology of pregnancy, be able to identify when the pregnancy deviates from the norm, and be able to refer to the appropriate practitioner.
- The antenatal period is an important window of opportunity for the midwife in terms of health promotion and the wider public health, from advising on smoking cessation, to diet and exercise.

REFERENCES

Adelson, P., Frommer, M. & Pym, M. (1992) Teenage pregnancy and fertility in New South Wales: an examination of fertility trends, abortion and birth outcomes. *Australian Journal of Public Health* **16**(3): 238–244.

Alexander, J. (1991) The prevalence and management of inverted and non-protractile nipples in antenatal women who intend to breastfeed. PhD Thesis. Southampton: University of Southampton.

American Institute of Medicine (1990) *Committee on Nutrition Status During Pregnancy and Lactation.* Washington: National Academy Press.

Association of Chartered Physiotherapists in Women's Health (ACPWH) (1996) *Symphysis Pubis Dysfunction Guidelines.* London: Chartered Society of Physiotherapy.

Barnet Health Authority (BHA) (2000) *Evaluation of Edgeware Birth Centre.* London: BHA.

Bastian, L., Nanda, K., Hasselblad, V. *et al.* (1998) Diagnostic efficiency of home pregnancy test kits. *Archives of Family Medicine* **7**(5): 465–469.

Binstock, M.A. & Wolde-Tsadik, G. (1995) Alternative prenatal care. Impact of reduced visit frequency, focused visits and continuity of care. *Journal of Reproductive Medicine* **40**(7): 507–512.

Bjorklund, K., Bergstrom, S., Nordstrom, M., Ulmsten, U. (2000) Symphyseal distention in relation to serum relaxin levels and pelvic pain in pregnancy. *Acta Obstetricia et Gynecologica Scandinavica* **79**: 269–275.

Black, M.C. & Mayou, C. (1995) Skin diseases in pregnancy. In: De Swiet, M. (ed) *Medical Disorders in Obstetric Practice*, 3rd edn. Oxford: Blackwell Scientific.

Blackburn, S.T. (2003) *Maternal, Fetal and Neonatal Physiology: A Clinical Perspective.* Philadelphia: W.B. Saunders.

Blair, P.S., Fleming, P.J., Bensley, D. *et al.* (1996) Smoking and sudden infant death syndrome results from 1993–95 case control study for confidential enquiry into stillbirths and deaths in infancy. *British Medical Journal* **313**(7051): 195–198.

Blondel, B. Pusch, D. & Schmidt, E. (1985) Some characteristics of antenatal care in 13 European countries. *British Journal of Obstetrics and Gynaecology* **6**: 65–68.

Borelli, B., Bock, B., King, T. *et al.* (1996) The impact of depression on smoking cessation in women. *American Journal of Preventive Medicine* **12**(5): 378–387.

British Nutrition Foundation (BNF) (1994) *Briefing Paper: Nutrition in Pregnancy.* London: BNF.

Broadhurst, M. (1988) Computers can improve the quality of care. *Nursing Times* **84**(48): 7.

Broussard, C.N. & Richter, J.E. (1998) Nausea and vomiting of pregnancy. *Gastroenterology Clinics of North America* **27**(1): 123–151.

Brucker, M.C. (1988) Management of common minor disorders in pregnancy. Part 3, Managing gastro-intestinal problems in pregnancy. *Journal of Nurse Midwifery* **33**(2): 67–73.

Campbell, J.M. (1924) *Maternal Mortality. Reports on Public Health and Medical Subjects,* No. 25. London: HMSO.

Campbell, J. (1986) Nursing assessment for risk of homicide with battered women. *American Journal of Nursing* 86(8): 910–913.

Campion, M. (1997) Disabled women and maternity services. *Modern Midwife* 7(3): 23–25.

Central Statistical Office (CSO) (1994) *Social Trends,* No. 24. London: HMSO.

Chamberlain, G. (1991) Abdominal pain in pregnancy. *British Medical Journal* 302: 1390–1394.

Chamberlain, G., Wraight, A. & Crowley, P. (1997) *Home Births. The Report of the 1994 Confidential Enquiry by the National Birthday Trust Fund.* Carnforth: Parthenon Publishing Group.

Charles, J. (1992) Pregnant pause. *Nursing Times* 88(34): 30–32.

Christoffel, K.K. & Salafsky, I. (1975) Fetal alcohol syndrome in dizygotic twins. *Journal of Paediatrics* 87(6 Pt 1) 963–967.

Chudleigh, P. & Pearce, M. (1994) *Obstetric Ultrasound,* 2nd edn. Edinburgh: Churchill Livingstone.

Clement, S., Candy, B., Sikorski, J. *et al.* (1999) Does reducing the frequency of routine antenatal visits have long term effects? Follow up of participants in a randomised controlled trial. *British Journal of Obstetrics and Gynaecology* 106(4): 367–370.

Cook, A.J.C., Gilbert, R.E., Buffolano, W. *et al.* (2000) Sources of toxoplasma infection in pregnant women: European multicentre case-control study. European Research Network on Congenital Toxoplasmosis. *British Medical Journal* 321(7254): 142–147.

Corkhill, A. (1995) Effectiveness of current antenatal care. *British Journal of Midwifery* 3(10): 528–532.

Culp, R., Appelbaum, M. & Osofsky, J. (1988) Adolescent and older mothers: comparison between prenatal variables and newborn interaction measures. *Infant Behaviour and Development* 11: 253–362.

Currell, R. (1990) The organisation of midwifery care. In: Alexander, J., Levy, V. & Roch, S. (eds) *Antenatal Care – A Research Based Approach.* Houndmills: Macmillan Educational.

Dawes, M.G. & Grudzinskas, J.G. (1991) Repeated measurement of maternal weight during pregnancy. Is this a useful practice? *British Journal of Obstetrics and Gynaecology* 98(2): 189–194.

Day, N.L., Richardson, G.A., Geva, D. *et al.* (1994) Alcohol. Marijuana, and tobacco: effects of prenatal exposure on offspring growth and morphology at age 6. *Alcoholism, Clinical and Experimental Research* 18(4): 786–794.

De Swiet, M. (1999) K5 rather than K4 for diastolic blood pressure measurement in pregnancy. *Hypertension in Pregnancy* 18(3): iii–v.

Department of Health (DoH) (1989) *Working together under The Children Act – A Guide to Arrangements for Inter-Agency Co-operation for the Protection of Children from Abuse.* London: HMSO.

Department of Health (DoH) (1992a) *Folic Acid and the Prevention of Neural Tube Defects. Report from the Expert Advisory Group.* London: HMSO.

Department of Health (DoH) (1992b) *Second Report of Maternity Services,* Vol. 1 (Winterton Report). London: HMSO.

Department of Health (DoH) (1992c) *The Health of the Nation. A Strategy for Health in England.* London: HMSO.

Department of Health (DoH) (1993) *Changing Childbirth,* Part 1. *Report of the Expert Maternity Group.* London: HMSO.

Department of Health (DoH) (1994) *Weaning and the Weaning Diet. 45. Report of the Working Group on the Weaning Diet of the Committee on Medical Aspects of Food Policy.* London: HMSO.

Department of Health (DoH) (1995a) *Sensible Drinking: The Report of an Interdepartmental Working Group.* London: HMSO.

Department of Health (DoH) (1995b) *Obesity – Reversing the Increasing Problem of Obesity in England. A Report from the Nutrition and Physical Activity Task Forces.* London: HMSO.

Department of Health (DoH) (1998) *Why Mothers Die. Report on Confidential Enquiries into Maternal Deaths in the United Kingdom, 1994–1996.* London: The Stationery Office.

Department of Health (DoH) (2000b) *The NHS Plan.* London: DoH.

Department of Health (DoH) (2001) *Scientific Advisory Committee on Nutrition Report on Obesity 'Quick think'.* Online. Available: http://www.doh.gov.uk/sacn/pdf/quickthinksacn0115.pdf, September 2001.

Department of Health (DoH) (2002) *National Services Framework for Diabetes.* London: DoH.

Department of Health (DoH) (2003) *The Pregnancy Book.* London: DoH.

Department of Health and Social Security (DHSS) (1970) *Domiciliary Midwifery and Maternity Bed Needs* (Peel Report). London: HMSO.

Department of Health and Social Security (DHSS) (1990) *Vitamin A and Pregnancy.* PL/CMO(90)10. 25 October. London: DoH.

Dimond, B. (2000) Implications of the Disability Discrimination Act. *British Journal of Midwifery* 8(9): 571–574.

Disability Discrimination Act 1995 London: HMSO.

Dodds, W.J., Dent, J. & Hogan, W. (1978) Pregnancy and the lower oesophageal sphincter. *Gastroenterology* 74(6): 1334–1336.

Dolby, E. (1998) Is sex education in the Netherlands better organised than in Britain? *British Journal of Midwifery* 6(2): 96–100.

Donnison, J. (1988) *Midwives and Medical Men.* London: Heinemann.

Dowell, A. & Price, H. (1998) Multi disciplinary teamwork in maternity care. In: Marsh, G. & Renfrew, M. (eds) *Community-based Maternity Care*. Oxford: Oxford University Press.

Drake, R. & Cullum, A. (1998) Don't ignore weight gain during pregnancy. *British Journal of Midwifery* 6(4): 211–214.

Driessen, F. (1987) Postpartum arthropathy with unusual features. *British Journal of Obstetrics and Gynaecology* 94(9): 870–872.

Earle, S. (2000) Pregnancy and the maintenance of self identity: implications for antenatal care in the community. *Health and Social Care in the Community* 8(4): 235–241.

Eastman, N.J. & Hellman, L.M. (1966) *Obstetrics,* 13th edn. New York: Appleton Century Crofts.

Eckardt, M.J., File, S.E., Gessa, G.L. *et al.* (1998). Effects of moderate alcohol consumption on the central nervous system. *Alcoholism, Clinical and Experimental Research* 22(5): 998–1040.

Enkin, M., Keirse, M., Neilson, J. *et al.* (2000) *A Guide to Effective Care in Pregnancy and Childbirth,* 3rd edn. Oxford: Oxford University Press.

Fawdry, R. (1994) Antenatal casenotes 1: comments on design. *British Journal of Midwifery* 2(7): 320–327.

Fitzpatrick, T.B., Freedburg, I.M., Eisen, A.Z. *et al.* (eds) (1999) *Fitzpatrick's Dermatology in General Medicine,* Vols 1 & 2. New York: McGraw-Hill.

Florey, C. du V., Taylor, D., Bolumar, F. *et al.* (eds) (1992) EUROMAC – a European concerted action: maternal alcohol consumption and its relation to the outcome of pregnancy and child development at 18 months. *International Journal of Epidemiology* 21(Suppl. 1): S82–S83.

Foster, K., Lader, D. & Cheesebrough, S. (1997) *Infant Feeding 1995*. Office for National Statistics. London: HMSO.

Fry, A. (1994) Effective communication with people with visual disabilities. *Nursing Times* 90(44): 42–43.

Gadsby, R., Barnie-Adshead, A.M. & Jagger, C. (1993) A prospective study of nausea and vomiting during pregnancy. *British Journal of General Practice* 43(371): 245–248.

Galloway, L. (1994) Knowing the form. *Modern Midwife* 4(9): 24–26.

Gamble, J.G., Simmons, S.C. & Freedman, M. (1986) The symphysis pubis. *Clinical Orthopaedics and Related Research* (203): 261–272.

Gardosi, J. & Francis, A. (1999) Controlled trial of fundal height measurement plotted on customised antenatal growth charts. *British Journal of Obstetrics and Gynaecology* 106(4): 309–317.

Gherman, R.B., Ouzounian, J., Incerpi, M., Goodwin, T. (1998) Symphyseal separation and transient femoral neuropathy associated with the McRoberts maneuver. *American Journal of Obstetrics and Gynecology* 178(3): 609–610.

Gibb, D.M.F. & Arulkumaran, S. (1997) *Fetal Monitoring in Practice,* 2nd edn. London: Butterworth-Heinemann.

Grieve, F. (1976) The sacroiliac joint. *Physiotherapy* 62: 386–399.

Guerri, S., Riley, E. & Strömland, K. (1999) Commentary on the recommendations of the Royal College of Obstetricians and Gynaecologists concerning alcohol consumption in pregnancy. *Alcohol and Alcoholism* 34(4): 497–501.

Haglund, B.C. & Cnattingius, S. (1990) Cigarette smoking as a risk factor for sudden infant death syndrome: a population based study. *American Journal of Public Health* 80(1): 29–32.

Hall, M.H., Chng, P.K. & MacGillivray, I. (1980) Is routine antenatal care worthwhile? *Lancet* ii(8185): 78–80.

Hall, M., MacIntyre, S. & Porter, M. (1985) *Antenatal Care Assessed: A Case Study of an Innovation in Aberdeen*. Aberdeen: Aberdeen University Press.

Hally, R., Bond, J., Crawley, J. *et al.* (1984) What influences a mother's choice of infant feeding method? *Nursing Times* 80(4): 65–68.

Hamlyn, B., Brooker, S., Oleinikova, K. *et al.* (2002) *Infant Feeding 2002*. London: The Stationery Office.

Harden, C. (1997) The National Maternity Record Project. *MIDIRS Midwifery Digest* 7(4): 419.

Hartrick, G. (1997) Women who are mothers: the experience of defining self. *Health Care for Women International* 18: 263–277.

Heagerty, B.V. (1996) Reassessing the guilty: the Midwives Act and the control of English midwives in the early 20th century. In: Kirkham, M. (ed) *Supervision of Midwives*. Hale: Books for Midwives.

Heckmann, J. & Sassard, R. (1994) Musculoskeletal considerations in pregnancy. *Journal of Bone and Joint Surgery* 76A(11): 1720–1730.

Henderson, C. (1997) Choices and patterns of care. In: Sweet, B. (ed) *Mayes' Midwifery,* 12th edn. London: Baillière Tindall.

Hoddinott, P. & Pill, R. (1999) Qualitative study of decisions about infant feeding among women in the East End of London. *British Medical Journal* 318(7175): 30–34.

Homer, C.S.E., Davis, G.K. & Everitt, L.S. (1999) The introduction of a woman-held record into a hospital antenatal clinic: the bring your own records study. *Australian and New Zealand Journal of Obstetrics and Gynaecology* 39(1): 54–57.

House of Commons (2003) Select Committee/Health Committee; fourth, eighth and ninth Reports of the Maternity Services. London: The Stationery Office.

Hughes, D.F.J. & Goldstone, L.A. (1989) Frameworks for midwifery care in Great Britain: an exploration into quality assurance. *Midwifery* 5(4): 163–172.

Hutton, E. (1994) What women want from midwives. *British Journal of Midwifery* 2(12): 608–611.

Hytten, F. (1990) The alimentary system in pregnancy. *Midwifery* 6(4): 201–204.

Jacobson, J.L., Jacobson, S.W. & Sokol, R.J. (1996) Increased vulnerability to alcohol related birth defects in the off-spring of mothers aged over 30. *Alcoholism, Clinical and Experimental Research* 20(2): 359–363.

Jewell, M. (1993) Antacid therapy for heartburn in pregnancy. In: Enkin, M.W., Keirse, M.J.N., Renfrew, M. et al. (eds) *Pregnancy and Childbirth Module. Cochrane Database of Systematic Reviews*, No. 06885. Cochrane updates on disk, Issue 1. Oxford: Update Software.

Jewell, D.J. & Young, G. (2001) Interventions for treating constipation in pregnancy. *The Cochrane Library,* Issue 2. CD001142. Oxford: Update Software.

Jewell, D.J. & Young, G. (2002) Interventions for nausea and vomiting in early pregnancy. *The Cochrane Library,* Issue 1, 2000. CD000145. Oxford: Update Software.

Jewell, D., Sharp, D., Sanders, J. et al. (2000) A randomised controlled trial in routine antenatal care. *British Journal of Obstetrics and Gynaecology* 107(10): 1241–1247.

Jones, S.V. & Black, M.C. (2002) Skin diseases in pregnancy. In: De Swiet, M. (ed) *Medical Disorders in Obstetric Practice*, 4th edn. Oxford: Blackwell Scientific.

Jones, K.L., Smith, D.W., Ulleland, C.N. et al. (1973) Pattern of malformation in offspring of chronic alcoholic mothers. *Lancet* 1(7815): 1267–1271.

Kelsall, J. (1993) Giving midwifery care for the deaf in the 1990s. *Midwives Chronicle* 106(1262): 80–83.

Kharrazi, F.D., Rodgers, W.B., Kennedy, J., Lhowe, D. (1997) Parturition-induced pelvic dislocation: a report of four cases. *Journal of Orthopaedic Trauma* 11(4): 277–282.

Kirkham, M.J. & Perkins, E.R. (eds) (1997) *Reflections on Midwifery*. London: Baillière Tindall.

Klebanoff, M.A., Koslowe, P.A., Kaslow, R. et al. (1985) Epidemiology of vomiting in early pregnancy. *Obstetrics and Gynecology* 66(5): 612–616.

Knowles, H. & Wilson, L. (1999) Baseline audit of an antenatal day assessment unit. *British Journal of Midwifery* 7(3): 181–184.

Kramer, M.S. (1987) Determinants of low birth weight: methodological assessment and meta-analysis. *Bulletin of the World Health Organization* 65(5): 663–737.

Kristiansson, P., Svardsudd, K., Von Scholtz, B. (1996) Serum relaxin, pain and back pain during pregnancy. *American Journal of Obstetrics and Gynecology* 175: 1342–1347.

Kowalk, D., Perdue, P., Bourgeois, J., Whitehill, R. (1996) Disruption of the symphysis pubis during vaginal delivery: a case report. *The Journal of Bone and Joint Surgery* (American Volume), Vol. 78-A(11) Nov: 1746–1748.

Kubitz, R.L., Goodlin., M.D. (1986) Symptomatic separation of the pubic symphysis. *Southern Medical Journal* 79(5): 578–580.

Lacroix, R., Eason, E. & Melzack, R. (2000) Nausea and vomiting during pregnancy: a prospective study of its frequency, intensity, and patterns of change. *American Journal of Obstetrics and Gynecology* 182(4): 931–937.

Larson, J., Patatanian, E., Miner, P.B. et al. (1997). Double blind, placebo-controlled study of ranitidine for gastroesophageal reflux symptoms during pregnancy. *Obstetrics and Gynecology* 90(1): 83–87.

Leap, N. & Hunter, B. (1993) *The Midwife's Tale: An Oral History from Handywoman to Professional Midwife*. London: Scarlet Press.

Lewis, G. (ed) (2001) *Why Mothers Die 1997–99: Fifth Report of the Confidential Enquiries into Maternal Deaths in the United Kingdom*. London: CEMD: associated with NICE, RCOG.

Lilford, R.J., Kelly, M., Baines, A. et al. (1992) Effect of using protocols on medical care: randomised trial of three methods of taking an antenatal history. *British Medical Journal* 305(6863): 1181–1184.

Lindsey, M.D., Leggon, R., Wright, D. et al. (1988) Separation of the symphysis pubis in association with childbearing. *Journal of Bone and Joint Surgery* 70-A(2): 289–292.

Llewellyn Jones, D. (1999) *Fundamentals of Obstetrics and Gynaecology*. London: Mosby.

Local Government Board (1918) *Forty Seventh Annual Report of the Local Government Board 1917–18*, Part 1Cd 9157, p. 19.

Lowe, S.W., House, W. & Garrett, T. (1987) A comparison of outcome of low risk labour in an isolated general practitioner maternity unit and a specialist maternity hospital. *Journal of the Royal College of General Practitioners* 37(304): 484–487.

Lumley, J., Oliver, S. & Waters, E. (2000) Interventions for smoking cessation during pregnancy. *The Cochrane Library,* Issue 2. CD001055. Oxford: Update Software.

McCandlish, R., Renfrew, M.J., Ashurst, H. et al. (1992) Getting results: the processes involved in organising and analysing data from the MAIN trial. *Research and the Midwife, Conference Proceedings*, Manchester, pp. 17–25.

McCourt, C. & Page, L. (1996) *Report on the Evaluation of One-to-one Midwifery*. London: Thames Valley University.

McDuffie, R.S., Beck, A., Bischoff, K. et al. (1996) Effect of frequency of prenatal care visits on perinatal outcome among low risk women. *Journal of the American Medical Association* 275(11): 847–851.

McFarlane, J., Parker, B. & Soeken, K. (1992) Assessing for abuse during pregnancy. *Journal of the American Medical Association* 267(24): 3176–3178.

McIntosh, J. (1985) Decisions on breast feeding in a group of first-time mothers. *Research and the Midwife Conference Proceedings*, Manchester, pp. 46–64.

McIntosh, J.M. (1993) Incidence of separated symphysis pubis. *Midwives Chronicle and Nursing Notes* 106(1260): 23–24.

McIntosh, J. (1995) Treatment note: an alternative pelvic support. *Journal of the Association of Chartered Physiotherapists in Women's Health* 76: 28.

McLeish, J. (2002) *Mothers in Exile: Maternity Experiences of Asylum Seekers in England.* London: Maternity Alliance.

McNeil, A., (1998) Smoking and pregnancy. *Family Medicine* 2(2): 21–22.

McVeigh, C. & Smith, C. (2000) A comparison of adult and teenage mothers self esteem and satisfaction with social support. *Midwifery* 16(4): 269–276.

Mallol, J., Belda, M.A., Costa, D. *et al.* (1991) Prophylaxis of striae gravidarum with a topical formulation. A double blind trial. *International Journal of Cosmetic Science* 13: 51–57.

Mansion, E.M. & McGuire, M.M. (1998) Factors which influence women in the choice of domino care. *British Journal of Midwifery* 6(10): 664–668.

Maternity Alliance (1994) *Disability Working Group Pack.* London: Maternity Alliance.

Mayes, G.E. (1987) Developing a model of care in Waltham Forest. *Midwives Chronicle* 100(1198): v–ix.

Methven, R.C. (1982a) The antenatal booking interview: recording an obstetric history or relating with a mother-to-be? *Research and the Midwife Conference Proceedings*, Glasgow, pp. 63–76.

Methven, R.C. (1982b) The antenatal booking interview: recording an obstetric history or relating with a mother-to-be? *Research and the Midwife Conference Proceedings*, Glasgow, pp. 77–86.

Methven, R.C. (1986) Care plan for a woman having antenatal care based on Orem's Self Care Model. In: Webb, C. (ed) *Woman's Health: Midwifery and Gynaecology.* Sevenoaks: Hodder & Stoughton.

Methven, R.C. (1989) Recording an obstetric history or relating to a pregnant woman? A study of the antenatal booking interview. In: Robinson, S. & Thomson, A. (eds) *Midwives, Research and Childbirth*, Vol. 1. London: Chapman & Hall.

Midgely, C. (1988) *Survey of use of models for nursing in midwifery.* BEd Dissertation. Huddersfield: Huddersfield Polytechnic.

MIDIRS/NHS Centre for Reviews and Dissemination (NHSCRD) (1999a) *Routine Ultrasound Scanning in the First Half of Pregnancy.* Informed Choice Leaflets for Women and Professionals. Bristol: MIDIRS.

MIDIRS/NHS Centre for Reviews and Dissemination (1999b) *Alcohol and Pregnancy.* Informed Choice for Professionals and Informed Choice for Women. Bristol: MIDIRS.

MIDIRS/NHS Centre for Reviews and Dissemination (1999c) *Breast or Bottle Feeding: Helping Women to Choose.* Informed Choice Leaflets for Women and Professionals. Bristol: MIDIRS.

MIDIRS/NHS Centre for Reviews and Dissemination (2002) *Alcohol and Pregnancy.* Topic 4: Informed Choice for Professionals and Informed Choice for Women. MIDIRS National Electronic Library for Health.

Mills, J.L., Graubard, B.I., Harley, E.E. *et al.* (1984) Maternal alcohol consumption and birthweight. How much drinking is safe? *Journal of the American Medical Association* 252(14): 1875–1879.

Ministry of Health (MoH) (1929) *Memorandum on Antenatal Clinics: Their Conduct and Scope.* Appendix to the Ministry of Health Report. 1930. London: HMSO.

Mooney, J. (1993) *The Hidden Figure of Domestic Violence in North London.* London: Islington Council.

Moore, J., Peters, A. & Frame, S. (1983) The relevance of shoe size to obstetric outcome. *Research and the Midwife, Conference Proceedings*, 53–68.

Musumeci, R., Villa, E. (1994) Symphysis pubis separation during vaginal delivery with epidural anaesthesia. A case report. *Regional Anaesthesia* 19(4): 289–291.

Narang, I. & Murphy, S. (1994) Assessment of the antenatal care for Asian women. *British Journal of Midwifery* 22(4): 169–173.

Neilson, J. (2000) Symphysis–fundal height measurement in pregnancy. *The Cochrane Library*, Issue 4. Oxford: Update Software.

Newton, M. (1952) Nipple pain and nipple damage; problems in the management of breast feeding. *Journal of Pediatrics* 41: 411–423.

NHS Centre for Reviews and Dissemination (NHSCRD) (1997) Preventing and reducing the adverse effects of unintended teenage pregnancies. *Effective Health Care Bulletin* 3(1): 1–12.

NHS Centre for Reviews and Dissemination (NHSCRD) (2000) Promoting the initiation of breastfeeding. *Effective Health Care Bulletin* 6(2): 1–12.

NHS Executive (NHSE) (1999) *Reducing Mother to Baby Transmission of HIV.* Health Service Circular (HSC 1999/183), 13 Aug 1999. London: NHS Executive.

Nolan, M. (1994a) Care for the deaf mother. *Modern Midwife* 4(7): 15–16.

Nolan, M. (1994b) Choice and control for the disabled mother. *Modern Midwife* 4(4): 10–12.

Nolan, M.L. (1998) Teenage pregnancy: a challenge for the Government and nation. *RCM Midwives Journal* 1(5): 152–154.

Nolan, M. & Hicks, C. (1997) Aims, processes and problems of antenatal education as identified by three groups of childbirth teachers. *Midwifery* 13(4): 179–188.

North Staffordshire Changing Childbirth Research Team (NSCCRT) (2000) A randomised study of midwifery caseload care and traditional 'shared-care'. *Midwifery* 16(4): 295–302.

Nursing and Midwifery Council (NMC) (2002) *Standards for Records and Record Keeping* (amended standards first published by UKCC 1998). London: NMC.

O'Brien, B., Relyea, J. & Lidstone, T. (1997) Diary reports of nausea and vomiting during pregnancy. *Clinical Nursing Research* 6(3): 239–252.

O'Dowd, M. & O'Dowd, T. (1985) Quickening – a re-evaluation. *British Journal of Obstetrics and Gynaecology* **92**(10): 1037–1039.

O'Leary, J.A. (1992) *Shoulder Dystocia and Birth Injury: Prevention and Treatment.* London: MacGraw-Hill.

Oakley, A. (1982) The relevance of the history of medicine to an understanding of current change: some comments from the domain of antenatal care. *Social Science & Medicine* **16**(6): 667–674.

Oakley, A., Rajan, L. & Grant, A. (1990) Social support and pregnancy outcome. *British Journal of Obstetrics and Gynaecology* **97**(2): 152–162.

ONS (2001) Childhood, infant and perinatal mortality series DH5, No. 34, Table 15, p. 70. Live births, stillbirths and linked infant deaths, birth weight and mother's country of birth. HMSO.

ONS (2004) Birth statistics: maternities, age of mother, occurrence within/outside marriage, number of live born children and place of confinement, 2002 series FM1, No. 31, Table 8.1, p. 38, HMSO.

Ogerek, C.P. & Cohen, S. (1989) Gastroesophageal reflux disease: new concepts in pathophysiology. *Gastroenterology Clinics of North America* **18**(2): 275–292.

Olsen, K. (1999) 'Now just pop up here dear'. Revising the art of abdominal palpation. *Practising Midwife* **2**(9): 13–15.

Parsons, W.D. & Perkins, E.R. (1982) *Why Don't Women Attend for Antenatal Care?* Leverhulme Health Education Project, Occasional Paper No. 23, University of Nottingham.

Petersen, L.K., Hvidman, L. Uldeberg, N. (1994) Normal serum relaxin levels in women with disabling pelvic pain during pregnancy. *Gynecologic and Obstetric Investigation* **38**: 21–23.

Plant M.L. (2000) Alcohol in pregnancy. *MIDIRS Midwifery Digest* **10**(4): 443–447.

Proud, J. (1997) *Understanding Obstetric Ultrasound*, 2nd edn. Cheshire: Books for Midwives Press.

Putschar, W.G.J. (1976) The structure of the human symphysis pubis with special consideration of parturition and its sequelae. *American Journal of Physical Anthropology* **45**(3 Pt 2): 589–594.

Redman, C. (1996) Why antenatal care must not be reduced. *Midwives* **109**(1303): 233.

Rogers, I., Emmett, P., Baker, D.G. *et al.* (1998) Financial difficulties, smoking habits, composition of the diet and birthweight in a population of pregnant women in the South West of England. *European Journal of Clinical Nursing.* **52**(4): 251–260.

Rosser, J. (2000) Calculating the EDD – which is more accurate, scan or LMP? *Practising Midwife* **3**(3): 28–29.

Rosser, J. (2001) Birth centres across the UK: a win/win strategy for saving normal birth. *RCM Midwives Journal* **4**(3): 88–89.

Rossner, S. & Ohlin, J. (1995) Pregnancy as a risk factor for obesity: lessons from the Stockholm pregnancy and weight development study. *Obesity Research* **3**(Suppl. 2): 267s–275s.

Royal College of Midwives (RCM) (1997) *Domestic Abuse in Pregnancy.* Position Paper 19. London: RCM.

Royal College of Midwives (RCM) (2000a). *Vision 2000.* London: RCM.

Royal College of Midwives (RCM) (2000b) Position Paper 11a. Maternity care for women with disabilities. *RCM Midwives Journal* **13**(2): 46.

Royal College of Midwives (RCM) (2001) *Clinical Risk Management Series: Shoulder Dystocia.* London: RCM.

Royal College of Midwives (RCM) (2002). *Helping Women Stop Smoking: A Guide for Midwives.* London: RCM.

Royal College of Obstetricians and Gynaecologists (RCOG) (1982) *Report from the RCOG Working Party on Antenatal and Intrapartum Care.* London: RCOG.

Royal College of Obstetricians and Gynaecologists (RCOG) (1995) *Organisational Standards for Maternity Services.* Report of a Joint Working Group. London: RCOG.

Royal College of Obstetricians and Gynaecologists (RCOG) (1999) *Alcohol Consumption in Pregnancy (9) Clinical Green Top Guidelines.* London: RCOG.

Royal College of Obstetricians and Gynaecologists (RCOG) (2000) *Alcohol Consumption in Pregnancy.* London: RCOG. Online. Available: http://www.rcog.org.uk/guidelines/alcohol.html.

Rubin, P. (1996) Measuring diastolic blood pressure in pregnancy. *British Medical Journal* **313**(7048): 4–5.

Ryan, P., Booth, R., Coates, D. *et al.* (1980) *Experiences of Pregnancy. Pregnant Pause Campaign.* Australia: Health Commission of New South Wales, Division of Drug and Alcohol Services.

Scott, P., Milsom, G. & Milsom, K. (1995) Teachers and parents too: an assessment of Dutch sexual health education. *British Journal of Family Planning* **21**(1): 20–21.

Scriven, M., Mcknight, L. & Jones, D. (1991) Diastasis of the symphysis pubis in pregnancy. *British Medical Journal* **303**(6793): 56.

Scriven, M., Mcknight, L. & Jones, D. (1995) The importance of pubic pain following childbirth: a clinical and ultrasonographic study of diastasis of the symphysis pubis. *Journal of the Royal Society of Medicine* **88**(1): 28–30.

Secretary of State for Health (2004) Government response to the Health Select Committee's fourth, eighth and ninth Reports of the Maternity Services. CM6140. London: The Stationery Office.

Shaw, R.W. (1978) Randomized controlled trial of Syn-Ergel and an active placebo in the treatment of heartburn in pregnancy. *Journal of International Medical Research* **6**(2): 147–151.

Shennan, A., Gupta, M., Halligan, A. *et al.* (1996) Lack of reproducibility in pregnancy of Korotkoff phase IV as measured by sphygmomanometry. *Lancet* **347**(8995): 139–142.

Shepherd, J. & Fry, D. (1996) Symphysis pubis pain. *Midwives* **109**(1302): 199–201.

Sikorski, J., Wilson, J., Clement, S. *et al.* (1996) A randomised controlled trial comparing two schedules of antenatal visits: The antenatal Care Project. *British Medical Journal* **312**(7030): 546–553.

Silverton, L. (1993) *The Art and Science of Midwifery.* London: Prentice Hall.

Smaill, F. (2001) Antibiotics for asymptomatic bacteriuria in pregnancy (Cochrane Review). *The Cochrane Library,* Issue 2. CD000490. Oxford: Update Software.

Snelling, F.G. (1870) Relaxation of the pelvic symphyses during pregnancy and parturition. *American Journal of Obstetrics and Gynecology* **2**(4): 561–596.

Social Exclusion Unit (SEU) (1999) *Teenage Pregnancy.* London: The Stationery Office. Online. Available: http://www.cabinet-office.gov.ok/seu/1999/ Teenpar/index.htm.

Springer, N.S., Bischoping, K., Sampselle, C.M. *et al.* (1992) Using early weight gain and other nutrition related factors to predict pregnancy outcomes. *Journal of the American Dietetic Association* **92**(2): 217–219.

Stammers, T., Ingham, R. (2000) For and against: doctors should advise adolescents to abstain from sex. *British Medical Journal* **321**(7275): 1520–1522.

Standing Nursing and Midwifery Advisory Committee (SNMAC) (1998) *Midwifery: Delivering Our Future.* London: DoH.

Tabberer, S., Hall, C., Prendergast, S. *et al.* (1999) *Teenage Pregnancy and Choice: Abortion or Motherhood: Influences on the Decision.* York: Joseph Rowntree Foundation.

Taylor, R.N. & Sonson, R.D. (1986) Separation of the symphysis pubis: an underrecognised peripartum complication. *Journal of Reproductive Medicine* **31**(3): 203–206.

Tew, M. (1998) *Safer Childbirth? A Critical Review of Maternity Care.* London: Free Association Books.

Thomas, C. & Curtis, P. (1997) Having a baby: some disabled women's reproductive experiences. *Midwifery* **13**(4): 202–209.

Thorley, K. & Rouse, T. (1993) Seeing mothers as partners in antenatal care. *British Journal of Midwifery* **1**(5): 216–219.

Tincello, D.G. & Richmond, D.H. (1998) Evaluation of reagent strips in detecting asymptomatic bacteriuria in early pregnancy: prospective case series. *British Medical Journal* **316**(7129): 435–437.

Too, S-K. (1996) Do birthplans empower women? A study of their views. *Nursing Standard* **10**(31): 33–37.

Toxoplasmosis Trust (2000) Fact sheets 1–6. Online. Available: http://www.toxo.org.uk 19 March 2001.

Tucker, J. & Hall, M. (1999) Latest views on antenatal care programmes. In: Marsh, G. & Renfrew, M. (eds) *Community-based Maternity Care,* Ch. 19, pp. 337–358. Oxford: Oxford University Press.

United Kingdom Central Council for Nursing, Midwifery and Health Visiting (UKCC) (1998) *Midwives Rules and Code Of Practice.* London: UKCC.

United Kingdom Central Council for Nursing, Midwifery and Health Visiting (UKCC) (2000) *Registrar's letter. Supporting women who wish to have a home birth.* London: UKCC.

Vause, S. Maresh, M. & Khaled, K. (1996) Study ignored influence of parity on women's needs. *British Medical Journal* **313**(7050): 167.

Villar, J. & Bergsjo, P. (1997) Scientific basis for the content of routine antenatal care: philosophy, recent studies, and power to eliminate or alleviate adverse maternal outcomes. *Acta Obstetricia et Gynecologica Scandinavica* **76**(1): 1–14.

Villar, J., Carroli, G., Khan-Neelofur, D. *et al.* (2001) Patterns of routine antenatal care for low-risk pregnancy. *The Cochrane Library* (4): CD000934. Oxford: Update Software.

Waldenstrom, U., Brown, S., McLachlan, H. *et al.* (2000) Does team midwife care increase satisfaction with antenatal, intrapartum and postpartum care? A randomised controlled trial. *Birth* **27**(3): 156–167.

Walker, J.J. (1993) Day care obstetrics. *British Journal of Hospital Medicine* **50**(5): 225–226.

Walsh, D. (2000) Evidence-based care series 2: Free-standing birth centres. *British Journal of Midwifery* **8**(6): 351–355.

Wand, J. (1990) Carpal tunnel syndrome in pregnancy and lactation. *Journal of Hand Surgery* **15-B**: 93–95.

Wardle, S.A., Wright, P.J. & Court, B.V. (1997) Knowledge of and preference for the DOMINO delivery option. *Midwifery* **13**: 149–153.

Warriner, S. (2000) Women's views on being weighed during pregnancy. *British Journal of Midwifery* **8**(10): 620–633.

Weeks, A.R.L. & Flynn, M.J. (1975) Engagement of the fetal head in primigravidae and its relationship to the duration of gestation and time of onset of labour. *British Journal of Obstetrics and Gynaecology* **82**(1): 7–11.

Wergeland, E., Strand, K. & Bjerkedal, T. (1996) Smoking in pregnancy: a way to cope with excessive workload. *Scandinavian Journal of Primary Health Care* **14**(1): 21–28.

Wheeler, M. (1999) Home and laboratory testing pregnancy testing kits. *Professional Nurse* **14**(8): 571–576.

Whitby, P. (2003) The agony of pelvic joint dysfunction. *The Practising Midwife* **4**(6): 14–16.

Whitford, H.M. & Hillan, E.M. (1998) Women's perceptions of birth plans. *Midwifery* **14**(4): 248–253.

World Health Organization (WHO) (1989) *The Reproductive Health of Adolescents – A Strategy for Action.* Geneva: WHO.

Wraight, A., Ball, J., Seccombe, I. *et al.* (1993) *Mapping Team Midwifery.* IMS Report Series 242. Brighton: Institute of Manpower Studies.

Yerby, M. (2000) *Pain Management in Childbearing.* Edinburgh: Baillière Tindall.

Young, G.L. & Jewell, D. (2000a) Creams for preventing stretch marks in pregnancy. *The Cochrane Library,* Issue 2. CD000066. Oxford: Update Software.

Young, G.L. & Jewell, D. (2000b) Interventions for varicosities and leg oedema in pregnancy. *The Cochrane Library,* Issue 2. CD001066. Oxford: Update Software.

Young, G.L. & Jewell, D. (2001) Topical treatment for vaginal candiasis in pregnancy. *The Cochrane Library,* Issue 4. CD000225. Oxford: Update Software.

Young, G.L. & Jewell, D. (2002a) Interventions for preventing and treating pelvic and back pain in pregnancy. *The Cochrane Library,* Issue 1. CD 001139. Oxford: Update Software.

Young, G.L. & Jewell, D. (2002b) Interventions for leg cramps in pregnancy. *The Cochrane Library,* Issue 1. CD000121. Oxford: Update Software.

Zeuner, D., Ades, A.E., Karnon, J. *et al.* (1999) Antenatal and neonatal haemoglobinopathy screening in the UK: review and economic analysis. *Health Technology Assessment* 3(11): i–v, 1–186.

FURTHER READING

Department of Health (DoH) (2000a) *Domestic Violence: A Resource Manual for Health Care Professionals.* London. DoH.

MacLennan, A.H. & MacLennan, S.C. (1997) Symptom giving pelvic girdle relaxation of pregnancy, pelvic joint syndrome and developmental dsysplasia of the hip. The Norwegian Association for women with pelvic girdle relaxation (Landforeningen for Kvinner Med Bekkenlosningsplager). *Acta Obstetricia et Gynecologica Scandinavica* 76(8): 760–764.
This study identifies the incidence and long-term morbidity associated with the condition and the limitations of current treatment therapies.

Siney, C. (ed) (1999) *Pregnancy and Drug Misuse.* Hale: Books for Midwives Press.
A very readable text with a sympathetic approach that discusses the obstetric, social and sexual problems of the pregnant drug misuser. The medical management of abuse and the outreach and support services are included.

Wheeler, M. (1999) Home and laboratory testing pregnancy testing kits. *Professional Nurse* 14(8): 571–576.
This useful review discusses home and laboratory pregnancy testing, how the tests work, their reliability and potential problems.

17

Maternal and Fetal Physiological Responses to Pregnancy

Mary McNabb

LEARNING OUTCOMES

After reading this chapter, you will be able to:

- understand the adaptations occurring in maternal organ systems in response to pregnancy
- appreciate the complex neurohormonal regulation of these adaptations that

accommodate the changing needs of the embryo and fetus.

In healthy, well-nourished women, extensive modifications occur in all bodily systems in response to the varying requirements of pregnancy and lactation. These changes begin to emerge during the luteal phase of the cycle, largely facilitated by rising levels of oestrogens, progesterone and deoxycorticosterone (DOC). In addition to the steroid-induced changes in the inner linings of the reproductive tract, oestrogens stimulate an increased retention of intravascular fluid and increase the capacity of intercellular connective tissues to retain water. The resulting fall in plasma osmolality stimulates a compensatory retention of sodium and water by the kidneys and the slight increase in intravascular fluid may also explain the rise in measures of glomerular filtration rate. At the same time, some of the increased progesterone is converted to DOC, a glucocorticoid hormone that acts on the distal tubule of the kidney to promote the reabsorption of sodium from the urine. The resulting shifts in fluid produce the slight tendency towards oedema that characterizes the second half of the cycle (Davison and Lindheimer, 1989; Davison and Noble, 1981; Schrier and Briner, 1991) (Fig. 17.1).

Premenstrual *engorgement of breast tissue* also results from local oedema and cell proliferation due to the activation of oestrogen and progesterone receptors in different sections of the mammary gland. A slight *hyperventilation* also develops during the luteal phase of the cycle and alveolar and arterial tensions of carbon

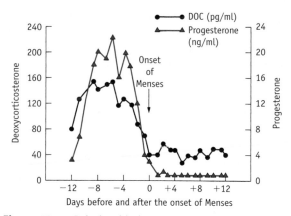

Figure 17.1 Relationship between mean plasma concentrations of deoxycorticosterone (DOC) and progesterone in women during the menstrual cycle. (Reproduced with permission from Parker *et al.*, 1981: 28.)

dioxide are lower than those observed prior to ovulation. Present evidence indicates that this occurs through the combined neuronal actions of oestrogens and progesterone within the respiratory centre in the medulla. Rising levels of oestrogens during the luteal phase stimulate the synthesis of progesterone receptors in these neurones, while the simultaneous increase in progesterone activates them by increasing their sensitivity to P_{CO_2}.

Following fertilization, these luteal changes are accentuated and gradually merge with others that arise in response to the complex patterns of hormonal interactions that characterize early pregnancy. In very early pregnancy, many women experience a *heightened sense of smell*, particularly of noxious substances like nicotine; a distaste for coffee and sugary foods; varying degrees of nausea and increased saliva and an overwhelming *desire for sleep*. Changes in smell, taste and saliva closely follow the pattern of human chorionic gonadotrophin (hCG) secretion and tend to diminish as levels of this hormone decline. The increased desire for sleep during the first trimester has been attributed to the predominant influence of progesterone on neuronal activity in the brain. Experiments on animals have demonstrated that progesterone diminishes excitatory neuronal transmitters while oestrogens increase brain receptors for progesterone as well as for other inhibitory and stimulatory neurotransmitter substances (Smith, 1991).

RENAL HAEMODYNAMIC CHANGES

Although the kidneys constitute less than 0.5% of total body weight in resting non-pregnant subjects, blood flow is equal to 25% of cardiac output, reflecting their key role in regulating fluid and electrolyte balance (Stanton and Koeppen, 1993: 720). From the mid-luteal phase of the cycle, significant changes occur in renal haemodynamics, as vascular resistance declines and plasma flow and glomerular filtration rate increase significantly by 6 weeks' gestation, compared to values obtained during the mid-follicular phase of the cycle. Minimal renal vascular resistance occurs at 8 weeks' gestation and this coincides with a peak rise in plasma flow of around 70%, which remains at slightly lower values for the remainder of pregnancy (Baylis and Davison, 1998; Chapman *et al.*, 1998).

Taken together, these findings suggest that hormonal changes in the corpus luteum before and after conception stimulate a primary fall in renal and systemic vascular resistance that initiates a chain of events leading to an early rise in cardiac output and plasma volume before any increase in basal metabolic rate. This temporal sequence of events indicates that a primary reduction in the vascular resistance of non-reproductive organs is initiated in preparation for the dramatic increase in uteroplacental blood flow during the second and third trimester. Considerable evidence suggests that *luteal* decline in vascular resistance and plasma osmolality and the subsequent rise in plasma volume and total body water are positive indicators of maternal adaptation to pregnancy because of their strong association with increased fetal growth and reduced perinatal mortality (Churchill *et al.*, 1997; Duvekot *et al.*, 1995; Steer *et al.*, 1995; Thompson *et al.*, 1967).

Hormonal regulation

Current findings suggest that the renal and systemic fall in vascular resistance and the rise in cardiac output are stimulated by the post-ovulatory increase in hCG, relaxin, oestrogens and progesterone from the corpus luteum followed by a significant rise in adrenomedullin, a long-lasting vasorelaxant, from a variety of tissues by 8 weeks' gestation (Coulson *et al.*, 1996; Hermsteiner *et al.*, 2002; Kristiansson and Wang, 2001; Nakamura *et al.*, 1988; Novak *et al.*, 2001; Sudhir *et al.*, 1995; Wu *et al.*, 2003). In human pregnancy, relaxin is detectable in the peripheral circulation 6 days after the mid-cycle LH/FSH surges. By 11 days, concentrations are significantly higher in fertile than in non-fertile cycles and concentrations increase rapidly up to 20 weeks' gestation (Johnson *et al.*, 1991; Stewart *et al.*, 1993). Experiments on rats have found that relaxin is a potent renal vasodilator and has a stimulatory effect on cardiac output (Coulson *et al.*, 1996; Novak *et al.*, 2001). More limited, human studies have demonstrated that higher plasma concentrations of relaxin and progesterone in early pregnancy are associated with lower mean systolic blood pressure in late pregnancy (Kristiansson and Wang, 2001). Recent evidence suggests that while oestrogens have a stimulatory effect on cardiac output and both oestrogens and progesterone have an important role in stimulating systemic and uterine vasodilatation, neither of these hormones seem to influence renal blood vessels which show a marked degree of dilatation following ovulation (Chapman *et al.*, 1997; Nakamura *et al.*, 1988; Sudhir *et al.*, 1995).

CARDIOVASCULAR ADAPTATIONS

Rise in cardiac output

The maternal cardiovascular system undergoes extensive changes in response to pregnancy. It is generally agreed that cardiac output rises by about 40% during pregnancy but uncertainty remains about the exact timing and pattern of the component changes and the underlying factors that bring them about (de Swiet, 1991b; Duvekot *et al.*, 1995).

Early studies using various invasive methods suggested that cardiac output increased gradually until the end of the second trimester and then declined towards non-pregnant values during the third trimester. This view was subsequently modified with the use of improved equipment and by taking measurements of women lying in a lateral rather than supine position in the third trimester. In general, these cross-sectional studies reported that cardiac output peaked before 30 weeks and plateaued over the remainder of pregnancy (de Swiet, 1991b).

More recent data have come from longitudinal studies using improved non-invasive techniques. While values for cardiac output vary considerably in different population groups, these studies generally suggest that it rises significantly during the first trimester, either peaks at 32 weeks with no significant changes thereafter, or continues to show further small rises until term (Mabie *et al.*, 1994). Measures of the pattern and relative contribution of heart rate and stroke volume to increased cardiac output suggest that heart rate is the more variable component in different population groups (Capeless and Clapp, 1989; Duvekot *et al.*, 1993; Robson *et al.*, 1989).

Stroke volume increases significantly by 8 weeks, peaks at 16–22 weeks and plateaus or shows further small increases during the third trimester. This represents a rise of 21–22% over pre-pregnant values. In different studies, heart rate has been found to increase significantly above pre-pregnant values by 5 and 16 weeks' gestation. Data on the remainder of pregnancy suggest that the increase peaks at 31–32 weeks and shows no significant change thereafter. Until more longitudinal studies are available, current evidence indicates that heart rate may increase by between 11 and 17% over pre-pregnant values (Capeless and Clapp, 1989; Duvekot *et al.*, 1993; Robson *et al.*, 1989).

Peripheral arterial vasodilatation

Studies suggest that cardiac output rises in early pregnancy in response to a fall in systemic vascular resistance that produces a reduced afterload in the myocardial fibres during left ventricular ejection. Decreases in both mean arterial pressure and total peripheral resistance are evident at 8 weeks' gestation and reach their lowest point by the middle of pregnancy, before returning to similar or slightly above pre-pregnant values at term. The decline in peripheral vascular resistance seems to be brought about by early relaxation in systemic, renal and pulmonary vascular tone and by the later development of new vascular beds in the placenta (Schrier and Briner, 1991).

The initial fall may be induced during the luteal phase of the cycle by rising levels of oestrogens and progesterone. Experimental studies in non-pregnant ovariectomized sheep have reproduced the characteristic

sequence of changes in vascular and fluid dynamics in early pregnancy by a gradual infusion of oestrogen into the systemic circulation. In addition, progesterone has been shown to reduce muscle tone in the vasculature (Magness and Rosenfeld, 1989; Omar *et al.*, 1995).

The current hypothesis suggests that when fertilization occurs, the further fall in peripheral vascular resistance creates a state of relative hypovolaemia that the heart attempts to modify by an increase in stroke volume and heart rate (Clapp *et al.*, 1988; Davison and Noble, 1981; Duvekot *et al.*, 1993; Schrier and Briner, 1991). This compensatory increase in cardiac output produces a rise in vascular filling state that is characterized by a rise in left atrial diameter, a rise in glomerular filtration rate and a fall in plasma renin, between the fifth and eighth week of gestation (Duvekot *et al.*, 1993). Studies on humans and animals have demonstrated that the fall in vascular resistance precedes the rise in circulating blood volume during pregnancy. This suggests that systemic vasodilatation may be a primary adaptation to pregnancy that initiates a rise in cardiac output and maintains overall tissue perfusion and blood pressure, prior to significant increases in circulating blood volume (Capeless and Clapp, 1989; Phippard *et al.*, 1986) (Fig. 17.2).

Blood volume

The increase in blood volume is composed of a maximum rise of 50% in plasma volume and a 20% rise in red cell volume. The time course of the increase in plasma volume is quite different from that of changes in red cell mass. Plasma volume begins to increase in the first trimester, increases more rapidly in the second and only slightly during the remainder of pregnancy. In contrast, expansion in red cell mass only begins in the second trimester and achieves highest increases in the third. Because of the different pace at which these changes proceed, haemoglobin concentration and haematocrit decline progressively until about 30 weeks' gestation. From then onwards, this trend is reversed, since increases in red cell volume outstrip those of plasma volume during the last trimester (Fig. 17.3).

Erythropoiesis

The increase in red cell mass during pregnancy is stimulated by erythropoietin. This glycoprotein hormone is synthesized in ground tissue, in the kidneys and to a lesser extent in the liver. Levels of serum immunoreactive erythropoietin remain at non-pregnant values during the first trimester, begin to rise during the second and reach maximum levels during the third trimester.

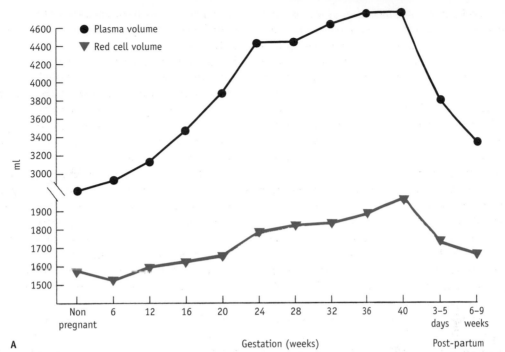

Figure 17.2   A. Mean total plasma and red cell volume during normal pregnancy. (Reproduced with permission from Lund and Donovan, 1967: 399.)

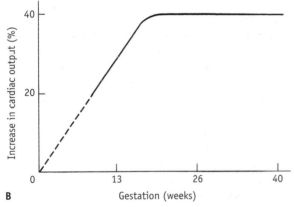

Figure 17.2   B. Changes in cardiac output through pregnancy. (Reproduced with permission from Hytten and Chamberlain, 1991: 8.)

Within the bone marrow, erythropoietin acts on erythrocyte colony-forming cells. These give rise to increasing numbers of mature erythrocytes within 2 days of increased levels of erythropoietin within the circulation.

At present, the precise mechanisms involved in stimulating erythropoietin during pregnancy remain unclear. The evidence suggests that components of the maternal plasma renin–angiotensin system may be involved. Angiotensinogen and erythropoietin share a number of similarities. Both compete for specific binding to

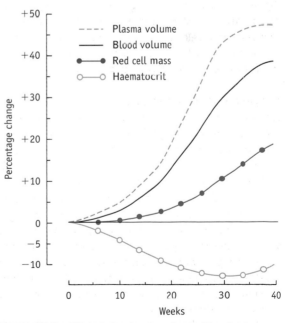

Figure 17.3   Changes in plasma volume, blood volume, red cell mass and haematocrit during normal pregnancy, expressed as a percentage of pre-pregnancy levels. (Reproduced with permission from Rosso, 1990: 25.)

erythropoietin receptors on human bone-marrow cells, and bone-marrow cells show binding of angiotensinogen that is inhibited by erythropoietin. This evidence suggests that angiotensinogen is a precursor for erythropoietin. In addition, animal experiments indicate that angiotensin II exhibits significant renal and extrarenal erythropoietin-stimulating activity. But while both components are increased in the maternal circulation during pregnancy, the timing and possible interactions between these components and erythropoietin remain to be clarified. A number of pregnancy hormones have both stimulatory and inhibitory influences on the actions of erythropoietin. Progesterone partly prevents the inhibitory influence of oestrogen on stem cell utilization of erythropoietin, while both placental lactogen and prolactin enhance the stimulatory action of erythropoietin on red cell production. At present, however, the precise significance of these hormonal actions remains unclear (Beguin *et al.*, 1990; Cotes *et al.*, 1983; Neng Lai and Fai Lui, 1993).

Renin–angiotensin system

Current evidence suggests that plasma volume expansion is primarily regulated by an oestrogen-stimulated rise in angiotensin II that activates the maternal vascular renin–angiotensin system as a result of the progressive rise of oestrogens in the maternal circulation (Skinner, 1993).

Evidence is accumulating to suggest that renin–angiotensin systems operate in a number of fetal and maternal sites during pregnancy. In embryonic and fetal tissues, components of the system have been found to accelerate cell growth and division and to stimulate the formation of blood vessels and tissue vascularization. In uteroplacental tissues, components of the system are thought to be involved in regulating local blood flow and liquor volume. Although many aspects of these findings remain uncertain, the emerging picture suggests that renin–angiotensin systems play an important role in creating conditions that enhance fetal growth (Broughton Pipkin, 1993; Downing *et al.*, 1995).

To date, greatest understanding has been gained of the vascular renin–angiotensin system. Its increased activity during pregnancy is initiated by the release of dehydroepiandrosterone (DHEAS) from the fetal zone of the adrenals. When it reaches the placenta, DHEAS is efficiently converted to a form that serves as substrate for the synthesis of oestrogens. Rising levels of oestrogens in the maternal circulation provide the main stimuli for the hepatic production of a specific globulin that circulates in plasma and acts as a substrate for renin. Angiotensinogen or renin substrate increases

very early in pregnancy and closely mirrors levels of oestrogens in individual women (Skinner, 1993).

Renin   Renin is a proteolytic enzyme that is synthesized and released mainly by specialized smooth muscle cells of afferent arterioles entering the glomeruli of the kidney. On reaching the blood stream, renin cleaves off part of angiotensinogen, triggering an enzymatic cascade that initially forms a biologically inactive peptide called angiotensin I. The next phase requires the action of angiotensin-converting enzyme, which circulates in plasma and is found in most tissues, but particularly high activities of the enzyme have been found in the lungs. This glycoprotein cleaves off part of angiotensin I to form the biologically active peptide angiotensin II that acts directly on the proximal tubules to enhance fluid reabsorption, and on the adrenal cortex to stimulate increased production of aldosterone.

Angiotensin II   By the second week of pregnancy, plasma levels of angiotensin II are double those in the non-pregnant state. Within the kidneys, angiotensin II stimulates increased fluid reabsorption in the proximal tubular cells, by enhancing the reabsorption of bicarbonate. Within the adrenals, angiotensin II stimulates cells in the outer zone of the cortex to secrete aldosterone. In the non-pregnant state, angiotensin II also acts on peripheral arterioles as a potent vasoconstrictor. During pregnancy, this pressor effect is thought to be counteracted by the vasodilatory activity of progesterone and oestrogens and by the vascular release of dilatory prostaglandins (Cook and Trundinger, 1993; Skinner, 1993).

Aldosterone

In situations of hypovolaemia, aldosterone acts mainly on the distal tubules to enhance the reabsorption of sodium. Plasma levels of aldosterone increase significantly by 12 weeks' gestation, and at 30 weeks reach a plateau that is three to five times higher than non-pregnant values. During the first half of pregnancy, effective renal plasma flow increases by 70–80% and then declines slightly in the third trimester, but still remains 50–60% above non-pregnant values, which is greater than occurs in any other physiological state. The resulting increase in glomerular filtration rate increases the sodium load from 20 000 to 30 000 mmol/day. Current evidence suggests that in these conditions, neither progesterone nor aldosterone has a major role in fluid regulation. Instead, fetal provision of increasing substrate for placental synthesis of oestrogens brings about

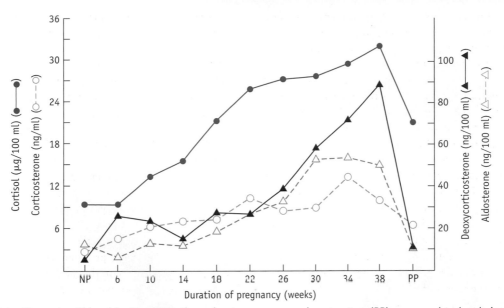

Figure 17.4   Mean steroid level in 11 women throughout pregnancy and postpartum (PP) compared to levels in non-pregnant (NP) women. (Reproduced with permission from Wintour *et al.*, 1978: 399.)

adaptive changes in maternal cardiovascular and renal capacity that provide the conditions needed to promote fetal growth and nutrition (Duvekot *et al.*, 1995; Longo, 1983; Pepe and Albrecht, 1995; Romen *et al.*, 1991; Skinner, 1993; Steer *et al.*, 1995).

Progesterone and deoxycorticosterone

In the non-pregnant state, progesterone acts to enhance the excretion of sodium by decreasing its reabsorption in the proximal sections of the tubules and by blocking the increased reabsorption of sodium by aldosterone in the distal tubules. At present it is not clear to what extent this progesterone action operates as a negative feedback element of the maternal plasma renin–angiotensin system during pregnancy. Some of the large increase in progesterone is converted to DOC, which acts on the distal tubules to promote the reabsorption of sodium. Rising levels of DOC occur by approximately 8 weeks' gestation and increase 10–15-fold, to a peak of approximately 100 mg/dl at term, which is higher than that of aldosterone. However, the salt-retaining properties of this hormone are 30–50 times less potent than those of aldosterone (Nolten and Rueckert, 1981; Skinner, 1993) (Fig. 17.4).

Atrial natriuretic peptide

The other main hormone that may influence renal handling of sodium during pregnancy is atrial natriuretic peptide (ANP). ANP is a peptide hormone produced in

the atrial chambers of the heart. Outside of pregnancy, secretion is primarily stimulated by stretching of the atrial wall that accompanies increases in blood pressure. ANP has been found to act in a number of ways to promote diuresis. Within the kidney, it directly inhibits both renin production and the tubular reabsorption of sodium and also acts on the adrenal glands to inhibit the production of aldosterone. In vitro studies have also shown that it produces marked relaxation of vascular smooth muscle.

Conflicting evidence currently exists on the pattern of ANP secretion during normal pregnancy. Plasma levels have been reported to decline from 20 weeks' gestation, reach lowest levels at 36 weeks and return to non-pregnant values by 12 weeks' postpartum. Another study has reported a gradual increase during the course of pregnancy to reach peak values at placental separation before declining significantly by 72 hours postpartum. Until more consistent data are obtained, it is not possible to identify the way in which this hormone participates in regulating fluid volume during pregnancy and the early postpartum period (Mukaddam-Daher *et al.*, 1995; Thomsen *et al.*, 1993; Yoshimura *et al.*, 1994).

ANATOMICAL RENAL ADAPTATIONS

All parts of the renal system are altered by a variety of different changes in pregnancy. The kidneys enlarge in

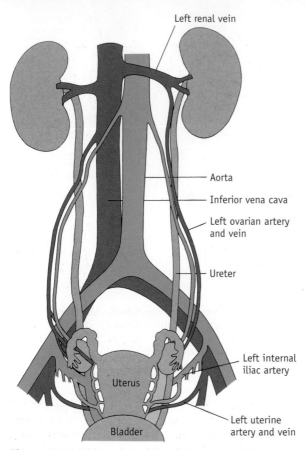

Figure 17.5 Obstruction of the right ureter at the pelvic brim by an enlarged ovarian vein. Note that the ovarian vein enters the vena cava by several trunks and the pelvic portion of the ureter is normal.

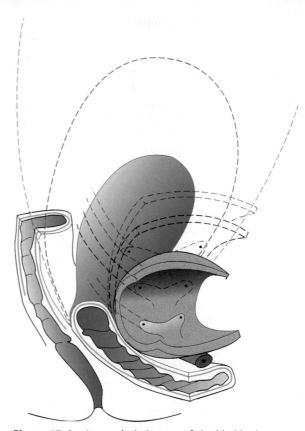

Figure 17.6 Anatomical changes of the bladder base with advancing pregnancy, showing elevation of the trigone and lateral displacement of the ureteral orifices. (Reproduced with permission from Mattingly and Borkowf, 1978: 869.)

response to increased vascular volume and the calyces, renal pelves and ureters dilate. Dilatation occurs during the first trimester and is always more prominent on the right. The common dilatory changes seem to occur in response to increased vascular volume and are not accompanied by reduced muscle tone. Progesterone has not been found to induce dilatation or to reduce peristalsis of the ureters. The more distinct dilatory changes on the right side have been explained by specific pressure on the ureter. A degree of obstruction seems to occur in the right ureter, as it crosses the enlarged iliac artery and ovarian vein almost at right angles, while the left ureter runs parallel to these vessels (Baylis and Davison, 1991; Marchant, 1978).

Real-time ultrasound studies on the kidney suggest that dilatation of the pelvis and calyces is accompanied by a progressive increase in urinary stasis. However, studies have found no evidence that this persists in the ureters. In contrast to earlier reports of their reduced

tone and motility, subsequent studies found hypertrophy of ureteric muscle and no changes in the intensity, frequency and tone of ureteral contractions during pregnancy (Cietak and Newton, 1985) (Fig. 17.5).

During pregnancy, the bladder is progressively elevated into the abdomen and the ureteral orifices are displaced laterally by the growing uterus. These changes may produce frequency of micturition and a degree of ureteral reflux. In early pregnancy, as the uterus occupies more space in the pelvic cavity, it may compress the bladder and cause frequency. Lateral displacement of the ureteral orifices is most pronounced during late pregnancy. It is thought to reduce intra-ureteral pressure, predisposing to backflow of urine through the ureteral orifice. Near term, engagement of the fetus within the pelvis may also exert upward pressure on the bladder, leading to increased frequency of micturition and discomfort (Marchant, 1978; Mattingly and Borkowf, 1978) (Fig. 17.6).

Tubular reabsorption of nutrients

The increased glomerular filtration rate also increases the load of other plasma constituents besides sodium. Urinary excretion of most amino acids increases by 200–700% above non-pregnant values, representing a loss of up to 2 g/day. In well-nourished women, this level of excretion is amply substituted by increased dietary intake (Baylis and Davison, 1991; Romen *et al.*, 1991).

The excretion of glucose increases progressively from 4 weeks' gestation until term. Serial studies have demonstrated that marked variations occur between and within individuals that are not related to blood sugar concentrations or to the length of gestation. In healthy women, glycosuria seems to occur primarily as a consequence of the 50% increase in glomerular filtration rate that is maintained throughout pregnancy (Lind and Hytten, 1972; Romen *et al.*, 1991).

VENTILATION

Extensive anatomical and functional changes occur in the respiratory system. These accommodate both the progressive increase in gas exchange required by the rising blood volume and the growing space occupied by the uterus. From early pregnancy onwards, the overall shape of the chest alters, by a flaring of the lower ribs that seems to occur independently of any mechanical pressure from the growing uterus. This progressively increases the subcostal angle, from 68 degrees in early pregnancy to 103 degrees at term and increases the transverse diameter of the chest by approximately 2 cm. Because of the flaring of the lower ribs, the diaphragm rises by a maximum of 4 cm while its contribution to the respiratory effort increases and shows no evidence of being impeded by the uterus. Studies on diaphragmatic movements during respiration either sitting or lying down have found them to be larger than in the non-pregnant state. This implies that breathing during pregnancy is more diaphragmatic than costal (de Swiet, 1991a; Romen *et al.*, 1991) (Fig. 17.7).

The main functional change that occurs within the lungs is the gradual increase in the amount of air that is inspired or expired with a normal breath. This functional capacity, called tidal volume, increases from 500 ml in the non-pregnant state to approximately 700 ml at term. As a result of this change, women breathe more deeply during pregnancy than in the non-pregnant state (Table 17.1).

Since the maximum amount of air that can be expired forcibly after maximum inspiration only increases by

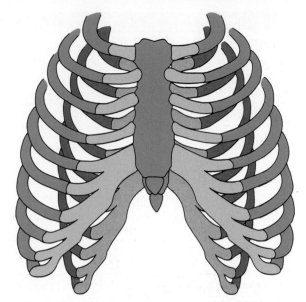

Figure 17.7 The ribcage in pregnancy (**coloured**) and the non-pregnancy state (**grey**) showing the increased subcostal angle, the increased transverse diameter and the raised diaphragm in pregnancy. (Reproduced with permission from de Swiet, 1991a: 88.)

100–200 ml, the increase in tidal volume is produced at the expense of the expiratory reserve volume. This means that a smaller amount of air remains in the lungs at the end of quiet expiration. As less residual air is mixed with the next inspiration of fresh air, this results in lower levels of P_{CO_2} that bring about a reciprocal rise in P_{O_2}. P_{CO_2} declines from approximately 39 mmHg in the non-pregnant state to 31 mmHg during pregnancy, while P_{O_2} increases from 93.4 to 101.8 mmHg, over the same period (de Swiet, 1991a) (Fig. 17.8).

Oxygen consumption

The progressive increases in cardiac output and pulmonary ventilation are proportionately greater than those occurring in maternal and fetal oxygen consumption during pregnancy. Oxygen consumption shows a linear increase with body weight as pregnancy advances. It is composed of the overall increase in tissue mass, the higher metabolic rate of fetal and placental tissue, along with that of some maternal organs, particularly the heart, lungs and kidneys. The maximum increase in oxygen consumption of 38 ml/min is 15% above average values in the non-pregnant state (de Swiet, 1991a) (Fig. 17.9).

This increase in oxygen consumption is facilitated by a 40–50% increase in ventilation and by an 18% increase in the oxygen-carrying capacity of the blood.

Table 17.1   Pulmonary adaptations in pregnancy (Gabbe *et al.*, 1991: 129)

Volumes/capacities	Definition	Changes
Respiratory rate	Number of breaths per minute	Unchanged
Vital capacity	Maximum amount of air that can be forcibly expired after maximum inspiration	Increases from mid-pregnancy by 100–200 ml
Inspiratory capacity	Maximum amount of air that can be inspired from resting expiratory level throughout pregnancy	Increases by 300 ml
Tidal volume	Amount of air inspired and expired with normal breath	Increases by 200 ml throughout pregnancy
Functional residual capacity	Amount of air in lungs at resting expiratory level	Decreases by 500 ml
Expiratory reserve volume	Maximum amount of air that can be expired from resting	Decreases by 200 ml throughout pregnancy
Residual volume	Amount of air in lungs after maximum expiration	Decreases by 300 ml throughout pregnancy
Total lung capacity	Total amount of air in lungs at maximum inspiration	Decreases by 300 ml throughout pregnancy

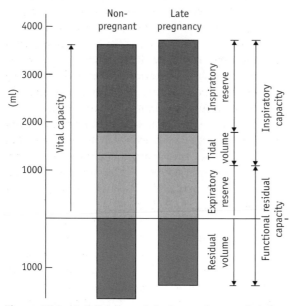

Figure 17.8   Subdivisions of the lung volume and their alterations in pregnancy. (Reproduced with permission from de Swiet, 1991a: 84.)

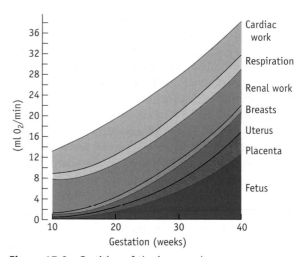

Figure 17.9   Partition of the increased oxygen consumption in pregnancy among the organs concerned. (Reproduced with permission from de Swiet, 1991a: 91.)

Because of this relative oversupply of oxygen, higher concentrations are returned to the heart from the venous circulation, making the arteriovenous oxygen difference significantly smaller than in the non-pregnant state. The extent of the arteriovenous oxygen difference is smallest in early pregnancy and does not reach average non-pregnant values until term (de Swiet, 1991a).

The increase in ventilation during pregnancy reduces alveolar and plasma concentrations of carbon dioxide. Studies have demonstrated that arterial partial pressure of carbon dioxide (P_{CO_2}) is about 30 mmHg in late pregnancy, compared to 39 mmHg during the follicular phase of the cycle. Since fetal P_{CO_2} remains at approximately 41 mmHg, the lower levels in the maternal circulation encourage the diffusion of CO_2 from fetal blood, across the placental membranes.

Hormonal regulation

The interdependent adaptations that develop within the cardiovascular and respiratory systems are regulated by a complex interplay between maternal, placental and fetal steroid hormones. Pulmonary changes are largely effected by progesterone, which resets the threshold at which the respiratory centre is stimulated. During pregnancy, a rise of 1 mmHg in P_{CO_2} increases ventilation by 6 litres/min, compared to 1.5 litres/min in the non-pregnant state (Bayliss and Millhorn, 1992; Romen et al., 1991).

Adaptations of the cardiovascular system include:

- enlargement of the heart
- peripheral vasodilatation
- development of new vascular beds in the placenta
- an increase in circulating blood volume, and
- a fall in plasma osmolality which is accompanied by a generalized oedema.

The increased size of the heart primarily affects the left ventricle. In animal experiments, this change has been shown to be stimulated by oestrogen. The accompanying changes in general systemic and uteroplacental vascular tone seem to be brought about by oestrogen and progesterone in conjunction with local vasodilatory agents (Morton, 1991; Pepe and Albrecht, 1995; Romen et al., 1991).

Peripheral vasodilatation is a very striking feature of pregnancy. Dilated veins appear on the surface of the breasts as well as on the hands, face and nasal mucous membrane. Experimental evidence suggests that this generalized tendency towards vasodilatation is brought about by a number of counteracting forces. These include the increased release of vasodilatory substances, prostacyclin and prostaglandin E_2 (PGE_2), by vascular endothelial cells. The combined actions of oestrogen and progesterone also depress vascular responses to the pressor effects of rising levels of angiotensin II which may also be involved in stimulating the release of prostaglandins. In addition, oestrogen has been found to depress the effects of sympathetic innervation, which tends to increase the general tone of the vascular system (Broughton Pipkin et al., 1982; Friedman, 1988; Pepe and Albrecht, 1995).

FETAL ADRENOPLACENTAL HORMONAL REGULATION OF CORTISOL

For most of intrauterine life, the fetus has a limited capacity to produce cortisol because the adult zone of the adrenal gland displays minimal activity until late in gestation. During the first half of pregnancy, the fetus is supplied with low levels of cortisol via the placenta. Cortisol metabolism within the placenta and in a variety of fetal tissues seems to be mediated by oestrogen through its regulation of two distinct isoforms of 11 β-hydroxysteroid dehydrogenase (11βHSD). Experimental findings suggest that up to mid-gestation, the predominant form of corticosteroid metabolism within the placenta is the reduction of cortisone to cortisol, which exceeds the oxidation of cortisol to inactive cortisone. This pattern of metabolism allows low quantities of biologically active maternal cortisol to enter the fetal compartment. Current evidence suggests that oestrogens regulate the latter but not the former reaction. Experiments have also shown that oestrogens increase the oxidation of cortisol to inactive cortisone in a variety of fetal organs. Together, these activities ensure that biologically active cortisol remains very low in fetal tissues and largely acts on the hypothalamus to suppress corticotrophin-releasing hormone (CRH). This in turn limits pituitary capacity for ACTH production, preventing growth and maturation of the adult cortisol-producing zone of the adrenal glands (Pepe and Albrecht, 1990, 1995; Stewart et al., 1995).

As synthesis of oestrogens increases with advancing gestation, oxidation of cortisol to cortisone becomes the predominant placental reaction. Research on the human placenta near term suggests that its capacity to convert cortisol to cortisone is four times higher than that required to inactivate its estimated exposure to 70 nmol maternal free cortisol/min. This shift in placental metabolism of maternal glucocorticoids has two major effects on the fetus. From mid-gestation onwards, cortisol of maternal origin decreases within the fetal compartment. Consequently, the earlier inhibitory action of maternal cortisol on growth and maturation of the adult zone is removed, while at the same time oestrogen activity within fetal tissues ensures that all organs are protected from the growth-retarding effects of cortisol. These conditions allow for the gradual maturation of the hypothalamic–pituitary–adrenal axis and the synthesis and release of fetal cortisol. Alongside the increasing capacity of the lungs and liver to convert cortisone to cortisol, production of cortisol by the fetal adrenals plays an important role in stimulating maturational changes in these organs in preparation for extrauterine development (Brown et al., 1993; Pepe and Albrecht, 1995; Pepe et al., 1988).

Research findings suggest that placental 11βHSD activity plays a crucial role in facilitating fetal growth and development during the second half of pregnancy. A variety of studies on humans and rats suggest that inappropriate exposure of fetal tissues to cortisol during their formative period of development creates a range of problems associated with impaired fetal growth and preterm labour. Increased release of maternal cortisol in response to social stress or poor nutrition may impose excessive demands on the capacity of 11βHSD to protect the fetal compartment from the growth-retarding effects of cortisol. Reduced growth implies lower levels of adrenal precursors for placental oestrogen, which in turn lowers its stimulatory effect on 11βHSD, thus further reducing the capacity of the placenta to inactivate cortisol (Blasco et al., 1986; Brown et al., 1993; Challis et al., 1995; Edwards et al., 1993; Godfrey and Barker, 1995; Hedegaard et al., 1993; Pepe and Albrecht, 1990; Seckl, 1994; Tangalakis et al., 1992).

MATERNAL HYPOTHALAMIC–PITUITARY–PLACENTAL AXIS

Gonadotrophin-releasing hormone, follicle-stimulating hormone and luteinizing hormone

The anterior pituitary undergoes significant anatomical adaptations during pregnancy. The gland increases in size by 30–50% and a redistribution occurs in the number and relative secretory activities of its distinct cell populations. In studies on women during the first and second trimester, basal concentrations of follicle-stimulating hormone (FSH) and luteinizing hormone (LH) are undetectable and significant short-term increases only occur in response to exogenous gonadotrophin-releasing hormone (GnRH) stimulation during the first trimester. Experiments on pituitary tissue from a variety of animal species have shown that these low concentrations of FSH and LH are accompanied by a progressive fall in the number, size and functional capacity of gonadotrophs during pregnancy (Jacobs, 1991; Shoupe and Kletzky, 1984; Wise et al., 1986).

Prolactin

At the same time a significant increase occurs in the number, size and secretory activity of prolactin-releasing cells. From 10–25% of the total population in the non-pregnant state, they grow to reach more than 50% during late pregnancy and lactation. Changes in this cell population are responsible for the overall increase in the size of the gland during pregnancy. Maternal serum levels are significantly elevated from early in the first trimester and continue rising progressively, reaching

up to 20 times non-pregnant values at term (Yen, 1991).

These distinct changes appear to be regulated by the increased placental release of oestrogens and progesterone. Prolonged elevation of oestrogen has been found to inhibit GnRH activity within the hypothalamus. This mode of action seems to be predominant in the first trimester. From the second trimester onwards, the higher level of oestrogens may also act directly to inhibit FSH and LH secretion from the anterior pituitary gland. The cellular changes that proceed simultaneously in lactotrophs are induced by steady increases in both oestrogen and progesterone, while the increased synthesis, storage and secretion of prolactin is stimulated by separate mechanisms that involve direct and indirect actions of oestrogen. Data from a number of experimental studies on animals suggest that synthesis and storage of prolactin is stimulated by a direct genomic action that takes place over 2–3 days, while prolactin secretion occurs within 2–3 hours and is mediated by oestrogen stimulation of a prolactin-releasing factor in either the hypothalamus or the posterior pituitary gland (Murai and Ben-Jonathan, 1990; Tong et al., 1990).

HYPOTHALAMIC–PITUITARY–ADRENAL–PLACENTAL AXIS

Maternal cortisol

In studies on plasma and saliva, total cortisol concentrations in pregnancy retain the daily variations that characterize the non-pregnant state (Fig.17.10). Continued diurnal variation of cortisol indicates its overall regulation by the hypothalamic–pituitary– adrenal (HPA) axis.

During pregnancy, daily patterns are largely similar to non-pregnant values, until approximately 12 weeks, when they begin to show a higher profile (Goland et al., 1990, 1992). By the last trimester, total cortisol levels are approximately three times non-pregnant levels (Allolio et al., 1990; Keller-Wood and Wood, 2001; Nolten et al., 1981) (Fig. 17.11). At present, it is thought that cardiovascular, metabolic and hormonal changes stimulate increasing concentrations of cortisol during pregnancy.

Placental steroids

Oestrogen has been found to enhance the production of a corticosteroid-binding globulin (CBG) that increases three-fold in the maternal circulation during pregnancy. While this increase in CBG could be expected to inactivate the higher levels of cortisol by increasing

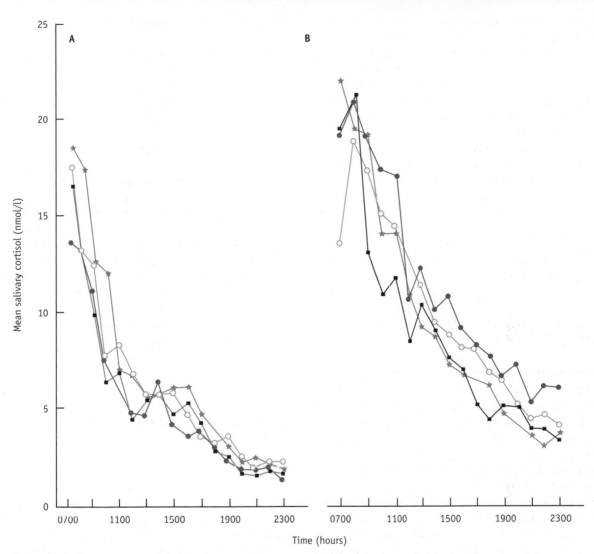

Figure 17.10 Salivary cortisol profiles throughout pregnancy in 10 healthy women (for clarity mean values are given). **A.** ■–■, 9–12; ●–●, 13–16; ★–★, 17–20; ○–○, 21–24: **B.** ■–■, 25–28; ●–●, 29–32; ★–★, 33–36; ○–○, 37–40 weeks of gestation. (Reproduced with permission from Allolio *et al.*, 1990: 281.)

its binding capacity, a number of studies have demonstrated that unbound, biologically active cortisol levels rise during the third trimester (Allolio *et al.*, 1990; Jones and Challis, 1990; Jones *et al.*, 1989).

The evidence suggests that this trend is influenced by the progressive increase in progesterone that has been found to compete with circulating cortisol for CBG-binding sites. This action is further confirmed by studies demonstrating that progesterone displays circadian variations during the second half of pregnancy that are inversely related to changes in cortisol. In contrast to cortisol, lowest levels of progesterone have been found at 08.00 and highest levels between 16.00

and 20.00 (Allolio *et al.*, 1990; Junkermann *et al.*, 1982) (Fig. 17.12).

This evidence of competitive binding between cortisol and progesterone has been used to explain increased tissue resistance to cortisol during pregnancy. If progesterone diminishes cortisol binding to specific glucocorticoid receptors, then higher levels of free cortisol may be stimulated to maintain its metabolic effects. In addition, the sustained increase in cardiac output and the lower levels of fasting glucose that characterize the latter half of pregnancy may also stimulate increased adrenal secretion of cortisol. Current evidence suggests that this is achieved by the increased release of placental

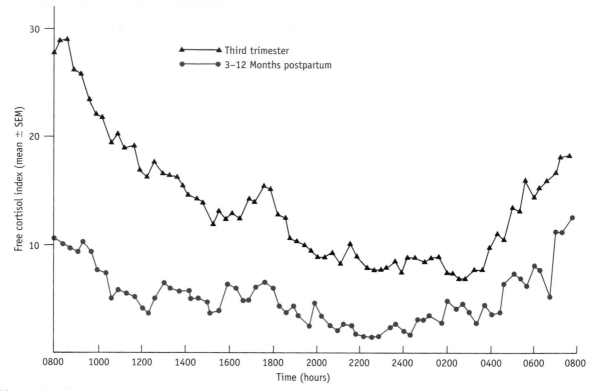

Figure 17.11 Patterns of mean free cortisol indexes measured at 20-minute intervals during a 24-hour period in seven third trimester gravid women and in three women who were 3–12 months postpartum. (Reproduced with permission from Nolten and Rueckert, 1981: 494.)

corticotrophin-releasing hormone (CRH) and adrenocorticotrophic hormone (ACTH) into the maternal circulation. Rising levels of CRH from the placenta seem to downregulate pituitary CRH receptors, reducing its stimulatory influence on ACTH. At the same time, placental ACTH may act as an additional stimulatory influence on maternal production of cortisol (Fraser, 1991; Goland *et al.*, 1990, 1992, 1994; Waddell and Atkinson, 1994; Waddell and Burton, 1993).

Corticotrophin-releasing hormone

Corticotrophin-releasing hormone is a neuropeptide synthesized mainly in the hypothalamus and released in response to different forms of physical and emotional stress. Its major site of action is the anterior pituitary, where it stimulates the release of ACTH, β-endorphin and other related peptides. Until the middle of the second trimester, plasma CRH remains at low or undetectable levels, similar to those in the non-pregnant state. Concentrations display a marked increase from 28 weeks and peak during labour. Present evidence strongly indicates that this rise is of placental rather than hypothalamic origin. In contrast to circulating

ACTH, no diurnal changes have been observed in plasma CRH. A low but detectable amount is present in the placenta and membranes until approximately 35 weeks, when it increases more than 20-fold during the remainder of pregnancy. Unlike that released from the hypothalamus, placental CRH is not subject to inhibition by glucocorticoids. In vitro findings suggest that glucocorticoids and oestrogen stimulate gene expression for CRH, while progesterone decreases levels of CRH and messenger ribonucleic acid (mRNA) in human placental tissue in culture (Chan *et al.*, 1993; Frim *et al.*, 1988; Goland *et al.*, 1992, 1994; Perkins and Linton, 1995; Robinson *et al.*, 1988; Vamvakopoulos and Chrousos, 1993; Warren and Silverman, 1995) (Figs 17.13 and 17.14).

Not all of the increase in circulating CRH is biologically active. A binding protein for CRH has been identified in plasma and found to inhibit its stimulatory effect on pituitary ACTH. During the first 25 weeks of pregnancy, maternal levels of CRH-binding protein remain similar to those in the non-pregnant state. Plasma concentrations decrease slightly from 26 to 30 weeks, then more rapidly, particularly over the last

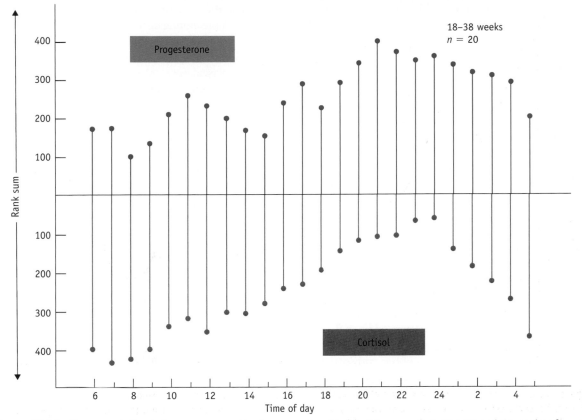

Figure 17.12 Inverse relation between serum progesterone and cortisol in 20 women between 18 and 38 weeks of pregnancy. Rank sums of cortisol and progesterone values are shown. (Reproduced with permission from Junkermann *et al.*, 1982: 103.)

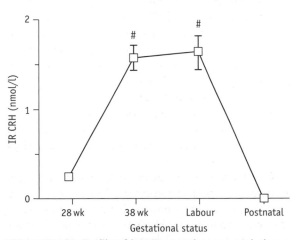

Figure 17.13 Profile of immunoreactive maternal plasma corticotrophin-releasing hormone (IR CRH) during pregnancy and parturition. (Reproduced with permission from Chan *et al.*, 1993: 341.)

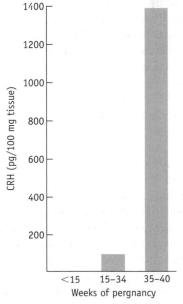

Figure 17.14 Changes in placental corticotrophin-releasing hormone peptide during pregnancy. (Reproduced with permission form Frim *et al.*, 1988: 290.)

5 weeks of gestation, to reach 33% of control values by term. This implies that concentrations of biologically active CRH rise significantly during the last trimester (Challis *et al.*, 1995; Perkins and Linton, 1995).

Adrenocorticotrophic hormone

Most studies have found that plasma ACTH remains fairly constant during pregnancy at a similar or slightly lower concentration than in the non-pregnant state. Like cortisol, the pattern of circulating ACTH shows daily variations indicating its regulation by the pituitary gland. However, between 20 and 40 weeks' gestation, afternoon values of ACTH are less suppressed than in the non-pregnant state, suggesting an additional non-pituitary source of secretion (Goland *et al.*, 1992).

During pregnancy, placental CRH stimulates the synthesis of ACTH alongside other related peptides, notably melanocyte-stimulating hormone (MSH) and β-endorphin. Unlike that released from the pituitary, placental ACTH is not subject to inhibition by glucocorticoids. Evidence suggests that this additional, independent source of ACTH may also act on the maternal adrenals. Despite the higher levels of free cortisol during the third trimester, there is no indication of a simultaneous decline in ACTH within the maternal circulation. At the same time the continued rise in placental CRH during the second half of pregnancy is not associated with a rising pattern of ACTH, suggesting a downregulation of pituitary CRH receptors. This hypothesis has been confirmed in experiments on baboons who showed a diminished response to exogenous CRH during the second half of pregnancy. Overall, these findings indicate that maternal cortisol production is regulated by placental and pituitary ACTH (Challis *et al.*, 1995; Goland *et al.*, 1990; Waddell, 1993).

Maternal and fetal significance

Current evidence suggests that these changes in the hypothalamic–pituitary–adrenal axis have a range of influences within the maternal, placental and fetal compartments during the second half of pregnancy. The rising pattern of cortisol in the maternal circulation coincides with the sustained mobilization of energy stores that is characterized by glucose resistance and hyperlipidaemia during the latter half of pregnancy. This suggests that placental CRH and ACTH may enhance the capacity of the maternal hypothalamic–pituitary–adrenal axis to meet the increased cardio-respiratory and metabolic activities that support rapid fetal growth in the second half of pregnancy (Waddell, 1993; Waddell and Atkinson, 1994).

Within the placenta, CRH, MSH and ACTH are involved in promoting different aspects of fetal growth. In vitro experiments on placental tissue have shown that CRH has a potent vasodilatory action on the fetal–placental vasculature. MSH directly stimulates fetal adrenal production of DHEAS and ACTH which does not cross into the fetal compartment and increases placental production of oestrogen and progesterone (Barnea *et al.*, 1986; Clifton *et al.*, 1995; Dupouy *et al.*, 1980; Pepe and Albrecht, 1990; Waddell, 1993).

Outside of these trophic influences, CRH has a range of activities within both placental and fetal compartments that may prepare a number of organs and tissues for the onset of labour. Placental CRH is secreted into the fetal circulation, reaching approximately 10% of maternal values at term. CRH-binding protein is also present in fetal plasma and follows a similar pattern to that found in the maternal circulation. The current hypothesis suggests that increased CRH in the fetal compartment assists in maturing the hypothalamic–pituitary–adrenal axis which stimulates cortisol production from the adult zone of the adrenal gland.

In the placenta, CRH is part of a number of positive feedback loops with factors that contribute towards the onset of labour. In vitro experiments have shown that CRH upregulates the production of prostaglandins from the placenta and membranes, while prostaglandins and other pro-inflammatory agents like interleukin-1 (IL-1) have a stimulatory influence on placental CRH. However, the significance of these and other similar findings remains to be identified in vivo, to take into account the modifying influences of the CRH-binding protein, the distribution of CRH receptors and the activity of hydroxyprostaglandin dehydrogenase (PGDH) which inactivates prostaglandins (Kelly, 1994; Perkins and Linton, 1995; Petragalia *et al.*, 1995; Wu *et al.*, 1995).

Endogenous opioids

It has been found that plasma concentrations of β-endorphin remain similar or lower than non-pregnant values until the third trimester, when concentrations increase significantly. During pregnancy, distinct pituitary and placental forms of β-endorphin have been identified. The pituitary source is mainly in an opioid active form, whereas that from the placenta contains little opioid activity. The pituitary form is predominant in the maternal circulation during pregnancy and its pattern of release maintains a daily rhythm that characterizes all hormones regulated by the hypothalamus. At the same time, significant correlations have

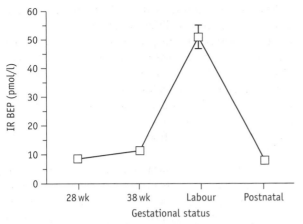

Figure 17.15 Profile of immunoreactive maternal plasma β-endorphin (IR BEP). (Reproduced with permission from Chan *et al*, 1993: 341.)

been found between plasma CRH and β-endorphin during the third trimester. This suggests that the enhanced release of pituitary β-endorphin may be influenced by placental CRH (Chan and Smith, 1992; Chan *et al.*, 1993) (Fig. 17.15).

Endogenous opioids and maternal pain threshold in late pregnancy

Findings in humans and other animals suggest that a distinct opioid pathway is activated in late pregnancy and labour that increases the maternal threshold for pain and discomfort. Observational studies on humans have reported a progressive rise in the pressure-induced pain threshold during the last 16 days of pregnancy. In daily tests on pregnant and non-pregnant women, discomfort thresholds also increased during the last 11 days of pregnancy and were higher than in those for non-pregnant women, whose responses remained unchanged throughout the course of the study. In experiments on rats, more direct evidence suggests that this analgesia of pregnancy may be mediated by a specific opioid system in the lumbar spine which is only activated during the latter part of pregnancy. Studies that have simulated the blood concentration profiles of oestradiol and progesterone during pregnancy have demonstrated that the spinal cord concentration of the opioid peptide dynorphin rises at steroid concentrations which correspond to the last week of pregnancy (Cogan and Spinnato, 1986; Medina, 1993; Sander *et al.*, 1988, 1989).

Endogenous opioids and oxytocin

From extensive studies on rats, an endogenous opioid input on oxytocin neurones has been found to be activated during the latter half of pregnancy. In this species there is evidence of a steroid-mediated increase in the synthesis of oxytocin during pregnancy and stores accumulate in the posterior lobe of the pituitary gland. From mid-pregnancy onwards, animals receiving intravenous injections of naloxone produce significantly higher plasma concentrations of oxytocin, compared to those receiving saline alone. This evidence of a restraining influence of opioids on oxytocin neurones is peculiar to periods of enhanced production of oxytocin. During pregnancy, this action is thought to be exerted by the depressive influence of opioids on the electrical activity of oxytocin neurones in the hypothalamus and by the co-release of opioids at oxytocin terminals in the posterior pituitary gland (Broad *et al.*, 1993; Douglas *et al.*, 1993).

THE MAMMARY GLAND

Pre-lactational adaptations

Maximum development of the mammary gland occurs during pregnancy. Blood flow starts to increase very soon after conception, as indicated by the early appearance of enlarged and distended veins beneath the skin. Estimates of mammary blood flow suggest that it rises from 1 to 2% of cardiac output, as pregnancy advances. The first 20 weeks are characterized by an intensification of the cell proliferation that begins during the luteal phase of the cycle. Growth of the ductal system is a predominant feature of the first half of pregnancy and is followed by enlargement and growth in the number of lobules from mid-pregnancy onwards. In this phase, new ducts are formed along with proliferation of adjoining clusters of alveoli. Towards the end of the first trimester, epithelial cells lining the alveoli also begin to differentiate from a double to a single layer of tissue. This change marks the emergence of secretory activity in the alveoli and is followed by the accumulation of secretory substances within the lumen of the alveoli during the second trimester (Fuchs, 1991; Russo and Russo, 1987).

In the third trimester, the secretory cells display an increased accumulation of lipids that are made available because of high levels of triglycerides in the maternal circulation. The process occurs through a tissue-specific increase in enzyme activity that augments the uptake of lipids from the circulation. As a result of this activity, an abundant supply of fat droplets accumulates in the secretory cells in preparation for the next phase of lactation. By the end of pregnancy, the secretory alveoli form the largest part of the gland. Connective and adipose tissue progressively diminish to form thin layers separating large, fully formed lobes of secretory cells (Russo and Russo, 1987).

The myoepithelial cells surrounding the alveoli also increase in size and number and form an open network around the epithelial cells. In rats, oxytocin receptors appear on the myoepithelial cells towards the end of pregnancy but functional capacity only develops with the onset of lactation. At this point the cytoplasm becomes packed with microfilaments that facilitate contractile activity within the cells (Fuchs, 1991).

Hormonal regulation

At present, most research has focused on the response of the mammary gland to a wide variety of external hormones. However, there is evidence from a variety of species for the synthesis of a range of hormones and growth factors within the gland. Current experimental findings suggest that the mammary gland operates as an endocrine organ in the luteal phase of the menstrual cycle as well as during pregnancy and lactation. While wide species variation is to be expected, some of these findings help to illuminate the complexity of hormonal interactions that have been identified in humans during pregnancy and lactation (Peaker, 1995).

In the presence of the anterior pituitary, placental steroids have been found to enhance cell proliferation, while growth hormone and prolactin have been shown to stimulate the uptake of lipids into mammary epithelial cells. Oestrogens specifically promote elongation of the ductal system and simultaneously increase receptor concentrations for progesterone, which stimulates ductal branching and development of lobes and alveoli (Fuchs, 1991; Haslam, 1987; Pepe and Albrecht, 1995; Thordarson et al., 1987).

In addition to these influences on mammary development, oestrogens stimulate the synthesis and release of increasing levels of prolactin from the anterior pituitary, while rising levels of progesterone inhibit the induction of lactose, lactalbumin and casein synthesis in the alveolar cells. Progesterone is thought to exert this effect by competing with cortisol for binding to alveolar receptors. In the presence of the high levels of progesterone that persist during pregnancy, prolactin seems to act within the mammary gland in conjunction with placental steroids to promote lobular and alveolar development and to stimulate the accumulation of lipid molecules in the secretory cells (Goodman et al.,

1983; Lee and Oks, 1992; Martin et al., 1980; Vonderhaar, 1987).

Besides these hormones, human placental lactogen (hPL) may also be involved in mammary development during pregnancy. In in vitro studies in humans, hPL has been found to induce substantial growth in ductal tissue that is independent of steroid hormones. However, it is not certain to what extent this occurs in vivo, as mammary development does not seem to be inhibited in women with very low levels of hPL during pregnancy. Uncertainties also exist on the timing of increased oxytocin receptor concentrations in the myoepithelial cells. Most studies in humans have found no increased sensitivity to exogenous oxytocin in pregnancy but marked increases have been reported in a number of studies following birth (Fuchs, 1991; Thordarson et al., 1987; Wiederman et al., 1964).

UTERINE ADAPTATIONS

Before pregnancy, the uterus is a small pelvic organ, with a cavity of around 10 ml and weighs approximately 50 g. By around 36 weeks, it is in contact with the anterior abdominal wall and extends as far as the xiphisternum. At this point, its weight has increased to an estimated 1100 g, representing almost a 20-fold increase in mass, and its average volume is 5 litres. During pregnancy, the uterus is a central recipient of the increases in circulating blood volume. In the non-pregnant state, uterine blood flow is approximately 10 ml/min. This changes very little during early pregnancy but rises sharply from about 20 weeks to reach 600–800 ml/min at term, when it receives nearly 20% of total cardiac output (Steer, 1991).

Myometrial changes

The bundles of smooth muscle fibres within the uterus are arranged in three or four layers embedded in a matrix of connective tissue which acts as intramuscular tendons. Two outer layers contain longitudinal and circular fibres that are partly continuous with the supporting ligaments. The middle layers that hold the vascular supply have a criss-cross pattern of fibres that run in all directions. Finally, the inner layer is composed of longitudinal fibres and covers the decidua (Steer, 1991).

Uterine growth occurs partly by cell division, particularly in early pregnancy, and by hypertrophy of existing cells during the remainder of pregnancy. Growth is stimulated by hCG and oestrogens and by the progressive distension exerted by the growing fetus. Both

A

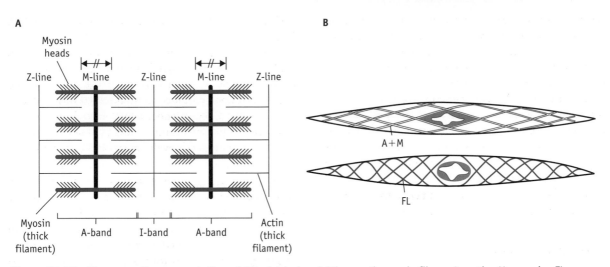

B

Figure 17.16   Diagrammatic representation of (**A**) striated and (**B**) smooth muscle fibres. A, actin; M, myosin; FL, filaments. (Reproduced with permission from Huszar and Roberts, 1982: 226.)

factors have been found to promote the synthesis of the contractile proteins, actin and myosin. During the first few months, growth is accompanied by increasing thickness of the myometrium in the corpus and the fundus. As the organ increases in length from around 12 weeks, the isthmus is gradually formed as an area containing a reduced density of muscle fibres (Steer, 1991).

The smooth muscle forming the myometrium does not have the precise transverse alignment of thick and thin filaments that characterizes the organization of skeletal fibres. Filaments of smooth muscle are situated in random bundles throughout the cells, and myosin filaments are arranged alongside actin in uninterrupted unidirectional order. In addition to these main contractile filaments, smooth muscle also contains intermediate filaments. These are attached to all areas of cell membrane which allows them to form networks across the cell. As a result of this organization, contractions can generate force in any direction and also produce a much greater degree of shortening than in skeletal muscle. For most of pregnancy, however, this action remains a local event, as few intracellular connections are formed until the last few weeks (Huszar and Roberts, 1982) (Fig. 17.16).

Influences of placental steroids

In addition to its structural differences with skeletal muscle, the myometrium has a number of additional features that distinguish it from smooth muscle in other parts of the body. Myometrial cells are uniquely regulated by oestrogens and progesterone. During pregnancy, oestrogen induces synthesis of structural and

contractile proteins and enzymes that supply energy for the process of contraction. Oestrogen also influences molecules within the plasma membrane that control its permeability for ions like sodium, potassium, calcium and chloride. These ion fluxes determine the resting potential and electrical excitability of myometrial cells (Fuchs and Fuchs, 1984; Pepe and Albrecht, 1995).

Besides having a direct effect on the structure of myometrial cells, oestrogens also regulate the formation of oxytocic and α-adrenergic receptors, both of which promote uterine contraction. During pregnancy, myometrial and decidual receptors for oxytocin increase from 27.6 fmol/mg DNA in the non-pregnant state, to 171.6 fmol/mg DNA, at mid-gestation and to 1391 fmol/mg DNA at term. Over the whole of pregnancy, this represents an 80–100-fold increase within the uterus. Some studies on women have reported an increase in α_1 receptors at term. β-adrenergic receptor formation is also stimulated by oestrogens. While static and decreasing concentrations have been reported at term, they do not appear to be activated prior to the onset of labour (Dahle *et al.*, 1993; Fuchs and Fuchs, 1991; Pepe and Albrecht, 1995; Wray, 1993).

Some, but not all, of the actions of oestrogens are modulated by progesterone. This hormone stimulates the synthesis of distinct and overlapping proteins and inhibits the production of oestrogen receptors and certain oestrogen-stimulated enzymes within myometrial cells. In direct contrast to oestrogens, progesterone stimulates the formation of β-adrenergic receptors which induce myometrial relaxation. But like the α-adrenergic receptors influenced by oestrogens, these are not activated before the onset of labour (Fuchs and Fuchs, 1991; Pepe and Albrecht, 1995; Wray, 1993).

Cervical changes

In nulliparous women, the cervix is largely composed of dense fibrous connective tissue, formed by thick, cross-linked collagen fibrils that are invested in a ground substance, composed of core proteins attached to large numbers of unbranched polysaccharide chains. These form an interconnecting lattice that actively binds to collagen fibrils in a way that positions them to provide maximal mechanical strength. The smaller muscle content is organized as a continuous external layer and scattered bundles are located internally. Few structural changes occur in the cervix until the latter part of pregnancy. There is an overall increase in the size of the cervix which is accompanied by a rise in total collagen content, some hypertrophy of external muscle fibres and a progressive rise in vascularity. As pregnancy advances, some biopsy studies have reported a gradual reduction in collagen density, a rise in polysaccharide chains and a possible redistribution of core proteins in favour of those that are highly absorbent. In addition to the increased vascularity, these findings may explain the increasing water content and the slightly softer consistency of the cervix during pregnancy (Hughesdon, 1952; Huszar and Walsh, 1991; Jeffrey, 1991; Uldbjerg *et al.*, 1983) (see Ch. 25).

MUSCULOSKELETAL ADAPTATIONS

Considerable alterations occur in the musculoskeletal system during pregnancy. From the first trimester onwards, rising levels of oestrogens and relaxin reduce the density of connective tissue, cartilage and ligaments and increase the quantity of synovial fluid. Taken together, these changes produce a greater degree of mobility and flexibility in the joints. During the second half of pregnancy, joint mobility may be reduced, particularly in ankle and wrist joints, by increasing fluid

retention in the surrounding connective tissue. At the same time, the woman's centre of gravity is displaced by the increasing size, weight and anterior orientation of the uterus as it expands into the abdominal cavity and, to a lesser extent, by the growing weight of the breasts. To compensate for the increased likelihood of tilting forward, the woman's centre of gravity is simultaneously displaced back over the pelvis, which tends to produce a progressive lordosis of the lumbar spine.

Pelvis – bones and ligaments

The pelvic girdle is uniquely formed to respond to hormonal and postural influences in pregnancy and labour. At birth, the bony pelvis is composed of a pair of coxal or hip bones which form the anterior and lateral walls of the pelvic cavity. The remaining wall is shaped by vertebrae which gradually fuse to form the sacrum and coccyx. Each coxal bone is made up of three adjoining bones. At birth, parts of these bones, together with their adjoining areas, are still composed of cartilage. Bone growth and ossification, together with joint fusion, continue throughout childhood, puberty and early adult life. Joint fusion is thought to be complete by approximately 25 years.

CONCLUSION

Adaptations in pregnancy affect all systems of the body. These are regulated by a complex series of hormonal interactions between maternal systems and the fetoplacental unit. This chapter has identified some of these and has demonstrated their importance for pregnancy, labour and lactation.

Reflective Activity 17.1

Review the information in this chapter and link it to your experiences and observations in encounters with women during pregnancy.

KEY POINTS

- Pregnancy is a period of structural and functional adaptations for all organ systems.
- These changes affect and are affected by neurohormonal interactions between mother and fetus.

- Neurohormonal regulation of maternal adaptations are critical to a successful pregnancy, followed by the onset of labour at term and the shift from placental to mammary nutrition immediately after birth.

REFERENCES

Allolio, B., Hoffmann, J., Linton, E.A. *et al.* (1990) Diurnal salivary cortisol patterns during pregnancy and after delivery: relationships to plasma corticotrophin-releasing-hormone. *Clinical Endocrinology* 33: 279–289.

Barnea, E.R., Lavy, G., Fakih, H. *et al.* (1986) The role of ACTH in placental steroidogenesis. *Placenta* 7: 307–313.

Baylis, C. & Davison, J. (1991) The urinary system. In: Hytten, F. & Chamberlain, G. (eds) *Clinical Physiology in Obstetrics*, pp. 245–302. Oxford: Blackwell Scientific.

Bayliss, D.A. & Millhorn, D.E. (1992) Central neural mechanisms of progesterone action: application to the respiratory system. *Journal of Applied Physiology* 73(2): 393–404.

Beguin, Y., Lipscei, G., Oris, R. *et al.* (1990) Serum immunoreactive erythropoietin during pregnancy and in the early postpartum. *British Journal of Haematology* 76: 545–549.

Blasco, M.J., Lopez Bernal, A. & Turnbull, A.C. (1986) 11β-hydroxysteroid dehydrogenase activity of the human placenta during pregnancy. *Hormone and Metabolic Research* 18: 638–641.

Broad, K., Kendrick, K.M., Sirinathsinghji, D.J.S. *et al.* (1993) Changes in oxytocin immunoreactivity and mRNA expression in the sheep brain during pregnancy, parturition and lactation and in response to oestrogen and progesterone. *Journal of Neuroendocrinology* 5: 435–444.

Broughton Pipkin, F. (1993) The fetal renin–angiotensin system. In: Robertson, J.I.S. s Nicholls, M.G. (eds) *The Renin–Angiotensin System,* Vol. 1, pp. 51.1–51.10. London: Gower Medical Publishers.

Broughton Pipkin, F., Hunter, J.C. & Turner, S.R. (1982) Prostaglandin attenuates the pressor response to angiotensin II in pregnant subjects but not in nonpregnant subjects. *American Journal of Obstetrics and Gynecology* 142(2): 168–176.

Brown, R.W. & Chapman Edwards, C.R.W. (1993) Human placental 11β-hydroxysteroid dehydrogenase: evidence for and partial purification of a distinct NAD-dependent isoform. *Endocrinology* 132(6): 2614–2621.

Capeless, E.L. & Clapp, J.F. (1989) Cardiovascular changes in early pregnancy. *American Journal of Obstetrics and Gynecology* 161(6): 1449–1452.

Challis, J.R.G., Matthews, S.G. & Van Meir, C. (1995) Current topic: the placental corticotrophin-releasing hormone–adrenocorticotrophin axis. *Placenta* 16: 481–502.

Chan, E-C. & Smith, R. (1992) β-endorphin immuno-reactivity during human pregnancy. *Journal of Clinical Endocrinology and Metabolism* 75(6): 1453–1458.

Chan, E-C., Smith, R., Lewin, T. *et al.* (1993) Plasma corticotrophin-releasing hormone, β-endorphin and cortisol inter-relationships during human pregnancy. *Acta Endocrinologica* 128: 339–344.

Chapman, A.B., Zamudio, S., Woodmansee, W. *et al.* (1997) Systemic and renal haemodynamic changes in the luteal phase of the menstrual cycle mimic early pregnancy. *American Journal of Physiology* 273(42): F777–F782.

Chapman, A.B., Abraham, W.T., Zamudio, S. *et al.* (1998) Temporal relationships between hormonal and hemodynamic changes in early pregnancy. *Kidney International* 54: 2056–2063.

Churchill, D., Perry, I.J. & Beevers, D.G. (1997) Ambulatory blood pressure in pregnancy and fetal growth. *Lancet* 349: 7–10.

Cietak, K.A. & Newton, J.R. (1985) Serial qualitative maternal nephrosonography in pregnancy. British Journal of Radiology 58(689): 399–404.

Clapp, J.F., Seaward, B.L., Sleamaker, R.H. *et al.* (1988) Maternal physiologic adaptations to early pregnancy. *American Journal of Obstetrics and Gynecology* 159(6): 1456–1460.

Clifton, V.L., Read, M.A. & Leitch, I.M. (1995) Corticotrophin-releasing hormone-induced vasodilatation in the human fetal–placental circulation: involvement of the nitric oxide-cycle guanosine 39,5-monophosphate-mediated pathway. *Journal of Clinical Endocrinology and Metabolism* 80(10): 2888–2893.

Cogan, R. & Spinnato, J.A. (1986) Pain and discomfort thresholds in late pregnancy. *Pain* 27: 63–68.

Cook, C. & Trundinger, B. (1993) Angiotensin sensitivity predicts aspirin benefit in placental insufficiency. *British Journal of Obstetrics and Gynaecology* 100: 46–50.

Cotes, M.P., Canning, C.E. & Lind, T. (1983) Changes in serum immunoreactive erythropoietin during the menstrual cycle and normal pregnancy. *British Journal of Obstetrics and Gynaecology* 90: 304–311.

Coulson, C.C., Thorp, J.M., Mayer, D.C. *et al.*, (1996) Central haemodynamic effects of recombinant human relaxin in the isolated, perfused rat heart model. *Obstetrics and Gynecology* 87(4): 610–612.

Dahle, L.O., Andersson, R.G.G., Berg, G. *et al.* (1993) Alpha-adrenergic receptors in human myometrium: changes during pregnancy. *Gynecologic and Obstetric Investigation* 36: 75–80.

Davison, J.M. & Lindheimer, M.D. (1989) Volume homeostasis and osmoregulation in human pregnancy. *Baillière's Clinical Endocrinology and Metabolism* 3(2): 451–472.

Davison, J.M. & Noble, M.C.B. (1981) Serial changes in 24 hour creatinine clearance during normal menstrual cycles and the first trimester of pregnancy. *British Journal of Obstetrics and Gynaecology* 88: 10–17.

De Swiet, M. (1991a) The respiratory system. In: Hytten, F. & Chamberlain, G. (eds) *Clinical Physiology in Obstetrics*, pp. 83–100. Oxford: Blackwell Scientific.

De Swiet, M. (1991b) The cardiovascular system. In: Hytten, F. & Chamberlain, G. (eds) *Clinical Physiology in Obstetrics*, pp. 3–38. Oxford: Blackwell Scientific.

Douglas, A.J., Dye, S., Leng, G. *et al.* (1993) Endogenous opioid regulation of oxytocin secretion through pregnancy in the rat. *Journal of Neuroendocrinology* 5: 307–314.

Downing, G.J., Poisner, A.M. & Barnea, E.R. (1995) First-trimester villous placenta has high prorenin and active renin concentrations. *American Journal of Obstetrics and Gynecology* 172(3): 864–867.

Dupouy, J-P., Chatelain, A. & Allaume, P. (1980) Absence of transplacental passage of ACTH in the rat: direct experimental proof. *Biology of the Neonate* 37: 96–102.

Duvekot, J.J., Cheriex, E.C. & Pieters, F.A.A. (1993) Early pregnancy changes in hemodynamics and volume homeostasis are consecutive adjustments triggered by a primary fall in systemic vascular tone. *American Journal of Obstetrics and Gynecology* 169(6): 1382–1392.

Duvekot, J.J., Cheriex, E.C., Pieters, F.A.A. *et al.* (1995) Maternal volume homeostasis in early pregnancy in relation to fetal growth restriction. *Obstetrics and Gynecology* 85(3): 361–367.

Edwards, C.R.W., Benediktsson, R., Lindsay, R.S. *et al.* (1993) Dysfunction of placental glucocorticoid barrier: link between fetal environment and adult hypertension. *Lancet* 341: 355–357.

Fraser, R.B. (1991) Carbohydrate metabolism. In: Hytten, F. & Chamberlain, G. (eds) *Clinical Physiology in Obstetrics*, pp. 204–212. Oxford: Blackwell Scientific.

Friedman, S.A. (1988) Preeclampsia: a review of the role of prostaglandins. *Obstetrics and Gynecology* 71(1): 122–137.

Frim, D.M., Emanuel, R.L., Robinson, B.G. *et al.* (1988) Characterisation of gestational regulation of corticotrophin-releasing hormone messenger RNA in human placenta. *Journal of Clinical Investigation* 82: 287–292.

Fuchs, A-F. (1991) Physiology and endocrinology of lactation. In: Gabbe, S.G., Niebyl, J.R. & Simpson, J.L. (eds) *Obstetrics, Normal and Problem Pregnancies*, pp. 175–205. New York: Churchill Livingstone.

Fuchs, A-F. & Fuchs, F. (1984) Endocrinology of human parturition: a review. *British Journal of Obstetrics and Gynaecology* 91: 948–967.

Fuchs, A-F. & Fuchs, F. (1991) Physiology of parturition. In: Gabbe, S.G., Niebyl, J.R. & Simpson, J.L. (eds) *Obstetrics, Normal and Problem Pregnancies*, pp. 147–174. New York: Churchill Livingstone.

Gabbe, S.G., Niebyl, J.R. & Simpson, J.L. (eds) (1991) *Obstetrics, Normal and Problem Pregnancies*. New York: Churchill Livingstone.

Godfrey, K. & Barker, D.J.B. (1995) Maternal nutrition in relation to fetal and placental growth. *European Journal of Obstetrics, Gynecology, and Reproductive Biology* 61: 15–22.

Goland, R.S., Stark, R.I. & Wardlaw, S.L. (1990) Response of corticotrophin-releasing hormone during pregnancy in the baboon. *Journal of Clinical Endocrinology and Metabolism* 70(4): 925–929.

Goland, R.S., Conwell, I.M., Warren, W.B. *et al.* (1992) Placental corticotrophin-releasing hormone and pituitary–adrenal function during pregnancy. *Neuroendocrinology* 56: 742–749.

Goland, R.S., Jozak, R.N. & Conwell, I. (1994) Placental corticotrophin-releasing hormone and the hypercortisolism of pregnancy. *American Journal of Obstetrics and Gynecology* 171(4): 1287–1291.

Goodman, G.T., Akers, R.M., Friderici, H. *et al.* (1983) Hormonal regulation of α-lactalbumin secretion from bovine mammary tissue cultured in vitro. *Endocrinology* 112(4): 1324–1330.

Haslam, S.Z. (1987) Role of sex steroid hormones in normal mammary gland function. In: Neville, M.C. & Daniel, C.W. (eds) *The Mammary Gland*, pp. 499–533. New York: Plenum Press.

Hedegaard, M., Henriksen, T.B., Sabroe, S. *et al.* (1993) Psychological distress in pregnancy and preterm delivery. *British Medical Journal* 307: 234–239.

Hughesdon, P.E. (1952) The fibromuscular structure of the cervix and its changes during pregnancy and labour. *Journal of Obstetrics and Gynaecology of the British Empire* 59: 763–776.

Huszar, G. & Roberts, J.M. (1982) Biochemistry and pharmacology of the myometrium and labour: regulation at the cellular and molecular levels. *American Journal of Obstetrics and Gynecology* 142(2): 225–237.

Huszar, G.B. & Walsh, M.P. (1991) Relationship between myometrial and cervical functions in pregnancy and labour. *Seminars in Perinatology* 15(2): 97–117.

Hytten, F. & Chamberlain, G. (eds) (1991) *Clinical Physiology in Obstetrics*. Oxford: Blackwell Scientific.

Jacobs, H.S. (1991) The hypothalamus and pituitary gland. In: Hytten, F. & Chamberlain, G. (eds) *Clinical Physiology in Obstetrics*, pp. 345–356. Oxford: Blackwell Scientific.

Jeffrey, J.J. (1991) Collagen and collagenase: pregnancy and parturition. *Seminars in Perinatology* 15(2): 118–126.

Johnson, M.R., Okokon, E., Collins, W.P. *et al.* (1991) The effect of human chorionic gonadotrophin and pregnancy on the circulating level of relaxin. *Journal of Clinical Endocrinology and Metabolism* 72(5): 1042–1047.

Jones, S.A. & Challis, J.R.G. (1990) Steroid, corticotrophin-releasing hormone, ACTH and prostaglandin interactions in the amnion and placenta of early pregnancy in man. *Journal of Endocrinology* 125: 153–159.

Jones, S.A., Brooks, A.N. & Challis, J.R.G. (1989) Steroids modulate corticotrophin-releasing hormone production in human fetal membranes and placenta. *Journal of Clinical Endocrinology and Metabolism* 68(4): 825–830.

Junkermann, H., Mangold, H., Vecsei, P. *et al.* (1982) Circadian rhythm of serum progesterone levels in human pregnancy and its relation to the rhythm of cortisol. *Acta Endocrinologica* 101: 98–104.

Keller-Wood, M. & Wood, C.E. (2001) Pituitary adrenal physiology during pregnancy. *Endocrinologist* 11: 159–170.

Kelly, R.W. (1994) Pregnancy maintenance and parturition: the role of prostaglandin in manipulating the immune and inflammatory response. *Endocrine Reviews* 15(5): 684–706.

Kristiansson, P. & Wang, J.X. (2001) Reproductive hormones and blood pressure during pregnancy. *Human Reproduction* 16(1): 13–17.

Lee, C.S. & Oks, T. (1992) Progesterone regulation of a pregnancy-specific transcription repressor to β-casein gene promoter in mouse mammary gland. *Endocrinology* 131(5): 2257–2262.

Lind, T. & Hytten, F.E. (1972) The excretion of glucose during normal pregnancy. *Journal of Obstetrics and Gynaecology of the British Commonwealth* 79(11): 961–965.

Longo, L.F. (1983) Maternal blood volume and cardiac output during pregnancy: a hypothesis of endocrine control. *American Journal of Physiology* 245: R720–R729.

Lund, C.J. & Donovan, J.C. (1967) Blood volume during pregnancy. *American Journal of Obstetrics and Gynecology* 98(3): 393–403.

Mabie, W., DiSessa, T.G., Crocker, L.G. *et al.* (1994) A longitudinal study of cardiac output in normal human pregnancy. *American Journal of Obstetrics and Gynecology* 170(3): 849–856.

Magness, R.R. & Rosenfeld, C.R. (1989) Local and systemic estradiol-17β: effects on uterine and systemic vasodilation. *American Journal of Physiology* 256: E536–E542.

Marchant, D.J. (1978) Alterations in anatomy and function of the urinary tract during pregnancy. *Clinics in Obstetrics and Gynaecology* 21(3): 855–861.

Martin, R.H., Glass, M.R., Chapman, C. *et al.* (1980) Human α-lactalbumin and hormonal factors in pregnancy and lactation. *Clinical Endocrinology* 13: 223–230.

Mattingly, R.F. & Borkowf, H.I. (1978) Clinical implications of ureteral reflux in pregnancy. *Clinics in Obstetrics and Gynaecology* 21(3): 863–873.

Medina, V.M. (1993) 17β-estradiol and progesterone positively modulate spinal cord dynorphin: relevance to the analgesia of pregnancy. *Neuroendocrinology* 58: 310–315.

Morton, M.J. (1991) Maternal hemodynamics in pregnancy. In: Mittelmark, R.A. & Wiswell, R.A. (eds) *Exercise in Pregnancy,* pp. 61–70. Baltimore: Williams & Wilkins.

Mukaddam-Daher, S., Gutkowska, J. & Tremblay, J. (1995) Regulation of renal atrial natriuretic peptide receptors in pregnant sheep. *Endocrinology* 136(10): 4565–4571.

Murai, I. & Ben-Jonathan, N. (1990) Acute stimulation of prolactin by estradiol: mediation by the posterior pituitary. *Endocrinology* 126(6): 3179–3184.

Neng Lai, K. & Fai Lui, S. (1993) Renin and erythropoietin. In: Robertson, J.I.S. & Nicholls, M.G. (eds) *The Renin–Angiotensin System,* Vol. 1, pp. 39.1–39.8. London: Gower Medical Publishers.

Nolten, W.E. & Rueckert, P.A. (1981) Elevated free cortisol index in pregnancy: possible regulatory mechanisms. *American Journal of Obstetrics and Gynecology* 139(4): 492–498.

Nolten, W.E., Holt, L.H. & Rueckert, P.A. (1981) Deoxycorticosterone in normal pregnancy: III. Evidence of a fetal source of deoxycorticosterone. *American Journal of Obstetrics and Gynecology* 139(4): 477–482.

Novak, J., Danielson, L.A., Kerchner, L.J. *et al.,* (2001) Relaxin is essential for renal vasodilation during pregnancy in conscious rats. *Journal of Clinical Investigation* 107(11): 1469–1475.

Omar, H.A., Ramirez, R. & Gibson, M. (1995) Properties of a progesterone-induced relaxation in human placental arteries and veins. *Journal of Clinical Endocrinology and Metabolism* 80(2): 370–373.

Parker, C.R., Winkel, C.A., Rush, J.A. *et al.* (1981) Plasma concentrations of 11-deoxycorticosterone in women during the menstrual cycle. *Obstetrics and Gynecology* 58(1): 26–30.

Peaker, M. (1995) Endocrine signals form the mammary gland. *Journal of Endocrinology* 147: 189–193.

Pepe, G.J. & Albrecht, E.D. (1990) Regulation of the primate fetal adrenal cortex. *Endocrine Reviews* 11(1): 151–176.

Pepe, G.J. & Albrecht, E.D. (1995) Actions of placental and fetal adrenal steroid hormones in primate pregnancy. *Endocrine Reviews* 16(5): 608–648.

Pepe, G.J., Brendan, J. & Waddell, S.J. (1988) The regulation of transplacental cortisol-cortisone metabolism by estrogen in pregnant baboons. *Endocrinology* 122(1): 78–83.

Perkins, A.V. & Linton, E.A. (1995) Placental corticotrophin-releasing hormone: there by accident or design? *Journal of Endocrinology* 147: 377–381.

Petragalia, F., Benedetto, C., Florio, P. *et al.* (1995) Effect of corticotrophin-releasing factor-binding protein on prostaglandin release from cultured maternal decidua and on contractile activity of human myometrium in vitro. *Journal of Clinical Endocrinology and Metabolism* 80(10): 3073–3076.

Phippard, A.F., Horvath, J.S. & Glynn, E.M. (1986) Circulatory adaptations to pregnancy – serial studies of haemodynamics, blood volume, renin, and aldosterone in the baboon. *Journal of Hypertension* 4: 773–779.

Robinson, B.G., Emanuel, R.L., Frim, D.M. *et al.* (1988) Glucocorticoid stimulates expression of corticotrophin-releasing hormone gene in human placenta. *Proceedings* of the National Academy of Sciences of the USA **85**: 5244–5248.

Robson, S.C., Hunter, S. & Boys, R.J. *et al.* (1989) Serial study of factors influencing changes in cardiac output during human pregnancy. *American Journal of Physiology* **256**: H1060–H1065.

Romen, Y., Masaki, D.I. & Mittelmark, R.A. (1991) Physiological and endocrine adjustments to pregnancy. In: Mittelmark, R.A. & Wiswell, R.A. (eds) *Exercise in Pregnancy,* pp. 9–29. Baltimore: Williams & Wilkins.

Rosso, P. (1990) *Nutrition and Metabolism in Pregnancy.* New York: Oxford University Press.

Russo, J. & Russo, I.H. (1987) Development of the human mammary gland. In: Neville, M.C. & Daniel, C.W. (eds) *The Mammary Gland,* pp. 67–93. New York: Plenum Press.

Sander, H.W., Portoghese, P.S. & Gintzler, A.R. (1988) Spinal κ-opiate receptor involvement in the analgesia of pregnancy: effects of intrathecal norbinaltorphimine, a κ-selective antagonist. *Brain Research* **474**: 343–347.

Sander, H.W., Kream, R.M. & Gintzler, A.R. (1989) Spinal dynorphin involvement in the analgesia of pregnancy: effects of intrathecal dynorphin antisera. *European Journal of Pharmacology* **159**: 105–109.

Schrier, R.W. & Briner, V.A. (1991) Peripheral arterial vasodilation hypothesis of sodium and water retention in pregnancy: implications for pathogenesis of pre-eclampsia. *Obstetrics and Gynecology* **77**(4): 632–639.

Seckl, J.R. (1994) Glucocorticoids and small babies. *Quarterly Journal of Medicine* **87**: 259–262.

Shoupe, D. & Kletzky, O.A. (1984) Priming with gonadotrophin-releasing hormone restores gonadotrophin secretion during first but not second trimester of pregnancy. *American Journal of Obstetrics and Gynecology* **150**(5): 460–464.

Skinner, S.L. (1993) The renin system in fertility and normal human pregnancy. In: Robertson, J.I.S. & Nicholls, M.G. (eds) *The Renin–Angiotensin System,* Vol. 1, pp. 50.1–50.16. London: Gower Medical Publishers.

Smith, S.S. (1991) Progesterone administration attenuates excitatory amino acid responses of cerebellar Purkinje cells. *Neuroscience* **42**(2): 309–320.

Stanton, B.A. & Koeppen, B.M. (1993) The kidney. In: Berne, R.M. & Levy, M.N. (eds) *Physiology.* St Louis: Mosby Year Book.

Steer, P.J. (1991) The genital system. In: Hytten, F. & Chamberlain, G. (eds) *Clinical Physiology in Obstetrics,* pp. 303–344. Oxford: Blackwell Scientific.

Steer, P., Ash Alam, M., Wadsworth, J. *et al.* (1995) Relation between maternal haemoglobin concentration and birth weight in different ethnic groups. *British Medical Journal* **310**: 489–491.

Stewart, D.R., Overstreet, J.W., Nakajima, S.T. *et al.* (1993) Enhanced ovarian steroid secretion before implantation in early human pregnancy. *Journal of*

Clinical Endocrinology and Metabolism **76**(6): 1470–1476.

Stewart, P.M., Fraser, M.R. & Mason, J. (1995) Type 2 11β-hydroxysteroid dehydrogenase messenger ribonucleic acid and activity in human placenta and fetal membranes: its relationship to birth weight and putative role in fetal steroidogenesis. *Journal of Clinical Endocrinology and Metabolism* **80**(3): 885–890.

Tangalakis, K., Lumbers, E.R. & Moritz, K.M. (1992) Effect of cortisol on blood pressure and vascular reactivity in the ovine fetus. *Experimental Physiology* **77**: 709–717.

Thordarson, G. *et al.* (1987) Role of the placenta in mammary gland development and function. In: Neville, M.C. & Daniel, C.W. (eds) *The Mammary Gland,* pp. 459–489. New York: Plenum Press.

Thompson, A.M., Hytten, F.E. & Billewicz, W.Z. (1967) The epidemiology of oedema during pregnancy. *Journal of Obstetrics & Gynaecology of the British Commonwealth* **74**: 1–10.

Thomsen, J.K., Fogh-Andersen, N., Jaszczak, P. *et al.* (1993) Atrial natriuretic peptide (ANP) decrease during normal pregnancy as related to hemodynamic changes and volume regulation. *Acta Obstetricia et Gynecologica Scandinavica* **72**: 103–110.

Tong, Y., Zhao, H.L. & Abrie, F. (1990) Effects of estrogens on the ultrastructural characteristics of female rat prolactin cells as evaluated by in situ hybridization in combination with immunogold staining technique. *Neuroendocrinology* **52**: 309–315.

Uldbjerg, N., Ulmsten, U. & Ekman, G. (1983) The ripening of the human uterine cervix in terms of connective tissue biochemistry. *Clinics in Obstetrics and Gynaecology* **26**(1): 14–26.

Vamvakopoulos, N.C. & Chrousos, G.P. (1993) Evidence of direct estrogen regulation of human corticotrophin-releasing hormone gene expression. *Journal of Clinical Investigation* **92**: 1896–1902.

Vonderhaar, B.K. (1987) Prolactin, transport, function, and receptors in mammary gland development and differentiation. In: Neville, M.C. & Daniel, C.W. (eds) *The Mammary Gland,* pp. 383–438. New York: Plenum Press.

Waddell, B.J. (1993) The placenta as hypothalamus and pituitary: possible impact on maternal and fetal adrenal function. *Reproduction, Fertility, and Development* **5**: 479–497.

Waddell, B.J. & Atkinson, H.C. (1994) Production rate, metabolic clearance rate and uterine extraction of corticosterone during rat pregnancy. *Journal of Endocrinology* **143**: 183–190.

Waddell, B.J. & Burton, P.J. (1993) Release of bioactive ACTH by perfused human placenta at early and late gestation. *Journal of Endocrinology* **136**: 345–353.

Warren, W.B. & Silverman, A.J. (1995) Cellular localization of corticotrophin releasing hormone in the human placenta, fetal membranes and decidua. *Placenta* **16**: 147–156.

Wiederman, J., Freund, M. & Stone, M.L. (1964) Oxytocin effect on myoepithelium of the breast throughout pregnancy. *Journal of Applied Physiology* 19(2): 310–315.

Wintour, E.M., Coghlan, J.P., Oddie, C.J. *et al.* (1978) A sequential study of adrenocorticosteroid level in human pregnancy. *Clinical and Experimental Pharmacology & Physiology* 5: 399–403.

Wise, M.E., Sawyer, H.R. & Nett, T.M. (1986) Functional changes in luteinizing hormone-secreting cells from pre- and postpartum ewes. *American Journal of Physiology* 250: E282–E287.

Wray, S. (1993) Uterine contraction and physiological mechanisms of modulation. *American Journal of Physiology* 264: C1–C18.

Wu, W.X., Unno, S. & Giussani, D.A. (1995) Corticotrophin-releasing hormone and its receptor distribution in fetal membranes and placenta of the rhesus monkey in late gestation and labour. *Endocrinology* 136(10): 4621–4628.

Yen, S.S.C. (1991) Endocrine metabolic adaptations in pregnancy. In: Yen, S.S.C. & Jaffe, R.B. (eds) *Reproductive Endocrinology,* pp. 936–981. Philadelphia: W.B. Saunders.

Yoshimura, T., Yoshimura, M., Yasue, H. *et al.* (1994) Plasma concentration of atrial natriuretic peptide and brain natriuretic peptide during normal human pregnancy and the postpartum period. *Journal of Endocrinology* 140: 393–397.

18

Antenatal Investigations

Maureen Boyle

LEARNING OUTCOMES

After reading this chapter you will be able to:

- understand the fundamental differences between screening and diagnostic tests used during the antenatal period
- discuss the range of routine and specialized tests available to the woman and her family during the antenatal period
- be familiar with the screening/diagnostic tests available to detect fetal anomalies, together with their limitations
- be aware of the research and evidence around screening and diagnostic tests, and the means by which the midwife and mother can access this information
- be conversant with the necessity and strategies for information sharing between the woman and midwife to ensure informed choice by the woman.

INTRODUCTION

The field of antenatal investigations has grown greatly in the past few years. Tests are being offered today – and decisions from women are becoming necessary – that would have been unthinkable to our mothers, or perhaps even our older sisters. There is also a wide variation in what tests are considered 'routine' in various parts of the UK, so a woman in London may find herself needing to make decisions about taking a test which her friend in another locale is not even offered. The increase in use of the Internet and other information technology has meant that women and their partners often have accessed much specialized information themselves, and this may shape their questions.

Therefore midwives need to have a better-than-ever knowledge of what tests are being offered, in order that they can ensure women are making their choices based on up-to-date and comprehensive information. They also need to be effective counsellors as it is acknowledged that the skills and attitudes of midwives influence the uptake of screening tests (Thornton *et al.*, 1995). The midwife should also appreciate that the complete clinical antenatal examination is one of the most effective and efficient screening and diagnostic tools, if undertaken skilfully and systematically.

SCREENING AND DIAGNOSIS

Although the meanings of screening and diagnosis are very different, they are often confused, and the midwife must ensure that the woman fully understands the difference.

Screening can be defined as determining the risk or likelihood of a condition, whereas a *diagnostic test* will give a definite answer. Sometimes action will be taken following the results of a screening test. For example a low haemoglobin (Hb) result in pregnancy may be assumed to be caused by pregnancy-induced anaemia and iron tablets will probably be given without further investigation, although in a few rare cases the anaemia may be caused by uncommon conditions, such as chronic renal infection, which would need further investigations to obtain a diagnosis. However, it would not be cost-effective to do an infinite range of investigations for every woman who presented with a positive screening test where the usual cause can be easily treated.

Some screening tests will produce results which mean an invasive test will be necessary to obtain a diagnosis. This needs to be made clear to the woman by the midwife counselling her – should a woman be undertaking a serum screening for Down's syndrome test if she would not undergo amniocentesis in the case of a 'high risk'

Table 18.1 Common procedures used for fetal assessment

Test		Time
Nuchal translucency (screening)	Chromosomal abnormality	10–14 weeks
Chorionic villus sampling (diagnostic)	Chromosomal abnormality Genetic disease Metabolic disorders Haemoglobinopathies Infection	>10 weeks
Amniocentesis (diagnostic)	Chromosomal abnormality Genetic disease Metabolic disorders Haemoglobinopathies Infection	10–14 weeks (early) 15–18 weeks
Ultrasound (screening and diagnostic)	Assess fetus (dates/growth/viability/number) Diagnosis of some abnormalities (e.g. structural) Screening for abnormalities (e.g. soft markers) Assessment of placental site Liquor volume	All gestations
Cordocentesis (diagnostic)	Obtain fetal blood sample	2nd/3rd trimester
Doppler (screening)	Assess fetal/placental/uterine blood flow	2nd/3rd trimester

result? Some tests, such as ultrasound, can be both screening and diagnostic (Table 18.1) – for example a scan can diagnose a missing limb or neural tube defect, but can also discover anomalies (e.g. 'soft markers') which would need further investigations to determine a diagnosis.

It is obviously not enough just to have the tests explained by the midwife – the implications of both positive and negative results also need to be explored before a woman can be said to be making an informed choice. As tests become more varied and complex, and midwives' time more limited, ensuring properly informed choice is becoming a greater challenge for midwives.

BLOOD TESTS

Blood is taken from a woman during pregnancy to detect conditions which may influence her well-being, that of the developing fetus, or indeed both.

Blood tests for assessment of maternal well-being (Table 18.2)

ABO and rhesus blood grouping
Blood is typed as A, B, AB or O depending on specific agglutinogens on the erythrocytes. The rhesus factor identifies the blood group as negative or positive depending on whether the rhesus factor antigen is present. Because of the risk of anaemia, haemorrhage or shock in pregnancy and during birth, and the possible need to provide transfusion, it is important that the blood group is identified early in the pregnancy.

Antibodies
Maternal blood is examined for the presence of antibodies, particularly rhesus antibodies if the woman is rhesus negative. If the fetus is rhesus positive, antibodies can be stimulated by the occurrence of a fetomaternal haemorrhage, when 'leaks' occur and some fetal rhesus positive cells pass into the maternal circulation. This can happen as pregnancy progresses, during procedures such as amniocentesis, chorionic villus sampling (CVS), external cephalic version, in situations such as an antepartum haemorrhage or at delivery. The rhesus-negative woman may respond by producing antibodies which may then cross the placenta, in this or subsequent pregnancies, to the fetal circulation and cause haemolysis in a rhesus-positive fetus. The administration of anti-D immunoglobulin is effective in preventing the production of these antibodies (MacKenzie *et al.*, 1991). Recent guidance has been provided by the National Institute for Clinical Excellence (NICE) that routine antenatal anti-D prophylaxis should be offered to all non-sensitized, rhesus-negative women. This may actually change some management in future screening. It is crucial that careful discussion takes place

Table 18.2 Normal laboratory values in non-pregnant and pregnant women (Blackburn, 2003: 214)

	Non-pregnant	Pregnant
General screening assays		
Haemoglobin	12–16 g/dl	11–13 g/dl
Packed cell volume (PCV)	37–45%	33–39%
Red blood cell count (RBC)	4.2–5.4 million/mm^3	3.8–4.4 million/mm^3
Mean corpuscular volume (MCV)	80–100 fl	70–90 fl
Mean corpuscular haemoglobin (MCH)	27–34 fl	23–31 fl
Mean corpuscular haemoglobin concentration (MCHC)	32–35 fl	32–35 fl
Reticulocyte count	0.5–1%	1–2%
Specific diagnostic tests		
Serum iron	50–100 µg/dl	30–100 µg/dl
Unsaturated iron binding capacity	250–300 µg/dl	280–400 µg/dl
Transferrin saturation	25–35%	15–30%
Iron stores (bone marrow)	Adequate ferritin	Unchanged
Serum folate	6–16 µg/ml	4–10 µg/ml
Serum vitamin B$_{12}$	70–85 ng/dl	70–500 ng/dl

regarding this prophylaxis, as the woman must appreciate that she is being given a blood product. She may also prefer to have anti-D only if necessary, i.e. after birth or any invasive procedures. There may also be the scenario of the woman who knows that the father of the child is rhesus negative also, which would make prophylaxis unnecessary (NICE, 2002).

ABO incompatibility and less common antibodies such as Kell, Duffy and Kidd (Hoffbrand and Pettit, 2000) can also affect the fetus or newborn.

Early identification can ensure that the levels in maternal serum during pregnancy are monitored. If the antibody titre is rising, early delivery or intrauterine exchange transfusion through the umbilical vessels may be considered.

Full blood count

Full blood counts are routinely done at booking and at intervals during pregnancy, mainly to detect a pathological fall in haemoglobin (Hb) which may indicate an iron-deficiency anaemia. No woman should reach term with a potentially dangerous anaemia because of the risk of excessive blood loss at delivery. It must be remembered, however, that other rare conditions may be discovered 'accidentally', for example a low white cell count may lead to a diagnosis of leukaemia. It is important therefore that no abnormal result ever be disregarded.

Haemoglobin (Hb)   Because of physiological changes in pregnancy, haemoglobin levels will normally reduce, with the lowest reading expected at about 34 weeks. The World Health Organization cites 11 g/dl as the lowest acceptable reading, although other authorities quote figures down to 10 g/dl. A low Hb reading needs further investigation to establish the cause, so that appropriate treatment can be commenced.

Serum ferritin levels and total iron-binding capacity (TIBC) may be assessed, and causes of insidious blood loss such as from chronic renal infection or parasitic infestation may be investigated.

In the past, iron supplements were routinely given to pregnant women, but this is no longer considered appropriate (Day, 1998).

Mean corpuscular volume (MCV)   The earliest effect of iron deficiency is a reduced MCV. MCV is also reduced with alpha and beta thalassaemia minor. A raised mean corpuscular volume is associated with folate deficiency (high alcohol intake can reduce absorption of folic acid) or B$_{12}$ deficiency.

Platelets   Platelets usually stay within the normal range for non-pregnant women, although levels may fall during pregnancy within this range. An abnormal fall could indicate various medical conditions and would need further investigation.

White cell count   The total number of white cells rises in pregnancy, mainly due to the increase of neutrophils. However, an abnormal rise could indicate an infection, and this cause needs additional exploration.

Haemoglobinopathies

Haemoglobinopathies are a diverse group of inherited single-gene disorders involving abnormal haemoglobin patterns which constitute two major conditions: thalassaemia (minor or major) and sickle cell disorders: sickle cell trait (SCT or HbAS); sickle cell haemoglobin C disease (HbSC); and sickle cell disease/anaemia (HbSS).

Both sickle cell disease and thalassaemia are recessive conditions, therefore only those inheriting an affected gene from each parent will have the disease. If a woman is found to be carrying either the HbS gene or the thalassaemia trait (thalassaemia minor), it is necessary to test her partner before a prediction about the baby's condition can be made. If both parents carry the gene, prenatal diagnosis can be made by chorionic villus sampling (CVS), cordocentesis or amniocentesis.

Thalassaemia is seen mainly in those of Mediterranean, Middle Eastern or South East Asian origin. Selective screening for sickle cell disorders has also traditionally been done according to the woman's origin: African, Caribbean, Mediterranean, Middle Eastern or Asian Indian. Although some laboratories test all blood samples with a low Hb or MCV, this system has not been effective in identifying all those at risk. It is recommended that districts with more than 15% antenatal population at risk for haemoglobinopathies should adopt a universal antenatal and neonatal strategy for screening (DoH, 1993).

However, with recent understanding of the changes in population and ethnicity it is worth the midwife asking the woman at the booking interview whether she herself knows whether her family background increases her risk of having any of these disorders.

Phenylketonuria (PKU)

Phenylketonuria is an inherited inborn error of metabolism whereby there is a deficiency of the enzyme *phenylalanine hydroxylase*. The condition can cause irreversible brain damage if untreated, due to a build-up of phenylalanine in the body, but can be managed by following a low-phenylalanine diet. Serum phenylalanine testing may be carried out on women with phenylketonuria to establish their serum phenylalanine levels as there is a high risk of miscarriage or transplacental fetal brain damage. It is recommended that these women follow a low-phenylalanine diet to reduce serum phenylalanine before conception to improve the outcome of pregnancy (Platt *et al.*, 2000).

Maternal infection screening

Rubella

This common viral infection is a significant condition in pregnancy because of the teratogenic effect on the developing fetus caused by transplacental transmission of the virus. Detection of rubella antibodies is carried out by serological testing to detect immunity (IgM and IgG antibodies).

The majority of women in the UK are immune as a result of routine vaccination against rubella at 11–14 years of age. However, since 1988, vaccination is now by measles, mumps and rubella (MMR) vaccine, usually administered before 15 months to male and female infants. It was hoped that with a universal take-up, rubella would be eradicated altogether. However, controversies over routine vaccination for infants reported in the media may compromise this.

All pregnant women are tested for rubella immunity at antenatal booking. Some women who have been previously vaccinated, and indeed previously tested as immune, have been known to become infected or test as susceptible, therefore testing in the preconception period is to be advised.

If a woman is not immune and comes into contact with rubella she may develop the disease. Rubella can cause the loss of the pregnancy or the birth of a rubella-infected baby with various physical and mental anomalies. The fetus is most vulnerable up until 16 weeks, but the infection can cross the placenta at any gestation. An infected baby can be infectious for up to 2 years. To avoid the danger of rubella in future pregnancies the non-immune woman is offered vaccination in the puerperium, together with contraceptive advice for a period of 3 months.

Hepatitis

Hepatitis means inflammation of the liver. There are several different viruses which affect the liver (A, B, C, D and E) but B and C are the types with the most direct relevance to midwives at present.

Hepatitis B (HBV)   Hepatitis B is an infectious blood-borne viral disease. It can cause a range of symptoms from very mild to life-threatening. About 10% of adults infected become chronic carriers and this may then progress to serious liver disease. Transmission is by contact with body fluids or vertically to the fetus. HBV is a potentially serious infection but it often only manifests with influenza-like symptoms. However, although there is a high chance of perinatal transmission, interventions after birth can greatly reduce the risk of the baby becoming a chronic carrier, and therefore identification of the mother's HBV status during pregnancy is important. In 1998 the Department of Health issued guidelines advising that all pregnant women should be screened for HBV infection (Winyard, 1998).

Because of its high level of infectivity, all healthcare workers (especially midwives) who have contact with body fluids should be vaccinated against HBV.

Hepatitis C (HCV)   Although HCV is very similar to hepatitis B, many more people infected with it will become chronic carriers and develop liver damage. There is no vaccine against HCV and because of its structure it is unlikely that one will be developed. At present universal antenatal screening for HCV is not undertaken, but recent research has demonstrated a 0.8% prevalence rate in inner London, and in this study the majority of the infected women had no identified risk factors (Ward *et al.*, 2000).

Human immunodeficiency virus infection (HIV)

Department of Health (1999) guidelines state that HIV testing should be recommended to all women as part of the routine antenatal testing, as there are now clearly identified strategies which can reduce transmission to the fetus. As with all tests, informed consent is necessary and the midwife should ensure her knowledge base in this very fast-changing area is up to date in order that she can offer explanations and answer questions. This is a condition where new research is almost continuously being published and therefore all maternity units should have an identified resource person to whom the more complex enquiries can be referred.

Toxoplasmosis

Toxoplasmosis is a parasitic infection caused by the protozoan *Toxoplasma gondii* which may cause congenital infection in the fetus. It can be transmitted from domestic cat faeces, soil, raw meat and unpasteurized milk. Pregnant women are also advised to avoid contact with sheep during lambing (DoH, 2000).

The test, which examines the immunity status of the woman by looking at IgG and IgM antibodies, should be performed in a toxoplasmosis reference laboratory as diagnosis is not straightforward. There is some evidence that if infected women receive antiparasitic treatment during pregnancy, this may offer some protection to the fetus (Foulon *et al.*, 1999).

Listeriosis

Listeriosis can cause upper respiratory disease, septicaemia and encephalic disease. In pregnancy it can result in preterm labour, stillbirth or meningitis (of mother or baby). It is caused by a common bacterium usually transmitted via contaminated food, and advice is given to pregnant women to specifically avoid soft cheeses and pâtés, and to ensure 'cook-chill' meals are well heated through. Pregnant women are advised to avoid contact with sheep during lambing (DoH, 2000). There have also been reports of the infection being passed by contaminated equipment. Diagnosis is made by culture of blood or cerebrospinal fluid.

Cytomegalovirus (CMV)

Cytomegalovirus is a herpes virus that can be passed on by many routes, including sexual activities. Cytomegalovirus can lie latent in maternal tissues and become reactivated during pregnancy. The presence of antibodies in the blood against cytomegalovirus is indicative of infection, and virus-specific IgM antibody is present in acute infections. It is the most common cause of intrauterine infection, and the fetus can be assessed by amniotic fluid studies (Antsaklis *et al.*, 2000).

Serology

Serological tests, both non-treponemal and treponemal, can be done in the antenatal period, and most women in the UK are routinely screened for syphilis at booking, as there is evidence this is still an appropriate test (Cameron *et al.*, 1998). It is possible to get false positive results with conditions such as malaria, tuberculosis and glandular fever, and those infected with pinta and yaws may test positive. Those who abuse narcotics can also test as a false positive (Ault and Faro, 1993).

Antenatal maternal blood tests to assess the fetus

Maternal serum screening for Down's syndrome (MSSDS) (also known as the triple test/double test/Bart's test)

In the late 1980s, workers at St Bartholomew's Hospital, London, developed a method of screening all women for the risk factor of Down's syndrome in a current pregnancy by means of a maternal blood test (Loncar *et al.*, 1995). The levels of:

- maternal serum alpha-fetoprotein (AFP): reduces in Down's syndrome, rises in neural tube defects

- maternal serum human chorionic gonadotrophin (hCG): increases in Down's syndrome
- maternal serum unconjugated oestriol: decreases in Down's syndrome

were examined, together with the mother's age (it has long been recognized that the incidence of Down's syndrome increases with the age of the woman) and these calculations resulted in an individual risk estimation.

This test is usually done at about 16 weeks and because accurate dates are important in the assessment of levels, a 'dating scan' is often offered at booking if the woman plans to have this test.

It is important the woman realizes that the outcome is only a risk assessment and if her result is considered a 'screen positive' (usually about 1 : 250 or higher) she will probably need an amniocentesis for a diagnosis. It is obviously also possible that a 'screen negative' may well occur despite an affected fetus, and this also needs to be made clear.

Many variations of this test are currently being used, or being researched. Some areas are omitting the maternal serum oestriol and/or assessing subunits of human chorionic gonadotrophin. There are also suggestions that the hormone inhibin A may be valuable as a second trimester marker (Wald *et al.*, 1996).

Work at present is concentrating on establishing earlier normal/abnormal levels, and determining if other substances can be used as markers in the first trimester, so the test can be offered before 16 weeks (Cuckle and van Lith, 1999). A combination of pregnancy-associated plasma protein-A (PAPP-A) and free beta-hCG levels from maternal serum and nuchal translucency ultrasound at about 11–14 weeks, is currently being introduced to practice (Nicolaides *et al.*, 2000).

An increased level of alpha-fetoprotein (AFP) has been previously used on its own as a screening test for neural tube defects (spina bifida and anencephaly), to be followed by amniocentesis to detect diagnostic levels in the amniotic fluid. Most neural tube defects are now diagnosed by ultrasound examination.

Not all pregnancies are suitable for routine MSSDS screening. Levels can be influenced by a multiple pregnancy, intrauterine bleeding, obesity or the woman being an insulin-dependent diabetic. Different values may also be necessary for IVF pregnancies (Wald *et al.*, 1999).

In the future, DNA analysis of fetal cells found in maternal blood may provide a diagnosis without depending on invasive tests (Verma *et al.*, 1998).

ASSESSMENT OF FETAL WELL-BEING

Fetal heart rate

In looking at the fetal heart rate as an indication of fetal well-being, it is usual practice to assess baseline heart rate, variability and alteration in heart rate in reaction to stress or movement.

The fetal heart rate varies through the antenatal period, and will range between 110–160 b.p.m., with an average baseline at 20 weeks of 155 b.p.m.; 30 weeks 144 b.p.m. and at term 140 b.p.m. During this time, variations around 20 b.p.m. above and below these baselines are considered normal, and signify changes in fetal oxygenation (Blackburn, 2003). Tachycardia is more common in the preterm fetus, but may also indicate fetal infection, reaction to maternal medication (i.e. β-sympathomimetic drugs), acute blood loss, fetal anaemia, or conditions such as Wolff–Parkinson–White disease. Tachycardia may be seen in fetal hypoxia, but not usually without other indications.

Bradycardia (heart rate under 110 b.p.m.) on the other hand is more likely to be caused by hypoxia, fetal heart block, hypothermia, and vagal nerve stimulation as seen during head compression during labour (Blackburn, 2003).

Fetal movements

Monitoring fetal movements as a test of fetal well-being was introduced by Sadovsky in the 1970s (Sadovsky and Polishuk, 1977; Sadovsky *et al.*, 1983), and this led to extensive use of the Cardiff 'Count to ten kick chart'. This required the woman to count 10 movements over a 12-hour period, with instructions to contact her GP, or midwife should the 10 movements not be achieved. Various problems with this method include non-compliance by women; or apparent compliance in which the woman completes the 'kick chart' in the antenatal clinic for the professionals' approval; or a concern that this monitoring may add to the pregnant woman's stress and anxiety levels, although research has indicated that stress levels are not significantly affected (Liston *et al.*, 1994). There may be difficulties for some women in understanding the purpose and process required, although this may be assisted by using pictorial instructions and information (Shafi *et al.*, 1989). The reporting of lack of or diminished fetal movements may be increased, and this may in itself lead to increased stress for the woman and family and has additional resource implications for the maternity services.

Fetal movements are deemed to be an effective means of assessing well-being, and reduced fetal activity as one of the most accurate means of identifying the fetus at risk of intrauterine death (James, 2002).

Maternity units and services have a variety of approaches, and some still use 'kick charts'. Whatever system is in place, it is important to encourage the woman to become familiar with her own baby's pattern of movement, and for her to be aware of what actions she should take should there be a significant change in the movements.

ULTRASOUND

Ultrasound scanning (USS) (Fig. 18.1) has become a routine part of antenatal care for women in the UK today, as well as being an integral part of many of the specialized investigations offered to individual women.

Ultrasound imaging is a non-invasive screening and diagnostic technique using sound waves with a frequency well above the range of human hearing. The use of ultrasound for medical purposes was developed from SONAR (*sound navigation and ranging*), a system used to detect submarines by emitting pulses of sound and evaluating echoes. It was introduced into obstetrics in the 1950s and although there is little or no evidence at the present time that it is harmful to mother or fetus (Proud, 1997), the issue of safety is still of concern as the use of ultrasound in pregnancy has never been fully evaluated (Wood, 2000). There is no doubt, however, that it is a popular test with pregnant women and there is some suggestion that it can provide a positive psychological benefit (Proud, 1997).

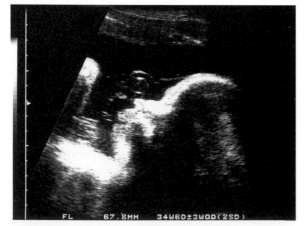

Figure 18.1 Ultrasound scan.

Method

Ultrasound scanning may be performed by a sonographer who may be a radiographer, doctor or midwife trained in the technique. The ability of the operator to give individualized attention is important, and the screen should be positioned so the woman can see it easily. A water-soluble gel is used to ensure contact of the ultrasound probe. If performed in early pregnancy the only discomfort experienced by the mother is that of a full bladder, which is necessary to raise the uterus out of the pelvis. Although at present the usual method of ultrasound scanning is abdominal, vaginal ultrasound, using a special probe, is becoming more common in early pregnancy.

Ultrasound scans can be performed for a variety of reasons, from the earliest gestation up to and including when in labour, as well as postnatally to detect complications in the mother (e.g. retained products of conception) or to assess the baby. However, antenatal USS is most common, and it is important to remember that a scan for any reason during this period may result in a finding apart from that for which it was being done – for instance a scan to assess the placental site may result in the discovery of a fetal abnormality. A woman undergoing ultrasound scanning should be aware of a scan's capabilities, and also that the finding of no abnormalities on USS is not a guarantee of no problems.

Reflective Activity 18.1

With the woman's and ultrasonographer's permission, sit in on some ultrasound scans at various gestations in pregnancy, so you can become familiar with the findings of the ultrasonographer and with the questions women may ask.

Indications for first trimester ultrasound

Booking/early/dating scans

Historically, first trimester scans were only routinely offered to women unsure of their last menstrual period, and therefore an estimated delivery date (EDD) was able to be calculated from fetal measurements taken during scanning. However, with the increase in MSSDS, where a 'dating' scan is often offered to ensure accurate timing of the test, even women sure of their dates may have a first trimester ultrasound scan.

Parameters which may be used to determine gestational age are crown–rump length, biparietal diameter, femur length, and head circumference. The gestational sac is sometimes assessed early in the first trimester to confirm an intrauterine pregnancy, to calculate the gestational age before the fetus is visible or to diagnose an anembryonic pregnancy (no embryonic tissue).

For accuracy, the measurements to assess gestational age should be done in the first or early second trimester, as prediction of gestational age by ultrasound scan cannot be accurately made after 24 weeks, because of the wide spread of normal measurements (Proud, 1997). Measurements will be recorded, to act as a baseline in case fetal growth needs to be monitored later in pregnancy.

Diagnosis of pregnancy

The embryonic sac may be identified as early as 5 weeks' gestation, using a transabdominal probe, and at 4 weeks with a transvaginal probe. Fetal heart movements can be visualized at 6–7 weeks' gestation and lack of fetal heart movement is a reliable method of diagnosing fetal death after this time. Actual movements of the fetus can be observed from 8–9 weeks. Doppler ultrasound equipment which produces amplified sound waves (i.e. Sonicaid/Doptone) may be used to hear the fetal heart after about 12 weeks' gestation, but failure to hear the fetal heart should not be assumed to indicate fetal death, and fetal viability should be checked by an ultrasound scan.

Ectopic pregnancy

This may be detected by ultrasound scan, the transvaginal route being more accurate than the abdominal route (Proud, 1997). Diagnosis is not always easy, but identification of high-risk groups, clinical examination and biochemical tests usually assist the diagnosis.

Missed abortion/miscarriage

If a woman reports no longer 'feeling pregnant', or there are no signs of expected growth, an ultrasound scan may show the fetal sac failing to grow and a visible fetal pole but no fetal heartbeat. During research, some hospitals have shown that if a scan is done routinely at 11–14 weeks, a rate of 2–3% missed miscarriages may be identified. An advantage of a routine early scan may be the avoidance of traumatic bleeding and possible emergency admission for these women (Economides *et al.*, 1999).

Hydatidiform mole

This can be accurately diagnosed by seeing a classic white mottled area 'snow-storm' appearance on scan, and by the lack of any recognizable structures. Ultrasound scan confirms the diagnosis following clinical signs such as painless vaginal bleeding, a large-for-dates uterus, hyperemesis gravidarum and absence of fetal heart sounds by 14 weeks' gestation using Doppler ultrasound.

Cervical incompetence

In some cases, serial ultrasound from about 14 weeks, can assess the condition of the cervical canal and detect shortening (Rocco and Garrone, 1999).

Multiple pregnancy

Multiple pregnancy can be identified by ultrasound from 4 weeks transvaginally, and 5 weeks abdominally (Proud, 1997). Initially it is suspected when more than one fetal sac is seen; the presence of two (or more) viable fetuses confirms the diagnosis.

Many twin pregnancies result in a singleton birth. Since the increased number of first trimester ultrasound scans, the 'vanishing twin' syndrome has been described, where twins are seen on an early scan but one is then lost – this is sometimes associated with vaginal bleeding, but often not. The figures for this are uncertain and range between 20–50% of twin pregnancies.

The early diagnosis of twins therefore has the potential to prove very distressing if the parents are then told one twin has died and they only have a singleton pregnancy – and in fact it has been suggested that the bereavement felt for the dead baby could outweigh the joy of having a healthy ongoing pregnancy (Proud, 1997). However, in the limited work available on this subject, most parents say they would prefer to know (Bryan, 1986). There would also be ethical considerations if professionals considered withholding information from parents.

Serial ultrasound scans to estimate fetal growth and development may be carried out throughout pregnancy, as complications are more likely to arise in a multiple pregnancy.

Vaginal bleeding

Vaginal bleeding is not uncommon in early pregnancy and often the cause is never determined. Ultrasound is extremely valuable in assessing fetal viability when bleeding occurs, to determine what action, if any, should be taken.

Since there is some evidence that seeing a live fetus on ultrasound scanning can relax a woman, many authorities will do regular routine scans for those with a history of recurrent miscarriages (Regan, 2000).

Fetal assessment

Nuchal translucency   Nuchal translucency measurement is done by ultrasound between 10–14 weeks' gestation. Fluid at the back of the fetus's neck is measured against the norm established, and the more fluid accumulated, the greater the risk of an abnormality being present. After 14 weeks the development of the lymphatic system and changes in the placental circulation will cause any excess fluid to drain away; therefore an abnormality may not be represented by an increased nuchal translucency measurement. Nuchal translucency scans were developed to detect chromosomal abnormalities, in particular trisomy 21, but can also indicate other abnormalities (Hyett and Thilaganathan, 1999), such as fetal cardiac anomalies.

It is suggested that by examining fetal anatomy as well as measuring nuchal translucency at 12–13 weeks, the majority of structural and chromosomal abnormalities can be detected. However, significant defects can be missed (such as some heart and spine abnormalities); therefore a later scan would also be recommended (Economides *et al.*, 1999).

Indications for second trimester ultrasound

Since the 1980s women have been offered routine ultrasound assessment between 18–20 weeks' gestation, often called the 'anomaly' or 'mid-trimester' scan. By this time most fetal organs are formed and many abnormalities can be seen. However, it must be stressed that not all structures and their functions can be assessed – some may need later scans, and many abnormalities may not be able to be assessed by ultrasound at all. In spite of this, women frequently see this routine scan as a signal that 'everything is alright' and a guarantee of a problem-free pregnancy and baby, and this can be a very misleading assumption.

Estimation of fetal age

If an earlier scan has not been done, the accuracy of the gestational age by dates can be confirmed by fetal measurements. These measurements are recorded at this time as a baseline to use if there is a suspected IUGR (previously 'intrauterine growth retardation', but now the terminology is changing to 'intrauterine growth restriction', owing to the misinterpretation often placed on the word 'retardation' by parents) later in pregnancy.

Placental location

During all ultrasound examinations, identification of the placenta is made, but it is routinely done during this scan. If the placental site is low in the mid-trimester scan, a repeat scan is often offered at about 32 weeks, and the woman is advised as to what to do in the case of bleeding prior to this. Only about 6% of placentae will fail to become fundal by 32 weeks (Proud, 1997) but if the placenta remains partially or wholly in the lower uterine segment it is a placenta praevia, and appropriate care must be instigated.

Identification of fetal anomalies

Although fetal anomalies can be detected during any ultrasound scan, the mid-trimester scan is used routinely for this examination.

Fetal anatomy is assessed and many conditions, mainly structural, can be diagnosed (although some may need referral to a specialist centre for a definitive diagnosis). In addition the ultrasonographer can also note any 'soft markers' – for example extra digits, choroid plexus cysts or talipes. These can be benign anomalies which either disappear (e.g. most choroid plexus cysts) or can be easily treated after birth. However, they can also be a manifestation of more serious underlying conditions such as a chromosomal abnormality, and an amniocentesis may be offered to exclude this. The use of soft markers is a controversial subject and can be a cause of great anxiety for many (Boyd *et al.*, 1998).

Indications for third trimester ultrasound

Assessment of fetal growth

Fetal growth is assessed clinically at every antenatal visit. If the midwife or doctor feels growth is suboptimal than a referral for ultrasound assessment is usually made to confirm the clinical findings.

To assess fetal growth by ultrasound, the age of the fetus must be accurately established before 24 weeks' gestation. Fetal growth may be monitored by serial ultrasound measurements of various parameters, every 2–4 weeks. Measurements of head and abdominal circumference are commonly used to estimate the growth in small-for-gestational-age fetuses, both asymmetrical and symmetrical, and large-for-gestational-age fetuses. In the symmetrical intrauterine growth restricted fetus the normal growth shows deviation in later pregnancy below the 5th (or 10th) centile. In the asymmetrical condition, the abdominal circumference growth is slow and may stop, and eventually the head circumference growth also slows. IUGR (intrauterine growth restriction) can be diagnosed by plotting serial scans along centile lines previously defined as the normal growth pattern for that

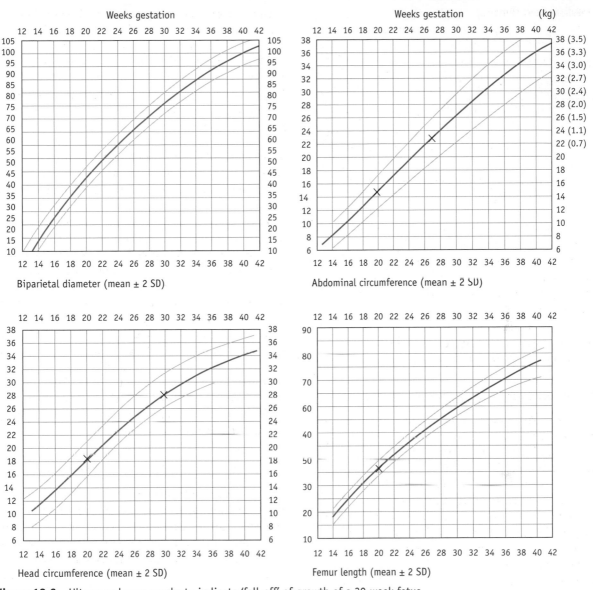

Figure 18.2 Ultrasound scan graphs to indicate 'fall-off' of growth of a 30-week fetus.

population. If IUGR occurs a fall-off of growth can be seen (Fig. 18.2). Growth acceleration (large abdominal circumference) above the 90th centile may be due to maternal diabetes mellitus, especially if associated with polyhydramnios and a large placenta.

Malpresentations/malpositions

Late in the third trimester an ultrasound scan can be used to confirm clinical findings regarding the presentation and position of the fetus (or each fetus in the case of a multiple pregnancy). This information can be used to help decision-making if there is a question over the mode of delivery.

Ultrasound will also be used to guide the clinician if external cephalic version (ECV) is undertaken to turn a breech presentation.

Additional uses for ultrasound

Tumours

Some tumours, such as maternal ovarian cysts and uterine tumours, may be detected by ultrasound scanning. The assessment of fibroids and any changes which may occur during pregnancy can also be made by ultrasound.

Fetal/infant therapy

Ultrasound may be used in conjunction with karyotyping and an echocardiogram, to establish accurate diagnosis of the fetal condition prior to selection of fetuses for possible therapy. In-utero fetal therapy is still in the experimental stage, but has been successfully used in the treatment of some renal conditions such as bilateral urinary tract obstruction.

Fetal anaemia, usually caused by alloimmunization, twin-to-twin transfusion or even trauma, can be treated by intravascular fetal transfusion. While there is a risk of pregnancy loss, in most cases it is the best option for saving the fetus's life.

Ultrasound scanning may be used to monitor the degree of various dysfunctions, and to aid decision-making regarding the time, place and mode of delivery to ensure the best possible after-care for the baby. Ultrasound scanning is used also after birth to aid in the management of certain conditions of the infant, such as congenital dislocation of the hips.

Selective fetal reduction

This can be done in a multiple pregnancy by identifying the individual fetus with ultrasound and injecting potassium chloride into the fetal heart.

Doppler ultrasound

As well as being used through a small machine to monitor the fetal heart (e.g. Sonicaids) this technique is also used to measure blood flow in the fetal and uterine/placental vessels from a waveform recording on a monitor screen. The blood flow pattern will change as an adaptation to poor placental function, so it is thought that alterations in the fetal umbilical blood flow may occur in early fetal compromise, and this test may be included routinely in the 18–20 weeks scan in some units. More commonly, however, women are referred for Doppler assessment in the second and third trimester because of oligohydramnios, differing growth in multiple pregnancies, IUGR or maternal conditions (e.g. hypertensive disorders of pregnancy). It may also form part of post-dates assessment, as there is research assessing uncomplicated post-term pregnancies which showed that those with abnormal Doppler results needed increased interventions during labour for fetal distress (Anteby *et al.*, 1994).

Uterine artery Doppler studies may also be used to predict pre-eclampsia or IUGR in some cases.

Biophysical profile

This is a non-invasive test of fetal well-being which was first described in the early 1980s, using ultrasound imaging and cardiotocography to measure five biophysical variables:

- fetal heart rate
- fetal tone
- somatic movements
- breathing movements
- amniotic fluid volume (James, 1993).

The variables are scored individually and totalled to give a biophysical score. The biophysical profile is concerned with detecting the 'at-risk' fetus.

Most clinicians would not consider the 1-centimetre pocket of amniotic fluid described in the original biophysical profile, as adequate, especially when assessing post-term pregnancies. It is also often considered that the amniotic fluid measurement is the most important component of this test and, in combination with CTG, Doppler studies and placental assessment, can be used as a post-dates assessment.

Alfirevic and Neilson (2003) suggested that at present there are insufficient data to be able to effectively evaluate the use of biophysical profiles.

Amniotic fluid measurement

As a routine clinical assessment during palpation, during the second and third trimester, amniotic fluid quantity can be estimated to be reduced (oligohydramnios) or increased (polyhydramnios), and both these conditions, if suspected, need to be referred for ultrasound evaluation. Oligohydramnios may be associated with various fetal abnormalities, or with fetal compromise. Polyhydramnios may also be associated with fetal abnormality, for example oesophageal atresia, or associated with maternal disease (e.g. diabetes mellitus) and a large fetus. All these conditions will need expert assessment, especially in determining timing and mode of delivery and planning aftercare.

Estimation of fetal weight

Estimation of fetal weight can be made by using measurements obtained during ultrasound assessment. For the preterm fetus, and especially very preterm and multiples, ultrasound estimation of weight is the method of choice, and may provide vital information when consideration is being given to expediting a premature delivery.

However, at term it has been shown that parous women can often estimate the weight of the fetus as accurately as doctors using palpation (Herrero and Fitzsimmons, 1999). Clinical assessment can also be as accurate as ultrasound (Raman *et al.*, 1992) in determining estimated fetal weight around term – however, research studying this has specified using experienced professionals to do the assessments. It may be that a generation of practitioners who are becoming increasingly dependent upon ultrasound in their practice, may not be able to replicate this research in the future. Since there will always be situations where ultrasound cannot be accessed, it is a reminder for all midwives to maintain their clinical skills of palpation and weight estimation.

Reflective Activity 18.2

When carrying out an antenatal check in late pregnancy or when caring for a woman in labour, try to estimate the fetal weight during your routine palpations. Check after the birth to assess your skill.

RADIOLOGICAL AND MAGNETIC VISUALIZATION TECHNIQUES

Ultrasound has replaced radiology as a mean of imaging in obstetrics since an X-ray is considered to be harmful to the fetus (Johnson, 1992). In a small number of cases X-ray pelvimetry may be performed, for example when considering a vaginal breech delivery, although pelvic measurements in pregnancy often provide inconclusive information for labour (Krishnamurthy et al., 1991).

If it cannot be avoided, radiology should generally be delayed until 30–32 weeks when it is less harmful to the fetus. There may be a case for an X-ray to assess previous injury such as a past fractured pelvis or spine.

However, if it is necessary for a pregnant woman to have a chest X-ray, the best time is between 14 and 24 weeks, after fetal organogenesis and before the uterus pushes the diaphragm upwards, causing compression of the lower lobe of the lungs.

Magnetic resonance imaging (MRI) is used as a diagnostic tool in medicine but research in obstetrics has shown that it is usually inferior to ultrasound as a means of imaging the fetus owing to fetal movement, and difficulties in selecting the plane of imaging, although MRI may provide fetal visualization when conditions (e.g. maternal obesity, oligohydramnios) make ultrasound imaging difficult. However, it has been found to be satisfactory for imaging maternal structures. Its uses include:

Maternal

- To assess the cervix in late pregnancy to help in predicting delivery time.
- To assess abnormalities in the liver in conditions such as HELLP syndrome (see Ch. 45).
- To evaluate third trimester bleeding.

Placental

- Possible antenatal diagnosis of placenta percreta.

Fetal

- To examine the fetal brain anatomy when there is difficulty in diagnosing fetal brain abnormality.
- To assess fetal lung maturity.
- To assess fetal fat and predict neonatal morbidity in pregnancy complicated by diabetes mellitus.

Neonatal

- Perinatal post-mortem examination.

INVASIVE TESTS

Chorionic villus sampling (CVS)

Chorionic villus sampling can be undertaken at any gestation, but it is seen primarily as a first trimester test. Following visualization of the placenta by ultrasound, chorionic villi are obtained, usually by syringe, and these can be analysed for fetal chromosomal abnormalities. A provisional result is usually available within a few days.

Depending on the position of the placenta, the procedure can be done either transabdominally (generally accepted as the safer route) or via the cervix.

The advantage of an early diagnostic test for chromosomal abnormality is that the woman would probably have the option of a first trimester termination, if that was her decision. Disadvantages include a rate of pregnancy loss quoted at about 2% (Alfirevic, 2000). Difficulty in analysing the miscarriage rate is, however, complicated by the higher rate of spontaneous miscarriage in the first trimester. There is also a risk of results failure and studies have indicated a link between CVS and limb abnormality, probably restricted to procedures undertaken before 10 weeks' gestation (Proud, 1997).

Following the procedure, rhesus-negative women will be given anti-D immunoglobulin to prevent possible isoimmunization.

Amniocentesis

Amniotic fluid can be used to test for fetal conditions such as chromosomal abnormalities, genetic diseases, or some fetal infections.

In the UK amniocentesis is usually performed at about 15–18 weeks' gestation, using ultrasound to visualize the uterus and its contents. A fine needle is passed through the abdominal wall into the uterus and about 20 ml of amniotic fluid is extracted. The fetal cells in the amniotic fluid must be cultured and the time taken for their growth (about 2–3 weeks) accounts for the wait for a diagnosis, which women find so difficult. Some amniocentesis will fail to give a result when the fetal cells do not grow, and the woman must be aware of this small risk (about 1 : 500), as well as the other disadvantages, before she can make an informed choice to have an amniocentesis.

Some tests on amniotic fluid, such as diagnosis of neural tube defects (which is now done by ultrasound) or assessing the lecithin : sphingomyelin ratio for fetal pulmonary maturity, are now no longer considered a reason for an invasive test.

After the procedure the fetal heart is auscultated or visualized on ultrasound and the woman should be allowed to hear/see this. She will usually be advised to rest for that day and avoid strenuous activity for a few days. Rhesus-negative women will receive anti-D immunoglobulin to prevent possible rhesus isoimmunization.

The risk of pregnancy loss following amniocentesis is about 0.5–1% but this can vary according to operator and centre. There is also a risk of infection following any invasive procedure.

There may be a possibility in the future of routinely using DNA analysis for all tests done on amniotic fluid, which would give a much quicker result (Verma *et al.*, 1998).

'Early' amniocentesis

Although in the UK amniocentesis is usually done at about 15–18 weeks, early amniocentesis (from about 10–14 weeks) is commonly undertaken in the USA. Potential problems include premature rupture of membranes, infection, and bleeding. An increased rate of talipes equinovarus has also been demonstrated (Alfirevic, 2000).

Compared with CVS there are fewer sampling failures but more pregnancy loss (Alfirevic, 2000). There is also a higher rate of pregnancy loss when compared with second trimester amniocentesis.

These disadvantages must be set against the obvious advantage of having a first trimester diagnosis, and each woman considering this test will make her choice based on her own individual priorities – the midwife's role will be to ensure her decision is an informed one, and then to offer support.

Cordocentesis

This is an invasive investigation performed using ultrasound imaging, whereby a sample of fetal blood is obtained from the umbilical cord or intrahepatic vein, usually in the second or third trimester of pregnancy. The site of sampling is selected on considerations of accessibility, quality of visualization, gestational age and safety. The investigation was developed from a number of earlier interventions, including fetoscopy, for the purpose of antenatal diagnosis.

Cordocentesis carries a risk of miscarriage and also a risk of maternal infection or haemorrhage.

Reflective Activity 18.3

Explore the provision of tests at your unit:

- What range of tests are there?
- When are they offered and to whom?
- What written information is available for women and their families – is it accessible? Up-to-date?
- How are the results conveyed?

You may find it useful to compile this information into a resource file for reference.

CONCLUSION

The suggestion of even a minor defect in the fetus can cause extreme anxiety for parents, especially as, even if all further tests are undertaken, no professional can guarantee a 'perfect' baby.

There is some evidence that the anxiety engendered on identification of a potential problem, does not go away even after a reassuring diagnosis (Lawrence, 1999), and also that maternal anxiety during pregnancy may affect the physiological development of the fetus (Teixeira *et al.*, 1999).

However, the concept of prenatal screening is popular with most women, and the ability to identify many abnormal fetuses leads to women having a choice of terminating the pregnancy. There are also many healthy children – and their mothers – alive today because of the provision of the tests described in this chapter.

The midwife's role is to ensure that the woman receives accurate, evidence-based and up-to-date information in language she can understand, in order to make an informed decision. Where possible, the midwife should provide written information to support any discussions, and should also be aware of other sources of information, which may be helpful, such as through the Internet, and through voluntary groups. Whatever range of tests the woman and her family choose to access, for whatever reason, the midwife should continue to provide support and respect throughout her care.

KEY POINTS

- Investigations offered to women in the antenatal period have increased in number and complexity.
- Midwives need to keep up to date in the changing field of antenatal investigations, and have access to contemporary sources of information.
- Antenatal tests, and their potential consequences, need to be fully understood by the woman before they are undertaken. Written information should support any verbal discussion where possible.
- The well-being of mother and baby, and the successful outcome of a pregnancy, can be dependent on antenatal investigations.

REFERENCES

Alfirevic, Z. (2000) Early amniocentesis versus transabdominal chorion villus sampling for prenatal diagnosis. *The Cochrane Library*, Issue 4. Oxford: Update Software.

Alfirevic, Z. & Neilson, J.P. (2003) Biophysical profile for fetal assessment in high risk pregnancies, *Cochrane Database Library*, Issue 1: CD000038. Oxford: Update Software.

Anteby, E., Tadmor, O., Revel, A. *et al.* (1994) Post term pregnancy with normal cardiotocographs and amniotic fluid columns: the role of Doppler evaluation in predicting perinatal outcomes *European Journal of Obstetrics and Gynecology and Reproductive Biology* 54(2): 93–98.

Antsaklis, A., Dkalaki, G., Mesogitis, S. *et al.* (2000) Prenatal diagnosis of fetal primary CMV infection. *BJOG* 107(1): 84–88.

Ault, K. & Faro, S. (1993) Viruses, bacterial and protozoans in pregnancy: a sample of each. *Clinics in Obstetrics and Gynecology* 36(4): 878–885.

Blackburn, S.T. (2003) *Maternal, Fetal and Neonatal Physiology: A Clinical Perspective*. Philadelphia: W.B. Saunders.

Boyd, P., Chamberlain, P. & Hicks, N. (1998) 6-year experience of prenatal diagnosis in an unselected population in Oxford UK. *Lancet* 352(9140): 1577–1581.

Bryan, E. (1986) The intrauterine hazards of twins. *Archives of Disease in Childhood* 61(II): 1044–1045.

Cameron, S., Young, H. & Liston, W. (1998) The usefulness of antenatal screening for syphilis. *Contemporary Reviews in Obstetrics & Gynaecology* 10(1): 33–38.

Cuckle, H. & van Lith, J. (1999) Appropriate biochemistry parameters in first trimester screening for Down syndrome. *Prenatal Diagnosis* 19(6): 505–512.

Day, L. (1998) Iron supplementation in pregnancy: can it be justified? *British Journal of Midwifery* 6(3 March): 180–183.

Department of Health (DoH) (1993) *Report of a working party of the Standing Medical Advisory Committee on Sickle Cell, Thalassaemia and other Haemoglobinopathies*. London: HMSO.

Department of Health (DoH) (1999) *Targets Aimed at Reducing the Number of Children Born with HIV: Report from an Expert Group*. UK Health Departments. London: DoH.

Department of Health (DoH) (2000) *Advice to pregnant women during the lambing season*. London: DoH.

Economides, D., Whitlow, B. & Braithwaite, J. (1999) Ultrasonography in the detection of fetal anomalies in early pregnancy *British Journal of Obstetrics and Gynaecology* 106(6): 516–523.

Foulon, W., Villena, I., Stray-Pedersen, B. *et al.* (1999) Treatment of toxoplasmosis during pregnancy: a multicenter study of impact on fetal transmission and children's sequelae at age one year. *American Journal of Obstetrics and Gynecology* 180(2 Pt 1): 410–415.

Herrero, R. & Fitzsimmons, J. (1999) Estimated fetal weight: maternal vs physician estimate. *Journal of Reproductive Medicine* 44(8): 674–678.

Hoffbrand, A. & Pettit, J. (2000) *Essential Haematology*, 4th edn. London: Blackwell Scientific Publications.

Hyett, J. & Thilaganathan, B. (1999) First trimester screening for fetal abnormalities *Current Opinion in Obstetrics & Gynecology* 11(6): 563–569.

James, D. (1993) Monitoring the biophysical profile. *British Journal of Hospital Medicine* 49(8): 561–563.

James, D. (2002) Assessing fetal health. *Current Obstetrics & Gynaecology* 12(5): 243–249.

Johnson, I. (1992) Radiological and magnetic visualisation techniques. In: Brock, D., Rodeck, C. & Ferguson-Smith, M.A. (eds) *Prenatal Diagnosis and Screening*. Edinburgh: Churchill Livingstone.

Krishnamurthy, S., Fairlie, F., Cameron, A. *et al.* (1991) The role of X-ray pelvimetry after caesarean section in the management of subsequent delivery. *British Journal of Obstetrics and Gynaecology* 98(7): 716–718.

Lawrence, S. (1999) Counselling for Downs syndrome screening. *British Journal of Midwifery* 7(6): 368–370.

Liston, R.M., Bloom, K. & Zimmer, P. (1994) The psychological effects of counting fetal movements. *Birth* 21(3): 135–140.

Loncar, J., Barnabei, J. & Larsen, J. (1995) Advent of maternal serum markers for Down syndrome screening. *Obstetrical & Gynecological Survey* 50(4): 316–320.

MacKenzie, I., Selinger, M. & Bowell, P. (1991) Management of red cell isoimmunisation in the 1990s. In: Studd, J. (ed) *Progress in Obstetrics and Gynaecology*, Vol. 9. Edinburgh: Churchill Livingstone.

National Institute for Clinical Excellence (NICE) (2002) *Guidance on the use of routine antenatal anti-D prophylaxis for RhD-negative women*. NICE Technology Appraisal Guidance No 41. London: NICE.

Nicolaides, K., Cicero, S. & Liao, A. (2000) One-stop clinic for assessment of risk of chromosomal defects at 12 weeks of gestation. *Prenatal and Neonatal Medicine* 5(3): 145–154.

Platt, L., Koch, R., Hanley, W. *et al.* (2000) The international study of pregnancy outcome in women with maternal phenylketonuria: report of a 12-year study. *American Journal of Obstetrics and Gynecology* 182(2): 326–333.

Proud, J. (1997) *Understanding Obstetric Ultrasound*, 2nd edn. Cheshire: Books for Midwives Press.

Raman, S., Urquhart, R. & Yusof, M. (1992) Clinical versus ultrasound estimation of fetal weight. *Australian and New Zealand Journal of Obstetrics and Gynaecology* 32(3): 196–199.

Regan, L. (2000) *Miscarriage*, revised edn. London: Orion.

Rocco, B. & Garrone, C. (1999) Can examination of the cervix provide useful information for prediction of cervical incompetence and following preterm labour? *Australian and New Zealand Journal of Obstetrics and Gynaecology* 39(3): 296–300.

Sadovsky, E. & Polishuk, W.Z. (1977) Fetal movements in utero: nature, assessment, prognostic value, timing of delivery. *Obstetrics and Gynecology* 50(1): 49–55.

Sadovsky, E., Ohel, G., Havazeleth, H. *et al.* (1983) The definition and the significance of decreased fetal movements. *Acta Obstetricia et Gynecologica Scandinavica* 62(5): 409–413.

Shafi, M.I., Dover, M.S., Dyer, C.A. *et al.* (1989) Pictorial fetal, movement charts in a multiracial antenatal clinic. *British Medical Journal* 298(6689): 1688.

Teixeira, J., Fisk, N. & Glover, V. (1999) Association between maternal anxiety in pregnancy and increased uterine artery resistance index: cohort based study. *British Medical Journal* 318(7177): 153–157.

Thornton, J., Hewison, J., Lilford, R. *et al.* (1995) A randomised controlled trial of three methods of giving information about prenatal testing. *British Medical Journal* 311(7013): 1127–1130.

Verma, L., Macdonald, F., Leedham, P. *et al.* (1998) Rapid and simple prenatal DNA diagnosis of Down's syndrome. *Lancet* 352(9121): 9–12.

Wald, N., Donsem, J., George, L. *et al.* (1996) Prenatal screening for Down's syndrome using inhibin-A as a serum marker. *Prenatal Diagnosis* 16(2): 143–153.

Wald, N., White, N., Morris, J. *et al.* (1999) Serum markers for Down's syndrome in women who have had IVF: implications for antenatal screening. *British Journal of Obstetrics and Gynaecology* 106(12): 1304–1306.

Ward, C., Tudor-Williams, F., Cotzias, T. *et al.* (2000) Prevalence of hepatitis C among pregnant women attending an inner London obstetrics department: uptake and acceptability of named antenatal testing. *Gut* 47(2): 277–280.

Winyard, G. (1998) *Screening of pregnant women for hepatitis B and immunisation of babies at risk*. HSC1998/127. 22nd July. Leeds: DoH, NHS Executive.

Wood, P. (2000) Safe and (ultra)sound – some aspects of ultrasound safety. *RCM Midwifery Journal* 3(2): 48–50.

19

Maternal Nutrition

Denise Tiran

LEARNING OUTCOMES

By the end of this chapter you will be able to:

- understand the basic principles of good maternal nutrition
- use a knowledge of nutrition to advise women about their diet during pregnancy
- appreciate the value of nutrition as a therapeutic intervention for specific conditions during pregnancy.

Nutrition is the sum of the processes involved in taking in nutrients, assimilating and utilizing them. Nutrients such as proteins, carbohydrates, fats, vitamins and minerals are necessary for development, growth, normal functioning and maintenance of life and, because the body cannot produce them, they need to be obtained from a variety of food sources.

Nutritional status is affected by the amount and quality of food eaten, the digestion, absorption and utilization of food nutrients, and by biochemical individuality. In westernized countries, eating enough food is not normally a problem. Nevertheless, many people do not eat the correct balance of nutrients, and malnourishment causes impairment of health, although for different reasons than in developing countries, where food is scarce. Food quality may be affected by nutrient-deficient soil in which crops are grown for human or livestock consumption, or by the use of pesticides. The addition of chemical preservatives, colourings and flavourings to ready-prepared food, and of antibiotics to meat, will also adversely influence nutrient absorption and utilization.

Digestion and absorption may be affected by general health or the combination of foods eaten. On the other hand, impaired absorption of certain nutrients may be iatrogenic, as when someone is taking specific drugs. Overindulgence in some foods can affect the body's ability to absorb essential nutrients; for instance, coffee and tea interfere with the absorption of zinc and iron from food. Similarly, abuse with other substances such as alcohol, cigarettes or recreational drugs will result in malnourishment as they prevent adequate absorption and utilization of nutrients from food. Environmental factors, including lead pollution, may predispose to nutritional inadequacies. Biochemical individuality means that each person has unique nutritional requirements, which will alter according to the person's age, gender, general health, level of activity, genetic influences and stressors, such as pregnancy.

Some people need professional help to direct them towards the most appropriate diet; this is usually because they suffer from conditions where diet plays a part in conventional management, such as in diabetes mellitus or coeliac disease. Patients will normally be advised by dieticians, who work from the premise that all necessary nutrients can be obtained solely from the food we eat and who advise people regarding relevant adaptations to their diet. Nutritional therapists go one step further by working on the basis of nutrition as a therapeutic intervention to assist in the overall health and well-being of the individual and may often prescribe additional supplements to balance the intake of dietary nutrients.

WHY IS GOOD NUTRITION IN PREGNANCY IMPORTANT?

Pregnancy is a time when women are receptive to advice about lifestyle changes, for they wish to be as healthy as possible for the sake of their babies. The midwife plays an important part in this process, as she is the health professional most frequently seen by the expectant mother. Encouraging women to adapt their diet to a more healthy one during pregnancy can have long-term benefits for the whole family for, as the mother is usually the main person responsible for the preparation of meals, she can influence the well-being of future generations by facilitating good eating habits in childhood (Harding, 1999). Impaired maternal nutrition may influence disease programming of the fetus for adult life, such as increasing the tendency to hypertension and cardiovascular disease (Barker, 1999).

Inadequate maternal nutrition during pregnancy and *prior* to conception may have an adverse effect on the fetus, with a higher than normal perinatal mortality and morbidity, and low birthweight or preterm infants, possibly owing to low placental weight, although Matthews *et al.* (1999) dispute this, at least in relation to women in industrialized countries. Birth defects may be more prevalent, such as neural tube defects as a result of low folic acid, and all women intending to become pregnant are advised to take routine folic acid supplements prior to pregnancy and during the first trimester. Other obstetric complications such as maternal pregnancy-induced hypertension and pre-eclampsia may also be precipitated by poor nutrition.

PERICONCEPTIONAL NUTRITION

Ideally, dietary advice should be given prior to conception, for it has been known since the famines of the Second World War that fetal outcome is worse if the mother is malnourished at the time of conception rather than at the time of delivery (Doyle *et al.*, 1999). A thorough investigation into the mother's diet and other aspects of her lifestyle would be a more efficient and cost-effective use of time at the booking appointment, than focusing purely on physiopathological history. This latter could be obtained via alternative means, such as a questionnaire sent to the woman in advance of her appointment. Time could then be spent by the midwife at the first meeting in discussing the concerns of the woman and offering her information and advice. Sujitor's paper (1994) discusses the need for standard procedures to incorporate nutritional assessment into the care of all expectant mothers, whilst Doyle *et al.* (1999) advocate counselling and advice on nutrition *between* pregnancies for women who have had previous low birthweight babies.

Infertility and subfertility are known to be exacerbated by poor nutrition, and dietary advice is a major component of preconceptional care where this is provided, for example for diabetic women. Ovulation (and therefore the ability to conceive) is dependent on the woman having a distribution of adipose tissue (fat) equal to at least 17% of her total body weight; anorexics and bulimic girls are thus less likely to conceive but also more likely to miscarry because of vitamin and mineral imbalances.

Male infertility may be triggered by, amongst other factors, poor sperm production, which is associated with deficiency of arginine, essential fatty acids, zinc, chromium, selenium and vitamins A, E, C and B.

Preconceptional nutritional advice should focus on encouraging a diet which is high both in beneficial nutrients and in those which suppress the effects of toxic elements caused by unavoidable factors such as environmental pollution. In addition, advice should be offered to assist women in reducing their intake of substances known to be detrimental to themselves and their fetus such as nicotine, tea, coffee, alcohol and drugs. Cigarette smoking is well known to interfere with nutrient intake and absorption, especially amongst young expectant mothers (Mathews *et al.*, 2000). The contraceptive pill interferes with the absorption of vitamin B_6 and zinc and should, where possible, be discontinued for at least 3 months before conception to avoid the woman commencing her pregnancy deficient in these nutrients which are essential for well-being, especially during the first trimester. Women who experience premenstrual syndrome are often deficient in magnesium, zinc and vitamin B_6 as well as other vital nutrients and would also benefit from preconceptional dietary changes to combat these. Many artificial preservatives can be harmful and pregnant women should be advised to eat as much fresh food as possible, with at least five portions of fruit, vegetables and salad daily. Organically grown foods may reduce the impact of fertilizer sprays used on crops but midwives need to mindful that it is usually more expensive and that the health benefits of organic foods have been questioned recently in the popular press.

The aetiology of recurrent spontaneous abortion is very complex but may predominate in women who are deficient in essential fatty acids, zinc, manganese and vitamin E, or in whom overload with toxic elements such as nicotine, alcohol, caffeine or other substances adversely affects the absorption of beneficial nutrients. There continues to be controversy regarding the amount of caffeine that is likely to provoke miscarriage, with some authorities suggesting that as little as one to two cups of coffee per day increases the risk (Fernandes, 1998). Eskenazi *et al.* (1999) highlighted the increased risk of low birthweight babies in women who drank caffeinated rather than decaffeinated coffee, although advice regarding decaffeinated coffee needs to be given with care as the process used to remove the caffeine may involve the addition of chemicals which can, in themselves, be harmful to pregnant women.

WEIGHT IN PREGNANCY

Most mothers are expected to gain between 11 and 15.75 kg (25–35 lb) (Kolassa and Weismiller, 1997) in weight during pregnancy, but this is dependent on maternal diet, activity, food availability (especially in the developing world), and gestational factors such as physiological sickness or multiple pregnancy. Attention to a balanced diet in the mother is more significant than concern about her weight gain, and is more likely to result in full-term babies of adequate birthweight. Preconceptional, gestational and lactational nutrition are known to affect the birthweight, well-being and long-term health prognosis of infants (Butte, 2000). Excessive weight gain in pregnancy also impacts on the mother's risk of obesity in later life (Reifsnider and Gill, 2000). Catalano (1999) identifies a wide range of additional energy requirements in pregnancy, according to nationality, but recognizes that recommendations for the most acceptable levels of fat and carbohydrate intake for individuals are difficult to specify.

There has also been some discussion regarding *restriction* of energy intake during pregnancy. Dieting to lose weight is not recommended during pregnancy, even for obese women, but they may wish to restrict calories moderately, particularly as the decrease in physical activity in the third trimester must be accounted for. In societies where energy intake is forcefully restricted because of lack of food, maternal metabolic adaptations are made to spare energy for fetal growth. However, care must be taken when advising immigrant women, such as those from the Indian subcontinent, who may, for a variety of genetic and diet-related factors, traditionally produce small babies. Encouraging them to consume a British type of diet and increase their weight beyond that which is culturally the norm could result in large babies and consequent cephalopelvic disproportion, with all its related problems (see Case scenario 19.1).

Case scenario 19.1

Yasmin had journeyed from Yemen to visit her brother in England when she was in the second trimester of her *13th* pregnancy. Her other 12 children, all born normally, were all alive except one, the fourth child having died at the age of 3 from measles. Yasmin planned to go home for the birth of her baby but was denied a flight by the airline so was committed to delivering in the UK. I met her at the booking clinic when she was 31 weeks' pregnant and found a petite frail-looking woman who was accompanied by her 15-year-old son as interpreter, which made obtaining a full medical history difficult as he refused to discuss intimate female issues.

Initial assessment by the (male Caucasian) doctor identified Yasmin as at risk of having a 'small for dates' infant and she was given standard dietary advice to help her put on more weight. She spent several weeks eating a western diet including more protein than she would normally eat at home and by her 38 week antenatal appointment was deemed to have increased her weight to more 'acceptable' levels. However, pelvic assessment by another (female Caucasian) doctor identified potential cephalopelvic disproportion, as the fetus was now larger than her pelvis could accommodate. Yasmin was booked for elective Caesarean section which, once she understood, caused her much distress and would have impacted on her stay in Britain. Fortunately for her, a new registrar arrived who himself came from Yemen and he met Yasmin just days before her scheduled surgery. Not only was he able to communicate with her but he also altered the management of her care, induced labour and very expertly conducted a ventouse extraction resulting in the birth of a live healthy baby and a mother who was saved from having a uterine scar.

Muslim women are required to fast during Ramadan and, although some exceptions are made, pregnancy is a normal physiological event and therefore women are expected to comply with total fasting, i.e. no food or drink from dawn till dusk. Midwives should be aware of current teachings regarding Ramadan, and they should ask Muslim women if they are fasting.

ESSENTIAL NUTRIENTS

Proteins and amino acids

Required for:

- development of cells, enzymes, hormones, antibodies, haemoglobin
- buffers, helping to regulate acid–base balance
- controlling osmotic pressure between body fluids
- assisting in the transport of lipids as lipoproteins, and of free fatty acids and bilirubin.

Foods which contain proteins:

- meats, poultry, fish
- cheese, milk, eggs and other dairy produce
- beans, peas and other legumes
- corn, wheat products
- grains, seeds, nuts
- brewer's yeast, soya.

Essential amino acids include leucine, lysine, methionine, cystine, phenylalanine, tryptophan and valine; non-essential amino acids include alanine, glutamic acid, glycine and tyrosine. Proteins are digested by being broken down into amino acids and transported to the liver, where enzymes called amino acid transferases convert them into a more usable form. This process requires vitamin B_6; consequently, a high protein intake will require an increase in vitamin B_6 intake. For example, pregnant women are known to have higher blood levels of tryptophan, an amino acid which is converted to serotonin and which acts as a calming and antidepressive agent. A woman who has recently discontinued the contraceptive pill, which inhibits the effects of vitamin B_6, may require supplements.

Certain protein foods may become sources of potential infection for pregnant women. Meat, in particular, may be contaminated and advice regarding cooking may help to prevent gastrointestinal disorders. In addition, raw meat may be contaminated by the *Listeria monocytogenes* bacterium or the parasite *Toxoplasma gondii*, so mothers should be advised against consuming raw or undercooked meat. *Listeria monocytogenes* may also be present in unpasteurized milk, and women are advised to refrain from eating soft cheeses, such as Brie, for this reason.

Essential fatty acids

Required for:

- energy, heat insulation
- production of active biological substances essential for normal body functioning

- facilitation of absorption of fat-soluble vitamins and calcium
- formation of cell walls throughout the body
- production of prostaglandins.

Foods which contain unsaturated fatty acids:

- vegetable oils, especially safflower and sunflower, but excluding coconut and palm oil, which are saturated
- fish oils.

Foods which contain saturated fatty acids:

- animal fats such as butter and lard, meat fat
- margarines and vegetable shortening.

Fats are composed of triglycerides – three fatty acids with a unit of glycerol – and are broken down into these components during digestion. Most fatty acids can be synthesized by the body, with the exception of linoleic acid, linolenic acid and arachidonic acid, which must be obtained from food. Fatty acids are composed of a chain of carbon atoms, with each atom having one or more free 'arms' or bonds to link with other atoms. Where one or more 'arm' is unattached, the fatty acid is unsaturated: if only one 'arm' is free it is mono-unsaturated; if more than one 'arm' is free it is poly-unsaturated. Unsaturated fatty acids are preferable to saturated ones, and poly-unsaturated are the most favourable as they are more readily converted into energy; however, a balance of each type is needed for adequate nutrition. Brooks *et al.* (2000) discuss the importance of one specific essential fatty acid, docohexaenoic acid (DHA) during pregnancy and lactation for adequate neurological functioning of the neonate.

Fatty acids depend on certain other nutrients for their metabolism, including zinc, magnesium, selenium, and vitamins B_3, C and E. There is a need for small additional quantities of fats during pregnancy, particularly for extra energy, to avoid protein calories being misused. An American investigation by Hachey (1994) explored the maternal and fetal outcomes related to fat consumption during pregnancy. The conclusion was drawn that while middle-aged multiparous mothers may be at increased risk of later developing angina or cholesterol gallstones due to the hypercholesterolaemia of normal pregnancy, this does not support a practice of low-fat diets during pregnancy. This is because serum lipids are reduced by poly-unsaturated fatty acids, some obstetric complications may be improved by n-3 fatty acids, and arachidonic acid may help visual and psychomotor development in the child.

Carbohydrates

Required for:

- calorie intake: 1 gram of carbohydrate provides 4 calories of energy
- regulation of gastrointestinal function
- balancing the growth of normal bacterial flora against undesirable flora.

Foods which contain carbohydrates:

- sugars, fruit sugars and foods which contain sugars, including 'hidden' sugars in savoury foods
- breads, pastas, flours, cereals
- potatoes, bananas
- beetroot
- dates, figs
- maple syrup
- sauces, flavourings.

Carbohydrates are classified as sugars (mono- and disaccharides) or starches and fibre (polysaccharides). They are the most easily digested of all nutrients, and can be stored in the body and released as energy when required, thereby preventing excessive oxidation of fats for energy. All carbohydrates are broken down partly in the mouth and mainly in the small intestine to the simplest compound, glucose; excess glucose is converted into glycogen to be stored by the liver. It is generally considered that carbohydrate intake should equate to approximately half of all food consumed, which in many people would indicate a need to increase starches and fibre and decrease fats and proteins.

Vitamins and minerals

Vitamin A

Required for:

- growth and repair of cells
- fighting infection
- synthesis of ribonucleic acid (RNA)
- healthy eyes, especially night vision
- protein metabolism
- aids in detoxification processes
- as an antioxidant.

Foods which contain vitamin A:

- liver and kidneys
- fish oils
- eggs and dairy produce
- apricots, carrots, other yellow vegetables
- broccoli, parsley, green leafy vegetables.

Deficiency of vitamin A may cause anaemias, blindness, skin disorders, tooth decay, allergies and gastrointestinal disorders. Absorption of vitamin A from the diet can be impeded by vitamin D deficiency, alcohol, coffee, mineral oil, nitrate fertilizers and strong glaring sunlight. While there is a need for adequate intake of vitamin A during pregnancy, birth defects have been found to occur in women taking supplements, or eating *excessive* amounts of vitamin A-containing foods such as liver during the first trimester, because of the presence of retinol. In 1990 the Department of Health stated that the recommended daily amount (RDA) of vitamin A in pregnancy (i.e. 2500 IU) should not be exceeded because higher intakes may pose a teratogenic risk (DHSS, 1990). It is now felt that pregnant women and those intending to become pregnant should not take *supplements* of vitamin A, but that the advice from the early 1990s to avoid liver and liver products such as pâté is no longer necessary. All women should be advised to eat all things in moderation and not to consume anything to excess.

Thiamin (vitamin B$_1$)

Required for:

- synthesis of acetylcholine within the cells
- maintenance of healthy nerves, cardiac muscle and digestive tissues
- digestion of carbohydrates.

Foods which contain thiamin:

- whole grains
- nuts and seeds, such as sunflower
- brewer's yeast
- fruit and green vegetables
- liver, kidneys
- fish
- eggs and milk.

Absorption of available thiamin from food will be impaired by stress, food additives, alcohol, coffee, excessive sugar consumption, overcooking of vegetables, especially boiling, and by some antibiotics. The need for thiamin increases during pregnancy and lactation, and long-term deficiency could lead to irritability, insomnia, weight loss, oedema, poor reflexes, and ultimately to impairment of the cardiovascular, nervous and gastrointestinal systems.

Riboflavin (vitamin B$_2$)

Required for:

- metabolism of fats, proteins and carbohydrates
- wound healing
- regulation of hormones
- growth and development of the fetus.

Foods which contain vitamin B$_2$:
- foods which also contain thiamin.

Absorption is adversely affected by antibiotics and the contraceptive pill. Deficiency may cause various external lesions, fatigue, personality disturbance, anaemia, digestive upset and hypertension.

Niacin (vitamin B$_3$)

Required for:
- conversion of food to energy
- metabolism of fats, proteins and carbohydrates
- regulation of hormonal and enzymal actions
- vasodilatation.

Foods which contain niacin:
- liver, lean meat
- poultry
- fish
- grains
- yeast
- butter
- nuts.

Absorption of niacin is antagonized by alcohol, stress, coffee, high carbohydrate intake, antibiotics and antitubercular drugs. A variety of skin and gastrointestinal disturbances may result from inadequate intake, as well as headache, memory loss, insomnia and poor appetite. If a mother is deficient in vitamin B$_6$ her needs for niacin will also increase.

Pyridoxine (vitamin B$_6$)

Required for:
- synthesis of proteins
- production of antibodies
- manufacture of erythrocytes
- enzyme reactions
- development of the nervous system
- healthy teeth and gums
- release of stored glycogen.

Foods which contain pyridoxine:
- foods which contain other B vitamins
- bananas, grapefruit
- prunes and raisins.

Absorption is affected by many drugs, including the contraceptive pill, cortisone, penicillamine and antitubercular treatments. Pyridoxine requirements increase during pregnancy and lactation, with insufficient intake leading to anaemia, neuritis, convulsions, depression, dermatitis and possibly renal calculi.

Cobalamin (vitamin B$_{12}$)

Required for:
- proper functioning of the bone marrow and erythrocytes
- nervous system, including myelin formation
- development of RNA and DNA
- regulation of normal blood ascorbic acid levels
- carbohydrate metabolism.

Foods which contain cobalamin:
- liver, kidney
- fish and shellfish.

Absorption may be adversely affected by aspirin, the contraceptive pill, codeine, alcohol and nitrous oxide. Deficiency can result in pernicious anaemia, poor growth, memory loss, nervous disorders and ataxia. Although requirements do not increase significantly during pregnancy, certain women are at risk of deficiency, including vegetarians, epileptics, those who have recently discontinued the contraceptive pill, and women with tapeworms. Neurological damage in the infants of vitamin B$_{12}$-deficient vegetarian mothers has been reported (Specker, 1994).

Folic acid

Required for:
- production of erythrocytes, in conjunction with B$_{12}$
- maintenance of the nervous system
- gastrointestinal tract functioning
- production of leucocytes
- production of choline and methionine
- development of the fetus.

Foods which contain folic acid:
- leafy greens
- whole grains, nuts
- oranges
- broccoli
- tuna
- liver and kidney.

The incidence of neural tube defects is increased when women are deficient in folic acid, both before and during pregnancy. Original research by Smithells *et al.* (1981) and by Laurence *et al.* (1981) highlighted this. The Department of Health subsequently recommended folate/folic acid supplementation of 0.4 mg daily for all women prior to conception and also during the first 12 weeks of pregnancy. To prevent recurrence of neural tube defects the dose of folic acid supplements should be increased to 4–5 mg daily. Czeizei (1995) suggests that folate supplementation may also reduce the incidence of other major congenital malformations, such as in the cardiovascular system and urinary tract, as well as limb abnormalities and congenital hypertrophic pyloric stenosis. In the mother, folic acid deficiency can lead to some anaemias, depression, nervousness, cell and tissue disruptions and premature greying or loss of hair.

Impaired absorption and utilization may occur if the woman is stressed, drinks alcohol, has recently discontinued the contraceptive pill, or is taking certain drugs such as aspirin, sulphonamides or anticonvulsants.

Vitamin C

Required for:

- cell, tissue, nerve, tooth and bone health
- wound healing
- metabolism of amino acids
- facilitation of iron absorption.

Foods which contain vitamin C:

- all citrus fruits
- berries
- melons
- tomatoes
- potatoes
- parsley
- green vegetables (although cooking will destroy it)
- blackcurrants.

Inadequate levels of vitamin C can lead to bacterial infections, bruising, oedema, haemorrhage, anaemia, poor digestion, tooth and gum disease and scurvy. Certain drugs, especially aspirin, anticoagulants, antibiotics, diuretics, cortisone, the contraceptive pill and antidepressants, can interfere with absorption, as can also pollution, industrial toxins and overcooking or poor storage of food sources.

Vitamin D

Required for:

- calcium absorption
- healthy bones and teeth
- renal, cardiac and nervous systems
- blood clotting.

Foods which contain vitamin D:

- fish liver oils
- liver
- brewer's yeast
- tuna
- avocados.

The main source of vitamin D is the sunshine, so women who are long-stay antenatal inpatients should be given the opportunity to sit outside as much as possible. Drugs such as laxatives and antacids inhibit absorption, so care must be taken not to overuse these for women with physiological constipation or heartburn. The mother and fetus both require additional vitamin D to prevent skeletal malformations, rickets, osteoporosis, poor muscle tone, and reduced function of the kidneys and parathyroid glands.

Vitamin E

Required for:

- maintenance of erythrocytes
- major bodily functions, including reproduction
- retarding ageing
- helping the body to respond to stress.

Foods which contain vitamin E:

- whole grains
- eggs
- leafy greens, broccoli, cabbage
- avocados
- nuts
- liver, kidneys
- cold-pressed vegetable oils.

Vitamin E is destroyed by food processing, rancid fats and oils and by inorganic iron. Absorption is adversely affected by mineral oil, the contraceptive pill, chlorine and thyroid hormone. Requirements for vitamin E increase during pregnancy: indeed, what was originally called vitamin E is now known to be a group of compounds called tocopherols, a name derived from two Greek words *tocos* (childbirth) and *pheros* (to bring forth), owing to the finding that animals deficient in vitamin E were unable to attain successful pregnancies. In humans, deficiencies are known to result in spontaneous abortion, preterm labour and stillbirths, as well as possible anaemia and muscular or cardiovascular diseases.

Calcium

Required for:

- formation of bones and teeth
- utilization of iron
- assisting coagulation
- regulation of cardiac rhythm.

Foods which contain calcium:

- milk and dairy products such as yogurt, egg yolk
- sardines and salmon with bones
- green beans

- bone marrow
- tofu and soya beans.

High-protein or high-phosphorus diets will antagonize absorption, as will either an excess or a deficit of physical activity, or stress. Drugs which affect absorption or utilization of calcium include antacids, laxatives, diuretics and anticonvulsants. Deficiencies may lead to bone disorders such as osteoporosis or osteoarthritis, dental problems, palpitations, hypertension, insomnia or muscle cramps. Routine calcium supplementation may be helpful in women at risk of pre-eclampsia or those who have an identified low level of calcium.

Zinc

Required for:

- cell development in the brain, thyroid gland, liver, kidneys, lungs and prostate gland
- skeletal growth, skin, hair, repair of body tissues, wound healing
- metabolism of proteins, carbohydrates and phosphorus
- facilitation of release of stored vitamin A.

Foods which contain zinc:

- herrings, oysters, fish bones
- liver, red meat, meat bones
- eggs, milk
- nuts, whole grains
- mushrooms, leafy green vegetables
- paprika.

Zinc requirements rise by approximately 30% during pregnancy, to provide for the development of the fetal central nervous system, and by 40% in lactating women. Absorption is enhanced by adequate intakes of calcium, copper, vitamins A, B_6, B_{12} and C and certain amino acids. Absorption and utilization are impaired by tea, coffee, alcohol, processed grains, iron tablets, the contraceptive pill, and by excess levels of phytates, found in bran, and calcium. Jewish women may be deficient in zinc, owing to the presence of phytates in unleavened bread.

Zinc neutralizes the toxic effects of cadmium, a contributory factor in hypertension, but, conversely, high levels of cadmium, found in large amounts in cigarettes, some processed and canned foods, some instant coffees and gelatine, will inhibit the action of zinc. Excessive sweating can cause a loss of up to 3 mg of zinc per day and zinc is lost in the urine at times of stress and during increased diuresis such as following high alcohol consumption.

Inadequate zinc levels can lead to retarded growth and mental development, delayed sexual maturity or sterility (normal semen contains large quantities of zinc). It may exacerbate pregnancy sickness and worsen the appearance of striae gravidarum. Women who are zinc deficient may have white spots on their fingernails, experience a metallic taste in the mouth and have a poor appetite. There is a risk of poor pregnancy outcome when intake is less than 6 mg daily, including low birthweight and preterm babies and impaired immune systems. Studies suggest that adequate zinc intake contributes to a reduction in the risk of neural tube defects in the fetus (Shaw *et al.*, 1999). Zinc is an antagonist to lead and cadmium, both of which have been found in higher than normal quantities in the bones of stillborn infants; by inference therefore, adequate zinc levels may decrease the risk of stillbirth caused solely by nutritional deficiencies.

Iron

Required for:

- manufacture of haemoglobin for oxygenation of the blood
- protein metabolism
- bone growth
- resistance to disease.

Foods which contain iron:

- red meats, liver
- sardines, pilchards, sprats, whitebait, cockles
- eggs, especially the yolks
- wholemeal bread, chapattis, oatcakes
- cereals
- potatoes, parsley, chives, spinach
- dried fruits, nuts and cherries
- soya beans, red kidney beans, lentils, chick peas.

It was widely regarded as good practice until the 1990s to provide all pregnant women routinely with iron supplements in order to prevent anaemia. However, gradually realization dawned that many women failed to take their tablets, which wasted resources, and that anaemia does not arise exclusively as a result of iron deficiency. Furthermore, the body is capable of absorbing only up to 3 mg of iron daily, including that taken in as food. There continues to be a practice in some units of encouraging women to take *double* iron tablets, without a fuller understanding of the pathology of anaemia, and the appreciation that advising women to take their tablets with a glass of orange juice (or other vitamin C-containing drink) will facilitate absorption of the iron, while over-consumption of tea will hinder its absorption.

An inadequate iron level will lead to anaemia, fatigue, headache, palpitations and heartburn and supplementation will be required to treat iron-deficiency anaemia. Dietary iron consumption will normally achieve sufficient serum levels of iron, although a high zinc intake, tea, coffee, intestinal parasites, antacids and tetracycline will interfere with absorption. Women who consume adequate amounts of foods containing vitamins C, E, B_6, B_{12}, folic acid, calcium, copper and other trace elements will normally be able to utilize efficiently the iron from dietary intake.

> ### Reflective Activity 19.1
>
> Make comprehensive lists of foods which contain certain minerals, e.g. magnesium, selenium, and identify what might happen if a mother were to be deficient in these elements.

NUTRITION AS A THERAPEUTIC INTERVENTION FOR DISORDERS OF PREGNANCY

Nausea and vomiting

Many women find that nausea is exacerbated by hypoglycaemia, especially if they are also tired, and advice can be given by the midwife to eat small frequent meals of high-carbohydrate foods but not those that are also high in sugar or salt. Sweet foods contain sugars that are easily digested and quickly utilized and will therefore result in a return to the hypoglycaemia and the nausea more quickly than if complex carbohydrates are taken. Bananas are a good source of carbohydrate, which will also help to prevent potassium deficiency. Sickness in pregnancy is worse if the woman is lacking in vitamin B_6, magnesium and zinc and she should be advised to eat foods rich in these substances or to take a good-quality supplement. Reducing the amount of dairy produce may also help, whilst increasing intake of citrus fruits or juices may improve the situation.

Constipation

This is automatically treated by advising women to increase the amount of high-fibre foods, but more importantly they must increase their fluid intake to at least 3 litres of water or fruit juice daily. Tea consumption should be decreased as tannin reduces peristalsis and inhibits the absorption of iron, which might result

in prescription of iron tablets that may, in turn, exacerbate the constipation. Women can be encouraged to eat plenty of fresh fruits, vegetables, unrefined carbohydrates, nuts, seeds, grains and pulses such as beans. Bran should be *avoided* as this absorbs fluid from the intestines, makes the stool hard and increases the severity of the constipation. Wheat and wheat products such as bread and cereals may increase bloating and abdominal discomfort, particularly if the problem was present before pregnancy, as it may be due to a wheat intolerance. Long term use of laxatives is to be discouraged as they will not treat the cause of the problem and can often create other side-effects. Vitamin C supplements may be necessary in some mothers. If iron tablets are prescribed for anaemia and found to exacerbate the problem, other sources of iron-containing foods should be advised and it may be necessary to suggest alternatives to medication such as herbal liquid preparations, available from healthfood stores.

Heartburn and indigestion

Advise the mother to eat small frequent meals and to avoid drinking with the meal but to maintain a high fluid intake between meals. She should avoid foods known to aggravate the condition, such as spicy or greasy foods, as well as coffee, tea, alcohol and cigarettes. Milk and milk products do not always help to relieve the symptoms, and may actually exacerbate them, as may sugar, sweet foods, wheat and bread. Excessive use of antacids should be avoided during pregnancy, especially those containing aluminium, as some of this may be absorbed and cause a degree of toxicity. A small amount of sodium bicarbonate (quarter of a teaspoonful) dissolved in water can be helpful but should not be taken at meal times or used frequently as it may neutralize gastric acid which is required for the absorption and digestion of essential nutrients. Using large quantities of garlic in cooking can be very helpful. It is best to use whole, peeled but uncut, cloves of garlic which, when cooked can be squashed and stirred into the food. In this way adequate quantities of the active ingredients, allicin and other sulphur-containing substances, will be consumed but there will be no excessively strong flavour nor the after-taste and halitosis of which many people complain.

Anaemia

Anaemia may be prevented, or the effects reduced, by encouraging the mother to eat foods which are rich in iron. Her diet should include plenty of fresh green leafy vegetables such as cabbage, spinach, watercress, plus parsley, spring onions, chives, sprouted grains and seeds. Seaweeds, nettle tops and dandelion leaves are also good sources of iron. Dried fruits such as prunes, raisins, figs and unsulphured apricots are helpful, as are blackcurrants, blackberries, cherries and loganberries. Wholegrain bread, oatcakes and chapattis should be eaten rather than highly refined carbohydrates. Pilchards, salmon and kippers and organic liver also provide good amounts of iron. Bran should be avoided as it inhibits the absorption of iron from foods. Tea and coffee, particularly when taken with meals, have similar effects. Vitamin C-containing fruits and vegetables which enhance the uptake of iron include kiwi fruits, oranges, rosehips, potatoes, cauliflower, broccoli, Brussels sprouts and parsley. If iron supplements are prescribed, the mother should be advised to take them with a glass of orange juice and avoid drinking too much tea or coffee.

Thrush

Candida albicans yeast infection is common in pregnancy and if left untreated can complicate delivery and may develop into a chronic condition. Women who have been on the contraceptive pill recently are more susceptible to thrush, as also are those on antibiotics, especially when there are recurrent infections or antibiotics are required long term. Zinc deficiency compromises the immune system, so infection is more likely and any nutritional deficiencies should be corrected, initially with an increase in foods containing the relevant minerals and vitamins, or, if necessary, with supplements. Refined carbohydrates and yeast-containing foods exacerbate the condition as they enable the multiplication of the candida. Therefore refined carbohydrates should be eliminated from the diet, especially white flour, white or brown sugar or any foods which contain these. Similarly, foods which contain yeast should be avoided such as bread, cheese, alcohol, Marmite, frozen or concentrated orange juice, grapes and grape juice, unpeeled fruits, raisins, sultanas and B vitamin supplements (unless they are specifically labelled as yeast-free). Food which is not absolutely fresh should also not be consumed. Foods which contain natural antifungal agents include garlic, other fresh herbs and spices and fresh green leafy vegetables and can be eaten frequently. For vaginal thrush, a whole peeled but uncut clove of garlic can be inserted into the vagina and will act as a local antifungal agent, but daily consumption of garlic in the food is also recommended.

> ### Reflective Activity 19.2
>
> Reflect on some of the women you have cared for during pregnancy and explore how you may have been able to help them to relieve their symptoms by a more efficient management of their diet.
>
> Keep a record during 1 week of your clinical practice to identify the dietary practices of the women you see: how many of them actively seek advice regarding their nutrition?

CONCLUSION

Adequate nutrition during pregnancy and lactation is vital for the continued good health of the mother and the fetus. The midwife is in an invaluable position to educate women and thereby influence family nutrition and health from the very beginning, in line with the Government's agenda for improving the health of the nation. This chapter has discussed the needs of normal women and no mention has been made of the special nutritional requirements of some mothers, for example diabetics. Midwives should have a basic knowledge of the main dietary needs of mothers, and be able to advise women accordingly. However, it is also important that midwives are able to identify those women more at risk of poor nutrition, so that they can be referred to a specialist nutritional therapist or dietician for the most appropriate information. It has not been possible here to provide more than a general introduction to the vast subject of nutrition but suggestions for further reading are made below.

KEY POINTS

- Good nutrition is essential both before and during pregnancy, and the midwife has a vital role to play in educating parents about good family nutrition.
- There is a correlation between poor nutritional status and physiopathological conditions in pregnancy, and nutrition can be used as a therapeutic tool to correct or treat some of these conditions.
- Midwives need a comprehensive understanding of what constitutes a balanced diet in order to advise women in their care accordingly.

REFERENCES

Barker, D.J.P. (1999) Foetal and childhood growth and cardiovascular disease in adult life. *Journal of Paediatrics, Obstetrics and Gynaecology* 25(6): 5–8.

Brooks, S.L., Mitchell, A. & Steffenson, N. (2000) Mothers, infants and DHA. *MCN – American Journal of Maternal and Child Nursing* 25(2): 71–75.

Butte, N.F. (2000) Dieting and exercise in overweight, lactating women. *New England Journal of Medicine* 342(10): 502–503.

Catalano, P.M. (1999) Pregnancy and lactation in relation to a range of acceptable carbohydrate and fat intake. *European Journal of Clinical Nutrition* 53(Suppl. 1): S124–S135.

Czeizei, A.E. (1995) Nutritional supplementation and prevention of congenital abnormalities. *Current Opinion in Obstetrics and Gynecology* 7(2): 88–94.

DHSS (Department of Health and Social Security) (1990) *Vitamin A and pregnancy*. PL/CMO (90) 11/PL/CNO (90) 10. London: DHSS.

Doyle, W., Crawford, M.A., Srivastava, A. *et al.* (1999) Interpregnancy nutrition intervention in mothers of low birthweight babies living in an inner city area: feasibility study. *Journal of Human Nutrition and Dietetics* 12(6): 517–528.

Eskenazi, B., Stapleton, A.L., Kharrazi, M. *et al.* (1999) Associations between maternal decaffeinated and caffeinated coffee consumption and fetal growth and gestational duration. *Epidemiology* 10(3): 242–249.

Fernandes, O. (1998) Moderate to heavy caffeine consumption during pregnancy and relationship to spontaneous abortion and abnormal fetal growth: a meta-analysis. *Reproductive Toxicology* 12: 435–444.

Hachey, D.L. (1994) Benefits and risks of modifying maternal fat intake in pregnancy and lactation. *American Journal of Clinical Nutrition* 59(2): 454–464.

Harding, J. (1999) Nutritional causes of impaired fetal growth and their treatment. *Journal of the Royal Society of Medicine* 92(12): 612–615.

Kolassa, K.M. & Weismiller, D.G. (1997) Nutrition during pregnancy. *American Family Physician* 56(1): 205–212.

Laurence, K.M., James, N., Miller, M.H. *et al.* (1981) Double-blind randomised controlled trial of folate treatment before conception to prevent recurrence of neural tube defects. *British Medical Journal* 282: 1509–1511.

Mathews, F., Yudkin, P. & Smith, R.F. (2000) Nutrient intakes during pregnancy: the influence of smoking status and age. *Journal of Epidemiology and Community Health* 54(1): 17–23.

Matthews, F., Yudkin, P., Neil, A. *et al.* (1999) Influence of maternal nutrition on outcome of pregnancy: prospective cohort study. *British Medical Journal* 319(7206): 339–343.

Reifsnider, E. & Gill, S.L. (2000) Nutrition for the childbearing years. *Journal of Obstetric, Gynecologic and Neonatal Nursing* 29(1): 43–55.

Shaw, G.M., Todoroff, K., Schaffer, D.M. *et al.* (1999) Periconceptional nutrient intake and risk for neural tube defect-affected pregnancies. *Epidemiology* 10(6): 711–716.

Smithells, R.W., Sheppard, S., Schorar, C.J. *et al.* (1981) Apparent prevention of neural tube defects by periconceptual vitamin supplementation. *Archives of Disease in Childhood* 56: 911–918.

Specker, B.L. (1994) Nutritional concerns of lactating women consuming vegetarian diets. *American Journal of Clinical Nutrition* 59(4): 1182–1186.

Sujitor, C.W. (1994) Nutritional assessment of the pregnant woman. *Clinical Obstetrics and Gynecology* 37(3): 501–514.

FURTHER READING

Davies, S. & Stewart, A. (1987) *Nutritional Medicine*. London: Pan.
Although this book is old it remains one of the most comprehensive dictionaries of nutrients, their purpose and the effects of deficiency, together with good application to a range of clinical conditions.

Worthington Roberts, B. & Rodwell Williams, S. (1993) *Nutrition in Pregnancy and Lactation*, 5th edn. St Louis: Mosby.
A comprehensive text with specific application to childbearing women.

20

Complementary Therapies in Childbearing

Denise Tiran

LEARNING OUTCOMES

By the end of this chapter you will be able to:

- provide women in your care with adequate information to make an educated choice regarding the use of complementary therapies for pregnancy and childbearing
- appreciate the need for research-based evidence to evaluate the safety and efficacy of complementary medicine, with particular reference to maternity care
- understand the specific issue of professional accountability in relation to complementary therapies within midwifery in order to determine personal limitations of practice.

INTRODUCTION

Complementary and alternative medicine (CAM) is any form of healthcare which is not part of mainstream care. The British Medical Association referred to this as 'unconventional' medicine (BMA, 1993) but increasingly it is becoming *integrated* into orthodox services (FIM, 1997). General practitioners and primary care groups have been issued with guidance to assist them in referring or recommending patients and clients to practitioners of complementary therapies (DoH, 2000a,b).

Within maternity care, pregnant women demand more choices and wish to remain in control of their bodies during a period when they can feel very vulnerable. Increasingly they request information and advice on natural remedies since they are unable to use pharmacological preparations to deal with the discomforts of pregnancy, labour and the puerperium. Enabling women to use complementary and alternative therapies empowers them in the childbearing process and provides them with additional resources, which are not only therapeutically effective but also often relaxing and calming.

Complementary medicine focuses on the holistic approach to care, which recognizes the interrelationship between body, mind and spirit of each individual. This is in keeping with the holistic approach of midwifery care, although it must be noted that service provision and limitations do not always facilitate fully holistic maternity care. A holistic framework can assist in achieving this (Tiran, 1999).

Women may come into contact with complementary medicine in several ways:

- They may have consulted a complementary practitioner before pregnancy.
- They may have utilized natural remedies themselves at home.
- They may wish to self-administer essential oils, herbal or homeopathic medicines whilst in labour.
- They may wish to be accompanied by an independent therapist in labour.
- They may be recommended to seek complementary treatment for a specific condition during pregnancy.
- They may be fortunate enough to be offered the services of a complementary therapist within the NHS.

PROFESSIONAL ACCOUNTABILITY OF THE MIDWIFE

The professional autonomy of midwives places them in an excellent position to offer women advice about complementary and alternative medicine and, if adequately and appropriately trained, to incorporate complementary therapies into their own practice. Over 34% of midwives have used some form of complementary therapy (NHS Confederation, 1997) and this number is growing all the time.

However, enthusiasm for integrating additional strategies into midwifery practice in order to enhance the care of expectant and labouring women must be balanced by comprehensive contemporary knowledge, which is research based where possible, so that efficacy can be measured and safety can be assured. Student and newly qualified midwives should acknowledge the need to consolidate conventional midwifery knowledge and skills before rushing to develop new techniques (Tiran, 2000c). Similarly, it must be remembered that each complementary therapy is a discreet discipline in its own right, the majority of the commonly used ones having their own body of knowledge, an expanding research base and professional practitioners educated at least to diploma level, and increasingly, to degree and postgraduate levels.

Midwives who have undergone an appropriate training programme are able to utilize aspects of complementary therapies in their work and do not necessarily need to be fully qualified practitioners of the therapy. An example of this might be the use of a limited number of essential oils for women in labour although the midwives using them are not fully trained aromatherapists. The Nursing and Midwifery Council (NMC, formerly the UKCC) supports the incorporation of new skills into practice but also specifies that midwives should not undertake any practices for which they have not previously received training (UKCC, 1998: Rule 40). It is not acceptable for midwives to 'dabble' in complementary medicine, for not only are they jeopardizing the health of women and babies but also risking their own professional careers. If, for example, you were asked by a pregnant woman if she should use raspberry leaf tea to prepare her body for labour, could you explain with the authority of adequate knowledge exactly how and when she should take it? If the answer is 'no', you should refrain from doing so but could refer her to a colleague with the relevant expertise. The development of a specific role as a complementary therapy clinical specialist midwife within each trust or area could assist in this process (Tiran, 1995).

The NMC (UKCC, 1998: Code of Practice, 22,23) identifies that some midwives utilize homeopathic and herbal preparations in their practice but refers them to the parameters of Rule 41. When midwives use complementary therapies in their own work they must be sure that the therapies are appropriate for the mother and any coexisting medical treatment (NMC, 2002). Midwives must recognize that women have the right to administer these substances to themselves, but if they are unfamiliar with the effects, indications, contraindications and side-effects, they should discuss this with the mother(s) and, if necessary, consult an appropriately trained practitioner of the relevant therapy. The NMC acknowledges that some midwives are qualified in other therapies, such as acupuncture, which they may wish to incorporate into their practice, but states that 'it is essential that practice … is based upon sound principles and … all available knowledge and skill' (UKCC, 1998: Code of Practice, 37). Informed consent from the women is vital and midwives must appreciate the limitations of their own professional practice.

The NMC exists to regulate the practice of nurses, midwives and health visitors, in order to protect the public and the statutory roles of its registrants. Therefore the NMC can *only* regulate midwives' use of complementary therapies when it relates to their *midwifery* practice – and it is *not* possible for qualifications in different therapies to be added to an individual's entry in the NMC register. Midwives who are fully qualified in a therapy which they also practise independently of their normal midwifery responsibilities need to separate the two and should not rely on their registration as a midwife to add credibility to their complementary therapy qualification (NMC, 2002).

IMPLEMENTATION OF COMPLEMENTARY THERAPIES IN MIDWIFERY PRACTICE

Availability of a complementary therapy service as part of maternity care may be dependent on local interest and demand from mothers and midwives, support from medical colleagues and relevant expertise. Most often, midwives who have trained in therapies such as aromatherapy or reflexology (sometimes at their own expense and in their own time) incorporate the therapy into their personal practice. Some units have established a more formal service with managers willing to send staff on courses or to appoint midwives with special responsibility for a particular therapy (Burns *et al.*, 1999; Tiran, 1995; Yelland, 1995).

Where obstetricians have seen the benefits to mothers – in increased satisfaction and physical comfort – and to the unit – in reduced costs of inpatient admissions and iatrogenic complications – they do not view the use of such therapies as a threat to their own position and are usually extremely supportive. It should

> **Box 20.1 Summary of issues for midwives incorporating complementary therapies into their practice (adapted from Tiran, 2000a)**
>
> - Adequate and appropriate education and training in the therapy
> - Recognition of professional accountability and service obligations
> - Advocacy for and rights of the mothers
> - Communication and collaboration with all colleagues
> - Maternal consent; comprehensive and contemporaneous record-keeping
> - Policies and protocols
> - Evaluation and audit of complementary therapy services and treatments
> - Research-based practice where possible

be emphasized, however, that it is *not* necessary to obtain consultant permission to utilize aspects of complementary therapy to deal with physiological symptoms of pregnancy or the puerperium, or in helping women to cope with pain in labour, as these are within the normal remit of responsibilities of the midwife. On the other hand, it *is* important to communicate adequately with all colleagues to avoid antagonism and conflict.

If midwives wish to consider links with independent complementary therapists who may provide care for women during the childbearing period, the law states that *only* midwives or doctors or those in training are permitted to provide sole care for women except in an emergency; therefore, any therapies offered to women must be *complementary* rather than *alternative* to conventional care.

The issues for midwives incorporating complementary therapies into their practice are summarized in Box 20.1.

Policies and protocols

It is vital that midwives and their managers and supervisors develop local policies or protocols regarding the use of complementary therapies in order to protect both clients and professionals. These may be in the form of 'standing orders' for limited specific elements, or lists of midwives named as adequately trained to use a whole or part of a therapy, or guidelines to assist midwives when caring for women who wish to utilize aspects of complementary therapy on their own account. It is not appropriate, however, for 'blanket' policies to be developed within a trust, for there will be specific

differences between clinical specialities which need to be identified. Neither is it acceptable for local trust policies to specify which complementary therapy training courses should have been undertaken by its staff in order for them to be allowed to use a therapy in their practice, as there is a vast range of standards with, in some therapies, no national minimum criteria for initial training. See also Tiran (2000a,b).

Professional indemnity insurance

If a midwife is appropriately trained and experienced in aspects of complementary therapy and has the permission of her employing authority to incorporate this into her practice, the Royal College of Midwives' and the Royal College of Nursing's personal professional indemnity insurance schemes are suitable cover. The vicarious liability cover of the employing authority will be invalidated unless the midwife has gained permission of the relevant authorities to use complementary therapies in her work. If the midwife also chooses to practise independently as a therapist, she should arrange additional insurance cover through one of the complementary therapy organizations.

> **Reflective Activity 20.1**
>
> Brainstorm with a colleague to find out how many different complementary therapies you can name.
> Conduct a survey amongst your midwifery and medical colleagues to determine their views and attitudes regarding complementary therapies.

THE MOST COMMONLY USED COMPLEMENTARY THERAPIES

There are well in excess of 200 complementary therapies in existence, all of which focus on the holistic concept of integration between body, mind and spirit. The British Medical Association (BMA, 1993) identified 10 therapies which have become almost mainstream within healthcare; the Foundation for Integrated Medicine (FIM, 1997) added a further four therapies to the list. Some therapies may be more appropriate for certain conditions than others and some therapists will combine the use of several therapies to achieve optimum care for the client. Care is based on involvement of clients in their own care and may involve lifestyle changes, dietary adaptations or other elements of self-care. Often there is a worsening of the condition before the person begins to feel better, for all complementary therapies work by triggering the body's innate self-healing capacity, which usually provokes a healing crisis as the body 'kick starts' itself into improving.

The following are the most commonly used complementary therapies:

- Osteopathy
- Chiropractic
- Homeopathy
- Medical herbalism
- Acupuncture
- Aromatherapy
- Reflexology
- Massage
- Shiatsu
- Hypnotherapy
- Yoga
- Alexander technique
- Nutritional therapies
- Relaxation therapies.

Osteopathy and chiropractic

These are related therapies in which manipulation of the musculoskeletal system helps to realign the body which is directly or indirectly attached to the spine. Osteopathy aims to restore and maintain balance within the body, particularly in the relationships between the neural, muscular and skeletal systems and by examining and maintaining the biomechanical functioning of the body. Osteopathy became one of the professions supplementary to medicine with the passing of the Osteopaths Act in 1993 and all practitioners are now statutorily regulated by the General Osteopathic Council. Osteopathy is particularly effective for the treatment of back pain in pregnancy but can be useful for other problems, for example heartburn or carpal tunnel syndrome.

An offshoot of osteopathy is craniosacral therapy or cranial osteopathy, which is a very gentle form of treatment involving minute manipulations of the head (cranium) and sacrum and the cerebrospinal fluid which flows between. Within maternity care it has become notable for its value in calming fractious babies delivered by forceps or those suffering from colic.

Chiropractic is similarly concerned with the relationship of the nervous system to the mechanical structure of the body and places emphasis on spinal joints as well as related muscles and ligaments. The therapy is also statutorily regulated since the Chiropractors Act was passed in 1994 and practitioners will be governed by the General Chiropractic Council. It is the largest system of healthcare in the world after conventional medicine and dentistry, with approximately 68 000 chiropractors practising throughout the world (Tellefsen, 2000). Like osteopathy, chiropractic is most appropriate for musculoskeletal conditions of pregnancy, especially symphysis pubis diastasis and sacroiliac joint pain.

Both osteopathy and chiropractic are safe throughout pregnancy, although some practitioners decline to treat women at around 16 weeks' gestation when there is a surge of relaxin and a rebalancing of other hormones.

Homeopathy

Homeopathy involves the use of minute doses of substances which, if given in their full dose, would actually cause the problems they are attempting to rectify. Although many of the preparations are in the form of tablets and oral granules, tinctures and liquids, it is not a system of medicine which works in the same way as pharmaceutical preparations, but is in fact part of the group of therapies known as vibrational or energy medicine. Remedies are totally individually prescribed and take into account not only the *exact* symptom picture, but also the personality of the person and the factors which make the symptoms better or worse. Despite using minute doses, however, it is a very powerful system of care and, although it offers a gentle and safe means of treating women during pregnancy and childbirth, it should not be considered to be totally harmless. Like any other form of complementary medicine, if homeopathy has the power to act therapeutically, it can, in the wrong hands, cause possible problems, side-effects or complications.

Practitioners of homeopathy are regulated either by the Faculty of Homeopathy at the Royal London Homeopathic Hospital (doctors, dentists and veterinary surgeons) or by the Society of Homeopaths (lay practitioners such as nurses, midwives and others). Homeopathy is the only therapy to have been available on the National Health Service since its inception and there remain five homeopathic hospitals in Britain.

If a woman wishes to treat herself with homeopathic substances she should ensure that, as nearly as possible, the most appropriate remedy has been selected. If the correct remedy has been selected there will be a change in the symptom picture, for better or worse, within 3 days; if no change occurs thereafter, it is probable that the wrong remedy has been used. Homeopathic tablets should always be taken when the mouth is clean from all food, drink, tobacco and toothpaste and should be handled as little as possible and only by the person who is to take them. The remedies should be stored away from strong-smelling substances, including essential oils which can act as antidotes, as also can others such as coffee and peppermint toothpaste. Proof that homeopathy is effective is difficult to demonstrate in randomized controlled trials because of the individual nature of prescribing, but a review of several studies was undertaken by Kleijnen *et al.* (1991). Many women use homeopathic arnica tablets for bruising after delivery and find it effective in reducing perineal discomfort, although a trial comparing arnica with placebo for post-hysterectomy patients did not support the claims for its use (Hart *et al.*, 1997).

A related therapy, based on the principles of using the minute dose, is Bach flower remedies, a range of liquid preparations which work on the concept of vibrational medicine to treat the emotional symptoms associated with disease and disorder. Rescue Remedy is perhaps the best known of these, for stress, panic and nervous tension, and could be useful for women in the transition stage of labour or for those who are frightened of having blood taken in the antenatal clinic.

Medical herbalism

This can be likened to the original pharmaceutical industry, for it involves the medicinal use of plants and plant substances. Various constituents of the plants are known to have a range of therapeutic effects but conversely can also be harmful if used inappropriately. Herbal remedies are taken in the form of tablets, tinctures, decoctions, teas and used fresh as whole herbs in cooking. The practitioner will also incorporate dietary adaptations into care. There are several herbal preparations which are contraindicated during pregnancy as they are known or thought to be abortifacient. However, remedies such as camomile tea are safe and versatile; its sedative, antispasmodic and anti-inflammatory chemicals make it a useful solution for insomnia, non-infective 'sticky' eyes in the neonate, gastrointestinal problems and pain relief in labour.

The majority of medical herbalists are registered with the National Institute of Medical Herbalists. There continues to be debate about the safety and efficacy of herbal remedies since the European Union has questioned whether those herbal products currently classified as foods should be considered as medicines, with the legal, financial and social implications of demonstrating 'scientifically' that they are safe as well as effective.

> ### Reflective Activity 20.2
>
> Keep a record of how often you are asked for information about raspberry leaf tea, arnica for bruising, or the safety of aromatherapy oils in pregnancy and labour.

Acupuncture/acupressure/shiatsu

Acupuncture is a part of traditional Chinese medicine in which care is based upon the principle that the body has energy lines, called meridians, running through it from top to toe, each of which passes through a major organ from which it takes its name. There are 365 meridians in the body, and along each there are various focal points where energy is concentrated – these are the acupuncture points into which acupuncture needles can be inserted, or to which thumb pressure can be applied (acupressure). When the body, mind and spirit are all in good health the energy in the meridians is able to flow without interruption, but disorders or disease can cause either blockages (stagnation) or over-stimulation of the energy levels, and treatment involves correction and rebalancing of the energy levels.

Other techniques are used within traditional Chinese medicine, including cupping (placing special cups over acupuncture points to draw out heat), moxibustion (the use of dried moxa sticks as a heat source over specific acupuncture points) and Chinese herbs. Auricular acupuncture is another form in which the ear has a complete set of acupuncture points. Within maternity care, acupuncture is extremely effective in treating a range of physiological disorders of pregnancy, labour and the puerperium and moxibustion has been used in several centres to turn breech presentation to cephalic.

Most practitioners in Britain are regulated by the British Acupuncture Council.

Shiatsu is the Japanese form of acupressure but it has evolved further and incorporates the use of simple pressure and holding techniques combined with gentle stretching. Touch is used as a means of adjusting the internal energies of the body, both in treating and preventing energy imbalances.

Aromatherapy

This involves the use of highly concentrated essential oils extracted from plants that are used, similarly to herbal medicine, for their chemical constituents, which have a variety of therapeutic purposes. The term 'aromatherapy' is a misnomer, for although the oils have various aromas, which can affect mood, the power of aromatherapy extends beyond simply the smell of the oils. Administration is usually in a carrier oil and given in the form of massage, in the bath, in compresses, suppositories, pessaries, creams, lotions or inhalations. Oral use is not encouraged in Britain as it is not possible to ascertain the doses, rate of absorption or effects on the gastrointestinal tract, although medically qualified aromatherapists in France use them as alternatives to medicines and administer them by mouth. With very few exceptions, essential oils should not be applied to the skin neat because some of the chemical constituents can precipitate skin reactions. Many essential oils are contraindicated during pregnancy, labour and breastfeeding and most should not be administered to neonates. Some essential oils are known to raise the blood pressure, whilst others lower it; some potentiate the action of certain drugs or alcohol; all have a range of anti-infective properties. Many oils are relaxing and some contain chemicals which are analgesic. Dosages should be kept as low as possible, preferably to below 2%. For a more detailed exploration of the research related to aromatherapy and its application to maternity care, see Tiran (2000b).

The main regulatory body is the Aromatherapy Organisations Council (AOC) to which most other groups and colleges belong.

Reflexology

This is based on the principle that the feet (and hands) represent a map of the rest of the body so that by working on specific areas of the feet, other parts of the body can be treated. It is not fully understood how reflexology works although it is thought to be related to acupuncture meridians. It is especially beneficial for stress-induced conditions and for disorders which involve structural 'blockages', such as constipation. Reflexology is not simply foot massage, and indeed, vigorous massage of the heels should be avoided during early pregnancy as this is the part of the foot which corresponds to the pelvic region. There is no evidence to suggest that reflexology will trigger miscarriage, which is a reaction of the body to a non-viable conceptus, but great caution should be used in the first trimester. Later in pregnancy, reflexology is effective for the relief of many of the physiological conditions of pregnancy as well as labour and the postnatal period (Tiran, 1996, 2000a,b).

Practitioners are usually registered with one of several bodies, all of which, at the time of writing, are discussing a combined organization similar to the Aromatherapy Organisations Council.

Massage

Massage, or healing touch, is already used spontaneously by many midwives in the delivery suite. Massage is the applied use of touch and is a means of relieving some of the effects of stress, aiding relaxation, reducing blood pressure and inducing sleep. Touch impulses reach the brain more quickly than pain impulses; therefore massage is effective in alleviating some of the discomfort of labour. Massage can also work to stimulate areas of the body, including excretory processes and the circulation.

There are few contraindications to the use of massage in pregnancy although care should be taken in the first trimester with sacral and suprapubic massage, and certain areas may precipitate preterm labour if acu pressure or reflex points are overstimulated. Massage should not be applied directly over varicosed areas to avoid the risk of dislodging clots into the bloodstream, but can be substituted by simple stroking over the skin.

Massage of the neonate has become increasingly popular and has been found to be of particular benefit for preterm babies (Acolet et al., 1993; Adamson Macedo and Attree, 1994; Adamson Macedo et al., 1997).

Hypnotherapy

This is the applied, medical use of a state of deep physical relaxation with an alert mind in order to access the subconscious mind and is often likened to daydreaming. It can be used to cause a change in behaviour in the client, such as habitual and addictive behaviours, and has been used to good effect to alter women's perceptions of labour pain.

Yoga

Yoga involves learning a series of postures and positions, often in conjunction with meditation, for relaxation and for the relief of various symptoms. For women who practise yoga during pregnancy, the positions encourage flexibility, suppleness and strength and are a valuable method of preparing for labour. Various breathing techniques are also used which can facilitate breath control during labour.

Alexander technique

An Australian actor, Frederick Alexander, devised the technique as a means of relieving the constant throat problems which adversely affected his ability to perform. He recognized that changes in his posture could reduce the physical tensions which accompanied his psychological nervousness, and went on to adapt the technique for other actors. The Alexander technique is more than a therapy, although it is used therapeutically, but actually becomes a way of life for many people. Teachers of the technique hold classes or one-to-one sessions to teach clients how they can alleviate problems such as backache, headaches, constipation and other conditions by adjusting the ways in which the body is held. It depends on a consciousness of oneself in order to 'unlearn' postures which have become constant through the years and to relearn more positive ones.

Nutritional therapy

Although there are many different types of nutritional therapies they all focus on the ways in which our nutritional status is affected not only by the quantity and quality of the food but also the absorption, metabolism, utilization and excretion of the nutrients. Simple dietary suggestions can be made to help pregnant women overcome some of the physiological discomforts of pregnancy, such as reducing tea intake for constipation or taking vitamin B$_6$ and zinc supplements if suffering from nausea and vomiting, especially if previously on the contraceptive pill (Davies and Stewart, 1987).

Relaxation therapies

This is a composite term which includes general physical exercises, breathing techniques and specific therapies such as Tai Chi and Qi Gong, which are elements of Chinese martial arts that have been formulated to appeal to a wider audience for relief of stress, both physical and mental. These latter therapies improve stamina and flexibility and assist in the promotion of general health and well-being.

Reflective Activity 20.3

Ask 10 women in your care what they understand by the term 'complementary therapies' and find out whether or not they have used any therapies or natural remedies.

THE USE OF COMPLEMENTARY THERAPIES DURING PREGNANCY

This section of the chapter aims to give a few examples of the ways in which complementary therapies may be

of use for women with physiological symptoms of pregnancy. It is not exhaustive and midwives should not normally attempt to utilize the suggestions in practice until they have received additional education to enable them to understand more fully the theories behind the particular therapies they wish to use. Conventional midwifery advice such as dietary changes or postural advice has largely been omitted from this chapter, as they can be found in Chapters 19 and 23, but would of course be incorporated into the full care provided, alongside the relevant therapy (see also Tiran and Mack, 2000).

Nausea and vomiting

One of the simplest techniques is to use a strategy from traditional Chinese medicine in which wrist bands or minute magnets are placed over the relevant acupuncture point, the Pericardium 6 (P6) on the inner wrist, approximately where the buckle of a watch strap might rest. It is important to use the mother's own fingers to measure three finger breadths up from the crease between hand and wrist, and to position the magnet or button (on the inside of the wristband) between the two tendons (see Fig. 20.1). Acupuncture, acupressure and shiatsu have been well researched as a means of treating nausea and vomiting, in pregnancy, postoperatively and following chemo- or radiotherapy (Barsoum *et al.*, 1990; Bayreuther *et al.*, 1994; Belluomini *et al.*, 1994; de Aloysio and Penacchioni, 1992; Dundee *et al.*, 1988; O'Brien *et al.*, 1996).

Nutritional therapists suggest excessive nausea and vomiting may be due to a deficiency of vitamin B$_6$ and zinc, and herbalists recommend the use of ginger capsules or tea made from fresh grated infused ginger but *not* ginger biscuits or beer as the sugar content may itself exacerbate the symptoms. Chamomile tea is also

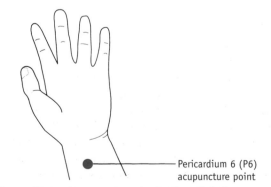

Pericardium 6 (P6) acupuncture point

Figure 20.1   Acupressure point P6 for relief of nausea and vomiting. The point is 2–3 finger widths below the wrist crease on the inner aspect of the arm.

worth trying and is a simple suggestion which mid-wives can make to women. Essential oils of peppermint or spearmint can be inhaled on a cotton wool ball (good also for nausea in labour) or ginger and lime can be tried, but care should be taken as the aromas themselves can make the nausea worse.

A homeopath would need to determine the exact nature of the symptoms but might prescribe nux vomica or sepia. Osteopathy or chiropractic can be extremely effective in reducing structural tensions in the body, commonly in the cervical vertebrae, which may be contributing to the nausea. Personal experience of this author has also found that reflexology is beneficial by working on the foot zones for the cervical vertebrae, as there appears to be a correlation between women with severe nausea and vomiting and a history of whiplash injury or other neck or back problem (Tiran, 2002).

Heartburn

In the absence of any indication for an alternative homeopathic remedy, pulsatilla can be tried for up to 3 days – it seems to be especially effective for women who also have haemorrhoids and/or varicose veins, either in the legs or the vulva. Other homeopathic remedies include capsicum, lycopodium or phosphorous. A shiatsu technique which the mother can try for herself is shown in Figure 20.2. Garlic capsules may reduce the severity of heartburn, and herbal remedies such as slippery elm tablets or dandelion tea can help (Stapleton and Tiran, 2000). Osteopathy or chiropractic are also effective by relaxing the diaphragm and realigning the ribcage and spine. Reflexology can temporarily relieve symptoms but usually requires repeated treatments to keep the problem under control.

Constipation

Simple natural strategies for helping women to reduce the effects of constipation in pregnancy include nutritional elements such as limiting the intake of tea, for the tannin reduces peristalsis, increasing the use of foods such as celery and artichokes, and adding linseeds or flax seeds to meals (Stapleton and Tiran, 2000).

Firm abdominal massage in a clockwise direction will encourage peristalsis (see Fig. 20.3), as will clockwise massage of the arches of the feet, utilizing a technique from reflexology. Essential oils such as grapefruit, mandarin, bergamot, lime and lemon can be applied in a carrier oil to assist the massage.

Acupuncture to the relevant points or acupressure/shiatsu may help (see Fig. 20.4); osteopathy and chiropractic can also be effective. Certain yoga positions can be learnt to prevent or treat the problem.

Haemorrhoids

Essential oil of cypress with its astringent properties can be added to the bath or bidet, or made into a compress as appropriate. Homeopathic pulsatilla 30C is the most versatile remedy and may be effective when there

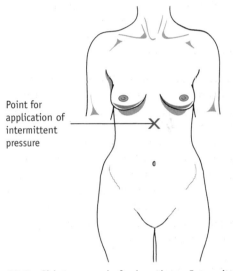

Point for application of intermittent pressure

Figure 20.2 Shiatsu remedy for heartburn. Intermittent pressure is applied at a point four fingers above the umbilicus.

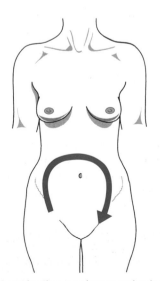

Figure 20.3 Constipation can be treated using abdominal massage in a clockwise direction.

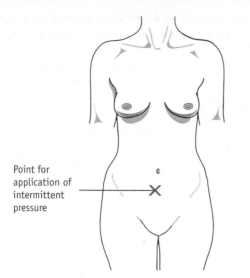

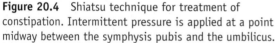

Point for application of intermittent pressure

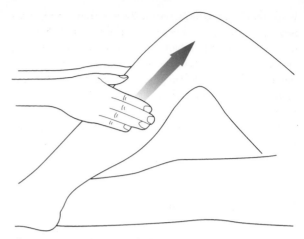

Figure 20.5 Direction of bimanual leg massage for the reduction of ankle oedema.

Figure 20.4 Shiatsu technique for treatment of constipation. Intermittent pressure is applied at a point midway between the symphysis pubis and the umbilicus.

is no reason to use an alternative (Geraghty, 1997). When haemorrhoids and constipation exist together, sepia may be a more appropriate remedy, and if the piles itch and accompanying constipation causes backache, nux vomica should be tried. One tablet three times daily should cause a change in the symptoms. Reflexology can treat the acute symptoms in the short term. Acupuncture or acupressure can also help. Applying hamamelis water directly to the external haemorrhoids causes a constriction of the veins and may be a temporary relief.

Oedema

Ankle and leg oedema respond well to bimanual massage moving upwards from ankle to knee, which may be enhanced by adding one drop of lemon essential oil and one drop of geranium to the carrier oil (see Fig. 20.5). It is also possible for the mother to learn some yoga poses which can increase circulation and prevent or reduce the severity of oedema. One of the most effective remedies for gestational and postnatal oedema is to apply dark green cabbage leaves (or rhubarb or olive) over the affected area. The leaves should be wiped clean but not allowed to get wet, then wrapped around the legs; excess fluid is drawn out into the leaves, which should be replaced with new ones when they become wet.

Backache, sciatica and associated discomforts

Osteopathy or chiropractic is by far the most effective therapy for backache especially when there have been

back problems prior to pregnancy. Symphysis pubis diastasis responds particularly well, as does sacroiliac joint pain (Conway, 2000; Daly *et al.*, 1991; Fallon, 1993; Hansen *et al.*, 1996; McMullen, 1995; Petersen *et al.*, 1994; Schauberger *et al.*, 1996; Stern *et al.*, 1993; Tellefsen, 2000). Reflexology can ease the symptoms but will not deal with the cause. Aromatherapy and massage should be used with care; sacral massage may not always be appropriate as there are several acupuncture points in the area which should not be stimulated during pregnancy, as they may initiate labour contractions. Alexander technique offers a means of re-educating the woman regarding her posture, but is usually a long-term commitment.

Headache

Headache in the first trimester of pregnancy is often a result of dilatation of the cerebral blood vessels under the influence of progesterone, and is very common. It may be associated with a history of neck or upper back problems prior to pregnancy or be compounded by sinus congestion or progress to a migraine. Headaches may be eased by a variety of massage techniques which often incorporate aspects of shiatsu. Simple application of one drop of neat lavender essential oil to the temples can be effective on isolated occasions, although there remains some controversy about the safety of lavender in early pregnancy (Tiran, 2000b). For a more diversified ache, firm scalp massage in a 'hairwashing' action can bring relief. This massage does not require the application of any oils and can be done by the woman herself or by a partner. Pressure of two fingers directly under the occiput will rebalance the meridians as there is an acupressure point there. Firm massage of the big toes, particularly if they feel painful to touch, will act on the reflex zone for the head and may be effective. More chronic headache for which no pathological cause has been found will benefit from osteopathy. Alternatively, the postural realignment of the Alexander technique may be of help.

Nutrition therapists suggest the elimination of stimulants such as tea, coffee, cola and chocolate from the diet as well as avoiding the food additives in the E200–E274 range.

Stress, anxiety and panic

Most pregnant women experience periods of anxiety, worry and fear about their impending labours and the advent of parenthood, and this will be worse if there have been complications in either this or a previous pregnancy. Many complementary therapies are relaxing and can be administered regularly throughout pregnancy, although women should be advised to consult a registered practitioner who is familiar with treating expectant mothers. Reflexology, massage, shiatsu, and aromatherapy are notably good or the mother may wish to attend yoga or Tai Chi classes, which will produce the additional benefit of relieving some of the physical discomforts of pregnancy as well as being relaxing.

Panic attacks are also common, although there appears to be no physiological reason why this should be so. The Bach flower remedy Rescue Remedy can be helpful and is a natural remedy which the woman can purchase from chemists or health stores. She should take four drops neat on her tongue as required, or, if the problem is persistent, Rescue Remedy can be taken on a regular basis, three to four times daily. This is also a valuable substance for the woman who is frightened of having blood taken in the antenatal clinic or when she is in labour for episodes of panic and for transition from first to second stage. As this is a homeopathic remedy, the dose of active ingredients is negligible and is not known to be harmful to the mother or fetus. It is, however, preserved in brandy and this needs to be explained to the mother in case she objects to alcohol. It is also useful prior to caesarean section, for although the remedy is taken by mouth, four drops makes little difference to her 'nil by mouth' status.

Breech presentation

Persistent breech presentation after 34 weeks' gestation can be corrected in almost 70% of cases using a technique from traditional Chinese medicine called moxibustion. This involves the application of a moxa stick containing dried mugwort, a herb, to the Bladder 67 acupuncture point at the base of the little toenails. The moxa sticks (two) are lit at one end and the flames are quenched but the tips will continue to smoke. They are then used as a heat source twice a day for 15 minutes for a maximum of 5 days. The treatment has been shown to stimulate myometrial sensitivity and contractility through adrenocortical stimulation and the effects on placental lactogens and prostaglandin levels which encourages fetal movement so that the fetus will, in most cases, turn itself (Cooperative Research Group of Moxibustion Version, 1984). A randomized trial in Italy by Cardini *et al.* (1991) showed promising results, and their follow-up study in China (Cardini and Weixin, 1998) compared three groups of women with breech presentation: a control group who received no treatment, a moxa group, and a third group who had external cephalic version. Despite the number of spontaneous resolutions of the breech in all three groups, the number of term cephalic vaginal deliveries was greatest in the moxa group. Budd (2000) discusses the technique further. Several maternity units in Britain now offer this treatment, which offers a cost-effective and safer alternative to caesarean section, and the technique could be easily learnt by experienced midwives as an adjunct to their normal practice.

Integration of complementary therapies in the antenatal clinic

This author, a practising midwife, runs a complementary therapy antenatal clinic in southeast London. Although women are usually referred for a specific reason, their care may extend to the management of a range of other physiological symptoms which arise during the course of treatment.

For example, Maddie was referred for severe constipation at 24 weeks of pregnancy. This was treated with a combination of reflexology with the addition of essential oils, dietary and herbal advice. During the course of three treatments given at weekly intervals, Maddie revealed that she was also suffering from haemorrhoids and heartburn, for which the midwife suggested a homeopathic remedy, which was effective.

Another expectant mother, Ann, was referred by the caseload midwife at 38 weeks' gestation for correction of a breech presentation, and was shown how to carry out moxibustion at home. This was effective within 3 days and Ann was delighted to be able to look forward to a normal birth. However, she returned at

41 weeks because she had still not started labour and was keen to avoid a medical induction. The complementary therapy midwife performed reflexology to the relevant points for the uterus and pituitary gland, acupressure to points on the toes, shoulders, hands and sacrum and gave Ann a blend of essential oils to take home to put in her bath. She also suggested a herbal remedy which tones up the uterus. Ann went into labour the following day and achieved a normal delivery.

Diana came for massage and reflexology relaxation therapy in an attempt to reduce her blood pressure at 33 weeks. Although she had been seen by her community midwife the previous day, she had denied that she was experiencing visual disturbances because she did not want to leave her three other children if she was admitted to hospital. However, during the reflexology, the complementary therapy midwife identified – from Diana's feet – that there was a change in her eyes. When she questioned her, Diana burst into tears and agreed that she was seeing 'spots in front of her eyes'. Her blood pressure was taken and the diastolic pressure was found to be 100 mmHg; she was taken to the delivery suite, where labour was induced and she delivered a small preterm infant 4 hours later.

These examples demonstrate the use of several complementary therapies in combination so that the most appropriate strategy can be implemented to deal with each individual condition. In addition, they highlight the value of the complementary practitioner also being a midwife, when dual knowledge can be used to optimum benefit of the mothers.

THE USE OF COMPLEMENTARY THERAPIES DURING LABOUR

Onset of labour

It is theoretically possible to encourage the onset of labour using a variety of complementary methods. However, midwives should take careful note that it is not within the remit of their role as practitioners of normal midwifery to interfere with natural physiological processes unless they have been properly taught to do so and have discussed the situation with the relevant medical staff. Many midwives have long advocated sexual activity as an aid to ripening the cervix, in the belief that prostaglandins in semen, local cervical stimulation and uterine contraction from orgasm will initiate labour. Nipple stimulation can also be used, both as a way of cervical ripening from about the 37th week (although only one breast should be massaged at a time

to avoid overstimulation) and to increase the length, strength and frequency of contractions in labour. This obviously increases pituitary output of oxytocin and can be very useful during the transition phase at the end of the first stage of labour, when contractions may slow down, or if there is delay in separation of the placenta during the third stage.

Phytotherapists (medical herbalists) recommend taking raspberry leaf tea. This has a toning effect on the uterus and can be drunk during the third trimester of pregnancy, as well as during labour to assist with contractions, and postnatally to aid involution of the uterus. Women who request advice about it in the antenatal clinic should be told to start after 28 weeks with one cup daily and increase gradually to three cups daily; tablets are also available but are not as effective as the dried raspberry leaf.

Homeopaths also have many remedies at their disposal, but as with any other situation the remedy must be appropriate for the individual. For example caulophyllum (blue cohosh), which stimulates uterine muscle, can be useful if the cervix is slow to dilate, contractions are weak or the mother is exhausted. Care should be taken with this remedy, however, for if it is inappropriately administered it may be so powerful that labour is short and violent, or it may work in reverse and, instead of accelerating labour, it could cause it to become protracted.

Aromatherapists may choose to massage the suprapubic and sacral areas with a blend of jasmine and lavender for a few days before labour as this will aid in strengthening the uterus, and its use can be continued into labour. Stimulation (by either acupuncture or acupressure) of the Bladder 67 point at the base of the little toenail can, in addition to turning a breech presentation to cephalic, enhance and coordinate uterine action during labour.

Reflexology can also be effective by stimulating the parts of the feet which relate to the pituitary gland and the uterus. Shiatsu to the Gall Bladder 21 point on the shoulders, the Large Intestine 4 point on the webbing between thumb and forefinger and the spread of acupuncture points around the sacral area can also encourage the onset of labour. It goes without saying, therefore, that many of these techniques are contraindicated during pregnancy as they could possibly trigger preterm contractions.

Pain and discomfort in labour

The relief of pain and discomfort in labour is one of the main areas of midwifery in which alternative treatments can truly act as a complement to any other conventional care, and is also an area in which midwives may feel deficient in what they have to offer women. The range of analgesia is limited in conventional terms, and many women find the available analgesics ineffective, unpleasant or possessing undesirable side-effects.

Mothers may wish to be accompanied in labour by an independent complementary therapist, and midwifery management and medical attendants should facilitate this. It may require a change in attitude for many doctors and midwives to accept that a different professional can be of help. Our aim in caring for childbearing women should be to relinquish control, and to provide choices and optimum care for each individual woman. Those midwives who feel unable to cope with a situation in which there is a complementary therapist in attendance should defer to another midwife to care for that mother. However, it is also incumbent upon us to increase our awareness and understanding of the various therapies in order to provide good-quality care and to assist those women who wish to administer natural remedies to themselves during labour.

Appropriately trained midwives may use essential oils of clary sage, lavender and jasmine, which not only strengthen the uterus but also alleviate pain, discomfort and anxiety. These can be massaged into the abdomen, put into a warm bath, used as a room spray or added to a cotton wool ball or piece of gauze for the mother to inhale. The concentration of jasmine should not be too high, however, as some women find its strong aroma rather cloying. Other oils that can be useful in relaxing both mother and father include rose, orange and geranium, and the oils selected should depend on the mother's preference. It is worth noting, however, that all essential oils are inhaled by everyone present in the room. It may be necessary to consider the effects that soporific oils can have on midwives who are required to make professional judgements, sometimes in an emergency, and, in the community, to drive cars.

A trial at the John Radcliffe Hospital in Oxford was one of the largest clinical aromatherapy trials ever undertaken and certainly the most significant study in relation to maternity complementary therapies. The researchers investigated the use of a range of essential oils for in excess of 8000 women over a period of 9 years and demonstrated their effectiveness in relieving pain, discomfort, anxiety and other symptoms in labour. Less than 1% of side-effects were reported, all were minor and none affected the neonates (Burns et al., 1999).

Simple massage of the abdomen without essential oils can also be effective in reducing the mother's perception of pain (see Massage, Ch. 27). Reflex zone therapy is relaxing and will increase uterine efficiency (Feder et al., 1993). Alternatively, either the midwife or the father could perform simple foot massage without reflexology which will redirect the mother's attention away from her contractions. It will also warm the mother's feet, for many women in labour literally have cold feet, and if done by the father, this will make him feel useful.

Hypnotherapy can be taught to the mother during pregnancy and self-induced during labour, or she may choose to have her hypnotherapist with her. Trials have shown that hypnotherapy can be particularly valuable in labour, without the danger of side-effects (Jenkins and Pritchard, 1993; Mairs, 1995).

Acupuncture has also been well documented for its use in labour in western cultures, although it is interesting to note that it is not used in China as a means of relieving pain in labour because contractions produce physiological rather than pathological discomfort (Budd, 2000).

A simple shiatsu technique to ease the pain of labour contractions, or of dysmenorrhoea, can be performed by midwives or taught to partners. For example: standing or kneeling behind the mother, the thumbs are pressed into the 'dimples' visible on either side of the spine, starting at the coccyx and working up intermittently to the lumbosacral area (i.e. from the coccyx to the waist). This should be done with a rocking motion with the fingers resting over the areas of the sacroiliac joints, and performed throughout each contraction (for dysmenorrhoea the procedure is carried out for about 5–10 minutes until relief is obtained, and repeated as necessary) (Fig. 20.6).

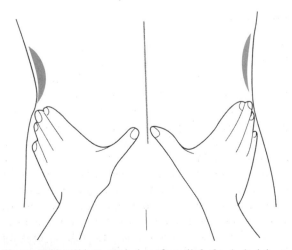

Figure 20.6 Shiatsu technique for relief of pain in labour.

Again, there are many homeopathic remedies which can be of use, but because of the changing nature of the process of parturition it is vital to have knowledge and experience of using them.

As mentioned previously, the Bach flower remedy Rescue Remedy is excellent for relieving panic, anxiety and hysteria and lends itself very well to use in labour, particularly during transition from the first to second stage. Many mothers have their own bottle but midwives may wish to consider stocking it for professional use. Although it is used by some midwives, further trials need to be carried out and published in accepted journals to promote more widespread use. Other Bach flower remedies can also be useful in labour (Mantle, 2000).

There are many herbal substances which are suitable for women in labour, including squaw vine and birth root, but qualified assistance is required to select the most appropriate one. However, the ubiquitous raspberry leaf tea is safe and can be drunk throughout labour, either hot or iced, to strengthen contractions and relieve the intensity of pain.

Other natural means of relieving pain and discomfort in labour include the use of warm water for bathing during the first stage (some mothers wish to remain in the water for the delivery) (Garland, 2000) and a range of relaxation techniques including visualization, meditation, music, yoga postures and breathing exercises. The midwife should consider the whole range at her disposal in order to offer a comprehensive choice to women. However, at present it is unlikely that any one midwife or maternity service will be able to provide the entire selection, as many depend on having appropriately trained practitioners within the area.

It would be preferable for each maternity services manager to identify the skills and knowledge available amongst the staff and to build on them in order to expand the facilities for the local clientele, focusing on a limited number of therapies. The unit to which this author is attached maintains a register of those midwives qualified in massage, aromatherapy and reflex zone therapy/reflexology and, within the restrictions laid down in the unit policy, allows those midwives to apply their skills to their normal midwifery practice.

There are other situations that occur during labour that can be adequately treated with various complementary therapies. Reflexology can be used to separate a retained placenta, saving time and money by avoiding the need for removal of placenta under anaesthetic. (This is effective in cases where the placenta has not yet separated, by stimulating uterine contraction, but will not deal with a morbidly adherent placenta.) Acupuncture can also be effective in promoting placental separation (Budd, 2000) as can homeopathic remedies such as pulsatilla (Geraghty, 1997), while phytotherapists might use myrrh, feverfew or raspberry leaf. Nipple stimulation can be advised and discreetly practised to increase the pituitary output of oxytocin, or of course the baby could be put to the breast. Jasmine essential oil has been found to be of use when massaged into the abdomen, and could be combined with massage over the area of the fundus to stimulate the uterus to contract (Tiran, 2000b).

THE USE OF COMPLEMENTARY THERAPIES IN THE POSTNATAL PERIOD

Much of our care in the puerperium revolves around helping the mother to return to her non-pregnant state both physically and mentally, as well as facilitating the establishment of a suitable feeding method for the baby. Complementary therapies have much to offer the mother at this time, especially for enhancing her confidence and self-esteem.

Postnatal mood changes

Those women who are susceptible to postnatal 'blues' or depression, because of either a previous personal or a family history, may benefit from the use of essential oils of jasmine, with its antidepressant properties, and rose, which has a particular affinity for the reproductive tract and can help to cleanse, tone and purify the uterus. Both of these oils are extremely expensive but only a few drops would be used and the effects are profound in some cases. The oils could be massaged into the back, abdomen and legs, added to bath water or sprayed around the room. Jasmine tea will also have some effect.

Agnus-castus or squaw vine may be advocated by herbalists for depression, and cups of camomile tea will calm the mother, help her to sleep and also act as a diuretic to cleanse the urinary tract (Stapleton and Tiran, 2000). The elimination of all sugars from the diet will enable the hormones to rebalance themselves, and nutrition therapists also suggest taking supplements of vitamin B_6 and zinc (Davies and Stewart, 1987).

Inadequate lactation

Where the mother has poor lactation, reflexology can be of enormous help. The part of the foot which relates to the breast is an area on the dorsum situated above the point where the toes join the foot. If this principle is related to the hand, the place in which an intravenous

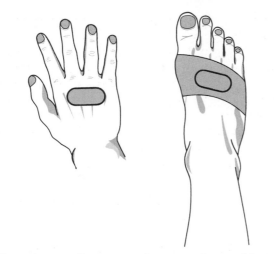

Figure 20.7 Reflex zones to breasts on dorsum of foot and back of hand. These areas can be massaged to stimulate lactation.

cannula may be sited lies directly over the zone for the breast, and the theory that women who receive intravenous fluids in labour may have impaired lactation would certainly be worth investigating. This then is the area which midwives could massage firmly on the hands and the feet in order to increase lactation. The mother could also be shown how to perform this for herself (Fig. 20.7).

Fennel and dill teas have been found to aid lactation and are now available as proprietary teas, although they can be high in sugar content.

Breast engorgement

Early breast engorgement responds well to the application of either dark green cabbage or rhubarb leaves. Although research has not supported the effects reported by women and midwives (see Ch. 41), what woman perceive as being beneficial may be the soothing action of the local application. The cabbage leaves are wiped clean and cooled in the refrigerator, then applied to the engorged breasts. Within minutes the leaves become soaking wet, after which time they are replaced with dry ones. This process is repeated until relief is obtained. The technique may also be of use when mothers wish to suppress lactation, and research by Shrivastav *et al.* (1988) demonstrated that jasmine flowers are also effective for this purpose. Homeopaths may recommend belladonna, particularly where the breasts have red streaks on them, or bryonia in cases where the discomfort is greater with movement. However Castro (1992)

advises that arnica tablets should be discontinued while the remedy for engorgement is used.

Nipple soreness may respond to Bach Rescue Remedy cream, calendula or camomile creams (now used in a proprietary form in many units) or phytolacca tincture.

Perineal problems

One of the commonest discomforts in the early postnatal period is that of the perineum while healing from lacerations, bruising or episiotomy. Dale and Cornwell's trial (1994) found that using lavender essential oil in the bath water did not significantly accelerate healing of the perineum, as anticipated. However, it was found to ease discomfort and relax the mothers, particularly between the third and fifth postnatal days.

If there is bruising of the buttocks and surrounding area, arnica homeopathic tables can be taken or arnica cream applied direct (although this should not be used on open wounds). Arnica is one of the few homeopathic remedies which can be universally used in cases of trauma, shock or bruising. Other homeopathic remedies suitable for perineal discomfort include hypericum, bellis perennis or nux vomica, but as with all other situations it is important to find the correct remedy for the individual. Phytotherapeutic marigold tincture may also be of use.

Various complementary strategies can also be utilized for other postnatal problems. For example, retention of urine in the early puerperium can be relieved with reflex zone therapy. This is useful also for easing the stiff neck and headache which occasionally follow epidural anaesthesia.

CONCLUSION

Within maternity care, complementary therapies can be extremely valuable in alleviating many of the physiological disorders of the childbearing period, and can be incorporated into midwifery practice relatively easily. The suggestion that all student midwives should receive an introduction to the subject during their initial education programmes, and proposals for the development of a new complementary therapy speciality within the midwifery profession, have been made (Tiran, 1995).

The explosion of interest amongst doctors, midwives and nurses will stimulate research projects, which will give further credibility to the practice of alternative therapies. Only in this way can there be any hope of those therapies which are currently 'alternative' becoming truly 'complementary' to the care on offer.

KEY POINTS

- Complementary therapies offer a range of additional strategies for helping women during pregnancy, childbirth and the puerperium.
- There are over 200 complementary therapies, many of which have now been classified by the House of Lords into three main groups.

- Midwives must be adequately and appropriately trained to use complementary therapies within their practice and must be able to justify their actions in accordance with the NMC regulations.

REFERENCES

Acolet, D., Modi, N., Giannakoulopoulos, X. *et al.* (1993) Changes in plasma cortisol and catecholamine concentrations in responses to massage in preterm infants. *Archives of Disease in Childhood* **68**(1): 29–31.

Adamson Macedo, E.N. & Attree, J.L.A. (1994) TIC TAC therapy: the importance of systematic stroking. *British Journal of Midwifery* **2**(6): 264–269.

Adamson Macedo E.N., de Roiste, A., Wilson, A. *et al.* (1997) Systematic gentle/light stroking and maternal random touching of ventilated preterm: a preliminary study. *International Journal of Prenatal and Perinatal Psychology and Medicine* **9**(1): 17–31.

Barsoum, G., Perry, E.P. & Fraser, I.A. (1990) Postoperative nausea is relieved by acupressure. *Journal of the Royal Society of Medicine* **83**(2): 86–89.

Bayreuther, J., Lewith, G.T. & Pickering, R. (1994) A double-blind cross-over study to evaluate the effectiveness of acupressure at pericardium 6 (P6) in the treatment of early morning sickness (EMS). *Complementary Therapies in Medicine* **2**: 70.

Belluomini, J., Litt, R.C., Lee, K.A. *et al.* (1994) Acupressure for nausea and vomiting of pregnancy: a randomized, blinded study. *Obstetrics and Gynaecology* **84**(2): 245–248.

BMA (British Medical Association) (1993) *Complementary Medicine – New Approaches to Good Practice.* Oxford: Oxford University Press.

Budd, S. (2000) Acupuncture. In: Tiran, D. & Mack, S. (eds) (2000) *Complementary Therapies for Pregnancy and Childbirth*, 2nd edn, Ch. 5, pp. 79–104. London: Harcourt Health Sciences.

Burns, E., Blamey, C., Errser, S. *et al.* (1999) *The Use of Aromatherapy in Intrapartum Midwifery Practice: an Evaluative Study.* Oxford: OCHRAD.

Cardini, F. & Weixin, H. (1998) Moxibustion for correction of breech presentation: a randomized controlled trial. *Journal of the American Medical Association* **280**(18): 1580–1584.

Cardini, F., Basevi, V., Valentini A. *et al.* (1991) Moxibustion and breech presentation: preliminary results. *American Journal of Chinese Medicine* **XIX**(2): 105.

Castro, M. (1992) *Homeopathy for Mother and Baby.* London: Macmillan.

Conway, P. (2000) Osteopathy during pregnancy. In: Tiran, D. & Mack, S. (eds) (2000) *Complementary Therapies for Pregnancy and Childbirth*, 2nd edn, Ch. 3, pp. 39–59. London: Harcourt Health Sciences.

Cooperative Research Group of Moxibustion Version of Jangxi Province (1984) Clinical observation on the effects of version by moxibustion. *Abstracts from the Second National Symposium on Acupuncture and Moxibustion and Acupuncture Anaesthesia, Beijing, China*, p. 150. All China Society of Acupuncture and Moxibustion.

Dale, A. & Cornwell, S. (1994) The role of lavender oil in relieving perineal discomfort following childbirth: a blind randomised clinical trial. *Journal of Advanced Nursing* **19**(1): 89–96.

Davies, S. & Stewart, A. (1987) *Nutritional Medicine.* London: Pan.

Daly, J.M., Frame, S.P. & Rapoza, P.A. (1991) Sacroiliac subluxation: a common treatable cause of low back pain in pregnancy. *Journal of Orthopaedic Medicine* **13**(3): 60–65.

De Aloysio, D. & Penacchioni, P. (1992) Morning sickness control in early pregnancy by Neiguan point acupressure. *Obstetrics and Gynaecology* **80**: 852–854.

DoH (Department of Health) (2000a) *Complementary Medicine Information Pack for Primary Care Groups.* London: DoH.

DoH (Department of Health) (2000b) *Complementary Medicine Information Pack for Primary Care Clinicians.* London: DoH.

Dundee, J.W., Sourial, F.B.R. & Ghaly R.G. (1988) P6 acupuncture reduces morning sickness. *Journal of the Royal Society of Medicine* **81**(8): 456–457.

Feder, E., Liisberg, G.B. & Lenstrup, C. (1993) Zone therapy in relation to birth. In: *Midwives: hear the heartbeat of the future. Proceedings of the International Confederation of Midwives 23rd International Congress*, Vol. 2, pp. 651–656. International Confederation of Midwives.

Fallon, J. (1993) Orthopaedic and neurological conditions of pregnancy and chiropractic management of care. *International Review of Chiropractic* 25–30.

FIM (Foundation for Integrated Medicine) (1997) *Integrated Healthcare: A Way Forward for the Next Five Years?* London: FIM.

Garland, D. (2000) The uses of hydrotherapy in today's midwifery practice. In: Tiran, D. & Mack, S. (eds) (2000) *Complementary Therapies for Pregnancy and Childbearing*, 2nd edn. London: Harcourt Health Sciences.

Geraghty, B. (1997) *Homeopathy for Midwives*. London: Churchill Livingstone.

Hansen, A., Vendelbo Jensen, D., Larsen, E. *et al.* (1996) Relaxin is not related to symptom giving pelvic girdle relaxation in pregnant women. *Acta Obstetricia et Gynecologica Scandinavica* **75**(3): 245–249.

Hart, O., Mullee, M.A., Lewith, G. *et al.* (1997) Double blind placebo-controlled randomised clinical trial of homeopathic arnica 30C for pain and infection after total abdominal hysterectomy. *Journal of the Royal Society of Medicine* **90**(2): 73–78.

Jenkins, M.W. & Pritchard, M. (1993) Practical applications and theoretical considerations of hypnosis in normal labour. *British Journal of Obstetrics and Gynaecology* **100**: 221–226.

Kleijnen, J. Knipschild, P. & Gerben, T.R. (1991) Clinical trials of homeopathy. *British Medical Journal* **302**(2): 316–321.

Mairs, D. (1995) Hypnosis and pain in childbirth. *Contemporary Hypnosis* **12**(2): 11.

Mantle, F. (2000) The role of hypnosis in pregnancy and childbirth. In: Tiran, D. & Mack, S. (eds) (2000) *Complementary Therapies in Pregnancy and Childbirth*, 2nd edn. London: Harcourt Health Sciences.

McMullen, M. (1995) Physical stresses of childhood that could lead to need for chiropractic care. *International Review of Chiropractic* 24–28.

NHS Confederation (1997) *Complementary Medicine in the NHS: Managing the Issues*. Birmingham: NHS Confederation.

Nursing and Midwifery Council (NMC) (2002) *Guidelines for the Administration of Medicines*. NMC: London.

Nursing and Midwifery Council (NMC) (2002) *Code of Professional Conduct*. NMC: London.

O'Brien, B., Relyea, M.J. & Taerum, T. (1996) Efficacy of P6 acupressure in the treatment of nausea and vomiting during pregnancy. *American Journal of Obstetrics and Gynecology* **174**(5): 708.

Petersen, K.L., Hvidman, L. & Uldbjerg, N. (1994) Normal serum relaxin in women with disabling pelvic pain during pregnancy. *Gynecological and Obstetric Investigations* **38**: 21–23.

Schauberger, C.W., Rooney, B.L., Goldsmith, L. *et al.* (1996) Peripheral joint laxity increases in pregnancy but does not correlate with serum relaxin levels. *American Journal of Obstetrics and Gynecology* **174**(2): 667–671.

Shrivastav, P., George, K., Balasubramaniam, N. *et al.* (1988) Suppression of puerperal lactation using jasmine flowers. *Australian and New Zealand Journal of Obstetrics and Gynaecology* **1**(28): 68–71.

Stapleton, H. & Tiran, D. (2000) Herbal medicine. In: Tiran, D. & Mack, S. (eds) *Complementary Therapies for Pregnancy and Childbirth*, 2nd edn, Ch. 6. London: Harcourt Health Sciences.

Stern, P.J., O'Connor, S.M. & Silvano, A.M. (1993) Symphysis pubis diastasis : a complication of pregnancy. *Journal of Neuromusculoskeletal System* **1**(2): 74–78.

Tellefsen, T. (2000) The chiropractic approach to health care during pregnancy. In: Tiran, D. and Mack, S. (eds) (2000) *Complementary Therapies for Pregnancy and Childbirth*, 2nd edn, Ch. 4, pp. 61–78. London, Harcourt Health Sciences.

Tiran, D. (1995) Complementary therapies education in midwifery. *Complementary Therapies in Nursing and Midwifery* **1**(3): 41–43.

Tiran, D. (1996) The use of complementary therapies in maternity care: a focus on reflexology. *Complementary Therapies in Nursing and Midwifery* **2**(1): 32–37.

Tiran, D. (1999) A holistic framework for maternity care *Complementary Therapies in Nursing and Midwifery* **5**(2): 127–135.

Tiran, D. (2000a) Incorporation of complementary therapies into maternity care. In: Tiran, D. and Mack, S. (eds) (2000) *Complementary Therapies for Pregnancy and Childbirth*, 2nd edn, Ch. 1, pp. 1–12. London: Harcourt Health Sciences.

Tiran, D. (2000b) *Clinical Aromatherapy for Pregnancy and Childbirth*. London: Harcourt Health Sciences.

Tiran, D. (2000c) Complementary therapies and the M25: Editorial. *Complementary Therapies in Nursing and Midwifery* **6**(3): 109–110.

Tiran, D. (2002) Reflexology in pregnancy and childbirth. In: Mackereth, P. & Tiran, D. *Clinical Reflexology*. London: Harcourt Health Sciences.

Tiran, D. & Mack, S. (eds) (2000) *Complementary Therapies for Pregnancy and Childbirth*, 2nd edn. London, Harcourt Health Sciences.

United Kingdom Central Council for Nursing, Midwifery and Health Visiting (UKCC) (1998) *Midwives Rules and Code of Practice*. London: UKCC.

Yelland, S. (1995) Using acupuncture in midwifery care. *Modern Midwife* **5**(1): 8–11.

FURTHER READING

Complementary Therapies in Maternity Care National Forum (1999) *Implementing Complementary Therapies within Maternity Care: a Guide for Professionals*. London: CTMC National Forum (available from Denise

Tiran (Chair), c/o School of Health, University of Greenwich, Eltham, London SE9 2UG; Tel: 020 8331 8494).

Tiran, D. (2000) *Clinical Aromatherapy for Pregnancy and Childbirth*. London: Churchill Livingstone.
A comprehensive exploration of the application of essential oils to the care of pregnant and childbearing women, written by a midwife who teaches aromatherapy and practises within an NHS clinic.

Tiran, D. & Mack, S. (eds) (2000) *Complementary Therapies for Pregnancy and Childbirth*, 2nd edn. London: Harcourt Health Sciences.

Offers a general introduction to the subject of using complementary therapies within maternity care; all contributors are either midwives qualified in a therapy or therapists who specialize in caring for pregnant and childbearing women.

West, Z. (2000) *Acupuncture in Pregnancy and Childbirth*. London: Harcourt Health Sciences.
The most up-to-date text specifically on using acupuncture and traditional Chinese medicine for expectant mothers written by a midwife practising acupuncture in the NHS.

ADDITIONAL RESOURCES

Complementary Maternity Forum
This is an independent multidisciplinary professional organization offering a source of networking and support to practitioners involved in or interested in complementary therapies specifically for pregnancy, labour and the puerperium. Further information may be obtained from: Denise Tiran (Chair), School of Health, University of Greenwich, Honeycomb Building, Mansion Site, Avery Hill Campus, Bexley Road, Eltham, London SE9 2UG; Tel: 020 8331 8494.
www.expectancy.co.uk

21

Health Promotion in Midwifery

Jacqueline Dunkley-Bent

LEARNING OUTCOMES

After reading this chapter you will be able to:

- appreciate the scope of health promotion in midwifery practice
- discuss the provision of health promotion within the context of inequalities in health and healthcare provision
- identify the emerging public health role of the midwife in the primary care setting
- apply the principles of health promotion to enhance the health of the woman and her family.

INTRODUCTION

The importance of the health promotion role of the midwife within the context of health and healthcare provision in the 21st century is crucial in enhancing the health and well-being of women and their families. The potential for health enhancement is a key focus for this chapter, utilizing midwifery practice as the vehicle for promoting health gain. The notion of health promotion is explored, enabling readers to develop firm foundations for effectively progressing their work in midwifery and their wider public health role.

THE MEANING OF HEALTH

It is difficult to promote health if a personal clarification of its meaning is not sought. Health is a state of being to which most people aspire, yet it is a concept which is difficult to define, as personal meanings are enshrined in social structure, culture and belief systems. In 1946, the World Health Organization described health as a state of complete physical, mental and social well-being and not merely the absence of disease or infirmity (WHO, 1946). Health is thus seen as an ideal state of being which may be impossible to achieve. In an attempt to clarify the meaning of health, Seedhouse (1997) suggests that health is determined by the individual's socioeconomic and cultural position, the context of which is determined by biological or chosen health potentials, which provides an opportunity for the individual to aspire to achieve good health within the context of that health potential. Lifestyle behaviours, personal habits and personal constructs of the health of individuals are major contributors to health and illness, and may be affected not just by the individuals' attitudes and beliefs, but by their culture, ethnicity, social class, religion, gender and economic status. It is crucial therefore that health professionals are aware of their own attitudes, beliefs and personal constructs of health prior to promoting the health of others.

For the purpose of this chapter, health will be viewed holistically, to involve dimensions of health that are inextricably linked and include physical, mental, emotional, societal, sexual and spiritual health. If one dimension is negatively affected, this will have an impact on other dimensions (Ewles and Simnett, 1998).

Reflective Activity 21.1

What does being healthy mean to you? Jot down your personal definition of 'being healthy'.

MODELS OF HEALTH

Health models have been developed to try to explain why some individuals indulge in healthy behaviour and others do not. Well-_____ models include the Health Belief Model, formul___ by Rosenstock in the 1960s and further developed by Becker in the 1970s (Becker *et al.*, 1977), and the Health Locus of Control proposed by Rotter (1966). The Health Belief Model was developed specifically to explain and predict preventive health behaviours. The Health Locus of Control refers to the personal control over events that people believe they possess and is commonly used to explore how people's beliefs about health and illness affect what they do. The reader is encouraged to explore this area in more detail by accessing the information provided in the Further reading list.

REDUCING INEQUALITIES IN HEALTH

Understanding the social, cultural and economic context of health and illness increases the potential for health promotion to be meaningful and effective. It is well established that poverty and deprivation are linked to poor health outcomes (DoH, 1999). In the UK the National Health Service (NHS) was set up in 1948 to provide a range of free medical care to the whole population and thereby achieve equality of access to health services for those in need. It was hoped that this would eliminate or greatly reduce inequalities in health. Unsurprisingly, this rather narrow approach to improving the health of those worst off in society did not succeed. The provision of health services cannot singularly solve inequality in health without addressing factors that influence ill-health.

Top-down commitment bottom-up approach?

The Black Report demonstrated substantial differences in mortality and morbidity rates of social class groups and made recommendations to address this (Black *et al.*, 1982). Unfortunately these recommendations were not endorsed. A pre-election promise in 1997 by the new Labour Government included an independent review of the inequalities in health, which highlighted increasing inequality in most aspects of health in the last few decades. The enquiry advanced 39 recommendations that focused on social justice (Acheson, 1998).

Saving Lives: Our Healthier Nation (DoH, 1999) embraces the recommendations by Acheson and the long-standing Black Report. It sets out a strategy to save lives, promote healthier living and reduce inequalities in health. The key aims are:

- to improve the health of the population as a whole by increasing the length of people's lives and the number of years people spend free from illness
- to improve the health of the worst off in society and to narrow the health gap.

This involves the local community, health professionals, local authorities and the Government playing a part, therefore encouraging a multi-agency approach to reducing inequalities in health and healthcare provision may be successful where other strategies have failed.

The report acknowledges the midwife's scope of practice, including the midwifery contribution to women's health, and makes a commitment to expand the midwife's health promotion role. Specific targets, including those set to be achieved by 2010, and those that relate to midwifery practice are detailed below. The NHS Plan (Secretary of State for Health, 2000) is the Government's 10-year programme of investment and reform to secure an NHS that is fit for the 21st century. The plan sets out a coherent framework and includes factors relating to high national standards, diversity, flexibility, more choices, reducing inequalities and improving the life chances of children. Midwives have a unique opportunity to work with key stakeholders and members of the multidisciplinary team to provide convenient high quality services that enable women to exercise greater choice (DoH, 2003).

WHAT IS HEALTH PROMOTION?

The World Health Organization (WHO, 1984) defines health promotion as the process of enabling people to increase control over their health, and improve it. Integral to this definition is the notion of empowerment. An example of empowerment in midwifery practice is the process by which the health professional uses strategies to enable the woman and her partner to lead and take control over their childbirth experience. The potential to transfer/develop these skills in everyday life can be achieved if the initial process of empowerment is successful.

The midwife's role encompasses a wide range of health promotion initiatives that may not involve behaviour change, including advice and guidance about baby care and parenting issues. Decision-making, empowerment, debriefing and health education are important aspects of health promotion in midwifery.

Health promotion needs to be addressed throughout pregnancy, childbirth and the puerperium, as a coherent whole, rather than an activity placed within 'parentcraft classes'.

Seedhouse (1997) suggests that the ultimate aim of health promotion is to provide opportunities for people to move within the context of their biological, intellectual and/or emotional potential. The momentum of the movement or indeed its maintenance is likely to be successful only if the most appropriate avenue has been chosen to promote health, one that is particular to or within the context of the individual's life. A realistic approach to health promotion for the midwife therefore, would include assessing the context of the woman's living experience and identifying with the woman, obstacles that inhibit the fulfilment of health potentials (see Case scenario 21.1).

Mental health promotion

Impaired mental health has a negative impact on emotional and physical health and reduces the individual's capacity to cope with everyday life activities. The process and impact of postnatal depression is one example of how physical, spiritual, emotional and mental health are affected (refer to Ch. 54 for further information).

Sexual health promotion

Addressing sexual health issues may contribute to the overall well-being of the woman, fetus and her family.

Case scenario 21.1

Alice is asked to attend the midwifery day assessment unit twice a week for blood pressure measurements. She is 32 weeks' pregnant and has a diastolic blood pressure of 100 mmHg (20 mmHg above her booking diastolic blood pressure). She is anxious and distressed because each time she attends the hospital she leaves her 3-year-old twin daughters in the care of her 10-year-old son.

- Consider the health deficits that inhibit the achievement of Alice's psychological and physical well-being.
- What actions could you take to ensure the achievement of health potentials in this situation?
- Identify foundations for health that Alice could achieve if antagonists were removed.

The midwife has an important role to play in this area of public health and should therefore understand the impact of sexually transmitted infections on the woman, fetus and infant (see Ch. 47).

Sexuality and pregnancy

Sexuality is influenced by health, personal circumstances, self-image and self-esteem. Physical, mental and emotional health have an impact on how individuals view their own sexuality. Pregnancy, childbirth and motherhood challenge personal concepts of sexuality and sexual expression, though the impact of physiological and psychological changes that occur during pregnancy is generally beyond personal control. Physiological effects of pregnancy include pelvic vasocongestion that occurs as a result of increases in the hormones oestrogen and progesterone. Vaginal congestion as a result of increased vascularity and venous stasis either results in a greater pleasurable experience from orgasm or may predispose to discomfort during sexual intercourse (Walton, 1994). The presence of vulval varicosities and haemorrhoids, which may be more prevalent or aggravated during pregnancy, renders sexual pleasure or the desire for sexual intercourse difficult. Changes in body image, including increased weight gain, loss of pre-pregnancy waistline, striae gravidarum, breast changes, leaking colostrum, tiredness and backache may all, or singularly, contribute to altered sexual expression.

Sexuality in pregnancy is an important aspect of health that is not always addressed appropriately. Some women may feel embarrassed broaching this topic and some midwives, fearing intrusion of privacy, may also be reticent about discussing the issue. There may be religious, cultural and social taboos about having sexual intercourse during pregnancy, but some couples may have anxieties that could be relieved through frank discussion.

Sexual intercourse

There is little evidence that sexual intercourse during a pregnancy with no identified related risk factors is harmful. Couples may benefit from reassurance in this area. As pregnancy advances, the woman will find intercourse more comfortable if positions are used which do not put undue pressure on her enlarging abdomen, such as lying side by side with her legs across her partner or the female-superior position (see Ch. 7). In the last weeks of pregnancy, sexual intercourse and orgasm may stimulate strong uterine contractions that can make the woman feel uncomfortable. Seminal fluid contains a large amount of prostaglandins and intercourse may help to ripen the cervix. These issues may be discussed at antenatal education forums or may be deemed more appropriate for one-to-one discussion.

Health promotion models

A model may be described as a conceptual framework for organizing and integrating information offering causal links among a set of concepts believed to be related to a particular problem (Seedhouse, 1997). Consider the well-known health model presented in Figure 21.1. This consists of three overlapping circles separately labelled: health education, prevention and health protection. The overlapping design of the model creates seven different sections, each represented by a number that refers to different combinations of health promotion approaches. For example section four involves health education, health protection and prevention of ill-health. It could be argued that all categories are inextricably linked and therefore cannot exist in isolation. Section six, health protection, may be difficult to achieve without section five, health education. When considering vaccination against childhood diseases section one, ill-health prevention, and section six, health protection, are effective but section five, health education, is essential. This model may be useful in helping those new to health promotion appreciate the scope of health promotion work. Unfortunately, sociocultural and economic factors that influence the health promotion approach taken are not represented.

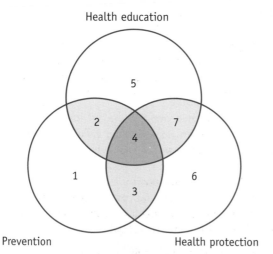

Figure 21.1 A model of health promotion.
(From Tannahill, 1985.)

Health promotion approaches

A health promotion approach can be described as the vehicle used to achieve the desired aim. An example would be the aim of raising awareness about the efficacy of vitamin K. The ultimate objective may be to enable the woman and her partner to make an informed choice about its use, but the health promotion approach may vary according to the woman, context and practitioner.

Ewles and Simnett (1998) identify five approaches to health promotion: the medical or preventive approach, behavioural change approach, educational, client-centred and the societal change approach (see Box 21.1 for practice application).

THE PUBLIC HEALTH ROLE OF THE MIDWIFE

It is important for the midwifery profession to have a clearly defined and identifiable public health role. *The NHS Plan* (Secretary of State for Health, 2000) and the *Supporting Families* initiative (Home Office, 1998) acknowledge the contribution that midwives make to the health of the nation, particularly in relation to the health of the next generation. The public health role of the midwife involves working with disadvantaged groups, including refugees and asylum seekers, teenage mothers and women who are involved in drugs, alcohol and substance misuse and domestic violence. The public health role also includes improving breastfeeding rates and improving screening for mental ill-health. The RCM position paper entitled 'The Midwife's Role in Public Health' provides further guidance (RCM, 2001).

> ### Reflective Activity 21.2
>
> Think about your midwifery practice over the past 2 months in terms of public health. How many public health activities have you been involved in?
>
> Reading the next section may increase the number of activities counted.

Health promotion – community action

The scope for midwifery health promotion has the potential to influence the health of the next generation and have a profound impact on reducing inequalities in health and healthcare provision. Work in the community has long been recognized as the main arena within which to tackle these issues (Gunning-Schepers and Gepkens, 1996). The statutory obligation to continue midwifery support until 28 days postpartum provides further scope for health promotion work to be practised, increasing the potential for health influence (Dunkley, 2000b). This freedom and flexibility is influenced by resource constraints.

The provision of maternity care to members of the travelling community and immigrant families presents challenges to the midwife's role in relation to equality of healthcare provision. Eviction orders, commonly associated with the travelling community owing to unlawful caravan parking, cause disruption in midwifery care provision. Local authorities proceeding with eviction orders are required to liaise with the relevant statutory agencies, to enable practitioners to fulfil statutory obligations, particularly where pregnant women and neonates are involved (DoH and Welsh Office, 1994). There are 13.2 million refugees worldwide, of whom 22% are women whose health needs are rarely catered for (Kealy, 1999). The Reproductive Health for Refugees Consortium made recommendations which included the need for culturally sensitive reproductive health, and appropriate referral systems should obstetric emergencies arise. The health of pregnant asylum seekers is frequently compromised by lack of antenatal care, stressful, torturous journeys from countries of origin, turmoil caused by war, oppression and poor nutrition. Their health disadvantage increases the risk of perinatal mortality and morbidity and renders them ill prepared for childbirth and parenting, particularly if antenatal care has been sparse. Midwives and other health professionals need to be aware of the difficulties and problems faced by travellers and immigrant communities and use opportunities for health promotion when they arise.

Health enhancement through community initiatives is well supported politically, including the development of Health Action Zones (DoH, 1999) and Sure Start programmes (Home Office, 1998). Funding support is limited and mainstream services are expected to absorb the cost of programmes once the initial funding ceases. The Sure Start programmes seek to improve the health of children and their families by providing a vehicle for achieving health and reducing inequalities (Roberts, 2000). Several target areas have been identified and include parenting support and information to be made available to all parents and identification and support for mothers with postnatal depression. The Sure Start initiative aims to achieve a 5% reduction in

---

Box 21.1 Health promotion in practice

Medical approach

Seeks to prevent and/or cure illness through medical intervention.

Example: the midwife may offer the woman who is non-immune to rubella the vaccination in the puerperium and contraceptive advice for a period of 3 months. Education and discussion should form part of this process. Didactic instruction should be avoided.

Behavioural change approach

Primary focus is on encouraging people to change their behaviour.

Example: dietary adjustment to include more fruit and vegetables. This may involve raising awareness through education, empowerment and decision-making. Client-centred work should form part of this strategy to ensure success.

Educational approach

Provision of information, tailored to meet the individual needs of the client.

Example: this approach is generally a precursor for other approaches. Methods that will progress the educational approach include group work, discussion methods and problem-solving.

Client-centred approach

This places the client at the centre of an interaction that is based on an equal partnership between the client and the professional. Empowerment is integral to this approach where individuals are encouraged to utilize personal strength toward health gain.

Example: making an informed decision about the uptake of antenatal screening tests, and behaviour change including stopping smoking.

Societal change approach

Health promotion initiatives are focused on societal health and involve, for example, policy planning and political action (Dunkley, 2000a).

Example: political and community action toward increasing the number of general practitioner services.

low birthweight babies and a 10% reduction in children admitted to hospital as an emergency with gastroenteritis (DfEE, 2000). The contribution by midwives to achieving the targets is paramount and as such, several Sure Start programmes have allocated resources to fund extra midwifery time.

Of the 39 recommendations made by the Acheson report (Acheson, 1998), several emphasize the need to support childbearing women and their families within the community setting. It is suggested that midwives can:

- target vulnerable groups, including single mothers and ethnic groups, through pregnancy clubs and link workers
- provide preconception counselling for prospective parents, with an emphasis on smoking cessation, alcohol and diet, thereby reducing the incidence of low birthweight and premature babies
- collaborate with health visitors on postnatal depression, breastfeeding and the implementation of best practice to reduce the incidence of sudden infant death syndrome.

The Royal College of Midwives (RCM) clearly emphasizes the strength of midwifery within the community setting and encourages the development of the midwife's public health role (RCM, 2000, 2001).

Preconception care

Preconception care is described as the passport to positive health during pregnancy. The aim of care is to optimize the chances of conception, ensure the maintenance of a healthy pregnancy and promote a healthy outcome for the mother and baby. This approach positively influences the health of the next generation.

Despite policy statements highlighting the need to secure this goal, resource allocation is not focused toward preconception care and it does not form part of routine primary care services. The *Foresight* organization is a registered charity that offers preconception services. Despite the exceptional benefits of the organization, equality in terms of availability and access is questionable. Leading health documents including *The NHS Plan* (Secretary of State for Health, 2000), *Supporting Families* (Home Office, 1998) and *Saving Lives: Our Healthier Nation* (DoH, 1999) do not directly identify preconception care as a focus area for enhancing the health of the next generation but rather favour a whole-population approach to enhancing health status, despite recommendations from the Acheson report (1998). Naturally the benefits of targeting the whole population can be clearly identified, particularly for those pregnancies that are unplanned. The magnitude of this approach may, however, reduce the impact on reproductive health and exclude the expertise of the midwife. Ensuring the best start in life for the next generation is clearly an integral part of the midwife's role. Preconception care should be recognized as the main practice for achieving this aim and be resourced accordingly.

HEALTH PROMOTION IN THE ANTENATAL PERIOD

Diet and nutrition

The midwife has an important role to play when advising the woman about diet and nutrition. Effective health education in this area may contribute to long-term healthy lifestyle changes. The health promotion approach chosen should include health education, empowerment and a client-centred approach. Behaviour change may also be necessary to promote immediate and long-term health. (Diet and nutrition are presented in detail in Ch. 19.)

Exercise during pregnancy

Most people are well aware of the benefits of exercise and sport and many women are fitness conscious. Exercise has many positive benefits for the individual including mental well-being, improvement in stamina and posture and maintenance of good muscle tone. In addition, exercise during pregnancy improves cardiovascular function and reduces excess weight gain (Clapp, 2000).

The American College of Obstetricians and Gynecologists (ACOG, 1994) issued guidelines to ensure the safety of pregnant women with no identified risk factors, taking exercise (see Box 21.2). It is important to adhere to safety principles during exercise to enable physiological adjustment to take place. Just as the maternal system copes with gradual respiratory and cardiac adjustment during pregnancy, so too can the body adjust during exercise in a pregnancy identified as low risk. The woman who leads a sedentary lifestyle before pregnancy should be encouraged to take part in gentle exercise during pregnancy. Aquanatal exercise may be the preferred option because of the benefits of non-weight-bearing activity, hydrostatic pressure, buoyancy and upthrust. In addition, the increased mobility experienced puts less strain on joints and may relieve backache (Dunkley, 2000a). Women who exercised prior to becoming pregnant and present with no risk factors should be encouraged to continue, but attention should be drawn to safety parameters (see Box 21.2) and any risk factors that occur during pregnancy. Generally, exercise to exhaustion should be avoided as this may cause blood flow diversion from the uterus, with resultant acute fetal hypoxia (Gilbert and Harman, 1998). Jumpy, jerky movements should also be avoided.

The ligaments that support joints are relaxed by the hormone relaxin in pregnancy and therefore minimum muscle tension during exercise should be employed to avoid overstretching the ligaments permanently. The rectus abdominis muscles are already stretched over the growing uterus, and women should not exercise to stretch them further. Stretching to increase flexibility should be avoided but short static stretches to relieve tension are relatively safe (Baddeley, 1999).

Most physically active sports become more difficult during pregnancy as weight increases and the breasts and abdomen enlarge. More stress is placed on weight-bearing joints and musculoskeletal injury becomes more common, and balance is naturally affected as the centre of gravity changes. Other physiological changes in pregnancy of raised cardiac output, reduced lung capacity and decreased agility, may encourage the pregnant woman to choose less active sports than those pursued when not pregnant. Any sport that causes undue fatigue, muscle cramps, or joint pain should be modified or discontinued, and women should avoid becoming overheated and dehydrated. Strenuous unaccustomed exercise and heavy lifting should be avoided in pregnancy. Pelvic floor exercises should be taught as early as possible during the antenatal period and encouraged as a life-time activity. It may be useful to explain the role of the pelvic floor, its position anatomically, the nature of the exercise, compliance testing and the benefits of pelvic floor exercises.

Box 21.2 Guidelines for exercise during pregnancy

1. During pregnancy, women can continue to exercise at mild to moderate levels regularly (at least three times a week). This is preferable to intermittent activity.
2. Women should avoid exercising in the supine position and avoid prolonged periods of motionless standing.
3. Pregnant women should stop exercising when fatigued and not exercise to exhaustion.
4. Weight-bearing exercises may be continued under certain circumstances, but should be maintained at intensities similar to pre-pregnancy and not increased.
5. Non-weight-bearing exercises reduce the risk of injury and facilitate the continuation of exercise during pregnancy.
6. Exercise which poses a risk to abdominal trauma should be avoided.
7. Women who exercise should ensure they take an adequate diet.
8. During the first trimester, attention should be paid to enhancing heat loss through appropriate clothing, adequate hydration, and optimal environmental conditions.
9. Postpartum exercise should be resumed gradually and determined by the woman's physical capability.

(American College of Obstetrics and Gynecology, 1994: 65–70)

Smoking in pregnancy

Smoking is the largest single preventable cause of mortality and is responsible for reducing the female advantage in life expectancy (Callum, 1998). It is a major cause of coronary heart disease, stroke and chronic bronchitis, lung and other cancers, and is also associated with reduced fertility and early menopause in women (DoH, 1999). In pregnancy, smoking is related to spontaneous abortion, placenta praevia, placental abruption, low birthweight and preterm labour (Dewan *et al.*, 2003; Lindley *et al.*, 2000). Other reports show an association between maternal smoking and wheeze during early childhood (Lux *et al.*, 2000).

24% of women smoke during pregnancy and only 33% of these give up whilst pregnant (Foster *et al.*, 1997). In the most recent survey, 20% of women smoked before or during pregnancy, and 44% gave up before or during pregnancy (BMRB Social Research, 2001).

Women from lower socioeconomic groups are more likely to smoke during pregnancy, which significantly increases the risk of perinatal and infant mortality. Children who are exposed in the home to cigarette smoke are more likely to develop otitis media and asthma and have higher hospitalization rates for severe respiratory illness. The publication *Smoking Kills* details the Government's commitment towards helping people quit smoking and reducing the prevalence of those who start. This identifies the provision of funding toward delivering expert help to those most in need and the phasing out of tobacco advertising by 2006 (Secretary of State for Health, 1998).

Smoking cessation: the midwife's role

The midwife plays a vital role during the woman's childbirth experience, and support, guidance and advice that she offers is generally well received and acted upon. This unique relationship provides a window of opportunity for health education which, if delivered appropriately, should not alter the dynamics of the midwife–woman relationship but form an integral part of practice. A client-centred approach and empowerment are more likely to secure and strengthen the midwife's relationship with the woman and ultimately achieve the health promotion goal, rather than persuasion, cajoling and scare-mongering.

At the first antenatal visit, the midwife should establish the smoking status of the woman, her partner and other members of her household. The dialogue should involve identifying the woman's readiness to change her smoking behaviour, and ideally should include the partner. Prochaska and Diclemente developed the behaviour change cycle to assist health professionals in identifying the readiness of clients to change their smoking behaviour (Prochaska *et al.*, 1993) (see Box 21.3).

The midwife should increase her understanding of the complex nature of nicotine addiction experienced by smokers and not view the process of cessation as simply as cutting down or stopping. Women who are highly dependent on tobacco may feel guilty and inadequate at not being able to give it up. The midwife should be encouraging and supportive and ready to offer help to women who express the desire to stop smoking. 10 minutes of counselling interaction may be sufficient as an effective intervention for smoking cessation (Lancaster *et al.*, 2000).

Box 21.3 The model of behaviour change in practice

Precontemplator

Not interested in stopping, has no intentions of stopping.

What can I do?
- Present the risk factors and offer damage-limitation advice.

Contemplator

Is thinking about stopping, may have been thinking about stopping for several years.

What can I do? Encourage the woman to:
- Explore reason for wanting to stop; explore barriers to stopping.
- Discuss preparation needed in order to stop – this may involve removing all ashtrays and similar appliances.
- Consider triggers to smoking, e.g. telephone, coffee, after a meal, and think of an alternative strategy.
- Consider substitutes for habitual feelings, e.g. something in the mouth or hand.
- Consider substitutes if smoking is regularly used as a relaxer, or ice melter.
- Consider strategies which may help to overcome the nicotine craving; think of times when the craving is

strongest and consider strategies which may help to overcome this.

Ready for action

Ready to stop – may need help and support in doing so.

What can I do? Encourage the woman to:
- Choose a time to give up when there are fewer triggers to smoke (e.g. stress).
- Set a date to stop and stick to it (make plans for stopping as detailed in the contemplator section).

Relapse

Stopped smoking but has re-started:

What can I do?
- Unsuccessful attempts to quit work toward successful quitting; the smoker may learn valuable lessons after each relapse episode which may increase the chances of future success.
- Make a list of everything that went wrong, think of strategies which may reduce the likelihood of relapse.

NB: Strategies must be client led and not prescribed by the midwife, whose role is primarily facilitating the discussion and offering support and guidance.

Reducing the number of cigarettes smoked should generally be discouraged, but praised if this action is taken prior to contact with the midwife. The nature of smoking behaviour whilst cutting down should be discussed with the woman. Whilst cutting down, people tend to drag on the cigarette more frequently than usual, inhale more deeply and smoke the cigarette as far to the end as is physically possible (Dunkley, 2000a). The amount of noxious chemicals inhaled may therefore be the same as the dose inhaled prior to cutting down, when the nature of the smoking behaviour was casual.

The midwife should have current knowledge of the support services available in the local area. Health education leaflets, the quit line number and self-help groups should be offered as additional support, but it is important that leaflets should not be used as a replacement for discussion, personal support and counselling. Nicotine gum and patches are contraindicated in pregnancy. Several GPs are now prescribing nicotine replacement therapy for women who are described as heavy smokers.

Damage limitation

Overwhelming evidence shows the association between passive smoking and sudden infant death syndrome (SIDS), suggesting that 30–40% of all cases of SIDS could be avoided if pregnant women stopped smoking (Wisborg et al., 2000). Further evidence points toward the long-term effects of postnatal neonatal exposure with associations made between passive smoking and heart disease. Parental smoking and the influence on asthma have been associated with increased hospital admissions in children under 5 years old (Secretary of State for Health, 1998). More recent reports show an association between passive smoking by the pregnant non-smoking mother and increased maternal circulating absolute nucleated red blood cell counts, which suggests there may be subtle negative effects on fetal oxygenation (Dollberg et al., 2000).

The midwife has a responsibility to provide health education to women and their families to reduce the damage to the fetus/infant. Women and their partners who have no intention of giving up smoking should not be persuaded to do so, as this may lead to resentment and feelings of guilt. Through two-way communication with the woman and her partner the midwife should establish the nature of the smoking behaviour. The provision of health information forms part of the discussion. Once the readiness to change has been established, for example the woman may decide not to

give up smo[...]
be offered [...]
reducing [...]
ing tha[...]
baby, [...]
win[...]
ex[...]
t[...]

Alcohol in[...]

Alcohol ingestion is [...] forms part of everyday soc[...] world. Over the past 30 years, [...] drinkers has increased much more t[...] 90% of the adult population consume alcoh[...] pregnancy this is reduced to 40–60% (RCOG, 1[...] Excessive alcohol intake is potentially lethal, affecting virtually every organ and system in the body, including the liver, gastrointestinal tract, cardiovascular and neurological systems. It affects nutrition by suppressing the appetite and by altering the metabolism, mobilization and storage of nutrients (Wardlow, 2000). Excessive or chronic alcohol abuse is associated with several vitamin and mineral deficiencies, including folic acid, vitamin B, magnesium and iron. Learning difficulties, loss of memory and other mental problems are associated with infants born to parents who have abused alcohol (Chang et al., 1998). Women cannot tolerate as much alcohol as men because of differences in body size, absorption and metabolism. They have a higher proportion of fat to water; therefore alcohol becomes more concentrated in body fluids and damaging effects such as gastritis, pancreatitis, peptic ulcers and malnutrition are more likely to develop.

Drinking excessively in pregnancy can adversely affect the pregnancy and fetal development and is associated with fetal alcohol syndrome and alcohol-related birth defects (see Ch. 36).

Antenatal screening

Despite numerous research studies, to date there is no universally acceptable safe measure of alcohol consumption during pregnancy. In the USA alcohol consumption of any amount during pregnancy is not recommended. The midwife has the dilemma of whether to encourage abstinence or not. The RCOG (1999) suggest that pregnant women should moderate their alcohol consumption to one alcoholic measure per day (maximum of 7 units per week). This level of

drinking appears to sho[...]
nancy outcome. [...]
At the first antenat[...]
woman if she dri[...]
include 'no', 'yes'[...]
enquiry must f[...]
ensure the de[...]
The respons[...]
mation ab[...]
who res[...]
ing be[...]
trend[...]
ide[...]

... no adverse effect on preg-

... visit, the midwife should ask the ...ks alcohol. Common responses ...'not really', or 'just socially'. Further ...llow to establish clear meaning and ...very of appropriate health promotion. ... of 'just socially' does not provide infor-...ut the number of units ingested. The person ...onds 'not really' may be comparing her drink-...aviour to that of an alcoholic. There is a general ... toward under-reporting, which will inhibit the ...tification of high-risk drinkers (Stoler and Holmes, ...99). Heavy drinkers may book late for maternity care and need intensive counselling and referral to specialist agencies to help them reduce alcohol consumption. Highlighting teratogenic effects on the fetus forms part of health education but midwives should be sensitive in ensuring that the information they provide is balanced and informed, and does not result in fear or guilt, as this may impede reducing drinking levels.

A useful way of taking a drinking history is to ask specifically about the preceding 7 days. If alcohol has been consumed, the amount in units should be recorded. If intake is higher than RCOG guidelines, the midwife should discuss this with the woman and explore ways of reducing the amount and nature of alcohol intake. Ingesting 7 units of alcohol over a week may be considered safe (RCOG, 1999), whereas this amount in one evening may not be. A screening tool to detect alcohol abuse recommended by the RCOG is the T-ACE questionnaire (Sokol *et al.*, 1989). This consists of four questions that assess tolerance of alcohol, other people's perceptions of the individuals drinking behaviour, thoughts about cutting down and the need for a drink first thing in the morning. High scores highlight problem drinking which should be explored sensitively and referral made to specialist local agencies, such as Alcoholics Anonymous (AA) or other self-help groups. The woman should be reassured of continued support regardless of the referral and close liaison should be maintained.

Drugs in pregnancy

Pregnant women should be advised to take only those drugs that are prescribed by a doctor. The British National Formulary (BMA and RPSGB, 2003) offers an excellent guide on drugs contraindicated in pregnancy. The reader is encouraged to refer to Chapter 71, and the recommended reading list for further information about drugs in pregnancy and drug misuse.

Domestic violence

Domestic violence poses a serious threat to women's health, and may be emotional, sexual, physical or financial abuse and may result in homicide. It is well established that violence towards women increases during pregnancy (DoH, 2000; Mezey, 1997). The perpetrator is usually the male partner or ex-partner, but domestic violence may occur in same sex relationships, or from other family members.

Abused women and abusers come from all cultural, educational, racial, religious and socioeconomic backgrounds. The Yale trauma study showed that victims of domestic violence are 15 times more likely to abuse alcohol, nine times more likely to abuse drugs, three times more likely to be diagnosed as depressed or psychotic and five times more likely to attempt suicide than women generally (Maryland Department of Health, 2001). Midwives should be able to recognize women at risk of abuse, and provide information and support, acting as a conduit to local resources, support networks and services which may be available. In some cases this will include working with other professional groups to provide and improve such services (RCM, 1999).

Prevalence

Research indicates that domestic violence is widespread in the UK but it is difficult to obtain reliable statistics, as it is generally under-reported and therefore a hidden crime. One in three women will experience domestic violence at some time in their lives. It is estimated that 30% of domestic violence starts in pregnancy (DoH, 2001). Reasons for this are numerous and may include feelings of overpossessiveness, jealousy and denial of the women having any other role than spouse. The perpetrator may feel jealous of the woman's ability to produce a child, or see the fetus as an intruder. He may also become violent because of strained finances or reduced sexual activity (Gaines, 1997).

Risk to the woman and fetus

The physical and psychological risks to the woman and fetus are overwhelmingly high, and the fetus may be injured or may die during the pregnancy. Depression, suicide and substance abuse (Lewis, 2001; Martin *et al.*, 1996) are not uncommon. 45 women whose deaths were investigated in *the Confidential Enquiries into Maternal Deaths in the United Kingdom* between 1997–1999 self-reported a history of domestic violence to a healthcare professional. Domestic violence was fatal for eight of these women. Recommendations including the health professional's role have been for-mulated as a result of these enquiries. The main points are included in Box 21.4.

The midwife's role

Questioning about domestic violence should form part of health education only if appropriate education and training has been provided, guidelines have been developed to support staff, and support/referral systems are current and reliable.

When abuse is suspected, the best way to confirm suspicion is by direct questioning, which may include the following questions:

- Has somebody been hurting you?
- Did somebody cause these injuries?
- Do you ever feel frightened of your partner, or other people at home?
- Have you ever been slapped, kicked or punched by your partner?

Box 21.4 Guidelines for health professionals

- Health professionals should make themselves aware of the nature of domestic violence, taking a non-judgemental and supportive stance.
- Disclosure of violence should always be taken seriously.
- Information about sources of help should be displayed in the antenatal clinic, ladies toilets and in printed form on all maternity records.
- Where an interpreter is required this should not be a partner, friend or family member. Link workers/interpreter services should be utilized.
- Local trusts and community teams should develop guidelines for the identification and provision of further support, and effective referral and multi-agency working.
- Enquiry about violence should be routinely included when taking a social history.
- If routine questioning is introduced, a strategy for referral must be in place and education provided for health professionals in collaboration with local groups. This should be supported by an effective education and training programme for practitioners, provided by people working in this area of practice.
- The woman should be seen at least once on her own during the antenatal period.

(Lewis, 2001: 241–242)

It may be useful to approach the subject by asking indirect questions first, which may include (DoH, 2000):

- Is everything all right at home?
- Do you get on well with your partner?

The woman may choose to deny being abused, but awareness that help is available is useful. The woman may disclose domestic violence at some stage during the childbirth experience. Pregnancy provides a unique opportunity for change for women suffering from domestic violence, and disclosure may therefore be likely (Mayer and Liebschutz, 1998).

Routine questioning of all antenatal women reduces the chances of targeting certain female and male groups that conform to personal stereotypes. However, there are difficulties in routine questioning:

- finding an appropriate time to ask the question, particularly when the woman is accompanied by her partner
- denial of abuse and subsequent non-attendance for antenatal care
- lack of supervision services for midwives who receive disclosure. (Without supportive structures in place direct questioning should be approached with caution.)

Fostering a nurturing environment during antenatal visits, including genuineness, positive regard, empathy and honesty, may provide the woman with an opportunity to seek help should she feel the need. Survivors of domestic violence often feel ashamed about being abused by their partner, have low self-esteem and have conflicting feelings about disclosure, including the repercussions of their actions. Very often leaving the abuser is not considered a favourable option at that time. Some women are financially and emotionally dependent on their abusers, who often have control over all domestic arrangements. Religious and cultural influences often encourage people to stay in abusive marriages where separation or divorce is considered unacceptable.

Reflective Activity 21.3

Refer to the signs of domestic violence (Box 21.5) and reflect on your antenatal and postnatal experiences for similar behaviour you may have observed. Think about possible ways of raising the issue of domestic violence when it is suspected. Do you have local practice unit policies for guidance? What resources are in place to support an abused woman?

Box 21.5 Possible signs of domestic violence

Possible signs of domestic violence include:

- frequently missed appointments
- appointments made for vague complaints or symptoms
- injuries that are not consistent with accidental causes – multiple injuries
- attempts made by the woman to minimize the extent of the injury
- signs of anxiousness, or depression
- an aggressive or over-dominant partner, reluctant to allow the woman to speak for herself.

(Adapted from DoH, 2000: 24)

The midwife should understand the nature of domestic violence, be sensitive to clues that may suggest abuse (see Box 21.5) and be aware of the impact of abuse on everyday life. Ensuring that all consultations with the woman offer quality time where a safe nurturing environment is perceived, is useful. When the woman and the midwife are not in the company of the partner, for example showing the woman where the toilet is, taking her to the weighing scales if they are outside of the consultation area, may provide an opportunity for the woman to disclose something about how she is feeling that may be indirectly related to the abuse. Although considered a viable approach, direct questioning should not be considered the *only* option for obtaining information. Some midwives may be reluctant to acknowledge domestic violence or ask questions about it because of their fear of offending; fear of disclosure; lack of knowledge of what action to take if this occurs; feeling that it is a private matter and belief that it is not a part of their role (Watts, 1998).

Staff should be trained in conflict avoidance to ameliorate the course of violence (Bewley and Gibbs, 1997), and this often increases their confidence.

Each maternity unit and independent midwifery group practice should have current details about domestic violence units and the Women's Aid Federation who provide a safe refuge for those who need it. The Samaritans, Relate and Victim Support all offer support services to survivors of domestic violence. The midwife should be able to supply the woman with relevant local telephone numbers and addresses.

Teenage pregnancy

Teenage pregnancy is generally seen as a major problem in the western world. In England and Wales, the rate of conceptions for teenagers under the age of 16 has risen steadily from the late 1950s, followed by a sharp increase after the Abortion Act of 1967. One of the targets of the Health of the Nation report was to halve the conception rate in girls under 16 by the year 2000 (DoH, 1993). Unfortunately this did not occur; despite some local benefits in improving sexual health services for young people, conception rates remained high. This failure may be attributed to the strategy of personal health services used to reduce a public health problem. Britain continues to have the highest teenage birth rate in Europe. The annual birth rate for teenagers (aged 15–19) in England and Wales was 30 per 1000 in 1997 (Office for National Statistics, 1998). Each year 90 000 teenagers become pregnant, of whom 70 000 are under 16 years of age and 2200 are girls aged 14 years and under (Turner, 1999).

Action to reduce the teenage conception rate

The Social Exclusion Unit (SEU) was commissioned by the Government to identify reasons for the high teenage pregnancy rate in England, advance recommendations for the reduction of teenage pregnancy and prescribe the way forward. After a rigorous consultation process, the SEU presented their findings, which suggested that teenagers who become pregnant tended to have low expectations of employment, were ignorant about contraception and relationship expectations, and received mixed messages from society, which they perceived to support sexual intercourse but turn away when they seek advice (SEU, 1999).

Risk factors associated with teenage pregnancies

The fetus is at increased risk of low birthweight, congenital malformation and perinatal death, which may be a consequence of low socioeconomic status, smoking, alcohol or drug abuse. Adolescent mothers may have poor dietary intake and need advice and guidance in this area, particularly if bone growth is not complete (Dunkley, 2000a). The death rate for babies of teenagers is 60% higher than for babies born of older mothers, and the incidence of low birthweight, childhood accidents and hospital admissions is also higher. Daughters of teenage mothers are also more likely to have babies during their teenage years.

The Government is committed to reducing teenage conception rates by 50% by the year 2010. Action for achievement includes:

- a national campaign involving government, media and the voluntary sector

- joined-up action, i.e. action at national and local level
- better prevention, which includes better education, and access to contraception
- a national helpline and child care support.

The midwife's role

The midwife should be sensitive to the needs and feelings of the pregnant teenager. It may be embarrassing and intimidating for the teenager to attend the antenatal clinic alongside more mature women. In some areas, midwives have set up teenage antenatal clinics and parent education classes which provide a system of peer support from other pregnant teenagers and potential for developing better social support networks. The midwife should ensure that appropriate referral systems enable teenagers to receive support from Sure Start programmes that are focused toward children under 4 and their families, providing support that meets their individual needs. Collaboration with Sure Start plus whoever provides exclusive services for pregnant teenagers across the childbirth continuum would be extremely useful.

Employment and health

For the majority of women, work during pregnancy does not pose a threat to their health or that of their babies. For some, it may be necessary to modify working practices to promote safety and comfort.

The pregnant woman should avoid heavy lifting. Seating for sedentary workers should be supportive to the back because of increased lumbar lordosis. Standing for long periods should be avoided and rest periods instituted because of the risk of development of varicosities. Smoky environments should be avoided because of the risks associated with passive smoking.

Some occupations may actually be hazardous to the health of the fetus and expectant mother, including exposure to toxic chemicals (e.g. lead and pesticides), anaesthetic gases and radiation (Bradley and Bennett, 1997). Utilization of protective clothing in the home and the workplace where appropriate, and adhering to safety parameters and work codes will minimize exposure to teratogenic hazards (Dunkley, 2000a). This makes it important for the midwife to establish the woman's normal working environment, identify any potential hazards, and provide a conduit for further information should this be required.

Travel

The midwife has a responsibility to raise awareness about travel and health. The most basic but essential information can reduce the risk of harm to the woman, fetus and infant. The Government has made a commitment to reducing the number of road traffic accidents by one-tenth by 2010 among children and young people in England. Health education during the antenatal period should include issues relating to car seats and the correct application of seat belts during pregnancy (DoH, 1999). Other travel advice given to pregnant women may need to include information about airline travel. Most airlines will not carry pregnant women after 32 weeks' gestation.

EVALUATION

Evaluation is the process by which criteria to determine the value of an idea or method are formulated. The aim of this is to demonstrate the success of the method based on designated aims and learning outcomes (Downie *et al.*, 1996).

Without the use of appropriate evaluation tools, the potential to challenge the efficacy of midwifery health promotion is reduced. Evaluation is a worthwhile process and should be used to demonstrate the impact and outcome of interventions deemed to enhance health. Knowledge about the most suitable methods of evaluation is not only essential in highlighting the most effective health interventions but also to demonstrate their efficacy to key stakeholders who influence resource allocation. Midwives may use qualitative or quantitative methods of data collection to formulate evaluation results (see Ch. 4).

Health promotion evaluation can be extremely difficult for the midwife, particularly when assessing long-term success of a health intervention or behaviour change. Other areas that present challenges in terms of evaluation include, awareness raising and empowerment.

> **Reflective Activity 21.4**
>
> Consider your own practice. There may be areas in which you have gathered considerable information and experience. How would you structure and evaluate this information to, for example, apply for a different role in your maternity service?

CONCLUSION

Health promotion is an integral part of the midwife's role, with many potential health-gain benefits for the childbearing population. Understanding the context of health and illness is a key factor in promoting health, and choosing the appropriate health promotion approach to achieve the desired aim is essential if the health promotion approach is to be effective. The midwives' scope of practice provides room for the public health role to be enhanced and community initiatives to be embraced. The midwife is a vital resource in terms of advice and information on diet, smoking and exercise,

and may be a useful means of promoting a healthy lifestyle. The woman may look at her midwife as a role model, and her attitudes and activities may carry as much weight as her words.

The current political health agenda recognizes the valuable contribution midwives make to the health of the nation. Rigorous robust evaluation of all health promotion activities will provide evidence of the impact of the midwife's work in terms of health gain.

KEY POINTS

- The concept of health and the meaning of health promotion are fundamental to the role of the midwife.
- The midwife needs to be aware of her own attitudes, behaviours and understanding of health in order to develop an effective health promotion approach to apply to midwifery practice.

- The midwife should expand her knowledge of women's health and screening to enable her to meet the public health agenda.
- It is important to provide realistic and appropriate health promotion strategies, and develop a mechanism for evaluation of their effectiveness.

REFERENCES

Acheson, D. (Chair) (1998) *Independent Inquiry into Inequalities in Health*. London: The Stationery Office.

American College of Obstetricians and Gynecologists (ACOG) (1994) *Exercise During Pregnancy and the Postpartum Period*. Technical Bulletin No. 189: 65–70. Washington DC: ACOG.

Baddeley, S. (1999) *Health Related Fitness During Pregnancy*. Wiltshire: Quay Books.

Becker, M.H., Haefner, D.P., Kasl, S.V. *et al.* (1977) Selected psycho-social models and correlates of individual heath-related behaviours. *Medical Care* **15**(5): 27–46.

Bewley, C.A. & Gibbs, A. (1997) The role of the midwife. In: Bewley, S., Friend, J. & Mezey, G. (eds) *Violence Against Women*, pp. 199–210. London: RCOG Press.

Black, D., Morris, J.N., Smith, C. *et al.* (1982) *Inequalities in Health: the Black Report*. Harmondsworth: Penguin.

BMRB Social Research (2001) *Infant Feeding 2000*. London: Department of Health.

Bradley, S. & Bennett, N. (1997) *Preparation for Pregnancy: an Essential Guide*. Scotland: Argyll Publishers.

British Medical Association (BMA) and Royal Pharmaceutical Society of Great Britain (RPSGB) (2003) *British National Formulary*, 46th edn. London: BMA and RPSGB.

Callum, C. (1998) *The United Kingdom Smoking Epidemic: Deaths in 1995*. London: Health Education Authority.

Chang, G., Wilkins-Haug, L., Berman, S. *et al.* (1998) Alcohol use and pregnancy: improving identification. *Obstetrics and Gynecology* **91**(6): 892–898.

Clapp, J.F. (2000) Exercise during pregnancy. A clinical update. *Clinics in Sports Medicine* **19**(2): 273–286.

Department for Education and Employment (DfEE) (2000) *Sure Start: a Guide*. London: DfEE.

Department of Health (DoH) (1993) *The Health of the Nation. Targeting Practice: the Contribution of Nurses, Midwives and Health Visitors*. London: DoH.

Department of Health (DoH) (1999) *Saving Lives: Our Healthier Nation: a Contract for Health*. London: The Stationery Office.

Department of Health (DoH) (2000) *Domestic Violence: a Resource Manual for Health Care Professionals*. London: NHS Executive.

Department of Health (DoH) (2003) *Delivering the Best; Midwives Contribution to the NHS Plan*. London: DoH.

Department of Health (DoH) and the Welsh Office (1994) *Gypsy Sites Policy and Unauthorised Camping*. DOE 18/94 and WO 76/94. London: HMSO.

Dewan, N., Brabin, B., Wood, L. *et al.* (2003) The effects of smoking on birthweight for gestational age curves in teenage and adult primigravidae. *Public Health* **117**: 31–35.

Dollberg, S., Fainaru, O., Mimouni, F.B. *et al.* (2000) The effect of passive smoking in pregnancy on neonatal nucleated red blood cells. *Paediatrics* **106**(3): E34.

Downie, R.S., Tannahill, C. & Tannahill, A. (1996) *Health Promotion Models and Values*, 2nd edn. New York: Oxford University Press.

Dunkley, J. (2000a) *Health Promotion in Midwifery Practice a Resource for Health Professionals.* Edinburgh: Baillière Tindall.

Dunkley, J. (2000b) The health promoting role of the midwife. *MIDIRS Midwifery Digest* 10(4): 430–434.

Ewles, L., Simnett, I. (1998) *Promoting Health, a Practical Guide,* 4th edn. London: Baillière Tindall.

Foster, K., Lader, D. & Cheesborough, S. (1997) *Infant Feeding 1995.* London: The Stationery Office.

Gaines, K. (1997) Abuse and pregnancy: What every childbirth educator/nurse should know. *Journal of Perinatal Education* 6(4): 28–39.

Gilbert, E.S. & Harman, J.S. (1998) *High Risk Pregnancy and Delivery,* 2nd edn. USA: Mosby.

Gunning-Schepers, L.J. & Gepkens, A. (1996) Review of interventions to reduce social inequalities in health: research and policy implications. *Health Education Journal* 55: 226–238.

Home Office (1998) *Supporting Families.* London: The Stationery Office.

Kealy, L. (1999) Women refugees lack access to reproductive health service. *Population Today* 7(1): 1–2.

Lancaster, T., Silagy, C. & Fowler, G. (2000) Training health professionals in smoking cessation. *Cochrane Database of Systematic Reviews* (3): CD000214. Oxford: Update Software.

Lewis, G. (ed) (2001) *Why Mothers Die 1997–99: Fifth Report of the Confidential Enquiries into Maternal Deaths in the United Kingdom.* London: CEMD: associated with NICE, RCOG.

Lindley, A.A., Becker, S., Gray, R.H. *et al.* (2000) Effect of continuing or stopping smoking during pregnancy. *American Journal of Epidemiology* 152(3): 219–225.

Lux, A.L., Henderson, A.J. & Pocock, S.J. (2000) Wheeze associated with prenatal tobacco smoke exposure: a prospective, longitudinal study. ALSPAC Study Team. *Archives of Disease in Childhood* 83(4): 307–312.

Martin, S.L., English, K.T., Anderson, K. *et al.* (1996) Violence and substance use among North Carolina pregnant women. *American Journal of Public Health* 6(7): 991–998.

Maryland Department of Health (2001) Pregnancy associated homicide. *Journal of the American Medical Association* 285: 1444–1449.

Mayer, L. & Liebschutz, J. (1998) Domestic violence in the pregnant patient: Obstetric and behavioural interventions. *Obstetrics and Gynaecology Survey* 53(10): 627–635.

Mezey, G.C. (1997) Domestic violence in pregnancy. In: Bewley, S., Friend, J. & Mezey, G. (eds) *Violence Against Women,* pp. 77–85. London: RCOG Press.

Office for National Statistics (1998) *Review of the Registrar General on Births and Patterns of Family Building in England and Wales.* London: The Stationery Office.

Prochaska, J., Diclemente, C. & Norcoss, C. (1993) In search of how people change: applications to addictive behaviours. *Addictions Nursing Network* 5(1): 3–16.

Roberts, H. (2000) What is Sure Start? *Archives of Disease in Childhood* 82: 435–436.

Rotter, J.B. (1966) Generalized expectancies for internal versus external control of re-enforcement. *Psychological Monographs* 80: 1–28.

Royal College of Midwives (RCM) (1999) *Position Paper: Domestic Abuse in Pregnancy.* London: RCM.

Royal College of Midwives (RCM) (2000) *Vision 2000.* London: RCM.

Royal College of Midwives (RCM) (2001) *Position Paper: The Midwife's Role in Public Health.* London: RCM.

Royal College of Obstetricians and Gynaecologists (RCOG) (1999) *Alcohol Consumption in Pregnancy Guideline.* London: RCOG.

Secretary of State for Health (1998) *Smoking Kills.* London: The Stationery Office.

Secretary of State for Health (2000) *The NHS Plan: a Plan for Investments. A Plan for Reform.* Cm4818-1. London: The Stationery Office.

Seedhouse, D. (1997) *Health Promotion Philosophy, Prejudice and Practice.* Chichester: John Wiley.

Social Exclusion Unit (SEU) (1999) *Teenage Pregnancy.* London: The Stationery Office.

Sokol, R.J., Martier, S.S. & Ager, J.W. (1989) The T-ACE questions: Practical prenatal detection of risk-drinking. *American Journal Obstetrics and Gynecology* 160: 863–870.

Stoler, J. & Holmes, L. (1999) Under-recognition of prenatal alcohol effects in infants of known alcohol abusing women. *Journal of Paediatrics* 135(4): 405–406.

Tannahill, A. (1985) What is health promotion? *Health Education Journal* 44: 167–168.

Turner, T. (1999) Too much too young. *Community Practitioner* 72(7): 196–197.

Walton, I. (1994) *Sexuality and Motherhood.* Books for Midwives Press: Hale.

Wardlow, G. (2000) *Contemporary Nutrition: Issues and Insights,* 4th edn. USA: McGraw Hill Higher Education.

Watts, S. (1998) *What are Effective Health Care Interventions in Response to the Needs of Victims of Domestic Violence?* Policy report prepared for MSc in Public Health. London: London School of Hygiene and Tropical Medicine.

Wisborg, K., Kesmodel, U., Henriksen, T.B. *et al.* (2000) A prospective study of smoking during pregnancy and SIDS. *Archives of Disease in Childhood* 83(3): 203–206.

World Health Organization (WHO) (1946) *Constitution.* New York: WHO.

World Health Organization (WHO) (1984) *Health Promotion: a Discussion Document on Concepts and Principle.* Geneva: WHO.

FURTHER READING

Dunkley, J. (2000) *Health Promotion in Midwifery: A Resource for Health Professionals*. Edinburgh: Baillière Tindall.
This text provides a comprehensive practical guide to health promotion in midwifery practice. Chapter 3 provides an overview of behaviour change theories.

Royal College of Midwives (RCM) (2002) *Helping Women Stop Smoking: a Guide for Midwives*. London: RCM.
This guide provides a useful resource package for midwives and other health professions and includes strategies for smoking cessation and supporting women.

Siney, C. (ed) (1999) *Pregnancy and Drug Misuse*. Hale: Books for Midwives Press.
This comprehensive text explores the management of drug-dependent women. Main features include medical and obstetric problems of mothers, the consequences for the child and outreach and counselling work.

ADDITIONAL RESOURCES

http://www.rcm.org.uk/
The website of the Royal College of Midwives – source of the most up-to-date midwifery issues, and a range of 'position papers' and other resources.

22

Education for Parenthood

Tandy Deane-Gray

LEARNING OUTCOMES

After reading this chapter you will be able to:

- define and focus a personal definition of parent education and parenting education in the light of current trends, to provide strength and direction for practice
- explore ways and methods of incorporating parenting skills into programmes delivered to parents
- utilize a range of formal and informal approaches to support and develop parents' understanding of

pregnancy, childbirth and neonatal care during the period of care
- outline the Government's initiatives that influence the provision of parent education
- practice appropriately in the delivery of parent education and leading of groups.

Parenting is one of the most important and challenging tasks that most of us will embark upon during our lives. To enable parents in their obligations, parents must be supported by society so they can fulfil their role with sufficient knowledge, understanding and enjoyment (Pugh *et al.*, 1994). Parents are the most important educator in any person's life and receive little support or training, yet they get most of the blame when things go wrong.

Reflective Activity 22.1

What do you see as the essential and desirable characteristics of a parent? Where do these skills get learned and developed?

If the job of parent were to be advertised, the advertisement might read:

A responsible person, male or female, to undertake a lifelong project. Candidates should be totally committed, willing to work up to 24 hours daily, including weekends during the initial 16-year period. Occasional holiday possible, but may be cancelled at no notice. Knowledge of health care, nutrition, psychology, child development, household management, and the educational system essential. Necessary skills: stress management and conflict resolution, problem solving, communication and listening, budgeting and time management, decision making, ability to set boundaries and priorities as well as providing loving support. Necessary qualities: energy, tolerance, patience, good self-esteem, self-confidence, and a sense of humour. No training or experience needed. No salary but very rewarding work for the right person.

(Pugh *et al.*, 1994)

The importance of work with parents cannot be overestimated. However, some of the assumptions underlying this quotation affect the people working with parents, particularly that the job of being a parent is self-evident; hence the neglect of coherent training for parents. Midwives are in a privileged position to support and work with parents during their transition to parenthood, particularly for those with little or no experience of parenting, but also for more experienced parents who may still need support and guidance with a new and/or needy baby. The Government's public health initiatives are congruent with roles which many midwives have undertaken for many years, but provide a fresh focus, and a new understanding of the importance of facilitating parenting skills, summed up by the term *parenting skills* rather than *parentcraft*

(RCM and DoH, 2000). The midwife works in partnership with other practitioners such as the health visitor, working towards a seamless provision of this aspect of care.

WHAT IS PARENT EDUCATION?

Reflective Activity 22.2

How would you define parent education? Is it about parenting classes? Talking to women during their antenatal examinations? Supervising parents doing tasks such as mixing and preparing a bottle feed? Think about some of the attributes you thought of earlier – how do these fit with your definitions?

To clarify what is meant by the terms, the current definitions will be discussed.

Parentcraft evolved to fulfil two main functions (Williams and Booth, 1980). Firstly, women were given instructions on hygiene and baby care, as an attempt to improve perinatal and maternal mortality. Secondly, they were given theoretical and practical training in preparation for labour, focused on the alleviation of pain, often using approaches such as psychoprophylaxis. This was provided by a childbirth trainer who was an 'expert' authority on preparation for childbirth.

Educating for healthy habits was indeed desirable; however, one of the benefits of parentcraft (as seen by a medical approach to childbirth) was that it increased client compliance. Parentcraft was taught in such a way that it was not uncommon for women to believe that an enema and shave were necessary prior to delivery. Fortunately, research-based practice has led to a questioning of care, with the move to a more client-centred approach (DoH, 1993).

Increasingly it has been recognized that emotional as well as physical needs should be addressed during sessions. The trend in classes is now to concentrate less on the 'craft' and more on sharing feelings, emotions and experiences, and 'parent education' has become the preferred term.

Crisp (1994) defines parent education and parenting education in the following paragraphs.

Parent Education began as antenatal education, education in preparation for birth, in the early part of this century. Today this is provided almost exclusively through the health service, with the main voluntary organisation providing services being the NCT. ... The classes concentrate on the physical aspects of pregnancy and care of baby. However, users of both statutory and voluntary services have also identified the opportunity to meet other parents as the main reason for attending classes.

Parenting education differs ... because its focus is on family relationships rather than physical care. It is mainly provided through the voluntary sector. Many of the areas explored within parenting education, such as stress management and negotiation, assertiveness and communication skills, are frequently provided by adult education classes. ... Parenting education builds on parents' own skills and abilities, rather than relying on the professional expert to tell parents what to do.

(Crisp, 1994)

Reflective Activity 22.3

Are these understandings of parenting education included in the classes provided in your area or unit? How could you include these features during a session or series of sessions?

There is a subtle difference between parent education and parenting, which includes stress management and negotiation, assertiveness and communication skills. But, also, parenting classes rely less on the 'telling expert', and more on building parents' own abilities and skills. One example is of relaxation, which has traditionally been taught as part of parentcraft as a way of coping with the stress of labour. A more useful approach is to view relaxation as an important means of stress management, and as a vital technique to utilize in a variety of different ways in daily life. This does require a different approach in teaching relaxation, and a move from teaching it in a quiet room with mats on the floor, to teaching women and their partners the skills in more realistic surroundings, and encouraging them to practice the skills whilst coping with a crying or fretful baby, or coping with being in a car in a traffic jam.

It could be argued that parenting skills can be part of parent education, and indeed a few midwives are practising in this way. But as Nolan's (1995) discussion paper identifies, many antenatal classes are inadequate in terms of realistic preparation for parenthood. Yet, contrary to popular belief, parents can see beyond labour. Grimshaw and McGuire (1998) found that parents were motivated to attend groups to break the mould of parenting set in their own childhood, to access support from other parents, and to gain ideas from which to choose to use if they want to.

Critiques of parent education (Coombes and Schonveld, 1992; Perkins, 1980) have suggested for the last two decades that those who facilitate parent education, have poor knowledge of teaching and poor facilitation of parent's emotional needs. Underdown (1998) pointed out that the teaching of group work skills is not a required part of the Midwifery or Health Visiting programmes. She found staff considered they had learned their skills by practical observation and training from their placement mentors, thus perpetuating a style of delivery that is directive rather than facilitative. Sadly, parent education is poorly delivered and is not necessarily given a priority in the provision of services for parents, which is contrary to the present Government initiatives (RCM and DoH, 2000).

GOVERNMENT INITIATIVES

Government initiates which sought to support and intervene in parenting occurred because of the dramatic changing social circumstances for families, which frequently put parenting under pressure. In the family today:

- Lone parenting is increasing and they are likely to be living in poverty.
- Child poverty has tripled since 1968.
- Childhood death has reduced in comparison with Europe, but it is still high.
- Poor children are four times more likely to die in an accident than those from affluent families.
- 20% of the UK's children and young people have mental health problems.
- Smoking and drinking alcohol is rising in young people.
- Every day one baby will be born to a notified drug user.
- The number of children and young people in prison is increasing.

(Kaufmann and Whelan, 1999)

The International Year of the Family in 1994 saw the setting up of the Parenting Education and Support Forum which would act as 'a focus for information and support, for debate, to support those working in the field, to network and to influence policy by building on good practice' (Pugh, 1999). Following this,

the Government agenda became focused on families and children.

The Government's consultative document 'Supporting Families' (Home Office, 1998) gave parenting education high priority, by identifying five main areas within the proposals:

- *Ensuring families have access to advice and support;* which led to the development of a national parenting helpline, The National Family and Parenting Institute, which replaced the Parenting Education and Support Forum. There was also an investment of £540 million on the initiation of 'Sure Start schemes'.
- *Better financial support for families;* which led to the Working Families Tax Credit, New Deal for Lone Parents and reform of the Child Support Agency.
- *Helping families balance work and home;* which brought the UK more into line with Europe in enabling employed parents to access parental leave.
- *Strengthening marriage;* which emphasized developing supporting relationships and reducing conflict in relationship breakdown.
- *Better support for serious family problems;* which covered dealing with truancy and school exclusion, work with children with behavioural problems, domestic violence, youth offending and teenage pregnancy.

Sure Start initiatives (DfEE, 1999) focused on early intervention and support for families with children under 3 years in 250 high-need areas. These are grounded in evidence from attachment theory, child development, and support of families in the community. All these services are directed towards the reduction of family breakdown, readiness of children for school, and in the long term prevention of social exclusion, regeneration of communities, and reduction of crime (Pugh, 1999).

Parenting education has been identified as a means of preventing difficulties in areas ranging from marital breakdown to juvenile crime, derived from evidence from several studies. The HighScope study is perhaps most widely quoted as it demonstrated that for every $1 spent $7 was saved in welfare costs (Schweinhart and Weikart, 1993). Pugh *et al.* (1994) state that evaluating the cost is not straightforward as each parent's needs are different. Prevention is difficult to identify as savings, because causal links are involved and complex. However, if crime alone is examined, a saving of £18 billion per year to the cost of the NHS could be realized.

In the UK, the Parents In Partnership – Parent Infant Network (PIPPIN) programme (Parr, 1996), which has a focus on parent–parent and parent–infant relationships, costs £100 per couple. It is currently the only such parenting programme that begins in the antenatal period.

The expenditure on education and support for parents is generally minimal. The report 'Life will never be the same again' (Coombes and Schonveld, 1992) criticized the managers of parenthood educators, reporting that support was lacking in key areas of training development and resources. This Government's white paper (DoH, 1999) has removed the internal market, though the funding for parent education in the health service is not clearly defined; but is simply part of antenatal care.

Parent education should be seen as part of a lifelong journey, and as a means of helping parents acquire understanding of their own social, emotional and psychological needs and those of their children. This would enhance relationships within the family, and also allow families to identify and take advantage of supportive networks within local communities (Smith, 1997). The Government have also recognized that fathers have a crucial role to play in their children's upbringing and the particular importance of their involvement to their sons.

Most parenting programmes use group work, and this could be more effectively facilitated in parent education.

PARENT EDUCATION AND GROUP WORK

More use of group work has been advocated for parent education (Coombes and Schonveld, 1992; Underdown, 1998), though it seems that the most favoured method of teaching is still the lecture. Most parent educators will begin their session with a short lecture, followed by a video and/or a discussion. Unfortunately it is hard to promote interaction on emotional and social issues using this approach. In a study on an evaluation of a group skills training course for antenatal educationalists, it was found that 'the teacher talked for about four-fifths of the class, the mothers contributed to less than one fifth, and the remainder of the time was spent in silence or confusion' (Murphy-Black and Faulkner, 1990).

Underdown (1998) found in her observation study of 10 midwives that 90% of classes were directive in approach, showing a high level of teacher input, and a low level of acceptance of ideas, behaviours and feelings. More than 75% of questions used were closed

and 78% of responses were restricted. This examination of the amount the leader speaks in relation to the group members is a useful indicator for all those delivering parent education.

Reflective Activity 22.4

Think about the last parenting session you led. How did you structure the session? What were the methods and approaches you used? For what sort of percentage of the time of a class did the clients talk? What do you think would have increased this percentage?

In exploring the ratio of time that the facilitator speaks to the time clients speak, if this mirrors the previous research, it may be that further development in group work skills are needed to be able to provide effective parent education programmes that can facilitate parents in their life journey.

There are many advantages of learning in groups. Group discussion helps to explore and clarify issues, clear up misunderstandings and resolve problems. There are also the social benefits; as group cohesion is established, mutual support is nurtured and group members are able to support each other rather than relying on the leader. Skilful, democratic leadership can promote a heightened sense of sensitivity to others within the group and a greater tolerance of other viewpoints. Motivation to learn is increased and parents develop insights into their own feelings and behaviours and those of others. All these factors help to promote effective learning in groups.

Burnard (1995) argues that 'much of what we need to know … is grounded in our own personal experience; we do not have to be taught it'. The implication is that the parent learners must be acknowledged as adults who bring a wealth of life experience to the group encounter. This should be identified and made relevant to the learners' educational development.

In this situation the teacher cannot claim full control but is a joint shareholder with the learner. The teacher adopts a non-directive role and aims to 'make it possible (through an enabling process) for another person to achieve goals' (Craddock, 1993). This is what is truly meant by facilitation.

Some of the characteristics of facilitation include:

- parent learners are entrusted with the responsibility for their own learning
- learning activities are centred on the needs of the parent learners; this means that the parent learner is

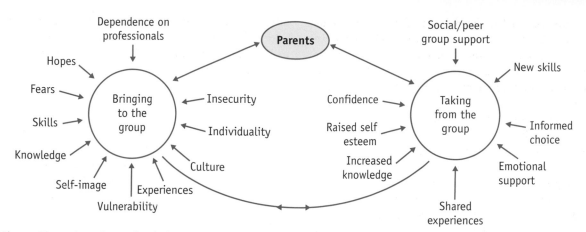

Figure 22.1 On-going cycle of what parents bring to and take from groups. (Based on Leslie-Green and Reavill, 1989, with permission of Central Nottinghamshire Healthcare (NHS) Trust.)

an equal partner in the planning and implementation of learning activities

- strategies or facilitation methods are geared to enquiry and discovery learning
- a role change or reversal can be observed with the facilitator becoming a senior learner and gaining as much from the encounter as the parent learner
- the focus shifts from controlling to fostering a behaviour where the emphasis is on building relationships, assessment of needs, encouraging independence of learning and providing an environment where individual differences are tolerated and positively encouraged.

(Honey, 1991)

These characteristics are congruent with adult learning theory, but do require a fundamental mental and cultural shift within power relationships. However, a more facilitative approach is more likely to result in the parent learners being able to:

- think for themselves
- develop curiosity and willingness to explore
- take account of all available relevant evidence before coming to conclusions
- develop creativity
- have the confidence to speculate without reliance on an expert telling them what to do
- achieve a degree of self-fulfilment.

These are the behaviours a parent educator should strive to facilitate in parent learners. It also implies that a more social model of care is adopted as the 'medical information' is less important and the parents' experiences are the focus. Parents as adult learners bring their previous knowledge and life experience

to a group as well as take from the group, as illustrated in Figure 22.1.

In order for parents to bring and share information as well as receiving from the group, the group needs to be client centred. An important factor in facilitating groups is the use of teaching methods that promote group sharing. A brief description of some of the appropriate methods are outlined here.

Buzz groups

Parents are asked to discuss a topic/issue in small groups of about three and then feed back to the whole group. An example might be what the parents' baby might look like. This method can also be used for negotiating the course content. In this way even the less-confident members of the group will contribute.

Quizzes

A fun set of questions can act as an icebreaker. Stocktaking worksheets can provide a starter for discussion. For example, to begin an infant feeding discussion, a list of questions on the facts, feelings and myths of breastfeeding can be posed, then responses shared with other members of the group. Another example might be who does what in the home before and after the arrival of the baby.

Stories and scenarios

These are used as case studies, and the facilitator can build up a 'library' of fictitious ones. Parts of the story are distributed and the parents are asked to discuss the circumstances. When they have discussed the situation fully, the next part of the story is given. This helps parents to consider realistic situations, test out ideas and explore attitudes. Topics that might suit this method include labour, or postnatal depression.

Problem solving

Realistic problems are posed for small groups of parents to solve. Examples of topics are: 'You have been told your breast milk is too thin. What do you do?'; 'Your baby only sleeps 2 hours at a time and is now 6 weeks old. What do you do?' This approach encourages self-direction and self-investigation of resources available.

Snowballing

The facilitator chooses a topic for discussion, and asks the group to discuss the topic in pairs, which then are grouped into fours, eights and even 16. Each stage has a discussion task, which builds on the one before. An example might be a discussion about pain and coping in labour. Individually, the parents are asked to consider their most painful experience. Then they share it with the person next to them and discuss their reactions to pain and physiological response. In groups of four, the parents then discuss labour and how they intend to cope with pain. If they have read about pharmacological methods prior to the session they can clarify their ideas with other parents. This is a good method of getting a quiet or reserved group to get to know one another.

Games

For parenthood education a variety of games has been developed to explore many topics. A popular variation is the 'grab bag', in which a selection of items of equipment used in labour (either real or cardboard cut-outs) are placed in a bag. Participants dip in the bag, pull out an item or piece of equipment (an amnihook, or a pair of shorts, for example), identify it and then discuss the item – what it might mean for them and their feelings. There are also a range of 'ice breaker' games which may be useful in establishing interaction and relationships between participants during the first few sessions.

With all these methods, facilitators need to be mindful of not answering all the questions themselves. Often because health professionals are used to giving information and advice, they automatically feed the information to parents. The skill of facilitation is to use communication skills that move the topic around the group, and the facilitator should develop a range of prompts to assist this:

- What happened during the activity?
- Thank you for that Mary. What do you think about this issue Jane?
- How did you feel?
- How does that fit with what I was saying?
- Can someone help me explain this?
- For you breastfeeding would be inconvenient for your lifestyle, I wonder if anyone else has a similar or different view?
- I can hear that there is a disagreement, is there some common ground we can agree on?
- I notice that the group feeling is that epidurals are scary, could you say more about that?
- If you were to come to a compromise, what would it be?
- I notice that several members have been quiet for some time now and others have a lot to say, and there is a difficulty in focusing on the topic tonight. I am wondering what the group want to do?
- Does anyone have a different point of view to those expressed so far?

These statements are some possible examples of moving the topic around the group, which also acknowledge some feelings and manage disagreements that are not unusual in open discussions.

Problems may arise in groups, and a skilful group leader should be perceptive to feelings and situations, and thus be both participant and observer. Occasionally there are one or two people who monopolize or dominate the group and this can give rise to feelings of frustration in other group members, especially if the facilitator does not intervene. Intervention may take the form of thanking the vocal parent for her or his contributions and then making it clear that you would like to give others the opportunity to express their views.

Another problem, which may occur, is a low level of participation from the group as a whole. This could be in response to a rather autocratic style of leadership, in which case the midwife needs to review her approach as a facilitator. Other reasons include talking about issues that are frightening, or seem irrelevant and unimportant to the group; or perhaps there is some conflict amongst members which has not been resolved. There are often one or two quiet or inarticulate members of a group who feel uncomfortable if forced to contribute to discussion before they feel ready, although they usually participate in work in pairs, buzz groups or other small group sessions.

The group process

Using methods that encourage small group work will help everyone to participate, and the start of this process lies in encouraging participation within a group of strangers. Utilizing 'icebreakers' will require some time, but can help with the initial difficulties, and will ensure that the participants get to know each other, and are more likely to continue to attend and fully participate in the parenting sessions.

In the first session it is useful to avoid sensitive topics until the parents know each other. The better people know one another, the more comfortable is the group. Asking people to give their names in turn can be threatening and may be ineffective for learning, particularly in groups larger than six (Brown, 1992). There are many exercises described for name games in Brandes' *The Gamesters Handbook* (1, 2 & 3) (1998), or Priest and Schott's *Leading Antenatal Classes* (1991), or Nolan's *Antenatal Education* (1998). The snowball method (as described earlier) can be used to warm up the group: first, two people introduce themselves to each other; then they build into fours to introduce the persons who have just met to the two joining. If there are men present, it is useful to have the same gender talking to each other, as their needs differ.

Edwards and Nichols (2000) adapt the Stanford and Roark model of group life to parent education. The process begins with a warm-up, proceeds to a middle work phase and ends with integration. In the warm-up phase the parent learners disengage from previous activities and tune in to the new situation. The work phase is where learning takes place and the parents focus on the task. The last integration phase requires reflection on personal meaning, integrating the understanding, significance and usefulness of the session for the future. These phases will be used to discuss the management and cooperation of groups.

Warm-up phase   This phase focuses attention on the group, providing a bridge between 'job' and group. The leader needs to get group members 'settled down' and 'tuned in' to the group. A low-threat beginning to each session contributes to continued building of the group (Edwards and Nichols, 2000). The leader could begin the session with an icebreaker and work with the group to develop group ground rules, and indeed a framework for the course. The leader could divide the group into smaller groups of six to eight people and invite them to brainstorm their hopes and fears for the course, or problems that might face them as parents. These will assist the group in beginning to move the focus of the group to the progress being made.

Work phase   During this phase, the topics to be covered during a session need to be structured by the leader. This work phase of the session incorporates the teaching plan, which includes a good structure and examination of the events occurring during learning (Frederick, 2000). The planning of an educational encounter is by necessity a dual responsibility – that of the teacher and the learners. However, a certain amount of decision making needs to be done by the leader. Obviously the needs of the parents and what parents bring to a group as in Figure 22.1, will form the basis of the objectives for the group. It is important to gain agreement from the parents so they feel committed to the session.

Group size may influence the choice of activity, but dividing the group into pairs enables parents to work with different people. This allows them to explore other views and work with all the members of the group (Rolls, 1992). Forming subgroups requires thought as to the balance and mix in terms of gender, ability and social status. For example, it may be important in one activity to have men working together, but, on another occasion an integrated group of men and women would be more appropriate. Mixing can be facilitated by asking members of the group to find someone wearing the same colour, with the same colour eyes, or perhaps finding the person with the nearest expected date of delivery to work with.

To get cooperation from the learners it is useful to share why the activity is useful and what is expected to be drawn from the experience. Some activities are easily explained verbally, but occasionally written instruction is helpful as back-up. Instructions may need repeating two or three times as it helps people to internalize what is being asked of them. Parents should be organized as required for the exercise chosen, and understanding checked before they begin the exercise. Before moving on, the facilitator should ensure that the group as individuals have completed the exercise to their satisfaction. This will provide a link to the next piece of work, or to an evaluation.

It is important that prior to selecting activities the facilitator considers any possible threat to self-esteem for individual members, and works to build on the existing knowledge of the parents. This will require a good deal of flexibility, as the facilitator may begin the session with one plan which has to be altered should the participants require more or less time or discussion than originally thought. It is useful to have a plan which allows for this, and have some 'spare' activities or discussion items as well as a varied format to take into account the energy and concentration levels.

Activities should direct the attention of the parents to achieve the task. During the activity the leader needs to watch, give attention to what is going on, use appropriate communication interventions, and manage time, thus promoting group participation. Generally the group leader manages the continuing tension between the task and group maintenance, keeping the boundaries for the members (Henderson, 1989). The relationship between the task and the individual is balanced with the building of the group as shown in Figure 22.2.

Integration phase   This phase is more than the end of the session. It is the achievement phase for the parents. The leader encourages and validates learning by giving feedback on aspects of performance and correction of misconceptions. It is useful to ask the parents

themselves what they have achieved at the end of a session, or simply summarize the session. Providing opportunities to rehearse the application of learning enhances retention of learning (Frederick, 2000). For example, after identifying the signs of labour, parents can be given a scenario of ruptured membranes in the supermarket. Parents could speculate on how their knowledge of coping with pain might have changed the way in which they coped in the past.

> ### Reflective Activity 22.5
>
> Find out some possible ice-breaker activities. Which activities would you use for your next session? Try one out at your next session, and consider how effective it is in getting the group 'warmed up'.

What should be the content of parent education programmes?

Currently most UK parenting programmes contain an integration of psychological approaches and have four key elements (Pugh, 1999):

- information
- skills learning
- sharing experiences
- opportunities to reflect on the past.

These key elements would be useful for any learning group as they address the three domains of learning:

- affective – feelings and attitudes
- skills – doing physical tasks
- knowledge – information and thinking.

These domains of the affective, skills and knowledge (ASK) are what define learning (Jarvis, 1995). A parent education session should therefore have a balance of the three domains of learning. Using them to consider content will encourage the full potential of parent learners. Also, any programme that is negotiated with parents is more likely to meet their needs.

A parent educator is unlikely to be able to solve all the problems of parents, or meet all their identified needs. This is becoming increasingly difficult as the number and length of classes are being reduced, and therefore parents' needs require prioritizing. This requires a process of needs identification by the facilitator and parents, and a plan of how these needs might best be met. Parents can thus be well supported and, should they require more information, directed to additional resources, and guided as to the best use of

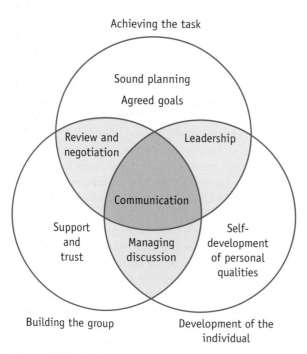

Figure 22.2   Activities contributing to development of groups. (Based on Rolls, 1992, with permission of the Health Education Authority.)

these by the facilitator. Giving information in advance of the group, by offering the loan of a book or video, or asking parents to do 'homework' of reading about a topic will often be a good way of directing the parents' learning, and may also save some time. Setting priorities without being biased about what you think they need to know (and feeling you must tell them all of it) is often difficult, but the learning is ultimately the responsibility of the parents.

Reflective Activity 22.6

How can priorities be set? To answer this, a brainstorm of educational needs must be prioritized.

Below are some educational needs of clients. Give each need a priority, listing it as 1 = high; 2 = moderate; 3 = low.

Information about obstetric care

Feelings of being unable to cope, stressed, and emotional

Work-related issues, hazards, posture, rest, maternity benefits

Physical discomforts, minor disorders of ante- or postpartum period

Issues which have influence on health, e.g. diet, smoking, alcohol, exercises

Behavioural skills, assertiveness, communication

Potential health problems, obesity, or HIV

How the body works, e.g. physiology of breastfeeding

In reviewing these priorities, it may be found that because of the influences of the origins of parent education the answers are favouring the process of childbirth and hygiene (Williams and Booth, 1980). Of course, all of the educational needs are important; perhaps the answer lies in the priority for the client.

Often, parenting sessions have been designed around what professionals think women and their partners need to know, and some programmes have a traditional structure, often centred on antenatal and labour issues, with some focus on infant care and feeding.

It is probable that this structure does not meet parents' needs, and the facilitator needs to consider a more flexible and consumer-focused programme, which would better fit the many and varied needs of women and their families in preparing for the transition to parenthood in the UK today.

The facilitator therefore needs to consider how best to conduct the session, what would be the proposed

structure and sequence and appropriate content for the women and partners in the client group being invited to the sessions. For example, the needs, content and delivery of material for a group of pregnant teenagers may be very different from those needed for a group of refugee women being taught with the support of a link worker or translator.

What is important is that the structure developed should provide the parents with a 'map' so that they can see where the session is taking them (Johnson, 1996). Organizing the content is often summarized by the following saying:

Tell 'em what you're going to tell 'em;
tell 'em;
then, tell 'em what you've told them.

This suggests the structure of the session has an introduction, middle and conclusion. The main section can be thought of as key points. The points can then be used as the main discussion and then drawn together in the conclusion of the session as in Table 22.1.

Before undertaking any form of teaching it is expected that the teacher understands the subject, and has a clear idea of the depth and breadth of the topic (Johnson, 1996). Any evidence or information presented should be critically appraised (Johnson, 1996). Schott's (1995) article entitled 'Cancel the labour talk' highlights the danger of overloading parents with the breadth and depth of information. Appropriate appraisal and selection of information to be presented to parents is vital to planning and preparation. Parents come from all sectors of society and will expect educators to have a depth of knowledge that will include the need for a literature search prior to teaching. It is also important to reflect on the session, and incorporate an evaluation of both the 'performance' and the achievement of the group outcomes in order to validate what has worked well, and what requires further development for the future.

The far-reaching changes within the family have led to parenting being high on the professional and political agenda. In many ways there is a great potential for midwives to have a key position in supporting families in their transition to parenthood. In order to achieve the most effective result, midwives need to be knowledgeable and up to date in the knowledge and information they are sharing; flexible and innovative in the way they share that knowledge and support parents; and committed to a continual process of reflection, evaluation and development.

Table 22.1 Structuring a parent education session

Prior to the session
What is the purpose of this session?
What do the parents want/need?
Do my needs match parents' needs? = Your *aims* for the session
What will the parents be able to do at the end of the session? = Your *objectives/outcomes* for the session

Phase of group	Possible ways of delivery	What the parents are doing
Beginning: warm-up (tell them what you are going to tell them)	Welcome/icebreaker – refreshments, toilets, etc. Set ground rules Develop programme with the group Address any issues from last week	Settling down Feeling they belong Beginning to work, taste topic
Middle: work phase (tell them, let them tell you, and listen)	Introduction/explain topic Group work on topic Facilitate discussion Break Trigger for a related or new topic Parents discuss Activity in which they participate Debrief/feedback	Parents engage with information and think for themselves Leader checks information, noticing how much parents talk Focus on new aspect, e.g. feelings on topic. Sharing experiences. Opportunities to reflect on the past Skills learning. Parents learn by doing
End: integration and conclusion	Evaluate: ask them to state what was achieved	Assimilate their learning Reinforce with hand-out
Prepare for next week	Summarize the session. Suggest reading for topic next week	Parents read pregnancy book during the week

KEY POINTS

- Midwives are in a privileged position to support parents in the transition to early parenthood, and this will be aided by a conceptual leap from 'parentcraft' to preparation for parenting education.

- The Government has given parenting a high priority, and this is congruent with the changing role of midwives in developing their public health role.

- Management systems need to be fully developed to resource and support parent education programmes and activities, allowing a cost benefit to long-term health and well-being of parents and their children.

- Good facilitation and group work will usually promote effective and meaningful learning and enable parents to access information, learn from a wide range of other parents and develop their repertoire of life skills.

- Midwives need to fully develop their facilitation and group growth skills to promote interaction and learning in groups.

- Groups require the leader to manage the balance between the building of the group and achievement of the task, and this must be supported by the use of evidence-based practice and reflective skills.

REFERENCES

Brandes, D. with Morris, J. (1998) *The Gamesters Handbook* (1, 2 & 3). London: Hutchinson.

Brown, A. (1992) *Groupwork*, 3rd edn. Hants, UK: Arena Ashgate Publishing.

Burnard, P. (1995) *Learning Human Skills: an experiential guide for nurses*, 3rd edn. Oxford: Butterworth & Heinemann.

Coombes, G. & Schonveld, D. (1992) *Life Will Never be the Same Again: A Review of Antenatal and*

Postnatal Education. London: Health Education Authority.

Craddock, E. (1993) Developing the facilitator role in the clinical areas. *Nurse Education Today* **13**: 217–224.

Crisp, S. (1994) *Counting on Families: Social Audit Report on the Provision of Family Support Services.* London: Exploring Parenthood.

Department for Education and Employment (DfEE) (1999) *Sure Start: Making a Difference for Children and Families,* London: DfEE.

Department of Health (DoH) (1993) *Changing Childbirth, The Report of The Expert Maternity Group.* London: HMSO.

Department of Health (DoH) (1999) *Making a Difference Strengthening the Nursing, Midwifery and Health Visiting Contribution to Health and Healthcare.* London: HMSO.

Edwards, M. & Nichols, F. (2000) Group process. In: Nichols, F. & Smith-Humenick, S. (eds) *Childbirth Education: Practice, Research, and Theory.* Philadelphia: W.B. Saunders.

Frederick, A. (2000) The teaching–learning process. In: Nichols, F. & Smith-Humenick, S. (eds) *Childbirth Education: Practice, Research, and Theory.* Philadelphia: W.B. Saunders.

Grimshaw, R. & McGuire, C. (1998) *Evaluating Parenting Programmes: A Study of Stakeholders.* London: National Children's Bureau.

Henderson, P. (1989) *Promoting Active Learning.* Cambridge: National Extension College.

Home Office (1998) *Supporting Families: A Consultative Document.* London: HMSO.

Honey, P. (1991) The learning organisation simplified. *Training and Development* July: 6–7.

Jarvis, P. (1995) *Adults and Continuing Education,* 2nd edn. London: Routledge.

Johnson, B. (1996) Seven secrets of successful presenters. *Business Life* April: 53–54.

Kaufmann, M. & Whelan, S. (eds) (1999) *Fact File 2000: Facts and Figures on Issues Facing Britain's Children.* London: NCH Action for Children.

Leslie-Green, B. & Reavill, E. (1989) *PIPSI Activity Pack.* Nottingham: Central Nottinghamshire Healthcare (NHS) Trust.

Murphy-Black, T. & Faulkner, A. (1990) Antenatal education. In: *Excellence in Nursing: The Research Route: Midwifery.* London: Scutari Press.

Nolan, M. (1995) Helping parents adapt to parenthood. *British Journal of Midwifery* **3**(1): 23–26.

Nolan, M. (1998) *Antenatal Education, a Dynamic Approach.* London. Baillière Tindall.

Parr, M. (1996) *PIPPIN: Support for Couples in the Transition to Parenthood.* PhD dissertation. University of East London: Department of Psychology.

Perkins, E. (1980) *Education for Childbirth and Parenthood.* London: Century Publishing.

Priest, J. & Schott, J. (1991) *Leading Antenatal Classes: A Practical Guide.* Oxford: Butterworth Heinemann.

Pugh, G. (1999) Parenting education and social policy agenda. In: Einzig, H. (ed) *Parenting Education and Support: New Opportunities.* London: David Fulton.

Pugh, G., De'Ath, E. & Smith, C. (1994) *Confident Parents Confident Children: Policy and Practice in Parenting Education and Support.* London: National Children's Bureau.

Royal College of Midwives (RCM) & Department of Health (DoH) (2000) *Midwives and the New NHS.* London: Royal College of Midwives Trust.

Rolls, L. (1992) *Team Development, a Manual of Facilitation for Health Educators and Health Promoters.* London: Health Education Authority.

Schott, J. (1995) Cancel the labour talk. *British Journal of Midwifery* **3**(10): 517–518.

Schweinhart, L. & Weikart, D. (1993) *A Summary of the Significant Benefits: The High/Scope Perry Pre School through Age 27.* Ypsilanti, USA, High/Scope.

Smith, C. (1997) *Developing Parenting Programmes.* London: National Children's Bureau.

Underdown, A. (1998) Investigating techniques used in parenting classes. *Health Visitor* **71**(2 February): 65–68.

Williams, M. & Booth, D. (1980) *Antenatal Education: guidelines for teachers,* 2nd edn. Edinburgh: Churchill Livingstone.

FURTHER READING

Nichols, H. & Smith Humenick, S. (2000) *Childbirth Education: Practice, Research and Theory,* 2nd edn. Philadelphia: W.B. Saunders.
The new edition includes childbirth preparation and parenting, and it addresses the transition to parenthood and the application of new-born behaviours and attachment theory.

Royal College of Midwives (RCM) (1999) *Transition to Parenting: An Open Learning Resource for Midwives.* London: The Royal College of Midwives Trust.

This is an excellent summary of the psychological issues for parent education. It includes reflections for professional development and has some examples of exercises that can be incorporated into parent education programmes.

Smith, C. (1997) *Developing Parenting Programmes.* London: National Children's Bureau.
A description of the current parenting programmes available is included in this publication.

ADDITIONAL RESOURCES

Parents in Partnership – Parent Infant Network
http://www.pippin.org.uk

The National Childbirth Trust
http://www.nct-online.org

Sure Start Forums
http://www2.dfee.gov.uk/3t/surestart/text/forum.cfm

23

Physical Preparation before Childbirth

Eileen Brayshaw

LEARNING OUTCOMES

After reading this chapter and practising the suggested activities, you will:

- have developed an increased knowledge of the anatomy and functions of the abdominal and pelvic floor muscles
- have increased your awareness of the effects on the musculoskeletal system of pregnancy, labour and the postpartum period
- understand possible long-term physical problems and when and to whom to refer clients for specialist therapy

- have become aware of the beneficial effects of exercise
- be able to teach specific exercises relevant to pregnancy, labour and the postpartum
- have gained knowledge for your own well-being in terms of back and pelvic floor care and dealing with stress.

Physical preparation for childbirth has been recommended for many years. Randall, a physiotherapist and midwife, introduced bed exercises for postnatal mothers as early as 1912 to help prevent the numerous problems arising from prolonged postpartum immobility. Following their success, she encouraged mobilizing exercises for pregnant women. Then in the 1930s, Randall and Grantly Dick-Read introduced the principles of relaxation and deep breathing into antenatal preparation classes. These classes were continued by Heardman, another well-known physiotherapist, and one of the founder members of what is now the Association of Chartered Physiotherapists in Women's Health (ACPWH).

It has been acknowledged by the Royal College of Midwives and the Health Visitors' Association (Brayshaw, 2003) that the obstetric physiotherapist is an invaluable member of the obstetric team. She is the ideal professional to help women to adjust to the physical changes which occur throughout pregnancy and the puerperium, to prepare them for labour using relaxation and breathing awareness, to teach postnatal exercises and to carry out specialized treatments where

necessary. However, obstetrics is no longer a core clinical speciality area of physiotherapy training and, as more and more women and couples are demanding antenatal education, there are insufficient numbers of obstetric physiotherapists. In some areas, midwives may be asked to teach antenatal and postnatal exercises and coping skills for labour.

WOMEN'S HEALTH PHYSIOTHERAPIST

Some maternity units have a designated women's health physiotherapist, which denotes a practitioner who has undertaken significant specialist postgraduate training in obstetric and gynaecological issues. Other units will have a physiotherapist who has an interest in obstetric and gynaecological physiotherapy. It should be noted that, currently, physiotherapy training does not automatically include obstetric problems and incontinence issues within the core curriculum, and therefore midwives cannot assume that all physiotherapists will have the requisite skills. Ideally, they would need to refer to an appropriately qualified practitioner, which may require referral to another unit.

In this chapter, the term physiotherapist will be used to describe the practitioner who is qualified to the appropriate level.

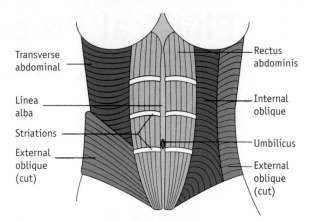

Figure 23.1   Anterior abdominal wall showing muscle layers and striations of the rectus muscle.

Reflective Activity 23.1

Find out where your nearest specialist women's health physiotherapist is based. Does she provide antenatal and postnatal education? Will she treat musculo-skeletal problems associated with pregnancy? Does she specialize in treatment of incontinence?

Having identified your contact, how can you refer patients to her? Can you ring her? Do you have to refer through a GP or does the woman have to be referred by a consultant? (The answers to these questions will vary considerably from one area to another.)

Record this information in your resource file/diary for future reference.

ANATOMY AND FUNCTIONS

Before teaching exercises for specific muscle groups, it is important to understand their anatomy and functions. The anatomy of the pelvic floor is explained in Chapter 28, but it is also useful to understand the role of the abdominal wall anatomy.

Anatomy of the abdominal muscles (Fig. 23.1)

The abdominal muscles form the anterior and lateral parts of the abdominal wall or corset and consist of three layers of muscle and fascia. The deepest muscle layer is formed by transversus abdominis, which runs in a horizontal direction from the thoracolumbar fascia, iliac crest and inguinal ligament at each side. It attaches to the inner surface of the lower six ribs and its aponeurosis inserts into the linea alba.

The next layer comprises two sets of oblique muscles. The deeper are the internal obliques which run upwards and inwards from the thoracolumbar fascia, iliac crest and inguinal ligament and insert into the inferior borders of the lower three ribs and by an aponeurosis into the linea alba. Directly superficial and running at right angles to these muscles are the external obliques. Their origin is the outer surface of the lower eight ribs and they insert into the anterior half of the iliac crest, pubic crest and by an aponeurosis into the linea alba. The lower border of each external oblique muscle forms the inguinal ligament.

The most superficial group of abdominal muscles are the recti abdominis which run in a vertical direction, are narrow and anterior, and are enclosed in the aponeuroses formed by the other abdominal muscles. This enclosure of the recti is known as the rectus sheath. The rectus muscles attach superiorly to the cartilages of the fifth, sixth and seventh ribs and to the xiphisternum and inferiorly to the crest of the pubis. The muscles have three fibrous bands known as tendinous intersections.

Functions of the abdominal muscles

The abdominal 'corset' provides support for the abdominal organs, the pelvis and spine. It helps control the intra-abdominal and intrapelvic pressures, thus aiding expulsive actions such as defecation and parturition, and, together with the diaphragm, helps with breathing and coughing. The abdominal muscles perform forward and side flexion and rotation of the trunk. With the hip and back extensors, they control the tilt of the pelvis and splint the spine, making a large contribution to body posture. The transversus, which is the deepest abdominal muscle attached to the lumbar fascia, together with the back muscles is particularly important in maintaining the stability of the lumbar spine. Research has pinpointed the transversus in being crucial to maintaining correct alignment of the spine and preventing long-term back problems (Richardson and Jull, 1995). This has major implications for antenatal and postnatal exercises.

Anatomy of the pelvic floor

Review Chapter 28.

Functions of the pelvic floor muscles

The two most important functions of the pelvic floor are control of the sphincters of the bladder and bowel and support of the pelvic contents in their correct anatomical position. However, the pelvic floor muscles also play a large part in both partners' sexual satisfaction during intercourse. Muscles with good tone will stretch and recoil more effectively than weak muscles and therefore will relax more easily.

PHYSIOLOGICAL EFFECTS OF PREGNANCY ON THE MUSCULOSKELETAL SYSTEM

The physiological effects on the musculoskeletal system in pregnancy are mainly due to the hormonal influence of oestrogen, progesterone and relaxin. Oestrogen is thought to help the action of relaxin which is produced at 2 weeks and is at its highest level in the first trimester (Weiss, 1984). Relaxin alters the composition of collagen, which is present in joint capsules, ligaments and fibrous tissue such as the linea alba. This collagen is remodelled, and has a higher water content which leads to greater pliability and extensibility. This means, however, that joints do not receive the same protection from the ligaments as before and become lax. Muscles which are intersected with fibrous bands, e.g. the recti, or those interspersed with fascial layers, e.g. the pelvic floor, are weakened.

An increase in joint laxity leads to an increase in joint range. Calguneri *et al.* (1982) have shown that this increase is greater in second pregnancies than in first pregnancies. Increased range in the pelvic joints, coupled with the weight of the developing uterus may cause backache and referred 'sciatica-like' pain down the leg. Posture is altered: the pelvis tips forward and the pregnant woman adopts a typical stance, with exaggerated spinal curves and protruding abdomen which again can produce backache (Fig. 23.2). The woman may also experience a dragging sensation in the lower abdomen as the weight of the uterus is transmitted through these muscles instead of the thighs. The centre of gravity is shifted further forward, causing the woman to be unbalanced.

CARE OF THE BACK DURING PREGNANCY

During pregnancy, the back is especially vulnerable. The stretching ligaments, increased joint range, extra weight and altered posture all mean that women should

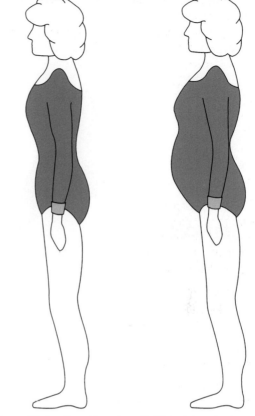

Figure 23.2 Normal posture (left) and posture in pregnancy (right).

pay particular attention to back care in order to avoid long-term back problems. They should be taught correct lifting, keeping the back straight and holding the object close (Fig. 23.3). If possible, lifting, and especially moving heavy objects should be discouraged.

Midwives can make sure that women know how to get up from the examination couch/bed and how to get up and down from the floor. Trying to sit up forwards from lying with legs straight is the same as performing sit-ups and puts a great strain on the abdominals as well as the back. Women should be shown how to bend the knees up, keep them together, roll over on to one side, and to push up on the upper hand and underneath elbow into a sitting position with the legs over the side of the bed before slowly standing. If on the

Reflective Activity 23.2

Try both methods of getting up from a lying position: i.e. as a 'sit up' and from the side-lying position. Compare the strain felt in your body.

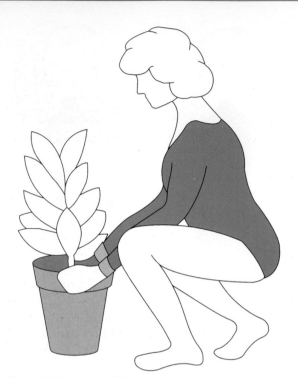

Figure 23.3 Correct lifting technique.

floor, women should go over on to their hands and knees before standing.

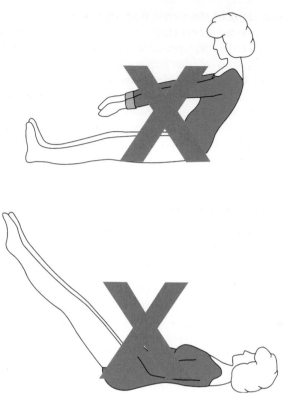

Figure 23.4 Exercises to avoid.

ANTENATAL EXERCISES

It is inadvisable for women to take up any new sporting activities in pregnancy (Sady and Carpenter, 1989) but it is usually considered safe to continue with familiar activities as long as these do not involve lifting or twisting. Swimming and walking are especially beneficial, but competitive or contact sports should be discontinued during pregnancy (Revelli *et al.*, 1992). If in doubt, the midwife or physiotherapist should be consulted.

The following exercises could lead to long-term back problems (Donovan *et al.*, 1988) and should be avoided at all times, but especially during pregnancy and the postnatal period:

- *Double leg lifting*: Lying on the back with both legs straight, lifting both legs up into the air, then lowering them back down.
- *Sit-ups*: Lying on the back with both legs straight, sitting up to touch the toes, then lowering the head and shoulders back down to the floor (Fig. 23.4).

The exercises described below are recommended during pregnancy and may be started in the first trimester unless the woman has specific orders to rest.

In the last two trimesters, women may suffer from supine hypotension so should never be asked to lie flat on their backs to exercise. Half-lying, i.e. lying with the back supported at an angle of 45 degrees, is a safe and comfortable position.

Circulatory exercises

Because of the hormonal effects and the increasing size of the baby, the circulation – particularly the venous return – becomes more sluggish. This may lead to foot and ankle oedema, varicose veins and cramp. The following exercises may help to alleviate these problems:

- *Ankle circling*: Sit or half-lie with legs stretched out and supported, circle both ankles round in a large circle keeping knees still. Do this at least 20 times in both directions.
- *Leg tightening*: In the same position, bend both feet upwards at the ankle and press the back of the knees down on to the underneath surface, tightening both calf and thigh muscles. Hold for a couple of seconds, breathing normally. Repeat 10 times.

Women will benefit from sitting with their legs supported and elevated whenever possible, and should avoid prolonged standing as this may compound circulatory stasis. If oedema is present, women may find it helpful to lie supported at an angle of about 45 degrees with legs elevated just higher than the level of the groin to aid drainage by gravity. Great care must be taken to ensure a wide angle at the groin to prevent circulatory stasis in that region.

Circulatory exercises are not a substitute for weight-bearing exercise, e.g. walking, which should be encouraged to improve the venous return.

Abdominal exercises

The transversus abdominis is the most important abdominal muscle to keep toned during pregnancy (Richardson and Jull, 1995) and the transversus exercise can be performed in any position (apart from supine in later pregnancy).

- *Transversus exercise*: Place both hands on the lower abdomen below the umbilicus, breathe in and on the outward breath pull in the abdomen towards the spine. Hold for up to 10 seconds, breathing normally. Repeat up to 10 times.

As already mentioned, the pelvis will tilt further forwards as pregnancy advances, putting a strain on the ligaments and joints of the pelvis and on the abdominal and back muscles. Tilting the pelvis in the opposite direction will help to alleviate this strain. The action involves all the abdominal muscles and the hip extensors so will help to maintain their tone and support for the pelvic joints as the ligaments stretch.

- *Pelvic tilting exercise*: Half-lie with knees bent up and feet resting on the floor, tighten and pull in the abdomen, tighten the buttock muscles and press the small of the back downwards on to the supporting surface. Hold for up to 10 seconds, breathing normally. Repeat up to 10 times (Fig. 23.5).

This exercise may be performed in a supported sitting position, prone kneeling or standing, but most pregnant women find it easier to learn the exercise in the half-lying position. Because of the hormonal effects on the linea alba, exercises which cause contraction of the muscles inserting obliquely into this area should be avoided in later pregnancy to minimize the risk of diastasis of the recti (Noble, 1995). These include rotation exercises and stronger abdominal exercises such as curl-ups.

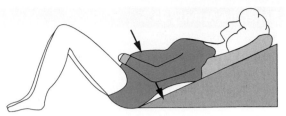

Figure 23.5 Pelvic tilting exercise in half-lying position.

Pelvic floor exercises

Wilson *et al.* (1996) and Mørkved and Bø (1999) report incontinence rates of 34% and 38% up to 3 months postpartum. Pelvic floor exercises should be introduced during pregnancy to maintain muscle tone and promote understanding of the effects of pregnancy on the functional ability of the pelvic floor postnatally. Few women will have performed pelvic floor exercises before coming to antenatal classes, so it is important to explain, in simple terms, the relevant anatomy and the importance of the muscles before embarking on the exercise itself.

Pelvic floor contractions can be performed in any position except with crossed legs. Probably the easiest position is sitting, leaning forwards with the legs slightly apart.

- *Pelvic floor exercise*: Close the back passage as though preventing a bowel action, close the middle and front passages too as though preventing the flow of urine, then draw up all three passages inside. Hold as strongly as possible for as long as possible up to a count of 10, breathing normally throughout. Relax and rest for 5 seconds. Repeat slowly up to a maximum of 10 repetitions. Then tighten and relax more quickly up to 10 times without holding the contraction.

The transversus and pelvic floor exercises can be practised together for greater impact and it is an excellent idea to relate the practice of these exercises to the performance of everyday activities, e.g. washing hands, after emptying the bladder, answering the telephone. This will establish a routine for postnatal practice.

Some women find the exercise difficult to comprehend at first and may need other suggestions to describe the sensation of tightening their pelvic floor. It may be helpful to try to stop the flow of urine midstream occasionally, but this is not advisable regularly as it is not good bladder training and could lead to urinary tract infection due to reflux of urine.

STRESS AND RELAXATION

Most people show signs of stress when problems accumulate, workloads increase and there are staff shortages. It is often a very insignificant factor which breaks the 'camel's back'. Pregnant woman may have many everyday stresses plus the added mental stresses, which even a planned and longed-for pregnancy can bring, let alone an unplanned and unsupported one. Pregnancy also brings additional physical stresses – fatigue, aching joints, reduced mobility. The whole process increases the work of every body system, so acquiring relaxation skills during pregnancy can be greatly beneficial.

The automatic reaction of the body to stress is the 'fight or flight' response. A tense position is assumed – hunched shoulders, elbows close to the body, hands clenched, legs crossed, feet pulled up and body leaning forward, frowning face, tense jaw and dry mouth. The heart beats faster, there may be sweating and shallow and rapid breathing. Adopting this position in itself increases tension and fatigue. The release of adrenaline may cause headaches following the stressful event.

Part of mastering relaxation techniques is gaining an awareness of the tense situation before it is too late and changing it to a position of ease. This position is the exact opposite of one of tension and allows all joints to assume a comfortable mid-position and the muscles around the joints to be as relaxed as possible.

Physiological relaxation, first taught by Mitchell (1988), works joints into positions of ease which the brain accepts as a neutral position. The method works on the principle of reciprocal innervation of opposite muscle groups, e.g. if one muscle group shortens or contracts, the opposite muscle group lengthens or relaxes allowing that action to take place. As the finger muscles flex to make a fist, the extensor muscles are stretched

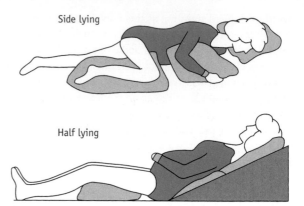

Side lying

Half lying

Figure 23.6   Relaxation in half-lying and side-lying positions.

or lengthened. Conversely, the flexors are stretched or lengthened as the fingers extend or straighten. This principle is applied to the tense muscles of each joint in the stressed position.

There are specific instructions for this method of relaxation:

1. Work the opposite muscle group to the tense ones strongly.
2. Stop the action of those muscle groups.
3. Pause to 'feel the difference' now the joint is in a position of ease.

Women need to be aware of the groups which exhibit tension, then work their way through the opposite ones. Relaxation can be practised in any comfortable supported position but half-lying and side-lying are often preferred in pregnancy (Fig. 23.6). For relaxation instructions, see Box 23.1.

Following the relaxation sequence, the circulation should be stimulated by stretching or moving feet and hands before sitting up slowly, then standing. Women should be encouraged to practise the relaxation technique every day of their pregnancy, either sitting supported in an armchair whilst watching the television, or lying on the bed for an afternoon rest or in bed before going to sleep. The importance and value of this relaxation sequence should be emphasized both for coping with normal life stresses and as an important preparation for labour.

Find other positions that are comfortable for you so you can suggest positions for pregnant women.

When you feel tense and uptight during a boring meeting or whilst in a traffic jam, follow the instructions for your shoulders and hands and breathing. This will reduce your tension and your oxygen need. Can you think of other activities in your everyday life when this relaxation technique might be useful?

Box 23.1 Relaxation exercise

- *Shoulders*: Pull your shoulders down towards your feet. Stop pulling your shoulders down. Your shoulders are now lower and your neck feels longer.
- *Elbows*: Move your elbows slightly away from your side. Stop moving your elbows. Be aware that your elbows are open and slightly away from your side.
- *Hands*: Stretch out and separate your fingers and thumbs. Stop stretching. Your fingers are fully supported. Feel the surface they are resting on.
- *Hips*: Roll your hips and knees outwards. Stop rolling outwards. Your legs are slightly apart and feel heavy.
- *Feet*: Push your feet away from your body. Stop pushing. Your feet feel loose and heavy.
- *Body*: Press your body into the support. Stop pressing. Feel your body resting on the surface.
- *Head*: Press your head into the pillow. Stop pressing. Your head is nestling comfortably in the hollow you have made.
- *Jaw*: Pull down your lower jaw. Stop pulling down. Your teeth are no longer touching and your tongue is resting on your lower jaw.
- *Eyes*: Close your eyes if you want to.
- *Forehead*: Imagine someone smoothing away your frown lines from your eyebrows up over to the top and the back of your head.
- *Breathing*: Give a big sigh out. Breathe fairly low down in your chest at your own natural resting breathing rate. To prevent your brain being too active during your relaxation think about something pleasant which helps you to feel comfortable.

COPING STRATEGIES FOR LABOUR

When asked their reasons for attending antenatal classes, women will usually cite their need to '*learn what to do in labour*' and their partners will express their need to help and share in the experience. Each couple is different and every labour unique, but there are common coping skills that couples can learn during pregnancy and put into practice in labour. The main tools are relaxation, breathing awareness and positions of ease. All three are interrelated and all can be practised at home.

Relaxation

The physiological method of relaxation lends itself very well to both first and second stages of labour. If women can conserve their energy during the first stage they can prepare themselves for the increased stress of the second stage, as well as ensuring that baby and uterus both receive sufficient oxygen. Any position which is comfortable is acceptable, allowing for the possibility of infusions or monitors being attached. Alteration of maternal position during the first stage encourages productive contractions (Roberts *et al.*, 1983), and suggestions for different positions appear in Chapter 26.

Breathing

The use of breathing has been the subject of much debate and criticism over the years. Levels of breathing and breathing patterns formed the basis of the psychoprophylaxis teaching in the 1960s. It has now been shown that these can cause hyperventilation which may be disadvantageous for both mother and baby. The emphasis nowadays on encouraging the woman to 'tune in' to her own natural breathing rhythm and to recognize times in labour when she may need to adapt this. This 'breathing awareness' is being accepted as non-interfering and is unlikely to lead to hyperventilation. It is the outward breath which is the relaxing phase of respiration, so women should be encouraged to concentrate on that when 'tuning in' to their breathing. They may also become aware of a slight pause at the end of the outward breath before the next inward breath follows. There is no need to instruct anyone to breathe in, as this happens automatically. It may be necessary, however, to encourage the breath out or to extend the expiratory phase.

Alteration in breathing is one of the first obvious signs of tension or panic. It becomes rapid and shallow involving only the upper part of the lungs and increasing tension in the shoulder muscles. If this continues, hyperventilation or hyperoxygenation may result – a state where too much oxygen has been inhaled and too much carbon dioxide has been exhaled.

The symptoms of hyperventilation are pallor, dizziness, sweating and pins and needles in the face and extremities. The woman feels very unwell and the baby's blood gases may also be compromised. The immediate remedy is to inhale carbon dioxide as soon as possible by breathing in and out of cupped hands until the blood gas levels are stabilized. To prevent hyperventilation, SOS breathing can be practised during the contraction. SOS stands for 'sigh out slowly' and is a relaxed breathing, exaggerating the outward breath by making a sighing noise. It slows down 'panic breathing' and relaxes the shoulder muscles. As SOS represents an emergency situation (as indeed hyperventilation would be) it is a useful phrase for couples to remember.

The transition period can be difficult for all women but particularly those who experience a premature urge to push. In addition to altering their position, these women can adapt their breathing to prevent themselves from pushing. To avoid fixing the diaphragm, breath-holding must be discouraged. Panting, as used at the crowning of the fetal head, would prevent pushing but may lead to hyperventilation. Instead, a modified panting breathing may be useful – breathing in threes with the emphasis on two short breaths out followed by a longer breath out. It may be called pant–pant–blow or puff–puff–blow breathing and can be practised for the length of a contraction without hyperventilation occurring.

Midwives will have their own ideas and policies on the management of second stage and the question 'to push or not to push' initiates much discussion. It is now known that the continued practice of the Valsalva manoeuvre when pushing could lead to loss of maternal consciousness if the woman's cerebral blood flow is already compromised (Bush, 1992). It is also documented that breath-holding for more than 5 or 6 seconds alters the blood gases in the placenta and may compromise the fetal circulation (Tucker Blackburn, 2003; Caldeyro-Barcia, 1979). Certainly, women are less exhausted when allowed to push whenever and for however long they choose.

Positions adopted for the second stage will also affect the outcome (Russell, 1982). Chapter 29 discusses practical positions for delivery. Note that if symphysis pubis dysfunction has presented antenatally, side-lying or kneeling may be the only safe positions (Fry *et al.*, 1997). Guidelines for the management of women with symphysis pubis dysfunction (SPD) have been developed by the Association of Physiotherapists in Women's Health in consultation with midwives, obstetricians and GPs (ACPWH, 2000) (see Ch. 16).

Reflective Activity 23.6

Make sure you have copies of SPD guidelines to give to any woman who is suffering from symphysis pain.

POSTNATAL EXERCISES

The overall aim of postnatal exercises is to restore the woman to the pre-pregnancy state as soon as possible.

Circulatory exercises

Women confined to bed may perform circulatory exercises described earlier and follow advice given to avoid sitting or lying with legs crossed.

Abdominal exercises

The abdominal corset has stretched to approximately twice its length and two-thirds of its girth by the end of pregnancy. The component muscles will need exercising to regain their former length and strength. However, because of their insertion into the linea alba and rectus sheath (see earlier in this chapter) the oblique muscles should not be exercised before checking for any undue diastasis of the rectus muscles. Up to two fingers' width is considered normal 48 hours after delivery, but if the gap is more than that, any exercises or activities which involve rotating the trunk should be avoided to prevent further separation of the rectus muscles (Noble, 1995).

Ideally the midwife should measure diastasis when checking the fundus on the third day postdelivery. The woman should lie on her back with knees bent up and feet flat on the bed. With the midwife's fingers pressed into the midline of the abdomen just above or below the umbilicus, the woman is asked to pull in the abdomen and lift head and shoulders off the pillow. If there is no undue diastasis, the rectus muscles will be felt taut either side of the fingers. If the rectus muscles cannot be felt until more than two fingers are inserted, only the transversus and pelvic tilting exercises should be performed until the gap is reduced (Fig. 23.7).

Reflective Activity 23.7

Test your own rectus muscles as follows. Lie on your back with knees bent up and feet on the floor, and place one finger widthways between your rectus muscles just below the umbilicus. Pull in the abdomen and lift your head and shoulders forward and feel whether you have a gap between your rectus muscles. If you have had a baby you will have a gap of one finger's width but no wider. Check colleagues who have had babies and compare.

The *transversus* and *pelvic tilting exercises* described earlier in this chapter can be started on the first or second day postdelivery. As well as toning up the abdominal muscles, these exercises will help to ease any postural backache which may be present after delivery. They should be encouraged in sitting and standing as well as lying and, as with the pelvic floor exercise, they can be related to activities to ensure frequent practice.

If there is no undue diastasis or when the gap has reduced, the following exercises can be started when the woman feels like it.

- *Curl-ups.* In back lying with knees bent up, the pelvis should be tilted back, the head and shoulders are then lifted forwards. This should be held for a few seconds before lowering down slowly, and repeated up to 10 times. NB: This exercise must always be done with knees bent and never without pelvic tilting first – the abdomen should remain flat throughout (Fig. 23.8).
- *Knee rolling.* In back lying with knees bent up, the abdomen should be pulled in and both knees rolled over to the left as far as possible, keeping shoulders flat (Fig. 23.9). The knees are then rolled to the centre and the abdomen relaxed. This can then be repeated, turning to the right, and finishing with the knees in central position.

Pelvic floor exercises (see p. 387)

These should be started as soon after delivery as possible to avoid disassociation by the brain (Shepherd, 1980). The woman should be warned that contracting the pelvic floor will be much more difficult postnatally because of the stretching that has taken place during delivery and possible discomfort from a bruised or sutured perineum. However, if these pelvic floor exercises are persevered with for several weeks, many urinary problems, prolapse and sexual problems may well be avoided (Mørkved and Bø, 1997, 2000). Frequent performance of the pelvic floor exercise is vital in the postnatal period – every hour or so – and its performance can be linked to baby activities, e.g. feeding, bathing, washing and also after bladder emptying. Stopping midstream during bladder emptying does not promote good bladder function and should be avoided. If a sore perineum makes the exercise difficult in sitting, then it could be done in prone, side-lying or standing.

Women can test the strength of their pelvic floor muscles 2–3 months postdelivery by stride jumping with a full bladder and coughing deeply twice whilst doing so. If any leakage occurs, the muscles have not regained their former strength and function and need further intensive exercising. The test can be repeated 4–6 weeks later and if there are still problems, women should be referred to the gynaecologist or a physiotherapist before embarking on any strenuous exercise or a subsequent pregnancy. Even when the muscles are functioning adequately, women are advised to continue regular pelvic floor contractions for the rest of

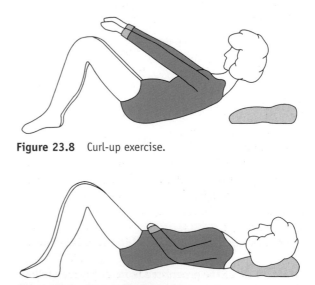

Figure 23.8   Curl-up exercise.

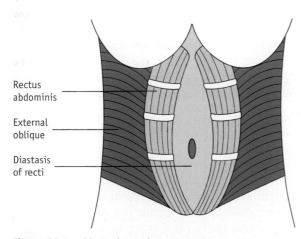

Rectus abdominis

External oblique

Diastasis of recti

Figure 23.7   Diastasis recti postpartum.

Figure 23.9   Knee rolling exercises.

their lives to prevent gynaecological problems in the future.

Reflective Activity 23.8

Test your own pelvic floor's capabilities. If you leak then seek the advice of your women's health physiotherapist.

CARE FOLLOWING CAESAREAN DELIVERY

Circulatory exercises and deep breathing (no more than three or four) are extremely important following caesarean delivery and should be performed regularly whilst women are relatively immobile. Women should be taught to move up and down the bed by bending the knees, curling forwards and pushing on hands and feet to move in a forwards or backwards direction. They should not attempt to sit up forwards from a lying position, but instead roll over on to their sides as described earlier in this chapter. This is also the easiest way of getting out of bed – pushing up into a sitting position on the edge of the bed.

If the woman needs to cough, she should bend her knees and support the wound with a pillow or hands whilst leaning forwards to prevent undue strain on sutures.

Transversus and pelvic tilting may be performed as soon as the woman feels able; the latter will relieve postural backache as well as helping to disperse wind. It is not possible to check for diastasis of the recti until about the fifth day postdelivery, so other abdominal exercises should be left until after this time, then progressed more gently than after a normal delivery.

Pelvic floor exercises should be performed regularly even though the muscles have not been stretched at birth as in a vaginal delivery. They have been subjected to pregnancy and it is still believed that hormonal influences during pregnancy are responsible for most urinary problems (Francis, 1960).

A caesarean birth has necessitated major surgery and these women will require more rest and more support at home. Many relatives do not appreciate this and the community midwife may need to emphasize the woman's needs.

CARE FOLLOWING INSTRUMENTAL DELIVERY

Exercises should be progressed more slowly than following a normal delivery with the emphasis on circulatory exercises if an epidural had been administered and pelvic floor exercises when the woman feels comfortable after adequate pain relief.

CARE OF THE BACK POSTNATALLY

The early postpartum period is when the woman's spinal and pelvic joints are at their least protected because the ligaments are at their most relaxed. Unfortunately this is the time when there are numerous objects to lift, e.g. baby bath, carrycot, and tasks which involve bending and stooping. The midwife must explain the underlying physiology and reinforce good back care routines both in hospital and at home, now and for the future.

Positions for feeding, bathing and nappy changing must be discussed (Fig. 23.10). To avoid slouching whilst feeding, women should sit well-supported with the baby resting on pillows. Baby bathing and nappy changing can be done on a surface at waist height if standing, or at coffee table height if kneeling, to avoid stooping. Lifting should be kept to an absolute minimum and, if unavoidable, only light objects lifted and held close to the body. The correct lifting procedures as described earlier should be followed to avoid back strain at this very vulnerable time.

DAILY ACTIVITIES

If possible, heavy housework, e.g. vacuuming, moving furniture, cleaning windows, should be avoided for several weeks after delivery to prevent back strain. Walking and swimming are good ways of supplementing the postnatal exercises, but more strenuous keep-fit classes, aerobics or competitive sports should be left for 10–12 weeks or even longer if there are any joint or bladder problems. Double leg lifting and sit-ups should never be performed (see Fig. 23.4).

POSTNATAL COMPLICATIONS

Pain from a bruised or oedematous perineum can be eased by the application of ice (Knight, 1989). Testing for diastasis recti has already been described. If a gap of more than two fingers' width is discovered, 'J' or 'K' size tubigrip applied from the xiphisternum to below the buttocks will give some support in the early stages. Advice about posture, getting out of bed and special exercises for the rectus muscles are all important and the physiotherapist can advise.

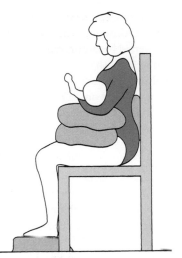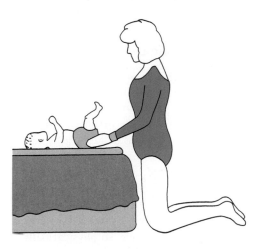

Figure 23.10 Positions for feeding and nappy changing.

Separated symphysis may require complete bedrest in the acute stage until the severe pain has subsided, then limited walking with the aid of a frame or crutches. Local pain relief will help (see Ch. 16 and ACPWH guidelines).

Backache is usually postural and advice on positions, transversus, pelvic tilting and lifting plus some local heat should ease it considerably. Women with long-term back problems should be referred for individual assessment by a physiotherapist.

Coccydynia (painful coccyx) can be incapacitating, women finding it impossible to adopt sitting positions. Pain-relieving therapies such as ice, therapeutic ultrasound or pulsed electromagnetic energy may help.

Urinary problems, such as stress incontinence, frequency and urgency, which do not respond to pelvic floor exercise, will require referral to the general practitioner/gynaecologist before a subsequent pregnancy compounds the problem.

Dyspareunia can often be treated successfully by physiotherapy (McIntosh, 1988), though some women may require psychosexual counselling.

Most women welcome the opportunity to return with their babies and discuss progress with their peers at a reunion session. It may be in this informal atmosphere that urinary and back problems are mentioned and referrals can be made to the appropriate professionals.

TEACHING PHYSICAL SKILLS

Before teaching physical skills, midwives must be proficient in those skills themselves, memorizing the appropriate instructions and practising teaching family members or a small group of colleagues.

Points to consider

- Is the room of adequate size with appropriate facilities for exercises, e.g. mats or carpeted floor, wedges and/or pillows?
- Can all individuals see the instructor and each other?
- Is the demonstration/description of the exercise clear?
- Have the purpose and benefits of the exercise been stated?
- Do the individuals know how many repetitions to perform?
- Does each individual understand the exercise/activity?
- Do you need to provide written or pictorial information to support the session and facilitate participants in their practice?
- Have they been told to practice at home?

Many midwives will find themselves battling for floor space in crowded community clinics and may have to adapt some of the above criteria. Some exercises could be taught in other positions or it may only be possible

---

Reflective Activity 23.9

Practice teaching each of the exercises to willing volunteers, bearing in mind the above teaching points. Reward your 'class' with a relaxation session.

Make sure you are familiar with all the instructions and do not need to read from a sheet.

to demonstrate a position or to use visual aids to show it, if space is limited.

When should women begin physical preparation?

This should begin as early as possible as long as there is no risk of miscarriage. It is much easier to teach good posture and back care in early pregnancy rather than trying to relieve back problems in later pregnancy. This might be learned in one-to-one or group sessions according to the woman's need.

Two or three early pregnancy classes for couples at 3–4 months of pregnancy are extremely useful, though many hospitals/clinics have only the resources to provide one evening session at this time, so physical skills priorities would be posture, working positions, lifting techniques, transversus and pelvic floor exercises.

Partners enjoy participating in the exercises and relaxation techniques at couples classes. They can be very supportive, helping with coping strategies and checking their partner's relaxation. It may be appropriate on occasions to divide couples so the women could cover such topics as pelvic floor problems whilst the men discuss worries with another member of the antenatal team.

Reflective Activity 23.10

Survey your couples to find out when and where they would like their classes – perhaps weekends would be a possibility for working couples.

If women have been attending daytime classes on their own, they should have an opportunity to have access to at least one evening session to practise coping strategies for labour with their partners.

Some women will prefer their antenatal preparation on a one-to-one basis because the group situation is not convenient or they have individual problems. In these cases the community midwife might provide the preparation in the woman's own home, or within the antenatal clinic setting.

Any woman with specific needs for a physical disability should be referred to the physiotherapist if at all possible for specialist support.

It may be necessary to hold separate or one-to-one tuition with women from different ethnic groups for whom English is not their first language, and this can be facilitated by local use of translators and link workers.

Leaflets with explanatory diagrams should also be available in different languages but these should be carefully vetted because there can be problems in directly translating English terms as many are not acceptable to all cultures. The use of pictures and diagrams may be useful for many women (whether English speaking or not), but these should be culturally and ethnically varied and appropriate to a range of women.

Aquanatal sessions

Aquanatal exercise can be seen as a 'fun' form of exercise both during pregnancy and afterwards. Many swimming pools offer special times for ante- and postnatal groups as well as sessions for mothers and babies. The water temperature should be at least 30°C as cooler than this does not allow for relaxation to be included. However, a hospital hydrotherapy pool at 37°C would be too warm to exercise in antenatally as there is risk of fetal abnormality if the woman's core temperature rises above 39.2°C (Artal and Buckenmeyer, 1995), though the woman would have to be exercising vigorously to cause this rise.

The buoyancy of water supports body weight, making it much easier to move and exercise without putting additional strain on joints. This increases general muscle tone, improves venous return and respiratory coordination as well as giving the women a sense of well-being, freedom and weightlessness whilst in the water (McMurray *et al.*, 1990). For some women there may be significant psychological effects from feeling less clumsy and awkward.

Women who swim may safely continue as long as they warm up gently beforehand and cool down afterwards. Some may find that breaststroke aggravates backache in pregnancy if they are in the habit of keeping their face out of the water, thus increasing the lumbar lordosis. Backstroke may therefore be more comfortable.

There are certain safety recommendations and contraindications to aquanatal therapy in pregnancy which must be observed by any professional wishing to set up aquanatal classes.

Safety precautions

Adequate staffing is essential – at least two professional staff and one lifeguard per session unless one professional has life-saving qualifications. The professionals may be a physiotherapist and a midwife or two midwives provided one has aquanatal qualifications and has discussed the exercise content with a physiotherapist.

The assistant midwife will be in the water with the women to facilitate and correct the exercises.

Women should be of at least 16 weeks' gestation, have written permission from their obstetrician and have none of the contraindications listed below. Comprehensive records of appropriate personal and obstetric details of each participant should be available.

Strict observation of the group is necessary at all times so numbers of participants should ideally be 8–12. To avoid fatigue and overheating, no more than 40 minutes of exercise should be performed, followed by relaxation if the temperature of the water is sufficient.

Exercises should avoid producing increased lumbar lordosis and should never cause pain. The pool surrounds must be safe and there must be access to an emergency telephone. A warm drink after the session will prevent the women feeling chilled.

Contraindications

These include heart or lung disease, infections, diabetes mellitus or epilepsy. Specific pregnancy-related conditions include history of spontaneous abortion, cervical cerclage, pregnancy-induced hypertension, antepartum haemorrhage, intrauterine growth restriction, ruptured membranes and history of preterm labour. However, if an earlier problem has settled and the obstetrician agrees in writing, then that woman may be included, but must be carefully observed. Postnatal contraindications would be an unhealed perineum, abnormal vaginal discharge or any infective condition.

If musculoskeletal problems present, the woman should be assessed by a physiotherapist before being accepted into the class.

Exercise-to-music

There is a growing demand for exercise-to-music classes from women who are not usually 'exercisers', as well as from those who are health conscious and want to keep fit with specific safe and effective exercises designed for pregnancy. There are both physical and psychological gains from these group sessions, which can be specially tailored for different stages of the childbearing year. During pregnancy the exercises can be gradually decreased in intensity then built up again in the postnatal weeks.

Special exercises for pregnancy, e.g. transversus, pelvic tilting and pelvic floor exercises described earlier, can be incorporated into the classes. Circulation will be improved and a greater awareness of good posture and body image will be promoted. General exercises improve mobility and help to maintain a feeling of well-being. It has been suggested that regular exercise may help prevent some problems developing in pregnancy, e.g. gestational diabetes.

Research is very limited in this area, but there is a growing acceptance of the gains from exercising to music and certainly women who are fit during pregnancy recover more quickly after the birth. Music can help motivation and increase the value of the exercise routine but needs to have a slower tempo than that used for normal movement to music classes for the non-pregnant population.

Such classes are intended to be complementary to conventional antenatal classes and should be led by teachers who are qualified to teach the specific exercises that are safe and appropriate for each stage of the childbearing year. Recognized courses are run by the YMCA and Royal Society of Arts (RSA) to train teachers to lead such exercise-to-music sessions.

Reflective Activity 23.11

Ask if you can participate in an aquanatal and exercise-to-music ante/postnatal class or at least observe one.

CONCLUSION

By encouraging physical skills in the antenatal period, good health and a sense of well-being during pregnancy are enhanced, which in turn increases the woman's confidence to cope in labour and facilitates a speedier return to normal after delivery. The midwife is the lead professional of a team of practitioners and will be asked to give advice about sport and exercise both during pregnancy and afterwards. This falls within the remit of health promotion encouraged in 'Making a Difference' (DoH, 1999). However, if there is any doubt about the suitability of any exercise or the physical fitness of the woman, then the midwife, after assessment of the situation, should refer to a physiotherapist or GP.

The midwife should encourage the practice of relaxation, back care and pelvic floor exercises, for her clients, far beyond pregnancy and childbirth, for herself and for her family and friends. In this way the midwife can support and facilitate the normal process of pregnancy and childbirth and have a profound effect on the health and well-being of society itself.

KEY POINTS

- Having a clear understanding of the anatomy and changing physiology of the abdominal and pelvic floor muscles and the musculoskeletal system enables the midwife to identify deviations from normal physiology and consult and refer appropriately to other practitioners such as the women's health physiotherapist.
- Learning about general exercise, back care and pelvic floor exercises will have long-term benefits for the midwife, and the woman, and enables both to work with the physiological changes in terms of exercise and relaxation approaches.
- It is important for the midwife to be able to provide individualized information and advice to women and their partners in preparing physically for pregnancy, childbirth and the puerperium, and to be able to support and facilitate the woman in coping with the normal physiological changes during this time.
- Developing the skills of relaxation will be of benefit for the midwife, and for her clients.
- Alternative approaches to exercise and well-being may be beneficial to many women, both physically and psychologically, and the midwife should be aware of what approaches are available and what might be appropriate to the woman and her partner.

REFERENCES

Association of Chartered Physiotherapists in Women's Health (ACPWH) (2000) *Symphysis Pubis Dysfunction Guideline*. London: Chartered Society of Physiotherapy.

Artal, R. & Buckenmeyer, P.J. (1995) Exercise during pregnancy and postpartum. *Contemporary Obstetrics/Gynecology* **40**(5): 62–90.

Brayshaw, E. (2003) *Exercises for Pregnancy and Childbirth: a Guide for Educators*, pp. x–xi. Oxford: Books for Midwives.

Bush, A. (1992) Cardiopulmonary effects of pregnancy and labour. *Journal of the Association of Chartered Physiotherapists in Obstetrics and Gynaecology* **71**: 3.

Caldeyro-Barcia, R. (1979) The influence of maternal bearing-down efforts during second stage on fetal well-being. *Birth and Family Journal* **6**: 17–22.

Calguneri, M., Bird, H.A. & Wright, V. (1982) Changes in joint laxity during pregnancy. *Annals of the Rheumatic Diseases* **41**(2): 126–128.

Department of Health (DoH) (1999) *Making a Difference*. London: The Stationery Office.

Donovan, G., McNamara, J. & Gianoli, P. (1988) *Exercise Danger*. Western Australia: Wellness Australia PTY.

Francis, W. (1960) The onset of stress incontinence. *Journal of Obstetrics and Gynaecology. British Empire* **67**: 899–903.

Fry, D., Hay-Smith, J., Hough, J. *et al.* (1997) Symphysis pubis dysfunction. *Physiotherapy* **83**: 41–42.

Knight, K.L. (1989) Cryotherapy in sports injury management. In: Grisogono, V. (ed) *Sports Injuries*. Edinburgh: Churchill Livingstone.

McIntosh, J. (1988) Research in reading into treatment of perineal trauma and late dyspareunia. *Journal of the Association of Chartered Physiotherapists in Obstetrics and Gynaecology* **62**: 7.

McMurray, R.G., Berry, M.J. & Katz, V. (1990) The beta endorphin response of pregnant women during aerobic exercise in water. *Medicine and Science in Sports and Exercise* **22**(3): 298–303.

Mitchell, L. (1988) *Simple Relaxation*, 2nd edn. London: John Murray.

Mørkved, S. & Bø, K. (1997) Effect of postpartum pelvic floor muscle exercise in the prevention and treatment of urinary incontinence. *International Urogynecology Journal* **8**: 217–222.

Mørkved, S. & Bø, K. (1999) Prevalence of urinary incontinence during pregnancy and postpartum. *International Urogynecology Journal* **10**(6): 394–398.

Mørkved, S. & Bø, K. (2000) Effect of postpartum pelvic floor muscle training in prevention and treatment of urinary incontinence: a one year follow-up. *British Journal of Obstetrics and Gynaecology* **107**(8): 1022–1028.

Noble, E. (1995) *Essential Exercises for the Childbearing Year*, 4th edn. Harwich MA; New Life Images.

Revelli, A., Durando, A. & Massobrio, M. (1992) Exercise and pregnancy: a review of maternal and fetal effects. *Obstetrical and Gynecological Survey* **47**(6): 355–367.

Richardson, C.A. & Jull, G.A. (1995) Muscle control – pain control. What exercises would you prescribe? *Manual Therapy* **1**(1): 2–10.

Roberts, J.E., Mendez-Bauer, C. & Wodell, D.A. (1983) The effects of maternal position on uterine contractility and efficiency. *Birth* **10**(4): 243–249.

Russell, J.G.B. (1982) The rationale of primitive delivery positions. *Journal of Obstetrics and Gynaecology* **89**(9): 712–715.

Sady, S.P. & Carpenter, M.W. (1989) Aerobic exercise during pregnancy: special considerations. *Sports Medicine* **7**(6): 357–375.

Shepherd, A. (1980) Re-education of the muscles of the pelvic floor. In; Mandelstam, D. (ed) *Incontinence and its Management*. London: Croom Helm.

Tucker Blackburn, S. (2003) *Maternal, Fetal and Neonatal Physiology: A Clinical Perspective*. London: W.B. Saunders.

Weiss, G. (1984) Relaxin. *Annual Review of Physiology* **46**: 42–52.

Wilson, P.D., Herbison, R.M. & Herbison, G.P. (1996) Obstetric practice and the prevalence of urinary incontinence 3 months after delivery. *British Journal of Obstetrics and Gynaecology* **103**(2): 154–161.

FURTHER READING

Brayshaw, E. (2003) *Exercises for Pregnancy and Childbirth: a Guide for Educators*. Oxford: Books for Midwives.
This book provides more depth of detail on all topics discussed in this chapter.

ADDITIONAL RESOURCES

Jackson, L. (2001) *Pilates in Pregnancy* (video). Wetherby: Enhance. **Association of Chartered Physiotherapists in Women's Health**
c/o The Chartered Society of Physiotherapy, 14 Bedford Row, London WC1R 4ED

PART 4

LABOUR AND DELIVERY

24. Place of Birth 401

25. Physiological Changes in Labour 410

26. Care in the First Stage of Labour 428

27. Relief of Pain During Labour 458

28. The Pelvic Floor 476

29. Care in the Second Stage of Labour 492

30. Care in the Third Stage of Labour 507

Place of Birth

Tina Heptinstall and Gay Lee

LEARNING OUTCOMES

By the end of this chapter the reader will be able to:

- discuss how the roles of midwives working in the community have changed over the last century, in terms of the focus and organization of their work
- evaluate the functions of antenatal and postnatal groups in maternity care

- critically evaluate the meaning of the concept of 'risk' when applied to birth at home
- debate the issues surrounding the choice of place of birth and the variety of skills needed by a midwife in order to provide good community-based care.

A HISTORICAL PERSPECTIVE

The role of the midwife working in the community in Britain has been constantly changing since the first Midwives Act was passed in 1902. At this time, the majority of midwives were working as independent practitioners in the community, taking responsibility for the total care of women who hired their services. Most babies were born at home and general practitioners were only called by midwives when problems occurred. Whilst antenatal care was virtually non-existent, the new professional midwives placed emphasis on the postnatal care of mothers and babies. Women were strictly 'confined to bed' for at least 10 days and postnatal care was characterized by elaborate, time-consuming rituals such as routine bed bathing (Leap and Hunter, 1993).

By 1937, the numbers of births at home had decreased as the percentage of births in institutions rose. Campbell and Macfarlane (1994) cite government records: in 1927, 15% of births took place in institutions. This rose to 24% in 1932 and to almost 35% by 1937. At this time the Midwives Act of 1936 charged local authorities in England and Wales with providing an adequate, salaried midwifery service. Most midwives became employees of local authorities and no longer had to purchase their own uniforms and equipment. For the first time they had 'off-duty', annual leave, pensions and financial security (Towler and Bramall, 1986). However, until the establishment

of the National Health Service in 1948, midwives still had to collect fees for their services from their clients, albeit on behalf of the local authorities.

After the Health Service Reorganisation Act of 1973 (implemented in 1974), local authorities no longer employed community midwives. They became employees of health authorities. The concept of the midwife being part of a team was developed and many community midwives became 'general practitioner (GP) attached' (Towler and Bramall, 1986). This reorganization resulted in a loss of autonomy for many community midwives.

Home births continued to decline until by the late 1980s, only 1% of births occurred at home. The decline was the result of successive government reports: the Cranbrook Report (Ministry of Health, 1959), the Peel Report (Standing Maternity and Midwifery Advisory Committee, 1970) and the Short Report (Social Services Committee, 1980). The overall message was that birth in hospital is safer than birth at home and that the reduction in stillbirths and neonatal deaths could be attributed to the increase in hospitalization for childbirth.

In a study of the personal registers of 300 midwives working during the years 1948–1972, Julia Allison analysed data on 35 000 home births (Allison, 1996). She identified that the rates of stillbirth and neonatal death were consistently less at home than in hospital, despite the fact that 50% of women who gave birth at home would be considered 'unsuitable' for home birth by current criteria. Also, as the percentage of these deaths fell at a similar rate for both home and hospital, she suggests that socioeconomic factors played a more important role than place of birth.

The decline of births at home meant that the focus of the community midwife's work centred on statutory postnatal visits. Some were able to develop their own antenatal clinics and in many areas the 'domino' ('domiciliary midwife in and out') scheme enabled community midwives to provide intrapartum care in hospital with an early transfer home. In the 1990s, the role of the community midwife continued to change. Early transfer home from hospital became normal practice for the majority of women and the number of postnatal visits for each community midwife increased. Antenatal care in the community also increased. At the time, Newson (1985) emphasized the importance of the need for a change in the attitude to care, not just a change in the organization of care:

> These [community-based antenatal] clinics are smaller, the waiting times shorter, and it is to be hoped that GP and midwife will be known to the mother. Low risk women can, therefore, be transferred from the hospital clinics to community clinics and this will lead to an improvement in care.
>
> Or will it? Does a reduction in travelling or waiting times combined with a known care-giver necessarily lead to an improvement in care? Or is it just possible that the only true improvement is the women receive inappropriate care more quickly?
>
> (Newson, 1985: 18)

The concept of midwifery practices based in the community with midwives providing continuity of care for women, regardless of place of birth, was first suggested in *The Vision*, a document published by the Association of Radical Midwives (ARM, 1986). The themes of continuity, choice and control were reiterated in the Winterton Report (House of Commons Health Committee, 1992) and in the Expert Maternity Group report *Changing Childbirth* (DoH, 1993). The report set indicators for success and action points for those providing maternity care. Community-based care and active user involvement in planning and reviewing services are central themes of this report:

In their book *Who's Left Holding the Baby?*, Ball *et al.* (1992) proposed a framework for change that would maximize midwifery skills. The establishment of midwifery group practices where midwives have

caseloads would be a key feature in the framework for change.

General conclusions about the benefits of these ways of organizing care are difficult because of the differences between schemes. Trying to examine both clinical and satisfaction outcomes complicates it. Economic outcomes of continuity of carer schemes are not always evaluated. Moreover, Green *et al.* (1998) comment that with the current level of knowledge of economic costs it is hard to ask meaningful questions of the costs and benefits of alternative ways of organizing midwifery services. The views and experiences of women and midwives of community-based schemes, particularly in relation to satisfaction, is a crucial part of any evaluation.

INITIATIVES IN THE COMMUNITY AND MODELS OF WORKING FOR MIDWIVES

Examples of some early community-based schemes include the Sighthill initiative in 1975 in Edinburgh (McKee, 1984). The scheme was concerned with the poor uptake of antenatal services and high perinatal mortality rate. A community-based service was introduced involving general practitioners and obstetricians. This met the needs of local women as well as providing more satisfaction for the midwives. The proportion of women booking in early in pregnancy was increased with improved attendance subsequently. There were improved outcomes of labour and a significant fall in the perinatal mortality over the next 5 years.

In a similar socially deprived area in Newcastle-upon-Tyne, a Community Midwifery Care project was set up in 1983 to assess the impact of midwives providing additional care to women in their own homes. The evaluation revealed an improvement in client satisfaction coupled with a greater partnership between the women and midwives. A survey of case notes revealed a reduction in the incidence of preterm labour and a reduction in the births of low birthweight babies (Davies, 1992). Davies revisits this study in her discussion of the experience of poverty among pregnant women and new mothers, and how this influences the midwife–mother relationship (Davies, 2000). Tyler (1994) has also pointed to the importance of midwives helping socially and politically disadvantaged women. She argues that resources, especially quality midwifery care, should be directed towards those in most need. Directing social care towards vulnerable women has significant positive outcomes, not only in terms of increasing women's self-confidence but also in reducing postnatal maternal and infant morbidity.

Oakley *et al.* (1990) conducted one of the most significant studies that examined the benefits of social support. The authors reported more positive pregnancy outcomes (physical and psychological health and use of health services) from a group of women who received social support intervention in pregnancy in contrast to a control group who received standard antenatal care. Furthermore, Oakley *et al.* (1996) conducted a follow-up survey of the same families and found that the intervention group, i.e. those who received social support in pregnancy, had better outcomes than those in the control group. The children had more favourable health and developmental outcomes and the mothers had better physical and psychological health.

In a randomized controlled trial of continuity of carer by a team of midwives, Flint *et al.* (1989) demonstrated that their scheme resulted in greater satisfaction, control and information for women compared to a control group. Quantitative data revealed that the women in the 'Know Your Midwife' ('KYM') group had fewer antenatal admissions, more spontaneous labours and less analgesia in labour than those in the control group. However, the authors say that 'it is not known how much the observed effects of this style of provision of perinatal care were due to the enthusiasm, personality and efficiency of the midwives' rather than the organization of care (Flint *et al.*, 1989: 15).

It has been suggested by some midwives that caseload practice is an ideal way to provide woman-centred continuity of midwifery care (Leap, 1994). A caseload is usually defined as a specific group of women, cared for predominantly by one midwife who usually has a reciprocal relationship with a midwife partner who gives care when the other is not available.

In 1994 the South East London Midwifery Group Practice became the first group of self-employed midwives to be contracted into the NHS. This group was one of three pilot schemes aimed at providing examples of how caseload practice can be implemented within a community setting (Reid, 1994).

Schemes such as those described above have demonstrated that midwifery practices based in the community provide an arena in which midwives are able to use and develop all their skills. Each of these schemes has developed a particular idea of how to practice but there is no organizational blueprint. In setting up practices, midwives need to take into consideration the needs of their local community, both socially and culturally. Undoubtedly, the community provides an ideal environment in which to develop new ways of working and the chance for midwives to develop more flexible and satisfying working patterns.

One of the most detailed studies of the organization of midwives' working lives was conducted by Sandall (1997). Her study raised interesting issues about midwives' occupational autonomy, developing meaningful relationships with women, and social support for midwives. Sandall (1997) also addressed the issue of 'burnout', which was the experience of some midwives working in continuity-of-carer schemes. This arose particularly when midwives worked in large teams with large caseloads and where they did not know the women. Midwives carrying their own smaller caseload suffered less burnout and experienced more satisfaction with their work.

Green *et al.* (1998) provide a critical review of the ways in which some maternity services have organized their midwifery care. In addition, Campbell and Garcia (1997) provide a valuable guide to the evaluation of maternity care from a number of different perspectives, such as safety, effectiveness, satisfaction and costs.

In summary, Flint's pioneering scheme was a catalyst for further change in the organization of midwifery care throughout the 1990s and many schemes were developed around the concept of continuity of carer. However, reflecting on the significance of the concept of continuity, Lee (1997) suggests that it is a concept that is not clear and has a range of meanings, not least to women who receive care from midwives. Furthermore, the term 'named midwife' and the meanings of 'care', 'carer', 'team', 'caseload' and women 'knowing' a midwife do not have universal agreement. In conclusion, Lee (1997) suggests that what women want is *good* care and that midwives should organize care in ways that increase the power of women, particularly the most vulnerable.

The organization of care also raises questions about whether it is the structure of the service or the individual qualities of the midwife that determine the quality of care. Quality of care is often explored using economic, satisfaction and clinical outcomes but these are just some perspectives. The final question here is – who should define quality and who has the power to do so?

For example, the epidural rate in one maternity unit might be 20%, but midwives, obstetricians, anaesthetists and women might each, as a group, evaluate this statistic differently. Which group might feel it reflected good-quality care and which group might feel it reflected poor-quality care? Which group perspective might be most influential in terms of reflecting an ideal maternity service?

WORKING IN THE COMMUNITY AND NETWORKING

In light of the current public health agenda there will be an increased need for midwives working in the community to liaise with other health and social care workers. Collaboration with other healthcare professionals in the community is a key feature of NHS reforms (DoH, 1999), and working with health visitors, GPs and others will increasingly be a feature of midwives' work. Initiatives such as 'Sure Start' are examples of collaboration that goes beyond arguments over which health professional provides which care.

Midwives are also well placed to forge links with community workers, youth workers and voluntary organizations. This may mean that midwives become involved with the work of local organizations such as women's groups and welfare rights projects. It could mean getting involved in the work of a Maternity Services Liaison Committee (MSLC), a local branch of the National Childbirth Trust (NCT) or the Stillbirth and Neonatal Death Society (SANDS) or a government-funded scheme, e.g. Sure Start.

Antenatal and postnatal education/support groups

In recent years the conventional model of 'parentcraft' has been challenged and there is a move away from formal antenatal 'classes' towards a more facilitative style within groups (Leap, 1991; MacKeith et al., 1991; Priest and Schott, 1991). Hospitals are no longer the primary setting for such groups and they may be successfully run in youth and community centres, health centres or leisure centres.

For midwives, networking is not only about building up their own relationships in the community or about using agencies; it is also about putting people in touch with each other. It is about linking people, particularly new mothers, in similar circumstances. Antenatal and postnatal groups provide an ideal forum for networking between women. Women who have made friendships within an antenatal group are well motivated to continue to meet where provision exists in the postnatal period (Leap, 1991). Midwives can

also support the establishment and continuation of new-mothers' groups by collaborating with other health professionals, voluntary organizations and with women themselves. Reducing isolation, loneliness and depression among new mothers is a key feature of postnatal care (Alabaster, 2000; MacInnes, 2000).

Priest and Schott (1991) do, however, emphasize that midwives need appropriate skills to run such groups, with the emphasis on building women's understanding and confidence; it is not simply about giving information. Antenatal and postnatal groups provide an opportunity for women to share their experiences and to learn from each other. Women set the agenda and they are encouraged to see themselves as 'the experts'. The midwives' skill in facilitating the group lies in listening and in ensuring that everyone is introduced and included. They need to know when to provide guidance and information and when it is more appropriate to enable group members to respond to each other (Leap, 1991; Priest and Schott, 1991).

In responding to local need, midwives may need to consider establishing women-only groups, evening groups that partners or friends can attend, or other groups such as those for young women (MacKeith et al., 1991) or for women who need interpreters. Consideration needs to be given to using images and audiovisual aids that are racially and culturally appropriate. There is also a need to resist using words and phrases that can trivialize or disempower women such as 'old wives' tales' and 'confinement'; and referring to women as 'girls' or 'ladies' (Leap, 1992b).

Reflective Activity 24.1

Arrange to meet a group (or a member of one) that involves childbearing women. For example:

- Maternity Services Liaison Committee
- an antenatal group
- a postnatal group.

Consider whether the needs of the women attending have been met.

Postnatal care

Midwives attend women and their babies in the postnatal period for a relatively short time, although this may change in the future. The key to postnatal care lies in providing support and encouragement to new parents, thus building self-confidence and minimizing dependency on professionals. The midwife can encourage parents to rely on their own common sense and intuition.

Where the midwife sees the mother as her baby's expert, she will avoid gratuitous advice and instructions. A directive approach may be appropriate in certain situations, such as when the mother asks for information or where there is a safety issue. For example, midwives need to inform mothers about the link between babies' sleeping positions, overheating and sudden infant death syndrome (SIDS). More recently the Foundation for the Study of Infant Deaths launched a campaign message; 'sleep on the back, play on the front and watch the world'. The latter advice relates to encouraging motor development in young infants (FSID, 2001). Additionally, midwives need to give clear advice about bed sharing and co-sleeping (Inch, 2003).

BIRTH AT HOME

Issues of safety

The issue of safety is at the heart of most debates on the choice of home birth. In spite of a culture that is dominated by images and acceptance of hospital birth as the norm the Winterton Report in 1992 commented that:

> There is no convincing and compelling evidence that hospitals give a better guarantee of the safety of the majority of mothers and babies. It is possible, but not proven, that the contrary may be the case.
>
> (House of Commons Health
> Committee, 1992: xii)

The statistics about the safety of home birth were first challenged in the late 1970s, particularly by statistician Marjorie Tew. A comprehensive summary of her analysis of the data is presented in *Safer Childbirth* (Tew, 1998). Although Campbell and Macfarlane (1994) challenged Tew's methodology, they also questioned the prevailing assumptions that had underpinned government policy since the 1960s. Their conclusions included the following statements:

> There is no evidence to support the claim that the safest policy is for all women to give birth in hospital (p. 119).

> The statistical association between the increase in the proportion of hospital deliveries and the fall in the crude perinatal mortality rate seems unlikely to be explained either wholly or in part by a cause and effect relationship (p. 119).

> For some women, it is possible, but not proven, that the iatrogenic risk associated with institutional delivery may be greater than any benefit conferred (p. 120).

Campbell *et al.* (1984) addressed the importance of distinguishing between planned and unplanned home births when interpreting data. They noted a difference in perinatal mortality according to the intended place of birth, ranging from 4.1/1000 in those booked for birth at home compared with 196.6/1000 in unbooked home births. They recognized that women booking a home birth are a selected group and that those transferred to hospital during labour would not have been included in the survey. Nevertheless, they concluded that perinatal mortality among births booked to occur at home was low, particularly for parous women.

When supporting women in making choices about the place of birth, midwives may like to consider the words of Nancy Stewart of the Association for Improvements in Maternity Services (AIMS):

> All of living involves some risk, and this applies to giving birth and being born, wherever the birth takes place. ... It is important to go beyond the statistics, to consider the real influences on safety for you and your baby. ... Where to give birth is not a matter of physical safety versus feelings. They are inextricably wrapped up together and you can trust the wisdom of your feelings in choosing where your baby is to be born.
>
> (AIMS Information Booklet, *Choosing a
> Home Birth*, undated)

So women's decisions about where to give birth are probably rarely based on objective statistical risk but on a woman's own understanding of that risk. They are also based on intuition and the way the midwife presents the pros and cons of home and hospital birth.

Facilitating home birth

Reasons given by women for choosing to give birth at home, apart from risk and safety, have included:

- family tradition
- personal control/privacy
- relaxed environment

- fear of hospitals and of unnecessary, routine intervention
- knowing the midwife
- intimacy with children and partners
- emotional and physical spontaneity.

(Chamberlain *et al.*, 1997; Kitzinger, 1991; Leap, 1992a; Wesson, 1996)

One of the critical reasons for women choosing, and midwives supporting, home birth is that women can have more control over the birth process. Midwives who regularly attend home births have noted that women are less likely to require pharmacological analgesia when they labour and give birth in their own homes (Cronk and Flint, 1989; RCM, 1993). Various authors have described the significance of the social environment of birth and its impact on labour (Gaskin 1990; Odent, 1984; Simkin, 1986). Arguably home birth provides the optimum chance for physiological processes to take place without disturbance. These may be among the reasons for the reported favourable outcomes for planned home births in the western world (Durand, 1992; Ford *et al.*, 1991; Tew and Damstra-Wijmenga, 1991).

Preparation for birth at home

If the midwife is not an employee of the hospital, but is, for example, an independent midwife, she may ask the supervisor of midwives to organize a contract to enable her to continue to provide midwifery care to the woman should transfer become necessary. When planning to attend a woman who has chosen to give birth at home, the midwife needs to notify her intention to practise to the supervisor of midwives for the area in which the woman lives if she has not already done so (UKCC, 1998). The situation is more straightforward if the midwife is an employee of a trust in the area. The supervisor of midwives should ensure that the midwife has access to referral for screening tests that are necessary and will provide forms such as the birth notification. She may also facilitate referral to an obstetrician or paediatrician when problems arise where the midwife does not have arrangements for direct referral.

Reflective Activity 24.2

Identify and justify the items that you as a midwife will need to take to a woman's home prior to and at the birth.

What will you advise her and her helpers to prepare?

Do you think midwives working in the community should be able to:

- resuscitate the newborn?
- undertake perineal suturing?
- insert an intravenous cannula?
- carry out a full physical examination of the newborn?

Give reasons for your answers.

Midwives attending home births will have considered their sources of support during the labour, particularly if events do not progress in a straightforward fashion. They need to remember Rule 40 in the *Midwives' Rules* (UKCC, 1998) to call for assistance of a qualified health professional if appropriate. These rules are currently being updated (NMC, 2003).

During the birth

The midwife's primary responsibility during the labour lies in ensuring that the woman can labour in a safe environment that encourages the normal physiological processes to work without disturbance. It is not about 'managing' the labour. It is about listening, watching, thinking, picking up cues and responding. At home, women are often less inhibited about moving around, making noise and behaving instinctively. This enables midwives to develop their skills in assessing the progress of labour without resorting to routine vaginal examinations.

The midwife can minimize disruption at a home birth by not turning the woman's home into a 'mini labour ward'. Non-essential equipment can often be left out of the immediate vicinity chosen by the woman for labour and birth. Since women often decide at the last minute where they will give birth, it can be practical to place all the essential equipment on a tray so that the midwife can follow the woman to the place of her choice. As part of the midwife's role is to ensure safety, she may need to improvise at a home birth, particularly where heating is concerned. For example, towels may be warmed on a hot water bottle, a radiator or a heating pad, ready for the baby. Essentially, midwives' skills relate to their own ability and being confident in the women's ability.

The experience of home birth

Women describe feeling empowered by giving birth at home. They also speak of a shift in the balance of power where the midwife is an invited guest in their homes:

> When you go into hospital it's their place, they know where the loo is and all that and you're standing around waiting for them to tell you what to do. Whereas at home, it's your place, you know where everything is and they have to ask you where things are.
>
> (Leap, 1992a)

CONCLUSION

While the focus of this chapter is on women who have their babies in the community, we acknowledge that the majority of women currently give birth in hospital. Inevitably the underlying context of other aspects of labour and birth is in hospital. Although many labour wards are designed in a 'home-from-home' style, fundamentally there is little point in changing the curtains if midwives' practice philosophy is not woman-centred or is based on a medical model of care (Kitzinger, 1991).

Ideally, midwifery care will follow the woman regardless of whether she needs or wants to give birth in hospital. Increasingly, midwives encourage women to see home birth as a safe choice for uncomplicated childbirth. This has meant an increase in the rate of birth at home. Final decisions about the place of birth can be left for the woman to make during labour, thereby ensuring that she keeps all her options open. All this means that midwives are moving more freely between hospitals and the community. Thus the conventional 'community midwife', as discretely different from her hospital counterpart, may disappear.

However, in contrast, Anderson (2000) suggests that the notion that midwives will be flexible, multi-skilled and be able to work in a range of settings at any one time is not so straightforward. She describes two distinct models of a midwife. The first model has highly developed social, interpersonal and networking skills, which are used most effectively in the community. The second model is more hospital based, where midwives have developed their technical skills to a high level and can provide care for women when pregnancy and labour become complicated. She poses the question, 'does it matter that there are two highly differing models of midwifery?' This is a challenging point in the context of the significant changes that have evolved within the past decade that have focused on integrated midwifery care.

Striking a balance between the organization of sustainable schemes that offer a high standard of care across a spectrum of need with good clinical and economic outcomes, and satisfaction for both women and midwives is likely to be the challenge of future midwifery practice.

KEY POINTS

- The structure of the midwifery service and the content of the community midwife's job has changed over the past century.
- There is no causal connection between the rise in hospital births and the decrease in perinatal mortality over the last few decades. Hospital birth has not been proven to be safer than birth at home, so doctors, midwives and mothers are rethinking the concept of 'risk' as applied to home birth.
- Whether birth takes place at home or in hospital, the experience can be an empowering and positive one for both mother and midwife if the midwife is well prepared and encourages the woman to have confidence in her own abilities to give birth.

REFERENCES

Association for Improvements in Maternity Services (AIMS) (undated) *Choosing a Home Birth*. London: AIMS.

Alabaster, M. (2000) Postnatal depression: working and learning with mothers *Community Nurse* 6(4): 39–40.

Allison, J. (1996) *Delivered at Home*. London: Chapman & Hall.

Anderson, T. (2000) What does a midwife do? *Practising Midwife* 2(1): 4–5.

Association of Radical Midwives (ARM) (1986) *The Vision: Proposals for the Future of the Maternity Services*. ARM, 62 Greetby Hill, Ormskirk, Lancashire, L39 2DT.

Ball, J., Flint, C., Garvey, M. *et al.* (1992) *Who's Left Holding the Baby? An Organisational Framework for Making the Most of Midwifery Services*. University of Leeds: The Nuffield Institute for Health Services Studies.

Campbell, R. & Garcia, J. (1997) *The Organisation of Maternity Care: A Guide to Evaluation.* London: Haigh & Hochland.

Campbell. R. & Macfarlane. A. (1994) *Where to be Born?: The Debate and the Evidence*, 2nd edn. Oxford: National Perinatal Epidemiology Unit.

Campbell, R., MacDonald Davies, I., Macfarlane, A. *et al.* (1984) Home births in England and Wales, 1979: perinatal mortality according to intended place of delivery. *British Medical Journal* 289: 721–724.

Chamberlain, G., Crowley, P. & Wraight, A. (1997) *Home Births. The Report of the 1994 Confidential Enquiry by the National Birthday Trust Fund.* London: Parthenon

Cronk, M. & Flint, C. (1989) *Community Midwifery: A Practical Guide.* London: Heinemann Medical Books.

Davies, J. (1992) The role of the midwife in the 1990s. In: Chard, T. & Richards, M.P.M. (eds) *Obstetrics in the 1990s.* London: Palgrave.

Davies, J. (2000) Being with women who are economically without. In: Kirkham, M. (ed) *The Midwife–Mother Relationship.* London: Macmillan.

Department of Health (DoH) (1993) *Changing Childbirth.* Report of the Expert Maternity Group. London: HMSO.

Department of Health (DoH) (1999) *Making a Difference. Strengthening the Nursing, Midwifery and Health Visiting Contribution to Health and Health Care.* London: DoH.

Durand, A.M. (1992) The safety of home birth: the Farm study. *American Journal of Public Health* 82(3): 450–453.

Flint, C., Poulengeris, P. & Grant, A. (1989) The 'Know your Midwife' Scheme – a randomised controlled trial of continuity of care by a team of midwives. *Midwifery* 5: 11–16.

Ford, C., Iliffe, S. & Franklin, O. (1991) Outcome of planned home births in an inner city practice. *British Medical Journal* 303: 1517–1519.

Foundation for the Study of Infant Deaths (FSID) (2001) Online. Available: http://www.sids.org.uk/fsid/

Gaskin, I.M. (1990) *Spiritual Midwifery*, 3rd edn. Summertown, TN: The Book Publishing Company.

Green, J., Curtis, P., Price, H. *et al.* (1998) *Continuing to Care: the Organisation of Midwifery Services in the UK: a Structured Review of the Evidence.* Hale, Cheshire: Books for Midwives Press.

House of Commons Health Committee (1992) *Maternity Services Second Report*, Vol. 1. (Chairman: Sir Nicholas Winterton) London: HMSO.

Inch, S. (2003) Bedsharing and co-sleeping in the UK – implications for midwives. *Midwives* 6(10): 425–427.

Kitzinger, S. (1991) *Homebirth and Other Alternatives to Hospital.* London: Dorling Kindersley.

Leap, N. (1991) Helping you to make your own decisions – antenatal and postnatal groups in South East London. VHS Video. Available from ACE Graphics: PO Box 173, Sevenoaks, Kent TN14 5ZT, UK. Tel: 01959 524622.

Leap, N. (1992a) Home birth your choice. VHS Video. Available from ACE Graphics: PO Box 173, Sevenoaks, Kent TN14 5ZT, UK. Tel: 01959 524622.

Leap, N. (1992b) The power of words. *Nursing Times* 88(21): 60–61.

Leap, N. (1994) Caseload practice within the NHS: are midwives ready and interested? *Midwives Chronicle* 107(1275): 130–135.

Leap, N. & Hunter, B. (1993) *The Midwife's Tale: An Oral History from Handywoman to Professional Midwife.* London: Scarlet Press.

Lee, G. (1997) The concept of continuity – what does it mean? In: Kirkham, M.J. & Perkins, E.R. (eds) *Reflections on Midwifery.* London: Baillière Tindall.

MacInnes, A. (2000) Findings of a community-based group for women with PND. *Community Practitioner* 73(99): 754–756.

McKee, I.H. (1984) Community antenatal care: the Sighthill Community Antenatal Scheme. In: Zander, L. & Chamberlain, G. (eds) *Pregnancy Care for the 1980s.* London: Royal Society of Medicine, Macmillan Press.

MacKeith, P., Phillipson, R. & Rowe, A. (1991) *45, Cope Street: Young Mothers Learning Through Group Work.* An evaluation report. Nottingham Community Health, Memorial House, Standard Hill, Nottingham, NG1 6FX.

Ministry of Health (1959) *Report of the Maternity Services Committee.* (Cranbrook Report: Chairman: Lord Cranbrook) London: HMSO.

Newson, K. (1985) Breaking away from routine care. *Nursing Mirror* 161(3): S18–S21.

Nursing and Midwifery Council (NMC) (2003) Press statement 18/2003. Online. Available: http://www. nmc-uk.org/pressstatements

Oakley, A., Rajan, L. & Grant, A. (1990) Social support and pregnancy outcome. *British Journal of Obstetrics and Gynaecology* 97: 155–162.

Oakley, A., Hickey, D., Rajan, L. *et al.* (1996) Social support in pregnancy: does it have long term effects? *Journal of Reproductive and Infant Psychology* 14: 7–22.

Odent, M. (1984) *Birth Reborn: What Birth Can and Should Be.* London: Souvenir Press.

Priest, J. & Schott, J. (1991) *Leading Antenatal Classes.* Oxford: Butterworth Heinemann.

Royal College of Midwives (RCM) (1993) *Audit of Independent Midwifery 1989–1991.* 15 Mansfield Street, London W1M 0BE: RCM.

Reid, T. (1994) A bid for independence. *Nursing Times* 90(30): 18.

Sandall, J. (1997) Midwives burnout and continuity of care. *British Journal of Midwifery* 5(2): 106–111.

Simkin, P. (1986) Stress, pain and catecholamines. *Birth* 13(4): 227–240.

Social Services Committee (1980) *Second Report from the Social Services Committee: Perinatal and Neonatal*

Oestrogens and oxytocin receptors

While progesterone inhibits oestrogen-induced formation of oxytocin receptors in the myometrium during the first trimester, myometrial and decidual receptors for oxytocin increase from 27.6 fmol/mg DNA in the non-pregnant state to 171.6 fmol/mg DNA at mid-gestation, and to 1391 fmol/mg DNA at term (Fuchs and Fuchs, 1991). This represents an 80–100-fold increase within the uterus. However, progesterone inhibits the production of myometrial ERa, which desensitizes this tissue to the contractile properties of oestrogens until the end of pregnancy (Mesiano, 2001, Mesiano et al., 2002).The capacity of progesterone to maintain uterine relaxation is also enhanced by functional inactivation of sympathetic nerves in the myometrium, and increased receptors for a large number of peptides and neurotransmitters that promote relaxation and inhibit the contractile effects of oxytocin (Casey et al., 1997; Dong et al., 1999, 2003; Ferguson et al., 1998; Grammatopoulos et al., 1996; Owman, 1981).

Uterine changes in preparation for labour

Current research suggests the emergence of a nocturnal surge in uterine activity as an early indication of maternal changes preparing for the onset of labour. From 30 weeks' gestation, progressive nocturnal increases in myometrial activity have been demonstrated in women, and nocturnal peaks in plasma concentrations of oxytocin have been found at 37 and 39 weeks' gestation (Fuchs et al., 1991; Germain et al., 1993; Moore et al., 1994).

Cervical and myometrial changes

From approximately 36 weeks onwards, structural alterations become apparent in cervical and myometrial tissues. Within cervical connective tissue, alterations occur in the composition and concentration of the gel-like material called ground substance (proteoglycans) in which connective tissue cells and fibres are embedded. At the same time an increase occurs in enzymes that degrade collagen. The concentration of ground substance relative to that of collagen is thought to reach a maximum during the process of cervical softening prior to the onset of labour. This overall increase is characterized by the emergence of a higher proportion of molecules that have a weaker affinity for collagen fibrils. During late pregnancy, the myometrial component of the cervix seems to contract in characteristic short, high-frequency pressure increases that are independent of the rest of the uterus. These contractions may stimulate local connective tissue changes in preparation for labour (Olah et al., 1993; Pajntar, 1994), and are followed by progressive dilatation of the external os during labour. This movement tends to occur slowly until approximately 3–4 cm and then more rapidly, until the cervix has passed over the presenting part of the descending fetus.

Changes in cervical tissue during this period are an acceleration of events in late pregnancy. During the latent phase of labour, a significant increase has been found in the concentration of a specific molecule called hyaluronic acid. In addition to its weak affinity for collagen, this molecule has a high water-binding capacity, which is thought to explain the swollen and fragile consistency of the cervix in labour. In addition, most studies report significant decreases in collagen content following labour, and the duration of cervical dilatation is significantly correlated with cervical collagen content prior to the onset of labour (Jeffrey, 1991; van Dessel et al., 1993).

In primiparous women, softening of cervical tissue proceeds alongside effacement and is thought to occur in response to an increase in the formation of gap junctions between adjacent cells in the myometrium of the uterine cavity. Gap junctions are composed of symmetrical portions of plasma membrane from adjacent cells. These form intercellular channels for the passage of ions and small molecules, facilitating rapid transmission of electrical impulses and chemical signals between cells. Gap junctions emerge in late pregnancy and undergo further increases in size and number during early labour. In animal studies, the formation and permeability of gap junctions are stimulated by oestrogens and prostaglandins and inhibited by progesterone and relaxin (Burghardt et al., 1993; Chow and Lye, 1994).

By facilitating the propagation of action potentials from cell to cell, gap junctions synchronize myometrial activity. Tension is transmitted from the myometrium by the outer layer of muscle in the cervix and by localized pressure on the lower uterine segment, which is exerted by the fetus, as the presenting part descends in the pelvis. These combined pressures produce a differential rate of tissue uptake in the cervix and the adjacent part of the uterus. Maximum uptake occurs at the lower peripheral end of the cervix, producing a gradual upward movement of soft cervical tissue that eventually merges with the lower uterine segment (Gee and Olah, 1993) (Fig. 25.1).

In a recent study on women following induction and augmentation of labour, a number of significant

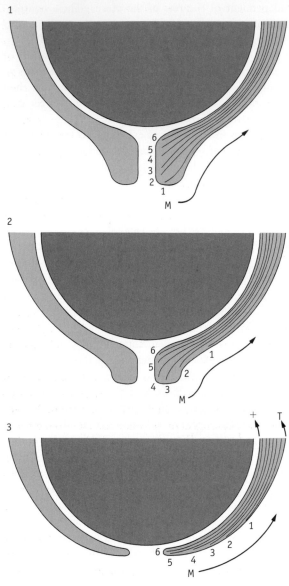

Figure 25.1 Diagram representing the differential movement of tissue planes at the time of cervical effacement and dilatation. M, direction of movement of collagen bundles; T, +, differential tension across the myometrium.

features were associated with the presence or absence of cervical contractions in response to myometrial activity. Cervical contractions predominantly occurred in women with lower measures of cervical effacement and dilatation and a longer latent phase, compared to those in whom cervical contractions were absent. While these findings do not reflect the sequence of events during spontaneous labour, they highlight the importance of effacement and suggest that cervical muscle is

actively involved in bringing it about (Olah *et al.*, 1993; Pajntar, 1994).

Tissue changes and inflammation

Local pro-inflammatory changes are thought to accompany the reorganization and stretching of cervical connective tissue that occurs in the latter part of pregnancy. The progressive release of a number of inflammatory mediators like prostaglandins and interleukins may gradually overwhelm the selective suppression of inflammatory and immune responses that is established from the beginning of pregnancy by progesterone. The reorganization of the cervical connective tissue and stretching of the lower uterine segment and the consequent disruption of fetal membranes is accompanied by local alterations in the relative activity of a number of mediators of inflammatory and anti-inflammatory reactions (Bennett *et al.*, 2001). These include increased synthesis of prostaglandins in the amnion during the third trimester and a simultaneous reduction in prostaglandin catabolism in the chorion surrounding the lower uterine segment (Bennett *et al.*, 2001). The enzymes that stimulate prostaglandin synthesis are regulated by a nuclear transcription factor that inhibits progesterone receptors, while the sharp increase in fetal cortisol at the end of pregnancy may act within the fetal membranes to reduce the activity of prostaglandin dehydrogenase (PGDH), the enzyme stimulated by progesterone that inactivates prostaglandins throughout pregnancy (Kelly, 1994; Patel *et al.*, 2003).

Progesterone

Progesterone has a range of inhibitory effects on mediators of the immune/inflammatory response. Some studies have demonstrated that progesterone plays a critical role in preventing immune rejection of the fetoplacental unit throughout pregnancy (Pepe and Albrecht, 1995). While no reduction in plasma concentrations of progesterone has been demonstrated consistently in humans, recent findings indicate that receptors for progesterone in the amnion may be downregulated in labour (Bennett *et al.*, 2001). This suggests that a local reduction in progesterone activity may occur at a time when tissue changes are stimulating a progressive rise in the synthesis of a large number of inflammatory mediators. Most research in this area has focused on prostaglandins, short-acting local hormones formed in cell membranes from arachidonic acid (Kelly, 1994; Siteri and Stites, 1982).

Prostaglandins

The placenta, decidua, myometrium and fetal membranes have varying capacities to synthesize prostaglandins, including $PGF_{2\alpha}$, PGE_2 and PGI_2. Both $PGF_{2\alpha}$ and PGE_2 stimulate myometrial contractions. PGE_2 is the most potent but unlike $PGF_{2\alpha}$, has a dual action that simultaneously desensitizes the myometrium to its stimulatory effects. PGI_2 is a potent vasodilator that relaxes smooth muscle.

$PGF_{2\alpha}$ and PGE_2 are produced in varying amounts in the placenta, decidua and fetal membranes, while PGI_2 is predominantly produced by the myometrium and to a much lesser extent in the amnion (Fuchs and Fuchs, 1991).

Decidual prostaglandins

The decidua is a major source of uterine prostaglandins during and after labour. Following spontaneous delivery, production rates of $PGF_{2\alpha}$ and PGE_2 in decidual cells, are reported to be approximately 30 times greater than those obtained following elective caesarean section, and this is accompanied by significantly greater concentrations of enzymes required for their production. Concentrations of $PGF_{2\alpha}$ are higher than those of PGE_2 (Skinner and Challis, 1985).

Levels of 6-keto-$PGF_{1\alpha}$ and 13,14-dihydro-15-keto-$PGF_{2\alpha}$ (PGFM) progressively increase up to full dilatation and further increase at delivery of the fetal head. Between birth and placental separation, additional increases occur, producing values that are double those at full dilatation. Further increases occur after delivery, to reach highest levels at 5 minutes following placental separation (Fuchs et al., 1983; Noort et al., 1989).

Amniotic prostaglandins

The amnion is composed of a single layer of cuboidal epithelial cells, supported by a thick basement membrane composed of collagen and fibroblasts. This avascular membrane shows a small but steady increase in a key enzyme involved in prostaglandin synthesis from the first trimester, followed by a much larger increase from 38 weeks' gestation and again following labour and birth (Bennett et al., 2001). Unlike decidual prostaglandins, those from the amnion do not have direct access to the myometrium. Once produced, they are subject to distinct paracrine influences as they move across the chorion and the decidua (Collins et al., 1992; Germain et al., 1994; Mitchell et al., 1993).

Amnion obtained following spontaneous labour at term has been found to produce higher levels of PGE_2, but no change in $PGF_{2\alpha}$ following exposure to term amniotic fluid, compared to membrane obtained following elective caesarean section at term but these changes only appear on the fetal amniotic side of the membrane. Isolated chorion/decidual membranes obtained after labour produce significantly higher levels of PGE_2 and $PGF_{2\alpha}$, compared to membranes obtained at term, but this does not occur when these are studied as intact membranes, intimately associated with the amnion, as they exist in vivo (Collins et al., 1992).

Action of the chorion

This difference seems to be due to varying levels of enzyme activity that metabolizes prostaglandins to their inactive metabolites. Amnion is characterized by a high capacity to synthesize and a low capacity to inactivate PGE_2. Chorion has a very low capacity to synthesize both PGE_2 and $PGF_{2\alpha}$ but, like the decidua, it contains high concentrations of PGDH that converts both groups of prostaglandins to inactive metabolites. The activity of this enzyme impedes the transfer of prostaglandins across intact amnio-chorio-decidua before and after the onset of labour (Germain et al., 1994).

Research findings suggest that the chorion contains enzymes that degrade prostaglandins and other molecules that stimulate myometrial contractions. Experiments on dispersed chorion before and after spontaneous labour at term show a high level of $PGF_{2\alpha}$ metabolism but no net production of either PGE_2 or $PGF_{2\alpha}$. The specific activities of PGDH were not found to be significantly different in samples taken before and after the onset of labour and similar findings were reported in the decidua (Germain et al., 1994; Skinner and Challis, 1985).

In addition to PGDH, the chorion contains high concentrations of a protein called gravidin that inhibits the release of arachidonic acid from decidual cells. The activity of this protein is significantly greater in chorion obtained following elective caesarean section, compared to that following spontaneous delivery at term. Another enzyme, phospholipase A_2, directly releases arachidonic acid from plasma membranes. Within the decidua, concentrations of this enzyme have been found to increase threefold during pregnancy. High concentrations of gravidin in the chorion may inhibit the activity of phospholipase A_2 in the adjoining decidua, and this may, with the onset of labour, have an inhibitory effect on decidual prostaglandins (Wilson et al., 1989).

Intact membranes

Experimental findings on the combined effects of intact membranes strongly indicate that they are ideally positioned to protect the fetus from locally produced prostaglandins and other inflammatory mediators that also have the capacity to stimulate the myometrium to contract. In a recent in vitro experiment, the presence of fetal membranes and decidua from term pregnancies following caesarean section or vaginal delivery produced a 40% decrease in spontaneous contractions of adjacent muscle fibres. Studies on the accumulation of prostaglandins in different compartments of amniotic fluid before, during and after labour suggest that it occurs as a constituent part of local tissue changes that are an integral part of labour (Collins *et al.*, 1992; MacDonald and Casey, 1993).

Rupture of the membranes

Findings on PGDH in decidua and chorion have led to suggestions that the increased production of PGE_2 in the amnion from 38 weeks and specific collagen degrading enzymes during labour may be involved in weakening the basement membrane and thickening the spongy layer that separates the amnion from the chorion, particularly at the site which overlays the cervix (Bennett *et al.*, 2001; Vadillo-Ortega *et al.*, 1995). Recent experiments have found that amnion obtained from spontaneous deliveries is 42% heavier than that obtained following elective caesarean sections. This is thought to result from an increase in hydrolysis of collagen that results in increased uptake of water in the collagen matrix. These structural changes are thought to facilitate the spontaneous rupture of membranes during labour.

Maternal oxytocin

For individual women, labour and birth are momentous life events and evidence suggests that all animals, including humans, are apprehensive and fearful at some point either before or during labour (Klaus *et al.*, 1986; Melender, 2002; Odent, 1992). A variety of studies have shown that neurohormonal mechanisms modulate the stress axis during late pregnancy, labour and lactation, and these changes appear essential for the enhanced accumulation of oxytocin during late pregnancy and its release during labour and lactation (Groer and Davis, 2002; Haddad *et al.*, 1985; Magiakou *et al.*, 1996).

Oxytocin neurones display a low level of electrical activity during pregnancy; then increased bursting behaviour during active labour and birth, followed by a pattern of episodic high-frequency-bursting behaviour during lactation (Fuchs *et al.*, 1991; Jiang and Wakerley, 1995; Matthiesen *et al.*, 2001).

Under the stimulatory influence of rising concentrations of oestrogens and progesterone, central and peripheral sensitivity to oxytocin is increased during pregnancy and labour by tissue-specific changes in oxytocin and oxytocin receptor mRNA in a number of brain regions and in the heart, kidneys, uterus and mammary gland (Fuchs *et al.*, 1984; Kimura *et al.*, 1996; Mitchell and Schmid, 2001; Mukaddam-Daher *et al.*, 2002).

Central and peripheral receptor activity is regulated by oxytocinase, an enzyme that rapidly degrades oxytocin. Placental oxytocinase is released into the maternal circulation during pregnancy to reach highest levels just before the onset of labour (Ito *et al.*, 2001). This enzyme prevents receptor desensitization during prolonged oxytocin release, as happens during labour and lactation, and may also suppress the pain of uterine contractions before and after birth, by rapidly inactivating oxytocin following its release (Jiang and Wakerley, 1995).

Myometrial oxytocin receptors gradually increase up to 36 weeks, then more rapidly until term, to reach peak values before active labour begins (Fuchs *et al.*, 1984; Kimura *et al.*, 1996; Wathes *et al.*, 1999). Because of the increase in oxytocinase before the onset of labour, receptor concentrations remain elevated for approximately 20 hours of labour before they begin to decline (Ito *et al.*, 2001).

Systemic oxytocin from late pregnancy to birth

From around 32 weeks the onset of increased nocturnal release of oxytocin coincides with decrease in the plasma oestrogen/progesterone ratio and the rise in oxytocin receptor density in the uterus. Under these conditions, a small rise in the pulsatile release of oxytocin seems to stimulate episodes of uterine contractions during the hours of darkness (Fuchs *et al.*, 1991; Germain *et al.*, 1993; Moore *et al.*, 1994). The expression of oestrogen-induced gap junction proteins in the myometrium also increases from around 37 weeks and these provide low-resistance pathways between smooth muscle cells that increase the coordination of contractile activity throughout the uterus (Chow and Lye, 1994). From around 36 weeks many women also display a slight increase in blood pressure, which is thought to increase placental blood supply to the fetus.

From pregnancy to labour

In women, the transition from nocturnal uterine contractions to latent labour is highly variable and influenced by a host of factors including fetal position and maternal cognitive activity (Haddad *et al.*, 1985; Wuitchik *et al.*, 1989). Research evidence indicates that low cognitive anxiety enables women to experience less discomfort during latent labour, which suggests that in the absence of stress the enhanced release of central oxytocin provides effective analgesia (Wuitchik *et al.*, 1989). During the transition from pregnancy to labour, oxytocin released from the median eminence into the anterior pituitary may indirectly enhance maternal comfort by increasing appetite, through its stimulatory action on prolactin (Noel and Woodside, 1993). For first-time mothers in particular, increased appetite during the latent phase of labour will induce comfort and sleep, which will enhance oxytocin release. Maintaining a calm, low-lit environment during labour also prevents a stress-induced rise in catecholamines which have been shown to inhibit oxytocin and attenuate uterine contractions (Levinson and Shnider, 1979; Peled, 1992; Wuitchik *et al.*, 1989).

The pattern of systemic oxytocin

The pattern of systemic oxytocin release in women has been identified from samples taken at 1-minute intervals over 30 minutes, in three groups, from late pregnancy until the expulsion of the placenta (Fuchs *et al.*, 1991). Group one were at term but not in labour; group two were in spontaneous labour with cervical dilatation of 2–5 cm; and group three were at various points in the second and third stages of labour. Basal levels of oxytocin were below detection limit of the assay, $0.17\,\mu U/ml$, in all women but the percentage of samples below the detection limit decreased from late pregnancy onwards, as pulse frequency increased significantly as labour progressed (Fuchs *et al.*, 1991) (Figs 25.2–25.4).

Labour is characterized by a highly individual pulsatile pattern in all groups. Pulses occur at irregular intervals with variable peak levels or amplitudes lasting 1–3 minutes. Mean pulse frequency and duration of pulses are lowest in group one and progressively increase as labour advances. No significant increase was evident in mean peak levels between labour and non-labour groups. Although highest peaks occurred in the second and third stage of labour, these were highly variable and not uniformly associated with contractions, birth or ejection of the placenta. (Fuchs *et al.*, 1991). During labour, basal plasma concentrations of oxytocin remain at $\sim 0.17\,\mu U/ml$, while pulse amplitude increases moderately from $0.92–1.4\,\mu U/ml$ as labour progresses and pulse frequency increases from 1.2/30 minutes at term, to 6.7/30 minutes during the second and third stage of labour (Fuchs *et al.*, 1991).

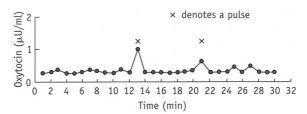

Figure 25.2 Daytime plasma oxytocin levels in one woman in late pregnancy not in labour. Samples were collected at 1-minute intervals from an indwelling catheter. (Reproduced with permission from Fuchs *et al.*, 1991: 1517.)

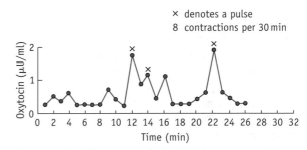

Figure 25.3 Plasma oxytocin levels in one woman during the first stage of labour (cervix 2–5 cm dilated). (Reproduced with permission from Fuchs *et al.*, 1991: 1517.)

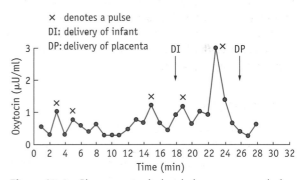

Figure 25.4 Plasma oxytocin levels in one woman during the second and third stages of labour. DI, delivery of infant; DP, delivery of placenta. (Reproduced with permission from Fuchs *et al.*, 1991: 1517.)

The systemic release of oxytocin from the neurohypophysis during labour occurs in response to neuronal feedback to the brainstem from the uterus, cervix and vagina. During late pregnancy and labour, innervation is low in the body of the uterus and significantly higher in the cervix, vagina and adjacent parts of the pelvic cavity. Stretching and distension of these areas has been found to activate sensory afferent nerve pathways that

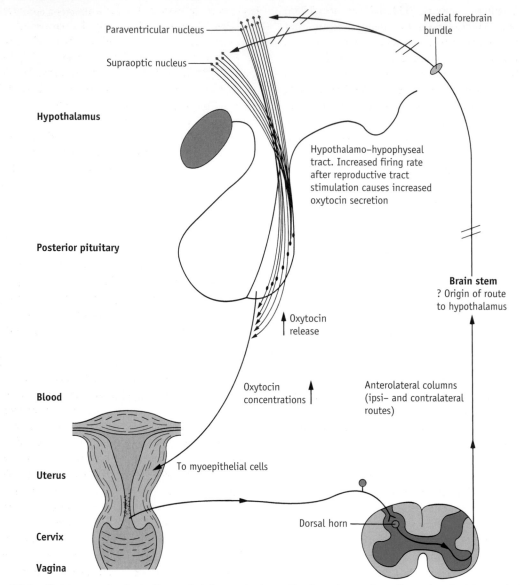

Figure 25.5   The neuroendocrine reflex underlying oxytocin synthesis and secretion. (Reproduced with permission from Johnson and Everitt, 1995: 299.)

transmit signals via the spinal cord and brainstem to oxytocin neurones in the hypothalamus. These respond with discrete bursts of accelerated discharge that transport the stored hormone along axons of hypothalamic neurones that terminate in the neurohypophysis. From here oxytocin is released into the general circulation (Antonijevic *et al.*, 1995) (Fig. 25.5).

Intrauterine oxytocin system

Oestrogen-induced intrauterine expression of oxytocin receptors operates locally to regulate uterine contractions during pregnancy and labour (Chibbar *et al.*, 1995; Mitchell and Schmid, 2001; Morel *et al.*, 2001; Wu *et al.*, 2001). In humans, a >300-fold increase in oxytocin receptor mRNA has been demonstrated in the myometrium at term, compared to non-pregnant values (Kimura *et al.*, 1996; Wathes *et al.*, 1999). These display a gradient expression, with highest and lowest concentrations in the fundus and cervix respectively, which may be one of the mechanisms involved in generating uterine polarity to assist fetal descent during labour and birth (Fuchs *et al.*, 1984;

Loup *et al.*, 1991; Wu *et al.*, 2001). Myometrial oxytocin receptor concentrations increase before and after the onset of labour but no increase has been observed in receptor concentrations in the lower segment (Waithes *et al.*, 1999). Consequently, during early labour, myometrial receptor concentrations are uniformly high in the upper segment and progressively lower in the isthmus and cervix, while those in the decidua are highest in the corpus, followed by the fundus and the isthmus (Fuchs and Fuchs, 1991; Fuchs *et al.*, 1984; Hirst *et al.*, 1993). Within the fetal membranes, increased oxytocin-receptor binding has also been found between late pregnancy and labour, with highest increases detected in the amnion (Takemura *et al.*, 1994).

Current experiments suggests that oxytocin mRNA is synthesized in epithelial, myometrium and in choriodecidual tissues between late pregnancy and birth (Chibbar *et al.*, 1995; Mitchell and Schmid, 2001; Morel *et al.*, 2001). Under the stimulatory influence of physiological doses of oestrogens, oxytocin mRNA and peptide increase significantly in choriodecidual tissues obtained after spontaneous labour but oxytocin concentrations in these tissues are not increased following labour; and in myometrial tissue from the lower uterine segment, oxytocin mRNA is low and does not increase in response to labour (Chibbar *et al.*, 1995).

Oxytocin in amniotic fluid is thought to flow directly from the umbilical circulation and fetal urine. Concentrations of oxytocin in amniotic fluid are higher in samples taken at delivery than during late pregnancy. Following spontaneous labour and delivery, significantly higher levels of oxytocin have also been found in the umbilical artery than in the umbilical vein. In contrast, no significant differences have been found following elective caesarean section (Benedetto *et al.*, 1990).

While some authors speculate that the initiation of labour in women may be stimulated by intrauterine oxytocin, at present there is insufficient evidence to support this view (Blanks and Thornton, 2003; Mitchell and Schmid, 2001; Russell *et al.*, 2002).

Central and systemic oxytocin during active labour

As labour progresses, increasing cervical stretching and myometrial contractions activate uterine afferent nerve pathways to the hypothalamus that stimulate both central and peripheral release of oxytocin (Antonijevic *et al.*, 1995; Neumann *et al.*, 1996). Once active labour begins, most women are overwhelmed by the increased intensity of uterine contractions.

There is a dramatic fall in food appetite and intestinal mobility, which is mediated by the pattern of central and peripheral oxytocin release that characterizes labour and birth (Diaz-Cabiale *et al.*, 2000; Morien *et al.*, 1999). On the basis of these findings on the activation of oxytocin systems during established labour, maternal food appetite can be expected to fall to nonexistent levels, towards the end of labour.

This effect of oxytocin on maternal appetite and gastrointestinal function complements changes in maternal energy requirements. In contrast to the need for rapid utilization of glucose for milk lactose secretion during lactation, the most energetically demanding phase of the reproductive cycle, myometrial contractions impose no additional demand on maternal energy stores (Odent, 1994; Steingrimsdottir *et al.*, 1993; Tigas *et al.*, 2002). The myometrium has a low energy requirement and considerable capacity for glycogen storage which increases up to 10-fold during pregnancy, peaks at term and is used as a predominant source of energy for contractions during and after labour (Steingrimsdottir *et al.*, 1993).

Skeletal muscle activity is characteristically reduced during active labour and maternal neocortical or higher brain requirements for glucose may also decline, as women tend to withdraw and become remote from verbal communications around them (Odent, 1992). This tendency for women to occupy 'another world' is particularly evident at home, in a warm low-lit environment, where labouring women lose all track of time, and the increased release of central oxytocin may also induce periods of sleep between contractions, particularly before the expulsive phase of labour. These profound alterations in the activity of oxytocin neurones enable women to get in touch with their instinctive behaviours and close down all forms of rational, neocortical activity (Odent, 1992; Uvnas-Moberg, 1994).

Contractions and spontaneous pushing

Around the transition to second stage, the frequency of contractions often slows down while their duration increases (Morrin, 1985). When maternal and fetal events are not completely synchronized, this often presents as a slowing down of the labour process and may require experimenting with different maternal positions to allow the fetus to fully descend into the pelvic outlet (see Chs 29 and 30). A slow pace of descent allows the simultaneous surge in fetal adrenaline to complete the removal of lung liquid which enhances respiratory adaptations immediately following birth (Bland, 2001).

Spontaneous breathing

To maintain uterine blood flow and adequate oxygenation to the fetus during the second stage of labour, maternal hyperventilation and breath holding need to be avoided during contractions. Over prolonged periods, breath holding (as in the Valsalva manoeuvre) increases intrathoracic pressure, which reduces venous return to the heart. Consequently, cardiac output falls and blood pressure drops leading to a reduction in uteroplacental perfusion (Blackburn, 2003).

Expulsive phase of labour

In biological terms, the second stage is reached when the cervix has completely dilated and has become incorporated into the lower uterine segment, which becomes progressively thinner, as expulsive contractions set up positive afferent nerve pathways to the hypothalamus. This reflexive mechanism stimulates increased central and peripheral release of oxytocin that reaches a high point in the peripheral circulation immediately following birth (Antonijevic et al., 1995; Sansone et al., 2002). With increasing flexion and anterior rotation of the fetal head, pressure from the vertex against the gutter-shaped pelvic floor muscles stimulates their stretch receptors that activate the neurohormonal stimulation of central oxytocin neurons (Antonijevic et al., 1995; Sansone et al., 2002).

Unresolved anxieties or perceived danger may stimulate catecholamines, particularly adrenaline, which inhibits the release of oxytocin leading to the decline or cessation of uterine contractions, excessive blood loss following birth and delay in the onset of suckling and lactation (Chen et al., 1998; Levison and Schnider, 1979; Odent, 1992; Peled, 1992). The downregulation of myometrial oxytocin receptor concentrations following very prolonged labour because of inhibition of oxytocin release, may result in atony of the myometrium and excessive blood loss following birth (Jouppila, 1995). Current evidence suggests that providing a private, warm, low-lit environment, will enhance oxytocin secretion and minimize the rise in maternal cortisol and catecholamines activated by heightened fear and anxiety that often occurs just before expulsive contractions begin (Chen et al., 1998; Levison and Schnider, 1979; Wuitchik et al., 1989). The expulsive phase of labour is accompanied by a physiological increase in catecholamine levels, particularly noradrenaline. This rise increases cardiac output and pulmonary circulation, providing the physical energy that usually coincides with the final moments of the expulsive phase of labour (Odent, 1987).

FETAL RESPONSES TO LABOUR AND BIRTH

The progressive nocturnal surge in uterine activity during the last trimester gradually shifts the fetus towards the lower pole of the uterus and allows the presenting part to descend into the pelvis. This allows the fetus to then increase flexion and descent and follow the curve of Carus (see Ch. 29).

Figure 25.6 illustrates the rise in catecholamine levels in the human fetus throughout labour, reaching 20 times adult resting values immediately following birth. The intermittent squeezing of the fetal head during human labour triggers a rapid surge in catecholamine release (Lagercrantz and Slotkin, 1986); free cortisol levels double in association with labour, rising further in the 1–2 hours following birth; and a dramatic surge in thyroid-stimulating hormone (TSH) at birth stimulates striking increases in thyroid hormones during the first 24 hours of neonatal life (Pearson Murphy and Branchaud, 1994).

Studies on the influence of labour on catecholamine production at term have found that umbilical arterial concentrations are four times higher in babies delivered vaginally, compared to those delivered by elective caesarean section. The increasing catecholamine output produces a variety of cardiorespiratory and metabolic adaptations during and after labour and key neurodevelopmental changes following birth (Lagercrantz and Slotkin, 1986; Lagercrantz and Herlenius, 2002).

Pulmonary

The fetus is subject to many different forms of stimulation from hormonal and mechanical changes that facilitate the onset and progress of labour. During the last couple of days before labour begins, breathing activity is reduced and lung fluid is produced at a gradually decreasing rate (Bland, 2001). Fetal breathing may be depressed by rising concentrations of PGE_2, while a decline in the volume of lung liquid is associated with increased production of catecholamines. Concentrations of catecholamines in amniotic fluid have been shown to rise from the second to the third trimester (Bland, 1992, 2001; Divers et al., 1981). Experimental evidence suggests that rising concentrations of adrenaline during labour positively correlate with the progressive reabsorption of lung liquid, and the composition of surfactant also matures and production levels increase following the administration of synthetic catecholamine preparations. The presence

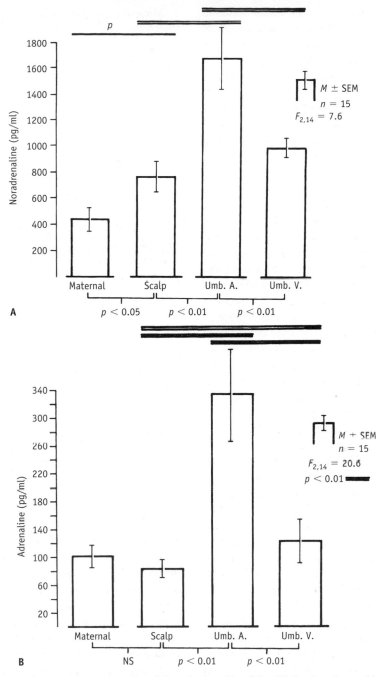

Figure 25.6 Comparison of maternal noradrenaline **(A)** and adrenaline **(B)** with fetal scalp, umbilical artery (Umb. A.) and vein (Umb. V.) noradrenaline and adrenaline. Bar graphs are linked by lines that illustrate significant statistical differences: *one line*, at 0.05 level; *two lines*, at 0.01 level. M, mean; SEM, standard error of the mean; n, sample size; F, variance ratio; p, probability; NS, not significant. (From Artal, 1980.)

of similar changes in humans are evident from studies comparing lung function in infants born vaginally, to those delivered by elective caesarean section. From measurements taken at 30 and 120 minutes after birth, tidal volume, minute ventilation and dynamic lung compliance were found to be significantly lower in the caesarean section group. Taken together, these results indicate that higher levels of surfactant are produced and a more rapid elimination of lung liquid occurs in response to the stimulatory influences of labour (Irestedt *et al.*, 1982; Mortola *et al.*, 1982; Oliver, 1981) (see Chs 31 and 35).

Cardiovascular

Contractions induce transient reductions in uteroplacental perfusion that alter the pattern of fetoplacental circulation. Ultrasonic studies suggest that at the beginning of a uterine contraction, maternal venous outflow is halted and the content of the uterine veins is expressed into the maternal circulation. Simultaneously, arterial inflow that coincides with the onset of contractions is retained within the intervillous space. During contractions, this blood forms an increased pool that creates marked distension and vascular engorgement in the intervillous space. Transient reduction in uteroplacental perfusion during contractions may be partly compensated by the increased volume of maternal blood made available for gaseous exchange. To ensure the perfusion of the placenta, maternal blood pressure and cardiac output also rise in response to contractions. During the phase of uterine relaxation following each contraction, an increased blood flow has been observed which may also compensate for decreased oxygen delivery during the preceding contraction (Bleker *et al.*, 1975; Robson *et al.*, 1987).

The circulation of a healthy fetus in spontaneous labour is not thought to be compromised by contractions. The umbilical circulation does not appear to be altered by changes in intrauterine pressure or by short-term changes in fetal or maternal–placental blood flow that accompany contractions. Fetal cardiac output rises in response to increased intrauterine pressure during contractions, which allows fetal blood pressure to maintain a relatively constant pressure difference between the inside and outside of its vascular system. Concurrently, raised levels of fetal adrenaline specifically act to facilitate increases in heart rate and blood pressure, both of which serve to increase the rate of fetoplacental blood flow between contractions. During the latter part of labour, selective pressure on the soft-walled umbilical vein has been reported to produce a net transfer of approximately 66 ml from fetus to placenta. While the fetal circulation remains attached to the high-capacity reservoir provided by the umbilical–placental unit, this redistribution of blood has no impact on the fetal circulation and only becomes relevant if the cord is clamped immediately after birth (Dunn, 1985; Reynolds, 1955).

The effect of fetal head pressure, and the resulting catecholamines activates the parasympathetic system and inhibits cardiac pacemakers, resulting in decreased cardiac output, slowing of the heart rate and reduced blood pressure. Slowing of the heart rate during contractions reduces the oxygen requirements of cardiac muscle. Parasympathetic influences on heart rate can be counteracted by adrenaline but not by noradrenaline. In the fetus at term, sufficient levels of adrenaline may be released to produce variable increases or decreases in heart rate, in response to uterine contractions (Lagercrantz and Slotkin, 1986; Reynolds, 1955).

BIRTH, MATERNAL–INFANT INTERACTIONS AND PLACENTAL EJECTION

Until birth, the fetus is essentially a parenterally nourished organism receiving a fairly constant supply of simple nutrients from the maternal circulation across the fetoplacental barrier (Blackburn, 2003). During this period of enhanced anabolic metabolism, the maternal circulation supplies the placenta with glucose, amino acids and relatively smaller amounts of essential and non-essential fatty acids for selective uptake and transfer to the fetus (Hay, 1995; Herrera, 2000). Soon after birth, placental transfer of nutrients and gaseous exchange between maternal and fetal circulatory systems comes to an end and the neonate undergoes neurodevelopmental, cardiovascular, respiratory and metabolic adaptations for the final phase of dependent growth and development that ends at spontaneous weaning.

As the fetus leaves the uterine cavity, the surface area of the contracting uterus declines rapidly to produce a uterine diameter of around 10 cm (Blackburn, 2003). This reduction encompasses the site of placental attachment to the decidual lining, leading to compression of placental tissue and the uteroplacental blood vessels, including approximately 100 spiral arteries that have been supplying blood to the placenta at a rate of 500–800 ml/min throughout the course of labour (Letsky, 1998). Myometrial compression of these blood vessels following birth is greatly facilitated by placental-induced adaptations in the constituents of decidual and myometrial segments of the spiral arteries. During the first and second trimester, structural transformations of the vessel walls replace elastic lamina and smooth muscle layers with a matrix containing fibrin (Matijevic *et al.*, 1996).

When the mother is free to reach down and take the baby into her arms at birth, she brings herself into an upright position. This prevents any compression of uterine blood flow returning to the heart via the inferior vena cava and allows gravity to assist the process of placental ejection, while the sight, sounds and sensory contact between mother and infant stimulate a significant increase in central and peripheral release of oxytocin, as the opioid restraint on maternal oxytocin neurones is removed immediately after birth (Jiang and Wakerley, 1995; Matthiesen *et al.*, 2001). Basal levels of oxytocin rise significantly and sensory stimulation and suckling increase pulse frequency and amplitude of oxytocin release, compared to labour and birth (Matthiesen *et al.*, 2001)

The enhanced release of oxytocin into the peripheral circulation following birth stimulates further intermittent contraction and retraction of the myometrium that squeezes the spongy placental tissue and forces blood in the collapsing intervillous spaces back into the veins

of the decidua. Meanwhile, the uninterrupted flow of blood through the intact umbilical cord further reduces placental size, by transferring approximately 120 ml blood into the neonatal circulation (Dunn, 1985). As illustrated in Figure 25.7, the intact cord continues to provide oxygenated blood to the infant, until placental separation is progressing. This allows volume adjustments to supply new capillary beds, which are opened by the dramatic fall in pulmonary vascular resistance following the rise in Po_2, as the lung capillaries dilate with the onset of ventilation immediately following birth (Boldt *et al.*, 1998; Dunn, 1985).

With further myometrial contractions, the congested decidual veins are severed and sealed by the shearing forces of the criss-cross network of muscle fibres surrounding them. As illustrated in Figure 25.8, the placenta is simultaneously torn from the uterine wall, at the line of the decidua basalis, and falls into

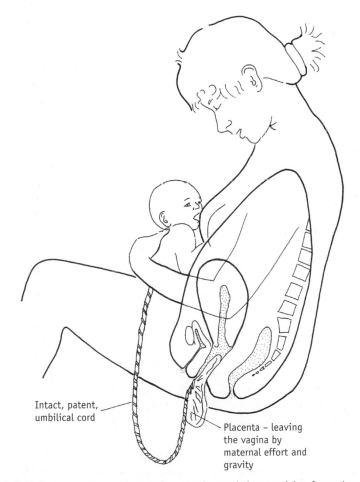

Intact, patent, umbilical cord

Placenta – leaving the vagina by maternal effort and gravity

Figure 25.7 Maternal–infant sensory contact, placental separation and the transition from placental to mammary nutrition. (From Inch, 1989.)

the uterine cavity, peeling off the membranes as it descends towards the cervix, and then is expelled into the vagina (Benirschke, 1992).

Placental separation leaves behind a surface wound of 300 square centimetres containing approximately 100 severed arteries in which maternal blood coagulates rapidly because of a major increase in the concentration of several coagulation factors and decreased fibrinolytic activity which characterizes pregnancy,

labour and the first couple of hours following birth (Letsky, 1998). Pregnancy is accompanied by marked increases in clotting factors VII, VIII, X and XII and by a significant rise in vascular and placental plasminogen activator inhibitors (PAIs) leading to a marked increase in plasma fibrinogen by the third trimester (Dalaker, 1986; Letsky, 1998).

Before and after birth, these systemic haemostatic changes are accompanied by a local activation of the

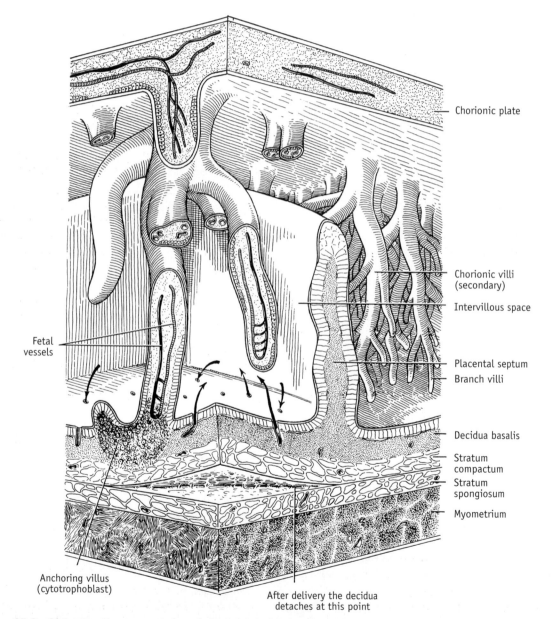

Chorionic plate

Chorionic villi (secondary)

Intervillous space

Placental septum

Branch villi

Decidua basalis

Stratum compactum

Stratum spongiosum

Myometrium

Fetal vessels

Anchoring villus (cytotrophoblast)

After delivery the decidua detaches at this point

Figure 25.8   Diagrammatic representation of placental decidual and myometrial tissue near term illustrating the line of placental separation. Arrows indicate maternal blood flow in the intervillous space. (From Duplessis, G.D.T. and Haegel, P. (1971) *Embryologie*. New York: Masson. English edition by Springer-Verlag; Chapman and Hall; and Masson (1972).)

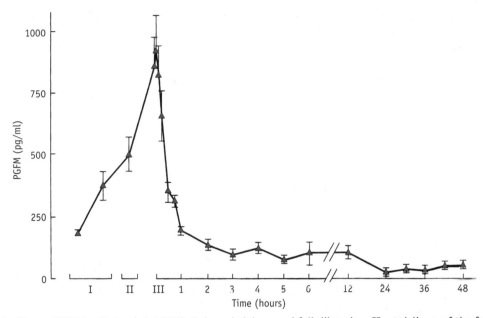

Figure 25.9 Plasma PGFM levels (pg/ml ±SEM). I: in early labour and full dilatation; II: at delivery of the fetal head; III: at placental separation and up to 48 hours afterwards. (Reproduced with permission from Noort *et al.*, 1989: 6.)

clotting factors V and VIII and increased levels of fibrinogen, which results in a pronounced shortening of whole blood clotting *time* that is more pronounced in uterine than in peripheral blood. Because of their combined effects, torn blood vessels are sealed and the site of placental separation is rapidly covered by a fibrin mesh that represents 5–15% of total circulating fibrinogen (Letsky, 1998). As illustrated in Figure 25.9, prostaglandin metabolites are simultaneously released into the general circulation from the torn surface tissues of the decidua basalis at the site of separation where they stimulate sustained uterine contractions (Noort *et al.*, 1989).

When women do not experience prolonged stress-induced catecholamine release or severe vaginal or perineal laceration during labour and birth, immediate blood loss from the vagina constitutes a small proportion of the increase in plasma and red cell volume that occurs during pregnancy. Under these conditions, most of the pregnancy-induced increase in blood volume is lost over a longer time period, through diuresis during the first 48 hours and lochia discharge from the placental site over the first 2 months postpartum (Hytten, 1995). While visual estimates of blood loss within the first hour following birth are highly inaccurate, the significance of estimated blood loss at birth needs to be judged in relation to the expansion in blood volume that occurred during pregnancy (Bloomfield and Gordon, 1990; Gyte, 1992).

The expression of innate mother–infant interactions particularly during the early weeks after birth is critical for the infant's long-term health and well-being (Stern, 1997). Close body contact reduces energy loss, regulates homeostatic mechanisms, promotes a physiological increase in glucocorticoid and mineralocorticoid brain receptors and prevents a rise in the infant's stress axis which is highly sensitive to periods of separation, particularly during the first 3 days after birth (Bystrova *et al.*, 2003; Christensson *et al.*, 1995; Hofer, 1994; Kehoe and Bronzino, 1999; Sarrieau *et al.*, 1988).

Reflective Activity 25.1

In your next span of care of a woman in labour, consider the environment you are providing and its effect on the woman and her labour.

Review the labour in relation to the neurohormonal interplay at work.

CONCLUSION

It is important that midwives are knowledgeable about the physiological basis of labour and birth, as this will provide an important reservoir of evidence on which to base appropriate and effective care for the woman, the fetus and baby.

KEY POINTS

- The hormonal basis of parturition commences during the third trimester.
- The process of the preparation for, initiation and continuation of labour is regulated by maternal, placental and fetal systems.
- Provision and maintenance of a quiet and private environment during labour will facilitate the spontaneous process of labour.

- An understanding of neurohormonal interactions assists in the provision of effective care for the woman and baby.

REFERENCES

Antonijevic, I.A., Leng, G., Luckman, S.M. *et al.* (1995) Induction of uterine activity with oxytocin in late pregnant rats replicates the expression of c-fos in neuroendocrine and brain stem neurons as seen during parturition. *Endocrinology* **136**(1): 154–163.

Artal, R. (1980) Fetal adrenal medulla. *Clinical Obstetrics and Gynecology* **23**(3): 825–836.

Benedetto, M.T., Di Cicco, F., Rossiello, F. *et al.* (1990) Oxytocin receptor in human fetal membranes at term and during labor. *Journal of Steroid Biochemistry* **35**(2): 205–208.

Benirschke, K. (1992) Placental separation at birth. In: Polin, R.A. & Fox, W.W. (eds) *Fetal and Neonatal Physiology*, pp. 95–96. Philadelphia: W.B. Saunders.

Bennett, P., Allport, V., Loudon, J. *et al.* (2001) Prostaglandins, the fetal membranes and the cervix. In: Smith, R. (ed) *The Endocrinology of Parturition. Basic Science and Clinical Application. Frontiers of Hormone Research*, Vol. 27, pp. 147–164. Basel: Karger.

Blackburn, S.T. (2003) *Maternal, Fetal and Neonatal Physiology*. Philadelphia: W.B. Saunders.

Bland, R.D. (1992) Formation of fetal lung liquid and its removal near birth. In: Polin, R.A. & Fox, W.W. (eds) *Fetal and Neonatal Physiology*, pp. 782–789. Philadelphia: W.B. Saunders.

Bland, R.D. (2001) Loss of liquid from the lung lumen in labour: more than a simple 'squeeze'. *American Journal of Physiology* **280**(4): L602–L605.

Blanks, A.M. & Thornton, S. (2003) The role of oxytocin in parturition. *British Journal of Obstetrics and Gynaecology* **110**(Suppl. 20): 46–51.

Bleker, O.P., Kloosterman, G.J., Mieras, D.J. *et al.* (1975) Intervillous space during uterine contractions in human subjects: An ultrasonic study. *American Journal of Obstetrics and Gynecology* **123**(7): 697–699.

Bloomfield, T.H. & Gordon, H. (1990) Reaction to blood loss at delivery. *Journal of Obstetrics and Gynaecology* **10**(Suppl. 2): S13–S16.

Boldt, T., Luuhleainen, P., Tyhrquist, F. *et al.* (1998) Birth stress increases adrenomedullin in the newborn. *Acta Paediatrica* **87**(1): 93–94.

Burghardt, R.C., Barhoumi, R. & Dookwah, H. (1993) Endocrine regulation of myometrial gap junctions and their role in parturition. *Seminars in Reproductive Endocrinology* **11**(3): 250–260.

Bystrova, K., Widstrom, A-M., Mattheisen, A-S. *et al.* (2003) Skin-to-skin contact may reduce negative consequences of 'the stress of being born': a study on temperature in newborn infants, subjected to different ward routines in St Petersburg. *Acta Paediatrica* **92**(3): 320–326.

Casey, M.L., Smith, J., Alsabrook, G. *et al.* (1997) Activation of adenylyl cyclase in human myometrial smooth muscle cells by neuropeptides. *Journal of Clinical Endocrinology and Metabolism* **82**(9): 3087–3092.

Chen, D.C., Nommsen-Rivers, L., Dewey, K.G. *et al.* (1998) Stress during labour and delivery and early lactation performance. *American Journal of Clinical Nutrition* **68**(2): 335–344.

Chibbar, R., Wong, S., Miller, F.D. *et al.* (1995) Estrogen stimulates oxytocin gene expression in human chorio-decidua. *Journal of Clinical Endocrinology and Metabolism* **80**(2): 567–572.

Chow, L. & Lye, S.J. (1994) Expression of the gap junction protein connexin-43 is increased in the human myometrium toward term and with the onset of labour. *American Journal of Obstetrics and Gynecology* **170**(3): 788–795.

Christensson, K., Cabrera, T., Christensson, E. *et al.* (1995) Separation distress call in the human neonate in the absence of maternal body contact. *Acta Paediatrica* **84**(5): 468–473.

Collins, P.L., Goldfien, A. & Roberts, J.M. (1992) Exposure of human amnion to amniotic fluid obtained before labour causes a decrease in chorion/decidual prostaglandin release. *Journal of Clinical Endocrinology and Metabolism* **74**(5): 1198–1205.

Dalaker, K. (1986) Clotting factor VII during pregnancy, delivery and puerperium. *British Journal of Obstetrics and Gynaecology* **93**: 17–21.

Diaz-Cabiale, Z., Narvaez, J.A., Petersson, M. *et al.* (2000) Oxytocin/alpha$_2$-adrenoceptor interactions in feeding responses. *Neuroendocrinology* **71**(3): 209–218.

Divers, W.A., Wilkes, M.M., Babakni, A. *et al.* (1981) An increase in catecholamines and metabolites in the amniotic fluid compartment from middle to late gestation. *American Journal of Obstetrics and Gynecology* **139**: 483–486.

Dong, Y.-L., Fang, L., Kondapaka, S. *et al.* (1999) Involvement of calcitonin gene-related peptide in the modulation of human myometrial contractility during pregnancy. *Journal of Clinical Investigation* **104**(5): 559–565.

Dong, Y.-L., Wimalawansa, S.J. & Yallampalli, C. (2003) Effects of steroid hormones on calcitonin gene-related peptide receptors in cultural human myometrium. *American Journal of Obstetrics and Gynecology* **188**(2): 466–472.

Dunn, P.M. (1985) The third stage and fetal adaptation. In: Clinch, J. & Matthews, T. (eds) *Perinatal Medicine: IX European Congress of Perinatal Medicine,* Dublin 1984, pp. 47–54. Lancaster: MTP Press.

Ferguson, J.F., Seaner, R.M., Bruns, D.E. *et al.* (1998) Expression and specific immunolocalization of the human parathyroid hormone/parathyroid hormone-related protein receptor in the uteroplacental unit. *American Journal of Obstetrics and Gynecology* **179**(2): 321–329.

Fuchs, A-F. & Fuchs, F. (1991) Physiology of parturition. In: Gabbe, S.G. (ed) *Obstetrics, Normal and Problem Pregnancies,* pp. 147–174. New York: Churchill Livingstone.

Fuchs, A-F., Goeschen, K., Husslein, P. *et al.* (1983) Oxytocin and the initiation of human parturition III Plasma concentrations of oxytocin and 13.14-dihydro-15-keto-prostaglandin $F_{2\alpha}$ in spontaneous and oxytocin-induced labour at term. *American Journal of Obstetrics and Gynecology* **147**(5): 497–502.

Fuchs, A.-R., Fuchs, F., Husslein, P. *et al.* (1984) Oxytocin receptors in the human uterus during pregnancy and parturition. *American Journal of Obstetrics and Gynecology* **150**(6): 734–741.

Fuchs, A.-R., Romero, R., Keefe, D. *et al.* (1991) Oxytocin secretion and human parturition: pulse frequency and duration increase during spontaneous labour. *American Journal of Obstetrics and Gynecology* **165**(5): 1515–1523.

Gee, H. & Olah, K.S. (1993) Failure to progress in labour. In: Studd, J. (ed) *Progress in Obstetrics and Gynaecology,* Vol. 10, pp. 159–181. Edinburgh: Churchill Livingstone.

Germain, A.M., Valenzuela, G.J., Ivankovic, M. *et al.* (1993) Relationship of circadian rhythms of uterine activity with term and preterm delivery. *American Journal of Obstetrics and Gynecology* **168**(4): 1271–1277.

Germain, A.M., Smith, J., Casey, M.L. *et al.* (1994) Human fetal membrane contribution to the prevention of parturition: uterotonin degradation. *Journal of Clinical Endocrinology and Metabolism* **78**(2): 463–470.

Grammatopoulos, D., Stirrat, G.M., Williams, S.A. *et al.* (1996) The biological activity of the corticotrophin-releasing hormone receptor–adenylate cyclase complex in human myometrium is reduced at the end of pregnancy. *Journal of Clinical Endocrinology and Metabolism* **81**(2): 745–751.

Groer, M.W. & Davis, M.W. (2002) Postpartum stress: current concepts and the possible protective role of breastfeeding. *Journal of Obstetric, Gynecologic, and Neonatal Nursing* **31**(4): 411–417.

Gyte, G. (1992) The significance of blood loss at delivery. *MIDIRS Midwifery Digest* **2**(1): 88–92.

Haddad, P.F., Morris, N.F. & Spielberge, C.D. (1985) Anxiety in pregnancy and its relation to use of oxytocin and analgesia in labour. *Journal of Obstetrics and Gynaecology* **6**: 77–81.

Hay, W.W. (1995) Metabolic Interrelationships of placenta and fetus. *Placenta* **16**(1): 19–30.

Herrera, E. (2000) Metabolic adaptations in pregnancy and their implications for the availability of substrates to the fetus. *European Journal of Clinical Nutrition* **54**(Suppl. 1): S47–S51.

Hirst, J.J., Chibbar, R. & Mitchell, B.F. (1993) Role of oxytocin in the regulation of uterine activity during pregnancy and in the initiation of labour. *Seminars in Reproductive Endocrinology* **11**(3): 219–233.

Hofer, M.A. (1994) Early relationships as regulators of infant physiology and behaviour. *Acta Paediatrica* **397**: 9–18.

Huszar, G. & Roberts, J.M. (1982) Biochemistry and pharmacology of the myometrium and labour: regulation at the cellular and molecular levels. *American Journal of Obstetrics and Gynecology* **142**(2): 225–237.

Hytten, F. (1995) *The Clinical Physiology of the Puerperium.* London: Farrand Press.

Inch, S. (1989) *Birthrights.* London: Green Print, Merlin Press.

Irestedt, L., Lagercrantz, H., Hjemdahl, P. *et al.* (1982) Fetal and maternal plasma catecholamine levels at elective cesarean section under general or epidural anaesthesia versus vaginal delivery. *American Journal of Obstetrics and Gynecology* **142**(8): 1004–1010.

Ito, T., Nomura, S., Okada, M. *et al.* (2001) Transcriptional regulation of human placental leucine aminopeptidase/oxytocinase gene. *Molecular Human Reproduction* **7**(9): 887–894.

Jeffrey, J.J. (1991) Collagen and collagenase: pregnancy and parturition. *Seminars in Perinatology* **15**(2): 118–126.

Jiang, Q.B. & Wakerley, J.B. (1995) Analysis of bursting responses of oxytocin neurons in the rat in late pregnancy, lactation and after weaning. *American Journal of Physiology* **486**(1): 237–248.

Johnson, M.H. & Everitt, B.J. (1995) *Essential Reproduction,* pp. 33–36. Oxford: Blackwell Science.

Jouppila, P. (1995) Postpartum haemorrhage. *Current Opinion in Obstetrics & Gynecology* **7**(6): 446–450.

Kehoe, P. & Bronzino, J.D. (1999) Neonatal stress alters LTP in freely moving male and female adult rats. *Hippocampus* **9**(6): 651–658.

Kelly, R.W. (1994) Pregnancy maintenance and parturition: the role of prostaglandin in manipulating the immune and inflammatory response. *Endocrine Reviews* **15**(5): 684–706.

Kimura, T., Takemura, M., Nomura, S. *et al.* (1996) Expression of oxytocin receptor in human myometrium. *Endocrinology* **137**(2): 780–785.

Klaus, M.H., Kennell, J.H., Robertson, S.S. *et al.* (1986) Effects of social support during parturition on maternal and infant morbidity. *British Medical Journal* **6547**(293): 585–587.

Lagercrantz, H. & Herlenius, E. (2002) Neurotransmitters and neuromodulators. In: Lagercrantz, H., Hanson, M., Evrard, P. *et al.* (eds) *The Newborn Brain*. Cambridge, Cambridge University Press.

Lagercrantz, H. & Slotkin, T.A. (1986) The 'stress' of being born. *Scientific American* **254**(4): 920–102.

Letsky, E.A. (1998) The haematological system. In: Chamberlain, G. & Broughton Pipkin, F. (eds) *Clinical Physiology in Obstetrics*, pp. 71–110. Oxford: Blackwell Science.

Levison, G. & Shnider, S.M. (1979) Catecholamines: the effects of maternal fear and its treatment on uterine function and circulation. *Birth and the Family Journal* **6**(3): 167–174.

Loup, F., Tribollet, E., Dubois-Dauphin, M. *et al.* (1991) Localization of high-affinity binding sites for oxytocin and vasopressin in the human brain. An autoradiographic study. *Brain Research* **555**(2): 220–232.

MacDonald, P.C. & Casey, M.L. (1993) The accumulation of prostaglandins (PG) in amniotic fluid is an after effect of labour and not indicative of a role for PGE_2 or $PGF_{2\alpha}$ in the initiation of human parturition. *Journal of Clinical Endocrinology and Metabolism* **76**(5): 1332–1339.

Magiakou, M-A., Mastorakos, G., Rabin, D. *et al.* (1996) The maternal hypothalamic–pituitary–adrenal axis in the third trimester of human pregnancy. *Clinical Endocrinology* **44**: 419–428.

Matijevic, R., Meekins, J.W., McFaden, I.R. *et al.* (1996) Physiological changes of spiral arteries and blood flow in the placental bed during early pregnancy. *Contemporary Reviews in Obstetrics and Gynaecology* **8**: 127–131.

Matthiesen, A-S., Ransjo-Arvidson, A-B.R., Nissen, E. *et al.* (2001) Postpartum maternal oxytocin release by newborns: effects of infant hand massage and suckling. *Birth* **28**(1): 13–19.

Melender, H-L. (2002) Fears and coping strategies associated with pregnancy and childbirth in Finland. *Journal of Midwifery & Women's Health* **47**(4): 256–263.

Mesiano, S. (2001) Roles of estrogen and progesterone in human parturition. *Frontiers of Hormone Research* **27**: 75–85.

Mesiano, S., Chan, E-C., Fitter, J.T. *et al.* (2002) Progesterone withdrawal and estrogen activation in human parturition are coordinated by progesterone receptor A expression in the myometrium. *Journal of Clinical Endocrinology and Metabolism* **87**(6): 2924–2930.

Mitchell, B.F. & Schmid, B. (2001) Oxytocin and its receptor in the process of parturition. *Journal of the Society for Gynecologic Investigation* **8**(3): 122–133.

Mitchell, B.F., Rogers, K. & Wong, S. (1993) The dynamics of prostaglandin metabolism in human fetal membranes and decidua around the time of parturition. *Journal of Clinical Endocrinology and Metabolism* **77**(3): 759–764.

Moore, T.R., Iams, J.D., Creasy, R.K. *et al.* (1994) Diurnal and gestational patterns of uterine activity in normal human pregnancy. *Obstetrics and Gynecology* **83**(4): 517–523.

Morel, G., Pechoux, C., Raccurt, M. *et al.* (2001) Intrauterine oxytocin system. *Cell and Tissue Research* **304**(3): 377–382.

Morien, A., Cassone, V.M. & Wellman, P.J. (1999) Diurnal changes in paraventricular hypothalamic α_1 and α_2-adrenoreceptors and food intake in rats. *Pharmacology, Biochemistry, and Behavior* **63**(1): 33–38.

Morrin, N. (1985) The second stage. *Nursing Mirror* **161**(3): S7–S10.

Mortola, J.P., Fisher, J.T., Smith, J.B. *et al.* (1982) Onset of respiration in infants delivered by caesarean section. *Journal of Applied Physiology* **52**(3): 716–724.

Mukaddam-Daher, S., Jankowski, M., Wang, D. *et al.* (2002) Regulation of cardiac oxytocin system and natriuretic peptide during rat gestation and postpartum. *Journal of Endocrinology* **175**: 211–216.

Neumann, I.D., Alison, J., Douglas, A.J. *et al.* (1996) Oxytocin released within the supraoptic nucleus of the rat brain by positive feedback action is involved in parturition-released events. *Journal of Neuroendocrinology* **8**: 227–233.

Noel, M. & Woodside, B. (1993) Effect of systemic and central prolactin injections on food intake, weight gain and estrous cyclicity in female rats. *Physiological Behaviour* **54**(1): 151–154.

Noort, W.A., van Bulck, B., Vereecken, A. *et al.* (1989) Changes in plasma levels of $PGF_{2\alpha}$ and PGI_2 metabolites at and after delivery at term. *Prostaglandins* **37**(1): 3–12.

Odent, M. (1987) The fetus ejection reflex. *Birth* **14**(2): 104–108.

Odent, M, (1992) *The Nature of Birth and Breastfeeding*, pp. 61–62. Westport, Connecticut: Bergin & Garvey.

Odent, M. (1994) Labouring women are not marathon runners. *Midwifery Today* **31**: 23–51.

Olah, K.S., Gee, H. & Brown, J.S. (1993) Cervical contractions: the response of the cervix to oxytocic stimulation in the latent phase of labour. *British Journal of Obstetrics and Gynaecology* **100**: 635–640.

Oliver R.E. (1981) Of labour and the lungs. *Archives of Disease in Childhood* 56: 659–662.

Owman, C. (1981) Pregnancy induces degenerative and regenerative changes in the autonomic innervation of the female reproductive tract. In: Elliot, K. & Lawrence, G. (eds) *Development of the Autonomic Nervous System,* pp. 252–279. London: Pitman Medical.

Pajntar, M. (1994) The smooth muscles of the cervix in labour. *European Journal of Obstetrics, Gynecology, and Reproductive Biology* 55(1): 9–12.

Patel, F.A., Funder, J.W. & Challis, J.R.G. (2003) Mechanism of cortisol/progesterone antagonism in the regulation of 15-hydroxysteroid dehydrogenase activity and messenger ribonucleic acid levels in human chorion and placental trophoblast cells at term. *Journal of Clinical Endocrinology and Metabolism* 88(6): 2922–2933.

Pearson Murphy, B.E. & Branchaud, C.L. (1994) The fetal adrenal. In: Tulchinsky, D. & Little, A.B. (eds) *Maternal–Fetal Endocrinology,* pp. 275–295. Philadelphia: W.B. Saunders.

Peled, G. (1993) Birth and the Gulf War. *MIDIRS Midwifery Digest* 3(1): 54.

Pelletier, G. & El-Alfy, M. (2000) Immunocytochemical localization of estrogen receptors α and β in the human reproductive organs. *Journal of Clinical Endocrinology and Metabolism* 85(12): 4835–4840.

Pepe, G.J. & Albrecht, E.D. (1995) Actions of placental and fetal adrenal steroid hormones in primate pregnancy. *Endocrine Reviews* 16(5): 608–648.

Reynolds, S.R.M. (1955) Circulatory adaptations to birth and their clinical implications. *American Journal of Obstetrics and Gynecology* 70(1): 148–161.

Robson, S.C., Dunlop W., Boys, R.J. *et al.* (1987) Cardiac output during labour. *British Medical Journal* 295(6607): 1169–1172.

Russell, J.A., Leng, G. & Douglas, A.J. (2002) The magnocellular oxytocin system, the fount of maternity: adaptations in pregnancy. *Frontiers in Neuroendocrinology* 249(1): 27–61.

Sansone, G.R., Gerdes, C.A., Steinman, J.L. *et al.* (2002) Vaginocervical stimulation releases oxytocin within the spinal cord in rats. *Neuroendocrinology* 75: 306–315.

Sarrieau, A., Sharma, S. & Meaney, M.J. (1988) Postnatal development and environmental regulation of hippocampal glucocorticoid and mineralocorticoid receptors. *Brain Research* 471: 158–162.

Siteri, P.K. & Stites, D.P. (1982) Immunologic and endocrine interrelationships in pregnancy. *Biology of Reproduction* 26: 1–14.

Skinner, K.A. & Challis, J.R.G. (1985) Changes in the synthesis and metabolism of prostaglandins by human fetal membranes and decidua at labor. *American Journal of Obstetrics and Gynecology* 151(4): 519–523.

Steingrimsdottir, T., Ronquist, G. & Ulmsten, U. (1993) Energy economy in the pregnant human uterus at term: studies on arteriovenous differences in metabolites of carbohydrate, fat and nucleotides. *European Journal of Obstetrics, Gynecology and Reproductive Biology* 51: 209–215.

Stern, J.M. (1997) Offspring-induced nurturance: animal–human parallels. *Developmental Psychobiology* 31: 19–37.

Takemura, M., Kimura, T., Nomura, S. *et al.* (1994) Expression and localization of human oxytocin receptor mRNA and its protein in chorion and decidua during parturition. *Journal of Clinical Investigation* 93: 2319–2323.

Tigas, S., Sunehag, A. & Haymond, M.W. (2002) Metabolic adaptation to feeding and fasting during lactation in humans. *Journal of Clinical Endocrinology and Metabolism* 87(1): 302–307.

Uvnas-Moberg, K. (1994) Role of efferent and afferent vagal nerve activation during reproduction: integrating function of oxytocin on metabolism and behaviour. *Psychoneuroendocrinology* 19(5–7): 687–695.

Vadillo-Ortega, F., Gonzalez-Avila, G., Furth, E.A. *et al.* (1995) 92-kd type IV collagenase (matrix metalloproteinase-9) activity in human amniochorion increases with labor. *American Journal of Pathology* 146(1): 148–156.

Van Dessel, T., Frijns, J.H. & Wallenburg, H.C. (1993) Prostaglandins and cervical dilatation. *Fetal Maternal Medicine Review* 5: 79–88.

Wathes, D.C., Borwick, S.C., Timmons, P.M. *et al.* (1999) Oxytocin receptor expression in the human term and preterm gestational tissues prior to and following the onset of labour. *Journal of Endocrinology* 161(1): 143–151.

Wilson, T., Liggins, G.C. & Joe, L. (1989) Purification and characterization of a uterine phospholipase inhibitor that loses activity after labour onset in women. *American Journal of Obstetrics and Gynecology* 160(3): 602–606.

Wuitchik, M., Bakal, D. & Lipshitz, J. (1989) The clinical significance of pain and cognitive activity in latent labour. *Obstetrics and Gynecology* 73(1): 35–42.

Wu, W.X., Ma, X.H., Zhang, Q. *et al.* (2001) Characterization of topology- gestation- and labour-related changes of a cassette of myometrial contraction-associated protein mRNA in the pregnant baboon myometrium. *Journal of Endocrinology* 171(3): 445–453.

26

Care in the First Stage of Labour

Denis Walsh

LEARNING OUTCOMES

After reading this chapter you will be able to:

- develop an awareness of the importance of the context of childbirth
- recognize the onset of labour and appreciate the normal physiology of labour
- provide research- and evidence-based care appropriate to the needs of the woman and her baby

- understand the value of principles such as woman-centred care
- have insight into the key roles of environment and relationships with carers
- have an awareness of the holistic elements of labour care.

INTRODUCTION

Labour and birth are an amazing integration of powerful physiological and psychological forces that bring a new human life into the world. It is difficult not to devalue labour and birth when it is analysed, dissected and examined in order to make it understood, as it works best as a coherent whole. There are key physical, emotional and social dimensions to the process of labour, in that the arrival of a baby also heralds the birth or extension of a family. Throughout history, labour and birth have had special meaning for every culture and their occurrence is often marked by spiritual and cultural symbols (Kitzinger, 2000). In the UK today, such rituals have been marginalized by the medical environment in which most parturition takes place, in that about 98% of birth occurs in hospital. For the midwife, a holistic understanding of labour and birth requires not only awareness of the physiological/psychological changes, but an ability to see these remarkable events as deeply social and even political. This perspective has as a starting point *a profound respect for and trust in women's innate ability to birth without technology or medical intervention*. The chapter will attempt to describe the changes, the events and the care from these philosophical positions.

Two birth stories (Case scenarios 26.1 and 26.2) reveal the complexity of labour and birth.

The midwife's description of these births shows how the experience of labour can vary for different women. The time spans were very different – the first was in excess of 24 hours and the second had a 'rest

---

Case scenario 26.1

Emily's birth story

Emily was a 'no-nonsense' sort of person. She approached the birth of her first baby in a straightforward way. 'I'll know what to do at the time,' she kept telling me. 'You just tag along and I'll ask if I need anything.' She called me out one Sunday morning and when I arrived told me her labour had started, and although she didn't want me to do anything, she asked me to stay for a few hours. Later, she said I could go as she had hours to go yet. She called me again early the next morning and said it was time for the baby to come. I drove over to her house, and 2 hours later her son was born into the birthing pool and there were tears all round. Emily was in tune with her body. She understood it and how the birth process would go for her far better than I did.

phase' of 4 hours prior to the birth. The women adapted to their experience in contrasting ways – one was confident and controlled, the other just felt swamped by the power of her labour. In neither case is the midwife's role described, but different strategies of support would have been required to care appropriately for each woman.

Other aspects are key to assisting our understanding of these births. Both babies were born at home. Both women had people in attendance whom they knew and had chosen to be there. Neither woman had any drugs nor common birth interventions. They did it 'naturally'. Yet their births were not typical of 21st century childbirth experience in the UK. More typically, childbirth occurs in hospital with carers who have not been previously met, using routine interventions like continuous electronic fetal monitoring. One in three will end in an instrumental vaginal delivery or a caesarean section (ENB, 2001; Thomas and Parenjothy, 2001).

Being in hospital requires conforming to an environment where the woman inevitably becomes a 'patient' and the carers assume the status of expert. Labour is expected to conform to protocols and policies designed for the 'average', which trigger a range of interventions if deviation occurs from this 'average'. This chapter explores normal labour and birth from the perspective of non-intervention and views the birth environment as crucial to physiological processes. Having a baby in hospital may be viewed as a 'care intervention', likely to upset a delicate balance of physical, psychological and social processes that need to work in harmony for birth to be humane and life-enhancing.

Case scenario 26.2

Judy's birth story

Judy just avoided induction of labour because she was 13 days past her due date when her waters broke. The contractions arrived 8 hours later and were huge from the start. Despite fantastic support from Ben, her partner, she felt out of control with the labour's intensity. Her cervix was 7 cm dilated when she requested a vaginal examination 2 hours later. After an hour her contractions became even more intense and I suspected she was approaching the pushing phase. Then suddenly, everything stopped. She dozed on and off for 4 hours when suddenly she was bearing down and the baby was born within two contractions. Judy felt traumatized by her rollercoaster ride, which she felt swept along by.

Reflective Activity 26.1

Ask your mother about your birth and note the phrases she uses to describe it, the memories that have stayed with her and the overall impression of the experiences that she communicates to you.

THE CONTINUUM OF LABOUR

Labour has been traditionally divided into stages but this demarcation has its origins in a preoccupation with the time duration of each stage and its historical link to complications for the mother and baby. When learning about labour, practitioners are introduced to notions of time at the outset, which is consistent with a biomedical understanding of parturition that anticipates pathology in an effort to treat it as early as possible.

An alternative approach is beginning to gain exposure through the writings of midwives in particular (Downe, 2000), seeing labour as a continuum from onset to completion, characterized by particular physiological and psychological behaviours at various points on that continuum. Some of these behaviours are anatomical changes, e.g. changes in the cervix, some are physiological, e.g. release of body hormones, and some psychological, e.g. an alertness and focusing just prior to birth. Individual behaviours and responses vary, and the importance of knowing and intuitively connecting with women is a key challenge for the midwife and allows care to be appropriate and tailored to individual need.

Although the demarcations of the stages of labour in the traditional biomedical model are intended to aid clarity in understanding physiology and care for the professional care-giver, they may also effectively silence the woman and discredit her version of events. For the woman, labour is seen as a continuing physiological, psychological and emotional experience, the culmination and main focal point of the reproductive process, where artificial compartmentalization may be neither relevant nor important. The significance of labour, a biologically and socially creative life event, is reflected in the minutiae of detail women can recall about their particular labour(s). Events that are relatively common and usual from a midwife's perspective, acquire much meaning and importance in the eyes of the woman and her family. To maximize the potential for a satisfactory outcome of labour it is therefore essential that women's stories and details of events are listened to and valued.

Finally if the midwife is anticipating a normal outcome to labour and birth, trusting that the woman's physiology will function optimally, this can impact positively on the woman's own attitude. Women who have an optimistic demeanour towards childbirth have better experiences and outcomes than those beset by anxiety and fear of what could go wrong (Green *et al.*, 1998). Midwives have therefore a key role in empowering women as they approach these events.

CHARACTERISTICS OF LABOUR

Normal labour naturally follows a sequential pattern that involves painful regular uterine contractions stimulating progressive effacement and dilatation of the cervix and descent of the fetus through the pelvis, culminating in the spontaneous vaginal birth of the baby, followed by the expulsion of the placenta and membranes (Gould, 2000). This definition provides an alternative model of understanding to the orthodox biomedical model. This 'social model' of childbirth contrasts with the traditional biomedical model, which divides labour into three stages:

- *First stage of labour:* from the onset of regular uterine contractions, accompanied by effacement of the cervix and dilatation of the os, to full dilatation of the os uteri.
- *Second stage of labour:* from full dilatation of the os uteri to the birth of the baby.
- *Third stage of labour:* from the birth of the baby to the expulsion of the placenta and membranes.

Within this definition, maximum time frames are designated for each phase depending on a woman's parity as shown in Table 26.1.

The social model identifies the *strenuous work* labour entails for these woman and the crucial role of *movement* (Gould, 2000). This highlights the courage and perseverance demonstrated by women as they 'work' during labour and the importance of an environment where movement will be facilitated. In fact the birth space needs to be one chosen specifically by the

woman – indeed many mammals choose privacy and darkness for birth.

PHYSIOLOGY OF LABOUR

Several physiological factors integrate as labour develops (Box 26.1), and these will be examined in turn.

Cervical effacement and dilatation

These occur as a result of contraction and retraction of the uterine muscle.

Effacement (taking up) of the cervix may start in the latter 2 or 3 weeks of pregnancy and occurs as a result of changes in the solubility of collagen present in cervical tissue. This is influenced by alterations in hormone activity, particularly oestradiol, progesterone, relaxin, prostacyclin and prostaglandins (Blackburn, 2003). Braxton Hicks contractions, which become stronger in the final weeks of pregnancy, may also enhance the process. Effacement is completed in labour, when the cervix becomes shorter, dilates slightly and then becomes funnel-shaped as the internal os opens to form part of the lower uterine segment (see Fig. 26.1).

Progressive dilatation of the cervix (see Fig. 26.2) is a definitive sign of labour.

When the cervix is dilated sufficiently to allow the fetal head to pass through, full dilatation has been achieved. Although this is usually 10 cm, it may be more or less depending on the size of the fetal head.

In primigravidae, effacement of the cervix usually precedes dilatation, but in multigravidae effacement and

---

Box 26.1 Summary of the physiological changes in the first stage of labour

- *Completion of effacement of the cervix* and *dilatation of the os uteri* caused by *uterine activity*:
  - Contraction and retraction of uterine muscles
  - Fundal dominance
  - Active upper uterine segment, passive lower segment
  - Formation of the retraction ring
  - Polarity of the uterus
  - Intensity or amplitude of contractions
  - Resting tone
- Formation of the bag of *forewaters* and the *hindwaters*
- *Rupture* of the membranes
- *Show*

Table 26.1   Approximate time taken for each stage of labour

	Primigravidae	Multigravidae
First stage	12–14 hours	6–10 hours
Second stage	60 minutes	Up to 30 minutes
Third stage	20–30 minutes, or 5–15 minutes with active management	20–30 minutes, or 5–15 minutes with active management

dilatation of the cervix normally occur simultaneously (Fig. 26.2).

Uterine contractions

Uterine contractions are responsible for achieving effacement and dilatation of the cervix and for the descent and expulsion of the fetus in labour. Contractions of the uterus in labour are:

- involuntary
- intermittent and regular, and
- in most labours, painful.

The cause of the pain may be due, in part, to ischaemia developing in the muscle fibres during contractions. The backache which may accompany cervical dilatation is caused by stimulation of sensory fibres which pass via the sympathetic nerves to the sacral plexus.

Coordination of contractions

Contractions start from the cornua of the uterus and pass in waves, inwards and downwards. In normal uterine action the intensity is greatest in the upper uterine segment and lessens as the contraction passes down the uterus. This is called *fundal dominance*. The upper segment of the uterus contracts and retracts powerfully, whereas the lower segment contracts only slightly and dilates. Between contractions the uterus relaxes. The coordinated uterine activity characteristic of normal labour occurs as a result of near-simultaneous

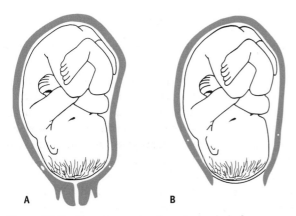

Figure 26.1 The uterus, showing: **A.** cervix before effacement; and **B.** effacement and dilatation of the cervix and the stretched lower uterine segment.

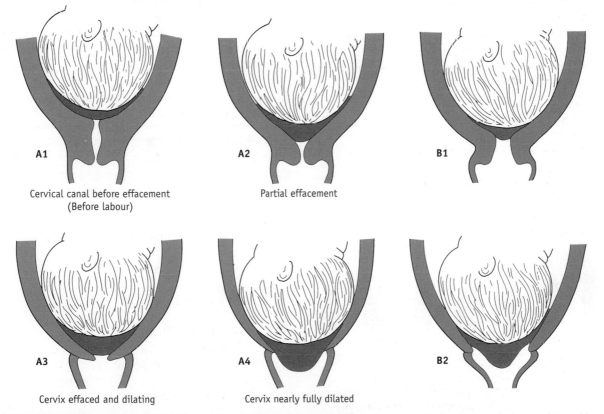

A1 — Cervical canal before effacement (Before labour)

A2 — Partial effacement

B1

A3 — Cervix effaced and dilating

A4 — Cervix nearly fully dilated

B2

Figure 26.2 Effacement and dilatation of the cervix: **A.** in a primigravida; **B.** occurring simultaneously in a multigravida.

contraction of all myometrial cells. During pregnancy increasing numbers of gap junctions form between the cells of the myometrium. These low-resistance communication channels enhance electrical conduction velocity and facilitate the coordination of myometrial contraction (Blackburn, 2003).

Retraction

Retraction is a state of permanent shortening of the muscle fibres and occurs with each contraction (see Fig. 26.3).

The muscle fibres gradually become shorter and thicker, especially in the upper uterine segment. This exerts a pull on the less-active lower uterine segment, the maximum pull being directed towards the weakest point, the cervix, and the os uteri. Hence the cervix is gradually 'taken up', or effaced, and the upward pull then dilates the os uteri. As the space within the upper uterine segment diminishes because of the contractions and retraction of the muscle fibres, the fetus is forced down into the lower segment and the presenting part exerts pressure on the os uteri. This aids dilatation, and also causes a reflex release of oxytocin from the posterior pituitary gland, promoting further uterine action. A ridge gradually forms between the thick, retracted muscle fibres of the upper uterine segment and the thin, distended lower segment. This is called a *retraction ring* and is a normal physiological occurrence in every labour.

Polarity

The coordination between the upper and lower segments is balanced and harmonious in normal labour. While the upper segment contracts powerfully and retracts, the lower segment contracts only slightly and dilates. This rhythmical coordination between the upper and lower uterine segments is called *polarity*.

Intensity or amplitude

Contractions cause a rise in intrauterine pressure. This is called the *intensity* or *amplitude* of contractions and can be measured by placing a fine catheter into the uterus and attaching it to a pressure-recording apparatus. Each contraction rises rapidly to a peak and then slowly declines to the resting tone. In early labour the contractions are weak, with an amplitude of about 20 mmHg, last 20–30 seconds and occur infrequently, about every 20 minutes. As labour progresses the contractions become stronger, longer and more frequent. At the end of the first stage they are strong, with an amplitude of 60 mmHg, last 45–60 seconds and occur every 2–3 minutes.

Resting tone

The uterus is never completely relaxed, and in between contractions a resting tone can be measured – usually between 4 and 10 mmHg. During contractions the blood flow to the placenta is curtailed; thus oxygen and carbon dioxide exchange in the intervillous spaces is impeded. The period of relaxation between contractions when the uterus has a low resting tone is therefore vital for adequate fetal oxygenation.

Formation of the forewaters and hindwaters (Fig. 26.4)

As the lower uterine segment stretches and the cervix starts to efface, some chorion becomes detached from the decidua and both membranes form a small bag containing amniotic fluid, which protrudes into the cervix. When the fetal head descends on to the cervix, it separates the small bag of amniotic fluid in front, the forewaters, from the remainder, the hindwaters.

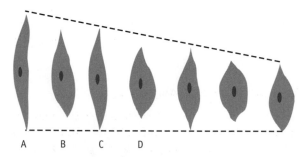

Figure 26.3   Retraction of the uterine muscle fibres: **A.** relaxed; **B.** contracted; **C.** relaxed but retracted; **D.** contracted but shorter and thicker than those in B.

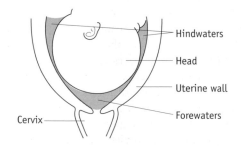

Figure 26.4   Formation of hindwaters and forewaters.

The forewaters aid effacement of the cervix and early dilatation of the os uteri. The hindwaters help to equalize the pressure in the uterus during uterine contractions and thereby provide some protection to the fetus and placenta.

Rupture of the membranes

The membranes are thought to rupture as a result of increased production of prostaglandin E_2 in the amnion in labour (McCoshen *et al.*, 1990) and the force of the uterine contractions, causing an increase in the fluid pressure inside the forewaters and a lessening of the support as the cervix dilates. In normal labour the membranes usually rupture towards the end of the first stage.

Show

The show is the operculum from the cervical canal which is shed per vaginam in labour. It is displaced when effacement of the cervix and dilatation of the os uteri occur and is usually mucoid and slightly streaked with blood due to some separation of the chorion from the decidua around the cervix.

There is increasingly awareness of the relationship between oxytocin release and the level of catecholamines (see Ch. 25). Anxiety and fear stimulate the release of adrenaline (epinephrine) and noradrenaline (norepinephrine), and inhibit oxytocin; hence the importance of birth environment and birth relationships in promoting calm and confidence in birthing women.

CARE DURING THE FIRST STAGE OF LABOUR

The aims of midwifery care in labour are to achieve a safe labour and birth for mother and baby, and a pleasurable, fulfilling experience of childbirth for the mother and her partner.

Now that deaths in childbirth for women and babies in the western world are rare, women's experience of childbirth has taken on greater significance and has become a major focus for the professionals assisting childbirth. The majority of research on labour and birth did not include an objective to explore women's experiences and has been based around the professionals' priorities and their interests. Fortunately, there is some evidence about women's experience of maternity care. Over the past 20 years, studies have been done to determine women's views on various aspects of care (DoH,

1992; Garcia *et al.*, 1997; Jacoby and Cartwright, 1990). It is now possible to summarize these themes under a number of headings:

- information that is full, accurate, evidence-based, individualized (Kirkham, 1989)
- choice (DoH, 1993)
- control (Oakley, 1984)
- continuity (Enkin *et al.*, 2000).

These themes should underpin the philosophy of care and shine through its application. They help define woman-centred care, which has been described and endorsed by those associated with maternity care provision.

In order to give woman-centred care, the midwife should:

1. assess the needs and expectations of each individual woman regarding labour and birth
2. plan care with each woman in labour that is tailored to meet her specific needs and expectations
3. put the care plan into practice, and
4. evaluate the care given to measure its effectiveness.

Partnership in care

The relationship between the woman and her midwife is ideally a partnership (Pairman, 2000) which should begin in pregnancy. It requires both members to have common aims and to seek ways of working together to achieve them. Page (1995) likened the relationship to 'skilled companionship' or the 'professional friend' to highlight its intimacy and reciprocity. The partnership ethos requires a social rather than a medical model of maternity care, endorsing the involvement of the woman and her partner in decision-making, and requiring the woman to be able to voice her needs and wishes freely. The midwife should strive to build a relationship of mutual trust and create an environment in which expectations, wishes, fears and anxieties can be readily discussed. This requires good communication, which results from a two-way interaction between equals.

Emotional and psychological care

It is important for the midwife to have a good understanding of a woman's feelings in labour. Attitudes and reactions to childbirth vary considerably and are influenced by differing social, cultural and religious factors. For a multigravida, the previous experience of birth will also be important.

Many women anticipate labour with mixed feelings of fear and excitement. Some may eagerly anticipate the birth, confident in their ability to cope, seeing birth as an emotionally fulfilling and enriching experience involving all immediate family members. They may have attended teaching sessions for natural or active childbirth and have a particular plan of action for their labour. Others may be excited at the prospect of actually seeing their baby, yet fearful of labour and anxious about their ability to cope with pain and 'perform' well. Some expect labour to be painful and unpleasant, controlled by obstetricians and midwives, and to be achieved with as little pain and active participation as possible.

The woman may be apprehensive about entering an unknown, and perhaps threatening, hospital environment and concerned about relinquishing her personal autonomy and identity. Alternatively, expectations of labour may be unrealistic, and may be unfulfilled, leading to feelings of disappointment, failure or loss. Multigravidae are often anxious about children they have left at home. The midwife can do much to alleviate these worries.

Birth partners may also have particular concerns which they feel unable to share. Reservations may be influenced by the role society attributes to gender, e.g. for a man, being strong and able to cope; or may be due to fear of the unknown and concern for someone who is loved. With a partnership and individual approach to care, particularly if established in the antenatal period, the midwife has a valuable opportunity to encourage the couple to voice their particular needs and anxieties, and explore and agree ways of dealing with them. Whatever the needs of the individual couple, they are usually influenced by the desire to do what is best for their baby and, if they are confident that the midwife will respect and comply with their wishes in normal circumstances, they will usually readily agree to modify expectations should problems arise.

Throughout labour there should be a free flow of information between the woman and her partner and the midwife, particularly in relation to examinations and their findings. Being fully informed and involved in decision-making helps the woman to retain a sense of autonomy and control (Flint *et al.*, 1987). Some professionals have difficulty in communicating with single women and those belonging to minority ethnic groups (Fleissig, 1993). The midwife should be aware that not all individuals may feel sufficiently secure or able to freely express fears or anxieties during labour.

Circumstances such as an unwanted pregnancy, fear or previously poor relationships with professional caregivers may engender feelings of unhappiness, hostility and resentment. The midwife needs to be particularly sensitive to non-verbal indicators of such feelings and give the necessary help and support needed by the woman.

The role of the birth supporter

Evidence from a number of studies indicates the positive effect of continuous support in labour (Hodnett, 2002a). Although it is usual in the UK for a couple to support each other in labour, in some instances the woman may choose to have a relative, friend or labour supporter from a voluntary organization such as the National Childbirth Trust (NCT) as a labour companion. Whoever has been chosen, the midwife should explore with supporters their experiences of childbirth, their role expectations during labour and their ability to undertake the supporter role. It has been suggested that if chosen supporters have had negative childbirth experiences, these need to be addressed by the midwife if they are not to hinder the supporting relationship with the woman.

The midwife involves the birth supporter as part of the team, with a defined role, which can include sponging the woman's face, massaging her back, abdomen or legs, helping her with breathing awareness and relaxation and offering drinks and other means of sustenance. Such activities, during a highly anxious time, can be very valuable in helping the partner to feel usefully occupied and involved in the birthing event.

The midwife needs to be sensitive to the possible need for personal space and privacy and should judge when, and if, it is appropriate to leave the woman and partner alone. This is usually more acceptable in early labour but less so when labour is strong and well advanced, when to be left alone might be frightening. If the midwife must leave for a short period then she must ensure that the couple can summon help if necessary. The midwife must also be sensitive to the emotional needs of the partner and other members of staff and recognize that, particularly during a long labour, a short break may be beneficial in helping to replenish energy levels.

Advocacy

For some women fear of the unknown, being cared for in hospital by unfamiliar people, greater pain than expected or the effect of analgesic drugs can give rise to feelings of vulnerability, loss of personal identity and powerlessness. This may be magnified for women for whom English is not their first language. Vulnerable individuals lose the ability to adequately express their needs, wishes, values and choices (Morrison, 1991) and therefore adopt a passive recipient role. In such circumstances, and as part of the supportive role, the midwife may need to act as advocate, in order to ensure that personal needs are met (Walsh, 1999). This includes informing, supporting and protecting women, acting as intermediary between them and obstetric and other professional colleagues, and facilitating informed choice. In order to act effectively as an advocate, the midwife must be professionally confident, have a clear awareness of the woman's needs, and be able to communicate these to other colleagues to ensure effective collaboration. Developing and trusting *intuition* is central to this activity. The midwife's rapport and connectedness with the woman she is caring for mean that appropriate decision-making and a facilitatory birth environment is more likely (Davis-Floyd, 1998). Using these skills, the midwife is more able to empower the woman and her partner so that they feel sufficiently informed and confident to participate in decision-making during this important life experience.

Reflective Activity 26.2

How would you describe the relationship you observe between midwives and the women they care for in labour? How would you describe the relationship between women and their birth partner?

ENVIRONMENT FOR BIRTH

Practitioners of normal birth and women themselves know how significant the birth environment is for the experience and outcomes of birth. It may seem unnecessary to research the relative merits of a clinical labour ward, within a large institution, full of strangers calling themselves experts compared with a homely, familiar environment surrounded by friends of one's own choosing.

Three dimensions of the birth environment will be examined: home, midwife-led care/birthing units and continuity of care.

Home

Home birth has long generated an intense debate, and birth at home has become a rallying point for midwives and women who endorse childbirth's essential normality

against those who can only view its normality retrospectively. Tew (1998) first challenged the dominant view of the 1970s and 1980s that the safest environment for birth was hospital. She exposed the fundamental flaw of assigning a single cause (hospitalization of birth) to a discrete effect (lowering perinatal mortality rates) without consideration of alternative explanations. This spurious logic drove a nationwide movement of birth to hospitals over these two decades before an alternative explanation gained credibility – that the fall was due to the dramatic improvement in the general health of women in the post-war period coupled with an even more dramatic rise in living standards (Campbell and McFarlane, 1994; Tew, 1998).

It is now acknowledged that current evidence does not provide justification for requiring that all women give birth in hospital (Olsen and Jewell, 2001) and that women should be offered an explicit choice when they become pregnant, of where they want to have their baby (DoH, 1993). Results from international studies in the 1990s (Olsen, 1997) indicated that perinatal mortality was not significantly different between hospital and home birth groups. Lower frequency of low Apgar scores (1 and 5 minutes) and fewer severe perineal lacerations in home birth groups were the principal differences. These groups also had fewer medical interventions including inductions, augmentations, episiotomies, assisted vaginal births and caesarean sections. It was also suggested that there might be clear benefit from aspects of the home birth 'package of care', including continuity of care during labour and birth and midwife-led care, both common aspects of home birth provision (Olsen, 1997).

Though official government policy during most of the 1990s was to offer women a choice about place of birth, national home birth statistics were still only about 2% compared with 25% in the early 1960s (Chamberlain *et al.*, 1997). Despite the rhetoric of choice, there are anecdotal stories of women being discouraged from choosing home birth. An NCT survey (1999) showed over 50% of GPs expressed reluctance to recommend home birth, and in many maternity services home birth provision is reactive rather than proactive (women have to ask, otherwise it is assumed birth will be in hospital).

One practical measure to reduce the bias to hospital birth may be to keep the option for home birth open till labour starts. Requiring a firm decision in early pregnancy regarding home birth may be problematic, as some women will develop complications during pregnancy which require hospital care. If women have access to midwifery support at home in early labour, they may prefer to stay there rather than face an uncomfortable journey to hospital. Finally, choice without flexibility may be nearly as bad as no choice at all if one is locked into a decision about care, when the care, by its very nature, is dynamic and changeable over time. Leap's (1996) midwifery group practice adopted this model and its essential rationality makes it a model worth replicating in other settings.

Many of the problems around home birth relate to unplanned birth at home or women giving birth at home who are at high obstetric risk (Bastian *et al.*, 1998). The debate over its relative safety continues despite the work of Tew, Campbell and McFarlane, and Olsen, and may be heavily influenced by issues of power and control: whoever controls the place of birth also controls maternity care.

Midwifery-led care in birthing units

Free-standing units

Free-standing birth centres as an option for women are especially relevant now. NHS trusts across the country are merging, driven by the growth of neonatal tertiary referral centres and by a rationalizing of management and clinical structures of individual trusts that are no longer seen as cost-effective if they remain separate. These pressures are leading to stakeholders often choosing to either combine birth facilities on one site together with neonatal services or retain present infrastructures and open midwifery-led units or birthing units. Already a trend is emerging in favour of the first option, which will result in further centralization of birth, in some areas up to 10 000 births in a single hospital. This mirrors the controversial process in the 1980s, during which many small hospitals and isolated GP units closed, and which midwives and user lobby groups have lamented ever since.

Some consultant units have developed into midwife-led units and there have been some high-profile successes, e.g. Bournemouth Midwifery Unit, Edgware Birth Centre and the midwife-led facility at Grantham. All of these units had to fight to be established, turning the lens squarely on the safety and effectiveness of free-standing birth units. Research and evaluation is needed to establish whether expansion is appropriate, as currently, practitioners are reliant on evidence drawn from abroad.

Albers and Katz (1991) reviewed the outcomes of free-standing birth centres in the USA and concluded that 'non-traditional birth settings present advantages for low risk women as compared with traditional

hospital settings: lower cost for maternity care, lower use of childbirth procedures, without significant differences in perinatal mortality' (p. 215). The largest published study, the National Birth Centre Study in the USA, involved 12 000 women in 84 free-standing birthing units (Rooks *et al.*, 1992). This was a prospective observational survey of antenatal, intrapartum and postnatal care, supported by a smaller prospective study of 2000 matched women at low obstetric risk who gave birth in standard maternity hospitals. These were not randomized designs and the first study only included about half the birth centres in existence at that time. Generalizability is therefore less certain, with trends rather than statistically significant differences being demonstrated, though the large sample size does add weight to the findings. Results indicated that birth centre women had fewer labour interventions (e.g. analgesia, inductions, continuous monitoring) with mortality and morbidity rates similar to women receiving conventional hospital care. Additionally, birth centres were cheaper and attracted a lower socioeconomic group who could not afford standard maternity care provision.

A retrospective German study compared births from free-standing birth centres with hospital deliveries in matched groups of women. Birth centre women had significantly fewer medical interventions and a similar perinatal mortality rate, and the conclusion was that if risk selection was thorough, there was no evidence of increased maternal or perinatal risk (David *et al.*, 1999).

Trying to draw substantive conclusions from quantitative studies in this area is difficult owing to the heterogeneity of studies, e.g. different countries, different entry criteria, different outcome measures and weak research designs. Qualitative research may assist in this. Esposito's 1993 ethnographic study of a birth centre in the USA situated in a deprived, inner-city area illuminates another dimension to birth centre care that may matter as much to women as quantitative process and outcome data. The birth centre had an explicit woman-centred, 'birth as normal' ethos and mainly served low income, minority groups. Esposito found that regardless of their prior beliefs about childbirth, women using the centre tended to adopt the philosophy and ethos of the centre over the months of contact. She describes the culture there as humanistic and woman-empowering with a distinct rapport with the local community and strong networks with other women's organizations (Esposito, 1993). Further qualitative work with a subset of these women who had had previous experience at a large maternity hospital in the same city demonstrated that key issues for the women were control of the birth environment, the opportunity to develop supportive interpersonal relationships with midwives, to have a safe birth and to be treated with dignity and respect – all of which were less evident within the hospital system (Esposito, 1999).

Though there is no research in this area, midwives working in existing birth centres report increased clinical freedom and accountability of their practice, and therefore the potential for increased autonomy does exist. Sandall's (1997) work emphasizes the role of occupational autonomy in midwifery job satisfaction, illustrating high rates of burnout in hospital-based midwives.

The development of robust process and outcomes measures with which to evaluate free-standing birth units in England and then prospective studies of their clinical effectiveness are urgently needed. Parallel to this work is the need for qualitative designs to explore the culture of these centres and the experience of women who give birth there and of the midwives who work in them.

> ### Reflective Activity 26.3
>
> During your course/practice, search out opportunities to see birth in alternative environments to hospital, such as in women's homes, birth centres or in midwifery-led units.

Integrated birthing suites

Integrated birthing suites and midwifery-managed units within the confines of consultant maternity units have been subjected to a number of good-quality randomized controlled trials (RCTs) and therefore do provide clearer recommendations for intrapartum care. Hodnett's (2001) systematic review of 'home-like' (birthing suites) versus conventional institutional settings for birth included five trials, three of them from the UK, and nearly 5000 women. Allocation to a home-like setting was associated with:

- less analgesia/anaesthesia
- fewer fetal heart abnormalities
- less augmented labour and immobility during labour
- greater maternal satisfaction with care.

There was a non-significant trend towards higher perinatal mortality in three of the studies.

Waldenstrom and Turnbull's (1998) systematic review of midwife continuity schemes that were all explicitly midwife-led included two studies from Hodnett's (2002b) review in addition to five other RCTs, two of which were from the UK. Their findings

were similar to those of Hodnett. Continuity of carer within the midwifery-led model resulted in similar outcomes to those listed above, but in addition included fewer inductions, less electronic fetal monitoring, and fewer episiotomies and assisted vaginal births than the conventional model of care, and there were no significant differences in neonatal or maternal morbidity or mortality.

The review did not address maternal satisfaction but at least three of the studies (Flint and Poulengeris, 1987; Rowley *et al.*, 1995; Shields *et al.*, 1998) independently reported that women were more satisfied with midwife-managed care.

Midwives working in units that provide birthing suite facilities stress the need to have this area both physically separate and philosophically different from conventional labour wards. The powerful culture of obstetrically dominated labour wards inevitably flows over to low-risk areas unless clear demarcation lines are drawn between the two (Hunt and Symonds, 1995). This typically manifests as inappropriate intrapartum interventions, e.g. routine electronic fetal monitoring on women in normal labour (Walsh, 1998). Simple measures like not including the birthing suite on obstetric ward rounds and having separate core staff for each area facilitate this demarcation.

The extent to which midwife-managed units and integrated birthing suites have spread during the 1990s, prompted by *Changing Childbirth* (DoH, 1993) indicators is difficult to assess, though most services have begun to address these areas (Garcia *et al.*, 1997). The evidence so far suggests that establishing this provision within local maternity services provides fewer interventions and a more satisfying birth experience.

Continuity of carer

There is a continuing debate about the value of continuity, and whether this applies to the whole continuum of pregnancy, labour and birth, or part of the experience. The preference for being cared for by a known midwife, rather than one not previously met, during such a stressful, intense experience as labour is a predictable finding (Walsh, 1999). Both RCTs (Hodnett, 2002a,b) and descriptive studies (Garcia *et al.*, 1997; Oakley *et al.*, 1990) repeatedly show that schemes offering continuity result in high maternal satisfaction, and the small number of schemes that extend this to labour and birth specifically reveal the same finding (North Staffordshire Changing Childbirth Research Team (NSCCRT), 2000; Page *et al.*, 1999; Walsh, 1999).

Hodnett's (2002b) review found women in continuity schemes had less need for pharmacological pain relief and their babies required resuscitation less often. The non-randomized, comparative studies of schemes delivering high levels of intrapartum continuity (NSCCRT, 2000; Page *et al.*, 1999) found lower epidural rates, less perineal trauma and a higher normal birth rate. The comprehensive systematic review of continuity of care by Green *et al.* (2000) concluded that women appear to value competence and sensitivity as much as continuity and suggested that a known midwife for intrapartum care should not be the main determinant of a service. Clearly, care from an insensitive, incompetent midwife is unacceptable even if that midwife has provided continuity of care. They highlight the difficulty of teasing out attributable aspects of quality in women's perception of care. It is a complex area, not least because women evaluate what they experience, as best (Porter and MacIntyre, 1984). More research into schemes offering a known midwife for labour and birth is required to ascertain impact on birth outcomes and birth experiences.

Despite the widespread concern expressed by midwives about working in continuity schemes (Warwick, 1997), Sandall's (1997) research showed that midwives who have control over their work patterns and can practice autonomously, are less prone to burnout than midwives working in traditional ways.

The value of continuous support from care-givers during childbirth itself has been demonstrated, illustrating clear clinical benefits of this aspect of care with remarkable consistency. The latest Cochrane Review (Hodnett, 2002a) included 14 RCTs and 5000 women from a diverse range of settings, i.e. different countries, different carers, over the past 25 years. Continuous support:

- reduces the need for pharmacological pain relief, operative vaginal delivery, and caesarean section
- reduces the frequency of low Apgar scores
- improves maternal childbirth experience
- has other benefits such as reduced augmentation of labour and improved breastfeeding rates.

These benefits seem so unequivocal that it is suggested that all services should implement the concept.

Reflective Activity 26.4

What are your views on this topic? Ask some of your clients whether continuity of care or carer matters to them.

THE ONSET OF LABOUR

Physiological changes that occur in late pregnancy have been described in Chapter 25, and give rise to signs that herald the onset of labour. While some women will follow a particular physiological pattern, allowance should be made for individual variations which may be associated with differences in pain perception and response, parity, and expectations of labour. These factors should be considered by the midwife in assisting the woman to recognize when she is in labour.

Uterine contractions

Generally women will be aware of the painless, irregular, Braxton Hicks contractions of pregnancy which increase as pregnancy advances. In labour these become regular and painful. Initially the woman may experience minimal discomfort and complain of sacral and/or lower abdominal pain, which she may not immediately associate with labour. Such discomfort may later be noted to coincide with tightening or tension of the abdomen, occurring at regular intervals of 20–30 minutes and lasting 20–30 seconds. These uterine contractions may be readily felt by the midwife on abdominal palpation. As labour progresses the contractions become longer, stronger and more frequent, resulting in progressive effacement and dilatation of the cervix.

Show

This mucoid, often blood-stained, discharge is passed per vaginam. It represents the passage of the operculum which previously occupied the cervical canal and is indicative of a degree of cervical activity, i.e. softening and stretching of tissues which causes separation of the membranes from the decidua around the opening of the internal os. The show is often the first sign that labour is imminent or has started.

Rupture of the membranes

Rupture of the membranes can occur before labour or at any time during labour (see Ch. 25). Although a significant occurrence, it is not a true sign of labour unless accompanied by dilatation of the cervix. It is estimated that 6–19% of women at term will experience spontaneous rupture of membranes before labour starts (Tan and Hannah, 2002). In 85% of women the membranes rupture spontaneously at a cervical dilatation of 9 cm or more (Schwarcz *et al.*, 1977). The amount of amniotic fluid lost when the membranes rupture depends to a great extent on how effectively the fetal presentation assists in the formation of the forewaters. In the presence of a normal amount of amniotic fluid, if the head is not engaged in the pelvis and the presenting part is not well applied to the os uteri, rupture of the membranes is easily recognized by a significant loss of fluid. However, in the presence of an engaged head and well-applied presenting part, rupture of the forewaters may give rise to minimal fluid loss. This is usually followed by further seepage of amniotic fluid which may be mistaken for urinary incontinence, which is not uncommon in late pregnancy. Usually the woman's history or evidence of amniotic fluid confirms the rupture of the membranes.

Contact with the midwife

Changing patterns of care enable more midwives to provide continuity of care. Consequently, there is an increased possibility that the woman will be cared for in labour, at home or in hospital, by a midwife known to her from the antenatal period. In keeping with the 'ten indicators of success' (DoH, 1993), every women should have the name of the midwife who works locally and is known to her. The woman should therefore be advised to contact the midwife when regular contractions are recognized, when the membranes rupture, or should she be concerned for any reason. Clear and written instructions, given well in advance of the expected date of birth, regarding relevant telephone numbers of the community or team midwives, and their location are necessary and useful for anxious partners/birth supporters. Any particular information which relates to home birth and/or care should be clarified.

If the woman does not know the midwife, the midwife must be aware of the sensitivity of the first meeting and the importance of the initial interaction with the woman, which will form the basis for their future relationship. As discussed earlier, women experience a variety of conflicting emotions and it is important that at the initial meeting the midwife makes a rapid assessment of the woman and context in order to prioritize her care.

Information should be calmly and sensitively sought, allowing sufficient time for the woman to express her feelings and identify needs. Kirkham (1989) found that the proforma used by midwives required only short answers, but that women gave lengthy replies to questions asked. It was noted that when the midwife filled in the form with a brief summary of each reply, the woman's responses eventually become shorter. The midwife can achieve a relaxed, confident and reassuring approach, while trying to acquire the necessary information and enable the woman's verbal contribution to be valued. This will do much to foster the desired supportive partnership in care.

Prior to examining the woman, the midwife should review the woman's notes and ensure that all required information is present and clear. It is often useful to clarify at this point, any issues which are not clear, or seek more information about previous history, and then seek a detailed history of events so far.

The birth plan should indicate the special needs and wishes of the woman and her partner and can assist in providing continuity of care and may provide reassurance to the woman that her particular needs and wishes are recorded for staff caring for her to see. Such plans may also be instrumental in enabling the woman to retain control of labour events and can provide the midwife with a valuable opportunity for health education in relation to birth.

OBSERVATIONS

General examination

The midwife should assess the woman's general appearance and demeanour, looking for features of general health and well-being. Observations of temperature, pulse, blood pressure and urinalysis are done to provide a baseline for the labour. Recommendations regarding the frequency of recording the vital signs in labour are based on tradition rather than evidence. Commonly, the temperature, pulse and blood pressure are recorded 4-hourly.

Abdominal examination

A detailed abdominal examination is carried out, between contractions, to determine the lie, presentation, position and engagement of the fetus. This should be a gentle process avoiding pain or discomfort and involving the couple as much as possible. The lie should be longitudinal. It is also important to determine the presentation and whether the presenting part is engaged, or will engage, in the pelvis. Auscultation of the fetal heart completes the abdominal examination. It should be strong and regular with a rate of between 110 and 160 beats per minute.

Vaginal examination

This procedure is one of the options to help confirm the onset of labour. However, it is invasive and often very uncomfortable for the woman and also poses a potential infection risk. Women may request it in seeking reassurance about the status of labour.

Records

When labour is established, all observations, examinations and any drug treatment should be recorded on the partogram which enables all observations to be detailed on one sheet. Specifically, it records the rate of cervical dilatation over time (see Fig. 26.5) The midwife's record of care constitutes a legal document, and throughout labour accurate, concise and comprehensive records must be maintained in accordance with the *Midwives Rules* (UKCC, 1998) and *Standards For Record Keeping* (NMC, 2002; UKCC, 1996). Such notations should be made at the time of the event, or as near to it as possible, and authenticated with the midwife's full and legible signature. In addition to fulfilling the legal requirements, contemporaneous records are

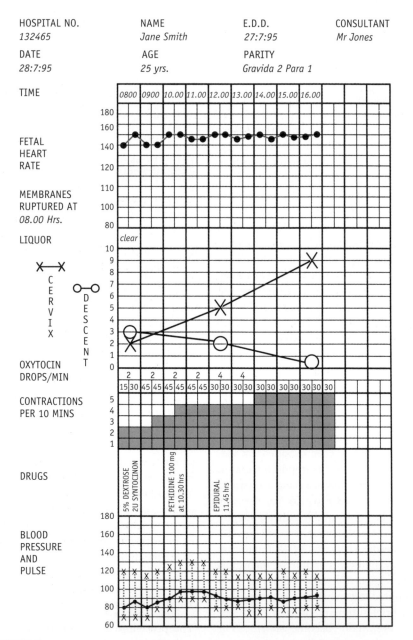

Figure 26.5 A partogram.

necessary to facilitate intelligent continuity of care in the event that care has to be transferred to another member of the team.

GENERAL MIDWIFERY CARE IN LABOUR

Assessment of progress

Because the environment has a significant impact on labour interventions, e.g. analgesia requirement, understanding of the progress of normal labour is best obtained in as woman-friendly a setting as possible. Large observational studies of women's behaviour at home birth, free-standing birth centres and midwife-led birthing suites may provide the data to understand the progress of normal labour and some parameters indicating a deviation from a spectrum of normality. However, much of the early work on labour progress has been done by obstetricians, usually exclusively in medicalized settings, and these findings have now found their way into midwifery textbooks as the official version of cervical dilatation patterns in labour.

Friedman is credited with a vast publication record in this area (over 200 papers) from the 1950s (Friedman, 1954) through to the 1990s (Friedman, 1995) and of devising the classic sigmoid-shaped curve of cervical dilatation (see Fig. 26.6).

He was the first to use the two terms – 'latent phase' and 'active phase' – of the first stage of labour and quantified their length in both nulliparous and multiparous women. The value of this research and that of other obstetricians, e.g. Philpott and Castle who invented the partogram (1972) or Studd (1973) who adapted it to British conditions, could be questioned, in that it is uncertain whether hourly vaginal examinations in hospital settings of large samples of women really reveal physiological markers of normal labour. There is still limited robust research data from alternative midwifery sources to question this current orthodoxy, apart from substantial anecdotal experiences of midwives and women.

Latent phase

Women's experience of early labour within the current maternity services throws up many of the 'old chestnuts' about midwifery care – lack of continuity, inappropriate medicalization and professional dominance. There are often still separate staffing arrangements for community and hospital, so women meet strangers when they come into hospital. The labour ward may be the wrong place to be for most women in early labour, and some women will find their subjective experience of contractions redefined as 'not in labour' or 'niggles' (Hunt and Symonds, 1995).

Friedman (1983) suggested that a prolonged latent phase was probably not clinically significant for how the active phase of labour developed and suggested care could either be supportive (rest and analgesia) or interventionist (artificial rupture of the membranes (ARM) and/or Syntocinon), though he cautioned against the latter because, in some women, this would amount to an induction of labour.

Evaluations of traditional DOMINO schemes in the 1980s where community midwives offered home assessment in early labour and then accompanied women into hospital at a later time indicated that these women experienced fewer labour interventions and spent less time on labour wards (Klein et al., 1983; Walsh, 1989). Hemminki and Simukka's (1986) study specifically examined time on admission and labour progress and suggested that later admission was linked to a lower caesarean section rate.

Independent midwives have promoted the inherent common sense of offering supportive care at home from a known midwife during the latent phase (Flint, 1986; Walmsley, 1999) but until the RCT of McNiven et al. (1998) there were no controlled prospective studies confirming what smaller studies and midwifery experience had been suggesting – delivery suites are not an appropriate environment for women in the latent phase of labour. Their study showed that women who were reviewed in a specifically designated early labour assessment facility rather than those sent directly to a delivery suite experienced:

● shorter labours
● fewer epidurals

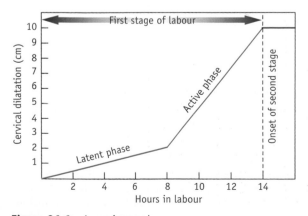

Figure 26.6 A cervicograph.

- less Syntocinon augmentation
- more positive births.

These studies demonstrate that the spectrum of presentation of the latent phase of labour varies greatly in different women and, as Koontz and Bishop (1982) argue, care must be tailored to individual need and not laid down in prescriptive protocols. Appropriate support is essential because of the balance of catecholamines required to optimize physiology.

Active phase

The monitoring of progress in labour has focused on what constitutes an acceptable cervical dilatation rate when women are in the active phase. Historically, obstetricians were driven by the significant morbidity and mortality associated with obstructed labour, particularly in developing countries, and it was in Africa that Philpott and Castle (1972) developed the first partogram that measured cervical dilatation over time. They were concerned about high caesarean section rates among women transferred from rural areas to provincial units, either because transfer was delayed or because intervention was too aggressive when women were transferred. This is an important point because they recognized that inappropriate intervention, e.g. recourse to early ARM and Syntocinon, may have iatrogenic effects. They drew an alert line at 1 cm dilatation/hour, and women who crossed it were transferred. Once at a provincial centre, women laboured until they crossed an action line set at 4 hours after the alert line when they received ARM and Syntocinon. With this protocol, caesarean sections rates were decreased significantly.

As partograms became widely adopted in the UK, a debate ensued as to when action for delay should begin (1, 2 or 4 hours to the right of the alert line) and whether 1 cm/hour represents an acceptable baseline for cervical dilatation or would 0.5 cm/hour be more clinically efficacious (Enkin *et al.*, 2000).

Active management of labour as a method to reduce caesarean section rates for dystocia has been largely discredited now, apart from the guarantee of the continuous presence of a midwife throughout labour and birth (McDonald, 1997; Thornton, 1996). A paradox in the active management debate is that such an interventionist approach to labour care, which never sought the views of women subjected to it during all the studies assessing its clinical value over 20 years, resulted in demonstrating that the only benefit is the 'soft' dimension of continuous support from carers (Frigoletto *et al.*, 1995).

Active management which endorses early ARM and aggressive use of Syntocinon has fuelled the debate over routine induced membrane rupture, which may be beginning to subside but which raged through the 1980s and early 1990s. Like episiotomy, it came to represent an 'intervention too far' as childbirth became medicalized over this period (NCT, 1989; Oakley, 1980). As with many intrapartum interventions, for years, research was inconclusive about benefits and risks leaving proponents and opponents free to champion their particular viewpoint. A meta-analysis of 10 trials up to 1995 by Goffinet *et al.* (1997) and another, later trial (Johnson *et al.*, 1997) conclude that there are both benefits (shorter labours in nulliparous women) and risks (possible increase in caesarean sections) and suggest amniotomy is probably more appropriately reserved for labours which are progressing slowly. Secondary analysis by Goffinet *et al.* (1997) of an earlier trial showed a link between early amniotomy and an increased frequency of severe variable fetal heart rate decelerations. Though there was no evidence of adverse neonatal outcome, the authors comment that the findings would increase the predilection for caesarean section. Meta-analysis by Fraser *et al.* (1998) of trials that included amniotomy and Syntocinon for delay in labour found that early augmentation (ARM and Syntocinon) did not provide benefit over more conservative forms of management in women with mild delay, but may reduce caesarean sections in women with established delay.

This requires a clear definition and understanding of what constitutes delay in labour. The World Health Organization (WHO, 1994) undertook a major multicentre trial in south-east Asia involving 35 000 women to test Philpott and Castle's 4 hour action line and found significant reductions in:

- prolonged labour
- caesarean sections
- augmentation.

More recently a well-designed British RCT compared an action line at 2, 3 or 4 hours and included maternal satisfaction as a primary outcome measure. There were no differences in the caesarean section rates between the 2-hour and 4-hour groups but women in the 2-hour group were more satisfied with their labour (Lavender *et al.*, 1999). The evaluation of maternal views is imperative when testing interventions with a major impact on women's experience, and the high profile of midwifery representation within the study possibly facilitated this; indeed it is one of the few trials in the field to include such an evaluation.

Bates (1997) highlights the feminist perspective on normal labour, arguing that the introduction of active management of labour and its subsequent influence on obstetric practice is a classic example of patriarchal control – a regime imposed by male obstetricians that appropriated the female domain of labour and birth for their practice – without any prior evaluation of women's views or consideration of its impact on midwifery independence. The debate over what constitutes normal progress in labour mirrors the wider struggle between the technocratic birth model, aligned with male power, and a woman-centred model, aligned with women's and midwives' autonomy (Davis-Floyd and Davis, 1997). Bates also discusses the power of language to perpetuate patriarchal control as it is the dominant discourse in maternity units throughout the country. This is typified by the mechanistic, victim-blaming rhetoric of 'uterine inertia' and 'failure to progress' and the medical language of case notes that becomes the 'official' record of the labour and birth events (Kirkham, 1997). Midwives need to be aware that the birth environment may be imbued with gender-mediated practices that do not place the woman at the centre of care, or consider her an equal partner in decision-making.

Vaginal examination

Vaginal examinations as the primary means of assessing progress in labour have been routine for some decades. Recently the impact of the procedure on some women has been brought to practitioners' notice. In Menage's (1993, 1996) study of a convenience sample of 500 women, 100 gave a history of an obstetrical or gynaecological procedure that was traumatizing and, of these, 30 fulfilled the criteria for a diagnosis of post-traumatic stress disorder. The descriptions of their experiences are harrowing.

Sexual abuse is especially relevant. Robolm and Buttenheim (1996) compared the effects of gynaecological examination on survivors of childhood sexual abuse with non-abused controls, and the former group reported more trauma-like responses including overwhelming emotions and unwanted, unpleasant memories and thoughts. Over 80% of this group had not been asked by the examiner about any history of sexual abuse or assault prior to examination. Bewley and Gibbs (2000) make some helpful comments, albeit under the more general heading of domestic violence, including cues that may indicate that screening is appropriate if it is carried out with sensitivity.

Bergstrom *et al.* (1992) highlight the cultural rationalization that the practitioner often takes on in undertaking the procedure, describing behaviours and language used surrounding vaginal examination which sanitize and make it socially acceptable when in just about every other context it is intimate, private and sexual. This is an example of how qualitative research, in this case an ethnographic study using videotaping as the data collection tool, can shed light on clinical events by challenging taken-for-granted assumptions about how those events are managed.

Devane's (1996) review of the research literature on the clinical benefits of vaginal examinations concludes along with Enkin (1992) that 'repeated vaginal examinations (in labour) are an invasive intervention of yet unproven value'. Spurious indications for routine examination include confirming the onset of the second stage of labour and assessing progress in normal labour.

Textbooks have outlined the detailed clinical information that can be gleaned from the examination (Bennett and Brown, 1999; Sweet, 1997) but the key question for the midwife as Warren (1999) argues is: What decision has to made at this time which requires information that can only be obtained from a vaginal examination?

In answering this question, an exploration of alternatives for obtaining the same information needs to be made. Warren is particularly challenging because she believes there is no place for routine vaginal examination in any labour and seeks to assess progress in labour by other means. McKay and Roberts (1990) describe behaviours and vocalizations indicative of the second stage of labour, and by analysing vocalizations, Baker and Kenner (1993) were able to ascertain the onset of transition. Hobbs (1998) describes the 'purple line', extending from the margin of the anus to the natal cleft at the top of the buttocks, said to be analogous to full cervical dilatation; the reliability of this has yet to be tested in a research setting.

Anecdotally, many midwives have developed sensitive 'antennae' which enable them to monitor progress in ways other than this procedure. However, the widespread practice of routine examinations of women in normal labour (CSAG, 1995) supports a belief that practitioners have an inherent distrust in women's ability to labour and birth and that the procedure is 'protocol driven'.

There are also iatrogenic risks. Imseis and colleagues (1999) showed conclusively that supposedly sterile digital examinations always introduced vaginal organisms into the cervical canal. This held true regardless of whether membranes were ruptured or not and supports earlier work revealing increased infection rates in women who had vaginal examinations after premature rupture of membranes (Lewis and Dunnihoo, 1995).

The issue of informed consent was starkly exposed by the practice of examinations under anaesthetic by medical students without a woman's prior agreement (Bewley, 1992). It seems incredible with hindsight that this practice was actually defended at the time (Cardozo, 1992) and reinforces the feminist view that practices propagated by reproductive medical specialities can objectify and dehumanize women (Greer, 1999). Sandelowski's (2000) exposé of the vaginal speculum and its historical role in the surveillance and therefore the controlling of women's reproductive health makes the same point. It is refreshing therefore to find that the Royal College of Obstetricians and Gynaecologists have produced sound guidelines for vaginal examinations which midwives will find helpful (RCOG, 1997).

Finally, when examination is clinically justifiable, can the findings be accepted with confidence? The poor inter-observer reliability of the procedure (Clement, 1994), illustrated by 'guesstimate' rather than 'estimate' scenarios of some clinical practice, may be assisted by practitioners ensuring that they undertake the examination systematically, and seeking a 'second opinion' should the findings be unclear.

It is imperative that midwives approach vaginal examinations guided by negotiated and explicit consent, clear clinical justification and with sensitivity for the discomfort and pain that may be caused.

Reflective Activity 26.5

Notice any feelings that arise in you about doing vaginal examinations. What have you observed about women's reaction to the examination in practice?

Indications for vaginal examination

1. To confirm the onset of labour and to establish a baseline for further progress.
2. To aid in assessing labour progress through determining the dilatation and condition of the cervix. (It is good practice to precede this with an abdominal examination to determine the fetal lie, presentation and position, the engagement or otherwise of the presentation and to auscultate the fetal heart.)
3. To diagnose the presentation, when this is in doubt.
4. To rupture the membranes when necessary.

Method

The woman is made comfortable in a semi-recumbent or lateral position with her legs separated and as relaxed as possible. She can be encouraged to practice relaxation exercises. Appropriate cleansing is carried out, then the examining fingers (index and forefinger) are generously lubricated and gently inserted into the vagina.

During the examination, the midwife should note any abnormalities or deviations from normal, such as vulval varicosities, lesions (such as warts or blisters), vaginal discharge/loss, oedema, and any previous scarring. She should also note the tone of the vaginal muscles and pelvic floor, and other characteristics such as vaginal dryness or excess heat which might indicate pyrexia.

Cervix

The cervix is assessed for consistency, effacement and dilatation. Changes which bring about initiation of labour and cervical effacement have been detailed in Chapter 25.

Consistency   The cervix is usually soft and pliable to the examining fingers. It may feel thick and is often described as having a consistency comparable to that of the lips.

Effacement and dilatation   The cervical canal, which usually projects into the vagina, becomes shorter, until no protrusion can be felt. This shortening is often referred to as the 'taking up' of the cervix which results from the dilatation of the internal cervical os, and the gradual opening out of the cervical canal. During and following effacement, the cervical consistency alters and it becomes progressively thinner. Complete effacement may be present in primigravidae prior to the onset of labour and prior to dilatation. In the multiparous woman, although a degree of effacement may be present prior to labour, completion of the process occurs simultaneously with cervical dilatation as labour advances.

A soft, stretchy cervix, closely in contact with the presenting part, indicates potential for normal cervical dilatation. A tight, unyielding cervix or one loosely in contact with the presenting part is less favourable and may be associated with long labour.

Membranes

In early labour the membranes can be difficult to feel as they are usually closely applied to the head. During a contraction the increase in pressure may cause the bag

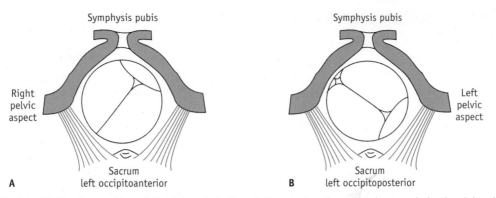

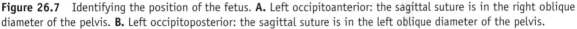

Figure 26.7 Identifying the position of the fetus. **A.** Left occipitoanterior: the sagittal suture is in the right oblique diameter of the pelvis. **B.** Left occipitoposterior: the sagittal suture is in the left oblique diameter of the pelvis.

of forewaters to become tense and bulge through the os uteri. The membranes may be inadvertently ruptured if pressure is applied at this time. If the head is poorly applied to the cervix, the bag of forewaters may bulge unduly early in the first stage and early rupture of membranes is likely to occur. This tends to occur with an occipitoposterior position.

Presentation

The presentation is normally the smooth round, hard vault of the head. Sutures and fontanelles can be felt with increasing ease as the os uteri dilates, thereby enabling confirmation of the presentation and determination of the position and attitude of the head. The degree of moulding of the fetal head can also be assessed. As labour continues, particularly if the membranes are ruptured, subsequent formation of a caput succedaneum may make recognition of sutures and fontanelles difficult and sometimes impossible. Rarely, a prolapsed cord may be felt as a soft loop lying in front of or alongside the fetal head. If the fetus is still alive the cord will be felt to pulsate.

Position

This can be determined by identification of the fontanelles and the sutures (Figs 26.7 and 26.8). An occipitoanterior position is identified by feeling the posterior fontanelle towards the anterior part of the pelvis. In an occipitoposterior position the anterior fontanelle will be felt anteriorly. The fontanelles are identified by the number of sutures which meet (see Ch. 15).

When the sagittal suture lies in the right oblique diameter of the pelvis (i.e. from the right posterior quadrant of the woman's pelvis to the left anterior quadrant) and the posterior fontanelle is felt anteriorly

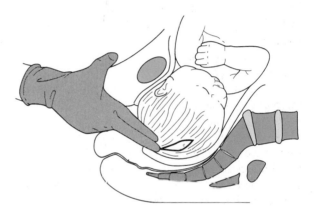

Figure 26.8 Identifying the sagittal suture and fontanelles during vaginal examination.

to the left, the position is the left occipitoanterior. When the sagittal suture is felt in the left oblique diameter of the pelvis (i.e. from the left posterior quadrant of the woman's pelvis) and the posterior fontanelle anteriorly to the right, the position is the right occipitoanterior.

If the sagittal suture is in the right oblique with the anterior fontanelle lying anteriorly to the left, the position is a right occipitoposterior, whereas when the sagittal suture is in the left oblique and the anterior fontanelle anteriorly to the right, the position is left occipitoposterior. Occasionally the sagittal suture is found in the transverse diameter of the pelvis between the ischial tuberosities. It is then necessary to identify one or both fontanelles to determine the position. It may also be possible to feel an ear under the symphysis pubis and this may give an indication of the position of the fetus. Prior to delivery, when the fetal head has

Table 26.2 Assessing the position of the fetus

Position of sagittal suture	Position of fontanelle	Position of fetus
Right oblique	Posterior fontanelle anteriorly to the left	LOA
	Anterior fontanelle anteriorly to the left	ROP
Left oblique	Posterior fontanelle anteriorly to the right	ROA
	Anterior fontanelle anteriorly to the right	LOP
Transverse diameter of the pelvis	Posterior fontanelle to the left	LOL
	Posterior fontanelle to the right	ROL
Anteroposterior diameter of the pelvis	Posterior fontanelle felt anteriorly	OA
	Anterior fontanelle felt anteriorly	OP

LOA, left occipitoanterior; LOL, left occipitolateral; LOP, left occipitoposterior; OA, occipitoanterior; OP, occipitoposterior; ROA, right occipitoanterior; ROP, right occipitoposterior; ROL, right occipitolateral

rotated on the pelvic floor, the sagittal suture should be in the anteroposterior diameter of the pelvis.

A summary of how to assess the position of the fetus is given in Table 26.2.

Flexion and station of the head

The fetal head may or may not be flexed at the onset of labour. However, in the presence of efficient uterine action and as a result of fetal axis pressure, the fetal head usually flexes, further facilitating a well-fitting presenting part. Unless the pelvis is particularly roomy or the fetal head small, deflexion of the head is indicated if the posterior and anterior fontanelles can be felt. This may be associated with malposition of the fetal head, poor cervical stimulation and prolongation of labour. The station or level of the presenting part refers to the relationship of the presenting part to the ischial spines. The maternal ischial spines are palpable as slight protuberances covered by tissue on either side of the bony pelvis. Descent in relation to the maternal ischial spines should be progressive and is expressed in centimetres as indicated in Figure 26.9.

Pelvic assessment

Prior to withdrawing the examining fingers, the midwife should estimate the size and shape of the pelvis, by comparing the size of the fetal presenting part with the space available at the pelvic outlet. If the head is not engaged, it may be possible to assess the curve of the sacrum. The ischial spines may also be felt, and assessed for undue prominence. As the examining fingers are withdrawn, the subpubic arch may be measured by being able to fit two fingers on the lower border of the symphysis pubis. Finally, after withdrawing the fingers, the intertuberous diameter can be established by placing

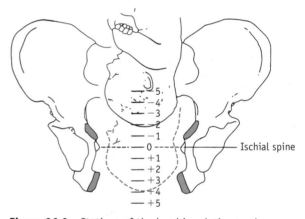

Figure 26.9 Stations of the head in relation to the pelvis. Descent in relation to the maternal ischial spines is expressed in centimetres.

the knuckles in between the two ischial tuberosities on the perineum.

The examination is completed by applying a vulval pad, changing any soiled linen and making the woman comfortable. The fetal heart is auscultated. All findings are recorded and the midwife must now analyse these findings to establish a total picture on which to make an accurate assessment of the progress of labour and to forecast how the labour is likely to advance. The midwife is able to relate to the woman and her partner the progress to date, and review with them the original birth plan for any adjustments which the woman and the midwife feel are necessary.

Psychological assessment

Many factors influence the manner in which the woman and her birth supporter respond to and deal with the pain and process of labour. Such factors include cultural and social differences, physiological factors which may influence the length of labour, the woman's reaction to pain, the woman's confidence in her own ability to cope with labour, her trust in her carers, how welcome the pregnancy is or how much the labour process is feared or welcomed. The midwife should note how the woman copes with each contraction and how well she relaxes between contractions. Additional relaxation techniques may be employed if relaxation during and between contractions is poor.

The hormone balance may be upset by anxiety and fear and this may slow the labour. Simkin and Ancheta (2000) outline some psychological interventions that can help restore this hormonal balance.

Uterine activity

The patterns of uterine contractions provide valuable information on which to determine the progress of labour. The frequency, strength and duration of the contractions are assessed at increasingly frequent intervals until in the late first stage they are assessed every 15 minutes. As the initiation point for contractions is in the uterine fundus, contractions are assessed by placing the hand lightly on the fundus of the uterus, which becomes increasingly firm as the contraction commences and reaches a peak, then diminishes. The normal resting tone of the uterus is between 4 and 10 mmHg and as pain is not felt until the contraction reaches 20 mmHg, the first and last few seconds of the contraction are pain free. The midwife will be able to feel the contraction for a few seconds before and after the woman feels pain. Some women do not like to be touched during contractions, and it is important to discuss the reasons for this touching with the woman and her partner and teach them the characteristics of uterine contractions. This facilitates their participation in the labour process and enables them to incorporate the information into relaxation techniques or self-administered methods of pain relief.

The total duration of the contraction should be timed. Frequency of the contractions is assessed by counting the interval from the onset of one contraction to the onset of the next. In between contractions the fundus will be soft and relaxed.

Loss per vaginam and rupture of the membranes

The time at which the membranes rupture should be recorded, together with the appearance of the liquor.

A minor amount of bloodstained loss is consistent with a show or detachment of the membranes which occurs with increasing cervical dilatation. A copious mucoid bloodstained loss may herald full cervical dilatation. A greenish colour is indicative of meconium staining sometimes associated with fetal distress. Frank bleeding per vaginam is abnormal, and if this occurs the midwife should consult with the obstetrician, who will ascertain the source, i.e. whether maternal or fetal, and determine the appropriate action. Measurement of loss and monitoring of the woman's condition is vital.

Bladder care in labour

The woman is encouraged to empty her bladder every 2 hours. A full bladder is uncomfortable and may delay the progress of labour by inhibiting descent of the fetal head if it is above the ischial spines. This will reflexly inhibit efficient uterine contractions and cervical dilatation. Pressure on the distended bladder by the fetal head may give rise to oedema and bruising, leading to possible difficulties in micturition in the early days of the puerperium.

Mobility and ambulation

Seven RCTs undertaken to evaluate ambulation all agree that there are no negative effects associated with mobility but there were varying conclusions as to benefit. Two studies (Flynn *et al.*, 1978; Read *et al.*, 1981) found the following advantages:

- greater uterine contractility
- shorter labours
- less oxytocin augmentation
- less need for pharmacological analgesia
- fewer operative deliveries
- less fetal distress.

MacLennan and colleagues' (1994) meta-analysis of their own trial with five others confirms the finding of reduced analgesia requirements and also notes that 46% of women in their study who declined entry to the trial did so because they did not want to lose the choice of ambulation. The most recent and largest trial (Bloom *et al.*, 1998) found that 99% of ambulant women would choose this mobility again. No other differences were noted compared with the recumbent group. An observational study by Albers *et al.*, (1997) of nurse-midwifery care for low-risk women at three different sites examined the specific association between ambulation and operative delivery. Women in the ambulation group had half the rate of operative birth.

The study allowed for a number of possible confounders, e.g. parity, which increases its validity but the authors also acknowledge the limitations of its non-randomized design.

Movement appears to be a central characteristic of normal labour (Gould, 2000). In an overview of trials of ambulation, Smith *et al.* (1991) found that when given the choice, women changed position an average of seven to eight times in the course of their labours.

Upright posture

Positive effects of gravity and lessened risk of aortocaval compression (and therefore improved fetal acid–base outcomes) have been described by Bonica (1967) and Humphrey *et al.* (1973). Mendez-Bauer *et al.* (1975) demonstrated stronger, efficient uterine contractions. Radiological evidence from the 1950s and 1960s showed larger anteroposterior and transverse diameters of the pelvic outlet in squatting and kneeling positions (Russell, 1969). Gupta and Nikodem's (2001) review of position in second stage seem to support these earlier findings.

Recumbent positions negatively affect these factors and may result in:

- supine hypotension (Johnstone *et al.*, 1978)
- less efficient uterine contractions
- less available space at the pelvic outlet.

Flint (1986) discussed the idea of midwives 'fitting around women', emphasizing that nearly all common procedures, e.g. fetal monitoring, vaginal examinations, could be done without asking the woman to get on the bed. Props such as bean bags and birth balls can be used to facilitate positional and posture changes, and Robertson (1997) elaborates on these through Active Birth Workshops. Given the paradoxical situation midwifery has found itself in, in having to justify mobility and upright birth posture, it may be time to remove the bed from the birth room. Certainly, the mass trend to lying down for childbirth, at least in western cultures, was never tested empirically and occurred largely to assist the birth practitioners to carry out technical interventions like forceps deliveries and the administration of anaesthetics (Donnison, 1988). This will continue to be tacitly endorsed by midwives as long as the 'bed birth myth' of childbirth remains. Some independent birth centres have replaced conventional beds with sofa beds and it may be time for delivery suites across the country to follow suit. This simple, cosmetic alteration would be deeply symbolic and may have a significant impact on birth positions. Figure 26.10 illustrates a variety of positions for the first stage of labour.

Moving and handling

Moving and handling concerns, and worries about back injuries, may preclude some midwives from assisting women who opt for an upright birth posture. If this is a real issue for practitioners, it may also have implications for assisting at recumbent births as well, as that sometimes requires awkward twisting and bending. Midwives are now usually trained in 'good back care' with mandatory moving and handling sessions run by hospitals. The application of these principles should not interfere with assisting women to birth in upright postures, not least because these postures probably also protect women's joints and backs more than conventional bed birth.

Home birth practitioners are familiar with birth taking place in living rooms as well as bedrooms, and with the restlessness of labour, during which women move freely within the privacy of their chosen birthing space, and may choose the bed only as a prop. It is probably time to expunge the term 'confinement' from the vocabulary of childbirth once and for all, and ensure that the environment 'belongs' to the woman and her partner.

> ### Reflective Activity 26.6
>
> Review the records of the births you have attended, and consider the positions women adopted. Begin to include this component of the birth in your records, and evaluate the effect on the woman and on you.

Prevention of infection

In labour both mother and fetus are vulnerable to infection, particularly when the membranes rupture. The possibility is increased when the immune response is undermined by suboptimal health, for example anaemia, malnourishment, chronic illness or when the woman is exhausted by a long and arduous labour. The hospital environment itself may increase the woman's risk of infection as she is exposed to a variety of unfamiliar organisms and possible sources of infection.

The midwife should ensure, as far as possible, a safe environment for the women and prevent infection and cross-infection. Such measures include good standards of hygiene and care, correct handwashing on the part of the carers before and after attending the woman, frequent changing of vulval pads, and meticulous aseptic

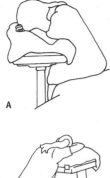
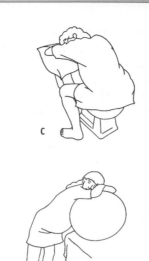
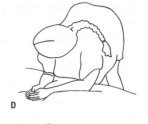
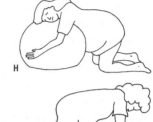
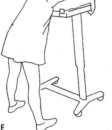
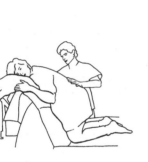
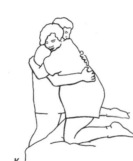
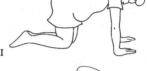
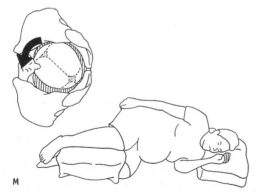
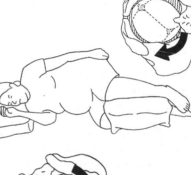
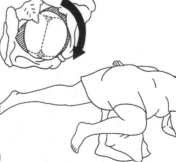

Figure 26.10   A variety of positions for the first stage of labour. **A.** Sitting, leaning on a tray table. **B.** Straddling a chair. **C.** Straddling toilet, facing backwards. **D.** Standing, leaning on bed. **E.** Standing, leaning on a tray table. **F.** Standing, leaning forward on partner. **G.** Standing, leaning on ball. **H.** Kneeling with a ball. **I.** On hands and knees. **J.** Kneeling over bed back. **K.** Kneeling, partner support. **L.** Pure side-lying on the 'correct' side, with fetal back 'toward the bed'. If the fetus is ROP, the woman lies on her right side. Gravity pulls fetal head and trunk towards ROL. **M.** Pure side-lying on the 'wrong' (left) side for an ROP fetus. Fetal back is 'toward the ceiling'. Gravity pulls fetal occiput and trunk towards direct OP. **N.** Semi-prone on the 'correct side' – with fetal back 'toward the ceiling'. If the fetus is ROP, the semi-prone woman lies on her left side. Gravity pulls fetal occiput and trunk towards ROL, then ROA. (From Simkin, P. & Ancheta, R. (2000) *The Labor Progress Handbook*, with permission of Blackwell Science, Ltd.)

techniques when undertaking vaginal examination and other invasive procedures such as catheterization.

General measures such as limiting the flow of traffic within the delivery area, meticulous cleansing of communal equipment such as beds, baths, toilets and trolleys, and increasing staff awareness of the potential for, and prevention of, infection should all be observed. A formal mechanism for infection control within hospitals should include maternity departments. One survey of surveillance of hospital-based obstetric and gynaecological infection showed a significant reduction in the incidence of infection when regular feedback to staff was implemented (Evaldon *et al.*, 1992).

NUTRITION IN LABOUR

Odent (1998) and Anderson (1998) have suggested that the smooth muscle structure of the uterus works much more efficiently than skeletal muscle and makes comparatively small energy demands, utilizing fatty acids and ketones readily as an energy source. It is also suggested that because the woman in physiological labour becomes withdrawn from higher cerebral activity and her skeletal muscles are at rest, her energy requirements are less than normal.

Considerable differences of opinion exist in relation to whether or not oral fluid and food in labour should be given. A survey conducted on the policies of various maternity units in England and Wales (Michael *et al.*, 1991) indicated that 79.5% of units had a policy on oral intake in labour and that 96.4% of units allowed women some form of oral intake. However, only 38.8% allowed food and drink, and, of these, 13.6% had a selection policy. Johnson and colleagues (1989) concluded that the risk of regurgitation and aspiration of gastric contents in labour is real and serious, and this is a recognized cause of maternal mortality (DoH, 1994). Such aspiration may include either food particles, which can obstruct the air passages and may result in atelectasis distal to the obstruction, with subsequent hypoxaemia, or aspiration of acidic stomach secretions and chemical burns of the airways (Mendelson's syndrome). Whilst recognizing this risk, incidents were almost entirely associated with the use of general anaesthetics and directly related to the frequency of general anaesthesia and the skill with which it was administered. Between 1991–1993 there were eight maternal deaths which were directly attributable to anaesthesia (DoH, 1996), though this reduced to three deaths in 1997–1999 (Lewis, 2001).

The confidential enquiries into maternal mortality have included fatal cases of Mendelson's syndrome and are often critical of the practice of medical practitioners, particularly anaesthetists. The incidence of Mendelson's syndrome in childbearing women is almost exclusively related to situations where women lose control of their airway, which occurs during the administration of general anaesthesia. This has three implications:

- Maternity departments should be staffed with senior anaesthetic practitioners.
- There should be strict protocols which include the application of cricoid pressure during the induction of general anaesthetic (for all pregnant women, from the first trimester of pregnancy to at least 48 hours postpartum).
- Midwives need to be fully involved in the policies and decision-making in this area because these have implications for all labouring women.

Discussions about reducing the risks of Mendelson's syndrome should centre on reducing the requirement for general anaesthetic risk as well as restricting food and drink to those labouring women who are likely to need a general anaesthetic. There remains the assumption that any labouring woman may need general anaesthesia.

Imposed fasting in labour for all women is questionable, particularly in the light of evidence which indicates that fasting in labour does not ensure an empty stomach or lower the acidity of stomach contents (Johnson *et al.*, 1989). Such restrictions may lead to dehydration and ketosis with a resultant need for intervention, and this should be weighed against the alternative course of allowing women to eat and drink as desired (Johnson *et al.*, 1989).

Advocates for providing oral nutrition in normal labour encourage frequent light meals, low in fat and roughage, which are easily absorbed (Johnson *et al.*, 1989). Such foods could include clear soup, jelly, ice cream, tea, toast and marmalade or jam, boiled egg, fruit juices or cooked fruit, or light cereals. Fluids as desired should be given to replace fluid lost through perspiration and other biological functions and to prevent dehydration. A small RCT (Riches, 1996) demonstrated that women who were allowed to eat and drink freely had significant differences in rates of intervention, increased mobility and shorter labours, and their babies had better Apgar scores, in comparison to women on a restricted intake. An interesting finding was that some women who were later 'nil by mouth', reported that they had eaten a wide variety of foods which may be considered unsuitable, e.g. kebab and chips.

Grant (1990) suggests that a rational plan for nutrition in labour, in the light of current evidence, should include the following:

- Where no risk of general anaesthesia or instrumental delivery exists, the woman should be allowed to eat a light diet and drink as required.
- When narcotic analgesia has been given, oral food should be withheld, and only sips of water given.

In further attempting to reduce the very real risk of regurgitation and inhalation, it is common practice in some maternity units and by some obstetricians and anaesthetists to deploy pharmacological agents such as magnesium trisilicate, cimetidine or ranitidine to increase the pH of the stomach contents and drugs such as metoclopramide to alter the rate of gastric emptying. However, utilizing such agents does not necessarily reduce the incidence and severity of Mendelson's syndrome (Johnson *et al.*, 1989).

Intravenous carbohydrate-containing solutions have been used in the prevention or treatment of ketoacidosis and have been evaluated in a number of controlled trials, which indicate that there may be undesirable effects such as fetal and early neonatal hyperinsulinaemia leading to a subsequent neonatal hypoglycaemia (Aynsley-Green and Soltesz, 1986; Johnson *et al.*, 1989).

Odent suggests that in the absence of a comprehensive understanding, practitioners should withdraw and leave it to labouring women to self-regulate food and fluid intake, and in the absence of sufficient evidence, this may be useful.

ASSESSING THE FETAL CONDITION

In order to interpret the fetal response to labour it is essential that the midwife understands the mechanisms which control fetal heart response. The cardioregulatory centre of the brain, situated in the medulla oblongata, is influenced by many factors. Baroreceptors situated in the arch of the aorta and carotid sinus sense alterations in blood pressure and transmit information to the cardioregulatory centre. Similarly, chemoreceptors situated in the carotid sinus and arch of the aorta will respond to changes in oxygen and carbon dioxide tensions. The cardioregulatory centre is controlled by the autonomic nervous system and, in response to varying physiological factors, either the sympathetic or parasympathetic nervous system will be stimulated. The sympathetic nervous system, via the sinoatrial node, causes an increase in heart rate while the parasympathetic nervous system

causes a rate reduction. The continuous interaction of these two systems results in minor fluctuations in the heart rate which is recognized as *variability*. Development of the sympathetic nervous system occurs early in fetal life, while the parasympathetic nervous response does not become pronounced until later in pregnancy. This accounts for the higher baseline rate of the fetal heart during early pregnancy and the lower rate at term.

Monitoring the fetal heart

The activity of the fetal heart may be assessed intermittently using the Pinard fetal stethoscope or a Sonicaid. This provides the midwife with sample information relative to the rate and rhythm of the fetal heart. At commencement of intermittent auscultation, it is important to distinguish the maternal pulse from the fetal heart as the former can mimic a fetal heart, and therefore can be falsely reassuring to the midwife. An understanding of the workings of the Sonicaid is useful, and reinforces the value of the use of the Pinard stethoscope at regular intervals even if the Sonicaid is used (Gibb and Arulkumaran, 1997).

Intermittent auscultation of the fetal heart is usually undertaken hourly in early labour, every 15 minutes as contractions increase, and after each contraction in the late first and second stages of labour. The National Institute for Clinical Excellence recommends intermittent auscultation and the abandoning of the admission trace for women in normal labour (NICE, 2001).

Healthy fetal heart patterns

The normal fetal heart has a baseline rate of between 110 and 160 beats per minute (b.p.m.). The baseline rate refers to the heart rate present between periods of acceleration and deceleration (NICE, 2001). Baseline variability refers to the variation in heart rate of 5–15 b.p.m., which occurs over a time base of 10–20 seconds. Figure 26.11 demonstrates normal baseline variability. The presence of good variability is an important sign of fetal well-being (NICE, 2001).

Acceleration patterns of the fetal heart of 15 b.p.m. from the baseline as shown in Figure 26.12 are often associated with fetal activity and stimulation and are thought to be useful indicators of absence of fetal acidaemia in labour (Spencer, 1993). They are not considered to be clinically significant if they are of short duration, that is 15 seconds. When two are present within a 20-minute period the trace is described as 'reactive' (Gibb, 1988). This is considered to be a positive

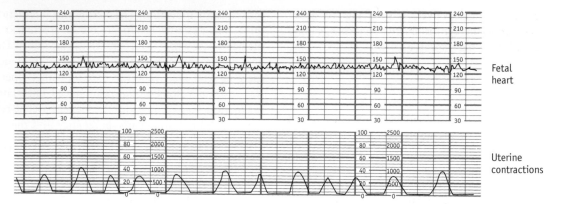

Figure 26.11   ECG trace showing baseline variability in fetal heart rate. (Courtesy of Sonicaid, Abingdon, Oxon.)

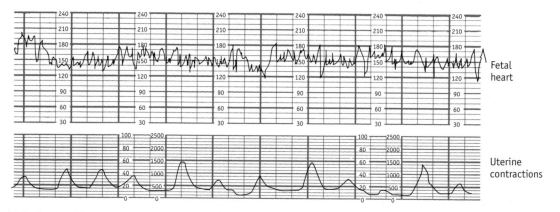

Figure 26.12   Fetal heart rate accelerations. (Courtesy of Sonicaid, Abingdon, Oxon.)

sign of fetal health, indicating good reflex responsiveness of the fetal circulation.

Electronic fetal monitoring

In normal labour, continuous electronic fetal monitoring (EFM) is not required as it results in more birth interventions without a demonstrable improvement in fetal outcome (NICE, 2001; Thacker *et al.*, 2001). In addition, inter- and intra-observer reliability is poor with EFM, and maternity units regularly update all delivery suite staff in the interpretation of traces as recommended by the Confidential Enquiry into Stillbirth and Neonatal Death (CESDI) (MCHRC, 1999).

NEW RESEARCH AND DEVELOPMENTS

Some midwives (Downe, 2001) are questioning whether much of the research around the physiology of birth needs to be redone in alternative birth settings to large

hospitals. Already, Albers' (1999) research is challenging the traditional length of the first stage of labour. Greater understanding of the delicate balance of hormones that facilitates optimum labour is supporting this rethinking. Midwifery needs midwives who want to research birth physiology to increase the knowledge base in this area and to blend it with women's experience of birth (sometimes called embodied knowledge) to help develop more holistic understanding.

CONCLUSION

Care during first stage of labour is as much about trusting the birth process and intuitively connecting with labouring women as it is about monitoring and understanding the physiology. A social model of birth emphasizes the relational aspects of this experience and the key role of birth environment. When these are understood and appropriately applied, physiology will be maximized and complications will occur in only a small minority of women. However, against the backdrop of increasing medicalization of childbirth, midwives may feel caught between the social and medical models and will need the support of each other if they are to facilitate empowering birth experiences for women in their care.

KEY POINTS

- Labour is an intense, individual event, in which the midwife can play a pivotal role in supporting normality, and enabling and facilitating birth to be a positive and empowering experience.
- The midwife should be knowledgeable about the psychological, physiological and social aspects of labour in order to work in partnership with the woman, and plan care appropriately.
- The midwife should be conversant with contemporary research and evidence, and committed to sharing this knowledge with the woman and her partner.
- Continuity of care and carer provides a valued model of care and improves the outcomes of labour, and where possible this should be worked towards. Effective use of notes and records, including partograms, is a crucial part of this.
- One-to-one care during the active phase of the first stage of labour should be utilized both as a means of monitoring maternal and fetal well-being and as an educational opportunity for the woman and her birth partner.
- New models of care such as birth centres, midwifery-led units and birthing suites provide an opportunity to develop women-centred care, and increase midwifery autonomy.

REFERENCES

Albers, L. (1999) The duration of labour in healthy women. *Journal of Perinatology* **19**(2): 114–119.

Albers, L. & Katz, V. (1991) Birth setting for low risk pregnancies: an analysis of the current literature. *Journal of Nurse-Midwifery* **36**(4): 215–220.

Albers, L., Anderson, D. & Cragin, L. (1997) The relationship of ambulation in labour to operative delivery. *Journal of Nurse-Midwifery* **42**(1): 4–8.

Anderson, T. (1998) Is ketosis in labour pathological? *Practising Midwife* **1**(9): 22–26.

Aynsley-Green, A. & Soltesz, G. (1986) Metabolic and endocrine disorder, Part 1, Disorders of blood glucose homeostasis in the neonate. In: *Textbook of Neonatology*. Edinburgh: Churchill Livingstone.

Baker, A. & Kenner, A. (1993) Communication of pain: vocalisation as an indicator of the stage of labour. *Australian and New Zealand Journal of Obstetrics and Gynaecology* **33**(4): 384–385.

Bastian, H., Kierse, M. & Lancaster, P. (1998) Perinatal death associated with planned home birth in Australia: population based study. *British Medical Journal* **317**(7155): 384–388.

Bates, C. (1997) Care in normal labour: a feminist perspective. In: Alexander, J., Levy, V. & Roth, C. (eds) *Midwifery Practice: Core Topics 2*. London: Macmillan.

Bennett, V. & Brown, L. (eds) (1999) *Myles Textbook for Midwives*. Edinburgh: Churchill Livingstone.

Bergstrom, L., Roberts, J., Skillman L. *et al.* (1992) 'You'll feel me touching you, sweetie'. Vaginal Examinations during the second stage of labour. *Birth* **19**(1): 10–18.

Bewley, S. (1992) The law, medical students and assault. *British Medical Journal* **304**(6841): 1551–1553.

Bewley, C. & Gibbs, A. (2000) Domestic violence in pregnancy: a midwifery issue. In: Alexander, J., Roth, C. & Levy, V. (eds) *Midwifery Practice: Core Topics 3*. London: Macmillan.

Blackburn, S.T. (2003) *Maternal, Fetal and Neonatal Physiology*, 2nd edn. Philadelphia: W.B. Saunders.

Bloom, S., McIntyre, D. & Beimer, M. (1998) Lack of effect of walking on labour and delivery. *New England Journal of Medicine* **339**(2): 76–79.

Bonica, J. (1967) *Principles and Practice of Obstetric Analgesia and Anaesthesia*. Philadelphia: F.A. Davis.

Campbell, R. & McFarlane, A. (1994) *Where to be Born: The Debate and the Evidence*, 2nd edn. Oxford: National Perinatal Epidemiology Unit.

Cardozo, L. (1992) Teaching vaginal examinations. *British Medical Journal* **305**(6845): 113.

Chamberlain, G., Wraight, A. & Crowley, P. (1997) *Home Births: The Report of the 1994 Confidential Enquiry by the National Birthday Trust Fund*. London: Parthenon.

Clement, S. (1994) Unwanted vaginal examinations. *British Journal of Midwifery* **2**(8): 368–370.

Clinical Standards Advisory Group (CSAG) (1995) *Report of a CSAG Committee on Women in Normal Labour.* London: HMSO.

David, M., Kraker von Schwarzenfeld, H., Dimer, J. *et al.* (1999) Perinatal outcome in hospital and birth centre obstetric care. *International Journal of Gynecology and Obstetrics* **65**(2): 149–156.

Davis-Floyd, R.E. (1998) Ritual in the hospital: giving birth the American way. *Birth Gazette* **14**(4): 12–17.

Davis-Floyd, R. & Davis, E. (1997) Intuition as authoritative knowledge in midwifery and homebirth. In: Davis-Floyd, R. & Sargent, C. (eds) *Childbirth and Authorative Knowledge,* pp. 315–349. London: University of California Press.

Department of Health (DoH) (1992) *Health Committee, Second Report, Sessions 1991–1992, Maternity Services.* London: HMSO.

Department of Health (DoH) (1993) *Changing Childbirth. Report of the Expert Maternity Group,* Part 1. London: HMSO.

Department of Health (DoH) (1994) *Report on Confidential Enquiries into Maternal Deaths in the United Kingdom 1988–1990.* London: HMSO.

Department of Health (DoH) (1996) *Report on Confidential Enquiries into Maternal Deaths in the United Kingdom 1991–1993.* London: HMSO.

Devane, D. (1996) Sexuality and midwifery. *British Journal of Midwifery* **4**(8): 413–420.

Donnison, J. (1988) *Midwives and Medical Men: A History of the Struggle for the Control of Childbirth.* London: Historical Publications.

Downe, S. (2000) A proposal for a new research and practice agenda for birth. *MIDIRS Midwifery Digest* **10**(3): 337–341.

Downe, S. (2001) Is there a future for normal birth? *Practising Midwife* **4**(6): 10–12.

English National Board for Nursing, Midwifery and Health Visiting (ENB) (2001) *Midwifery Practice in Action: Report of the Board's Midwifery Practice Audit 2000/2001.* London: ENB.

Enkin, M. (1992) Commentary: Do I do that? Do I really do that? Like that? *Birth* **19**(1): 19–20.

Enkin, M., Kierse, M., Neilson, J. *et al.* (2000) *A Guide to Effective Care in Pregnancy and Childbirth.* Oxford: Oxford University Press.

Esposito, N. (1993) Giving back the body: ethnography of a birthing center. New York: Columbia University, Teachers College.

Esposito, N. (1999) Marginalised women's comparisons of their hospital and free-standing birth centre experience: a contract of inner-city birthing centres. *Health Care for Women International* **20**(2): 111–126.

Evaldon, G.R., Frederici, H., Jullig, C. *et al.* (1992) Hospital-associated infections in obstetrics and gynaecology. Effects of surveillance. *Acta Obstetricia et Gynecologica Scandinavica* **71**(1): 54–58.

Fleissig, A. (1993) Are women given enough information by staff during labour and delivery? *Midwifery* **9**(2): 70–75.

Flint, C. (1986) *Sensitive Midwifery.* London: Heinemann.

Flint, C. & Poulengeris, P. (1987) *The Know Your Midwife Report.* London: South West Thames Regional Health Authority and the Wellington Foundation. Available from 46 Peckerman Rd, London.

Flint, C., Poulengeris, P. & Grant, A.M. (1987) The 'Know Your Midwife' scheme: a randomised trial of continuity of care by a team of midwives. *Midwifery* **5**: 11–16.

Flynn, A., Hollins, K. & Lynch, P. (1978) Ambulation in labour. *British Medical Journal* **2**(6137): 591–593.

Fraser, W., Vendittelli, F., Krauss, I. *et al.* (1998) Effects of early augmentation of labour with amniotomy and oxytocin in nulliparous women: a meta-analysis. *British Journal of Obstetrics and Gynaecology* **105**(2): 189–194.

Friedman, E. (1954) The graphic analysis of labour. *American Journal of Obstetrics and Gynecology* **68**: 1568–1575.

Friedman, E. (1983) Dysfunctional labour. In: Cohen, W. & Friedman, E. (eds) *Management of Labour.* Baltimore: University Press.

Friedman, E. (1995) Comment: physiology of cervical change over the course of labour. *European Journal of Obstetrics and Gynecology and Reproductive Biology* **61**(2): 179–180.

Frigoletto, F., Lieberman, E. & Lang, J. (1995) A clinical trial of active management of labor. *New England Journal of Medicine* **333**: 745–750.

Garcia, J., Redshaw, M., Fitzsimons, B. *et al.* (1997) *First Class Delivery: Audit Commission Report on the Maternity Services Part 1.* Oxford: Audit Commission.

Gibb, D. (1988) *A Practical Guide to Labour Management.* London: Blackwell Scientific.

Gibb, D.M.F. & Arulkumaran, S. (1997) *Fetal Monitoring in Practice,* 2nd edn. London: Butterworth-Heinemann.

Goffinet, F., Fraser, W., Marcoux, S. *et al.* (1997) Early amniotomy increases the frequency of fetal heart abnormalities. *British Journal of Obstetrics and Gynaecology* **104**(5): 548–553.

Gould, D. (2000) Normal labour: a concept analysis. *Journal of Advanced Nursing* **31**(2): 418–427.

Grant, J. (1990) Nutrition and hydration in labour. In: Alexander, J., Levy, V. & Roch, S. (eds) *Intrapartum Care – A Research-Based Approach.* London: Macmillan.

Green, J., Coupland, B. & Kitzinger, J. (1998) *Great Expectations: A Prospective Study of Women's Expectations and Experiences of Childbirth.* Cambridge: Child Care and Development Group.

Green, J., Renfrew, M. & Curtis, P. (2000) Continuity of carer: what matters to women. *Midwifery* **16**(3): 186–196.

Greer, G. (1999) *The Whole Woman.* London: Doubleday.

Gupta, J. & Nikodem, V. (2001) Woman's position during second stage of labour (Cochrane Review). *The Cochrane Library,* Issue 2. Oxford: Update Software.

Hemminki, E. & Simukka, R. (1986) The timing of hospital admission and progress of labour. *European Journal of Obstetrics and Gynecology and Reproductive Biology* **22**: 85–94.

Hobbs, L. (1998) Assessing cervical dilatation without VEs. *Practising Midwife* **1**(11): 34–35.

Hodnett, E.D. (2001) Home-like versus conventional birth settings (Cochrane Review). *The Cochrane Library*, Issue 4. Oxford: Update Software.

Hodnett, E.D. (2002a) Caregiver support for women during childbirth (Cochrane Review). *The Cochrane Library*, Issue 1. Oxford: Update Software.

Hodnett, E.D. (2002b) Continuity of caregivers during pregnancy and childbirth (Cochrane Review). *The Cochrane Library*, Issue 3. Oxford: Update Software.

Humphrey, M., Hounslow, D. & Morgan, S. (1973) The influence of maternal posture at birth on the fetus. *Journal of Obstetrics & Gynaecology of the British Commonwealth* **80**: 1075–1080.

Hunt, S. & Symonds, A. (1995) *The Social Meaning of Midwifery*. Basingstoke: Macmillan.

Imseis, H., Trout, W. & Gabbe, S. (1999) The microbiologic effect of digital cervical examination. *American Journal of Obstetrics and Gynecology* **180**(3): 578–580.

Jacoby, A. & Cartwright, A. (1990) Finding out about the views and experiences of maternity service users. In: Garcia, J., Kilpatrick, R. & Richards, M. (eds) *The Politics of Maternity Care*. Oxford: Clarendon Paperbacks.

Johnson, C., Kierse, M.J.N.C., Enkin, M. *et al.* (1989) Nutrition and hydration in labour. In: Chalmers, I., Enkin, M. & Kierse, M.J.N.C. (eds) *Effective Care in Pregnancy and Childbirth*, Vol. 2. Oxford: Oxford University Press.

Johnson, N., Lilford, R., Guthrie, K. *et al.* (1997) Randomised trial comparing a policy of early with selective amniotomy in uncomplicated labour at term. *British Journal of Obstetrics and Gynaecology* **104**: 340–346.

Johnstone, F., Aboelmagd, M. & Harouny, A. (1978) Maternal position in the second stage of labour and fetal acid base status. *British Journal of Obstetrics and Gynaecology* **94**(8): 753–757.

Kirkham, M. (1989) Midwives and information giving during labour. In: Robinson, S. & Thompson, A. (eds) *Midwives, Research and Childbirth*, Vol. 1. London: Chapman and Hall.

Kirkham, M. (1997) Stories and childbirth. In: Kirkham, M. & Perkins, E. (eds) (1997) *Reflections on Midwifery*. London: Baillière Tindall.

Kitzinger, S. (2000) *Rediscovering Birth*. London: Simon & Schuster.

Klein, M., Lloyd, I. & Redman, C. (1983) Comparison of low risk pregnant women booked for two systems of care: shared care (consultant) and integrated general practitioner unit: labour and delivery management and neonatal outcomes. *British Journal of Obstetrics and Gynaecology* **90**: 123–128.

Koontz, W. & Bishop, E. (1982) Management of the latent phase of labour. *Clinical Obstetrics and Gynecology* **25**: 111–114.

Lavender, T., Wallymahmed, A. & Walkinshaw, S. (1999) Managing labour using partograms with different action lines: a prospective study of women's views. *Birth* **26**(2): 89–96.

Leap, N. (1996) Persuading women to give birth at home – or offering real choice. *British Journal of Midwifery* **4**(10): 536–538.

Lewis, D. & Dunnihoo, D. (1995) Digital vaginal examinations after PROM: what consequences? *Contemporary Ob/Gyn* **40**(1): 33–34, 37, 40.

Lewis, G. (ed) (2001) *Why Mothers Die 1997–99: Fifth Report of the Confidential Enquiries into Maternal Deaths in the United Kingdom*. London: CEMD: associated with NICE, RCOG.

McCoshen, J.A., Hoffman, D.R. & Kredenster, J.V. (1990) The role of fetal membranes in regulating production, transport and metabolism of prostaglandin E_2 during labour. *American Journal of Obstetrics and Gynecology* **163**(5): 1632–1640.

McDonald, S. (1997) Active management of labour. In: Alexander, J., Levy, V. & Roth, C. (eds) *Midwifery Practice: Core Topics 2*. London: Macmillan.

McKay, S. & Robert, J. (1990) Obstetrics by ear – maternal and caregivers' perceptions of the meaning of maternal sounds during second stage of labour. *Journal of Nurse-Midwifery* **35**(5): 266–273.

MacLennan, A., Crowther, C. & Derham, R. (1994) Does the option to ambulate during spontaneous labour confer any advantage or disadvantage? *Journal of Maternal and Fetal Medicine* **3**(1): 43–48.

McNiven, P., Williams, J., Hodnett, E. *et al.* (1998) An early labour assessment program: a randomised controlled trial. *Birth* **25**(1): 5–10.

Maternal and Child Health Research Consortium (MCHRC) (1999) *Confidential Enquiry into Stillbirths and Deaths in Infancy: 6th Annual Report*. London: MCHRC.

Menage, J. (1993) Post-traumatic stress disorder in women who have undergone obstetric and/or gynaecological procedures. A consecutive series of 30 cases of PTSD. *Journal of Reproductive and Infant Psychology* **11**: 221–228.

Menage, J. (1996) Post-traumatic stress disorder following obstetric/gynaecological procedures. *British Journal of Midwifery* **4**(10): 532–533.

Mendez-Bauer, C., Arroyo, J. & Garcia-Ramos, C. (1975) Effects of standing position on spontaneous uterine contractility and other aspects of labour. *Journal of Perinatal Medicine* **3**: 89–100.

Michael, S., Reilly, C.S. & Caunt, J.A. (1991) Policies for oral intake during labour. A survey of maternity units in England and Wales. *Anaesthesia* **46**(12): 1071–1073.

Morrison, A. (1991) The nurse's role in relation to advocacy. *Nursing Standard* **5**(41): 37–41.

National Childbirth Trust (NCT) (1989) *Rupture of the Membranes in Labour: Women's Views.* London: NCT.

National Childbirth Trust (NCT) (1999) Fifty per cent of doctors oppose home birth – results of survey of NCT branches. *Press Release* London, 23rd August.

National Institute of Clinical Excellence (NICE) (2001) *The Use of Electronic Fetal Monitoring.* Online. Available: http://www.nice.org.uk.

North Staffordshire Changing Childbirth Research Team (NSCCRT) (2000) A randomised study of midwifery caseload care and traditional 'shared-care'. *Midwifery* **16**(4): 295–302.

Nursing and Midwifery Council (NMC) (2002) *Code of Professional Conduct.* London: NMC. Online. Available: http://www.nmc-uk.org.

Oakley, A. (1980) *Women Confined.* London: Robertson.

Oakley, A. (1984) *The Captured Womb: A History of the Medical Care of Pregnant Women.* Oxford: Basil Blackwood.

Oakley, A., Rajan, L. & Grant, A. (1990) Social support and pregnancy outcome. *British Journal of Obstetrics and Gynaecology* **97**(2): 152–162.

Odent, M. (1998) Labouring women are not marathon runners. *Practising Midwife* **1**(9): 16–18.

Olsen, O. (1997) Meta-analysis of the safety of home birth. *Birth* **24**(1): 4–13.

Olsen, O. & Jewell, M. (2001) Home versus hospital birth (Cochrane Review). *The Cochrane Library*, Issue 1. Oxford: Update Software.

Page, L. (1995) Putting principles into practice. In: Page, L. (ed) *Effective Group Practice in Midwifery: Working with Women.* Oxford: Blackwell Science.

Page, L., McCourt, C., Beake, S. *et al.* (1999) Clinical interventions and outcomes of one-to-one midwifery practice. *Journal of Public Health Medicine* **21**(3): 243–248.

Pairman, S. (2000) Women-centred midwifery: partnerships or professional friendships? In: Kirkham, M. (ed) *The midwife–mother relationship.* London: Macmillan.

Philpott, R. & Castle, W. (1972) Cervicographs in the management of labour on primigravidae 1. The alert line for detecting abnormal labour. *Journal of Obstetrics & Gynaecology of the British Commonwealth* **79**: 592–598.

Porter, M. & MacIntyre, S. (1984) What is, must be best: A research note on conservative or deferential responses to antenatal care provision. *Social Science and Medicine* **19**(11): 1197–1200.

Read, J., Miller, F. & Paul, R. (1981) Randomised trial of ambulation versus oxytocin for labour enhancement: a preliminary report. *American Journal of Obstetrics and Gynecology* **139**: 669–672.

Riches, L. (1996) *A Comparative Study on the Effects of Eating and Drinking Versus a Restricted Food and Fluid Intake During Labour.* MSc Dissertation. Guildford: University of Surrey.

Robertson, A. (1997) *The Midwife Companion.* Sydney: ACE Graphics.

Robolm, J. & Buttenheim, M. (1996) The gynaecological care experience of adult survivors of childhood sexual abuse: a preliminary investigation. *Women and Health* **24**(3): 59–75.

Rooks, J., Weatherby, N. & Ernst, E. (1992) The National Birth Centre Study. Part 11 – intrapartum and immediate postpartum and neonatal care. *Journal of Nurse-Midwifery* **37**(5): 301–330.

Rowley, M., Hensley, M., Brinsmead, M. *et al.* (1995) Continuity of care by a midwife team versus routine care during pregnancy and birth: a randomised trial. *Medical Journal of Australia* **163**: 289–293.

Royal College of Obstetricians and Gynaecologists (RCOG) (1997) *Intimate Examinations: Report of a Working Party.* London: RCOG Press.

Russell, J. (1969) Moulding of the pelvic outlet. *Journal of Obstetrics & Gynaecology of the British Commonwealth* **76**: 817–820.

Sandall, J. (1997) Midwives burnout and continuity of care. *British Journal of Midwifery* **5**(2): 106–111.

Sandelowski, M. (2000) 'This most dangerous instrument': propriety, power and the vaginal speculum. *Journal of Obstetric, Gynecologic, and Neonatal Nursing* **29**(1): 73–82.

Schwarcz, R., Diaz, A.G., Fescina, R. *et al.* (1977) Latin American collaborative study on maternal posture in labour. *Birth Family Journal* **6**(1): 1979.

Shields, N., Turnbull, D. & Reid, M. (1998) Satisfaction with midwife managed care in different time period: a randomised controlled trial of 1299 women. *Midwifery* **14**: 85–93.

Simkin, P. & Ancheta, R. (2000) *The Labor Progress Handbook.* London: Blackwell Science.

Smith, M., Acheson, L., Byrd, J. *et al.* (1991) A critical review of labour and birth care. *Journal of Family Practice* **35**: 107–115.

Spencer, J.A. (1993) Clinical overview of cardiotocography (Review). *British Journal of Obstetrics and Gynaecology* **100**(Suppl. 9): 4–7.

Studd, J. (1973) Partograms and nomograms of cervical dilatation in management of primigravid labour. *British Medical Journal* **4**: 451–455.

Sweet, B. & Tiran, D. (eds) (1997) *Mayes' Midwifery: A Textbook for Midwives,* 12th edn. London. Baillière Tindall.

Tan, B.P. & Hannah, M.E. (2002) Oxytocin for prelabour rupture of membranes at or near term (Cochrane Review). (Substantive update: 28 August 1996) *The Cochrane Library,* Issue 3. Oxford: Update Software.

Tew, M. (1998) *Safer Childbirth? A Critical History of Maternity Care.* London: Free Association Books.

Thacker, S., Stroup, D. & Peterson, H. (2001) Continuous electronic fetal heart monitoring during labour.

(Cochrane Review) *The Cochrane Library,* Issue 1. Oxford: Update Software.

Thomas, J. & Parenjothy, S. (CESU) (2001) *The National Sentinel Caesarean Section Audit.* London: RCOG Press.

Thornton, J.G. (1996) Active management of labour. *British Medical Journal* 313(7054): 378.

United Kingdom Central Council for Nursing, Midwifery and Health Visiting (UKCC) (1996) *Standards for Records and Record Keeping.* London: UKCC. Now replaced by the NMC (2002) reprint *Guidelines for Records And Record Keeping.* London: NMC.

United Kingdom Central Council for Nursing, Midwifery and Health Visiting (UKCC) (1998) *Midwives Rules and Code of Practice.* London: UKCC.

Waldenstrom, U. & Turnbull, D. (1998) A systematic review comparing continuity of midwifery care with standard maternity services. *British Journal of Obstetrics and Gynaecology* 105: 1160–1170.

Walmsley, K. (1999) Caring for women during the latent phase of labour. *Practising Midwife* 2(2): 12–13.

Walsh, D. (1989) Comparison of management and outcome of labour under two systems of care. *Midwives Chronicle* 102(1211): 270–273.

Walsh, D. (1998) Electronic fetal heart monitoring: revisited and reappraised. *British Journal of Midwifery* 6(6): 400–404.

Walsh, D. (1999) An ethnographic study of women's experience of partnership caseload midwifery practice: the professional as friend. *Midwifery* 15(3): 165–176.

Warren, C. (1999) Invaders of privacy. *Midwifery Matters* 81: 8–9.

Warwick, C. (1997) Open dialogue. Can continuity of care be the only answer? *British Journal of Midwifery* 5(1): 6.

World Health Organization (1994) World Health Organization partograph in management of labour. *Lancet* 343(8910): 1399–1404.

FURTHER READING

Davis, E. (1997) *Heart and Hands: A Midwife's Guide to Pregnancy and Birth.* Berkeley: Celestial Arts.
Well-illustrated combination of text and women's guide, includes the emotions and lived experience of childbirth.

Lavender, T., Alfirevic, Z. & Walkinshaw, S. (1998) Partogram action line study: a randomised trial. *British Journal of Obstetrics and Gynaecology* 105(9): 976–980.

National Institute of Child Health and Human Development Research (1997) Electronic fetal heart monitoring: research guidelines for interpretation. *American Journal of Obstetrics and Gynecology* 177(6): 1385–1390.

Robertson, A. (1997) *The Midwife Companion.* Sydney: ACE Graphics.
Practical tips for assisting birthing without medical interventions from an internationally known childbirth educator committed to an active birth philosophy.

Walsh, D., Harris, M. & Shuttlewood, S. (1999) Changing midwifery birthing practice through audit. *British Journal of Midwifery* 7(7): 432–435.

ADDITIONAL RESOURCE

http://www.fons.org/networks/ebm/guidesm.pdf
Evidence-based midwifery guidelines for midwifery-led care in normal labour produced by the Evidence Based Midwifery Network. Useful resource for different aspects of care.

27

Relief of Pain During Labour

Helen Bryant and Margaret Yerby

LEARNING OUTCOMES

After reading this chapter you will:

- understand the physiological aspect of pain processes in labour and its effect on the woman, and how this knowledge can be used in planning management of pain and discomfort
- appreciate the impact of psychological interactions on the pain process in labour and how this impacts on the woman's perception of pain

- be aware of the effect of culture and environment on the birth process
- understand the nature of support and its relationship to women's coping mechanisms
- be familiar with the range of contemporary approaches available to the woman for the control and management of pain during labour.

INTRODUCTION

The 9 months of pregnancy culminate in birth, an experience that many women fear because the process of birth is painful. Pain is generally a warning to the individual to protect an injury or slow down in order to be aware of some mishap in the body and seek help to diagnose the ailment. When labour commences it enables the woman to prepare for the coming events, to travel or move to her chosen place for giving birth. Today this is generally the hospital unit. Often women are worried about being able to reach the hospital in time, about getting in contact with their partner, and organizing childcare, and this can often create anxiety which is hard to adequately dispel. The hospital may also create anxiety, as the woman has to adapt to a sometimes alien environment, and this may distract her from identifying and adopting her own coping mechanisms during labour. Some of the strategies would assist the woman's own physiology, and are often used by women in the more homely surroundings of the home or birth centre. Women birthing in hospitals may therefore be more likely to opt for pharmacological preparations such as Entonox, pethidine, or local anaesthetic delivered via an epidural catheter.

Reflective Activity 27.1

Compare your experiences of caring for women during labour in different environments. Would you agree that more women rely more on pharmacological methods of pain relief in society today than in the past? Is this actually true and evidence based?

DEFINITION OF PAIN

Pain is a sensation distinct from touch, warmth, or cold; it may change the person's behaviour and is associated with tissue changes (Keele *et al.*, 1983). Pain is a complex, personal, subjective, multifactorial phenomenon, which is influenced by psychological, physiological and sociocultural factors, and, although pain is universally experienced and acknowledged, it is not completely understood (Lowe, 1991; Walding, 1991). Women in labour will react in different ways, and will feel pain differently, according to their emotional status, as stress and anxiety potentiate pain mechanisms. Walding (1991) confirmed the relationship between pain, anxiety and powerlessness and agreed that active participation by the woman may reduce the perception of pain. In particular, the anticipation of pain increases anxiety levels and hence the pain experienced (Melzack and Wall, 1996). This linked with earlier work into the cycle of fear and tension and its impact on the perception and experience of pain (Dick-Read, 1944).

PSYCHOLOGY OF PAIN

Whereas it might be easier for health professionals to acknowledge physical pain, midwives and other health professionals need to appreciate that pain also has a psychological component, although this may not be so easy to quantify. Atkinson *et al.* (1990) state that pain is as much a matter of the mind as of sensory reception. The perception of pain will vary among women even when the pain stimuli are similar.

The psychological perception of pain remains poorly understood (Sherr, 1995), and consideration should be given to the many intervening variables such as previous experience, personal emotional feelings and expectations of the childbirth experience. Raphael-Leff (1993) supports this view stating that responses to pain are influenced by cultural norms and expectations and that the perceived pain of any individual will depend on how it is personally constructed by them. The experience of pain may also be determined by concurrent emotional factors such as anxiety, uncertainty, fatigue, depression and panic, as well as personality, inappropriate behaviours and incorrect cognitive processes (Raphael-Leff, 1993; Symonds, 1998).

Women's expectations and understanding of pain are intertwined with their view of the quality, as well as the degree, of pain and how it can, or should, be relieved (Green *et al.*, 1998). In this study, pain was viewed positively by these women as something they had chosen to experience, knowing that their labour was progressing with the build-up of regular contractions and ultimately looking forward to the birth of their baby.

One of the first theories to encapsulate the idea that pain had a psychological perspective originated from Melzack and Wall (1965) when they discussed their gate control theory, referred to later in this chapter. No alternative model has as yet been proposed to rival the gate theory; it remains unchallenged, with little analysis or assessment in the available literature (Yerby, 2000).

ANTENATAL EDUCATION/PREPARATION FOR CHILDBIRTH

The need for antenatal education and preparation for childbirth was initially highlighted by Grantly Dick-Read

in 1944. Through observation and perseverance he recognized that the anxiety state of women in childbirth could have a detrimental effect on the outcome of their birth experience and he suggested that possible benefits could be gained by preparing women for childbirth. He proposed that if women were better prepared, then they would feel less anxious and therefore less fearful about the event. He was one of the first in the field of medicine to begin to question the practice of administering strong analgesia to labouring women. Through his observation he considered fear to be one of the underlying factors influencing the severity of the pain perceived by women. He believed that childbirth was inherently painless if a women's culturally conditioned fear of giving birth could be controlled through techniques of breathing and relaxation. His aim was to encourage women to communicate with their care-givers and he proposed that pain might be controlled by using psychophrophylaxis. Psychophrophylaxis was seen as a means of regaining control of childbirth by women (Nolan, 2000). This promotes a belief that information imparted through the communication of women and their care-givers can help to reduce anxiety and fear.

The learning of relaxation and relaxation techniques has been included in parentcraft classes, in the belief that it may obviate use of pain-relieving drugs. Earlier research proposed that knowledge imparted in these classes led to less anxious, more self-reliant and confident mothers when compared to non-attendees at classes (Quereshi *et al.*, 1996). This investigation also identified that although significantly more non-attendees were admitted to hospital during their pregnancy there was no significant difference in the use or type of analgesia used. They also reported that 94% of attendees had found attending preparation for childbirth classes useful (Quereshi *et al.*, 1996).

Reflective Activity 27.2

Consider your own experience of childbirth. This might be the birth of your own children or of assisting friends or family members through the process. Do you believe childbirth is a life crisis or a natural physiological and psychological process? How do you think this view influences the way you function as a midwife?

According to Moore (1997), childbirth can either be seen as a time of increased anxiety, 'a period of crisis involving profound psychological changes' and of major life transition, or a natural occurrence in procreation of the human species in which 'pregnancy, childbirth and motherhood are an intrinsic part of a woman's experience.'

Negative feelings surrounding the perception of pain are often associated with anxiety during pregnancy. Reading and Cox (1985) found anxiety occurring after 32 weeks of gestation was a predicator of a more painful labour. Subsequently they found that labour was a predictor of postnatal mood changes and that severe pain experienced in labour could inhibit maternal emotions. This suggests that events during the childbearing process could have a detrimental effect on parent–infant attachment (Bowlby, 1969; Condon, 1993; Robson and Kumar, 1980).

The focus on pain relief during labour needs to move from pain medication to providing strategies to assist woman to maximize their own resources for coping with pain (Nolan, 2000). Rather than discussing psychological approaches or education regarding the physiology of pain, as suggested by Robertson (2000), Nolan's study found that women discussed their choices regarding methods of pain relief and their views apparently remained the same before and after antenatal classes. Nolan suggested that this might indicate that women may be unable to make choices because they are ignorant of their own body's resources for coping with pain, such as the existence of endorphins, and how these can enable the mechanics of labour to work more efficiently. Although all subjects in this study were keener to try non-invasive methods, this was not often reflected in the choices they made when admitted to the labour ward. This highlights the need for childbirth educators to present a realistic picture of labour. In order to make informed choices, women need to be educated regarding the physiology of pain and how they can harness their own internal resources, and be given practical tips on how to achieve comfort during labour (Robertson, 2000). The role of endorphins should be explained during the discussion about pain, and the teacher should be positive, presenting pain as protective and diagnostic in labour. Participants should have the time to explore their fears and base new perspectives on more positive views.

Melzack *et al.* (1981) demonstrated that prepared childbirth training designed to reduce fear, anxiety and tension, did decrease the pain women felt in labour. Women who received parent education were less likely to require pain relief in labour, though this was dependent on the personality and enthusiasm of the instructor. This was disputed by a later study which showed no evidence to support that attendance at parent education classes was linked to an actual reduction in pain; however, there was some evidence suggesting that attendance was associated with a reduction in the use of pain medication (Simkin, 1995). Studies by Hillan (1992) and Simkin (1995) do reflect the statement made by Melzack *et al.* (1981) in that it was the quality, rather than the provision, of parent education classes that impacted on the experience of pain and amount of pain relief required.

In preparing for labour, women should practice coping strategies, for example relaxation techniques, which could increase their confidence and reduce the amount of pain relief required. The provision of a culture of good education and support enabling women to foster a more positive approach to labour may be superior to the encouragement of the use of pain relief with its many side-effects (Crafter, 2000).

Reflective Activity 27.3

Observe an antenatal/parent education class, and consider the following:

- How was pain relief approached and discussed by the facilitator of the class?
- Do you feel that this antenatal education regarding the relief of pain in labour prepared women and their partners psychologically for the reality of childbirth?
- How would you plan and deliver an appropriate session?

PAIN: PHYSIOLOGICAL EFFECTS ON THE BODY

Pain causes an increase in catecholamine secretion, thus increasing levels of adrenaline. The result is an increase in cardiac output, heart rate, and blood pressure, giving rise to hyperventilation, which decreases cerebral and uterine blood flow by vasoconstriction (Bonica, 1994). Nausea and vomiting may occur and uterine activity may be disrupted (Heywood and Ho, 1990; Reynolds, 1998). This may alter the acid–base balance of the blood, giving rise to maternal alkalosis, which may in turn cause fetal hypoxia (see Fig. 27.1).

TOWARDS AN EXPLANATION OF PAIN

The origins of labour pain are centred on the tremendous physiological changes which take place during labour.

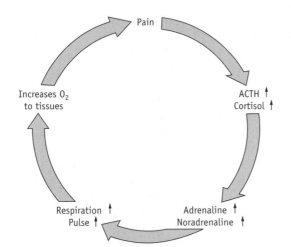

Figure 27.1 Homeostasis in labour. (Reprinted from *Pain in Childbearing*, Yerby, M. (ed) 2000 by permission of the publisher Baillière Tindall.)

During pregnancy women experience Braxton Hicks contractions or 'practice contractions', during which the uterus contracts. These can be as strong as labour contractions but are usually only felt as tightenings rather than pain (Gibb, 1993). Effacement and dilatation cause the stripping of membranes away from the cervix and often cause the 'show' of early labour (Bonica, 1994). This causes prostaglandin release, which then aids cervical softening and uterine contractility. Prostaglandins are made in the fetal membranes and maternal decidua (Gibb, 1998; Fuentes *et al.*, 1996), particularly in spontaneous labour. The research by Fuentes and colleagues (1996) examined amnions of labouring and non-labouring women and found that the amnions of labouring women had a twofold increase in cyclo-oxygenase, the precursor enzyme, which converts arachidonic acid into prostaglandins (Box 27.1). Bonica (1994) cites research by Moir (1939) and Javert and Hardy (1950) that links the pain of labour directly to the stretching of the cervix and lower uterine segment.

The action of prostaglandins in labour is to increase the contractility of the myometrium, playing an important role in the initiation of labour (Vander *et al.*, 2000). In practical terms this can be seen in labour when a vaginal examination is performed. Manipulation of the cervix to ascertain effacement and dilatation causes the membranes to be loosened or stripped from the cervix and also directly stimulates the production of prostaglandins (Keele *et al.*, 1983). An antenatal 'stretch and sweep' will act in the same way, and in this situation may well induce labour to commence in a natural way. Nerve endings are stimulated and a form of inflammatory

Box 27.1 Prostaglandins (PG) – eicosonoids

- Substances often termed tissue hormones found in all tissues of the body
- Usually metabolized locally
- Capable of being synthesized rapidly
- Precursors: linoleic and arachidonic acids
- Large family: PGA, PGE, PGF mostly – PGF is specific to the reproductive system
- Play a key function during pregnancy and labour
- Aspirin inhibits their production

response is produced in the tissues, creating pain signals. This response produces substances – histamine, serotonin and bradykinins – that stimulate the nociceptors in the cervix, setting up pain sequences. This stimulates an action potential in the nerve, setting up a chain reaction to the spinal cord and the higher centres in the brain (Bullock, 1992; Tortora and Grabowski, 2000; Yerby, 2000). The nervous system has a network of nerve fibres carrying electrical impulses throughout the body in order to transfer information, rather like the wiring circuit in a house (Bloom and Lazerson, 1988).

Uterine nerve supply

The autonomic nervous system serves the uterus with sympathetic and parasympathetic nerve fibres. The nerves which supply the uterus are ill-defined, but nerve pathways are known (Williams *et al.*, 1989). Nerve pathways supplying the uterus and cervix arise from afferent fibres of the sympathetic ganglia. Nociceptive (i.e. pain receptive) nerve endings in the uterus and cervix pass through the cervical and uterine plexuses to the pelvic plexus, the middle hypogastric plexus the superior hypogastric plexus and then to the lumbar sympathetic nerves to eventually join the thoracic 10, 11, 12 and lumbar 1 spinal nerves (Fig. 27.2). Signals are then received at the dorsal horn of the spinal column (Bonica, 1994) and then via the spinothalamic tract to the higher centres of the brain to become a conscious pain sensation. The nerve supply to the perineum and lower pelvis from the second and third sacral nerve roots meets the plexuses from the uterus at the Lee–Frankenhäuser plexus at the uterovaginal junction (Stjernquist and Sjöberg, 1994).

Nerve transmission

Nerve transmission is along fibres that conduct sensations in different strengths and at different speeds.

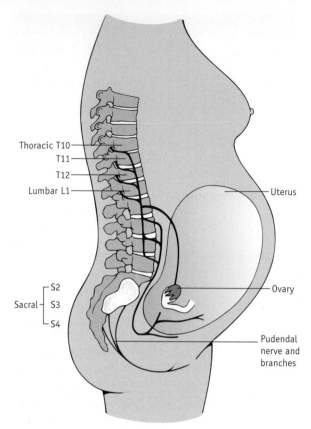

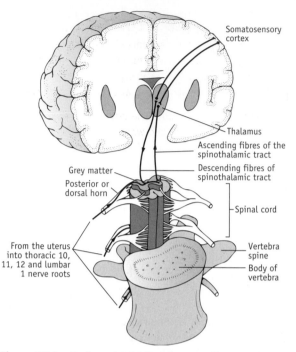

Figure 27.3 Brain and spinal cord connections. (Reprinted from *Pain in Childbearing*, Yerby, M. (ed) 2000 by permission of the publisher Baillière Tindall.)

Figure 27.2 Pain pathways. (Reprinted from *Pain in Childbearing*, Yerby, M. (ed) 2000 by permission of the publisher Baillière Tindall.)

These fibres are either *A delta*, thinly myelinated fibres, or C fibres, which are unmyelinated. It is the smaller C fibres which are found in the deep viscera such as the uterus that give rise to the deep prolonged pain of labour when stimulated by muscular contraction and chemical substances (Whipple, 1990). Pain sensation is transferred by action potentials along the nerve fibres to the dorsal horn of the spinal cord and thence via upward tracts to the central nervous system (Fig. 27.3). As a result of the release of bradykinins and histamines and other pain-inducing substances at tissue level, 'substance P' is also released. This is a neuropeptide and is released from the afferent nerves (Vander *et al.*, 2000) as part of the 'signalling process' of pain on its way to the dorsal horn of the spinal cord; it could be termed a potentiator of pain sensation. As the action potentials from the afferent neurones meet the spinal cord they enter by the posterior (dorsal) root and are transferred to the substantia gelatinosa at laminae (or layers) II and III of the grey matter of the spinal cord. These laminae decode various types of stimulus and

transfer sensations to the higher centres of the brain via the anterior and lateral spinothalamic tracts, which cross to the opposite side of the cord before ascending (Barasi, 1991; Whipple, 1990). Descending tracts from the brain, returning to the spinal cord, may have a modulating effect on the nerve transmission of pain (Fig. 27.3). Naturally occurring endorphins at the spinal level act like exogenous opioids by modulating pain response (Barasi, 1991; Hung, 1987).

Pain gate theory

Melzack and Wall provided greater understanding of the ability of the body to control pain mechanisms by their proposition that at spinal cord level there is a mechanism for modulating pain. The 'gate control theory' was based on experiments in animals using electrical impulses and testing their reaction to painful stimuli under certain conditions. Opioid-like substances, namely endorphins and enkephalins, were found to occur naturally within the body. These substances are neurotransmitters and neuromodulators, and are found principally in the sensory pathways where pain is relayed (Melzack and Wall, 1965). As highly effective pain-modulating substances they also play a role in pleasure, learning and memory (Tortora and Grabowski, 2000).

Reflective Activity 27.4

Next time you care for a woman in labour who is coping without pain relief, observe her reactions both during labour, and after delivery. Often women will exhibit a 'spaced-out' feeling or look on their faces.

Alternatively, think about the last time you yourself experienced bad pain, and what you experienced physiologically when the pain disappeared.

The gate theory suggested a mechanism which prevents the transfer of nerve stimuli to the higher centres of the brain where they are perceived and become a conscious feeling of pain. At the dorsal horn root in the substantia gelatinosa area of the spinal cord it was proposed that substances could be blocked by a 'gating' mechanism. When the 'gate' is open, pain sensations reach the higher centres. When the 'gate' is closed, pain is blocked and does not become part of the conscious thought, and therefore pain is less. With greater understanding of endorphins and their opiate-type properties it was noted that they dampened the effect of substance P. These nerves can be excitatory and modulatory and by the competition of these actions, pain can be inhibited. The descending pathways from the brain are also said to be inhibitory in action and modulate pain sensations (Jacques, 1994).

The opportunity for women to develop coping mechanisms for dealing with labour may be limited, and this may be exacerbated by the approach taken during antenatal clinic visits and in parenting sessions, where time and attention is often focused on epidurals, pethidine and/or Entonox. It may also be difficult for women to develop a trusting relationship with the midwife when many systems of care are fragmented, and where they may meet several different practitioners during pregnancy, childbirth and the puerperium. Even if continuity is provided by a parenting education midwife, they may not see this midwife at any other time, i.e. during the birth or postnatal period. If a partnership *is* developed between the midwife and client antenatally, the woman will feel more positive about herself and her own ability to travel through labour in a positive manner (Page *et al.*, 2000). Hughes (1999) suggests that midwives may assist women to cope in natural ways by being relaxed themselves, fostering a quiet and calm atmosphere, and making the woman the centre of attention. This is more easily achieved in the home setting, but as many births take place in hospital, greater effort may be required from the midwife

to achieve the same effect. Nevertheless the principle still applies; each woman needs to feel supported and cared for. If the labour continues over a length of time and the woman increasingly begins to require pharmacological pain relief, then the midwife needs to support her in her decisions.

CULTURAL ASPECTS OF PAIN

In responding to the individual needs of women, midwives should acknowledge that the definition, understanding and manifestation of pain will be influenced by cultural experiences. Hayes (1997) suggests that there is private and public pain, in that reactions to pain are not simply involuntary or instinctive, but take place within a social context and therefore could be considered to have a voluntary component.

The amount and quality of the pain felt by the individual is determined by previous experiences and how well these are remembered, and by the ability to understand the cause of the pain and grasp its consequences. Culture plays an important role in how pain is felt and responded to by the individual (Melzack and Wall, 1996; Moore, 1997). Culture also mediates the inference of that pain by care-givers, who will have their own definitions and understandings of pain, which in turn reflects upon their support to the woman in coping with the pain during labour. It is also crucial that the midwife is aware of how interpersonal impact may have a powerful influence on the expression and meaning of pain for that woman (Weber, 1996).

In labour and birth, part of the culture is expressed through the environment and the organization within that environment (Crafter, 2000). The Peel Report (DHSS, 1970) changed the place of birth for women, who had traditionally had their babies at home. Hospitalization altered the women's view of birth, and led to more medicalized birth with greater use of drugs for pain relief, which many women accepted as a normal part of the new environment.

The high rate of hospital birth has other effects. Crafter (2000) suggested that furnishings within the room may give women subliminal messages about how the presiding culture, i.e. birth at home or in hospital, expects them to behave within that environment. Crafter also postulated that the place of birth might have a significant impact on the experience of pain. There are some studies which suggest that women who give birth at home use less pharmacological pain relief, though these studies *do not* tend to state that women suffer less pain, but rather that perhaps the supportive environment usually found in a home birth makes the pain more manageable.

Reflective Activity 27.5

Observe the environment within your hospital, trying to see how it might appear to the woman. What subliminal message do you think that the furniture and setting provides?

Think about how this might affect cultural needs and expectations of birth.

Culture is known to affect the perception of pain for both the woman and the midwife. It is for this reason that midwives need to develop an understanding of how culture affects perceived pain. Weber (1996) considered that the pain threshold might differ because of culturally learned pain responses.

Rajan (1993) focused on the differing perceptions of individual women's experience of pain and pain relief amongst women and the professionals who attended them in labour. Attempts to draw meaningful conclusions about the cognisance of pain perception proved difficult, with discrepancies highlighted about perceived effectiveness of pain relief between the women and the midwife who cared for her.

In understanding the role culture plays in perceptions and experience of pain, the midwife needs to be aware of the many cultural assumptions that are made, which like any assumptions may prevent individualized and appropriate care.

THE USE OF WATER AS PAIN RELIEF

It is well known that a warm bath is useful for relaxation, and is a simple means of reducing muscular aches and pains. Some evidence and anecdotal reports suggest that water may help to relieve some of the pain in labour, improve the woman's mobility, increase the level of relaxation and reduce the use of augmentation and pharmacological agents (Active Birth Centre, 2002), though more research is needed (Nikodem, 2002). The perinatal outcomes of actual water birth are similar to those from low-risk deliveries (Gilbert and Tookey, 1999). In recent years, hospital units have improved their services, and many now provide water pools for use during labour and delivery. Evidence suggests that more women use water as a means of pain relief or

relaxation than for actual delivery, though this may be affected by unit policies (RCM, 2000).

Ideally, the woman should have access to a designated 'birth pool' rather than a bath (though this may be the only available hydrotherapy unit), as this will usually cover issues of safety and permit a deeper level of water, allowing the woman to submerge her body above the level of the fundus. The temperature should be maintained at 36–38°C, to ensure that the woman does not become hyperthermic, as this may have adverse effects on the fetus.

Women often become very drowsy whilst in the water, and the midwife should ensure a woman's safety, particularly should she require additional analgesia, i.e. Entonox, when she should not be left unattended in the water pool.

SELF-HYPNOSIS

This builds upon the original work around psychoprophylaxis and may be useful for some women. To use it successfully, it is useful to have discussed it antenatally, and be familiar with the purpose and support of the method. This can include Lamaze preparation (Lamaze International, 2001) and 'hypno-birthing' (Hypno-birth, 2002), and therefore can vary from simple patterns of practised breathing to visualization, in which the woman focuses on an object and develops a process of self-hypnosis.

Self-hypnosis develops the individual's skills in maintaining awareness of physiological processes, whilst increasing the level of control and reducing the pain experienced (Oster, 1994). Some practitioners believe that it can be developed to a degree that individuals can influence their physiology to control bleeding, aid healing and later develop lactation (Lifeforce, 2002), and these skills, like relaxation, can be used in other parts of life (Oster, 1994).

Midwives will often use elements of hypnosis in working with the woman prior to labour in preparing for the birth, and during labour, talking her through breathing techniques and ensuring the woman is as calm as possible. Using any formal hypnosis technique requires commitment and preparation and should be seen as a holistic method focusing on the woman in context.

POSITIONS AND MASSAGE

An important part of dealing with pain is the ability to find a comfortable position, according to the person's individual needs. For some women this may mean using the bed, and for others using upright positions and aids such as birthing balls, birthing chairs, rocking chairs and the physical support of their birth partner. Though upright positions may increase the intensity of contractions, the feeling of control, and the ability to use strategies such as pelvic rocking, may add considerably to the woman's feeling of well-being, and thus the degree to which she can cope with the pain (MacLennan *et al.*, 1994). The use of massage may also be helpful for some women. This may vary from firm back massage, to stroking of the woman's abdomen or feet, and it is important to establish with the woman what is helpful. Massage may be used during or between the actual contractions.

Using a variety of different positions and movements may also provide a useful element of distraction and activity (see Ch. 26).

Reflective Activity 27.6

When you are next caring for a woman during labour, consider suggesting that she try different positions to cope with contractions. Which positions are the most effective? After the delivery, discuss the woman's opinion of what difference this made to her perception of pain.

TRANSCUTANEOUS ELECTRICAL NERVE STIMULATION (TENS)

Transcutaneous electrical nerve stimulation (TENS) has assisted many women seeking a natural alternative to enable them to cope with the pain of labour. Some women may complete labour successfully with TENS exclusively, whilst others may choose to supplement it with other methods of relief such as Entonox and pethidine, and if their labour is long and protracted, an epidural (Chamberlain *et al.*, 1993).

TENS is the application of pulsed electrical current through surface electrodes placed on the skin parallel to and on each side of the spine (Fig. 27.4). The first pair reaches from the 10th thoracic to the 1st lumbar vertebra and treats the pain associated with the first stage of labour, and the second pair extends from the 2nd to the 4th sacral vertebra and treats the pain of the second stage.

TENS is thought to assist in the prevention of the perception of pain sensations based upon the gate control theory. Small electrical sensations at the site of the surface electrodes stimulate the large peripheral nerve fibres and close the gate to pain, blocking pain sensations from reaching the higher brain centres. It is said to stimulate release of the naturally occurring endorphins (Simkin, 1989), which are produced at the spinal cord level.

The advantages of TENS are that it is a non-invasive form of pain relief, which can be used effectively whether the mother is mobile or in bed, and there is no effect on the fetus or the woman systemically. The woman is also in control of the apparatus. Used early in labour when contractions first commence, it enables the endorphins to build up naturally as labour progresses and becomes more effective (Price, 2000). It takes about 40 minutes for the maximum endorphin level to be reached (Salar *et al.*, 1981).

Placed in the correct position, the electrodes supply a residual voltage, which can be boosted by the woman during a contraction. This provides the woman with

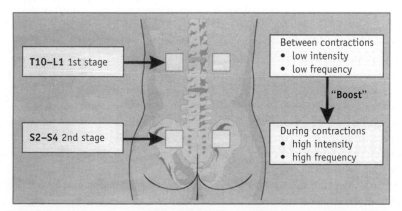

Figure 27.4 TENS electrode positioning for use during labour. (From Johnson 1997, with permission of Mark Allen Publishing Ltd.)

autonomy and helps her achieve greater emotional fulfilment from the experience of childbirth (Cluett, 1994).

Research into the use of TENS is scanty, and it may not be a method appropriate for a long difficult labour. Women using TENS often resort to the use of more powerful analgesia as labour progresses (Reynolds, 1993b). In the National Survey conducted by the National Birthday Trust only 5.5% of women reported using TENS (Chamberlain *et al.*, 1993). This survey suggested that whatever the pain relief chosen most women will describe their labour as exceedingly painful.

Some hospital physiotherapy units hire out TENS machines and most women would be encouraged at around 37 weeks to commence their hire period so that they can get used to it. This is also a good opportunity for partners to learn their role in placing the electrodes in the correct positions on their partner's back. Machines may also be bought from chemist outlets, and generally are accompanied by a video, are self-explanatory and very easy to use.

In 1991 the UKCC approved that midwives may on their own responsibility manage pain relief in labour by the use of TENS provided that:

- they have received adequate and appropriate instruction, which is a matter to be determined by agreed local policy
- safety standards conform to those laid down by the Department of Health Medical Devices Directorate in England, or equivalent body in Scotland, Wales or Northern Ireland.

CONCEPT OF SUPPORT IN LABOUR

It is important that women are supported and feel 'cared for' during labour, and if this is provided, it may result in a shorter duration of labour, more positive experience of childbirth, and a positive attitude towards motherhood. Social support has an important role to play in the process of adapting to stressful life events of which childbirth is one. Tarkka and Paunonen (1996) define social support as an intentional human interaction involving one or more of the following elements: appreciation, love or respect, and sense of security. They suggested that midwives provide most support in the domain of affect. During labour the main source of emotional support or affect for the mothers was the midwife, who helped to provide a sense of security. Findings suggest that this may be responsible for a positive and less painful birth experience. Mothers attached

much importance to the presence of the midwife, to the encouragement the midwife offered them. The support of significant others was also considered important but less so than the presence of a professional.

Kaufman (1993) asserts that midwives should seek to increase a woman's knowledge and sense of control through a relationship built on trust and confidence. Labour is experienced through a continuum of care where information and choices have been discussed and where the capabilities of each person are known to each other. The relationship between the midwife and the mother should provide a context for the use and development of high-level clinical skills, including the ability to make clinical decisions, to comfort and to alleviate pain and distress, to counsel, to advise and teach (Page, 1993).

In a phenomenological study of women's experiences of birth, researchers were able to conclude that women's expectations could influence their perceptions of the birth experience. Women identified a need for a sense of control and when this was achieved women felt strong and unafraid. Their perception of the journey through labour focused mainly on their perceptions of pain and hard work (Halldorsdottir and Karlsdottir, 1996). A later qualitative phenomenological study by Lundgren and Dahlberg (1998) studied nine women between the ages of 23–31 who had spontaneous vaginal births. Four were primiparous and five multiparous and all used varied methods of pain relief in labour.

Themes which emerged were:

- pain is hard to describe and is contradictory
- trust in oneself and one's body
- trust in the midwife and husband.

Hutton (1994) suggests that by providing explanation, encouragement and progress reports throughout labour, the midwife can demonstrate a commitment to attending to the woman's needs, and also that consulting with the woman throughout the labour will ensure that she feels that her wishes are being acknowledged. Hutton demonstrated that if a woman was being supported by a midwife known to her, she required less pain relief because of the trust that had developed.

Hodnett (1997) reported that all indicators of maternal satisfaction favoured continuity of care and caregiver and that continuity of care by the midwife was associated with the increased likelihood of a woman labouring and giving birth without using any analgesia. This suggested that the attendance of a familiar caregiver provided more support or was viewed as more supportive of women in labour, ultimately resulting in the decreased need for pharmacological pain relief.

In a further systematic review Hodnett (2000) looked at care-giver support for women during childbirth, assessing the effects of continuous support during labour, provided by both health professionals and lay people. The results of 14 trials involving 5000 women suggested that the continuous support of a care-giver reduced the likelihood of medication for pain relief as well as facilitating a number of other beneficial outcomes of the birth. This supported evidence in previous research by Hodnett, reported in Fridh *et al.* (1990).

Other evidence suggests that the support does not have to be provided by a health professional. Currently there is a resurgence of female birth companions, who may be female family members, friends or trained supporters such as doulas (Anderson 1996). The continuous presence of a trained support person with no previous social bond with the woman may reduce the requirement for pain relief. This suggested that the provision of such emotional support and physical comfort may enable a woman to cope better with labour pain by reducing fear and anxiety (Hutton, 1994).

Women's overall perception of 'helpfulness' may be influential in the reporting of modulation of pain. Women accompanied by their husbands often judge their presence to be helpful. A helpful husband was one whose presence was comforting – someone familiar, someone to hold on to (Niven, 1994). However it should not be assumed that all men desire to be present at the birth. There is evidence to suggest that being present at the birth can have adverse effects on the relationship (O'Driscoll, 1994).

Reflective Activity 27.7

When you are next on the labour ward, take an opportunity to observe the level of support a woman receives during labour and from whom.

What effect do you observe on the process of labour, and on the outcome?

Was the quality and quantity of support the same as you would observe in a home setting, or birth centre? If not, what were the key factors influencing this?

The current framework for midwifery practice encompasses a belief that all women should be the recipients of individualized care, with midwives acknowledging a woman's physical, social, educational, spiritual and psychological needs (Moore, 1997). Furthering knowledge of some of the psychological factors associated with pain and pain relief in labour could, according to Moore (1997), potentially increase understanding and appreciation of the unique birth experience for each woman. In understanding these events it is clear that not all women can cope without some form of systemic pain relief and midwives need to advise them as to which path to take when pain becomes unbearable.

PHARMACOLOGICAL PAIN RELIEF

A midwife must keep up to date with current medications and their side-effects and be able to give sound advice to women in labour. The unit policies should be adhered to at all times (NMC, 2002; UKCC, 1998). An understanding of pharmacokinetics, and the changing drug absorption, metabolism, distribution and excretion in both the woman's body and that of her fetus and baby, is important in providing information and advice to the woman regarding choices of pain relief (see Ch. 71).

Nitrous oxide

The use of inhalation analgesia for pain relief in childbirth originated from the work of Simpson of Edinburgh in 1847, who introduced chloroform for anaesthetic purposes (Ostheimer, 1992). In 1853 Queen Victoria used chloroform during the birth of her seventh child, Prince Leopold, and was greatly pleased with the relief it gave. However, anaesthesia not only relieves pain but also produces loss of consciousness with its associated risks (Ostheimer, 1992).

Nitrous oxide is sometimes known as 'laughing gas' and can be used in labour in a mixture of 50% nitrous oxide and 50% oxygen (Entonox: produced by BOC UK). It can be supplied in small portable cylinders (Fig. 27.5) or piped directly to the delivery suite, which is common in most units today. If the temperature of the gas in cylinders falls below −8°C the gases separate, leaving nitrous oxide at the bottom of the cylinder. This may be easily remedied by inverting the cylinder before use.

Entonox has a sedative effect in use but is not an analgesic. It is self-administered by the use of a mouthpiece or mask and will only cause unconsciousness if the woman is hypoxic or the partner is assisting in holding the apparatus, and continuous aspiration occurs. Although the effect of Entonox is limited, many women like the control it provides. The effects are quite rapid, commencing 20 seconds after administration

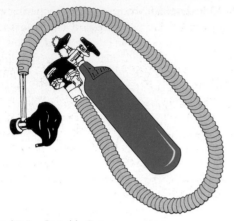

Figure 27.5   Portable Entonox apparatus.

with a maximum effect at 60 seconds. It is essential that the breathing technique is correct: short panting breaths are not effective, whereas deep breathing at the normal rate is effective. To obtain effective relief from pain, inhalation should begin before the contraction begins, then at the height of contraction when it is most painful the Entonox has had time to produce an effect. A fit healthy person will get beneficial absorption and excretion with few side-effects; however, there is complete absorption through the placenta (Carson, 1996). The amount absorbed by the mother rapidly gains equilibrium in the fetus but, equally so, it is rapidly cleared from the fetal system when the mother stops inhalation. Entonox has no effect on uterine contractility (Jayaram, 1997). Modified respiratory effort in the mother may decrease uteroplacental perfusion to the fetus by constriction of the placental vessels; this may occur when she commences self-administration because of a poor technique and altered breathing patterns (Gamsu, 1993). It may cause hallucinations in some women.

In the NBT survey (Chamberlain *et al.*, 1993) Entonox was available in 99% of the units included in the study. 60% of women had used Entonox and it was the most frequently used form of analgesia, except where the epidural rate was higher than 50%. The majority of the women who used it rated it as 'useful' or 'highly useful'.

Systemic analgesia

Pethidine

Analgesia is defined as reduced sensibility of pain, without loss of consciousness and sense of touch being necessarily affected (Dickersin, 1989). The objective of using analgesic drugs in labour is to achieve an acceptable level of pain relief without compromising the health of mother or fetus. There should be minimal effect on physiological processes, such as uterine activity, and minimal side-effects.

Opioid analgesics include the morphine-like substances derived from the opium poppy (*Papaver somniferum*) which induce 'euphoria, analgesia and sleep' (Rang *et al.*, 1995). These have been widely used in midwifery for women in labour since the 1950s (Bradford and Chamberlain, 1995), mainly because they are readily available and easy to administer by intramuscular injection. They may be given by a midwife under Standing Orders (now replaced by Patient Group Directives in some units) in the delivery suite without the requirement for a prescription from a medical practitioner (Reynolds, 1993a). The derivative most commonly used in the 1990s was pethidine (meperidine in America), and it is still used today by midwives, although less often as the epidural rate rises.

Pethidine is a synthetic substance, shorter acting than morphine with the effect of producing euphoria and sometimes dysphoria. Its effect is rapid and lasts for approximately 3–4 hours. It may be given intramuscularly or as an intravenous injection or in an infusion, which may be self-administered. In practice, this is rarely done and more often it is administered as a bolus intramuscular injection. The dose ranges from 50–200 mg and is dependent on the route of administration, the woman's weight, degree of pain, stage of labour and the rate of progress. The side-effects may be nausea, loss of self-control, reduction in blood pressure and sweating. Its pain-relieving properties in labour are disputed by many women who do not like the side-effects it produces. In the NBT survey 1990 (Chamberlain *et al.*, 1993), as the labour length increased so the use of pethidine decreased and women turned to other methods of pain relief such as epidural. Olofsson *et al.* (1996) compared the pain-relieving properties of morphine and pethidine in a double-blind randomized trial of 20 multiparous women – 10 in each group. The women had high pain scores and were well sedated but woke to uterine contractions. The researcher's conclusions were that they felt it unethical to use pethidine or morphine as a pain-relieving agent, as it was only useful for its sedative effect.

Physiological action on the mother   Pethidine binds to receptor proteins to diffuse through cell membranes to exert its effect within the central nervous system. Its action at the cellular level alters potassium and calcium channels, affecting ion exchange in the neuronal membrane and calming the excitability of the nerve as it reacts to the pain-producing substances. It acts on efferent nerve pathways descending from the brain at the dorsal horn, thus playing a role in the 'gating' of pain at the spinal column level (Rang et al 1995, Scrutton 1997). It is metabolized by the liver to *norpethidine* (normeperidine in America) by a process termed *n*-demethylation, which produces a substance that has half the potency of the original and has a stimulant, convulsive effect (Jayaram, 1997).

Physiological effects on the fetus Diffusion across the placenta occurs readily, and equilibrium between maternal and fetal levels is easily achieved. This depends on the lipid solubility of the drug and its molecular weight. The lower pH levels of the fetus relative to the mother would suggest a greater transfer of the active drug (Low, 1963, cited in Burt, 1971). The route of administration is also important when considering fetal effects. Following an intravenous dose of pethidine, it has been found in the cord blood within 2 minutes (Crawford and Rudofsky, 1966, cited in Briggs *et al.*, 1994). Tests on maternal and fetal blood following the administration of intramuscular pethidine showed that 2 hours after administration pethidine began to pass back to the mother via the placenta (Cawthra, 1986). Undoubtedly pethidine passes from mother to fetus very readily as does the metabolite norpethidine, and this is dose dependent. The fetus will also produce norpethidine, and the levels in the fetal circulation may be higher than in the mother. The fetus may be more susceptible to the effects of this type of medication because of the immaturity of the blood–brain barrier and the fetal bypass of the liver where it would normally be metabolized (Burt, 1971).

Pethidine tends to result in respiratory depression in the baby at birth but the peak effects of the drug on the baby were observed on and after the 7th day of age (Rosenblatt *et al.*, 1981). Babies were found to be less alert, quicker to cry when disturbed, more difficult to quieten and less able to settle. When the birth of the baby follows within 2–5 hours of administration, there may well be more respiratory depression in the neonate and, although this is the peak time range for neonatal effect, it may also occur if delivery occurs prior to 2 hours (Belfrage *et al.*, 1981). Plasma half-life of pethidine in the maternal systems is 3–4 hours, whereas the levels in the infant's plasma are still significant at 13–23 hours with the metabolite norpethidine still being present at 62 hours (Righard and Alade, 1990).

Antagonist to pethidine Naloxone is commonly given to the baby where there is an observed effect, such as low Apgar scores or difficulty in establishing breathing following the administration of pethidine to the mother. It is an antagonist, blocking the receptors that pethidine binds to and thus blocking the action of pethidine and its consequent depressant effect on respiration. It is comparatively safe for the neonate and may be given via the intramuscular route in doses of 1 mg per kg of body weight.

It is important, however, that the midwife is aware that naloxone has a short half-life, which means that the effects may wear off around about an hour after administration, and therefore careful observation should be made of neonatal behaviour and vital signs for at least 2 hours after administration. It is also important, if naloxone is administered during resuscitation, that an adequate heart rate is present, as otherwise the drug will not be effectively metabolized.

Meptazinol (Meptid)

Meptazinol has been used as an alternative to pethidine in some units. It has little effect on cardiovascular and respiratory function. The usual dose is 100–150 mg and it is administered intramuscularly (Heywood and Ho, 1990). Some preliminary trials have shown that meptazinol gives better analgesia than pethidine and causes no known adverse effects on the fetus (Jackson and Robson, 1980, 1983). However, a comparative study by Sheikh and Tunstall (1986) showed no significant differences in the analgesic and side-effects of the two drugs, although meptazinol is more likely to cause vomiting in the mother. This must be balanced against the fact that Apgar scores of the baby are improved (Reynolds, 1998).

The structure of meptazinol makes neonatal naloxone unnecessary, and indeed naloxone is not usually an effective antagonist of meptazinol.

The lumbar epidural

The epidural has saved many women from a long-drawn-out, painful labour. The midwife can observe the change in a woman's whole demeanour following effective and total pain removal. It is, however, an invasive technique that requires an anaesthetist. The midwife needs expertise to help her client understand the whole process, which will enable the woman to maintain control in labour (Mander, 1997).

Epidural induction and the anatomy of epidural analgesia

The risks and the benefits must be fully discussed and understood by the woman, in order for her to make an informed decision. The midwife must record all discussions and the course of events in the notes (UKCC, 1998). Russell (1997) suggested that the anaesthetist should also sign these records.

The epidural is commenced by locating the space between the 2nd and 3rd lumbar vertebrae, and this is made easier by increasing the flexion of the spine. Following cleansing of the skin and application of local anaesthetic to the skin, a Tuohy needle is carefully inserted. This is a large-bore needle with centimetre marking to aid insertion (Fig. 27.6). The tough ligamentum flavum has to be overcome prior to the insertion of the needle into the 4-mm thick potential epidural space (Fig. 27.7). This space contains blood vessels, nerve roots and fat (Russell and Reynolds, 1997).

At the level of the 1st lumbar vertebra the spinal cord becomes a collection of nerve fibres termed the *cauda equina*, which as its Latin name suggests resembles a horse's tail (Tortora and Grabowski, 2000: 414). The injection of bupivacaine into this potential space at this level will block the autonomic nerve pathways that supply the uterus. Although anatomically the epidural space runs the length of the spinal column, occasionally the epidural injection is unsuccessful and it is believed that there may be folds in this membrane diverting the flow of analgesia away from the nerves (Russell and Reynolds, 1997). Throughout the induction procedure the midwife should support the woman and her partner both physically and psychologically. Record-keeping must be maintained.

Physiological effects of the epidural

The epidural analgesic lowers the blood pressure by its action on the sympathetic nervous system by altering adrenaline and noradrenaline levels in the blood (May, 1994). Lederman *et al.* (1978) suggested that by decreasing the levels of these catecholamines, uterine activity may be improved, as high levels tend to lengthen labour. As the woman relaxes, hyperventilation is prevented, maintaining normal blood gases and thus helping the fetus. Cortisol levels are lower, which helps to decrease adrenaline levels and keep the woman calm (Jowitt, 1993).

The effect on the autonomic nervous system produces vasodilatation in the peripheral circulation, causing the extremities to feel warm, a good test that the epidural is working. However, pooling of the circulation in the

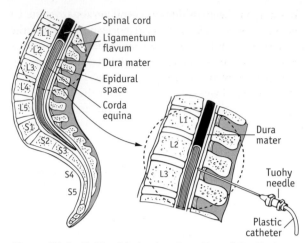

Figure 27.6   Epidural induction: insertion of the Tuohy needle. (Reprinted from *Pain in Childbearing*, Yerby, M. (ed) 2000 by permission of the publisher Baillière Tindall.)

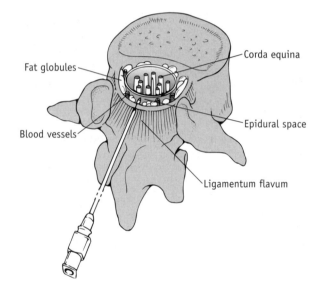

Figure 27.7   Epidural induction: Tuohy needle positioned in the epidural space. (Reprinted from *Pain in Childbearing*, Yerby, M. (ed) 2000 by permission of the publisher Baillière Tindall.)

periphery may cause hypotension, as there is a loss of peripheral resistance in the lower limbs. Aortocaval compression is always a risk from 20 weeks of gestation; therefore position in labour is important and the left lateral tilt would be favoured at all times. Blocking the sympathetic system should, in theory, improve fetal blood flow (Reynolds, 1993b).

Disadvantages of an epidural

In the normal course of events the urinary bladder should be emptied regularly in labour. When an epidural is in place it may be more difficult to micturate as sensation is poor. A full bladder during birth may delay the progress of labour and may also lead to bladder damage if an instrumental delivery is required, or postnatal urinary problems causing a transient incontinence (Russell, 1997).

Progress of labour Women usually request an epidural because they cannot cope with the pain. This may be due to a malpresentation of the fetus causing a longer labour, though there is debate about whether the use of an epidural lengthens labour. Zhang *et al.* (1999) and Beilin *et al.* (1999) made extensive studies of the controversies surrounding the use of epidural analgesia and its side-effects: long labour, instrumental delivery, and increased caesarean section rate. Despite these controversies, however, many women still prefer a pain-free birth and could relate good experiences.

Complications Women who choose an epidural immediately often need technological support in the form of electronic fetal monitoring, intravenous infusion, further epidural top-ups (which can be administered by the midwife) and medical intervention. This includes acceleration of labour and referral to the anaesthetist as required.

Hypotension is a real risk at the induction of an epidural; it is controlled by increasing intravenous fluids.

Respiratory arrest may be caused by the accidental induction of a high nerve block or the injection of bupivacaine into a vein. The first sign will be a tingling tongue and a rapid deterioration, and therefore the midwife needs to be prepared for immediate resuscitation.

Dural tap may occasionally occur, causing a loss of pressure in the circulating cerebrospinal fluid, resulting in the woman complaining of headaches. Rest is important prior to and following the procedure to prevent more spinal fluid leakage increasing headaches, until the dura is healed. It can be treated with an autologous blood patch of 20 ml of the patient's own blood injected near the site of the epidural to seal the dura (Crawford, 1980; Reynolds, 1997).

Long-term problems Holdcroft *et al.* (1995) estimated the risk of serious neurological complications as 1 : 2530, whereas 1 : 13 007 had a prolonged paraesthesia of a nerve root. As always when medical interventions go wrong, the resulting media headlines often cause women concern, and emotionality often takes precedence over calculated risk.

Long-term backache During pregnancy and labour, ligaments are altered by the hormones of pregnancy, permitting some movement to increase pelvic size to facilitate birth. Backache is a common complaint in pregnancy and following birth. MacArthur and colleagues (1990) studied 1634 women who had an epidural during labour and reported backache following birth. The analysis showed that there was an association between normal birth and backache but not caesarean birth and backache. Their conclusions were that the lack of sensation permitted unusual strain on bones and ligaments during labour, which possibly created long-term backache following birth. Research continues in this area and is not conclusive (Russell *et al.*, 1993, 1996).

Mobile epidural

In the past, epidural anaesthesia produced good pain relief but had the distinct disadvantage of causing a profound motor block, causing the woman in labour to be practically immobile. In order to prevent this, a group of anaesthetists developed the 'mobile epidural' (Collis *et al.*, 1993). This entailed giving a small spinal dose of bupivacaine 2.5 mg and fentanyl 2.5 μg and then an epidural catheter was inserted into the epidural space as normal and left in situ for subsequent top-ups. Full pain relief occurred in 5 minutes and once all observations were normal the women were permitted to walk around with an attendant. Women in the study liked the ability to be mobile although they did not actually walk far. They also had better control as they were better able to push in the second stage. In most units today this form of administration has been discontinued in favour of the combined use of bupivacaine with fentanyl into the epidural space, a low dose of analgesia creating less of a motor block (Eisenach, 1999).

Reflective Activity 27.8

Think about your own experience of supporting women in using different methods of pain relief.

- What do you find the most useful facts and information to give women when they use each method?
- What do you feel is the most useful method, and why?
- What sort of side-effects or disadvantages have you noted?

CONCLUSION

Pain is a multifaceted phenomenon of pregnancy, without which women would not know they were in labour. Psychological factors affect women's perception of pain in labour, and though education helps to decrease anxiety it has not been proved by research to lessen women's pain. Support has been shown to be valuable, whether by partner or midwives, and the latter is valued more when care is continuous from a known midwife. Women with better support seem to require less pain relief but when labours become long and pain increases, women tend to require systemic pain relief. Pethidine seems to be used less often in today's delivery suites in favour of the more effective epidural analgesia, though both methods of pain relief have side-effects. Research should continue to investigate women's needs and the production of systemic analgesia that is safe in labour for both mother and fetus. Midwives should continue to develop their skills in supporting women in labour whether with or without pain relief.

KEY POINTS

- An understanding of what pain is and how it may be experienced is influenced by the women's expectations, previous experience and the effect of childbirth education on women's experiences and the fear–pain–anxiety triangle.
- The midwife must take account of the physiological aspects of pain, its transmission, pain substances and the gate control theory of pain control.
- The cultural and social aspects of pain will influence the environment and coping mechanisms of women in labour, and how they can be supported by their families and friends.
- There is a wide range of pain-management strategies, from the use of distractive techniques or TENS to pharmacological methods of pain relief, including Entonox, pethidine and epidural analgesia.

REFERENCES

Active Birth Centre (2002) How to use water during labour. Online. Available: www.activebirthcentre.com June 2002.

Anderson, T. (1996) Support in labour. *Modern Midwife* **6**(1); 7–11.

Atkinson, R.L., Atkinson, R.C., Smith, E.E. *et al.* (1990) *Introduction to Psychology.* San Diego: Harcourt Brace Jovanovich.

Barasi, S. (1991) The Physiology of Pain. *Surgical Nurse* **4**(5): 14–20.

Beilin, Y., Leibowitz, A., Bernstein, H. *et al.* (1999) Controversies of labour – epidural analgesia. *Anaesthesia and Analgesia* **89**(4): 969–980.

Belfrage, P., Boreus, L.O., Hartvig, P. *et al.* (1981) Neonatal depression after obstetrical analgesia with pethidine. The role of the injection–delivery time interval and plasma concentrations of pethidine and norpethidine. *Acta Obstetricia et Gynecologica Scandinavica* **60**(1): 43–49.

Bloom, F.E. & Lazerson, A. (1988) *Brain, Mind and Behaviour,* 2nd edn. New York: W.H. Freeman.

Bonica, J.F. (1994) Labour pain. In: Wall, P.D. & Melzack, R. (eds) *Textbook of Pain,* Ch. 34. Edinburgh: Churchill Livingstone.

Bowlby, J. (1969) *Attachment and Loss: Attachment,* Vol. 1. London: Hogarth Press.

Bradford, N. & Chamberlain, G. (1995) *Pain Relief in Childbirth.* London: Harper Collins.

Briggs, G.G., Freeman, R.K. & Yaffe, S.J. (1994) *Drugs in Pregnancy and Lactation,* 4th edn. Baltimore: Williams & Wilkins.

Bullock, B.L. (1992) Pain. In: Bullock, B.L. & Rosendahl, P.P. (eds) *Pathophysiology: Adaptations and Alterations in Function,* 3rd edn, Ch. 51. Philadelphia: J.B. Lippincott.

Burt, R.A.P. (1971) The fetal and maternal pharmacology of some of the drugs used in the relief of pain in labour. *British Journal of Anaesthesia* **43**(9): 824–833.

Carson, R. (1996) The administration of analgesics. *Modern Midwife* **6**(11): 14–16.

Cawthra, A.M. (1986) The use of pethidine in labour. *Midwives Chronicle and Nursing Notes* **99**(1183): 178–181.

Chamberlain, G., Wraight, A. & Steer, P. (1993) *Pain and its Relief in Childbirth: The Results of a National Survey Conducted by the National Birthday Trust.* Edinburgh: Churchill Livingstone.

Cluett, E. (1994) Analgesia in labour: a review of the TENS method. *Professional Care of Mother and Child* **4**(2): 50–52.

Collis, R.E., Baxandall, M.L., Srikantharajah, I.D. *et al.* (1993) Mobility during labour with combined analgesia. *Lancet* **341**(8847): 767–768.

Condon, J.T. (1993) The assessment of antenatal emotional attachment: development of a questionnaire instrument. *British Journal of Medical Psychology* **66**(Pt 2): 167–183.

Crafter, H. (2000) Psychology of pain in labour. In: Yerby, M. (ed) *Pain in Childbearing*, Ch. 4. London: Baillière Tindall.

Crawford, J.S. & Rudofsky, S. (1966) Some alterations in the pattern of drug metabolism associated with pregnancy oral contraceptives and the newly born. *British Journal of Anaesthesia* 38(6): 446–454.

Crawford, S.J. (1980) Experiences with epidural blood patch. *Anaesthesia* 35(5): 513–515.

Department of Health and Social Security (DHSS) (1970) *Domiciliary and Maternity Bed Needs. Report of the Sub-committee of the Standing Midwifery and Maternity Advisory Committee* (Peel Report). London: HMSO.

Dickersin, K. (1989) Pharmacological control of pain during labour. In: Chalmers, I., Enkin, M. & Keirse, M.J.N.C. (eds) *Effective Care in Pregnancy and Childbirth*, Vol. 2. Oxford: Oxford University Press.

Dick-Read, G. (1944) *Childbirth Without Fear*. New York: Harper Row.

Eisenach, J. (1999) Combined spinal epidural analgesia in obstetrics. *Anaesthesiology* 91(1): 299–302.

Fridh, G. & Gaston-Johansson, F. (1990) Do primiparas and multiparas have realistic expectations of labor? *Acta Obstetricia et Gynecologica Scandinavica* 69(2): 103–109.

Fuentes, A., Spaziani, E.P. & O'Brien, W.F. (1996) The expression of cyclo-oxygenase-2 (COX-2) in amnion and deciduas following spontaneous labour. *Prostaglandins* 52(4): 361–367.

Gamsu, H. (1993) The effect of pain relief on the baby. In: Chamberlain, G., Wraight, A. & Steer, P. (eds) *Pain and its Relief in Childbirth,* Ch. 9. Edinburgh: Churchill Livingstone.

Gibb, D.M.F. (1993) Measurement of uterine activity in labour. *British Journal of Obstetrics and Gynaecology* 100(Suppl. 9): 28–31.

Gibb, W. (1998) The role of prostaglandins in human parturition. *Annals of Medicine* 30(3): 325–341.

Gilbert, R.E. & Tookey, P.A. (1999) Perinatal mortality and morbidity among babies delivered in water: surveillance study and postal study. *British Medical Journal* 319(7208): 483–487.

Green, J.M., Coupland, V.A. & Kitzinger, J.V. (1998) *Great Expectations*. Hale, Cheshire: Books for Midwives Press.

Halldorsdottir, S. & Karlsdottir, S.I. (1996) Journeying through labour and delivery: perceptions of women who have given birth. *Midwifery* 12(2): 48–61.

Hayes, L. (1997) Cultural experience of pain. In: Moore, S. (ed) *Understanding Pain and its Relief in Labour,* Ch. 6. Edinburgh: Churchill Livingstone.

Heywood, A.M. & Ho, E. (1990) Pain relief in labour. In: Alexander, J. Levy, V. & Roch, S. (eds) *Intrapartum Care: A Research Based Approach*. London: Macmillan.

Hillan, E.M. (1992) Research and audit; women's views of caesarean section. In: Roberts, H. (ed) *Women's Health Matters*, Ch. 9, pp. 157–175. London: Routledge.

Hodnett, E.D. (1997) Continuity of caregivers during pregnancy and childbirth. In: Neilson, J.P., Crowther, C.A., Hodnett, E.D. *et al.* (eds) *Pregnancy and Childbirth Module. Cochrane Database of Systematic Reviews* (updated 04 March 1997). Oxford: Update Software.

Hodnett, E.D. (2000) Caregiver support for women during childbirth (Cochrane Review). *The Cochrane Library,* Issue 2. Oxford: Update Software.

Holdcroft, A., Gibberd, F.B., Hargrove, R.L. *et al.* (1995) Neurological complications associated with pregnancy. *British Journal of Anaesthesia* 75(5): 522–526.

Hung, T.T. (1987) The role of endogenous opioids in pregnancy and analgesia. *Seminars in Reproductive Endocrinology* 5(2): 161–168.

Hughes, D. (1999) Midwives and women coping with pain together. *Practising Midwife* 2(5): 12–13.

Hutton, E. (1994) What women want. *British Journal of Midwifery* 2(12): 608–611.

Hypno-birth (2002) Pregnancy and birth – the feel good factor. Online. Available: http://www.hypno-birthing.org.uk/ June 2002.

Jackson, M.B. & Robson, P.J. (1980) Preliminary experience of the use of meptazinol as an obstetric analgesic. *British Journal of Obstetrics and Gynaecology* 87(4): 296–301.

Jackson, M.B. & Robson, P.J. (1983) Preliminary clinical and pharmacokinetic experiences in the newborn when meptazinol is compared with pethidine as an obstetric analgesic. *Postgraduate Medical Journal* 59(Suppl. 1): 47–51.

Jacques, A. (1994) Physiology of pain. *British Journal of Nursing* 3(12): 607–610.

Javert, C.T. & Hardy, J.D. (1950) Measurement of pain intensity in labour and its physiologic, neurologic, and pharmacologic implications. *American Journal of Obstetrics and Gynecology* 60: 552–563.

Jayaram, A. (1997) Practical obstetric pharmacology. In: Dewan, D. & Hood, A. (eds) *Practical Obstetric Anesthesia*. London: W.B. Saunders.

Johnson, M.I. (1997) Transcutaneous electrical nerve stimulation in pain management. British Journal of Midwifery 5(7): 400–405.

Jowitt, M. (1993) *Childbirth Unmasked*. Bodmin: Harnells.

Kaufman, K.J. (1993) Effective control or effective care? *Birth* 20(3): 156–158.

Keele, C.A., Neil, E. & Joels, N. (1983) *Samson Wright's Physiology,* 13th edn. Oxford: Oxford Medical Publications.

Lamaze International (2001) Position Paper – Lamaze for the 21st Century. Online. Available: http://lamaze.org/2000/home.htm June 2002.

Lederman, R.P., Lederman, E., Work, B. *et al.* (1978) The relationship of maternal anxiety, plasma catecholamines, and plasma cortisol to the progression in labour. *American Journal of Obstetrics and Gynecology* 132(5): 495–500.

Lifeforce (2002) Online. Available: http://lifeforce.co.uk/review.html June 2002.

Low, J.A. (1963) Acid base assessment of the fetus in the normal obstetric patient. *Obstetrics and Gynecology* **22**: 15.

Lowe, N.K. (1991) Maternal confidence in coping with labour. *Journal of Obstetric, Gynecologic and Neonatal Nursing* **20**(6): 457–463.

Lundgren, I. & Dahlberg, K. (1998) Women's experience of pain during childbirth. *Midwifery* **14**(2): 105–110.

MacArthur, C., Lewis, M., Knox, E.G. *et al.* (1990) Epidural and long term backache after childbirth. *British Medical Journal* **301**(6742): 9–12.

MacLennan, A., Crowther, C., Derham, R. (1994) Does the option to ambulate during spontaneous labour confer any advantage or disadvantage? *Journal of Maternal and Fetal Medicine* **3**(1): 43–48.

Mander, R. (1997) *Pain in Childbearing and its Control.* Oxford: Blackwell Science.

May, A. (1994) *Epidurals for Childbirth.* London: Oxford University Press.

Melzack, R., Taenzer, P., Feldman, P. *et al.* (1981) Labour is still painful after prepared childbirth training. *Canadian Medical Association Journal* **125**(4): 357–363.

Melzack, R. & Wall, P. (1996) *The Challenge of Pain.* London: Pelican.

Melzack, R. & Wall, P. (1965) Pain mechanisms: a new theory. *Science* **150**(699): 971–979.

Moir, C. (1939) The nature of the pain of labour. *Journal of Obstetrics and Gynaecology. British Empire* **46**: 409–424.

Moore, S. (1997) Psychology of pain in labour. In: Moore, S (ed) *Understanding Pain and its Relief in Labour*, Ch. 4. Edinburgh: Churchill Livingstone.

Niven, C. (1994) *Coping with Labour Pain; the Midwife's Role.* London: Chapman and Hall.

Nikodem, V.C. (2002) Immersion in water in pregnancy, labour and birth (Cochrane Review). *The Cochrane Library*, Issue 2. Oxford: Update Software.

Nolan, M. (2000) The influence of antenatal classes on pain relief in labour. *Practising Midwife* **3**(6): 26–31.

Nursing and Midwifery Council (NMC) (2002) *Guidelines for the Administration of Medicines.* London: NMC.

O'Driscoll, M. (1994) Midwives, childbirth and sexuality; men and sex. *British Journal of Midwifery* **2**(2): 74–76.

Olofsson, C.H., Ekblom-Ordeberg, G., Helm, A.H. *et al.* (1996) Lack of analgesic affect of systemically administered morphine or pethidine for labour pain. *British Journal of Obstetrics and Gynaecology* **103**(10): 968–972.

Oster, M.I. (1994) Psychological preparation for labor and delivery using hypnosis. *American Journal of Clinical Hypnosis* **37**(1): 12–21.

Ostheimer, G.W. (1992) *Manual of Obstetric Anaesthesia.* New York: Churchill Livingstone.

Page, L. (1993) Redefining the midwife's role; changes needed in practice. *British Journal of Midwifery* **1**(1): 21–24.

Page, L.A., Cooke, P., Percival, P. (2000) Providing one-to-one practice and enjoying it. In: Page, L.A. (ed) *The New Midwifery*, Ch. 6. Edinburgh: Churchill Livingstone.

Price, S. (2000) Pain relief: a practical guide to obstetrics TENS machines. *British Journal of Midwifery* **8**(9): 550–552.

Quereshi, N.S., Scofield, G., Papaioannou, S. *et al.* (1996) Parentcraft classes: do they effect outcome in childbirth? *Journal of Obstetrics and Gynaecology* **16**: 358–361.

Rajan, L. (1993) Perceptions of pain and pain relief in labour: the gulf between experience and observation. *Midwifery* **9**(3): 136–145.

Raphael-Leff, J. (1993) *Psychological Processes of Childbearing.* London: Chapman and Hall.

Rang, H.P., Dale, M.M. & Ritter, J.M. (1995) *Pharmacology*, 3rd edn. Edinburgh: Churchill Livingstone.

Reading, A.E. & Cox, D.N. (1985) Psychological predictors of labour pain. *Pain* **22**(3): 309–315.

Reynolds, F. (1991) Pharmacokinetics. In: Hytten, F. & Chamberlain, G. (eds) *Clinical Physiology in Obstetrics*, Ch. 10. London: Blackwell Scientific Publications.

Reynolds, F. (1993a) Pain relief in labour: a review. *British Journal of Obstetrics and Gynaecology* **100**(11) 979–983.

Reynolds, F (1993b) *Effects on the Baby of Maternal Analgesia and Anaesthesia.* London: W.B. Saunders.

Reynolds, F. (1997) They think its all over. In: Reynolds, F. (ed) *Pain Relief in Labour*, Ch. 12. London: BMJ Publishing Group

Reynolds, F. (1998) Effects of analgesia on the baby. *Fetal and Maternal Medicine Review* **10**: 45–59.

Righard, L. & Alade, M.O. (1990) Effect of delivery rooms routines on the success of first breast-feed. *Lancet* **336**(8723): 1105–1107.

Robertson, A. (2000) Tell me about the pain. *Practising Midwife* **3**(7): 46–47.

Robson, K. & Kumar, R. (1980) Delayed onset of maternal affection after childbirth. *British Journal of Psychiatry* **136**: 347–353.

Rosenblatt, D., Belsey, E.M., Lieberman, L. *et al.* (1981) The influence of maternal analgesia on neonatal behaviour: II Epidural bupivacaine. *British Journal of Obstetrics and Gynaecology* **88**(4): 407–413.

Royal College of Midwives (RCM) (2000) *The Use of Water in Labour and Birth.* Position Paper. London: RCM.

Russell, R. (1997) Practical procedures. In: Reynolds, F. (ed) *Pain Relief in Labour*, Ch. 10. London: BMJ Publishing Group.

Russell, R. & Reynolds, F. (1997) Neuroscientific aspects. In: Reynolds, F. (ed) *Pain Relief in Labour*, Ch. 7. London: BMJ Publishing Group.

Russell, R., Groves, P., Taub, N. *et al.* (1993) Assessing long term backache after childbirth. *British Medical Journal* **306**(15): 1299–1303.

Russell, R., Dundas, R. & Reynolds, F. (1996) Long term backache after childbirth: prospective search for causative factors. *British Medical Journal* **312**(7043): 1384–1388.

Salar, G., Job, I., Mingrino, S. *et al.* (1981) Effect of transcutaneous electrotherapy on CSF beta-endorphin content in patients without pain problems. *Pain* 10(2): 169–172.

Scrutton, M. (1997) Systemic opioid analgesia. In: Reynolds, F. (ed) *Pain Relief in Labour,* Ch. 5. London: BMJ Publishing Group.

Sheikh, A. & Tunstall, M.E. (1986) Comparative study of meptazinol and pethidine for the relief of pain in labour. *British Journal of Obstetrics and Gynaecology* 93(3): 264–269.

Sherr, L. (1995) *The Psychology of Pregnancy and Childbirth.* Oxford: Blackwell Science.

Simkin, P. (1989) Non-pharmacological methods of pain relief during labour. In: Chalmers, I., Enkin, M. & Keirse, M.J.N.C. (eds) *Effective Care in Pregnancy and Childbirth,* Vol. 2, pp. 893–912. Oxford: Oxford University Press.

Simkin, P. (1995) Psychologic and other non-pharmacologic techniques. In: Bonica, J.J. & McDonald, J.S. (eds) *Principles and Practices of Obstetric Analgesia and Anaesthesia.* Baltimore, MD: Williams & Wilkins.

Stjernquist, M. & Sjöberg, N.O. (1994) Neurotransmitters in the myometrium. In: Chard, T., Grudzinskas, J.G. (eds) *The Uterus,* Ch. 9. Cambridge: Cambridge University Press.

Symonds, T. (1998) Pain: psychological aspects. In: Pitts. M., Phillips, K. (eds) *The Psychology of Health,* Ch. 6. London: Routledge.

Tarkka, M.T. & Paunonen, M. (1996) Social support and its impact on mothers' experiences of childbirth. *Journal of Advanced Nursing* 23(1): 70–75.

Tortora, G.J. & Grabowski, S.R. (2000) *Principles of Anatomy and Physiology,* 7th edn. New York: Harper Collins College Publications.

United Kingdom Central Council for Nursing Midwifery and Health Visiting (UKCC) (1991) *Registrar's Letter 8/91. Transcutaneous Nerve Stimulation in Labour.* London: UKCC.

United Kingdom Central Council for Nursing Midwifery and Health Visiting (UKCC) (1998) *Midwives Rules and Code of Practice.* London: UKCC.

Vander, A.J., Sherman, J.H. & Luciano, D.S. (2000) *Human Physiology,* 7th edn. Boston: McGraw-Hill.

Walding, M.F. (1991) Pain, anxiety and powerlessness. *Journal of Advanced Nursing* 16(4): 338–397.

Weber, S.E. (1996) Cultural aspects of pain in childbearing women. *Journal of Obstetric, Gynecologic and Neonatal Nursing* 25(1): 67–72.

Whipple, B. (1990) Neurophysiology of pain. *Orthopaedic Nursing* 9(4): 21–25.

Williams, P.L., Warwick, R., Dyson, M. *et al.* (eds) (1989) *Gray's Anatomy,* 37th edn. Edinburgh: Churchill Livingstone.

Yerby, M. (ed) (2000) *Pain in Childbearing.* Edinburgh: Baillière Tindall.

Zhang, J., Klebanoff, M. & DerSimonian, R. (1999) Epidural analgesia in association with the duration of labour and mode of delivery: a quantitative review. *American Journal of Obstetrics and Gynecology* 180(4): 970–977.

FURTHER READING

Bannister, C. (1997) *The Midwife's Pharmacopoeia.* Hale, Cheshire: Books for Midwives Press.
A very readable book useful for quick reference, clearly set out.

Briggs, G., Freeman, R., & Yaffe, S.J. (eds) (1998) *Drugs in Pregnancy and Lactation,* 5th edn. Philadelphia: Lippincott Williams & Wilkins.
A comprehensive and fully referenced text, with detail of drugs used in pregnancy and their effect on the fetus and neonate.

de Swiet, M. & Chamberlain, G. (1992) *Basic Science in Obstetrics and Gynaecology,* 2nd edn. Edinburgh: Churchill Livingstone.

An advanced level of physiology with particular application to obstetrics and gynaecology; well referenced. A book written for doctors as preparation for Part 1 of the MRCOG. It has many relevant chapters from which midwives could benefit.

Yerby, M. (ed) (2000) *Pain in Childbearing.* Edinburgh: Baillière Tindall.
The content covers in detail aspects of pain in childbearing, including antenatal, labour and postnatal pain in the context of physiology, psychology and sociological issues. Chapters on fetal and neonatal pain are included.

ADDITIONAL RESOURCES

http://www.doh.gov.uk/
National Health Service circular (HSC 2000/26) clarifies the legal issues in the administration of drugs. Issued August 2000.

http://www.groupprotocols.org.uk/
Gives guidance on the use of Patient Group Directives that replace Standing Orders for the administration of drugs.

http://www.hypno-birthing.org.uk/
A website for parents to learn about 'hypno-birthing', a self-hypnotherapy programme.

28

The Pelvic Floor

Chris Kettle

LEARNING OUTCOMES

After reading this chapter you will:

- have enhanced your knowledge and understanding of the anatomy and function of the pelvic floor in relation to trauma and repair
- understand the short- and long-term morbidity associated with perineal trauma

- be able to base practice on current research
- be aware of employing authorities' policies and guidelines and understand the legal implications associated with inadequate or incorrect repair of the perineum.

INTRODUCTION

Historical studies have shown that perineal injury has occurred during childbirth throughout the ages and that various methods and materials were used by accoucheurs in an attempt to restore the integrity of severely traumatized tissue. The earliest evidence of extensive perineal injury sustained during childbirth exists in the mummy of Henhenit, a Nubian woman aged approximately 22 years, from the harem of King Mentuhotep II of Egypt, 2050 BC (Derry, 1935; Graham, 1950; Magdi, 1949). Despite the fact that maternity care has greatly improved over the past decade women continue to suffer the consequences of pelvic floor damage resulting from childbirth.

THE PELVIC FLOOR

The development of the upright posture in humans has been the dominant factor in the evolution of the pelvic floor (Benson, 1992). Its main function is to provide support for the pelvic and abdominal organs, which lie in the cavity above. Therefore, it must be strong to oppose the forces of gravity and increases in abdominal pressure. Unfortunately, childbirth is a known source of pelvic floor damage, causing muscle weakness, incontinence, and prolapse of the pelvic organs.

It is extremely important that the midwife has a sound understanding of both the structure and function of the pelvic floor so that she can apply her knowledge in order to minimize any associated morbidity during the process of childbirth.

Structure

The ischial spines are key landmarks in understanding the location and structure of the pelvic floor. They lie laterally, in a plane which spans the pelvic cavity where many important parts of the pelvic floor are attached (Benson, 1992). The soft tissues, which form the pelvic floor, fill the outlet of the bony pelvis forming a 'sling', which is higher posteriorly (Verralls, 1993). In the female, the urethra, vagina, and rectum pass through its structures. It consists of the following six layers extending from the pelvic peritoneum above to the skin of the vulva, perineum, and buttocks below:

- pelvic peritoneum
- pelvic fascia
- deep muscles
- superficial muscles
- subcutaneous fat
- skin.

Pelvic peritoneum

This forms a smooth covering over the uterus and fallopian tubes. Anteriorly it forms the uterovesical pouch and covers the upper surface of the bladder. Posteriorly it forms the pouch of Douglas. Laterally it covers the fallopian tubes and forms the broad ligaments, but in spite of their name they do not act as supports.

Pelvic fascia

This is connective tissue, which fills the space between the pelvic organs and lines the walls of the pelvic cavity. Its function is to provide support for the organs, whilst at the same time allowing them to move within the limits of normal function (Verralls, 1993). In areas where extra support is needed it thickens to form the pelvic ligaments:

- *Transverse cervical ligaments.* These form the principal, direct supports of the uterus and are also known as the cardinal or Mackenrodt's ligaments. They are attached to the vaginal vault and supravaginal cervix and extend transversely in a fan-like way across the pelvic floor to the white line of fascia on the lateral pelvic walls.
- *Uterosacral ligaments.* These are attached to the vaginal vault and supravaginal cervix and pass backwards and upwards from the cervix to the lateral border of the sacral body.
- *Round ligaments.* These originate just below the cornua of the uterus, passing through the inguinal canal and anterior abdominal wall to become inserted into each labium majus. They assist in keeping the uterus in its normal anteverted (forward tilted) anteflexed (bent on itself) position.
- *Pubocervical ligaments.* These are attached to the inner part of the pubic bones and run posteriorly to form attachments to the bladder, vault of vagina and supravaginal cervix. They provide support for the bladder (Verralls, 1993).

Deep muscle layer

This is formed from a group of muscles, which are approximately 3–5 cm in depth and are collectively known as the levator ani. They arise at the inner circumference of the true pelvis from the white-line of the obturator fascia and decussate midline between the urethra, vagina, and rectum. The muscle fibres pass downwards and backwards and are inserted medially into the upper vagina, perineal body, anal canal, anococcygeal body, coccyx, and lower borders of the sacrum. The levator ani when viewed from above look like two joined cupped hands.

The main function is to provide a strong sling to support the pelvic organs and to counteract any increase in the intra-abdominal pressure during coughing and laughing. When the levator ani is contracted the pelvic floor and perineum are lifted upwards, which is an important mechanism to maintain continence.

The deep muscles are named after the corresponding fused bones of the innominate bone (pubis, ilium and ischium) (Fig. 28.1):

- *Pubococcygeus muscles.* These arise from the inner surface of the pubic bones and pass posteriorly below

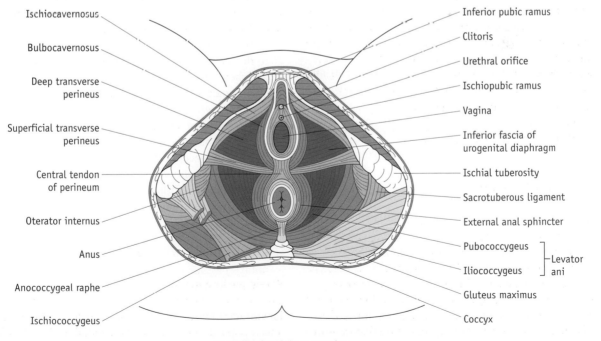

Superficial and deep muscles

Figure 28.1 Muscles of the pelvic floor seen in the female perineum. (From *Principles of Anatomy and Physiology*, 7th edn, by Tortora, G.J. and Grabowski, S.R. Copyright © 1993 John Wiley & Sons. Reprinted by permission of John Wiley & Sons, Inc.)

the bladder on either side of the urethra, upper vagina and anal canal to the anococcygeal body and coccyx. Fibres cross medially and join those from the opposite sides to form U-shaped slings around the urethra, vagina, and rectum. The part that forms a loop around the anorectal junction is called the puborectalis muscle and its posterior fibres communicate with the external anal sphincter. The medial part is attached to the vagina but there is no direct attachment to the urethra. On dissection, they appear paler in colour suggesting they are fast-twitch muscle capable of rapid contraction (Benson, 1992). The function of these muscles is to provide support to the urethra, vagina, and rectum and control micturition and defecation.

- *Iliococcygeus muscles.* These arise from the inner border of the white line of fascia on the inner aspects of the iliac bones and from the ischial spines. They join midline and are inserted posteriorly into the anococcygeal raphe and coccyx. On dissection, they appear darker in colour suggesting they are slow-twitch muscles (Benson, 1992).
- *Ischiococcygeus muscles.* These are triangular sheets of muscle and fibrous tissue, which arise from the ischial spines and pass downwards, and inwards to be inserted into the coccyx and lower part of the sacrum. They are sometimes referred to as the coccygeus muscles. Their main function is to stabilize the sacroiliac and sacrococcygeal joints.

Blood, lymph and nerve supply

- Blood is supplied from the pudendal arteries and branches of the internal iliac artery and venous drainage is into corresponding veins.
- Lymphatic drainage is into the inguinal and external internal iliac glands.
- Nerve supply is from the third and fourth sacral nerves.

Superficial perineal muscles

These are less important than the levator ani muscles; however, they do contribute to the overall strength of the pelvic floor and are likely to be damaged during vaginal delivery (Fig. 28.1):

- *Bulbocavernosus muscles.* These extend from a central point in the perineal body and encircle the vagina and urethra before inserting anteriorly into the corpora cavernosa of the clitoris. Posteriorly some fibres merge with the superficial transverse muscle and external anal sphincter. Situated beneath bulbocavernosus are the vestibular bulbs

anteriorly and the Bartholin's glands posteriorly. Its main function is to cause erection of the clitoris and contraction of the vagina during sexual activity.

- *Ischiocavernosus muscles.* These arise from the ischial tuberosities and pass upwards and inwards along the pubic arch to be inserted into the corpora cavernosa of the clitoris. Some fibres interweave with those forming the membranous sphincter of the urethra.
- *Transverse perineal muscles.* These arise from the ischial tuberosities and pass transversely to converge in a central point of the perineum. Fibres of each transverse muscle unite and interweave with the superficial tissue of the perineal body and external anal sphincter. They provide additional support transversely across the perineal region and help fix the position of the perineal body.

Sphincters

- *Membranous sphincter of the urethra.* This arises from one pubic bone and passes above and below the urethra to the opposite pubic bone. It is not a true sphincter; however, it is capable of contracting to occlude the lumen of the urethra.
- *External anal sphincter.* This is a teardrop-shaped circle of muscle, which surrounds the anus and is subdivided into three parts (subcutaneous, superficial and deep) which are not easily defined during dissection. The deep external sphincter is inseparable from the puborectalis muscle and is shorter anteriorly in the female (Sultan *et al.*, 1994a). Posteriorly, it is attached to the coccyx by some of its fibres. The circular striated (voluntary) muscle of the external anal sphincter when dissected or torn looks similar to 'dark red meat'. Its main function is to close the lumen of the anal canal and control the voluntary passage of faeces and flatus.
- *Internal anal sphincter.* This is a condensation of the circular smooth muscle of the rectum and is approximately 3 cm long and 5 mm thick. It is not easily defined and on dissection is paler in colour than the external anal sphincter. Its main function is to close the lumen of the anus and to prevent involuntary passage of faeces and flatus, which is very important when sleeping.

Ischiorectal fossa   This is a deep wedge-shaped area, which is filled with fat and is bounded by the gluteus maximus, anal sphincter, transverse perinei and bulbocavernosus muscles. It is a potential area for haematoma formation.

Blood, lymph and nerve supply

- Blood is supplied from branches of the internal iliac arteries and venous drainage is into corresponding veins.
- Lymphatic drainage is into the internal iliac glands.
- Nerve supply is from the third and fourth segments of the sacral plexus and pudendal nerve.

Subcutaneous fat and skin

Neither of these has any supporting function.

Perineal body

This is a triangular-shaped structure consisting of muscular and fibrous tissue. It is situated between the vagina and the anal canal, with the ischial tuberosities laterally. Each side of the triangle is approximately 3.5 cm in length with the base being the perineal skin and the apex pointing inwards. It is an integral part of the pelvic floor, since it is the central point where both the levator ani and most of the superficial muscles unite. Blood is supplied by the pudendal arteries and venous drainage is into the corresponding veins. Lymph drains into the inguinal and external iliac glands. The nerve supply is derived from the perineal branch of the pudendal nerve.

Reflective Activity 28.1

Can you name the pelvic floor muscles that converge at the central point of the perineum?

Discussion

The primary function of the pelvic floor is to support the pelvic organs, namely the vagina, uterus, bladder and rectum. During pregnancy the body releases a hormone called relaxin which softens the pelvic muscles and ligaments, allowing them to stretch during childbirth. After delivery, the pelvic floor is able to resume its original supporting function in a surprisingly short time because of its remarkable elasticity. However, prolonged, repeated or extreme stretching of the pelvic floor muscles may cause permanent damage, resulting in loss of tone and elasticity. If these muscles fail to support the pelvic organs, prolapse results. These problems may not manifest until later life when postmenopausal oestrogen deficiencies may predispose to muscle weakness (Haadem et al., 1991). Another factor to consider is that the life expectancy of women in the developed world has doubled, which has contributed to the increasing number of women being affected

(Sultan et al., 1996). Defects in connective tissue, which may be caused by congenital conditions such as Ehlers–Danlos syndrome, are also important in the aetiology of genital prolapse and stress incontinence (Sultan et al., 1996). Postnatal pelvic floor exercises may promote the return of effective function and help to prevent any long-term urinary problems and uterovaginal prolapse (Brayshaw and Wright, 1994; Hay-Smith et al., 2001).

PERINEAL TRAUMA

Definition

Anatomically, the perineum extends from the pubic arch to the coccyx and is divided into the anterior urogenital and posterior anal triangle. Anterior perineal trauma is defined as any injury to the labia, anterior vagina, urethra, or clitoris and is associated with less morbidity. Posterior perineal trauma is defined as any injury to the posterior vaginal wall, perineal muscles, anal sphincters (external and internal) and may include disruption of the rectal mucosa. Perineal trauma may occur spontaneously during vaginal birth or a surgical incision (episiotomy) is made intentionally by the midwife or obstetrician to increase the diameter of the vulval outlet and facilitate delivery.

Prevalence

Over 85% of women who have a vaginal birth will sustain some form of perineal trauma (McCandlish et al., 1998) and up to 69% of these will require stitches (McCandlish et al., 1998; Sleep et al., 1984). These rates will vary considerably according to individual practices and policies of hospitals throughout the world. This is illustrated by wide variations in episiotomy rates in different countries, ranging from 8% in the Netherlands, 13% in England, 43% in the USA to 99% in the Eastern European Countries (Graham and Graham, 1997; Graves, 1995; Statistical Bulletin, 2003; Wagner, 1994).

Midwives should be aware that certain intrapartum interventions or alternative forms of care may also affect the rate and extent of perineal trauma; for example, continuous support during labour, position for delivery, epidural anaesthesia, style of pushing, restricted use of episiotomy and ventouse delivery (Kettle, 1999, 2001).

Aetiology and risk factors

Perineal trauma occurs during spontaneous or assisted vaginal delivery and is usually more extensive after the first vaginal birth (Sultan et al., 1996). Women who have no visible damage may be subject to transient pudendal or peripheral nerve injury due to prolonged active pushing or pressure exerted by the fetal head on the surrounding structures (Allen *et al.*, 1990).

Associated risk factors include parity, size of baby, mode of delivery, malpresentation and malposition of the fetus. Other maternal factors that may contribute to the extent of trauma are ethnicity, age, tissue type, and nutritional state (Renfrew *et al.*, 1998). Smoking is thought to affect the rate of perineal wound healing by causing vasoconstriction and tissue ischaemia (Mikhailidis *et al.*, 1983).

Short- and long-term effects

In the UK approximately 23–42% of women will have perineal pain and discomfort up to 10–12 days following vaginal delivery and 7–10% of these women will continue to have long-term pain up to 18 months postpartum (Glazener *et al.*, 1995; Gordon *et al.*, 1998; Grant, 2001; McCandlish *et al.*, 1998; Mackrodt *et al.*, 1998; Sleep *et al.*, 1984). Research carried out by Gordon *et al.* (1998) and Mackrodt *et al.* (1998) found that 44–46% of women who had resumed intercourse at 3 months postpartum experienced superficial dyspareunia, and 15–19% continued to have pain.

It is difficult to estimate the extent of urinary and faecal incontinence owing to under-reporting of these problems (Sultan *et al.*, 1996). A survey carried out by MacArthur *et al.* (1993) found that 15.2% of the participating women (*n* = 1782) reported stress incontinence which started for the first time within 3 months of the baby's birth, and 75% of these still had problems over a year later.

Very few studies have examined the prevalence of faecal incontinence following childbirth. Sleep *et al.* (1987) and MacArthur *et al.* (1997) found that up to 4% of women reported occasional loss of bowel control, but this is probably grossly underestimated as a result of under-reporting due to the sensitive nature of this complaint.

Antenatal preparation

The midwife can contribute to reducing the extent and rate of perineal trauma by reviewing the woman's lifestyle and giving appropriate advice regarding diet, smoking, exercise, and perineal massage. A healthy, well-nourished body should ensure optimum condition of the perineal tissue prior to labour. Current evidence supports the use of antenatal perineal massage for preserving the integrity of the perineum particularly in women having their first vaginal birth (Labrecque *et al.*,

2000, 2001). Women wishing to carry out this practice should be instructed to perform perineal massage from 34–35 weeks' gestation for 5–10 min daily using sweet almond oil (Labrecque *et al.*, 1999; Shipman *et al.*, 1997). Midwives should also instruct and encourage women to carry out regular antenatal pelvic floor exercises to strengthen the muscles in preparation for childbirth. Women should also be informed of the importance of continuing these exercises postnatally to reinnervate and increase the tone of the pelvic floor muscle in order to reduce any associated morbidity such as stress incontinence (Mason *et al.*, 2001).

Spontaneous trauma

This can be classified as:

- First degree, which may involve:
  - the skin and subcutaneous tissue of the anterior or posterior perineum
  - vaginal mucosa
  - a combination of the above resulting in multiple superficial lacerations.
- Second-degree tears, which may involve:
  - superficial perineal muscles (bulbocavernosus, transverse perineal)
  - perineal body
  - deep perineal muscle (pubococcygeus).

  Tears usually extend downwards from the posterior and/or lateral vaginal walls, through the hymenal remnants, midline downwards towards the anal margin, in the weakest part of the stretched perineum. Less frequently, they occur in a circular direction, behind the hymenal remnants extending bilaterally upwards towards the clitoris and detaching the lower third of the vagina from the underlying structures (Sultan *et al.*, 1994a). This type of complex trauma causes vast disruption to the perineal body and muscles but the perineal skin may remain intact, making it difficult to repair.
- Third-degree tears, which involve the superficial and/or deep perineal muscles and anal sphincter/s. More recently, third-degree tears have been subclassified as:
  (3a) less than 50% of the external anal sphincter (EAS) torn
  (3b) more than 50% of the EAS torn
  (3c) to include internal anal sphincter (IAS) torn (Keighley *et al.*, 2000).
- Fourth-degree tears, which involve the same structures as above, including disruption of the EAS and/or IAS and anorectal epithelium.

Cervical tears

If an instrumental delivery (forceps or ventouse) is attempted before the cervix is fully dilated, a cervical tear may occur. Similarly, a tear may result if the woman forcibly pushes the fetus through a cervix, which is incompletely dilated (Llewellyn-Jones, 1990). Bleeding is usually very severe and will persist despite the uterus being well contracted. Postpartum haemorrhage (PPH) resulting from a cervical tear must be managed appropriately and efficiently according to individual unit guidelines, as mismanagement can cause maternal mortality. Once the maternal condition has been stabilized, a skilled operator should repair the cervical tear in a theatre with good lighting, appropriate assistance, and adequate anaesthesia.

> ### Reflective Activity 28.2
>
> What is the definition of a PPH? Find out what your unit's guideline is for the management of this obstetric emergency.

Surgical incision (episiotomy)

Episiotomy is defined as a surgical incision of the perineum made to increase the diameter of the vulval outlet during childbirth. Midwives have been permitted to carry out this procedure in the UK since 1967. The incision is made with either sharp scissors or a scalpel.

Straight, blunt-ended Mayo episiotomy scissors are usually used because it is thought that there is less risk of accidental damage to the baby, and haemostasis of the cut tissue is promoted by the crushing action as the incision is made. Those professionals who favour the scalpel feel that it minimizes trauma to the tissues and allows better healing of the perineal wound. However, there are no data to support the validity of either of these claims (Sleep *et al.*, 1989).

The decision to perform an episiotomy must be made on an individual basis, taking the woman's wishes and obstetric history, and clinical judgement into consideration. It is essential that the midwife gives the woman information regarding the rationale for performing an episiotomy, during the antenatal period. This should enable the woman to make an informed decision regarding this procedure if needed during labour.

There are two main types of incision:

- *Mediolateral or posterolateral.* The incision starts midline at the fourchette, avoiding damage to the Bartholin's gland. It is then directed diagonally to the right or left side of the posterior perineum to a point midway between the anus and ischial tuberosity, avoiding the anal sphincter. In the UK most midwives and obstetricians perform a right mediolateral episiotomy (Fig. 28.2).
- *Midline.* The incision starts in the midline position at the fourchette and is made vertically towards the anus.

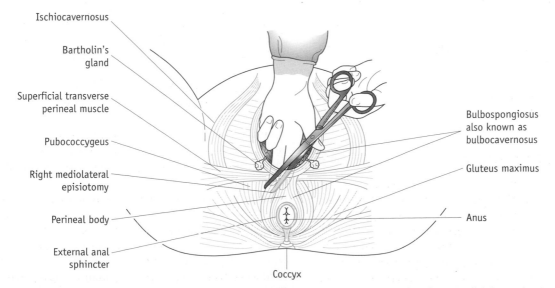

Figure 28.2 Diagrammatic representation of a right mediolateral episiotomy showing the superficial muscles involved when the incision is made.

Reflective Activity 28.3

Can you describe what anatomical structures are involved when a right mediolateral episiotomy is made?

Timing of the incision

An episiotomy must only be made when the presenting part is distending the perineal tissues; otherwise it will fail to accelerate delivery and excessive bleeding may occur.

Indications

The following are not absolute, and clinical discretion should always be used.

An episiotomy may be performed to:

- Aid delivery if the perineal tissue is very rigid causing serious delay in the second stage.
- Reduce prolonged maternal 'pushing' efforts in cases of severe hypertensive or cardiac disease.
- Accelerate spontaneous vaginal delivery in cases of fetal distress.
- Prevent severe perineal trauma during instrumental delivery (forceps or ventouse) or when the baby is in the direct occipitoposterior position.
- Facilitate safe delivery in cases of shoulder dystocia.

NB: There is no scientific evidence to support the routine procedure of episiotomy to prevent intracranial haemorrhage in preterm deliveries (Woolley, 1995).

Risks

- Liberal use of episiotomy increases the overall rate of posterior perineal trauma.
- It may contribute to an increase in intrapartum maternal blood loss.
- Midline episiotomies increase fourfold the risk of anal sphincter damage (Coats *et al.*, 1980; Thacker and Banta, 1983).
- It may increase the risk of postpartum pain and perineal infection.
- It is associated with a reduction in pelvic floor muscle function.
- It increases the risk of vertical transmission of the human immunodeficiency virus.

NB: The risks are clearly increased with a high episiotomy rate.

Procedure

Prior to performing the episiotomy, the midwife must prepare the delivery trolley and equipment according to the practice policies and guidelines of the individual employing authority. Safety glasses and gloves must be worn during all obstetric procedures to protect the operator against HIV and hepatitis infection. The woman's dignity and comfort must be maintained throughout the procedure. The stages of the procedure and the rationale for each stage are listed in Table 28.1.

Complications

Incisions that begin laterally will not increase the diameter of the vulval outlet and may cause damage to the Bartholin's gland. This could predispose to cyst formation or a decrease in vaginal lubrication leading to sexual difficulties. Lateral episiotomies are very painful and difficult to repair.

If the episiotomy is too small, the diameter of the vulval outlet will not be sufficiently increased to facilitate delivery and the incision may extend downwards into the ischiorectal fossa and anal sphincter/s.

Episiotomy rate

There seems to be no consensus as to the recommended episiotomy rate. The World Health Organization recommends that an episiotomy rate of 10%, for normal deliveries, would be 'a good goal to pursue' (WHO, 1996).

Reflective Activity 28.4

Find out what the episiotomy rate is for spontaneous vaginal deliveries in the maternity unit where you are working.

Discussion

Women often describe episiotomy as the unkindest cut of all and yet it is one of the most frequent obstetric operations performed. It was first introduced over 250 years ago (Ould, 1742) but most obstetricians only came to favour the procedure at the beginning of the 20th century. It was postulated that all primigravidae should receive an episiotomy to protect the fetal head and preserve the integrity of the pelvic floor (DeLee, 1920; Pomeroy, 1918). During the 1930s it became a routine procedure in most American hospitals but it was not widely used in Britain until the 1950s when childbirth became increasingly medicalized (Tew, 1990). By the 1970s, rates were as high as 91% in some UK hospitals (Thacker and Banta, 1983). Major variations

Table 28.1 Procedure for mediolateral episiotomy

Action	Rationale
1. Explain the procedure and indications to the woman and her partner	1. To reassure the woman and confirm consent
2. Place the woman in a comfortable position with her legs open	2. To ensure that the whole perineal area is accessible
3. Cleanse the perineal area using the agreed aseptic technique	3. To minimize infection
4. Place the index and middle fingers into the vagina between the presenting part and perineum. Insert the needle fully into the perineal tissue starting at the centre of the fourchette and directing it midway between the ischial tuberosity and anus	4. To protect the baby from accidental damage
5. Draw back the plunger of the syringe prior to injecting 5–10 ml of local anaesthetic 1% (lidocaine (lignocaine)) slowly into the tissue as the needle is withdrawn	5. To check that the lidocaine (lignocaine) is not accidentally injected into a blood vessel and provide effective anaesthesia to facilitate a pain-free incision
6. Insert the middle and index fingers into the vagina and gently pull the perineum away from the presenting fetal part	6. To protect the presenting fetal part from accidental damage
7. Perform the incision when the presenting part has distended the perineum	7. To minimize pain and blood loss
8. Insert the open scissors between the two fingers and make the incision in one single cut	8. To ensure a straight cut, minimize severe perineal damage and facilitate optimum anatomical realignment
9. Perform the incision – it should extend at least 3–4 cms into the perineum. The incision should start midline from the centre of the fourchette and then extend outwards in a mediolateral direction, avoiding the anal sphincter/s Withdraw the scissors carefully	9. To increase the vulval outlet and facilitate delivery
10. Control delivery of the presenting part and shoulders	10. To prevent sudden expulsion of the presenting part and extension of the episiotomy incision
11. Apply pressure to the episiotomy incision between contractions if there is a delay in delivering the baby	11. To control bleeding from the wound
12. Thoroughly inspect the vagina and perineum following completion of the third stage	12. To identify the extent of trauma prior to repair

in current national rates may indicate uncertain justification for this practice (Audit Commission, 1997).

It is evident that this procedure was introduced without substantial scientific evidence to support either its benefits or risks, and its efficacy remains a centre of controversy. Some argue that episiotomy causes more pain, weakens the pelvic floor structures, interferes with breastfeeding and increases sexual problems (Greenshields and Hulme 1993; Kitzinger and Walters 1981). Others argue that the procedure actually reduces the incidence of severe perineal trauma and prevents overstretching of the pelvic floor muscles, which could lead to long-term problems such as stress incontinence and uterine prolapse (Donald, 1979; Flood, 1982). However, more recent research carried out by Klein and co-workers (1994) found that women who delivered with an intact perineum or tear had less pain, stronger pelvic floor muscles, and better sexual function when compared to those with an episiotomy at 3 months postpartum.

Midwives should restrict the use of episiotomy to specific fetal and maternal indications. Previous randomized controlled trials comparing restricted to liberal use of episiotomy found that a restricted policy is associated with lower rates of posterior perineal trauma, less suturing, and reduction in pain and healing complications

(Carroli and Belizan, 2001). This results in a lower rate of maternal morbidity associated with this procedure and may have significant cost-saving implications for suture materials (Carroli and Belizan, 2001; Sleep *et al.*, 1984).

The question of whether an episiotomy incision should be mediolateral or midline is still relatively unanswered (Carroli and Belizan, 2001). Midline episiotomy is easily repaired and is associated with less blood loss, fewer healing complications, and less pain than a mediolateral incision. However, it has an increased risk of extending and causing damage to the anal sphincters and rectal epithelium (Coats *et al.*, 1980; Klien *et al.*, 1994; Thacker and Banta, 1983). In comparison, an 'appropriate' mediolateral episiotomy is thought to reduce the risk of anal sphincter damage (de Leeuw *et al.*, 2001).

Suturing the perineum

In the UK the theory and technique of perineal repair has been part of the midwifery curriculum since 1983 when midwives were permitted to perform the procedure following appropriate instruction and practical experience (Silverton, 1993). By 1986, midwives were repairing perineal trauma in over 60% of consultant units in England and Wales (Garcia *et al.*, 1986). This practice is associated with many advantages, some of which include continuity of care, prompt sensitive repair, and increased job satisfaction.

Suture materials for primary repair of perineal trauma

The ideal suture material should cause minimal tissue reaction and be absorbed once it has served its purpose of holding the tissue in apposition during the healing process (Taylor and Karran, 1996). Well-aligned perineal wounds heal by primary intention with minimal complications, usually within 2 weeks of suturing. However, if the stitches remain in the tissues for longer than this period, they act as a foreign body and may impair healing and cause irritation. Local infection of the stitches will prolong the inflammatory phase and cause further tissue damage, which will delay collagen synthesis and epithelialization (Flanagan, 1997).

There is also good evidence that perineal repair with an absorbable synthetic material, such as polyglactin 910 (*Vicryl*) or polyglycolic acid (*Dexon*) reduces short-term pain. However, the long-term effects are less clear and there are some concerns regarding the need to remove sutures up to 3 months after delivery (Kettle and Johanson, 2001a).

Recently a new suture material, *Vicryl Rapide*, has become available which has all the properties of other synthetic materials, but because of changes in the manufacturing process its tensile (breaking) strength is lost by 10–14 days and it is totally absorbed by 42 days (Ethicon, 1991). Two studies carried out by Masson *et al.* (1988) and Gemynthe *et al.* (1996) found no short-term adverse effects associated with this new material. More recently, a large randomized controlled trial ($n = 1542$), carried out in the UK, which compared *Vicryl Rapide* with *Vicryl* found no significant differences in short- or long-term pain or wound breakdown (Kettle *et al.*, 2002). However, there was a significant reduction in pain when walking in the *Vicryl Rapide* group, which mirrors the findings of the small study by Gemynthe *et al.* (1996). More importantly, *Vicryl Rapide* was associated with a significant reduction in suture removal. Given that this was the main previous concern with absorbable synthetic sutures, it would appear that *Vicryl Rapide* is the ideal material for perineal repair.

Suture techniques for primary repair of perineal trauma

A systematic review of four randomized controlled trials (Kettle and Johanson, 2001b) found that a continuous subcutaneous technique of perineal skin closure, when compared to interrupted, transcutaneous stitches, was associated with less short-term pain. However, many midwives and students are still taught the interrupted suturing technique, because it is considered easier to learn and may cause fewer problems in the hands of the inexperienced or novice operators (Grant, 1989). In 1990, Fleming published her experience of using a simple non-locking, loose, continuous suturing technique with subcutaneous stitches placed well below the perineal skin surface, thus avoiding the profusion of nerve endings. She found that the continuous method was simple to perform and could easily be taught to relatively inexperienced operators. Women reported low levels of pain following this type of repair and the cosmetic results were good; however, her findings were purely observational. More recently a large randomized controlled trial ($n = 1542$) carried out in the UK compared the loose continuous technique with the more traditional interrupted method (Kettle *et al.*, 2002). The trial found that there was a highly significant reduction in short-term pain associated with the continuous suturing technique, but there was no difference in superficial dyspareunia at 3 or 12 months postpartum.

Non-suturing of perineal skin

A large randomized controlled trial, which compared suturing the vagina and muscle, but leaving the skin unsutured, to the conventional method, whereby the skin was repaired, found no significant difference between groups in short-term pain. However, there was a reduction in dyspareunia at 3 months postpartum (Gordon *et al.*, 1998).

Procedure

Perineal tears and episiotomies are repaired under aseptic conditions with a good source of light and the mother in a comfortable position so that the trauma can be easily visualized. It is not necessary to use lithotomy poles to support the woman's legs during the repair. The act of restraining the woman's legs in stirrups during suturing may bring back locked in memories of sexual abuse making her feel helpless and out of control (Walton, 1994). Furthermore, as suggested by Borgatta (1989) leg restraints (lithotomy poles) cause flexion and abduction of the woman's hips which results in excessive stretching of the perineum, causing the episiotomy

or tear to gape. This, apart from being uncomfortable for the woman, can make the trauma difficult for the operator to realign and suture. There is no need to use a tampon.

If the woman has a working epidural it may be topped-up to give an effective anaesthesia to the perineal area instead of injecting local anaesthetic. However, Khan and Lilford (1987) recommend that even if an epidural is used, the perineal wound should be infiltrated with normal saline or local anaesthetic to mimic tissue oedema and prevent overtight suturing.

Prior to performing the repair, the midwife must prepare the suturing trolley and check equipment according to individual employing authorities' practice policies and guidelines. The woman's comfort and dignity must be maintained throughout the procedure.

The area is usually cleaned with an antiseptic solution but a recent study found that tap water was just as effective as chlorhexidine antiseptic (Calkin, 1996).

The method of performing the repair is shown in Figure 28.3 and the rationale for each stage of the process is given in Table 28.2.

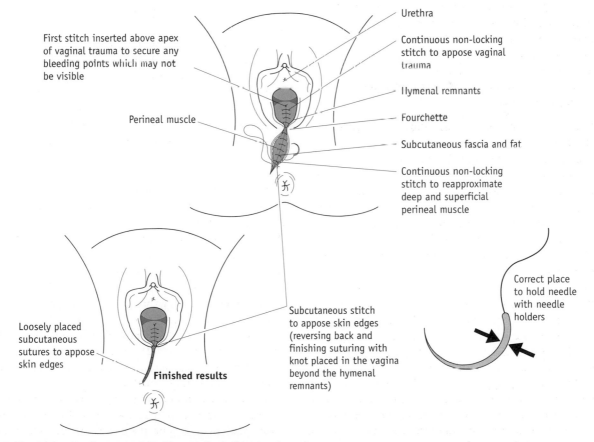

Figure 28.3 Continuous non-locking method of perineal repair.

Table 28.2 Procedure for continuous method of perineal repair

Action	Rationale
1. Explain the procedure to the woman and her partner	1. To reassure the woman and confirm consent
2. Check maternal baseline observations and PV blood loss	2. To ensure that the woman's general condition is stable prior to commencing the repair
3. Assess the extent of perineal trauma	3. To ensure the repair is not beyond the operator's level of competence
4. Ensure that the woman is in an appropriate position	4. To ensure that the whole perineal area is accessible
5. Cleanse the vulva and perineal area. Drape the area with a sterile lithotomy towel	5. To minimize risk of infection.
6. Identify anatomical landmarks. These may include hymenal remnants and tissue of different colour	6. To aid the operator to correctly align and approximate the traumatized tissue *NB*: Misalignment may cause long-term morbidity such as dyspareunia
7. Draw back the plunger of the syringe prior to injecting 10–20 ml of local anaesthetic 1% (lidocaine (lignocaine)) slowly into the traumatized tissue, ensuring even distribution	7. To check that the lidocaine (lignocaine) is not accidentally injected into a blood vessel and to provide effective anaesthesia to facilitate a pain-free repair
8. Identify the apex of the vaginal trauma and insert the first stitch 5–10 mm above this point	8. To ensure haemostasis of any bleeding vessels that may have retracted beyond the apex
9. Suture posterior vaginal trauma using a loose continuous non-locking stitch. Continue to the hymenal remnants taking care not to make the stitches too wide	9. To appose the edges of traumatized vaginal mucosa and muscle without causing shortening or narrowing of the vagina
10. Ensure that each stitch reaches the trough of the traumatized tissue	10. To close dead space, achieve haemostasis and prevent paravaginal haematoma formation
11. Visualize the needle at the trough of the trauma each time it is inserted	11. To prevent sutures being inserted through the rectal mucosa *NB*: A recto-vaginal fistula may form if this occurs
12. Bring the needle through the tissue underneath the hymenal ring and continue to repair the deep and superficial muscles using a loose continuous stitch	12. To realign the perineal muscles, close the dead space, achieve haemostasis and minimize the risk of haematoma formation
13. Reverse the stitching direction at the inferior aspect of the trauma and place the stitches loosely in the subcutaneous layer, approximately 5–10 mm apart	13. To appose skin edges and complete the perineal repair
14. Do not pull the stitches too tight	14. To prevent discomfort from overtight sutures if reactionary oedema and swelling occur
15. Complete the subcutaneous repair to the hymenal ring, swing the needle under the tissue into the vagina and complete the repair using a terminal loop knot	15. To secure the stitches
16. Inspect the repaired perineal trauma	16. To ensure the trauma has been sutured correctly and that haemostasis has been achieved. Check that there is no excessive bleeding from the uterus
17. Insert two fingers gently into the vagina	17. To confirm that the introitus and vagina have not been stitched too tightly
18. Perform a rectal examination	18. To confirm that no sutures have penetrated the rectal mucosa
19. Cleanse and dry the perineal area. Apply a sterile pad	19. To minimize infection
20. Check and record that all swabs, needles and instruments are correct	20. To confirm that all equipment and materials used are complete and accounted for
21. Place the woman in the position of her choice	21. To ensure that the woman is made comfortable following the procedure
22. Complete the appropriate documentation	22. To fulfil statutory requirements and to provide an accurate account of the repair

On completion of perineal repair the woman should be given advice regarding:

- extent of trauma
- what to expect during the healing process
- methods of pain relief
- personal hygiene
- diet and rest
- pelvic floor exercise
- avoidance of constipation
- who to contact in case of long-term perineal pain/dyspareunia or incontinence.

Labial lacerations

These are usually very superficial but they can be very painful. Some practitioners do not recommend that they are sutured but if the trauma is bilateral, the lacerations can sometimes heal together over the urethra and the woman presents with voiding difficulties.

Tissue adhesive

There have been two small trials, which have looked at the use of tissue adhesive for closure of perineal skin following second-degree tear or episiotomy (Adoni and Anteby, 1991; Rogerson et al., 2000). Both trials claim that this method is effective but results must be interpreted with caution owing to the poor methodological design of these studies and the small number of participants included.

Non-suturing of perineal trauma

The effects of not suturing deeper perineal trauma such as second-degree tears or episiotomies have not yet been evaluated in robust clinical trials. However, there appear to be increasing numbers of midwives in the UK adopting a non-suturing policy without reliable evidence to support their practice. The small studies, which have been undertaken, have been of poor methodological quality (Clement and Reed, 1998; Head, 1993; Lundquist et al., 2000) and their results must be interpreted with caution. More recently, an RCT carried out in Scotland (n = 74 primiparous women) found no significant difference between non-suturing and suturing of first and second degree tears in terms of perineal pain. However, significantly more women in the non-sutured group had poorer wound approximation at 6 weeks postpartum compared to the sutured group (Fleming et al., 2003). None of the research to date has examined the long-term effects of this practice relating to alterations in sexual and pelvic floor muscle function. Until sound evidence is available to support this controversial practice midwives must be cautious about leaving trauma other than small first-degree tears unsutured unless it is the explicit wish of the woman. Practitioners must base their practice on scientific principles and sound evidence rather than just personal preference.

Third- and fourth-degree tears

The reported incidence of clinically detectable anal sphincter injuries following childbirth ranges from 0.5–3% (Sultan et al., 1994b; Tetzschner, 1996); however, the full extent of the problem is probably underestimated. Recent research carried out at Queen Charlotte's Hospital has highlighted that a number of third-degree tears are not recognized following vaginal delivery (Groome and Paterson Brown, 2000). They found that with increased vigilance, the diagnosis of anal sphincter disruption could be vastly improved. If this type of trauma is not recognized at the time of delivery, women can be left with long-term problems such as incontinence of faeces and flatulence. The rate of anal incontinence following anal sphincter injury varies between 7–59% (Goffeng et al., 1998; Kamm, 1994; Tetzschner, 1996) but realistically it is probably much higher because women feel embarrassed to disclose their problems. In one study only one-third of the participants with faecal incontinence had ever discussed their problem with a physician (Johanson and Lafferty, 1996).

Midwives and medical staff must be aware of this type of trauma and be adequately trained to identify anal sphincter injuries when they occur.

Associated risk factors are:

- first vaginal delivery
- forceps delivery, which has a higher risk of resulting in severe perineal trauma than vacuum extraction (Johanson et al., 1993; Sultan and Kamm, 1993; Sultan et al., 1994b)
- birthweight greater than 4 kg
- prolonged duration of the second stage of labour (de Leeuw et al., 2001; Wood et al., 1998)
- direct occipitoposterior position at delivery (Sultan et al., 1994b)
- midline episiotomy.

All perineal trauma must be thoroughly examined with the aid of a good light source and the extent of injury must be accurately documented in the hospital case notes. When assessing perineal injury after delivery, a rectal examination should be routinely performed to avoid missing trauma to the anal sphincters.

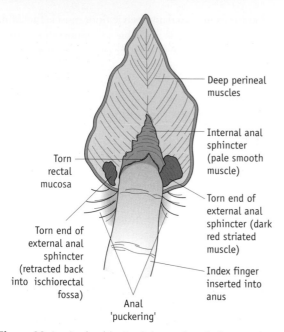

Figure 28.4 Anal sphincter injury – fourth-degree tear.

If a third- or fourth-degree tear is suspected it should be checked by an independent experienced practitioner.

Identification of anal sphincter injury

- Look for absence of 'puckering' around the anterior section of the anus.
- Observe if the trauma extends down to the anal margin.
- Perform a digital rectal examination and ask the woman to contract the anal sphincter. If the external anal sphincter (EAS) is damaged, the torn ends will be observed retracting backwards towards the ischiorectal fossa (Fig. 28.4).

NB: Damage to the internal anal sphincter is much more difficult to detect, as this is a less well-defined paler muscle.

Repair of third/fourth-degree tears

An experienced practitioner who has received specialized training and is competent to carry out the procedure must repair this type of severe trauma. It should be performed as soon as possible, under a general or spinal anaesthetic, in an operating theatre and with appropriate assistance. There are no randomized controlled trials to provide reliable evidence regarding the best method or material for repair of third- and fourth-degree tears. Broad-spectrum antibiotics and a stool softener such as lactulose and a bulking agent (Fibogel) should be prescribed following the repair.

It is important that the woman is given a full explanation of the injury sustained and a contact number to ring if she has any problems during the postnatal period. Follow-up should be provided at specialist clinics so that problems can be sensitively identified and promptly treated. Women with persistent anal problems must be referred for anal manometry, ultrasound scan, and consultation with a colorectal surgeon.

The appropriate management of women who have had previous third-degree tears still remains uncertain. There is no evidence to suggest that performing an episiotomy prophylactically will prevent recurrence of a third-degree tear (Sultan *et al.*, 1994a). Women with long-term problems should be assessed and a joint decision made regarding the mode of delivery for subsequent deliveries.

Professional and legal issues

Litigation or the threat of it is a major concern for all practitioners; however, a competent midwife has little to fear if she works within the parameters of employing authorities' policies, guidelines, and the UKCC *Midwives Rules and Code of Practice* (1998). In an action for damages, practitioners may be held personally liable if it can be shown that they failed to exercise properly the skills expected of them or that they under-took activities outside their level of competence or scope of practice.

Recommendations for future research

There is an urgent need for a large randomized controlled trial to be undertaken comparing non-suturing versus suturing of second-degree perineal trauma with long-term follow-up.

CONCLUSION

Mismanagement of perineal trauma has a major impact on women's health and has significant implications for health service resources. Midwives must base their practice on current research evidence and be aware of problems associated with perineal trauma and repair. Careful identification and repair of trauma by a skilled practitioner may avoid problems. Furthermore, it is important that prompt sensitive treatment is provided for those women with problems in order to reduce the morbidity associated with perineal injury following childbirth.

KEY POINTS

- A restricted episiotomy policy reduces the rates of posterior perineal trauma.
- The use of absorbable synthetic suture material (*Dexon* and *Vicryl*) for repair of perineal trauma is associated with less short-term pain but increased suture removal when compared to catgut. Current evidence indicates a more rapidly absorbed synthetic suture material (*Vicryl Rapide*) when compared to standard material (*Vicryl*) is associated with significantly less perineal pain when 'walking' and suture removal up to 3 months postpartum.
- The loose, continuous non-locking suturing technique for repair of vaginal tissue, perineal muscle and skin is associated with a significant reduction in pain and suture removal compared to the traditional interrupted method.
- It is important to recognize when anal sphincter injury has occurred.
- Pelvic floor exercises during pregnancy and following childbirth help to reduce morbidity.

REFERENCES

Allen, R.E., Hosker, G.L., Smith, A.R.B. *et al.* (1990) Pelvic floor damage and childbirth: a neurophysiological study. *British Journal of Obstetrics and Gynaecology* **97**: 770–779.

Adoni, A. & Anteby, E. (1991) The use of Histoacryl for episiotomy repair. *British Journal of Obstetrics and Gynaecology* **98**: 446–478.

Audit Commission (1997) *First Class Delivery: Improving Maternity Services in England and Wales.* London: Audit Commission Publications.

Benson, J.T. (1992) *Female Pelvic Floor Disorders, Investigation and Management.* London: Norton Medical Books.

Borgatta, L. (1989) Association of episiotomy and delivery position with deep perineal laceration during spontaneous delivery in nulliparous women. *American Journal of Obstetrics and Gynecology* **160**(2): 294–297.

Brayshaw, E. & Wright, P. (1994) *Teaching Physical Skills for the Childbearing Year*, pp. 82–83. Hale: Books for Midwives Press.

Calkin, S. (1996) Chlorhexidine swabbing in labour. *Modern Midwife* **1**: 28–33.

Carroli, G. & Belizan, J. (2001) Episiotomy for vaginal birth (Cochrane Review). *The Cochrane Library*, Issue 1. Oxford: Update Software.

Clement, S. & Reed, B. (1998) To stitch or not to stitch? A long term study of women with unsutured perineal tears. *Practising Midwife* **2**(4): 20–28.

Coats, P.M., Chan, K.K., Wilkins, M. *et al.* (1980) A comparison between midline and mediolateral episiotomies. *British Journal of Obstetrics and Gynaecology* **87**: 408–412.

DeLee, J.B. (1920) The prophylactic forceps operation. *American Journal of Obstetrics and Gynaecology* **1**: 34–44.

de Leeuw, J.W., Struijk, P.C., Vierhout M.E. *et al.* (2001) Risk factors for third degree perineal ruptures during delivery. *British Journal of Obstetrics and Gynaecology* **108**: 383–387.

Derry, D.E. (1935) Notes on five pelves of women of the eleventh dynasty in Egypt. *Journal of Obstetrics and Gynaecology. British Empire* **13**: 490–495.

Donald, I. (1979) *Practical Obstetric Problems.* London: Lloyd-Luke.

Ethicon (1991) *A Unique Product Completes the Family: Ethicon VICRYL Rapide.* Edinburgh: Ethicon.

Flanagan, M. (1997) *Wound Management*, p. 30. New York: Churchhill Livingstone.

Fleming, N. (1990) Can the suturing method make a difference in postpartum, perineal pain? *Journal of Nurse-Midwifery* **35**(1): 19–25.

Fleming, E.M., Hagen, S., Niven, C. (2003) Does perineal suturing make a difference? The SUNS trial. *British Journal of Obstetrics and Gynaecology* **110**: 684–689.

Flood, C. (1982) The real reasons for performing episiotomies. *World Medicine* **6**: 51.

Garcia, J., Garforth, S. & Ayers, S. (1986) Midwives confined? Labour ward policies and routines. *Research and the Midwife Conference Proceedings* 2–30.

Gemynthe, A., Langhoff-Ross, J., Sahl, S. *et al.* (1996) New VICRYL formulation: an improved method of perineal repair? *British Journal of Midwifery* **4**: 230–234.

Glazener, C.M.A., Abdalla, M., Stroud, P. *et al.* (1995) Postnatal maternal morbidity: extent, causes, prevention and treatment. *British Journal of Obstetrics and Gynaecology* **102**: 286–287.

Goffeng, A.R., Andersch, B., Andersson, M. *et al.* (1998) Objective methods cannot predict anal incontinence after primary repair of extensive anal tears. *Acta Obstetricia et Gynecologica Scandinavica* **77**: 439–443.

Gordon, B., Mackrodt, C., Fern, E. *et al.* (1998) The Ipswich Childbirth Study: 1. A randomised evaluation of two stage postpartum perineal repair leaving the skin unsutured. *British Journal of Obstetrics and Gynaecology* **105**: 435–440.

Graham, H. (1950) *Eternal Eve.* London: William Heinemann Medical Books.

Graham, I.D. & Graham, D.F. (1997) Episiotomy counts: trends and prevalence in Canada, 1981/1982 to 1993/1994. *Birth* **24**: 141–147.

Grant, A.M. (1989) Repair of perineal trauma after childbirth. In: Chalmers, I., Enkin, M. & Keirse, M.J.N.C. (eds) *Effective Care in Pregnancy and Childbirth*, Vol. 2, pp. 1170–1181. Oxford: Oxford University Press.

Grant, A., Gordon, B., Mackrodt, C. *et al.* (2001) the Ipswich childbirth study: one year follow up of alternative methods used in perineal repair. *British Journal of Obstetrics and Gynaecology* **108**: 34–40.

Graves, E.J. (1995) 1993 summary: National Hospital Discharge Survey. *Advance Data* May 24 (264): 1–11.

Greenshields, W. & Hulme, H. (1993) *The Perineum in Childbirth: A Survey of Women's Experiences and Midwifery Practices*. London: National Childbirth Trust.

Groome, K.M. & Paterson-Brown, S (2000) Third degree tears. are they clinically underdiagnosed? *Gastroenterology International* **13**(2): 76.

Haadem, K., Ling, L., Ferno, M. *et al.* (1991) Estrogen receptors in the external anal sphincter. *Obstetrics and Gynecology* **164**: 609–610.

Hay-Smith, E.J.C., Bø, K., Berghmans, L.C.M. *et al.* (2001) Pelvic floor muscle training for urinary incontinence in women (Cochrane Review). *The Cochrane Library*, Issue 1. Oxford: Update Software.

Head, M. (1993) Dropping stitches. Do unsutured tears to the perineum heal better than sutured ones? *Nursing Times* **89**(33): 64–65.

Johanson, J.F. & Lafferty, J. (1996) Epidemiology of faecal incontinence: the silent affliction. *American Journal of Gastroenterology* **91**: 33–36.

Johanson, R.B., Rice, C., Doyle, M. *et al.* (1993) A randomised prospective study comparing the new vacuum extractor policy with forceps delivery. *British Journal of Obstetrics and Gynaecology* **100**: 524–530.

Kamm, M.A. (1994) Obstetric damage and faecal incontinence. *Lancet* **344**: 730–733.

Keighley, M.R.B., Radley, S. & Johanson, R. (2000) Consensus on prevention and management of post-obstetric bowel incontinence and third degree tear. *Clinical Risk* **6**: 211–217.

Kettle, C. (1999) *Perineal Tears*. Nursing Times Clinical Monograph. London: Nursing Times Books.

Kettle, C. (2001) Perineal care. In: BMJ *Clinical Evidence – A Compendium of the Best Available Evidence for Effective Health Care*. London: BMJ Publishing Group.

Kettle, C. & Johanson, R.B. (2001a) Absorbable synthetic vs catgut suture material for perineal repair (Cochrane Review). *The Cochrane Library*, Issue 1 (Updated Quarterly). Oxford: Update Software.

Kettle, C. & Johanson, R.B. (2001b) Continuous versus interrupted sutures for perineal repair (Cochrane Review). *The Cochrane Library*, Issue 1 (Updated Quarterly). Oxford; Update Software.

Kettle, C., Hills, R.K., Jones, P. *et al.* (2002) Continuous versus interrupted perineal repair with standard or rapidly absorbed sutures after spontaneous vaginal birth: a randomised controlled trial. *Lancet* **359**(9325): 2217–2223.

Khan, G.Q. & Lilford, R.J. (1987) Wound pain may be reduced by prior infiltration of the episiotomy site after delivery under spinal epidural anaesthetic. *British Journal of Obstetrics and Gynaecology* **94**(4): 341–344.

Kitzinger, S. & Walters, R. (1981) *Episiotomy – Physical and Emotional Aspects*. London: National Childbirth Trust.

Klein, M.C., Gauthier, R.J., Robbins, J.M. *et al.* (1994) Relationship of episiotomy to perineal trauma and morbidity, sexual function, and pelvic floor relaxation. *American Journal of Obstetrics and Gynecology* **171**(3): 591–598.

Labrecque, M., Eason, E., Marcoux, S. *et al.* (1999) Randomised controlled trial of prevention of perineal trauma by perineal massage during pregnancy. *American Journal of Obstetrics and Gynecology* **180**: 593–600.

Labrecque, M., Eason, E. & Marcoux, S. (2000) Randomised trial of perineal massage during pregnancy: perineal symptoms three months after delivery. *American Journal of Obstetrics and Gynecology* **182**: 76–80.

Labrecque, M., Eason, E. & Marcoux, S. (2001) Women's views on the practice of perineal massage. *British Journal of Obstetrics and Gynaecology* **108**: 499–504.

Llewellyn-Jones, D. (1990) *Fundamentals of Obstetrics and Gynaecology, Volume 1 Obstetrics*, 5th edn. London: Faber and Faber.

Lundquist, M., Olsson, A., Nissen, E. *et al.* (2000) Is it necessary to suture all lacerations after a vaginal delivery? *Birth* **27**(2): 79–85.

MacArthur, C., Bick, D. & Keighley M.R. (1997) Faecal incontinence after childbirth. *British Journal of Obstetrics and Gynaecology* **104**: 46–50.

MacArthur, C., Lewis, M. & Bick, D. (1993) Stress incontinence after childbirth. *British Journal of Midwifery* **1**(5): 207–215.

McCandlish, R., Bowler, U., van Asten, H. *et al.* (1998) A randomised controlled trial of care of the perineum during second stage of normal labour. *British Journal of Obstetrics and Gynaecology* **105**: 1262–1272.

Mackrodt, C., Gordon, B., Fern, E. *et al.* (1998) The Ipswich Childbirth Study: 2. A randomised comparison of suture materials and suturing techniques for repair of perineal trauma. *British Journal of Obstetrics and Gynaecology* **105**: 441–445.

Magdi, I. (1949) Obstetric injuries of the perineum. *Journal of Obstetrics and Gynaecology. British Empire* **49**: 697–700.

Mason, L., Glenn, S., Walton, I. *et al.* (2001) The instruction in pelvic floor exercises provided to women during pregnancy or following delivery. *Midwifery* **17**: 55–64.

Masson, F., Bilweis, J., Di Lucca, D. *et al.* (1988) Interest in the new future material for 2000 episiotomy repairs: polyglactin 910. 19/21 Rue du Bois d'Amour 93700, Drancy: Clinique Gynaecologique et Obstetricale.

Mikhailidis, D.P., Bauadas, M.A., Jeremy, J.Y. *et al.* (1983) Cigarette smoking inhibits prostacycline. *Lancet* **2**: 627.

Ould, F. (1742) *A Treatise of Midwifery*. Dublin: Nelson and Connor.

Pomeroy, R.H. (1918) Shall we cut and reconstruct the perineum for every primipara. *American Journal of Obstetric Disease of Women and Child* **78**: 211–220.

Renfrew, M., Hannah, W., Albers, L. *et al.* (1998) Practices that minimize trauma to the genital tract in childbirth: a systematic review of the literature. *Birth* **25**(3): 143–159.

Rogerson, L., Mason, G.C. & Roberts, A.C. (2000) Preliminary experience with twenty perineal repairs using Indermil tissue adhesive. *European Journal of Obstetrics and Gynecology and Reproductive Biology* **88**(2): 139–142.

Shipman, M., Boniface, D., Tefft, M. *et al.* (1997) Antenatal perineal massage and subsequent perineal outcomes: a randomised controlled trial. *British Journal of Obstetrics and Gynaecology* **104**: 787–791.

Silverton, L. (1993) *The Art and Science of Midwifery*. Prentice Hall, London.

Sleep, J., Grant, A., Garcia, J. *et al.* (1984) West Berkshire perineal management trial. *British Medical Journal* **298**: 587–690.

Sleep, J., Roberts, J. & Chalmers, I. (1989) Care during the second stage of labour. In: Chalmers, I., Enkin, M.W. & Keirse, M.J.N.C. (eds) (1989) *Effective Care in Pregnancy and Childbirth*, pp. 1129–1141. Oxford: Oxford University Press.

Statistical Bulletin (2003) *NHS Maternity Statistics, England: 2001–2002*. London: DoH.

Sultan, A.H. & Kamm, M.A. (1993) Ultrasound of the anal sphincter. In: Schuster, M.M. (ed) *Atlas of Gastrointestinal Motility in Health and Disease*, pp. 115–121. Baltimore: Williams & Wilkins.

Sultan, A.H., Kamm, M.A., Bartram, C.I. *et al.* (1994a) Perineal damage at delivery. *Contemporary Review of Obstetrics and Gynaecology* **6**: 8–24.

Sultan, A.H., Kamm, M.A., Hudson, C.N. *et al.* (1994b) Third degree anal sphincter tears: risk factors and

outcome of primary repair. *British Medical Journal* **308**: 887–891.

Sultan, A.H., Monga, A.K. & Stanton, S.L. (1996) The pelvic sequelae of childbirth. *British Journal of Hospital Medicine* **55**(9): 575–579.

Taylor, I. & Karran, S.J. (eds) (1996) *Surgical Principles*, p. 28. London: Oxford University Press.

Tetzschner, T., Sorenson, M., Lose, G. *et al.* (1996) Anal and urinary incontinence in women with obstetric anal sphincter rupture. *British Journal of Obstetrics and Gynaecology* **103**: 1034–1040.

Tew, M. (1990) *Safer Childbirth? A Critical History of Maternity Care*, p. 116. London: Chapman and Hall.

Thacker, S.B. & Banta, D. (1983) Benefits and risks of episiotomy: an interpretative review of the English language literature 1860–1880. *Obstetrics and Gynaecological Survey* **38**(6): 322–335.

United Kingdom Central Council for Nursing, Midwifery and Health Visiting (UKCC) (1998) *Midwives Rules and Code Of Practice*. London: UKCC.

Verralls, S. (1993) *Anatomy and Physiology Applied to Obstetrics*, 3rd edn. London: Churchill Livingstone.

Wagner, M. (1994) *Pursuing the Birth Machine: The Search for Appropriate Birth Technology*, pp. 165–174. Camperdown: ACE Graphics.

Walton, I. (1994) *Sexuality and Motherhood*, p. 125. Hale: Books for Midwives Press.

Wood, J., Amos, L. & Rieger, N. (1998) Third degree anal sphincter tears: risk factors and outcome. *Australian and New Zealand Journal of Obstetrics and Gynaecology* **38**: 414–417.

Woolley, R.J. (1995) Benefits and risks of episiotomy: a review of the English-language literature since 1980. Part II. *Obstetrics and Gynaecology Survey* **50**(11): 821–835.

World Health Organization Maternal and Newborn Health/Safe Motherhood Unit (1996) *Care in Normal Birth: A Practical Guide Report of a Technical Working Group*, p. 29. Doc. No. WHO/FRH/MSM/96.24. Geneva: World Health Organization.

FURTHER READING

Kettle, C. (1999) *Perineal Tears*. Nursing Times Clinical Monograph. London: Nursing Times Books.
This is an overview of perineal trauma and repair following childbirth. Midwives can accrue 5 study hours toward PREP by reading and reflecting on this monograph.

Kettle, C. (2001) Perineal care. In: BMJ *Clinical Evidence – A Compendium of the Best Available Evidence for Effective Health Care*. London: BMJ Publishing Group.
This is an up-to-date overview of the best available evidence on intrapartum interventions relating to perineal trauma.

Kettle, C., O'Brien, S. (2000) *Methods and Materials Used in Perineal Repair*. Royal College of Obstetricians and Gynaecologists Guidelines No 23. London: RCOG.

Woolley, R.J. (1995) Benefits and risks of episiotomy: a review of the English-language literature since 1980. Part II. *Obstetrics and Gynaecology Survey* **50**(11): 821–835.
This is an excellent review covering many controversial aspects of episiotomy.

29

Care in the Second Stage of Labour

Soo Downe

LEARNING OUTCOMES

After reading this chapter you will:

- understand the maternal behaviours associated with transition and the expulsive stage of labour
- have enhanced your knowledge of the basic physiology of transition and the second stage
- appreciate some of the techniques which are currently used in childbirth
- recognize that many midwifery practices in the area of physiological birth are based on empirical but not formal evidence
- understand the importance of clear, comprehensive, accurate record-keeping.

INTRODUCTION

The anatomical second stage of labour has been traditionally defined as the period from full dilatation of the os uteri to the birth of the baby. However, women do not experience labour and birth by its anatomical divisions, or by the dilatation of the cervix. In addition, labours do not usually progress at a uniform rate. Often there is more rapid progress towards the end of the first stage. This leads to distinctive maternal behaviours.

The phase marked by these changes is traditionally defined as 'transition'. There is very little formal evidence about the nature of transition, although some observational studies have noted the fluid nature of the end of the first and beginning of the second stage of labour (Cosner and deJong, 1993; Crawford, 1983; Roberts and Woolley, 1996). Either during this phase, or following on from it, the woman begins to feel a variable urge to bear down. Anecdotal evidence indicates that it is not uncommon for midwives to offer women pain relief if the urge to bear down follows soon after a vaginal examination which has suggested that the anatomical second stage is still some way off. The woman may then be found to have a fully dilated cervical os soon after the pain relief has been administered,

with the consequence that she is less able to respond to the natural urge to bear down actively. It is thus essential that midwives know how to recognize and support women through the transitional phase of labour.

The period during which this bearing down becomes organized and sustained, until the birth of the baby, has been referred to as the expulsive phase of the labour (Cosner and deJong, 1993).

SIGNS OF PROGRESS

Transition

Transition is a phase of the labour which occurs at variable times between the late first stage and early second stage of labour. It is recognizable by a change in the behaviour of the woman, and, sometimes, by a change in the nature of the contractions she is experiencing. Anecdotal accounts by mothers and by on-lookers observing labour indicate that any or all of the following may be noted:

- loss of control; panic
- belief that she cannot carry on
- fearfulness (sometimes of dying)
- disorientation
- nausea

- uncontrollable shivering
- demands for pain relief
- a need to shout and scream
- a slowing of contractions
- a heavy 'show' – a loss per vaginum which is usually a mixture of blood and mucus
- a period when the woman dozes, and goes 'inside herself' (the so-called 'rest and be thankful' phase)
- a variable urge to bear down or to push.

If a vaginal examination is undertaken, the mother's cervical os will typically be found to be between 7 and 9 cm dilated. There have been occasional reports of transition, as evidenced by an early pushing urge, occurring when the cervical os is less than 7 centimetres dilated (Roberts *et al.*, 1987).

Expulsive phase

The strength and consistency of the pushing urge will usually vary in intensity to begin with, becoming more consistent over time. The woman will usually make a characteristic grunting noise at the height of the contraction. She may feel that her bowels are emptying, which may be very embarrassing for her. The midwife will observe the external signs of full dilatation. The perineum bulges and is stretched thin as it is distended by the descending fetus. The anus initially pouts and then dilates with contractions. The vagina begins to gape and finally the presenting part is visible.

Some midwives have also noted another sign of full dilatation, namely the appearance of a rounded area at the level of the lower back, the so-called 'rhomboid of Michaelis' (Burnett, 1969; Sutton and Scott, 1996). Jean Sutton and Pauline Scott, who term this phenomenon the 'rhombus of Michaelis', note that it is caused by 'the pressure of the fetal head [which] … lifts the sacrum and the coccyx out of the way'. They also record their observations that a woman's instinctive reaction to the descent of the fetus is to arch her back, push her buttocks out (or off the bed if she is semi-recumbent) and throw her arms back to grasp on to any fixed object behind them. They hypothesize that this is a physiological response, since it causes a lengthening and straightening of the curve of Carus, optimizing the fetal passage through the birth canal.

Others have noted anecdotally that women who have an epidural in situ often have a sense of discomfort under the ribs as the baby uncurls. This tends to coincide with full cervical dilatation. The efficacy of these observations in predicting the onset of the anatomical second stage of labour remains to be researched.

If necessary, the midwife can carry out a vaginal examination to confirm full dilatation of the os uteri. If no cervix is felt, there is positive confirmation of the onset of the anatomical second stage of labour.

PHYSIOLOGY OF THE SECOND STAGE OF LABOUR

Contractions

On average, at this stage, studies have indicated that contractions have an amplitude of 60–80 mmHg, occur every 2–3 minutes and last for 60–70 seconds, although other patterns of second stage contractions can be effective. Marked retraction of the uterus further aids the descent of the fetus through the birth canal. There is no appreciable fall in the height of the fundus, however, because the fetal back tends to uncurl from its flexed attitude and the lower uterine segment stretches. The force of the uterine contractions and secondary powers is transmitted down the fetal spine to its head. This is called fetal axis pressure and helps the descent of the fetus through the birth canal.

Secondary powers

The expulsion of the fetus is further aided by the voluntary muscles of the diaphragm and abdominal wall. As the presenting part descends to approximately 1 cm above the level of the ischial spines, pressure from the fetal presentation stimulates nerve receptors in the pelvic floor, and the woman experiences the desire to bear down. This is termed the 'Ferguson reflex' (Ferguson, 1941). This sensation may occur prior to the end of the anatomical first stage of labour, or some time after the cervix is found to be fully dilated. The voluntary muscles of the chest and abdominal wall act reflexively in concert with the uterine contractions to overcome the resistance of the vagina, pelvic floor muscles, and external parts. During this process, the diaphragm is lowered and the abdominal muscles contract.

Displacement of the pelvic floor

The advancing fetus gradually stretches the vagina and displaces the pelvic floor. Anteriorly the pelvic floor is pushed up and the bladder is drawn up into the abdomen where it is less likely to be damaged. Posteriorly the pelvic floor is pushed down in front of the presenting part. The rectum is compressed; thus any faecal contents will be expelled. The perineal body becomes elongated and paper-thin as it is flattened by the advancing fetus.

Mechanism of labour

As labour progresses the fetus is moved through the birth canal and induced to make various twists and turns due to the various forces which occur. These movements are called, collectively, the mechanism of labour. They are necessary because the fetus has to adapt to the changing shape of the mother's pelvis during the passage through the birth canal. An understanding of these movements is important to the midwife so that she can assess progress in labour, anticipate the movements of the baby at the time of the birth and recognize when she needs to offer a physiological intervention, or call for assistance.

The widest diameter of the brim of the pelvis is the transverse, whereas the widest diameter of the outlet is the anteroposterior. To make the best use of available space, therefore, the widest presenting diameter of the fetal head enters the pelvis in the transverse diameter. During its passage through the pelvis, first the fetal head and then the shoulders rotate to emerge in the anteroposterior diameter because that is the largest diameter of the pelvic outlet. There is a mechanism for every presentation and position. The commonest presentation is cephalic, with the area of the vertex the presenting part and the position either left or right occipitoanterior. The mechanism for this presentation is as follows:

The lie is longitudinal, the presentation is cephalic and the presenting part is the area of the vertex. The attitude is one of flexion and therefore the denominator is the occiput. The engaging diameter is the suboccipitobregmatic which, on average, measures approximately 9.5 cm. The position may be either right or left occipitoanterior.

Descent

Descent is the process whereby the fetal head becomes engaged in the pelvis (Fig. 29.1). This is more likely to occur prior to the onset of labour in nulliparous women. In multigravid women engagement may not occur until labour is established. This is due to a certain degree of laxity of the uterine and abdominal muscles following previous births. Further descent takes place throughout labour. The pressure of the uterine contractions pushes the fetus down the birth canal.

Flexion

At the beginning of labour the head is usually in an attitude of natural flexion. Flexion is further increased as labour progresses when the head meets the resistance of the birth canal. When the fetal head is flexed, fetal axis pressure is transmitted through the occiput.

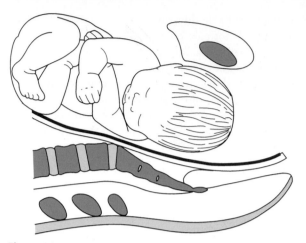

Figure 29.1   Descent of a fetus with a well-flexed head presenting. The sagittal suture is in the transverse diameter of the pelvis.

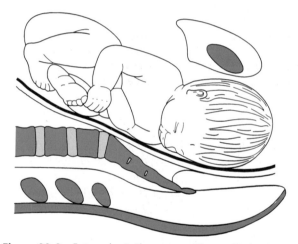

Figure 29.2   Internal rotation occurs. The sagittal suture is in the oblique diameter of the pelvis.

As a result, the occiput is pushed down lower and the forehead is pushed upwards by the resistance of the soft parts, and so complete flexion is obtained.

Internal rotation

When the occiput meets the resistance of the pelvic floor it rotates forward 45°; that is, one-eighth of a circle (Fig. 29.2). The slope of the pelvic floor aids this rotation forwards. Internal rotation allows the head to emerge in the longest diameter of the pelvic outlet; that is, the anteroposterior diameter (Figs 29.3 and 29.4). The occiput then escapes under the pubic arch and the head is crowned.

Crowning of the head

The head is crowned when it has emerged under the pubic arch and no longer recedes between contractions,

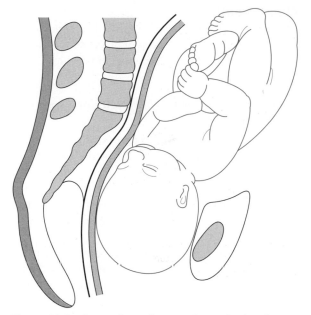

Figure 29.3   Internal rotation complete – further descent occurs. The sagittal suture is now in the anteroposterior diameter of the pelvis. As the head deflexes slightly with descent, the sacrum and coccyx are displaced posteriorly.

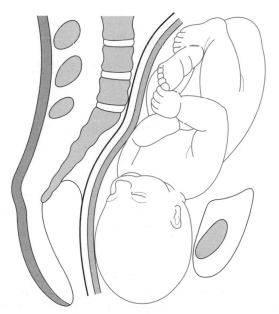

Figure 29.4   The head descended to the vulval outlet.

because the widest transverse diameter of the head (the biparietal diameter) is born (Fig. 29.5).

Extension

Once the head is crowned, extension takes place to allow the bregma, forehead, face and chin to pass over the perineum.

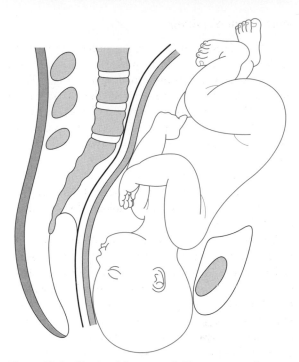

Figure 29.5   The head is crowned. The sacrum and coccyx regain their normal position.

Restitution

When the head is born it rights itself with the shoulders (Fig. 29.6). During the movement of internal rotation the head is slightly twisted because the shoulders do not rotate at that time. The baby's neck is untwisted by restitution.

Internal rotation of the shoulders

The shoulders undergo an internal rotation similar to that of the head and then lie in the anteroposterior diameter of the outlet. The head, being free outside the birth canal, moves 45° at the same time, so internal rotation of the shoulders is accompanied by external rotation of the head. Rotation follows the direction of restitution; thus the occiput turns to the same side of the maternal pelvis as it was at the beginning of labour (Fig. 29.7).

Lateral flexion

In most supine or semi-recumbent maternal birthing positions, the anterior shoulder is born under the pubic arch first, then the posterior shoulder passes over the perineum. If the woman is in a position in which she is leaning forwards, the posterior shoulder may be born first because of the action of gravity and the effect of the curve of the birth canal (known as the curve of Carus). This curve causes the trunk of the baby to flex sideways as it is born.

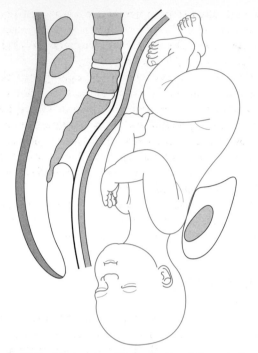

Figure 29.6 The head restitutes to the oblique, in line with the position of the shoulders.

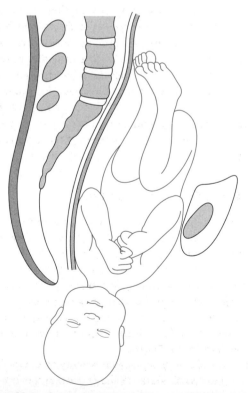

Figure 29.7 Internal rotation of the shoulders leads to external rotation of the head.

After the birth

Once the baby is born, there is a marked retraction of the uterus which starts the process of placental separation. This is completed in the third stage of labour.

DURATION OF THE SECOND STAGE OF LABOUR

The midwife should be aware of the rapidity with which the second stage can progress. Particular care should be taken when supporting multiparous women, since their second stage sometimes lasts only a few minutes. The woman should not be left alone in the late first stage, during the passive second stage or the expulsive stage of labour.

Evidence from research findings indicates that the traditional rigid time limitations set for the second stage are invalid and do not provide a sound guide for practice. It is now generally accepted that in the presence of effective uterine activity, where there is progressive descent of the presenting part and the condition of the mother and fetus does not give rise for concern, time alone does not provide sufficient grounds for curtailment of the second stage (Enkin *et al.*, 2000: 293). Intervention should be based on the rate of progress and the condition of the mother and baby rather than on the time which has elapsed since full dilatation of the cervix.

Many midwives take note of the pattern of progress in previous labours if the woman is multigravid. Some midwives also pay attention to the pattern of labour in the sisters and mothers of the labouring woman. This concept has not yet been tested in formal research studies.

Factors that may slow the progress of the active second stage but which can be corrected by time or by technique include a malpositioned or deflexed fetus (see Case scenario 29.1), and use of pain relief (particularly pethidine or epidural analgesia). Corrective techniques for the former include the use of optimal fetal positioning (Sutton and Scott, 1996). The effect of pethidine will ameliorate with time. Effective corrective techniques for the effects of epidural analgesia include the use of oxytocin in the second stage of labour (Saunders *et al.*, 1989); delaying the onset of active pushing until the fetal head has descended to the perineum (Fraser *et al.*, 2000); changing the concentration of the local anaesthetic (Turner *et al.*, 1988) and letting the epidural wear off in the late first stage (Phillips and Thomas, 1983). This last approach is disliked by many women since the returning sensation of pain is very unpleasant. The use of the lateral position in the passive second stage of labour has been shown to reduce the risk of instrumental birth

Case scenario 29.1

Rose is in labour with her first baby. She has progressed well in the first stage of labour, but the second stage is taking longer than expected. She is coping well, as is the baby. After an hour and a half of good contractions and spontaneous pushing, the vertex still is only just visible. The midwife checks the position of the baby, and finds that it is rather deflexed. As she is establishing this, she feels the head flexing under the pressure of her fingers. Rose experiences a strong contraction and pushes hard, and the midwife feels the head descend significantly. As soon as the midwife has finished her examination, the labour ward coordinator knocks, obtains permission, and enters the room. She states that Rose has been in the second stage long enough, according to the local guidelines, and that it is time to consider calling a doctor to undertake a vacuum extraction. If you were the midwife in this situation, what would you do now?

for a particular sample of nulliparous women using epidural analgesia for pain relief (Downe, 1999) but the generalizability of this finding is not clear.

POSITIONS IN THE SECOND STAGE OF LABOUR

If left to their own devices, most women will move around during their labour and birth, as they instinctively adapt to the position of the baby and the progress of the labour. A woman's choice of birth position may vary from the left lateral in bed, to kneeling or squatting on the bed or on the floor, or supporting herself on her hands and knees. Others may elect to use a birthing chair, ball, or stool, and most maternity units have equipment which will meet some or all of these needs.

The effect of different positions on the length and outcome of labour has been the subject of much interest and investigation in recent years. Gupta and Nikodem (2000) undertook a meta-analysis of controlled studies of positions in the second stage of labour. They noted that in all the parameters they assessed except one, a policy of upright positions led to benefits for women. The exception was an increased risk of estimated blood loss above 500 ml. In interpreting these findings, it should be noted that 'upright' included kneeling, squatting, sitting, use of a birthing chair, and use of a lateral tilt, while 'recumbent' included supine, lithotomy, lateral (without a tilt) recumbent and semi-recumbent, and

dorsal. It has also been observed that where maternal preference was elicited, the most frequent positive responses were from those women who had used an upright position (Sleep *et al.*, 1989).

If the woman does choose to adopt a semi-recumbent position she should be well supported by pillows and perhaps a wedge to prevent her from sliding down and eventually adopting the dorsal position. Should this happen, the heavy gravid uterus is likely to compress the vena cava causing subsequent hypotension, reduced placental perfusion and fetal hypoxia (Humphrey *et al.*, 1974; Johnstone *et al.*, 1987).

Whatever position the woman chooses, the midwife should be able to adapt the principles of care in labour and management of birth appropriately.

MIDWIFERY CARE

During this highly charged period of maximum exertion, the woman should be praised for her efforts and both she and her partner should be kept fully informed of progress made. Information should be given between contractions, when the woman can relax and attend to what is being said. The midwife can help to promote confidence and allay anxiety by adopting a quiet, calm manner. This is further expressed in the midwife's tone of voice, tactile gestures and other non-verbal means of communication. Privacy is essential, and unnecessary intrusion by other care-givers, which may interrupt the woman's concentration, should be avoided. It may help to have a 'do not disturb' sign on the door. Casual conversation between staff over the woman is never acceptable, and is particularly disrespectful at this time.

Hygiene and comfort measures

The extreme exertion of the woman during the second stage of labour is likely to make her feel hot and sticky. She may appreciate having her face and hands sponged frequently to remove perspiration. However, some women find this distracting as it breaks their concentration: it is very much a matter of personal choice. The woman may find drinks of iced water welcome and refreshing. If oral fluids are contraindicated, mouthwashes should be offered.

It is not uncommon for the woman to complain of leg cramps, particularly if she is tensing her muscles during bearing-down efforts, and utilizing the common practice of pulling her knees to her chest. This may be relieved by massage and by extending the leg and dorsiflexing the foot; that is, bending it upwards.

A full bladder will delay progressive descent of the fetus and the bladder may also be damaged by pressure as the fetus advances. Occasionally, if the fetal head has descended deeply into the pelvis and has caused upward displacement of the maternal urinary bladder, the woman may be unable to pass urine and the midwife may also find the passage of a catheter difficult. For this reason it is advisable to encourage regular micturition throughout labour, and especially once the midwife recognizes that the expulsive stage of labour is imminent.

Close attention to the individual nature of the labour enables the midwife to recognize the onset of the transitional phase of labour through the changing behaviour of the woman. The development of expulsive contractions can then be anticipated. Constant observation and care is now necessary and the woman will need the emotional support and skilled care of an attentive midwife.

Support during transition

This phase of labour is very difficult for those attending and supporting the women, as well as for the woman herself. The midwife needs to be a calm and reassuring presence at this time. She also needs to assess each woman carefully, since individuals react in extremely diverse ways at this time. It is important that the midwife responds to the transitional phase appropriately in each individual case. The aim is to enable the woman to regain her ability to cope and to trust in her own ability to birth her baby, so that she can take a positive approach to the active second stage of labour. The midwife should also pay attention to the woman's other birth companions, to ensure that they are reassured that this is a normal part of labour and an indication that the birth of the baby is not far away.

Reflective Activity 29.1

Next time you are with a woman in transition and/or the expulsive phase of labour, ask yourself the following questions. If the answers conflict with local guidelines, or with the usual actions midwives are expected to take locally, consider how these guidelines or informal expectations can be examined by you and your colleagues, with a view to revision.

- Does she want/need pain relief? Could reassurance, support, and faith in her capacity to birth the baby be just as effective?

- Will shouting be helpful for her, or will it increase her panic?
- Are the contractions dying off for pathological reasons, or is it only part of a physiological transition? Is she hungry?
- Is she well hydrated?
- Does she want to be touched or not?
- Is the early pushing urge being felt because of fetal malposition, or is the head just descending very rapidly? Should she push spontaneously if you are not sure the cervical os is fully dilated?
- Is she enabled to adopt any position she wants? What would you do if she throws her arms back and brings her hips forward when she begins pushing?
- Is it difficult not to say 'hold your breath and *push*'?

Support during the expulsive phase of labour

Early bearing-down efforts

It has been traditional for midwives to discourage women from bearing down until the cervical os is known to be completely dilated, particularly in the case of the primigravid woman. This has usually been advised on the assumption that active pushing prior to full cervical dilatation may cause oedema of the os uteri, which will impede or prevent the vaginal birth of the baby. However, a small observational study undertaken with nulliparous women by Roberts *et al.* (1987) found that over half of the participants experienced the desire to bear down prior to full dilatation of the cervix.

Petersen and Besuner (1997) reported on the effects of disseminating a protocol based on the findings of Roberts and colleagues, and of later authors. The protocol was disseminated via the American Association of Women's Health, Obstetric and Neonatal Nurses. A before and after survey indicated a change towards a more liberal response to early bearing-down efforts, with 'no untoward clinical problems'.

The most authoritative advice to date, based on the studies undertaken by Roberts and her colleagues, states that: 'If the cervix is less than 8 cm dilated, the woman should be asked to … try to resist the urge to push …' (Enkin *et al.*, 2000). However, this statement, and the American protocol, are based on very small studies to date. Techniques for helping women to minimize the bearing-down urge include the use of Entonox; the adoption of the left lateral position; controlled breathing techniques; or, at the extremes, the administration of pain relief, including the siting of an epidural. The impact of these techniques, and the consequences of either a liberal or a conservative approach to early bearing down, remain to be tested in larger studies.

Delayed bearing-down efforts

On the other hand, some women may feel little or no desire to bear down when the cervix is fully dilated. This sensation does not usually develop until the fetal presentation descends to compress the tissues of the pelvic floor. There has been recent recognition that some women experience a physiological early or passive phase of the second stage of labour, in contrast to the later active or perineal phase when the woman experiences the irresistible urge to bear down (Roberts and Woolley, 1996).

The role of the midwife in this situation is to ensure that the woman is well hydrated and not ketotic, and to ensure that maternal and fetal well-being are maintained. Assuming all is well, a watch and wait policy can be adopted until the woman begins to experience the bearing-down sensation. For some women, this can be optimized by a change to a more upright position, to encourage descent and the activation of the Ferguson's reflex (Ferguson, 1941).

Case scenario 29.2

Rashida was in labour with her fifth baby. She was attended by a midwife, and an interpreter who was also acting as a labour supporter. The midwife was not really sure if labour was established – however, Rashida was obviously in some pain with the occasional contractions she was experiencing. Through the interpreter, the midwife requested permission to assess the progress of labour by vaginal examination. Rashida indicated that she understood, and was in agreement. The midwife was very surprised to find that the cervical os was soft, but that it only admitted a finger. After discussion, Rashida indicated that she would like an epidural, as she had had one before, and had found it useful. By the time the anaesthetist was in attendance, Rashida was extremely agitated, and beginning to bear down occasionally. The epidural was sited with difficulty. Rashida was still experiencing discomfort, this time under her ribs. The midwife obtained permission to check again for progress. She was astonished to find that no cervix could be felt, and the baby's head was in the mid-cavity of the pelvis. At this point, Rashida found it very difficult to push. The baby was born an hour later, after a lot of hard work with the support of the midwife.

Pushing technique

Organized sustained 'pushing' with contractions, which involves breath-holding (closed glottis pushing, known as the Valsalva manoeuvre) is still practised by some midwives in the belief that it reduces the duration of the second stage of labour and therefore the period of highest risk to the fetus. This practice has been challenged intermittently since the late 1950s (Beynon, 1957). The most recent authoritative statement on the subject, based on a synthesis of the evidence to date, concludes that 'there are no data to support a policy of directed pushing during the second stage of labour, and some evidence to suggest that it may be harmful. The practice should be abandoned' (Enkin *et al.*, 2000).

In the absence of epidural analgesia, the woman should push spontaneously when she feels the irresistible urge to do so and to a self-determined pattern. The observation that the woman tends to push her pelvis forward and arch herself backwards during the second stage of labour throws into question the common practice in many consultant maternity units of encouraging women who use the semi-recumbent position to abduct their legs by bending them and pushing them towards their hips, and to lean forwards as they push. This practice, and the alternatives, require more examination.

There is as yet no good evidence on the optimum advice for women who have an epidural in situ during the second stage of labour. However, in the absence of maternal sensation, some degree of direction from the midwife is probably necessary. Any advice given in this respect should taken note of the evidence that prolonged breath-holding during pushing may be harmful to the fetus (Aldrich *et al.*, 1995).

Perineal practices

A number of practices are used by midwives in an effort to minimize trauma to the perineum. These include the use of hot or cold compresses or of perineal massage as the fetal head advances, and guarding with a gentle, or, in some cases, firm pressure, to maintain fetal flexion, and to support the perineal tissues as they stretch. There is very little evidence for the benefits or risks of hot compresses and perineal massage, or of the various oils and techniques used.

One large trial has been conducted to assess the effect of guarding the perineum (McCandlish *et al.*, 1998). This found a small increase in mild pain at 10 days postpartum in the control group, where guarding was not employed. This finding can be generalized to other similar settings. However, over two-thirds of the women in the study adopted a semi-recumbent or lying down position for the birth of their baby. It is therefore not clear whether the hands-on or hands-poised techniques, as used in the study, would benefit women using other positions in labour.

Assessing the need for episiotomy

An episiotomy is a surgical incision of the perineum to enlarge the vulval orifice. The midwife should be aware that pelvic floor and perineal trauma may have long-term implications for the woman and her partner (Sleep and Grant, 1987). Second-degree lacerations heal as well as episiotomies (Sleep et al., 1984).

Many factors influence the maintenance of perineal integrity, including the condition of both mother and baby and the length of labour. As the head distends the perineum, the midwife may decide that an episiotomy is necessary to prevent a severe perineal laceration, or to expedite the birth if there are definite indications of severe fetal hypoxia. This intervention should not be performed as a routine (Carroli and Belizan, 2000). The possibility of perineal trauma should be discussed with the woman prior to the labour, and her informed choices for this element of labour should be recorded. If an episiotomy becomes necessary, she should be informed, and the midwife should only proceed with her consent. If an episiotomy is considered essential, the perineum should be infiltrated with a local anaesthetic such as 10 ml of lidocaine (lignocaine) 0.5% (i.e. 50 mg) before the episiotomy is performed (see Ch. 28).

OTHER MIDWIFERY TECHNIQUES

Optimal fetal positioning

In recent years, the technique of optimal fetal positioning has become increasingly popular (Sutton and Scott, 1996). This is based on the theory that the modern habit of sitting for much of the day in seating which tips the pelvis back below the level of the knees is contributing to fetal malposition. The protagonists of the technique maintain that teaching women to adopt positions in pregnancy which keep the knees lower than the hips, and which tip the uterus forward, will encourage the fetus to settle in the anterior position prior to labour.

Techniques are also proposed for shifting a baby which is malpositioned or asynclitic in labour. Although most of these are applicable in pregnancy or in the first stage of labour, delay due to malposition in the second stage may be susceptible to one of the interventions

proposed, which involves raising one hip, or rotating the hips, to change the angles of inclination of the pelvis. Sutton and Scott also propose that a woman's instinct to throw her hips forward and her arms back during active pushing should be respected, since this straightens the curve of Carus and optimizes maternal effort. All these observations and techniques have empirical credibility, but remain to be tested formally for their efficacy.

Waterbirth

The therapeutic use of water in childbirth is a relatively new concept which has grown in popularity as some women seek alternative methods of relieving the pain and discomfort of labour. Some women may wish to spend most of their labour and birth in the water pool, others choose to spend short periods and some women may wish to leave the water for the actual birth of the baby and birth of the placenta.

In response to women's requests for this way of labouring and giving birth, many maternity units have installed a purpose-built bath or pool in the labour area. If a home birth is planned, equipment can be hired, structure of the building permitting. Alternatively, use can be made of the domestic bath, although this may not allow maximum freedom of movement for the woman and may also restrict the midwife's activity because of its relatively small size.

As there is as yet no firm research evidence to guide the midwife, it will be necessary to determine the benefits and risks of waterbirth by a careful individual assessment of each woman. In accordance with the midwives' rules and code of practice (UKCC, 1998), the midwife must ensure that she is adequately prepared and competent to undertake this type of labour care. The midwife should also be familiar with the UKCC's current position statement on waterbirths (UKCC, 1996).

A number of theoretical and empirically observed benefits have been identified in association with waterbirths, although some of the evidence is conflicting (Nikodem, 2000). Caution has also been expressed, particularly in respect to the temperature of the water, the risk of maternal or fetal infection, the risk of inhalation if the baby is hypoxic, and the theoretical risk of a water embolus if the mother births the placenta under water. Nikodem's meta-analysis concludes that 'there is not enough evidence to evaluate the use of immersion in water during labour'.

There are now a number of publications which set out the current evidence and the techniques and cautions which carers should pay heed to (Balaskas and

Gordon, 1992; Beech, 1996; Garland 2000). The essential issues to consider are as follows:

Temperature of the water

Respiratory efforts are not initiated until the baby emerges from the water and experiences external stimuli (Jackson *et al.*, 1989). If the water is kept at a constant temperature of 36.5–37.5°C the baby will not lose body heat (Deans and Steer, 1995). A higher water temperature is uncomfortable for the woman and may cause a fetal tachycardia (Nightingale, 1994). Water which is too cool may induce respiration before the baby has been brought to the surface.

Time of entry to water

Balaskas and Gordon (1992) suggest that because relaxation is maximized, too-early immersion in water may inhibit uterine activity. Therefore, unless the contractions are particularly strong or painful, some midwives recommend that the woman should refrain from entering the water before the os uteri is 4–5 cm dilated (Brown, 1998; Nightingale, 1994).

Infection of mother or baby

In her audit of 1082 women booked for a waterbirth, 343 of whom gave birth in the pool, Brown (1998) noted one infected mother and five infected babies. There were no reports of serious morbidity as a consequence. It is possible that such risks may be reduced by using disposable bath linings where possible and by cleaning of the bath after use in accordance with current methods of prevention of cross-infection, such as washing with a sanitizing agent and drying after use. Any faeces which contaminate the water should be removed using a simple plastic strainer. This should be disinfected after use. Once the membranes have ruptured the protection afforded by the intact amniotic sac is missed. Waldenstrom and Nilsson (1992) found that, although there was no statistical difference with respect to infection, respiratory difficulties and signs of maternal amnionitis; babies born more than 24 hours after rupture of the membranes had significantly lower Apgar scores than those born to women who had not had a waterbirth.

The question of hepatitis B or HIV transmission is discussed by Garland (2000) who suggests that, although there is a theoretical risk of transmission to birth attendants, the viruses are fragile, and the effect of water dilution and pool temperature should minimize any risks. Garland also points out that pool births are normally held to be 'no touch' procedures.

Water embolism

Although there is no evidence confirming the risk of water embolism, in theory it may occur when maternal placental bed sinuses are torn in the third stage of labour. Water may then enter the circulation. For this reason it is deemed advisable for the third stage of labour to be conducted out of the water. Any oxytocic preparation, if used, should be given when the woman has left the water.

Perineal trauma

The possibility of perineal trauma should be borne in mind. The midwife should ensure that she is able to provide sufficient verbal support to enable the woman to control her birth, allowing the head and shoulders to emerge slowly during the perineal phase of the second stage of labour.

Monitoring maternal and fetal health

Observations of maternal and fetal well-being are made as for any labour. The fetal heart can be auscultated using an underwater ultrasonic monitor, or a Pinard's stethoscope. The woman should be asked to raise her abdomen clear of the water to aid auscultation. If pain relief is required, inhalational analgesia (Entonox) is suitable. The woman should not be left unattended while using inhalational analgesia during a waterbirth. If narcotic analgesia is required, the woman should be asked to leave the water as the drowsiness induced by the drugs compromises safety.

The baby

The baby should be brought to the surface immediately after birth. The umbilical cord should not be clamped and cut while the baby is still under water because the sudden reduction in placental–fetal blood flow may initiate respiration, and thus water inhalation. When the baby's head is above the surface of the water the cord may be divided. If the umbilical cord needs to be cut prior to the birth of the baby, the woman should be asked to stand with the baby's head clear of the water so that the cord may be clamped and cut before the birth of the shoulders.

PREPARATION FOR THE BIRTH

This is a time of great anticipation and it is now that the true value of the midwife–woman relationship, the strength of the mother, and the skills of the midwife are demonstrated. If the midwife has established a good relationship with the woman and her partner, has enabled the woman to work through her labour with confidence, and has kept the woman and her supporting companions informed of progress and what to expect in the second stage, then the woman and her companions can approach the actual birth with confidence. The atmosphere in the birth room should be calm and unhurried, so that the woman can emerge from the experience with positive memories and intact self-respect. Privacy for the mother must be ensured because it is embarrassing and stressful for her if people repeatedly enter her room.

If the woman is multigravid, the midwife should prepare for birth as soon as she suspects that the second stage is imminent. The primigravid woman usually progresses more slowly and final preparations can therefore be made later during the second stage.

The room should be clean and warm for the birth of the baby. A warm cot is prepared and resuscitation equipment is checked.

THE ACTIVITIES OF THE MIDWIFE DURING THE BIRTH

The actual methods of supporting women during birth can be learned only by experience. However, the principles remain the same and can be applied to whatever position the woman adopts for birth. She should be kept informed at all times, and her wishes must be respected.

A clean area is prepared, including a sterile gown and gloves for the midwife. To prevent contamination from blood or liquor splashes, and the risk of diseases such as HIV, the midwife should also wear unobtrusive eye protection such as plain spectacles. Any other person likely to come into contact with blood or other body fluids should be similarly protected.

Local anaesthetic and syringe are made available for infiltration of the perineum prior to an episiotomy, should it be necessary. If the mother has consented to active management of the third stage of labour a suitable oxytocic drug such as Syntometrine 1 ml or Syntocinon 5–10 units is checked and drawn up in readiness for use. Discussion should have taken place previously regarding active and expectant management (see Ch. 30).

If the woman is recumbent, the vulva is usually washed with warm solution, the birth area draped with clean or sterile towels, and a clean pad placed on the rectum to minimize faecal contamination.

The midwife should be ready to guide the mother's pushing as the head crowns if this is needed, and to cup her hand over the head and the perineum to provide gentle counterpressure if rapid progress seems to be threatening the integrity of the perineum. When women adopt a semi-recumbent position, most midwives maintain flexion by placing the palm of the hand lightly on the head with fingers pointing to the sinciput. However, the head should not be held back by excessive pressure, since this risks overstretching and tearing of the deeper structures of the pelvic floor.

Until the head crowns it will recede between contractions. It crowns when the widest transverse diameter, the biparietal diameter, distends the vulva, and then no longer recedes. During the birth of the head the mother is usually asked to breathe steadily in and out to prevent the birth taking place too quickly. She may use inhalational analgesia if required. Once crowned, the remainder of the head is born by extension. The midwife may change hand position to grasp the parietal eminences to assist in extending the head, if necessary.

When the child's head is born most midwives will check to see if the cord is round the baby's neck. If so, it is normal practice to free the cord, or to make a loop large enough for the shoulders to pass through. There is, however, no evidence that this improves fetal oxygenation, and some midwives report that they will not check for the cord unless the birth seems to be impeded. Rarely, if the cord is so tightly round the neck or shoulders as to prevent the birth of the baby, two pairs of artery forceps must be applied 2–5 cm apart, and the cord cut between them and unwound. However, this procedure should only be performed when absolutely necessary since, once the cord is severed, the baby is no longer oxygenated, and the loss of placental blood flow may further compromise the baby if there is any subsequent delay with the shoulders.

If necessary, such as in the presence of meconium or maternal faecal matter, the babies nose and mouth can be gently suctioned, and the eyes swabbed, from within out, using one swab for each eye. If the woman is in an upright position, any mucus will usually drain spontaneously as the head rests on the perineum prior to internal rotation of the shoulders. At this stage some mothers like to be helped into a position to see their baby's head and watch, or perhaps assist with, the birth of the trunk.

Following restitution and external rotation of the head, the shoulders will normally be in the anteroposterior diameter of the pelvis, although some babies are born with the shoulders in the oblique. If the mother is in the semi-recumbent position, and if the midwife is sure that internal rotation of the shoulders has occurred, the midwife can assist the mother by placing one hand each side of the baby's head. With the next contraction gentle downward traction may be applied to the baby's head. The anterior shoulder will then come down below the symphysis pubis.

If the mother has consented to active management of the third stage of labour, an oxytocic is given as the anterior shoulder is born. The posterior shoulder is then born by guiding the head in an upward direction and the baby's trunk is carried towards the mother's abdomen, being born by lateral flexion. The baby can then be placed on the mother's abdomen, or in her arms, where she can immediately see and touch it. The time of birth is noted.

If the mother is in an upright forward-leaning position, the posterior shoulder will normally be born first, following the curve of Carus. In this circumstance, the midwife usually only needs to be in a position to receive the baby to ensure that it is brought safely to the ground, or into its mothers arms.

For most babies, nasopharyngeal suctioning is unnecessary. However, in the presence of meconium or of excessive mucus, this may be required. There is some debate as to whether the umbilical cord should be cut before or after the vessels have finished pulsating (Enkin *et al.*, 2000: 303–304). Whenever it is severed, it is first clamped with two artery forceps. It is cut between the forceps with blunt-ended scissors, and then sealed close to the umbilicus, usually with a plastic clamp. Once the cord is cut, the mother can then hold her baby more comfortably in her arms. It is important to ensure that the baby is gently dried and covered warmly to prevent excessive heat loss, while maintaining the skin-to-skin contact with its mother which appears to be an important component of early breastfeeding success (Bier *et al.*, 1996). This is an ecstatic moment for the parents and the midwife is privileged to share their joy in the birth of their baby.

OBSERVATIONS AND RECORDINGS

Transition and the second stage of labour are very demanding for both the woman and the fetus. It is a time when the possibility of fetal hypoxia in a previously compromised baby increases as the alteration in uterine activity reduces placental–fetal oxygenation (Katz *et al.*, 1987). It is also a time when the capacity of the woman to birth her baby is most tested. It is therefore important to continually assess the well-being of mother and fetus.

Recordings should include any discussions with the mother, and any decisions she has taken about the way the labour is conducted. The decisions and actions of the midwife must also be recorded. The woman's general condition and state of mind are noted. Her pulse is taken regularly (usually every 15-minutes) to rule out rare acute problems such as intrauterine infection, or a concealed intrapartum haemorrhage. Provided the blood pressure has been within normal limits, and there is no history of hypertension, it does not need to be recorded unless there is cause for concern, or the second stage is prolonged. The frequency, strength and duration of uterine contractions are observed, as well as the relaxation of the uterus between contractions. Any sustained loss of uterine activity will result in delayed progress. The midwife will need to reassess the situation to establish the likely cause, and either remedy the situation or seek assistance if necessary.

The fetal heart is auscultated towards the end of each contraction. If continuous electronic fetal heart monitoring is in progress, the cardiotocograph trace should be analysed and the midwife should assess its normality. The amniotic fluid is observed for meconium staining. In a breech presentation thick fresh meconium is commonly passed at this stage owing to the immense pressure exerted on the breech. There is some debate about the significance of meconium in cephalic presentations. While all authorities agree that thick fresh meconium in a cephalic presentation is a serious sign of fetal hypoxia, and that it poses a major risk of meconium aspiration syndrome for the neonate, the significance of the presence of thin, old meconium is subject to more controversy (Enkin *et al.*, 2000: 268–269).

All observations, including the timing of the various stages and phases of the labour, must be recorded in locally approved labour records. Independent midwives are advised to agree their records in collaboration with their local supervisor of midwives. All actions taken by the midwife must be noted. Each entry must be dated, timed, and signed legibly.

FUTURE RESEARCH IN THIS AREA

There has been an increase in interest in the nature of normal birth and its consequences over the last few years. Some examples of the areas of research which are likely to grow over the next few years are given below:

Physiological and biochemical outcomes of neonates and infants: comparisons between physiological birth and elective caesarean section   Studies in this area have already found differences in neonatal and infant parameters such as phagocyte function (Gronlund *et al.*, 1999), persistent pulmonary hypertension (Levine *et al.*, 2001), gut flora colonization (Hall *et al.*, 1990) and stress response (Taylor *et al.*, 2000). Such research is very likely to expand in the near future.

Studies of techniques in the second stage of labour
Participants are currently being recruited in Australia for a large randomized study looking at the efficacy of optimal fetal positioning. A further large Canadian study is at the design stage. An RCT assessing the use of topical analgesia for perineal discomfort in the late expulsive stage of labour is currently recruiting in Bristol.

Studies of the nature of and culture around normal birth   An increasing interest in this area is likely to attract research from those working in a wide range of disciplines in order to assess the normal physiology of labour, and the short- and longer-term physiological, psychological, social, and emotional effects on mother and baby (Downe, 2000).

CONCLUSION

For many years it has been assumed that the second stage of labour can be strictly delimited and predicted. Increasing attention to the actual experiences of women has led to more formal recognition of the fluidity of the phases of labour, and to an acknowledgement of the nature of transition. While many of these hypotheses about transition and the second stage remain to be tested by formal research, they have strong observational and anecdotal validity. Whatever the eventual findings of future research in this area, transition and the expulsive stage of labour remain times of intense hard work, profound psychological impression, and great exhilaration for the mother, her partner, and possibly her baby. The empathetic and skilled midwife is an essential companion on the journey to motherhood which is represented by this stage of labour.

KEY POINTS

- Transition and second stage can be very intense, both physically and emotionally. Maternal behaviour is usually a good indication of progress during this time.
- It is an essential midwifery skill to understand the physiology and the mechanisms of this phase of labour, and to be able to apply this knowledge in different situations.
- A skilled midwife can offer unobtrusive support and care while ensuring the well-being of the mother and baby.

- Clear, comprehensive record-keeping is essential.
- Empirical evidence indicates that traditional and new midwifery skills can be beneficial, but there are many gaps in the research evidence in this area, and in understanding the nature of normal birth.
- Such studies as there have been in this area generally indicate that the second stage of labour can generally be left to progress according to the pattern and activities of the individual woman.

REFERENCES

Aldrich, C.J., D'Antona, D., Spencer, J.A. *et al.* (1995) The effect of maternal pushing on fetal cerebral oxygenation and blood volume during the second stage of labour. *British Journal of Obstetrics and Gynaecology* **102**(6): 448–453.

Balaskas, J. & Gordon, Y. (1992) *Waterbirth*. London: Thornson Publishers.

Beech, B.A.L. (ed) (1996) *Water Birth Unplugged: Proceedings of the First International Water Birth Conference*. Cheshire: Books for Midwives Press.

Beynon, C.L. (1957) The normal second stage of labour: a plea for reform of its conduct. *Journal of Obstetrics and Gynaecology. British Empire* **64**: 815–820.

Bier, J.A., Ferguson, A.E., Morales, Y. *et al.* (1996) Comparison of skin-to-skin contact with standard contact in low-birth-weight infants who are breast-fed. *Archives of Pediatrics and Adolescent Medicine* **150**(12): 1265–1269.

Brown, L. (1998) The tide has turned: audit of water birth. *British Journal of Midwifery* **6**(4): 236–243.

Burnett, C.W.F. (1969) *The Anatomy and Physiology of Obstetrics: A Short Textbook for Students and Midwives.* London: Faber and Faber.

Carroli, G. & Belizan, J. (2000) Episiotomy for vaginal births (Cochrane Review). *The Cochrane Library,* Issue 4. Oxford: Update Software.

Cosner, K.R. & deJong, E. (1993) Physiologic second-stage labor. *Maternal–Child Nursing Journal* 18: 38–43.

Crawford, J.S. (1983) The stages and phases of labour: an outworn nomenclature that invites hazard. *Lancet* 2(8344): 271–272.

Deans, A.C. & Steer, P.J. (1995) Labour and birth in water. Temperature of pool is important. (Letter) *British Medical Journal* 311(7001): 390–391.

Downe, S. (1999) *Reducing the Risk of Adverse Outcome for Nulliparous Women using Epidural Analgesia in Labour.* PhD thesis. Derby: University of Derby.

Downe, S. (2000) A proposal for a new research and practice agenda for birth. *MIDIRS Midwifery Digest* 10(3): 337–340.

Enkin, M., Keirse, M.J.N.C., Neilson, J. *et al.* (2000) *A Guide to Effective Care in Pregnancy and Childbirth,* 3rd edn. Oxford: Oxford University Press.

Ferguson, J.K. (1941) A study of the motility of the intact uterus at term. *Surgical Gynaecology and Obstetrics* 73: 359–366.

Fraser, W.D., Marcoux, S., Krauss, I. *et al.* (2000) Multicenter, randomized, controlled trial of delayed pushing for nulliparous women in the second stage of labor with continuous epidural analgesia. *American Journal of Obstetrics and Gynecology* 182(5): 1165–1172.

Garland, D. (2000) *Waterbirth: An Attitude to Care,* 2nd edn. Oxford: Books for Midwives Press.

Gronlund, M.M., Nuutila, L.P., Pelto, L. *et al.* (1999) Mode of delivery directs the phagocyte functions of infants for the first 6 months of life. *Clinical and Experimental Immunology* 116: 521–526.

Gupta, J.K. & Nikodem, V.C. (2000) Woman's position during second stage of labour (Cochrane Review). *The Cochrane Library,* Issue 4. Oxford: Update Software.

Hall, M.A., Cole, C.B., Smith, S.L. *et al.* 1990 Factors affecting the presence of faecal lactobacilli in early infancy. *Archives of Disease in Childhood* 65(2): 185–188.

Humphrey, M.D., Chang, A., Wood, E.C. *et al.* (1974) A decrease in fetal pH during the second stage of labour when conducted in the dorsal position. *British Journal of Obstetrics and Gynaecology. British Commonwealth* 81(8): 600–602.

Jackson, V., Corsaro, M., Niles, C. *et al.* (1989) Incorporating waterbirths into nurse-midwifery practice. *Journal of Nurse–Midwifery* 34(4): 193–197.

Johnstone, F.D., Aboelmagd, M.S. & Harouny, A.K. (1987) Maternal posture in second stage and fetal acid–base status. *British Journal of Obstetrics and Gynaecology* 94(8): 753–757.

Katz, M., Lunenfeld, E., Meizner, I. *et al.* (1987) The effect of the duration of the second stage of labour on the acid–base state of the fetus. *British Journal of Obstetrics and Gynaecology* 94(5): 425–430.

Levine, E.M., Ghai, V., Barton, J.J. *et al.* (2001) Mode of delivery and risk of respiratory diseases in newborns. *Obstetrics and Gynecology* 97(3): 439–442.

McCandlish, R., Bowler, U., van Asten, H. *et al.* (1998) A randomised controlled trial of care of the perineum during second stage of normal labour. *British Journal of Obstetrics and Gynaecology* 105(12): 1262–1272.

Nightingale, C. (1994) Waterbirth in practice. *Modern Midwife* 4(1): 15–19.

Nikodem, V.C. (2000) Immersion in water in pregnancy, labour and birth (Cochrane Review). *The Cochrane Library,* Issue 4. Oxford: Update Software.

Petersen, L. & Besuner, P. (1997) Pushing techniques during labour: issues and controversies. *Journal of Obstetric, Gynecologic and Neonatal Nursing* 26(6): 719–726.

Phillips, K.C. & Thomas, T.A. (1983) Second stage of labour with or without extradural analgesia. *Anaesthesia* 38(10): 972–976.

Roberts, J. & Woolley, D. (1996) A second look at the second stage of labor. *Journal of Obstetric, Gynecologic and Neonatal Nursing* 25(5): 415–423.

Roberts, J.E., Goldstein, S.A., Gruener, J.S. *et al.* (1987) A descriptive analysis of involuntary bearing down efforts during the expulsive phase of labour. *Journal of Obstetric, Gynecologic and Neonatal Nursing* 16(1): 48–55.

Saunders, N.J. St. G., Spiby, H., Gilbert, L. *et al.* (1989) Oxytocin infusion during second stage of labour in primiparous women using epidural analgesia: a randomised double blind, placebo controlled trial. *British Medical Journal* 299(6713): 1423–1426.

Sleep, J. & Grant, A. (1987) West Berkshire Perineal Management Trial: a three year follow-up. *British Medical Journal* 295(6601): 749–751.

Sleep, J., Grant, A., Garcia, J. *et al.* (1984) West Berkshire Perineal Management Trial. *British Medical Journal* 289(6445): 587–590.

Sleep, J., Roberts, J. & Chalmers, I. (1989) Care during the second stage of labour. In: Chalmers, I., Enkin, M. & Keirse, M. (eds) *Effective Care in Pregnancy and Childbirth,* Vol. 2. Oxford: Oxford University Press.

Sutton, J. & Scott, P. (1996) *Understanding and Teaching Optimal Fetal Positioning,* 2nd edn. Tauranga, NZ: Birth Concepts.

Taylor, A., Fisk, N.M. & Glover, V. (2000) Mode of delivery and subsequent stress response. *Lancet* 355: 120.

Turner, M.J., Sil, J.M., Alagesan, K. *et al.* (1988) Epidural bupivacaine concentration and forceps birth in primiparae. *Journal of Obstetrics and Gynaecology* 9(2): 122–125.

United Kingdom Central Council for Nursing, Midwifery and Health Visiting (UKCC) (1998) *Midwives Rules and Code of Practice.* London: UKCC.

United Kingdom Central Council for Nursing, Midwifery and Health Visiting (UKCC) (1996) *Waterbirths: The Current Position*. London: UKCC.

Waldenstrom, U. & Nilsson, C.A. (1992) Warm tub bath after spontaneous rupture of membranes. *Birth* **19**(2): 57–63.

FURTHER READING

Davis, E. (1992) *Heart and Hands: a Midwife's Guide to Pregnancy and Birth*, 2nd edn. Berkeley, Celestial Arts.
This is a manual of midwifery based on the skills and experiences gained by lay midwives working in America. It offers some unique tips and insights.

Floyd-Davis, R. & Sargent, C.F. (1997) *Childbirth and Authoritative Knowledge: Cross-Cultural Perspectives*. California: University of California Press.
A seminal work, which explores how authority is given to certain kinds of knowledge, and how the knowledge and expertise of women and of less dominant cultures is not privileged, even in the area of childbirth, and even in the face of the evidence.

Leap, N. & Hunter, B. (1993) *The Midwife's Tale: An Oral History from Handywoman to Professional Midwife.* London, Scarlet Press.
This is an historical account of trained midwives and laywomen practising in the 1950s. The stories of their experiences and responsibilities while attending women in labour are fascinating. The final chapter offers some accounts of labours from the point of view of women themselves.

30

Care in the Third Stage of Labour

Tina Harris

LEARNING OUTCOMES

At the end of this chapter the reader will be able to:

- describe the physiology of the third stage of labour
- explore the concept of choice in relation to management of the third stage
- differentiate between expectant and active management

- outline the development of active management within the UK
- explore the debate between active and expectant management and implications for midwifery practice
- identify how to examine the term placenta and membranes.

INTRODUCTION

The period from the birth of the baby until expulsion of the placenta and membranes is known as the third stage of labour. It is during this phase of the birthing process that mother and child meet face to face for the first time – a moment long anticipated. From frantic activity to quiet contemplation, at last the woman giving birth has the opportunity to welcome her baby; to touch and explore and reassure herself that the child has coped well with the rigours of the birthing process. It is a time of great importance, when the actions of those present can have a long-term effect on developing family relationships and successful breastfeeding (Righard and Alade, 1990). It is also a time when the placenta will separate from the uterine wall, descend into the lower uterine segment and be expelled together with the membranes.

The skill and expertise of the midwife continue to be needed to support this special time between mother, baby and family whilst monitoring successful completion of the childbirth process.

Traditionally this period of childbirth has been regarded as 'hazardous' because of the risk of excessive bleeding. Haemorrhage is the commonest cause of maternal death in the world (WHO, 1994) and in the early 20th century was a significant cause of maternal

death in the UK (DoH, 1957). However, currently within the UK, a very small number of women die as a result of excessive bleeding and these cases are usually associated with medical or childbirth complications (DoH, 2001). This low rate of haemorrhage has been attributed to the prophylactic or routine use of active management in the third stage of labour for all women.

Active management is a package of care which includes the administration of an oxytocic drug such as Syntocinon or Syntometrine, early clamping and cutting of the cord and the speedy delivery of the placenta, usually by cord traction.

While the benefits of active management cannot be questioned for women at risk of postpartum haemorrhage, its indiscriminate use for women at low risk experiencing normal birth has been challenged (Harris 2001; Odent, 1998; WHO, 1999). Active management is not without risk and the component of active management which reduces blood loss has still not been clearly identified. The WHO suggest that the 'use of routine oxytocin and/or controlled cord traction be used with caution until further research can be carried out as there is currently insufficient evidence to support a clear recommendation' (WHO, 1999: 50).

An alternative to active management is expectant management. Also called 'passive', 'physiological', or 'natural' management. This is a package of care where there is no active intervention in the normal physiological processes. It is characterized by activity on the part of the woman in birthing the placenta and membranes herself; the midwife's role is one of 'watchful waiting'.

The role of the midwife during the third stage of labour is:

- to offer women a choice of care relevant to their individual needs
- to support and monitor the normal physiological, sociological and psychological processes at work
- to detect those women who deviate from the normal and offer appropriate care which may include active management of the third stage.

In achieving this, midwives need to have an understanding of the physiology of the third stage and be able to develop partnerships with women to achieve successful delivery of the placenta and membranes with the appropriate rather than indiscriminate use of intervention.

CHOICES FOR THE THIRD STAGE OF LABOUR

It is suggested that women often are not given information about the third stage and do not choose how it will be managed. If women are to benefit from controlling their birth experience then this should include the third stage of labour.

Ideally, discussion about the third stage should take place antenatally to allow the woman and her partner to consider the information given and to make an informed choice. Following the discussion, the woman's choice should be recorded clearly in her notes.

Checklist of issues to be discussed when talking about management of the third stage of labour:
- What is meant by the third stage of labour.
- What happens during the third stage of labour.
- Meeting the infant for the first time – importance of close contact.
- Expulsion of the placenta and membranes.
- Discussion regarding the ways in which the third stage of labour is managed: benefits/limitations of each approach.
- Situations in which expectant and active management may be appropriate.

The midwife needs to pay careful attention to offering women clear information, which should be as value free as possible.

Reflective Activity 30.1

Take a few minutes to jot down notes on your feelings about the third stage of labour and how it should be managed in women experiencing normal birth. How may your personal feelings influence a woman's choice of management for the third stage?

Some midwives struggle in offering women this choice for a variety of reasons.

- Current evidence appears to support the continued use of prophylactic active management for all women (Prendiville *et al.*, 2000).
- The majority of midwives in practice will have trained during the period when active management was regarded as appropriate for all women and to be recommended (Harris, 2001).
- Some midwives may have either little or no experience of managing the third stage of labour expectantly and lack confidence in this form of care (Featherstone, 1999).

If women are to have a real choice, then consideration needs to be given to educating and supporting midwives in clinical practice and in developing a reflective analytical approach to discussions about the third stage which take place between midwives and women.

PHYSIOLOGY OF THE THIRD STAGE

The third stage of labour is not really a stage at all. It is an extension of what has gone before (i.e. the process of giving birth) and what will happen afterwards (the control of bleeding and the return of the uterus to its non-pregnant state). During labour the uterine muscles contract and retract under the influence of naturally produced oxytocin. These muscles continue to contract and retract during the third stage to expel the placenta and membranes. The control of bleeding is brought about by the same physiological processes.

Separation of the placenta usually begins with the contraction which delivers the baby's trunk and is completed with the next one or two contractions. As the baby is delivered, there is a marked reduction in the size of the uterus because of the powerful contraction and retraction which take place. The placental site therefore greatly diminishes in size. Initially, placental separation was thought to be brought about by the bursting of decidual sinuses under pressure and the

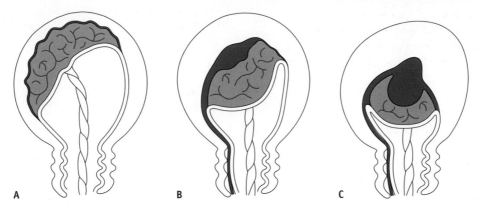

Figure 30.1   Phases in the third stage of labour. **A.** *Latent phase*: characterized by a thick placenta-free wall and thin placental site wall. **B.** *Detachment phase*: characterized by a gradual thickening of the uterine wall over the site of placental attachment. This process can be monophasic (a constant shearing off movement) or multiphasic (which is characterized by pauses between phases of active detachment). **C.** *Expulsion phase*: the uterine wall is uniformly thickened and drives the placenta into the lower segment for expulsion.

subsequent forming of a retroplacental blood clot which tore the septa of the spongiosa layer of the decidua basalis, detaching the placenta from the uterine wall (Brandt, 1933). However, Dieckmann *et al.* (1947) and more recently Herman *et al.* (1993) suggest separation is caused by the active placental site uterine wall thickening and reducing in size, causing the placenta to 'shear off'. It is suggested that blood collecting on the maternal surface of the placenta as it separates is an incidental finding. Krapp *et al.* (2000) described three phases to the third stage of labour (Fig. 30.1). These three phases have now been widely accepted as describing the process of placental detachment and expulsion (Herman, 2000).

- *Latent phase*: period of time from delivery of the infant until the beginning of placental separation. During this phase the placenta-free uterine wall thickens under the influence of intermittent contractions, with minimal thickening of the uterine wall over the placenta. Median duration 141 seconds (range 5–790).
- *Detachment phase*: period of placental separation and detachment from the uterine wall. This is brought about by gradual thickening of the uterine wall over the site of placental attachment. The myometrium adjacent to the lower edge of the placenta contracts, thickens and reduces its surface area overall, which leads to a shearing off of the placenta in that area. This wave of placental wall thickening and placental separation continues upwards and outwards until the whole placenta is detached. Median duration 50

seconds (range 15–100). Separation of the placenta from the uterine wall is normally achieved within 3 minutes.

- *Expulsion phase*: period from complete separation of the placenta to vaginal expulsion. The upper uterine segment contracts strongly, forcing the placenta to fold in on itself and descend into the lower segment and from there to the vagina. Gravity and sometimes maternal effort brought about by stimulation of the pelvic floor, lead to expulsion of the placenta and membranes. Median duration 80.5 seconds (range 2–385).

In the work by Krapp *et al.* (2000) median length of the third stage was calculated to be approximately 6 minutes in both active and expectant management. (See Fig. 30.2)

Cord clamping   If the umbilical cord remains intact during the 3rd stage, blood can pass to and from the infant until cord pulsation has ceased. The amount of blood gained or lost by the baby will depend on its position (above, at, or below the level of the uterus) and uterine activity (Harris, 2001). The infant can gain up to 80 ml of blood in this way (Yao and Lind, 1974). It is suggested that if the cord is clamped early the resulting extra fetal blood retained in the placenta prevents it from being so tightly compressed by the uterus. As a result, contraction and retraction of the uterus may be less effective, and maternal blood loss increased, leading to a greater retroplacental blood clot being formed. Botha (1968) does not consider the

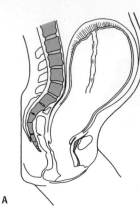
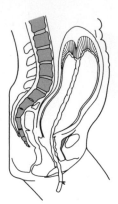

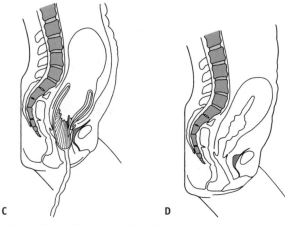

Figure 30.2   The mechanism of placental separation. **A.** The placenta before the child is born. **B.** The placenta partially separated immediately after the birth of the child. **C.** The placenta completely separated. **D.** The placenta expelled and the uterus strongly contracted and retracted.

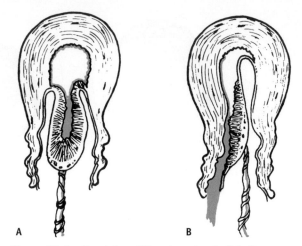

Figure 30.3   Expulsion of the placenta: **A.** Schultze method; **B.** Matthews Duncan method. (From Bennett and Brown 1999.)

- Abdominally, the uterus rises up to sit on top of the descended placenta, which can resemble a full bladder as it lies in the lower uterine segment (sign of descent).
- The cord lengthens (sign of descent).

Presentation of the placenta at the vulva

During the expulsive phase, the placenta may appear at the vagina in one of two ways (Fig. 30.3).

Schultze   The placenta appears fetal surface first like an inverted umbrella with the membranes trailing behind. Any blood lost during the third stage will collect on the maternal surface of the placenta and be encased by the membranes. Over 80% of placentae are delivered in this way (Akiyama *et al.*, 1981).

Matthew Duncan   Less commonly, the placenta slips from the vagina sideways and the maternal surface appears at the vulva first. Midwives often use the term 'dirty Duncan' for this type of presentation because more bleeding is seen vaginally – blood escapes immediately from the placental site because it is not encased in the membranes. This is often associated with slower separation of the placenta and ragged membranes.

Control of bleeding

Following placental expulsion, several mechanisms come into play to control bleeding from maternal sinuses at the site of placental attachment.

formation of a retroplacental blood clot a physiological process. Rather it occurs as a result of intervention, in this case the clamping of the cord.

Detachment of the membranes begins in the first stage of labour, when separation occurs around the internal os. In the third stage complete separation takes place assisted by the weight of the descending placenta, which peels them from the uterine wall.

During the process of separation descent and expulsion of the placenta, a number of clinical signs may be seen.

- A small amount of blood oozes from the placental bed and tracks down between the membranes and appears as a gush of blood per vagina (sign of separation).

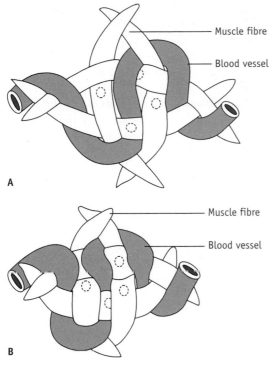

A

B

Figure 30.4 How the blood vessels run between the interlacing muscle fibres of the uterus. **A.** Muscle fibres relaxed and blood vessels not compressed. **B.** Muscle fibres contracted, blood vessels compressed and bleeding arrested.

1. The empty uterus fully contracts and the uterine walls come into apposition.
2. The myometrium continues to contract and retract intermittently. The interlacing muscle fibres (known as living ligatures) constrict the torn blood vessels sealing them (see Fig. 30.4).
3. The process of blood clotting at the site of placental attachment is initiated and the area quickly becomes covered with a fine protective mesh.

Any factor which interferes with the normal physiological processes can influence the outcome of the third stage of labour (see Box 30.1). This includes a variety of complications of pregnancy and childbirth (Gilbert *et al.*, 1987) as well as the action of individual midwives (Logue, 1990). Oxytocic drugs given prior to and during the third stage of labour also influence events. A woman's ability to avoid complications will also be based on her general health and by avoiding predisposing factors such as anaemia, ketosis, exhaustion and hypotonic uterine action.

Box 30.1 Factors that may interfere with the physiological processes of the third stage of labour

- Previous postpartum haemorrhage
- Anaemia
- Clotting disorders
- Pregnancy-induced hypertension
- Overdistended uterus as in polyhydramnios, twins, fibroids
- Grand multiparity
- Induction/augmentation of labour
- Poor uterine action during labour and delivery
- Long first or second stage of labour
- Instrumental delivery
- Oxytocic drugs
- Dehydration during labour
- Full bladder at onset of the third stage of labour
- How the third stage of labour is managed

Reflective Activity 30.2

As a midwife supporting a woman during the third stage of labour, how might you detect the difference between the latent phase, the contraction phase and the expulsive phase of the third stage of labour?

MANAGEMENT OF THE THIRD STAGE OF LABOUR

Commonly, midwives describe two ways of managing the third stage: active management and expectant management. However, difficulties remain in defining what these terms mean, as midwives practice both methods in a variety of different ways (Harris, 2000). The most commonly described form of each management will be outlined here with discussion about where variation may take place. The woman in conjunction with her midwife will have discussed options for the third stage during the antenatal period and again during labour and made a decision over which management she would like.

Expectant management

Expectant management is one of 'watchful anticipation' and draws upon the normal physiological processes to bring about expulsion of the placenta and membranes. The woman is active during this process and the midwife's role is a passive one involving close observation and encouragement.

Principles of expectant management

Positioning the baby after birth Whichever position a woman chooses to give birth in, the newborn infant will be placed either on the bed/floor between the woman's legs or on the woman's abdomen, depending on her choice. Early skin-to-skin contact is advantageous in maintaining the infant's temperature, in promoting successful breastfeeding and in supporting development of mother–infant attachment. The midwife then steps back to leave the woman and her family to experience undisturbed the powerful first meeting with their new baby, while continuing to observe the well-being of the infant and maternal vaginal blood loss.

When to cut the cord There is some debate about when the cord should be clamped and cut, with a need for further study of this area of practice (Enkin *et al.*, 2000). In accordance with the principles of non-intervention in expectant management, Inch (1985) suggests that ideally the cord should be left intact until the placenta and membranes are completely expelled as this enables compaction and compression of the placenta and retraction of muscle fibres to occur unhindered. There may also be beneficial effects of continued delivery of oxygenated blood to the newborn infant via the cord (Harris, 2001), particularly in those born prematurely or asphyxiated. In a study of premature infants conducted by Kinmond *et al.* (1993), a 30-second delay in cord clamping with the infant held 20 cm below the introitus was associated with improved outcome for the baby. It results in a higher initial packed cell volume and therefore a reduced need for red cell transfusions. Higher arterial–alveolar oxygen tensions were also noted in the first 24 hours, which indicates less right-to-left shunting of deoxygenated blood. Early cord clamping has also been associated with fetomaternal transfusion, of particular importance in women who are rhesus negative (Lapido, 1972). Enkin *et al.* (2000) suggest that free bleeding of the cut end of the severed umbilical cord reduces the risk of fetomaternal transfusion. If the cord is short this may prevent a woman from holding her baby. In these circumstances the woman may choose to have the cord clamped and cut once it has stopped pulsating (approximately 5–10 minutes after the baby is born).

Position of the woman during the third stage of labour Whichever position a woman gives birth in, usually she will choose to sit once the baby is born. This allows her the opportunity to touch, hold and examine her baby. If she chooses to breastfeed she may wish to do so at this point. This also aids separation and expulsion of the placenta and membranes by the release of additional amounts of naturally produced oxytocin from stimulation of the breast.

Detection of separation and descent of the placenta As the uterus begins to contract again, the woman will usually indicate this and may have an urge to bear down. The midwife may also notice abdominal changes; the fundus rises up and becomes more globular. The separated placenta may be seen as a bulge, similar to a full bladder, just above the symphysis pubis with the well-contracted uterus sitting above it. In addition, a gush of blood per vagina and cord lengthening may occur. There is no necessity to palpate the abdomen unless there is cause for concern or the midwife suspects there may be some delay. Encouraging the woman to adopt an upright position at this time will lead to rapid expulsion of the placenta and membranes (Botha, 1968). Care needs to be taken when assisting the woman to move into another position as she will have the baby in her arms. Standing, squatting and sometimes using a toilet, bucket or bedpan can be used.

Delivery of the placenta and membranes The placenta is delivered by maternal effort. Normally, the woman in an upright position will feel the placenta as it descends to the pelvic floor, which will trigger an urge to push, or the placenta under the influence of gravity will just fall out. The midwife's role is to let the woman know what is happening (that the placenta is now separated and is waiting to be delivered), to encourage her to adopt an upright position, and to advise her to listen to what her body is saying (to push or bear down if she wants to). A flat hand placed across the lower abdomen may assist the woman to birth the placenta as the counterpressure compensates for poor muscle tone. The placenta and membranes are then delivered either on to the bed/floor or into a bedpan/toilet/bucket. If the membranes trail behind they can be eased out of the vagina in a number of ways. By turning the placenta to make a rope of the membranes, by applying gentle traction on the membranes with the fingers (usually in an up and down motion), or by asking the woman to cough. Once the placenta is completely expelled, the time is noted to calculate the length of the third stage for recording later. The midwife then palpates the abdomen to ensure the uterus is well contracted and there is no excessive bleeding. The placenta and membranes can then be checked in front of the parents if they wish and any cord blood taken if the woman is rhesus negative.

It is suggested by midwives that this process normally takes between 5 and 15 minutes but can take up to an hour (Harris, 2000). Whilst some authors suggest the length of the third stage is longer with expectant management than active management (Prendiville et al., 1988; Rogers et al., 1998), other authors looking specifically at ultrasound images suggest there is no difference (Herman et al., 1993; Krapp et al., 2000). If physiologically the length of the third stage is similar for both active and expectant management, perhaps time differences may be attributed to the actions of either the midwife or the woman. It has been noted that the use of an upright posture following separation appears to reduce blood loss and the length of the third stage in expectant management (Rogers et al., 1998).

Active management

Active management is an intervention in the normal physiological processes. The administration of oxytocic drugs at the end of the second stage of labour combined with early cord clamping and cord traction are used to bring about delivery of the placenta and membranes. The woman for the most part is a passive participant in this process.

History of active management

Active intervention in the third stage of labour is not new. Aristotle referred to cord traction 2000 years ago (see Hibbard, 1964) and manipulation of the uterus to deliver a separated placenta was commonly taught at the beginning of the 20th century (Jellett, 1901). However, active management did not become popular until after the isolation of ergometrine (Dudley and Moir, 1935) and the development of synthetic oxytocin (Syntocinon) (du Vigneaud and Tippett, 1954). Initially ergometrine was used as a treatment for postpartum haemorrhage (PPH), and it was then given following the third stage to prevent PPH. In the 1950s it became popular to give ergometrine at crowning of the baby's head (Moir, 1955). Syntometrine (a mixture of Syntocinon and ergometrine) was marketed in the 1960s (Embrey et al., 1963). This was given with the birth of the baby's anterior shoulder and followed by cord traction. This package of care became known as active management and its popularity quickly spread. It has been so successful that it has become normal practice throughout the UK (Garcia and Garforth, 1989). As Moore highlights: 'As so often with developments

in obstetrics all mothers come to be treated in the same manner irrespective of the degree of risk' (Moore, 1977: 120).

Uterotonic drugs

Uterotonic drugs (drugs that make the uterus contract) are used during the third stage in three ways:

- *as a prophylaxis* to prevent postpartum haemorrhage irrespective of the risk status of the woman
- *as a planned treatment* when a risk of postpartum haemorrhage has been identified, for example when a woman has a low haemoglobin level or a history of previous postpartum haemorrhage
- *as treatment in an emergency* when uncontrolled bleeding occurs as a result of uterine atony.

While the benefits of oxytocic drugs in controlling atonic postpartum haemorrhage are recognized, their routine use in preventing the problem has been the subject of much debate and various clinical trials. A systematic review of four studies comparing active management with an expectant or physiological approach, supports the prophylactic use of active management in a hospital birth situation (Prendiville, et al., 2000). The implications for home birth are less clear (Enkin et al., 2000). The review concluded that there was an overall reduction in maternal blood loss of less than 100 ml in women having an active third stage of labour over expectant management (mean weighted difference −79.33 ml; 95% confidence interval −94.29 to −64.37) (Prendiville et al., 2000). The review also highlights that certain uterotonic drugs have been associated with raised blood pressure, nausea, vomiting and headaches (Prendiville et al., 2000). Higher rates of retained placenta in active management have also been reported (Begley, 1990) along with more serious complications such as postpartum eclampsia and cardiac disorders (WHO, 1999). It has been suggested that Syntocinon replace Syntometrine as the drug of choice in active management as some of the complications above have been associated with the ergometrine component of Syntometrine (McDonald et al., 1993, 2000).

Critics of these research studies highlight a number of factors that may have influenced the results achieved.

Lack of skill in expectant management among midwives

Three out of four studies were conducted in hospitals where active management was the norm (Gyte, 1994). Whilst the latest study was conducted at Hinchingbrooke (Rogers et al., 1998), where expectant management was said to be more common, statistics are not available as to the rate of expectant management before the trial began. Milner suggests that this was 15–20% in the mid-1980s (Milner, 1989), which does not necessarily mean all midwives were skilled in expectant management techniques at the start of the study.

Difficulty in defining what constitutes excessive blood loss

It is well recognized that blood loss estimation is inaccurate, with high loss often being underestimated (Brant, 1967; Razvi et al., 1996). In addition, as the reduced loss associated with active management has become the norm, midwives may interpret the slightly higher blood loss rate in expectant management as abnormal. Currently a postpartum haemorrhage is defined as a blood loss in excess of 500 ml. In some countries this is 1000 ml, and Gyte (1992) suggests that healthy women appear to cope well with the loss of such amounts. If this more generous definition had been used in the Hinchingbrooke study, no statistically significant difference in postpartum haemorrhage rates would have been found between expectant and active management approaches (Rogers et al., 1998). In the Netherlands only 10% of midwives routinely use oxytocic prophylaxis for the third stage (de Groot et al., 1996) and rates of home birth are much higher than in the UK. Results from the Lente study comparing active and expectant management of the third stage among Dutch midwives are eagerly awaited; initial findings point to no difference in blood loss rates in excess of 1000 ml for active and expectant management arms of the trial (Herschderfer, 1999). This may add weight to the growing evidence that for low-risk women an expectant management approach may not significantly increase blood loss following birth, making it a realistic option.

More recently it has been suggested that whilst oxytocics may appear to reduce blood loss at delivery in the short term, when the action wears off on the postnatal ward the blood will be lost then (Wickham, 1999). Wickham observed that following active management, women often experienced a heavy blood loss when going to the bathroom for the first time. She suggests this heavy loss does not occur in women who have had expectant management. Is the use of uterotonics during the third stage merely delaying blood loss until a time when it is less likely to be noticed? Perhaps women are supposed to lose blood at this time as they no longer require such a high circulating blood volume to supply the placental bed, and the haemodilution of pregnancy may support a woman's ability to cope with this.

Further studies are required to look at what constitutes normal blood loss following childbirth and the implications of actively reducing it.

Variation in practice When comparing research protocols of published trials no consensus can be reached on a definition of what constitutes active and expectant management, which implies that there is variation in practice (Begley, 1990; Prendiville et al., 1988; Rogers et al., 1998; Thilaganathan et al., 1993). Gyte (1994) suggests that a 'piecemeal' approach, a combination of active and expectant management techniques, was used by a significant number of midwives within the Bristol trial. Currently a study is underway exploring with midwives their practice during the third stage of labour, and initial results support variation in practice (Harris, 2000). This highlights the difficulty in evaluating the results of comparative studies where variation in practice could have occurred.

Logue (1990) looked at PPH rates among doctors and midwives and found considerable variation, with some individuals having consistently much higher rates of PPH than others. Logue (1990) proposes that when managing the third stage, 'more conservative and patient operators show the lowest PPH rates compared with the more impatient and heavy-handed who show the highest rates' (Logue, 1990: S11). This implies that the action or inaction of practitioners may have a direct impact on the outcome of the third stage and requires further exploration. This is supported in the literature by reference to the potential dangers of fundal fiddling and inappropriate cord traction leading to uterine inversion (McDonald, 1999). It would be interesting to see an analysis of PPH rates for active and expectant management in individual midwives within the published trials.

Currently, the following uterotonic drugs are available to manage the third stage of labour:

Intramuscular Syntometrine 1 ml This preparation is usually given with the birth of the anterior shoulder or shortly after. Syntometrine contains ergometrine 500 μg and oxytocin 5 units in 1 ml. The oxytocin fraction induces strong, rhythmic contraction of the muscle fibres of the upper segment of the uterus within 2–3 minutes of administration. Its effect lasts for approximately 5–15 minutes (Baskett, 1999). This rapid-acting, short-duration component is designed to initiate strong uterine action, which is sustained by the action of the ergometrine fraction, which will induce a strong, non-physiological spasm of uterine muscle within 6–8 minutes (Sorbe, 1978). The effect of ergometrine is maintained for approximately 60–90 minutes (Baskett, 1999). Because of the spasm-inducing properties of ergometrine there is a theoretical risk of retained placenta and therefore the midwife should aim to deliver the placenta before ergometrine takes effect. Syntometrine becomes inactive at high temperatures.

Syntocinon   Syntocinon is a synthetically produced form of oxytocin, which can be given intravenously (5 IU) or intramuscularly (5–10 IU). It can be given at crowning of the head, with delivery of the anterior shoulder or shortly after the birth. Intramuscular Syntocinon acts within 2–3 minutes of administration. It is considered the oxytocic drug of choice if there is a history of pre-existing hypertension (DoH, 1994). Whilst Syntometrine remains the most effective oxytocic in reducing blood loss (McDonald *et al.*, 2000), it may cause nausea, vomiting and hypertension, making Syntocinon, which has fewer side-effects, an appropriate alternative. Syntocinon becomes inactive at high temperatures.

Intramuscular ergometrine 500 μg   This will cause a strong, sustained uterine contraction. If intramuscular ergometrine is administered instead of Syntometrine it is given a little earlier, at the crowning of the head, as it takes longer to act, 6–8 minutes. The WHO (1999) do not support its use for routine management in the third stage owing to its effect on blood pressure.

Intravenous ergometrine 250–500 μg   This takes effect approximately 45 seconds after administration. It is usually given by a doctor but may be given by a midwife in an emergency situation, usually to control postpartum bleeding.

Prostaglandins

There is currently some interest in exploring the use of a prostaglandin E_1 analogue (misoprostol) for management of the third stage. Misoprostol (in doses of 400–600 μg) can be given orally or rectally, needs no equipment to administer and does not become inactive at high temperatures. This makes it an ideal therapy for third world countries where refrigeration and health services are limited. However, it is associated with shivering and transient pyrexia. A study comparing the administration of an oral dose of misoprostol 600 μg with intramuscular Syntometrine 1 ampoule suggests there are no significant differences between the two groups in the mean blood loss, the incidence of PPH and the fall in haemoglobin administration, though the need for additional oxytocic injection was significantly higher in the misoprostol group (Ng *et al.*, 2001).

Nipple stimulation

A simple alternative to parenteral oxytocics for the third stage of labour is nipple stimulation which, according to Irons *et al.* (1994), tends to reduce the length of the third stage and the amount of blood loss. This was a small study, however, and larger trials are needed.

Principles of active management

Positioning the baby after birth   Where the infant is placed at birth will depend on the position the woman chooses to give birth in. As discussed previously, there are significant benefits for both mother and child of early skin-to-skin contact. There is also a need to provide a warm draught-free environment.

When to give the oxytocic   Traditionally it was recommended that Syntometrine 1 ml IM be given with the birth of the baby's anterior shoulder. However, if a midwife is alone she is unable to do this. In these circumstances the oxytocic is given immediately following the birth of the baby. Midwives have identified that this may occur before or after the cord is clamped and cut (Harris, 2000).

When to cut the cord   The umbilical cord is clamped and cut as soon as possible after the birth of the baby to prevent an excess of placental blood being forced into the infant's circulation under the influence of the administered oxytocic. This has the potential to cause hypervolaemia and hyperbilirubinaemia in the neonate. Clamping may occur before or shortly after the administration of Syntometrine.

Position of the woman during the third stage of labour   As with expectant management, irrespective of the position a woman gives birth in, she will usually choose to sit once the baby is born. In addition, the midwife often wishes to gain access to the woman's abdomen for palpation and delivery of the placenta and therefore may encourage a woman to do so.

Detection of separation and descent of the placenta
In active management it is normally the midwife who detects the first uterine contraction following the baby's

birth by placing a hand on the woman's abdomen and waiting for the uterus to rise up and contract beneath it. Midwives are often warned at this time of the dangers of fundal fiddling, which may lead to partial separation of the placenta, with the potential for excessive bleeding to occur. Therefore the hand rests gently at the fundus and does not move, until the uterus contracts and there are signs of separation and descent. Although cord traction as described by Spencer (1962) should be commenced as soon as the uterus contracts, Levy and Moore (1985) suggest waiting until signs of separation are present. This study found no significant difference in the incidence of postpartum haemorrhage, or the length of the third stage, between those who started controlled cord traction as soon as the uterus contracted and those who waited for signs of separation. However, the rate of postpartum haemorrhage appeared to be significantly higher when the midwife unsuccessfully used controlled cord traction without awaiting signs of separation.

Signs of separation and descent As the uterus contracts and the placenta separates, the fundus rises up and becomes more globular. The separated placenta may be seen as a bulge similar to a full bladder just above the symphysis pubis, with the well-contracted uterus sitting above it. Combined with the abdominal findings, the midwife may notice that there is a gush of blood per vagina and that the cord lengthens. The woman may experience pain at this time and also feel the urge to bear down as the placenta enters the vagina.

Delivery of the placenta and membranes The placenta is delivered by cord traction with the woman in a sitting/semi-recumbent position. The midwife either wraps her fingers around the cord or uses a clamp to apply downward sustained traction until the placenta appears at the vulva. When the placenta becomes visible, traction is applied upwards following the curve of Cares to extract the placenta from the vagina (Spencer, 1962). The placenta is delivered into the midwife's hands or into a bowl placed close to the introitus. Care is taken with the membranes, which may trail behind. Some midwives ask women to cough gently, particularly if the membranes appear caught in the cervix.

Whilst applying cord traction, some midwives place a hand above the symphysis pubis and push the uterus upwards (known as 'guarding of the uterus') (Fig. 30.5). This is said to prevent uterine inversion. However, there is currently no evidence available to support this practice. Some midwives use this hand as counterpressure

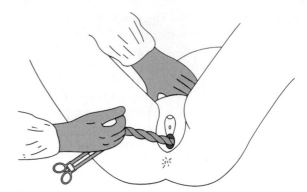

Figure 30.5 Controlled cord traction while guarding the uterus.

when applying cord traction and others suggest it provides valuable information on descent, as the placenta can be felt beneath the hand, moving down into the vagina (Harris, 2000).

In some units women are encouraged to deliver the placenta by maternal effort (see Expectant management).

Following placental delivery the length of the third stage is noted for recording later. The midwife palpates the abdomen to ensure the uterus is well contracted and notes vaginal blood loss. The average length of the third stage is 6–8 minutes (Krapp *et al.*, 2000; Rogers *et al.*, 1998).

Examination of the placenta and membranes

The placenta and membranes are carefully examined as soon after delivery as possible so that, if incomplete, action can be taken immediately. The examination is to determine completeness, and to detect any abnormalities, which may suggest problems in the neonate.

Initially the placenta is held up by the cord to view the membranes; a discrete hole, which the baby passed through, may be seen. Sometimes membranes are ragged and every attempt should be made to piece them together to ensure completeness.

The placenta is placed on a flat surface and thoroughly examined in a good light. The amnion is stripped from the chorion up to the umbilical cord to confirm that both membranes are present. The maternal surface is wiped clear of blood clots and carefully examined to ensure all the cotyledons are present. Any areas of infarction (firm whitish patches) are noted and the placental edge examined for blood vessels running into the membranes. These vessels may track back to the placenta (an erratic vessel) or go to an accessory lobe in the membranes (a succenturiate lobe). If a vessel ends at a hole in the membranes (Fig. 30.6), a succenturiate

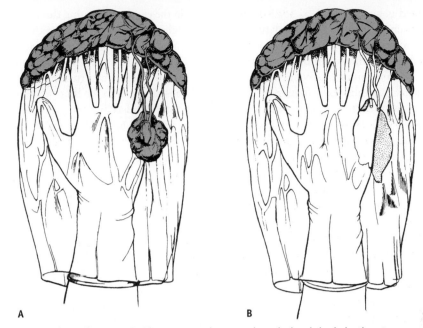

Figure 30.6 **A.** Succenturiate placenta. **B.** The torn membrane – the missing lobe is in the uterus.

lobe may have been left behind in the uterus and the woman will need referral to an obstetrician. The cord is then examined, noting its insertion and length (though this is no longer measured) and the number of umbilical vessels. Usually the cord insertion is central and the length is approximately 50 cm. Occasionally only one umbilical artery is present; this is associated with congenital anomalies, especially renal agenesis (absence of kidneys). The paediatrician is informed and a detailed examination of the newborn requested. The placenta is usually weighed; weight at term is usually about one-sixth of the baby's birthweight. Early cord clamping increases the placental weight as it contains a greater residual blood volume (Prendiville and Elbourne, 1989).

Finally, any blood loss collected is measured and added to the estimated amount of loss which has soaked into linen and pads. An accurate assessment is necessary to determine whether the loss was excessive and is likely to have a detrimental effect on maternal well-being. Particular care is needed in estimating losses in excess of 300 ml, when amounts are often underestimated (Levy and Moore, 1985), with the level of error increasing with the amount lost.

The findings are recorded in the mother's notes. Immediate referral to a doctor is made if it is thought that a piece of placental tissue has been retained.

CARE FOLLOWING BIRTH (THE FOURTH STAGE)

Following delivery of the placenta and membranes, the midwife palpates the woman's abdomen to ensure the uterus is well contracted, assesses vaginal blood loss and examines the woman for any soft tissue damage which may require repair. The midwife makes the mother comfortable. It is an ideal time for the midwife to share the couple's delight in their baby and to encourage any questions. This can be a good opportunity for health education and may also facilitate the development of parent–baby attachment. Most women will enjoy this early contact with their baby and there is evidence that this early and unhurried contact significantly affects maternal emotional well-being when measured 6 weeks postnatally (Ball, 1994). The father too usually wishes to share this time with his family and should be encouraged to do so. This should be given priority over the many routine procedures. Sensitivity is required in caring for women who appear to show little interest in their baby at birth.

Women who plan to breastfeed should be encouraged to do so soon after birth, usually within the first hour. At this time the baby usually displays a strong urge to suck and a successful feed benefits both mother and baby. The mother is encouraged to breastfeed and evidence suggests she is more likely to be successful for longer if an early feed is given (Salariya, 1978). The baby receives colostrum, a high-protein meal that is easily digestible. An additional benefit is the release of oxytocin during suckling, which stimulates uterine contractions and helps to maintain haemostasis.

Ongoing care includes regular examination of the woman's abdomen to ensure the uterus remains contracted and observation of the lochia. The woman is encouraged to pass urine, as a full bladder predisposes to a relaxed uterus and heavy blood loss. If this occurs, the midwife can massage the fundus of the uterus to stimulate a contraction. Observation of the infant will include colour, respirations, and general activity. The umbilical cord is checked to ensure the cord clamp is firmly in place and that there is no bleeding. Care is taken to ensure that the baby does not become chilled; body temperature can be maintained by skin-to-skin contact or warm wrapping and cuddling by the parents. The midwife should remain in the birthing room for at least 1 hour after delivery, whether at home or in hospital.

RECORDS

A complete and accurate account of labour must be recorded. Such notations must be sufficiently comprehensive to enable other carers to have a clear picture of events, thus facilitating communication and avoiding discontinuity of care (NMC, 2002).

Statute requires that a birth notification form be completed. This is normally undertaken by the midwife and sent, within 36 hours of the birth, to the medical officer of the district in which the birth took place (UKCC, 1998b).

THE PLACENTA AT TERM

At term, the placenta is flat and round or oval in shape. It is 18–20 cm in diameter and about 2.5 cm thick in the centre, becoming thinner towards the edges. Its weight is about one-sixth of the weight of the fetus and it is usually situated on the anterior or posterior wall of the uterine cavity, near the fundus. The placenta has two surfaces, maternal and fetal. The *maternal surface* is attached to the uterine decidua, is deep red in colour and divided by deep grooves or sulci into about 15–20 irregular lobes. These lobes (called cotyledons) contain masses of chorionic villi. On examination after birth a thin greyish layer, part of the basal decidua, can be seen (Fig. 30.7). It may feel gritty due to the presence of lime salts. The *fetal surface* lies adjacent to the fetus and has a pearly white appearance as it is covered with amnion. From the insertion of the cord, which is usually situated centrally, blood vessels can be seen radiating to the periphery, like the roots of a tree. These vessels give off branches which penetrate into the substance of the placenta, each cotyledon having its own supply of fetal blood. In the centre of each cotyledon there is a main branch of the umbilical artery and vein.

Abnormalities of the placenta

Succenturiate lobe

A succenturiate lobe (Fig. 30.8) is a small portion or lobe of placenta which is separated from the main body. This is formed from some of the villi of the chorionic membrane which have continued to develop instead of becoming atrophied. It is attached to the main placenta by blood vessels which pass through the membrane. A succenturiate lobe may be retained in the uterus after the placenta has been expelled; this can cause postpartum haemorrhage and sepsis. When there is a small hole in the fetal membranes with placental vessels running towards it, a retained succenturiate lobe may be suspected and the woman should be referred to an obstetrician for assessment.

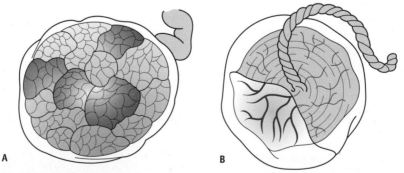

Figure 30.7   The placenta. **A.** The maternal surface, showing the cotyledons. **B.** The fetal surface.

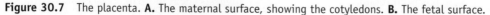

Circumvallate placenta

In this type of placenta the chorion is attached not to the edge of the placenta, but to the fetal surface at some distance from the edge (Fig. 30.9). A thickened ring of membrane is seen on the fetal surface.

Bipartite placenta

This is a placenta divided into two main lobes.

Placenta accreta

This is a placenta which becomes abnormally adherent to the uterine muscle over the whole or part of its surface. It is very rare.

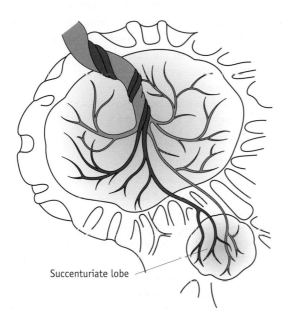

Succenturiate lobe

Figure 30.8 Succenturiate placenta.

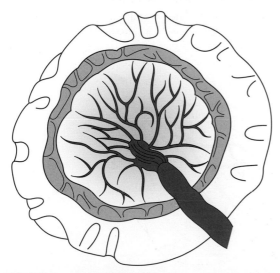

Figure 30.9 Circumvallate placenta.

Infarcts

These are red or white patches sometimes seen on the maternal surface of the placenta. They are caused by localized death of placental tissue due to interference with the blood supply.

Infarcts are red at an early stage of their development; later they become white and appear as patches of white fibrous tissue. They may be seen occasionally in any placenta, but they are often associated with pre-eclampsia.

Calcification

On the maternal surface of the placenta small greyish-white patches are often to be seen, particularly on the postmature placenta. These are deposits of lime salts. They convey a gritty sensation to the fingers and are not significant.

FETAL MEMBRANES

There are two fetal membranes: the chorion and the amnion.

The chorion is the outer membrane, continuous with the edge of the placenta and derived from the tropho-blast. It is opaque, thick but friable and roughened by tiny pieces of decidua adherent to it. It lines the uterine cavity.

The amnion is the inner membrane, derived from the inner cell mass. It is smooth, transparent and the stronger membrane of the two. The two membranes lie over each other, but can be separated; the amnion may be stripped back to the insertion of the cord. The amnion secretes amniotic fluid or liquor amnii which at term measures 1000–1500 ml.

UMBILICAL CORD

The umbilical cord (Fig. 30.10) or funis connects the placenta to the fetus. The cord is about 50 cm long and 2 cm thick. It is composed of a jelly-like substance known as Wharton's jelly; this is a primitive connective tissue, primary mesenchyme. The cord is covered externally by amnion. It supports and protects three blood vessels: one large umbilical vein carrying oxygenated blood to the fetus, and two umbilical arteries winding around the vein carrying deoxygenated blood from the fetus to the placenta. The absence of a vessel may be associated with fetal abnormalities. The cord has a spiral twist; this torsion gives a certain amount of protection from pressure.

The function of the cord ceases as pulmonary respiration is established shortly after birth. Lacking a blood supply, the cord becomes dead tissue and quickly atrophies, as do the internal structures continuous with it. It

can provide access for bacteria to enter the body, therefore care needs to be taken to keep it dry until the cord stump separates (between 5 and 10 days postnatally).

Abnormalities of the umbilical cord

The cord may be too short (which may cause delay during labour) or too long when there is a risk of cord prolapse. Occasionally it is very thick or very thin; in either case great care is required in tying the cord and subsequently watching for haemorrhage. Rarely a piece of fetal intestine may protrude into the cord; the possibility of this abnormality will be suspected if the cord is swollen close to the umbilicus, the size of the swelling depending on the amount of intestine which has protruded. Knots are caused by movements of the fetus before birth, the baby slipping through a loop of the cord. False knots may be due to the blood vessels being longer than the actual cord, and so doubling back upon themselves in the Wharton's jelly, or to irregularities and the formation of nodes.

Abnormalities of insertion

The cord may be attached to one side of the placenta (an eccentric insertion) or to the margin of the placenta (a battledore insertion), or the vessels of the cord may break up and run into the membrane before reaching the placenta (a velamentous insertion) (Fig. 30.11). This is particularly dangerous if the unprotected blood vessels should lie near the internal os. This very rare condition is called vasa praevia (vessels in advance of the fetus). Should a blood vessel so situated be compressed when the membranes rupture, the fetus will suffer hypoxia. If such a vessel should actually rupture, blood will be lost from fetal vessels in the membrane. Such fetal haemorrhage is dangerous and could lead to stillbirth.

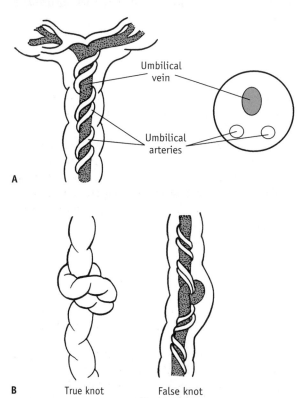

Figure 30.10 **A.** The umbilical cord in side view and cross-section, showing the one umbilical vein with the two umbilical arteries twisting spirally around it. The vein and arteries lie in Wharton's jelly; the cord is enclosed within the amnion. **B.** True and false knots.

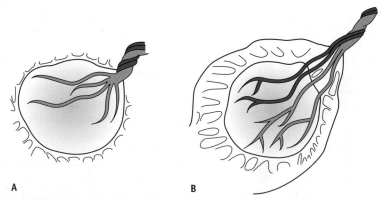

Figure 30.11 Abnormal insertions of the cord: **A.** battledore; **B.** velamentous.

CONCLUSION

The third stage of labour is an important period for mother and baby, when the importance of their first meeting cannot be overestimated. The midwife supports this special time while monitoring successful delivery of the placenta and membranes. Currently women appear to have little choice about how the third stage is managed, with active management being used indiscriminately. If midwives are to offer women a choice for the third stage, skills in both active and expectant management are required with a body of knowledge which enables the detection of those women who deviate from the normal, in whom active management may be the most appropriate form of care. In this way, women at low risk may be spared unnecessary intervention in the normal process of giving birth.

KEY POINTS

- The third stage of labour is a time of great importance when mother and baby meet face to face for the first time.
- The skill and expertise of the midwife is needed to support this special time while monitoring successful completion of the childbirth process with delivery of the placenta and membranes.
- Care will be based upon knowledge of the normal physiological, sociological and psychological processes at work and the effect of interventions on that process.

- The indiscriminate use of active management for women experiencing normal birth has been challenged.
- The challenge for midwives is to change the focus for the third stage to one of normality and re-skill in expectant management techniques to include the ability to detect women deviating from the normal perspective in whom active management may be appropriate.

REFERENCES

Akiyama, H., Kohzu, H. & Matsuoka, M. (1981) An approach to detection of placental separation and expulsion with new clinical signs: a study based on haemodynamic method and ultrasonography. *American Journal of Obstetrics and Gynecology* **140**(5): 505–511.

Ball, J.A. (1994) *Reactions to Motherhood*, pp. 113–115. Hale: Books for Midwives Press.

Baskett, T.F. (1999) *Essential Management of Obstetric Emergencies*, 3rd edn. Bristol: Clinical Press.

Begley, C. (1990) A comparison of 'active' and 'physiological' management of the third stage of labour. *Midwifery* **6**(1): 3–17.

Bennett, V. & Brown, L. (eds) (1999) *Myles Textbook for Midwives*. Edinburgh: Churchill Livingstone.

Botha, M.A. (1968) The management of the umbilical cord in labour. *South African Journal of Obstetrics and Gynaecology* **16**(2): 30–33.

Brandt, M. (1933) The mechanism and management of the third stage of labour. *American Journal of Obstetrics and Gynecology* **23**: 662–667.

Brant, H.A. (1967) Precise estimation of postpartum haemorrhage: difficulties and importance. *British Medical Journal* **1**(537): 398–400.

De Groot, A.N., van Roomaleb, J. & van Dongen, P.W. (1996) Survey of the management of third stage of labour in the Netherlands. *European Journal of Obstetrics and Gynecology and Reproductive Biology* **66**(1): 39–40.

Dieckmann, W.J., Odell, L.D., Williger, W.M. *et al.* (1947) The placental stage and postpartum hemorrhage. *American Journal of Obstetrics and Gynecology* **54**: 415–427.

Department of Health (DoH) (1957) *Confidential Enquiries into Maternal Deaths, 1952–4.* London: HMSO.

Department of Health (DoH) (1994) *Confidential Enquiries into Maternal Deaths in the UK, 1988–90.* London: HMSO.

Department of Health (DoH) (2001) *Why Mothers Die: Report on Confidential Enquiries into Maternal Deaths in the United Kingdom, 1997–9.* London: HMSO.

du Vigneaud, V.R.C. & Tippett, S. (1954) The sequence of amino acids in oxytocin with a proposal for the structure of oxytocin. *Journal of Biological Chemistry* **205**: 949.

Dudley, H.W. & Moir, J.C. (1935) The substance responsible for the traditional clinical effect of ergot. *British Medical Journal* **1**: 520–523.

Embrey, M.B., Barber, D.T.C. & Scudamore, J.H. (1963) The use of Syntometrine in prevention of post partum haemorrhage. *British Medical Journal* **1**(5342): 1387–1389.

Enkin, M., Keirse, M.J.N.C., Neilson, J. *et al.* (2000) The third stage of labour. In: *A guide to Effective Care in Pregnancy and Childbirth*, 3rd edn, Ch. 33. Oxford: Oxford University Press.

Featherstone, I.E. (1999) Physiological third stage. *British Journal of Midwifery* 7(4): 216–221.

Garcia, J. & Garforth, S. (1989) Labour and delivery routines in English consultant maternity units. *Midwifery* 5(4): 155–162.

Gilbert, L., Porter, W. & Brown, V.A. (1987) Postpartum haemorrhage – a continuing problem. *British Journal of Obstetrics and Gynaecology* 94(1): 67–71.

Gyte, G. (1992) The significance of blood loss at delivery. *MIDIRS Midwifery Digest* 2(1): 88–92.

Gyte, G. (1994) Evaluation of the meta analyses on the effects, on both mother and baby, of the various components of 'active' management of the third stage of labour. *Midwifery* 10(4): 183–199.

Harris, T. (2000) *Midwifery Practice in the Third Stage of Labour.* A conference paper at Midwives Marking the Millennium Conference: the Diversity of Practice, 2-day international conference, 8–9th June, Bournemouth.

Harris, T. (2001) Changing the focus for the third stage of labour. *British Journal of Midwifery* 9(1): 7–12.

Herman, A. (2000) Complicated third stage of labor: time to switch on the scanner. *Ultrasound in Obstetrics and Gynecology* 15(2): 89–95.

Herman, A., Weinraub, Z., Bukovsky, I. *et al.* (1993) Dynamic ultrasound imaging of the third stage of labour: new perspectives into third stage mechanisms. *American Journal of Obstetrics and Gynecology* 168(5): 1496–1499.

Herschderfer, K. (1999) *Results of RCT Expectant versus Active Management within Setting of Dutch Midwives' Independent Practices (Home Births).* Presented at National Study Day on Third Stage Issues, Manchester.

Hibbard, B. (1964) The third stage of labour. *British Medical Journal* 1(5396): 1485–1488.

Inch, S. (1985) Management of the third stage of labour – another cascade of intervention. *Midwifery* 1(2): 114–122.

Irons, D.W., Sriskandabalan, P. & Bullough, C.H. (1994) A simple alternative to parenteral oxytocics for the third stage of labour. *International Journal of Gynecology and Obstetrics* 46(1): 15–18.

Jellett, H. (1901) *A Short Practice of Midwifery for Nurses.* London: J and A Churchill.

Kinmond, S., Aitchison, T.C., Holland, B.M. *et al.* (1993) Umbilical cord clamping and preterm infants: a randomised trial. *British Medical Journal* 306(6871): 172–175.

Krapp, M., Baschat, A.A., Hankeln, M. *et al.* (2000) Grey scale and color doppler sonography in the third stage of labour for early detection of failed placental separation. *Ultrasound in Obstetrics and Gynecology* 15(2): 138–142.

Lapido, O.A. (1972) Management of third stage of labour with particular reference to reduction of feto-maternal transfusion. *British Medical Journal* 1(5802): 721–723.

Levy, V. & Moore, J. (1985) The midwife's management of the third stage of labour. *Nursing Times* 81(39): 47–50.

Logue, M. (1990) Management of the third stage of labour: a midwife's view. *Journal of Obstetrics and Gynaecology* 10(Suppl. 2): 10–12.

McDonald, S. (1999) Physiology and management of the third stage of labour. In: Bennett, V.R. & Brown, L.K. (eds) *Myles Textbook for Midwives*, 13th edn, Ch. 25. London: Churchill Livingstone.

McDonald, S.J., Prendiville, W.J. & Blair, E. (1993) Randomised controlled trial of oxytocin alone versus oxytocin and ergometrine in active management of labour. *British Medical Journal* 307(6913): 1167–1171.

McDonald, S., Prendiville, W.J. & Elbourne, D.A. (2000) Prophylactic Syntometrine versus oxytocin for delivery of the placenta. *The Cochrane Library*, Issue 3. Oxford: Update Software.

Milner, I. (1989) Personal communication cited in Levy, V. (1990) The midwife's management of the third stage of labour. In: Alexander, J., Levy, V. & Roch, S. (eds) *Midwifery Practice Volume 2: Intrapartum Care.* London: Macmillan.

Moir, J.C. (1955) The history of present day use of ergot. *Canadian Medical Association* 72: 727–734.

Moore, W.M.O. (1977) In: Chard, T. & Richards, M. (eds) *Benefits and Hazards of the New Obstetrics.* London: Heinemann.

Ng, P.S., Chan, A.S., Sin, W.K. *et al.* (2001) A multi centre controlled trial of oral misoprostol and IM Syntometrine in the management of the third stage of labour. *Human Reproduction* 16(1): 31–35.

Nursing, Midwifery and Health Visiting (NMC) (2002) *Guidelines for Records and Record Keeping.* London: NMC.

Odent, M. (1998) Don't manage the third stage of labour. *Practising Midwife* 1(9): 31–33.

Prendiville, W.J. & Elbourne, D. (1989) Care during the third stage of labour. In: Chalmers, I., Enkin, M. & Keirse, M.J.N.C. (eds) *Effective Care in Pregnancy and Childbirth*, Vol. 2. Oxford: Oxford University Press.

Prendiville, W.J., Harding, J.E., Elbourne, D.R. *et al.* (1988) The Bristol Third Stage Trial: Active versus physiological management of the third stage of labour. *British Medical Journal* 297(6659): 1295–1300.

Prendiville, W.J., Elbourne, D. & McDonald, S. (2000) Active versus expectant management of the third stage of labour. *The Cochrane Library*, Issue 3. Oxford: Update Software.

Razvi, K., Chua, S., Arulkumaran, S. *et al.* (1996) A comparison between visual estimation and laboratory determination of blood loss during the third stage of labour. *Australian and New Zealand Journal of Obstetrics and Gynaecology* 36(2): 152–154.

Righard, L. & Alade, M.O. (1990) Effect of delivery room routines on success of first breast-feed. *Lancet* 336(8723): 1105–1107.

Rogers, J., Wood, J., McCandlish, R. *et al.* (1998) Active versus expectant management of the third stage of labour: the Hinchingbrooke randomised controlled trial. *Lancet* **351**(9104): 693–699.

Salariya, E.M., Easton, P.M. & Cater, J.I. (1978) Duration of breast feeding after early initiation and frequent feeding. *Lancet* **2**(8100): 1141–1143.

Sorbe, B. (1978) Active pharmacologic management of the third stage of labor. *Obstetrics and Gynecology* **52**(6): 694–697.

Spencer, P.M. (1962) Controlled cord traction in management of the third stage of labour. *British Medical Journal* **1**(5294): 1728–1732.

Thilaganathan, B.C.A., Cutner, A., Latimer, J. *et al.* (1993). Management of the third stage of labour in women at low risk of postpartum haemorrhage. *European Journal of Obstetrics and Gynaecology and Reproductive Biology* **48**(1): 19–22.

United Kingdom Central Council for Nursing, Midwifery and Health Visiting (UKCC) (1998b) *Midwives Rules and Code of Practice.* London: UKCC.

World Health Organization (WHO) (1994) *Mother–Baby Package. Implementing Safe Motherhood in Developing Countries.* Maternal Health and Safe Motherhood Programme, Division of Family Health, WHO/FHE/MSM/94:11: Geneva: WHO.

World Health Organization (WHO) (1999) *Care in Normal Birth: A Practical Guide.* Report of the Technical Working Group. Geneva. Online. Available: http://www.who.int/rht/documents/MSM96-24/msm9624.htm.

Wickham, S. (1999) Further thoughts on the third stage. *Practising Midwife* **2**(10): 14–15.

Yao, A.C. & Lind, J. (1974) Placental transfusion. *American Journal of Diseases in Children* **127**(1): 128–141.

FURTHER READING

Edwards, N. (2000). *Delivering Your Placenta: The Third Stage.* London: AIMS.
This easy-to-read booklet adds depth to the discussion about active versus expectant management.

Enkin, M., Keirse, M.J.N.C., Neilson, J. *et al.* (2000) The third stage of labour. In: *A Guide to Effective Care in Pregnancy and Childbirth*, 3rd edn, Ch. 33. Oxford: Oxford University Press.
This chapter provides the obstetric point of view on how the third stage of labour should be managed.

Harris, T. (2001) Changing the focus for the third stage of labour. *British Journal of Midwifery* **9**(1): 7–12.
This article provides a critique of active management for low-risk pregnant women.

ADDITIONAL RESOURCES

A qualitative study exploring midwifery practice in the third stage of labour is currently nearing completion with findings being available later this year. Information about the study is available from Tina Harris, Faculty of Health and Life Sciences, De Montfort University, Hawthorne Building, Leicester LE1 9BH.

PART 5

THE NEWBORN BABY

31. Physiology, Assessment and Care 527

32. Thermoregulation 573

33. Infant Feeding 591

34. The Preterm Baby and the Small Baby 628

35. Respiratory and Cardiac Disorders 649

36. Congenital Anomalies, Fetal and Neonatal Surgery, and Pain 670

37. Neonatal Jaundice 684

38. Metabolic and Endocrine Disorders 696

39. Infections 703

40. Sudden Infant Death Syndrome 715

THE NEWBORN BABY

Physiology, Assessment and Care

Stephanie Michaelides

LEARNING OUTCOMES

At the end of this chapter, you will have:

- a clear understanding of the physiology of the neonate, and the transition from fetal life
- an understanding of the importance of providing evidence-based and physiologically appropriate care and management to the neonate

- a commitment to allocating the same time and attention to the assessment and examination of the newborn as to the woman/mother
- a framework for undertaking an assessment of the newborn, and of educating the woman about her baby's needs and how they might be met.

INTRODUCTION

Providing the woman with support and guidance in her adjustment to motherhood is an important aspect of the midwife's role, and the midwife works with a range of agencies and professionals in order that this support is a seamless process from the antenatal period through to bringing up children. Statutory and voluntary services can assist in helping children to develop to their full potential through education and health services and providing specialist help and support to those at time of need.

As well as being a screening test, examination of the newborn enables the woman and her partner to learn to understand their own unique baby and facilitates maternal/paternal–infant interaction through the understanding of the baby's development and behaviour.

The baby as an individual

In the past it is likely that the attention given to the baby and his assessment, even on a day-to-day basis, has been a fraction of that paid to the woman. This focus on the woman, and making her the centre of care has been an important development in providing choice, continuity and control to women and their families. However, it is crucial that babies are viewed as individuals in their own right, and that midwives allocate the same attention to their assessment and care.

This requires in-depth knowledge of neonatal psychological and physiological development. Rather than relying on verbal responses, the midwife communicates with the baby via sight, touch and hearing. This must be a focused activity in order to absorb all of the information provided by the baby's responses and behaviour. Upon completion of the examination, the findings must be discussed with the parents, so that the baby's management and care can be planned as a partnership.

The baby is recognized as a person (Children Act, 1989) with individual needs that require the midwife to act as an advocate and provide duty of care for those needs. Prior to the examination, the midwife must gain consent from the legal guardian. If a woman who is not married is unable to give consent, then it has to be gained from the woman's next of kin. This should be discussed with the woman when she first attends for care, so that she can provide information which may be required in an emergency.

If consent is withheld, then further information, support of a peer, or medical advice may be sought. The consent needs to be obtained by the person providing the care, i.e. if the baby deviates from normal, the decision of how to proceed must be made in partnership with a senior neonatologist.

If the woman wishes the baby to be given oral or no vitamin K preparation, under statute (UKCC, 1998a) the midwife has a duty to ask the paediatrician to see the baby, and ensure that whatever decision is made is recorded in the baby's notes. If invasive treatment is required, the consent needs to be obtained by the person implementing the invasive procedure so that the parents can be given as much information as they need. If the parents feel that they have not been given adequate information the consent may not be valid (DoH, 2001).

If the parents refuse life-saving care for the baby, the midwife needs to work with the appropriate professionals (the GP, or a senior neonatologist) to enable the parents to understand the severity of the situation. It is important to record what information has been given.

The midwife should document clearly the decisions and justification of actions and omissions, providing a clear picture of the transitional events which occurred at birth and during the first 28 days of postnatal life.

Assessment of the newborn

This assessment is not a 'one-off' assessment, but a complex, dynamic and continuous activity which begins in the antenatal period and is followed through the birth and neonatal period. Quick recognition and appropriate referral of the fetus/neonate with deviations from normal, result in an enhanced quality of life for that baby and family.

In order to achieve this, a formalized communication system between the baby and midwife is vital and should include a thorough understanding of fetal and neonatal anatomy and physiology, thus assisting the detection of deviations from the norm.

For a period of 9 months the fetus has been in a safe, untouched and warm environment in which every need is catered for, free movement is allowed and psychological attachment to the mother is developed.

The long-term effects of the birth experience and transition from this safe environment are unknown, and it is imperative that the birth attendants consider the baby and the environment he has recently left with as much empathy and care as are lavished on the mother.

PHYSIOLOGY

The midwife's knowledge of the transitional events which occur at birth and the changes to the neonate's physiology can be applied to recognition of normal and abnormal events at birth and the difference between primary and secondary apnoea and their management. In this way the midwife is able to provide thoughtful and reasoned practice and justify all actions.

Respiratory system

In this section, the embryological development of lungs, role of lung fluid, fetal breathing movements, and development and function of surfactant will be explored. The transitional events that take place in order for the baby to take the initial breath change the lungs from being passive organs filled with fluid to structures which play a vital role in aerobic metabolism.

The respiratory system consists of:

● upper respiratory tract: the nasal cavity, pharynx and associated structures
● lower respiratory tract: the larynx, trachea, bronchi and lungs.

In uterine life the fetus obtains oxygen and excretes carbon dioxide via the placenta. Although the lungs are not used for gaseous exchange, the healthy fetus makes breathing movements 80% of the time in utero to exercise the muscles of respiration.

The pneumocyte is the only cell in the body that changes function from being a secretary cell producing lung fluid in utero, to becoming an absorbent cell in postnatal life.

Development
Prenatal lung growth occurs in four stages:

● embryonic
● pseudoglandular
● canalicular
● terminal air sac.

Embryonic stage (0–5 weeks)   At the end of this stage, the lobular divisions of the lung are beginning to appear – three on the right of the lung and two on the left. The embryological development is significant in that later fetal and neonatal well-being hinge on the normal process. However, the most significant development is that of the terminal air sacs.

Pseudoglandular stage (5–17 weeks)   A tree of narrow tubules begins to form. These tubules have thick epithelial walls, made of columnar or cuboidal cells. Towards the end of this stage, cartilage, connective tissue, muscle, blood vessels and lymphatic system can be identified.

Canalicular stage (13–25 weeks)   A rich vascular supply develops, and the blood supply is brought closer to the airway epithelial cells. Primitive respiratory bronchioles are beginning to appear.

Babies born at this stage can survive but lung ventilation and sustaining respiration are difficult. At this gestation, chest movement will not be observed as the lungs are very stiff. In order to ascertain whether the baby is breathing, the heart rate must be auscultated. Careful and lengthy auscultation should be carried out to avoid a false diagnosis of neonatal death, and a senior neonatologist may be needed to confirm this. If a midwife is present at a birth deemed pre-viable, she will need to be aware of existing indicators of gestational age, such as ultrasound scans (accurate within ±2 weeks), and be conversant with the physiological differences that gestational age presents – which include lung maturity.

Resuscitation of premature babies should fall to a consultant neonatologist, who will be knowledgeable in premature physiology and experienced in intubation (CESDI, 2003). The development of neonatal networks should further ensure that women at this early gestation will give birth with the relevant support present.

Terminal air sac stage (24/26–37 + weeks) Terminal air sacs develop and multiply to form many pouches or alveoli, similar to bunches of grapes, leading to the alveolar duct then to the bronchioles and ultimately to the bronchi (Inselman *et al.*, 1981). The epithelial surface of these alveolar sacs becomes thinner at the same time as vascular proliferation increases. As a result, capillaries are brought into close proximity to the developing airways, forming the future blood–gas interface. As this process continues, there is an effective fusion of the basement membranes between the endothelium and the epithelium.

These primitive alveoli will continue to deepen and multiply after the baby is born until around 8 years of age. A newborn at term has 20–24 million alveoli compared with 296–300 million in the adult (Hand *et al.*, 1990). Even though the lung may be damaged by technological means to sustain life, it can regenerate to sustain breathing and, providing there is no brain damage, long-term outcomes from prolonged ventilation are good.

The epithelial lining of the primitive alveoli of the lung is formed from two types of pneumocyte:

- type 1 cover the alveolar surface, forming a thin and elastic layer facilitating gaseous exchange
- type 2 are thought to produce and secrete surfactant, the biochemical synthesis and stability of which determine how well the lung functions (Brian and

Brian, 1978: 269–281). They are first seen between 20–24 weeks' gestation – alveolar stability occurs around 33–36 weeks.

Surfactant
Surfactant is a lipoprotein which allows:

- a decrease in surface tension at the end of expiration
- an increase in surface tension during lung expansion.

This prevents atelectasis at the end of expiration and accommodates elastic recoil of the lungs at the last stage of inspiration.

Surfactant biosynthesis is a complex process, not yet fully understood, but thought to be affected by temperature and acidosis. Therefore premature newborns and those of 38 plus weeks who become hypothermic may be severely affected. A term baby who is hypothermic may exhibit expiratory grunting – where the epiglottis closes prematurely – and does not exhale all carbon dioxide. If this is not treated promptly by increasing the baby's temperature, respiratory acidosis will result, followed by metabolic acidosis and collapse.

Lung fluid
Lung fluid is not to be confused with surfactant. It is a silky clear fluid, which may be seen draining from the baby's mouth at delivery. If the secretion is appropriate and clear, the baby's mouth can be cleared with gauze rather than suction.

The function of lung fluid appears to be mainly for cell proliferation and differentiation. At birth the lungs must switch function from the secretion of fluid to absorption of gasses. The catecholamine surge, which occurs at delivery, is probably the final catalyst to complete this change (Milner and Vyas, 1982). Some lung fluid is swallowed and then excreted via the fetal kidneys and into the amniotic fluid. At term, 10–25 ml/kg body weight of liquid remains, which must be either expelled via the upper airways or absorbed via the lymphatic system of the lungs. This is said to commence when labour begins and is completed at birth (Taeusch *et al.*, 1991).

If delivered by elective lower section caesarean section (ELSCS), the burst of catecholamines provided by the onset of labour will not occur and therefore lung fluid will be unabsorbed and present at birth. Neither will the lungs have been compressed to expel any lung fluid. Therefore the midwife will need to observe the baby closely for signs and symptoms of *transient tachypnoea of the newborn* (TTN) (see Ch. 35).

Factors affecting lung maturity

Influencing factors on lung maturity are **hormones**:

- *Steroids* accelerate fetal lung growth and are given to women antenatally to prevent respiratory distress syndrome in the newborn (see Ch. 50).
- *Insulin* is thought to delay maturation of type II cells and therefore has an effect on surfactant production, and low phosphatidylglycerol may result in lung disease of infants of diabetic mothers.
- *Prolactin* is said to be present at higher levels in girls than in boys. If prolactin does enhance biosynthesis of surfactant, this may in part explain the slight edge on survival which girls appear to have over boys.
- *Thyroxine* is thought to increase the rate of phospholipid synthesis. Thus a baby with reduced T_3 or T_4 may be at a greater risk of respiratory distress syndrome (RDS), though the mechanism is not fully understood.

Catecholamines are substances normally released in adults at times of stress, and in the fetus, may be identified around the onset of labour. These have a twofold action on the alveoli: increasing the lecithin:sphyngomyelin ratio to enhance synthesis of surfactant; and decreasing lung fluid production and increasing absorption of lung fluid during the labour process.

Fetal breathing movements

Fetal breathing movements occur from as early as 11 weeks of gestation. As the fetus grows, the strength and frequency of fetal breathing movements increases, until they are present between 40–80% of the time, at a rate of 30–70 breaths per minute (Davis and Bureau, 1987: 551–579).

Respiration in the neonate

Rib cage and respiratory musculature   The newborn rib cage shape and musculature are immature and will continue to develop into adulthood (Harris, 1988). The neonate uses the diaphragm and abdominal muscles for respiratory movement. When counting respiratory rate it may be difficult to see movement of the chest; however, a hand placed gently on the baby's abdomen will detect the rise and fall, allowing respirations to be counted.

Because of the anatomical structure of the air passages and neurological development, for the first 2–3 months the baby breathes through the nose.

Breathing rate   The respiratory rate is usually between 40 and 60 breaths per minute. All infants are periodic rather than regular breathers and premature infants more so than full-term infants. The neonate may have periods of very even breathing and periods when the respirations are uneven and there are long gaps between breaths. The breathing rate is a simple guide to well-being and cannot be used to validate normality without considering the baby's behaviour. A baby that has recently been very active or crying may have a respiratory rate above 70–80 per minute, and in a sleeping baby the rate may be less than 40.

Tachypnoea is a result of increased carbon dioxide and baroreceptors providing the information to the medulla; thus an increased respiratory rate may reduce the respiratory acidosis (see Ch. 35).

Breathing movements

Chest moving symmetrically   Babies can generate spontaneous pressures above $70\,cmH_2O$ and thus can develop a spontaneous pneumothorax; therefore symmetrical movement of the chest validates normality.

Diaphragm moving symmetrically   Babies mainly use the diaphragm to aid breathing. Symmetrical movement of the diaphragm confirms phrenic nerve integrity. Damage to the phrenic nerve can occur following shoulder dystocia and it is important to validate normality at an early stage to avoid later respiratory arrest.

Abnormal signs

Stridor   The presence of stridor alerts the practitioner to upper airway obstruction, which could be due to oedema or abnormal growths.

Expiratory grunting   This is a problem with lower airway function, such as surfactant not functioning appropriately or meconium inhalation into the alveoli.

Nasal flaring   The baby is able to increase its ability to inhale oxygen by flaring the nostrils.

Cyanosis in room air   This is a late sign indicating that the baby has large amounts of unsaturated *haemoglobin* and is thus short of oxygen. Cyanosis is best observed by looking at the central circulation such as in the gums and tongue, since they are more likely to show the level of central perfusion. A baby that is cyanosed needs to be close to resuscitation equipment, as reserves to sustain breathing are at a minimum.

Control of respiration

The control of the respiratory system is mainly autonomic, involving the cortex, brainstem, airways, aortic/carotid chemoreceptors and central control by the medulla. The development and maturity of the central nervous system influence control of respiration, as also do temperature, drugs, hypoxia, acidosis and the sleep state of the infant.

At birth the umbilical cord is clamped and cut; this causes major circulatory changes which divert the blood to the fetal lungs rather than to the placenta for oxygenation.

Cardiovascular system (CVS) in the embryo and fetus

The CVS is composed of the heart and blood vessels, and is a closed system that continuously circulates a given blood volume. It is the first functioning system in the embryo. Blood can be seen circulating in the body by the end of 3 weeks.

Fetal circulation

The structure of the heart provides a circulatory process that is very different from that needed to maintain cardiovascular function after birth. There is low systemic pressure and an increased pulmonic pressure leading to very little blood flow to the lungs, which are non-functional in utero. The fetal brain requires the highest oxygen concentration, and the fetal circulation is designed to provide the vital organs such as the brain, liver and tissues with the maximum concentration of vital materials.

Reflective Activity 31.1

Look at the diagram of fetal circulation in Chapter 14 (Fig. 14.4, p. 210), and review your understanding of it. You may find it helpful to trace the process through, from when the blood carrying oxygen and nutrients travels through the umbilical vein to its return to the placenta via the umbilical arteries.

Note the three main shunts/temporary structures which are affected by transitional events at birth.

Within the fetal system, oxygen content varies throughout the circulation and is lower than in the neonate or adult, but as the concentration of fetal haemoglobin is 18–20 g/dl, fetal blood has a high affinity for oxygen.

Changes at birth

At term, only 5–10% of the cardiac output perfuses the lungs to meet the needs of cellular nutrition, because of pulmonary vascular resistance, the *patent ductus arteriosus* and low resistance of the placental component of the systemic circulation.

With the clamping of the cord, the right atrial pressure is lowered and the left atrial pressure is increased slightly, making the *foramen ovale* close. Aeration of the lungs opens up the pulmonary capillary bed, lowering vascular resistance and increasing the pulmonary bed blood flow. The neonate can generate a pressure of up to 70 cmH$_2$O during inspiration, and 20–30 cmH$_2$O on expiration (Strang, 1977). This is thought to be mainly to force fluid out of the lungs to overcome the high resistance and surface tension of the alveoli, and to be necessary to establish lung volumes and distribute gas through the lungs.

Oxygenation and the reduction of endogenous prostaglandins from the maternal circulation further *reduce* the vascular resistance and initiate the closure of the *ductus arteriosus*. As a result of pressure changes within the heart, the *foramen ovale* closes functionally at or soon after birth from compression of the two portions of the atrial septum. The *ductus arteriosus* is closed functionally by the fourth day, and it closes structurally later when fibrin is laid down – this can take several months to complete.

These physiological changes normally take place when the neonate takes the first breath. The neonatal brain must be functioning adequately in order for the baby to continue to breathe at a sufficient rate to allow homeostasis of oxygen and carbon dioxide within the body.

The vessels which in intrauterine life carried deoxygenated blood to the placenta, the umbilical and *hypogastric arteries*, and those which conveyed oxygenated blood from the placenta to the fetus, namely the *umbilical vein* and the *ductus venosus*, also close and in time become ligaments.

These circulatory changes are not completed immediately after birth, but take place over a period of hours or even days. Respiratory and cardiac disorders accompanied by hypoxia and acidosis may delay, or even reverse, the circulatory changes in the heart and lungs.

Changes in the blood

At birth the baby has a high haemoglobin concentration (about 17 g/dl) most of which is of the fetal type, HbF. This high concentration of HbF is required in utero to increase the oxygen-carrying capacity of the blood, since oxygenated blood from the placenta is soon mixed with deoxygenated blood from the lower part of the fetus. The overall oxygen saturation of the fetal blood is therefore reduced.

After birth the high number of red blood cells is not required, so haemolysis of excess red blood cells takes place. This may result in physiological jaundice of the newborn within 2–3 days of birth (Ch. 37). By the age of 3 months the haemoglobin has fallen to about 12 g/dl. The conversion of fetal haemoglobin to adult haemoglobin (HbA) starts in utero and is completed during the first year or two of life.

At birth the prothrombin level is low because of lack of *vitamin K*, which is required as a cofactor for the activation of several clotting proteins in the blood. A deficiency may result in spontaneous bleeding in the newborn between the third and sixth day of life. The administration of vitamin K can rapidly correct such a clotting problem. By the fifth or sixth day, milk feeding is usually established and the bacteria necessary for the synthesis of vitamin K are present in the intestine.

Temperature control

After birth the baby must adjust to a lower and labile environmental temperature. The heat-regulating mechanism in the newborn is inefficient and the body temperature may drop unless great care is taken to avoid chilling. Heat is lost by radiation, convection, evaporation and conduction. These can be reduced if the baby is born into a warm environment of 26°C, dried carefully and wrapped warmly or provided with skin-to-skin contact with the mother (see Ch. 32).

Skin

The full-term newborn's skin is well developed, opaque with few veins visible, has limited pigmentation and wrinkles around joints.

The layers of the skin include the epidermis, dermis, and subcutaneous layer. The epidermis is a thin but effective barrier, preventing penetration and absorption of potential toxins and microorganisms and retaining water, heat, and other substances. Keratinocytes are the major cells of the epidermis. The dermis is composed predominantly of collagen and elastin fibres enclosed in a gel continuum of mucopolysaccharides; it contains mast and inflammatory cells, blood supply, lymph vessels and cutaneous nerves. The strength and elasticity of the dermis enable it to extend over the joints. The subcutaneous layer is made up of fatty connective tissue, and during the last trimester additional fat is laid down, acting as insulation and a calorific reservoir (Weston *et al.*, 1996).

The skin of full-term newborns is covered with a varying amount of vernix caseosa, a thick white, creamy substance. This forms between 17–20 weeks' gestation and by 40 weeks is found primarily in creases such as axilla, neck and groins, acting as protection during uterine life (Moore and Persaud, 1998). Vernix is a perfectly balanced moisturizer and any surplus should be massaged gently into the baby's skin after the birth.

Gastrointestinal system

Part of the cycle of amniotic fluid is via the fetal gastrointestinal (GI) system, and this is achieved by swallowing (beginning at 10–14 weeks). This process prepares the development of the oesophagus to pass food into the stomach through peristaltic movement. Gut-regulating polypeptides appear by 6–16 weeks and intestinal villi develop at 14–19 weeks. Glucose from the mother is the major source of fetal energy and growth.

Normal function of the gastrointestinal system should be established prior to artificially feeding the newborn baby. This can be achieved through reviewing the woman's history, and antenatal profile. Polyhydramnios, for example, may indicate some disruption of the GI tract.

The midwife also needs to understand glucose metabolism of the fetus and newborn in order to support the woman in feeding her baby, whatever method is chosen (de Rooy and Hawdon, 2002) (see Ch. 33).

After birth the maturation of the GI tract is stimulated by specific peptides: enteroglucagon stimulates intestinal mucosa to develop and motilin encourages gut motor activity.

The baby at 38 plus weeks' gestation has the following features:

- The ability to swallow, digest, metabolize and absorb proteins, simple carbohydrates and emulsified fats.
- Moist and pink mucous membranes in the mouth, and some drooling of mucus in the first few hours following birth.
- Full and well-developed cheeks, with sucking pads.
- Intact hard and soft palate.
- Retention cysts (Epstein's pearls) may be present and disappear some time later. Occasionally the neonate may have one or more teeth.
- Sucking, swallowing and breathing take place in small bursts of three to four sucks at a time and occur very soon after birth. The newborn is unable to move food from the lips to the pharynx; hence normally the nipple is drawn deeply into the mouth.
- Uncoordinated peristaltic activity in the oesophagus in the first few days of life.

- Occasional regurgitation may be noted, as the cardiac sphincter and nervous control of the stomach are immature at the time of birth and take months to mature. (If this is a problem, the baby can be positioned on the right side, and the head end of the cot mattress may be raised to aid stomach emptying. Pillows must never be used under the baby's head.)

Nutritive/non-nutritive sucking is the baby's main pleasure, and may be satisfied by breast- or bottlefeeding alone. Babies will find solace, perhaps following a difficult labour or delivery, in sucking their fingers or thumbs, or suckling at the breast. Mothers need to understand why the baby is frequently feeding so that they are reassured and not concerned they have insufficient milk to satisfy their baby.

Artificially fed babies cry longer than those who are breastfed and may therefore ingest more food and air, and because of inadequate peristalsis in the neonatal period, become uncomfortable as their intestines become full of air and milk. Women need to be taught how to prevent overfeeding and how to improve the baby's comfort, such as by massaging the baby's abdomen in circular motion. Strategies such as frequent stopping, and the use of a smaller hole in the teat, or firmer teat, can slow the feed.

The woman should avoid changing the baby's napkin soon after a feed, as the knee-to-abdomen position increases abdominal pressure and may cause vomiting of newly ingested food. However, this position, 3–4 hours following feeds, can aid the baby to open the bowels if constipated, as also can the intake of extra water with feeds. The supporting gastric and intestinal musculature of the newborn is relatively deficient, shown by the reduced peristaltic movement and the tendency towards distension. The use of pethidine or morphine during labour may decrease peristalsis and in some cases increase regurgitation for several days following birth. Stomach capacity varies between 30–90 ml depending on the size of the baby, and stomach emptying time varies greatly from 1–24 hours.

The gut is sterile at birth, but soon after birth, oral and anal orifices allow bacteria and air to enter and bacteria are found in the large bowel. Bowel sounds can be heard 1 hour after birth.

Meconium is a soft, greenish-black viscid substance, which has gradually accumulated in the intestine from about the 16th week of intrauterine life. It consists of mucus, epithelial cells, swallowed amniotic fluid, fatty acids and bile pigments. Meconium is passed for about 2 days after birth, the first stool being passed within the first 48 hours. The passage of meconium indicates that the lower bowel is patent, though certain conditions, such as a fistula connecting the urethra and anus and absence of the anus, may still result in the passage of meconium. As the baby takes food the residue mixes with the remaining meconium and the stool changes to a greenish-brown colour (*changing stool*). This indicates that the whole gastrointestinal tract is patent. By the fourth or fifth day the stools become yellow. The breastfed baby passes soft, bright yellow inoffensive stools, and may pass stools as often as five or more times a day as lactation is establishing. After 3 or 4 weeks, when lactation is fully established, the baby may only pass one soft yellow stool every 2 or 3 days, as there are few waste products from breast milk. The artificially fed baby passes paler, more formed stools with a slightly offensive odour, and this may occur more regularly when feeding is established, though the baby is more likely to become constipated.

Renal system

The fetus passes urine into the amniotic fluid during pregnancy, and oligohydramnios may indicate renal abnormalities. At term the kidneys are relatively immature, the renal cortex being more immature than the medulla. Glomerular filtration rate and ability to concentrate urine are limited. Relatively large amounts of fluid are required to excrete solids.

The baby should pass urine within 24 hours of birth. Initially urinary output is about 20–30 ml per day, rising to 100–200 ml daily by the end of the first week as fluid intake increases. The urine has a low specific gravity.

If the baby becomes dehydrated, excretion of solids such as urea and sodium chloride is further impaired. Dehydration in the baby can be recognized by a sunken fontanelle, dry mouth, reduced urine output and skin inelasticity.

Glucose metabolism

In utero the fetus relies for growth and development on the intravenous transfer of glucose and other nutrients via the umbilical vein. Under abnormal circumstances such as intrauterine growth restriction (IUGR) the fetus may experience profound hypoglycaemia (Soothill *et al.*, 1987). This may be a factor in children found to be handicapped despite a lack of any hypoxic or traumatic event at birth or during the postnatal period. Fetal metabolism is directed to anabolism under the influence of insulin, utilizing glycogen, fat and protein. Insulin, the main fetal anabolic hormone, can be identified as early as 8–10 weeks of gestation. Cells secreting somatostatin, glucagon and pancreatic polypeptide are also found in the normal mature islet of Langerhans. Whilst the enzymes involved in gluco-neogenesis and glycogenolysis are also present, there is little evidence that either process is active before birth during normal pregnancy. The fetal endocrine pancreas ensures that there is a high circulating insulin : glucagon ratio, favouring anabolism and the formation of glycogen, protein and adipose tissue (Aynsley-Green, 1985).

Metabolic adjustments after birth

After birth, normoglycaemia must be maintained, to protect brain function and to adapt to the intermittent delivery of milk into the gut for nutritional needs. The normal term neonate is able to adapt physiologically to episodes of starvation by utilizing ketone bodies, and this is reflected in a postnatal fall in blood glucose concentration, which may be wrongly viewed as patho-logical and managed accordingly (de Rooy and Hawdon, 2002). The fall in blood glucose coincides with an increase in plasma glucagon levels (Bloom and Johnston, 1972), and may also be due to a cat-echolamine surge and increased activity of the sympa-thetic nervous system. Circulating growth hormone concentration is also high at birth. Following birth the breakdown of glucose continues under the influence of insulin, but about 8 hours after birth the baby begins to switch to glucagon metabolism.

Musculoskeletal system

The musculoskeletal system provides stability and mobility for all physical activity, and includes the bones, joints, and supporting and connecting tissue. This provides a means of protection for vital organs (brain, spinal cord), mineral storage (calcium, phos-phorus) and production of red blood cells. Compared with the skeleton of an adult or a child, the newborn's skeleton is flexible, the bones mainly consisting of cartilage; the joints are elastic, facilitating the passage through the birth canal.

Normal variations in shape, size, contour, or movement may be due to position in utero or genetic factors, and should be distinguished from congenital anomalies and birth trauma. Early diagnosis of dis-orders and early intervention often prevent long-term deformity and the need for surgery.

Central nervous system

The development of the neurological system commences 18 days post-conception and continues until the child is 10 years old. There are three stages of development: neurulation, secondary canalization and retrogressive differentiation, which take place from 18 days. This complex process goes through the development of the brain and spinal cord, and problems in correct fusing may occur comparatively early resulting in myelomeningocele or anencephaly. Neurological devel-opment, specifically brain growth of the fetus/new-born, continues with a further two stages which lay the foundation of the very intricate and yet not fully understood system of the human brain. Stage I occurs from 10–18 weeks of pregnancy and stage II from 20 weeks' gestation to 2 years of age. During stage I the number of nerve cells that an individual will have is being developed; however, environmental factors can affect this development. Stage II marks the spurt in growth of the dendrites of the cortex. After birth the brain continues to grow rapidly within the first year of life, follows a more gradual growth rate until the age of 10 and then there is minimal growth to adolescence. Physiological and psychological well-being are vital to the development of full neurological potential.

At term, babies are born with the ability to be active participants in their environment and are capable of social interaction. It has been shown that they are able to mimic the expression of their carers and are able to some extent to self-regulate themselves.

At birth, the baby's autonomic system functions, maintaining homeostasis of all major organs in order to maintain temperature and regulate cardiorespira-tory function. The well newborn will have mature autonomic and motor systems which can be assessed by the ability to maintain stable cardiorespiratory function. If the baby is unwell or premature, handling will stress the autonomic system and the baby can become cyanosed and bradycardic (Roberton and Rennie, 2001).

State of consciousness in the newborn is influenced by the reaction to stimuli, and it is important to under-stand the baby's level of consciousness in order to pro-vide more sensitive care and management in assisting him in adapting to a given environment and to advance through stages of consciousness gently. Providing this information to the mother, also assists her in caring for her baby, and may help in feeding (see Box 31.1). This ensures that the baby's energy and available resources are utilized effectively.

> **Box 31.1 States of consciousness in the newborn (Brazelton and Nugent, 1995)**
>
> **Sleep states**
>
> 1. *Deep sleep.* Hard to waken, eyes closed, some jerky movements.
> 2. *Light sleep.* Eyes closed, moves from deep to light sleep, light sleep to drowsy state – may be sucking present.
>
> **Awake states**
>
> 3. *Drowsy or semi-dozing.* Eyes open or closed, reacts to source of sensory stimuli, minimal motor activity, eyes with bright look.
> 4. *Quite alert.* Focuses on stimuli source, minimal motor activity in relation to stimuli, may or may not be fussing.
> 5. *Active alert.* Much motor activity, increased startles or activity in relation to stimuli, may or may not be fussing.
> 6. *Crying.* Difficult to get a response to stimuli, will need to bring infant down to state 5 to begin response to stimuli or to feed baby.

Babies are able to 'tune out' noxious stimuli and this occurs through the process of habituation. The baby stores the memory of the stimulus and with repeated episodes learns not to respond to it.

The newborn baby has very poor motor development compared with other mammals but highly developed senses (sight, hearing, taste, smell); hence the importance of picking babies up, talking to them and stroking them to stimulate and evoke response. Maternal–infant interaction is facilitated by eye-to-eye contact with the mother. A 12-day-old baby is able to imitate the facial and manual gestures of adults and this may operate as a positive feedback mechanism to care-givers.

Protection against infection

In utero the fetus is protected from infection by the intact amniotic sac and the barrier mechanism of the placenta, although certain microorganisms do cross the placenta and infect the fetus (see Ch. 39). During the last trimester of pregnancy there is a transplacental transfer of IgG from the mother to the fetus, which provides protection against the infectious diseases to which the mother has antibodies. These antibodies give the baby passive immunity for about 6 months (Remington and Klein, 2000).

The newborn baby has no immunity to the common organisms, and when exposed to them for the first time at birth, is highly susceptible to infection. Soon after birth the baby becomes colonized by the mother's set of microorganisms, which is facilitated by early and frequent contact. Clinical infection occurs when the number and virulence of the organisms overwhelm the poorly developed defence mechanisms of the baby. Breastfeeding encourages specific bacteria to multiply in the bowel and the acid conditions that result from this may help to prevent the overgrowth of potential pathogens, providing some protection from infection.

PREPARATION FOR BIRTH

The midwife is obliged to support the birth of any baby showing signs of life at any gestation – in all environments including outside hospital. It is crucial that midwives are knowledgeable about the physiology of the baby born after 37 weeks, but they also need to be aware of the physiology of babies born at a lower gestation, who may require different care and management prior to transfer to an appropriate acute neonatal unit.

Preparations should have been made prior to the baby's birth, and these include identifying women whose babies are at increased risk or who will require specialist care following delivery. The midwife must be prepared to provide care for what may be considered 'high-' and 'low-risk' women (see Box 31.2), though research indicates that the classification of risk factors remains a debatable area. This ensures that information and preparation are given to the mother and her partner so that she is prepared for a birth rather than a 'normal delivery' of a perfect baby.

The development of complications during labour and birth is recognized as a major contributor towards an increase in neonatal mortality and morbidity (MCHRC, 2001). The midwife is in the prime position to identify that all is normal, but can also detect deviations from normal and make appropriate referral or alter management of care appropriately.

This action plan needs to begin in the antenatal period in order to educate the woman to take control of her body and pregnancy so that she feels confident in the knowledge of normality and seeks appropriate support should deviations occur.

Whether or not problems are anticipated, the midwife should ensure that an area has been identified that can be used for resuscitation of the newborn. In the hospital this may be the resuscitaire; in the home an area needs to be prepared, taking into consideration height of the working surface, adequate space for

working, and light – which may be an Anglepoise lamp or large torch should the mother have requested dimmed lights.

Consideration should be given to the ease with which equipment can be reached and used without detriment to the midwife or the neonate. Some midwives may be surprised to see a laryngoscope included in the list of equipment but this is essential if the baby requires resuscitation as recommended by the UK Resuscitation Council (2002) (see Ch. 35).

Whilst undertaking this vital part of their role, it is a useful time for midwives to discuss with the mother and partner what is being done and why. If sufficient information is given, simply and clearly, the parents will be reassured by the knowledge that the midwife is able to deal with an emergency situation competently and confidently. Although two midwives are not required throughout labour unless support is required for the newly qualified midwife, at the time of birth, one midwife will be required to provide duty of care to the woman and one midwife to provide equal time and duty to the newborn baby.

Box 31.2 Risk factors for specialist care (Levene and Tudehope, 1993)

High-risk pregnancy
- Rhesus isoimmunization
- Moderate to severe pre-eclampsia
- Growth-restricted fetus
- Insulin-dependent diabetes (mother)
- Antepartum haemorrhage
- Prolonged rupture of membranes

Abnormal labour
- Fetal distress
- Deep transverse arrest
- Cephalopelvic disproportion

Abnormal delivery
- Caesarean section
- Moderate or heavy meconium staining of liquor
- Prolapsed cord
- Vacuum or high, medium forceps

Abnormal presentation
- Breech
- Face
- Brow
- Compound/shoulder

Abnormal gestation
- Pre-term delivery

Abnormal fetus
- Hydramnios
- Known abnormality
- Past history of abnormality
- Multiple births

THE APGAR SCORE

The Apgar score was devised by Virginia Apgar in 1953 (Levene and Tudehope, 1993) and is a commonly used quantitative measure of the neonate's well-being at and around birth. Five indicators are used to measure this: heart rate, respiratory effort, colour, muscle tone and response to stimuli (Table 31.1).

This remains a universally useful measure of neonatal condition at birth, though criticized for its simplicity. Each score indicates a physiological state. Recording the numerical score alone provides insufficient information concerning the neonatal condition and may in fact be meaningless. The important factor is that the neonate's physiological condition and progress is recorded verbally and in writing until the neonate is in a good condition.

Table 31.1 The Apgar score

Sign	Score		
	0	**1**	**2**
Heart rate	Absent	Slow < 100	Fast > 100
Respiratory effort	Absent	Slow irregular	Good/crying
Muscle tone	Limp	Some flexion of extremities	Active
Reflex irritability	No response	Grimace	Cry, cough
Colour	Pale blue	Body pink, extremities blue	Completely pink

It is also advisable, if more than one practitioner is present at a delivery where resuscitation is undertaken, that the baby's Apgar score is agreed between practitioners prior to the formal record being made. If there is disagreement regarding the score, the midwife should discuss this with her supervisor and the senior neonatologist. It is important for the future management of the newborn's well-being that an accurate assessment is given.

The most important measures within this scoring system are the heart and respiratory rate. These will indicate the nature and timing of active resuscitation.

An Apgar score of 8–9 indicates that the neonate is in good condition. The midwife should expect that most neonates would obtain a score of about 9 as the baby of above 38 weeks' gestation will have a mature neurological system restricting blood flow to the extremities in order to supply the brain and other major organs with extra oxygenated blood. Therefore the baby will have acrocyanosis, and this condition tends to remain until after 24 hours because of a poor peripheral circulation.

TRANSITIONAL EVENTS

At birth the fetus has to make the transition to independent life, and this requires a significant physiological shift (see above).

If the lungs are unable to inflate, this sequence of events will be impeded whilst the cells in the neonate's body continue to need oxygen and glucose. If ventilation is still not achieved, not only will the ductus arteriosus remain patent, but the foramen ovale will also remain open, allowing a right-to-left shunting of blood. This is an attempt by the neonate's body to conserve energy and reduce oxygen consumption and will result in less oxygen being supplied to the tissues.

An elevated carbon dioxide level will cause a *respiratory acidosis*, in which the pH is low, the CO_2 level is high and the base deficit is normal. *Metabolic acidosis* occurs when a cycle of anaerobic (without oxygen) metabolism takes place. This means that the glycogen stores from the neonate's muscles and fat will be utilized for energy, to be concentrated on the neonate's vital centres such as the heart and the brain. Other organs such as the gut, skin and renal systems will receive a reduced blood supply. The by-product of such metabolism is lactic acid, which is the cause of the acidosis. The blood does contain buffering agents, such as bicarbonate, but these are quickly used up.

This can be described as *respiratory and metabolic acidosis*.

Preparation for resuscitation

It is important that the mother and the midwife are fully prepared for the management of the asphyxiated baby. The midwife needs to ensure that the mother understands that no matter how normal her pregnancy and labour may be, there is still a chance of a problem occurring that will necessitate some action from the midwife. The mother must be given factual, accurate and research-based information in a sensitive manner. Phrases such as 'the baby is a little tired, can you turn on your side' can be seen as matriarchal and protective of the woman. This does not adequately respect her as an autonomous person, nor provide her with the knowledge that she requires to prepare herself psychologically and physically for what may lie ahead.

During the pregnancy, the midwife must allocate a period of time to discuss place of birth and what preparations must be made for the birth. In the community setting the midwife and mother should designate an area to be set aside for resuscitation, whether the birth is planned to take place in the home, hospital or GP unit. The midwife can then assist the mother and her partner to become familiar with the equipment at the same time as ensuring that the equipment and resources are available and are not going to be a health and safety risk. The use of oxygen cylinders and their positioning are important considerations.

The midwife can also prepare a small card to be available for use by a relative or friend should an emergency occur (see Box 31.3). During an emergency, it is normal for those involved to become frightened and anxious and forget simple details; such a card may save a few valuable minutes.

Should the woman have an at-risk pregnancy or labour, the midwife should also ensure that relevant

Box 31.3 **Emergency card**	
Emergency number:	*999*
Name:	*Mrs Bloggs*
Address:	*123 The Street*
	Anytown
	Happy County
Telephone number:	*0181 1234*
Midwife:	*Mary Smith*

colleagues are kept informed including the supervisor of midwives, the neonatologist/paediatrician, the obstetrician and the staff in the neonatal unit.

CARE AT BIRTH

It is the midwife's duty to:

> Examine and care for the new-born infant: to take all initiatives which are necessary in case of need and to carry out where necessary immediate resuscitation …
>
> care for and monitor the progress of the mother in the post-natal period and to give all necessary advice on infant care enabling her to ensure the optimum progress of the new-born infant.
>
> (UKCC, 1998a)

Initially, the midwife will dry the baby's skin with a warmed towel, which is then discarded and the neonate wrapped in another warm towel. The midwife should then use the stethoscope over the apex of the baby's heart to establish and assess cardiac well-being.

Once the heart rate is identified, it will be the greatest indicator of the neonate's needs and the method of resuscitation (for resuscitation, see Ch. 35).

Maternal–infant relationship

The relationship between mother and baby begins at birth and the experience of the pregnancy may act as a positive or negative foundation for early extrauterine relationship. The mother's apparent reaction to her baby will vary greatly according to her culture, experience, expectations and environment and will be affected by her physical and emotional well-being at that time. In some cultures the mother will wish to have immediate and close contact with her baby from the moment of birth. Others will want the baby cleansed and presented in a more restrained way. It is therefore vital that the midwife has discussed the mother's wishes, expectations and fears prior to the labour and delivery so that individual needs can be appropriately met.

'Bonding' is a term to be used with caution as it may imply an immediate and strong relationship at the moment of first sight. This may be very threatening and inhibiting for some mothers who will build up their relationship with their new baby in a slower and less obvious way, though the end result is as enduring and strong.

Research into mothers' reactions to their newborn infants has shown a similar pattern, in that the mother's first response is to touch her baby (easier if the baby is naked) with fingertips and this changes to a protective caressing movement. The mother will often then move the neonate to a position in which she can have face-to-face and thus eye contact. Throughout this time she talks to the baby in a higher-pitched voice than is normal for her (Klaus and Kennell, 1976). Early research suggested the existence of a 'sensitive time' around the birth at which the mother and baby should be encouraged to be together. It was suggested that women missing this sensitive time were at risk of neglecting or abusing their infants. This has since been refuted by Brazelton who postulated that even if the parent and child have to be separated, if the attendants ensure that the mother has photographs of her baby and is involved in the baby's management and care, cuddling or even just touching her child, the relationship can be effectively preserved and nurtured (Brazelton, 1983).

Warmth (see Ch. 32)

The baby has been accustomed to a constant intrauterine temperature of 37.8°C and is born into a much cooler atmosphere, if well prepared, of 26°C. At birth, the baby should be dried to prevent evaporation from his wet skin and then given to his mother who will keep him warm. Warm wrappers are placed over the baby if necessary for skin-to-skin contact. Later the baby is dressed and covered appropriately and placed in a preheated cot. Unnecessary exposure should be avoided. Within an hour of birth the baby's axillary temperature is taken using a low-reading thermometer.

Identification

Two labels record date of birth and sex. An indelible pen should be used and the writing should be clear and legible. These should be shown to the mother or partner and applied to the baby's ankles or wrists whilst in the mother's presence. Should a label become detached, a replacement should be completed and placed on the baby using the same procedure. Ideally the labels should not be removed until the baby is in his own home. The midwife should inspect these labels as part of the daily examination: for cleanliness; for number (i.e. two); and that they are neither too tight nor too loose for the baby's wrist or ankle.

Several maternity units have developed systems to ensure that babies are properly identified and secure and these include the taking of footprints and handprints. These should be prepared showing the names of the mother and baby (if the mother wishes the baby's name to be included).

Ideally, a resuscitaire should be situated in the delivery room, as, should the baby need resuscitation, to remove him from his parents can add significantly to their distress. If the baby does have to be separated from the mother, one midwife should remain with the baby until he returns to the mother, and/or is properly labelled.

Vitamin K

The Department of Health has advised that all babies should be given vitamin K. The Drugs and Therapeutics Bulletin (http://www.dtb.org.uk/dtb/index.html) and local guidelines and leaflets should provide information to the parents on whether or not to give vitamin K and the route of administration.

Excessive bleeding following trauma

Following birth, free circulating vitamin K is low, decreasing during the first few days of life and gradually rising after 3–4 days. This may result in excessive bleeding if trauma occurs, for example during instrumental delivery.

Haemorrhagic disease

Haemorrhagic disease of the newborn (HDN) is a bleeding tendency, which results from a lack of ability in the newborn to utilize vitamin K (see Ch. 34).

Signs and symptoms include bleeding from:

- the GI tract
- the intracranial space
- generalized petechiae
- mucosal surfaces
- circumcision site
- venepuncture site
- heel-prick sites
- the umbilical stump (delayed).

Oral use of vitamin K

Absorption from the gastrointestinal tract is erratic in the newborn and there is possibility of regurgitation and therefore loss of vitamin K and inhalation. More work needs to be done before firm recommendations can be made concerning the optimal dose and form of the vitamin K. Motohara *et al.* (1987) reported that oral prophylaxis with a single 2 mg dose of vitamin K_2 given at birth did not completely prevent the findings of raised PIVKA-II (protein induced by vitamin K absence or antagonist-II) levels at 1 month of age and that levels were also raised in some babies who received a second dose at 1 week of age.

Prophylaxis against late-onset HDN Three babies have been reported to have developed HDN (late onset) after being given vitamin K at birth, therefore it is not yet known how best to prevent late onset of HDN.

The Guthrie test provides a simple method for assessing HDN. Pressure should be applied to the puncture wound after taking the blood sample, and a note made of the time taken for the bleeding to stop. Plasters damage the baby's skin and should not be used unless absolutely necessary.

Education of the parents can also support the midwife in preventing haemorrhagic disease.

Examination of the newborn

It is the midwife's responsibility to undertake a thorough examination of the neonate soon after birth. The later examination by the neonatologist/paediatrician or general practitioner (GP) includes heart and lung sounds, full central nervous system examination, abdominal examination and examination of the neonate's hips. The main aim of the examination by the doctor is to detect abnormalities and reassure the parents.

Since 1994 midwives have emerged not only as lead professionals for the woman but also for the baby, and many midwives are now undertaking this kind of examination rather than their medical colleagues. This provides more continuity of care as recommended by *Changing Childbirth* (DoH, 1993), facilitates the midwife's self-audit, and has the potential for improving interprofessional partnerships (Hall, 1999).

The midwife's initial examination includes a physiological assessment of the newborn, using the senses of hearing, vision and touch supported by the intuitive knowledge obtained from experience. This provides an excellent opportunity for the midwife to continue to support the parents in their new role as carers to the new addition to their family.

The first examination will be undertaken sometime after the birth and, depending on the depth and findings of that examination, a decision will be made as to when and what the aim of the next examination will be. During the postnatal period the midwife will be able to assess the parent–infant interaction. The midwife provides the parents with the relevant information for them to appreciate their baby's individuality, guiding them to recognizing when their baby is not well and how to seek appropriate help when necessary. Accurate record-keeping of each visit and also the aim and goal of the next visit will enable continuity of carers within a midwifery team.

Following the birth the first question the parents wish to have answered is whether or not their baby is 'normal'. They unwrap and examine the baby from head to toe in minute detail equal to that of any dedicated professional. Therefore the midwife's examination is undertaken with the history of that first examination undertaken by the parents. It is important, prior to any examination, that the parents' participation is welcomed and that any concerns they have are identified and discussed.

To assist the midwife's examination, a clinical assessment tool (Examination of the Newborn Tool) has been designed to assess the physiological and behavioural cues that can validate normality and assist the practitioner to recognize deviations from normal (Michaelides, 1994).

The tool includes important information that is gained through assessment and analysis of the woman's history, verbally and through her records. A systematic framework is provided, consisting of examination of the heart at the beginning while the baby is quiet to the most intrusive, such as testing the Moro reflex and measuring the head circumference, which are left to the end of the examination. The latter is undertaken last as the baby will find it uncomfortable and will require to be comforted upon completion.

The tool consists of 26 criteria (A–Z; see Figs 31.5–31.21), and the number of these that will be fully examined at each examination will depend on the experience and training of the midwife. The full examination of the criteria needs to be undertaken sometime after birth and again at 28 days prior to discharge and transfer to the care of health visitor and GP. In between those two examinations, the midwife will assess each baby on its individual history, past and

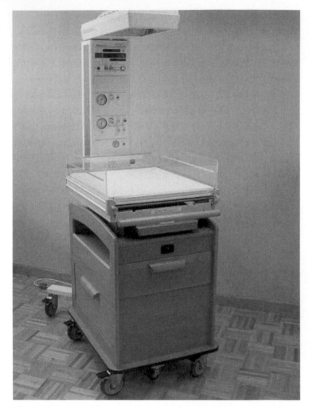

Figure 31.1 Apparatus for examining babies.

present, prior to deciding which criteria need to be validated during physical examination and which will require to be validated through observation alone.

It is recognized that the hips are best examined in the first 24 hours, whereas the cardiovascular system requires continual evaluation until the ductus arteriosus closes (after 48 hours following birth).

Prior to examination, the midwife discusses the examination with the mother and partner, ensuring that they understand the reasons for the examination, and obtaining informed consent. The neonate should have had some time to recover after birth, and therefore the examination should not be undertaken for at least 1 hour following birth. This allows the mother and baby time to adapt to physiological changes and gives time for the baby to adapt to the environment and, if breastfeeding, time to feed successfully.

Preparation is vital so that the process is smooth and effective. An area needs to be set aside for the examination, which provides privacy and a controlled environment. An examining table with an overhead heater and light source can be utilized effectively to examine babies at a height that will prevent

> **Box 31.4 Resources and equipment required to undertake the examination**
>
> - Firm surface
> - Sheets and blankets
> - A spare nappy
> - Cleaning equipment (bowl and cotton wool)
> - Ophthalmoscope (cleaned and pre-set to the practitioner's eyesight)
> - Stethoscope
> - Small torch
> - Tape measure
> - Thermometer
> - Mediswabs
> - Gloves
> - Cord clamp remover
> - Bag for used nappy
> - Non-stretchable tape measure
> - Scales
> - Supine stadiometer/roll measuring mat

practitioner back strain. It provides a safe environment for the baby (see Fig. 31.1) and space for equipment (see Box 31.4) to be stored safely. In the home environment the midwife can use the changing mattress or table (or similar surface area) covered with a warm sheet/towel to examine the baby.

On completion of the examination, the midwife must explain what has been examined and why. This may involve the use of 'link workers', family members or translators for those women who are unable to speak English. The midwife must also demonstrate an ability to communicate with the neonate and an understanding of his 'language', which at this time is used merely to observe and take note of his physiological and behavioural well-being.

PHYSICAL ASSESSMENT OF THE NEWBORN

The baby enters postnatal life with a prior knowledge of a quiet, dark, warm, wet environment with set boundaries provided by the uterus, and enters a whole new world into the confident hands of the midwife or, in some cases, the doctor, and in even fewer, a paramedic or the mother herself. While drying the baby or, in the case of waterbirth, when the baby reaches the surface, the midwife is assessing adaptation to extrauterine life by undertaking the Apgar score

assessment (p. 536) at 1 minute and again at 5 minutes, and a brief physical assessment to exclude gross structural abnormalities.

In that first hour of life the baby is given to the mother or father and their interaction begins. As the baby is alert in this first hour, the mother should be supported to give the baby a first feed by the breast. If the baby is to be given a bottle, the midwife needs to undertake a fuller assessment of the gastrointestinal system. The baby who will breastfeed will take in a small but valuable quantity of colostrum but a baby given a bottle is likely to take an amount of fluid which, if the GI tract is incomplete, such as in cleft palate or imperforate anus, may cause preventable damage.

The formal assessment of the newborn

The assessment includes the criteria in the Examination of the Newborn Tool (Michaelides, 1994). For ease of discussion this is divided into systems and areas of assessment, but would be integrated into a more concise format for the practitioner to use in the practice area.

The completion of this assessment tool will depend on the knowledge and experience of the midwife. For example, full cardiac assessment, listening to heart sounds and feeling brachial and femoral pulses may not be a practice every midwife can currently undertake and the examination may have to be undertaken by another midwife or a doctor or neonatal nurse.

The physical examination of the newborn baby should be performed in a systematic fashion, examining each physiological system to ensure that nothing is forgotten. This involves primarily the skills of observation, palpation and, where relevant, auscultation. Each system should be critically evaluated, normality validated and deviations from normality recognized. Where deviations occur, the midwife needs to ascertain the severity in order to plan appropriate management and where necessary, transfer to the care of the neonatologist.

It is important that the parents recognize that assessment of well-being is a continual process and, as such, one examination only validates normality for that moment in time. With continual observation and care, and professional support through education and physical assessment, there is a growing reassurance.

Using the examination tool, the assessment is as shown in Box 31.5 for areas A–F.

Box 31.5 Examination of the Newborn Tool: A–F

A Identifying data
- Mother's name
- Date of birth
- Baby's hospital/NHS No.
- Sex

B Maternal history
- Age
- Gravida
- Para
- LMP
- EDD
- Abnormalities of previous pregnancies (describe)
- Significant medical, surgical, gynaecological history
- Medication during pregnancy

C Laboratory findings
- Maternal blood type
- Rh factor
- Most recent MCV
- PCV: haemoglobin (Hb)
- HbsAg
- HIV
- Rubella
- Serology
- Other significant

D Family history
- Diabetes
- TB
- Congenital anomalies
- Other significant
- Health status of newborn's siblings

Social history
- Ethnic group
- Single mother/stable relationship
- Type of occupation

E Labour and birth history
- Date/time of birth
- Amniotic fluid colour
- Membranes ruptured
- Length of 1st stage
- Length of 2nd stage
- Hours prior to birth
- Complications of labour
- Complications of birth
- Type of birth
- Perineal status
- Drugs given during labour, and time
- Anaesthesia type and time

F Immediate neonatal period
- Apgar – 1 minute
- Apgar – 5 minutes
- Resuscitation used (facial oxygen, bag and mask or IPPV with mask/endotracheal tube)
- Period of apnoea
- Cord gases
- Blood type
- Rh factor
- Coombs' test
- Antibodies
- Placenta or cord abnormalities
- Medication given

Importance of history

The examination of the newborn commences in the antenatal period. The midwife should review the family history, including the previous medical and obstetric history of the mother and partner. An effective review of the present pregnancy, labour and prenatal period should be undertaken to identify any risk factors which may affect the neonate.

It is important when obtaining a history from women that the communication process is interactive rather than using closed questions that elicit either a 'yes' or 'no' answer. The women should be given the reasons why certain questions are asked and how this affects the care provided. For example, in asking about infectious diseases, the woman would be asked whether she has experienced flu-like symptoms during pregnancy. Many viral infections are not detected because their signs and symptoms can be confused with those of flu or a minor virus. It is vital for the woman to be informed of the importance of pyrexia during the antenatal period in a sensitive way so as not to cause undue anxiety.

Laboratory results need to be assessed by the midwife for their relevance to the assessment of the newborn. For example, a group O positive mother with a baby who is jaundiced may suggest the need to consider ABO incompatibility.

Kell antibodies can attack the bone marrow and reduce red cell production with the result that the baby may be anaemic at the time of birth. Anaemia in the newborn will render the baby hypoxic and require resuscitation at the time of birth and the administration of fresh blood. The affected fetus may require specialist care including resuscitation and blood transfusion following birth.

Sexually transmitted diseases, if not treated in the antenatal period, may affect the baby postnatally and thus the baby will need to be observed for signs of infection (Ch. 47).

Health education is important, but it is not always possible to reduce at-risk behaviour of women, and a non-judgemental and supportive approach is required in obtaining true and accurate information to facilitate appropriate care. Informing the woman of drug withdrawal and its effect on the newborn may encourage her to provide correct information at some point during her pregnancy so that substance withdrawal can be swiftly recognized and treatment instigated.

Information such as the date of the first day of the last menstrual period (LMP) and the estimated date of conception (EDC) is crucial in the calculation of gestational age, which is an important aspect of management of care.

It is of paramount importance to sensitively inform the woman antenatally that no test can guarantee normality for her baby, it can only provide a guide within set criteria.

When undertaken correctly, fetal monitoring (Ch. 26) can assist the midwife to have the relevant practitioners present at the birth of the baby.

The type of birth may affect the management of the baby. A baby who has had a very long labour and birth may be traumatized and may require an initial superficial examination to validate well-being, followed by a full examination when signs of recovery are apparent. Minimal handling may assist the shocked newborn to recover.

Maternal concerns are an important guide to the focus of the examination, as the majority of women will spend some time examining their baby, feeling, stroking and counting fingers and toes, and they will have a good idea in the majority of the cases if their baby deviates from normal.

General appearance (Box 31.6)

Both age and gestation of the baby will influence his general appearance.

The time of the last feed will also affect the behaviour of the baby. A hungry baby will be difficult to

---

Box 31.6 Examination of the Newborn Tool: G

G General appearance
- Well/not well
- Weeks of gestation
- Age at examination (hours/days)
- Weight: which centile?
- Length
- Position
- Posture and state of consciousness
- Spontaneous activity
- Body proportions
- Facial expressions
- Cry
- Vital signs: temperature and respirations

---

examine as the majority of the examinations require a quiet calm baby who will be able to tolerate handling for 10–15 minutes in order to complete the physical examination. Ideally, the examination should not last longer than 15 minutes.

Type of birth and postnatal age of the baby can affect the behaviour. A baby who has had a difficult birth may be very irritable or be in a deep sleep (State 1 – see Box 31.1), and the behaviour of the baby will inform practice. The physical examination can be delayed until the baby is able to tolerate handling and the examination of the baby is undertaken by observation of well-being.

Observation

Observation of the baby is undertaken with a 'hands-off' approach, in the position that the baby is in at that moment in time. The baby of above 38 weeks' gestation will display a flexed posture indicating good muscle tone (Fig. 31.2). Facial features are noted, to see whether the baby has dysmorphic features.

Gestational assessment

In the past, the weight designated term and preterm babies. For example a baby weighing below 2500 g was deemed to be premature and below term. Further research (Battaglia and Lubcjemco, 1967) showed that gestational age and whether the baby's growth is appropriate for that age was a greater predictor of outcome.

Assessment tools such as the Dubowitz scoring system (Dubowitz et al., 1970) are used to assess the gestational age of the newborn using a neurological scale (see Ch. 34). This assessment is used if the baby is deemed to be less than 38 weeks' gestation. The main assessment of gestational age can be carried out using approximate estimates of fetal development, these being the LMP, the estimated date of delivery (EDD), ultrasound and physical characteristics.

Table 31.2 shows physical characteristics of the newborn at two gestations.

Graphs are now available (see Ch. 34) that are used to plot the baby's weight, length and head circumference against age, to assess whether the baby is average for gestational age (AGA) and born above 38 weeks' gestation, when problems are least likely. Babies also born above 38 weeks' gestation but with measurements below the 9th centile line on the graph are deemed to be small for gestational age (SGA). Large-for-gestational-age (LGA) babies are those whose measurements lie above the 97th centile, and they are deemed to need extra attention because they are likely to have more sequelae.

Weight   The baby should be placed on scales that are regularly maintained for accurate measurement and recording. They are zeroed after a warmed sheet or blanket has been placed in the scales to prevent heat

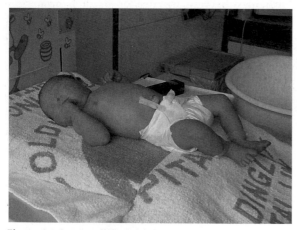

Figure 31.2   A well-flexed baby.

loss prior to the baby being weighed and to provide comfort. Care must be taken to ensure that the neonate's surroundings are warm and free from draughts and that he can be safely placed in the scales.

The weight can then be plotted on the centile chart, and babies who are small or large for gestational age identified and a plan agreed. Babies below the 9th centile have reduced glycogen stores and may be more prone to hypothermia and hypoglycaemia, so thermoregulation and feeding need to be given extra attention.

The baby will lose 5–10% of body weight in the first week of life, then steadily gain at an average rate of 25–30 g per day until 6 months of age (Wilkinson, 1997).

Length   There is debate as to whether or not babies should be measured. Historically, the neonate was lifted by the ankles and suspended while being stimulated to breathe by administration of a sharp slap, and measured in the same position. However, in order for length measurement to be deemed correct we need to use a supine stadiometer (Wilkinson, 1997) newborn length instrument, as used by some maternity units, or a rollamat (Fig. 31.3). Both methods require the baby to be stretched, and therefore two persons are needed to undertake these measurements effectively.

Head circumference   This measurement is taken with a non-stretchable tape applied closely around the scalp, using the frontal and parietal eminences and the occiput as markers. The largest estimate of three is taken. Immediately following birth the measurement may be increased by oedema or caput, and thus it needs to be repeated when the swelling has subsided.

Vital signs

The temperature is measured as the respiratory rate is counted. If the baby is cold (less than 36.5°C) the

Physical characteristic	36 weeks' gestation	40 weeks' gestation
Ear cartilage	Ear less complicated in character	Pinna firm and springs back firmly when folded
Breast tissue	Nodule present 1–2 mm in diameter	Nodule present 6–7 mm in diameter
Male genitalia	Rugae not fully present	Covered in rugae
Female genitalia	Labia majora cover labia minora	Clitoris covered by labia majora
Plantar surface	Some creases present	Creases cover the sole

Table 31.2   Physical characteristics of the newborn at 36 and 40 weeks' gestation

examination may be discontinued or the baby is placed under the radiant heater for the rest of the assessment.

The respiratory rate is usually between 40 and 60 breaths per minute although, as discussed earlier, the baby's behaviour prior to counting the respiratory rate needs to also be taken into account. All infants are periodic rather than regular breathers and premature infants are more so than full-term infants. This means that the neonate may have periods of very even breathing and periods when the respirations are uneven and there are long gaps between breaths.

In a warm infant there should be no expiratory grunting and little or no flaring of the nostrils. As a general rule, if the infant has good colour and appears in no respiratory distress, it is of no further benefit to percuss the chest.

Skin (Box 31.7)

The skin is a large organ which not only protects the baby against infection but also enables communication. The sensations of touch, pressure, temperature and pain are received by 1 million nerve endings. When the newborn baby has been rubbed dry, touching and picking up are procedures that need to be undertaken gently to minimize discomfort to the baby. The skin also enables maternal–infant interaction to take place through gentle soothing touch or massage.

The epidermis of the skin of a newborn is thin and delicate and in postmature babies is dry and sometimes peeling. The colour of the baby's skin is pink, red or pale. Pink is the normal colour of newborns. Red/plethoric colour which, when the baby cries, becomes a dusky/purple, may be due to an excessively high packed cell volume (PCV) and is deemed to be pathological as it may indicate polycythaemia. The thickening of the blood can cause clots in the blood vessels to the main organs such as bowel, liver or brain and may also affect glucose metabolism in the newborn. Pale skin or pallor is an indication of poor perfusion and anaemia. Infants of diabetic mothers tend to be pinker than average and 'postmature' infants are paler. The best environment to observe colour of the baby is in natural daylight, as artificial light can affect the depth of colour observed.

Asian and dark-skinned babies may have blue naevi scattered around any area of the body, and what are referred to as Mongolian spots may be mistaken for bruises. Parents are sometimes concerned and need to be told that this deep pigmentation of the skin will disappear in a few months.

Petechiae are normally caused through traumatic delivery, for example a tight cord around the neck; they should disappear within 24–48 hours. If this does not happen and they appear to multiply, the baby needs to be referred for diagnosis of the pathological cause.

Jaundice may occur physiologically after 48 hours because of extra red cell breakdown in combination with an immature liver which cannot metabolize all unconjugated bilirubin; the latter leaks under the skin and gives a jaundiced colour. Utilizing the Kramer tool (see Ch. 37) supports estimation of jaundice.

The common variations of the skin include tiny milia on the nose (plugged sweat glands).

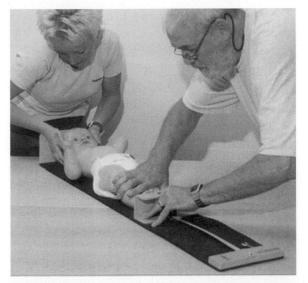

Figure 31.3 Measurement of height. (From Jokinen, 2002.)

Box 31.7 Examination of the Newborn Tool: H

H Skin
- Colour: changes during activity
- Staining: meconium/blood/jaundice
- Presence and location of oedema
- Presence, condition and shape of nails
- Texture
- Lesions/peeling

Variations: milia, acrocyanosis, Mongolian spots, erythema toxicum, forceps marks, bruising

Abnormalities: haemangiomas, pustules, many petechiae, plethora

Erythema toxicum may be noted. These papular lesions with an erythematous base are found more on the trunk than on the extremities and fade away without treatment by 1 week of age. Occasionally their profusion is alarming.

Haemangiomata

- *Vascular naevi* are superficial capillary haemangiomata, which may occur over the upper eyelids and the nape of the neck, sometimes hidden by the hairline. These diminish in size and fade by 1 year of age.
- *Capillary (strawberry) hemangioma* usually presents between birth and 2 months of age. These are most common on the face, scalp, back or chest. This hemangioma enlarges prior to diminishing by 1 year of age and disappears by the age of 5–7 years.
- *Port wine stain (naevus flammeus)*, if situated on an area of skin over a nerve pathway, such as the trigeminal area on the face, may be associated with meningeal haemangioma (Sturge–Webber syndrome). Large areas of discoloration may require laser treatment.

The skin is observed daily for soreness, rashes and septic spots. The midwife should make every effort to avoid trauma to the baby's skin or indeed to any superficial tissues.

Cardiorespiratory system (Box 31.8)

The heart and lung assessments are interlinked in order to reduce handling and ascertain how both function, to distinguish between heart and lung physiology and pathology.

Observation

Colour The infant's colour is probably the single most important index of the function of the cardiorespiratory system. 'Good' colour in Caucasian infants means a reddish pink hue all over, except for possible cyanosis of the hands, feet, and occasionally the lips (acrocyanosis). The mucous membranes of dark-skinned babies are more reliable indicators of cyanosis (and degree of jaundice) than the skin.

The baby's colour should be assessed at regular intervals in the postnatal period. The examinations, whenever possible, should be undertaken with the baby naked, in order to ascertain symmetry of colour from head to toe.

Chest cavity The general appearance of the chest is noted, observing the neck and collarbone area. The chest and abdomen are examined, which gives the midwife the opportunity to observe respirations. The position of the nipples is noted and the presence of skin tags, accessory nipples, or skin discoloration recorded.

Box 31.8 Examination of the Newborn Tool: I

I Chest – respiratory

The respiratory system is best assessed early in the examination to take advantage of the quiet state of the neonate.

Lungs
- Respirations (recession, rate, depth, type, type of breathing periodic/shallow)
- Shape/symmetry
- Symmetrical expansion
- Symmetrical diaphragmatic movement

Variations: breast engorgement, supernumerary nipples, placement of nipples, 'witches' milk
Abnormalities: tachypnoea at rest, recession, retractions, grunting, inaudible breath sound, and asymmetry of diaphragmatic movement, apnoeic episodes, cyanosis in air

I Chest – cardiac

The cardiac examination is best carried out early in the examination to take advantage of the quiet state of the neonate.

Heart
- Colour of infant
- Symmetry of colour from head to toe
- Central perfusion
- Peripheral perfusion
- Thrills and heaves
- Capillary filling time
- Point of maximum impulse, lower left sternal edge, pulmonic area, aortic area and between scapulae
- Rate, rhythm, character
- Presence, quality and symmetry of pulses:
  a. brachial
  b. femoral

Abnormalities: presence of cyanosis when quiet or crying, visible pulsations over precordium, heaves, thrills, presence of murmurs, absent femoral pulses, delay in brachial and femoral pulses

- The chest should be rounded, and the left and right sides of the chest cavity should be moving symmetrically, with breathing being mainly via the action of the diaphragm and abdominal muscles.
- The respiratory rate and pattern are observed to confirm symmetrical movement of the diaphragm. Asymmetrical movement of the diaphragm should alert the midwife to possible phrenic nerve damage. Although babies may have periodic breathing, episodes of true apnoea are deemed abnormal and may indicate neurological damage or abnormality.
- The baby should be able to sustain breathing without the use of accessory muscles; indrawing of intercostal or subcostal muscles and signs of accessory muscle use should be recognized as severe respiratory distress.
- The baby's breathing should be quiet – audible sounds are a sign of deviation from normal. The type of sound can help to identify the origins of respiratory difficulty. For example, inspiratory grunting could indicate a problem in the upper airway, i.e. oedema or mass. An expiratory grunt suggests the cause is in the lower airways and may be due to hypothermia, surfactant deficiency or meconium aspiration.

Palpation

The chest is palpated gently as there may be breast enlargement due to maternal hormones, and pressure can cause discomfort and pain.

The position of the heart is checked to see whether it is on the left or right side of the chest. This is best done by auscultation (see below), but it can be confirmed occasionally by palpation. This is followed by validation of the absence of heaves and thrills and identification of the point of maximum impulse.

Capillary filling time is also measured using applied pressure on the chest or squeezing of the ear lobe or toe and expecting the blood flow to return within 3 seconds.

Brachial and femoral pulses are identified and palpated for strength, rhythm and volume. The femoral pulses should be felt for, although often they feel quite weak in the first day or two. Dorsalis pedis pulses may be substituted. Femoral pulses are best palpated when the baby is quiet, as it is vital to the assessment of cardiovascular function for their presence to be validated.

Auscultation

Breath sounds – whether normal or abnormal – may be noticed by the practitioner prior to the use of the paediatric stethoscope, which may then identify heart and breath sounds. This can be done after a period of observation which can enhance the examiner's perception, knowledge of and communication with the neonate. A stethoscope with a double-headed chest piece with an open bell and a closed diaphragm should be used. Warming the chest piece by applying friction to the stethoscope head reduces disturbance of the baby and thus makes auscultation easier.

Auscultation of breath sounds in the newborn is easier than in a child, as breath sounds are being established, with absence of crackles and wheezes (see Fig. 31.4).

The heart should be examined. It is important that the limitations of this examination are kept in mind and it is used in conjunction with examination of other aspects such as femoral pulses. It should be determined whether the heart is on the right or left side, and the examiner should observe precordial activity, rate, rhythm, quality of the heart sounds and the presence or absence of murmurs.

It is difficult to try to examine the heart of a 'fussy' or crying baby. When the baby is peaceful the rate, rhythm and presence of murmurs can be determined much more easily. The midwife could encourage the mother to pacify the baby by the use of her little finger or a dummy.

The heart rate is normally between 120 and 160 beats per minute, and varies with gestational and chronological age and changes with activity.

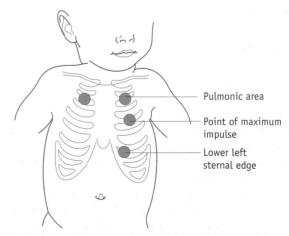

Figure 31.4 The areas of auscultation of heart and lung sounds.

Murmurs mean less in the newborn period than at any other time. A neonate may be found to have an extremely serious heart anomaly without any murmurs (Hall, 1996). A closing ductus arteriosus may cause a murmur that, in retrospect, is only transient, but at the time is very loud, worrisome, and misleading. Gallop sounds may be an ominous finding, while the presence of a split 'S2' (i.e. lub dub dub) may be reassuring. If new to auscultation of heart sounds, it is difficult to ascertain SI and S2. However, if the brachial pulse is palpated simultaneously with auscultating the lub dub, the identification of sounds becomes easier.

The stethoscope may aid assessment of the cardiovascular system. However, by far the best assessment is to observe, or obtain an accurate history of, the baby's behaviour. A baby who has been active but suddenly becomes lethargic and appears to have less tone, is not interested in feeding, or is tachypnoeic on effort, needs urgent referral and admission by ambulance to the nearest acute neonatal unit. As major congenital abnormalities can be duct dependent, most cardiac conditions will be diagnosed in the community. Therefore it is important for the parents to understand the normal behaviour of the newborn in order to seek advice if the baby deviates from what is expected.

The cardiovascular assessment is not complete until the liver is palpated and deemed to be of normal size.

Morphological examination (Boxes 31.9–31.14)

Accurate assessment of the morphological system is essential for identifying the baby who will need more thorough examination, medical/support services or family counselling. External assessment of dysmorphic features offers clues to the presence of internal anomalies. The morphological examination requires a systematic approach to assessment, including observation and palpation.

The head (Box 31.9)   The shape of the head following birth can be round, bullet-shaped or an elongated oval. Parents can be very disturbed and worried on first viewing their baby, and need to be reassured that the baby's head will assume its natural shape, given time. This needs to be noted, as the measurement of the head circumference will differ from birth to the one taken 4 or 5 days later. The average full-term head circumference should be approximately 33–38 cm

---

Box 31.9 Examination of the Newborn Tool: J–K

J Head
- Head circumference
- Shape/symmetry
- Anterior fontanelle
- Posterior fontanelle
- Palpate sutures:
  a. open
  b. width
  c. prematurely fused
  d. overriding
- Skull depressions or irregularities

K Hair
- Texture
- Distribution/direction of swirl
- Scalp lesions

Variations: moulding, caput succedaneum

Abnormalities: coarse hair, cephalhaematoma, macrocephaly, hydrocephaly, craniotabes

---

when measured around the occipital–frontal diameter, avoiding the ears.

The vault of the head is held in the midline while the size, shape and symmetry is assessed.

The infant's scalp and face should be inspected for cuts, abrasions or bruises. Sites of trauma such as fetal blood sample site should be identified and recorded.

The presence of caput succedaneum or cephalhaematoma should be noted (see Ch. 15).

The mobility and width of the suture lines are noted, and also the degree and direction of moulding of the skull bones. The fontanelles are examined. Large fontanelles may reflect a delay in ossification of bones and may be associated with hypothyroidism. The anterior fontanelle can provide valuable information on the well-being of the baby. In its normal state it is flat and at the same level as the surrounding bones. A sunken fontanelle can be one of the symptoms of dehydration, and a full and bulging fontanelle and wide sutures are characteristic of hydrocephalus.

The hair (Box 31.9)   The condition and amount of hair is also noted as this can be affected by certain metabolic disturbances (e.g. hypothyroidism).

Box 31.10 Examination of the Newborn Tool: L–M

L Face
- Symmetry
- Expression
- Shape

M Eyes
- Symmetry: shape and size
- Pupils react to light
- Sclera
- Bilateral red reflex
- Presence of lashes and brows
- Lacrimal process

Variations: strabismus, subconjunctival haemorrhages

Abnormalities: prominent, narrow, flat forehead, micrognathia, paralysis, epicanthal fold, cataracts, bushy eyebrows, very long eyelashes, exudate, setting sun sign, jaundice, Brushfield's spots, repetitive movement of the eyelids, erythema of the conjunctiva, eyes do not react to light and incomplete red reflex

Box 31.11 Examination of the Newborn Tool: N

N Ears
- Symmetry/alignment
- Hearing
- Shape

Variations: preauriculur sinus, overly prominent ears, Darwin's tubercle, absent anthelix

Abnormalities: low-set, large, flabby ear; abnormal attachment, absent external meatus, does not respond to loud noises, secretion of fluid (blood or serous)

The face (Box 31.10) is examined for normal appearance and symmetry of eyes, ears and features during crying and rest.

The eyes (Box 31.10) should be checked for congenital cataracts, and any small haemorrhages under the eyes or within the conjunctiva noted for size and severity. The eyes may be tested for the red reflex by means of an ophthalmoscope. When examined, the retina is seen as clear and red; the amount of red pigment is dependent on race.

The ears (Box 31.11) are examined for symmetry and normal position on the baby. An imaginary line is drawn from the inner canthus of the eye to the posterior fontanelle, and the helix of the ear should be above the line to validate normality. The pinna of the ear should be flexible and recoil easily (Tappero and Honeyfield, 1993: 47/8). Accessory auricles and skin tags should be noted. The midwife should examine the ears closely, including the backs of the ears for small spots or skin tags.

Hearing Sensitivity to sounds should be noted. The ability to hear enables babies to commence communication and learn about the world they live in. However, one baby will sleep through the loudest music and another will be startled by someone speaking softly. Therefore the best time to assess whether babies can hear or not is when they are fully awake. Hearing could be tested by observing the baby when a loud noise is made, but hearing can and should be tested fully at a later date.

The mouth (Box 31.12) should be checked, and the midwife should ensure that there are neither hard nor soft palatal clefts (Bannister, 2001). Both the hard and soft palates should be palpated and visualized. The rooting and sucking reflexes are elicited (see p. 559). The gums are examined for clefts and to ensure that there are no deciduous teeth present. Epstein's pearls (small white inclusion cysts clustered about the midline at the juncture of the hard and soft palate) are a normal finding. Tongue-tie, in which the frenulum restricts the movement of the tongue, should be identified.

The mouth should be examined at regular intervals to validate normality and exclude infection, for example thrush.

The nose (Box 31.12) is examined for normal position and the presence of nares and possible choanal atresia. This may or may not be easily identifiable.

Suctioning of babies is no longer advisable unless in specific circumstances of meconium or blood being present at birth. If the baby has a suction catheter introduced into the nasal passages, the baby may become snuffly due to damage to the epithelial lining and dissection of the mucous glands. Unless the baby has a problem with breathing, time will heal the

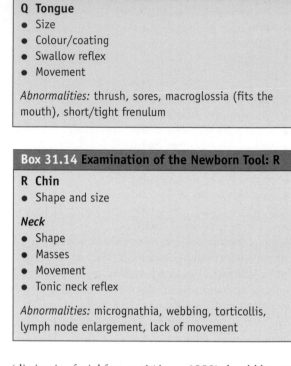

> **Box 31.12 Examination of the Newborn Tool: O–P**
>
> **O Mouth**
> - Symmetrical grimace
> - Arched palate
> - Lips/gums
>
> **P Nose**
> - Size
> - Placement
> - Symmetry
> - Patency of nares
>
> *Variation:* Epstein's pearls, sucking tubercle, premature dentition
>
> *Abnormalities:* choanal atresia. Cleft soft/hard palate, high palate arch, profuse saliva, unable to suck, swallow and breath, abnormal masses

> **Box 31.13 Examination of the Newborn Tool: Q**
>
> **Q Tongue**
> - Size
> - Colour/coating
> - Swallow reflex
> - Movement
>
> *Abnormalities:* thrush, sores, macroglossia (fits the mouth), short/tight frenulum

> **Box 31.14 Examination of the Newborn Tool: R**
>
> **R Chin**
> - Shape and size
>
> *Neck*
> - Shape
> - Masses
> - Movement
> - Tonic neck reflex
>
> *Abnormalities:* micrognathia, webbing, torticollis, lymph node enlargement, lack of movement

damage and breathing should be normal within several days.

The neck (Box 3.14) The neck is passively examined for rotation and for anterior and lateral flexion and extension. In anterior flexion, the chin should touch or almost touch the chest, and on extension, the occipital part of the head should touch or almost touch the back of the neck. When there is asymmetrical rotation or lateral flexion or when range of motion is limited, it is recognized as abnormal. The neck should be examined for goitre and thyroglossal or brachial arch sinus tracks.

The spaces hidden by creases should be examined for evidence of septic spots or irritated skin.

Sharing information with parents

If on completion of the morphological examination there are concerns that the baby is dysmorphic it is important to communicate the concerns to the parents. One useful way to begin the discussion is to ask the parents whom the baby resembles. The parents may then feel they can disclose their concerns. On the other hand, it may be that the baby does have a resemblance to other members of the family, but this does not exclude a genetic abnormality, and the baby should be referred to a neonatologist for follow-up. The words we use to describe a dysmorphic baby need to accentuate the positive; therefore words such as

'distinctive facial features' (Aase, 1990) should be used rather than 'abnormal' or 'deformed'.

Musculoskeletal system

History

Prenatal history is vital to the musculoskeletal assessment because the uterine environment affects the musculoskeletal development of the fetus. Any event or condition that changes the intrauterine environment can alter fetal growth, movement or position. Factors such as oligohydramnios, breech presentation, abnormal growth patterns and exposure to teratogenic agents may adversely affect the development and maturation of the musculoskeletal system in utero. The skeletal system is interlinked with the neurological system and therefore factors such as possible birth trauma need to be considered when analysing the facts.

The history of the birth, such as duration of labour, signs of fetal distress, type of birth (vaginal or caesarean), have a bearing on conditions such as cerebral palsy and brachial palsy.

In multiple gestations, the birth order is also worth noting because there is a higher incidence of congenital hip dysplasia in first-born children.

An accurate gestational age assessment is necessary for assessment of the infant's posture and muscle tone.

Careful scrutiny of the musculoskeletal system during the newborn's physical examination is imperative because the information recorded during the first examination forms the database for all future examinations.

Examination

Ideally, a thorough physical examination of the skeletal system should be done within the first 24 hours after delivery. The musculoskeletal examination must be done systematically. The examination should include the skull, clavicles, upper limbs, legs, spine and finally the hips. The rationale that supports the given systematic framework is based on the fact that if an abnormality of the spine is noted, the senior neonatologist will undertake the hip examination, thereby limiting the stress to the newborn. As with other systems, skeletal examinations are undertaken while watching the newborn or while examining other systems.

A thorough evaluation of the musculoskeletal system includes an appraisal of:

- posture, position, and gross anomalies
- discomfort from bone or joint movement
- range of joint motion
- muscle size, symmetry, and strength
- the configuration and mobility of the back.

Observation

Observation should proceed from the general to the specific. General inspection includes observation for symmetry of movement as well as size, shape, general alignment, position and symmetry of different parts of the body.

Soft tissue and muscles should be observed for swelling, muscle wasting and symmetry. In the extremities no asymmetry of length or circumference, constrictive bands, or length deformities should be noted.

The ratio of extremity length to body length is also observed.

Palpation

This technique, along with inspection, is used on each extremity to identify component parts (for example, the two bones in the forearm), function and normal range of motion.

Upper extremities (Box 31.15)

Clavicle   The clavicles are inspected and palpated for size, contour and crepitus (grating that can be felt or

---

> **Box 31.15 Examination of the Newborn Tool: S**
>
> **S Upper extremities**
> - Movement
> - Clavicle
> - Radius and ulna
> - Finger length/movement
> - Nails: shape and size
> - Grasp reflex
> - Length
>
> *Variations:* single simian crease without any other signs
>
> *Abnormalities:* single simian crease, syndactyly, polydactyly, fisted hands, abnormal shape/position of digits, paranychia

---

heard on movement of ends of broken bone). A broken clavicle is one of the most common birth injuries in newborns, which can be very uncomfortable and painful.

A fractured clavicle should be suspected when there is a history of a difficult delivery, irregularity in contour, shortening, tenderness or crepitus on palpation.

Humerus   Length and contour of the humerus should be noted. A fractured humerus should be suspected if there is a history of difficult delivery. A mass due to haematoma formation may also be noted, or signs of pain during palpation.

Elbow, forearm, and wrist   The elbow, forearm, and wrist are examined for size, shape and number of bones as well as for range of joint motion.

Hands   The hands should be examined for shape, size and posture, while the fingers are examined for number, shape and length. Inspection of palm creases should also be included. Although a single simian crease across the palm is usually associated with Down's syndrome, it is often found in normal babies.

The fingers are usually flexed in a fist with the thumb under the fingers.

Examine the nails for size and shape. The nails are usually smooth and soft and extend to the fingertips. The mother needs to be told how to cut the nails to avoid causing infection to the nail bed, which can cause septicaemia.

Whilst dressing or undressing the newborn the midwife should note any apparent discomfort.

Abdomen (Box 31.16)

History

During fetal life the fetus relies on the placenta for food and elimination of waste products. Following birth, in order to sustain life, the newborn baby must adapt to the intermittent intake of nutrients necessary for the body's metabolic requirements of growth, replacement and energy production, followed by their digestion and utilization, and the excretion of waste products. The baby is able to suck and swallow but the digestion process and glucose metabolism take time to adapt to postnatal life.

Physical assessment of the gastrointestinal system therefore commences with the mouth and completes on examination of the anus to confirm normality prior to the baby being able to undertake artificial feeding, as this entails a comparatively large intake volume.

The shape of the abdomen should be rounded, soft, symmetrical and slightly protruding. Fullness of the abdomen will depend to some degree on the time the baby has last fed. A flat abdomen may signify decreased tone and may herald the presence of abdominal contents in the chest cavity through a diaphragmatic hernia or abnormalities of the abdominal musculature.

Abdominal skin in the term baby is smooth and opaque, with a medium-thick texture. Post-term babies have thick, parchment-like skin with superficial or sometimes deep cracking in the creases of the skin, and no vessels seen over the trunk.

Midline defects such as omphalocele or gastroschisis may be seen at birth, and the immediate management is to avoid fluid loss and maintain a clean environment; therefore the baby's body is placed in a special plastic bag and tied below the arms, or wrapped in cling film from below the arms. Diastasis recti (separation of the rectus muscles) is a common finding in the newborn. Another midline malformation is an umbilical hernia which reduces spontaneously within 2 years. However, if it is large it will require surgical treatment.

Umbilical cord

The umbilical cord is examined prior to cutting it (Fig. 31.5) and applying the Hollister clamp, to exclude herniation of intestine into the cord itself and to visualize the presence of three vessels. Two vessels, one artery and a vein, sometimes indicate renal anomaly (Thummala *et al.*, 1998). The cord is a bluish white colour and gelatinous at birth. The quantity of Wharton's jelly affects the thickness of cord. Large-for-gestational-age infants have thick, gelatinous cords. Babies with congenital syphilis may also have thick cords. Thin small cord is another indication of intrauterine growth restriction.

The cord darkens and shrivels as it dries, and falls off within 10–14 days. The cord should be dry and not have drainage of any type. Drainage of any colour before or after separation is deemed a deviation from normal; for example clear discharge indicates a patent urachus or omphalomesenteric duct (see Tappero and Honeyfield, 1993: 84, Fig. 7-6).

The area around the cord is observed for any redness, which needs to be dealt with quickly to avoid serious septicaemia. The mother needs to understand

---

Box 31.16 Examination of the Newborn Tool: T

T Abdomen
- Shape/size: symmetry
- Movement
- Bowel sounds
- Umbilicus
- Femoral pulse
- Liver size
- Kidney felt/not felt
- Spleen felt/not felt
- Bladder felt/not felt
- Masses

Variations: diastasis recti, umbilical hernia

Abnormalities: distension, ascites, umbilical discharge/odour, flare, enlarged liver, spleen or kidney, masses – abdominal or in groin area

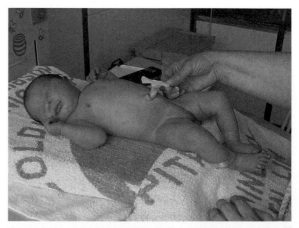

Figure 31.5   The correct length for clamping and cutting the cord.

the potential for infection from urine and faeces if the umbilical cord is placed inside the nappy, and the midwife can support the mother by showing her how to place the nappy so that the cord is always on the outside (Zupan and Garner, 2001).

Cleaning the cord   A good handwashing technique is essential before attending to the cord, otherwise there may be a spread of *Staphylococcus aureus*, which can be highly dangerous. The umbilical cord is inspected daily by the midwife for signs of infection and separation. It separates by a process of dry gangrene, usually between the fifth and seventh day. If the cord is soiled by a dirty nappy, it should be cleaned with water only and dried with cotton wool swabs.

The application of spirit and powder or antiseptic sprays was shown to delay separation of the cord as far back as the early 1980s (Barr, 1984; Lawrence, 1982, Magowan *et al.*, 1980). In these studies, cords not treated or treated only with an antibacterial powder separated by the seventh day and showed no increase in infection. A larger, more recent study confirmed the finding that there is no increase in infection when the umbilical cord is not treated with alcohol wipes and hexachlorophene powder (Dore *et al.*, 1998).

Peristaltic movement

The observation of movement needs to be undertaken from the side of the abdomen and at eye level. The midwife should observe for patterns and shape of movement. Normal abdominal movements are synchronous with chest movements. After 1 hour of life, intermittent peristaltic movement is visible. Continuous peristaltic movement can imply obstruction.

It is important for the midwife to auscultate numerous neonatal heart and bowel sounds in order to be confident in validating normality.

Palpation

Before palpating the abdomen, the midwife needs to check that the baby has not been fed a large amount prior to the examination because such a baby will not be able to tolerate deep palpation. The midwife should stand at the side of the baby and, as with the rest of the examination, the hands must be warm and the nails short to enable palpation of the deep organs to take place without discomfort to the newborn. Ideally the baby should be lying supine and be relaxed. Palpation should be light at first, progressing to deep palpation. The baby's facial expression needs to be observed for signs of discomfort or pain, and to validate that the

liver and spleen are not enlarged, the baby's respirations need to be synchronized with the palpation. Flexing the baby's knee at the hip can allow the abdominal muscles to relax and aid palpation.

Light palpation of the four quadrants assesses the texture and warmth of the skin; it also reveals tenderness and guarding. Deep palpation identifies the absence of masses. Faecal masses may sometimes be felt along the descending colon or in the suprapubic area.

The liver is a superficial organ and palpation needs to take that into consideration. The liver edge should not be more than 2 cm inferior to the right costal margin. Babies in heart failure do not become oedematous but the liver acts as a sponge for fluid, and a baby in heart failure will have an enlarged liver which can be palpated more than 2 cm below the costal margin. Slight oedema can sometimes also be seen around the eyelids.

The spleen is a deep organ; thus firm pressure needs to be applied in order to confirm normality. As with other systems, not being able to palpate the spleen equates to normality.

The abdominal area overlying the kidneys is also ballotted, applying firm even pressure. The kidney should not be felt.

Vomiting

Most babies vomit at some time and mostly this is unimportant (Orenstein, 1999). However, there are circumstances when the type of vomiting is important, the main one being green bile. It cannot be assumed that this is meconium which was ingested at birth; the baby should be discussed with a senior neonatologist so that an obstruction can be excluded. Usually, the origin of blood is clear from the history but if there is any doubt the laboratory can perform an Apt test (blood mixed with sodium hydroxide), which distinguishes fetal from adult haemoglobin.

Possets   Small, frequent vomits are referred to as 'possets'. Possetting is particularly common in the first few days after birth, especially if the baby has swallowed any blood or meconium. It is also common when the milk flow is excessive. Most babies cope with these episodes quite well and either swallow the regurgitated contents or cough them out. The parents need to be informed how to manage these episodes. The baby should be left slightly on his side while the posset is wiped away gently. The baby should not be lifted or patted on the back as both will overstimulate the baby and may affect the coordination of sucking, swallowing and breathing.

If the baby has inhaled a large amount of vomit, appropriate resuscitation needs to take place (Page and Jeffery, 2000). Prior to any resuscitation involving mask ventilation and when the baby has had a feed, the midwife needs to be prepared to pass a nasogastric tube to empty the contents of the stomach to avoid inhalation.

Examination of the groin

In the baby lying quietly the groin is flat, and if the baby is thin, visible pulsation of the femoral pulse may be noted. Any visible swelling on crying or on palpation must be referred urgently for diagnosis and management. The diagnoses that could be made are inguinal hernia or undescended testis in the male or female, leading to questioning the sex of the baby.

Genitourinary (Box 31.17)

Male infant genitalia
Scrotum   All embryos are initially female. Then, under the influence of testosterone, the labia enlarge to become a scrotum. It has a brownish pigmentation and should be fully rugated.

Testes   The testes should be palpated. Normally, the testes of a full-term newborn are approximately 1.5–2 cm in length (Conner, 1993) and when palpated have a consistency similar to that of a pea. If the

---

Box 31.17 Examination of the Newborn Tool: U
U Genitourinary
• Appropriateness of genitals for sex of infant
• Male scrotal size
• Testes
• Urethral opening
• Female clitoral size
• Hymen
• Passage of urine (within 24 hours)
• Passage of stool (within 48 hours)
Variations:
Male: priapism, adherent foreskin, skin rugae
Female: mucoid vaginal discharge
Abnormalities:
Male: epispadias, hypospadias, hydrocele, chordee
Female: enlarged clitoris, inperforate hymen

---

scrotum appears discoloured and the testes feel solid, urgent referral is required.

The differential diagnosis for the presence of a solid scrotal mass includes testicular torsion, scrotal haematoma and testicular infarction (Diamond and Gosalbez, 1998).

Hydrocele   The signs of a hydrocele include palpation of a cystic mass in the scrotal pouch. The whole scrotum appears swollen and firm – like a balloon filled with water – and it allows the passage of light from a torch (transillumination) (Diamond and Gosalbez, 1998). Hydroceles are not uncommon but unless they are communicating types, they will disappear in time.

Undescended testes   (UDT) is a common finding in the neonatal period. In most cases the aetiology is unknown. There is an increased risk of infertility and testicular cancer in men with a history of UDT. The testes are very sensitive to temperature and can sometimes be seen moving up the inguinal canal. If a testis is not readily identified, a finger sweep should be performed from the anterior iliac crest along the inguinal canal. It can take up to 3 years for UDT to descend; therefore the baby will be followed-up until the testes have descended.

Hypospadias   It is important to recognize that congenital abnormalities rarely appear singly; therefore if the baby is noted to have UDT extra vigilance is required to validate that the urethral opening is central on the glans. In hypospadias the opening is found on the under surface and in epispadias it is above. Observing the baby pass urine is a good method of observing normality.

The penis shape and length are noted. Chordee is a lack of ventral tissue on the penis leading to it being curved ventrally. Surgery is required to correct the condition.

Female infant genitalia
In the female newborn the labia majora cover the labia minora and the clitoris.

Before designating a sex to an apparently female infant, the labia majora must be parted and the clitoris observed to be an appropriate size. The hymen should be perforated and this is validated by a discharge from the vagina. The discharge is usually creamy white in colour and consistency, is commonly found at birth, and is occasionally replaced after the second day by pseudomenses. If the hymen is not perforated, it appears like a tiny smooth bald head.

Ambiguous genitalia

If there is doubt as to the sex of the baby, it is important that the concerns are discussed sensitively with the parents (Ahmed and Hughes, 2002). Parents will often be very distressed and will continually apply pressure to be told the sex of the baby. The parents will take on board any terminology used so it is important to avoid the terms 'he' or 'she' or 'it'. At the same time, the sex of the baby cannot be entered on the birth certificate until further investigations have been undertaken to designate a sex to the baby. If the 'wrong' sex is registered it is an extremely difficult and lengthy process to correct the mistake (Reiner, 1999).

Anus and rectum

The anus and rectum should be checked carefully for patency and position. The use of a clinical thermometer for ensuring anal patency is now considered to be outmoded practice. The anal sphincter is assessed by gently touching the anus and eliciting the anal 'wink', which is the contraction and retraction of the muscle proving the anus is patent. If further proof is needed, anal patency can be more effectively proved by the passing of a lubricated catheter or awaiting the passage of meconium. This observation is considered to be as effective and may indeed prevent the trauma that may be caused by passing a thermometer via an anal obstruction. It is postulated that 94% of babies will pass meconium, thus proving anal patency, soon after birth (Gryboski and Walker, 1983). The use of a thermometer may be indicated in the case of hypothermia, and should be preceded by the passage of a soft rubber catheter.

Stools   A record is made of the number and character of all stools passed.

Constipation   Constipation most commonly occurs in babies who are artificially fed. Extra water may be given. Breastfed babies may not pass a stool for 2 or 3 days once feeding is established but this is quite normal providing the stools are the usual soft, yellow consistency.

Urinary output   A record is made of the number of wet napkins in each 24-hour period. The odour and colour of the urine are also noted. Occasionally a red stain is found on the napkin due to urates colouring the urine.

Lower extremities (Box 31.18)

When the baby is viewed, the position of the lower limbs will give a picture of the position the baby adopted in utero. The majority of babies would lie with the legs folded on the abdomen and appearing externally rotated and bowed with everted feet. The baby delivered in a breech presentation often has flexed, abducted hips and extended knees. This positional adaptation of the lower limbs should not be confused with congenital malformations; however, a midwife who is in doubt should refer to a peer or a neonatologist for a second opinion.

The midwife should examine the baby for normal appearance, for length, shape and movement of limbs, ensuring that the baby is able to utilize each limb fully and thus that the joints are functional. The legs are palpated to ascertain the presence of the femur, tibia and fibula. Femoral length can be observed by straightening both legs together and noting the length or by testing for the *Allis sign* as follows. Keeping the feet flat on the bed and the femurs aligned, flex both of the baby's knees. With the tips of the big toes in the same horizontal plane, face the feet, bend so that the baby's knees are at eye level and note the height of both knees. It will be apparent if one knee is higher than the other, a positive Allis sign. A positive Allis sign may indicate developmental hip displacement.

The feet should be examined for shape, size and posture, i.e. that the baby is using both feet and when at rest a normal position is adopted.

Box 31.18 Examination of the Newborn Tool: V

V Lower extremities
- Leg length
- Allis sign
- Movement
- Tibia and fibula
- Ankle dorsiflection
- Position of feet relative to ankles
- Babinski reflex
- Toes: length/movement
- Nails: shape and size
- Creases on feet

Variation: bowed legs

Abnormalities: syndactyly, pes cavus, pes valgus, pes varus, rocker-bottom feet

Ankles and feet   Examination of the ankles and feet includes observation of resting and active movement. Passive motion of the ankle in dorsiflexion and plantar flexion varies depending on the infant's position in utero. For example, ankle and forefoot adduction, a positional deformity, can be differentiated from congenital equinovarus (clubfoot) malformation by passively positioning the foot in the midline and gently applying pressure to dorsiflex the foot to form a square window.

A clubfoot or other structurally abnormal foot and ankle will not have a full range of motion and will resist dorsiflexion and not be able to form a square window.

The toes should be examined for number, position and spacing between them. Note should be taken of whether webbing is present between the toes and whether the nails are a normal shape and appearance. The soles of the feet should be inspected as part of the gestational age assessment. The feet should therefore each be opened fully. This part of the examination is undertaken when eliciting the Babinski reflex (see below).

Assessment of the back (Box 31.19)

Spine   The detection of neural tube defects frequently occurs before delivery, as a result of maternal AFP measurement or ultrasound examination. Therefore the birth will take place in the appropriate unit and the relevant staff, neonatologist and neonatal nurses, will be present to support the midwife at the birth of the baby. However, not all women choose to go for antenatal screening and some women may not have presented for antenatal care; thus spinal neural defects could still present without warning.

On completing the examination of the lower limbs, the baby is lifted and held suspended with the examiner's hand under the chest. In this position the back is observed, to see the curvature of the spine and also the baby's ability to lift the head. The spine should be straight, excluding scoliosis, kyphosis and lordosis.

The back continues to be observed with the baby lying prone. The spine is then examined from the base of the skull to the coccyx, noting any skin disruption, tufts of hair, soft or cystic masses, haemangioma, pilonidal dimple cysts or sinus tract. These deviations from normal may be signs of congenital spinal anomaly.

The position of the scapulae should also be noted while the infant is in the prone position to rule out Sprengel's deformity, a winged or elevated scapula.

The entire length of the spine should be gently palpated to ensure that it is complete and that there is no sign of pain.

If birth takes place in the home and meningocele (herniation of meninges) is noted, the midwife must refer this to the appropriate personnel and transport the baby safely into hospital. Before and during transport, the lesion, especially if ruptured, should be covered with a sterile, non-adherent dressing. If that is not available, gently place sterile gauze soaked in normal saline and wrap gently in cling film. Pressure on the affected area must be avoided, and the baby should be nursed in the prone position and gently driven into hospital.

Hips (Box 31.20)

History

Developmental dysplasia of the hip (DDH) is the preferred term for the disease previously referred to as congenital dislocation of the hip (CDH). The new term takes into consideration that dislocation of the hip can develop after birth, and although the hips can be deemed to be normal at birth, the baby can later have a positive screening for a dislocated or dislocatable hip joint. The pelvic girdle of the neonate is not fully ossified and does not have the same characteristics as the adult pelvic girdle. Notably, the acetabula are shallower

---

Box 31.19 Examination of the Newborn Tool: W
W Back
• Spinal curve: (corrects with lifting the baby, or not)
• Spine integrity
• Anal patency
• Gluteal folds
• Trunk incurvation
• Reflex
Abnormalities: cysts, dimples, hair tufts, pilonidal sinus, nevus pilosus, scoliosis

---

Box 31.20 Examination of the Newborn Tool: X
X Hips
• Barlow test
• Ortolani test
Variation: audible click
Abnormalities: pain on attempting to abduct and resistance, audible clunk, dislocated and dislocatable hip/s, difference in leg length, difficulty in abducting hip to 90 degrees

than in the adult. The acetabulum is still developing and thus it is quite possible for the femoral head to be able to move outside the acetabulum (luxation or dislocation) or through an abnormality within the acetabulum (subluxation or partial dislocation).

Early detection is vital, since if DDH is left untreated the hip joint develops abnormally and surgical reduction is required. If the abnormality is diagnosed early, the use of splints allows the hip joint to develop normally and avoids surgical intervention.

Examination

The ideal time for the examination of the hip (Fig. 31.6) is within the first 24 hours of life if the baby's condition allows. Incidence of dislocatable hips is higher in the first 24 hours when the neonate's muscles and ligaments are still developing and not strong enough to always support this joint.

High-risk factors for DDH include (Keay and Morgan, 1982: 269):

- family history of DDH
- abnormal rotation of the developing hip during the first trimester
- neuromuscular disease, especially in the second trimester
- abnormal mechanical forces, e.g. oligohydramnios
- breech presentation in utero for a significant part of fetal life
- female infants (who are more susceptible to the maternal hormone relaxin).

The left hip is more frequently affected than the right.

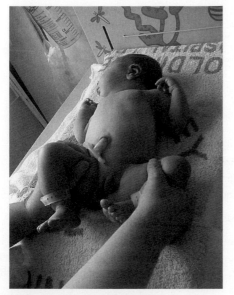

Figure 31.6 Examination of the hips.

Care that can prevent DDH includes postnatal application of mechanical forces associated with the baby being able to fully abduct the hips:

- being allowed to lie in the prone position when awake
- being carried in a sling with hips fully abducted – African babies whose mothers transport them in this way have a low incidence of DDH.

The hips should be examined at regular intervals for congenital dislocation, which may be identified by the use of one of two tests – the Ortolani test or the Barlow test:

- the Ortolani test detects a dislocated hip reducing during the examination
- the Barlow test detects a hip dislocating or subluxing during the examination.

A distinctive 'clunk', if felt, is of significance. However, 'clicks' are often felt while performing these tests and are not predictive of DDH but can be confusing for someone who is inexperienced in undertaking hip examinations.

Ideally, examination of the hips should be undertaken at the end of the examination as it is often disruptive and uncomfortable for the neonate.

Practitioners who undertake the examination of the hips need to have undertaken training in that area, during which they have been both shown and observed by an expert in the examination. The practitioner can practice the tests on the 'Baby Hippy' manikin prior to undertaking them on a baby. An inexperienced practitioner can cause damage to the baby by failing to diagnose a false negative test, because of poor practice, or use excessive force on a dislocated hip during abduction, causing damage to blood supply and ligaments around the joint.

Observation

Firstly the midwife should observe the neonate and note any difficulties with abduction. For example, if the baby found the procedure of examining the femoral pulses distressing or the Allis sign was positive, the practitioner will have an indication that the right or left hip may be dislocated.

Ortolani and Barlow tests

The baby should be lying relaxed on a flat, firm surface. The environment should be warm and free from draughts.

It is vital that unless the practitioner is expert at examining hips, only one hip is examined at a time. This way the practitioner is able to focus fully on undertaking the manoeuvre correctly.

The Ortolani test
- Stabilize one hip by bending the knee and hip, keeping the pelvis stable and firmly on the mattress (Fig. 31.6).
- Bend the other knee and hip.
- Place two fingers over the greater trochanter (outer upper leg).
- Position the thumb on the inner trochanter.
- Attempt to abduct (away from the midline of the body) the thigh to 90 degrees by applying pressure with the two fingers on the greater trochanter.

It must be noted that if the hip is dislocated, it will not be possible to abduct it and the neonate will keep the thigh at an angle less than expected. This angle is noted and recorded.

The Barlow test
- Continue to stabilize one hip, keeping the pelvis stable and firmly on the mattress (Fig. 31.6).
- Once again, bend the other knee and hip.
- Place two fingers over the greater trochanter (outer upper leg).
- Position the thumb on the inner trochanter.
- This time, the thigh is lifted and adducted (moved towards the midline of the body).
- With pressure applied with the thumb laterally, the femur is telescoped several times to note any movement of the head of the femur away from the acetabulum. Normality is confirmed when no movement is noted.

These two manoeuvres are then repeated with the other hip joint.

If any deviations from normal are noted, the examiner should refer the baby for examination by a senior medical practitioner.

Additional investigations
X-rays are unhelpful in assessment, as the femoral head is cartilaginous until 6 months of age. Ultrasound examination of the hips is undertaken as part of screening for DDH; however, its effectiveness is not recognized by all.

The Ortolani and Barlow manoeuvres remain the best screening method for DDH if undertaken by a competent practitioner.

Neurological examination (Box 31.21)
Assessment of neurological function is the initial step in evaluating a neonate's responses to the transition from extrauterine life and environmental factors in the perinatal period that may have caused a pathological response of the central and peripheral nervous system. Assessment of neurological function and identification of deviations from normal is an important area of midwifery practice in order not only to reduce mortality but also to improve the quality of life for the newborn and his family.

The Apgar score and its running commentary may indicate a baby that requires focus on neurological well-being. The type of delivery, such as in shoulder dystocia, can cause brachial plexus damage, facial and Erb's palsy, paralysed vocal cords and damage to the phrenic nerve, all of which need to be excluded. Thus it can be seen that the examination of the neurological system is in large part undertaken by examining the other systems.

Physical examination
Probably the most reliable information that can be obtained quickly from a neurological evaluation is gained while discussing the baby's behaviour with the mother and handling the infant during the preceding parts of the physical examination.

Box 31.21 Examination of the Newborn Tool: Y

Y Neurological system
- Activity
- Tone
- Posture
- Response to stimuli
- Sucking reflex
- Movements:
  a. normal/abnormal
  b. spontaneous
  c. symmetrical/asymmetrical
- Pull to sit manoeuvre
- Reflexes: rooting, sucking, tonic neck, palmar grasp, stepping/placing, Babinski, trunk incurvation, anal wink, Moro

Variation: jittery

Abnormalities: floppy tone, drowsy/passive response, abnormal rhythmic sustained movements of extremities (e.g. fits), fits, high-pitched cry, absent sucking reflex, jittering does not respond to pressure

Level of consciousness One of the most important parts of the examination is the neonate's alertness and interaction with his mother, his overall behaviour and movement preceding and during the examination.

Mental status

Cry is the main method of communication for the baby to alert the carers to pain, hunger, discomfort or suffering. When listening to the sound of crying, it is important to note a clear tone without hoarseness or nasal tone. It is important that the carers understand the types of crying in order to give appropriate care. For example, for a baby in pain, the type of pain and whether or not the baby requires pain relief needs to be established and may require change, i.e. from an uncomfortable position to a soothing bath, massage, sucking on a finger or breast, as feeding alone will not dissipate the pain. It takes time and skill to interpret the different sounds, and conscious effort needs to be given to listening and observing babies in order to perfect this form of communication.

Head shape and size, fontanelle and suture size are examined as stated during the morphological examination. Cranial bruit may indicate an intracranial vascular malformation.

Face Facial dysmorphism may indicate a genetic syndrome such as trisomy 18, and also the facial features are observed during crying for facial palsy.

Eye examination The baby's pupil should be equal and reacting to light, and the red reflex should be present and completely round in shape.

Skin Cutaneous birthmarks such as café au lait spots may indicate presence of genetic disorder such as neurofibromatosis.

Skeletal system The skeletal and neurological systems are interlinked and thus examination of the baby can indicate an abnormality, e.g. a hair tuft over the spinal region may indicate a degree of spina bifida.

Tone The strength and reflexes of limbs can indicate normal or abnormal movements indicating neurological damage.

Reflexes

A well-known philosopher stated that human beings came into this word in 'tabula rasa' meaning as empty vessels; however, it is now known that babies are aware of the environment in utero, and at birth they are equipped for survival. The baby at birth can hear, smell and taste, and see up to a distance of 30 cm (Wilkinson, 1997) and favours the colours black and white. The majority of reflexes are deemed to be primitive, involving the brainstem and spinal cord.

- *Sucking reflex*. This can be tested by placing a clean, little finger into the baby's mouth or observing the baby feeding. The baby will tend to make sucking efforts, whether hungry or not. This will illustrate the baby's ability to coordinate breathe, suck and swallow, making this an important measure of neural integrity.
- *Rooting reflex*. This is a primitive survival reflex in which a touch on the baby's cheek will cause him to move his mouth to the site of touch, searching for food. When the upper lip is touched the mouth will open. These are useful reflexes for the mother to utilize when preparing the baby for feeding, whether breast, bottle or cup feeding.
- *Grasp reflex*. This can be tested by brushing the infant on the back of the hand. The hand will then open to grasp an offered finger. The midwife should then extend the baby's arms and lift the baby gently, observing the head and how well controlled or lax is the way in which it is held. This will also test the *traction reflex*. This reflex will also need to be checked after a traumatic birth to note nerve damage that may not be obvious by observing the tone and position of the arms.
- *Moro reflex* (startle reflex). This can be observed physiologically or tested for. The baby may already have demonstrated this reflex during the examination, and therefore a further demonstration is not required. If it has not been seen, the midwife can test the reflex by first ensuring the baby is calm and at rest. The midwife supports the baby's head with the left hand from the neck to the lower back and brings the baby's chin to his chest. The baby is then elevated several centimetres off the bed and the baby's head allowed to drop gently to the right supporting hand. The baby will throw his arms back and then forwards towards his chest, allowing his fists to close. He may also cry. The aim of this examination is to enable the baby's head to appear to fall into an empty space; it is not to fall from a height and the head must never touch the mattress. This procedure must not be undertaken if the baby is not relaxed.

- *Asymmetrical tonic neck reflex*. The baby will extend his limbs on the side of the body his head is turned towards.
- *Stepping or walking reflex*. The baby is supported by the practitioner with the soles of his feet flat against the mattress. This will encourage the baby to put one foot in front of the other, straighten his spine and attempt to 'walk'.
- *Babinski reflex*. The baby's foot is supported in the left hand and pressure is applied with the index finger of the other hand on the outer part of the sole of the foot up to the small toe and across to the big toe. The normal response is for the baby to extend and fan the toes and finally to flex them. The midwife can take the opportunity to note webbing of the toes when eliciting this reflex.

The complete behavioural examination is quite dependent on infant–examiner interaction, and thus the midwife should aim to examine the baby with gentleness and respect, communicating with him on both verbal and non-verbal levels.

Cranial nerves

The 12 pairs of cranial nerves are referred to by name or roman numerals (Table 31.3). They originate from different parts of the brain, and assessment of their function confirms normality and recognizes deviations from normal.

Assessment of the autonomic nervous system

The autonomic nervous system is involved in a complex of reflex activities essential to sustain life and these are dependent on sensory input to the brain or spinal cord. Normal autonomic function in a baby at term is well developed and it can be observed through the following reflex actions:

- the ability to adapt temperature to the environment
- respiratory rate and heart rate changes with physical activity
- responses of the pupils to light
- contraction of the external anal sphincter (anal wink) in response to touch or when air is blown over it – the muscular opening of the anus should have a firm appearance and not be distended and lax
- skin – harlequin sign – when the baby is lying on one side, the upper area is light and the lower area dark red.

Identifying and managing pain and stress in the term newborn

Until the 1980s it was thought that babies did not feel pain, and therefore pain relief was rarely given.

Dummies laced with brandy and sugar were sometimes used to pacify a very distressed newborn; however, procedures which required pain relief in children or adults were undertaken on newborns without pain relief. Today from numerous studies (mainly on rats) we understand the physiology of the pain pathway in

Table 31.3   Cranial nerves

No.	Name	Type and function
I	Olfactory	Sensory: smell; able to smell mother's breast pads
II	Optic	Sensory: vision
III	Oculomotor	Motor, autonomic: eye movement
IV	Trochlear	Motor: eye movement
V	Trigeminal	Sensory, motor, autonomic: rooting, sucking reflex or blink of the eye
VI	Abducens	Motor: eye movement; optical blink, notes face, follows object; doll's eyes – normal if when the head is turned to one side, the eyes move in the opposite direction
VII	Facial	Motor: facial movement; facial movements when crying; wrinkled brow – smooth if paralysed
VIII	Vestibular	Sensory: hearing and balance; response to sound
IX	Glossopharyngeal	Somatic/autonomic, motor to tongue, soft palate and pharynx; tongue movement and gag reflex; correct position of the uvula
X	Vagus (cranial)	Autonomic motor/sensory soft palate, pharynx and larynx: swallowing; hoarse voice or stridor; ability to swallow present or absent
XI	Accessory	Motor: neck and shoulder; head turns from side to side; shoulder height
XII	Hypoglossal	Motor: tongue movements; gag or suck reflex; atrophy of the tongue

babies and we now recognize that the baby's spinal sensory nerve cells are more excitable than those of adults. Midwives, doctors and nurses rely on patients to report their pain and its severity. The baby is unable to speak, so practitioners need to be aware of evidence of pain and obtain experience of the normal behaviour of the baby. The time spent observing babies is invaluable, not least when trying to understand how to adapt the care provided in order to minimize stress and pain to the newborn.

The physiological response to painful stimulus in the baby is greater and lasts for a longer period of time than in the adult. Adults have a sophisticated nerve pathway which can narrowly pinpoint the area of painful stimulus. In the newborn this pathway is still developing, which means the baby is unable to localize pain but can feel pain in response not only to painful stimuli but also to touch over a wide area of the body (Anand and Scalzo, 2000). Damaged skin, either from a heel prick or ventouse or other instrumental birth, will be very sensitive to touch.

Newborns feel pain (Anand, 2001), and therefore procedures that can cause pain should be kept to a minimum. Following birth, giving the baby to his mother instantly provides human contact. Being stroked gently and given the opportunity to suck at the breast will reduce the newborn's pain and discomfort (Carbajal et al., 2003). Bathing or washing the baby for whatever reason needs to be delayed until the baby has had time to recover and for his skin to heal prior to pressure being applied to broken or bruised skin. It is important to note that damage to the skin at birth or soon after can cause the damaged area to be oversupplied with sensory nerve terminals, which will leave the area hypersensitive to touch for some weeks after the wound has heeled. This information needs to be shared with parents for them to have an insight into the baby's behaviour when that area is handled.

Causes of pain   The effect of certain procedures needs to be considered in relation to the amount of pain caused to the baby, for example:

- long/precipitate labour – headache
- type of labour, e.g. occipitoposterior position
- instrumental birth – bruising/trauma from ventouse cap
- heel pricks undertaken for the Guthrie test, etc.
- removal of plasters
- insertion of intravenous needles for antibiotic therapy

- delivery of fluid to the subcutaneous tissue following blockage of an intravenous cannula.

Signs of pain   One of the best indicators is vocal expression, heard in long-lasting crying. Facial expressions – brow bulge, eye squeeze and nasolabial furrow – are also reliable indicators of pain (Stevens and Johnston, 1993). Other behavioural signs of pain include pedalling movement of the legs, toes spread, legs tensed and pulled up, agitation of arms, and a withdrawal reaction.

Sucrose administration   The majority of research regarding non-pharmacological analgesia was performed on babies at term undergoing a heel prick procedure to obtain blood. Prior to this procedure, the baby should, if possible, be held by the mother if breastfeeding to establish sucking for several minutes, or the baby can be given a dummy/finger to suck throughout the procedure (Carbajal et al., 2003). If possible/available, sucrose should be given to reduce pain.

One study has shown that breastfeeding alone can reduce crying; however, a number of randomized controlled trials provide unequivocal evidence that babies cry less when given a combination of nutritive or non-nutritive sucking and sucrose (Carbajal et al., 2003). 2 ml of 12–25% sucrose is administered and the baby is able to suck for 2 minutes before being subjected to a painful procedure.

It is recognized in many cultures that the taste of sweetness reduces pain. Also, massage, speaking to the newborn and obtaining eye contact are methods that can reduce pain.

Research on pain has been undertaken on the Guthrie and venepuncture procedures, which are recognized as being very painful for the newborn and for the parents observing a distressed newborn. There needs to be clear evidence of why we need to undertake every heel prick procedure.

The inability to communicate in no way negates the possibility that the baby is experiencing pain and is in need of appropriate pain-relieving treatment. The issue is no longer that neonates are incapable of feeling pain but how the carers minimize procedures that cause pain and, when that is not possible, recognize pain and provide appropriate pain relief (Carbajal et al., 2003).

Jitteriness versus seizures

Jitteriness, although not a type of seizure, is a movement disorder that is characterized by movements with qualities primarily of tremulousness but occasionally also of clonus. It is important to distinguish jitteriness from seizures. If the limb that is tremulous is pressed down against the mattress and the tremors stop, seizure is excluded; if movement continues, it is a positive sign of seizure. It is important for the midwife to call for help and stay with the baby to observe the progress and length of seizures. Staying with the baby is also important in order to provide support if the respiratory system is involved.

Assessment of feeding (Box 31.22)

The final part of the assessment is that of feeding, and this is a crucial part of ascertaining well-being. A baby who has been feeding well and who becomes tachypnoeic on feeding will require urgent further assessment.

Mother–baby attachment

Parent–infant interaction is believed to play a central role in the infant's social, emotional and physiological development. The quality of the interaction between mother and baby can provide the baby with an environment for optimal development and growth. The foundation of this relationship is trust and affection. If there is failure to develop this relationship, the baby is at risk of delays in neurological developmental, child abuse, neglect and failure to thrive (Pridham *et al.*, 1999). Research has shown that educating the mother to understand her baby and his behaviour can have a positive effect on maternal–infant interaction (Anderson, 1981).

> **Box 31.22 Examination of the Newborn Tool: Z**
>
> **Z Feeding**
> - Pattern
> - Number of feeds per 24 hours
> - Baby waking up/woken up for feeds
> - Amount/timing
> - Settles after feeds
> - Vomiting
>
> *Variation:* reluctance to feed, small posits, urates
>
> *Abnormalities:* Noticeable change in feeding pattern: green vomit, perfusion changes during feeding, tachypnoea with feeds, regurgitation or vomit, vomiting, failure to gain weight, delay in passing meconium, blood in stools, dark urine and pale stools

---

Today, women stay in hospital less than 24 hours for a non-complicated birth, and therefore teaching opportunities are limited. Antenatal classes can provide the ideal opportunity for women to receive the necessary education and this serves as a valuable health-promotion tool to effect positive parenting beginning at birth.

After the time of prolonged contact at birth, mother and baby should be kept together as much as possible during the early neonatal period when they are getting to know one another and mothering skills are developing. This is not a problem if the birth takes place in the home. If birth takes place in hospital, the Maternity Services Advisory Committee 1985 advocated that the baby's cot remains beside the mother's bed. Restricted contact between mother and baby in the early postnatal period is associated with less affectionate maternal behaviour and maternal feelings of incompetence and lack of confidence (Thomson and Westreich, 1989). Maternal–infant attachment established from birth is strengthened by the woman getting to understand her newborn baby, and because handling her baby can aid this process, the mother is encouraged to care for her baby soon after birth. The use of strategies such as the shortened Brazelton Neonatal Behavioural Assessment scale can assist parents to learn more about their baby's capabilities (Nugent, 2004). Unrestricted access allows her freedom to respond to her baby whenever he is awake. Although it is recognized that this is an important aspect of initiating the relationship between mother and baby, the ability to enhance that relationship is to some extent dependent on the mother's physiological well-being.

In order for interaction to take place between mother and baby there needs to be a means of communication between them. The mother must be able to respond to the cues given by the baby, the baby needs to respond to the cues given by the mother, and the environment must be such as to facilitate that interaction. It is difficult for a woman who has had a difficult delivery to respond physically to her baby if she is unable to move and handle her child. The midwife needs to provide the response to the cues given by the baby while allowing the mother to recover from her difficult delivery, and in doing so, acts as a role model, educating the woman about the different cues the baby provides, such as cues to hunger, boredom, discomfort and pain. A crying baby can overwhelm the woman's psychological well-being at this vulnerable time following birth. The father, too, should be involved in his child's care and progress, otherwise he may feel neglected and become jealous of the close relationship developing between mother and baby.

Three stages have been described in the maternal–infant attachment process.

- The first is when the mother and baby first become acquainted and involves early physical contact.
- The next is the care-taking relationship when the mother learns to care for her baby, to feed, change, wash and bath him.
- The final stage is called identity, when the child is incorporated into the family. To reach this final stage mother and baby grow to know and love each other as they interact. The newborn may initiate interaction by crying. The mother responds by rocking the cot or picking him up and cuddling him. This is the expression of a normal mother's instinct to tend and protect her child and it should be encouraged rather than repressed. The baby stops crying when he is picked up and becomes alert and responsive, so the mother should be encouraged to talk and establish eye-to-eye contact with him. In turn the baby gazes at his mother and responds; thus mother–baby interaction is synchronized and attachment develops.

In some situations mother and child have to be separated because of maternal illness or the need for special and intensive care of the newborn and most mothers are likely to overcome any adverse effects of this separation (Thomson and Westreich, 1989). Some consider that the degree to which a mother perceives separation as having an adverse effect on her mothering ability may be related to the outcome (Richards, 1978; Ross, 1980) and also the contact between mother and baby while the baby is in hospital (Moore and Nelson, 2003). It is possible that women of low socioeconomic status who have low social support may be more adversely affected by restricted contact with their baby than their more affluent counterparts (Thomson and Westreich, 1989). This was demonstrated in a study by Anisfeld and Lipper (1983) and highlights the benefits to women with low social support and their babies when they have early and prolonged contact soon after birth. Those with high levels of social support of course also benefit, but usually form close attachments to their babies whether or not they have early contact.

Some mothers are, not uncommonly, worried because they do not feel a maternal instinct or that they really love their baby during the early days of motherhood. They need reassurance that their feelings are quite normal and that, as they learn to know their baby and he them, they will gradually fall in love with him.

Each society and culture has its own set of behaviours and what is accepted as normal and appropriate maternal–infant interaction and it is important to acknowledge these differences.

Newborn behaviour

For the first 6 weeks of life the baby does not distinguish night from day and spends day and night sleeping, waking, crying, feeding and sleeping again. The baby will, on the whole, feed every 3–4 hours. What parents find difficult is that the baby is awake at night and asleep during the day. Newborns have a very small stomach and require regular intake of food. Babies move from one sleep state to another, from quietly looking around, actively responding to sounds, to crying. Parents are sometimes concerned not to spoil their babies and therefore delay in answering their baby's cries. Prior to 6 months of age the neural processes are not mature enough to enable the baby to manipulate the carer; the baby is unable to think 'if I cry I will get my mother to come to see to me'; the baby is not able to lie. If and when the baby cries, it is for a reason such as hunger, fear, discomfort, pain or boredom. Rather than spoiling the baby, if the mother/carer answers the cries immediately the baby will develop securely, knowing his needs will be answered (Bell and Ainsworth, 1972).

A baby's primary needs are for food, fluid, sleep, warmth, security and love. His method of expressing those needs is crying, which is a signal to the carer to communicate with the baby through recognizing the cry and meeting the need. However, this is something that parents and practitioners need time to understand and interpret. Parents need to be given this information to recognize the newborn baby's needs and know what to do to help the baby calm down. When responding to the baby's cry, the mother/carer must be 10–12 inches in front of the baby, establish eye contact and at the same time find a way to control his flailing arms and legs while firmly and gently talking to the baby (Ludington-Hoe et al., 2002). The baby can alternatively be held against the mother's body and be talked to gently.

Another method of satisfying the baby is to provide non-nutritive sucking either by putting the baby to the breast or giving him fingers to suck or providing a dummy. Teaching the baby the difference between night and day is also helpful. That could be accomplished by placing the baby in an environment of normal sounds and light during the day, and making sure the room is dark, or the lights are dimmed, and sounds are gentle at night. Parents need to understand that they will not always succeed immediately in stopping the baby from crying; however, a variety of methods should be tried until the baby stops crying. Scientifically it is recognized that crying in the newborn can cause pathological changes to the cardiorespiratory system (Anderson, 1988); therefore listening to the baby crying without taking action to stop the crying is no longer an acceptable practice.

Placing the cot near the bed will make access to the baby easier at night-time. The baby will develop an organized pattern of sleep by the age of 16 weeks (Matsuoka *et al.*, 1991). At 6 weeks the baby should begin to smile, and at 3 months take note of his surroundings. At 6 months he should be sitting up but still needing support; at 9–10 months crawling; and at about a year he should be starting to walk. It must be emphasized that these 'milestones' are only approximate and that many perfectly normal babies show wide variations from this pattern.

Bad news

Prior to any practitioner undertaking the examination of the newborn it is important to have had training in how to provide bad news. It is important to recognize that what the practitioner deems good news may not produce the same reaction in the parents. A girl rather than a boy is a disaster for some parents. The smallest of deformities such as an extra digit can cause major concerns for parents who wished for the 'perfect' baby. For major congenital abnormalities it is important to know specialists' centres in the area and the latest management and treatment in order to have some insight when the parents start asking questions about the well-being of their baby.

For this reason it is important that the examination of the newborn is undertaken where privacy is guaranteed and the parents do not feel that they cannot ask questions or feel that they do not have the professionals' full attention, as would be the case in a four-bedded or Nightingale ward. If the midwife is not able to convey bad news, the examination should be delayed until the support of a senior colleague who has had training and experience in undertaking the process is available.

Sleep versus play time

Following any physical examination the baby is gently dressed and given to a parent to hold. When the baby is placed in the cot, the position of the baby in the cot is informed by the 'Back to Sleep' campaign to prevent sudden infant death syndrome (SIDS) (see Ch. 40). It is important to recognize that the baby is positioned on the back for sleep but when the baby is awake evidence recommends that he is able to play in the prone position for 15 minutes each day. This can prevent conditions such as delays in motor skills, positional plagiocephaly (flattening of the occipital region of the head), positional torticollis (contracture of the sternocleidomastoid muscle) and shoulder retraction. None of these is life-threatening or should lead to abandoning the back to sleep position (Fig. 31.7). However, parents need to be aware of the problems and encouraged to have the baby in the prone position for 15 minutes each day while they are playing with him.

Reflective Activity 31.3

How would you communicate this to women for whom English is a second language?

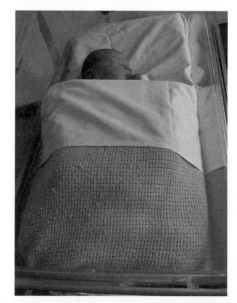

Figure 31.7 Baby in cot in the recommended position for sleep.

POSTNATAL CARE

Care of the newborn is based on the philosophy of providing a continuum of quality care that commences with antenatal and intrapartum care. The care begins with getting to know the fetus both antenatally and during the intrapartum period, and that knowledge informs the management of care given to the baby from the moment of birth to 28 days.

Preparation of the parents is vital to early detection of deviations from normal and management of the newborn wherever the birth takes place. It is expected that preparation for parenthood has taken place, in order to reduce the psychological stress to both the baby and family.

The UK is a multicultural society, and in order for a partnership of care to be developed with parents, the cultural norms of the ethnic groups need to be understood. Many traditional practices need to be understood rather than feared, as they are on the whole beneficial or harmless and can be learned from. One of these practices which is utilized effectively today in neonatal units is cup-feeding, which was brought into the UK from Africa where the survival of high-risk newborns has been achieved by cup-feeding well before it was introduced into the UK. The midwife of today needs to make links with women's ethnic groups and religious leaders in order to learn and understand traditional practice so that safe care can be provided to the newborn by supporting and, where necessary, sensitively changing practice.

Follow-up of the baby

The care of the baby is transferred from the midwife to the health visitor between the 10th and 28th days after birth. The health visitor usually visits the mother and baby at home on or around the 11th day. The health visitor discusses problems with the mother, gives advice on topics such as childcare and family planning, and encourages the mother to take her baby to the child health clinic or to her general practitioner regularly. The baby's development will be followed closely by initiating the vaccination programme and developmental assessments. The general practitioner is responsible for general medical care but some babies with medical problems are also followed-up by a neonatologist/paediatrician.

Hygiene

Because newborn infants have little resistance to microorganisms, they are highly susceptible to infection.

An apparently mild infection can rapidly become a serious condition in the newborn, so every effort must be made to protect them from infection.

There are three main factors concerned in avoiding infection:

1. Keep the baby's skin in a healthy condition and intact so that if bacteria should be deposited upon it there is no portal of entry for invasion of tissues.
2. Limit the bacteria in the baby's surroundings.
3. Adopt a barrier-nursing technique to avoid cross-infection.

Sources of infection   The infant may be infected in a number of ways:

Attendants   The nose, throat or skin of those dealing with the baby may harbour dangerous organisms (staphylococci and streptococci). This includes not only the midwife and doctor but the parents themselves.

Hands and clothing   Facilities for washing the hands must be available both after personal toilet and in the nursery and wards. Preferably, disposable hand towels should be used. The hands must be washed before and after attending each baby. Antiseptic hand cream applied to the hands after washing is valuable. Long fingernails not only hinder many examination procedures but can also cause the baby discomfort and harbour infection.

Dust   The air and dust in maternity wards and nurseries contain many bacteria, one of which, *Staphylococcus aureus*, is most liable to cause infection. The ward and nursery should be adequately ventilated. Cleaning must be thorough but it should be done in such a way that dust is not scattered around the room. Floors are cleaned using vacuum cleaners with filters preventing bacteria passing out of the machine into the air. Damp dusting is advisable. Cots, trolleys and tables can be wiped over with dilute antiseptic and dried well.

Fomites   Infection may be spread by unsterilized instruments, bowls and dressings. Clothing and napkins may be the source. Before the era of prepacked feeds and disposable bottles and teats in hospitals, inadequately sterilized bottles and teats were a source of infection. This may still be the case in some homes.

Cross-infection   Rooming-in, whereby the baby is nursed beside the mother's bed, is the usual practice nowadays. This not only aids the bonding process but also reduces the risk of cross-infection. Overcrowding in wards and nurseries should be avoided. Individual equipment for bathing and changing should be provided, disposable articles being used whenever possible. Prepacked artificial feeds and disposable bottles and teats help to reduce the risk of infection in babies who are not being breastfed. Any baby suspected of infection should be isolated from other babies.

The main routine care of the baby involves changing the napkins, washing or bathing, and feeding. Soiled linen and napkins should be handled as little as possible and placed in bags. The bag should be closed while it is carried to the waste bin.

Bathing the baby   Today, the issue of transmission of human immunodeficiency virus (HIV) through maternal vaginal secretions has encouraged the practice of the baby being given a bath soon after birth. As yet, there are no studies to support the reduction of HIV with the bathing of babies. Vernix is deemed to protect the skin, and may act as an antibacterial agent and promote healing from the trauma of birth. Bathing the baby removes vernix and with it the protection that nature has provided. From the work undertaken so far, it is important that the newborn's condition and temperature have stabilized in the normal range for 2–4 hours prior to the bath being given in order to avoid hypothermia (see Ch. 32).

Bath time in the home offers the parents a time to get to know their baby through tactile interaction.

In order to protect the skin pH, it is important that any cleansing agents that are used have a neutral pH and minimal dyes and perfumes, and that the baby's skin is rinsed well to reduce the risk of allergic sensitization (Cetta *et al.*, 1991).

Whilst the baby is being bathed, care must be taken to prevent abrasions of the skin which might allow entry of bacteria. Great care must also be taken with the eyes and cord, which are both sites of potential infection.

Chafing or intertrigo   This is caused by friction between two skin surfaces and is usually seen in the groin or axilla and in the folds of the neck. It indicates that the child's skin has not been adequately dried after being washed or bathed. The energetic removal of vernix caseosa may also be the cause. After a bath, a dabbing movement with a soft towel should dry the folds in the skin. Where chafing has occurred, drying and a very light dusting with an antiseptic powder will heal the lesion.

Newborn screening tests

Various tests and examinations may be carried out in the early neonatal period to detect the presence of specific abnormal conditions. Early diagnosis and treatment may ameliorate the effects of many conditions. Thus, some inborn errors of metabolism may be managed with diet and/or drugs. The traditional criteria for deciding what conditions to screen for are as follows:

1. Significant incidence of disease.
2. The consequences of failure to diagnose the condition until it declares itself clinically must be serious and costly.
3. Effective treatment must be available only if it is commenced before the onset of symptoms.
4. A satisfactory screening test must be available; it must be simple, cheap, specific (few false positives) and sensitive (few false negatives).

The aim of screening is not always to diagnose and treat, as some conditions are not treatable; however, an early diagnosis is of importance to the parents and extended family.

In the UK, screening programmes for phenylketonuria and congenital hypothyroidism have achieved their aim and objectives and are deemed to be cost-effective. The health benefits of early diagnosis and treatment of these conditions are the prevention of mental retardation, severe neurological disease and death.

Test for the diagnosis of phenylketonuria
Guthrie test   The Guthrie test and what is tested vary between regions and countries. With four completely filled blood circles, the baby can be tested for phenylketonuria and hypothyroidism, which is universal, and some regions will also test for haemoglobinopathies such as thalassaemia and sickle cell disease, cystic fibrosis and muscular dystrophy. In England the Guthrie test offers an opportunity for anonymous testing of HIV to take place. This highlights the areas where resources need to be applied to support families with HIV. It is therefore prudent that a midwife who is going to undertake the test has up-to-date information as to what the Guthrie test will elicit and what each one of the conditions entails. This is of major importance to providing information and obtaining consent that is valid.

The Guthrie test for the detection of phenylketonuria is carried out between the 6th and 14th day, by which time the baby should be well-established on milk feeds (see Ch. 33). When the bacterial inhibition test is to be used, sampling must be deferred if the baby is receiving antibiotics, because they will destroy *Bacillus subtilis* and a false result is likely. Nowadays the specific fluorometric method is more commonly used. A level of 4 mg/100 ml (240 mmol/l) or more is considered positive for phenylketonuria, and further investigations would then be carried out. If the diagnosis is confirmed, instigation of early treatment can prevent brain damage leading to severe mental retardation.

Test for the diagnosis of hypothyroidism   The baby is also screened for hypothyroidism by measuring the level of thyroxine or thyroid-stimulating hormone (TSH) in the Guthrie blood sample. Further investigations of thyroid function will be required if the test result is abnormal. If the condition is confirmed, early treatment with levothyroxine (thyroxine) sodium will prevent mental handicap and promote normal growth (Kelnar *et al.*, 1995).

Tests for the detection of cystic fibrosis   If there is family history of cystic fibrosis, chorionic villus sampling can be undertaken. This will involve taking a biopsy from the placenta. The Government is now encouraging that cystic fibrosis be screened nationally as part of the Guthrie test.

Immunoreactive trypsin (IRT) test   The immunoreactive trypsin test on blood obtained from a heel prick is the most reliable test that is available at the moment for the detection of cystic fibrosis. A positive result would be followed by a sweat test to confirm the diagnosis. Early diagnosis of cystic fibrosis improves the prognosis.

Tests of hearing
Recent technological advances have led to improved screening methods that can identify the majority of children with impaired hearing and it is recommended that babies should be screened before leaving hospital.

The test is non-invasive and involves the measurement of oto-acoustic emissions (OAE), which are low-level inaudible sounds produced by the inner ear. The screening of newborns forms part of the continuum of early childhood hearing tests in order to screen and diagnose children early to improve the early identification of hearing impairment in young children.

The value of such a test is that children with hearing impairments can be given extra help at an early age to develop speech, as the critical period for language and speech development is generally regarded as the first 2 years of life.

Minor disorders in the postnatal period

Dermatitis of the groin, buttocks and anus
Redness and excoriation may be produced around the groin, anus and buttocks. The development of this condition may be influenced by wetness of the skin.

When the skin is exposed to urine the pH rises and changes from acid to alkaline. This change in the pH enables penetration of microorganisms into the building blocks of the stratum corneum. When the skin changes from acid to alkaline it loses the protection from faecal enzymes that can cause injury to the area in contact with urine and faeces (Buckingham and Berg, 1986).

Using appropriate barrier creams containing petrolatum (soft paraffin) can protect the skin and maintain the acid pH and aid healing. Generous application of zinc oxide can enable the skin to heal and can prevent further injury. Keeping the buttocks exposed without a covering or skin barrier does not aid healing, as contact of faecal matter with the injured skin will continue to damage the skin structure. It is not necessary or desirable to completely remove skin barriers with every nappy change because this may disrupt healing tissue. Instead, as much urine and faeces as possible should be removed and the barrier cream reapplied to the affected areas.

If *Candida albicans* is suspected, the baby's mouth should be inspected and the mouth and groin/buttock area involved should be swabbed and sent for culture and sensitivity testing. While awaiting results an antifungal ointment or cream should be used. If the dermatitis is both fungal and a contact irritant dermatitis, it may be necessary to apply a layer of antifungal powder or cream under the zinc and castor oil-based skin barrier ointment.

Dermatitis is a very painful condition and great care is needed in its treatment. The affected area should be washed with soft absorbent cotton wool and well dried with gentle dabbing. There is no need to use soap or other cleaning substances as they also may cause irritation to the skin. Treatment includes finding the cause and maintaining high standards of hygiene.

RECORD-KEEPING

Record-keeping is an important aspect of care given to the newborn. The baby continually changes from the moment of birth and the majority of changes are physiological; however, on a rare occasion a baby that is deemed normal at birth may later be diagnosed with major congenital abnormality. The examination that is undertaken needs to be recorded along with the underpinning rationale for present and future management (UKCC, 1998b).

Record-keeping for the newborn commences with completing the case notes and birth notification, which needs to be completed within the first 36 hours and sent to the appropriate medical officer. Important information needs to be recorded in the notes, such as whether or not the baby has fed and whether urine and meconium have been passed, in order to form a baseline for further assessments.

It is also important on transfer from labour ward to postnatal ward or on completion of duty that the named midwife documents who will be carrying the care forward.

IN-UTERO TRANSFER

In-utero transfer is frequently undertaken by midwives. However, it is important to recognize the problems that could arise. Travel can accelerate labour and there is much anecdotal evidence of women giving birth to very premature newborns in transit, and the midwife and woman need to be prepared for this eventuality.

The transport team members should possess the combined expertise to assess actual and potential problems of the baby during inter/intrahospital transport, and plan and implement interventions effectively.

Action plan

All transport should be conducted by a team whose members possess the combined expertise necessary to safely transport neonates within the inter/intrahospital settings.

The transport team may be composed of any combination of the following personnel:

- midwife
- neonatologist/obstetrician
- neonatal nurse practitioner
- paramedic.

To work effectively the team need to consider the role that each will undertake during transit.

Consideration will be given to the following factors when determining team composition for any given transport:

- established local guidelines
- the degree of supervision required by and available to the transporting team members

- the complexity of the patient's condition and transport care required
- the anticipated degree of progression of illness prior to and during transport
- the type of technology to be employed during the transport
- legal scope of practice of potential team members.

Note   The lead professional in situations where a midwife and paramedic are present is always the midwife. The midwife is accountable and holds duty of care to both mother and baby despite the experience of paramedic staff. Its also recognized that if only one midwife is present the mother and baby must be kept together. An ambulance is always used to transport a newborn that is deemed to require admission to hospital.

An obstetrician/neonatologist should be designated and be available for consultation by telephone or radio where it is deemed that medical staff should not accompany the woman in transit. This arrangement needs to be documented in the notes.

NEONATAL TRANSPORT

Neonatal transport team members are expected to routinely provide care to neonatal patients on transport. Each NHS trust should incorporate guidelines for midwives to transport babies from home or accident and emergency departments to hospital.

In order for transport to be safe, guidelines need to be established that will ensure that team members are provided with an orientation based on predetermined criteria (as developed by the midwifery/medical/nursing staff) necessary to meet basic neonatal standards of care prior to participating in neonatal transport activities.

Questions regarding neonatal transfer from home to hospital include:

- What criteria will be used to dictate whether or not a doctor needs to accompany the woman?
- Who will produce the guidelines for this area of practice?
- What quality standard will practice in this area be audited against?

Characteristics required by the midwife undertaking neonatal transport include, but are not limited to, the following:

- educational and experiential background
- leadership skills

- critical thinking skills
- good communication and interpersonal skills.

The midwife should be able to demonstrate competency in the following neonatal content areas, including, but not limited to:

- newborn life support skills, by undertaking a neonatal resuscitation course such as the UK Resuscitation Council course in newborn life support (NLS)
- understanding of maternal physiological and pharmacological factors affecting the neonate
- neonatal assessment, which will include:
  - physical examination
  - gestational age assessment
  - oxygen monitoring
  - thermoregulation
- knowledge of anatomy, pathophysiology, assessment, and treatment for the following neonatal conditions:
  - acute respiratory diseases
  - cardiovascular abnormalities
  - infectious diseases
  - musculoskeletal abnormalities
  - neurological and spinal cord injuries
  - prematurity
  - gastrointestinal emergencies such as severe dehydration and exomphalos
  - genetic or other disorders noted by dysmorphic features.

The baby is best transported within a transport incubator, and the midwife needs to feel confident in its use, because paramedics have no training in its working function except on how to secure it appropriately within the ambulance.

If a transport incubator is not used, the midwife can utilize a baby changing mat with babies who require facial oxygen nursed prone. In this position, babies are able to splint the diaphragm and to breathe longer than if they were nursed supine. On the other hand, if the baby requires mask ventilation then the ambulance needs to be travelling at a speed that allows the midwife to undertake mask ventilation and support the airway. If the baby requires resuscitation in transit, it is imperative that the ambulance is stopped while the midwife stabilizes the baby before continuing the journey to the hospital.

At all times it is important to avoid heat loss by using a space blanket and keeping the temperature of the ambulance at a high level.

Skin-to-skin contact is an excellent way to maintain thermoregulation but this requires the baby to be able to maintain his own airway without difficulty and at the same time enable the midwife to continually observe the baby's well-being.

The midwife should systematically evaluate and continually reassess the efficacy and outcome of interventions throughout the transport process.

The newborn status will be monitored continuously, with documentation written a minimum of every 30 minutes, based on the baby's condition. The midwife will evaluate progress, analyse data and modify the planning and implementation of care, based on the baby's response to care.

On arrival at the hospital, the midwife should be able to give a thorough report supported by the written transport record-keeping.

It is important that the midwife utilizes a variety of forums, such as midwifery supervision, medical or neonatal nursing staff and peers, to discuss and evaluate care given while transporting the newborn from home to hospital.

Midwives need to feel confident in the legality and scope of their practice if they are to carry out the transport process confidently.

Support of parents whose baby needs to be transported to hospital

Any parent whose baby needs to be admitted to hospital will be very anxious, and the midwife needs to have a family-centred approach during this time of crisis in order to minimize harm and support not only for the baby but also for the parents.

The midwife and referring hospital nursing staff should provide appropriate educational and psychosocial support to families of infants requiring transport (Hubner, 1983). The parents need to be given information as to the reason for transport and an overview of the transport process.

The receiving and referring hospital staff should communicate as needed to remain knowledgeable of the infant's medical condition/status following transport, to ensure that appropriate psychosocial and educational support is provided to the family during the mother's hospitalization.

If the transport of the baby follows a birth that was not a planned home birth and little is known, the midwife must obtain any relevant information from the parent(s) and/or significant others. It is important to do so in order to plan and implement a comprehensive plan of care for stabilization of the infant requiring transport. The information that should be obtained includes, but is not limited to:

- maternal medical disease(s)
- past and current obstetrical history/complications

- maternal medications/substance abuse
- labour and delivery history
- social support systems (married, other children, including the presence of language barriers, ethnic and religious factors)
- bottle- versus breastfeeding plans for the infant.

The parents may also need to know the hospital to which the baby will be transported, and the ward, and be given appropriate travel direction for the father/relatives following the ambulance, and also the relevant telephone numbers.

Depending on the baby's condition the parents should be given an opportunity to see and touch the baby prior to transfer, if possible.

If the parents do not speak English the midwife needs to find mechanisms, or request the appropriate interpreter to be available on arrival at the hospital, in order to minimize the language barrier.

Record-keeping

The midwife is required to document the cultural and spiritual background of the parents, as well as their understanding of the baby's condition and their consent to the baby being transported to the nearest acute neonatal unit.

Environmental factors such as home/general living conditions need to be documented, where relevant, because they would support later management of the baby's care and give a holistic picture of the family. This will also support the social workers who may be required to support the family unit.

The transport process should be systematically evaluated for effectiveness through quality monitoring and research methods.

CONCLUSION

The aim of this chapter has been to introduce the reader to physiology applied to the examination of the newborn and the care given to newborn babies and their families. For more detail, the reader is referred to several excellent texts (see list of further reading) which will provide the in-depth knowledge required to undertake the examination of the newborn.

KEY POINTS

- The transition from fetus to neonate is a complex progression, and the midwife needs to be knowledgeable about fetal and neonatal physiology to recognize that the progression has been completed.
- Care of the neonate should be based upon supporting and enhancing normal transition, and in early identification of deviations from normal and appropriate management and referral.
- Midwives should allocate the same time and attention to the examination and assessment of the neonate, as they provide for the woman.
- Midwives should have a clear understanding of neonatal anatomy, physiology and behaviour in order to help the women understand the behaviours, responses and care needs of the newborn baby.
- Clear, accurate and contemporaneous record-keeping is essential in ensuring continuity of care, and effective information to the parents and carers of the neonate.

REFERENCES

Aase, J.M. (1990) *Diagnostic Dysmorphology*. New York: Plenum Medical Book Company.

Ahmed, S.F. & Hughes, I.A. (2002) The genetics of male undermasculinization. *Clinical Endocrinology* (Oxford) **56**(1): 1–18.

Anand, K.J. & International Evidence-Based Group for Neonatal Pain (2001) Consensus statement for the prevention and management of pain in the newborn. *Archives of Pediatrics & Adolescent Medicine* **155**: 173–180.

Anand, K.J. & Scalzo, F.M. (2000) Can adverse neonatal experiences alter the brain development and subsequent behaviour? *Biology of the Neonate* **77**: 69–82.

Anderson, C.J. (1981) Enhancing reciprocity between mother and neonate. *Nursing Research* **30**: 89–93.

Anderson, G.C. (1988) Crying, foramen ovale shunting, and cerebral volume. *Journal of Pediatrics* **113**(2): 411–412.

Anisfeld, E. & Lipper, E. (1983) Early contact, social support and mother–infant bonding. *Pediatrics* **72**: 79–83.

Aynsley-Green, A. (1985) Metabolic and endocrine interrelations in the human fetus and neonate. *American Journal of Clinical Nutrition* **41**(2 Suppl.): 399–417.

Bannister, P. (2001) Early feeding management. In: Watson, A.C.H., Sell, D.A. & Grunwell, P. (eds) *Management of Cleft Lip and Palate*, pp. 137–147. London: Whurr.

Barr, R.J. (1984) The umbilical cord: to treat or not to treat? *Midwives Chronicle* July: 224–226.

Bell, S.M. & Ainsworth, M.D. (1972) Infant crying patterns and maternal responsiveness. *Child Development* 43(4): 1171–1190.

Bloom, S.R. & Johnston, D.L. (1972) Failure of glucagon release in infants of diabetic mothers. *British Medical Journal* 4(838): 453–454.

Brazelton, T.B. (1983) *Infants and Mothers.* New York: Delacourt Press.

Brazelton, T.B. (1992) *Touchpoints.* London: Viking.

Brazelton, T.B. & Nugent, J.K. (1995) *Neonatal Behavioral Assessment Scale.* Cambridge: Mac Keith Press.

Brian, A.C. & Brian, M.H. (1978) Control of respiration in the newborn. *Clinics in Perinatology* 5: 269–281.

Buckingham, K.W. & Berg, R.W. (1986) Etiologic factors in diaper dermatitis: the role of feces. *Pediatric Dermatology* 3(2): 107 112

Carbajal, R., Veerapen, S., Couderc, S. *et al.* (2003) Analgesic effect of breast feeding in term neonates: randomised controlled trial. *British Medical Journal* 326(7379): 13.

Cetta, F., Lambert, G.H. & Ros, S.P. (1991) Newborn chemical exposure from over-the-counter skin care products. *Clinical Pediatrics* 30(5): 286–289.

Children Act 1989 London: HMSO.

Confidential Enquiry into Stillbirths and Deaths in Infancy (CESDI) (2003) *Project 27/8: an Enquiry into the Quality of Care and its Effect on the Survival of Babies Born at 27–28 Weeks.* London: The Stationery Office.

Conner, G.K. (1993) Genitourinary assessment. In: Tappero, E.P. & Honeyfield, M.E. (eds) *Physical Assessment of the Newborn.* Petuluma, USA: NICU Ink.

Davis, G.M. & Bureau, M.A. (1987) Pulmonary and chest wall mechanics in the control of respiration in the newborn. *Clinical Perinatology* 14(3): 551–579.

Department of Health (DoH) (1993) *Changing Childbirth. Report of the Expert Maternity Group.* London: HMSO.

Department of Health (DoH) (2001) *Reference Guide to Consent for Examination or Treatment.* London: DOH.

De Rooy, L. & Hawdon, J. (2002) Nutritional factors that affect the postnatal metabolic adaptation of full-term small- and large-for-gestational-age infants. *Pediatrics* 109(3): e42.

Diamond, D.A. & Gosalbez, R. (1998) Neonatal urologic emergencies. In: Walsh, P.C., Retik, A.B., Vaughan, E.D. *et al.* (eds) *Campbell's Urology,* 7th edn, pp. 1629–1654. Philadelphia: W.B. Saunders.

Dore, S., Buchan, D., Coulas, S. *et al.* (1998) Alcohol versus natural drying for newborn cord care. *Journal of Obstetric, Gynecologic, and Neonatal Nursing* 27(6): 621–627.

Dubowitz, L.M., Dubowitz, V. & Goldberg, C. (1970) Clinical assessment of gestational age in the newborn infant. *Journal of Paediatrics* 77(1): 1–10.

Gryboski, J. & Walker, W.A. (1983) *Gastrointestinal Problems in the Infant,* 2nd edn. Philadelphia: W.B. Saunders.

Hall, D.M.B. (1996) *Health for all Children. Report of the Third Joint Working Party on Child Health Surveillance.* Oxford: Oxford University Press.

Hall, D.M.B. (1999) The role of the routine neonatal examination. *British Medical Journal* 318: 619–620.

Hand, I.L., Shepard, E.K., Krauss, A.N. *et al.* (1990) Ventilation–perfusion abnormalities in the preterm infant with hyaline membrane disease: a two-compartment model of the neonatal lung. *Pediatric Pulmonology* 9(4): 206–213.

Harris, T.R. (1988) Physiologic principles. In: Goldsmith, J. & Karotkin, E. (eds) *Assisted Ventilation of the Neonate,* 2nd edn. Philadelphia: W.B. Saunders.

Hubner, L. (1983) Neonatal transport: the psychosocial impact on the family. *Neonatal Network* 1(4): 8–13.

Inselman, L.S. & Mellins, R.B. (1981) Growth and development of the lung. *Journal of Pediatrics* 98(1): 1–15.

Jokinen, M. (2002) Measuring newborns: does size really matter? *RCM Midwives Journal* 5(5): 186–187.

Keay, A.J. & Morgan, D.M. (1982) *Craig's Care of the Newly Born Infant,* 7th edn. Edinburgh: Churchill Livingstone.

Kelnar, J.H., Harvey, D. & Simpson, C. (1995) *The Sick Newborn Baby.* London: Baillière Tindall.

Klaus, M.H. & Kennell, J.H. (1976) *Maternal–Infant Bonding.* St Louis: Mosby.

Lawrence, C.R. (1982) Effect of two different methods of umbilical cord care on its separation time. *Midwives Chronicle and Nursing Notes* June: 204–205.

Levene, M. & Tudehope, D. (1993) *Essentials of Neonatal Medicine.* Oxford: Blackwell Scientific.

Ludington-Hoe, S.M., Cong, X. & Hashemi, F. (2002) Infant crying: nature, physiologic consequences and select interventions. *Neonatal Network* 21(2): 29–36.

Magowan, M., Andrews, A. & Pinder, B. (1980) The effect of an antibiotic spray on the umbilical cord separation times. *Nursing Times* 16 October: 1841.

Maternal and Child Health Research Consortium (MCHRC) (2001) *Confidential Enquiry into Stillbirths and Deaths in Infancy: 8th Annual Report.* London: MCHRC.

Matsuoka, M., Segawa, M. & Higurashi, M. (1991) The development of sleep and wakefulness cycle in early infancy and its relationship to feeding habits. *Tohoku Journal of Experimental Medicine* 165: 147–154.

Michaelides, S. (1994) Clinical assessment tool. In: *Neuro Behavioural Physiological Assessment of the Newborn Module Handbook.* London: North London College of Health Studies (Now Middlesex University).

Milner, A.D. & Vyas, H. (1982) Lung expansion at birth. *Pediatrics* 101(6): 879–886.

Moore, K.L. & Nelson, A.M. (2003) Transition to motherhood. *Journal of Obstetric, Gynecologic, and Neonatal Nursing* 32: 465–477.

Moore, K.L. & Persaud, T.V.N. (1998) *The Developing Human: Clinically Oriented Embryology,* 6th edn. Philadelphia: Saunders.

Motohara, K., Endo, F. & Matsuda, I. (1987) Screening for late neonatal vitamin K deficiency by acarboxypro-thrombin in dried blood spots. *Archives of Disease in Childhood* 62(4): 370–375.

Nugent, J.K. (2004) *A Relationship-building Approach to Family Centred Care* at Enriching Early Parent–infant Relationships conference. London: Brazelton/JJP.

Orenstein, S.R. (1999) Gastroesophageal reflux. *Pediatrics in Review* 20: 24–28.

Page, M. & Jeffery, H. (2000) The role of gastro-oesophageal reflux in the aetiology of SIDS. *Early Human Development* 59: 127–149.

Pridham, K., Kosorok, M.R., Greer, F. *et al.* (1999) The effects of prescribed versus ad libitum feedings and formula caloric density on premature infant dietary intake and weight gain. *Nursing Research* 48(2): 86–93.

Reiner, W.G. (1999) Assignment of sex in neonates with ambiguous genitalia. *Current Opinion in Pediatrics* 11(4): 363–365.

Remington, J.S. & Klein, J.O. (2000) *Infectious Diseases of the Fetus and Newborn Infant,* 5th edn. Philadelphia: W.B. Saunders.

Richards, M.P.M. (1978) Possible effect of early separation on later development. In: Brimblecombe, F.S.W., Richards, M.P.M. & Roberton, N.R.C. (eds) *Early Separation and Special Care Nurseries.* Clinics in Developmental Medicine. London: SIMP/Heinemann Medical Books.

Roberton, N.R.C. & Rennie, J. (2001) *A Manual of Neonatal Intensive Care.* London, Hodder Arnold.

Ross, G.S. (1980) Parental responses to infants in intensive care: a separation issue re-evaluation. *Clinics in Perinatology* 7: 47–61.

Soothill, P.W., Nicolaides, K.H. & Campbell, S. (1987) Prenatal asphyxia, hyperlacticaemia, hypoglycaemia, and erythroblastosis in growth retarded fetuses. *British Medical Journal Clinical Research Edition* 294(6579): 1051–1053.

Stevens, B. & Johnston, C.C. (1993) Pain in the infant: theoretical and conceptual issues. *Maternal–child Nursing Journal* 21(1): 3–14.

Strang, L.B. (1977) Pulmonary circulation at birth. In: *Neonatal Respiration, Physiological and Clinical Studies,* pp. 111–137. Oxford: Blackwell Scientific Publications.

Taeusch, W.H., Ballard, R.A., Avery, M.E. *et al.* (1991) *Diseases of the Newborn.* Philadelphia: W.B. Saunders.

Tappero, E.P. & Honeyfield, M.E. (eds) (1993) *Physical Assessment of the Newborn.* Petuluma, USA: NICU Ink.

Thomson, M. & Westreich, R. (1989) Restriction of mother–infant contact in the immediate postnatal period. In: Chalmers, I., Enkin, M. & Keirse, M.J.N.C. (eds) *Effective Care in Pregnancy and Childbirth,* p. 1324. Oxford: Oxford University Press.

Thummala, M.R., Raju, T.N. & Langenberg, P. (1988) Isolated single umbilical artery anomaly and the risk for congenital malformations: a meta analysis. *Journal of Pediatric Surgery* 33(4): 580–585.

Tiller, C. & Perry, S.E. (1999) Assessment and care of the newborn. In: Lowdermilk, D.L., Perry, S.E. & Bobak, I.M. (eds) *Maternity Nursing,* 5th edn. St. Louis: Mosby.

Weston, W.L., Lane, A.T. & Morelli, J.G. (1996) *Color Textbook of Pediatric Dermatology,* 2nd edn. St. Louis: Mosby.

Wilkinson, A. (1997) *Infants and children.* In: Epstein, O., de Bono, D.P., Perkin, G.D. *et al.* (eds) *Clinical Examination,* 2nd edn. St. Louis: Mosby.

United Kingdom Central Council for Nursing, Midwifery and Health Visiting (UKCC) (1998a) *Midwives Rules and Code of Practice.* London: UKCC.

United Kingdom Central Council for Nursing, Midwifery and Health Visiting (UKCC) (1998b) *Guidelines for Records and Record Keeping.* London: UKCC.

United Kingdom Resuscitation Council (2002) *Resuscitation at Birth.* Newborn Life Support Provider Course Manual. London: Resuscitation Council UK.

Zupan, J. & Garner, P. (2001) Topical umbilical cord care at birth (Cochrane Review). *The Cochrane Library,* Issue 2. Oxford: Update Software.

FURTHER READING

Blackburn, S.T. (2002) *Maternal, Fetal and Neonatal Physiology.* Philadelphia: W.B. Saunders.

Tappero, E.P. & Honeyfield, M.E. (1993) *Physical Assessment of the Newborn.* Petuluma, USA: NICU Ink.

ADDITIONAL RESOURCES

http://www.neoreviews.aappublications.org
American Academy of Pediatrics' online-only journal, focusing on neonatal and perinatal topics.

http://www.neonatology.org/syllabus/index.html
Neonatology on the Web: teaching files, outlines, and guidelines.

32

Thermoregulation

Stephanie Michaelides

LEARNING OUTCOMES

After reading this chapter you will be able to:

- describe the mechanisms of heat loss and gain, and identify examples of each
- define neutral thermal environment and the appropriate environment for the newborn infant
- identify signs and symptoms of cold stress
- identify methods of preventing and correcting hypothermia and hyperthermia
- include information and advice regarding thermoregulation in antenatal and parenting education.

INTRODUCTION

Practitioners involved in the care of the newborn need to master the art of thermoregulation to support and maintain an environment suitable for the baby's well-being, achieve safe and competent practice and provide information and advice for parents and other relevant persons involved in the baby's care.

No newborn baby can afford the effects of cold stress. Those least able to tolerate hypothermia include pre-term and/or growth-restricted and ill babies. Maintenance of an optimal thermal environment is a vital part of neo-natal care, and studies have shown that environmental conditions influence growth and survival of the neonate.

HISTORICAL BACKGROUND

Wrapping and swaddling

The Bible and some ancient Greek texts describe the process of cleansing newborn babies by rubbing salt into the skin and then wrapping them in swaddling clothes. The custom of using salt on the baby's skin was later discontinued because it was found to cause skin irritation, although it remained popular in some parts of England as late as the 18th century. A Dr Buchan advised midwives that, following birth, it was better to wash the baby in warm water (Dick, 1987). A midwife of that time, Mrs Sharpe, washed healthy babies in wine,

though she preferred to use warm water if the child showed signs of weakness. Afterwards she would rub the skin with acorn oil prior to swaddling. Both wine and salt have mild antiseptic properties which would have helped to protect babies exposed to the unhygienic practices of those times, and the acorn oil would have helped to insulate the baby's skin against the cold (Dick, 1987).

Swaddling was used primarily to counteract the limb deformities resulting from rickets caused by malnutrition, and involved wrapping cloth around the baby in a bandage-like fashion, often so tightly that the skin became excoriated, the compressed flesh became gangrenous and the circulation was affected (Dick, 1987). By the end of the 18th century the practice of swaddling babies had become unfashionable in England and America, though it continued in France and Germany until the 19th century. In some parts of the world, such as Sparta, Greece and in the Scottish Highlands, rather than swaddling, babies were exposed to severe hardening practices such as being carried naked, even in the winter. This was considered a way of ensuring that only the fittest and strongest individuals survived.

Modified swaddling, i.e. wrapping the baby in a tight bundle, is still practised today in many countries and cultures, though the rationale has changed as nutrition has improved and the focus has moved to the need to keep the baby warm and comfortable. Whether the baby is more comfortable in restraining folds of cloth is debatable and the practice owes more to history than to reasoned judgement. The best insulator of heat is warm air around the body, which swaddling excludes, thus reducing an efficient method of insulation for the baby. Respiratory distress may also result from the inability of the baby to expand the lungs fully (Yurdakok et al., 1990).

Comparisons have been made between the progress and well-being of sick neonates clothed and warmly wrapped and those nursed naked in incubators. The most effective means of maintaining the temperature and reducing energy loss was to dress the baby and nurse him in an incubator (Sinclair, 1992). This reduces heat loss by hindering excessive movement by the baby and thus conserves energy whilst preventing heat loss via conduction and radiation.

Temperature control

By 1870 it was recognized that temperature played a part in the survival of babies, although the methods used to keep babies warm were sometimes less than satisfactory. One method involved placing the baby into a pot stuffed with poultry feathers placed near a fire. The inflammable nature of the feathers and the proximity of the open fire proved rather hazardous and resulted in many babies being burned (Dick, 1987). Another dangerous method was to place the cot by the fireside at night.

The use of sheepskin or other animal skins was one of the more successful developments (Dick, 1987), and the use of artificial and real sheepskins continues to be an effective means of keeping the neonate warm and comfortable.

In 1878 the first incubator was developed in Paris by Tarnier, in collaboration with a zoo keeper. At that time incubated babies were put 'on show' as exhibits for the general public – the objective being to provide entertainment rather than increasing babies' survival rates – indeed few babies did survive.

An understanding of the thermal requirements of the high-risk baby was slow to develop. Budin worked with Tarnier to highlight the clinical importance of the thermal environment. In his pioneering book *The Nursing* (1907), he emphasized the need for temperature control after noting an increased survival rate for babies nursed in temperatures between 36–37°C. He recommended an air temperature of 30°C for the small (1 kg) fully clothed baby. These observations were not fully understood or developed until the latter half of the last century.

Between 1926 and 1933, Blackfan and Yaylou showed that for babies weighing 1360–2270 g, being nursed in high humidity and air temperature of 25°C was the ideal environment (Dick, 1987). Significant but unstudied changes were made in the baby's thermal environment during the next 29 years. At one point the humidity was increased to the point that it was impossible to see the babies in the incubators.

In the 1940s in a bid to improve observation, the baby was nursed naked without increasing the incubator temperature. The importance of incubator temperature and humidity was finally resolved by Silverman in 1957, who noted a striking difference in survival rates with an increase in incubator temperature alone.

In the late 1950s Dr June Hill found that in 20% oxygen, oxygen consumption and rectal temperature varied with the environmental temperature. She noted a set of thermal conditions at which heat production (measured as oxygen consumption) was minimal, yet core temperature was within the normal range – known as the *neutral thermal environment*. She also showed that, oxygen consumption would not increase if the environmental temperature was lowered beyond a certain limit, and that a baby given less oxygen (12%) would fail to maintain an adequate core temperature.

This work and others demonstrated that the human baby is a homeotherm (Greek: *homoios* – 'similar', *therme* – 'heat'); that is, the human organism can maintain its core body temperature within narrow limits in spite of large variations in environmental temperature (Dunn et al., 1994: 238). These observations became the basis of our understanding of temperature control today (Klaus et al., 1993).

PHYSIOLOGY OF THERMOREGULATION

Information from temperature receptors distributed widely in many parts of the body is transmitted to the hypothalamus where autonomic responses are coordinated and to the cerebral cortex where behavioural responses are coordinated.

When the body temperature rises, the typical human autonomic response is peripheral vasodilatation and sweating to cool the skin, whilst the behavioural response is to seek a cooler environment and remove clothing. When body temperature falls, the typical responses are peripheral vasoconstriction and shivering and for the individual to seek warmth and put on more clothing. These responses affect heat loss or heat production, and in either case the responses act to prevent or reverse the temperature changes that initiate them.

Normal thermoregulatory function ensures that over a wide range of ambient temperatures, body core temperature is controlled at a relatively stable level – generally between 36.5–37.5°C (Blackburn, 2003). The ambient temperature range over which normal body temperature is achieved with minimal activation of metabolic and evaporative process, is called the thermoneutral zone. For a naked adult, this zone is between approximately 27–33°C. Deviations of body temperature may take three forms:

1. Heat gain can exceed heat loss despite compensatory reactions. Body temperature rises and *hyperthermia* occurs.
2. Heat loss can exceed heat gain. Body temperature falls and *hypothermia* occurs.
3. The control mechanisms may break down and temperature alters according to environmental factors. If the rectal temperature rises above 40.8°C or falls lower than 35.8°C, there is increasing malfunction and risk of tissue damage and ultimately death.

The fetal perspective

During pregnancy, the heat generated by the mother increases by 30–35% and thus the woman can be expected to have a temperature of 37.5°C during pregnancy. This response is due to the effect of progesterone on metabolism and basal metabolic rate (BMR). This leads to the perception of the mother being more comfortable in a cool environment and being intolerant of heat. In the maternal system, there is an increase of four to seven times the cutaneous blood flow and activity of sweat glands.

Fetal temperature is inevitably tightly linked to the maternal temperature regulation and cannot be autonomously controlled by the fetus. This has been referred to as the *heat clamp*. The fetal temperature is generally about 0.3–1.0°C above maternal body temperature (Liebeman *et al.*, 2000) – usually 37.6–37.8°C (Blackburn, 2003; Polin and Fox, 1998).

The placenta is an effective heat exchanger for the fetus, who totally relies on the mother for thermoregulation. The placental role in thermoregulation is influenced by:

- fetal and placental metabolic activity
- thermal diffusion capacity of heat exchange within the placenta
- rates of blood flow in the placental and intervillous spaces (Adamsons, 1966).

It is also thought that some of the fetal generated heat is dissipated into the amniotic fluid via the umbilical cord (Morishima *et al.*, 1977). Transfer of heat is facilitated by the maternal–fetal gradient, which is significant when the mother is exposed to changes in temperature, either during exercise or illness or through environmental factors such as taking a sauna.

Unstable uterine temperature, especially in the embryological state, can cause teratogenic abnormalities in the newborn (Chambers *et al.*, 1998). In these cases the gradient may be reversed or reduced which can lead to the fetal temperature rising. Changes in fetal temperature will, however, tend to follow at a slower pace than maternal changes owing to the insulatory effects of the amniotic fluid (Blackburn, 2003).

The neonatal perspective

Thermoregulation is a critical physiological function in the neonate and is closely linked to survival and health status. Birth precipitates the baby into a harsh and cold environment in which major physiological adaptations and changes, including thermoregulatory independence, must be made; this is additionally difficult for newborn babies who are less efficient than adults in their ability to thermoregulate. Since the ability to generate heat depends on body mass and heat loss to the environment, the large surface-area-to-mass ratio (about three times higher than in the adult) leads to difficulty in maintaining body temperature in a cold environment.

Babies with a low body mass are more at risk. Although a full-term baby has control over peripheral vascular circulation equal to that of an adult, the autonomic thermoregulatory responses are not fully developed. The healthy baby can increase basal heat production by 2.5 times in response to cold within 1–2 days of birth, though this is less so in the first 24 hours. Newborn babies are rarely able to shiver, and the increased heat comes from the noradrenergic lipolysis of the brown fat deposits, characteristic of the neonate and activation of specially adapted mitochondria in the brown fat to produce heat.

The most dangerous time for the newborn to lose heat is during the first 10–20 minutes of life, and if measures are not taken to halt heat loss the baby will become hypothermic (i.e. with a temperature less than 36.5°C) soon after birth. A premature or sick baby who becomes hypothermic will be at risk of developing health problems and of dying (CESDI, 2003) but the chances of survival are greatly increased if temperature stays above 36°C, and therefore, birth should always take place in an environmental temperature above 25°C.

The most common thermal hazard facing a newborn baby is that of hypothermia. However, hyperthermia or a temperature above 37.5°C can also occur and in extreme cases can cause death within the first 24 hours after birth. Hyperthermia increases the metabolic rate, leading to increased oxygen and glucose consumption plus water loss through evaporation which can cause hypoxia, metabolic acidosis and dehydration. A core temperature above 42°C may lead to neurological damage (WHO, 1994).

Hyperthermia can be caused by infection and it is not possible to distinguish between infection and environmental factors by measuring the body temperature or by clinical signs. Therefore a temperature above 37.7°C in the newborn is a deviation from normal and it is important to refer the baby to the neonatologist for diagnosis and management.

Internal and external gradients

The *internal gradient* is the temperature differential between the core of the body and the skin, and results in the transfer of heat from within the body to its surface. This process relies on an effective and extensive blood flow in capillaries and venous plexi, influenced by tissue insulation provided by subcutaneous fat and the convective movement of heat through the blood. Heat conduction is under sympathetic control that results in changes in the skin blood flow by vasoconstriction and vasodilatation.

Heat loss through this gradient is increased in the neonate because of the thinner layer of subcutaneous fat and a larger surface-to-volume ratio than in the adult (Blackburn, 2003).

The *external gradient* results in heat loss from the body surface to the environment. The rate of heat loss is directly proportional to the difference between skin temperature and the environment.

Heat transfer by the external gradient is increased in the neonate because of an increased surface area and an increased thermal transfer coefficient. Therefore, the neonate maintains his temperature by means of the external gradient, i.e. the temperature changes of the skin, whereas the adult uses the internal gradient. This is especially significant for the preterm baby for which the control and effects of changes in the environment temperature are more profound.

The external and internal gradients are interdependent.

Heat loss and gain

As a rule, babies at term are treated as homeotherms; meaning having the ability to produce heat to maintain body temperature within a comparatively narrow range. The newborn cannot regulate body temperature as well as an adult can, and when the environment becomes too cold or too hot, is not able to respond and maintain temperature, and thus can only tolerate a limited range of environmental temperatures. Thermal stability improves gradually as the baby increases in weight and age.

There are four main routes of heat loss (Hammarlund and Sedin, 1986):

- *Evaporation*: heat loss occurs through evaporation of water from the skin and respiratory tract, and is highest immediately following delivery and bathing. Heat loss can be reduced if:
  - the baby's head is dried after birth and following a bath
  - a hat is put on the baby
  - wet towels are removed quickly following birth
  - the bath is delayed until the baby's temperature is stable and above 36.8°C.
- *Convection*: heat is lost to moving air or fluid around the neonate. The amount of heat lost depends on the difference between the skin and air or fluid temperature, the amount of body surface exposed to the environment, and the speed of air or fluid movement. Heat loss can be prevented by:
  - increasing the birthing room temperature
  - keeping room temperature above 25°C when the baby is naked
  - covering the baby with a blanket.
- *Radiation*: heat is radiated from the skin to surrounding colder solid objects such as windows or incubator walls. This is the predominant mode of heat loss after the first week of life in babies born before 28 weeks and in all other babies throughout the neonatal period. Heat loss can be prevented by keeping the baby away from windows and draughts.
- *Conduction*: babies conduct heat to cold objects they come into contact with such as a cold mattress, scales and radiograph plates (Avery *et al.*, 1994). Heat loss can be prevented by:
  - warming the resuscitaire and bedding
  - covering the scale with a sheet or blanket prior to weighing the baby (Hackman, 2001).

Other significant heat loss factors *Insensible water loss* (i.e. loss through the skin, urine, faeces and respiratory tract) is increased in preterm and low birthweight babies (Rutter, 1985) because of the large ratio of surface area to body mass; small amount of subcutaneous fat; immature structure of the epidermal skin layer: and increased body water content. This risk is increased in environments where insensible water loss is increased, as 0.58 kcal of heat is lost with each gram of water lost through evaporation (Hammarlund and Sedin, 1986).

The appropriate temperature of a baby is dependent on the baby's age, gestation and weight. If left wet and naked, the newborn infant cannot cope with an environmental temperature of less than 32°C. If a thermometer is not available in a room, the practitioner must assess the environment through personal comfort – what appears warm and uncomfortable for an adult dressed in thin clothes with short sleeves is likely to be appropriate for the newborn.

Heat production in the neonate

Metabolism is measured by the consumption of glucose and oxygen by all the cells in the body. A standardized estimate of metabolism is basal metabolic rate (BMR) – the minimal rate of energy output in an awake individual. The BMR is affected by the ambient temperature and energy balance, obtained from daily intake of food balanced by the energy used to maintain aerobic metabolism of cellular function.

The hypothalamus, the autonomic and sympathetic nervous systems are important aspects of maintaining the temperature within narrow set limits of 36.5–37.7°C in the newborn. Constant body temperature is achieved by a functioning neurological system balancing heat gain with heat loss effector systems.

In the newborn, heat production is a result of metabolic processes that generate energy by oxidative metabolism of glucose, fats and proteins. The organs that generate the greatest energy are the brain, heart and liver. To maintain a constant body temperature, heat loss from the surface of the body must equal heat gain. This stability involves heat production by metabolic processes, chemical and physical mechanisms. In the baby, though the hypothalamus will receive cold alert messages from the skin, abdomen, spinal cord and internal organs to regulate temperature stimuli from other areas of the body, the most sensitive receptors are contained within the trigeminal area of the face (Hackman, 2001).

The responses of the skin surface are determined by the skin temperature, the rate and direction of temperature change and size of area stimulated. In the human newborn, cooling of the skin has been shown to increase metabolic heat production without any change in the core temperature (Darnal, 1987). The posterior hypothalamus is thought to be the area which processes signals from the various thermal sensors located over the body.

Physical mechanisms include involuntary reactions such as shivering and voluntary reactions in the form of muscular activity, for example crying, restlessness and hyperactivity. These responses can be affected by anaesthetics, damage to the brain or drugs such as muscle relaxants or sedatives.

The baby may generate heat by crying and becoming hyperactive when cold stress is severe enough to cause jitteriness although shivering does not appear. If cold stress is not eliminated at this point the baby may become extremely hypothermic, hypoglycaemic, hypoxic, acidotic, lethargic and eventually death will ensue, caused by cold injury. The full-term baby can flex the body into the 'fetal' position, which can provide some protection against cold stress. However, the lack of muscle tone and flaccid posture of an immature or ill baby results in a higher heat loss. Babies can also reduce shunting of internal heat to body surfaces by constricting peripheral vessels.

Chemical or *non-shivering thermogenesis* is the process by which the neonate generates heat through an increase in the metabolic rate and through brown adipose tissue (BAT) metabolism. This process can be utilized by adults and neonates but in the adult the metabolic rate can be increased by about 10–15%, whereas the neonate can increase metabolic rate by up to 100% (Guyton, 1979).

Heat production and brown adipose tissue (BAT)

A cold-stressed baby depends primarily on mechanisms that cause chemical thermogenesis. In the neonate the main process of heat production is by non-shivering thermogenesis. When the baby becomes hypothermic, noradrenaline and thyroid hormones are released inducing lipolysis in brown fat. This process can be affected by pathological events such as hypoxia, acidosis and glycaemia.

Brown adipose tissue is believed to constitute 2–7% of the newborn's weight depending on gestation and weight. Brown fat starts to be deposited in the fetus from 26 weeks' gestation (Bruck, 1978). The brown adipocyte is uniquely suited to its role in newborn thermogenesis. This tissue differs from white adipose tissue because it is capable of rapid metabolism, heat production and heat transfer to the peripheral circulation.

The total amount of heat produced in the neonate is unknown, but may be up to 100% of its requirements (Blackburn, 2003). The sympathetic nervous system stimulates the adrenal gland to release adrenaline, which increases the metabolism of brown fat and catecholamines resulting in an increase in available glucose required for these metabolic processes. The thyroid gland is also stimulated by the pituitary to release thyroid-stimulating hormone and then produces thyroxine (T_4), which is known to enhance heat production from BAT.

Heat production within BAT is not fully known or understood but what is known is that BAT tissue contains a high concentration of complex mitochondria, stored triglycerides, sympathetic nerve endings, and a rich capillary network to carry heat around the body. The presence of an uncoupling protein within the mitochondria of brown fat cells supports the combustion of fatty acids to produce heat.

BAT is especially prominent in the mammalian fetus, and the anatomical distribution is important to its function. The largest mass of tissue envelops the kidneys and adrenal glands; smaller masses are present around the blood vessels and muscles in the neck and there are extensions of these deposits under the clavicles and into the axillae. Further extensions accompany the great vessels entering the thoracic inlet. The proximity of brown adipose tissue to large blood vessels and vital vascular organs provides the ability for rapid transfer of heat to the circulation (Okken, 1995; Polk, 1988). The activation of BAT metabolism *only* occurs following birth. During intrauterine life, maternal prostaglandins and adenosine do not allow non-shivering thermogenesis to take place. With the clamping of the cord, this mechanism is blocked, enabling the hypothalamus to react to hypothermia (Box 32.1).

Feeding

From birth, the baby requires water, glucose and certain electrolytes, and calories are utilized for growth and energy in order to maintain body temperature and metabolism. The method of feeding the neonate, whether orally, by nasogastric tube or intravenously, and the frequency and volume of feeds depends on gestational age and physical condition. When gastric feeds have to be delayed for days, and certainly if for more than a week as in a case of a baby with severe respiratory distress, parenteral nutrition will be required to ensure adequate calorific intake. Milk contains far more

> ### Box 32.1 Production and journey of heat
>
> Think of non-shivering thermogenesis as similar to a home heating system. The boiler (BAT) generates heat using oil or gas (glucose and oxygen). For the central heating to be switched on, the thermostat (hypothalamus) is required to pick up the temperature in each room. When the boiler is switched on, it heats up the water (blood) and sends it around the house (body) via the pipes (blood vessels). Touching the radiators (back of the neck, between the scapula and axilla) can let you know whether the system is on or off.

calories than dextrose given intravenously or orally (Klaus *et al.*, 1993).

Drugs

Medication given to pregnant women can affect thermoregulation. Analgesia in labour such as pethidine given intramuscularly or intravenously and the use of bupivacaine for epidurals, will cause vasodilatation and heat loss in the mother which in turn is passed to the fetus rendering it vulnerable to heat loss after birth. Other drugs which may adversely affect the neonate's temperature control are tranquillizers, antidepressants and hypnotics in large doses. These drugs will tend to affect the neonate's muscle activity and thus lead to flaccidity and a resulting hypothermia. General anaesthetics and muscle relaxants during caesarean section produce the same effect.

Babies of women addicted to drugs are often hyperactive with a higher metabolic rate, which can upset the thermoregulatory balance – potentially leading to hyperthermia.

THE ROLE OF THE MIDWIFE

Midwives are in control of the neonatal environment, and therefore the actions that they take prior to labour and delivery determine the well-being of the newborn baby. Attention must be paid to the temperature of the delivery room; warmth of the towels used for wrapping the baby; and also other factors which may affect the neonate's well-being.

During pregnancy

The midwife should counsel and advise the woman on maintaining a stable temperature, especially during the period of cell division and differentiation in the first trimester of pregnancy.

There is a higher risk of delivering a baby with congenital abnormalities in women who use a sauna, especially if this is a new activity to which the mother's physiology has not adapted (Cohen, 1987; Smith *et al.*, 1988; Tikkenhan and Heinonen, 1991). Care should be taken with other activities such as hectic exercise which significantly increase the maternal temperature.

Many women complain of the heat during their pregnancy, and the midwife can offer realistic and practical advice to the woman; including wearing natural fabrics such as cotton, thin wool, silk or linen and having cool baths/showers. The midwife should also assess the woman's health, excluding infection and/or pyrexia, and taking appropriate and swift action should either be identified.

Labour and birth

The temperature should be monitored on a regular basis, usually 4-hourly, and recorded on the mother's partogram. Any deviations from normal should be acted upon. A raised temperature may be an indication of infection or maternal ketosis (see Ch. 26) and may have implications for mother, fetus and neonate.

Waterbirth

The use of warm water as pain relief during labour and for giving birth in has become increasingly popular. It is believed that warm water can improve uterine perfusion and uterine contractions leading to a less painful birth.

The temperature of the water must be comfortable for the woman and should not rise above 37°C as this may cause hypotension in the woman and reduced blood flow to the fetus; therefore water temperature should be frequently measured and recorded. When the baby is delivered in warm water it is believed that breathing will not be initiated until the baby's head is lifted above the water. However, if the baby is asphyxiated or the water cold, then the baby may inhale some pool water (Gilbert and Tookey, 1999).

Delivery room

Whether the woman has her baby at home or in hospital, the midwife should ensure that all professionals, as well as the woman and her family, know the importance of preparing the birthing room in terms of warmth and absence of draughts from open windows, doors or from fans. The room temperature should be 25–28°C.

It is good practice to record the temperature of the birthing room in maternal and neonatal notes in order to audit care regarding thermoregulation (WHO, 1997).

Reflective Activity 32.1

Monitor and record the environmental temperature of 10 births, and reflect on the knowledge gained and how it will affect your future practice.

The midwife should prepare warmed soft towels, blankets and baby clothing (including a hat) by using the radiant heater of the resuscitaire, radiator, or warming pad. If there is a clean microwave oven available, this can be used to warm clothes quickly. The midwife must ensure that the blankets are warm prior to use, but not hot enough to cause any trauma to the neonate.

In preparing for the birth, the resuscitaire should be checked for cleanliness and all equipment should be made ready; this should include putting the radiant heater on pre-warmed mode, and heating sheets and blankets. The portable incubator/transport incubator should always be fully charged and heated, with additional warmed blankets, ready to go at short notice.

It is also helpful to discuss skin-to-skin contact for warmth after delivery, with the parents.

Risk factors in labour

The fetus is monitored for signs of hypoxia or distress in order to effectively prepare for delivery. The following aspects may lead to neonatal hypothermia or hyperthermia:

- maternal distress – resulting in pyrexia
- maternal infection resulting in pyrexia or hypothermia
- epidural anaesthesia in labour
- substance abuse.

If the neonate is considered to be at high risk, the midwife will need to inform the paediatrician and the staff in the special care baby nursery before delivery.

Initial care of the newborn

Midwives should utilize their knowledge of physiology to understand the implications of the neonate being exposed to heat or cold stress, and provide care accordingly.

The midwife should dry the neonate's head as it enters the cooler birthing environment or this could be done by the mother or father while the midwife checks the neck for the presence of the umbilical cord. The neonate's head is the largest surface area and liable to rapid heat loss. The temperature of a full-term baby may drop by 1–2°C within 30 minutes of birth if heat loss is not prevented (Fanaroff and Martin, 2001).

As the neonate is helped into the world he may, if the mother wishes, be placed on her abdomen. This is a source of heat and probably comfort to the newborn baby, and is an effective method of preventing heat loss in newborns whether full-term or preterm. The midwife then supervises the drying of the baby's skin, covers the baby with a second warm towel and applies a hat while the parents provide skin-to-skin contact to reduce heat loss (Vohra et al., 1999).

If the parents feel skin-to-skin contact is not acceptable, the baby should be dried, wrapped and placed into the mother's or father's arms (Karlsson, 1996).

A baby of less than 31 weeks' gestation will have inadequate keratinization of the skin, which enables evaporation of water and heat to be lost through the skin (Avery et al., 1994). To reduce the effect, some units place the baby up to the neck in a special plastic bag after being dried. The plastic bag can also be used to prevent heat and fluid loss in babies born with congenital abnormality such as exomphalos (see Ch. 36).

The first hour following birth

Care given in the first hour of life is important to the physiological well-being of the newborn baby, and equally important is the care he receives to remove fear, discomfort and pain from the strange environment in which he now finds himself. Supporting the woman to breastfeed her baby within the first hour of birth can provide the same human contact that the baby has known for the previous 40 weeks of gestation and enables the development of maternal–infant interaction (Lamb, 1983).

Nutritional needs

It is widely accepted that breast milk is the ideal food for babies (see Ch. 33). Colostrum is rich in nutrients and antibodies and is already warmed and calorie controlled perfectly to fulfil the neonate's nutritional requirements. It is also immediately metabolized and therefore available to the neonate as energy for cellular function.

The ideal time to feed the neonate is in the wakeful period after birth, though the intranatal history will need to be assessed prior to feeding. A growth-restricted baby, with limited stores of glycogen who has been asphyxiated and required resuscitation, may become hypothermic during the resuscitation process. A blood glucose assessment is undertaken and the result will determine whether the baby is fed either gastrically or intravenously supported by maternal consent. The follow-up management of a high-risk newborn will need to be developed in a partnership of parents, senior neonatologist and midwife/neonatal nurse, based on the individual baby's history.

Bathing

The timing of the first bath has on the whole depended on the culture of the hospital and its carers as well as the wishes of the parents. Babies can be bathed soon after birth or initially wiped clean and bathed a few days later.

Awareness of blood as a potential risk for hepatitis B virus and human immunodeficiency virus (HIV) (Hudson, 1992) has led to many hospitals encouraging staff to routinely bathe babies very soon after birth in order to reduce exposure to blood-borne pathogens for healthcare workers and family members (Varda and Behnke, 2000).

Midwives owe a duty of care to the newborn, and should work towards providing individualized care to both mother and baby. Care should be driven by the needs of the neonate and his mother, rather than routine practice and 'care by the clock'. Prolonged hypothermia can cause irreversible harm, and therefore bathing should not be undertaken unless the baby's temperature is stable. Factors that can affect the baby's ability to tolerate the bathing process include the assessment of well-being, though research so far has been undertaken on healthy babies of above 38 weeks gestation (Penny-MacGillivray, 1996).

Premature babies may also be unable to tolerate the additional oxygen and glucose demands of maintaining a temperature above 36.5°C, and may become cold stressed.

Before bathing the baby, the midwife should assess his well-being, considering factors which have been excluded from research because they were themselves risk factors for hypothermia (Varda, 2000):

- maternal history of pyrexia during labour and following birth
- prolonged rupture of membranes, >24 hours
- polyhydramnios
- oligohydramnios

- maternal use of medication such as aspirin to decrease body temperature, diazepam and antihypertensives such as magnesium sulphate
- maternal diabetes
- maternal use of illicit drugs
- any baby who has had fetal distress
- gestational age < 38 weeks
- birthweight < 2500 g
- Apgar scores of below 7 at 1 and 5 minutes
- evidence of respiratory disease.

When the baby has been assessed as being well, the midwife will then need to consider *where*, *when* and *how*.

Where   Bathing the baby prior to transfer to the postnatal ward exposes the baby to a greater risk of hypothermia, as differences in air temperature from one area to another may be greater than a newly bathed baby can tolerate. If mother and baby remain in the same room (as in a home birth or birth centre) this is less of a problem.

When   Nutrition takes priority over cleanliness. The mother should be supported to breastfeed, as this will facilitate successful breastfeeding. The baby's baseline observations need to be within normal criteria (see Ch. 31). Research indicates that the baby's temperature prior to bathing should be 36.7°C or above.

Studies thus far into the timing of the bath have recommended that the baby's temperature is monitored and recorded in the first few hours of life (Varda and Behnke, 2000).

How   The ambient temperature needs to be between 25–28°C, to minimize evaporative, conductive, convective and radiant heat loss. The water temperature should be 36.7°C and a radiant heater should be available to increase the environmental air temperature. After the bath, the baby should be dressed appropriately and given to parents or placed in a warmed cot.

The baby requiring resuscitation

Home environment   The area prepared for resuscitation should be warm. A changing mat can be used, with a nest of warm towels in which the baby is placed after being dried and the wet towel discarded. This can be achieved by the use of heat pads or water bottles but it is important that the heat source is removed as it can burn the baby.

Radiant heat   All resuscitaires have an overhead radiant heater which can work from three different settings:

- *Prewarm* – used prior to birth to warm the mattress and towels
- *Manual mode* – the heat output is manually controlled from 0–100% heat output
- *Baby mode/skin probe* – the temperature is controlled by a pre-set setting usually 36.5°C.

All practitioners who use resuscitaires should be competent in their use. Thermoregulation is a life or death issue to the premature infant and it has been recommended that 'all labour ward and paediatric staff should be trained in the thermal care of the infants at resuscitation' (CESDI, 2003).

The moment the baby is placed on the resuscitaire and under the radiant heater, the midwife needs to set the setting on either manual or servocontrol. When servo-controlled baby mode is used, the practitioner will first need to set the temperature setting to 36.8°C. A small area on the left side of the baby's abdomen is cleaned of vernix using a Mediswab and the silver side of the probe is placed against the abdominal skin and positioned in place using a reflective disc. This protects the probe from the infrared heat source and ensures that the probe does not overheat and provide the wrong information to the computerized sensor, causing the baby to become hypothermic as the radiant heat source output is reduced. Care needs to be taken to observe regularly that the probe remains attached to the skin of the abdomen, as this can cause the baby's temperature to be unstable. Technology is only as good as the practitioner using it and interpreting the findings.

The baby should be positioned to ensure that the whole of the body is under the heat – the baby may move down the table away from the radiant heater as resuscitation is taking place. It is also important not to occlude the radiant heat source.

Poor use of the radiant heater can lead to the baby becoming hyperthermic and dehydrated, or hypothermic, which causes respiratory and metabolic acidosis, increasing morbidity and mortality of the infant.

Warm gel pads can be used to provide conductive heat gain and support thermoregulation when transferring the newborn from labour ward to neonatal intensive care unit (NICU).

Oxygen therapy   Oxygen is cold and it is important when administered facially that a flow of 1–2 litres only is used with the mask firmly over the baby's face, avoiding the whole face/head becoming cold. In some units, resuscitaires have humidifiers attached to the resuscitaire which replace fluid lost and also provide warmed oxygen.

The baby's temperature should be recorded at 30 minutes of age in order to take appropriate action if heat is being lost rapidly (CESDI, 2003).

Examination of the neonate

As soon as the baby is given to the parents, they will often wish to uncover him and examine him carefully from head to toe. As long as the room is maintained at 25–28°C and the baby is dry, the parents can be left to get to know their newborn baby.

The midwife usually performs an examination of the neonate soon after birth. A warm and draught-free environment is essential during this examination, as the baby is usually exposed (Fanaroff and Martin, 2001). A superficial examination can be performed whilst the neonate is in his mother's or father's arms, which keeps the neonate warm through the warmth of his parent's skin, and provides an opportunity for the midwife to educate the parents about what is being looked for and why. This is a time for parents to wonder at the miracle that is their baby and for the midwife to assist in this and not to rush or bustle or make it seem an everyday episode in their lives. Parents can express their fears and anxieties and these can be discussed and usually alleviated. If done well and thoroughly, the parents can use the framework provided by the midwife to examine their baby and thus work in partnership with the midwife in the hospital or community.

The more in-depth examination requires a safe surface area, and will be undertaken with the baby naked; therefore it needs to be carried out under a radiant heater and on a firm mattress at the correct height (see Ch. 31).

Temperature   The baby's temperature will begin to adjust to the environment outside the uterus within a fairly short timescale. If the maternal temperature is 37.8°C immediately following the birth, the neonate could be expected to reflect that and a temperature of 38.8°C would therefore be acceptable.

Using the rectal route for routine measurement of the temperature is no longer a justifiable procedure. Historically this was carried out to confirm the patency of the anus, which is now examined visually by observing whether the anus is midline and patent (see Ch. 31). The measuring of temperature via the axilla is now considered to be preferable. However, if the baby shows signs of hypothermia the distribution of BAT will dictate

that the temperature is taken rectally (see Monitoring, below).

If the baby is cold, BAT will be metabolizing and thus the area of BAT concentration will be warm, and this can give a false positive reading to the practitioner. Temperature alone cannot confirm core temperature – the baby as a whole needs to be assessed, as a normal temperature may be a result of BAT metabolism being switched on, adequately maintaining temperature for that moment in time only.

Transfer

When the neonate is moved from one environment to another, there is an increased risk of temperature loss in transit. Transferring the baby from the labour ward to the postnatal ward is best done by placing the baby next to the mother covered loosely. If transported in the cot, the baby needs to be dressed appropriately, including a hat. If the woman has not brought clothes for the baby, the neonatal unit always has clothing which can be utilized on the postnatal ward.

The best method to transport sick and premature babies to the neonatal unit is to place the baby in a stable environment such as the transport incubator, which provides a warm environment that also allows observation and care.

If accompanying a woman with an in-utero transfer, the midwife must be prepared for the birth, and should have towels and space blankets available to minimize heat loss while in transit.

If the baby requires transfer from home to hospital, the ambulance should be sufficiently warm to allow observation of colour and respiratory effort. If the baby has no breathing problems, skin-to-skin contact can be used to support thermoregulation.

The midwife should record the temperature before leaving one area for another, be it one ward to another or home to hospital. The neonate's cot should also be placed away from draughts and large expanses of window.

MONITORING AND MAINTAINING TEMPERATURE

Monitoring

Devices with mercury are gradually being removed from the clinical area and replaced by infrared or electronic probes and very occasionally tympanic thermometers. Electronic and infrared thermometers predict the temperature within 60 seconds (Leick-Rude and Bloom, 1998). Servocontrol is used to reduce handling and maintain an automatic response to temperature changes in the baby.

The *rectal temperature* is one of the most accurate measurements, though psychologically from the neonate's point of view this is not the most ideal welcome to the world. The probe should not be inserted more than 3 cm (Blackburn, 2003; Fleming *et al.*, 1983) into the rectum of the term baby and no more than 2 cm in the preterm. It should be well lubricated with Vaseline or soft paraffin prior to insertion (see above). The midwife needs to recall that the rectum bends sharply to the right and thus the passing of a hard, 3 cm long object may cause a perforation. Stool in the rectum can influence the accuracy of readings.

Core temperature drops only when the baby's effort to produce heat has failed. A rectal temperature in the normal range does not therefore indicate that a baby is not cold stressed, it may mean that the baby has activated brown fat metabolism and is producing chemical heat to maintain its temperature. This means that the hypothalamus has recognized a temperature of less than 36.0°C in the newborn baby and has switched on the 'central heating' in the form of non-shivering thermogenesis. The cause of the hypothermia needs to be isolated and removed prior to the baby utilizing brown fat stores and becoming a cold-stressed sick newborn.

Axillary temperature is the preferable site to use. The axilla contains a large area of brown fat tissue which, when non-shivering thermogenesis takes place, releases chemical energy, causing the area to become warmer than core temperature. Thus, when using this site to assess the temperature of the baby, the reading will be higher than the core in a hypothermic baby (Bliss-Holtz, 1991). The difference could be as high as 0.49°C from the core temperature providing a false positive result. This may make it difficult to recognize hypothermia. Therefore midwives need to assess the temperature of the baby through behavioural and physiological signs and symptoms of cold stress. Babies must be assessed on an individual basis to ascertain which site is best used to monitor temperature. If the routine practice is to take axillary temperature, it does not preclude the midwife taking a rectal reading if the baby is assessed to be in danger of being hypothermic.

The use of the *inguinal site* may be useful, as there is a good blood flow and no brown adipose tissue to confuse readings, but research has yet to validate it as an accurate means of monitoring temperature in the newborn.

Tympanic temperature appears to be an excellent and accurate way to take the temperature of children and adults, but is *less accurate* for newborn babies, as the reading is affected by environmental temperature. Research has shown that when the environment was higher than 30°C tympanic readings were 0.5–1.0°C higher than the core temperature, and when less than 30°C the readings were 0.5–1.0°C lower, suggesting that this method of monitoring temperature in the newborn is inaccurate and its use questionable (Wells *et al.*, 1995).

The majority of babies maintain their temperature well but there are times that parents become concerned about their baby and need to be taught a safe method to assess their baby's temperature in order to detect hypothermia or hyperthermia early. This can be done by using a thermometer or by feeling the baby's skin (touch assessment) and observing other signs.

Skin sites that are useful are the abdomen and comparing the area between the scapulae. The feet are a useful indication of temperature to a trained professional, though it is a difficult skill to teach mothers, as extremities in the normal newborn are cooler than the rest of the body and therefore changes can be difficult to detect. However, if the feet are red and hot, the face is flushed and the baby restless, the baby could be overheated.

Another non-invasive method for taking temperature of the baby is the *Thermospot* – a 12 mm sticky black disc that changes to a 'smiley' face when the reading is complete. Parents are asked to place this high in the axilla or over the liver area in the epigastrium. This is not reliable if the temperature of the baby is below 35.5°C (Morley and Blumenthal, 2000).

Maintaining temperature

The mother is a great source of heat to her baby when he is in her arms. The midwife should therefore encourage the mother to hold her baby close to her body to promote warmth and also engender a greater sense of intimacy. This method of maintaining temperature was investigated in a study performed at the Hammersmith Hospital in 1987 and earned the term 'Kangaroo care' when used for very small neonates (Whitelaw *et al.*, 1988). A similar approach to care was used in a study in Colombia, in which very preterm and small-for-gestational-age babies were nursed inside their mothers' clothing between their breasts (Sleath, 1985). There was a 95% survival rate for babies of 500–2000 g; improved rate of breastfeeding and closer maternal–baby interaction. Similar good outcomes have been found by using the same approach in London.

The surgical patient

All known general anaesthetics inactivate the thermoregulatory system and the patient becomes poikilothermic. During the operation, the neonate should be nursed on heat pads and parts of the body not being operated on should be carefully covered. The environmental temperature needs to be maintained between 25.0–28.0°C

The artificial cooling of the neonate during a surgical procedure such as open-heart surgery will have little long-term effect on the neonate's well-being, owing to the rapid and well-controlled cooling of the baby. Therefore there is little risk of actual tissue damage. This is a similar mechanism to that found in cases where children or babies have been accidentally immersed in freezing water and have 'miraculously' survived.

MINIMIZING THE RISKS OF HYPOTHERMIA

Wrapping and swaddling

Warm towels or blankets and clothing for the baby are a necessity; but tight swaddling which restricts movement should be discouraged. When the baby is left in a cot, it should not be swaddled as this may have a detrimental effect on thermoregulation and respiration when the baby is asleep.

The silver swaddler is used when transporting a baby from one place to another and retains body heat. The midwife must ensure that the silver swaddler is used correctly as it can cause damage by cutting into the baby's skin. The baby should be dried, wrapped in a warmed blanket or towel and then wrapped in the silver swaddler, ensuring there are no sharp edges in contact with the baby's skin. The swaddler maintains rather than increases the temperature of the neonate as it will not allow heat transfer either in or out. Even placing the neonate in a warmed incubator will not affect the temperature if he is wrapped in a silver swaddler. Space blankets are now available and better assist in covering and transporting the baby.

The very premature baby also needs to be protected from water loss and this is another situation in which the baby can be placed up to the shoulders in special plastic bags to conserve heat loss through evaporation.

Hats and clothes

The use of hats for the newborn, especially those that are small for gestational age and preterm, and babies who are being resuscitated has proven effective in reducing heat loss from the largest surface area of the baby.

If the baby is wearing clothes, the midwife should ensure that these are of natural fabrics and are not too close-fitting. It is better to use several layers of thin clothing rather than one or two thick layers. The midwife needs also to ensure that there are no loose threads which may become wrapped around the neonate's fingers or toes, as these can cause considerable trauma if not discovered quickly.

Hot water bottles

Hot water bottles should only be used to warm a cot and must never be left with the baby in the cot. The midwife should explain the use of hot water bottles to the mother and partner and establish the rationale for removing them prior to putting the baby in the cot.

Daily bathing

Bathing the baby cleanses and provides an opportunity to assess and validate the baby's well-being by observing his physiological behavioural patterns. The bath time is also an excellent time for the baby and his family to interact (Karl, 1999) and adjust to each other. It may be viewed by some midwives as a time-consuming or mundane task within a busy day, which could be delegated to a healthcare support worker. If midwives make this choice, they must ensure that the person providing care is able to assess the well-being of the baby prior to the bath, and provide information and advice at an appropriate level to the parents. Throughout the bath, the baby's well-being should be assessed following the cues the baby is providing and pointing these out to the mother (Ch. 31).

Education of parents

Educating parents in the care of their babies at home includes giving advice on suitable clothing for the baby with regard to the material and the number of layers required to maintain both heat and ventilation. The midwife may find a checklist useful for educating parents of small babies going home which includes practical advice on helping babies keep warm indoors and outdoors (see Box 32.2). This should be translated into the appropriate language for those whose first language is not English, particularly for those who have little knowledge of caring for neonates in the UK climate.

Teamwork involves liaison with the community healthcare professionals. Social workers can be mobilized in circumstances where financial help is needed to assist with heating bills and adequate home insulation or ventilation.

Box 32.2 Advice sheet to mothers on the prevention of hypothermia

It is well recognized that small or preterm babies need careful protection against getting cold. What is less well known is that the normal term baby can become seriously cold in the first weeks of life and that this can be, in extreme cases, fatal.

Babies are most at risk during the winter and spring months, or when it is particularly cold. It is important to be aware of the temperature inside and outside the home.

All babies lose heat easily and have rather poor food and fat stores in the early days of life. They also cannot shiver and tend to lie immobile for a large part of the day. Activities such as feeding, crying and limb movements normally increase heat production. Therefore tight swaddling should be avoided, especially when the baby is sleeping.

Serious chilling

Temperature may fall to below 32°C (90°F) or lower. The baby may become:

- difficult to rouse
- difficult to feed
- cold to touch.

Unfortunately the baby's skin may appear quite pink or red, which may mask the seriousness of the situation. This can mislead parents who mistake the rosy appearance for a healthy glow.

Babies who have an infection or who are feeding poorly, are more prone to chilling.

Prevention

The house, or at least the preterm baby's room, should be kept evenly warm, if possible at 21°C (70°F). Draughty windows and doors should be attended to, and additional background heating provided. Insulation can be provided by stretching 'clingfilm' over the windows in the baby's room. Social services can give financial assistance for heating the home in cases of need.

The cot should not be placed by an outside wall or by a large window, as heat may be lost. Warm light cot coverings and clothing for the baby should be used and extra clothing put on the baby if taken outside or to a colder room.

As babies lose heat through the large surface area of the head, in cold weather it is advisable for the baby to wear a hat if taken outside.

The baby should be bathed in a thoroughly warm room and dried very thoroughly and dressed in warm clothes immediately afterwards. Baths should not be given if the baby is unwell in any way. The room temperature should not be allowed to fall too low during the night hours.

Never:

- put a hot water bottle or heat pad in the cot *with* the baby; only use to heat the cot and remove *before* the baby is placed in the cot
- use unguarded open fires or paraffin heaters
- use mittens where an unstitched seam can damage the baby's fingers.

NB: If you are at all worried about your baby, contact your general practitioner, midwife or health visitor.

Reflective Activity 32.2

Are the guidelines which support the care given in regard to thermoregulation in your area based on up-to-date evidence? If not, what do you feel needs to be added or removed to provide the professional with support to practise safely when considering thermoregulation?

THE SICK NEONATE

Hypothermia

The definition of hypothermia is a temperature less than 36.5°C. The first 12 hours following birth is the time interval that the baby is at risk of becoming hypothermic, though this can occur at other times during the neonatal period.

Signs and symptoms of cold stress in the newborn are non-specific and may indicate other severe diseases and can be confused with bacterial infection. Hypothermic babies have decreased sucking ability; impaired feeding will lead to decreased heat production due to reduced energy intake. As the body temperature continues to decrease, the baby becomes less active, lethargic, hypotonic and the effort to cry becomes weaker. Respiration becomes shallow and slow and the heart rate decreases.

If the cause is not discovered at this point the baby will develop *sclerema*, which is hardening of the skin, and the face and extremities become red. This can be

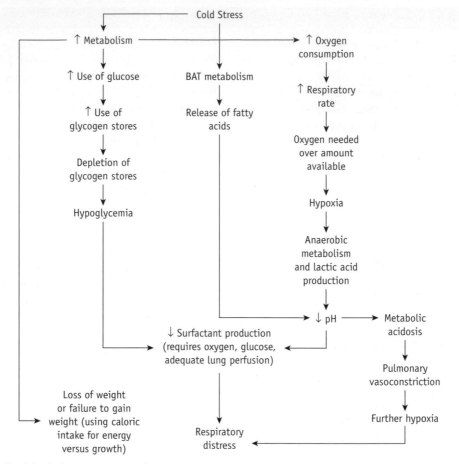

Figure 32.1   Physiological consequences of cold stress. BAT, brown adipose tissue. (From Blackburn, 2003.)

confusing, as superficially the baby appears rosy and this is associated with health.

As the baby utilizes oxygen to metabolize brown fat, it reaches its limit and as the baby is already hypoxic it may lead to impaired cardiac function and haemorrhage (especially pulmonary). Cellular function switches from aerobic to anaerobic metabolism and the end product is the production of lactic acid and metabolic acidosis (Fig. 32.1). Hypoglycaemia can also cause acidosis, and since the brain does not tolerate lack of glucose, neurological damage can occur. If severe cold stress is not treated the baby develops kernicterus and clotting disorders and dies (Blackburn, 2003).

Management

There is no general agreement on the management of hypothermia, but prevention is the best treatment. Rewarming the mildly hypothermic neonate is no great problem but debate continues about the virtues of rapid versus slow rewarming and their respective advantages and disadvantages in severe cold stress. Slow rewarming is the usual practice.

Moderate hypothermia   The temperature is between 32–35.9°C. The baby is placed clothed, but not covered, under the radiant heater or in an incubator set at a temperature of 35–36°C.

An alternative apparatus to warm the baby can be a gel- or water-filled mattress set at 36.5°C, with the room temperature set at 32–34°C.

In the home environment, the baby, if clinically stable, should be given skin-to-skin contact with the mother in a room with a temperature of at least 25°C.

Severe cold stress   The main aim is to maintain a thermal environment in which the baby is not required to increase its basal metabolic rate. The baby is rewarmed slowly to avoid hypotension due to vasodilatation of the peripheral circulation and acidosis.

Apnoea and cardiac failure may be induced by rapid rewarming. Because oxygen consumption is minimal with gradients of less than 1.5°C, the incubator temperature is set at 1.5°C higher than the baby's core temperature and adjusted every 15–30 minutes. The baby must be naked to allow the heat from the incubator or radiant warmer to warm him. The baby should preferably not be fed gastrically as hypothermia reduces evacuation of gastric contents and reduces peristalsis. Intravenous fluids ensure adequate fluid and glucose intake; however, it is important to warm all fluids given to the baby prior to administration.

Hyperthermia

Hyperthermia is a temperature of more than 37.8°C. This is a less common complication in the care of the neonate but can still be problematic. The pyrexia may be due to excessive environmental temperatures, incubator overheating (or the greenhouse effect of an incubator in the sunlight), overdressing the baby, infection, dehydration or a change in central control by drugs or cerebral damage.

As with cold stress, hyperthermia results in increased metabolism and oxygen consumption. It is important that the baby is cooled slowly. This means removing woollens or leaving the baby with only one blanket. Extreme measures, such as leaving the baby in thin clothes and only one sheet, should be avoided.

Reversal of heat stress

The aim in reversing hyperthermia is to reduce metabolic heat production. The baby will attempt to assume an extended position, allowing heat loss via the external gradient to the environment, and to aid this process the baby should have most of his clothes removed. Damp-sponging babies is not recommended as this encourages rapid heat loss, which may then lead to cold stress and shock (Kenner et al., 1993).

Once the cause of the hyperthermia is corrected the temperature should return to normal within 1 hour. If improvement is not noted within that hour, the baby remains pyrexial and looks unwell, infection is the first to be excluded and also brain damage needs to be investigated.

Effects and signs of hyperthermia

Hyperthermia increases the metabolic rate and rate of water loss by evaporation, which can cause dehydration. The baby is unable to fully utilize the mechanism of sweating to reduce heat. However, the exception is the baby born to a mother with substance abuse and that baby is and does become sweaty and wet when stressed and hyperactive. In the normal term baby the only area of the body on which sweating takes place is the head, and in times of shock the palms of the hands appear to be sweating.

Signs of hyperthermia are not easily apparent; they consist of the newborn being restless and crying. As a result of metabolic rate increases, there may be tachypnoea and tachycardia. The baby's face and extremities are red because of vasodilatation. This is a serious sign of hyperthermia and needs to be acted upon to reverse heat gain by isolating the cause. If this does not occur and the temperature rises above 42°C the baby will go into shock; convulsions and coma may occur.

As with hypothermia the main cause of hyperthermic stress in the newborn is caused by misinterpreting the environmental temperature and its effect on the baby. This can result from leaving the baby in a closed car on a hot and sunny day; overdressing the baby on a cold day, whilst inside; or putting the baby too close to a heat source.

EQUIPMENT

Equipment should be used appropriately and with consideration of the thermoregulatory effect.

Weighing scales   Should be used with a towel or sheet to prevent heat loss. The apparatus used needs to meet the approved standards set by the Medical Devices Unit in the UK.

Incubators   Should be used only for those babies who are ill, likely to become ill, or less than the 9th centile.

Modern incubators now have double walls to stop radiant heat loss. The air temperature can be controlled manually or automatically. Incubators and radiant warmers also have an automatic servocontrol skin probe attachment.

The addition of sterile water to the incubator humidity reservoir is not generally necessary or recommended because it can cause the growth of hydrophilic organisms such as Pseudomonas. Sterile water may need to be added for temperature stabilization of the baby weighing less than 1 kg; this is best accomplished by a humidifier system that can be changed daily.

The transport incubator   This is more familiar to the neonatal nurse than to the midwife, and provides the means of monitoring and supporting the small or sick neonate. The midwife should, however, gain a basic understanding of this equipment and its use (Crawford, 1994). This is the ideal mode of transport, and although used to transport babies from one unit to another or from labour ward to neonatal unit, it is seldom used in the transport of the baby from home to hospital. Babies, regardless of gestation and respiratory difficulty, are transported in midwives' arms or laid down on the ambulance stretcher. With clinical risk management and evidence-based practice, this approach to transfer is likely to be addressed when Neonatal Networks are implemented and regional flying squad teams are set up.

Heated mattress   Two types of mattress are used:

- *gel filled*: these have heat-conducting properties and are surrounded by a soft film which does not irritate the baby's skin
- *water filled*: when used in the cot, it should have holes in the base in case there is an accidental slow leak and there needs to be an outlet for the water.

Both mattress are electronically controlled, can be set to be heated to a required temperature, and are ideal for babies who need supplemented heat source to maintain temperature but are too big to be placed in an incubator. Incubators may also reduce the potential for maternal–infant interaction.

Phototherapy   Current practice allows phototherapy to be delivered to the baby in an incubator, cot or open bassinet with a servocontrolled overhead radiant heating source. The midwife should ensure that the neonate's temperature remains stable as the baby can become hyper- or hypothermic during this treatment. Axillary temperature should be checked and recorded every 3–4 hours.

Heat shields   Modern incubators have reduced the need for these, but if used, should be checked to see that they are not cracked and are wide enough to allow the baby to move inside, and they must be positioned correctly to avoid injury to the baby. Heat shields should be used when nursing a baby naked in an incubator, as well as in other situations to prevent, or help treat, hypothermia.

Oxygen therapy   When oxygen is given in percentages greater than 30% it should be humidified and warmed.

If given via an endotracheal tube, it should be given at body temperature; if given via a head box, it should be at the same temperature as the incubator to avoid causing physiological confusion.

CONCLUSION

Although a homeotherm in the true sense of the word, the neonate has higher heat and water losses compared to those of the adult, which require the carer to provide a thermal environment that allows a minimal resting metabolic rate. Midwives caring for neonates must give special attention to the maintenance of a 'normal' temperature particularly in the 'at-risk' neonate. Therefore an understanding of the physiology of temperature control, and of calorific intake and application to practice is vital for the midwife and includes the means of providing a safe transition to extrauterine life.

Midwives will apply their knowledge of physiology to monitor normal temperature variations, and identify when these become abnormal and the possible causes of the deviations from normal. These include sepsis, cerebral malfunction or simply an inadequately stable thermal environment.

They should have a clear and in-depth understanding of thermoregulation and all that it entails, including the use of equipment and monitoring devices that support a neutral thermal environment in hospital and at home. The midwife is only with the baby a short space of time; the main carer for the baby is the mother and it is important that the midwife has modified an educational plan which commences in the antenatal period to support the woman in her role as lead carer for the thermoregulation of her baby. Included in this educational role is up-dating and auditing the effectiveness of the midwife's practice in providing care and education of the woman and other support workers involved.

Midwives need to pay the same attention to the care of the neonate as they do to that of the mother. If there is a problem, a worry or individual needs, the woman has to be given the opportunity to express them. The neonate is not able to speak and sometimes not able to cry. He is at the mercy of those who care for him to recognize his needs and meet them. It is therefore important to learn to understand the language of the neonate through physiology and his behaviour in order to fulfil his needs.

KEY POINTS

- Thermoregulation is a crucial part of ensuring neonatal well-being, regardless of gestation and risk factors.
- The midwife oversees the environment, and should work towards providing a neutral thermal environment.
- An important part of the midwife's role is in educating and preparing parents and other professionals regarding the thermoregulatory needs of the neonate, integrating this into a framework of care which allows parents to learn more about their child.
- Appropriate and effective management of hypothermia and hyperthermia will reduce long-term morbidity and mortality.

REFERENCES

Adamsons, K. (1966) The role of thermal factors in fetal and neonatal life. *Pediatric Clinics of North America* **13**: 599.

Avery G., Fletcher, M.A. & MacDonald, M.G. (1994) *Neonatology: Pathophysiology and Management of the Newborn*. Philadelphia: Lippincott Williams and Wilkins.

Blackburn, S.T. (2003) *Maternal Fetal and Neonatal Physiology, A Clinical Perspective*, 2nd edn. Philadelphia: Saunders.

Bliss-Holtz, J. (1991) Determining cold stress in full term newborns through temperature site comparisons. *Scholarly Inquiry for Nursing Practice* **5**(2): 113–123.

Chambers, C.D., Johnson, K.A., Dick, L.M. *et al.* (1998) Maternal fever and birth outcome: a prospective study. *Teratology* **58**(6): 251–257.

Cohen, F.L. (1987) Neural tube defects: epidemiology, detection and prevention. *Journal of Obstetric, Gynecologic, and Neonatal Nursing* **16**(2): 105–115.

Confidential Enquiries into Stillbirth and Deaths in Infancy (CESDI) (2003) *Project 27/28. An Enquiry into Quality of Care and its Effect on the Survival of Babies Born at 27–28 weeks*. London: The Stationary Office.

Crawford, D. (1994) Resuscitation – flying squad transfer. In: Crawford, D. & Morris, M. (eds) *Neonatal Nursing*, pp. 43–59. London: Chapman & Hall.

Darnal, R.A. (1987) The thermophysiology of the newborn infant. *Medical Instrumentation* **21**(1): 16–22.

Dick, D. (1987) *Yesterday's Babies*. London: Bodley Head.

Dunn, P.A., York, R., Cheek, T.G. *et al.* (1994) Maternal hypothermia: implications for obstetric nurses. *Journal of Obstetric, Gynecologic, and Neonatal Nursing* **23**(3): 238–242.

Fanaroff, A.A. & Martin, R.J. (2001) *Neonatal–Perinatal Medicine: Diseases of the Fetus and Neonate*. St Louis: Mosby.

Fleming, M., Hakansson, H. & Svenningsen, N.W. (1983) A disposable temperature probe for skin measurement in the newborn nursery. *International Journal of Nursing Studies* **10**(2): 89–96.

Gilbert, R.E. & Tookey, P.A. (1999) Perinatal mortality and morbidity among babies in water: national surveillance study. *British Medical Journal* **319**(7208): 483–487.

Guyton, A.C. (1979) *Textbook of Medical Physiology*, 8th edn. Philadelphia: W.B. Saunders.

Hackman, P.S. (2001) Recognizing and understanding the cold-stressed term infant. *Neonatal Network* **20**(8): 35–41.

Hammarlund, K. & Sedin, G. (1986) Heat loss from the skin of preterm and full term newborn infants during the first weeks after birth. *Biology of the Neonate* **50**(1): 1–10.

Hudson, C.N. (1992) HIV infection in obstetrics and gynaecology. *Baillière's Clinical Obstetrics and Gynaecology* **6**(1): 137–148.

Karl, D. (1999) The interactive newborn bath: using infant neurobehavior to connect parents and newborns. *MCN. The American Journal of Maternal Child Nursing* **24**(6): 280–286.

Karlsson, H. (1996) Skin to skin care: heat balance. *Archives of Disease in Childhood* **75**(2): F130–F132.

Kenner, C., Brueggemeyer, A. & Gunderson, L.P. (1993) *Comprehensive Neonatal Nursing: a Physiologic Perspective*. Philadelphia: W.B. Saunders.

Klaus, M.H., Fanaroff, A.A. & Martin, R.J. (1993) The physical environment. In: Klaus, M.H. & Fanaroff, A.A. (eds) *Care of the High Risk Infant*. Philadelphia: W.B. Saunders.

Lamb, M.E. (1983) Early mother–neonate contact and mother child relationship. *Journal of Child Psychology and Psychiatry* **24**(3): 487–494.

Leick-Rude, M.K. & Bloom, L.E. (1998) A comparison of temperature taking methods in neonates. *Neonatal Network* **17**(5): 21–37.

Liebeman, E., Lang, J., Richardson, D.K. *et al.* (2000) Intrapartum maternal fever and neonatal outcome. *Pediatrics* **105**(1): 8–13.

Morley, D. & Blumenthal, I. (2000) A neonatal hypothermia indicator. *Lancet* **355**(9204): 659–660.

Morishima, H.O., Yeh, M.N., Niemann, W.H. *et al.* (1977) Temperature gradient between fetus and mother as an index for assessing intrauterine fetal condition. *American Journal of Obstetrics and Gynecology* **129**: 443.

Okken, A. (1995) The concept of thermoregulation. In: Okken, A. & Koch, J. (eds) *Thermoregulation of*

Sick and Low Birth Weight Neonates. Berlin: Springer-Verlag.

Penny-MacGillivray, T. (1996) A newborn's first bath. When? *Journal of Obstetric, Gynecologic, and Neonatal Nursing* 25: 481–487.

Polin, M.D. & Fox, W.W. (1998) *Fetal and Neonatal Physiology,* 2nd edn. Philadelphia: W.B. Saunders.

Polk, D-H. (1988) Thyroid hormone effects on neonatal thermogenesis. *Clinics in Perinatology* 12: 151–156.

Rutter, N. (1985) The evaporimeter and emotional sweating in the neonate. *Clinics in Perinatology* 12: 63–77.

Sinclair, J.C. (1992) Management of the thermal environment. *Effective Care of the Newborn Infant.* Oxford: Oxford Medical Publications.

Sleath, K. (1985) Lessons from Colombia. *Nursing Mirror* 160(14): 14–16.

Smith, M., Upfold, J. & Edwards, M. (1988) The dangers of heat to the newborn. *Patient Management* 3: 157–165.

Tikkenhan, J. & Heinonen, O. (1991) Maternal hyperthermia during pregnancy and cardiovascular malformations in the offspring. *European Journal of Epidemiology* 7(6): 628–635.

Varda, K.E. & Behnke, R. (2000) The effect of timing of initial bath on newborn's temperature. *Journal of Obstetric, Gynecologic, and Neonatal Nursing* 29(1): 27–32.

Vohra, S., Frent, G., Campbell, V. *et al.* (1999) Effect of polyethylene occlusive skin wrapping on heat loss in very low birth weight infants at delivery: a randomized trial. *Journal of Pediatrics* 134(5): 547–551.

Wells, N., King, J., Hedstom, C. *et al.* (1995) Does tympanic temperature measure up? *MCN. The American Journal of Maternal Child Nursing* 20: 95–100.

Whitelaw, A., Heisterkamp, G., Sleath, K. *et al.* (1988) Skin to skin contact for very low birthweight infants and their mothers. *Archives of Disease in Childhood* 63: 1377–1381.

World Health Organization (WHO) Division of Reproductive Health (Technical Support), Maternal and Newborn Health/Safe Motherhood (1994) Thermal protection and/or management of neonatal hypothermia and hyperthermia. Report of a Technical Working Group. In: *Essential Newborn Care.* Geneva: WHO.

World Health Organization (WHO) (1997) *Thermal Protection of the Newborn: A Practical Guide.* Geneva: WHO.

Yurdakok, K., Yavuz, T. & Taylor, C.E. (1990) Swaddling and acute respiratory infections. *American Journal of Public Health* 80(7): 873–875.

FURTHER READING

Blackburn, S.T. (2003) *Maternal Fetal and Neonatal Physiology, A Clinical Perspective,* 2nd edn. Philadelphia: Saunders.

An excellent text providing in-depth physiology well applied to clinical practice.

33

Infant Feeding

Belinda Ackerman

LEARNING OUTCOMES

At the end of this chapter, the reader will:

- understand the nutritional requirements of the normal term neonate, and the physiology of the neonatal digestive system
- be conversant with the anatomy and physiology of lactation, and its variants
- be aware of the importance of breastfeeding, including the advantages to both the woman and

baby and the impact on their long-term health, and proficient in its promotion
- be knowledgeable about artificial feeding
- have a clear understanding of the role of the midwife in infant feeding, and be able to apply this in health promotion and public health activities.

INTRODUCTION

This chapter will present the anatomy and physiology of infant feeding, including the maternal breast and hormonal influences and neonatal nutritional needs. Whilst it is appreciated that human milk is the superior food for the neonate and that breastfeeding is recommended by the midwife, there are some women who will choose, for a variety of reasons, not to breastfeed. It is the midwife's role to provide a facilitative non-judgemental environment for discussing the woman's views and expectations around infant feeding and factual, unbiased, evidence-based information in order that an informed decision about infant feeding can be made. It is vital that women are educated in the principles of safe preparation and administration of artificial feeds should they be unable or choose not to breastfeed.

GOLD STANDARD

Human milk is the gold standard for nutrition of the human infant (Lawrence, 1997). It contains unique constituents valuable for brain growth such as cholesterol, omega 3 fatty acids, the amino acid taurine, together with immune properties that cannot be matched with any substitutes. It is the standard all

health professionals should endeavour to achieve for the neonate, through the information given to women and their families.

In 1989 the World Health Organization and United Nations Children's Fund produced a joint statement on: *Protecting, Promoting and Supporting Breast-feeding: The Special Role of Maternity Services* (WHO/UNICEF, 1989). This was adopted as a global initiative by policy makers at a meeting in Florence, and has since been referred to as the Innocenti Declaration (Henschel and Inch, 1996) (see Box 33.1). In June 1991 the Baby-Friendly Hospital Initiative (BFHI) was launched at the International Paediatric Association Conference, Ankara, to provide a global focus for the intent of the Innocenti Declaration. The principles of the declaration were embodied in the 'Ten Steps to Successful Breastfeeding' (Box 33.2) which are designed as a set of standards that can be followed by maternity units all over the world and audited to demonstrate measurable improvements.

The *UK Baby Friendly Initiative* (UK BFI) launched in 1994, is a programme of the UK Committee for UNICEF and aims to ensure that all mothers and babies receive the health and social benefits provided by breastfeeding. The UK BFI encourages and assesses hospitals to become 'baby friendly' by implementing the 'Ten Steps' (Box 33.2).

Box 33.1 Innocenti Declaration (Henschel and Inch, 1996)

The Innocenti Declaration on the protection, promotion and support of breastfeeding recognizes that breastfeeding is a unique process that:

- Provides ideal nutrition for infants and contributes to their healthy growth and development
- Reduces incidence and severity of infectious diseases, thereby lowering morbidity and mortality
- Contributes to women's health by reducing the risk of breast and ovarian cancer, and by increasing the spacing between pregnancies
- Provides social and economic benefits to the family and the nation
- Provides most women with satisfaction when successfully carried out

and that

- Recent research has found that these benefits increase with the increased exclusiveness of breastfeeding during the first 6 months of life, and thereafter with increased duration with complementary foods
- Programme interventions can result in positive changes in breastfeeding behaviour.

We therefore declare that:

As a global goal for optimal maternal and child health and nutrition, all women should be enabled to practice exclusive breastfeeding and all infants should be fed on breast milk from birth to 4–6 months of age. Thereafter, children should continue to be breastfed, while receiving appropriate and adequate complementary foods for up to 2 years of age or beyond. This child feeding ideal is to be achieved by creating an appropriate environment of awareness and support so that women can breastfeed in this manner.

This declaration was adopted by the participants at the WHO/UNICEF meeting *Breastfeeding in the 1990's: A Global Initiative*, co-sponsored by the United States Agency for International Development (USAID) and the Swedish International Development Agency (SIDA) held at the Spedale degli Innocenti, Florence, Italy on 30 July–1 August 1990.

Box 33.2 The Ten Steps to Successful Breastfeeding (WHO/UNICEF, 1989)

All providers of maternity services should:

1. Have a written breastfeeding policy that is routinely communicated to all healthcare staff.
2. Train all healthcare staff in the skills necessary to implement the breastfeeding policy.
3. Inform all pregnant women about the benefits and management of breastfeeding.
4. Help mothers initiate breastfeeding soon after birth.
5. Show mothers how to breastfeed and how to maintain lactation even if they are separated from their babies.
6. Give newborn infants no food or drink other than breast milk, unless medically indicated.
7. Practice rooming in, allowing mothers and infants to remain together 24 hours a day.
8. Encourage breastfeeding on demand.
9. Give no artificial teats or dummies to breastfeeding infants.
10. Foster the establishment of breastfeeding support groups and refer mothers to them on discharge from the hospital or clinic.

Institutions which fully implement all Ten Steps can apply to be assessed and accredited as 'baby friendly'. A first step towards accreditation is the Certificate of Commitment, which is awarded to units which implement Steps 1,7 and 10 and adopt an action plan to meet the requirements of the remaining steps.

BREASTFEEDING AND PUBLIC HEALTH ISSUES

The Department of Health (DoH) set a target to reduce health inequalities in children under 1 year by 2010 'to reduce by at least 10% the gap in mortality between routine and manual groups and the population as a whole' (DoH, 2002). Promotion of health through breastfeeding is an important contribution to achieving this target by its major role in the protection of infants against infection, allergy, insulin-dependent diabetes and obesity, according to the Health Development Agency (Protheroe *et al.*, 2003). *Saving Lives: Our Healthier Nation* also promoted breastfeeding, by developing specific recommendations (DoH, 1999a, 1999b).

The DoH infant feeding survey conducted in 2000 reported that the incidence of breastfeeding in the UK was 69% at birth, 28% at 4 months, 21% at 6 months and 13% at 9 months. The population of women was found to be older (e.g. in England and Wales 46% of women were aged 30 or over compared with 40% in 1995) and better educated (e.g. in England and Wales 28% of women completed their education at 19 or above). There was a rise in initial breastfeeding from women in social class V, now at 57% (up from the previous survey), and in social class I the rate was 91% (Hamlyn *et al.*, 2002).

Not all units in the UK audit their breastfeeding statistics (Audit Commission, 1997) as recommended by the National Breastfeeding Working Group in 1994 (DoH, 1994). The DoH 'local infant feeding audit' was launched by the National Infant Feeding Advisors in May 2000 (RCM *et al.*, 2000) as a means of helping to monitor breastfeeding rates and demonstrate the impact of local breastfeeding promotion, with potential links to the ONS statistics. Low breastfeeding rates have huge implications for a nation's health and finance – illustrated by the USA where medical treatment of diarrhoea, respiratory disease, insulin-dependent diabetes and otitis media in non-breastfed babies was estimated to add an extra $1 billion to healthcare costs (Riordan, 1997).

The Scientific Advisory Committee on Nutrition (SACN) agreed at its September 2001 meeting, to recommend exclusive breastfeeding for 6 months (http://www.doh.gov.uk/sacn/meetingsept01mins.htm).

The UK had already supported the following WHO resolution on infant and child nutrition adopted at the World Health Assembly in May 2001: 'to protect, promote and support breastfeeding for six months as a public health recommendation …'. The WHO resolution was based on a commissioned, systematic review (Kramer and Kakuma, 2002). The WHO global strategy on infant and young child feeding reiterated this as a guide for action (WHO, 2002).

The Health Development Agency (Protheroe *et al.*, 2003) suggest attention is paid to individual and group health education on breastfeeding for specific ethnic and low income groups in antenatal and postnatal periods. Peer counsellors were found to enhance the effectiveness of sessions in the antenatal and postnatal period for women who planned to breastfeed. Early initiation of breastfeeding and 'rooming in', combined with education, improved the duration of breastfeeding, and local media campaigns improved breastfeeding rates (Protheroe *et al.*, 2003).

Midwives should expand their public health role in educating women and their families in the value of breastfeeding, and in encouraging women to breastfeed. In addition, they can reduce inequalities and social deprivation by working closely with health visitors (HVs) to support women who choose to breastfeed to continue to do so (DoH, 1999c). A multidisciplinary and longsighted approach is required which commences preconceptually, and develops and supports during pregnancy and through into the first few months of neonatal life. Working with Sure Start practitioners, HVs, and other midwives ensures a seamless, holistic support system in line with the NHS Plan (DoH, 2000; NHS Centre for Reviews and Dissemination, 2000).

NUTRITIONAL REQUIREMENTS OF THE FULL-TERM NEONATE

Calorific requirements were based traditionally on volumes of formula required by artificially fed babies (Auerbach and Riordan, 1998). The calorific requirement for term infants is thought to average 440 kJ per kilogram of body weight per day (110–120 kcal/kg/day) depending on gestational age (Blackburn, 2003).

Breast milk (or infant formulae) contains approximately 275 kJ (65 kcal) per 100 ml (Auerbach and Riordan, 1998). A baby weighing 3.5 kg requires approximately 1540 kJ in 24 hours – about 525 ml milk per day. This amount varies depending on the gestation of the baby, and volume and content will vary from feed to feed. A meta-analysis of the volume of milk secreted by exclusively breastfeeding women around the world found this to be constant at around 800 ml per day. The volume of milk transferred from the breast to the baby is less than 100 ml per day for the first 24–36 hours, then gradually increases to 500 ml from 36 hours (Neville, 1999).

There is no evidence to suggest that healthy term infants require larger volumes of fluid any earlier than they are made available (Williams, 1997). In fact the low volume of colostrum is important for optimal physiological adaptation of the neonate, and health professionals need to appreciate that bioavailability of breast milk's 200 known constituents identifies its superiority over formula milk. Therefore, forced breast feeds or excessive volumes of formula milk in the first few days of life must be discouraged, as they are unnecessary and can be harmful.

In human milk the calorific value is derived from the carbohydrate and fat content that is absorbed easily through the gut, while cows' milk has a higher proportion of protein that is less easily digestible.

The content of breast milk changes throughout a feed and during the day and night *so can never be directly compared with cows' milk or formula milk*. The ratio of total solids to fluid is 12 : 88 which enables the neonate to receive its total fluid requirements from its mother's milk (Henschel and Inch, 1996).

Midwives should be conversant with the relevant Department of Health guidelines (COMA Working Group, 1994; Statutory Instrument 77, 1995) and the WHO Global Strategy on Infant and Young Child Nutrition (WHO, 2002), as knowledge of basic nutrition has been found to be very poor amongst health professionals (Hyde, 1994).

PHYSIOLOGY OF THE GASTROINTESTINAL TRACT

The maturation of the neonatal gut is stimulated by initiation of feeding, milk composition, hormonal regulation and genetic encoding (Blackburn, 2003). Initiation of early feeding is a major stimulus for the increase of plasma concentrations of peptide hormones, e.g. *enteroglucagon*, which stimulates growth of the intestinal mucosa; *gastrin*, which stimulates growth of the gastric mucosa and exocrine pancreas; and *motilin* and *neurotensin*, which stimulate gut activity. Colostrum stimulates epithelial cell turnover and maturation. In addition, epidermal growth factor and *cortisol* assist in the growth and development of the neonatal gastrointestinal system. None of the above is available in formula milk.

Breast milk aids the passage of meconium through the gut, whereas formula milk does not. Delayed passage of meconium is associated with elevated bilirubin levels owing to reabsorption of unconjugated bilirubin and recirculation to the liver; therefore physiological jaundice may be problematic in formula-fed infants.

Until the baby is 9 months old, intake of formula milk stimulates a greater insulin response than intake of breast milk (Blackburn 2003), thus initiating an unnecessary increase in the metabolism of glucose stores.

One of the most notable actions is that of *secretory IgA*, which has important antitoxic and antiallergic properties. These properties serve to protect the neonatal gut from bacteria, viruses and other harmful organisms and can never be replicated in artificial formulae.

NORMAL NEONATAL METABOLISM

The immature exocrine pancreatic function of the neonate is a major factor in the digestion of foods in the first few weeks of life. The neonate relies on alternative/additional means for digestion of proteins, carbohydrates and fats, and compensation occurs by use of enzymes in the saliva, intestine and breast milk.

Protein digestion in the neonate is disadvantaged owing to the limited production of gastric pepsin (a mere trace in some) with pancreatic enterokinase output less than 10% of adults. The greater percentage of whey to casein proteins in breast milk is more easily digested (Hamosh, 1998).

Neonatal *carbohydrate digestion* relies on amylase in breast milk which remains high during the first 6 weeks of lactation. Neonatal salivary amylase is only one-third of adult levels, while pancreatic amylase represents only 2.5–5% of adult levels.

Fat digestion has been shown to be greater in breastfed versus formula-fed preterm neonates (Hamosh, 1998). Though the neonate has raised gastric lipase, there is reduced pancreatic lipase for fat digestion. This is compensated by the stimulus of suckling at the breast, stimulating secretion of lingual lipase in the neonate (Blackburn, 2003).

Colostrum and breast milk are uniquely tailored to assist the neonate in independent metabolism and this should be explained to the woman.

CONSTITUENTS OF COLOSTRUM AND BREAST MILK

Colostrum is produced from 16 weeks' gestation and continues for the first 3–4 days postpartum until replaced by milk. It is a yellow-orange, thick sticky fluid that assumes its colour from beta carotene (Lawrence and Lawrence, 1998) with a lower calorific value than breast milk (approx 67 kcal/100 ml versus 75 kcal/100 ml for breast milk).

The daily volume ranges from 2–29 ml per feed, and protein, fat-soluble vitamins and mineral percentages are higher than in breast milk, with lower levels of carbohydrate and fat. It is unique in its high concentration of protective constituents – immunoglobulins, macrophages, lymphocytes, neutrophils, and mononuclear cells – which give it a higher protein content. The concentration of growth factors is up to five times higher in colostrum than in mature milk.

Transitional breast milk is produced between colostrum (from 3–4 days) and mature milk and lasts for approximately 10 days to 2 weeks postpartum (Lawrence and Lawrence, 1998). During this time, protein and immunoglobulin levels decrease while carbohydrate and fat levels increase. Water-soluble vitamins increase and fat-soluble vitamins decrease.

Mature breast milk contains approximately 90% water with 10% proteins, carbohydrate and fats with vitamins and minerals. The main solid constituent is the fatty acid component that provides 50% of the calorific requirements. Fat content varies at and during each feed according to the neonate's requirement.

Protein

0.9% of breast milk is protein, which includes the easily digested non-casein or whey portion which makes up approximately 70% of the proteins. The main components are alpha-lactalbumin, beta-lactoglobulin, serum albumin, immunoglobulins, lactoferrin and lysozyme. Casein constitutes the other 30% of the protein. In cows' milk the protein content is reversed, with an approximately 80% casein to 20% whey ratio (Lawrence and Lawrence, 1998). Out of the 20 amino acids present, eight are essential and provide the important nitrogen content required by the neonate. Two of the most abundant amino acids are cystine and taurine. Taurine is absent from cows' milk but plays an important role in brain maturation and is thought to function as a neurotransmitter. It was originally presumed to be involved only in conjugation of bile acids. Cystine is essential for somatic growth (Auerbach and Riordan, 1998).

Carbohydrates

The carbohydrate portion comprises mainly lactose with small quantities of oligosaccharides, galactose and fructose. Lactose increases calcium absorption and is readily metabolized into galactose and glucose (assisted by the intestinal enzyme, lactase), providing the necessary energy to feed the growing brain (Auerbach and Riordan, 1998). These levels remain constant and are unaffected in malnourished women (Lawrence and Lawrence, 1998).

Some oligosaccharides promote the growth of *Lactobacillus bifidus*, which increases the acidity of the neonatal gut and protects it from invasion by pathogens (Kunz *et al.*, 1999).

Fats

The fat content is variable at different times of the day and during a feed, with higher amounts towards the end of a feed (Kunz *et al.*, 1999). Preterm fat concentrations are reported to be 30% higher (Auerbach and Riordan, 1998) though others did not detect any major differences in lipid composition between term and preterm breast milk apart from more medium- and intermediate-chain fatty acids (Rodriguez-Palmero *et al.*, 1999). Long-chain polyunsaturated fatty acids (LCPUFA) are important for normal visual and brain development and are absent from formula milk. Addition of LCPUFA to formula milk in one very small study was found to improve IQ at 10 months of age (Williatts *et al.*, 1998).

The majority of long-chain polyunsaturated acids are derived from maternal body stores rather than diet. It is suggested that maternal diet directly affects the fatty acid composition of breast milk (Kunz *et al.*, 1999). Women who are vegetarians are able to maintain high milk content of arachidonic (AA) and docosahexaenoic (DHA) acids. DHA is the LCPUFA associated with improved visual and neurological function (Makrides *et al.*, 1995).

98% of the fat components are triglycerides that are broken down to fatty acids and glycerol by the enzyme lipase, found in breast milk itself. The remaining fats are phospholipids (0.7%), cholesterol (0.5%) and other lipolysis products. Digestion of triglycerides is initiated in the stomach where gastric lipase commences lipolysis, and this is continued in the intestine by pancreatic lipase. The resulting monoglycerides have potent bactericidal properties and maintain infection control in the stomach and small intestine (Rodriguez-Palmero *et al.*, 1999).

Vitamins

Water-soluble vitamins C (ascorbic acid), B_1 (thiamine), B_2 (riboflavin and niacin), B_6 (pyridoxine), folate (pteroylglutamic acid), B_{12} (cobalamin), pantothenic acid and biotin are all present in breast milk. Only niacin and B_{12} can be increased by maternal intake if found to be deficient (Rodriguez-Palmero *et al.*, 1999).

Fat-soluble vitamins A (retinol), beta-carotene (carotenoids), D (cholecalciferol), E (alpha-tocopherol) and K (phylloquinone) are all present in breast milk.

Minerals

These include sodium, potassium, chloride, calcium, magnesium, phosphorus, free phosphate and sulphur.

Citrate binds some minerals and is soluble in water so has a part to play, despite not being a mineral. Trace elements such as iron, zinc, copper, manganese, selenium iodine and fluorine are all present in breast milk, though the latter two are absent from colostrum (Rodriguez-Palmero *et al.*, 1999).

The uptake of iron in breast milk is facilitated by the high levels of lactose and vitamin C enabling up to 70% of absorption to take place. Absorption of exogenous iron from formula milk is limited and can adversely affect the action of lactoferrin from breast milk in the gut if the woman is mixed-feeding (see Table 33.1).

Unabsorbed iron is a contributory factor to the increased incidence of gastroenteritis in formula-fed infants.

Defence agents

These can be divided into four groups, though some have multiple roles (Rodriguez-Palmero *et al.*, 1999); see Table 33.1.

ADVANTAGES OF BREASTFEEDING

The normal neonate

The value of breast milk to the neonate is well documented (Lawrence, 1997; NHS Centre for Reviews and Dissemination, 2000; MIDIRS/NHS Centre for Reviews and Dissemination, 1999; Riordan, 1997) and the importance of 'exclusive' breastfeeding is

Table 33.1 Defence agents in breast milk

Substance and production	Action
1. Antimicrobial agents Immunoglobulins	
Neonate produces minimal amounts of these in the first few months of life	Proteins produced by plasma cells in response to an antigen – located in the lactoglobulin fraction of breast milk
Secretory IgA – most abundant immunoglobulin IgG, IgM, IgD and IgE	Important in providing passive immunity More resistant to proteolytic enzymes Provides resistance to a range of pathogens in gastrointestinal and respiratory tract Neutralizes viruses and toxins from microorganisms such as *Escherichia coli*, *Salmonella*, *Clostridium difficile*, rotavirus and *Vibrio cholerae* (Auerbach and Riordan, 1998; Rodriguez-Palmero *et al.*, 1999) These are other immunoglobulins found in breast milk in small amounts
Lactoferrin – an iron-binding glycoprotein	Competes with bacteria for iron thus depriving bacteria of nutrients for proliferation Enhances iron absorption in neonate's intestinal tract An essential growth factor for B and T lymphocytes (Auerbach and Riordan, 1998)
Lysozyme – a whey protein	Acts with peroxide and ascorbate to destroy Gram-positive and other bacteria in the gut and respiratory system Increases progressively after 6 months' lactation
Bifidus factor – nitrogen-containing carbohydrate	Promotes growth of anaerobic lactobacilli in the neonatal gut, providing a protective acid medium (Auerbach and Riordan, 1998; Newman, 1995)
B_{12} binding protein	Deprives bacteria of vitamin B_{12}

(continued)

Table 33.1 (*continued*)

Substance and production	Action
Oligosaccharides – carbohydrates (monosaccharides)	Act by blocking antigens from attaching to the epithelium of the gastrointestinal tract Prevent the attachment of pneumococci (Auerbach and Riordan, 1998)
Fatty acids	Disrupt membranes surrounding certain viruses and destroy them
Complement (C3 and C4 components)	Has the ability to fuse bacteria bound to a specific antibody and destroy them through lysis (Lawrence and Lawrence, 1998)
Fibronectin	Facilitates the uptake of bacteria by mononuclear phagocytic cells
Mucins – protein and carbohydrate molecules	Adhere to bacteria and viruses (including HIV) and prevent them from attaching to mucosal surfaces (Lawrence and Lawrence, 1998; Newman, 1995)
2. Anti-inflammatory factors Secretory IgA, lactoferrin and lysozyme	Multipurpose anti-inflammatory role Lactoferrin inhibits the complement system and suppresses cytokine release from macrophages that have been stimulated by bacteria (Rodriguez-Palmero *et al.*, 1999)
Antioxidants (alpha-tocopherol, beta-carotene, cystine, ascorbic acid)	Absorbed into the circulation and have systemic anti-inflammatory effects (Rodriguez-Palmero *et al.*, 1999)
Epithelial growth factors	Enhance maturation of the neonatal gut and limit entry of pathogens
Other anti-inflammatory factors include platelet-activating factor, antiproteases (alpha-antichymotrypsin and alpha-antitrypsin) and prostaglandins	
3. Immunomodulators Nucleotides, cytokines and anti-idiotypic antibodies	Appear to promote development of the neonatal immune system
4. Leucocytes (white blood cells) Approximately 90% of leucocytes in breast milk are *neutrophils* and *macrophages* 80% of the *lymphocytes* are T cells, though the cytotoxic capacity of these cells is low (Rodriguez-Palmero *et al.*, 1999)	Eliminate bacteria and fungi by phagocytosis

promoted by the DoH. The UK Scientific Advisory Committee on Nutrition supported the WHO resolution passed in May 2001, which recommended 'exclusive breastfeeding for six months with the introduction of complementary foods and continued breastfeeding thereafter' (SACN, 2002). In addition, breastfeeding itself has a beneficial effect on the psychological and physical well-being of mother and baby.

The action of sucking at the breast helps to initiate production of saliva that increases absorption of carbohydrate and fat. The saliva of the neonate contains amylase that assists in glucose absorption and lipase that increases uptake of fatty acids (Blackburn, 2003). These enzymes will be reduced if the baby is preterm and unable to suckle, as tube-feeding bypasses this process, so it is important for the midwife to assist the women to initiate suckling as soon as the reflex is present.

Breast milk's immune properties have been specifically highlighted (Hanson, 1998a; Mannick and Udall, 1996; Newman, 1995; Orlando, 1995). It provides protection from leukaemia (Davis, 1998; Shu *et al.*, 1999); rotavirus infection (Newburg *et al.*, 1998); gastrointestinal infections (Dewey *et al.*, 1995; Golding *et al.*, 1997; Mannick and Udall, 1996); respiratory tract infection (Lopez-Alarcon *et al.*, 1997; Repucci, 1995); *Haemophilus influenzae* meningitis (Silfverdal *et al.*, 1999); urinary tract infection (Pisacane *et al.*, 1992); otitis media (Dewey *et al.*, 1995; Duncan *et al.*, 1993) and necrotizing enterocolitis (Lucas and Cole, 1990).

Others have demonstrated improved motor/personal and social development (Wang and Su, 1996); improved IQ (Florey *et al.*, 1995; Lucas *et al.*, 1992); protection from non-insulin-dependent diabetes mellitus (Cavallo *et al.*, 1996; Drash *et al.*, 1994; Pettitt *et al.*, 1997); eczema, asthma, and food allergies (Coutts, 1998; Hanson, 1998b; Oddy, 2000; Saarinen and Kajosaari, 1995); and from cardiovascular disease in later life (Ravelli *et al.*, 2000).

Other benefits of breastfeeding include possible protection from schizophrenia (McCreadie, 1997); juvenile rheumatoid arthritis (Mason *et al.*, 1995); Crohn's disease and coeliac disease (Hanson, 1998a; Koletzko *et al.*, 1989); development of the physiological integrity of the oral cavity, ensuring alignment of teeth and fewer problems with malocclusions (Palmer, 1998); and protection from sudden infant death has been suggested by McVea *et al.* (2000). The action of breastfeeding has beneficial effects on dental caries, mouth and jaw development, and reduces the risk of childhood obesity.

The preterm neonate

Breastfeeding confers all of the above advantages and because of the reduced capability of the immune system, is vital for early protection against infection. Preterm infants are particularly vulnerable to necrotizing enterocolitis so it is very important that women are supported to breastfeed fully (Lucas and Cole, 1990). Women who give birth prematurely provide perfectly balanced breast milk for their babies – the non-protein nitrogen content is 20% higher than in those who give birth at term, providing the necessary free amino acids essential for growth (Auerbach and Riordan, 1998). Preterm breast milk contains higher concentrations of polymeric immunoglobulin A (pIgA), lactoferrin, lysozyme and epidermal growth factor. In addition, the numbers of macrophages, neutrophils and lymphocytes are higher in the colostrum (Xanthou, 1998).

Lingual lipases will be reduced if the baby is preterm and unable to suckle, as tube-feeding bypasses this process.

The woman

Studies have demonstrated protection from premenopausal breast cancer (Buchanan and Sachs, 1998; Enger *et al.*, 1997; Katsouyanni *et al.*, 1996; Michels *et al.*, 1996; UK National Case-Control Study Group, 1993) and premenopausal ovarian cancer (Siskind *et al.*, 1997). Re-analysis of data from 47 epidemiological studies in 30 countries on pre- and postmenopausal breast cancer in women concluded that the longer women breastfeed the more they are protected against breast cancer (Collaborative Group on Hormonal Factors in Breast Cancer, 2002). Positive effects on bone density during the postmenopausal period have also been described (Cumming and Klineberg, 1993; Melton *et al.*, 1993).

Lactational amenorrhoea has been demonstrated to be an effective postpartum contraceptive during 'total' breastfeeding (Gross, 1999; Rogers, 1997; WHO Task Force, 1999), having the added advantage of delaying menstruation and reducing anaemia (Wang and Fraser, 1994).

CONTRAINDICATIONS TO BREASTFEEDING

There are very few absolute contraindications to breastfeeding.

HIV

HIV may be transmitted through breast milk. The increased risk of vertical transmission by this route is estimated to be about 1 in 7 for women with established infection (Baby Milk Action, 2001).

In the UK, women with HIV are advised against breastfeeding and are informed of the risks of vertical transmission to the baby in accordance with the WHO/UNICEF/UNAIDS consensus statement, DoH guidance and the Royal College of Midwives (RCM) (DoH, 1997, 1999d; NHS Executive, 1999; RCM, 1998; RCM and DoH, 1999, 2000; WHO, 1997; World Bank Symposium, 1998).

Though it has been suggested that breastfeeding in developing countries is more beneficial, this has been challenged. Research on the effects of exclusive breastfeeding by HIV-affected women in a cohort study in

South Africa demonstrated that babies were not protected against common childhood illnesses or failure to thrive, neither was there a significantly delayed progression to AIDS in HIV-infected babies (Bobat *et al.*, 1997).

More recently, studies have compared exclusive breastfeeding with mixed feeding in terms of mother-to-child transmission of HIV and have found reduced transmission with exclusive breastfeeding (Coutsoudine *et al.*, 1999). Millar and colleagues postulated that breast milk erythropoietin protects mammary epithelium and/or neonatal intestinal epithelial integrity thus reducing the viral load to the neonate (Miller *et al.*, 2002). However, more research is required in this area before policy changes are made by the DoH.

Hepatitis C

A small study of the breast milk of seropositive women indicated that there is a very low risk of transmitting the virus to the baby (Zimmermann *et al.*, 1995).

Drugs

Certain drugs pass through breast milk and may be harmful to the neonate, and temporary or permanent avoidance of breastfeeding may be recommended, depending on the prescription of drugs currently in use by the woman (e.g. antipsychotic, anticarcinogenic, iodides). Midwives can update their knowledge using the most recent British National Formulary (BNF) or the local pharmacy drug information service within their trust. The National Childbirth Trust guide to drugs in breast milk (NCT, 1996) gives an excellent overview for a quick reference guide, and the Breastfeeding Network can be contacted by phone or through the Internet for quick reference for women (see Additional resources, p. 627).

This knowledge must be taken into account when advising women about the behaviour of their baby following certain types of analgesia used during labour. Narcotics and drugs used in epidural/spinal analgesia interfere with the spontaneous breastfeeding movements and the temperature of the neonate at birth (Ransjo-Arvidson *et al.*, 2001).

Pollutants in breast milk

There are a variety of pollutants in the environment and some may arise in breast milk. These should not prevent breastfeeding or its promotion, as breastfeeding itself offers a degree of protection against many pollutants.

The Committee on Toxicity of Chemicals in Food, Consumer Products and the Environment examined the high quantities of polychlorinated biphenyls (PCBs) and dioxins present in breast milk and concluded that the advantages of breastfeeding still outweighed the risks (Mitchell, 1997). Intake of organochlorines measured in breast milk set against the WHO acceptable daily intakes failed to demonstrate an unacceptable intake for the baby (Quinsey *et al.*, 1996). The pesticide, DDT, was measured in breast milk fat and demonstrated a decline in most areas of the world (Smith, 1999), and guidance on the implications of exposure to cadmium, lead and mercury resulted in encouragement of breastfeeding under 'most circumstances' (Abadin *et al.*, 1997).

THE ROLE OF THE MIDWIFE

Knowledge of breastfeeding

- Midwives should be aware of their own attitudes towards and beliefs about breastfeeding prior to advising others. In her breastfeeding workshop pack, Jamieson suggested midwives complete their own 'lifeline' in order to review the influences in their own lives and help make sense of any deep-rooted beliefs about breastfeeding (Clifton and Long, 1992).
- In-depth knowledge about the physiology of lactation is crucial in order to teach women the fundamentals of supply and demand and the stages of breast milk production (Auerbach and Riordan, 1998; Blackburn 2003; Lawrence and Lawrence, 1998). Professional ignorance is unacceptable when information is so readily available in different forms and accessible to the general public via the media and electronic means.
- Midwives should work within the framework set out in the *Ten Steps to Successful Breastfeeding* (Saadeh and Akre, 1996; Woolridge, 1994; WHO, 1998) (see Box 33.2). This was developed from the joint World Health Organization (WHO) and United Nations Children's Fund (UNICEF) statement on protecting, promoting and supporting breastfeeding (WHO/UNICEF, 1989). It incorporates the responsibility for training *all* healthcare staff and ensuring there is a written breastfeeding policy in each unit (UNICEF UK BFI, 1998a; WHO, 1998). The subsequent community seven-point

plan (Box 33.3) provides guidance to healthcare professionals in the community (incorporating the Ten Steps). It sets out the gold standard for care of breastfeeding mothers in the community and should be followed by all midwives and trusts within the UK (UNICEF UK BFI, 2001).

- Knowledge shared with women and their families must be evidence based and linked to research as far as is possible. Where there is no research, this should be made explicit in the discussion in order to ensure informed decision-making (MIDIRS/NHS Centre for Reviews and Dissemination, 1999; UNICEF UK BFI, 2001).
- Midwives require the skills and ability to share their knowledge on breastfeeding with enthusiasm (Inch, 1996b).

- Midwives should be able to confidently promote breastfeeding for its public health benefits to the woman and baby (NHS Centre for Reviews and Dissemination, 2000; UNICEF UK BFI, 1996, 1998b).
- Midwives need to recognize the value and importance of breastfeeding for both the woman and her baby. They must be able to give practical support and advice to the woman and be sensitive to cultural issues and traditions surrounding breastfeeding (Kendall, 1995; Vincent, 1999).

Reflective Activity 33.1

How do you meet the criteria as listed above?

Do you have breastfeeding guidelines in your trust, and if so, are they audited regularly? Do you have a personal copy of the guidelines?

Is there a breastfeeding working group in your trust, and if so, are you a member?

Do you have a copy of the *Ten Steps to Successful Breastfeeding*?

Box 33.3 The seven-point plan for the protection, promotion and support of breastfeeding in community healthcare settings (UNICEF UK BFI, 2001)

All providers of community healthcare should:

1. Have a written breastfeeding policy that is routinely communicated to all healthcare staff.
2. Train all staff involved in the care of mothers and babies in the skills necessary to implement the policy.
3. Inform all pregnant women about the benefits and management of breastfeeding.
4. Support mothers to initiate and maintain breastfeeding.
5. Encourage exclusive and continued breastfeeding, with appropriately timed introduction of complementary foods.
6. Provide a welcoming atmosphere for breastfeeding families.
7. Promote cooperation between healthcare staff, breastfeeding support groups and the local community.

The seven-point plan is the result of a widespread consultation procedure involving health professionals, service providers, mother support groups, professional organizations and other interested parties. It therefore reflects consensus in the UK as to what constitutes best practice in the care for and support of breastfeeding mothers and babies by the community health services.

ANATOMY OF THE BREAST

Definition

The breasts are two mammary glands situated on either side of the anterior chest wall between the second and the sixth rib. They are covered with skin, and loose connective tissue attaches them to the deep fascia covering the pectoralis muscle.

Embryological development

- Week 4: Thickened ectoderm appears bilaterally in the pectoral region.
- Week 6: Pectoral thickenings enlarge and grow into the underlying mesenchyme. Secondary cords grow out into the surrounding mesenchyme to form *lactiferous ducts*.
- Week 13: The epidermis at the origin of the mammary gland becomes depressed to form a mammary pit.
- Week 32–36: Downgrowths and cords become canalized. Mesenchyme forms the fat and fibrous connective tissue.
- The nipples form and the skin becomes elevated just prior to birth.

Structure of the breast

The mammary gland is composed of glandular and contractile cells lying within a supportive framework of connective and adipose tissue that carries the vascular supply, nerve cells, and lymphatic vessels. Glandular tissue is organized into numerous ducts that drain clusters of 10–100 alveoli (acini) that are formed into lobules. Contractile tissue is made up of myoepithelial cells covering the alveoli and small ducts, together with smooth muscle that surrounds the large ducts and blood vessels. The small ducts are lined by secretory cells, whereas larger ducts and sinuses are lined by non-secretory cuboidal epithelium. Each alveolus consists of a hollow ball of secretory cells surrounded by a network of contractile myoepithelium and capillaries. The collections of alveoli, or lobules, are grouped into 15–20 lobes and drain into a single lactiferous duct. Adjacent lobes are separated by layers of connective and adipose tissue (Fig. 33.1).

The nipple is composed of connective tissue and smooth muscle fibres, and contains openings for approximately 15–20 lactiferous ducts, which form into lactiferous sinuses, or ampullae, that act as small milk reservoirs during lactation. The surrounding area, known as the areola, is darker pigmented skin that accommodates sweat and sebaceous (Montgomery's) glands. These glands become enlarged and lubricate the nipple during pregnancy and lactation.

Blood supply is from the internal and external mammary and upper intercostal arteries. Venous blood is transported away from the breast by circular veins behind the nipple, then into the internal mammary and axillary veins.

Lymphatic drainage is extensive and the systems of both breasts communicate freely.

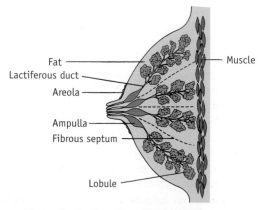

Fat
Lactiferous duct
Areola
Ampulla
Fibrous septum
Muscle
Lobule

Figure 33.1 Sagittal section of the breast.

Nerve supply is from branches of the fourth, fifth and sixth thoracic nerves. The nipple and areola are very sensitive and have a rich source of sensory nerves (Henschel and Inch, 1996). The breast is controlled by hormone action.

PHYSIOLOGY OF LACTATION

Puberty to pregnancy (mammogenesis)

At puberty, oestrogen and growth hormone stimulate the growth of the mammary ducts. In the second half of the menstrual cycle, progesterone stimulates development of the lactiferous ducts and alveoli. Proliferation of the epithelial tissue is a gradual process at each menstrual cycle.

In the first trimester of pregnancy, the myoepithelial cells hypertrophy and the blood vessels become more prominent under the influence of oestrogen, with a 50% increase in blood flow to the breast (Blackburn, 2003). In the second trimester, secretion of colostrum is facilitated. In the third trimester, progesterone and human placental lactogen ensure that the alveoli mature and milk is produced. Progesterone circulates in high concentrations in pregnancy and prevents milk secretion until the birth takes place (Neville, 1999).

Prolactin is a single-chain peptide hormone released from the anterior pituitary gland, and serum levels increase during pregnancy. It is thought to be essential for the development and final stages of the differentiation of the alveoli and ducts in pregnancy (Blackburn, 2003; Neville, 1999).

In addition, prolactin-inhibiting factor, produced by the hypothalamus, maintains low prolactin levels to prevent milk secretion in pregnancy.

Oxytocin is an octapeptide hormone produced in the hypothalamus and stored and secreted in the posterior pituitary gland (Blackburn, 2003). It is produced in low levels during pregnancy; this is thought to be due to the action of a placental enzyme. It stimulates electrical activity and muscle contractions in the myometrium during labour and is critical in the milk ejection reflex postpartum.

Other hormones such as human placental lactogen (hPL), human chorionic gonadotrophin (hCG), growth hormone and adrenocorticotrophic hormone (ACTH) act synergistically with prolactin and progesterone to influence the growth of the glandular tissues of the alveoli to promote mammogenesis (Blackburn, 2003). hPL assists in mobilization of free fatty acids and inhibition of peripheral glucose utilization and stimulates mammary growth. ACTH stimulates the adrenals to secrete corticosteroids.

Initiation of lactation (lactogenesis)

Lactogenesis is the initiation of milk production and involves a complex interaction of several hormones and factors. Following the birth, oestrogen and progesterone levels decline rapidly, allowing a rise in *prolactin* and *oxytocin* levels. Prolactin, released from the anterior pituitary gland, stimulates the alveolar cells to produce milk while acting synergistically with growth hormone, insulin, cortisol, and thyrotrophin-releasing hormone (TRH) (Blackburn, 2003).

Oxytocin, released from the posterior pituitary gland, stimulates contraction of the myoepithelial cells surrounding the alveoli. This causes an ejection reflex and milk is propelled down the lactiferous ducts to the ampulla.

The action required to stimulate both of these hormones is known as the *neurohormonal reflex* (or 'let-down' reflex). This stimulus is controlled by the effect of the neonate sucking at the breast, but may also be stimulated by the mother seeing, smelling, touching and hearing her baby.

Suckling stimulates prolactin release from the anterior pituitary gland, and therefore it is imperative that the midwife assists the woman to breastfeed as soon as possible after the birth. It is suggested that sucking movements reach a peak at 45 minutes and decline within 2–2.5 hours after the birth (Righard and Alade, 1990; WHO/UNICEF, 1989) in line with a physiological reduction in adrenaline levels (Widstrom *et al.*, 1990). Lack of 'priming' the alveolar prolactin-receptor cells may result in shut-down and reduction of milk supply. Sensory nerve endings are activated in the nipple and areola area and this stimulates the hypothalamus via the spinal cord. As a result, oxytocin is released, prolactin-inhibiting factor is suppressed and prolactin is released. The levels of prolactin are increased towards the end of a feed, after approximately 20–30 minutes following a feed and at night, thus maintaining a diurnal increase (Blackburn, 2003). The midwife needs to explain to women that breastfeeding at night promotes and stimulates the production of prolactin for the next day and should be encouraged.

Prolactin release works on a supply and demand principle. When the baby suckles at the breast, prolactin-releasing factor is released by the hypothalamus

and stimulates prolactin release from the anterior pituitary gland. When the baby stops suckling, a negative feedback *prolactin-inhibiting factor* is released by the hypothalamus, usually by half an hour after a feed (Prentice *et al.*, 1989; Wilde *et al.*, 1995), and this inhibits prolactin supply (Fig. 33.2).

Prolactin-inhibiting factor (PIF) is a protein secreted in the breast milk itself which increases in amount as breast milk accumulates in the breast. Its function is to exert negative feedback to block future milk production when there is ineffective milk removal from the breast. Whilst prolactin and oxytocin are released systemically, therefore influencing milk production in both breasts, PIF build-up can occur in one breast, only affecting milk production in that breast. Therefore if a baby is incorrectly attached and unable to effectively remove milk from the breast, the build-up of PIF will ultimately result in a reduced milk supply. Similarly milk production can be stepped up again by effectively removing milk from the breast, thereby reducing the amount of circulating PIF in the breast milk.

As prolactin can also be inhibited by oestrogen, a woman wishing to use oral contraception following the birth must be advised to take the 'progesterone-only' pill while she continues to breastfeed.

If the women 'complements' with formula milk following breastfeeds the baby's suckling may be reduced at subsequent feeds, which ultimately interferes with the body's ability to produce the required amount of breast milk.

It is vital that the midwife discusses the physiology of lactation with the woman to dispel any fears or myths about breastfeeding.

Maintenance of established lactation (galactopoiesis)

This phase is reliant on an intact hypothalamic–pituitary axis regulating prolactin and oxytocin levels and maintenance of frequent sucking and removal of milk by the neonate (Blackburn, 2003). Growth hormone, corticosteroids, thyroxine and insulin continue to play an important part in maintaining established lactation.

The volume of milk produced commences at approximately 50 ml per day and increases to around 500 ml per day (double for twins) by 36 hours and up to 800 ml per day by 3 months (Neville, 1999). Sodium and chloride levels in breast milk fall in the first few days, followed by an increase in lactose concentrations. Lactoferrin and secretory IgA rise immediately then fall with the increase in volume in the first few days.

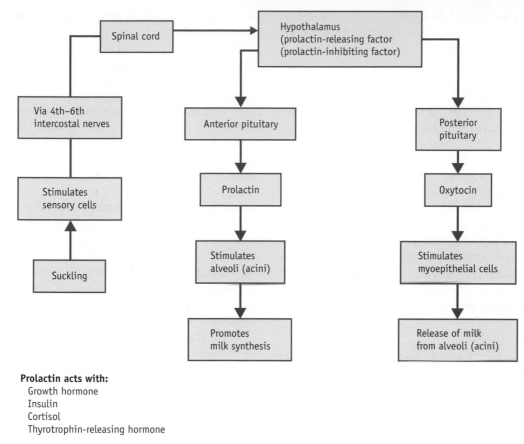

Prolactin acts with:
Growth hormone
Insulin
Cortisol
Thyrotrophin-releasing hormone

Figure 33.2 Physiology of breastfeeding – overview (neurohormonal reflex).

Regular suckling suppresses luteinizing hormone (LH) while follicle-stimulating hormone (FSH) may return to normal due to the pulsatile secretions of gonadotrophin-releasing hormone (GnRH) by 4 weeks postpartum (Neville, 1999). This may have an impact on the woman's fertility.

ASSISTING THE WOMAN TO BREASTFEED

Midwives' contribution to the support and education of women in the antenatal and immediate postnatal period has an enormous effect on the woman's satisfaction, with breastfeeding success and on breastfeeding rates overall.

Additional support has a positive effect on the duration of breastfeeding, demonstrated by a Cochrane database review (Anderson, 1999). This includes a range of activities, with face-to-face support in the antenatal and postnatal periods demonstrating the most positive effect 2 months postnatally. One Australian study used antenatal sessions on positioning and attachment of the baby and concluded that the experimental group women were better able to position and attach their babies; had less nipple pain and trauma in the first 4 postnatal days; and breastfed an average 6 weeks longer than the control group (Duffy et al., 1997).

Early initiation of breastfeeding 'It is important that skin-to-skin contact takes place in an unhurried environment for an unlimited period immediately (or as soon as possible) after delivery' (UNICEF UK BFI, 1998a). Early skin-to-skin contact and the opportunity to breastfeed within the first half an hour is supported by the BFI (WHO, 1998): it increases the duration of breastfeeding (Perez-Escamilla et al., 1994; Righard and Alade, 1990), maternal–infant interaction

(Ali and Lowry, 1981; de Chateau, 1980; de Chateau and Wilberg, 1977; Renfrew and Lang, 1999; Widstrom *et al.*, 1990), neonatal temperature, and glucose levels at 90 minutes; and reduces crying of the neonate (Christensson *et al.*, 1992).

This period of skin-to-skin contact and feeding is a precious one, and should be as unhurried and 'baby-led' as possible, as some babies will take slightly longer to seek the breast. Feeding is infrequent in the first 24 hours (Yamauchi and Yamanouchi, 1990).

A recent Cochrane review of early initiation of breastfeeding demonstrated that there is no statistical evidence to suggest that the duration of breastfeeding will be shorter if a mother does not feed her baby immediately after the birth (Renfrew and Lang, 1999). However, the increases in mother–infant interaction following early contact were found to be beneficial.

Midwives should ensure that they document and audit the timing and initiation of breastfeeding following all births.

Positions for feeding and good attachment/ latching-on

These have been cited as the key to successful breastfeeding (Fisher, 1994; RCM, 2002; UNICEF UK BFI, 1998b). The midwife needs to provide the woman with simple but helpful advice on positioning and attachment. These two aspects of breastfeeding can cause major problems if they are not addressed from the birth.

Preparation of the mother is important, either sitting or lying down using cushions or pillows to support the back (Henschel and Inch, 1996). Preparation of the baby so that she or he is unwrapped, with hands free (and mittens removed) enables the baby to experience touch, thus stimulating the neurological system and myelinization (Blackburn, 2003).

Positioning ('nose to nipple')   The baby needs to be supported to face the mother, parallel to the mother's chest. The baby's neck (rather than head) should be supported enough to allow the head to extend backwards as necessary (Fig. 33.3A). The mother should then bring the baby's nose in line with her nipple and ensure the rooting reflex is triggered, causing the mouth to 'gape' (RCM, 2002).

The consequences of ineffective suckling due to poor attachment on the breast have been linked to 'failure to thrive' (Morton, 1992) and early cessation of breast-feeding (Campbell, 1997; Righard and Alade, 1992).

The use of a pacifier (dummy) can cause confusion and should be discouraged, as the baby is more likely

to 'nipple-suck', and also may lead to reduced milk production (Neifert *et al.*, 1995; Righard and Alade, 1992; UNICEF UK BFI, 1998a). One randomized controlled trial (RCT) found a strong observational association between pacifier use and early weaning (Kramer *et al.*, 2001) though researchers were unable to determine whether the cause was poor motivation to breastfeed or the actual use of the dummy. It is suggested that continued support, promotion and encouragement of breastfeeding should be provided to avoid women requiring such 'props'.

Attachment ('baby to breast')   The baby should be brought up to the breast quickly to ensure correct attachment, rather than the breast brought down to the baby, which encourages bad maternal posture and poor attachment (RCM, 2002). The baby approaches the breast leading with the chin, which enables use of the tongue and lower jaw to 'scoop' up the breast tissues and access the lactiferous sinus and ampullae.

When the baby is attached to the breast properly 'his mouth is wide open and he has a big mouthful of breast; his chin is touching the breast; his bottom lip is curled back' (UNICEF UK BFI, 1998b). The correctly attached baby will take long deep sucks with pauses, and the ear will be seen visibly moving during the process (Fig. 33.3B).

If the baby is attached correctly (Fig. 33.4) there should be no friction of the tongue or gum on the nipple and no movement of the breast tissue in and out of the baby's mouth (RCM, 2002). The midwife should share this knowledge with women and help to reduce the confusion that can occur from poor positioning, or if bottle feeds are given as a complement to breast milk.

Expressing

> ... mothers should be shown how to express their milk or given written information on expression and/or advised where they could get help ... staff should teach mothers positioning, attachment, and techniques for manual expression of breast milk.
>
> (WHO, 1998)

This standard allows women to manage their own breastfeeding. Professionals who have adopted this practice have found that empowering women to offer hand-expressed breast milk to reluctant feeders dramatically reduces the need for supplementation with

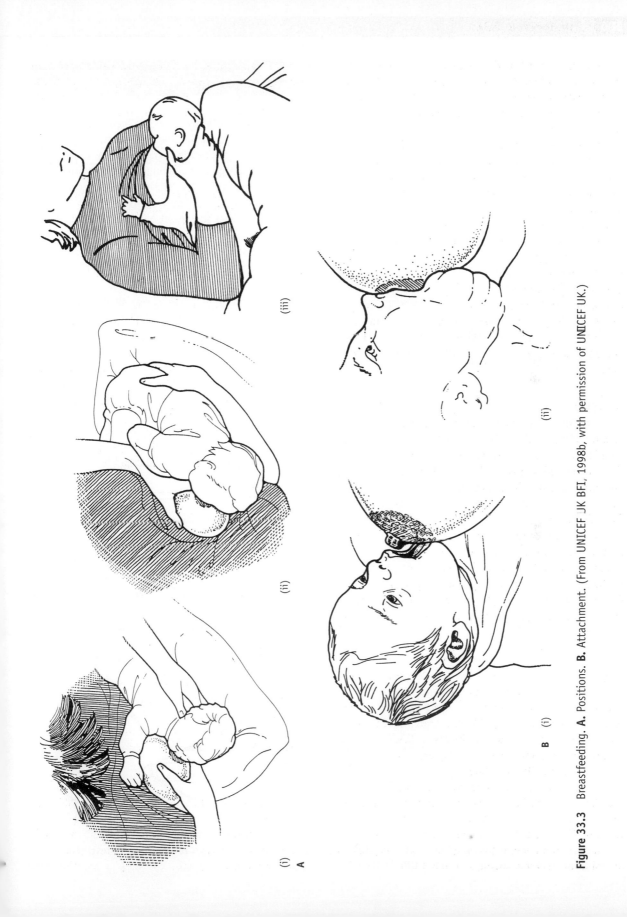

Figure 33.3 Breastfeeding. **A.** Positions. **B.** Attachment. (From UNICEF JK BFI, 1998b, with permission of UNICEF UK.)

formula milk. Manual expression (Box 33.4 and Fig. 33.5) has been demonstrated to be more effective than using a handpump (Fig. 33.6) as it provides a greater stimulus to prolactin levels (Howie, 1985; Howie *et al.*, 1980; Zinaman *et al.*, 1992).

Information on expression of breast milk should include clear guidelines on how often to express, and the importance of handwashing prior to expressing (Ackerley, 1996). A frequency of from six to eight times in 24 hours including once at night is advisable to optimize breast milk supply.

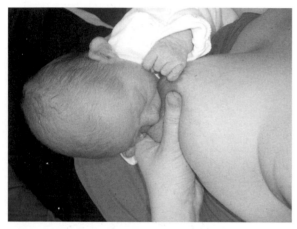

Figure 33.4   Breastfeeding.

> ## Box 33.4 Techniques for manual expression (UNICEF UK BFI, 1998b)
>
> ### Technique 1
> 1. Place your first finger under the breast, towards the edge of the areola, and your thumb on top of the breast opposite the first finger (Fig. 33.5A). If you have a large areola, you may need to bring your fingers in slightly. Your other fingers can be used to support the breast.
> 2. Gently compress the breast between the first finger and thumb.
> 3. Keep pressing and releasing, pressing and releasing. The milk will start to drip and then may spurt.
> 4. Press the areola in the same way all around the breast to make sure that the milk is expressed from all the lobes.
>
> ### Technique 2
> 1. Place your fingers in the same position as for technique 1.
> 2. Gently press your thumb and first finger back towards the chest wall as you press and release the breast tissue (Fig. 35.5B). This movement has been described as 'like easing a golf ball along a hosepipe'.

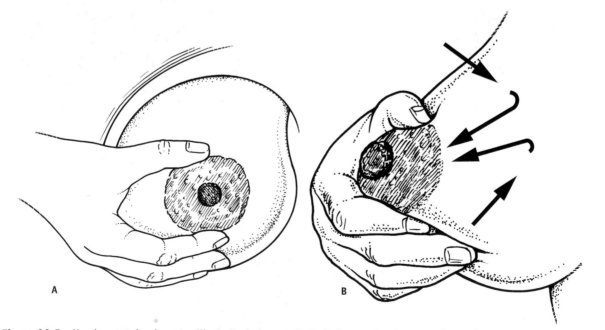

Figure 33.5   Hand-expressing breast milk. **A.** Technique 1. **B.** Technique 2. See Box 33.4 for explanatory text. (From UNICEF UK BFI, 1998b, with permission of UNICEF UK.)

Women should also be shown 'how to breastfeed and maintain lactation even if they should be separated from their infants' (WHO, 1998).

Frequent expression of breast milk has been associated with increased milk production (de Carvalho *et al.*, 1983) and should be recommended by midwives who are supporting women with preterm babies. Double-pumping (pumping both breasts simultaneously) encourages greater efficiency for mothers of preterm infants (Auerbach, 1990a; Hill *et al.*, 1996; Lang 1997).The sodium content of hand-expressed milk has been found to be higher than that of pump-expressed milk thus potentially reducing the amount of sodium supplementation required by preterm infants (Lang *et al.*, 1994).

Storage of milk

Expressed breast milk (EBM) should be collected in a sterilized container and covered. It can be stored in the refrigerator for up to 48 hours (RCM, 2002; see also http://www.ukamb.org), and in the freezer for 3 months, following which it must be thoroughly defrosted prior to use.

Warming to body temperature can be achieved by standing the EBM container in a jug of warm water. Milk should not be left standing at room temperature

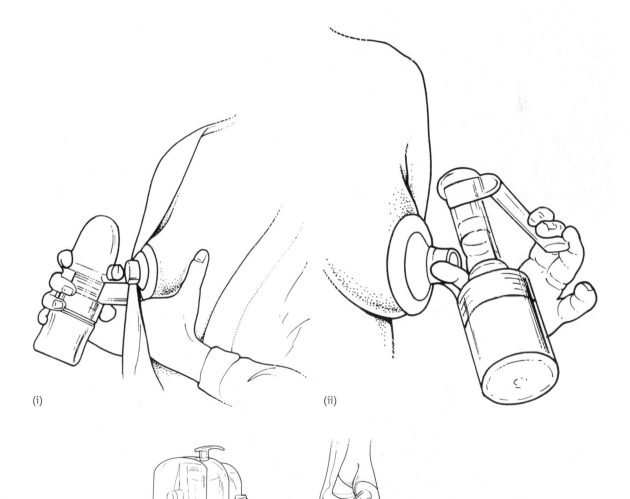

(i)   (ii)

(iii)

Figure 33.6   Handpumps and electric pumps. (From UNICEF UK BFI, 1998b, with permission of UNICEF UK.)

for longer than 1 hour, to prevent bacterial growth (Ackerley, 1996).

Neonatal nutrition

The midwife needs to have adequate knowledge of the constituents of breast milk (Henschel and Inch, 1996; RCM, 2002). A term breastfed baby should have adequate nutrition through breastfeeding on demand. A preterm neonate (less than 37 completed weeks of gestation) or small-for-gestational-age baby will have different demands and the midwife should seek guidance from a neonatologist on frequency and volume of feeds, as this is outwith normal midwifery practice (Lang, 1997; UKCC, 1998). The advantages of breast milk for a preterm baby are extremely important, and alternatives to suckling for the immature neonate will be discussed later. The fat content of breast milk promotes ketogenesis and reduces glucose oxidation (WHO, 1997).

Public health issues

Smoking carries higher risks for the infant (Becker *et al.*, 1999), and smoking during pregnancy and in the postnatal period reduces the volume of breast milk in addition to reducing the birthweight of the baby (Vio *et al.*, 1991), and this needs to be discussed with the woman.

The baby sharing the parents' bed has some physical and psychological advantages, including a better night's sleep for the woman, and perhaps a reduction in breastfeeding problems, sudden infant death syndrome and postnatal depression (Davies, 1995). However, the midwife needs to discuss the benefits and contraindications, such as if parents are heavy smokers, have drunk alcohol or have taken drugs that make them drowsy (Carpenter *et al.*, 2004; FSID and DoH, 2003; UNICEF UK/BFI/FSID, 2003).

Maternal nutrition during breastfeeding may vary according to cultural and religious differences, such as the use of 'hot' and 'cold' foods across cultures (Vincent, 1999), vegetarianism and fasting.

The lactating woman should aim for a diet containing no less than 1800 kcal with a recommended average intake of at least 2200 kcal (Lawrence and Lawrence, 1998). Women have enhanced metabolic efficiency due to hormonal influences during pregnancy and in the early postnatal period which enables them to utilize their normal diet to produce an adequate milk supply for their baby.

Dietary restriction during lactation should be discouraged (Butte, 2000), but midwives should be cautious about assuming that a poor diet will result in insufficient breast milk, which can undermine a woman's belief in her own body.

> ### Reflective Activity 33.2
>
> Consider the different management issues and how they apply to your practice, i.e. encouraging early skin-to-skin contact between mother and baby, positioning and attachment, and antenatal breastfeeding workshops. Are these part of your practice, and if not, how could you incorporate them?

COMMON PROBLEMS WHILST BREASTFEEDING

Insufficient milk

The woman's perception of the lack of an adequate milk supply, due to common myths rather than the reality, is the most notable explanation for this problem (Marasco, 1998). Woolridge (1995) has suggested that 'true' milk insufficiency occurs in as little as 2% of women.

The most common cause for insufficient milk is poor attachment, ineffective milk removal and infrequent feeding.

Women who have received continuous support are more likely to have a positive attitude to breastfeeding (Hillervik-Lindquist *et al.*, 1991). Lack of support and advice from the midwife, or from her immediate family and friends, can undermine the woman and lead to psychological and even 'iatrogenic' problems. It is helpful for the midwife to have discussed breastfeeding in the antenatal period and be aware of whether the woman actually planned to breastfeed or if she is 'under duress' from family members. Stress can inhibit oxytocin but should not be severe enough to inhibit lactation (Powers, 1999).

There are few physical causes for inadequate milk supply, and these need to be identified and rectified by midwives and the multiprofessional team. The principles of the physiology of lactation should be discussed with the woman to ensure she is positioning the baby for adequate and frequent milk 'removal' (Powers, 1999).

Certain drugs reduce lactation (oral contraceptives containing oestrogen, bromocriptine, thiazide diuretics) and should therefore be avoided. Smoking and alcohol consumption can reduce the milk supply (Horta *et al.*, 1997; Mennella, 1997), and women at risk should be identified in the antenatal period and offered appropriate advice and support.

Anaemia may affect the milk supply, shorten the length of breastfeeding and lower the age of weaning (Henly *et al.*, 1995). Women who experienced postpartum haemorrhage of between 500–1500 ml were found to have insufficient milk supply, with infants showing failure to thrive (Willis and Livingstone, 1995). An early review and treatment of such women is recommended.

Breast surgery may cause decreased milk production where the ducts have been severed, as in breast reduction (Neifert *et al.*, 1990). However, surgery for breast enhancement involving silicone implants does not normally cause nerve and duct damage as the prosthesis is implanted beneath the pectoral muscle (Berlin, 1994). The type of surgery should normally be identified by the midwife in the antenatal period and a plan of action documented.

Nipple shields, especially the non-silicone variety prevent the neonate from applying the stimulus required for effective milk removal from the lactiferous ducts and ampulla and may therefore reduce the milk supply.

Medical disorders such as hyperthyroidism or hypothyroidism can affect milk supply. Hypopituitarism (Sheehan' syndrome) affects the supply of hormones from the anterior pituitary gland and therefore prevents prolactin production. All such medical conditions require prompt referral and investigation.

Engorgement – venous/milk

Venous retention may occur because of the increase in blood and lymph circulation when the milk 'comes in' causing tenderness (Hill and Humenick, 1994) but this should not be confused with 'engorgement'.

Engorgement of the breast is a pathological condition whereby oedema causes poor milk flow by constricting the milk ducts. It is caused by infrequent, ineffective milk removal and is preventable by good breastfeeding practices such as correct positioning and attachment advice. Secondary vascular and lymph stasis may occur (Hill and Humenick, 1994).

Both milk and venous engorgement will cause distension of the breast tissue, impede the release of milk, and prevent the baby from 'latching on'. Engorgement may occur at any time during the first 2 weeks postpartum but is likely to peak at around the third to sixth day after delivery, or may occur following transfer home from hospital (Hill and Humenick, 1994). It may last for 48 hours, during which time the woman will experience discomfort and is at risk from development of mastitis and subsequent breast abscess (Auerbach, 1990b).

Warm flannels or a hot shower or bath may improve the milk flow by increasing the blood supply around the alveoli. Gentle hand (or pump) expression will help to release the milk flow and therefore the tension around the nipple and areola in order to attach the baby more easily. If the baby is separated from the woman, then hand-expressing or a breast pump needs to be used regularly.

A Cochrane review reported that treatments using cold cabbage leaves or cabbage leaf extract, ultrasound versus a placebo, and oxytocin and cold packs had no demonstrable effect on the symptoms. Use of Danzen (serrapeptase – an anti-inflammatory agent) and bromelain/trypsin complex improved the overall symptoms compared to a placebo (Snowden *et al.*, 2002).

There is limited evidence surrounding the practical relief of engorgement, and midwives should be aware that it is imperative to prevent such a condition occurring in the first place, by providing advice and support with regard to correct positioning, flexible feeding arrangements and completion of suckling on one breast at a time in order to ensure adequate milk removal (Renfrew *et al.*, 2000).

Sore/cracked nipples

The most common cause of sore or cracked nipples is incorrect attachment – preventable by good midwifery support, education and advice (Amir *et al.*, 1996; Inch and Fisher, 2000; Renfrew *et al.*, 2000; RCM, 2002). Poor attachment and soreness are created as the neonate compresses the end of the nipple against the hard palate causing damage, instead of taking the entire nipple in as far as the soft palate (Inch and Fisher, 2000).

Women with sore or cracked nipples are often prompted to wean their babies, as the pain can be unbearable. The psychological impact of nipple pain can cause high levels of emotional distress, and may affect the mother–child relationship, though both will resolve once the pain is removed (Amir *et al.*, 1996).

Problems in the neonate such as a short frenulum (ankyloglossia), or breast engorgement, should be identified by the midwife as these will create difficulties for the neonate in latching on (Amir *et al.*, 1996).

Occasionally the woman may suffer from a condition known as *Raynaud's phenomenon*. First described by Maurice Raynaud in 1862, this is intermittent ischaemia commonly affecting the fingers and toes and is more prevalent in women in a ratio of 9:1. It has been reported as affecting the nipples, causing blanching during and after feeds with acute pain (Lawlor-Smith and Lawlor-Smith, 1997), but can be minimized by correct attachment.

Other conditions causing pain may present as eczema or psoriasis on the nipple or areola. Fungal infections such as *Candida albicans* (thrush) can cause burning or shooting pain sensations, and need to be identified and treated with the appropriate medication (Amir *et al.*, 1996). Aggressive treatment with antibiotics to treat colonization of cracked nipples with *Staphyloccocus aureus* was found to improve healing and decrease the risk of developing mastitis in a randomized comparative study of 84 breastfeeding mothers in Canada (Livingstone and Stringer, 1999). Midwives must be vigilant in identifying and screening for differential diagnoses rather than assuming conservative treatment is all that is required.

The use of moisture to aid healing of wounds is the current treatment of choice in the form of hydrogel/lanolin/paraffin gauze dressings (Cable *et al.*, 1997; Inch and Fisher, 2000). Cracked nipples need a moist environment for epithelial growth and repair. An important benefit is that it offers immediate pain relief (Huml, 1999).

The midwife should assess the damage to the nipple for:

- location
- depth of tissue destruction
- size
- visible and non-visible characteristics of the wound
- appearance of the surrounding tissue.

A knowledge and application of current evidence-based practice will reduce conflicting advice to women. The midwife needs to be familiar with the principles of moist 'healing'. The methods employed in the past – drying the nipples through exposure to air or using a hair-dryer – are now known to cause scab formation and delayed healing by unnaturally drying the skin in an area that is normally moist (Inch and Fisher, 2000).

The three phases of healing are as follows:

- *Inflammatory phase* – 0–3 days after the trauma. Vasodilatation occurs, the tissues are red, warm and painful. Prevention of infection is vital during this time as a clot is formed to control the bleeding episode. Moisture decreases the amount of dead tissue and therefore reduces bacteria.
- *Proliferative phase* – occurs from 3–24 days. Moisture increases proliferation and migration of epithelial cells across the wound bed and protects the nerve endings from external stimuli.
- *Maturation phase* – final phase of healing (can last up to 2 years). The newly formed tissue is fragile. Moisture aids healing by decreasing tissue drying and bacterial invasion (Cable *et al.*, 1997; Huml, 1999).

Other suggested treatments using moisture but not demonstrating significant benefits include the application of teabags or warm water compresses (Lavergne, 1997); USP-modified lanolin cream and water compresses or air (Pugh *et al.*, 1996). Application of expressed breast milk uses the physiological knowledge of healing through growth and repair of skin cells but could attract yeast growth from the lactose content (Renfrew *et al.*, 2000).

The effectiveness of silicone nipple shields has been demonstrated in case studies and retrospective data following the establishment of the milk supply, but only as a last resort (Bodley and Powers, 1996; Brigham, 1996; Elliott, 1996; Pessl, 1996). They may cause a diminishing milk supply and exacerbate engorgement (Inch and Fisher, 2000) so should be treated with caution and never used as a substitute for teaching correct attachment.

Treatments that have not been proven to be effective include chlorhexidene spray (Renfrew *et al.*, 2000) and other creams (Inch and Fisher, 2000).

Mastitis, abscess

Mastitis is a pathological condition that occurs as a result of poor breastfeeding practice and is prevented by the midwife giving correct attachment advice, and advising a good technique when handling the breasts and positioning the baby; and by the mother wearing an adequately fitting bra (RCM, 2002).

It is defined as an inflammation of the breast, ranging from a localized area to a wedge-shaped segment or involving the whole breast. It can include the occurrence of systemic symptoms including pyrexia, rigors, and flu-like symptoms (Renfrew *et al.*, 2000). There are two types: *infective* and *non-infective mastitis*.

Non-infective mastitis is usually caused by milk stasis causing increased pressure in the alveoli due to non-removal of milk, often caused by engorgement related to poor attachment of the baby to the breast.

The pressure builds up forcing the milk out into the surrounding tissues (RCM, 2002). It is associated with increased levels of stress and blocked ducts in women with other children, and restriction from a tight brassiere and nipple pain during a feed in first-time mothers (Fetherstone, 1998).

Infective mastitis is caused by bacterial invasion, usually via a cracked nipple. Staphylococci or streptococci are the most common organisms and these act on the milk forced outside the alveoli into the surrounding cells.

Diagnosis is made by the flu-like signs and symptoms and pyrexia which present. A reddened area appears around the infected breast or segment and if left untreated it may give rise to an abscess. Treatment is with antibiotics and drainage of the abscess as appropriate.

Half of all mastitis cases are non-infective (Inch and Fisher, 1995), and the midwife's skill of preventing stasis of milk by advice on positioning, importance of emptying each breast, correct handling of the breasts and prevention of clothing restrictions will ensure good practice prevails and transmits a positive public health message.

Neonatal problems

Tongue tie (ankyloglossia)

A short frenulum may present the neonate with difficulty in attaching and suckling at the breast. The tongue is unable to move forward and cup the nipple and thus stimulate release of milk from the breast. One of the first signs is sore nipples and poor weight gain due to lack of adequate milk supply, in spite of regular feeds (Auerbach and Riordan, 1998).

Treatment consists of cutting the frenulum and thus freeing up the movement of the tongue (Marmet *et al.*, 1990) or waiting to see if the frenulum extends or tears off spontaneously (Renfrew *et al.*, 2000).

The problem needs to be identified and referred as soon as possible by the midwife in order to prevent poor feeding and possible failure to thrive. Hand expressing or use of the breast pump to ensure continued stimulation of the milk supply may be useful in the interim period.

Cleft lip and palate

Cleft lip and palate are congenital malformations characterized by incomplete fusing of the lip and upper jaw (Auerbach and Riordan, 1998). This may involve the lip, or may extend to the soft and hard palate, and may be unilateral or bilateral.

Surgical repair of the lip is carried out early, around 3 weeks of age. Breastfeeding during this time is possible if only the lip is involved. The mother is taught to press the cleft as tightly to the breast as possible and place a thumb or index finger over the cleft (Auerbach and Riordan, 1998).

If there is involvement of the soft or hard palate, breastfeeding is more problematic owing to regurgitation of the milk through the nose. The nose must be sealed from the mouth creating a negative pressure in the oral cavity. A dental prosthesis (palatal obturator) can be made to occlude the cleft in the palate pending surgery at 6 months to 3 years of age.

A plan for feeding should be made by the team. The mother should be taught to hold the nipple and areola between the finger and thumb, known as the 'Dancer hold' (Lawrence and Lawrence, 1998). This will enable the baby to milk the areola and nipple with the tongue pressing it against the roof of the mouth.

Trying different positions for feeding, such as sitting the baby upright facing the mother with legs astride her waist or leaning over the baby and letting the breast fall directly into the baby's mouth can be helpful in successful breastfeeding (Lang, 1997).

Down's syndrome

This congenital anomaly, characterized by heart defects, a protruding or large tongue and hypotonicity can be challenging for breastfeeding. Manual expressing or pumping is often required because of inadequate stimulation of the let-down reflex by the baby.

The women will need encouragement and advice for positioning the baby, with the emphasis on firm support of the breast and baby's head with use of pillows. Success of breastfeeding is most likely to be dictated by the severity of the cardiac abnormality which will affect the respirations and tire the baby easily (Renfrew *et al.*, 2000).

Breastfeeding the preterm baby

Breast milk is the optimum nutrition for the preterm infant – it provides additional immunity to the immature system, such as IgA, lactoferrin, lysozyme and oligosaccharides, stimulates maturation of the gastrointestinal tract and reduces necrotizing enterocolitis (Kunz *et al.*, 1999; Rodriguez-Palmero *et al.*, 1999).

Breast milk expression should be commenced as soon as possible following the birth in order to stimulate prolactin production (Daly and Hartmann, 1995; Prentice *et al.*, 1989). This necessitates teaching the woman hand expressing as well as use of the breast pump (WHO, 1998). Pumping from both breasts simultaneously can help increase stimulation of prolactin and therefore milk supply (Jones *et al.*, 2001). However, it should be explained to the woman that prolonged use of a breast pump, which provides 'negative' pressure, is less effective than hand expressing, which provides 'positive' pressure and is a more effective stimulus for oxytocin production (Jones and Spencer, 2002c).

Supplementer tubes connected to a breast milk supply from a bottle have been used to provide extra volume to a preterm baby who is slow to suck. Careful supervision is needed to ensure that the baby does not learn to suck the tube like a straw and fail to learn correct sucking techniques (Powers, 1999).

Use of metoclopramide 10 mg three times daily for 7–14 days to stimulate milk supply and increase prolactin levels has been tried as a last resort in cases when a woman's milk supply has diminished (Powers, 1999).

Preterm breast milk contains higher concentrations of long-chain polyunsaturated fats, proteins, sodium and fats than term breast milk (Jones and Spencer, 2002a), and higher levels of sodium were identified in hand-expressed breast milk (Lang *et al.*, 1994). It is therefore important that preterm babies receive their mother's preterm milk, which is more suited to their growing needs than 'term' breast milk. Freshly expressed milk is the most suitable, as storage and light can alter the immunological content (Jones and Spencer, 2002a). The fat content can become separated and adhere to the feeding tube and collection containers, so the contents should be thoroughly shaken before use.

For some time there has been fortification of preterm formula milk and human milk with proteins and fats to improve growth; however, the argument for fortifying human milk with long-chain polyunsaturated fats is less clear and requires further evidence (Koletzko and Agostoni, 2001; Kuschel and Harding, 2002). It is thought that the addition of nutrients may reduce the immunological content.

Cup-feeding (Fig. 33.7) can be used as an alternative method if a baby is unable to breastfeed immediately or when a nasogastric tube is 'temporarily or permanently inappropriate' (Lang, 1997). This provides an oral experience for the baby who is unable to breastfeed and stimulates the development of the suck–swallow reflexes, though it should never be used instead of a breastfeed. It is usually only appropriate when 2- or 3-hourly bolus tube feeds are introduced (Lang, 1997).

The neonate is neurologically and developmentally able to suck and swallow at 32 weeks' gestation

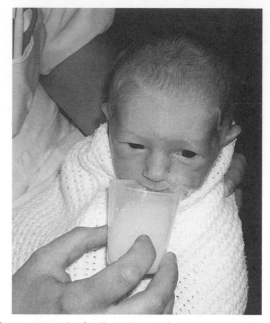

Figure 33.7 Cupfeeding. (From Johnston *et al.*, 2003.)

(RCM, 2002). The midwife should therefore encourage women who wish to breastfeed to have early frequent contact with their baby. Early skin-to-skin contact with the preterm baby promotes maternal production of specific antibodies against nosocomial pathogens in the neonatal environment (Jones and Spencer, 2002a). Massaging the breast prior to a feed as well as this contact with the baby encourages the let-down reflex (oxytocin production) and ensures that the milk is readily available, thus conserving the baby's energy (Jones and Spencer, 2002c).

The midwife can demonstrate techniques of holding and cup-feeding the baby by use of videos for the parents. Demonstration of correct use of the breast pump and technique for hand expressing form a major part of the midwife's role in supporting women.

Reflective Activity 33.3

Review the advice and support you have provided for women who have experienced feeding problems. Was your advice:

- research and evidence based
- consistent with physiological principles and the advice of others
- clearly recorded in the woman's notes
- given in a way that reinforces the woman's belief in herself and her ability to breastfeed successfully.

Breastfeeding twins and triplets

The Multiple Births Foundation produces a booklet for professionals and parents with advice and information on breastfeeding for multiples. This includes the importance of getting help and support for domestic chores as well as extra help for positioning the babies at each feed and especially at night. Cup feeding is suggested if the babies are born early (from 30 weeks' gestation) and are unable to feed at the breast initially.

Going back to work

The current recommendation is for all babies to be exclusively breastfed for 6 months (WHO, 2002). Many women need to return to work before this time and should be encouraged and supported by the midwife to continue breastfeeding before and after work, and to express either at work (dependent on facilities) or home and leave the EBM with the childminder.

There is no statutory right to paid breastfeeding breaks or a shorter working day in the UK but there is some legal protection under the health and safety laws, i.e. The Management of Health and Safety at Work Regulations 1992 and the Employment Rights Act 1996 (Maternity Alliance, 1999). If women work in the public sector they are protected under European law. The Pregnant Workers Directive (1992) says that 'if your work affects your breastfeeding' the public sector employer must temporarily alter the working conditions and/or hours of work to protect breastfeeding or give alternative work (Maternity Alliance, 1999).

Breastfeeding support groups

Providing improved support for women who breastfeed may ensure that women breastfeed for at least 2 months (Sikorski and Renfrew, 1999).

La Leche League's (LLL) Peer Counsellor programme, first introduced to the UK in the early 1990s from the USA, has been successfully replicated throughout the UK. Local women who have successfully breastfed are selected by midwives and health visitors and are trained by LLL breastfeeding counsellors to support women who wish to breastfeed, particularly in deprived areas.

Other groups such as Breastfriends Doncaster 2000, trained by health visitors and midwives, have repeated the concept and work in the local community

to support breastfeeding women and give feedback to midwives and student midwives about unhelpful advice (Kirkham, 2000).

Sure Start initiatives have set up paid peer support programmes for breastfeeding women in order to reduce childhood disadvantages and poverty (RCM et al., 2000).

Midwives need to be aware of local community initiatives for breastfeeding support, and ensure they work with peer groups to reinforce breastfeeding as the optimum nutrition for neonates. For many specialist problems, there are useful groups who can provide valuable advice and support to the woman and her baby (see Additional resources, p. 627).

Reflective Activity 33.4

Discuss the availability of long-term support for breastfeeding mothers with your community colleagues – and ensure that you have contact details for local groups in your resource file/diary.

ARTIFICIAL FEEDING

Although the DoH Infant Feeding Survey 2000 (Hamlyn et al., 2002) illustrated a small rise in breastfeeding, around 31% of babies were fed artificially. The midwife needs to be conversant with the equipment and information required for artificial feeding.

Many people (including midwives) believe that bottlefeeding is a safe alternative to breastfeeding. However, a large and growing body of research now exists which shows this is not the case. Babies who do not receive breast milk are at risk of serious consequences. The health of the woman may also be compromised if she does not breastfeed her baby (MIDIRS/NHS Centre for Reviews and Dissemination, 1999). For a comparison of breastmilk with infant formula, see Table 33.2.

Reasons why some women may artificially feed their baby

Some women may be unable to breastfeed their baby if they have HIV or are taking certain drugs (see Contraindications to breastfeeding, above). Other women may be unsupported by their families, be suffering from

Table 33.2   Comparison of breast milk with infant formula (DoH, 1994: 55; Inch, 1996a: 82–83; MIDIRS/NHS Centre for Reviews and Dissemination, 1999; Statutory Instrument 77, 1995)

Values (per 100 ml)	Mature breast milk	Infant formula	Effect in formula milk
Energy	70 kcal (293 kJ)	60–65 kcal (250–315 kJ)	
Protein (g)	1.3	1.2–1.95	Elevated blood urea and amino acid levels result in higher renal solute load and subsequent increased metabolic stress. Can provoke antigenic responses in those prone to asthma and eczema. Can also trigger IDDM
Fat (g)	4.2	2.1–4.2	Limited number of fatty acids. May compromise optimal brain growth and development of the CNS
Carbohydrate (g) Lactose	7	4.6–9.1	Energy requirements less efficiently met. Higher pH – greater risk of invasion from bacteria, e.g. *Escherichia coli*
Whey proteins Alpha-lactalbumin Beta-lactoglobulin Lactoferrin Immunoglobulins Lysozyme	Present (70%) Absent Present Present, mainly IgA Present	Bovine (20%) Present Trace Trace Trace	
Casein Micelle structure	Forms soft curds (30%)	Forms hard curds (80%)	Remains in stomach longer and requires high expenditure of energy to digest. May cause an intestinal obstruction
Essential amino acids Cystine : methionine ratio	1.3 : 1	0.7 : 1	Higher amino-acid levels may reduce health effects
Lipids Cholesterol	16 mg	Absent	
Essential fatty acids Linoleic : alpha-linolenic ratio Docosahexaenoic acid and arachidonic acid	9.1 : 1 Present	10.5 : 1 Added	
Minerals Calcium : phosphorus ratio Zinc : copper ratio Sodium (mg) Potassium (mg) Chloride (mg) Calcium (mg) Iron (µg)	2.3 : 1 7.6 : 1 15 60 43 35 76	1.5 : 1 10.0 : 1 13–39 39–94 32.5–81 19.5 325–975	Calcium less efficiently absorbed May disturb copper or iron absorption

Only 10% iron in formulae is absorbed |

(continued)

Table 33.2   *(continued)*

Values (per 100 ml)	Mature breast milk	Infant formula	Effect in formula milk
Vitamins			
A (μg)	60	39–117	All added
B$_6$ (μg)	6	22.8	
B$_{12}$ (μg)	0.01	0.07	
Total folate (μg)	5.0	2.6	
Thiamin (μg)	16	265	
Riboflavin (μg)	30	39	
Niacin (μg)	620	163	
C (mg)	3.8	5.2	
D (μg)	0.01	0.65–1.63	
E (μg)	0.35	>0.33	
K (μg)	0.21	2.6	
Digestive enzymes, e.g. bile salt simulated lipase – to complete fat digestion	Present	Absent	
Anti-infective factors			
Secretory IgA	Present (varied amounts)	Absent	Higher incidence of infection, e.g. gastroenteritis, respiratory infection, otitis media, UTI, NEC, IDDM, atopic disease – asthma, eczema
White cells	Present	Absent	Higher incidence of infection
Antibacterial, e.g. lactoperoxidase glycoproteins	Present (varied amounts)	Absent	Higher incidence of infection
Antiviral, e.g. ribonuclease oligosaccharides	Present (varied amounts)	Absent	Higher incidence of infection
Antiparasitic, e.g. lipid (free)	Present (varied amounts)	Absent	
Growth factors	Present (varied amounts)	Absent	

postnatal depression or post-traumatic stress disorder or simply be subjected to 'peer' pressure to artificially feed their babies.

Regulations surrounding infant formulae

Infant formulae are artificial feeds that are manufactured to take the place of human milk in providing a sole source of nutrition for the young infant (Hamlyn *et al.*, 2002; White *et al.*, 1992). The essential composition of these formulae was set down as a Parliamentary Statute, or law, which came into force in March 1995 (Statutory Instrument 77, 1995).

Midwives need to be aware of the WHO International Code of Marketing of Breastmilk Substitutes (WHO, 1981), the aim of which is to ensure that infants receive safe and adequate nutrition, through the marketing and practices surrounding breast milk substitutes, advertising and donation of free samples or equipment directly to the general public.

The majority of infant formula brands can be divided into two groups: *whey* dominant and *casein* dominant. When whey is the dominant protein the whey : casein ratio is closer to that of human milk. Casein-dominant formulae have a whey : casein ratio closer to that of cows' milk (Hamlyn *et al.*, 2002; White *et al.*, 1992).

Table 33.3 Infant formulae

Whey-dominant formulae	Casein-dominant formulae
SMA Gold	SMA White
Farleys First Milk	Farleys Second Milk
Cow and Gate Premium	Cow and Gate Plus
Milupa Aptamil	Milupa Milumil
Boots Formula 1	Boots Formula 2

Types of feed available

Examples of formulae available in the UK for infant feeding are given in Table 33.3.

Some manufacturers claim that casein-dominant formula is more satisfying for the baby than whey-dominant formula. White *et al.* (1992) suggest that, although there is no firm evidence to show that this formula is more suitable, parents may well be influenced by such claims.

Soya milk formulae

Some soya-based milk substitutes conform to the compositional guidelines (DHSS, 1988; Statutory Instrument 77, 1995). They have been approved for prescription in the NHS for established forms of milk intolerance (DHSS, 1988). Soya-based formulae of entirely plant origin are acceptable to vegans. Some 2–3% of infants are fed on soya-based formula (White *et al.*, 1992).

'Follow-on' milks

'Follow-on' milks may be used by some parents to provide the drink element of a more diversified diet in an infant of more than 6 months of age (DoH, 1994; Statutory Instrument 77, 1995).

Ready-to-feed formulae

Some formula milks are available in a liquid or ready-to-feed format. The liquid formula requires decanting into a sterile feeding bottle. Although more costly than the powdered formula, it is useful when travelling.

Methods of artificial feeding

The most common method of feeding a term baby with formula milk is via the bottle (Fig. 33.8). There is a range of bottles to choose from and teats that mimic the shape of the nipple. The midwife needs to have a good knowledge of how to teach women to make up feeds correctly (see Fig. 33.10).

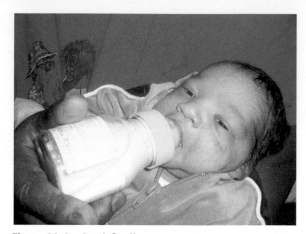

Figure 33.8 Bottlefeeding.

For babies born early and whose sucking reflex is not yet developed, tube feeding will be the method of choice to ensure adequate nutrition. As fat particles tend to adhere to the plastic tube, this needs to be taken into account when calculating daily intake.

Cup feeding

Cup feeding has been found to be a useful alternative to bottlefeeding for preterm babies in neonatal intensive care units (Gupta *et al.*, 1999). It must only be used when a baby has demonstrated that the suck–swallow reflex is present. It is a useful alternative to tube feeding until the baby is able to suck adequately at the breast for nutritional purposes and helps to prevent 'nipple confusion' by avoiding the use of a bottle.

Its advantages include the stimulation of saliva and lingual lipases and stimulation of the suck–swallow reflexes, yet very little energy is used in the process (Lang, 1997).

The baby should be wrapped securely to prevent use of his hands, which may knock over the cup. He should be supported in an upright or sitting position and the cup tipped against his lips. The baby will drink in his own time rather than milk being poured into the mouth (Lang, 1997).

Syringe feeding

Syringes are rarely used for feeding, but if used the syringe should be squeezed as the baby is sucking but not swallowing, to avoid choking. It should be aimed at the inside of the baby's cheek not directly down the throat, to prevent aspiration (Lang, 1997).

Supplement Nursing System (SNS)

This is a device that may be used if there is insufficient milk supply, breast surgery or following adoption.

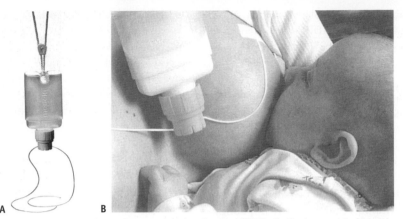
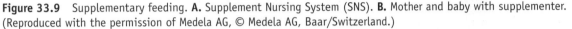

Figure 33.9 Supplementary feeding. **A.** Supplement Nursing System (SNS). **B.** Mother and baby with supplementer. (Reproduced with the permission of Medela AG, © Medela AG, Baar/Switzerland.)

It may also be used if the baby is preterm or has a weak suck because of neurological or chromosomal damage (Lang, 1997).

The supplementer tube (size 0.4–0.8 feeding tube) is attached to the breast/nipple at one end and at the other end is placed into the milk supply (Fig. 33.9). The baby can suck on the breast without exerting any effort and still get adequate milk supply. Once the milk supply has been re-established or the baby is strong enough to suck, the supplementer can be withdrawn (Lang, 1997).

Complementary/supplementary feeds

Supplementary feeds (food given to replace breast milk) and complementary feeds (food given as a substitute for breast milk) have no place in the care of a healthy term baby who is breastfeeding as they interfere with the breastfeeding physiology (MIDIRS/NHS Centre for Reviews and Dissemination, 1999). It is important that women understand the physiology of breastfeeding.

Ecology of artificial feeding

The dairy industry requires 10 000 square metres of pasture for each cow to produce milk. There are many countries clearing rainforests in order to meet this demand, causing an increase in greenhouse gases, soil erosion and a reduction in animal and plant species (BFHI, 1994).

In addition, the plastic bottles produced cannot be recycled. Factories producing such equipment consume energy, release pollutants into the atmosphere and create wasteful packaging (BFHI, 1994).

> **Box 33.5   Risk factors for infections/disorders requiring hospital admission or medical treatment**
>
> **Twice as likely**
> - Respiratory infection
> - Otitis media
> - Atopic disease: eczema or a wheeze
> - Diabetes mellitus: juvenile onset of insulin-dependent diabetes mellitus (IDDM)
>
> **Five times more likely**
> - Gastroenteritis
> - Diarrhoea
> - Urinary tract infection
>
> **20 times more likely**
> - Necrotizing enterocolitis: (preterm babies < 30–36 weeks' gestation)

Disadvantages of artificial feeding

Artificial feeding has been described as a risk behaviour (Minchin, 2000). The scientific dangers of artificial feeding are well known amongst health professionals and the midwife should share the information with women before a decision is made to feed artificially. Babies who are artificially fed are at risk of several infections and disorder as shown in Box 33.5.

Other risks of bottlefeeding currently being researched include childhood lymphomas, inflammatory bowel disease, multiple sclerosis, dental occlusions, coronary heart disease, autoimmune thyroid disease, coeliac disease,

Kawasaki disease, lower IQ, risk of sudden infant death syndrome and obesity (MIDIRS/NHS Centre for Reviews and Dissemination, 1999; Odent, 1996).

Advantages of artificial feeding

- If the woman is HIV positive it reduces the risk of acquired HIV infection.
- It reduces the risk of other harmful viruses such as hepatitis B and hepatitis C, and in addition Z and T cell leukaemia (HTLV-1).
- It may reduce the risk of haemorrhagic disease of the newborn as vitamin K is an additive (if pharmacological vitamin K is unavailable).
- It is the appropriate feeding method if the woman is an IV drug user or is taking medication that would be contraindicated in breastfeeding, e.g. diamorphine or anticancer drugs (MIDIRS/NHS Centre for Reviews and Dissemination, 1999).
- Allows others to participate in feeding the baby.

The role of the midwife in artificial feeding

The midwife needs to be:

- up to date in knowledge of the constituents of breast milk in comparison to artificial milk
- conversant with the physiology of the neonatal digestive system in relation to artificial milk and able to discuss this with the woman
- knowledgeable about the disadvantages and advantages of artificial feeding and able to convey this information in a factual manner so that the woman can make a truly informed choice
- sensitive to the many factors that influence a woman's choices, such as her partner's attitude, her cultural background and her level of education
- conversant with the equipment required, hygiene and methods of sterilization of equipment (Ackerley, 1996; Drane, 1996)
- expert in terms of safe storage of milk (Rotolli *et al.*, 1997; UNICEF UK Baby Friendly Initiative, 2001).

Preparation of feeds

All parents should be shown how to prepare artificial feeds and how to clean and sterilize the utensils. Ideally there should be an opportunity to practise with the midwife present so that any queries can be discussed. Women who have other children to care for may be rushed into taking shortcuts whilst making up their

baby's feeds. Mistakes such as using the wrong scoop for the brand of milk, over- or underfilling the scoop, adding too little or too much water and adding sugar or cereals to the feed are more common in parents with more than one child than in first-time parents and occur in all social classes. Hence, it is not safe to assume that multiparae or those in the higher social groups will make up feeds accurately. All parents need careful teaching and demonstrations for making up feeds by the midwife. See Figures 33.10 and 33.11.

The midwife should work in tandem with the health visitor and GP to provide a seamless service with regard to advice on infant feeding. Depending on the practice within the primary care trust, the midwife will probably 'transfer' the care of the mother and baby to the health visitor 10 days after the birth. The mother is invited to attend 'baby' clinics at the local health centre or GP surgery where she will get advice about feeding, weaning and immunizations. By 28 days postnatally, the midwife completes the legal requirement to provide care for both the women and her baby and will discharge them to the care of the health visitor (NMC, 1998).

> ### Reflective Activity 33.5
>
> Teach a woman who plans to artificially feed how to make up a feed from dried milk. Ensure you include sterilizing of equipment. Carry this out in the woman's home if possible during an antenatal visit, then follow up postnatally.

> ### Reflective Activity 33.6
>
> Consider how you discuss the issues around infant feeding with women and families. Are you up to date with current research and evidence? Are you able to provide unbiased information in an accessible way? Ask a colleague to observe you discussing this with a woman and to give you feedback.

> ### Reflective Activity 33.7
>
> Look at the information and resources available locally and whether they are 'baby friendly' and also woman friendly, i.e. in clear and accessible language and in a variety of languages. How could you contribute to the development of these resources?

Preparing a bottle feed using baby milk powder

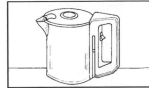

1 Boil some fresh tap water in a kettle or saucepan and let it cool. Do not use bottled or artificially softened water.

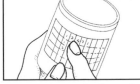

2 The amount of milk per feed suggested on the tin or packet is only a guide. Your baby may want more or less according to appetite.

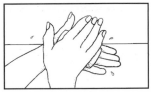

3 Wipe clean an area on which to prepare the feed. Wash your hands very well with soap and water.

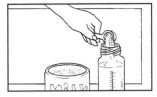

4 If using a chemical sterilising solution, remove the lid and turn it upside down. Remove the teat and cap and place them on the upturned lid. If you wish to rinse them, use cooled boiled water, not tap water.

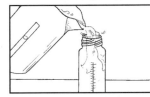

5 Remove the bottle(s), rinse if wished (with cooled boiled water), stand on a clean flat surface and pour cooled boiled water into the bottle up to the required mark.

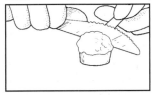

6 Measure the exact amount of powder using the scoop provided with the milk. Level the powder in the scoop using the plastic knife or the spatula supplied with the milk powder or steriliser.

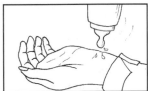

7 **Add the powder to the water in the bottle.** All baby milks in Britain now use one scoop to 1oz (30 mls) water. *Do not add extra powder (or anything else) to the feed as this may make your baby ill.*

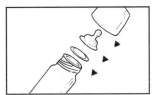

8 Place the disc supplied on the top of the bottle, followed by the teat and cap.

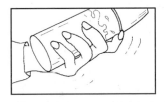

9 Screw the cap on tightly and shake well until all the powder has dissolved. Store the bottle(s) in the coldest part of the fridge (not in the door) if the milk is not being used straight away.

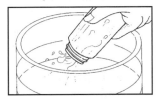

10 The feed should be warm before it is given to your baby. If it has been in the fridge, place it in a container of warm water until it has warmed through. Never heat milk (or baby food) in a microwave oven.

11 Check the temperature of the feed before giving it to your baby by dripping a little onto the inside of your wrist. It should feel slightly warm.

12 After the feed, throw any unused milk away and clean the bottle.

Additional tips:

- If your powder does not come with a spatula, you should sterilise a plastic knife and dry it on clean tissue paper. You can then keep it in the powder with the scoop.
- You can make up a day's supply of feeds in advance. They will keep for 24 hours in a fridge. Shake each bottle well before using.
- Almost all baby milk powders are made from **cows' milk** which has been processed to make it suitable for babies. **Whey based** (first) milks are more easily digested by a young baby. **Casein** based (second) milks take longer to digest and are not recommended for young babies. Ordinary cows' milk should not be given until your baby is at least a year old.
- Do not use soya based milks without medical advice.

Reproduced by the UNICEF UK Baby Friendly Initiative, with thanks to the Women's Centre, Oxford Radcliffe Hospital NHS Trust.

Figure 33.10 Preparing a bottle feed using formula milk powder. (From UNICEF UK BFI, with permission of UNICEF UK.)

Sterilising baby feeding equipment

It is very important to keep any equipment used for feeding your baby either formula or breastmilk (such as bottles, teats and breast pumps) completely clean. This will help to protect your baby against infection, particularly tummy bugs (diarrhoea and vomiting).

To do this you need to sterilise your equipment after you have washed it thoroughly. You will need to continue to do this until your baby is a year old.

There are several ways of sterilising equipment. You could use :

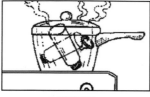 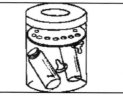 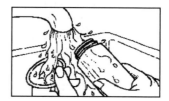

a saucepan   **a chemical steriliser**   **a steam steriliser**
              (not suitable for metal items)

You could also use a special microwave bottle steriliser in a microwave oven, but this is not suitable for metal items or certain types of plastic.

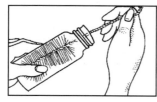 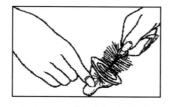 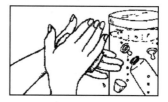

1 Wash all bottles and other equipment thoroughly in hot soapy water using a bottle brush. Scrub the inside and outside of the bottle to remove fatty deposits. Pay particular attention to the rim.

2 Use a small teat brush to clean the inside of the teat; *or* turn it inside out and wash in hot soapy water. Salt, if used to clean latex teats, should always be rinsed off completely.

3 Rinse all your washed equipment thoroughly before sterilising.

Check teats and bottles regularly for signs of deterioration. If you are unsure about a bottle or teat, it's safer to throw it away.

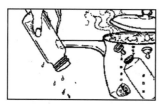 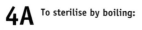 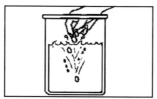 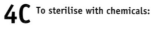 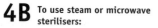

4A **To sterilise by boiling:**

Put the equipment into a large pan filled with water. Make sure there is no air trapped in the bottles or teats. Cover the pan with a lid and bring to the boil. **Boil for at least 10 minutes.** Make sure that the pan does not boil dry.

Keep the pan covered until the equipment is needed.

4B **To use steam or microwave sterilisers:**

Follow the manufacturer's instructions.

4C **To sterilise with chemicals:**

Make up the solution, using tablets or liquid, following the manufacturers' instructions. Submerge the equipment in the solution, making sure there is no air trapped in the bottles or teats. Your sterilising tank should have a plunger to keep all equipment under the water – or you can use a plate. **Leave in solution for at least 30 minutes.**

If you wish to rinse your equipment before using, use water that has been boiled and allowed to cool.

Make up a fresh solution every 24 hours.

5 Always wash your hands before removing equipment from your steriliser. Take care when handling equipment which may be hot.

Reproduced by the UNICEF UK Baby Friendly Initiative, with thanks to the Women's Centre, Oxford Radcliffe Hospital NHS Trust.

Breastfeeding is the healthiest way to feed your baby and it doesn't cost anything. If you use baby milk powder, it is very important for your baby's health that you follow all instructions carefully. It is possible, but difficult, to reverse a decision not to breastfeed or to re-start breastfeeding once you have stopped. Introducing partial bottle feeding will reduce a mother's breastmilk supply. Breastfeeding mothers do not need to eat any special foods but, just like everyone else, they are advised to follow a healthy diet. (Infant formula & follow-on formula regulations 1995)

Figure 33.11   Sterilizing baby feeding equipment. (From UNICEF UK Baby Friendly Initiative 2001, with permission of UNICEF UK.)

CONCLUSION

The mother's choice of feeding method, and her success with her chosen method, have long-term implications for the health of herself and her baby, and therefore for the health of the community as a whole. The importance of providing evidence-based, up-to-date and accurate information and sensitive support to women prior to the birth of the baby, and during the neonatal period, is fundamental to the woman's psychological well-being and to her view of herself as a mother. Time invested by the midwife can therefore pay huge dividends and should be seen as a priority.

KEY POINTS

- Midwives are key professionals in providing information, education and support to the woman, her baby and family regarding infant feeding.
- The knowledge provided must be up to date, research and evidence based, and provided in an accessible, supportive and non-judgemental manner.
- It is important that midwives are aware of their own biases and opinions regarding feeding choices in order to minimize the effect of both on the advice and support they provide.

- Midwives should work with professional and lay colleagues within the community to provide additional support to women and their families, whatever the method of feeding.
- Women who have chosen to bottlefeed their infant should be supported, and taught the principles of correctly making up the feeds, and choosing the most appropriate milk for their baby.
- Midwives should teach all parents the principles of cleaning and sterilizing feeding equipment.

REFERENCES

Abadin, H.G., Hibbs, B.F. & Pohl, H.R. (1997) Breastfeeding exposure of infants to cadmium, lead and mercury: a public health viewpoint. *Toxicology and Industrial Health* **13**(4): 495–517.

Ackerley, L. (1996) Home hygiene with a baby: the new approach to advising parents. *Professional Care of Mother and Child* **6**(4): 99–102.

Ali, Z. & Lowry, M. (1981) Early maternal–child contact: effects on later behaviour. *Developmental Medicine and Child Neurology* **23**: 337–345.

Amir, L.H., Dennerstein, L., Garland, S.M. *et al.* (1996) Psychological aspects of nipple pain in lactating women. *Journal of Psychosomatic Obstetrics and Gynaecology* **17**(1): 53–58.

Anderson, T. (1999) Support for breastfeeding mothers. *Practising Midwife* **2**(9): 10–12.

Audit Commission (1997) *First Class Delivery. Improving Maternity Services in England and Wales*. London: Audit Commission.

Auerbach, K.G. (1990a) Sequential and simultaneous breastpumping: a comparison. *International Journal of Nursing Studies* **27**: 257–265.

Auerbach, K.G. (1990b) Breastfeeding fallacies: their relationship to understanding lactation. *Birth* **17**(1): 44–49.

Auerbach, K. & Riordan, J. (eds) (1998) *Breastfeeding and Human Lactation*. Boston, Mass: Jones and Bartlett.

Baby-Friendly Hospital Initiative (BFHI) (1994) Bottle feeding is an environmental hazard. *BFHI News* January/February. 3.

Baby Milk Action (2001) *HIV and Infant Feeding – Issue Paper*. Cambridge: Baby Milk Action.

Becker, A.B., Manfreda, J. & Ferguson, A.C. (1999) Breastfeeding and environmental tobacco smoke exposure. *Archives of Pediatrics & Adolescent Medicine* **153**(7): 689–691.

Berlin, C.M. (1994) Silicone breast implants and breastfeeding. *Pediatrics* **94**: 547–549.

Blackburn, S.T. (2003) Maternal, Fetal and Neonatal Physiology – A Clinical Perspective. Philadelphia: W.B. Saunders.

Bobat, R., Moodley, D., Coutsoudis, A. *et al.* (1997) Breastfeeding by HIV infected women and outcomes in their infants: a cohort study from Durban, South Africa. *AIDS* **11**: 1627–1633.

Bodley, V. & Powers, D. (1996) Long term nipple shield use – a positive perspective. *Journal of Human Lactation* **12**(4): 301–304.

Brigham, M. (1996) Mothers' reports of the outcome of nipple shield use. *Journal of Human Lactation* **12**(4): 291–297.

Buchanan, P. & Sachs, M. (1998) Breastfeeding and breast cancer: research review. *RCM Midwives Journal* **1**(1): 306–309.

Butte, N.F. (2000) Dieting and exercise in overweight, lactating women. *New England Journal of Medicine* **342**(7): 502–503.

Cable, B., Stewart, M. & Davis, J. (1997) Nipple wound care: a new approach to an old problem. *Journal of Human Lactation* **13**(4): 313–318.

Campbell, C.M.A. (1997) Early breastfeeding failure. *Update* **55**(9): 722, 724, 726–727.

Carpenter, R.G., Irgens, L.M., Blair, P.S. *et al.* (2004) Sudden unexplained infant death in 20 regions in Europe: case control study. *Lancet* **363**: 185–191.

Cavallo, M.G., Fava, D., Monetini, L. *et al.* (1996) Cell mediated response to beta casein in recent onset insulin dependent diabetes: implications for disease pathogenesis. *Lancet* **348**(9032): 926–928.

Christensson, K, Siles, C., Moreno, L. *et al.* (1992) Temperature, metabolic adaptation and crying in healthy full-term newborns cared for skin-to skin or in a cot. *Acta Paediatrica* **81**: 488–493.

Clifton, A. & Long, L. (1992) *Bloomsbury Breastfeeding Workshop Evaluation Project.* London: UCH.

Collaborative Group on Hormonal Factors in Breast Cancer (2002) Breast cancer and breastfeeding: collaborative reanalysis of individual data from 47 epidemiological studies in 30 countries, including 50,302 women with breast cancer and 96,973 women without the disease. *Lancet* **360**(9328): 187–195.

COMA Working Group on the Weaning Diet (1994) *Weaning and the Weaning Diet.* London: HMSO.

Coutsoudine, A., Kuberdean, P., Spooner, E. *et al.* (1999) Patterns in early mother to child transmission of HIV-1 in Durban, SA. A prospective study. *Lancet* **354**: 471–476.

Coutts, A. (1998) Pregnancy, lactation and avoidance of food allergy in the infant. *British Journal of Midwifery* **6**(10): 622.

Cumming, R.G. & Klineberg, R.J. (1993) Breastfeeding and other reproductive factors and the risk of hip fractures in elderly women. *International Journal of Epidemiology* **22**(4): 684–691.

Daly, S.E.J. & Hartmann, P.E. (1995) Infant demand and milk supply. Part 1: infant demand and milk production in lactating woman. *Journal of Human Lactation* **11**: 21–26.

Davies, L. (1995) Babies co-sleeping with parents. *Midwives* **108**(1295): 384–386.

Davis, M.K. (1998) Review of the evidence for an association between infant feeding and childhood cancer. *International Journal of Cancer* **11**(Suppl.): 29–33.

De Carvalho, M., Robertson, S., Friedman, A. *et al.* (1983) Effect of frequent breastfeeding on early milk production and infant weight gain. *Pediatrics* **72**(3): 307–311.

De Chateau, P. (1980) The first hour after delivery – its impact on synchrony of the parent–infant relationship. *Paediatrician* **9**: 151–168.

De Chateau, P. & Wiberg, B. (1977) Long term effect on mother–infant behaviour of extra contact during the first hour post partum II. A follow-up at three months. *Acta Paediatricia Scandinavica* **66**: 137–151.

Department of Health and Social Security (DHSS) (1988) *Present Day Practice in Infant Feeding: Third Report.* London: HMSO.

Department of Health (DoH) (1994) *Breastfeeding: Good Practice Guidance to the NHS.* London: DoH.

Department of Health (DoH) (1997) *Better for your Baby, the Facts about HIV Antenatal Testing.* London: DoH.

Department of Health (DoH) (1999a) *Saving Lives: Our Healthier Nation.* London: The Stationery Office.

Department of Health (DoH) (1999b) *Reducing Health Inequalities: An Action Report. Our Healthier Nation.* London: The Stationery Office.

Department of Health (DoH) (1999c) *Making a Difference.* London: DoH.

Department of Health (DoH) (1999d) *HIV and Infant Feeding. Guidance from the UK Chief Medical Officers' Expert Advisory Group on AIDS.* London: DoH.

Department of Health (DoH) (2000) *The NHS Plan.* London: The Stationery Office.

Department of Health (DoH) (2002) *Health Inequalities; National Targets on Infant Mortality and Life Expectancy; Technical Briefing.* London: DoH.

Dewey, K.G., Henig, J. & Nommsen-Rivers, L.A. (1995) Differences in morbidity between breastfed and formula fed infants. *Journal of Pediatrics* **126**(5): 696–702.

Drane, D. (1996) The effective use of dummies and teats on orthodontic development. *Breastfeeding Review* **4**(2): 59–64.

Drash, A.L., Kramer, M.S., Swanson, J. *et al.* (1994) Infant feeding practices and their possible relationship to the etiology of diabetes mellitus. *Pediatrics* **94**(5): 752–754.

Duffy, E.P., Percival, P. & Kershaw, E. (1997) Positive effects of an antenatal group teaching session on postnatal nipple pain, nipple trauma, and breastfeeding rates. *Midwifery* **13**(4): 189–196.

Duncan, B., Ey, J., Holberg, C.J. *et al.* (1993) Exclusive breast-feeding for at least 4 months protects against otitis media. *Pediatrics* **91**(5): 867–872.

Employment Rights Act 1996. London: HMSO.

Elliott, C. (1996) Using a silicone nipple shield to assist a baby unable to latch. *Journal of Human Lactation* **12**(4): 309–313.

Enger, S.M., Ross, R.K., Henderson, B. *et al.* (1997) Breastfeeding history, pregnancy experience and risk of breast cancer. *British Journal of Cancer* **76**(1): 118–123.

Fetherstone, C. (1998) Risk factors for lactation mastitis. *Journal of Human Lactation* **14**(2): 101–109.

Fisher, C. (1994) Resolving and preventing mothers' problems with breastfeeding. *Modern Midwife* **4**(2): 17–19.

Florey, C.D., Leech, A.M. & Blackhall, A. (1995) Infant feeding and mental and motor development at 18 months of age in first born singletons. *International Journal of Epidemiology* **24**(3 Suppl. 1): S21–S26.

Foundation for the Study of Infant Deaths (FSID) & Department of Health (DoH) (2003) *Reduce the Risk of Cot Death. An Easy Guide.* DoH. Online. Available: http://www.sids.org.uk.

Golding, J., Emmett, P.M. & Rogers, I.S. (1997) Gastroenteritis, diarrhoea and breastfeeding. *Early Human Development* 49(Suppl.): S83–S103. Gastroenteritis, diarrhoea and breast feeding.

Gross, B. (1999) Breastfeeding – natural fertility control/LAM: an effective option? *Breastfeeding Review* 7(3): 21–24.

Gupta, A., Khanna, K. & Chattree, S. (1999) Cup feeding: an alternative to bottle feeding in a neonatal intensive care unit. *Journal of Tropical Pediatrics* 45(2): 108–110.

Hamlyn, B., Brooker, S., Oleinikova, K. *et al.* (2002) *Infant Feeding 2000.* London: The Stationery Office.

Hamosh, M. (1998) Protective function of proteins and lipids in human milk. *Biology of the Neonate* 74(2): 163–176.

Hanson, L.A. (1998a) Non breastfeeding: the most common immunodeficiency. *ALCA Galaxy* 9(3): 15–18.

Hanson, L.A. (1998b) Breastfeeding provides passive and likely long lasting active immunity. *Annals of Allergy, Asthma & Immunology* 81(6): 523–537.

Henly, S.J., Anderson, C.M., Avery, M.D. *et al.* (1995) Anemia and insufficient milk in first-time mothers. *Birth* 22(2): 87–92.

Henschel, D. & Inch, S. (1996) *Breastfeeding. A Guide for Midwives.* Hale, Cheshire: Books for Midwives Press.

Hill, P.D. & Humenick, S.S. (1994) The occurrence of breast engorgement. *Journal of Human Lactation* 10(2): 76–86.

Hill, P.D., Aldag, J.C. & Chatterton, R.T. (1996) The effect of sequential and simultaneous breast pumping on milk volume and prolactin levels: a pilot study. *Journal of Human Lactation* 12(3): 193–199.

Hillervik-Lindquist, C., Hofvander, Y. & Sjolin, S. (1991) Studies on perceived breast milk insufficiency. III. Consequences for breast milk consumption and growth *Acta Paediatricia Scandinavica* 80(3): 297–303.

Horta, B.L., Victor, C.S. & Menezes, A.M. (1997) Environmental tobacco smoke and the breastfeeding duration. *American Journal of Epidemiology* 146: 128–133.

Howie, P.W. (1985) Breastfeeding – a new understanding. *Midwives Chronicle and Nursing Notes* 98(1170): 184–192.

Howie, P.W., McNeilly, A.S., McArdle, T. *et al.* (1980) The relationship between suckling induced prolactin response and lactogenesis. *Journal of Clinical Endocrinology and Metabolism* 50: 670–673.

Huml, S. (1999) Sore nipples: a new look at old problems through the eyes of a dermatologist. *Practising Midwife* 2(2): 28–31.

Hyde, L. (1994) Knowledge of basic infant nutrition amongst community health professionals. *Maternal and Child Health* 19(1): 27–32.

Inch, S. (1996a) Breastmilk and formula milk – what's the difference? *MIDIRS Midwifery Digest* 6(1): 80–84.

Inch, S. (1996b) The Importance of breastfeeding. *MIDIRS Midwifery Digest* 6(2): 208–212.

Inch, S. & Fisher, C. (1995) Mastitis: infection or inflammation? *Practitioner* 239: 472–475.

Inch, S. & Fisher, C. (2000) Breastfeeding: early problems. *Practising Midwife* 3(1): 12–15.

Johnston, P.G.B., Flood, K. & Spinks, K. (2003) *The Newborn Child.* Edinburgh: Churchill Livingstone.

Jones, E. & Spencer, A. (2002a) Promoting successful preterm breastfeeding Part 1. *Practising Midwife* 5(4): 18–20.

Jones, E. & Spencer, A. (2002c) Promoting successful preterm breastfeeding Part 3. *Practising Midwife* 5(6): 18–19.

Jones, E., Dimock, P.W. & Spencer, S.A. (2001) A randomised controlled trail to compare methods of milk expression after preterm delivery. *Archives of Disease in Childhood* 85: F91–95.

Katsouyanni, K., Lipworth, L., Trichopoulou, A. *et al.* (1996) A case control study of lactation and cancer of the breast. *British Journal of Cancer* 73(6): 814–818.

Kendall, S. (1995) Cross-cultural aspects and breastfeeding promotion. *Health Visitor* 68(11): 450–451.

Kirkham, M. (2000) Breastfriends Doncaster 2000. *Practising Midwife* 3(7): 20–21.

Koletzko, B. & Agostoni, C. (2001) Long chain polyunsaturated fatty acids (LC-PUFA) and perinatal development. *Acta Paediatrica* 90(4): 460–464.

Koletzko, S., Sherman, P., Corey, M. *et al.* (1989) Role of infant feeding practices in development of Crohn's disease in childhood. *British Medical Journal* 298(6688): 1617–1618.

Kramer, M.S. & Kakuma, R. (2002) *The Optimal Duration of Exclusive Breastfeeding, A Systematic Review.* Department of Nutrition for Health and Development. Geneva: WHO.

Kramer, M.S., Barr, R.G. & Dagenais, S. (2001) Pacifier use, early weaning and cry/fuss behaviour: a randomised controlled trial. *Journal of the American Medical Association* 286(3): 322–326.

Kunz, C., Rodriguez-Palmero, M., Koletzko, B. *et al.* (1999) Nutritional and biochemical properties of human milk, part 1: general aspects, proteins, and carbohydrates. *Clinics in Perinatology* 26(2): 307–333.

Kuschel, C. A.& Harding, J.E. (2002) Fat supplementation of human milk for promoting growth in preterm infants. *The Cochrane Library,* Issue 3. Oxford: Update Software.

Lang, S. (1997) *Breastfeeding Special Care Babies.* London: Baillière Tindall.

Lang, S., Lawrence, C.J. & Orme, R.L.E. (1994) Sodium in hand and pump expressed human breast milk. *Early Human Development* 38: 131–138.

Lavergne, N.A. (1997) Does application of teabags provide effective relief? *Journal of Obstetric, Gynecologic and Neonatal Nursing* 26(1): 53–58.

Lawlor-Smith, L. & Lawlor-Smith, C. (1997) Vasospasm of the nipple – a manifestation of Raynaud's phenomenon: case reports. *British Medical Journal* 314: 644–645.

Lawrence, R.A. (1997) Breastfeeding is more than just good nutrition. *International Journal of Childbirth Education* 12(1): 16.

Lawrence, R.A. & Lawrence, R.M. (1998) *Breastfeeding. A Guide for the Medical Profession*, 5th edn. St Louis: Mosby.

Livingstone, V. & Stringer, L.J. (1999) The treatment of *Staphylococcus aureus* infected sore nipples: a randomised comparative study. *Journal of Human Lactation* 15(3): 241–246.

Lopez-Alarcon, M., Villalpando, S. & Fajardo, A. (1997) Breastfeeding lowers the frequency and duration of acute respiratory infection and diarrhoea in infants under six months of age. *Journal of Nutrition* 127: 436–443.

Lucas, A. & Cole, T. (1990) Breastmilk and neonatal necrotising entero-colitis. *Lancet* 336(8730): 1519–1523.

Lucas, A., Morley, R., Cole, T.J. *et al.* (1992) Breast milk and subsequent intelligence quotient in children born preterm. *Lancet* 339: 261–264.

McCreadie, R.G. (1997) The Nithsdale Schizophrenia Surveys. 16. Breastfeeding and schizophrenia: preliminary results and hypotheses. *British Journal of Psychiatry* 170: 334–337.

McVea, K.L.S.P., Turner, P.D. & Peppler, D.K. (2000) The role of breastfeeding in sudden infant death syndrome. *Journal of Human Lactation* 16(1): 13–20.

Makrides, M., Neumann, M. & Simmer, K. (1995) Are long chain polyunsaturated fatty acids essential nutrients in infancy? *Lancet* 345(8963): 1463–1468.

Management of Health and Safety at Work Regulations 1992. London: HMSO.

Mannick, E. & Udall, J.N. (1996) Neonatal gastrointestinal mucosal immunity. *Clinics in Perinatology* 23(2): 287–304.

Marasco, L. (1998) Common breastfeeding myths. *Leaven* 34(2): 21–24.

Marmet, C., Shell, E. & Marmet, R. (1990) Neonatal frenotomy may be necessary to correct breastfeeding problems. *Journal of Human Lactation* 6: 117–121.

Mason, T., Rabinovich, C.E., Fredrickson, D.D. *et al.* (1995) Breastfeeding and the development of juvenile rheumatoid arthritis. *Journal of Rheumatology* 22: 1166–1170.

Maternity Alliance (1999) *Having it All – A Woman's Guide to Combining Breastfeeding and Work*. London: Maternity Alliance.

Melton, L.J. 3rd, Bryant, S.C., Wahner, H.W. *et al.* (1993) Influence of breastfeeding and other reproductive factors on bone mass in later life. *Osteoporosis International* 3: 76–83.

Mennella, J.A. (1997) Infants' suckling responses to the flavor of alcohol in mothers' milk. *Alcoholism, Clinical and Experimental Research* 21: 581–585.

Michels, K.B., Willett, W.C., Rosner, B.A. *et al.* (1996) Prospective assessment of breastfeeding and breast cancer incidence among 89,887 women. *Lancet* 347(8999): 431–436.

MIDIRS/NHS Centre for Reviews and Dissemination (1999) *Breastfeeding or Bottlefeeding: Helping Women to Choose*, 2nd edn. Bristol: MIDIRS.

Miller, M., Iliff, P., Stoltzfus, R.J. *et al.* (2002) Breast-milk erythropoietin and mother-to-child HIV transmission through breastmilk. *Lancet* 360(9341): 1246–1248.

Minchin, M. (2000) Artificial feeding and risk: the last taboo. *Practising Midwife* 3(3): 18–20.

Mitchell, P. (1997) Pollutants in breast milk cause concern, but breast is still best. *Lancet* 349(9064): 1525.

Morton, J.A. (1992) Ineffective suckling: a possible consequence of obstructive positioning. *Journal of Human Lactation* 8(2): 83–85.

National Childbirth Trust (NCT) (1996) *Drugs in Breastmilk: a compendium*. London: NCT.

National Childbirth Trust (NCT) (2000) *Breastfeeding – How to Store your Milk*. London: NCT.

Neifert, M., DeMarzo, S. & Seacat, J. (1990) The influence of breast surgery, breast appearance, and pregnancy-induced breast changes on lactation sufficiency as measured by infant weight gain. *Birth* 17: 31–38.

Neifert, M., Lawrence, R. & Seacat, J. (1995) Nipple confusion – towards a formal definition. *Journal of Paediatrics* 126: S125–S129.

Neville, M. (1999) The physiology of lactation. *Clinics in Perinatology* 26(2): 251–279.

Newburg, D.S., Peterson, J.A., Ruiz-Palacios, G.M. *et al.* (1998) Role of human-milk lactadherin in protection against symptomatic rotavirus infection. *Lancet* 351(9110): 1160–1164.

Newman, J. (1995) How breastmilk protects newborns. *Scientific American* Dec: 58–61.

NHS Executive (1999) Reducing mother to baby transmission of HIV. HSC 1999/183. London: DoH.

NHS Centre for Reviews and Dissemination (2000) Promoting the initiation of breastfeeding. *Effective Health Care Bulletin* 6(2): 1–12.

Oddy, W.H. (2000) Breastfeeding and asthma in children: findings from a West Australian study. *Breastfeeding Review* 8(1): 5–11.

Odent, M. (1996) Multiple sclerosis and cow's milk. *Primal Health Research* 4(1): 1–2.

Orlando, S. (1995) The immunologic significance of breastmilk. *Journal of Obstetric, Gynaecological and Neonatal Nursing* 24(7): 678–683.

Palmer, B. (1998) The influence of breastfeeding on the development of the oral cavity: a commentary. *Journal of Human Lactation* **14**(2): 93–98.

Perez-Escamilla, R., Pollitt, E., Lonnerdal, B. *et al.* (1994) Infant feeding policies in maternity wards and their effect on breastfeeding success: an analytical overview. *American Journal of Public Health* **84**(1): 89–97.

Pessl, M.M. (1996) Are we creating our own breast-feeding mythology? *Journal of Human Lactation* **12**: 271–272.

Pettitt, D.J., Forman, M.R., Hanson, R.L. *et al.* (1997) Breastfeeding and incidence of non-insulin dependent diabetes mellitus in Pima Indians. *Lancet* **350**(9072): 166–168.

Pisacane, A., Graziano, L., Mazzarella, G. *et al.* (1992) Breastfeeding and urinary tract infection. *Journal of Pediatrics* **120**(1): 87–89.

Powers, N.G. (1999) Slow weight gain and low milk supply in the breastfeeding dyad. *Clinics in Perinatology* **26**(2): 399–430.

Prentice, A., Addey, C.V.P. & Wilde, J. (1989) Evidence for local feedback control of human milk secretion. *Biochemical Society Transactions* **17**: 489–492.

Protheroe, L., Dyson, L., Renfrew, M. *et al.* (2003) *The effectiveness of public health interventions to promote the initiation of breastfeeding. Evidence Briefing*, 1st edn. London: Health Development Agency.

Pugh, L.C., Buchko, B.L., Bishop, B.A. *et al.* (1996) A comparison of topical agents to relieve nipple pain and enhance breastfeeding. *Birth* **23**(2): 88–93.

Quinsey, P.M., Donohue, D.C., Cumming, F.J. *et al.* (1996) The importance of measured intake in assessing exposure of breast-fed infants to organochlorines. *European Journal of Clinical Nutrition* **50**(7): 438–442.

Ransjo-Arvidson, A.B., Matthieson, A.S., Lilja, G. *et al.* (2001) Maternal analgesia during labour disturbs newborn behaviour: effects on breastfeeding, temperature and crying. *Birth* **28**(1): 5–12.

Ravelli, A.C.J., van der Meulen, J.H.P., Osmond, C. *et al.* (2000) Infant feeding and adult glucose tolerance, lipid profile, blood pressure and obesity. *Archives of Disease in Childhood* **82**(3): 248–252.

Renfrew, M.J. & Lang, S. (1999) Early initiation of breastfeeding. *The Cochrane Library*. Issue 1. Oxford: Update Software.

Renfrew, M., Woolridge, M. & Ross McGill, H. (2000) *Enabling Women to Breastfeed*. London: The Stationery Office.

Repucci, A.H. (1995) Effect of breastfeeding on hospitalization rates for lower respiratory infections. *Journal of Pediatrics* **127**(4): 667.

Righard, L. & Alade, M.O. (1990) Effect of delivery room routines on success of first breastfeed. *Lancet* **336**(8723): 1105–1107.

Righard, L. & Alade, M.O. (1992) Sucking technique and its effects on success of breastfeeding. *Birth* **19**: 185–189.

Riordan, J.M. (1997) The cost of not breastfeeding: a commentary. *Journal of Human Lactation* **13**(2): 93–97.

Rodriguez-Palmero, M., Koletzko, B., Kunz, C. *et al.* (1999) Nutritional and biochemical properties of human milk: II. Lipids, micronutrients, and bioactive factors. *Clinics in Perinatology* **26**(2): 335–359.

Rogers, I.S. (1997) Lactation and fertility. *Early Human Development* **49**(Suppl. 29): S185–S190.

Rotolli, A., Decarlis, S. & Gianni, M.L. (1997) Influence of a mineral water on the rheological characteristics of reconstituted infant formulas and diluted cow's milk. *Journal of International Medical Research* **25**(5): 275–284.

Royal College of Midwives (RCM) (1998) *HIV & AIDS*. Position Paper No. 16a. London: RCM.

Royal College of Midwives (RCM) (2002) *Successful Breastfeeding*, 3rd edn. London: RCM, Churchill Livingstone.

Royal College of Midwives (RCM) and Department of Health (DoH) (1999) *HIV testing in pregnancy*. London: RCM.

Royal College of Midwives (RCM) and Department of Health (DoH) (2000) *HIV and Infant Feeding*. Report of a Seminar, 30th June 2000. London: RCM.

Royal College of Midwives (RCM), National Childbirth Trust (NCT), Royal College of Nursing (RCN) *et al.* (2000) *Barriers to Breastfeeding*. Conference report. London: DoH.

Saadeh, R. & Akre, J. (1996) Ten Steps to Successful Breastfeeding: a summary of the rationale and scientific evidence. *Birth* **23**(3): 154–160.

Saarinen, U.M. & Kajosaari, M. (1995) Breastfeeding as prophylaxis against atopic disease: prospective follow up study until 17 years old. *Lancet* **346**(8982): 1065–1069.

Scientific Advisory Committee on Nutrition (SACN) (2002) *Minutes from SACN 27th March Meeting*. Online. Available: http://www.sacn.gov.uk/meeting2002march.htm

Shu, X.O., Linet, M.S., Steinbuch, M. *et al.* (1999) Breastfeeding and risk of childhood acute leukaemia. *Journal of the National Cancer Institute* **91**(20): 1765–1772.

Sikorski, J. & Renfrew, M. (1999) Support for breastfeeding mothers (Cochrane Review). *The Cochrane Library*, Issue 2. Oxford: Update Software.

Silfverdal, S.A., Bodin, L. & Olc, N.P. (1999) Protective effect of breastfeeding: an ecologic study of *Haemophilus influenzae* meningitis and breastfeeding in a Swedish population. *International Journal of Epidemiology* **28**(1): 152–156.

Siskind, V., Green, A., Bain, C. *et al.* (1997) Breastfeeding, menopause, and epithelial ovarian cancer. *Epidemiology* **8**(2): 188–191.

Smith, D. (1999) Worldwide trends in DDT levels in human breast milk. *International Journal of Epidemiology* 28(2): 179–188.

Snowden, H.M., Renfrew, M.J. & Woolridge, M.W. (2002) Treatments for breast engorgement during lactation. *The Cochrane Library*, Issue 1. Oxford: Update Software.

Statutory Instrument No. 77 (1995) Food. The Infant Formula and Follow-on Regulations. London: HMSO.

UNICEF UK Baby Friendly Initiative (BFI) (1996) *Information Sheet*. London: UK BFI.

UNICEF UK Baby Friendly Initiative (BFI) (1998a) *Implementing the Ten Steps to Successful Breastfeeding: A Guide for UK Maternity Service Providers Working towards Baby Friendly Accreditation*. London: UNICEF UK BFI.

UNICEF UK Baby Friendly Initiative (BFI) (1998b) *Breastfeeding your Baby*. London: UNICEF UK BFI.

UNICEF UK Baby Friendly Initiative (BFI) (1999) *Towards National, Regional and Local Strategies for Breastfeeding*. London: UNICEF UK BFI.

UNICEF UK Baby Friendly Initiative (BFI) (2001) *Implementing the Baby Friendly Best Practice Standards*. London: UNICEF UK BFI.

UNICEF UK Baby Friendly Initiative with the Foundation for the Study of Infant Deaths (UNICEF UK/BFI/FSID) (2003) *Sharing a Bed with your Baby*. London: UNICEF BFI with FSID.

United Kingdom Central Council for Nursing, Midwifery and Health Visiting (UKCC) (1998) *Midwives Rules and Code Of Practice*. London: UKCC.

United Kingdom National Case-Control Study Group (1993) Breastfeeding and risk of breast cancer in young women. *British Medical Journal* 307(6895): 17–20.

Vincent, P. (1999) *Feeding our Babies*. England: Hochland and Hochland.

Vio, F., Salazar, G. & Infante, C. (1991) Smoking during pregnancy and lactation and its effects on breast-milk volume. *American Journal of Clinical Nutrition* 54(6): 1011–1016.

Wang, I.Y. & Fraser, I.S. (1994) Reproductive function and contraception in the postpartum period. *Obstetrical & Gynecological Survey* 49(1): 56–63.

Wang, Y.S. & Su, S.Y. (1996) The effect of exclusive breastfeeding on development and incidence of infection in infants. *Journal of Human Lactation* 12(1): 27–30.

White, A., Freeth, S. & O'Brien, M. (for OPCS) (1992) *Infant Feeding 1990*. London: HMSO.

Widstrom, A.M., Wahlberg, V. & Matthieson, A.S. (1990) Short term effects of early suckling and touch of the nipple on maternal behaviour. *Early Human Development* 21: 153–163.

Wilde, C.J., Addey, C.V.P., Boddy, L.M. *et al.* (1995) Autocrine regulation of milk secretion by a protein in milk. *Biochemical Journal* 305: 51–58.

Williams, A.F. (1997) *Hypoglycaemia of the Newborn – Review of the Literature*. Division of Child Health and Development and Maternal and Newborn Health/Safe Motherhood. Geneva: World Health Organization.

Williatts, P., Forsyth, J.S., DiModugno, M.K. *et al.* (1998) Effect of long-chain polyunsaturated fatty acids in infant formula on problem solving at 10 months of age. *Lancet* 352: 688–691.

Willis, C.E. & Livingstone, V. (1995) Infant insufficient milk syndrome associated with maternal postpartum hemorrhage. *Journal of Human Lactation* 11(2): 123–126.

Woolridge, M. (1994) The Baby Friendly Hospital Initiative UK. *Modern Midwife* 4: 32–33.

Woolridge, M.W. (1995) Breastfeeding: physiology into practice. In: Davies, D.P. (ed) *Nutrition in the Normal Infant. Nutrition in Child Health*, Ch. 2, pp. 13–30. London: Royal College of Physicians.

World Health Organization (WHO) (1981) *International Code of Marketing of Breastmilk Substitutes*. Geneva: WHO.

World Health Organization (WHO) (1997) *Hypoglycaemia of the Newborn – Review of the Literature*. Division of Child Health and Development and Maternal and Newborn Health/Safe Motherhood. Geneva: WHO.

World Health Organization (WHO) (1998) *Evidence for the Ten Steps to Successful Breastfeeding* (revised). Family and Reproductive Health, Division of Child Health and Development. Geneva: WHO.

World Health Organization (WHO) (2002) *Infant and Young Child Nutrition – Global Strategy on Infant and Young Child Feeding*. Fifty-fifth World Assembly, A55/15 16th April. Geneva: WHO.

World Health Organization/United Nations Children's Fund (WHO/UNICEF) (1989) *Protecting, Promoting and Supporting Breastfeeding: The Special Role of Maternity Services. A Joint WHO/UNICEF Statement*. Geneva: WHO.

WHO Task Force on Methods for the Natural Regulation of Fertility (1999) The World Health Organization multinational study of breastfeeding and lactational amenorrhea. III. Pregnancy during breastfeeding. *Fertility and Sterility* 72(3): 431–440.

World Bank Symposium (1998) World bank symposium encourages breastfeeding by HIV-positive mothers. *Action News* January: 7.

Xanthou, M. (1998) Immune protection of human milk. *Biology of the Neonate* 74(2): 121–133

Yamauchi, Y. & Yamanouchi, I. (1990) Breastfeeding frequency during the first 24 hours after birth in full term neonates. *Pediatrics* 86(2): 171–175.

Zimmermann, R., Perucchini, D. & Fauchere, J.C. (1995) Hepatitis C virus in breastmilk. *Lancet* 345(8954): 928.

Zinaman, M.J., Hughes, V., Queenan, J.T. *et al.* (1992) Acute prolactin and oxytocin responses and milk yields to infant suckling and artificial methods of expression in lactating women. *Pediatrics* 89(3): 437–440.

ADDITIONAL RESOURCES

Association of Breastfeeding Mothers
PO Box 207, Bridgewater, Somerset TA6 7YT
Website: http://www.clara.net/abm/

Cleft Lip and Palate Association (CLAPA)
235–237 Finchley Road, London NW3 6LS
Tel: 0207 431 0033
Email: info@clapa.com
Website: http://www.clapa.com

Down's Syndrome Association
155 Mitcham Road, London SW17 9PG
Tel: 0208 682 4001
Website: http://www.dsa-uk.com

Foundation for the Study of Infant Deaths
Artillery House, 11–19 Artillery Row, London SW1 1RT
Tel: 0870 787 0554
Website: http://www.sids.org.uk

La Leche League
Breastfeeding Help and Information, BM 3424, London
WC1N 6XX
Tel: 0207 242 1278
Website: http://www.laleche.org.uk

National Childbirth Trust
Breastfeeding Promotion Group

Alexandra House, Oldham Terrace, Acton, London W3 6NH
Tel: 0870 770 3236
Website: http://www.nctpregnancyandbabycare.com

The Breastfeeding Network
PO Box 11126, Paisley, PA2 8YB
Website: http://www.breastfeedingnetwork.org.uk

The Multiple Births Foundation
Hammersmith House, Level 4, Queen Charlotte's and
Chelsea Hospital, Du Cane Road, London W12 OHS
Tel: 0208 383 3519
Email: mbf@ic.ac.uk
Website: http://www.multiplebirths.org.uk

Twins and Multiple Births Association (TAMBA) (for
parents)
2 The Willows, Gardner Road, Guildford, Surrey GU1 4PG
Tel: 0870 770 3305
Email: enquiries@tamba.org.uk
Website: http://www.tamba.org.uk

UK Association for Milk Banking (UKAMB)
The Milk Bank, Queen Charlotte's and Chelsea Hospital,
Du Cane Road, London W12 OHS
Tel: 0208 383 3559
Website: http://www.ukamb.org

34

The Preterm Baby and the Small Baby

Carol Simpson

LEARNING OUTCOMES

At the end of this chapter, you will have:

- an understanding of classification and definitions of low birthweight infants
- knowledge of common causes of preterm and small-for-gestational-age babies and the implications for antenatal care
- an understanding of complications relating to preterm delivery and low birthweight
- knowledge of long-term outcomes for these babies.

INTRODUCTION

For the purpose of classification, management and research studies, newborn babies are considered according to their gestation, their birthweight relative to their gestation (centiles) and their actual birthweight. The midwife's role centres on the prevention of prematurity, on preparing parents for identifying risk factors antenatally, and, in the event of a preterm birth, in working with the caring team to support parents in the neonatal period.

Gestation

Antenatally, gestation is estimated from the date of the last menstrual period and the woman's normal cycle, clinical examination and early ultrasound scan measurements and uterine growth. It is important for midwives to obtain an accurate menstrual history from women and to recommend an early ultrasound scan to ascertain the gestation, if uncertain.

There are many scoring systems available to help estimate the gestation of the neonate following delivery, and generally a neonatal unit will use one, or an adaptation of one or two of the common ones. The improved accuracy of antenatal ultrasound scans has led to less reliance on these scales. The Dubowitz scale (Dubowitz *et al.*, 1970) (see Fig. 34.1) is the most widely used in the UK and, providing the baby is well and examined within a few hours of delivery, is accurate to within 2 weeks. It involves scoring the baby on its neurological state as well as external criteria, and may therefore be inappropriate for use with sick or ventilated neonates.

A more recent scoring system has been suggested by Ballard, which is an adaptation of the Dubowitz score (Fig. 34.2).

These scoring systems require that careful examination of the baby is carried out, looking at characteristics of appearance, reflexes and behaviour which gives an indication of whether the baby is small or premature.

- Post-term: >42 completed weeks of gestation
- Term: 37–42 completed weeks of gestation
- Preterm: <37 completed weeks of gestation.

Reflective Activity 34.1

Examine a healthy newborn baby and assess the gestational age using the Dubowitz and Ballard scoring systems.

Centiles

Using an appropriate centile chart, the weight, head circumference and length of the baby are plotted

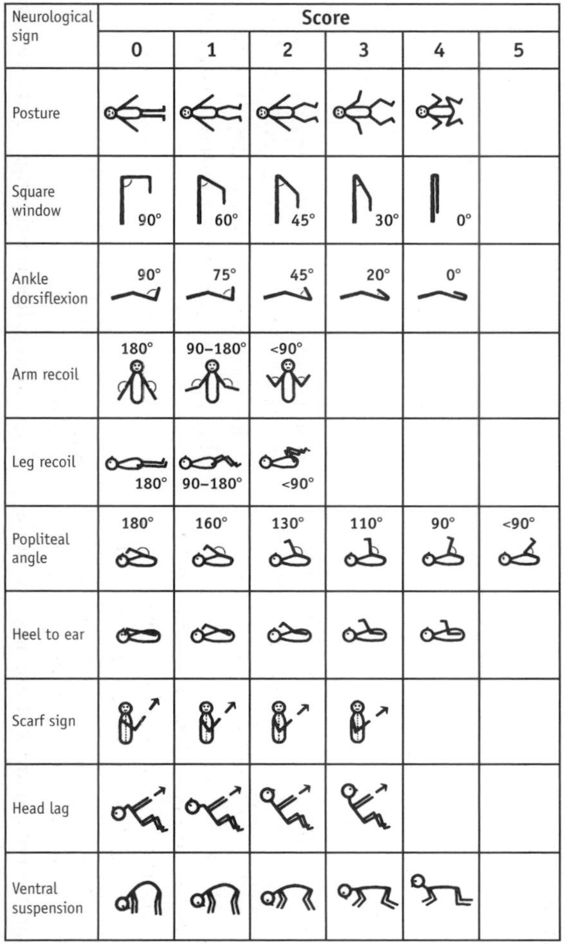

Neurological sign

Neurological sign	Score 0	1	2	3	4	5
Posture						
Square window	90°	60°	45°	30°	0°	
Ankle dorsiflexion	90°	75°	45°	20°	0°	
Arm recoil	180°	90–180°	<90°			
Leg recoil	180°	90–180°	<90°			
Popliteal angle	180°	160°	130°	110°	90°	<90°
Heel to ear						
Scarf sign						
Head lag						
Ventral suspension						

Physical (external) criteria

External sign	Score 0	1	2	3	4
Oedema	Obvious oedema hands and feet; pitting over tibia	No obvious oedema hands and feet; pitting over tibia	No oedema		
Skin texture	Very thin, gelatinous	Thin and smooth	Smooth, medium thickness. Rash or superficial peeling	Slight thickening. Superficial cracking and peeling, especially hands and feet	Thick and parchment-like. Superficial or deep cracking
Skin colour (infant not crying)	Dark red	Uniformly pink	Pale pink, variable over body	Pale. Only pink over ears, lips, palms or soles	
Skin opacity (trunk)	Numerous veins and venules clearly seen, especially over abdomen	Veins and tributaries seen	A few large vessels clearly seen over abdomen	A few large vessels seen indistinctly over abdomen	No blood vessels seen
Lanugo (over back)	No lanugo	Abundant, long and thick over whole back	Hair thinning, especially over lower back	Small amount of lanugo and bald areas	At least half of back devoid of lanugo
Plantar creases	No skin creases	Faint red marks over anterior half of sole	Definite red marks over more than anterior half. Indentations over more than anterior third	Indentations over more than anterior third	Definite deep indentations over more than anterior third
Nipple formation	Nipple barely visible, no areola	Nipple well defined, areola smooth and flat, diameter <0.75 cm	Areola stippled, edges not raised: diameter <0.75 cm	Areola stippled, edge raised: diameter >0.75 cm	
Breast size	No breast tissue palpable	Breast tissue or one or both sides <0.5 cm diameter	Breast tissue both sides, one or both 0.5–1.0 cm	Breast tissue both sides, one or both >1 cm	
Ear form	Pinna flat and shapeless, little or no incurving of edge	Incurving of part of edge of pinna	Partial incurving whole of upper pinna	Well-defined incurving whole of upper pinna	
Ear firmness	Pinna soft, easily folded, no recoil	Pinna soft, easily folded, slow recoil	Cartilage to edge of pinna but soft in places, ready recoil	Pinna firm, cartilage to edge, instant recoil	
Genitalia • Male	Neither testes in scrotum	At least one testis high in scrotum	At least one testis right down		
• Female (with hips half abducted)	Labia majora widely separated, labia minora protruding	Labia majora almost cover labia minora	Labia majora completely cover labia minora		

Figure 34.1 The Dubowitz score: graph for reading gestational age from total score. (From Dubowitz et al., 1970, with permission.)

Neuromuscular maturity

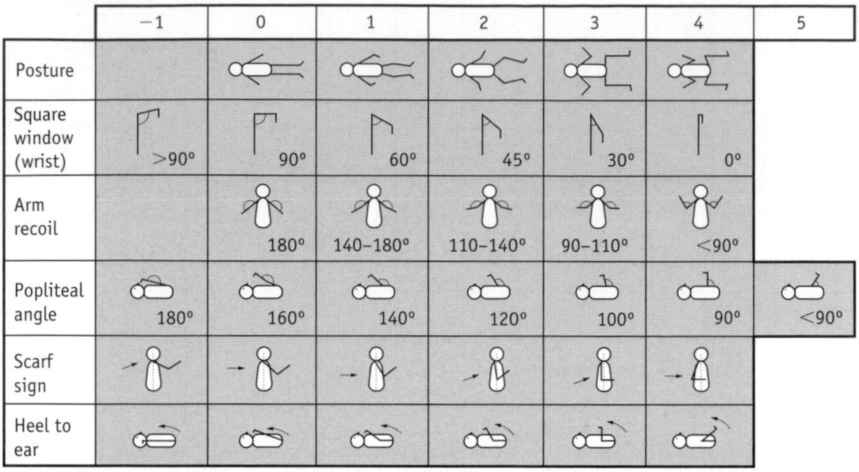

Physical maturity

	−1	0	1	2	3	4
Skin	Sticky friable transparent	Gelatinous red, translucent	Smooth pink, visible veins	Superficial peeling &/or rash, few veins	Cracking pale areas rare veins	Parchment deep cracking no vessels	Leathery cracked wrinkled
Lanugo	none	sparse	abundant	thinning	bald areas	Mostly bald	
Plantar surface	heel-toe 40–50 mm:−1 <40 mm:−2	>50 mm no crease	faint red marks	anterior transverse crease only	creases ant. 2/3	creases over entire sole	
Breast	imperceptible	barely perceptible	flat areola no bud	stippled areola 1–2 mm bud	raised areola 3–4 mm bud	full areola 5–10 mm bud	
Eye/ ear	lids fused loosely:−1 tightly:−2	lids open pinna flat stays folded	sl. curved pinna; soft; slow recoil	well-curved pinna; soft but ready recoil	formed & firm instant recoil	thick cartilage ear stiff	
Genitals (male)	scrotum flat, smooth	scrotum empty faint rugae	testes in upper canal rare rugae	testes descending few rugae	testes down good rugae	testes pendulous deep rugae	
Genitals (female)	clitoris prominent labia flat	prominent clitoris small labia minora	prominent clitoris enlarging minora	majora & minora equally prominent	majora large minora small	majora cover clitoris & minora	

Maturity rating

Score	Weeks
−10	20
−5	22
0	24
5	26
10	28
15	30
20	32
25	34
30	36
35	38
40	40
45	42
50	44

Figure 34.2   The Ballard score. Each of the clinical and neurological features is assessed and scored. The gestational age is determined by comparing the total score with the maturity rating grid. (From Johnston *et al.*, 2003: 109.)

against the gestation and an assessment made of the growth. The centile chart forms an important part of providing a dynamic growth record and a link to the neonatal management (see Ch. 31). There has been considerable controversy over the best centile chart to use, and currently the Child Growth Foundation chart (Fig. 34.3) has been approved as the optimum record from preterm to childhood.

- Large for gestational age (LGA): >90th centile
- Appropriate for gestational age (AGA): 10th to 90th centile
- Small for gestational age (SGA): <10th centile.

These classifications rely on an accurate assessment of the gestational age at delivery.

Birthweight

Babies may be grouped according to their birthweight, which is especially useful when the gestation is unknown. Many studies relate to birthweight rather than gestation as it is a better predictor of outcome. The World Health Organization (WHO) definition of low birthweight (WHO, 1977) is internationally adopted, with further subdivisions as shown below:

- Low birthweight (LBW): lower than 2500 g at birth
- Very low birthweight (VLBW): lower than 1500 g at birth
- Extremely low birthweight (ELBW): lower than 1000 g at birth.

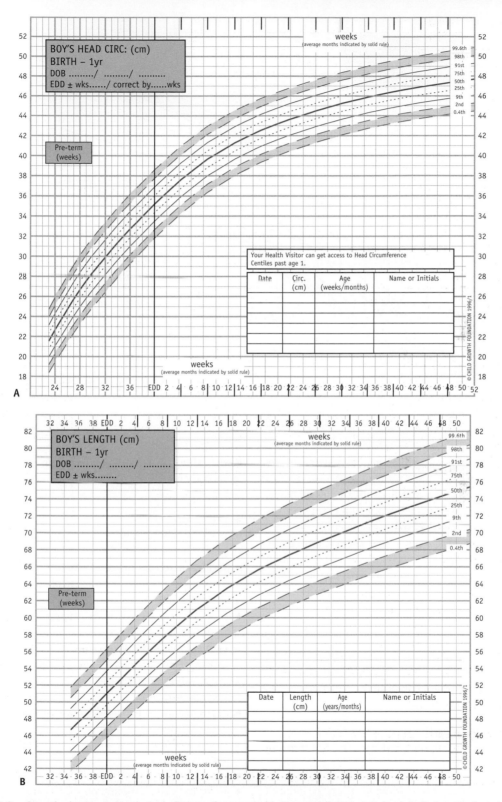

Figure 34.3 Growth charts. **A.** Head circumference from preterm (24 weeks) to 1 year (male). **B.** Length from term birth to 1 year (male). (Courtesy of the Child Growth Foundation, 2001; © Child Growth Foundation.)

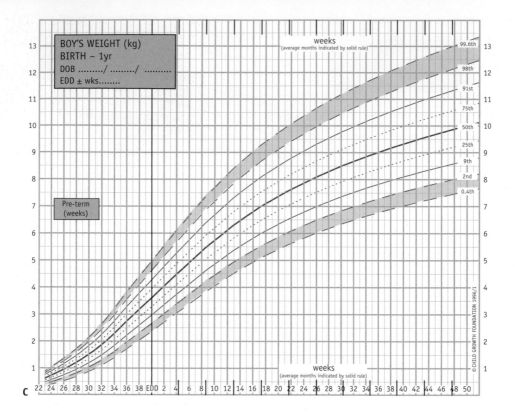

Figure 34.3 (*continued*) **C.** Weight from 23 weeks to 1 year (male).

The rapid developments in neonatology, particularly over the past decade, have resulted in the survival of LBW infants above 1500 g becoming commonplace. High mortality rates are found predominantly in the VLBW group and particularly those of ELBW. In 2000 in England and Wales, 7.6% of babies born were LBW, with 1.2% less than 1500 g (ONS, 2000a). LBW babies in general made up 72% of all neonatal deaths, whilst the VLBW group alone accounted for 60% of the deaths (ONS, 2000b).

Preterm and SGA babies are considered separately in this chapter, although there is much overlap in their causes, management and complications. A baby may be preterm, SGA and LBW and will therefore need consideration from all of these perspectives.

THE PRETERM BABY

Causes

Preterm delivery can occur spontaneously or be induced for maternal or fetal health problems. The aetiology is unknown in around 40% of spontaneous preterm births, although certain predisposing factors may be identified antenatally. The causes are often multifactorial and include:

- pre-eclampsia
- placental abnormalities – antepartum haemorrhage, placenta praevia
- serious maternal diseases – acute or chronic, such as pyelonephritis, chronic nephritis or essential hypertension
- illnesses associated with maternal pyrexia and infection
- cervical incompetence (history of repeated mid-trimester miscarriages) – incidence may be reduced with careful use of tocolytics and first trimester cervical suturing
- maternal alcohol or substance abuse – including cigarette smoking
- overdistension of the uterus – multiple pregnancies, polyhydramnios
- poor obstetric history
- maternal age <20 years or >35 years
- certain congenital anomalies
- social classes IV or V.

Some of these problems can be addressed antenatally, and a crucial part of the midwife's role is in educating the woman about normal pregnancy features and what should be reported to the healthcare team.

Characteristics [(Fig. 34.4)]

Preterm babies are immature and not ready to adapt to extrauterine life. Their appearance will depend on their maturity, but generally, the head is large in proportion to the body and the baby has a small triangular face with a pointed chin. If very immature, the eyelids may be fused. Owing to poor ossification, the sutures and fontanelles are widely spaced and skull bones soft. Because of the absence of subcutaneous fat, the skin is pinkish/red and surface veins are prominent. The body is covered with varying amounts of soft downy hair, called *lanugo*, and a protective creamy white substance, *vernix caseosa*. The limbs are thin, the nails soft, the chest small and narrow with little or no breast tissue, the abdomen large and the umbilicus appears to be low-set. The genitalia are not fully developed; the labia majora do not cover the labia minora and the testes may not have descended into the scrotum. Muscle tone is poor and the more immature the baby, the greater the degree of extension of the arms and legs. The baby has an incoordinated suck and swallow reflex.

Management

There are many physiological functions a preterm baby is unable to perform adequately due to immaturity. Neonatal care attempts to compensate for these deficiencies until such time as the infant is able to cope unaided. Accurate assessment of the baby's condition at birth and prompt resuscitation are therefore essential. Subsequent meticulous care and close observation are required to detect even small departures from normal physiological function, which can lead to serious complications.

Labour and delivery

If preterm labour is anticipated, every effort should be made to deliver the mother in a maternity unit with appropriate neonatal intensive care facilities. If possible, midwives should avoid giving the mother narcotics during labour, as these may depress the fetal respiratory centre, further compromising the baby's breathing following birth. They should ensure that the

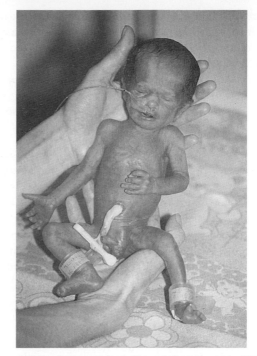

Figure 34.4   Preterm infant. (From Johnston *et al.*, 2003.)

resuscitaire is fully functional and equipped with the correct equipment prior to the birth.

An experienced paediatrician and midwife or neonatal nurse must be present at delivery to ensure immediate and expert resuscitation. Some paediatricians advocate elective intubation immediately following delivery for resuscitation of all very preterm and VLBW babies, especially those of 28 weeks' gestation and less.

The temperature of the delivery room should be increased to 26°C prior to delivery. The radiant heater of the resuscitaire must be calibrated to help prevent cold stress, which increases the baby's oxygen requirements. The neonate must be dried quickly and thoroughly with warm towels, paying particular attention to the head, as up to 80% of heat loss occurs from this area.

Common problems

Respiratory

The most common problems for preterm babies are respiratory disorders. These conditions are discussed more fully in Chapter 35.

The more preterm the baby, the less developed the physiological functions. The baby born at term has strong respiratory muscles and the nerve centre in the medulla controlling respiration is fully developed. In the preterm baby the muscles are weak and the respiratory centre immature; thus it may, in the first place, be difficult to establish respiration, especially if respiratory depressant drugs, such as narcotics, are given to the mother in labour.

In some circumstances the baby may initially appear well, breathing regularly and becoming pink, but later develop expiratory grunting, apnoeic episodes and cyanosis, deteriorating in condition rapidly.

Apnoeas   Many preterm babies have apnoeas associated with their prematurity and require constant monitoring; it is important that the parents understand the reasons for this and that they will resolve as the baby matures. Apnoea monitors should be removed several days prior to discharge so that the parents gain confidence and do not become reliant on them. Caffeine is given as a stimulant until these apnoeas of prematurity resolve.

Oxygen therapy   Oxygen is frequently required to relieve cyanosis in the neonate. However, oxygen is a dangerous drug when given in excessive or fluctuating quantities, and it is one major factor in the aetiology of retinopathy of prematurity (Whitfill and Drack, 2000), which can result in blindness. However, inadequate oxygenation may result in hypoxic brain damage; therefore careful administration and monitoring is essential, including during resuscitation.

Transient tachypnoea of the newborn (TTN)   Prior to birth the lungs are fluid-filled. With the first breath and the aid of surfactant, air replaces the fluid, some of which gets absorbed into the lymphatic system and some of which is physically squeezed from the respiratory tract during the process of a vaginal birth (see Ch. 31) and to a lesser extent during caesarean section.

TTN occurs when fluid is slow to clear from the lungs following birth and is fairly common in babies born by caesarean section. High maternal prostaglandin levels produced in labour halt the production of lung fluid and this does not occur to the same degree in babies born by caesarean section. It may also be the result of asphyxia which temporarily impairs cardiac function. This condition is characterized by expiratory grunting, nasal flaring, intercostal and sternal recession. The paediatrician should be informed and careful observation maintained. It usually resolves within a few hours of birth, but the baby may need oxygen therapy in the meantime. If still grunting at 4 hours of age, the baby should have a chest X-ray to eliminate other, more serious, respiratory conditions and may require an infection screen.

Temperature control

Although brown fat is utilized during cold stress, very low birthweight and preterm infants often have little or no brown fat stores to maintain the core temperature. The high surface area of preterm infants in relation to their size, and their thin skin, facilitate rapid heat loss.

Infants born before 30 weeks' gestation also have thin, porous skin, which allows evaporation of fluids, thereby increasing heat loss even further. Radiant heaters may exacerbate the problem by increasing the evaporative heat loss and their use is inappropriate for very small babies, who should be nursed in a humidified incubator for the first week of life.

At home, following an emergency or unexpected preterm birth, if no resuscitation is required, the midwife can place the baby on the mother's abdomen or chest for skin-to-skin contact, once dried. The baby's head should be covered and the mother and baby well wrapped in dry blankets. The aim is to maintain body temperature in the thermoneutral range, at which energy requirements are reduced to a minimum and oxygen consumption is less.

Hypoglycaemia

This is a common problem for preterm babies in the first 48–72 hours, as stores of brown fat, white fat and glycogen are too small to maintain their blood sugar level at a time when energy requirements are particularly high. Because of the heat loss from their large surface area, increased effort of breathing that accompanies respiratory difficulties and greater rate of growth, more energy is expended for their weight than in their term counterparts. Asphyxia and hypothermia aggravate this condition.

Blood sugar levels should be checked every 4–6 hours during the first 48–72 hours after birth using Dextrostix or BM Stix. Controversy still surrounds the clinical definition and significance of hypoglycaemia, but it is now generally accepted that the neonatal brain can be damaged by hypoglycaemia, whether symptomatic or not (Duvanel *et al.*, 1999). Current recommendations are to maintain serum blood glucose levels above 2.6 mmol/l (Cornblath *et al.*, 2000).

Jaundice

Physiological jaundice is exacerbated in preterm babies as the liver is immature and therefore conjugation of bilirubin is further delayed (see Ch. 37).

Another factor increasing the severity of jaundice, is that the passage of meconium in preterm babies may be delayed, particularly if enteral feeds are not commenced for several days, or with respiratory distress syndrome. This delay can contribute to hyperbilirubinaemia as the bilirubin in meconium may be reabsorbed.

Patent ductus arteriosus

The ductus arteriosus fails to close in a number of very preterm and low birthweight babies, partly because of immaturity and partly because the chemical conditions are not suitable in babies who are hypoxic and acidotic. A course of indometacin is commonly prescribed to facilitate closure, but surgical ligation of the duct is sometimes necessary.

Nutrition

Choice of milk

The rate of growth in preterm babies is greater than that in their mature counterparts and thus they require a greater energy intake. To achieve a rate of growth similar to that in utero, the preterm baby needs 540–600 kJ/kg/day. This equates to approximately 180–200 ml/kg/day of breast milk or standard formula milk. This may be achieved by giving smaller volumes of low birthweight formula milk, or by adding calorific supplements to breast milk. Larger babies will gain weight on smaller volumes but may also need over 200 ml/kg/day.

Wherever possible a mother's own fresh expressed breast milk is the milk of choice, as the milk the mother produces will be tailor-made to her baby's requirements, and this is especially pertinent to the preterm infant (Blackburn, 2003) (see Ch. 33).

The mother should be encouraged to breastfeed, if possible, or start expressing milk within a few hours of delivery and a minimum of six times every 24 hours. The sooner this is initiated, the greater the chance of establishing breastfeeding successfully. Midwives should teach all mothers how to express milk by hand and pump and how to store breast milk safely. Many mothers find breastfeeding a preterm baby rewarding, but very time-consuming and tiring. They should be advised that stress and fatigue can adversely affect milk production, and be provided with a range of advice on ways to increase their supply should it diminish, including getting sufficient rest, using hand and machine expression and ensuring an adequate diet (see Ch. 33).

The advantages of breast milk over formula milk for both term and preterm babies are widely documented, particularly in terms of immunological properties (Hanson, 1999). Research also suggests that breast milk is advantageous in the development of the central nervous system and subsequent intelligence quotient in preterm infants (Horwood et al., 2001).

Several centres have now reintroduced the use of human milk banks, with strict guidelines for the preparation of donor milk, heat treatment and pasteurization.

Reflective Activity 34.2

What facilities exist in your local neonatal unit for supporting breastfeeding? Is there a local milk bank and what policies and procedures exist to support bank breast milk? If donor milk is not used in your unit, look into its feasibility.

Low birth weight formula milks are available, the constitution of which provides the baby with more energy, protein, vitamins and minerals per millilitre than term formula milks or breast milk. These have long-chain polyunsaturated fatty acids (LCPFA) added to them, as these have been identified in human milk, term and preterm, as being important for normal development of the brain, retina and neural tissue in particular.

Methods of feeding

The method of feeding depends on the size, maturity and condition of the baby. Sucking is seen in the fetus as early as 13 weeks' gestation (Hafstrom and Kjellmer, 2000), although the suck and swallow coordination is not efficient until nearer term. Well babies of any size or gestation showing signs of sucking may therefore be tried with breast, cup or bottle feeds (see Ch. 33). The correct cup-feeding technique should be taught to parents. Careful supervision will be necessary to ensure that the fluid intake is adequate and that the baby is not becoming too tired by prolonged attempts at feeding.

Immature babies have an increased risk of aspiration and should be closely monitored. Small babies tire easily and may benefit from a regime of mixed breast/cup/bottle and tube feeds initially, until they can cope with more. Non-nutritive sucking during gastric feeding has been shown to facilitate the development of sucking behaviour (Pinelli and Symington, 2000); putting the baby to the breast at these times can be beneficial to the mother, baby and for the establishment of lactation.

Intravenous feeding   Ventilated babies may be fed by the intravenous route initially for four principal reasons:

- There is a substantial risk of milk aspiration which intubation does not abolish, as neonatal endotracheal tubes are uncuffed.
- A neonate with respiratory distress syndrome may have a paralytic ileus for the first few days. Any milk placed in the stomach or small bowel will accumulate, as if the bowel were obstructed. Therefore the residual volumes in the stomach should be checked, and feeding discontinued if accumulating.
- Milk in the stomach increases the respiratory effort. In infants suffering from respiratory distress, any factor that impairs respiration or increases oxygen demand should be avoided.
- During the course of respiratory distress syndrome, many infants have periods of hypotension and/or hypoxia. This is hazardous in any circumstances, but if bacteria proliferate in the bowel following oral feeds, the risks of septicaemia or necrotizing enterocolitis are greatly increased.

If ventilation or the condition of the baby does not allow oral feeds for a prolonged period, total parenteral nutrition is commenced. This contains the necessary nutrients and calories, individually tailored for each baby based on serum electrolyte results.

Naso/orojejunal feeding   Rarely, VLBW babies on long-term ventilation may be fed via a transpyloric or jejunal tube, which places milk directly into the bowel (Fig. 34.5), minimizing respiratory embarrassment by keeping the stomach empty. Once the baby's condition has improved, naso/orogastric feeding is commenced.

Naso/orogastric feeding   A naso/orogastric tube is used when the baby's suck is too weak or incoordinated to feed by breast, cup or bottle. Prior to each feed the position of the tube must be checked, either by checking the acidity of the fluid in the stomach, or by blowing a small amount of air into the stomach whilst listening with a stethoscope. Babies often pull them fully or partially out, causing an even greater risk of aspiration. Milk is given slowly via the tube using a syringe and positioning the baby at the breast during tube feeds may encourage rooting and early sucking.

The cardiac sphincter is poorly developed in the preterm baby and thus, if the stomach is overdistended, regurgitation and inhalation can occur, especially as the cough reflex is poorly developed or may be absent. Small frequent feeds are therefore advisable, initially

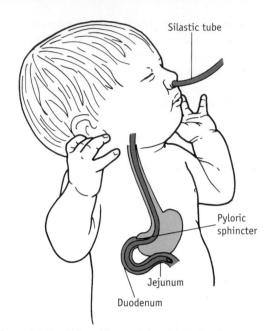

Figure 34.5   Baby with nasojejunal tube in situ.

hourly, gradually increasing to 3-hourly. Intermittent, as opposed to continuous feeding, has the advantage of encouraging normal hunger responses. VLBW and very preterm babies often tolerate continuous feeding better.

Minerals and nutritional supplements

Although preterm breast milk has a higher sodium content than mature breast milk, it may lack adequate energy, protein and some minerals to be the sole diet of very preterm and low birthweight infants. Human milk fortifiers containing carbohydrate, protein, vitamins and minerals may be used for these babies to supplement expressed breast milk, though only after consultation with the mother.

Current Department of Health recommendations are that all infants should receive daily vitamin supplements, such as children's vitamin drops (vitamins A, C and D) from the age of 1 month to 2 years. These are especially important for preterm babies as they have small stores of fat-soluble vitamins and are at risk of vitamin deficiency.

Vitamin C is required for efficient iron absorption as well as for growth and healing. Preterm babies have inadequate stores of iron at birth, which become depleted further as the baby grows. There is also a delay in the production of red blood cells by the immature bone marrow. All preterm babies are therefore supplemented with iron from the age of 4 weeks and this continues until they are weaned onto solid foods. Excessive or early iron supplementation can be harmful, since free iron in the bowel reverses the anti-infective properties of lactoferrin, enabling *Escherichia coli* to multiply. Very preterm and ill babies may need frequent blood transfusions, but whilst these boost the haemoglobin level they may also temporarily further suppress the formation of new red blood cells by the baby.

Very preterm babies of low birthweight also require folic acid to prevent macrocytic anaemia developing later. Blood alkaline phosphatase, calcium and phosphate levels should be regularly checked in very preterm babies, as they are at risk of developing osteopenia or metabolic bone disease (rickets of prematurity). Extra vitamin D, calcium and phosphate supplements may be needed, particularly in babies fed exclusively on breast milk. Calcium and phosphate supplements are continued until 42–43 weeks post-term, as there is an increased rate of bone mineralization at this stage.

Parent–baby relationship

It is crucial that the parents have an opportunity to see and hold their baby, even if only briefly, before transfer to the neonatal unit. The paediatrician must see the parents later to give them an account of their baby's condition, care and prognosis. A mother may feel quite bereft in a postnatal ward, especially when surrounded by other mothers who have their babies beside them and are busily involved in their care. It is common for parents to display signs of grief at this time, as they mourn the healthy baby they expected and fear getting attached to the small or ill baby they actually have. There must be good communication between the neonatal unit and the postnatal ward staff to ensure the family have the support they need.

The parents and siblings are encouraged to become involved in their baby's care as much as possible, from the earliest days, even if the baby is being ventilated. Very few babies are too sick to be cuddled for a short while or gently stroked by parents, although minimal handling techniques are generally applied to their care.

Many preterm babies are in hospital for several weeks or months before they are ready to be discharged home. During this time the parents participate in an increasing amount of their baby's care and will gradually gain confidence. Before discharge, they often find it helpful to stay in hospital to care for their baby day and night, either on the neonatal unit or in a transitional care ward.

> ### Reflective Activity 34.3
> Review the facilities for parents and siblings of babies in your neonatal intensive care unit.

Complications of prematurity

Several complications occur more commonly in the preterm baby than in the mature infant, relative to the degree of immaturity of the various systems or nerve centres controlling them. Extreme prematurity is a major cause of perinatal death, thus it is important to prevent complications occurring, where possible, and to detect early and treat those which cannot be prevented.

Respiratory distress syndrome (RDS)

Respiratory distress syndrome is uncommon in babies after 37 weeks' gestation and develops when there is insufficient surfactant, causing the alveoli in the lungs to collapse. Increasing effort is required to reinflate the alveoli after each breath and this is demonstrated by worsening tachypnoea, intercostal and sternal recession, expiratory grunting and characteristic X-ray changes.

Preterm babies may have a lack of surfactant as they miss out on the surge in surfactant levels normally seen at 32–35 weeks' gestation.

Many preterm babies develop respiratory difficulties at birth or within the first hours. In the very preterm, e.g. 24 weeks' gestation, this may be a result of the lungs not being sufficiently developed to support life without assistance. Gaseous exchange is insufficient, as the alveoli are lined by cuboidal epithelium and surrounded by an inadequate capillary network.

Over the past decade, many different ventilation methods and regimes have been utilized, in order to provide the necessary respiratory support for RDS, whilst reducing the iatrogenic damage due to the pressures and duration of ventilation.

Chronic lung disease (CLD)

Chronic lung disease (previously known as *bronchopulmonary dysplasia*) most commonly occurs in preterm and low birthweight babies and is defined clinically, as the sustained need for oxygen supplementation after 4 weeks of age when oxygen has been required since birth. In this condition there is serious disruption of lung growth, with X-rays and lung specimens showing a loss of alveoli, interstitial oedema, patches of collapse and fibrosis. The lungs are stiff and difficult to ventilate. High concentrations of oxygen, the need for prolonged ventilatory support and high ventilator pressures all contribute to the aetiology of CLD.

The survival of babies with a birthweight of 500–750 g is now approximately 50%, with 50% of these displaying CLD (Stevenson *et al.*, 1998). Many will be discharged from hospital still receiving continuous oxygen supplements for many months or even years, until the proportion of new lung tissue developing is adequate to sustain oxygenation without assistance. Practical and psychological support are required for parents of these babies, and close monitoring of the baby's lung function, growth and development.

Infection

A preterm infant is more vulnerable to infections than its term counterpart because:

- maternal IgG levels are low
- skin is a less efficient barrier to invading bacteria
- tears and saliva are less copious and contain fewer antibacterial factors
- stomach produces less protective acid
- immune cells are less numerous and efficient, and thus do not respond so effectively to stress
- the baby is subject to more invasive procedures and to multiple contacts with hospital staff.

In order to protect preterm babies as much as possible the following guidelines should be followed:

- *Handwashing* remains one of the biggest preventive measures staff and families can implement to reduce the risk of cross-infection. Parents, visitors and new staff need to be taught correct handwashing techniques to perform before and after handling the baby, using an antiseptic soap such as chlorhexidine.
- Every baby should have its own individual equipment, including stethoscope and thermometer, which should be thoroughly cleaned between use.
- The incubator or cot should be cleaned daily with soap and water – inside and out – and after use should be dismantled, thoroughly cleaned and aired before use.
- The unit should be cleaned and well ventilated, and soiled dressings or material placed in disposable bags and removed as soon as possible.
- All staff members, family and visitors caring for a neonate must be free from any signs of infection, including active cold sores (herpes simplex virus), coughs and sore throats.
- Preterm babies should be handled as little as possible and by as few people as possible. Parents are

involved in all aspects of their care as soon as their condition permits.

- The baby, if able, should have a gentle wash with warm water of the face, hands and skin folds, when necessary. The nappy area needs particular attention, as the skin is often friable and breaks down quickly when left in contact with urine or faeces.
- Oral hygiene is necessary for babies with an endotracheal tube in situ and for those unable to suck or receiving tube feeds.
- Antibiotic use may render the baby susceptible to candida infection and prophylactic treatment or early identification and treatment of this is important.
- Breastfeeding is encouraged and supported by midwives and neonatal staff, wherever possible. Consideration should be given to the use of donor breast milk, where milk bank facilities are available.

Hypocalcaemia

Early hypocalcaemia due to stress or illness may occur within the first 72 hours of life in preterm babies, infants of diabetic mothers and in those suffering from asphyxia, respiratory distress syndrome or sepsis. Asphyxia results in the excretion of high levels of calcitonin from the parathyroid glands and this reduces calcium mobilization from the bones. Vitamin D, which is required for parathyroid hormone action on bones and the gut, is also deficient in the preterm baby. Supplementation may be necessary.

Hypoxic ischaemic encephalopathy (HIE) (birth asphyxia)

The fetus only begins to lay down stores of brown fat from 22 weeks, white fat from 28 weeks, and glycogen from 36 weeks. Therefore, perinatally, the preterm infant has little energy reserve if there is any interruption to the oxygen supply, and in this event the heart will not continue pumping for long. Cardiac glycogen stores allow the heart to continue in cases of asphyxia, and continued cardiac function is required to remove the accumulated lactic acid from the brain. Since glycogen stores are reduced, the capacity of the preterm baby to withstand asphyxia is reduced.

The clinical presentation of the baby with HIE varies with severity. Six aspects of clinical presentation are assessed and may be predictive of outcome:

- level of consciousness
- tone and posture – neuromuscular indicator
- primitive, complex reflexes
- presence of seizures

- autonomic functions
- duration of symptoms.

Treatment is aimed at minimizing further cerebral damage, alleviating symptoms and early detection of any complications, such as cerebral haemorrhage or hydrocephalus. Drugs are given to maintain cerebral perfusion and blood pressure, to reduce cerebral oedema and control seizures.

Investigations to assess the severity of damage include ultrasound, CT scanning and EEG recordings. Prognosis depends on the severity of the insult, but may result in severe neurological damage. Hearing should be carefully screened, particularly if HIE is associated with seizures, associated organ damage or in a small for gestational age baby (Mencher and Mencher, 1999).

Cerebral haemorrhage and associated lesions

The incidence of neonatal cerebral haemorrhages in preterm and very low birthweight babies has declined in the past decade, partly due to the use of prophylactic antenatal steroids (Cooke, 1999). Cranial ultrasound scanning (see Fig. 34.6) is routinely performed on all preterm babies and small bleeds are commonly found within a few hours of birth, even after what seemed an easy delivery. These are classified depending on their site and severity. Major haemorrhages may cause ischaemic changes in the white matter around the ventricles, which can result in the formation of cysts. This is called periventricular cystic leucomalacia (PVL) and has major neurological implications. Whilst the rate of

periventricular haemorrhage (PVH) has reduced, the incidence of these ischaemic lesions appears to have increased, with implications for the morbidity of preterm and very low birthweight infants.

Causes Intrapartum events can predispose to the onset of PVH and PVL, which emphasizes the importance of preventing perinatal hypoxia. Poor skull ossification, fragile blood vessels and episodes of hypotension, hypertension or hypoxia are all risk factors for cerebral haemorrhage. Midwives need to closely monitor the fetus during a preterm labour for early signs of any degree of compromise. It should be remembered that the fetus does not pass meconium in utero prior to 34 weeks' gestation, so clear liquor is not necessarily an indicator of fetal well-being. In the neonatal unit, it is important to prevent fluctuations of blood pressure and heart rate, through gentle handling and good pain management.

Management Perinatal management is centred on preventing the occurrence of a major PVH or the extension of an existing bleed. It may be possible to prevent further haemorrhage by providing excellent postnatal supportive care, including control of blood pressure, blood gases and coagulation. The prevention of asphyxia at delivery and of respiratory failure at any time is crucial. Active resuscitation of all very low birthweight babies at birth and elective ventilation of most of these babies has proved helpful. Prevention of pneumothoraces is another factor of great importance – as episodes of deterioration associated with a pneumothorax lead to the extension of PVH.

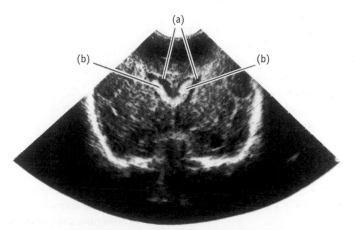

Figure 34.6 Coronal cranial ultrasound showing intraventricular haemorrhages (b) in dilated lateral ventricles (a). (From Kelnar et al., 1995.)

Complications Complications of PVH include shock, disseminated intravascular coagulation and pressure on parts of the brain linked with the autonomic system, thereby influencing respiration, blood pressure and temperature control. Hydrocephalus develops when blood in the ventricles clots and obstructs the flow of cerebrospinal fluid, or when the viscosity of the cerebrospinal fluid is altered by debris from the haemorrhage. Certain drugs can reduce the rate of cerebrospinal fluid production, thereby reducing hydrocephalus. Regular lumbar punctures may be performed to relieve excess pressure, but if the problem persists the surgical insertion of ventricular shunts may be necessary, to drain the fluid into the abdomen.

There is still a high incidence of cerebral palsy associated with periventricular cysts, but the prophylactic use of antenatal steroids has significantly reduced the incidence by more than 50% in preterm babies (Canterino *et al.*, 2001).

Anaemia

Anaemia is common in preterm babies. The shorter intrauterine period prevents the accumulation of an adequate iron store and the immature gastrointestinal system does not easily digest iron supplements. The underactive bone marrow is unable to keep up sufficient red blood cell production to match the rapid rate of growth and increase in circulation. Ill babies require frequent blood tests and may have had much blood removed for sampling. Blood transfusions are often necessary, although some babies make good progress in spite of a low haemoglobin level.

Vitamin K deficiency bleeding (VKDB)

Newborn babies are at risk of developing this haemorrhagic disease, previously known as haemorrhagic disease of the newborn (HDN) (Sutor *et al.*, 1999). It is caused by an accentuation of the normal neonatal deficiency of the vitamin K-dependent clotting factors, including prothrombin and factors VII, IX and X. Vitamin K is synthesized by the gut flora, which does not colonize until feeding has been established. There is substantially more vitamin K in formula milk than breast milk.

VKDB is classified according to the timing of onset:

- Early: within the first 24 hours
- Classic: 1–7 days
- Late: 8 days – 6 months.

Early VKDB is rare and is seen in babies of mothers taking certain drugs, such as vitamin K-antagonist anticoagulants (warfarin), some antituberculosis medication (isonazid) and some anticonvulsants (phenobarbital or phenytoin). At booking, the midwife should ask about any medicines the mother is taking and refer her to an obstetrician to review these. Unlike warfarin, heparin does not cross the placenta and is the anticoagulant of choice during pregnancy, particularly in the third trimester. In addition, women who continue these medications require oral vitamin K supplementation for the last couple of weeks of their pregnancy, as a prophylaxis. An unexpected preterm labour therefore results in a baby who is much more at risk of VKDB. Early VKDB is not preventable by postnatal vitamin K administration.

Classic VKDB is preventable by the recommended schedule of vitamin K 1 mg intramuscularly at birth (Puckett and Offringa, 2002).

Late VKDB occurs almost exclusively in breastfed babies and is more likely to present as intraventricular or pulmonary bleeding than gastrointestinal, with an associated high morbidity rate of up to 33% (Bor *et al.*, 2000). The cause is multifactorial, often related to hepatic disease or malabsorption syndrome. Repeated transfusions of blood, plasma and/or clotting factors are given and vitamin K is administered, in an attempt to treat the condition successfully.

Prophylactic vitamin K is recommended for all neonates at birth, although the optimal route, dosage and frequency of administration are still subject to debate (Autret-Leca and Jonville-Bera, 2001). The considerations centre on the efficacy of prophylaxis for the different classifications of VKDB, the most efficient regime for high-risk babies and the possible link between intramuscular administration and a potential increased risk of childhood leukaemia (Roman *et al.*, 2002). Midwives need to discuss individual risk factors with parents and obtain informed consent for vitamin K administration.

Repeated oral dosage requires compliance from parents to be effective and has not yet undergone randomized controlled trials to assess efficiency against classic or late VKDB (Puckett and Offringa, 2002). A commonly used regime is 2 mg oral vitamin K at birth, repeated for breastfed babies on day 7 and again at 6 weeks of age. The midwife needs to ensure these are documented clearly.

Babies in the high-risk group include those born with VLBW, preterm, hypoxic or as a result of a difficult or instrumental delivery. Currently, vitamin K 1 mg given intramuscularly, perinatally is recommended for this group (Sutor *et al.*, 1999).

Retinopathy of prematurity (ROP)

ROP is a disease of the developing retinal blood vessels and is a major complication for preterm and low birthweight babies surviving neonatal intensive care. Over recent years the incidence has increased as greater numbers of low birthweight babies are surviving (Whitfill and Drack, 2000). One major risk factor is oxygen exposure in excessive or fluctuating quantities. This results in retinal hyperoxia, which causes normal vascularization to cease. Following this there is a *rebound retinal hypoxia*, which stimulates the growth of new, but abnormal, blood vessels in the retina and these extend into the vitreous body. In advanced stages, opaque, fibrous tissue forms in the vitreous body, behind the lens, and retinal detachment may ensue. Visual impairment or total blindness are the worst outcomes.

Babies born before 32 weeks and those under 1000 g birthweight are at the greatest risk, with ROP rates of up to 60% in this latter group (Termote *et al.*, 2000). Screening programmes focus on these babies and involve regular checks by an ophthalmologist, until they are term.

Preventive care involves reducing the incidence of preterm and low birthweight babies and continuing with high-quality, controlled neonatal intensive care. Various treatments have been tried, but success is limited. Vitamin E supplementation and the reduction of ambient light have proved ineffective, but surfactant therapy has been shown to decrease the risk of severe ROP (Termote *et al.*, 2000).

Interventions that have been shown to be effective in some cases include cryotherapy and laser ablation, but generally, poor outcomes still persist. Microsurgical techniques have also had some limited success. Research continues into the environmental factors of the neonatal intensive care unit (NICU) that could be manipulated to have an impact on this disease.

Necrotizing enterocolitis (NEC)

Necrotizing enterocolitis is an inflammatory disease of the bowel normally associated with septicaemia. It is thought to occur as a result of bacteria proliferating in the bowel and then penetrating the wall at points where it has suffered ischaemic damage. Oedema, ulceration and haemorrhages of the bowel wall are found, which may progress to perforation or peritonitis.

The condition typically develops in preterm and low birthweight babies who have been ill with asphyxia, respiratory distress, hypoglycaemia, hypothermia or cardiovascular disease. Predisposing factors include variations in bowel perfusion associated with exchange transfusion, hypotension, patent ductus arteriosus, polycythaemia (when the blood is too thick to flow readily) and thrombosis or spasm of the mesenteric vessels from an umbilical catheter.

The problem usually manifests itself within a few days of starting milk feeds, as it is then that colonization of the intestine is more likely. It may present with non-specific malaise and indications of sepsis, with apnoea or septic shock or with abdominal signs such as distension, bile-stained aspirate or the passage of blood and mucus per rectum. The diagnosis is confirmed by the appearance of the bowel on radiography (Fig. 34.7). This will show thickening of the bowel wall due to oedema, a pattern of bowel obstruction, excessive or deficient quantities of gas within the bowel or the presence of gas bubbles in the bowel wall. This last feature is diagnostic of necrotizing enterocolitis.

Breast milk does afford some protection against NEC (Dai and Walker, 1999) and is the milk of choice when commencing feeds. If any baby develops early signs of sepsis or of NEC in particular, milk feeds must be stopped, parenteral nutrition resumed, infection screening performed and antibiotics commenced. Isolation may be used to prevent cross-infection. Further radiographs will be required to detect any early signs of bowel perforation.

Surgery is required in cases of bowel perforation but extensive resection leads to problems of short bowel malabsorption syndrome. Another possible late complication is stricture of the bowel as a result of scar formation and this may also require surgical treatment.

Necrotizing enterocolitis is now one of the commonest causes of neonatal surgery and is associated with a mortality of up to 40%. It is therefore essential to try to prevent the onset of the condition where possible or, failing that, to detect the earliest signs so that early treatment can be instigated to prevent extensive damage and long-term problems. Midwives should promote breastfeeding for all babies, but it is particularly important for sick, low birthweight and preterm babies. Human milk banks are increasing in number again in the UK, enabling the usage of appropriately screened and treated donor breast milk.

The neonatal intensive care unit (NICU) environment

The NICU is a busy, bright, harsh and noisy environment that could not be further from the circumstances experienced in utero. One of the aims of neonatal care is to achieve similar rates of growth and development

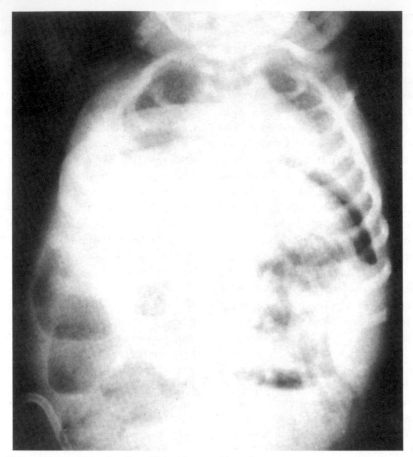

Figure 34.7   Necrotizing enterocolitis showing dilated loops of bowel.

of the baby to those that would have been attained in utero, and practitioners need to be aware of the impact of surroundings, interventions, care and treatments undertaken for the neonate's well-being.

Developmental care programmes are practised in many units, giving consideration to control of external stimuli, clustering of nursing activities and positioning of the neonates, particularly the preterm. There are many reports regarding the effects of high-intensity noise levels (Graven, 2000), night and day patterns (Rivkees and Hao, 2000), minimal handling (Slevin *et al.*, 2000) and the impact of the NICU in general on the neonate (Blackburn, 1998).

Such interventional programmes appear to demonstrate some benefits to preterm babies in terms of short-term growth, decreased respiratory support, decreased length of hospital stay and improved neurological outcomes at 2 years corrected age (Symington and Pinelli, 2001). However, many studies into developmental care have small sample sizes and include multiple interventions, making interpretation difficult.

SMALL-FOR-GESTATIONAL-AGE (SGA) BABIES

Incidence

One-third of all babies of low birthweight fall into this category and the majority of SGA babies are mature, having a gestational age of 37 weeks or more.

Causes

It is not uncommon for preterm babies to also be SGA and many of the predisposing factors are the same in both situations.

In many cases of placental insufficiency and subsequent SGA, there is no cause identified. However, this condition occurs more commonly in mothers in social classes IV and V and the effects of socioeconomic factors are great.

The growing fetus is entirely dependent upon the placenta for nutrition, elimination and respiratory exchange. Placental dysfunction is associated with maternal diseases such as pre-eclampsia, essential hypertension, chronic renal failure and nephritis. In all these conditions, spasm of the spiral arterioles reduces the intervillous blood flow and so reduces the exchange of nutrients and oxygen across the placental barrier. Other maternal conditions such as severe anaemia, as found in sickle cell disease, and phenylketonuria are also associated with SGA babies.

Following threatened abortion or antepartum haemorrhage, the fetus has to exist on less placental tissue and therefore fetal growth is likely to be restricted. SGA babies are common in multiple births, where there is an unequal distribution of placental flow or tissue.

Many substances, viruses and drugs, either prescribed or abused, have a small molecular size, allowing them to pass freely across the placental barrier where they may have a teratogenic or toxic effect, resulting in reduced growth. These include nicotine, alcohol, rubella, toxoplasmosis, cytomegalovirus, some steroids, anticonvulsants, antihypertensives, cytotoxics, cocaine and heroin.

Characteristics

Owing to lack of subcutaneous fat, the head appears large in relation to the wasted appearance of the body and limbs. The ribs are easily visible and the abdomen hollowed. The skin tends to be dry and loose and may be peeling and stained with meconium. Similarly, the umbilical cord is thin and may also be meconium-stained. The baby often appears wizened and old with an anxious, wide-awake expression. Muscle tone is usually good and the baby is active and tends to suck a fist as though ravenously hungry. Neurological responses usually correspond to gestational age.

Babies who are SGA are categorized into two groups according to whether they are affected by asymmetrical or symmetrical growth restriction.

Asymmetrical growth restriction

In cases of asymmetrical growth restriction, growth is normal until about the third trimester of pregnancy when complications such as pre-eclampsia develop. These adversely affect placental function and thereby lead to reduced growth as a result of malnutrition. It is thus a relatively late phenomenon and the degree of growth restriction depends on the severity of the causative condition.

The head circumference and length are within normal limits for the gestational age of the baby, but birthweight is low in proportion to head circumference when plotted on a centile chart.

Symmetrical growth restriction

The main underlying causes of symmetrical growth restriction are early intrauterine infections, such as cytomegalovirus, rubella or toxoplasmosis, maternal substance abuse (e.g. fetal alcohol syndrome) and other drugs taken early in the pregnancy. As described above, these have a toxic or teratogenic affect on the placenta, and fetal growth is therefore affected from the time these substances were introduced in the pregnancy. Some chromosomal anomalies and malformations also result in symmetrical SGA babies.

The appearance of the baby is similar to that described above, but the head circumference is in proportion to the overall size and weight. The prognosis for these babies is poorer than those asymmetrically grown, since they have been compromised for a much longer period.

Management

A detailed booking history is essential, as it may identify risk factors associated with intrauterine growth restriction (IUGR). Careful assessment of the uterine size and growth is important to enable early detection of a slow or reducing rate of growth of the fetus, possibly indicating the need for a more detailed assessment of fetal well-being.

A great deal of the care required by SGA babies in the first 48 hours following birth, centres around prevention and early recognition of any possible complications. In most cases, therefore, these babies can be cared for in normal postnatal wards with their mothers and do not need admission to a neonatal intensive or special care unit. Transitional care wards are an ideal place to care for those babies with minor problems such as poor temperature control.

Labour and delivery

The growth-restricted fetus is chronically hypoxic and consequently tolerates the stresses of labour and delivery poorly, as the blood supply to the placenta is further interrupted during each contraction. The midwife should anticipate the possibility of fetal distress and perinatal asphyxia. Close fetal monitoring and observation of the liquor for meconium during labour are imperative. A paediatrician should be present at the birth if the baby is known to be significantly small or compromised. Expert and urgent resuscitation is vital, if required, particularly if there is meconium-stained liquor. This will prevent further hypoxia and respiratory complications that may result in long-term neurological damage.

SGA babies have only a thin layer of subcutaneous fat and a relatively large surface area; they therefore lose heat very rapidly. The room temperature must be raised prior to delivery and the baby dried and wrapped in warm blankets quickly following birth. Since 80% of heat loss occurs through the head, a hat should be placed on the baby once the head is dry.

If the baby is well enough, early feeding is important as hypoglycaemia is a common result of insufficient energy stores in these babies.

Complications

Hypoxic ischaemic encephalopathy (HIE) (birth asphyxia)

This condition is mainly avoidable in countries with good antenatal care. The midwife must facilitate close and careful monitoring during labour and early intervention to expedite delivery in the event of fetal distress. Even modern methods of assessing fetal well-being are relatively insensitive and the midwife needs to be vigilant. SGA babies have limited reserves to cope with perinatal asphyxia and are at high risk. Mild symptoms of HIE may resolve after a few days with little or no residual cerebral damage. More severe injuries may result in neonatal fits and cerebral palsy.

Meconium aspiration syndrome

SGA babies do not tolerate perinatal stress and hypoxia well. Hypoxia causes relaxation of the anal sphincter allowing meconium to be passed into the liquor. Asphyxiated fetuses gasp in utero and will inhale the liquor and meconium into the bronchial tree, then further into the trachea, with the first breath at delivery. This clogs the lungs and commonly leads to pneumonitis, pneumothoraces or a secondary bacterial pneumonia.

Skilled resuscitation at delivery is vital. If the baby *does not breathe*, the nares and oropharynx should be suctioned prior to bag and mask resuscitation. If examination with a laryngoscope (which must be undertaken by a skilled practitioner) shows meconium in the larynx, the baby should be intubated and the trachea suctioned through the endotracheal tube. If the baby *does breathe* spontaneously and is vigorous, suction and intubation are unlikely to be helpful. Close observation of the baby is imperative for the first 24 hours following meconium staining of the liquor, to identify early signs of any respiratory problems or infection.

Hypothermia

As with preterm babies, the growth-restricted baby has a deficit of both subcutaneous and brown fat. Hypothermia is a risk because of the relatively high surface-area-to-bodyweight ratio. It is critical that the baby is dried and wrapped quickly following birth and the axillary temperature monitored carefully in the first 48 hours. If necessary, the baby may be nursed in an incubator next to the mother in the postnatal or transitional care ward. Skin-to-skin contact with the mother may help to maintain and stabilize the temperature.

Hypoglycaemia

This is a common problem for SGA babies and in most cases can be prevented with early and regular feeding. These babies particularly benefit from the advantages afforded by breastfeeding, as they are also at a greater risk of neonatal necrotizing enterocolitis. Low birthweight formula milks are now widely used with the advantage for these small babies that they are more energy-dense than regular formula milk.

SGA babies have small livers and correspondingly small glycogen stores. Large proportions of these energy reserves are used during labour, particularly if it is prolonged or difficult. Asphyxia and hypothermia will exacerbate the problem of hypoglycaemia. Frequent recordings of the blood glucose level are important within the first 48 hours, at least 4-hourly until they are stable and maintained above 2.6 mmol/l.

Polycythaemia

This is defined as a venous packed cell volume of >65% and occurs in these small babies as a consequence of chronic intrauterine hypoxia. To improve the oxygen-carrying capacity of the blood, the haemoglobin level may have risen to more than 20 g/dl. Haemoconcentration takes place, leading to a high proportion of red blood cells and therefore increased viscosity of the blood. This situation results in high jaundice levels and, in extreme cases, cerebral irritation may result. In this event an exchange plasma transfusion may be necessary, where 20–30 ml/kg of arterial blood is removed and replaced with fresh plasma into a peripheral vein. The viscosity of the blood is reduced and this can help to alleviate some of the symptoms of respiratory distress and cerebral irritation.

Polycythaemia is also a risk factor for necrotizing enterocolitis, especially when combined with perinatal asphyxia. The introduction of feeds is therefore often delayed in low birthweight SGA babies and intravenous fluids prescribed to prevent dehydration and hypoglycaemia.

Poor feeding

This is not usually a problem for asymmetrically growth-restricted babies, who tend to feed eagerly and thrive from birth. Symmetrically growth-restricted babies, however, who have been starved for a prolonged period in utero, often continue the slow rate of growth postnatally and may remain small, although a degree of catch-up growth is often evident.

Pulmonary haemorrhage

This rare complication associated with small babies has an uncertain aetiology. It may be due to left ventricular failure or a coagulation disorder, but appears to be largely preventable by eliminating other risk factors such as hypoglycaemia, perinatal asphyxia and hypothermia.

Substance abuse

Babies born to substance-abusing mothers are often growth restricted, particularly following the prolonged use of heroin, alcohol and nicotine (Bennett, 1999). It is often very difficult to obtain an honest and accurate history of drugs taken during pregnancy from the woman. These babies, as well as being at risk of withdrawal symptoms and future developmental problems, are often poor at withstanding labour and may suffer perinatal hypoxia, with all its added complications.

It is important that the baby of a narcotic-abusing mother is *not* given neonatal naloxone during resuscitation, as this will initiate rapid withdrawal symptoms as any narcotics in the baby's circulation are rapidly broken down. Implementing a scoring system for the frequency and severity of withdrawal symptoms, such as hyperactivity, irritability, high-pitched cry, sneezing and poor feeding, provides a framework for levels of treatment and interventions. These include nursing in quiet darkened surroundings, swaddling, and possibly medication.

FOLLOW-UP CARE FOR SMALL AND PRETERM BABIES

The paediatrician usually follows up preterm and SGA babies after discharge from hospital to assess progress, development, and general condition. Midwives, health visitors and general practitioners will see the infant more frequently and have a big role to play in the early recognition of associated complications, or deviations from normal development. It is important to be familiar with perinatal events, to enable vigilance relative to specific problems. Symmetrically growth restricted and neurologically damaged babies will need particularly close follow-up for several years in paediatric outpatient clinics.

Hearing must be carefully checked and most neonatal units now perform hearing tests routinely for preterm, sick and SGA babies. Babies are at particular risk of hearing impairment if they have experienced hypoxia, sepsis, hyperbilirubinaemia or received certain drugs (e.g. gentamicin, furosemide (frusemide)).

Some areas now employ specialized NICU liaison nurses or midwives to monitor these small babies in the community. They offer advice and support to the parents and other health professionals, maintain continuity of advice and prevent readmission to hospital by early recognition and treatment of minor problems.

Outcomes

Low birthweight babies have an increased risk of long-term problems, including a higher incidence of sudden infant death syndrome. With recent advances and developments in neonatal care, babies above 32 weeks' gestation and above 1500 g now have a much greater chance of intact survival than previously.

However, although the number of very low birthweight babies surviving is increasing, the percentage with major disabilities appears to have changed little. Continuing studies into the mortality and morbidity rates for this group of babies may help to identify significant perinatal findings that will enable a more accurate prediction of outcomes to be made.

The prognosis is dependent on many factors, including the cause of prematurity or poor growth and the severity and duration of any complications experienced. The effects of prematurity and intrauterine growth restriction differ; preterm babies generally display more motor deficits, whilst SGA babies have poorer cognitive skills.

45% of preterm babies showing neurological abnormalities in the neonatal period still show abnormalities at the age of 8 years (McGrath *et al.*, 2000). Studies have shown that over 50% of infants under 26 weeks' gestation still require oxygen at their due date, 14% have required treatment for ROP and 17% have PVL or hydrocephalus (Costeloe *et al.*, 2000).

In one small study, one-third of babies born at 23[+3] weeks' gestation survived to be discharged from hospital, but none were free from substantial morbidity, most commonly PVL, chronic lung disease, ROP or NEC (McElrath *et al.*, 2001).

The brain undergoes a growth spurt during the last trimester of pregnancy and is therefore particularly vulnerable to neurological damage at this time, as a result of prolonged or severe hypoxia and malnutrition. The outcome for SGA infants is not as good as that of babies of the same weight or gestation who are appropriately grown (Gutbrod *et al.*, 2000). The perinatal mortality rate increases with decreasing birthweight, regardless of gestation.

Epidemiological studies have demonstrated SGA babies to be at an increased risk in adult life of coronary heart disease and strokes (Rich-Edwards *et al.*, 1997); showing that poor intrauterine growth has major implications for mortality and morbidity throughout an individual's life.

The midwife can play a crucial role in health education and informed encouragement to reduce risk factors for prematurity and growth restriction, both preconceptually and during the antenatal period.

ETHICAL ISSUES

Complex ethical issues arise in the care of very preterm and VLBW babies, especially when complications substantially increasing the risk of long-term handicap arise, or if chromosomal abnormalities or major congenital malformations are present. A significant number of these babies die despite the efforts made to save them. Difficult decisions arise when the baby is surviving solely because of the supportive care being given, yet the risk of handicap is known to be extremely high. Both professionals and parents then need time to discuss the situation openly. Space is required to reflect on the possible consequences of continuing full intensive care as long as it is required, or of withdrawing such care to allow the baby to die in peace and dignity. This is one of the most agonizing and difficult decisions

both parents and professionals have to face. Having decided on what appears to be the best course of action, it is important for parents to accept that they made the best decision possible given the information and advice available at the time. Situations change and retrospectively they may be besieged by doubts and intense feelings of guilt if their baby dies, or perhaps survives despite discontinuing intensive care, and is severely handicapped.

Cultural factors and the individual's personal values and beliefs are deeply challenged at times like this and will influence the decisions made. Sometimes parents appreciate the opportunity to discuss the situation with a minister of religion, or with a counsellor who is not directly involved in the care of their baby. Such help can be invaluable during this extremely stressful period.

CONCLUSION

Many mothers feel extremely guilty when they give birth to a preterm or low birthweight baby, often blaming themselves for actions taken or omitted during the pregnancy. Midwives must offer as much support as possible during these times.

Individuals react differently to stress and midwives and neonatal staff need to learn to recognize the signs in parents and develop appropriate skills to enable families to cope during this difficult time. They must also recognize the signs of stress in themselves and in colleagues. Opportunities to share and discuss problems can be of immense benefit to all concerned. Effective personal coping strategies are therefore essential for those working with families with preterm, sick and VLBW babies.

Midwives are a key part of the team providing care to these small babies and their parents, and need to work closely with their colleagues to ensure a seamless, sensitive and high-quality service both initially and on a long-term basis.

KEY POINTS

- The causes of preterm labour and low birthweight are closely linked, with social factors playing a large role.
- Breastfeeding can make a significant difference to the short- and long-term health of these groups of babies, reducing the risk of complications associated with their small size or early gestation.

- Parents will require much support from the midwife, both practical and psychological, when they give birth to a very small or preterm baby. Close liaison between hospital and community staff is vital.

REFERENCES

Autret-Leca, E. & Jonville-Bera, A.P. (2001) Vitamin K in neonates: how to administer, when and to whom. *Paediatric Drugs* 3(1): 1–8.

Bennett, A.D. (1999) Perinatal substance abuse and the drug-exposed neonate. *Advance for Nurse Practitioners* 7(5): 32–36.

Blackburn S. (1998) Environmental impact of the NICU on developmental outcomes. *Journal of Pediatric Nursing* 13(5): 279–289.

Blackburn, S.T. (2003) *Maternal, Fetal and Neonatal Physiology: A Clinical Perspective*. Philadelphia: W.B. Saunders.

Bor, O., Akgun, N., Yakut, A. *et al.* (2000) Late haemorrhagic disease of the newborn. *Pediatrics International* 42(1): 64–66.

Canterino, J.C., Verma, U., Visintainer, P.F. *et al.* (2001) Antenatal steroids and neonatal periventricular leukomalacia. *Obstetrics and Gynecology* 97(1): 135–139.

Cooke, R.W.I. (1999) Trends in incidence of cranial ultrasound lesions and cerebral palsy in very low birthweight infants 1982–93. *Archives of Disease in Childhood Fetal and Neonatal Edition* 80(2): F115–117.

Cornblath, M., Hawdon, J.M., Williams, A.F. *et al.* (2000) Controversies regarding the definition of neonatal hypoglycaemia: suggested operational thresholds. *Pediatrics* 105(5): 1141–1145.

Costeloe, K., Hennessy, E., Gibson, A.T. *et al.* (2000) The EPICure study: outcomes to discharge from hospital for infants born at the threshold of viability. *Pediatrics* 106(4): 659–671.

Dai, D. & Walker, W.A. (1999) Protective nutrients and bacterial colonization in the immature human gut. *Advances in Pediatrics* 46: 353–382.

Dubowitz, L.M.S., Dubowitz, V. & Goldberg, C. (1970) Clinical assessment of gestational age in the newborn infant. *Journal of Pediatrics* 77(1): 1–10.

Duvanel, C.B., Fawer, C-L., Cotting, J. *et al.* (1999) Long-term effects of neonatal hypoglycaemia on brain growth and psychomotor development in small-for-gestational-age preterm infants. *Journal of Pediatrics* 134(4): 492–498.

Graven, S.N. (2000) Sound and the developing infant in the NICU: conclusions and recommendations for care. *Journal of Perinatology* 20(8 Pt 2): S88–93.

Gutbrod, T., Wolke, D., Soehne, B. *et al.* (2000) Effects of gestation and birth weight on the growth and development of very low birthweight small for gestational age infants: a matched group comparison. *Archives of Disease in Childhood Fetal and Neonatal Edition* 82(3): F208–214.

Hafstrom, M. & Kjellmer, I. (2000) Non-nutritive sucking in the healthy pre-term infant. *Early Human Development* 60(1): 13–24.

Hanson, L.A. (1999) Human milk and host defence: immediate and long-term effects. *Acta Pediatrica* (Suppl.) 88(430): 42–46.

Horwood, L.J., Darlow, B.A. & Mogridge, N. (2001) Breast milk feeding and cognitive ability at 7–8 years. *Archives of Disease in Childhood Fetal and Neonatal Edition* 84(1): F23–27.

Johnston, P.G.B., Flood, K. & Spinks, K. (2003) *The Newborn Child*, 9th edn. Edinburgh: Churchill Livingstone.

Kelnar, C.J.H., Harvey, D. & Simpson, C. (1995) *The Sick Newborn Baby*, 3rd edn. London: Baillière Tindall.

McElrath, T.F., Robinson, J.N., Ecker, J.L. *et al.* (2001) Neonatal outcome of infants born at 23 weeks' gestation. *Obstetrics and Gynecology* 97(1): 49–52.

McGrath, M.M., Sullivan, M.C., Lester, B.M. *et al.* (2000) Longitudinal neurological follow-up in neonatal intensive care unit survivors with various neonatal morbidities. *Pediatrics* 106(6): 1397–1405.

Mencher L.S. & Mencher G.T. (1999) Neonatal asphyxia, definitive markers and hearing loss. *Audiology* 38(6): 291–295.

Office for National Statistics (ONS) (2000a) *Birth Statistics 1999*. Series FM1, No. 28. London: The Stationery Office.

Office for National Statistics (ONS) (2000b) *Live births, stillbirths and linked infant deaths: birthweight by age of mother, numbers and rates, 1999*. Series DH3, No. 32. London: The Stationery Office.

Pinelli, J. & Symington, A. (2000) Non-nutritive sucking for promoting physiologic stability and nutrition in preterm infants. *Cochrane Database of Systematic Reviews* (2): CD001071. Oxford: Update Software.

Puckett, R.M. & Offringa, M. (2002) Prophylactic vitamin K for vitamin K deficiency bleeding in neonates. *Cochrane Database of Systematic Reviews* (4). Oxford: Update Software.

Rich-Edwards, J.W., Stampfer, M.J., Manson, J.E. *et al.* (1997) Birth weight and risk of cardiovascular disease in a cohort of women followed up since 1976. *British Medical Journal* 315(7105): 396–400.

Rivkees, S.A. & Hao, H. (2000) Developing circadian rhythmicity. *Seminars in Perinatology* 24(4): 232–242.

Roman, E., Fear, N.T., Ansell, P. *et al.* (2002) Vitamin K and childhood cancer: analysis of individual patient data from six case-controlled studies. *British Journal of Cancer* 86(1): 63–69.

Slevin, M., Farrington, N., Duffy, G. *et al.* (2000) Altering the NICU and measuring infants' responses. *Acta Pediatrica* 89(5): 577–581.

Stevenson, D.K., Wright, L.L., Lemons, J.A. *et al.* (1998) Very low birth weight outcomes of the National Institute of Child Health and Human Development Neonatal Research Network. *American Journal of Obstetrics and Gynecology* 179(6 Pt 1): 1632–1639.

Sutor, A.H., von Kries, R., Cornelissen, E.A. *et al.* (1999) Vitamin K deficiency bleeding (VKDB) in infancy. ISTH Pediatric/Perinatal Subcommittee. International Society on Thrombosis and Haemostasis. *Thrombosis and Haemostasis* **81**(3): 456–461.

Symington, A. & Pinelli, J. (2001) Developmental care for promoting development and preventing morbidity in preterm infants. *Cochrane Database of Systematic Reviews*, Issue 1. Oxford: Update Software.

Termote, J., Schalij-Delfos, N.E., Brouwers, H.A. *et al.* (2000). New developments in neonatology: less severe retinopathy of prematurity? *Journal of Pediatric Ophthalmology and Strabismus* **37**(3): 142–148.

Whitfill, C.R. & Drack, A.V. (2000) Avoidance and treatment of retinopathy of prematurity. *Seminars in Pediatric Surgery* **9**(2): 103–105.

World Health Organization (WHO) (1977) *Manual of International Statistical Classification of Diseases, Injuries and Causes of Death*, Vol. I. : Geneva. WHO

FURTHER READING

Goldson, E. (1999) *Nurturing the Premature Infant: Developmental Interventions in the Neonatal Intensive Care Nursery.* Oxford: Oxford University Press.
A very helpful text detailing some of the research into managing small and preterm babies in neonatal units.

Lang, S. (2002) *Breastfeeding Special Care Babies*, 2nd edn. London: W.B. Saunders.
A helpful guide including the physiology, management and support of breastfeeding the baby requiring special care.

Roberton, N.R.C. & Rennie, J. (2001) *A Manual of Neonatal Intensive Care.* London: Hodder Arnold.
This is a useful reference book for explaining the management of babies requiring intensive care.

35

Respiratory and Cardiac Disorders

Carol Simpson

LEARNING OUTCOMES

After reading this chapter you will be able to:

- have an understanding of fetal circulation and the circulatory and respiratory changes at birth
- appreciate the factors involved in the initiation and establishment of respiration
- describe the actions to be taken when resuscitating a neonate
- describe the aetiology of cardiac lesions

- be aware of the most common types of cardiac lesions and their prognosis
- discuss the most common cardiac investigations in the neonatal period
- have an overview of some of the common neonatal respiratory disorders.

INTRODUCTION

The neonate has to make significant adaptations in the transition from fetal to independent life. It is important that midwives understand the anatomy and physiology of the fetal circulation and its linkage with the respiratory system. They need to appreciate and recognize the momentous changes made at transition. This allows a validation of normality and swift recognition of potential problems, which then can be managed appropriately and effectively. This chapter will review the anatomy and physiology, present the transitional changes, cover resuscitation of the newborn, and complete with some of the cardiac anomalies which midwives may meet in their practice.

FETAL CIRCULATION

In order to recognize and understand the presentation and implications of cardiac conditions, it is important for midwives to have an understanding of fetal circulation and the changes that take place after birth (see fetal circulation in Chs 14 and 31).

In utero the fetal lungs are filled with fluid and are not functional for gaseous exchange. The majority of the circulating blood is diverted through the heart, bypassing the lungs. Oxygenation, nutrition and elimination of toxins are the functions of the placenta.

Blood, rich in nutrients and oxygen, travels from the placenta via the *umbilical vein*, along the underside of the liver and links with the inferior vena cava via the *ductus venosus* (see Fig. 14.4, p. 210). The liver receives a minimal blood supply from a small branch of the umbilical vein, which joins the portal vein.

In the inferior vena cava, oxygenated blood from the umbilical vein mixes with deoxygenated blood returning to the heart from the lower limbs, then enters the right atrium. Most of this mixed blood bypasses the lungs, flowing through the *foramen ovale* (an aperture in the atrial septum), into the left atrium. It is then pumped into the left ventricle and out via the aorta, as normal.

Deoxygenated blood from the upper body returns to the right atrium, via the superior vena cava. From here it passes into the right ventricle, then out through the *ductus arteriosus* into the aorta. The flow of blood and high levels of circulating prostaglandins maintain the patency of the ductus. A small quantity of blood passes through the pulmonary artery to nourish the lung tissue.

From the aorta, the blood passes into the internal iliac arteries, which branch off to form the *hypogastric arteries* and return to the placenta. These are renamed the umbilical arteries once they enter the umbilical cord.

THE FETAL RESPIRATORY SYSTEM

At around 4–6 weeks' gestation, embryonic lung buds begin to differentiate and formation of the diaphragm begins. The lungs start as epithelial tubes surrounded by mesoderm and develop into primitive bronchioles and terminal air sacs by around 16 weeks. By 24–26 weeks the capillary network is growing and alveoli are forming from the terminal air sacs. The lungs are now capable of some gaseous exchange but this may still not be adequate to support life.

Fetal lung fluid is produced from about 13 weeks' gestation by the alveolar epithelium. It plays an important role in normal lung tissue development. From around 36 weeks, in preparation for the imminent changes at birth, evidence suggests there is either a reduction of lung fluid production or a diminished lung fluid volume (Kalache *et al.* 2002).

As development proceeds, the strength and frequency of fetal breathing movements increase from 11 weeks until they are present between 40–80% of the time by term. The biophysical profile, performed by ultrasound scan, uses the presence of one or more 30-second episodes of fetal breathing in 30 minutes, as one of five criteria to assess fetal well-being.

Surfactant

At about 22 weeks, *surfactant*, a complex lipoprotein, begins to be produced and secreted into the lung fluid by the alveolar epithelial cells. The two main functions of surfactant are to reduce the surface tension in the alveoli, allowing them to expand more easily, and to help prevent atelectasis at the end of expiration.

The amount of surfactant continues to increase until birth, with a surge in production at around 33–35 weeks' gestation, which explains why respiratory distress syndrome (RDS) is rarely seen in near-term babies. Severe anaemia, polyhydramnios, hypothyroidism, isoimmune disease, toxoplasmosis and renal disease can lead to the chemical structure being affected and making the surfactant less efficient in its functions.

Surfactant production is stimulated by the release of glucocorticosteroids during episodes of fetal stress, in situations such as severe intrauterine growth restriction, prolonged premature rupture of membranes, certain haemoglobinopathies and pre-eclampsia. In an attempt to copy this natural phenomenon and boost surfactant production, antenatal corticosteroids are given to mothers in preterm labour. This has been shown to reduce the incidence and severity of respiratory distress syndrome. However, evidence from animal studies suggests that repeated doses (i.e. more than the recommended two injections) are linked to possible neurological problems and an increased incidence of childhood onset of diabetes. Therefore using these drugs requires caution and informed consent from the mother, should more than one dose be used. A trial is currently underway to find the correct dose to be given. There remains controversy over whether repeated doses are more beneficial than a single dose (Murphy and Aghajafari, 2003).

Surfactant may be natural or artificial, with the two main sources of natural surfactant being bovine or porcine. Consideration must be given to the cultural and religious beliefs of families (e.g. Hindus and Muslims) and consent must be obtained from parents prior to using these therapies.

TRANSITION TO NEONATAL LIFE

At birth, with the first breath and expansion of the lungs, pulmonary vascular resistance falls, resulting in a five-fold increase in pulmonary circulation. This increases the blood flow from the lungs to the left atrium, raising the pressure on the left side of the heart and closing the *foramen ovale*, then known as the *fossa ovalis*.

The placental circulation ceases with its separation from the uterine wall. As blood stops flowing through the *umbilical vein*, *ductus venosus* and *hypogastric arteries*, these structures constrict and eventually close, as blood is redirected through the liver. These first two vessels become ligaments, the *ligamentum teres* and *ligamentum venosum*, whilst the *hypogastric arteries* become the *obliterated hypogastric arteries*.

As the vascular resistances change within the heart, blood flows from the right ventricle into the pulmonary artery, rather than through the ductus arteriosus. Prostaglandin levels fall sharply once the placenta is delivered and these factors together promote closure of the ductus arteriosus. In healthy term babies, closure takes between 15–24 hours, but preterm babies may have a patent ductus arteriosus (PDA) for many weeks. A characteristic PDA murmur is therefore a common finding at the initial midwife's examination, but should resolve after 24 hours.

The functional changes to these fetal structures take place within the first week of life. Complete anatomical closure of these vessels and pathways, however, may take many weeks to complete.

Establishing respiration

Transition from placental to pulmonary oxygenation at birth depends on the rapid removal of fetal lung fluid from the developing alveoli. Prior to birth there is around 80–100 ml of fluid in the lungs of a term, healthy fetus. It is displaced from the respiratory tract by several different mechanisms:

- Catecholamines are released at the commencement of labour because of stress in the woman, and this increases the absorption of lung fluid in early labour; and at birth an extra surge causes the lungs to switch from secretion to a rapid absorption of the remaining lung fluid. This mechanisms does not occur with elective lower segment caesarean section (LSCS) and thus babies born this way are not able to clear all the fluid. They may have retention of fluid causing transient tachypnoea of the newborn.
- Around one-third is squeezed out of the alveoli, into the upper respiratory tract, by the action of uterine contractions during labour and the passage of the fetal chest through the birth canal.
- As the chest is delivered, it expands, drawing in air, increasing the surface area of the lungs by expanding the alveoli and displacing a further third of the fluid volume.

During the latter part of labour the fetus is relatively hypoxic. Once the placenta separates, the oxygen content of the blood begins to decrease further, whilst carbon dioxide tension rises. This causes chemoreceptors in the carotid arteries to set up a reflex stimulus in the respiratory centre, causing the baby to inspire. The presence of surfactant aids the distension of the air sacs, facilitating the uptake of oxygen. In addition, peripheral stimulation from handling and the relatively cool temperatures of the birthing room, encourage the baby to take the first gasp.

With the clamping of the cord, right atrial pressure is reduced and left atrial pressure increased, resulting in closure of the foramen ovale. This ensures that blood is directed to the lungs for oxygenation, rather than the placenta, following birth. With increasing oxygenation, the pulmonary vascular resistance reduces and this, in turn, initiates closure of the ductus arteriosus.

Hypoxia is the main stimulant to inspiration, but in a minority of babies the degree of hypoxia is so great that it depresses rather than stimulates the respiratory centre and asphyxia occurs.

In order to maintain effective oxygenation there are four essentials:

1. clear air passages
2. adequate respiratory exchange in the alveoli, facilitated by alveolar expansion and lack of barriers between air and the epithelium
3. adequate circulation to transport oxygen to the vital centres
4. intact neurological system with an active respiratory centre (undamaged and unaffected by drugs).

The care given during labour and at delivery is all directed to this end.

ASPHYXIA

Asphyxia occurs when there is a depletion of oxygen and an accumulation of carbon dioxide in the bloodstream, leading to acidosis. Unless respiratory function is quickly established the degree of asphyxia will continue to worsen. In many instances, this condition can be anticipated by events during labour. It is imperative at all births that at least one staff member present is proficient in neonatal resuscitation. All midwives must maintain their resuscitation competency and skills, as this situation may present unexpectedly.

Causes

- Preterm birth:
  - inadequate surfactant
  - weak respiratory muscles
  - immature respiratory system.
- Obstruction:
  - trachea and bronchi blocked by mucus, meconium, blood or liquor
  - aspiration of any of these substances into the alveoli
  - structural anomalies, such as choanal atresia.
- Certain drugs – respiratory depression from general anaesthetic, sedatives or narcotics.
- Congenital anomalies – hypoplastic lungs, anencephaly, diaphragmatic hernia.
- Cerebral damage – trauma or congenital anomalies.
- Infection – severe septicaemia or congenital pneumonia.
- Haemorrhage – resulting in hypovolaemic shock or raised intracranial pressure.
- Pneumothorax – resulting from over-vigorous resuscitation or meconium aspiration.
- Pharyngeal suctioning – may cause a reflex apnoea

Primary and secondary apnoea

Previously, birth asphyxia was classified according to the colour of the baby (blue or white). Whilst this may be a good clinical indicator of the severity of respiratory depression, a more definitive and meaningful distinction is *primary* or *secondary* (*terminal*) *apnoea*.

Asphyxia in a fetus or neonate results in a well-defined sequence of events, with four characteristic phases if hypoxia is prolonged or ongoing:

1. a brief period of hyperventilation
2. primary apnoea – respiratory effort ceases, heart rate falls, blood pressure rises gradually and the baby's tone decreases
3. deep, irregular gasping respirations, getting progressively weaker, further decrease in heart rate, falling blood pressure; the baby is virtually flaccid and takes a final gasp
4. terminal (secondary) apnoea – the baby is unresponsive to stimulation and the heart rate, blood pressure and oxygen levels in the blood continue to fall.

If resuscitation is instigated during a period of primary apnoea, with stimulation and exposure to oxygen, the baby will usually start breathing again. However, a baby in terminal (secondary) apnoea will die unless urgent, significant assisted ventilation and resuscitation measures, with oxygen, are commenced. The longer the delay before initiating resuscitation during this time, the longer it will take to establish respiration and the greater the risk of neurological damage.

As it is difficult to immediately distinguish between these two states, the midwife should always assume that a baby with a slow heart rate requires resuscitation and call for assistance and start appropriate resuscitative measures.

NEONATAL RESUSCITATION

Midwives must always be prepared for the possibility that the baby will require resuscitation at birth. All community midwives should carry a 500 ml resuscitation bag and mask system and 00 and 01 size masks, as part of their emergency equipment. Whilst severe birth asphyxia is uncommon in well-planned home births, unexpected births do occur in the community, often preterm or following a precipitate labour. If better equipment is not available, mouth–nose breathing should be attempted by the midwife. The baby's nostrils may be pinched to prevent air escaping through

> **Box 35.1 Equipment for resuscitation**
>
> - Area identified for resuscitation – table or resuscitaire
> - Source of warmth
> - Stethoscope
> - Source of oxygen
> - 500 ml self-inflating resuscitation bag with attached face mask sizes 0, 01
> - Suction unit and catheters 8 and 10 FG
> - Nasogastric tubes – 8 and 10 FG
> - Oropharyngeal airways 0, 00 and 000
> - Laryngoscope
> - Possibly endotracheal tubes 2.5, 3.0 and 3.5 sizes

the nose, if mouth-to-mouth resuscitation is preferred. Care should be taken that the breaths given are at an appropriate depth to avoid causing damage to lungs by overinflation.

Before each delivery the resuscitation equipment should be checked and prepared for use (see Box 35.1). Thorough antenatal assessments and careful monitoring during labour can help to identify those babies particularly at risk of perinatal asphyxia. These babies should be delivered in a tertiary unit, with immediate access to neonatal specialists. A neonatologist/paediatrician, neonatal nurse practitioner or midwife competent at neonatal resuscitation must be present at the birth where fetal distress is identified or suspected.

At birth, whatever the degree of asphyxia the initial treatment should be as follows (Resuscitation Council (UK), 2001):

- As the head is delivered onto the perineum, wipe the baby's face gently, to clear the nares and mouth of fluid or debris.
- **Call for assistance as early as possible.**
- Handle the baby gently and skilfully, and deliver into warm, dry towels. Since cold stress increases the oxygen requirements of a baby, the room temperature must be raised to 26 °C prior to delivery.
- While drying the baby assess the situation:
  - colour
  - tone
  - breathing
  - heart rate.
- **At regular intervals – usually after each cycle, assessment of the vital signs is undertaken – the ABC:**
  A   Airway

B Breathing: look at the rate and pattern of chest movement

C Circulation: listen for the heart rate with a stethoscope.

- Note the time as the baby is born and start the stop-watch if available, to enable the baby's condition to be assessed at specific times and recording made of the timing of any interventions.
- Clamp and cut the cord, ensuring that it is double clamped on the placental side, to facilitate accurate venous and arterial blood samples being taken for pH and gas analysis.
- Transfer the baby to the resuscitaire or prepared area in the home and place under a radiant heater, in the supine position, with the head nearest the resuscitator.
- Remove wet towels and rewrap in dry, prewarmed towels.
- Deep suction is no longer given to babies unless it is under direct vision, because suction can cause vagal stimulation, with reflex bradycardia and apnoea resulting. The aim of care should be to support and open the airway by positioning the baby.

Airway management

An important part of inflating the lungs is to use mask inflation successfully and this can only be achieved if the airway is sufficiently opened. The baby has a large occiput which may, when the baby is unconscious, force the chin towards the chest. The pharynx has a tendency to collapse and the tongue falls back and obstructs the airway. In order to open the airway the practitioner needs to undertake the following.

Opening the airway
- Place the baby on its back on a flat surface with a folded sheet (approx. 2 cm thickness) under the baby's shoulders, enabling the chin to be lifted off the chest.
- Hold the head in the neutral position with chin support (sniffing position) (see Fig. 35.1).
- Support the chin by using a finger on the bony part of the chin near the tip.

Bag and mask ventilation

Bag and mask ventilation is indicated if the baby is apnoeic or gasping; the heart rate is slow or around 100 beats per minute (b.p.m.) or less and falling. The Ambu-bag should have an oxygen reservoir, be

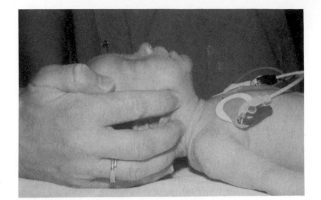

Figure 35.1 Neutral position. (Courtesy of UK Resuscitation Council.)

capable of providing 90–100% oxygen and *must* have a pressure-limiting valve attached. This reduces the risk of pneumothoraces from overinflation of the lungs. A range of face masks should be available and it is important to select the appropriate size, to ensure a good seal is formed around the nose and mouth.

The mask should then be applied – five inflation breaths are given, each lasting 2–3 seconds. Inflation breaths are like blowing up a balloon for the first time. Therefore, it is important to apply slow and sustained pressure by the Ambu-bag slowly and gently to effect a rise in the chest wall. If the Ambu-bag is squeezed forcefully and quickly the pressure-limiting device will become inoperable and pressure could reach above 60 cmH$_2$O.

The first two or three breaths will replace lung fluid with air without changing the volume of the chest; therefore the chest will not move until the fourth or fifth breath.

If the chest is moving and the heart rate is above 100 b.p.m continue to ventilate until the baby has a good tone, indicating that the acidosis has been reversed and the baby can continue to breathe spontaneously.

If the baby's chest is not moving and the heart rate is slow or falls, then other methods of opening the airway must be attempted.

Jaw thrust In the unconscious and asphyxiated baby the pharynx has a tendency to collapse and the tongue may block the airway. To clear the airway the practitioner gently pulls the jaw forward and also holds the baby's head in neutral position and maintains a good seal with the mask while the second person concentrates on providing five inflation breath

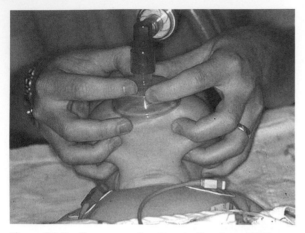

Figure 35.2   Two-person jaw thrust. (Courtesy of UK Resuscitation Council.)

either with the T piece or by squeezing the Ambu-bag (see Fig. 35.2).

Usually, if this method is used correctly the majority of babies will respond and begin to breathe spontaneously. However if the baby's chest is not moving and the heart rate is slow or falling, further action will be required.

Suction under direct vision and the insertion of a Guedel airway

If there is still no chest movement after five or six inflation breaths, the airway may be blocked. Visualization of the larynx and applying suction if necessary can be used at this point prior to introducing a Guedel airway, which will then maintain the airway. This does require the skill of using the laryngoscope.

The laryngoscope has been considered a part of advanced resuscitation and the skills to use it correctly have been partially lost. Most current resuscitation training includes the whole process from maintaining the airway through to using the laryngoscope for inserting airways and intubation where required.

The Guedel airway can be used if there is no second person to assist with the two-person jaw thrust. The airway should be measured from the middle of the mouth to the angle of the jaw, as it is crucial that the airway is the correct size and fit. The laryngoscope is used to aid the introduction of the airway, which should be inserted in the position that it will take in the baby's mouth. Inserting the airway upside down then turning it in the baby's mouth (as done for the adult or child) can damage the hard and soft palate of the newborn.

Following suction under direct vision and insertion of the airway, another five inflation breaths are given and the baby is assessed once again.

If the chest is still not moving, intubation is required.

Endotracheal intubation

Endotracheal intubation is indicated when prolonged bag-and-mask ventilation is required or ineffective, or when suctioning is required where meconium is present, or for resuscitation of a baby with a diaphragmatic hernia.

Significant damage can be caused to the baby's larynx by inexperienced attempts at intubation. Bag-and-mask ventilation is usually adequate, when performed correctly, to sustain respiration until further assistance is available. It is therefore not recommended that staff attempt intubation unless trained and competent at this procedure.

The laryngoscope is passed just beyond the base of the tongue to the posterior pharynx. As the blade is lifted, the epiglottis and glottis should come into view. If the epiglottis cannot be seen easily, gentle cricoid pressure may be applied, or the blade inserted further and lifted forward with slightly more firmness whilst it is slowly withdrawn. The epiglottis will then usually slip into view (Fig. 35.3). Further aspiration of fluid or mucus can then be carried out under direct vision.

An endotracheal tube (ETT) of the appropriate size should be introduced through the glottis. Markings on the side of the tube indicate the expected level of the vocal cords, giving a guide as to how far to advance the ETT. The laryngoscope can then be removed and the ETT connected to the resuscitation bag and oxygen supply.

Laryngeal mask airway (LMA)

The skill of intubation needs continuous practice and experience in order to undertake successful intubation within 30 seconds. If the procedure is taking longer, the practitioner needs to revert to giving five inflation breaths using the mask prior to attempting intubation once again.

If the chest is moving and the heart is slow, cardiac massage will need to be considered.

The LMA a relatively new device in neonatal resuscitation, not yet recommended for routine use as its efficacy is still being evaluated (Grein and Weiner, 2002). It consists of a small mask, inserted into the baby's mouth, with an inflatable cuff that seals off the oesophagus when blown up. In the middle of the mask is a silicone airway tube, which is positioned over the larynx and can be connected to a resuscitation bag or ventilator, as required. It does not allow the airway to

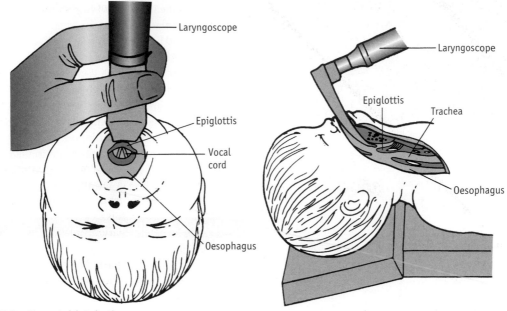

Figure 35.3 Neonatal intubation.

be suctioned once in place and is therefore not appropriate for use when meconium is present. It may, however, facilitate effective ventilation when bag-and-mask resuscitation is inadequate or it has not been possible to intubate the baby.

Cardiac massage (Box 35.2)

Irrespective of the heart rate, chest compression is useless if the chest is not moving and the lungs are not inflated. Therefore the lungs require inflation prior to cardiac massage being instigated in the ratio of 3 : 1 (3 compressions to 1 breath). The aim of cardiac massage is to apply appropriate chest compression and recoil in order to move the oxygenated blood from the pulmonary veins to the coronary arteries – a short distance of about 5 cm.

Assess ABC every 30 seconds. Unlike that of the adult, the baby's heart is usually a physiologically well organ and, as such, the aim is to 'bump start' the heart in the same way as the engine of a car with a flat battery. The heart needs to be made to beat in order to provide oxygen to the heart and vital centres. Once oxygen is supplied to the heart muscle, the heart rate and rhythm will improve.

Cardiac compressions should be commenced if the baby's heart rate is below 60 b.p.m., or is falling from a baseline of 60–100 b.p.m., despite 30 seconds of efficient ventilation with 100% oxygen being established.

Box 35.2 Cardiac massage technique

- Press down firmly and then release the pressure
- Aim to reduce the AP diameter of the chest by one-third with each compression.
- Pause briefly after each release allowing the blood to reach the coronary arteries.

There are two recommended methods, one using the tips of the middle and index fingers (Fig. 35.4B) and the other using the balls of the thumbs, whilst the hands encircle the baby's body (Fig. 35.4C). The former method is useful when there is only one person resuscitating. The latter method produces more efficient systolic pressure, but there is a risk of squeezing the baby too hard, causing internal injuries.

- Position the baby on a firm surface, with the neck slightly extended as for ventilation.
- Place two fingers, or the two thumbs, just below the middle of an imaginary line drawn between the baby's nipples, on the lower third of the sternum (Fig. 35.4A).
- Compress the sternum by a third of the depth of the chest, at a rate of three compressions to one breath every 2 seconds, resulting in 90 compressions and 30 ventilations per minute.

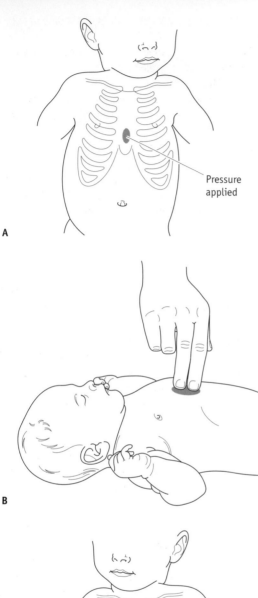

Pressure applied

A

B

C

Figure 35.4 Cardiac compression. **A.** Position for applying pressure. **B.** Using two fingers. **C.** Using two thumbs with the hands encircling the chest.

- Check the heart rate and respiratory effort every 30 seconds. If the heart rate is:
  - below 60 b.p.m., continue cardiac compressions and ventilation, consider drugs
  - 60 b.p.m. and falling, continue cardiac compressions and ventilation, commence drugs
  - 60 b.p.m. and increasing or above 60 b.p.m., discontinue cardiac compressions and assess the need for ongoing ventilation.

Resuscitative measures should be continued until further assistance arrives or the decision to discontinue is made by an attending doctor.

Reflective Activity 35.1

Have you attended a neonatal resuscitation update within the past 12 months? If not, ensure that you have booked in for the next available one.

Meconium

If meconium is present in the liquor, *whatever its consistency*, the following additional actions should be performed:

- If the baby is vigorous following birth, no further action is warranted. Tracheal suctioning under these circumstances is of limited value (Wisewell, 2000).
- If the baby is not breathing, intubation should be carried out (if possible with an ET tube designed for meconium aspiration), and direct suction applied to the endotracheal tube or as it is withdrawn from the airway. If the baby's condition permits, this may need to be repeated, until as much of the meconium as possible has been removed.
- If the practitioner is unable to intubate, the airway is cleared under direct vision and five inflation breaths undertaken. It is now known that in many cases, meconium will have been inhaled into the main bronchi and lungs during in-utero hypoxia. Therefore suction is unlikely to clear the lungs effectively. The aim should be to clear enough meconium to allow the passage of oxygen through to the lungs and thus the brain and main organs.
- Further resuscitation should then be commenced, following the steps as in Box 35.3.

The baby must be kept warm throughout. The parents should be comforted and kept informed of events. Apgar scores are assessed at 1 and 5 minutes of age and thereafter at 5-minute intervals until the baby is

---

Box 35.3 Steps to successful resuscitation

- Dry the baby and remove wet towel, take the baby to the resuscitation area and cover – assess as you dry.
- Call for help.
- Start the clock or stopwatch.
- Place the head in neutral position and give five inflation breaths.
- Assess ABC.
- If the chest is not moving and the heart is very slow
  - apply a small sheet under the baby's shoulder and provide five inflation breaths.
- Assess ABC.
- If the chest is not moving and the heart continues to be very slow
  - undertake a two-person jaw thrust and give five inflation breaths.
- Assess ABC.
- If the chest is not moving and the heart is very slow
  - suction under direct vision, measure and introduce in place a Guedel airway, and give five inflation breaths.
- Assess ABC.

- If the chest is not moving, intubate the baby and give five inflation breaths.
- Assess ABC.
- Once the chest is moving and the heart is slow
  - give cardiac massage at 3 : 1 ratio for 30 seconds.
- Assess ABC.
- If the chest is moving and the heart is above 60 b.p.m.
  - continue giving ventilation breaths, assessing every 30 seconds until the baby is PINK – HEART RATE FAST – BREATHING SPONTANEOUSLY – GOOD TONE.
- Stop ventilating, provide facial oxygen at 2 litres per minute.
- Assess ABC.
- If baby remains well
  - give the baby several minutes without handling to recover from the resuscitation process while you discuss with the parents what took place.
- Give baby to mother and handle gently. Remember the baby has undergone a major trauma – treat with respect.
- Complete record-keeping.

---

breathing spontaneously. The Apgar score at 5 minutes is considered of particular value in forecasting the long-term prognosis. Cord blood pH is also helpful in assessing the degree of intrapartum asphyxia.

Drugs and fluids in resuscitation

Naloxone hydrochloride (Narcan)

Respiratory depression may occur in the neonate as a result of narcotics (e.g. pethidine or morphine) given to the mother, most commonly within 4 hours of delivery. Narcan is *not* a resuscitative drug and thus it should not be used until the baby has been fully resuscitated and is able to sustain respirations. It is a narcotic antagonist, which can be administered to reverse the effects of narcotics. 0.1 mg/kg should be given via the umbilical vein or ETT for most rapid results, or intramuscularly for a slower effect.

Since narcotics have a longer half-life than naloxone, close observation of the baby is important to ensure that respiratory depression does not recur. Repeated doses may be required in this event. Once given, respiratory observations must be undertaken every 30–60 minutes until the baby is 6 hours of age.

Under no circumstances should Narcan be administered to the baby of an opiate-abusing mother, as it can precipitate a rapid withdrawal.

Adrenaline (epinephrine hydrochloride)

Adrenaline is a potent cardiac stimulant, given when the baby has no heart rate or when the heart rate remains below 60 b.p.m., following at least 30 seconds of ventilation and cardiac compressions. It increases the rate and strength of cardiac contractions and causes peripheral vasoconstriction. Adrenaline may be administered via the ETT or intravenously, at a dosage of 0.1–0.3 ml/kg of a 1 : 10 000 concentration solution. This can be repeated every 3–5 minutes, if necessary.

Volume expanders

These may be required in the event of a suspected, or actual, fetal or neonatal haemorrhage. Once delivered, the midwife should lower the baby as much as possible, to maximize the transfusion of blood from the placenta before clamping the cord.

Volume expanders increase the circulating blood volume and tissue perfusion, reducing metabolic acidosis. The fluids of choice are 0.9% normal saline solution or Ringer's lactate solution. Fresh whole O rhesus negative blood can be given if there is definite evidence of a haemorrhage. 10 ml/kg of fluid should be administered intravenously over 5–10 minutes.

There has been evidence of an increased mortality associated with the use of plasma substitute solutions, as well as a risk of infectious disease transmission. These are therefore not recommended for use during neonatal resuscitation (Cochrane Injuries Group Albumin Reviewers, 1998).

Sodium bicarbonate

Using sodium bicarbonate to counteract metabolic acidosis is controversial and no longer recommended in the acute resuscitation setting. It has been previously linked to an increased rate of intraventricular haemorrhage in neonates and its only use is in prolonged resuscitation attempts, where there has been no response to adequate ventilation, cardiac compressions and other medications. In this event, 2 mEq/kg of 4.2% sodium bicarbonate is given slowly, intravenously. It is imperative that adequate ventilation is established prior to sodium bicarbonate administration, to help correct metabolic acidosis.

ACIDOSIS

Acidosis is the presence of excess hydrogen ions in the body, the concentration of which is directly related to the ratio of carbon dioxide to bicarbonate; the more carbon dioxide, or the less bicarbonate, the lower the pH and the more acid the fluid. The normal blood pH in adults is 7.35–7.45 and in the fetus 7.30–7.35, showing that it is a slightly alkaline fluid. Relatively small alterations of pH are associated with serious disorders of metabolism.

There are two types of acidosis:

- *Metabolic acidosis* results from the loss of bicarbonate, caused either by the accumulation of acids in the body during anaerobic metabolism (e.g. lactic acid), or by renal problems which prevent their excretion or allow urinary leakage of bicarbonate.
- *Respiratory acidosis* results from the accumulation of carbon dioxide as a waste product of aerobic metabolism; the circulation of the fetus, or the ventilation of the neonate, has allowed oxygen to enter but is unable to remove the carbon dioxide produced.

Acidosis of a single type can be compensated for. Whilst the lungs are central in the control of carbon dioxide levels (respiratory acidosis), the kidneys are central to the regulation of bicarbonate levels (metabolic acidosis). If excess carbon dioxide is retained, the kidneys will increase the bicarbonate level present in body fluids, restoring the hydrogen ions and thereby the pH, to normal. These buffering systems (lung and kidney, respiratory and metabolic) may fail to cope in neonates, since acidosis at birth tends to be mixed (respiratory and metabolic) and the whole metabolism is so fragile. During periods of hypoxia or anoxia, there is initially a pure respiratory acidosis. However, as the metabolism changes to be anaerobic, lactic acid accumulates and a metabolic acidosis also develops.

Fetal blood sampling may be performed in an attempt to quantify any acidosis where intrapartum asphyxia is suspected, and assists in appropriate decision-making when deciding on any interventions necessary, such as caesarean section or instrumental delivery. Following any degree of fetal distress, umbilical cord venous and arterial pH measurements should be obtained as soon as possible.

Samples are taken and analysed quickly, to prevent haemolysis. Together with the Apgar scores, cardiotocograph recording and clinical presentation of the baby, this helps to assess the degree of asphyxia and can be useful in determining the prognosis (Steer *et al.*, 1989).

MECONIUM ASPIRATION SYNDROME

From 11 weeks' gestation the fetus shows signs of breathing movements, which increase over the subsequent trimester and are seen as a sign of fetal wellbeing. Hypoxia results in a reduced rate, or complete cessation, of these movements. It also increases gut peristalsis and relaxes the anal sphincter, allowing meconium to be passed into the liquor. The asphyxiated fetus gasps in utero, which causes the thick, tenacious meconium to be inhaled into the bronchial tree.

It is important to have a paediatrician, midwife or nurse skilled in resuscitation present at the delivery of all babies where there is meconium-stained liquor (see above).

Meconium liquor is evident in around 10–15% of all labours, but meconium aspiration syndrome occurs in only 1–5% of all live births. Meconium is rarely passed in utero prior to 34 weeks' gestation (Steer *et al.*, 1989); thus this syndrome is more common in near-term or term infants, especially small-for-gestational-age and postmature babies. Studies show surfactant therapy can help to reduce the severity of respiratory problems in babies with meconium aspiration syndrome (Merrill and Ballard, 2003).

TRANSIENT TACHYPNOEA OF THE NEWBORN (TTN)

This condition is commonly found in near-term or term babies and is thought to result from a mild surfactant deficiency, or failure to adequately absorb lung fluid following birth. Typically it presents in babies delivered by caesarean section, where the physical compression of the chest experienced during vaginal delivery, does not occur. In addition, the surge of catecholamines to initiate a switch in the lungs from secretion to absorption of lung fluid can be impaired by an operative delivery.

Following birth, the baby presents with a respiratory rate of more than 60 per minute, flaring of the nostrils, sternal or intercostal recession, expiratory grunting and possibly cyanosis. The baby is placed in an incubator, or with skin-to-skin contact with the mother, to maintain its temperature, as oxygen requirements are increased by hypothermia. Minimal handling is important and oxygen administration may be required to relieve cyanosis. An urgent neonatal/paediatric opinion will be necessary.

The symptoms usually resolve within 24 hours, although tachypnoea alone may persist a little longer. It is important to determine that infection is not the cause and further investigations will be performed if the tachypnoea persists beyond 4 hours. A chest X-ray shows enlarged lymph vessels as characteristic streaks and signs of oedema between the lung lobes. Blood gases and cultures may also be necessary and the neonate will require observation in a neonatal unit (NNU) or special care baby unit (SCBU).

Parents will need a full explanation of the situation and likely course of this disorder. There are no long-term complications associated with this condition.

RESPIRATORY DISTRESS SYNDROME (RDS)

Respiratory distress syndrome is the result of insufficient surfactant, resulting in alveolar collapse and inadequate oxygenation. It most commonly affects preterm babies, especially those of less than 34 weeks' gestation, infants of diabetic mothers and those born by caesarean section or following antepartum haemorrhage. Gestational age correlates with the incidence of RDS, with those of lowest gestational age being at greatest risk.

Surfactant reduces the surface tension in the alveoli, facilitating lung expansion and preventing complete alveolar collapse during expiration. Its deficiency leads to more respiratory effort to inflate the lungs with each breath. As the neonate quickly becomes exhausted, the alveoli collapse and hypoxaemia results. This in turn, stimulates prostaglandin production in the wall of the ductus arteriosus and prevents its closure. Blood therefore continues the right-to-left shunt, reducing blood flow to the lungs, further reducing oxygenation. The baby's condition will continue to deteriorate as surfactant production is also increasingly impaired by hypoxaemia. A vicious circle ensues and, unless appropriate respiratory support is instituted quickly, the metabolism spirals out of control. Ventilatory support may need to be continued for a considerable time, but should be reduced as soon as possible to prevent further lung damage. There is a significant morbidity associated with RDS and complications are common. The severity of these complications, together with the birthweight and gestation of the baby, will influence the outcome.

The initial signs and symptoms of RDS occur within 4 hours of birth and are the same as those of TTN, though RDS is rarely seen in neonates over 37 weeks' gestation and persists beyond 24 hours of age. Crepitations and reduced breath sounds are heard on auscultation. The diagnosis is confirmed by a chest X-ray which shows a fine ground-glass mottling throughout both lung fields and, in contrast, a clear outline of the bronchial tree.

At post-mortem, areas of atelectasis are found in the lungs and hyaline membranes, formed by plasma leakage from the pulmonary capillaries, line the alveoli and small bronchioles. These findings are known as hyaline membrane disease, the clinical syndrome of which is respiratory distress syndrome.

Prevention

It is recommended that antenatal corticosteroids are administered to all women in preterm labour before 34 weeks' gestation to boost fetal surfactant production. This reduces the incidence and severity of respiratory distress syndrome, intraventricular haemorrhage and mortality in the neonate (Murphy and Aghajafan, 2003). The optimal regime and number of doses is still a matter of debate. Animal studies currently conclude that multiple courses of corticosteroids appear to offer no additional benefits to a single course of treatment, but appear to be associated with greater developmental problems in the baby. These complications include intrauterine growth restriction, diabetes in childhood and altered brain development (Newnham *et al.*, 2002).

Improved ultrasound scanning accuracy for assessing gestational age means that, it is now rarely necessary to perform fetal lung maturation tests prior to elective preterm delivery. Analysis of a sample of amniotic fluid determines the relative ratios of lecithin (L) and sphingomyelin (S), two surfactant phospholipids. An L:S ratio greater than 2 indicates a low risk of RDS; less than 1.5, a high risk. Contamination of the sample with blood or meconium and conditions such as maternal diabetes can make this test unreliable; thus the presence of phosphatidylglycerol (PG), as a definitive marker of lung maturation, is also sought.

Following the birth of a preterm baby, prophylactic administration of surfactant via an endotracheal tube may improve the prognosis and course of RDS significantly (Soll and Morley, 2001). Multiple doses have been demonstrated to reduce the risk of pneumothoraces, chronic lung disease and mortality, more than a single dose (Soll, 2000). Active resuscitation of neonates less than 30 weeks' gestation at birth, using early intubation, surfactant therapy and continuous positive airway pressure, reduces the need for, and duration of, mechanical ventilation (Verder *et al.*, 1999).

CHRONIC LUNG DISEASE (CLD)

Chronic lung disease is defined as the continuing need, in preterm infants, for supplemental inspired oxygen at 36 weeks postconceptional age. It is considered to be a more sensitive indicator of ongoing lung problems than the previous definition of bronchopulmonary dysplasia (BPD). BPD is defined as the need for supplemental oxygen to maintain normal arterial oxygenation at 28 days of age, with radiological changes in the lung. The wide range of different findings on X-ray often made the diagnosis difficult.

Risk factors for CLD are:

- prematurity/pulmonary immaturity
- endotracheal intubation
- high ventilator peak inspiratory pressures
- oxygen toxicity

- low birthweight neonates with mild RDS in association with patent ductus arteriosus and nosocomial infections.

Surfactant therapy and new ventilation techniques have had an impact on reducing the severity of CLD, but as prematurity is a major factor, this needs to be addressed through careful history-taking, a high standard of antenatal care, and addressing issues around socioeconomic deprivation.

Treatment of CLD is aimed at reducing the baby's requirements for supplementary oxygen and high ventilatory pressures, as soon as possible. The early administration of postnatal dexamethasone has been shown to help achieve this, but studies demonstrate an associated increased risk of neurodevelopmental impairment (Shinwell *et al.*, 2000).

Many babies with CLD will require low-flow oxygen for several months, until new lung tissue develops that is able to support adequate oxygenation. Care can be provided at home, with adequate specialist follow-up, monitoring and support for the parents.

PNEUMOTHORAX

A pneumothorax occurs when alveoli in the lungs rupture, allowing air to escape into the pleural cavity, restricting the expansion of the lungs. It may be spontaneous as some babies can generate a pressure of above $60\,cmH_2O$, following meconium aspiration, or it may be a complication of high ventilator pressures, and is most frequently seen in babies with CLD, or following overzealous resuscitation. It is suspected when there is a sudden rapid deterioration in the baby's condition.

In the preterm baby, a quick diagnosis can be made using a fibreoptic light to transilluminate the chest, showing a dark shadow of trapped air. A chest radiograph will confirm the diagnosis. In mild cases the lung will re-expand spontaneously within a few days, or the air can be aspirated by inserting a needle into the pleural cavity. Larger pneumothoraces will require an underwater drain to be inserted. Adequate local anaesthesia must be given prior to these procedures. In an emergency, while on the resuscitaire on the labour ward, a 21 gauge butterfly needle may be used to aspirate the trapped air with the aid of a three-way tap and 10 ml syringe.

DIAPHRAGMATIC HERNIA (SEE CH. 36)

This is a congenital condition which presents as an emergency at birth. There is a defect in the diaphragm, usually on the left side, through which abdominal viscera herniate into the thoracic cavity. The developing lung on the affected side is often hypoplastic as a result of compression from these displaced organs (Jesudason *et al.*, 2000). Immediate intubation for resuscitation is vital; bag and mask ventilation will inflate the bowel in the thorax, causing increasing respiratory difficulty.

A right-sided diaphragmatic hernia does not have the same dramatic signs and symptoms and may initially be missed. The main sign is tachypnoea at rest. If not recognized, the baby's condition will deteriorate as loops of small intestine are inhaled into the chest cavity and severe respiratory distress develops.

Surgery is required to return the gut and any abdominal organs to their correct place and repair the diaphragmatic defect. Ongoing respiratory support may be necessary until lung growth occurs and the baby can maintain adequate oxygenation. Fetal surgery is currently being attempted in order to minimize the lung damage and facilitate lung growth, but these techniques are not yet perfected.

RESPIRATORY SUPPORT

A baby with respiratory problems can appear frightening to parents, who will require a great deal of support and a full explanation of the treatment and monitoring equipment used. Where full ventilation is necessary, the neonate may be sedated and parents need to be prepared for this.

Women whose babies are designated as high risk, should be given information and advice as soon as possible in order to be prepared for the birth and early neonatal period. Organizations such as BLISS produce booklets giving parents information regarding care the baby will receive on an NNU. Parents also value support from parents who have coped with similar experiences, either from local or national help groups.

Oxygen therapy

The concentration of oxygen administered to babies must be closely monitored, including during resuscitation. Both hyperoxaemia and hypoxaemia can result in long-term disabilities for the neonate. Sufficient should be given to maintain arterial oxygenation within normal limits, but excessive and fluctuating concentrations of oxygen are implicated in the aetiology of retinopathy of prematurity (Whitfill and Drack, 2000). All babies of less than 32 weeks' gestation must have regular eye examinations until they reach term, to enable early identification of any retinal damage. Regular monitoring of blood gases and percutaneous oxygen saturation levels is imperative.

Intermittent positive-pressure ventilation (IPPV)

Very small babies, or those with severe respiratory distress syndrome, may require virtually all the work of breathing to be done for them. Neonatal ventilators differ from those used for adults in that the controls preset the pressures generated, rather than the volume of each inflation. Since cuffed endotracheal tubes are not used, there is an unavoidable and variable leak around the endotracheal tube and a fixed-volume machine would be unreliable. The flow through a neonatal ventilator circuit is constant, while the pressure in the circuit is controlled at a valve on the gas return port of the ventilator. The pressure required to open this valve varies with the ventilator settings, and determines the pressure generated in the endotracheal tube.

The small airways of a baby with respiratory distress syndrome collapse at the end of each breath and require excessive effort to reinflate them. Babies with respiratory distress adopt a strategy that reduces this collapse somewhat by grunting. This is a partial Valsalva manoeuvre (breathing out against a closed larynx) that maintains a positive pressure in the chest even during exhalation, i.e. a positive end-expiratory pressure (PEEP). Intubation prevents the baby from generating this PEEP and causes a disadvantage unless positive pressure is applied externally; an endotracheal tube must never be left in place without a source of pressure applied.

The ventilation of such babies may require a moderately high pressure for about 1 second at a rate of about 30 per minute, the pressure being adjusted to maintain the P_{CO_2} in a satisfactory range, and to ensure adequate oxygenation. In between these inflations, a PEEP is applied to prevent alveolar collapse.

High pressures, particularly when sustained for relatively long periods of the respiratory cycle, cause damage to the lungs and may result in chronic lung disease or pneumothoraces. These conditions, in turn, lead to a greater incidence of periventricular haemorrhage and the resulting sequelae.

Many other types of ventilation are now available.

Continuous positive airways pressure (CPAP)

Some babies with respiratory distress require more help than additional oxygen and need to have the work of breathing done for them to some extent. This can be achieved with CPAP, which may also be used in preference to mechanical ventilation for babies with normal lungs who are having frequent apnoeic attacks.

CPAP prevents collapse of the alveoli on expiration by maintaining a positive pressure of about 5–10 cmH$_2$O in the airways whilst the baby breathes spontaneously. This effectively splints the airways open, thereby saving the baby much inspiratory effort and reducing the oxygen requirements (Morley, 1999). It is most commonly administered via nasal prongs, or through a short nasopharyngeal tube. A gastric tube must be left in place (oral or nasal) to prevent air accumulating in the stomach, causing gastric distension which further compromises respiratory effort.

Possible complications associated with CPAP are pneumothoraces and ulceration of the nasal passages, if prongs are used for a prolonged period.

Synchronous intermittent mandatory ventilation (SIMV)

SIMV is a form of trigger ventilation, which responds to a pressure change in the baby's airway, causing the ventilator to produce an inspiration in time with the baby's own breathing pattern. It can be helpful when weaning the neonate off mechanical ventilation and can be set to trigger a breath should long apnoeic periods occur. SIMV also reduces the risk of lung damage from high pressures.

High-frequency oscillatory ventilation (HFOV)

High-frequency ventilation delivers short bursts of high pressure, with rates exceeding 60 per minute. A high-frequency oscillation can be used, with rates over 1000 per minute, reducing damage to the lung tissue.

Nitric oxide

Inhaled nitric oxide (iNO) is used as a vasodilator in persistent pulmonary hypertension of the newborn (PPHN), which is associated with a variety of respiratory diseases. It has been shown to improve arterial oxygenation and reduces the amount of ventilatory support required (Sadiq et al., 2003), particularly when combined with high-frequency oscillatory ventilation (HFOV).

Extracorporeal membrane oxygenation (ECMO)

ECMO is often seen as a rescue treatment in severe cases of meconium aspiration syndrome, persistent pulmonary hypertension, diaphragmatic hernia or RDS which do not respond well to other methods of ventilation. It is an extension of cardiac bypass techniques. The right internal jugular vein is cannulated for drainage of blood, which is then circulated through an oxygenator before being returned to the baby via the right common carotid artery.

This extreme form of intervention carries a high risk of neurological damage from respiratory disorders and associated complications. Debate exists over whether ECMO further increases this risk and current studies are centred on minimizing potential damage by inducing hypothermia, which is known to be protective in hypoxic neonates (Ichiba et al., 2003).

Partial liquid ventilation (PVL)

PVL, using perfluorocarbon (PFC) or Perflubron liquids, has been extensively trialled in animal models since the mid 1960s. It shows favourable results regarding improved oxygenation and the possibility of anti-inflammatory properties, particularly when used in conjunction with other therapies, such as HFOV, surfactant or nitric oxide (Ricard and Lemaire, 2001).

Recent human trials in both adults and preterm neonates, also demonstrate certain advantages of PVL over traditional gaseous ventilation in cases of severe RDS unresponsive to surfactant therapy (Leach et al., 1996). These include reinflation and utilization of alveoli collapsed by atelectasis, providing more effective gaseous exchange and enabling lower ventilatory pressures to be used.

Reflective Activity 35.2

Identify the different techniques of ventilation utilized in your NICU.

Ventilation techniques and respiratory support of preterm babies is a highly specialized and rapidly advancing area of neonatology. Parents of these preterm babies inevitably become caught up in a 'high-tech', and often bewildering, world of machines, technical language and tests. Midwives need to support the family through these traumatic times, advocating for them where necessary and explaining procedures and events in plain language.

CARDIAC ABNORMALITIES

Cardiac conditions are the commonest single group of congenital abnormalities and account for about 30%

of all congenital malformations (Office for National Statistics, 1999). The prevalence is between 3–8 per 1000 live births, with about a third of these being mild defects requiring no treatment.

The cardiovascular system is the first system to be functional in utero, with blood beginning to circulate by the end of the 3rd week of gestation. Development is rapid and complex, making it susceptible to teratogenic insults. The effects of these depend on the toxicity of the teratogen, duration and dose of exposure and the parts of the system that are forming at that time.

90% of cardiac anomalies have a multifactorial aetiology; 8% are caused by genetic factors; and 2% can be traced to teratogens, such as rubella infection in early pregnancy or the effects of drugs, such as Ecstasy (McElhatton *et al.*, 1999).

Around 40% of babies with Down's syndrome have a congenital cardiac malformation (Freeman *et al.*, 1998). Diabetes in pregnancy significantly increases the risk of congenital anomalies, of which a third are cardiovascular (Schaefer-Graf *et al.*, 2000). Poor blood glucose control in the first trimester is particularly implicated, highlighting the importance of preconceptual counselling and stabilization of diabetes prior to pregnancy, where possible. Siblings of an affected child and offspring of a parent with a heart defect, also have an increased risk of a congenital cardiac lesion. A comprehensive booking history should identify these risk factors.

Prenatal diagnosis

Despite great advances in ultrasonography over the past decade, routine antenatal scanning at 18–22 weeks still fails to identify 60–80% of all cardiac defects (Grandjean *et al.*, 1999).

Nuchal translucency thickness measurement, performed by ultrasound scanning at 10–14 weeks, has been recommended as a sensitive screening method for major defects of the heart and great arteries (Huggon *et al.*, 2002). Subcutaneous oedema in the neck region is found in association with most of these anomalies, with an increasing prevalence of defects with increasing measurements.

Examination

More than half of all cases of congenital cardiac disease diagnosed in infancy, are missed at the initial examination and more than a third are missed at the 6-week check (Ainsworth *et al.*, 1999).

Obvious clinical signs are not always present in the early neonatal period, although many lesions present within the first few weeks with subtle signs or murmurs. Early signs of cardiac failure may be the first presentation of an anomaly, with persistent, unexplained tachypnoea, tachycardia, hepatomegaly, dyspnoea, feeding difficulties and vomiting. Cardiomegaly, sweating and excessive weight gain from peripheral oedema, are late signs. Careful, repeated examinations by the midwife (see Ch. 31) are important, specifically after 48 hours of age, in order to validate normality and recognize deviations from normal during this period. A key assessment is that of the baby's feeding pattern – if the baby is not feeding well, a full examination of the cardiovascular system, including checking peripheral pulses, auscultation and palpation of the liver should be carried out. Any concerns arising from this must be referred urgently to a paediatric cardiologist.

Abnormal heart sounds may be identified on auscultation. Blood flowing through a hole or malformed valve causes murmurs and approximately half of these are indicative of an underlying cardiac lesion (Ainsworth *et al.*, 1999).

Chest X-ray

The position, size and shape of the heart are noted on chest X-ray. An assessment of the relative positions and sizes of the heart chambers and great vessels can be made to aid diagnosis.

Electrocardiography (ECG)

An ECG recording should be taken when the baby is quiet, preferably asleep. Accurate interpretation provides information about the haemodynamic state and severity of the lesion.

Echocardiography

Transvaginal, intrauterine and three-dimensional ultrasound scans are all widely used diagnostic tools (Budorick and Millman, 2000). Doppler echocardiography allows measurement of the rate and direction of blood flow through the heart, detecting obstructions and shunting of blood through septal defects.

Magnetic resonance imaging (MRI)

MRI scanning gives much clearer, high-quality images of the anatomy of the heart, but is not as convenient as ultrasound scanning as it cannot be performed at the cotside.

Cardiac catheterization

As the quality of information available from non-invasive diagnostic techniques continues to improve, cardiac catheterization is being more widely used as a method of *treatment* for conditions such as valve stenosis. It allows the identification of abnormal tracts and the measurement of blood pressure and oxygen saturation levels within the heart and great vessels. The procedure is performed under general anaesthetic and involves passing a catheter through the femoral vein into the right side of the heart, pulmonary arteries and its branches. In neonates it is often possible to pass the catheter into the left side of the heart through the foramen ovale or a ventricular septal defect (VSD), if one is present.

TYPES OF CONGENITAL HEART DISEASE

Congenital cardiac lesions may be separated into two groups – acyanotic and cyanotic. Cyanosis is not always present at birth, but may develop later as the ductus arteriosus closes.

Acyanotic lesions

Patent ductus arteriosus (PDA)

The ductus arteriosus diverts blood from passing through the lungs in utero into the descending aorta. Specialized contractile tissue, formed from 25 weeks' gestation, enables it to close spontaneously, but is not fully mature and functional for about 3 months. This partly explains the high incidence of PDA in preterm babies. In the term infant the ductus normally closes at 15–24 hours of age, and spontaneous closure after 2 weeks is rare. In preterm infants, depending on the gestation, it may take up to 3 months as the contractile tissue develops.

PDA is the most common cause of congestive cardiac failure in the neonate, with symptoms occurring at about 3–10 days of age. The baby appears tachypnoeic, dyspnoeic and lethargic, with bounding pulses and audible systolic and diastolic murmurs. Midwives should be alert for these signs and make urgent referral for readmission to hospital when necessary. Treatment includes restricting fluids and eliminating hypoxia, which maintains the patency of the ductus. Indometacin may be prescribed for preterm babies. Surgical ligation of the duct is rarely necessary but may be indicated if medical management fails.

Ventricular septal defect (VSD)

This is the commonest single cardiac defect presenting in childhood, accounting for about 40% of all lesions (Bosi *et al.*, 1999). There is a hole in the ventricular septum allowing a left-to-right flow of blood through it. A VSD may be one component of a complex heart defect or other congenital anomaly.

The clinical presentation and prognosis depend on the size and position of the defect (Turner *et al.*, 1999). A small hole may be asymptomatic and the characteristic murmur is often not heard until the baby is a few weeks old. No treatment is needed for these, as the vast majority of them close spontaneously over a period of several years. Larger defects can cause dyspnoea and difficulty with feeds in the early weeks of life and surgical repair may be necessary if the symptoms are severe.

Atrial septal defect (ASD)

There are two types of atrial septal defects:

1. *Simple defects* in which there is a hole in the atrial septum. These very rarely give rise to symptoms until adult life and account for almost 9% of all cardiac lesions. Surgery to repair small lesions is carried out at 4–5 years of age, earlier if the mitral valve is involved, as deterioration is more likely.
2. *Complex defects* (*atrial ventricular septal defect, AVSD*) where there is also involvement of the mitral valve and in severe cases the ventricular septum, mitral and tricuspid valves. AVSD has a poor prognosis and there is a high mortality associated with surgery. In around 50% of cases there is an associated chromosomal abnormality (Huggon *et al.*, 2000). Babies usually present in the first few weeks with dyspnoea, poor feeding and failure to thrive, often initially identified by the midwife. Mild cyanosis may occur and there are abnormal heart sounds including a systolic murmur.

Coarctation of the aorta

In this condition, which accounts for 6% of all cardiac defects, there is a narrowing of the aorta where the ductus arteriosus joins the aorta. Associated lesions are present in more than 50% of cases, most commonly VSD, aortic stenosis and mitral valve abnormalities. A small narrowing may not produce symptoms for several years.

More severe strictures cause a neonatal emergency. There is a sudden onset of symptoms as the ductus arteriosus closes, usually between days 2–10. The baby becomes dyspnoeic and tachypnoeic with hepatomegaly and signs of renal and cardiac failure. The baby needs urgent treatment with prostaglandins to maintain the PDA and subsequent circulation. Surgery involves widening the constricted segment.

Pulmonary valve stenosis

A narrowing of the pulmonary valve in isolation accounts for about 8% of cardiac conditions. Even when severe narrowing occurs the only symptom in neonates is often a murmur. Mild stenosis usually improves with growth, but treatment, if needed, is surgical.

Aortic valve stenosis

A narrowing of the aortic valve causes restricted blood flow from the left ventricle into the aorta. Isolated cases account for 6% of cardiac conditions but this abnormality also occurs in association with other conditions, especially coarctation of the aorta. Mild or moderate stenosis is usually asymptomatic in neonates, although a murmur may be present.

A severe obstruction may cause sudden collapse, and urgent surgery is required, with subsequent valve replacement often necessary later in childhood.

Cyanotic lesions

Cyanosis is not always present at birth, but may develop later as the ductus arteriosus closes.

Transposition of the great arteries

This defect accounts for 4% of all lesions. The pulmonary artery arises from the left ventricle and the aorta from the right ventricle, thus producing two independent circulations (Fig. 35.5). A chest X-ray shows a typical 'egg-on-side' appearance of the heart, owing to the aorta overriding the pulmonary artery, and enlargement of the right ventricle.

Closure of the ductus arteriosus results in severe, worsening cyanosis, dyspnoea and cardiac failure. Urgent treatment with prostaglandins is needed to maintain a PDA. This may be followed by definitive surgery in the next few days when the vessels are 'switched' back to their normal anatomical positions.

Tetralogy of Fallot

Tetralogy of Fallot accounts for approximately 5% of cardiac lesions. This consists of four abnormalities (Fig. 35.6):

1. pulmonary stenosis
2. VSD
3. right ventricular hypertrophy
4. overriding aorta, across the ventricular septal defect.

In the neonatal period this condition often presents with symptoms of a VSD and mild pulmonary stenosis. The baby is pink at birth, gradually developing cyanosis on crying. Dyspnoea starts as the pulmonary stenosis worsens, which may take several months. Many present at 4–6 months with cyanotic episodes, often in the morning, resulting in a loss of consciousness.

Surgery is required to correct the abnormalities and the timing will depend on the severity of the defects and symptoms produced.

Hypoplastic left heart syndrome

This is the commonest cause of cardiac failure in the first 2–3 days of life and symptoms present much earlier than in other cardiac conditions. The whole of the

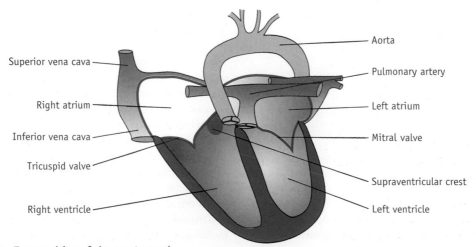

Figure 35.5 Transposition of the great vessels.

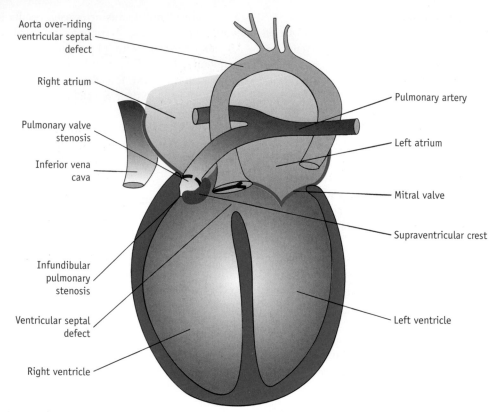

Aorta over-riding ventricular septal defect

Right atrium

Pulmonary valve stenosis

Inferior vena cava

Infundibular pulmonary stenosis

Ventricular septal defect

Right ventricle

Pulmonary artery

Left atrium

Mitral valve

Supraventricular crest

Left ventricle

Figure 35.6 Tetralogy of Fallot.

left side of the heart is underdeveloped – the ascending aorta and coronary arteries are hypoplastic, with blood passing into the aorta through the PDA (see Fig. 35.7). As the ductus closes there is increasing cyanosis and dyspnoea. The majority of babies die within the first week, although prenatal diagnosis enables early postnatal management. Heart transplantation offers these babies the best chance of survival, but many die awaiting a suitable organ.

Follow-up and support

Many babies are discharged home whilst awaiting non-urgent cardiac surgery; some will be cyanosed. Dyspnoea and tiredness may make feeding difficult and many babies require nasogastric tube feeds. Weight gain is often slow but may be improved by offering small, frequent feeds or by adding calorific supplements to the milk. Early involvement of a dietician is important and the family will require much support. Local and national cardiac support groups can provide longer-term support and information for families.

> **Reflective Activity 35.3**
>
> What facilities and information do you have in your unit and your own resources, which would assist in supporting women and their families who are coping with a baby with respiratory or cardiac problems?

CONCLUSION

The midwife is often the practitioner who will identify the woman and baby at risk. Information, education and support must be provided to properly prepare the woman and her family for different interventions and care which may be required, during pregnancy and following birth. The midwife should be skilled and knowledgeable in the effective resuscitation of the newborn, and be able to validate normality in the newborn baby, whilst ensuring that the woman is equipped to identify deviations from normal in her own baby.

This whole process ensures that women and their families are empowered and properly supported, and are able to participate in their care as true partners.

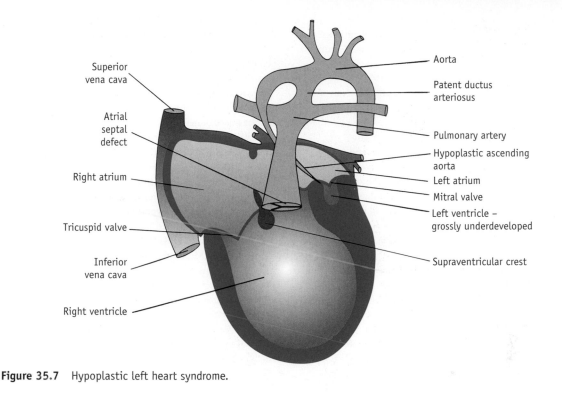

Figure 35.7 Hypoplastic left heart syndrome.

KEY POINTS

- Midwives need an understanding of transitional changes from fetal to neonatal circulation, in order to recognize potential cardiac problems.
- Midwives should recognize the changes required to take place before respiration can be successfully established in the neonate.
- All staff must maintain their competency in neonatal resuscitation and be prepared for the need to use these skills, even following an apparently uncomplicated labour.
- Respiratory problems of preterm babies remain one of the greatest challenges for neonatologists.

Many new techniques are currently being trialled, in an attempt to minimize complications and iatrogenic damage associated with these treatments.

- Cardiac anomalies are the commonest group of congenital abnormalities. Their aetiology is often multifactorial; they occur very early in the first trimester and are often complex.
- Midwives must be alert for early signs of cardiac problems and be able to recognize abnormal heart sounds in the neonate.

REFERENCES

Ainsworth, S., Wyllie, J.P. & Wren, C. (1999) Prevalence and clinical significance of cardiac murmurs in neonates. *Archives of Disease in Childhood* 80(1): F43–F45.

Bosi, G., Scorrano, M., Tosato, G. *et al.* (1999) The Italian Multicentric Study on Epidemiology of Congenital Heart Disease: first step of the analysis. Working Party of the Italian Society of Pediatric Cardiology. *Cardiology in the Young*; 9(3): 291–299.

Budorick, N.E. & Millman, S.L. (2000) New modalities for imaging the fetal heart. *Seminars in Perinatology* 24(5): 352–359.

Cochrane Injuries Group Albumin Reviewers (1998) Human albumin administration in critically ill patients: systematic review of randomised controlled trials. *British Medical Journal* 317: 235–240.

Freeman, S.B., Taft, L.F., Dooley, K.J. *et al.* (1998) Population-based study of congenital heart defects in Down syndrome. *American Journal of Medical Genetics* 80(3): 213–217.

Grandjean, H., Larroque, D. & Levi, S. (1999) The performance of routine ultrasonographic screening of pregnancies in the Eurofetus Study. *American Journal of Obstetrics and Gynecology* 181(2): 446–454.

Grein, A.J. & Weiner, G.M. (2002) Laryngeal mask airway versus bag–mask ventilation or endotracheal intubation for neonatal resuscitation *Cochrane Database of Systematic Reviews. The Cochrane Library,* Issue 1. Oxford, Update Software.

Huggon, I.C., Cook, A.C., Smeeton, N.C. *et al.* (2000) Atrioventricular septal defects diagnosed in fetal life: associated cardiac and extra-cardiac abnormalities and outcome. *Journal of the American College of Cardiology* 36(2): 593–601.

Huggon, I.C., Ghi, T., Cook, A.C. *et al.* (2002) Fetal cardiac abnormalities identified prior to 14 weeks' gestation. *Ultrasound in Obstetrics and Gynecology* 20(1): 22–29.

Ichiba, S., Killer, H.M., Firmin, R.K. *et al.* (2003) Pilot investigation of hypothermia in neonates receiving extracorporeal membrane oxygenation. *Archives of Disease in Childhood* 88(2): F128–F133.

Jesudason, E.C., Connell, M.G., Fernig, D.G. *et al.* (2000) Early lung malformation in congenital diaphragmatic hernia. *Journal of Pediatric Surgery* 35(1): 124–127.

Kalache, K.D., Chaoui, R., Marks, B. *et al.* (2002) Does fetal tracheal fluid flow during fetal breathing movements change before the onset of labour? *British Journal of Obstetrics and Gynaecology* 109(5): 514–519.

Leach, C.L., Greenspan, J.S., Rubenstein, S.D. *et al.* (1996). Partial liquid ventilation with Perflubron in premature infants with severe respiratory distress syndrome. *New England Journal of Medicine* 335(11): 761–767.

McElhatton, P.R., Bateman, D.N., Evans, C. *et al.* (1999) Congenital anomalies after prenatal Ecstasy exposure. *Lancet* 354(9188): 1441–1442.

Merrill, J.D. & Ballard, R.A. (2003) Pulmonary surfactant for neonatal respiratory disorders. *Current Opinion in Pediatrics* 15(2): 149–154.

Morley, C. (1999) Continuous distending pressure. *Archives of Disease in Childhood Fetal and Neonatal Edition* 81(2): F152–F156.

Murphy, K. & Aghajafari, F. (2003) Single versus repetitive courses of corticosteroids: what do we know? *Clinical Obstetrics and Gynecology* 46(1): 161–173.

Newnham, J.P., Moss, T.J.M., Nitsos, I. *et al.* (2002) Antenatal corticosteroids: the good, the bad and the unknown. *Current Opinion in Obstetrics and Gynecology* 14(6): 607–612.

Office for National Statistics (1999) *Congenital Anomaly Statistics. Notifications 1999.* Series MB3(4). London: The Stationery Office.

Resuscitation Council (UK) (2001) *Resuscitation Handbook.* London: Resuscitation Council (UK).

Ricard, J-D. & Lemaire, F. (2001) Liquid ventilation. *Current Opinion in Critical Care* 7(1): 8–14.

Sadiq, H.F., Mantych, G., Benawra, R.S. *et al.* (2003) Inhaled nitric oxide in the treatment of moderate persistent pulmonary hypertension of the newborn: a randomized controlled, multicenter trial. *Journal of Perinatology* 23(2): 98–103.

Schaefer-Graf, U.M., Buchanan, T.A., Xiang, A. *et al.* (2000) Patterns of congenital anomalies and relationship to fasting glucose levels in pregnancies complicated by type 2 and gestational diabetes. *American Journal of Obstetrics and Gynecology* 182(2): 313–120.

Shinwell, E.S., Karplus, M. & Reich, D. (2000). Early postnatal dexamethasone treatment and increased incidence of cerebral palsy. *Archives of Disease in Childhood (Fetal and Neonatal Edition)* 83(3): F177–F181.

Soll, R.F. (2000) Multiple versus single dose natural surfactant extract for severe neonatal respiratory distress syndrome. *Cochrane Database of Systematic Reviews*: CD000141. Oxford: Update Software.

Soll, R.F. & Morley, C.J. (2001) Prophylactic versus selective use of surfactant in preventing morbidity and mortality in preterm infants. *Cochrane Database of Systematic Reviews*: CD000510. Oxford: Update Software.

Steer, P.J., Eigbe, F., Lissauer, T.J. *et al.* (1989) Interrelationships among abnormal cardiotocograms in labor, meconium staining of the amniotic fluid, arterial cord blood pH and Apgar scores. *Obstetrics and Gynecology* 74: 715–721.

Turner, S.W., Hunter, S. & Wyllie, J.P. (1999) The natural history of ventricular septal defects. *Archives of Disease in Childhood* 81(5): 413–416.

Verder, H., Albertsen, P., Ebbesen, F. *et al.* (1999) Nasal continuous positive airway pressure and early surfactant therapy for respiratory distress syndrome in newborns of less than 30 weeks' gestation. *Pediatrics* 103(2): E24.

Whitfill, C.R. & Drack, A.V. (2000) Avoidance and treatment of retinopathy of prematurity. *Seminars in Pediatric Surgery* 9(2): 103–105.

Wisewell, T.E. (2000) Meconium in the delivery room trial group: delivery room management of the apparently vigorous meconium-stained neonate: results of the multicenter collaborative trial. *Pediatrics* 105(1): 1–7.

FURTHER READING

Clarke, E.B., Clarke, C. & Neill, C.A. (eds) (2001) *The Heart of a Child: What Families Need to Know about Heart Disorders in Children,* 2nd edn. Baltimore: Johns Hopkins University Press.
A useful text written by paediatric cardiologists and a neonatal nurse, primarily as a resource for parents.

Sinha, S. & Donn, M. (eds) (2003) *Manual of Neonatal Respiratory Care.* Massachusetts: Blackwell Publishing.
Helpful reference text, detailing the anatomy and physiology of lung development, the pathophysiology of respiratory disorders and how these are managed.

36

Congenital Anomalies, Fetal and Neonatal Surgery, and Pain

Carol Simpson

LEARNING OUTCOMES

After reading this chapter you will be able to:

- recognize the common congenital anomalies
- have an understanding of the aetiology and risk factors for congenital anomalies
- appreciate the principles and problems of fetal and neonatal surgery
- have an understanding of the issues surrounding fetal and neonatal pain.

INTRODUCTION

Congenital anomalies are defects present at birth. They occur in approximately 2–3% of babies, although it is hard to ascertain precise figures as many are not diagnosed until later in life. Figures appear to have risen in recent years, which can partly be attributed to improved notification to the National Anomaly System (ONS, 2000).

Parents generally expect the experience of pregnancy and birth to be a safe and happy event, with a normal, healthy baby as the result. Whilst this occurs in the majority of cases, there are no guarantees of normality. Midwives can facilitate the early identification of abnormalities and identify such conditions at their initial neonatal examination. They must be sensitive and honest when discussing these with the parents, and urgent referral to a neonatologist is imperative.

Congenital anomalies fall into two groups:

- *Malformation* – a primary defect of organ or tissue development in the embryo or fetus
- *Deformation* – damage caused by external factors influencing a previously normal structure.

Malformations and deformations occur in a ratio of ? and such conditions account for about 26% of infant deaths in England and Wales (ONS, 1999), with regional variations.

Careful and sensitive questioning at antenatal booking is important to ensure genetic, cultural and environmental risk factors are identified. Informed parental choice is an important factor when considering screening. Midwives should offer pre- and post-test counselling, discussing the risk factors, possible results, implications, prognosis and management options for any conditions screened for.

AETIOLOGY

In up to 80% of congenital anomalies the aetiology is unknown. The causes may be genetic, teratogenic, iatrogenic or a combination of these.

Mothers at the extreme ends of the childbearing age range have an increased risk of having a baby with a trisomy abnormality, such as Down's syndrome. The incidence of complex abnormalities is also increased with certain maternal diseases, such as unstable diabetes (Farrell *et al.*, 2002), or phenylketonuria.

Genetic factors

Each human cell has a total of 46 chromosomes arranged in 23 pairs, one of the pair from each parent.

Every chromosome carries a unique blueprint of its parent's characteristics in the form of genes. There are two sex chromosomes (X from the mother and either X or Y from the father); the remainder are called autosomes.

Genes may be dominant or recessive:

- Dominant genes will display their trait whenever they are present on just one chromosome – examples include osteogenesis imperfecta and achondroplasia.
- Recessive genes need to be present on both chromosomes of the pair – for example phenylketonuria and cystic fibrosis.

Teratogenic factors

Examples of well-documented teratogens are:

- maternal infections – including rubella, toxoplasmosis, cytomegalovirus, syphilis
- drugs – heroin, cocaine, nicotine, some anticonvulsants, anticoagulants, alcohol, streptomycin, tetracycline, thalidomide
- environmental – pesticides, dioxins, radiation
- sustained hyperthermia (therefore saunas during pregnancy are discouraged, as well as exercise which might raise the maternal temperature)
- maternal febrile illness in the first trimester is linked to an increase in congenital heart defects (Botto *et al.*, 2001).

Iatrogenic factors

Congenital constriction band (amniotic band) syndrome is a rare but potentially fatal condition, in which early amniotic rupture results in a constrictive band forming, occluding some part of the fetal body. Although often considered in relation to intrauterine limb amputations, its effects vary in severity and location and may cause major craniofacial deformities, or even fetal death.

> ### Reflective Activity 36.1
>
> Find out if your area has a high prevalence of any particular congenital anomalies and consider any known aetiological factors.

CENTRAL NERVOUS SYSTEM ANOMALIES

Spina bifida and anencephaly are the commonest neural tube defects, affecting up to 1 : 1000 pregnancies. Improved antenatal detection, therapeutic termination and routine vitamin supplementation (specifically folic acid 400 μg daily for 1 month preconceptually and for the first 12 weeks of pregnancy) have accounted for a dramatic drop in the incidence in the last decade. Since over half of all conceptions are unplanned, all women of childbearing age should be informed of the benefits of vitamin supplements and encouraged to take them. 50–70% of all neural tube defects could be prevented by this simple measure alone (Hasenau, 2002).

Spina bifida

This is a congenital defect of the posterior laminae and spinous processes of one or more vertebrae. The midwife must examine the spine carefully following birth, as a sacral dimple or hairy patch can be suggestive of an underlying lesion. There may be a simple bony defect, as in spina bifida occulta, giving rise to no symptoms and occasionally only found accidentally on X-ray in later life.

Spina bifida cystica involves the protrusion of the meninges covered by the meningeal membrane (meningocele), or, more commonly, of the cord and meninges (myelomeningocele). The latter is more serious, as areas of spinal cord are found in isolated patches in the protruding meninges. Fetal surgery involving myelomeningocele closure shows promising short-term results (Sutton *et al.*, 2001). The defect can occur anywhere from the head (encephalocele) to the sacrum, but most commonly affects the lumbosacral region of the spine, with talipes, paraplegia and neurological symptoms. Cerebrospinal fluid may leak from the swelling, posing the risk of meningitis.

In-utero transfer to a specialist centre should be considered for any baby with a neural tube defect, and it is useful to seek advice from such a centre – such as Great Ormond Street. At birth, the meningocele should be enclosed within a sterile bag, or 'cling film', to minimize fluid loss, prevent garments sticking to the lesion and reduce the risk of infection. Adequate analgesia must be administered to the baby.

Anencephaly

This condition, mainly affecting females, manifests as the absence of the vault of the skull and almost no development of the exposed brain. It can be detected by antenatal ultrasound scanning. Second trimester screening for abnormally elevated maternal serum alpha-fetoprotein and low oestriol concentration, has been cited as highly predictive of lethal defects, particularly anencephaly (Benn *et al.*, 2000).

The baby has large protruding eyes and wide shoulders, the face presents during labour and polyhydramnios is found in about 50% of cases. The incidence of anencephaly is approximately 1:1000 and it is often associated with spina bifida. Only 25% of the babies are born alive and this condition is incompatible with sustained life, most babies dying within a week. Parents require sensitive counselling once this condition is identified and many elect for termination of the pregnancy.

Hydrocephalus

An excess of cerebrospinal fluid, caused by an obstruction or overproduction, distends the ventricles of the brain. Antenatal diagnosis is usually by ultrasound scan, but a breech presentation or a large head palpating above the pelvic brim may alert the midwife. In severe cases, obstructed labour necessitates a caesarean section.

The head circumference of a hydrocephalic baby is at least 2 cm larger than the 90th centile for gestational age, the cranial bones are soft, fontanelles large and the sutures wide. This highlights the importance of accurate measurements at birth, which should be plotted on the appropriate centile chart.

Postnatal surgery, with the insertion of a shunt to drain fluid from the lateral ventricle into the peritoneal cavity, has proved a successful palliative treatment in more severe cases.

Microcephaly

Microcephaly is defined simply as a very small vault to the skull. There are two types, one in which the brain has failed to grow and the other in which the sutures have ossified prematurely and constricted the growth of the brain. The former type may be caused by intrauterine infections such as rubella, cytomegalovirus or toxoplasmosis, or by severe intrauterine hypoxia. These babies are usually mentally impaired and there is a high association with other abnormalities.

ABNORMALITIES OF THE RESPIRATORY SYSTEM

Diaphragmatic hernia

The incidence of diaphragmatic hernia is approximately 1:2000–5000 neonates; it is more common in male babies born at term. This condition develops as the result of a defect in the formation of the diaphragm, usually on the left side. The bowel and abdominal viscera herniate through the diaphragm and continue to develop in the thoracic cavity. These organs compress the developing lung and, together with abnormal branching of the airways, can result in pulmonary hypoplasia (Jesudason *et al.*, 2000).

This abnormality may be identified by early ultrasound scanning. Prenatal counselling should prepare parents for high mortality and morbidity rates – only approximately 50% survive. Herniation of the liver predisposes to a poorer outcome. In-utero transfer to a specialist centre, planned delivery and prompt, appropriate respiratory support improve the chances of survival.

With a left-sided anomaly, at delivery, the hypoplastic lung fails to inflate and the baby presents with increasing dyspnoea and cyanosis. Bowel sounds are heard in the chest and the heartbeat can be auscultated on the right-hand side as the inflated bowel displaces it. The abdomen appears hollow. Elective endotracheal intubation and ventilation are imperative for these babies, who present one of the most urgent neonatal emergencies. Bag and mask resuscitation should not be used as it will overdistend the stomach and bowel with air, further restricting breathing. However, if it is necessary for any period, a 10 FG nasogastric tube should be passed to alleviate the distension. Chest X-ray will confirm the diagnosis.

More rarely, a right-sided herniation occurs and tachypnoea may be the only presenting feature at birth. Careful monitoring of vital signs by the midwife may enable early detection of this condition.

Postnatal surgery involves replacing the bowel, stomach and any other herniated viscera into the abdominal cavity and repairing the diaphragmatic defect. Postoperative care centres on maintaining adequate oxygenation and respiratory support while pulmonary growth occurs. Repair by open fetal surgery has not improved survival and less invasive prenatal interventions, such as tracheal occlusion to facilitate lung growth, are currently being tried.

Choanal atresia

The posterior nasopharynx is blocked, unilaterally or bilaterally, by a membranous or bony septum. This causes acute respiratory problems from birth, as neonates breathe mainly through their nose. Dyspnoea and cyanosis relieved by crying are classic symptoms, since only in this circumstance can the baby inspire adequately. Diagnosis is confirmed by being unable to pass a nasal catheter, and immediate treatment is the insertion of an oral airway. Surgical correction is necessary.

ABNORMALITIES OF THE ALIMENTARY SYSTEM

Cleft lip and cleft palate

Cleft lip, with or without cleft palate, is one of the most common structural birth defects with an incidence of 1 : 700 neonates. It may be unilateral or bilateral and can involve the soft palate, hard palate, or both. The incidence of cleft palate alone is 1 : 2000 births. Great care and a good light source should be used during the midwife's initial examination of the neonate, as a slight deformity can easily be missed.

There is often a family history of such abnormalities, and prenatal genetic counselling should be offered in such cases. Clefts can result from both teratogenic and genetic factors. They are more common in Asian families. Studies have shown a correlation between an increased risk of these anomalies and maternal cigarette smoking (Chung *et al.*, 2000) and unstable diabetes mellitus (Spilson *et al.*, 2001).

A cleft lip is one of the most immediately noticeable and distressing of the congenital abnormalities. The midwife should reassure parents that with modern surgical techniques these can be repaired extremely skilfully. The initial reaction of those present at delivery can have a great influence on the parents' acceptance of the baby. Prolonged feelings of guilt, rejection and grief are common.

Feeding problems frequently occur, often related to the baby being unable to form a seal around the nipple or teat. Breastfeeding is not impossible and should be encouraged and assisted wherever possible, with referral to a lactation specialist (see Ch. 33).

There is debate over the optimum timing for surgical repair (Molsted, 1999). Advocates of early closure put a high priority on early speech function and the tendency for babies to heal well at this age. Advocates of delayed closure (12–15 months) prefer to wait for the maxilla to grow, which may lead to a smaller defect. Further research is required to ascertain which gives better results in terms of aesthetics and function. Early involvement of the orthodontist and speech therapist is vital. Fitting an orthodontic plate may help feeding and assist in controlling growth of the upper jaw. The parents will require on-going support and may benefit from information about local and national self-help organizations.

Pierre Robin syndrome

A midline cleft of the soft palate, without a cleft lip, micrognathia (small mandible) and abnormal tongue musculature (glossoptosis) are the main features of this syndrome. Until the defect is repaired, the baby must be nursed in the prone position to prevent the tongue protruding through the cleft and obstructing the airway. In severe cases a nasal airway or dental prosthesis will need to be kept in situ until surgical repair. There is a high incidence of aspiration pneumonia and feeding difficulties, but if the baby survives the neonatal period, the prognosis is good.

Oesophageal atresia (OA) and tracheo-oesophageal fistula (TOF)

OA affects about 1 : 4000 neonates. In this malformation there is a blind ending to the upper end of the oesophagus, usually at the level of the third or fourth vertebra (see Fig. 36.1). In about 90% of cases there is also an oesophageal fistula, where there is a connection between one or both portions of the oesophagus and the trachea. Associated anomalies are present in 50% of cases.

Polyhydramnios should always alert the midwife to the possibility of this condition, as the fetus is unable to swallow amniotic fluid, leading to its accumulation.

At birth there are often copious, frothy oral secretions and, if a fistula is present, aspiration will cause cyanotic episodes. If this condition is suspected and in all cases of polyhydramnios, the midwife should pass a 10 FG nasogastric tube to assess the patency of the oesophagus before oral feeds are given; the prognosis

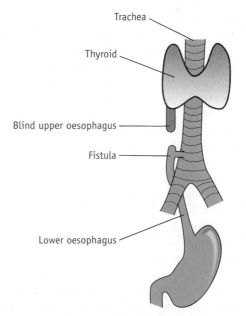

Figure 36.1 Tracheo-oesophageal atresia with fistula.

is much worse if milk is aspirated. The tube should not be too soft (or small) as it may curl in the back of the throat or in the blind pouch, whilst appearing to reach the stomach. If in doubt an X-ray should be taken.

The baby should be nursed with the head elevated and a double lumen (Replogle) tube in the upper pouch with continuous suction applied, to prevent collection and aspiration of the saliva. Surgery involves anastomosis of the ends of the oesophagus and division of any fistula. If the gap between the oesophageal ends is too wide, a portion of the colon or jejunum may be grafted on. Gastrostomy feeds will be necessary until repair is complete.

Survival rates are now more than 90%, with associated cardiac and chromosomal abnormalities being responsible for most of the early deaths and respiratory complications. These babies often need frequent dilatations of the oesophagus as they grow, because of scar tissue restricting the lumen. Complications include cough, wheeze, aspiration pneumonia, vomiting and feeding difficulties, which are most pronounced in the first 3 years and can be extremely wearing for parents.

Duodenal atresia

The incidence of duodenal atresia is 1 : 6000, making it the commonest site of atresia. In one-third of cases it is associated with Down's syndrome. The patency of the duodenum is interrupted and projectile, bile-stained vomiting occurs within 24 hours of feeds being commenced. An abdominal X-ray shows a classic 'double bubble' appearance. Surgical correction is required.

Congenital hypertrophic pyloric stenosis

The incidence of pyloric stenosis is approximately 1 : 500 and it is four times more common in boys than in girls. At booking, the midwife may find a family history of this condition. The muscle of the pylorus, in the stomach, hypertrophies over a number of days or weeks, causing increasing obstruction. The baby begins to posset regularly and this gradually worsens until projectile vomiting occurs immediately after all feeds. This can begin within the first week but more commonly presents at the age of 3–6 weeks.

Midwives should be alert to this condition in any baby who fails to thrive and presents with constipation. Peristalsis is often visible during feeds and a mass can be felt at the site of the obstruction. Surgery is performed to divide the relevant muscle thus resolving the problem.

Imperforate anus

The incidence of imperforate anus is approximately 1–3 : 5000 births. There is a high association with other anomalies, with genitourinary abnormalities present in almost half of cases. As part of the midwife's initial neonatal examination, the anus must be visually examined for signs of patency. No objects should be inserted, but an urgent paediatric referral made if there is any doubt. It is important that the midwife notes when meconium is first passed, and referral for further investigation should be made if this does not occur by 24–36 hours. Meconium-stained liquor is not indicative of a patent anus, as a fistula may be present. In the absence of a fistula the baby will fail to pass meconium, there will be abdominal distension and bile-stained vomiting. Surgical repair involves the formation of a temporary colostomy, which can be very distressing for parents.

Hirschsprung's disease

This is an inherited disorder, involving several different genes (Martucciello *et al.*, 2000), with an incidence of 1 : 5000 neonates. It is four times more common in male infants. There is an absence of ganglion cells in the nerve supply that controls peristalsis in the rectum and distal colon.

Diagnosis is often made by the delayed passage of meconium, subsequent infrequent, offensive stools, abdominal distension and vomiting. Any baby who has not passed meconium within 24–36 hours should be referred to a paediatrician for further investigations.

Surgical repair forms a temporary colostomy and removes the aganglionic segments of bowel. Less invasive, one-step surgical procedures are currently being tried, with some favourable results.

Exomphalos and gastroschisis

The incidence of these conditions is approximately 1 : 5000–6000 neonates. Both anomalies occur at the end of the first trimester and involve a herniation of abdominal contents, either through the base of the umbilical cord (exomphalos), or through a defect in the anterior abdominal wall (gastroschisis). There are raised maternal serum alpha-fetoprotein levels and diagnosis can be confirmed early by ultrasound scan.

Exomphalos has a covering of fused peritoneum and amnion, which may rupture during delivery. In up to 75% of cases there are associated chromosome or congenital abnormalities, particularly involving the alimentary tract, heart and genitourinary system.

The herniated viscera in *gastroschisis* are not protected by a covering sac and may appear oedematous or inflamed at birth. The blood supply can be disrupted to parts of the gut, resulting in necrosis, necessitating resection. If large lengths of bowel are involved, malabsorption syndrome may result. Teratogens have been implicated in its aetiology.

Following delivery, ideally in a specialist centre, the defect should be covered with sterile 'cling film', or the baby's legs and abdomen placed in a special surgical plastic bag up to the armpits. The main aims are to avoid overhandling of the herniated contents, prevent infection and reduce heat and evaporative fluid loss.

Surgery will attempt to replace as much of the abdominal contents as possible, but may need to be performed in stages over subsequent months or years. Survival rates for these conditions are 90–100% in the absence of other anomalies.

ABNORMALITIES OF THE GENITOURINARY SYSTEM

Undescended testes

The testes are normally present in the scrotum by 36 weeks' gestation. If they are undescended at the initial examination, the midwife should record this and recheck at 6 weeks postpartum. If they are still not palpable by 4 months of age in a term baby, or 6 months of age in a preterm baby, a paediatric referral and further investigation is warranted, as they are then unlikely to descend spontaneously.

Hypospadias and epispadias

Hypospadias is a malformation in which the urethral meatus opens on the ventral surface of the penis or, in severe cases, on the perineum. The rarer condition, epispadias, where the meatus opens on the dorsal surface, is usually part of a bladder exstrophy syndrome. Surgical correction is required in both cases and circumcision should not be performed prior to this, as the tissue will be required for repair. The nearer the meatus is to the tip of the penis, the less severe the problem and less urgent the surgery, providing there is no urinary obstruction. The midwife should observe the stream of urine to ensure it is not impeded.

One study (Wennerholm *et al.*, 2000) cites a fivefold increased risk of hypospadias in male infants conceived by in vitro fertilization, thought to be related to maternal progesterone administration.

Chordee

This condition frequently coexists with hypospadias and epispadias. There is penile curvature as a result of a tight skin attachment, but it is important to see the penis erect before making a diagnosis, as it may straighten at this time. Surgery will be required.

Autosomal polycystic kidney disease (APKD)

There are two main types of autosomal polycystic kidney disease – recessive (ARPKD) and dominant (ADPKD).

ARPKD occurs in 1 : 20 000 live births and the fetus presents in utero with enlarged, echogenic kidneys and oligohydramnios. Approximately 30% of these neonates die following birth, from associated pulmonary hypoplasia. Survivors display a range of renal and hepatic symptoms, the severity of which dictates the course of their condition.

ADPKD is more common, occurring in 1 : 500–1000 neonates, and typically involves progressive cyst formation in many organs, particularly the kidneys and liver, and results in renal failure in late middle age.

Renal agenesis

This is the developmental absence of a kidney as a result of failure of the ureteral bud to develop embryologically, or regression of a dysplastic kidney. It is found in approximately 1 : 1500 antenatal ultrasound scans and is usually asymptomatic in the neonate.

There is a high association with other congenital anomalies, particularly of organs that develop at the same time – genitourinary and musculoskeletal. Diagnosis is often incidental in the investigation of other disorders. Extra strain is placed on the solitary kidney, which commonly results in renal damage.

Urethral valves

This defect almost exclusively affects male infants. It is characterized by valves in the urethra that prevent the flow of urine from the bladder, resulting in bladder distension and back-pressure on the kidneys, leading to hydronephrosis. If undetected by antenatal ultrasound, severe renal damage may occur. Fetal surgery can alleviate the blockage, eliminating the need for elective preterm delivery.

Ambiguous genitalia

True hermaphroditism, in which both male and female genital organs are present, is very rare. In pseudo-hermaphrodites a small penis can be confused with a large clitoris, while a bifid scrotum may resemble the labia majora. One cause may be congenital adrenal hyperplasia, an autosomal recessive condition in which the adrenal gland produces an excessive quantity of androgens. If the genitalia appear to be ambiguous the midwife should inform a senior paediatrician, to have the baby examined as a matter of urgency. Chromosome analysis is necessary to establish the sex of the baby, which should *never* be assumed.

The parents will require great sensitivity and support from the midwife during this time, and information needs to be simple, non-judgemental and factual.

ABNORMALITIES OF THE LIMBS

Talipes

This deformity is due to the contraction of certain muscles or tendons. In mild cases it is positional, related to the fetal position in utero or restriction of movement from conditions such as oligohydramnios or multiple pregnancy. If passive movement cannot correct the deformity it may be of genetic origin.

There are three types:

- *Talipes equinovarus* – the commonest form, where the foot points downwards and inwards (Fig. 36.2). A higher incidence has been noted following first trimester amniocentesis (Wilson, 2000). Usually mild and easily correctable, this deformity requires physiotherapy and possibly splinting. The midwife should teach parents the passive movements required.
- *Talipes calcaneovalgus* – less common, with the foot pointing upwards and outwards (Fig. 36.3). An underlying lesion may be present, and prolonged splinting or surgical correction is more likely.
- *Talipes metatarsus varus* – affects only the forefoot, which turns inwards.

Syndactyly and polydactyly (Fig. 36.4)

There is a tendency for these abnormalities to be hereditary. The midwife should review the woman's notes prior to the initial newborn examination, and include a careful scrutiny of the hands and feet.

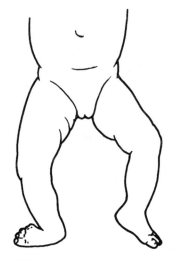

Figure 36.3   Talipes calcaneovalgus.

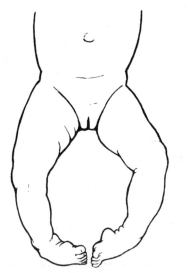

Figure 36.2   Talipes equinovarus.

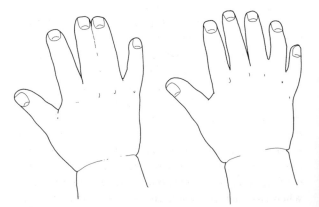

Figure 36.4   Syndactyly (*left*) and polydactyly (extra digit) (*right*).

Syndactyly is a condition in which the toes or, more commonly, the fingers are webbed. Plastic surgery will be required to separate the digits and in severe cases there is bony fusion requiring surgical separation.

Polydactyly is the presence of one or more extra digits, which may or may not have bones. If no bone is present, ligation can be undertaken, after which the digit will necrose and fall off leaving a small scar. Surgical removal is necessary if there is a bone.

Limb reduction deformities

In minor cases these deformities are confined to one or more digits. More severe deformities may involve the majority or whole of a limb. Teratogenic drugs taken in early pregnancy have been cited as a common cause – the best known of these being the antiemetic drug, thalidomide, from the 1950s. Congenital constriction band syndrome is another possible cause.

Some terms which may be used are:

- *Amelia:* absence of one or more limbs
- *Ectromelia:* absence of part of a limb
- *Phocomelia:* absence of the long bones of a limb – there may be a rudimentary or well-developed hand or foot present.

Congenital dislocation of the hip (CDH)

In this condition, one or both hips are abnormally developed with the head of the femur partially or wholly displaced from the acetabulum. Incidence is approximately 1:1500 births and the condition is of genetic origin, more prevalent in girls, children of affected families, primigravida and the left hip. It can also be associated with environmental factors such as breech presentation and oligohydramnios.

Ortolani and *Barlow* tests assess the hips for flexion and abduction to 90 degrees, without dislocation. 80% of hips are dislocatable at birth but normalize by 2 months of age. These tests should be carried out by a practitioner trained and skilled in this examination – increasingly midwives are undertaking this (see Ch. 31).

Early detection of CDH is essential to avoid long-term problems when the child begins to walk. Late diagnosis may necessitate 6 months to a year in a hip spica or, in the older child, long periods of traction or an open hip reduction. Ultrasound scanning of the hip joint confirms diagnosis and should routinely be performed when risk factors are present or this condition is suspected. An early orthopaedic referral is important, as a neonatal splint may be required. Parents will require

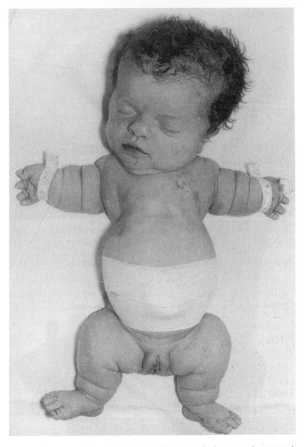

Figure 36.5 Achondroplasia. (From Beischer *et al.*, 1997.)

guidance from the midwife on how to maintain good standards of hygiene while the baby is in the splint.

Osteochondrodysplasias

Achondroplasia (dwarfism) (Fig. 36.5) is the commonest form of this group of disorders, which are characterized by abnormal growth of cartilage and bone and occur in approximately 1:3750 births. The clinical features of achondroplasia, an autosomal dominant disorder, vary little between patients. They are short in stature, short limbed and have a relatively large head, which may be worsened by hydrocephalus. Neurological problems exist in 20–40% of cases, but intelligence is usually normal. Growth hormones have been used with some good effect.

ABNORMALITIES OF THE SKIN

Most skin lesions are harmless in the neonate but can cause great distress to the family if large or clearly visible.

Parents need much reassurance and support. Early referral to a dermatologist may be appropriate and treatment options include steroids, laser treatment and cryotherapy.

Capillary haemangiomas

These fall under three main descriptions:

1. *Strawberry naevi* are caused by dilatation of capillaries in the skin and initially appear as small, red, raised blemishes, which are clearly outlined. They usually appear at about term and parents should be told that they will continue to grow over the next year. They do resolve to some extent following this but may not completely disappear.
2. *Naevus simplex* ('stork bite') is present at birth and presents as a flat, red area on the nape of the neck and upper eyelids and in a V shape on the forehead. These are extremely common, of no clinical significance and most will fade completely.
3. *Port-wine stains* are flat, purplish, well-defined and dense forms of capillary haemangiomas, often extensive. They are more common in girls and do not disappear. Laser surgery is being widely used with good success (Sheehan-Dare, 2001).

Pigmented naevi

Common brown moles, which vary in size, are present at birth and may be flat or raised. They can appear anywhere on the body. These grow with the child, do not resolve, and do not normally require treatment. As in adults, some may be precursors to melanoma and any clinical change in size or shape necessitates further investigation.

Bullae/blisters

If present at birth these may be due to a rare inherited disorder of the epidermis, epidermolysis bullosa, some forms of which are fatal. If they appear after birth they could be staphylococcal in origin and should be investigated.

CHROMOSOMAL ABNORMALITIES

Down's syndrome (trisomy 21)

This is a genetic disorder resulting in well-recognized clinical features and varying degrees of intellectual

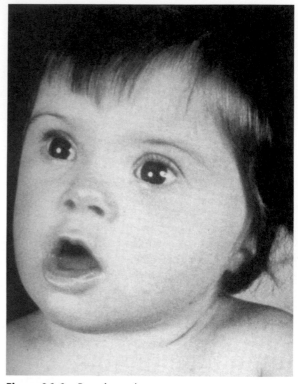

Figure 36.6 Down's syndrome.

disability. The incidence is 1 : 700 live births, but is known to increase significantly with increasing maternal age and amongst very young mothers. There are three recognized forms:

1. Most commonly there is an extra chromosome 21, making 47 chromosomes in total.
2. Chromosome 21 may translocate and become attached to another chromosome pair. In these cases there are still only 46 chromosomes in total.
3. 1–2% exhibit mosaicism where both normal and trisomic cells are present, suggesting abnormalities in the cell division processes. These individuals usually display milder intellectual disability.

The characteristic features of a baby with Down's syndrome (Fig. 36.6) are:

- wide-set, obliquely slanted eyes and prominent epicanthic folds
- white flecks in the iris – Brushfield's spots
- small head with a flattened occipital region
- increased fat pad on the neck
- small, droopy mouth
- generalized hypotonia
- protruding tongue
- broad, flat nose

- short hands, particularly the terminal phalanx of the little finger and a deep single palmar crease
- short, broad feet with a wide deviation of the great toe and a strong plantar crease between the first and second toes.

Feeding difficulties are common. New growth charts have recently been produced as standard reference for children with uncomplicated Down's syndrome in the UK and Ireland (Styles *et al.*, 2002). Associated anomalies, such as duodenal atresia, occur frequently and about 44% of these babies have congenital heart defects (Freeman *et al.*, 1998). Children with Down's syndrome have learning difficulties ranging from mild to severe, some needing care or supervision all their lives.

Midwives need to carefully explain the uses and limitations of antenatal screening tests such as nuchal translucency, serum alpha-fetoprotein levels, chorionic villus sampling and amniocentesis. Effective antenatal counselling and screening of women has led to increased and earlier detection of fetuses with Down's syndrome, enabling parents to make informed decisions. This is a life-changing diagnosis for parents and much sensitivity and support is required whenever this condition is suspected.

Edward syndrome (trisomy 18)

Edward syndrome has an incidence of about 1 : 5000. It results in well-recognized clinical features, where the baby is small for gestational age, with a poorly developed jaw and often a cleft palate. The ears are malformed and low-set, the occiput prominent and the fingers are characteristically crossed and flexed. The baby also displays prominent heels and 'rocker-bottom' feet. Most of these children have severe congenital heart disease and gastrointestinal anomalies. All are mentally retarded and most die within the first year. Careful examination of the cord and placenta are important as most have a single umbilical artery, which may alert the midwife.

Patau's syndrome (trisomy 13)

Patau's syndrome is relatively rare with an incidence of about 1 : 14 000. The face is abnormal with a sloping forehead, bilateral cleft lip and/or palate and malformed ears. Polydactyly is a common feature and the infant has prominent heels, rocker-bottom feet and a single umbilical artery. The brain is poorly developed and cardiac anomalies are common.

The prognosis for these children is poor, with few living beyond 3 years.

Potter's syndrome

This condition is incompatible with sustained life. Typical features include low-set ears, furrows under the wide-set eyes, a beaked nose and a failure to pass urine following birth owing to renal agenesis. There are only two vessels in the umbilical cord. Associated pulmonary hypoplasia frequently manifests itself in asphyxia at birth.

Turner's syndrome

Turner's syndrome – XO – only affects female infants and occurs in approximately 1 : 2500 live female births. One of the X chromosomes is missing or abnormal, which manifests itself with short stature, underdeveloped ovaries and infertility. Many of these fetuses will spontaneously abort. Those who do survive are of low birthweight, have a webbed neck and oedema of the lower limbs. They demonstrate normal intelligence, but have a reduced life expectancy that may be related to an increased incidence of congenital heart disease, particularly coarctation of the aorta.

Cri du chat syndrome

This is caused by deletion of a portion of chromosome 5, and is manifested by a typical mewing cry during infancy, caused by softening of the larynx. The baby has a moon-shaped face, with wide-set eyes, small jaw and low-set ears, and will have learning disabilities.

ABNORMALITIES OF THE HEART AND BLOOD VESSELS

These anomalies are described fully in Chapter 35.

Reflective Activity 36.2

Compile an up-to-date list of local and national contacts for parents of babies with specific conditions.

FETAL SURGERY

Fetal surgery is still in its infancy and is controversial. It is attempted in conditions where prenatal repair or intervention will significantly reduce the mortality or morbidity of that fetus. By far the greatest problems associated with these procedures are the high risks of precipitating preterm delivery and fetal loss (Kimber *et al.*, 1997). Maternal morbidity is also a major concern, with open surgical procedures requiring a classical caesarean section and necessitating a repeat caesarean section for delivery. Laparoscopic techniques are being developed for many conditions.

Animal experiments continue to develop techniques and technology for prenatal surgery. Long-term risks and benefits are not yet known for these procedures but trials are in progress. Myelomeningocele reconstruction is one of the most reviewed operations and has shown some neurological benefits in survivors (Sutton *et al.*, 2001).

To facilitate lung growth, in-utero tracheal occlusion, using clips or a balloon, is now the favoured procedure for severe congenital diaphragmatic hernia. In order to reverse the occlusion prior to delivery, the ex-utero intrapartum treatment (EXIT) procedure was developed. Just the baby's head is delivered through a hysterotomy incision, allowing removal of the occlusion and intubation prior to delivery of the body. This technique assures that placental circulation is maintained during intubation (MacKenzie *et al.*, 2002). It is also used when the airway is compromised, such as with laryngeal atresia and cystic hygroma.

Another condition that benefits from fetal surgery is posterior urethral valves, where a catheter is passed from the bladder into the amniotic fluid, bypassing the obstruction and reducing or preventing renal damage.

The physiology of wound healing in a fetus is known to be different from that of adults and results in scarless wound repair (Samuels and Tan, 1999). Animal studies suggest the advantages of this are particularly relevant in the repair of cleft lips and other disfiguring anomalies (Weinzweig *et al.*, 1999).

NEONATAL SURGERY

Many of the major anomalies requiring surgical correction can be identified within the first or early second trimesters, by ultrasound scanning. A family history of certain conditions, or specific problems identified in the pregnancy, may indicate to the midwife the need for more detailed investigation. Early diagnosis will enable counselling of the parents regarding the prognosis, allow informed choices regarding the pregnancy and enable specialist perinatal care to be planned.

To ensure optimal outcomes, in-utero transfer of the baby is recommended, if possible, to ensure that delivery takes place in a regional, specialist centre. In many instances this will mean the family travelling many miles to be with their baby and every neonatal unit should have facilities for families to be resident.

General preoperative care

Neonatal conditions requiring surgery fall into two main categories:

1. those which are life-threatening and need immediate surgery
2. those which may be postponed until the baby is in the optimum condition for surgery.

With modern technological advances, most procedures can be delayed for a short while, allowing the baby's condition to be stabilized. The better the condition of the baby at the time of surgery, the better the chances of survival.

Much of the preoperative care will be specific to the condition, but the general principles are as follows (not in order of priority):

- Stabilize the temperature. Hypothermia and hyperpyrexia have dramatic effects on metabolism, with cold stress in particular greatly increasing oxygen requirements.
- Stabilize the respiratory state; correct acidosis or electrolyte imbalances.
- Ensure good hydration with the administration of intravenous fluids.
- Ensure vitamin K is consented and administered.
- Screen for infection and begin antibiotics, if appropriate.
- Ensure adequate preoperative and postoperative analgesia are prescribed and administered.
- Check consent forms are signed and contact telephone numbers obtained from the parents.
- Explain all events and situations to the family using appropriate terminology. A brief antenatal tour of the neonatal unit is beneficial, where possible.
- Be aware of the family's religious and cultural beliefs. For example, Jehovah's Witnesses do not allow blood or blood products to be transfused, and artificial substitutes should be available.
- Encourage the parents to touch or cuddle their baby before surgery. In the event of the baby dying, this contact will have great significance in their memories.

Postoperative care

The principles of postoperative care are very similar to those of preoperative care, particularly with regard to involvement of the family. The mother should be encouraged to express her breast milk for the baby, as it is much better tolerated than formula milk and has been shown to significantly reduce the risk of necrotizing enterocolitis. The main aims are to:

- promote a good recovery
- identify and treat complications early
- prevent infection
- establish adequate nutrition
- promote parental involvement and interaction
- ensure the baby is pain free.

PAIN

There is controversy amongst clinicians, both scientific and emotional, on the subject of fetal and neonatal pain. It is comparatively recently that neonatal pain has been generally acknowledged and managed, but the gestational implications are still contentiously debated. The Royal College of Obstetricians and Gynaecologists working party (1997) recommend that consideration should be given to analgesia and sedation for fetuses 24 weeks or over during fetocide or invasive procedures, including intubation.

Many of the arguments centre on the topic of what constitutes pain. Not all stimuli are painful; some may cause discomfort or a disturbance as opposed to an actual pain. Examples in the neonate would include heel pricks as painful, physical examination as a discomfort and bright lights as a disturbance. These considerations are as relevant to the midwife caring for a healthy neonate at home as to those nursing a sick infant in the neonatal intensive care unit (NICU). Babies can manifest pain and disturbance following traumatic delivery such as ventouse, forceps delivery or shoulder dystocia.

Responses to pain

Although considerable maturation of the central nervous system takes place postnatally, basic pathways between the spinal cord and primary sensory neurones are present in the early stages of fetal development. From the 18th week of gestation the fetus has an independent noradrenaline response to invasive procedures, such as

umbilical blood sampling (Giannakoulopoulos et al., 1999). Redistribution of cerebral blood flow is another indicator of fetal stress and has been demonstrated, using Doppler studies, from as early as 18 weeks (Glover and Fisk, 1996).

Neonatal responses may be behavioural, physiological or metabolic. Numerous pain assessment tools are available (Abu-Saad et al., 1998), using scoring systems for varying degrees of one or more of these responses, in an attempt to quantify pain.

- Behavioural effects include crying, grimacing, increased agitation, withdrawal of limbs, Moro reflex and acute irritability.
- Physiological changes include tachycardia or bradycardia, tachypnoea, hypertension, increased oxygen requirements and palmar sweating in babies over 37 weeks' gestation.
- Metabolic changes include increased fat and carbohydrate metabolism and the release of corticosteroids, leading to hyperglycaemia, glycosuria, proteinuria, ketonuria and a raised urine pH.

Pain relief

There are many methods of relieving pain and discomfort. Careful attention to the environment, expertise at performing techniques and careful choice of equipment can all help. High levels of noise and bright lights are known to disturb neonates in the NICU and should be kept to a minimum.

Midwives should always use automated machines for heel-prick tests, as they initiate less pain response than manual sampling. Interventional techniques used during and following such procedures, which can be taught to parents, include comfortable positioning, kangaroo care, talking, gentle massage, cuddling and breastfeeding or non-nutritive sucking. Sucrose is widely used, and has been shown to be an effective analgesic agent during procedures such as venepuncture and heel lancing (Stevens and Ohlsson, 2000).

Pharmacological methods of alleviating pain should be considered where appropriate. The dose, method and frequency of administration of each drug will depend on the gestation, age, weight and condition of the baby, as these all affect the half-life and absorption rates of a drug. Some form of anaesthesia should routinely be given prior to any invasive procedure and adequate analgesia given postoperatively as a matter of course, as with adults.

CONCLUSION

The midwife's role is important in initially interviewing the woman, assessing her risk factors and ensuring that she is prepared for the birth – and not 'the perfect birth of the perfect baby'. In supporting the parents of a baby with a congenital anomaly, requiring surgery or pain management, midwives need to ensure that they are skilled at discussing the short- and long-term implications of congenital anomaly, being realistic and honest. In dealing with an unsuspected anomaly, they need to bring the whole gamut of their counselling and caring skills to the fore, and ensure that the woman and family are provided with information and support, and that long-term services are involved at the earliest stage.

KEY POINTS

- Midwives play a pivotal role in the provision of individualized screening, counselling and on-going support for families. Careful history-taking will help facilitate early identification of risk factors for certain anomalies.
- Antenatal identification of fetal anomalies allows preparation of the family and planned delivery in the optimal conditions for specialist neonatal care.

- Fetal surgery is in its relative infancy, but already contributes greatly to improved mortality and morbidity rates for several serious conditions.
- Consideration should always be given to the prevention and management of pain and discomfort of neonates during examinations or procedures.

REFERENCES

Abu-Saad, H.H., Bours, G.J., Stevens, B. *et al.* (1998) Assessment of pain in the neonate. *Seminars in Perinatology* **22**(5): 402–416.

Beischer, N., Mackay, E. & Colditz, P. (1997) *Obstetrics and the Newborn.* London: W.B. Saunders.

Benn, P.A., Craffey, A., Horne, D. *et al.* (2000) Elevated maternal serum alpha-fetoprotein with low unconjugated estriol and the risk for lethal perinatal outcome. *Journal of Maternal–Fetal Medicine* **9**(3): 165–169.

Botto, L.D., Lynberg, M.C. & Erickson, J.D. (2001) Congenital heart defects, maternal febrile illness and multivitamin use: a population-based study. *Epidemiology* **12**(5): 485–490.

Chung, K.C., Kowalski, C.P. & Kim, H.M. (2000) Maternal cigarette smoking during pregnancy and the risk of having a child with cleft lip/palate. *Plastic and Reconstructive Surgery* **105**(2): 485–491.

Farrell, T., Neale, L. & Cundy, T. (2002) Congenital anomalies in the offspring of women with type 1, type 2 and gestational diabetes. *Diabetic Medicine* **19**(4): 322–326.

Freeman, S.B., Taft, L.F., Dooley, K.J. *et al.* (1998) Population-based study of congenital heart defects in Down syndrome. *American Journal of Medical Genetics* **80**(3): 213–217.

Giannakoulopoulos, X., Teixeira, J., Fisk, N. *et al.* (1999) Human fetal and maternal noradrenaline responses to invasive procedures. *Pediatric Research* **45**(4 Pt 1): 494–499.

Glover, V. & Fisk, N. (1996) Do fetuses feel pain? *British Medical Journal* **313**(7060): 796.

Hasenau, S.M. (2002) Neural tube defects: prevention and folic acid. *MCN The American Journal of Maternal Child Nursing* **27**(2): 87–91.

Jesudason, E.C., Connell, M.G., Fernig, D.G. *et al.*(2000) Early lung malformation in congenital diaphragmatic hernia. *Journal of Pediatric Surgery* **35**(1): 124–127.

Kimber, C., Spitz, L. & Cuschierei, A. (1997) Current state of antenatal in-utero surgical interventions. *Archives of Disease in Childhood* **76**(2): F134–F139.

MacKenzie, T.C., Crombleholme, T.M. & Flake, A.W. (2002) The ex-utero intrapartum treatment. *Current Opinion in Pediatrics* **14**(4): 453–458.

Martucciello, G., Ceccherini, I., Lerone, M. *et al.* (2000) Pathogenesis of Hirschsprung's disease. *Journal of Pediatric Surgery* **35**(7): 1017–1025.

Molsted, K. (1999) Treatment and outcome in cleft lip and palate: issues and perspectives. *Critical Overviews in Oral Biology and Medicine* **10**(2): 225–239.

Office for National Statistics (ONS) (1999) *Live Births, Stillbirths and Linked Infant Deaths.* ONS Cause Groups Series DH3, No. 32. London: The Stationery Office.

Office for National Statistics (ONS) (2000) *Congenital Anomaly Statistics 1999*. Series MB3, No. 14. London: The Stationery Office.

Royal College of Obstetricians and Gynaecologists (RCOG) (1997) *Fetal Awareness. Working Party Report*. London: RCOG Press.

Samuels, P. & Tan, A.K. (1999) Fetal scarless wound healing. *Journal of Otolaryngology* **28**(5): 296–302.

Sheehan-Dare, R.A. (2001) The use of lasers in dermatology. *Hospital Medicine* **62**(1): 14–17.

Spilson, S.V., Kim, H.J. & Chung, K.C. (2001) Association between maternal diabetes mellitus and newborn oral cleft. *Annals of Plastic Surgery* **47**(5): 477–481.

Stevens, B. & Ohlsson, A. (2000) Sucrose for analgesia in newborn infants undergoing painful procedures. *Cochrane Database of Systematic Reviews* (2): CD001069. Oxford: Update Software.

Styles, M.E., Cole, T.J., Dennis, J. *et al.* (2002) New cross sectional stature, weight and head circumference

references for Down's syndrome in the UK and Republic of Ireland. *Archives of Disease in Childhood* **87**(2): 104–108.

Sutton, L.N., Sun, P. & Adzick, N.S. (2001) Fetal neurosurgery. *Neurosurgery* **48**(1): 124–144.

Weinzweig, J., Panter, K.E., Pantaloni, M. *et al.* (1999) The fetal cleft palate: II. Scarless healing after in-utero repair of a congenital model. *Plastic and Reconstructive Surgery* **104**(5): 1356–1364.

Wennerholm, U.B., Bergh, C., Hamberger, L. *et al.* (2000) Congenital malformations in children born after intracytoplasmic sperm injection (ICSI). *American Journal of Obstetrics and Gynecology* **182**(1 Pt 2): S182.

Wilson, R.D. (2000) Amniocentesis and chorionic villus sampling. *Current Opinion in Obstetrics & Gynecology* **12**(2): 81–86.

FURTHER READING

Sparshott, M. (1997) *Pain, Distress and the Newborn Baby*, 1st edn. Boston: Blackwell Science.
This is a practical and thoughtful text which is useful in exploring the physiology of neonatal pain and some of the complex knowledge required in caring for babies, and their parents.

Stevenson, R.E., Goodman, R. & Hall, J.G. (eds) (1993) *Human Malformations and Related Anomalies*. New York: Oxford University Press.

A large well-referenced and illustrated two-volume text containing information on congenital anomalies, incidence, recognition and management.

Wynbrandt, J.M. & Ludman, M.D. (1999) *The Encyclopedia of Genetic Disorders and Birth Defects*. New York: Facts on File Inc.
Comprehensive text outlining the history, diagnosis and prognosis of genetic disorders.

37

Neonatal Jaundice

Maggie Meeks and Stephanie Michaelides

LEARNING OUTCOMES

After reading this chapter you will be able to:

- understand the normal physiology of bilirubin metabolism
- identify common causes of unconjugated hyperbilirubinaemia
- make an assessment of jaundice and monitor its progress
- appreciate the principles of care of the jaundiced baby in the community
- understand the role and risks of phototherapy and exchange transfusion
- interpret the results of urine dipstick tests
- recognize the clinical signs of conjugated hyperbilirubinaemia
- plan and manage appropriate feeding regimes
- define the acute and chronic complications of kernicterus.

INTRODUCTION

Neonatal jaundice is common and occurs as a normal physiological event in up to 60% of full term infants (American Academy of Pediatrics (AAP), 1994). However, it is also important to be aware of the serious complications of severe jaundice and the variety of medical diseases that can cause it:

- High levels of bilirubin within the bloodstream can cause damage to the basal ganglia (kernicterus) and deafness with long-term neurodevelopmental complications.
- An infant that is jaundiced at <24 hours after birth always requires further investigation.
- Prolonged jaundice of the conjugated type is always pathological and needs to be investigated.

An understanding of the normal physiology of bilirubin metabolism allows recognition of why jaundice is so common in newborn infants and explains the mechanism of jaundice in many diseases. A basic knowledge of the rare genetic diseases may also allow a greater depth of understanding of normal physiology and these will be mentioned where appropriate. This chapter will therefore begin by discussing the physiology of bilirubin metabolism.

PHYSIOLOGY

Bilirubin is formed from the breakdown of an iron-containing molecule called *haem* that is an essential component of cytochromes, myoglobin and haemoglobin. The majority of bilirubin is produced as a consequence of haemoglobin breakdown within the spleen. At the end of their lifespan red blood cells are sequestered by the spleen and the haemoglobin is broken down into its component parts of haem and globin. The iron molecule is then removed from the haem to be recycled and the haem molecule is oxidized to biliverdin, which is reduced to form bilirubin (Dennery *et al.*, 2001).

Increased red cell breakdown will therefore lead to increased levels of unconjugated bilirubin. This is a lipid-soluble molecule that is insoluble in water. The lipid solubility means that it has the potential to cross the blood–brain barrier and enter into brain cells to cause kernicterus. The insolubility in water means that bilirubin needs to be transported to the liver linked to albumin within the plasma to prevent it precipitating. In this protein-bound state bilirubin is not available to be filtered by the glomerulus or to enter into tissues.

On arrival at the liver *unconjugated bilirubin* is transported into the liver cells and is converted into *bilirubin diglucuronide (conjugated bilirubin)* by the enzyme *UDP-glucuronyl transferase*. Conjugated bilirubin is water-soluble and is actively excreted by the liver cells into the intrahepatic bile ducts together with bile salts, cholesterol and phospholipids. This bile then flows down the extrahepatic ducts and into the small intestine. Within the colon some of the conjugated bilirubin is hydrolysed back to unconjugated bilirubin, while the remaining is metabolized into *stercobilinogen* and *urobilinogen*. Stercobilinogen is a brown pigment that is excreted within the faeces. Urobilinogen is reabsorbed in the enterohepatic circulation to be converted back to unconjugated bilirubin. A small amount of urobilinogen is carried in the bloodstream and excreted by the kidneys.

Reflective Activity 37.1

The imaginary journey of bilirubin

Imagine the bilirubin as a passenger undertaking a journey. This journey commences when the bilirubin leaves home (red blood cell) on its way to the train station. In order for the passenger to get to the station he has to catch a bus (albumin). The bus takes the passenger to the train station where he enters the train (liver). In order to arrive at his destination (nappy) the passenger will require the sustenance of food (glucose) and air (oxygen) in order to arrive safely (as water soluble bilirubin).

PHYSIOLOGICAL JAUNDICE

Physiological jaundice is the term used to describe jaundice that occurs as a consequence of the changeover from intrauterine to extrauterine life. The fetus requires a large number of red blood cells in order to attract oxygen from the placental circulation. The newborn infant therefore begins life with 6–7 million/mm^3 red cells which needs to reduce to the adult level of 5 million/ mm^3. The cells also contain fetal haemoglobin, which is gradually replaced by adult haemoglobin. These factors lead to increased red cell breakdown and an increased bilirubin load on the immature liver.

In addition, intestinal transit is slow until enteral feeds have been established, and this may lead to increased reabsorption of bilirubin via the enterohepatic circulation. Supplementing breastfeeding with water or glucose does not appear to have any effect on bilirubin levels in healthy newborns (Nicoll *et al.*, 1982) and thus should be avoided. Physiological jaundice is

characteristically noted around day 3 of life, peaks at day 5 and then slowly disappears. This jaundice is not associated with anaemia, and though not as alert as normal, the baby is usually well and the feeding pattern is satisfactory.

It may be exacerbated in situations that lead to an increased bilirubin production (e.g. polycythaemia, bruising) or decreased bilirubin excretion (poor feeding with delayed intestinal transit) and should be assessed on an individual basis and managed appropriately.

EVALUATION OF JAUNDICE

Prior to examination of the newborn to evaluate jaundice, the practitioner needs as much information as possible in order to assess and plan the management required. It is important to ascertain the severity of jaundice in order to refer appropriately. Although jaundice progresses from head to toe, it disappears from toe to head. Therefore observation of the colour of the sclera is not as useful in assessing improvement, as is observing the gums and tongue. This is informative in all babies regardless of ethnic background.

It is important to take into consideration the behaviour and feeding pattern of the baby – a baby who is alert and feeding well is less of a concern than one who is sleepy and not interested in feeding. Urine and bowel activity is also a strong indication of well-being.

Measurement of bilirubin

Jaundice becomes clinically apparent when the serum bilirubin (SBr) rises above 85 μmol/litre, and

---

Box 37.1 Taking blood for serum bilirubin measurement

In order to take a heel specimen correctly, the baby's foot needs to be lower than his body and the heel needs to be warm. A simple way to warm the foot if cold, is to use a gauze swab soaked in warm water wrapped around the heel and secured with cling film. The temperature of the gauze needs to be tested against the inner aspect of the practitioner's arm.

It is easier to scald the baby by dipping the foot in warm water, especially if the water temperature is tested by hand.

transcutaneous measuring devices have been developed that correlate well with serum bilirubin measurements (Rubaltelli *et al.*, 2001). The total serum bilirubin level can usually be measured on a capillary blood sample (Box 37.1) using a simple bilirubinometer that utilizes a spectroscopic (light absorptive) technique. It is important that these are regularly serviced and calibrated and in cases of significant jaundice a laboratory sample should always be sent to confirm the level of hyperbilirubinaemia and to quantify the unconjugated and conjugated proportions. Measurement of bilirubin is as a concentration in μmol/litre or mg/dl.

Light can alter the blood bilirubin; therefore it is important to transport blood specimens in a dark and safe environment. Because it is a blood product, the specimen should be carried in a container which avoids cross-contamination as well as protecting the specimen itself. The phototherapy light should also be switched off prior to the specimen being taken.

Recording the bilirubin result

In order to assess the situation and review management choices the bilirubin results need to be sequentially recorded. Graphs are available both for preterm and term infants and this allows the bilirubin levels to be plotted against the time the blood sample was taken. This can inform the practitioner at which level phototherapy should be commenced and also when exchange transfusion may be indicated. These charts enable the practitioner to view the progress of the jaundice and are a useful adjunct to the decision-making process for the jaundiced baby.

Urine dipstick testing shows a positive urobilinogen and negative bilirubin result and indicates an unconjugated hyperbilirubinaemia.

UNCONJUGATED HYPERBILIRUBINAEMIA

Unconjugated hyperbilirubinaemia has three main causes that can be predicted from an understanding of the physiology:

- increased red cell breakdown (haemolysis)
- failure of the ability to conjugate bilirubin
- increased enterohepatic circulation.

Increased red cell breakdown

Increased red cell breakdown occurs most commonly in the neonate because of infection, bruising (e.g. after ventouse or forceps delivery), polycythaemia and haemolytic disease of the newborn.

Haemolytic disease of the newborn

Haemolytic disease of the newborn is the term used to describe immune-mediated red cell breakdown such as occurs in rhesus disease and ABO incompatibility (this should not be confused with haemorrhagic disease of the newborn which refers to vitamin K deficiency). The maternal immune system is 'immunized' against aspects of the infant's blood group (see Fig. 37.1). This 'immunization' usually occurs because of a previous pregnancy or miscarriage when fetal blood cells have been transported into the maternal circulation, but in some patients it may have occurred following a blood transfusion and in ABO incompatibility IgM antibodies occur naturally.

Rhesus factor is the term used to describe the rhesus C, D and E antigens which are expressed on red blood cells, and it is the D antigen that is most likely to cause isoimmunization. An individual who is 'rhesus negative' does not express the D antigen and has the genotype dd. An individual who is rhesus positive does express the D antigen and can be heterozygous (Dd) or homozygous

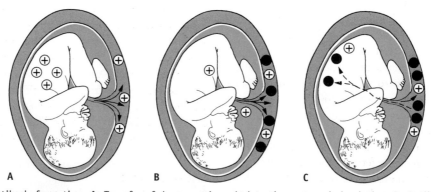

Figure 37.1   Antibody formation. **A.** Transfer of rhesus antigen (+) to the maternal circulation. **B.** Antibody formation (•) in the rhesus-negative mother. **C.** Transfer of rhesus antibody to the fetus.

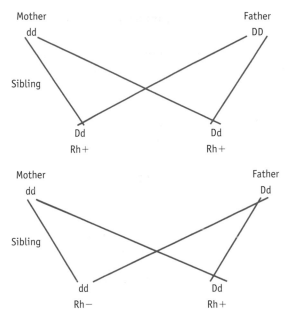

Figure 37.2 Inheritance of the rhesus factor.

(DD) for the rhesus antigen D genes. The risk of alloimmunization in a rhesus-negative mother will depend on the infant's genotype, which itself will be determined by the father's genotype, as shown in Figure 37.2.

In rhesus disease the haemolysis secondary to IgG that crosses the placenta can be severe enough to result in fetal anaemia and a need for intrauterine blood transfusions to prevent the development of *hydrops fetalis*. The aim is therefore to prevent alloimmunization by the administration of anti-D immunoglobulin to women at risk. This can be given antenatally and postnatally and will form complexes with the red cells to prevent the women's immune system from mounting its own immune response. Recent advice from the National Institute for Clinical Excellence (NICE) has supported the routine administration of antenatal anti-D prophylaxis to rhesus-negative women (NICE, 2002). However, anti-D is a blood product and prior to giving this drug the rules that follow the administration of blood products must be adhered to. Informed consent must be obtained and the administration of anti-D must be prescribed on the woman's drug chart by a medical practitioner (NMC, 2002).

Women and babies at risk can be identified by taking cord and maternal blood after delivery to determine the infant's blood group and Coombs' test result, and measure the presence of fetal blood cells and antibodies in the maternal system, as in Box 37.2.

Severe haemolysis is less common with ABO incompatibility (IgM antibodies do not cross the placenta): ABO blood group refers to the pattern of expression of the A and B antigens on the red blood cells. A mother of blood group O may have antibodies against the A and B antigens, a mother with blood group A against the B antigen and a mother of blood group B against the A antigen. These last two examples are extremely rare and ABO incompatibility is most common in a mother who has blood group O. It can occur with the first pregnancy and does not increase in severity with subsequent pregnancies.

ABO incompatibility in the newborn will usually manifest when the baby is less than 36 hours old – though it may not become obvious until after 48 hours. A history of a mother's blood group being O positive should alert the midwife to the possibility of ABO incompatibility. With the aid of the Kramer (1969) tool, the advancement of dermal icterus can be assessed in the jaundiced baby. Clinical evaluation of jaundice requires that the baby is undressed, and cephalocaudal progression of jaundice is evaluated using the five zones as in Figure 37.3. This clinical evaluation may be hindered if the baby has dark skin. The judicious use of this tool will assist the recording and monitoring of the progress of jaundice, and a baby advancing down the Kramer scale at a rapid rate can be referred swiftly to the neonatologist for diagnosis and treatment.

A baby who has been diagnosed and has received treatment for rhesus disease or ABO incompatibility needs to be closely observed for signs of 'late' anaemia. This may occur because the lifespan of the antibody is such that it will continue to haemolyse the red cells, causing the anaemia. Symptoms may include lethargy, pallor and poor feeding history. The baby will be under the neonatal team and may require iron or folate supplements or a possible blood transfusion. The continuity that is gained by the midwife providing care for up to 28 days can be very helpful in this sort of case.

Genetic causes

Biochemical or structural abnormalities of red cells may lead to a shortened lifespan with increased red

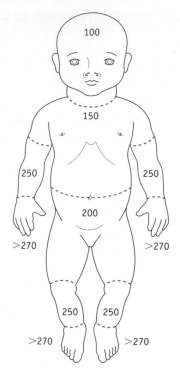

Jaundice which terminates at the neck – 100 μmol/l

Jaundice terminating at the umbilicus and upper arms – 150 μmol/l

Jaundice from umbilicus to knees – 200 μmol/l

Lower the arms and below the knees to the point of the wrist and ankles – 250 μmol/l

Jaundice from top to toe – above 250 μmol/l

Figure 37.3 The Kramer tool. Estimates of serum bilirubin (μmol/l) are obtained by assessing distal progression of jaundice. (Adapted from Kramer, 1969, with permission.)

cell turnover and jaundice. Some examples of inherited defects of red cells are listed below with their mode of inheritance:

- glucose-6-phosphate dehydrogenase (G6PD) deficiency
  - X-linked (males affected)
  - common in Mediterranean and Asian racial groups
- spherocytosis
  - autosomal dominant
- pyruvate kinase deficiency
  - autosomal recessive.

G6PD deficiency has been recognized since the time of Pythagoras, the Greek mathematician who warned his followers of the dangers of eating fava beans (broad beans). Today it is known that a variety of drugs, infection and the eating of fava beans may trigger G6PD deficiency.

Failure of conjugation

The ability to conjugate bilirubin may be immature in a newborn infant because of deficiency in the enzyme UDP-glucuronyl transferase. One of the explanations for a prolonged unconjugated hyperbilirubinaemia secondary to breastfeeding is that this enzyme is inhibited by breast milk.

There is no specific test for this condition and diagnosis is made when all the other causes have been excluded. The management is dependent on the baby's condition which on the whole is good, i.e. the baby is active and feeds well but the jaundice is prolonged and can take up to 6 weeks to resolve.

If the baby is well and all other causes have been excluded, the management is to encourage frequent breastfeeds as 'breastfeeding jaundice' rarely requires phototherapy treatment. Because of the benefits of breastfeeding, the mother should be encouraged and enabled to continue to breastfeed. Previously practitioners have advised the discontinuation of breastfeeding in order to confirm diagnosis, but this tends to provide negative feedback to the mother on her ability to feed and nurture her baby, so should be avoided.

Genetic reasons

There are a variety of genetic conditions that affect an individual's ability to conjugate bilirubin and these are listed below with their mode of inheritance:

- Gilbert syndrome: autosomal recessive

- Crigler–Najjar type I syndrome (bilirubin encephalopathy/kernicterus – common): autosomal recessive
- Crigler–Najjar type II syndrome (bilirubin encephalopathy/kernicterus – rare): autosomal recessive.

There is increasing molecular genetic evidence that Gilbert syndrome and Crigler–Najjar syndrome are allelic, that is, they both result from different mistakes (mutations) in the same gene, uridine diphosphate glycosyltransferase 1. This is the gene that codes for UDP-glucuronyl transferase and is found on chromosome 2. Gilbert syndrome is more common than Crigler–Najjar, and recent research suggests that significant hyperbilirubinaemia is only likely in Gilbert syndrome when G6PD deficiency is also present (Kaplan *et al.*, 1997). Gilbert syndrome alone does not result in a prolonged unconjugated hyperbilirubinaemia.

Increased enterohepatic circulation

Delayed intestinal transit will increase the enterohepatic circulation of bilirubin and lead to an increased level of unconjugated bilirubin. In a normal newborn infant, intestinal peristalsis develops over the first few days as enteral feeds are established, and delay in establishing feeds can exacerbate jaundice. The most common medical reason for delayed intestinal transit is *congenital hypothyroidism*. Infants diagnosed with congenital hypothyroidism must be commenced on levothyroxine sodium (thyroxine sodium) as soon as the diagnosis has been confirmed, to minimize the complication of neurodevelopmental delay. Infants are normally screened for this by measuring thyroid-stimulating hormone (TSH) on the Guthrie card.

The role of the midwife is to support the appropriate feeding of the newborn infant. The enzymes in colostrum encourage the passage of meconium (see Ch. 33), and the midwife can do much to support the woman in successfully breastfeeding in order for the baby to access colostrum and avoid dehydration. The midwife will note when the passage of meconium occurs as this is an important part of the assessment of the baby's progress and well-being. If the newborn does not pass meconium within 48 hours, referral should be made to a neonatologist to exclude congenital abnormalities.

Complications of unconjugated hyperbilirubinaemia

Kernicterus

Kernicterus is the term that describes yellow staining of the basal ganglia that is usually seen on post-mortem in infants who have had significant jaundice. The development of kernicterus is influenced by a number of factors (Pearlman *et al.*, 1980) which include the rate of rise of the bilirubin level as well as its maximum level. Other factors that affect an individual's susceptibility are:

- gestational age – preterm infants are more susceptible
- postnatal age – increasing postnatal age is protective
- albumin level – a normal albumin level is protective
- medication that interferes with bilirubin excretion – salicylates, sulphonamides, heparin, diazepam, chloramphenicol
- hypoxia/acidosis – both of these may reduce the effectiveness of the blood–brain barrier
- bacterial infection – e.g. group B sepsis, urinary tract infections.

There are also likely to be individual genetic factors affecting sensitivity to hyperbilirubinaemia that have not yet been identified (Hansen, 2000a).

Kernicterus is rare in Europe and the USA (Dodd, 1993; Newman and Maisels, 1992) but it appears to be increasing in incidence and this has paralleled the less aggressive management of jaundice and earlier hospital discharge of newborn infants, including those born at less than 37 weeks' gestation (Seidman *et al.*, 2001).

The symptoms of kernicterus can be divided into those that occur acutely and those that occur as long-term complications. Up to 15% of infants may be asymptomatic in the acute stage. The acute symptoms may also be reversible and without long-term complications if appropriately managed (Harris *et al.*, 2001). The common acute symptoms are summarized in Table 37.1.

Table 37.1 Acute symptoms of kernicterus

Age	Acute symptoms
1–2 days	Poor suck, hypotonia, stupor, seizures
3–7 days	Increased tone in extensor muscles, opisthotonos, fever
>1 week	Hypertonia

The long-term complications develop over the first 2 years of life with hypotonia and delayed motor development progressing to movement disorders such as choreoathetosis in association with a sensorineural hearing loss. Magnetic resonance imaging (MRI) can be used to guide prognosis, as the signal intensity in the globus pallidus reflects the deposition of bilirubin within basal ganglia (Harris *et al.*, 2001).

Management of unconjugated hyperbilirubinaemia

The recent trend towards home deliveries and early hospital discharge has been associated with increased readmission for jaundice and an increased risk of kernicterus (Newman and Maisels, 1990; Maisels and Newman, 1995). In some cases infants known to be at high risk can be identified (Box 37.3) and discharge may be delayed when appropriate. In most cases there should be active breastfeeding support and careful monitoring of the jaundice within the community by parents and community staff, and early hospital review where necessary (Bhutani and Johnson, 2000; 2001).

The initial assessment of an infant with significant jaundice is aimed at establishing the general condition and the most appropriate investigations and management that are required. General supportive measures may include the administration of antibiotics and the correction of dehydration. These are often required in the management of unconjugated hyperbilirubinaemia because meningitis and septicaemia are both more common during the first month of life than at any other time during childhood, and dehydration commonly exacerbates jaundice. In some situations it may also be important to correct acid–base defects and hypoxia, since both may increase the risk of kernicterus, and the administration of albumin may also reduce the amount of free bilirubin available to cross the blood–brain barrier (Ahlfors, 1994).

Specific treatments for unconjugated hyperbilirubinaemia are *phototherapy* and *exchange transfusion*. The exact level of bilirubin that causes bilirubin encephalopathy and kernicterus and at what stage these treatments

should be commenced, remains contentious. Bilirubin encephalopathy is rare in full-term infants without underlying pathology but a relaxation of treatment guidelines has led to an increase in the number of infants developing this complication (AAP, 2001; Hansen, 2000b). The aim of treatment should be to identify those infants at specific risk (Bhutani and Johnson, 2000) and to prevent kernicterus without exposing many more infants to unnecessary or potentially harmful treatment.

The American Academy of Pediatrics (AAP) has issued guidelines for starting phototherapy and exchange transfusion in healthy term infants >37 weeks' gestation and these are shown in Table 37.2.

Phototherapy

The effect of light on the excretion of bilirubin has been known since the 1950s (Cremer *et al.*, 1958), and phototherapy is an artificial method that provides light of a specific wavelength to enhance bilirubin excretion. The fat-soluble unconjugated bilirubin is converted into water-soluble lumirubin that can be excreted through the kidneys. The most effective light spectrum for converting the yellow bilirubin pigment to the photoisomer lumirubin is blue light and the wavelength of blue light is in the 425–475 nm range.

The other factors that influence the effectiveness of phototherapy are:

- total dose of light delivered
- energy output of light source
- number of light sources
- distance of light source(s) from infant
- maximum skin surface area exposed to those lights.

The two main ways of delivering phototherapy are the conventional overhead units (Fig. 37.4) and from light sources situated below the baby, either a fibreoptic device in contact with the baby's skin (biliblanket, Fig. 37.5) or a fluorescent lamp mounted beneath a light-permeable support (bilibed, Fig. 37.6). The term 'double phototherapy' refers to the combination of two phototherapy units (biliblanket and overhead

---

Box 37.3 Risk factors for developing significant unconjugated jaundice post-discharge

- Moderately preterm (35–37 weeks' gestation)
- Breastfeeding
- Jaundice <24 hours (haemolytic disease)
- Asian race
- Bruising/cephalhaematoma
- Infection
- Polycythaemic infants:
  - small-for-gestational-age infants
  - large-for-gestational-age infants, e.g. infant of diabetic mother
  - infants with chromosomal abnormalities, e.g. trisomy 21.

Table 37.2 Guidelines for phototherapy and exchange transfusion (AAP, 2001)

Age of baby	Phototherapy μmol/l (mg/l)	Exchange transfusion μmol/l (mg/l)
24–48 hours	>260 (15)	340 (20)
49–72 hours	>310 (18)	430 (25)
>72 hours	>340 (20)	430 (25)

or two overheads) placed at different positions above the infant. This has been demonstrated to significantly increase the excretion of bilirubin (Holtrop *et al.*, 1992) though 'triple phototherapy' does not appear to increase bilirubin excretion further.

It is important to be aware that the overhead units have incorporated or attached UV light filters that are designed to protect the infant from harmful rays and that manufacturers' guidelines for use of different phototherapy units (e.g. distance of the overhead from the infant) may vary. There have been reports of infants suffering UV burns as a direct consequence of phototherapy. Placing an infant under an overhead phototherapy unit also has the following implications for other aspects of care:

- Significant disruption of normal mother–infant interaction – the biliblanket is obviously less disruptive.
- Temperature regulation – infant temperature must be regularly monitored.
- Loose stools – there is a significant increase in fluid loss in the stools because of an associated decreased intestinal transit time.
- Nutrition and hydration – it is important to continue to establish demand feeding and to prevent dehydration. Extra fluids do not need to be routinely prescribed but the infant should be regularly assessed for signs of dehydration.
- Eye protection – the eyes must be protected as a precaution against possible damage (Fig. 37.7).
- Maternal anxiety – it is important to ensure that the woman understands the reasons for her baby requiring treatment and its basic principles.

Once phototherapy has commenced it is no longer possible to assess the degree of jaundice by looking at the skin and the serum bilirubin should be measured at least twice daily. On stopping phototherapy it is important to check the serum bilirubin at 4–6 hours to ensure that there has not been a significant rebound in hyperbilirubinaemia which may require further treatment.

Exchange transfusion

Exchange transfusion involves removing the baby's blood, with the maternal antibodies and bilirubin, and replacing it with fresh, rhesus-negative blood. During this procedure, up to 90% of the blood may be replaced. This was the first treatment to be successfully used in

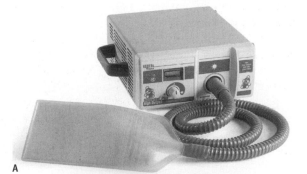

A

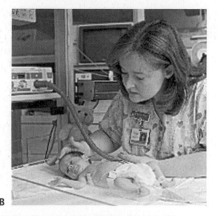

B

Figure 37.5 The Ohmeda Biliblanket. **A.** The phototherapy unit. **B.** Baby being nursed in a high-dependency setting. (Courtesy of Ohmeda Medical.)

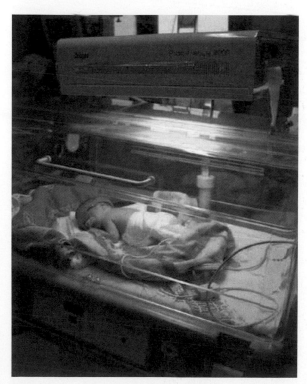

Figure 37.4 Baby receiving phototherapy.

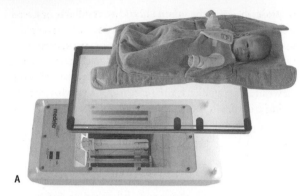

A

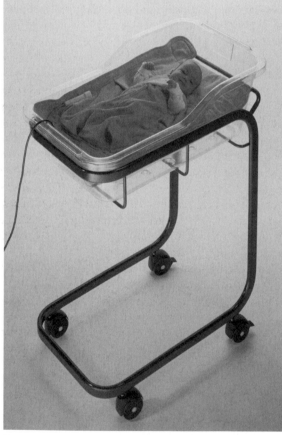

B

Figure 37.6 The Medela Bilibed. **A.** Phototherapy source, light-permeable support and baby in therapy blanket. **B.** Baby in crib with unit in position. (Courtesy of Medela AG.)

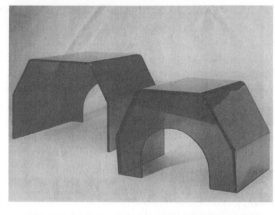

A

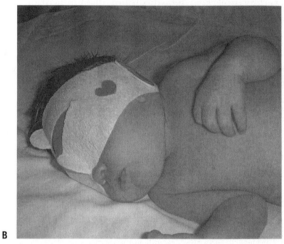

B

Figure 37.7 Viamed phototherapy lightshield (**A**) and eye protection (**B**). (Courtesy of Viamed Ltd.)

- anaemia
- oedema
- cardiac failure
- significant hyperbilirubinaemia
- hyperbilirubinaemia uncontrolled by phototherapy
- hyperbilirubinaemia associated with polycythaemia.

In most cases a two-volume exchange is performed, in which 160 ml/kg of the circulating blood volume is removed and this is replaced with transfused whole blood (more commonly packed red cells and 0.9% saline or 4.5% albumin nowadays since whole blood is difficult to obtain). The procedure should be conducted slowly under strict aseptic conditions with detailed recording of the amount of blood removed as well as the amount infused. There are two main ways in which the procedure is conducted, single site and two site method.

The *two site method* is preferred and involves aspirating blood from a peripheral artery or umbilical artery at a similar rate to the infusion rate of a transfusion that is being delivered through a peripheral vein. The

severe neonatal jaundice. It is particularly useful in haemolytic disease since both red blood cells and the red cell antibodies causing their breakdown are removed from the neonatal circulation.

The main indications for exchange transfusion are:

- severe haemolytic disease
- hypoproteinaemia

single site method involves cannulation of the umbilical vein with aspiration of 5–10 ml of blood through a three-way tap followed by infusion of the same quantity of donor blood. This can result in significant changes in central venous pressure and intravascular volume and is also associated with the complications of umbilical venous cannulation.

The complications of exchange transfusion are more common than those of phototherapy and include electrolyte imbalance, thrombocytopenia, infection, cardiac failure and necrotizing enterocolitis. An exchange transfusion should therefore only be performed in an infant that is at significant risk of kernicterus in whom the benefits of transfusion outweigh the risks of these complications (Ahlfors, 1994). The risks can be minimized by intensively monitoring the infant's electrolytes and platelets throughout the procedure and by minimizing the changes in circulating blood volume during the procedure.

Once the exchange transfusion has been completed the infant should continue to be monitored under phototherapy until the hyperbilirubinaemia has begun to decrease and phototherapy is no longer needed. Some infants require more than one exchange transfusion but in most cases an exchange transfusion followed by double phototherapy should be sufficient.

Immunoglobulin

The use of intravenous immunoglobulin as an additional form of treatment in haemolytic jaundice has also been described (Alpay *et al.*, 1999; Ergaz and Arad, 1993). The effect of this treatment is to reduce ongoing haemolysis although the exact mechanism remains unclear.

Follow-up

All infants who have had significant unconjugated hyperbilirubinaemia should be reviewed on at least one occasion following discharge. This enables the results of the investigations to be reviewed, further investigations to be arranged if appropriate and the infant's clinical condition to be reassessed. Since one of the complications of hyperbilirubinaemia is sensorineural hearing loss, these infants should also have formal hearing tests performed, e.g. auditory brainstem response (ABR), auditory evoked response (AER).

Neonates that have had evidence of haemolytic jaundice require early review and regular follow-up for the first 3 months of life, since the other effect of haemolysis is anaemia. The infant should be seen at less than 2 weeks of age to review its clinical condition and to perform a full blood count. This investigation will provide information about the extent of the ongoing haemolysis (haemoglobin) and the infant's bone marrow response and ability to compensate (reticulocyte count). Some infants may require a blood transfusion but the indications for this will include the infant's clinical condition and should be discussed with the parents.

Infants that had clinical evidence of kernicterus will require continued neurodevelopmental follow-up and further investigations such as MRI to establish a guide to prognosis.

CONJUGATED HYPERBILIRUBINAEMIA

A conjugated hyperbilirubinaemia is always pathological and refers to a situation where >15% of the total bilirubin is in the conjugated or 'direct-reacting' form. It occurs as a direct consequence of an interruption in the normal excretion of bilirubin diglucuronide and results from an obstruction at any point along the pathway from the hepatocyte to the intestine. The process of bilirubin conjugation within the liver is often able to continue even in the presence of significant liver damage but the excretion of the conjugated bilirubin into intrahepatic bile ducts may become obstructed. Consequently the concentration of bilirubin diglucuronide within the hepatocytes will then continue to increase and eventually it will diffuse into the bloodstream.

An understanding of the normal physiology of bilirubin and the pathophysiology of conjugated hyperbilirubinaemia enables one to predict that a conjugated jaundice can be suspected clinically in an infant with pale stools (absent stercobilinogen) and dark urine (bilirubin present). Urine dipstick test will be positive for bilirubin.

These are very important clinical features to note since this jaundice may initially be subtle and easily missed, and therefore always requires further assessment.

Some of the main causes of a conjugated jaundice are summarized below:

- Hepatitis with cholestasis:
  - prolonged total parenteral nutrition (TPN)
  - congenital infection, e.g. CMV, toxoplasmosis, rubella
  - metabolic disease, e.g. α_1-antitrypsin deficiency
  - galactosaemia
- Abnormality of bile ducts:
  - intrahepatic biliary atresia, e.g. Alagille syndrome (autosomal dominant)
  - extrahepatic biliary atresia.

In a term infant without any perinatal concerns conjugated jaundice most commonly presents as prolonged jaundice. Any infant that remains jaundiced at 10 days to 2 weeks of age should be investigated for this type of jaundice by examining the stools and taking blood for a split bilirubin (direct and indirect bilirubin), packed cell volume (PCV) and G6PD test. A midstream urine (MSU) may also be indicated (Hannam *et al.*, 2000). Those infants with extrahepatic biliary atresia need to be identified as early as possible since they have an improved prognosis if surgery is performed at 4–6 weeks of age.

Complications of conjugated hyperbilirubinaemia

The complications that are associated with conjugated hyperbilirubinaemia can be considered as general or specific complications of the underlying disease itself rather than direct complications of the conjugated jaundice. The general complications include deranged clotting with bleeding concerns and hypoglycaemia as a result of underlying hepatic dysfunction. In addition, the absorption of fat-soluble vitamins such as vitamins A, D and K may be reduced and the infant may need to be commenced on IV/IM vitamin K and appropriate vitamin preparations such as Ketovite. Specific complications include septicaemia and cataracts in galactosaemia, and microcephaly in congenital infection.

Management of conjugated hyperbilirubinaemia

The main objective in the management of an infant with conjugated hyperbilirubinaemia is to establish the cause of the jaundice. Neither phototherapy nor exchange transfusion has a role in this type of jaundice. Phototherapy is ineffective because conjugated bilirubin is already water-soluble and the inappropriate use of phototherapy may lead to the 'bronzed baby'

syndrome. Exchange transfusion is not indicated for conjugated hyperbilirubinaemia because conjugated bilirubin is not lipid-soluble in the same way as unconjugated bilirubin and will not cause kernicterus.

Examination of an infant suspected to have a conjugated jaundice may identify petechiae, bruising, bleeding or hepatomegaly and the first-line investigations should include a blood glucose measurement, liver function tests and clotting studies. Early advice should be sought from a paediatric hepatologist so that the most appropriate investigations and subsequent management can be arranged.

CONCLUSION

Jaundice is a common problem of the newborn infant. An understanding of the normal physiology of bilirubin metabolism enables the midwife to both predict the risk factors for developing an unconjugated hyperbilirubinaemia and the clinical signs suggestive of a conjugated hyperbilirubinaemia. The aim is to prevent infants from developing a severe unconjugated hyperbilirubinaemia that may lead to kernicterus and to identify those infants that need further medical investigation.

The midwife will often be the person who will identify the jaundice, and will also be the person who will continue to provide care and support to the woman, her baby and family, and needs to be knowledgeable about the different aspects of care and management, and be able to provide accurate and evidence-based information to the woman, ensuring she feels informed and confident in the professionals providing care to her baby.

ACKNOWLEDGEMENT

We are indebted to Dr Richard Thompson for his knowledge of paediatric liver disease.

KEY POINTS

- Jaundice is the clinical consequence of a high level of bilirubin, which may be unconjugated or conjugated.
- Jaundice is common but must always be investigated when it is noted at < 24 hours of age or is prolonged for more than 2 weeks.
- A significant unconjugated hyperbilirubinaemia must be treated with phototherapy or exchange

transfusion to prevent the acute complications of kernicterus and long-term complications of deafness and athetoid cerebral palsy.
- An infant that is jaundiced with pale stools and dark urine requires urgent assessment and referral to a paediatric hepatologist.

REFERENCES

Ahlfors, C.E. (1994) Criteria for exchange transfusion in jaundiced newborns. *Pediatrics* **93**(3): 488–494.

Alpay, F., Sarici, S.U., Okutan, V. *et al.* (1999) High-dose intravenous immunoglobulin therapy in neonatal immune hemolytic jaundice. *Acta Paediatrica* **88**(2): 216–219.

American Academy of Pediatrics (AAP) (1994) Practice parameter management of hyperbilirubinemia in the healthy term newborn. Provisional Committee for Quality Improvement and Subcommittee on Hyperbilirubinemia. *Pediatrics* **94**(4 Pt 1): 558–565.

Bhutani, V.K. & Johnson, L.H. (2000) Managing the assessment of neonatal jaundice: importance of timing. *Indian Journal of Pediatrics* **67**(10): 733–737.

Bhutani, V.K. & Johnson, L.H. (2001) Jaundice technologies: prediction of hyperbilirubinemia in term and near-term newborns. *Journal of Perinatology* **21**(Suppl. 1): S76–82; discussion S83–87.

Cremer, R.J., Perryman, P. & Richards, D. (1958) Influence of light on the hyperbilirubinemia of infants. *Lancet* **1**: 1094–1097.

Dennery, P.A., Seidman, D.S. & Stevenson, D.K. (2001) Neonatal hyperbilirubinemia. *New England Journal of Medicine* **344**(8): 581–590.

Dodd, K.L. (1993) Neonatal jaundice – a lighter touch. *Archives of Disease in Childhood* **68**(5 Spec. No.): 529–532.

Ergaz, Z. & Arad, I. (1993) Intravenous immunoglobulin therapy in neonatal immune hemolytic jaundice. *Journal of Perinatal Medicine* **21**(3): 183–187.

Hannam, S., McDonnell, M. & Rennie, J.M. (2000) Investigation of prolonged neonatal jaundice. *Acta Paediatrica* **89**(6): 694–697.

Hansen, T.W. (2000a) Kernicterus in term and near-term infants – the specter walks again. *Acta Paediatrica* **89**(10): 1155–1157.

Hansen, T.W.R. (2000b) Bilirubin oxidation in brain. *Molecular Genetics and Metabolism* **71**: 411–417.

Harris, M.C., Bernbaum, J.C., Polin, J.R. *et al.* (2001) Developmental follow-up of breastfed term and near-term infants with marked hyperbilirubinemia. *Pediatrics* **107**(5): 1075–1080.

Holtrop, P.C., Ruedisueli, K. & Maisels, M.J. (1992) Double versus single phototherapy in low birth weight newborns. *Pediatrics* **90**(5): 674–677.

Kaplan, M., Renbaum, P., Levy-Lahad, E. *et al.* (1997) Gilbert syndrome and glucose-6-phosphate dehydrogenase deficiency: a dose-dependent genetic interaction crucial to neonatal hyperbilirubinemia. *Proceedings of the National Academy of Sciences USA* **94**(22): 12128–12132.

Kramer, L.I. (1969) Advancement of dermal icterus in the jaundiced newborn. *American Journal of Diseases of Children* **118**: 454–458.

Maisels, M.J. & Newman, T.B. (1995) Kernicterus in otherwise healthy, breast-fed term newborns. *Pediatrics* **96**(4 Pt 1): 730–733.

National Institute for Clinical Excellence (NICE) (2002) *Technology Appraisal Guidance No. 41: Guidance on the Use of Routine Antenatal Anti-D Prophylaxis for Rhesus Negative Women*. London: NICE.

Newman, T.B. & Maisels, M.J. (1990) Does hyperbilirubinemia damage the brain of healthy full-term infants? *Clinics in Perinatology* **17**(2): 331–358.

Newman, T.B. & Maisels, M.J. (1992) Evaluation and treatment of jaundice in the term newborn: a kinder, gentler approach. *Pediatrics* **89**(5 Pt 1): 809–818.

Nicoll, A., Ginsburg, R. & Tripp, J.H. (1982) Supplementary feeding and jaundice in newborns. *Acta Paediatricia Scandinavica* **71**(5): 759–761.

Nursing and Midwifery Council (NMC) (2002) *Guidelines for the Administrations of Medicines*. (First published October 2000 by UKCC.) London: NMC.

Pearlman, M.A., Gartner, L.M., Lee, K. *et al.* (1980) The association of kernicterus with bacterial infection in the newborn. *Pediatrics* **65**(1): 26–29.

Rubaltelli, F.F., Gourley, G.R., Loskamp, N. *et al.* (2001) Transcutaneous bilirubin measurement: a multicenter evaluation of a new device. *Pediatrics* **107**(6): 1264–1271.

Seidman, D.S., Paz, I., Armon, Y. *et al.* (2001) Effect of publication of the 'Practice Parameter for the management of hyperbilirubinemia' on treatment of neonatal jaundice. *Acta Paediatrica* **90**(3): 292–295.

FURTHER READING

Blackburn, S.T. (2003) *Maternal, Fetal and Neonatal Physiology: a Clinical Perspective*. Philadelphia: W.B. Saunders.
This book is invaluable in the presentation of fetal and neonatal physiology, underpinning problems the neonate may experience.

Ives, N.K. (1997) Neonatal jaundice. *Current Paediatrics* **7**(2): 67–72.
This is a brief and accessible summary of jaundice, is easily readable and reviews the physiology, aetiology and treatment of jaundice.

38

Metabolic and Endocrine Disorders

Carol Simpson

LEARNING OUTCOMES

At the end of this chapter, you will have:

- developed your knowledge of the features of the common metabolic and endocrine disorders
- an understanding of inherited conditions, their recognition and their relevance to antenatal care and screening
- an understanding of screening and treatment options for common metabolic and endocrine disorders of the neonate.

INTRODUCTION

Midwives have a key role in providing information and advice to women and their families concerning the possibilities of metabolic and endocrine disorders, and how these might be detected and screened for. From careful questioning at booking to pre- and post-test counselling and support, midwives are a conduit for education and information. They need to be able to provide clear, up-to-date, simple and unbiased information to women and their families on which they can base an informed choice.

SCREENING

To enable parents to make informed choices, before any screening programme, they need to have full details of the test procedure, the conditions tested for, their implications, treatments and possible outcomes.

When a specific family trait or condition is identified, genetic counselling and gene mapping, from blood samples of the parents, may help to identify the risk of a fetus being affected. Other antenatal screening methods, such as amniocentesis and chorionic villus sampling, can test the individual fetus for such disorders.

Midwives must obtain informed consent for neonatal screening and should discuss all the conditions tested for by the laboratories. Ethical, financial, regional and political factors influence the range of conditions screened for in different areas, with some obtaining anonymous population data for HIV from Guthrie samples (Tappin *et al.*, 1991).

In many countries worldwide, routine neonatal screening (Guthrie test) is performed for phenylketonuria and congenital hypothyroidism, and has significantly reduced the long-term effects of phenylketonuria. This test involves biochemical testing of dried capillary blood spots obtained by a heel-prick, at least 48 hours after milk feeds are established. These blood spots can also be used to test for a number of other endocrine and metabolic disorders (Clague and Thomas, 2002) including galactosaemia, G6PD deficiency, congenital adrenal hyperplasia and amino-acidaemias (Matern, 2002). DNA extraction from these samples also enables identification of Duchenne muscular dystrophy, cystic fibrosis and haemoglobinopathies such as sickle cell anaemia.

In undertaking the Guthrie test, the midwife should also be alert to the possibility of conditions such as haemorrhagic disease which may be detected after the test. After taking the blood sample it is normal practice to apply pressure to the puncture wound on the heel. Prolonged bleeding should alert the midwife to potential problems. It is also useful to be aware that the use of sticking plaster should be restricted, as in removing the plaster the first layer of epidermis may also be removed.

Reflective Activity 38.1

Find out what disorders are routinely screened for from Guthrie cards in your area.

INBORN ERRORS OF METABOLISM

Phenylketonuria (PKU)

PKU is an autosomal recessive disorder occurring in about 1:10 000 births; more commonly in the Irish population where the incidence is about 1:4000.

There is a deficiency of the enzyme *phenylalanine hydroxylase*, which converts phenylalanine, an amino acid found in most foods, into tyrosine. Once milk feeds are established, blood levels of phenylalanine start to rise, together with a by-product of its metabolism, phenylpyruvic acid, which is toxic to the neonatal brain and causes irreversible neurological damage. Features, which present at around 3 months of age, include persistent vomiting, eczema and a characteristic musty smell to the urine. Early neonatal diagnosis using the Guthrie test and treatment with a phenylalanine-restricted diet have led to excellent outcomes for PKU. It is now rare to see older children or adults with the long-term effects of seizures, developmental delay and severe eczema.

Phenylpyruvic acid is excreted in the urine and can be used to test for PKU in pregnancy. A permanent low-phenylalanine diet is recommended, but is imperative preconceptually. High phenylalanine levels before and early in pregnancy result in an increased incidence of congenital heart defects, particularly hypoplastic left heart syndrome and coarctation of the aorta (Levy *et al.*, 2001).

Galactosaemia

Galactosaemia is an autosomal recessive disorder, occurring in about 1:40 000–60 000 babies. There is a deficiency of the enzyme *galactose-1-phosphate uridyltransferase*, required to metabolize galactose into glucose in the intestine. The resulting accumulation of galactose and galactose-1-phosphate in erythrocytes can cause liver cirrhosis, intellectual disability and cataract formation. Diagnosis is confirmed by the estimation of galactose-1-phosphate in the Guthrie blood spots.

A baby with this condition will present signs of failure to thrive, vomiting, persistent jaundice, sepsis and hepatosplenomegaly within the first week. Treatment is with a galactose-free diet, usually with the substitution of soya milk. The prognosis is improved with early diagnosis and treatment, since sepsis and damage to major organs may be prevented.

Glucose-6-phosphate dehydrogenase (G6PD) deficiency

G6PD deficiency is an X-linked recessive disorder, prevalent throughout tropical and subtropical regions of the world, where it affords some protection against malaria. Extremely high incidences have been reported in the Philippines and Taiwan, and midwives should consider ethnic origins when advising families of screening programmes. G6PD is a red blood cell enzyme found in all tissues and is involved in erythrocyte metabolism. When it is deficient, haemolysis occurs more readily, resulting in jaundice and potentially kernicterus. This affects males more than females.

Diagnosis can be made from Guthrie samples or cord blood. Common triggers for this disorder include infection, exposure to naphthalene vapour (e.g. moth balls) and ingestion of fava (broad) beans. Treatment involves avoidance of these triggers and alleviating symptoms with phototherapy, blood transfusion and prophylactic antioxidants, such as vitamin E.

Spherocytosis

This condition is characterized by spherical rather than biconcave red blood cells, leaving the baby at greater risk from anaemia and jaundice.

> **Reflective Activity 38.2**
>
> Find out what provisions your area has for preconceptual care and genetic screening.

ACQUIRED ERRORS OF METABOLISM

Hypoglycaemia

There is much debate over what constitutes a normal plasma glucose value for infants of different gestations and birthweight, and therefore what constitutes a finite biochemical definition of hypoglycaemia (Cornblath *et al.*, 2000). It is now accepted that damage to the neonatal brain does occur as a result of hypoglycaemia (Duvanel *et al.*, 1999), but the duration and severity needed to cause this remain unclear (Hawdon *et al.*, 1994). However, it is generally agreed that high-risk infants should be closely monitored and the plasma glucose levels maintained above 2.6 mmol/l.

Causes and risk factors

Hypoglycaemia is a complication of many conditions in the neonate and high-risk groups include:

- Preterm babies – the bulk of glycogen and fat stores are laid down in the fetus during the third trimester; thus preterm babies lack these energy stores.
- Small-for-gestational-age babies (SGA) – intrauterine malnutrition uses up energy reserves leaving these babies vulnerable to hypoglycaemia.
- Large-for-gestational-age babies (LGA) – these babies rapidly utilize stores and require regular feeding to prevent hypoglycaemia.
- Infants of diabetic mothers – overproduction of insulin continues for several hours following birth, utilizing glycogen stores.
- Babies with inborn errors of metabolism – for example galactosaemia, congenital hyperinsulinaemia, G6PD deficiency.
- Babies with specific anomalies – Beckwith–Weidemann syndrome, pancreatic tumours, pituitary insufficiency.
- Other miscellaneous conditions – feeding difficulties, hypothermia, cerebral damage, infection, severe rhesus haemolytic disease.

Prevention

Prevention centres on identifying babies at risk. This should begin during the antenatal period when women with problems such as diabetes should be identified, carefully monitored and a plan for the care and management of the baby agreed. This includes regular monitoring of blood sugar levels and early and regular feeding. Capillary blood glucose levels should be frequently checked using Dextrostix or BM Stix, particularly over the first 24–48 hours of life. The frequency will depend on the condition and risk factors of the individual baby. A healthy baby who is between the 10th and 90th percentiles generally does not require glucose analysis. A venous blood sample should be taken for a more accurate estimation if these readings are low.

Signs, symptoms and management

Hypoglycaemia may be asymptomatic but still requires treatment. Where signs are present they are often non-specific and include lethargy, poor feeding, hypotonia and jitteriness. Left untreated, convulsions, cyanosis and apnoea may occur, possibly resulting in neurological damage, coma and even death.

In mild or asymptomatic cases of hypoglycaemia, the baby should be fed immediately and at frequent regular intervals thereafter. Blood glucose estimation should be repeated 1 hour after feeding and, if still low, may warrant further investigation or intravenous fluids. Severe, prolonged or recurrent hypoglycaemia is most likely due to a metabolic disorder.

> ### Reflective Activity 38.3
>
> Locate and review your local guidelines for the definition and management of hypoglycaemia in term and preterm infants – are these up to date and based on research and evidence?

Neonatal convulsions

These are frequently a presenting feature of metabolic disorders, as well as of neurological problems. Neonatal convulsions are more subtle than those seen in adults and therefore not always obvious. Signs may include:

- cycling movements of limbs
- recurrent apnoeas and cyanosis
- jerky, rhythmic movements
- hypertonia
- rapid eye movements
- intense sucking.

If there is any doubt, an urgent paediatric opinion should be sought and blood samples taken for glucose and electrolyte measurements.

Hyperglycaemia

This is a blood glucose level greater than 8 mmol/l and occurs more commonly in preterm babies. It is associated with a decreased renal threshold for glucose, often found with infections, stress and postnatal steroid administration. Hyperglycaemia may result in osmolar diuresis and dehydration, requiring fluid replacement.

Hypocalcaemia

Hypocalcaemia (neonatal tetany) is a blood calcium level less than 1.7 mmol/l. Levels normally fall over the first 48 hours of life, then rise and stabilize in response to an increase in parathyroid hormone concentration. Persistent or severe neonatal tetany beyond this stage may be associated with maternal hyperparathyroidism.

Transient hypocalcaemia is relatively common in the first few days and is exacerbated in low birth-weight babies, infants of diabetic mothers and following exchange transfusions. Vitamin D deficiency and resulting hypocalcaemia are common in some immigrant populations and are risk factors for neonatal tetany. In many developing countries, hypocalcaemia is seen in association with feeding babies unmodified cow's milk, which is high in phosphorous.

Signs and symptoms include irritability followed by twitching, periods of apnoea and convulsions. Treatment with oral calcium is very effective. Intravenous calcium is for emergency use and must be administered slowly with the baby closely monitored, as bradycardias and arrhythmias can occur. It is also important to prevent extravasation as this causes severe skin necrosis.

The only sequela to this condition seems to be hypoplasia of the dental enamel in the first teeth, which predisposes to dental caries.

Hypomagnesaemia

Hypomagnesaemia is defined as a serum magnesium level less than 0.6 mmol/l.

Magnesium and calcium levels are closely linked and treatment of one deficit often relieves the other. Congenital (primary) hypomagnesaemia with secondary hypocalcaemia is a rare autosomal recessive condition which presents with recurrent tetany or convulsions in the early neonatal period. High-dose magnesium supplementation will be required for life but the long-term outcome for this condition appears to be good (Shalev *et al.*, 1998).

Hyponatraemia

Hyponatraemia is a serum sodium level of less than 130 mmol/l. This is a common condition affecting up to a third of all very low birthweight infants in the first week of life. Impaired reabsorption of sodium in the immature kidneys and insensible water loss are major causes of sodium depletion in preterm neonates. Routine sodium supplementation is given to premature babies, although the timing and duration of this is controversial (Hartnoll *et al.*, 2001). Chronic hyponatraemia is associated with poor neurodevelopmental outcome (Al-Dahhan *et al.*, 2002).

Hypernatraemia

A plasma sodium level above 143 mmol/l defines hypernatraemia.

In preterm babies this may be caused by a failure to compensate adequately for large fluid losses, for example from radiant heaters, phototherapy or during episodes of diarrhoea. The neonatal kidneys are immature and cannot cope with excess sodium. Correct technique and quantities must be used when reconstituting baby milk powder, and it is important to teach parents to do this correctly. Putting powder in the bottle prior to water, or using heaped, tightly packed, or extra scoops all increase the sodium content of the feed.

Early signs of hypernatraemia are that the baby becomes increasingly fretful, thirsty, dehydrated and pyrexial. Generalized oedema develops and cerebral oedema can lead to convulsions and irreversible neurological damage.

Treatment involves correction of dehydration by feeding with breast milk or low-solute artificial milk. Another preventive measure is delaying the introduction of solids until after 4–6 months of age, which also reduces the solute load to the kidneys.

EXOCRINE DISORDERS

Cystic fibrosis

Cystic fibrosis (CF) is an autosomal recessive condition associated with chromosome 7. It is the most common lethal genetic disorder within Caucasian populations, particularly northern Europeans, with an incidence of approximately 1 : 2500–3500 babies. Carriers are common (1 : 40) and preconceptual or antenatal testing is available for parents.

This is an abnormality of the exocrine mucus-secreting glands throughout the body, particularly the intestine, lungs and pancreas. The protein required to carry chloride ions, part of salt, across cell membranes, is absent. This causes the formation of thick mucus, which distends and dilates the affected areas, ultimately leading to obstruction and fibrosis.

About 15% of babies with CF will present with meconium ileus due to abnormally thick meconium; subsequent stools may be pale and hard. The passage of the first stool and its consistency are therefore important observations for the midwife to note. Most children are not diagnosed until infancy, following recurrent chest infections and failure to thrive.

Guthrie samples can be screened for *immunoreactive trypsinogen* levels, which are elevated in babies with CF. A sweat test is then carried out, measuring the salt content of the sweat, to confirm diagnosis. Early diagnosis and treatment can greatly improve the prognosis; thus routine neonatal screening is recommended by many clinicians.

There is no cure for CF and the international median life expectancy is currently about 30 years (Chini, 2002). Treatment is aimed at preventing complications and maintaining optimal growth and development. The control of infection, especially respiratory tract infection, is most important. Long-term antibiotics may be prescribed together with mucus-thinning agents and regular physiotherapy to try to minimize lung damage. Lung transplants are offered in some areas but survival after transplantation remains poor (Aurora *et al.*, 1999). Pancreatic enzyme replacements and vitamin supplements are prescribed and have improved the prognosis for these children.

ENDOCRINE DISORDERS

Congenital adrenal hyperplasia (CAH)

This is the most common cause of genital ambiguity in neonates. This autosomal recessive disorder is caused by an enzyme deficiency in the synthesis of aldosterone and cortisol. In its mild form it occurs in about 1 : 1000 births and in its classic, more severe form, 1 : 15 000 births. Diagnosis can be made from biochemical analysis of the Guthrie samples.

The mild disorder causes varying degrees of virilization, with reduced fertility in affected females and some signs of androgen excess in male children. Often no treatment is necessary, but the midwife must take care when examining the baby and not guess the sex if it is unclear (Fig. 38.1). Chromosomal analysis will be required.

The more severe form results in a potentially lethal electrolyte imbalance and dehydration from an acute salt-losing crisis at 1–2 weeks of age. Steroids are required to suppress adrenal androgen secretion and will need to be continued for life. Occasionally, plastic surgery is required to correct the virilization effects in females.

Prenatal treatments involving maternal dexamethasone administration are being researched but there are safety concerns (Merke and Kabbani, 2001). Adverse effects on the brain and kidneys from high doses of dexamethasone in the second trimester have been shown in animal studies.

If the genitalia are ambiguous, the midwife must involve a senior paediatrician as soon as possible, as the long-term psychological impact of providing wrong information to families can be devastating.

Congenital hypothyroidism

This is a relatively common (1 : 3500 neonates) and potentially severe disorder for which several genes have been implicated (Vilain *et al.*, 2001). Screening for this is included in the Guthrie test and midwives need to explain this to parents.

There are two types:

- *Thyroid dysgenesis* – hypoplastic, ectopic or absent thyroid gland accounts for most cases.

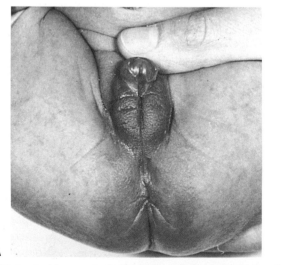
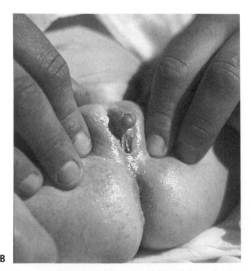

A   **B**

Figure 38.1   Ambiguous genitalia. **A.** In an infant with congenital adrenal hyperplasia. **B.** In a baby with androgen insensitivity. (From Johnston *et al.*, 2003.)

- *Hormonal dysfunction* – resulting in a defect in the synthesis of thyroid hormone. This can be caused by maternal antithyroid therapy, may cause goitre and demonstrates autosomal recessive inheritance.

Presentation varies depending on the severity of the disease. Signs and symptoms include prolonged jaundice, poor feeding, lethargy and delayed maturation of tibial and femoral epiphyses, found on X-ray. Clinical signs of a severely affected neonate include coarse facial features, a low hairline, a short, thick neck and flat nasal bridge, with intellectual and motor impairment. Treatment with levothyroxine sodium (thyroxine sodium), started during the first month of life, dramatically improves the neurological outcome.

Neonatal thyrotoxicosis

This is a severe, but rare, disorder with a high mortality, associated with maternal hyperthyroidism (Graves' disease). It precipitates neonatal symptoms in the first few days including weight loss, vomiting, thirst, irritability, goitre, cardiomegaly, hydrops and tachycardia. This can progress to cardiac failure and collapse if untreated. Diagnosis can be made from Guthrie test or cord blood. Treatment is with antithyroid drugs and rehydration.

Vitamin K deficiency bleeding (VKDB)

Newborn babies are at risk of developing this haemorrhagic disease, previously known as haemorrhagic disease of the newborn (HDN) (Sutor *et al.*, 1999). It is caused by an accentuation of the normal neonatal deficiency of the vitamin K-dependent clotting factors, including prothrombin and factors VII, IX and X. Vitamin K is synthesized by the gut flora, which do not colonize the gut until feeding has been established. This condition is discussed more fully in Chapters 31 and 34.

CONCLUSION

It is crucial that midwives are knowledgeable and up to date about metabolic and endocrine disorders which may affect the neonate. This should be linked to a knowledge of screening and its implications for the woman and baby. This will assist in identifying potential problems, and in the provision of information and support to the woman and her family. Midwives can access further information and support from a variety of sources, including the supervisor of midwives, link educationalists and colleagues in the neonatal and paediatric units.

KEY POINTS

- Midwives must take a detailed medical, family and obstetric history, in order to identify risk factors for specific diseases and facilitate genetic counselling and appropriate investigations.
- It is now possible to screen for a wide variety of neonatal conditions from Guthrie blood spots.
- Midwives must ensure that parents receive adequate information prior to screening, to enable them to make objective choices.

- Whilst most conditions are still relatively rare, early diagnosis and treatment can have a tremendous impact on their outcome.
- The midwife is a key practitioner in the identification of some of these disorders, and should be knowledgeable about the recognition of these, their management and sequelae in order to support and inform parents.

REFERENCES

Al-Dahhan J., Jannoun, L. & Haycock, G.B. (2002) Effects of salt supplementation of newborn premature infants on neurodevelopmental outcome at 10–13 years of age. *Archives of Disease in Childhood Fetal and Neonatal Edition* 86(2): 120–F123.

Aurora, P., Whitehead, B., Wade, A. *et al.* (1999) Lung transplantation and life extension in children with cystic fibrosis. *Lancet* 354(9190): 1591–1593.

Chini, B.A. (2002) Update on cystic fibrosis. *Current Opinion in Otolaryngology and Head and Neck Surgery* 10(6): 431–434.

Clague, A. & Thomas, A. (2002) Neonatal biochemical screening for disease. *Clinica Chimica Acta; International Journal of Clinical Chemistry* 315(1–2): 99–110.

Cornblath, M., Hawdon, J.M., Williams, A.F. *et al.* (2000) Controversies regarding the definition of neonatal hypoglycaemia: suggested operational thresholds. *Pediatrics* **105**(5): 1141–1145.

Duvanel, C.B., Fawer, C-L., Cotting, J. *et al.* (1999) Long-term effects of neonatal hypoglycaemia on brain growth and psychomotor development in small-for-gestational-age preterm infants. *Journal of Pediatrics* **134**(4): 492–498.

Hartnoll, G., Betremieux, P. & Modi, N. (2001) Randomised controlled trial of postnatal sodium supplementation in infants of 25–30 weeks gestational age: effects on cardiopulmonary adaptation. *Archives of Disease in Childhood Fetal and Neonatal Edition* **85**(1): F29–32.

Hawdon, J.M., Ward-Platt, M.P. & Aynsley-Green, A. (1994) Prevention and management of neonatal hypoglycaemia. *Archives of Disease in Childhood Fetal and Neonatal Edition* **70**(1): F60–65.

Johnston, P.G.B., Flood, K., Spinks, K. (2003) *The Newborn Child*, 9th edn. London: Churchill Livingstone.

Levy, H.L., Guldberg, P., Guttler, F. *et al.* (2001) Congenital heart disease in maternal phenylketonuria: report from the Maternal PKU Collaborative Study. *Pediatric Research* **49**(5): 636–642.

Matern, D. (2002) Tandem mass spectrometry in newborn screening. *Endocrinology* **12**(1): 50–57.

Merke, D. & Kabbani, M. (2001) Congenital adrenal hyperplasia: epidemiology, management and practical drug treatment. *Paediatric Drugs* **3**(8): 599–611.

Shalev, H., Phillip, M., Galil, A. *et al.* (1998) Clinical presentation and outcome in primary familial hypomagnesaemia. *Archives of Disease in Childhood* **78**(2): 127–130.

Sutor, A.H., von Kries, R., Cornelissen, E.A. *et al.* (1999) Vitamin K deficiency bleeding (VKDB) in infancy. ISTH Pediatric/Perinatal Subcommittee. International Society on Thrombosis and Haemostasis. *Thrombosis and Haemostasis* **81**(3): 456–461.

Tappin, D.M., Girdwood, R.W., Follett, E.A. *et al.* (1991) Prevalence of maternal HIV infection in Scotland based on unlinked anonymous testing of newborn babies. *Lancet* **337**(8757): 1565–1567.

Vilain, C., Rydlewski, C., Duprez, L. *et al.* (2001) Autosomal dominant transmission of congenital thyroid hypoplasia due to loss-of-function mutation of PAX8. *Journal of Clinical Endocrinology and Metabolism* **86**(1): 234–238.

FURTHER READING

Freshwater, D. (2003) *Counselling Skills for Nurses, Midwives and Health Visitors*. Buckingham; Philadelphia: Open University Press.
A useful text which includes a contemporary review of the philosophy, theory and practice of counselling.

Wald, N. & Leck, I. (eds) (2000) *Antenatal and Neonatal Screening*, 2nd edn. Oxford: Oxford University Press.
This text provides a useful and logically structured resource for the midwife. It takes a critical viewpoint of the different conditions which might be screened for and presents an evidence-based approach to guide practice.

39

Infection

Carol Simpson

LEARNING OUTCOMES

After reading this chapter you will be able to:

- have a clear understanding of the neonatal immune system
- apply this knowledge to practice, in order to prevent infection

- discuss common neonatal infections, their port of entry, treatments and outcomes
- appreciate the appropriate use of antibiotics.

INTRODUCTION

Neonatal infections can be fatal, especially in sick and preterm babies. They are still a significant cause of infant death and long-term morbidity. Prevention, early detection and prompt treatment of infections all have an important place in the care of pregnant women and neonates. Midwives must be vigilant in recognizing risk factors and early symptoms of infection, which are often non-specific in neonates.

Newborn babies are particularly prone to infections because of several physiological characteristics. They are relatively immunodeficient at birth, with some degree of natural immunity and acquired immunity if born at term. It is also said that male babies are more prone to infections than are females (Johnstone *et al.*, 2003).

Because much of the acquired immunity is transferred after 32 weeks' gestation, preterm infants are even more vulnerable. Their immune system is particularly immature and they may be subjected to many more invasive procedures, longer hospital stays and numerous care-givers.

NEONATAL DEFENCES

Some passive immunity is afforded to the neonate in the first few months of life by maternal *immunoglobulin*, IgG. This is the only immunoglobulin with a small enough molecular size to cross the placenta; it does so in the third trimester and confers some immunity to specific viral infections.

IgM is not passed transplacentally, but is synthesized by the fetus in small amounts. It takes approximately 2 years to attain adult IgM levels and babies are therefore more susceptible to Gram-negative organisms, causing gastrointestinal infections during this period. Elevated IgM levels at birth may therefore be indicative of an intrauterine infection.

IgA gives some protection against respiratory and gastrointestinal infections, but is relatively deficient at birth. IgA molecules are too big to be transferred across the placenta, though serum levels rise following birth. Breast milk, particularly colostrum, is rich in secretory IgA and *interferon*, which significantly enhance the baby's resistance to enteric infections (Kelly and Coutts, 2000). Several studies show that breast milk may actively stimulate the neonate's immune system (Oddy, 2001).

Further passive immunity is given to the baby from breast milk in the forms of *IgD*, *lactoferrin*, *Lactobacillus bifidus* and *lysozyme*, an anti-infective agent. These help to ensure the gut is colonized with relatively harmless Gram-positive bifidobacteria, as opposed to coliforms and enterococci found in formula-fed infants (Dai and Walker, 1999). *Lactoferrin* affects iron absorption, depleting *Escherichia coli* of the iron it needs to replicate.

Lymphocytes are produced in the thymus gland, which is fairly large at birth. The quantity and quality of neutrophils in the neonate are relatively low compared with older babies. Breastfeeding, particularly in the early weeks, can improve these levels, as breast milk is especially rich in neutrophils and macrophages.

Complement consists of substances which affect the cell membranes of organisms that have invaded the individual, and therefore assist in their destruction by the other mechanisms of the body. It is present only in small amounts in the neonate.

PREVENTION OF INFECTION

Preconceptual and antenatal care

Public health strategies need to target women of childbearing age with education and screening for sexually transmitted diseases and the prevention of conditions affecting the fetus. Vaccination programmes address some conditions, such as hepatitis B and rubella, and research into vaccines for other pathogens continues.

At booking, midwives should ensure sensitive questioning reveals any risk factors for infections. Immigrants and refugees from different countries may not have had rubella vaccinations or may come from areas with a high incidence of tuberculosis or HIV, for example. Easy access to translators and leaflets in a variety of languages, may help. Identification of the need to screen for nosocomial infections such as methicillin-resistant *Staphylococcus aureus* (MRSA) and other virulent pathogens, is also paramount. Babies of women who arrive for care late in pregnancy or in labour and who have not received antenatal assessment or screening, may also be at a higher risk and it is important that in these cases, the midwife undertakes an assessment and plans care accordingly, referring swiftly when required.

> ### Reflective Activity 39.1
>
> Check the availability of educational leaflets in languages relevant to your local client population. What facilities, i.e. translators/link workers, are available to assist staff in communicating with women?

As a part of antenatal care and education, midwives must ensure women are advised regarding dietary restrictions and safe practices in pregnancy, as many perinatal infections are preventable.

Handwashing

Contaminated hands are still one of the greatest risks for transmission of infections. Everyone who handles the baby must be taught correct handwashing techniques, using an antibacterial soap such as chlorhexidine. Midwives can teach parents by example, by washing their hands before and after handling each baby, particularly following nappy changes. Minimal handling of small and preterm neonates in hospitals reduces the risks of cross-infection. Of particular interest to community midwives is a recent small study which showed that rubbing hands with an alcohol-based solution between patients is more efficient in reducing hand contamination than washing with an antiseptic solution (Girou *et al.*, 2002).

Equipment

In hospital, each baby should have its own equipment. Any items that are shared must be thoroughly cleaned between each use, including stethoscopes, auroscopes, weighing scales, cots and resuscitaires. Parents must be taught effective sterilization methods for bottles, teats, expressing equipment and pacifiers, and the importance of hygiene must be emphasized. Correct storage and the prompt use of milk once prepared, is also important.

Though waterbirth should not pose an infection problem in healthy, low-risk women and neonates (Mackey, 2001), strict cleaning protocols need to be enforced for the pool and associated equipment to reduce the risk of infection from organisms such as *Pseudomonas aeruginosa*, *Klebsiella pneumoniae* and *Cryptosporidium*.

Environment

Adequate spacing of beds and cots in multi-bedded wards helps to significantly reduce cross-infection risks. Rooming-in practices in hospitals also help, by reducing the number of carers for each baby as well as helping the establishment of breastfeeding.

Any mother or baby with a known contagious disease or admitted from another hospital, should be initially isolated until screened. Strict isolation procedures, including use of gowns, gloves and masks where appropriate, must be followed.

Invasive procedures

Invasive procedures should be kept to an absolute minimum, to reduce pain, discomfort and the risk of infection to the neonate. When performing such procedures, for example the Guthrie test, good clinical practices and techniques reduce the need for them to be repeated. Very low birthweight and preterm babies have thin, friable skin that is easily traumatized and frequently require several invasive procedures. Aseptic techniques and gloves must be used appropriately and strict attention to wound care is imperative.

Illness of carers

Because of the relatively immunodeficient status of neonates, they are susceptible to pathogens. Midwives and others should avoid caring for babies if they have contagious infections, such as colds, active cold sores, influenza or gastroenteritis.

Breastfeeding

Exclusive breastfeeding should be encouraged wherever possible. The immunological benefits have already been highlighted (see Ch. 33) and these are even more important in preterm or compromised babies. Adequate time, consistent information and support must be given to all mothers, to enable them to succeed.

RECOGNITION OF INFECTION

The presentation of infection is highly variable in the newborn and is often subtle and difficult to recognize. It is important that midwives detect early signs to aid prompt diagnosis and treatment, educate mothers to recognize these variations, and ensure they are aware of the need to report any deviations from normal and contact their doctor.

Subtle presentations

The baby may initially show very few signs, which can include one or more of the following:

- reluctance to feed
- lethargy
- irritability
- poor temperature control – usually hypothermic or unstable (except meningococcal septicaemia – which is characterized by pyrexia around the 9th or 10th day)
- vomiting
- loss of weight/failure to thrive
- an 'anxious look'
- pale, grey or mottled skin
- persistent jaundice.

Apnoea and bradycardia are abnormal in the term neonate and should always be taken seriously. Urgent referral for further investigations is imperative as babies often deteriorate rapidly when ill.

Dramatic presentations

These mainly present as episodes of 'collapse'. The baby becomes pale or cyanosed, hypotonic or hypertonic and apnoeic. These signs may be the result of sepsis or due to other serious conditions such as hypoglycaemia, aspiration of milk, congenital heart disease or an inborn error of metabolism. Management is by resuscitation as appropriate and urgent transfer to hospital. Midwives must maintain their competency in neonatal resuscitation techniques, and community midwives should carry a bag and mask as part of their emergency equipment.

Management

Treatment for specific conditions is included under the appropriate illnesses, but the principles of care are outlined here. Community midwives should be aware of their scope of expertise and refer babies to their GP or paediatrician if concerned. In hospital, if infection is suspected, a full infection screen will be carried out. This includes taking relevant swabs (nose, throat, skin, umbilical or wound), collecting urine and stool samples, taking blood for culture and electrolytes and performing a lumbar puncture to eliminate meningitis as a cause.

PRENATAL INFECTIONS

The fetus is normally protected from extrauterine infection by the cervical mucus plug, intact amniotic sac and the placenta, which act as a barrier to most bacterial conditions. Because of their small molecular size, certain protozoa and viruses can cross the placenta and cause teratogenic effects and infections (see Ch. 16).

The acronym TORCH was devised to list some of them:

T   *Toxoplasma gondii*
O   Other, e.g. syphilis, HIV, hepatitis B
R   Rubella
C   Cytomegalovirus
H   Herpes.

These infections present in one of several ways:

- Widespread and severe – stillbirth or malformation
- Systemic – anaemia, jaundice, purpura, enlarged liver and spleen

- Central nervous system – encephalitis, meningitis, ocular involvement
- Mild – isolated features, such as skin or bone involvement
- Intrauterine growth restriction
- Subclinical – problems with vision, neurological state, deafness, seizures or microcephaly, for example, may arise later in infancy.

Even when curative treatment is not possible, early postnatal treatment can have a beneficial effect on the course of many of these diseases in the neonate.

Toxoplasmosis

Toxoplasmosis is a protozoal infection caused by the organism *Toxoplasma gondii* (see Ch. 16). The incidence of this infection is much higher in continental Europe than in the UK because of the cultural preference for rare meat. Preventive education given by the midwife should include advice on hygiene and safe preparation of food.

Most women with toxoplasmosis infection are asymptomatic, though some may experience a flu-like illness and such symptoms should alert the midwife to assess the risks for this disease. Screening is by detecting anti-toxoplasmosis IgM antibodies in the blood. The greatest risk of transmitting this infection to the fetus is when acute maternal infection occurs in the third trimester (Jones *et al.*, 2001). However, maternal infection in the first half of the pregnancy, particularly weeks 10–24, has the worst outcome, with intrauterine fetal death and subsequent abortion common.

Up to 85% of congenitally infected neonates are asymptomatic at birth, but most will develop complications later in life. Prenatal antibiotics appear to have no effect on the transmission rates for this disease, but do reduce the incidence of severe sequelae such as blindness from chorioretinitis and deafness (Jones *et al.*, 2001). Ultrasound can identify certain patterns of abnormalities associated with toxoplasmosis, which include cerebral ventricular dilatation, and intracranial and liver calcifications (Crino, 1999). Clinical signs in the neonate include low birthweight, hepatosplenomegaly, jaundice and anaemia.

Syphilis

The incidence of syphilis, caused by the spirochaete *Treponema pallidum*, is increasing worldwide, with recent epidemics in several developed countries including

the UK. In 1991 the World Health Organization (WHO) recommended that all women have serological testing for syphilis at their first antenatal appointment and again in the third trimester. This regime would identify both pre-existing syphilis and acute infections and may be prudent in view of the current trends. Serological screening using the *Treponema pallidum* haemagglutination assay (TPHA) has some advantages over the Venereal Disease Research Laboratory (VDRL) test, with less false positives and the identification of latent syphilis.

Early treatment of the mother with intramuscular *benzathine penicillin G* is important and effective in the prevention of congenital syphilis. Infection of the fetus does not occur before the 16th week, but after this time can result in abortion, stillbirth, preterm delivery or congenital syphilis. Neonatal symptoms, when present, include hepatosplenomegaly, skin lesions, maculopapular rashes, eye infections and jaundice. Many affected babies are asymptomatic at birth, with serious complications involving the nervous and skeletal systems arising later.

Human immunodeficiency virus (HIV)

The finding that sperm-associated HIV can be transmitted to oocytes following IVF (Douglas *et al.*, 1998) has heightened awareness of the many routes of transfer of infection. In approximately two-thirds of mothers who are HIV-positive the fetus is seropositive. The risk of fetal infection is greater if the mother has acquired immune deficiency syndrome (AIDS), rather than being HIV-positive alone. The presence of other sexually transmitted diseases facilitates HIV transmission and highlights the importance of sexual health education and screening in women of childbearing age.

Maternal–fetal transfer of HIV early in pregnancy appears to be rare. The times of greatest risk, and therefore the most effective times for prophylactic treatment, are in the third trimester, during labour and birth and in the postnatal period. Transmission rates can be reduced from around 15–20% in untreated mothers, to less than 2% with the use of antiretroviral therapy at these times, elective caesarean section for delivery and no breastfeeding (Anonymous, 2002). Universal HIV screening for pregnant women has been shown to be cost-effective and is recommended (Ades *et al.*, 1999). Midwives should ensure that women obtain appropriate pre- and post-test counselling and that adequate resources and supports are identified for the family in the event of a positive test result.

Mothers who breastfeed are about four times more likely to infect their baby (European Paediatric Hepatitis C Virus Network, 2001), with mastitis being associated with a higher risk (Semba, 2000). In the developed world, breastfeeding is usually discouraged for HIV-positive mothers, as the transmission risks are considered unnecessary. In developing countries, however, where antiretroviral drugs are not always accessible, the risks of using formula milk may be greater than the risk of HIV transmission, because of unclean water, inability to read the preparation directions and the inability to afford or obtain regular supplies of artificial milk. In these cases, and for those women who choose to breastfeed, exclusive breastfeeding and abrupt cessation on weaning may be recommended. Changes to the gut flora from the introduction of solids or formula milk increase the risk of HIV transmission.

Babies infected with HIV are often asymptomatic at birth, although common clinical features include intrauterine growth restriction, microcephaly and a high incidence of congenital malformations. A proportion of these babies will go on to develop AIDS, usually within 6–8 months of birth. Exact figures are uncertain as no universal screening policies exist and the incidence varies between countries. Intravenous antiretroviral agents are being used for neonates, but long-term studies are required to assess the risks and benefits of these.

Listeriosis

Listeriosis, one of the major pathogens of food-borne illness, is caused by the Gram-positive bacillus, *Listeria monocytogenes*, and is significantly more prevalent in pregnant women than in the general population. The mother will present with a history of a non-specific febrile illness with flu-like symptoms, which should alert the midwife to consider further serological investigations, stool and urine cultures (see Ch. 16). High-dose ampicillin antenatally is the treatment of choice.

Intrauterine infection results in spontaneous abortion or stillbirth in around 20% of cases. In the remaining cases, preterm labour and amnionitis are common. It can cause a green staining of the liquor, which may be mistaken for meconium. Since meconium is not normally passed prior to 34 weeks' gestation, this finding should alert the midwife to the possibility of listeriosis in a preterm labour.

Neonates usually develop severe pneumonia within the first week and this, together with general sepsis and meningitis, account for a 50% mortality rate and 50% of survivors having significant handicaps. Symptoms

at birth include maculopapular and petechial rashes, hepatosplenomegaly, leucopenia and thrombocytopenia.

Varicella zoster

This virus is responsible for chickenpox infection and causes congenital varicella syndrome in about 2–5% of neonates, if contracted in the first half of pregnancy. Chorioretinitis, skin lesions, skeletal abnormalities, encephalitis and neurological damage may result. About 30% of babies with these lesions will die in the first few months (Sauerbrie and Wutzler, 2000).

Maternal infections developing within 7 days before and 28 days after delivery, are more serious, with almost a quarter of these babies developing the infection. Neonatal varicella zoster immunoglobulin is recommended and can reduce the risk of serious complications, such as hepatic disorders and pneumonia. Breastfeeding should be encouraged.

Rubella

Rubella causes a mild, non-specific illness in adults, characterized by a measles-like rash, fever and an upper respiratory tract infection. Most countries now have rubella vaccination programmes in place for infants and women of childbearing age and it is part of preconceptual screening. Antenatal mothers are routinely tested for rubella antibodies and, if non-immune, are offered rubella virus vaccination in the early postnatal period. Recent evidence suggests that pregnancy following rubella vaccination may not be as dangerous as was thought and current recommendations are the avoidance of pregnancy for 28 days, rather than the 3 months previously advised (Centers for Disease Control and Prevention, 2002).

First trimester infections are the most serious, with up to 85% of babies being infected. The fetus develops a viraemia, which inhibits cell division and causes defects of the developing organs. Fetuses infected within the first 8 weeks of pregnancy, therefore, have a high risk of multiple defects affecting the eyes, cardiovascular system, ears and nervous system. Spontaneous abortion may occur. Sensorineural deafness often results from infection after 14 weeks' gestation and there is a risk of fetal damage up to 24 weeks. At birth, intrauterine growth restriction is common with hepatitis, thrombocytopenia and neurological disorders such as microcephaly or hydrocephaly.

These babies are very infectious and may excrete rubella virus in the urine for up to 12 months. They pose a cross-infection risk to other neonates as well as pregnant women. Isolation is necessary in hospital and great care required at home. Close follow-up is required, as neurological disorders, which are usually significant, may not be immediately obvious.

Cytomegalovirus (CMV)

CMV is the commonest perinatal infection, 0.4–2.3% of all births (Witters *et al.*, 2000), causing a mild, flu-like illness in the mother but possibly resulting in severe abnormalities in the fetus. The rate of in-utero transmission increases with gestational age. Where the mother has a primary infection, 30–40% of babies will have congenital infections (Gaytant *et al.*, 2002). Over 50% of women are already immune to CMV, and reactivated infections do not pose the same degree of risk to the fetus, with less than 1% resulting in congenital infection. The risk of acquiring a neonatal CMV infection during delivery or from breastfeeding is minimal.

Up to 90% of babies are asymptomatic at birth but 5–15% of these will develop visual or auditory defects, usually within 2 years. Symptoms include intrauterine growth restriction, hepatitis, with or without jaundice, thrombocytopenia and meningoencephalitis. For these babies, mortality from disseminated intravascular coagulation, sepsis or liver problems is 20–30%. The majority of the remaining survivors will have severe neurological morbidity. These babies remain infectious for many months, excreting the virus in their urine, and can be a risk to pregnant mothers.

Hepatitis

Six types of blood-borne hepatitis virus have so far been identified: A, B, C, D, E and G. Neonatal infections may arise from in-utero infection or exposure during birth. Transplacental infection from hepatitis A and E are very rare (Duff, 1998) but can result in fetal abnormalities. Hepatitis D requires simultaneous infection with hepatitis B to replicate and the hepatitis B vaccine is therefore effective against both diseases. The effects of these diseases in the fetus are compounded by their coexistence. Hepatitis G is related to hepatitis C, but little is known at present about its effects on the fetus.

80–90% of babies born to mothers who are chronically infected with hepatitis B and are positive for the hepatitis B e antigen (HBeAg), will become chronically infected themselves (Shiraki, 2000), with the risk of

hepatic carcinoma in later life. Routine antenatal testing identifies those at risk and the midwife must ensure that the baby receives hepatitis B immunoglobulin (100 IU) and hepatitis B vaccination (5 μg) within 12 hours of birth. Parental education and consent are vital and will help to ensure compliance with the full vaccination schedule, which comprises further hepatitis B vaccinations at 6 weeks and 3 months of age. On discharge, the midwife must ensure that the GP and health visitor are notified of the vaccinations given and the planned schedule. Serology testing of the baby will be required at around 5 months of age, to ensure immunity has been achieved.

Hepatitis C is far more prevalent than HIV and can result in liver cirrhosis, hepatic carcinoma, liver failure and death. It is common amongst intravenous drug users. The rate of maternal–fetal transfer of hepatitis C is approximately 5% (Zanetti *et al.*, 1999) and up to 10% in women co-infected with HIV. There is no indication for delivery by caesarean section or avoiding breastfeeding for hepatitis C alone (European Paediatric Hepatitis C Virus Network, 2001). Midwives should avoid unnecessary invasive techniques during labour and birth, to reduce the risk of maternal and fetal blood mixing. This includes artificial rupture of membranes and the use of fetal scalp electrodes. Washing the baby in a chlorhexidine-based solution soon after delivery may also reduce the transmission risk.

Reflective Activity 39.2

Review your local policies and procedures relating to the management of women with hepatitis B and C in pregnancy and the immediate postnatal care of the baby.

PERINATAL INFECTIONS

Invasive prenatal procedures

Organisms may be introduced during procedures such as amniocentesis, chorionic villus sampling, fetoscopy, cordocentesis, intrauterine blood transfusion and fetal surgery. Intrauterine pneumonia is the commonest effect, but it depends on the pathogens introduced. Strict aseptic techniques must be assured.

Ascending infections

Ascending infections most commonly occur once the membranes have ruptured. Repeated vaginal examinations can introduce infections if not carried out under strict aseptic conditions and should be avoided unless absolutely necessary. The application of a fetal scalp electrode or fetal blood sampling in labour may result in abscess formation.

Group B streptococcus (GBS) and *E. coli* are the commonest pathogens identified. GBS is a leading cause of neonatal bacterial sepsis, pneumonia and meningitis, with an incidence of up to 4 : 1000 births. Maternal risk factors include imminent preterm delivery, ruptured membranes for more than 18 hours at any gestation, fever and maternal chorioamnionitis. In these cases, prophylactic intrapartum antibiotics are recommended. There remains a lack of consensus on the efficacy of screening all women for GBS late in pregnancy, to prevent neonatal sepsis (Wendel *et al.*, 2002).

Infections acquired during delivery

Most of these infections are sexually transmitted and treatment should be given to the mother, partner and neonate, where appropriate. Midwives may refer women to sexual health clinics to facilitate full sexual health screening and contact tracing, as co-infections are common.

Gonorrhoea

The organism *Neisseria gonorrhoeae* typically produces severe bilateral conjunctival inflammation in the neonate, with a purulent discharge within 48 hours of birth. Oropharyngeal and systemic infections are also common. This infection is increasing in incidence. It used to be an important cause of blindness because, if not treated, it causes corneal scarring. Treatment is with antibiotics – penicillin 50 mg/kg intramuscularly at birth – if the mother is known to have the infection, or following investigation. This includes a direct Gram stain and culture to establish antibiotic sensitivity.

Chloramphenicol eyedrops can be administered and may initially need to be given every 15 minutes to act against the infection and complemented with intramuscular penicillin for 7 days. If the infection is penicillin resistant, intravenous cefotaxime may be used.

Chlamydia

Chlamydial conjunctivitis is the largest single cause of blindness in the world and usually appears around the 5th to 10th days of life. It is also readily treatable with systemic antibiotics such as erythromycin and with 1% chlortetracycline eye ointment five to six times a day for 2 weeks. Tetracycline may also be indicated. Unless eradicated, this organism, *Chlamydia trachomatis*, can cause neonatal pneumonia and otitis media. It can also result in infertility in women, if recurrent or left untreated. Antenatal screening may be undertaken using a cervical swab, or urine sampling if the mother has not voided for at least 2 hours.

Herpes simplex virus (HSV)

HSV infections are associated with active maternal genital herpes and can cause a range of illnesses in the neonatal period, from skin blisters to overwhelming viraemia and encephalitis. The baby may also develop chronic and progressive disorders of the brain, liver, eyes and adrenal glands. HSV can be acquired transplacentally, but the more common manner of infection is during birth. With primary lesions at birth there is a 50% risk of infection, reducing to about 5% with recurring lesions. Caesarean section may be the mode of delivery of choice when there are active herpetic lesions. Diagnosis requires culture of the virus from the affected skin, and treatment should be commenced as soon as the infection is identified. Infected neonates need supportive measures and systemic acyclovir.

Candida (thrush)

Candida albicans is the commonest cause of fungal infections in infants. It may be acquired at delivery if the mother has a vaginal infection, from poor hygiene practices or as a result of reduced resistance during antibiotic therapy. Midwives must teach parents sterilization techniques for equipment and good nappy changing practices.

Oral infection appears as white patches on the tongue, gums and palate; if the patches are removed, they leave a raw red area. If the mother is breastfeeding, her nipples should also be treated to prevent reinfection. Infection in the nappy area presents with a generalized papular or vesicular rash and antifungal preparations are effective treatments.

Disseminated candidiasis is an overwhelming septicaemia, usually found in preterm, very low birthweight and compromised babies in association with invasive procedures. There is significant associated morbidity and mortality because this serious disease can affect all the major organs. Infection of the central nervous system has a poor outcome for extremely low birthweight babies, with over 40% having severe disabilities at 2 years of age (Friedman *et al.*, 2000). Aggressive intravenous treatments with both antifungal and antibacterial agents are required. Fluconazole is an antifungal agent increasingly used, instead of amphotericin B and flucytosine, and may be given orally or intravenously in the management of neonatal *C. albicans* infection.

POSTNATAL INFECTIONS

Mild eye infection

Mild eye infections and 'sticky eyes' are not uncommon in the newborn. Singh *et al.* (1982) suggested the use of colostrum for sticky eyes and conjunctivitis, and some women may prefer to use this rather than conventional treatments. However, in the presence of aggressive infection, antibiotic treatment will be required.

It is important to teach the woman and her family good hygiene and care if the baby does have either problem. The hands should be washed prior to and after cleaning the eyes. The eyes can be cleaned with cool, boiled water, or sterile saline, using sterile cotton wool swabs – cleaning the eyes from the inner aspect to the outer, discarding the swab after one sweep. If only one of the baby's eyes is affected, the baby's head should be positioned with the sticky eye downmost, so that secretions do not run into the unaffected eye.

Ophthalmia neonatorum

This term is used to describe a discharge from the eyes of an infant within 21 days of birth. It became a notifiable condition in England and Wales in 1914 when it was the cause of 50% of blindness in children. Mild ophthalmia neonatorum is common and in many cases no bacteria are found. With modern antibiotics, the incidence of severe ophthalmia has greatly diminished. This presents as a purulent discharge from one or both eyes, oedema and erythema of the eyelids. The most commonly identified organisms include *E. coli*, *Streptococcus pneumoniae*, *N. gonorrhoeae* and *Chlamydia trachomatis* and these indicate the need for maternal screening. It is crucial that careful informed consent is obtained from the woman, and that appropriate tests (usually skin scrapings from the inner eyelid) are undertaken by a specialist practitioner.

Omphalitis

Severe cord sepsis is uncommon and with good standards of hygiene it can be prevented. Signs of infection include periumbilical inflammation, a moist, offensive smelling cord and delay in separation. The inflammation may be transported through the umbilical vein to the liver. The organism most commonly responsible is *Staph. aureus* and antibiotics are required. Parents must be taught cord care and the midwife should check this area regularly.

Gastroenteritis

This is highly infectious and carries a high risk of mortality for compromised babies. For this reason an outbreak in a neonatal intensive care unit (NICU), special care baby unit (SCBU) or nursery is a catastrophe. The neonate can become very ill and dehydrated within a short space of time. Electrolyte imbalance leads to tachycardia, hypotension and collapse if not speedily treated. There are a number of possible causative organisms including *Salmonella*, *Shigella* (a form of *E. coli*), echovirus type II and rotavirus. Isolation of infected babies is important to prevent cross-infection. The baby's electrolyte and urea levels require monitoring, and careful measurement of input and output should be undertaken. Intravenous fluids may be required. Preventive measures are of the utmost importance and exclusive breastfeeding should be encouraged, where possible. High standards of hygiene must be maintained and effective handwashing practices are vital.

Necrotizing enterocolitis (NEC)

This is an inflammatory disease of the bowel, mainly found in very low birthweight babies, associated with septicaemia and a mortality of up to 40%. Its aetiology is not fully understood but is associated with hypoxic episodes and ischaemia of the bowel, enabling pathogenic organisms to proliferate. Symptoms develop once feeding is commenced, with sepsis, abdominal distension and blood and mucus in the stools. Breastfeeding affords some protection (Dai and Walker, 1999).

Radiography will identify distended loops of gut, and cysts full of hydrogen, methane and carbon dioxide. Early diagnosis and treatment is imperative; enteral feeds are ceased and antibiotics and intravenous fluids given until recovery is noted. Surgical intervention may be required.

Neonatal pneumonia

Organisms that do not usually cause pneumonia, such as *E. coli*, *Staph. pyogenes* and *Strep. viridans*, can become extremely pathogenic in the neonate. One study into the causes of death in extremely low birthweight infants, showed amniotic fluid infections leading to pneumonia as the commonest cause. Most of these organisms were fungal and nosocomial (Barton *et al.*, 1999).

Midwives must confirm preterm rupture of membranes promptly and monitor neonates closely in this event for early symptoms of illness.

Urinary tract infections

Urinary tract infections vary in severity and may go undetected or cause serious illness. Untreated, these may cause pyelonephritis and/or long-term renal damage. The causative organism is usually *E. coli*, and occasionally other Gram-negative organisms. The baby can present with non-specific symptoms such as reluctance to feed, failure to thrive and occasionally pyrexia and sometimes jaundice. Uncontaminated urine should be cultured.

A urine sample can be collected by means of clean catch using a galipot and positioning the baby as appropriate. It can also help to smooth a cool wet swab across the pubic area, as this will often stimulate micturition. Alternatively an MSU bag can be used, though often this can result in a contaminated sample. Occasionally suprapubic aspiration is required in the neonatal intensive care unit. Pus cells of $25 \times 10^6/l$ (male) and $50 \times 10^6/l$ (female) are suggestive of infection.

Antibiotic therapy should be commenced prior to urine culture should the baby be unwell – cefotaxime, gentamycin or amoxicillin may be used, and the course should extend to 2 weeks, with some follow-up, which should include ultrasound examination and possibly a cystogram.

Pyelonephritis

This may be the result of a bacterial infection, such as *E. coli*, or a congenital malformation of the urinary tract, such as urethral valves. The signs are often non-specific in the neonate, with general malaise, lethargy, loss of appetite and possibly jaundice. Diagnosis is made on microscopy of a sterile urine sample (as above); suprapubic aspiration may be necessary to achieve this.

Recovery from this infection is usually rapid once appropriate treatment is commenced. Ultrasound examination of the urinary tract is indicated whenever a urinary tract infection is diagnosed. Long-term antibiotics may be prescribed until it is certain that the renal tract is normal.

Pyoderma

Small spots or pustules appear on the skin as a result, almost always, of staphylococcal infection. They must not be disregarded as they may spread rapidly,

especially in a preterm or ill baby, and may be a source of cross-infection. The baby should be treated with antibiotics once diagnosis is confirmed.

Paronychia

This is a staphylococcal infection of the nail bed of the fingers or toes and is usually caused by *Staph. aureus*. If the infection is on the hand, the baby should be prevented from sucking the fingers, by applying loose mittens. Antistaphylococcal cream applied locally, and occasionally antibiotics, will be required to control the infection.

Pemphigus neonatorum

This is a potentially fatal staphylococcal infection. Because of its highly contagious character and severe effects, it is wise for the midwife to consider any skin lesion associated with the formation of a blister or pus as a possible case of pemphigus.

Blisters, which fill with pus and burst leaving a raw surface, appear on the head or trunk. This is often called the *staphylococcal scalded skin syndrome* since the appearance mimics that of a scald. As the infection spreads in the superficial tissue, large areas become involved. Complications may arise since staphylococci can also affect the lungs, gut and liver.

Treatment is with systemic antibiotics such as flucloxacillin, which are given intravenously. It is also important to monitor for dehydration and other complications from fluid loss.

Arthritis and osteitis

These uncommon infections are usually caused by staphylococci and often present with general malaise, localized swelling and redness of the skin, or crying when the affected limb is disturbed. There may also be fever. Although early diagnosis is difficult, early treatment is necessary to prevent joint destruction. Changes will be seen on X-ray. Flucloxacillin may be used systemically over a period of weeks.

Otitis media

This is another condition that is difficult to diagnose in the neonate. Babies who have a nasotracheal tube in situ are at particular risk, as it blocks the eustachian tube. Chlamydial infection can also cause this condition.

Septicaemia

Septicaemia is the growth of bacteria in the bloodstream, as distinct from their presence in the blood (bacteraemia), which can be a transient phenomenon. The cause of septicaemia is not always clear but it generally occurs when infection spreads from localized sites to the bloodstream. It indicates a failure of the baby's defences, either at the site of infection or of the immune system as a whole. The organisms most commonly found in blood culture are *E. coli*, *Staph. aureus*, Group B β-haemolytic streptococcus, *Proteus*, *P. aeruginosa* and *L. monocytogenes*. Complications of septicaemia include disseminated intravascular coagulation and meningitis, and treatment depends on the causative organism. This may involve commencing antibiotic treatment prior to the identification of the specific organism, and often a combination of antibiotics such as gentamycin and penicillin will be used. Careful monitoring of temperature, fluid and electrolytes and glucose levels needs to be undertaken.

Meningitis

Group B streptococcus, *E. coli* and *L. monocytogenes* are the most common causative organisms of neonatal meningitis, which may follow septicaemia. Vomiting, a high-pitched cry, raised anterior fontanelle, convulsions and neck rigidity will present at some stage, although initial symptoms are often non-specific (reluctance to feed, temperature instability, listlessness and vomiting). Diagnosis is made by lumbar puncture and the condition is treated with intravenous or intrathecal antibiotics. Unless meningitis is diagnosed and treated early there is a high risk of permanent brain damage or even death.

Malaria

This is not commonly seen in neonates; however, it may occur if the woman has a history of being in a country with malaria during her pregnancy. The *Plasmodium falciparum* parasites may affect the placenta, causing growth restriction and in some cases, preterm labour. An affected neonate will be well at birth, with the development of fever, jaundice and splenomegaly within 10–20 days of the birth. Cloroquine is given orally.

Tuberculosis (TB)

Neonatal TB is not common, though there has been an increase in the rates of TB in the UK during the last decade. TB can be contracted during the early neonatal period and may be seen some 6 weeks postnatally. Symptoms include lethargy, reluctance in feeding, weight loss and pyrexia. Diagnosis is usually through chest X-ray – tuberculin tests are not useful as the neonate is unlikely to react. Treatment includes izoniazid and rifampicin, and should continue over 6 months.

Women who are at risk will have the immunization offered to their babies (0.05 ml BCG vaccine intradermally), and this is usually administered during the neonatal period.

Antibiotics

One study has shown that nearly half of all pregnant women receive antibiotics prior to delivery (Mercer *et al.*, 1999). With increasing use of antibiotics, both prophylactic and therapeutic, more resistant strains of organisms are developing and the clinical picture of causative organisms is changing. It is important to use specific antibiotics where possible, to eradicate the overuse of others, which leads to more resistance.

Reflective Activity 39.3

Audit antenatal notes for your caseload to determine the rate of antibiotic use in pregnancy.

General guidelines for safe use of antibiotics in the neonate are:

- Only treat sepsis, not colonization with bacteria
- Do not use prophylactic antibiotics without evidence that they are effective
- Use narrow-spectrum antibiotics where possible
- Keep broad-spectrum antibiotics as a back-up
- Stop antibiotics as soon as systemic blood cultures are negative.

A proactive approach should be taken to risk-identification, screening and treatment of infections in women, preconceptually and antenatally, in order to reduce fetal and neonatal mortality and morbidity. The majority of these conditions are preventable, and midwives can do much to reduce their incidence and severity with education, awareness, early diagnosis and treatment.

KEY POINTS

- Midwives need to ensure they identify individual risk factors for infections for each woman, through careful history-taking. Education and advice regarding diet and lifestyles can help to prevent certain infections.
- Many maternal infections have disastrous effects on the fetus or neonate, but can be effectively treated if diagnosed antenatally.

- Early signs of infection are often subtle in neonates, and midwives must seek further advice if at all concerned.

REFERENCES

Ades, A.E., Sculpher, M.J., Gibb, D.M. *et al.* (1999) Cost effectiveness analysis of antenatal HIV screening in the United Kingdom. *British Medical Journal* 319(7219): 1230–1234.

[Anonymous] (2002) Pregnancy and HIV infection: a European consensus on management: Executive summary. *AIDS* 16(2): S1–S18.

Barton, L., Hodgman, J.E. & Pavlova, Z. (1999) Causes of death in the extremely low birthweight infant. *Pediatrics* 103(2): 446–451.

Centers for Disease Control and Prevention (2002) Revised ACIP recommendations for avoiding pregnancy after receiving rubella-containing vaccine. *Journal of the American Medical Association* 287(3): 311–312.

Crino, J.P. (1999) Ultrasound fetal diagnosis of perinatal infection. *Clinical Obstetrics and Gynecology* 42(1): 71–80.

Dai, D. & Walker, W.A. (1999) Protective nutrients and bacterial colonization in the immature human gut. *Advances in Pediatrics* 46: 353–382.

Douglas, G.C., Fazley, F. & Hu, J.J. (1998) Transmission of HIV to the placenta, fetus and mother and implications of gametic infection. *Journal of Reproductive Immunology* 41(1–2): 321–329.

Duff, P. (1998) Hepatitis in pregnancy. *Seminars in Perinatology* 22(4): 277–283.

European Paediatric Hepatitis C Virus Network (2001) Effects of mode of delivery and infant feeding on the risk of mother-to-child transmission of hepatitis C virus. *British Journal of Obstetrics and Gynaecology* 108(4): 371–377.

Friedman, S., Richardson, S.E., Jacobs, S.E. *et al.* (2000) Systemic candida infection in extremely low birth weight infants: short term morbidity and long term neurodevelopmental outcome. *Pediatric Infectious Disease Journal* 19(6): 499–504.

Gaytant, M.A., Steegers, E.A.P., Semmekrot, B.A. *et al.* (2002) Congenital cytomegalovirus infection: review of the epidemiology and outcome. *Obstetrical & Gynecological Survey* 57(4): 245–256.

Girou, E., Loyeau, S., Oppein, F. *et al.* (2002) Efficacy of handrubbing with alcohol based solution versus standard handwashing with antiseptic soap: randomised clinical trial. *British Medical Journal* 325(7360): 362.

Johnstone, P.G.B., Flood, K. & Spinks, K. (2003) *The Newborn Child*, 9th edn. Edinburgh: Churchill Livingstone.

Jones, J.L., Lopez, A., Wilson, M. *et al.* (2001) Congenital toxoplasmosis: a review. *Obstetrical & Gynecological Survey* 56(5): 296–305.

Kelly, D. & Coutts, A.G. (2000) Early nutrition and development of immune function in the neonate. *Proceedings of the Nutrition Society* 59(2): 177–185.

Mackey, M. (2001) Use of water in labor and birth. *Clinical Obstetrics and Gynecology* 44(4): 733–749.

Mercer, B.M., Carr, T.L. & Beazley, D.D. (1999) Antibiotic use in pregnancy and drug-resistant infant sepsis. *American Journal of Obstetrics and Gynecology* 181(4): 816–821.

Oddy, W.H. (2001) Breastfeeding protects against illness and infection in infants and children: a review of the evidence. *Breastfeeding Review* 9(2): 11–18.

Sauerbrie, A. & Wutzler, P. (2000) The congenital varicella syndrome. *Journal of Perinatology* 20(8): 548–554.

Semba, R.D. (2000) Mastitis and transmission of human immunodeficiency virus through breast milk. *Annals of the New York Academy of Sciences* 918: 156–162.

Shiraki, K. (2000) Perinatal transmission of hepatitis B virus and its prevention. *Journal of Gastroenterology and Hepatology* 15(Suppl.): E11–E15.

Singh, M., Sugathan, P.S. & Bhujwala, R.A. (1982) Human colostrum for prophylaxis against sticky eyes and conjunctivitis in the newborn. *Journal of Tropical Pediatrics* 28(1): 35–37.

Wendel, G.D., Leveno, K.J., Sanchez, P.J. *et al.* (2002) Prevention of neonatal group B streptococcal disease: A combined intrapartum and neonatal protocol. *American Journal of Obstetrics and Gynecology* 186(4): 618–626.

Witters, I., Van Ranst, M. & Fryns, J.P. (2000) Cytomegalovirus reactivation in pregnancy and subsequent isolated hearing loss in the infant. *Genetic Counseling* 11(4): 375–378.

World Health Organization (WHO) (1991) *Maternal and Perinatal Infection: Report of a WHO Consultation.* Geneva: WHO.

Zanetti, A.R., Tanzi, E. & Newell, M.L. (1999) Mother-to-infant transmission of hepatitis C virus. *Journal of Hepatology* 31(1): 96–100.

FURTHER READING

Isaacs, D. & Moxon, E.R. (1999) *Handbook of Neonatal Infections. A Practical Guide.* London: W.B. Saunders.
A very useful text including the management and treatment of neonatal infection. Includes sections on immunization schedules, and antibiotic regimes and interactions.

Remington, J.S. & Klein, J.O. (eds) (2000) *Infectious Diseases of the Fetus and Newborn Infant*, 5th edn. Philadelphia: W.B. Saunders.
A key text which includes a description of the microbiology, pathogenesis, diagnosis, treatment, prevention and prognosis of each disease, and contains contemporary management and approaches to neonatal infection. There are also useful sections on international issues, clinical guidelines and decision-making processes.

40

Sudden Infant Death Syndrome

Carol Simpson

LEARNING OUTCOMES

After reading this chapter you will be able to:

- understand the risk factors associated with sudden infant death syndrome (SIDS)
- appreciate the history, aetiology and incidence of SIDS
- be conversant with what information and advice should be given to parents and families to reduce the risk of SIDS.

INTRODUCTION

The diagnosis of sudden infant death syndrome (SIDS) is one of exclusion, where the sudden death of an infant under 1 year of age remains unexplained after a post-mortem, a review of the clinical history and examination of the death scene. The Foundation for the Study of Infant Deaths (FSID) uses a definition of death up until 2 years of age, though the numbers do decline over 1 year (http://www.sids.org.uk).

It is a subgroup classification of sudden unexpected deaths in infancy (SUDI), otherwise referred to as cot deaths, which also include accidental deaths and those due to non-accidental injuries.

Midwives have a major role to play both antenatally and postnatally, in ensuring all parents receive and understand current information regarding SIDS. This includes identifying risks, educating and advising families on an individual basis and providing appropriate written materials. Consideration must be given to cultural differences and beliefs.

INCIDENCE AND TRENDS

During the 1970s and early 1980s in the UK, interest in the topic of SIDS increased considerably. Deaths previously attributed to other causes, particularly unspecified respiratory illnesses, were more frequently

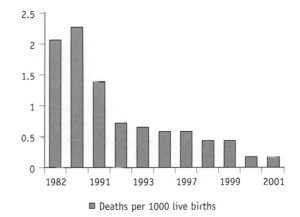

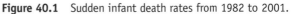

Figure 40.1 Sudden infant death rates from 1982 to 2001.

attributed to SIDS on death certificates, leading to a rise in the rate for England and Wales, to a peak rate of 2.3 per thousand live births in 1988 (Fig. 40.1).

At the end of 1991, the 'Back to Sleep' campaign was launched by the Foundation for the Study of Infant Deaths and the Department of Health, following research findings which illustrated that ensuring babies were placed on their backs or sides resulted in a significant reduction in cot deaths (Fleming *et al.*, 1990; Mitchell *et al.*, 1991). This aimed at educating parents and professionals about reducing known risk factors, making four main recommendations:

1. Place babies on their backs to sleep
2. Do not expose babies to cigarette smoke

3. Do not overheat babies
4. Seek medical advice early if babies are unwell.

Between 1991 and 1992 there was a 47% reduction in the UK SIDS rate; by 1993 it was 0.7 per 1000 live births – a reduction of 72% from 1988 – and it fell to 0.21 per 1000 in 2001.

The incidence of SIDS varies widely throughout the UK and worldwide, although all areas have shown great reductions in their SIDS rates on implementing similar educational campaigns. In 2000 the rate for the Maori population of the South Island of New Zealand was one of the highest in the world (1.04/1000 live births), compared to a very low rate in Hong Kong (0.1/1000 live births) (http://www.sidsinternational.minerva.com.au).

Reflective Activity 40.1

Compare your local SIDS rate with the national rate.

Since the success of the 'Back to Sleep' campaign, it has become clear that some of the epidemiological characteristics of SIDS have changed (Leach *et al.*, 1999). Families involved tend to come from more disadvantaged circumstances and the high number of SIDS cases usually noted during winter months is less obvious.

The majority of SIDS deaths occur in the postneonatal period (1 month to 1 year), with a peak incidence at around 2–4 months of age and 90% occurring within the first 6 months (http://www.sids.org.uk).

RISK FACTORS

The aetiology of SIDS is multifactorial and not yet fully understood, although much research has been, and continues to be, undertaken. Many interrelated physiological, social and environmental factors have been identified, which result in particular babies being more susceptible. Midwives need to identify these factors in each family and support the family in making the necessary changes, where possible (RCM, 2003). They include the following.

Sleeping position

This was first considered in 1965 (Carpenter *et al.*, 1965), but the association of sleeping position and SIDS was not found to be statistically significant at this time. In the 1970s in the Netherlands, prone sleeping became popular and there was a corresponding threefold increase in their SIDS rate. Subsequent studies have consistently shown this association, with one (Fleming *et al.*, 1990) demonstrating the risk to be 8.8 times higher if a baby sleeps prone, compared to supine.

Although safer than prone sleeping, babies lying on their sides appear to have almost twice the risk of SIDS than when supine (Fleming *et al.*, 1990). This is partly attributed to them rolling on to their stomachs from this position. Midwives must advise parents to only place babies on their backs to sleep, from birth.

As a result of supine sleeping, more babies are now presenting, in the first few months, with a misshapen head (plagiocephaly); commonly occipitoparietal flattening. This is due to persistent pressure on a specific area of the malleable skull bones and is emphasized more in preterm babies (Sweeney and Gutierrez, 2002). It is also important to consider normal hip development of the neonate, which may be affected by supine sleeping. To prevent or minimize these effects, midwives should encourage parents to vary the head position when putting their babies down to sleep, support the head in the midline position when using a car seat, and ensure they play with the baby in the prone position when awake.

Sleeping environment

A recent study into sleeping practices has identified important issues (Blair *et al.*, 1999), though the incidence of SIDS appears to be reduced when babies sleep in the same room as their parents for the first 6 months. Bed sharing has different risks dependent on the circumstances and should be avoided with babies under 14 weeks of age, and at any age if either parent has consumed alcohol, used drugs, smokes or is extremely tired (RCM, 2003). Sleeping together with an infant on a sofa is consistently associated with a significantly high risk of SIDS and midwives should advise parents against this practice at all times.

Bedding

Fleming *et al.* (1990) demonstrated that SIDS babies in their study were more likely to have been heavily wrapped, sleeping prone and to have had heating on all night. The risk from such overheating was found only to be significant in babies over 2 months of age. Each of these situations is recognized as a risk factor on its own, but when combined with one or more other factors becomes significant.

Overheating can occur if:

- the room temperature is inappropriately high
- there is an excessive amount of clothing or bedding, or
- if the baby's ability to lose heat is impaired – such as when swaddled tightly, owing to illness or pyrexia, when sleeping prone, or when the baby's head is covered by bedding.

Parents should be advised by the midwife about how many layers of clothing or bedding are appropriate and advised against using soft bedding, such as duvets, quilts and pillows, for babies under 1 year of age. The baby's temperature can be monitored by touch and thermometer, if necessary, and medical advice sought if there are any signs of illness. Room temperatures should not exceed 18°C and the cot must not be placed next to a radiator or fire. To prevent the baby wriggling under the bedding, the baby's feet should be at the foot of the cot, with bedding reaching shoulder level only.

Smoking

Smoking during pregnancy and following birth are widely acknowledged as major independent risk factors for SIDS (McMartin *et al.*, 2002). The baby of a mother who smokes is three times more likely to die from SIDS than the baby of a non-smoking mother, even after allowing for other influencing factors. Midwives should encourage parents to reduce or stop smoking during the pregnancy and have resources to offer them to help achieve this. Further studies are required to ascertain whether passive smoking poses a significant SIDS risk to babies (Dybing and Sanner, 1999).

Illness

Bacterial toxins, specifically of *Staphylococcus aureus*, are found in many SIDS babies at post-mortem (Blackwell *et al.*, 2002). A relatively large number of babies have a history of a recent hospital admission, or symptoms, commonly gastrointestinal or respiratory, in the weeks prior to death (Ford *et al.*, 1997). *Babycheck* provides a scoring system of signs and symptoms which can assist in identifying babies who may be at risk (Morley *et al.*, 1991).

Feeding method

Breastfeeding is associated with a lower risk of SIDS compared to formula feeding. The protection afforded may be related to IgA antibodies found in breast milk, which fight off bacterial toxins (Gordon *et al.*, 1999).

Weight and weight gain

Low birthweight is a known factor associated with SIDS, with the risk increasing significantly as birthweight falls. Poor or static postnatal weight gain has also been shown to be a strongly associated factor for normal birthweight babies (Blair *et al.*, 2000).

Pacifiers/dummies

Evidence regarding any effect on the prevalence of SIDS and the regular use of pacifiers is not conclusive (Fleming *et al.*, 1999) and further research is required in this area. As a measure to reduce the SIDS risk, current advice is not to start pacifier use, but if a pacifier is already used regularly, this should not be discontinued.

Immunization

There has been recent speculation that the accelerated immunization programme for diphtheria, tetanus, polio and pertussis, commenced in 1990, may be associated with a higher SUDI risk, of which SIDS is a subgroup. Further studies have shown that this is not the case and that it may even be a protective factor (Fleming *et al.*, 2001).

Other factors

Characteristic epidemiological features of SIDS include a higher number of male infants, low birthweight babies, those of short gestation and with neonatal problems. Single mothers, young maternal age, high parity (Froen *et al.*, 2002) and multiple pregnancies also correlate strongly. Research continues into the possibility of similarities between the mechanisms involved in SIDS and late antenatal stillbirths.

Reflective Activity 40.2

Does your unit have a range of leaflets and information available for women? Is the issue of SIDS, and the measures which can be taken to reduce the risks, discussed with women?

APNOEA ALARMS

There is no evidence that the use of apnoea monitors at home reduces the incidence of SIDS. It is widely accepted that monitoring normal, healthy babies is impractical and undesirable. There is a high rate of false alarms with apnoea monitors, which heighten anxieties. Many parents become reliant on the monitors as a measure of the well-being of their baby and may miss early signs of illness. Resuscitation of an apnoeic baby is not always successful and some will have sustained irreversible brain damage by this time. The FSID recommend all parents are taught general neonatal resuscitation skills. Voluntary bodies such as the St John's Ambulance Brigade or Red Cross may facilitate this.

Reflective Activity 40.3

What resuscitation courses are available in your local area for parents? Are they available to all parents?

APPARENT LIFE-THREATENING EVENTS

The breathing patterns of babies are erratic and short apnoeic spells are normal. Occasionally babies have longer periods of apnoea, which result in a degree of hypoxia. These are known as apparent life-threatening events (ALTEs) and it may require stimulation or resuscitation to correct them. Not all of these episodes are associated with prolonged apnoeic periods; some are caused by infection or aspiration of feed or vomit. Their relevance with regard to SIDS is uncertain; however, ALTEs are also more common in male infants and preterm babies, and occur more frequently in the same age ranges. Any baby having an ALTE should have an urgent medical review.

CARE OF THE FAMILY

SIDS is a tragedy that brings devastation to a family and the professionals involved with them. The unexpected nature of the death, usually of an apparently healthy baby, and the lack of explanation as to the cause, deepen the distress. Those professionals in contact with the family require great sensitivity at this time. It is useful to review the guidelines produced by the FSID. For fuller details on bereavement care, see Chapter 3.

The investigative procedure that follows an infant death is detailed, invasive and needs careful explanation to the parents. In the UK, a coroner investigates all sudden infant deaths and if the death occurred at home, the police will interview the parents and visit the home. They may remove bedding and clothing for further examination. A post-mortem examination will be necessary and these events should be sensitively explained to the family, in terms of the benefits of having a definite diagnosis.

The cultural, religious and personal beliefs of the family must be considered at all times. Many people find it helpful to talk to a social worker or minister of religion at this time. Advice on funeral arrangements, registering the death and financial issues may also be required. It is important to notify the members of the primary healthcare team of the baby's death as soon as possible, so that continued support can be given and insensitive errors, such as sending immunization reminders, prevented. Siblings and grandparents will also need support and explanations. Their grief is different from that of the parents and they are all too often forgotten. Support groups, locally or nationally, may be helpful to the family.

Reflective Activity 40.4

Go to the FSID website and access the guidelines for supporting parents following SIDS – you may find it useful to put a copy in your resource folder.

Follow-up

Parents will have many questions about their baby's death and it is important that they have the opportunity to discuss these. Once all the results of the tests and post-mortem examination are available, the parents should be offered an appointment with the paediatrician. It is very common for parents of SIDS babies to feel that their care was in some way inadequate and that they caused the death of their baby. Where possible, reassurances must be given that this was not the case.

Subsequent pregnancies

Families who have suffered the death of a baby often have mixed feelings about subsequent pregnancies. The pregnancy and first few months after the birth can be very anxious times, particularly around the age when the last baby died. The FSID have set up a programme of support for these families called 'Care of Next Infant' (CONI). This uses the skills and support of the paediatrician, obstetrician, family doctor, midwife, health visitor and a local CONI coordinator. The parents themselves decide the level of care they require throughout the pregnancy and following months. The support offered may include discussion and advice about antenatal and postnatal risk factors, weekly visits to the health visitor, a set of weighing scales to monitor the baby's weight regularly, a wall thermometer to monitor the room temperature, a symptom diary for the parents to note any changes in their baby and an apnoea monitor.

Reflective Activity 40.6

Who is your local CONI team? Ensure that you have contact details in your diary/resource file.

CONCLUSION

Losing a child so suddenly is a major trauma to parents and to the professionals providing care. Occasionally a baby may die whilst in the hospital environment and this will be immensely difficult for the staff and for the parents. The midwife can contribute to the prevention of such a tragedy and can provide support and care should this occur. Skills in dealing with loss and bereavement, and sensitive management are crucial in the support of parents and colleagues.

KEY POINTS

- Although the aetiology of SIDS is still unclear, specific predisposing factors have been clearly identified. Midwives must provide individualized antenatal and postnatal advice to families regarding these.
- Smoking and prone sleeping are two of the most significant and avoidable risk factors for SIDS.
- Stop-smoking programmes should be accessible for all prospective parents.
- Parents should be taught basic resuscitative measures.
- Multiprofessional working is crucial in providing seamless and appropriate care in preventing and managing SIDS.

REFERENCES

Blackwell, C.C., Gordon, A.E., James, V.S. *et al.* (2002) The role of bacterial toxins in sudden infant death syndrome (SIDS). *International Journal of Medical Microbiology* **291**(6–7): 561–570.

Blair, P.S., Fleming, P.J., Smith, I.J. *et al.* (1999) Babies sleeping with parents: case-controlled study of factors influencing the risk of the sudden infant death syndrome. *British Medical Journal* **319**(7223): 1457–1461.

Blair, P.S., Nadin, P., Cole, T.J. *et al.* (2000) Weight gain and sudden infant death syndrome: changes in weight z scores may identify infants at increased risk. *Archives of Disease in Childhood* **82**(6): 462–469.

Carpenter, R.G. & Shaddick, C.W. (1965) Role of infection, suffocation and bottlefeeding in cot death. An analysis of some factors in the histories of 110 cases and their controls. *British Journal of Preventive & Social Medicine* **19**(1): 1–7.

Dybing, E. & Sanner, T. (1999) Passive smoking, sudden infant death syndrome (SIDS) and childhood infections. *Human & Experimental Toxicology* **18**(4): 202–205.

Fleming, P.J., Gilbert, R., Azaz, Y. *et al.* (1990) Interaction between bedding and sleeping position in sudden infant death syndrome: a population based case-control study. *British Medical Journal* **301**(6743): 85–89.

Fleming, P.J., Blair, P.S., Pollard, K. *et al.* (1999) Pacifier use and sudden infant death syndrome: results from the CESDI/SUDI case control study. *Archives of Disease in Childhood* **81**(2): 112–116.

Fleming, P.J., Blair, P.S., Platt, M.W. *et al.* (2001) The UK accelerated immunisation programme and sudden unexpected death in infancy. *British Medical Journal* **322**(7290): 822–825.

Ford, R.P.K., Mitchell, E.A., Stewart, A.W. *et al.* (1997) SIDS, illness and acute medical care. *Archives of Disease in Childhood* **77**(1): 54–55.

Froen, J.F., Arnestad, M., Vege, A. *et al.* (2002) Comparative epidemiology of sudden infant death syndrome and sudden intrauterine unexplained death. *Archives of Disease in Childhood Fetal and Neonatal Edition* **87**(2): F118–F121.

Gordon, A.E., Saadi, A.T., MacKenzie, D.A. *et al.* (1999) The protective effect of breast feeding in relation to sudden infant death syndrome (SIDS): III. Detection of IgA antibodies in human milk that bind to bacterial toxins implicated in SIDS. *FEMS Immunology & Medical Microbiology* **25**(1–2): 175–182.

Leach, C.E., Blair, P.S., Fleming, P.J. *et al.* (1999) Epidemiology of SIDS and explained sudden infant deaths. CESDI SUDI Research Group. *Pediatrics* **104**(4): e43.

McMartin, K.I., Platt, M.S., Hackman, R. *et al.* (2002) Lung tissue concentrations of nicotine in sudden infant death syndrome. *Journal of Pediatrics* **140**(2): 205–209.

Mitchell, E.A., Scragg, R., Stewart, A.W. *et al.* (1991) Cot death supplement. Results from the first year of the New Zealand cot death study. *New Zealand Medical Journal* **104**(906): 71–76.

Morley, C.J., Thornton, A.J., Cole, T.J. *et al.* (1991) Baby check: a scoring system to grade the severity of acute systemic illness in babies under six months old. *Archives of Disease in Childhood* **66**(1): 100–105.

Royal College of Midwives (RCM) (2003) *Bed sharing: Briefing*. London: RCM.

Sweeney, J.K. & Gutierrez, T. (2002) Musculoskeletal implications of preterm infant positioning in the NICU. *Journal of Perinatal & Neonatal Nursing* **16**(1): 58–70.

FURTHER READING

http://www.sids.org.uk/fsid/pubslistfull.htm. FSID website: wide range of downloadable resources for parents and professionals, including research statistics, posters, leaflets and advice on prevention, management and care.

Horchler, J.N. & Rice, R. (2003) *SIDS & Infant Death Survival Guide: Information and Comfort for Grieving Family & Friends & Professionals Who Seek to Help Them.* London: SIDS Educational Services.

A resource containing journal entries, stories, and essays written by parents, grandparents, and professionals dealing with the emotional and practical issues of losing a child to SIDS.

PART 6

THE PUERPERIUM

41. Content and Organization of Postnatal Care 723

42. Morbidity Following Childbirth 736

PART 6

THE PUERPERIUM

Content and Organization of Postnatal Care

Debra Bick

LEARNING OUTCOMES

After reading this chapter, you will:

- be aware of the importance of providing postnatal care tailored to individual women's needs
- ensure that the woman is involved in discussions about the content and timing of her postnatal care
- understand the range of physical and psychological health problems women may experience
- be knowledgeable about the evidence base for the management of some postnatal health problems.

INTRODUCTION

The postnatal period or the 'puerperium' is traditionally defined as the time from immediately after the end of labour until the reproductive organs have returned as nearly as possible to their pregravid condition, a period estimated to be around 6–8 weeks, although the evidence base to support this duration is lacking. Recent studies suggest that, for some women, adaptation to motherhood and recovery from childbirth can take much longer than this (Bick and MacArthur, 1995a; Brown and Lumley, 1998; MacArthur *et al.*, 1991).

AIMS OF POSTNATAL CARE

The following are some of the aims of postnatal care, the successful achievement of which will result from the contribution to care made by the midwife and other members of the multidisciplinary healthcare team.

- To help the woman adapt to and successfully fulfil the role and responsibilities of motherhood
- To promote and monitor the woman's and the infant's physical well-being
- To promote and monitor the woman's psychological well-being

- To assist the woman with the successful establishment of her infant feeding
- To foster the development of maternal–infant chosen method of attachment
- To foster good family relationships
- To educate the woman and her family in the needs and development of the infant
- To enhance the woman's confidence in her ability to fulfil her role as a mother
- To promote health education.

PHYSIOLOGICAL HEALTH CHANGES DURING THE POSTNATAL PERIOD

During the puerperium the following physiological changes take place in all women as the body returns to its pre-pregnant state:

- involution of the uterus and other soft parts of the genital tract
- commencement of lactation
- physiological changes in other systems of the body.

It is important that the midwife is familiar with these to ensure that appropriate care and advice are given.

Involution of the uterus

After the birth of the baby and the expulsion of the placenta, the muscles of the uterus constrict the blood vessels, so that the blood circulating in the uterus is considerably reduced. This is known as *ischaemia*. The vagina, the ligaments of the uterus and muscles of the pelvic floor return to their pre-pregnant state. The term *involution* describes the return of the uterus to a pelvic organ, the next stage during the process of recovery. Redundant muscle, fibrous and elastic tissue has to be disposed of. The phagocytes of the bloodstream deal with the last two by phagocytosis, but the process is usually incomplete and some elastic tissue remains, so that a uterus which has once been pregnant never returns to its nulliparous state. Muscle fibres are digested by proteolytic enzymes, a process known as *autolysis*. The lysosomes of the cells are responsible for this process. The waste products then pass into the bloodstream to be eliminated by the kidneys.

The decidual lining of the uterus is shed in the *lochia*, which also contains blood and serum. A new endometrium grows from the basal layer, beginning to be formed around the tenth postnatal day and estimated to be completed in about 6 weeks, although the evidence base for this is absent. Variations in the duration of shedding of lochia have been reported in midwifery textbooks, with a range of 4–8 weeks (Abbott *et al.*, 1997; Silverton, 1993), although duration of loss appears to be based on assumption rather than evidence. The changes in lochia have been described in three stages: *lochia rubra* (red), *lochia serosa* (pink) and *lochia alba* (white). These terms describe changes in the colour of the lochia, which together with the assumed duration of loss, have formed the basis for current practice.

Lactation

The secretion of prolactin from the anterior pituitary gland initiates lactation. Levels of prolactin increase during pregnancy. After delivery, progesterone and oestrogen levels fall abruptly but prolactin levels continue to increase, stimulating milk secretion from the glandular epithelial cells within the breast. An increase in the concentration of oxytocin contracts the cells around the alveoli and milk ducts, raising the intra-alveolar pressure that propels milk along the ducts. The release of oxytocin may be experienced by the woman as a 'tingling' sensation in the breast and a cramping pain in the abdomen (as a result of uterine contraction). These are both normal reactions when feeding takes place. Once lactation commences, it is maintained by the baby suckling. This provides the natural stimulus for the release of prolactin.

Physiological changes in other systems of the body

Circulatory system   The volume of blood in the circulatory system decreases to pregravid levels and the blood regains its former viscosity. Smooth muscle tone in the vessel walls improves, cardiac output returns to normal and the blood pressure returns to its pre-pregnant level.

Respiratory system   Changes in the respiratory system are effected by the full ventilation of the basal lobes of the lungs which are no longer compressed by the enlarged uterus.

Musculoskeletal system   The musculoskeletal system returns gradually to its pregravid state over a period of around 3 months following delivery. The abdominal and pelvic floor muscles gradually regain tone, a process which may be promoted with the assistance of postnatal exercises (see later). The rectus abdominis muscles may remain separated at the midline, a condition known as *diastasis recti*, which is most likely to occur in grande multiparous women or in those who have had a multiple pregnancy or polyhydramnios. Low backache, a common postnatal problem, is discussed in more detail later.

Gastrointestinal system   The falling progesterone levels affect the alimentary tract. The smooth muscle tone gradually improves throughout the body, and symptoms of heartburn the woman may have experienced should resolve. Constipation may, however, remain a common problem during the postnatal period (see below and Ch. 42).

Reproductive system   The ovaries and uterine tubes become pelvic organs again. Following the delivery of the placenta, the circulating levels of oestrogen and progesterone fall. Eventually negative feedback mechanisms trigger the release of follicle-stimulating hormone and luteinizing hormone, responsible for the resumption of the ovarian menstrual cycle. Ovulation takes place before menstruation, so that a woman may become pregnant again before she has a period; thus all women should be advised within 1–2 weeks of delivery of the need to use contraception prior to resuming sexual intercourse.

Urinary system   Changes in the urinary tract include a marked *diuresis* after delivery which lasts for 2–3 days. This is due to the reduction in blood volume occurring in the immediate postnatal period. The dilatation of the urinary tract, which occurs in pregnancy due to increased vascular volume, resolves and the renal organs gradually return to their pregravid state.

THE ROLE OF HEALTH PROFESSIONALS DURING THE POSTNATAL PERIOD

The role of the midwife

The pattern and content of midwifery postnatal care have changed little during the course of the last century. The first Midwives Act was passed in 1902, when there was concern about the continuing high maternal mortality rate, due mainly to puerperal infection, when the death rate among the general population from infectious diseases had been falling. The 1902 Act instigated the establishment of the Central Midwives Board in 1905, which published the first edition of the Midwives Rules, and established the precedent for a proscriptive pattern and content of postnatal care, focused on the identification of infection.

The maternal mortality rate declined steeply at around the time of the onset of the Second World War, but despite this, the only changes to affect postnatal midwifery care in more recent times have been the introduction in 1986 of selective home visiting and earlier hospital discharge (see below). There continues to be very little guidance for midwives on the pattern and content of postnatal care, despite changing health needs and demographic trends that have affected women and their families in the UK. In the most recent Midwives Rules, issued nearly a century after the first edition, the postnatal period continues to be defined as: 'a period of not less than ten and not more than 28 days after the end of labour, during which time the continued attendance of a midwife on the mother and baby is requisite' (UKCC, 1998).

The role of the GP

As part of routine postnatal care offered by the GP, a woman may receive up to five home visits and a final consultation at 6–8 weeks, following which she is discharged from the maternity services. Despite this being a routine part of care for around 50 years, the evidence of the contribution of GPs to routine community-based maternity care is hard to quantify and anecdotally there is wide variation in the extent to which GPs delegate their responsibilities to midwives (Smith and Jewell, 1998). No studies have examined the benefit to women's well-being of routine GP home visits and whether they are an appropriate use of GP time and skills. The few studies that have examined the 6–8 week check found that the routine content and timing may not be appropriate to meet women's health needs (Bick and MacArthur, 1995b; Sharif et al., 1993), although the generally high uptake suggests women value a consultation for themselves after childbirth. Discussion of contraception is routinely included as part of the 6–8 week consultation; however, one recent study found more than half of postnatal women had resumed sexual intercourse within 6 weeks of the birth (Glazener, 1998), indicating that a discussion of contraception at this consultation is too late. These findings and the need to inform women of when ovulation may recommence highlights the importance of midwives providing appropriate advice on contraception in the immediate postnatal period.

The role of the health visitor

The health visitor will visit the woman and her infant during the postnatal period and for a number of years afterwards, until the child reaches school age. The health visitor may commence home visits whilst the midwife is still attending the woman. The health visitor's role is generic and will combine health surveillance, health promotion and diagnostic health screening. In many areas of the UK, health visitors routinely administer the Edinburgh Postnatal Depression Scale (EPDS) to postnatal women (Cox et al., 1987) which will assist in the identification of those at risk of developing depression.

CONTENT OF MIDWIFERY POSTNATAL CARE

The routine observations and examinations performed to monitor recovery from the birth will be the same in hospital as in the community. These are presented in Box 41.1.

> **Box 41.1 Routine postnatal observations and examinations**
>
> - Recording maternal temperature
> - Recording maternal blood pressure
> - Abdominal palpation
> - Observation of lochia
> - Examination of the perineum
> - Examination of the legs
> - Observation/examination of the breasts
> - Observation of abdominal wound (if present)

Although some or all of the observations in Box 41.1 are routinely performed at each postnatal examination, evidence is now available to suggest that they may not identify health problems commonly experienced by women after childbirth (see below), suggesting that midwives should only perform them as appropriate to take into account individual women's health needs.

Care of women's physical health during the postnatal period

Uterine involution and vaginal loss

The progress of involution is usually assessed by the midwife during the postnatal period by measuring the distance between the uterine fundus and the symphysis pubis, either with a tape measure or by simple abdominal palpation. There is little evidence as to which method is the more accurate, and variance in the rate of involution has been described. In a study to describe the rate of involution in a small ($n = 28$) sample of primiparae who had a spontaneous vaginal delivery, Cluett et al. (1997) found a considerable variability in the pattern of uterine involution. This occurred not only in the daily rate of decline in individual women, but also between women. At least one episode of 'slow decline' (defined as a decline in the SF-D of <1 cm over 3 or more days) was reported for 22 women at some time during the puerperium. In an earlier study by the same researchers (Cluett et al., 1995) intra-observer variability was assessed, where the same midwife measured the same women using a tape measure, and inter-observer variability, where different midwives measured the same women. The results showed disparity between both groups, indicating that the measurement of uterine involution is unreliable. The authors concluded that using a tape measure was not precise enough to enable a clinical decision to be taken about normal or abnormal progress of uterine involution. In order to ascertain if involution is associated with morbidity, other factors such as pyrexia, offensive lochia and maternal well-being should also be taken into account.

Recent studies have suggested that the normal duration and composition of vaginal loss is much more varied than was previously assumed, as described earlier (Marchant et al., 1999; Visness et al., 1997). A prospective study of breastfeeding women from the Philippines examined their experiences of postnatal loss and compared results with the duration of the stages of lochia described in a commonly cited obstetric textbook

(Visness et al., 1997). The study was undertaken as part of a randomized controlled trial of the effectiveness of the lactational amenorrhoea method of contraception. 477 women who had chosen this method of contraception, had a vaginal delivery and had previously breast-fed for a minimum of 12 months, were followed up for 1 year by means of a calendar on which the woman was to record a daily description of her vaginal loss. The duration of lochia as reported by the women ranged from 5–90 days (median 27 days) and did not vary by any of the maternal or obstetric characteristics included in the analysis. A quarter of the women reported that their blood loss stopped and recommenced.

Marchant et al., (1999) in the Blood Loss in the Postnatal Period (BLiPP) study aimed to describe as the first of a three-stage study, the range of normal postnatal vaginal loss from 24 hours after the birth until 3 months. To do this, a prospective survey of 524 women who gave birth between 1995–1996 was undertaken. Women were asked to complete two questionnaires and two diaries at intervals up to 16 weeks after delivery to record details of their vaginal loss and their experiences and expectations of the amount, colour and duration of loss. The first questionnaire, returned by 350 women (67%), was completed between 48 hours and 5 days of the birth; 318 women (61%) completed the first diary between days 2–10 and 284 (54%) the second diary on the 14th, 21st and 28th postnatal days. At 3 months postpartum, 325 (62%) women returned the second questionnaire. The findings were similar to those of the study described above, that postnatal vaginal loss was much more varied in amount, duration (median 21 days) and colour than described in commonly used midwifery textbooks.

Reflective Activity 41.1

Keep a record of the rate of involution and lochial loss of primigravid and multigravid mothers for as many days as possible. Are there many differences in the pattern of involution and lochial loss between the women?

Perineal pain

The majority of women who have had a vaginal delivery, with or without perineal trauma, will experience some degree of perineal pain and will require effective pain relief. A survey of midwives' management of postpartum perineal pain revealed that the first line of management in most cases was oral analgesia, most commonly paracetamol (Sleep and Grant, 1988). However, it is important that midwives monitor the effect of this, in order that the woman can be referred if stronger analgesia is required.

In addition to oral analgesia, midwives have also used local applications. Ice packs were the most commonly used local application in a survey of perineal care carried out by the National Childbirth Trust (Greenshield and Hulme, 1993), but these will only provide short-term relief and may burn the skin if applied directly. Other local applications include witch hazel and pramoxine and hydrocortisone spray (Epifoam). Moore and James (1989) compared topical pain relief applications (Epifoam, ice and witch hazel) in a randomized controlled trial (RCT) of 300 women who had an episiotomy for instrumental delivery. At delivery, women were randomized to one of three groups and the first application of the agent applied following repair of the episiotomy. Complete data were only available on 205 women who had an inpatient assessment of pain; 126 were seen at 6 weeks for a hospital appointment, when the perineal wound was examined. The results showed no difference in pain relief achieved amongst the groups on the first postnatal day, and at 6 weeks, of those who attended the outpatient appointment, there were no differences in resumption of intercourse or resolution of perineal pain.

Electrical therapies such as ultrasound and pulsed electromagnetic energy may also be used to relieve perineal pain, but further evidence of benefit is required. The effectiveness of diclofenac suppositories used prophylactically for those who have sustained perineal trauma was examined in two RCTs. Yoong et al., (1997) randomly allocated 110 women who had had an episiotomy for a spontaneous vaginal delivery to receive a diclofenac suppository ($n = 56$) or placebo ($n = 54$) immediately following the repair. At 24 hours, women given diclofenac had less perineal pain, as recorded on a visual analogue scale (VAS), but there were no differences in VAS scores at 48 hours. Searles and Pring (1998) randomly allocated 100 women who had a sutured second-degree perineal tear or episiotomy to receive a diclofenac suppository or placebo immediately following the repair and 12 hours later. Results were based on 89 women for whom there was complete follow-up. The level of pain was based on scores which ranged from '0' = no pain to '5' = worst pain possible, at 12, 24, 48 and 72 hours after delivery. At each time interval, the mean pain score was less in the diclofenac group. Larger studies are necessary to confirm this effect and whether administration of rectal

suppositories provides better and longer-lasting pain relief than oral administration. Some women may find bathing soothes their perineal pain, although this will only provide short-term relief. Additives to the bath water, such as salt, will not improve perineal-healing rates. It is important that midwives acknowledge women's pain-relief needs. Perineal hygiene should be discussed with women as and when appropriate.

Micturition and bowels

Various urinary symptoms may present in the postnatal period and it is important that the midwife is able to identify these in order to implement appropriate management and referral. Occasionally the bladder is numbed by injury or pressure during labour and the woman is unaware that it needs emptying. The bladder can only contain a certain amount of urine even when distended and once that capacity is reached, the sphincter of the bladder relaxes and urine escapes. This is referred to as *retention with overflow*, although the incidence of this condition postpartum is not known because 'retention' is defined in many ways. Yip et al. (1997) defined it as residual urinary volume of 150 ml or more, and Lee et al. (1999) as residual volume exceeding 200 ml on day 2 postpartum. Examination of the abdomen may show the presence of a soft rounded suprapubic swelling which may displace the uterus upwards and to the right side. Catheterization may be necessary, but it should be avoided if possible because of the risk of infection.

Other urinary symptoms that may present postnatally include stress urinary incontinence and urinary tract infection, the risk factors and symptoms of which are described in Chapter 42. The midwife should ask women about urinary symptoms and, if present, obtain a description of these, which will assist diagnosis and management. Midwives should be familiar with the teaching of pelvic floor exercises (PFE), in order to advise women on how to perform them correctly. Outcomes of studies that have investigated the benefit of performing PFE are described in Chapter 42. If a woman has a suspected UTI, she should be prescribed antibiotics.

Constipation and *haemorrhoids* are common symptoms after birth that more often than not will present in the immediate postnatal period either as new symptoms or as symptoms which have persisted from pregnancy (MacArthur et al., 1991). It could be 2–3 days after delivery before a woman has a bowel movement, especially if she has a painful perineum and/or inadequate dietary intake during labour. There is a dearth of research into the most effective management of postnatal constipation. Dietary bran and wheat supplements were the most effective treatment in one systematic review of interventions for constipation in pregnancy (Jewell and Young, 2002); however, this was based on only one trial of 40 women. Postnatal constipation may be associated with the development of *anal fissure* (see Ch. 42), which is why it is so important that midwives accurately identify and assess the problem by sensitive questioning of the woman.

Haemorrhoids can range in severity depending upon the degree of prolapse. Treatment will depend on severity, but for most women treatment with application of topical creams may be beneficial. Women who have haemorrhoids that do not return to the anal canal require immediate GP referral for appropriate treatment.

Symptoms of *faecal incontinence* after childbirth are more commonly experienced than previously considered. This is probably due to a number of factors, including lack of studies investigating the incidence and prevalence of the symptoms; reluctance of women to spontaneously report symptoms; and lack of awareness among health professionals (see Ch. 42). It is imperative that midwives ask women about symptoms in order that appropriate referral for specialist management can be made. Symptoms can include urgency (not being able to defer the urge to defecate), soiling or staining of underwear, loss of flatus and frank faecal incontinence.

Breastfeeding

Breastfeeding rates in the UK have remained fairly static, ranging from 65% in 1980 to 68% in 1995 (Foster *et al.*, 1997). Despite the strong evidence of the benefits of breastfeeding for both the woman and the infant, many women give up breastfeeding well before the end of the recommended 6-month period (WHO, 2001). One of the most important aspects of midwifery care is providing accurate and consistent advice on how to prevent breastfeeding problems and, if problems do occur, how to overcome them, in order to reduce early cessation of breastfeeding. If a baby is able to feed efficiently and effectively from the first feed, it is likely that postnatal breastfeeding problems can be prevented (Inch, 1999).

The World Health Organization (WHO) recommended that all babies should have skin contact with their mothers within half an hour of the birth. However, a recent Cochrane systematic review of early versus delayed commencement of breastfeeding (defined as breastfeeding within 30 minutes of the birth compared with breastfeeding within 4–8 hours of the

birth) which included 209 women from three RCTs, found no differences in the numbers of women who continued breastfeeding (Renfrew *et al.*, 2001).

The baby should be breastfed on demand with no limit on the frequency and duration of feeds. Initially the woman may require help and supervision from the midwife to position her baby correctly at the breast. The baby should be held close to the woman with his head and shoulders facing her breast, head slightly extended and nose at the level of her nipple. As he opens his mouth and begins to root, he is moved onto the breast with his mouth wide open and lower lip well below the nipple. The nipple and as much of the areola as possible should be in the baby's mouth, as the ampullae where the milk is stored lie within the areola, and it is the rhythmical, rolling action of the baby's tongue on the ampullae that expresses the milk into the baby's mouth. The nipple lies passively well back in the baby's mouth at the junction of the hard and soft palates and, when correctly positioned there, is not damaged by any friction from the gums (Inch, 1990). Described below are some of the more frequently reported problems and their management. Midwives should be aware of how to prevent problems and how to manage them if they do occur in order to inform and support women appropriately.

Frequently reported problems

Pain   Pain from nipple damage is one of the most frequently cited reasons for early cessation of breastfeeding. It is unlikely to occur if the baby is attached correctly, as described above. If pain is experienced, it is essential to remove the baby from the breast and check that both the position of the baby and attachment to the breast are correct, otherwise nipple pain and damage will occur.

Engorgement   This is most likely to present when the breast milk comes in, and occurs when the volume of milk exceeds the capacity of the alveoli to store it. As a result, milk seeps into the surrounding breast tissue, triggering an inflammatory response. Women may report red, tender and full breasts and on examination, may be pyrexial and tachycardic. Opinions vary as to what causes engorgement, although it is likely that previous implementation of restrictive feeding practices in hospital would have contributed to the incidence of the symptom (Snowden *et al.*, 2001). A recent Cochrane systematic review of interventions to relieve symptoms of engorgement during lactation, based on eight trials involving 424 women, found no overall benefit on symptoms of using cabbage leaves or cabbage leaf extracts, or oxytocin and cold packs. Use of ultrasound treatment and placebo were equally effective, whilst use of an anti-inflammatory agent (Danzen) significantly improved symptoms compared to a placebo, as did bromelain/trypsin complex (Snowden et al., 2001). Allowing the baby unrestricted access to the breast while correctly positioned will help to relieve symptoms as well as prevent them from occurring in the first instance (Enkin et al., 2000).

Insufficient milk   This was the most common reason for early cessation of breastfeeding in the most recent OPCS survey of infant feeding (Foster et al., 1997). The importance of explaining the physiological processes of breastfeeding is imperative. Objective evidence of insufficient milk is difficult to obtain; however, a prospective cohort study of over 600 women found an association with anaemia in the immediate postnatal period and insufficient milk (Henley et al., 1995).

Blocked milk duct   A blocked milk duct may occur as a result of pressure placed on the breast, for example from a badly fitting bra, or ineffective positioning of the baby on the breast. As a result, the woman may report a hard lump, which could be painful. In the absence of evidence of effective management, best practice recommends that the woman be shown how to gently 'massage' the lump during a feed to assist drainage of the breast.

Mastitis   Pressure placed on the breast may also result in mastitis, an inflammatory reaction, which can be infective or non-infective. Women require advice to ensure effective feeding from the affected breast, but if symptoms do not resolve within 6–8 hours of this, GP referral should be made, as there is a risk of the woman developing a breast abscess.

Additional breastfeeding support will be required in certain circumstances, for example if a woman is breastfeeding twins or higher birth order, if her infant has developed jaundice, if the infant is premature or if there are concerns about infant weight loss.

Suppression of lactation   Lactation can be suppressed naturally or pharmacologically. Natural suppression involves not putting the infant to the breast. As prolactin is not released, owing to lack of stimuli, the breasts will eventually stop secreting milk. The breasts may still become engorged on around the third to fourth day, so the woman will need to wear a good supporting bra. Simple pain relief (for example, paracetamol) may be required if the breasts are uncomfortable. Two

drugs, bromocriptine and cabergoline, are used to suppress lactation pharmacologically. Both drugs have similar actions, although owing to adverse side-effects on the cardiovascular and cerebrovascular systems reported in women who took bromocriptine, the drug of choice should be cabergoline, although further information is necessary on the most appropriate dose and timing of administration (Enkin et al., 2000).

Backache

No studies have been carried out to determine the most appropriate management of postnatal backache. It is important that the midwife asks about the presence of backache as part of postnatal care and determines, as far as possible, the onset of the symptom, as general population studies show conservative management is likely to be more successful if commenced within 6 weeks of onset. It is possible that the woman will require pain relief, usually paracetamol in the first instance, but GP referral may be required if this is not adequate. Several trials based on general population groups have shown that bedrest is not an effective treatment for backache and advice to continue with normal activities may contribute to faster recovery and less time away from paid employment (NHS Centre for Reviews and Dissemination, 2000).

Symphysis pubis dysfunction (S-PD)   This results from separation of the symphysis pubis increasing the gap between the pubic bones (normally between 4–9 mm), producing a gliding action, which on weight-bearing is extremely painful. Some women suffer from S-PD during pregnancy, and it then persists into the postnatal period, whilst for other women it is a symptom that occurs for the first time after the birth. As with management of postnatal backache, no studies have evaluated treatment for S-PD although there are some case studies. These suggest that conservative management which could include analgesia, pelvic support and bedrest (with the hips adducted and the woman lying on her side – not recommended for women with backache) is usually beneficial. GP referral should be made as soon as the midwife suspects a woman has S-PD, in order that adequate pain relief and physiotherapy support can be provided.

Pain relief

Many women experience significant pain and discomfort in the postnatal period, even if they have had a spontaneous vaginal delivery with an intact perineum (Dewan et al., 1993; Mander, 1998), but as with much of the area of postnatal care, there is little evidence of the most appropriate management of postnatal pain, other than some studies that have assessed pain relief for perineal trauma as described earlier. In the first 3 or 4 days after delivery, pain can arise from perineal trauma and bruising, abdominal wounds, 'after pains' as a result of uterine cramps, haemorrhoids, the breasts and musculoskeletal system (Mander, 1998). Many women will report pain persisting well beyond the immediate postnatal period and it is important that the midwife continues to ask about pain relief needs and ensures that these are adequately managed. Further research is urgently required on this very important, but neglected area of postnatal health and care.

Care of women's psychological health

Pregnancy and childbirth are often described as major life events (Clement and Elliot, 1998), and in addition to physical health changes, emotional and psychological changes are also commonly experienced. However, there is concern that they remain unidentified by health professionals and unreported by women. Midwives have an important role in the early detection of psychological health problems and, as part of a multidisciplinary team, ensuring that women receive appropriate support and care.

Postpartum psychological problems are divided into three main conditions: the 'blues', depression and puerperal psychosis.

Postpartum blues   This transient, self-limiting condition usually occurs between the third and tenth day after delivery and is considered a normal reaction to childbirth, estimated to be experienced by around 50–80% of all postnatal women (Ball, 1994; Paykel et al., 1980). Commonly reported symptoms include tearfulness, irritability and lability of mood (Hannah et al., 1992). Although most women recover within a day or two, studies have shown a higher incidence of blues among women who suffer from postnatal depression (Beck et al., 1992). Women often require emotional support from the midwife and reassurance that this is a common symptom, of short duration.

Postnatal depression   The incidence of postnatal depression and associated risk factors are described in more detail in Chapters 42 and 54. It is a condition sometimes difficult to define and recognize, but its clinical features are similar to depression occurring among the general (i.e. not postpartum) population. Symptoms can include feelings of hopelessness, lethargy, tearfulness, anxiety, guilt and disturbed sleep patterns. The midwife should be alert to the onset of symptoms of depression, and if concerned, referral to the woman's GP or health visitor should be made after discussing this with the woman.

Puerperal psychosis   This is the most severe form of psychiatric morbidity, but with an incidence of 1 in 500 women, it is also the most uncommon. It is characterized by a sudden onset, typically after a period of well-being (Riley, 1995). Symptoms may be characterized by obsessional thoughts and behaviour – for example, women may believe that their baby is dead or deformed. If puerperal psychosis is suspected, the midwife should refer the woman to the GP immediately.

Postnatal debriefing and psychosocial support

There has been considerable debate in the midwifery press as to the appropriateness of implementing postnatal debriefing. 'Debriefing' is considered to be beneficial, particularly for women who have had a traumatic labour and/or delivery, although there is limited evidence of the appropriateness of this intervention (Alexander, 1999) and debate as to whether this is the correct terminology to describe the active 'listening' that midwives may implement. Two recent trials which evaluated the benefit of debriefing by midwives to prevent postnatal depression (Lavender and Walkinshaw, 1998; Small et al., 2000) did not show any benefit, the findings of the second study indicating that debriefing could in some cases contribute to emotional health problems. Further research is required.

Oakley et al. (1994) described social support as listening, responding, informing when asked and helping whenever and however appropriate. All women should be asked about the level of social support available to them, to enable postnatal care to be planned to provide this if required. A randomized controlled trial was recently completed in two London boroughs to assess whether additional social support improves health outcomes for socially disadvantaged women and their infants. Routine postnatal care is being compared with additional social support from either a community group or research health visitor, tailored to individual need (Wiggins, 2000). Publication is awaited.

ORGANIZATION OF MIDWIFERY POSTNATAL CARE

Postnatal care commences in hospital for the majority of women, and for those who do not experience any labour or delivery complications, length of stay can range from 6 hours to 2–3 days, with longer stays for women who have had operative delivery. The average length of postnatal stay following a normal delivery has gradually decreased, from 5.4 days in 1981 (Rider, 1994) to 2.5 days in 1997 (Audit Commission, 1997), although figures vary from region to region. The 'Changing Childbirth' report (DoH, 1993) recommended that as far as is practicable, the length of hospital stay should be discussed and agreed with the woman. The Audit Commission report 'First Class Delivery', published in 1997, which presented the findings of a large survey of the maternity services in England and Wales identified that although the majority of 2375 women questioned about their stay in hospital considered this to have been 'about right', 25% reported they were dissatisfied. The Audit Commission recommended that hospital stay should be flexible and women consulted on how long they wanted to stay, but there is little evidence of this being adopted as routine practice.

The majority of women who choose to breastfeed will commence this whilst still in hospital (although lactation may not be established until they are home); however, the environment and routine pattern of care on a postnatal ward have frequently been cited as reasons for the low uptake and early cessation of breastfeeding. In the 1995 infant feeding survey (Foster et al., 1997), 12% of women who commenced breastfeeding gave up whilst still on the postnatal ward. In a recent survey by the NCT (Singh and Newburn, 2000), many women complained about the care they received in hospital, in particular inadequate support for breastfeeding and feeling left to cope alone. Women who delivered by caesarean section reported having too few staff available on the wards to assist them with physical tasks, made difficult when recovering from major abdominal surgery. There is an urgent need to review the provision of postnatal care in hospital.

The organization of community-based midwifery postnatal care varies throughout the UK, with little information on the most appropriate organization of care in terms of effect on women's well-being and use of resources. As referred to earlier, in 1986 the UKCC introduced the policy of 'selective' home visits; however, there was little evidence of guidance on how midwives should change the pattern of visits and no evidence to support the alteration of care. A survey of all then existing health districts in England undertaken in 1991 found that the extent to which selective visiting occurred in practice was variable and in many districts change in visit pattern was minor (Garcia et al., 1994).

Hamilton (1998) carried out a small ethnographic study of women's and midwives' views of the pattern of postnatal visiting which highlighted discrepancies between the opinions of the 'providers' and the 'users' of the service. Midwives considered that selective visiting enhanced the postnatal care they gave, but in contrast, women reported that they were not always informed that they could be involved in decisions regarding the frequency and duration of postnatal visits and did not consider that selective visiting enhanced their care.

Twaddle et al., (1993) undertook a small pilot pro-ject in Glasgow to examine if planning care based on women's individual needs reduced the number of postnatal maternal and infant health problems and increased continuity of care, satisfaction with care and cost savings to the NHS. The intervention comprised a brief agenda for action, which required the midwife to plan ongoing care with the woman at the first home visit. Assessments performed after implementing this agenda found that even with such a minimal plan, midwives made significantly fewer visits and improved continuity of midwifery care. The majority of women were satisfied with their care and the proportion who felt they required a daily visit decreased significantly.

Marsh and Sargent (1991) in a study in the Lothian Region of Scotland identified 10 factors which independently influenced the duration of postnatal visits. The factors were grouped as:

- 'time-consuming procedures' (physical examination of the mother, physical examination of the baby, performing a phenylketonuria (PKU) test)
- 'administration related' (liaison with the GP, health visitor or both; the total number of visits to be made in the same day; the waiting time to see the woman; previous contact between the woman and the midwife)
- 'feeding related' (breastfeeding problems, previous experience of breastfeeding); and 'delivery related' (delivery complications).

That the midwives in this study appeared to concentrate on physical tasks implies that this was a reflection of their perception of the needs of the women, rather than identifying the actual needs of the women.

COULD POSTNATAL CARE BE MORE EFFECTIVE?

Maternity care accounts for 5% of the total hospital and community health service expenditure, yet there has been very little evaluation of its cost-effectiveness, especially during the postnatal period (Winter et al.,

2000). Recent studies have shown significant levels of physical and psychological morbidity following childbirth (see Ch. 42) which suggests that current care is not meeting women's health needs. Randomized controlled trials have recently been completed in the UK and Australia aimed at improving the health of women, and some have also assessed if alteration to postnatal care makes more effective use of health service resources.

Reflective Activity 41.2

Find out the extent of postnatal visiting in your own unit. How effective do you think it is? What are the most common problems that women experience during this period?

Trials of postnatal care

As part of a randomized controlled trial, Gunn and colleagues (1998) in Victoria, Australia, assessed if a visit to the GP 1 week after hospital discharge resulted in:

- less postnatal depression
- increased breastfeeding rates
- improved maternal well-being, and
- increased satisfaction with care from the GP compared with the routine 6 week check.

683 women who gave birth at one rural hospital and one urban hospital between February and December 1995 were recruited on the 2nd or 3rd day after giving birth and randomized to the intervention (1 week GP visit) or control group (6 week GP visit). Outcomes were assessed at 3 and 6 months via a postal questionnaire which included the SF36 (a scale of general well-being) and the EPDS. There were no differences between the groups at both time periods in any of the outcomes. The authors concluded that to make clinically important improvements in maternal health, more than early postnatal review is required.

Morrell and colleagues (2000) undertook a randomized controlled trial of community support workers (CSWs) in an area of Sheffield, UK, to measure the effect and resource use and costs to the NHS of providing postnatal support in the woman's home, an intervention based on the Dutch maternity nurse model. The CSWs were to help women recover from the birth by providing practical and emotional support, based on the woman's needs and worked alongside existing midwifery postnatal services. 623 women were recruited, 311 randomized to the intervention and 312 to the control. Outcomes were assessed at 6 weeks and 6 months, using the SF36, the EPDS and the Duke Functional Social Support Scale (DUFSS). At 6 weeks and 6 months there were no differences in any of the health measures used and no differences in the use of NHS services, although three-quarters of the women who received the intervention were very satisfied with the community support worker.

MacArthur *et al.* (2002) in a cluster randomized controlled trial, implemented and evaluated a new model of midwifery-led postnatal care (the IMPaCT study). 36 general practice clusters randomly selected from within the West Midlands health region, UK, were randomized to the intervention ($n = 17$) or control ($n = 19$) group. The midwives attached to these clusters provided either the new model of care or current care. Midwives in the intervention clusters used symptom checklists at the first visit and at visits on the 10th and 28th postnatal day and at 10–12 weeks, and also administered the EPDS on the 28th day and at 10–12 weeks to identify commonly experienced physical and psychological health problems. Midwifery care was extended for all women to include a visit at about 28 days and a discharge consultation at 10–12 weeks (instead of the GP 6–8 week check). Evidence-based guidelines, with clear criteria for GP referral, enabled the midwife to implement primary management of symptoms identified from the checklist, observed by the midwife or spontaneously reported by the woman. GP contact was based on need, not routine. A total of 2064 women were recruited, with 1087 receiving new model care and 977 current care. The main outcome measures were the physical and mental health summary component scores (PCS and MCS) of the SF36 and the EPDS. Secondary outcomes were women's views of the care they received.

At 4 months, both of the mental health measures were significantly better among the intervention women compared with controls. There were no differences in the physical health measures. Women who received the new model of care were significantly more likely to rate their care as better than expected and scored the planning of their care significantly more highly. They were also significantly more likely to report that they could talk to their midwives about most or all of their health problems and to have experienced no difficulty in this. Outcomes at 12 months postpartum will be reported shortly.

IMPLICATIONS FOR MIDWIVES

One reason for continued adherence to a traditional content and pattern of midwifery postnatal care was the assumption that this was meeting women's needs. However, the findings of studies described in this and the following chapter on maternal morbidity highlight the need for midwives to evaluate the care they currently provide, in order to assess if this is appropriate. There will continue to be situations where the performance of routine observations and examinations are needed, but these should not continue to be the main focus of postnatal care. The results of ongoing research and the establishment of the All Party Parliamentary Committee on Maternity will continue the debate about the future direction of maternity care, including care provided after the birth. In the meantime, all midwives should ensure they are familiar with the research findings and evidence-based resources that are now available, as lack of awareness is not an acceptable reason for continuing to provide postnatal care which may not be appropriate.

KEY POINTS

- All women are entitled to postnatal care, which is provided by a range of healthcare professionals in both hospital and community settings.
- The provision of postnatal care has been a statutory part of midwifery practice for over a century, when it was introduced in an attempt to reduce the, then, high maternal mortality rate.
- Midwives have little information to guide the pattern and content of the postnatal care they provide.

- Recent studies have highlighted the long-term morbidity of childbirth, which current postnatal care may not address.
- More information is required on how to provide care that is effective and beneficial to women's well-being.

REFERENCES

Abbott, H., Bick, D. & MacArthur, C. (1997) Health after birth. In: Henderson, C., Jones, K. (eds) *Essential Midwifery*. London: Mosby.

Alexander, J. (1999) Can midwives reduce postpartum psychological morbidity? A randomized trial (Comments). *MIDIRS Midwifery Digest* 9: 730–731.

Audit Commission (1997) *First Class Delivery: Improving Maternity Services in England and Wales*. London: Audit Commission.

Ball, J.A. (1994) *Reactions to Motherhood. The Role of Postnatal Care*, 2nd edn. Hale: Books for Midwives Press.

Beck, C.T., Reynolds, M.A. & Rutowski, P. (1992) Postpartum depression. *Journal of Obstetric, Gynecologic, and Neonatal Nursing* 21: 287–293.

Bick, D. & MacArthur, C. (1995a) Extent, severity and effect of health problems after childbirth. *British Journal of Midwifery* 3: 27–31.

Bick, D. & MacArthur, C. (1995b) Attendance, content and relevance of the 6 week postnatal examination. *Midwifery* 11: 69–73.

Brown, S. & Lumley, J. (1998) Maternal health after childbirth: results of an Australian population based survey. *British Journal of Obstetrics and Gynaecology* 105: 156–161.

Clement, S. & Elliot, S. (1998) Psychological health before, during and after childbirth. In: Marsh, G. & Renfrew, M. (eds) *Community-based Maternity Care*, Ch. 18. Oxford: Oxford University Press.

Cluett, E.R., Alexander, J. & Pickering, R.M. (1995) Is measuring postnatal symphysis–fundus distance worthwhile? *Midwifery* 11: 174–183.

Cluett, E.R., Alexander, J. & Pickering, R.M. (1997) What is the normal pattern of uterine involution? An investigation of postpartum uterine involution measured by the distance between the symphysis pubis and the uterine fundus using a paper tape measure. *Midwifery* 13: 9–16.

Cox, J.L., Holden, J.M. & Sagovsky, R. (1987) Detection of postnatal depression. Development of the 10-item Edinburgh Postnatal Depression Scale. *British Journal of Psychiatry* 150: 782–786.

Department of Health (DoH) (1993) *Changing Childbirth, the Report of the Expert Maternity Group*. London: HMSO.

Dewan, G., Glazener, C. & Tunstall, M. (1993) Postnatal pain: a neglected area. *British Journal of Midwifery* 1: 63–66.

Enkin, M., Keirse, M.J.N.C., Neilson, J. *et al.* (2000) *A Guide to Effective Care in Pregnancy and Childbirth*, 3rd edn. Oxford: Oxford University Press.

Foster, K., Lader, D. & Cheesbrough, S. (1997) *Infant Feeding 1995*. London: The Stationery Office.

Garcia, J., Renfrew, M.J. & Marchant, S. (1994) Postnatal home visiting by midwives. *Midwifery* 10: 40–43.

Glazener, C.M.A. (1998) Sexual function after childbirth: women's experiences, persistent morbidity and lack of professional recognition (Letter). *British Journal of Obstetrics and Gynaecology* 105: 243–244.

Greenshield, W. & Hulme, H. (1993) *The Perineum in Childbirth. A Survey of Women's Experiences and Midwives' Practices*. London: National Childbirth Trust.

Gunn, J., Lumley, J., Chondros, P. *et al.* (1998) Does an early postnatal check-up improve maternal health: results from a randomised controlled trial. *British Journal of Obstetrics and Gynaecology* 105: 991–997.

Hamilton, M. (1998) Patterns of postnatal visiting: the views of women and midwives. *British Journal of Midwifery* 6(1): 15–18.

Hannah, P., Adams, D., Lee, A. *et al.* (1992) Links between early post-partum mood and post-natal depression. *British Journal of Psychiatry* 160: 777–780.

Henley, S.J., Andersson, C.M., Avery, M.D. *et al.* (1995) Anemia and insufficient milk in first-time mothers. *Birth* 22(2): 87–92.

Inch, S. (1990) Postnatal care relating to breastfeeding. In: Alexander J., Levy V. & Roch, S. (eds) *Postnatal Care: A Research Based Approach*. London: Macmillan.

Inch, S. (1999) Breast feeding update. In: Alexander, J., Roth, C. & Levy, V. (eds) *Midwifery Practice. Core Topics 3*. Basingstoke: Macmillan

Jewell, D.J. & Young, G. (2002) Interventions for treating constipation in pregnancy (Cochrane Review). *The Cochrane Library*, Issue 3. Oxford: Update Software.

Lavender, T. & Walkinshaw, S.A. (1998) Can midwives reduce postpartum psychological morbidity? A randomized trial. *Birth* 25: 215–219.

Lee, S.N.S., Lee, C.P., Tang, O.S.F. *et al.* (1999) Postpartum urinary retention (Brief communication). *International Journal of Gynecology and Obstetrics* 66: 287–288.

MacArthur, C., Lewis, M. & Knox, E.G. (1991) *Health After Childbirth*. London: The Stationery Office.

MacArthur, C., Winter, H.R., Bick, D.E. *et al.* (2002) The effects of re-designed community postnatal care on women's health at four months after birth: a cluster randomised controlled trial. *Lancet* 359(9304): 378–385.

Marchant, S., Alexander, J., Garcia, J. *et al.* (1999) A survey of women's experiences of vaginal loss from 24 hours to three months of childbirth (the BLiPP study). *Midwifery* 15: 72–81.

Marsh, J. & Sargent, E. (1991) Factors affecting the duration of postnatal visits. *Midwifery* 7: 177–182.

Mander, R. (1998) *Pain in Childbearing and its Control*. Oxford: Blackwell Science.

Moore, W. & James, D.K. (1989) A random trial of three topical analgesic agents in the treatment of episiotomy

pain following instrumental vaginal delivery. *Journal of Obstetrics and Gynaecology* 10: 35–39.

Morrell, C.J., Spiby, H., Stewart, P. *et al.* (2000) Costs and effectiveness of community postnatal support workers: randomised controlled trial. *British Medical Journal* 321: 593–598.

NHS Centre for Reviews and Dissemination (2000) Acute and chronic low back pain. *Effective Health Care Bulletin*, Vol. 6(5). York: University of York.

Oakley, A., Hickey, D. & Rigby, A.S. (1994) Love or money? Social support, class inequality and the health of women and children. *European Journal of Public Health* 4: 265–273.

Paykel, E.S., Emms, E.M., Fletcher, J. *et al.* (1980) Life events and social support in puerperal depression. *British Journal of Psychiatry* 136: 339–346.

Riley, D. (1995) Postnatal depression. In: *Perinatal Mental Health: A Sourcebook for Health Professionals*, Ch. 4, pp. 51–73. Oxford: Radcliffe Medical Press.

Renfrew, M.J., Lang, S. & Woolridge, M.W. (2001) Early versus delayed initiation of breastfeeding (Cochrane Review). *The Cochrane Library*, Issue 2. Oxford: Update Software.

Rider, A.C.E. (1994) Management – a manager's approach to the organisation of normal postnatal care. *Midwives Chronicle* ii: ix.

Searles, J.A. & Pring, D.W. (1998) Effective analgesia following perineal injury during childbirth: a placebo controlled trial of prophylactic rectal diclofenac. *British Journal of Obstetrics and Gynaecology* 105: 627–631.

Sharif, K., Clarke, P. & Whittle, M. (1993) Routine six weeks postnatal examination: to do or not to do? *Journal of Obstetrics and Gynaecology* 4(13): 251–252.

Silverton, L. (1993) *The Art and Science of Midwifery*. New York: Prentice Hall.

Singh, D. & Newburn, M. (2000) *Access to Maternity Information and Support. The Experiences and Needs of Women Before and After Giving Birth*. London: NCT.

Sleep, J. & Grant, A. (1988) The relief of perineal pain following childbirth: a survey of midwifery practice. *Midwifery* 4: 118–122.

Small, R., Lumley, J., Donohue, L. *et al.* (2000) Randomised controlled trial of midwife led debriefing to reduce maternal depression after operative childbirth. *British Medical Journal* 321: 1043–1047.

Smith, L. & Jewell, D. (1998) General practitioners' contributions – what's really going on? In: Marsh, G. & Renfrew M. (eds) *Community Based Maternity Care*, Ch. 4. Oxford: Oxford University Press.

Snowden, H., Renfrew, M.J. & Woolridge, M.W. (2001). Treatments for breast engorgement during lactation (Cochrane Review). *The Cochrane Library*, Issue 2. Oxford: Update Software.

Twaddle, S., Liao, X.H. & Fyvie, H. (1993) An evaluation of postnatal care individualised to the needs of the woman. *Midwifery* 9: 154–160.

United Kingdom Central Council for Nursing, Midwifery and Health Visiting (UKCC) (1998) *Midwives Rules and Code of Practice*. London: UKCC.

Visness, C.M., Kennedy, K.I. & Ramos, R. (1997) The duration and character of postpartum bleeding among breast-feeding women. *Obstetrics and Gynecology* 89: 159–163.

Wiggins, M. (2000) Psychosocial needs after childbirth. In: *Life After Birth – Reflections on Postnatal Care. Report of a Multi-disciplinary Seminar*. London: Royal College of Midwives.

Winter, H.R., MacArthur, C. & Bick, D.E. (2001) Postnatal care and its role in maternal health and well-being. *MIDIRS Midwifery Digest* 11(Suppl. 1): S13–S16.

World Health Organization (WHO) (2001) *The Optimal Duration of Exclusive Breastfeeding*. A systematic review. Geneva: WHO.

Yoong, W.C., Biervliet, F. & Nagrani, R. (1997) The prophylactic use of diclofenac (Voltarol) suppositories in perineal pain after episiotomy. A random allocation double-blind study. *Journal of Obstetrics and Gynaecology* 17: 39–41.

Yip, S-K., Brieger, G., Hin, L-Y. & Chung, T. (1997) Urinary retention in the post-partum period. The relationship between obstetric factors and the post-partum post-void residual bladder volume. *Acta Obstetricia et Gynecologica Scandinavica* 76: 667–672.

FURTHER READING

Bick, D.E., MacArthur, C., Knowles, H. *et al.* (2001) *Postnatal Care – Evidence and Guidelines for Practice*. London: Churchill Livingstone.
Full evidence-based guidelines and a 'What to do' summary for practice.

Enkin, M., Keirse, M.J.N.C., Neilson, J. *et al.* (2000) *A Guide to Effective Care in Pregnancy and Childbirth*, 3rd edn. Oxford: Oxford University Press. Essential reading.

MacArthur, C., Winter, H.R., Bick, D. *et al.* (2002) *Redesigning Postnatal Care: a Randomised Controlled Trial of Protocol-based Midwifery-led Care Focussed on Individual Women's Physical and Psychological Health Needs*. Health Technology Assessment.
Copies are available from the National Coordinating Centre for Health Technology Assessment (email hta@soton.ac.uk) or can be printed off the Web at http://www.ncchta.org.

Royal College of Midwives (RCM) (2000) *Midwifery Practice in the Postnatal Period. Recommendations for Practice*. London: Royal College of Midwives.
Informative advice covering a range of postnatal areas.

42

Morbidity Following Childbirth

Christine MacArthur

LEARNING OUTCOMES

After reading this chapter you will:

- be knowledgeable about the different health problems that women can experience after childbirth
- understand the childbirth-related risk factors of the various health problems
- realize the necessity of systematic identification of postpartum morbidities, since midwives are

not always aware of them and women often do not report them
- consider the possible effects on women's physical and psychological well-being if postpartum problems are not identified or managed.

INTRODUCTION

The postnatal examination offered to all women in the UK 6–8 weeks after childbirth is considered to mark the end of the puerperium and a woman's routine contact with the maternity services. Although childbirth-related problems are known to occasionally occur after this time, some even requiring readmission to hospital, only in the last decade have there been systematic investigations of longer-term postpartum morbidity. Several large studies, in the UK (Bick and MacArthur, 1995; Glazener *et al.*, 1995; MacArthur *et al.*, 1991) and elsewhere (Brown and Lumley, 1998; Saurel-Cubizolles *et al.*, 2000), have investigated the occurrence and persistence of a range of health problems following childbirth. All these studies have identified substantial postpartum ill-health, much of which persists well past the end of the puerperium and is often not reported to health professionals, nor observed by them. Smaller studies and investigations of particular symptoms have demonstrated a similar pattern. It is important to remember that not all the problems experienced following childbirth are attributable to the birth itself. Some morbidity is likely to be associated with the delivery and some with the pregnancy, but some will be due to the life-event changes of childcare and some unrelated to any of these events, occurring as part of a general

background of morbidity present at any time in any population. Particular childbirth-related causal factors have been investigated in some of the studies and these will be described in the relevant sections.

EXTENT OF LONGER-TERM MORBIDITY

A study in Birmingham (MacArthur *et al.*, 1991) obtained information on the health problems of 11 701 women between 1 and 9 years after childbirth. This information was from postal questionnaires to all women who delivered in one hospital during a defined period and was linked to their maternity case-note data, enabling associations to be made between the women's symptoms and their obstetric circumstances and procedures. Since one of the main objectives of the study was to investigate childbirth-related health and potential causal relationships, the analysis to examine associations was restricted to symptoms not previously experienced before the birth and starting within 3 months of it. Almost half of the women in the sample (47%) reported at least one symptom defined in this way that had lasted for longer than 6 weeks. If recurrent symptoms were also included, this total rose to almost two-thirds of the sample (64%). Most symptoms lasted much longer than 6 weeks: 35% of the women reported new symptoms lasting over a year and 31% still had unresolved symptoms at the time of questioning, indicating that many women experience childbirth-related morbidity that becomes chronic. Since the recall period in this study was lengthy for some women, it is likely that some health problems that lasted for only a few weeks or were relatively minor may not have been reported. Analyses of the 5119 women who had delivered only 1–2 years previously showed that this group did generally report higher rates of symptoms. A subsequent study of a sample of 1278 women from the same hospital as in the above study but contacted by postal questionnaire at 6–7 months then interviewed at 9–10 months postpartum, confirmed these levels of morbidity (Bick and MacArthur, 1995).

A longitudinal study in Scotland (Glazener *et al.*, 1995), recruited a 20% sample of all births over a year within one region (*n* = 1249) and surveyed the women three times. They were asked to complete a questionnaire whilst in hospital, and at 8 weeks post-delivery; then at 12–18 months those who had delivered in the second half of the study (*n* = 438) completed a further postal questionnaire, providing information on longer-lasting problems. The symptom prevalence included all symptoms, irrespective of previous occurrence and duration, experienced at some time during the defined period. At all times considerable morbidity was identified, with the prevalence of some symptoms reducing substantially over time but not that of others. 76% of the women surveyed at 12–18 months reported one or more problems that had occurred between then and the completion of their questionnaire at 8 weeks.

Brown and Lumley (1998), in a population-based sample of all births over 2 weeks in one large region of Australia, contacted women by postal questionnaire at 6–7 months postpartum. Again, substantial morbidity was reported, although prevalences were generally lower in this study, probably because the questions asked were about symptoms that had been 'a problem for them' since the birth. A European longitudinal study of health after birth and mothers' work, collected data from 697 women in Italy and 589 in France who had delivered in eight different maternity units (Saurel-Cubizolles *et al.*, 2000). The women were interviewed whilst in hospital, at which time information on pre-pregnancy health was obtained, then again at 5 and 12 months, when information on a range of health problems present at the time of the interview was obtained. This study generally found very high symptom prevalences and for most symptoms these had increased at 12 months.

The design of these studies has been described in some detail here because they are large epidemiological studies documenting health generally after birth and will be referred to throughout the chapter in relation to the specific symptoms. Examples of the symptoms or problems reported by the women in these studies include urinary stress incontinence and other bladder problems, haemorrhoids, faecal incontinence and other bowel problems, perineal pain and dyspareunia, backache, headache, depression and fatigue, all of which are described in more detail later.

The types of symptoms experienced after childbirth are rarely life-threatening but they can have an effect on the quality of life. The second study in Birmingham also investigated the severity and impact of symptoms on the women's lives. This showed that although some were minor and non-problematical, others were more severe, and many symptoms were present on a daily basis and some affected various aspects of the women's lives (Bick and MacArthur, 1995). A recent study in Australia has demonstrated a relationship between physical health after birth and postnatal depression and fatigue (Brown and Lumley, 2000).

MEDICAL CONSULTATION

Even though studies have shown that many women experience health problems after childbirth, it has consistently been shown that these are often not reported to a relevant health professional (Brown and Lumley, 1998; Glazener *et al.*, 1995; MacArthur *et al.*, 1991). The proportion of women in the Birmingham study (MacArthur *et al.*, 1991) who said they had consulted a doctor varied for different symptoms, but on average only about a third had been reported to a doctor. There could be many reasons for this lack of consultation. The symptom might only be mild or occur infrequently; the problem might be considered by the woman as 'normal' after having a baby; or she may have thought that there is nothing that a doctor could do. Whatever the reason, the effect of this lack of consultation is that the full extent of the postpartum morbidity has remained unrecognized by health professionals, and women are left with unmet health needs.

URINARY PROBLEMS

Symptoms of stress incontinence are the most common of the urinary problems that occur in association with childbirth but some women also have retention and voiding difficulties or urinary tract infection.

General population studies have shown that urinary stress incontinence, defined as the involuntary leakage of urine usually on exertion, is widely experienced among women. It is more prevalent in parous than nulliparous women and childbirth is generally considered to be the most common cause (Assassa *et al.*, 2000; Yarnell *et al.*, 1982). The prevalence of postpartum stress incontinence varies in studies according to the population included, the timing of questioning and the wording used, but a prevalence of around 20% has been commonly reported. Wilson *et al.* (1996), using a postal questionnaire at 3 months postpartum, found that 24% of 1505 women in New Zealand reported stress incontinence. MacArthur *et al.* (1991) in Birmingham found that 15% reported new stress incontinence persisting for more than 6 weeks, and a further 5% reported similar ongoing symptoms. Over a third of these still had stress incontinence symptoms at questioning at least a year later, yet only just over 10% had consulted a doctor about this. A randomized controlled trial of two different perineal management regimes in which stress incontinence was one of the outcome measures, found a prevalence of stress incontinence of 23% in both trial groups at 3 months and again at 3-year follow-up (Sleep *et al.*, 1984; Sleep and Grant, 1987a). Brown and Lumley (1998), in their Australian study of health at 6–7 months postpartum, found a symptom prevalence of 11%, lower than in the other studies. However, their question asked the women whether they had had stress incontinence 'as a problem' since the birth, and there is evidence to suggest that postpartum women do not always consider this symptom to be a problem (see below).

The precise role of pregnancy and of different delivery factors in the aetiology of stress incontinence remains unclear, but it is generally considered to be linked to pelvic floor innervation damage (Allen *et al.*, 1990). Urodynamic investigations of women after birth have consistently found pelvic floor innervation damage to be more common after a longer second stage labour and the delivery of a bigger baby, but the findings relating to the effect of forceps have been inconsistent. MacArthur *et al.* (1991) and Brown and Lumley (1998) in epidemiological studies, found stress incontinence symptoms to be more common after forceps delivery and a longer second stage labour, but the two are closely interrelated and the effect of forceps disappeared (MacArthur *et al.*, 1991) or became only marginally significant (Brown and Lumley 1998) after taking this into

account, suggesting that long second stage may have the greater effect. Increasing maternal age, heavier infant birth weight and larger head circumference have also been identified as risk factors in epidemiological studies (MacArthur *et al.*, 1991; Wilson *et al.*, 1996; Yarnell *et al.*, 1982). Delivery by caesarean section is generally associated with a lower prevalence of stress incontinence, which occurs about half as often as when delivery is vaginal (Assassa *et al.*, 2000; MacArthur *et al.*, 1991; Wilson *et al.*, 1996). Wilson *et al.* (1996), however, found that a reduced occurrence only applied to women who had up to two caesarean sections: women who had three or more sections had no reduced risk. MacArthur *et al.*, (1991) found that when delivery was abdominal, heavier infant birth weight was no longer associated with greater symptom occurrence, but the association with increasing maternal age remained (MacArthur *et al.*, 1991, 1993c), suggesting that the age effect may be unrelated to delivery factors.

The severity of postpartum stress incontinence and its effect on lifestyle seems to be variable. In the study by Sleep and Grant (1987a), at 3 months postpartum most (62%) of the symptomatic women had experienced stress incontinence less than once in the past week, although more than a quarter had found the problem sufficiently severe to have to wear a pad at some time. Another study found that 25% of the women who reported stress incontinence experienced this at least daily; 30% said it had an effect on their activities and 47% had needed to wear pads at some time to protect against leakage. Measured on a visual analogue scale, however, 59% of the women rated it in the lowest quartile, suggesting that most cases were not seen as severe. 'Not being bad enough' was the most common reason given by the women for not consulting a doctor (Bick and MacArthur, 1995).

Pelvic floor exercises are generally recommended and sometimes taught to postpartum women to strengthen the perineal muscles and minimize the likelihood of stress incontinence occurring. A randomized controlled trial of additional education on pelvic floor exercises, found no differences in subsequent incontinence between the groups at 3 months postpartum (Sleep and Grant, 1987b). Many women, however, practice pelvic floor exercises ineffectively and some not at all, since they compete with all the other demands in the immediate postnatal period. A more recent trial of treatment using pelvic floor exercise education given to women who still had stress incontinence at 3 months postpartum (rather than all women in the previous trial) found a significant reduction in those who still had the symptoms at 12 months (Glazener *et al.*, 2001). The intervention in this study comprised a symptom assessment from a specially trained nurse who visited the home at 5, 7 and 9 months postpartum and provided detailed pelvic floor muscle training and bladder training. It is likely that pelvic floor muscle exercises will be more effective if performed correctly, and adequate advice is necessary for this (Mørved and Bø, 1996).

Urinary voiding difficulties and retention are generally immediate post-delivery complications. Glazener *et al.* (1995) found, however, that in 2% of women, difficulties in voiding still occurred between 1 and 8 weeks postpartum. Risk factors of voiding problems are considered to be caesarean section, instrumental delivery and prolonged labour (Saultz *et al.*, 1991).

Urinary tract infections are common in pregnancy, but there is more limited information on postpartum occurrence. Glazener *et al.* (1995) found that 5% of women reported a urinary tract infection some time during the first postpartum year. A review of urine samples from all deliveries over a 2-year period in a Norwegian hospital found bacteriuria in 3.7%, although only 21% of these had dysuria (Stray-Pederson *et al.*, 1990). A postpartum urinary tract infection is more common after a caesarean section, and a recent Cochrane systematic review has shown that prophylactic antibiotics for women who have abdominal deliveries are effective in reducing the occurrence of this (Smaill and Hofmeyr, 2001).

BOWEL PROBLEMS

Constipation and haemorrhoids are well known to be common after childbirth, and more recent studies have shown faecal incontinence as well as anal fissure to sometimes occur.

Constipation is common during pregnancy owing to the hormonal relaxation of the bowel, and following delivery, the pain of perineal trauma or reduced dietary intake in labour can also predispose to constipation. The few studies that have documented the prevalence of constipation have indicated that it occurs at some time following about 15–20% of deliveries (Glazener *et al.*, 1995; Saurel-Cubizolles *et al.*, 2000). It has been shown to be more common after instrumental delivery than after spontaneous vaginal or caesarean deliveries (Glazener *et al.*, 1995).

Haemorrhoids are common in association with childbirth because of the action of progesterone on the bowel during pregnancy and as a consequence of pelvic

pressure and straining during labour, exacerbated if the woman also has constipation. Haemorrhoids can be extremely painful but it has generally been considered that most cases regress within a few days of the birth. More recently, however, studies have shown that childbirth-associated haemorrhoids can be longer lasting, with between 15 and 20% of women reporting these symptoms at about 2 months after the birth (Glazener *et al.*, 1995; MacArthur *et al.*, 1991). MacArthur *et al.* (1991) found that two-thirds of the women with haemorrhoids still had them at least a year after giving birth, indicating that complete resolution of childbirth-related haemorrhoids is not common. The severity of persisting symptoms, however, is not known. Longer second stage of labour, instrumental delivery and heavier infant birth weight are associated with an increased likelihood of haemorrhoids (MacArthur *et al.*, 1991). Glazener *et al.* (1995) found that haemorrhoids were more than twice as common after instrumental compared with spontaneous vaginal delivery. Women are much less likely to experience haemorrhoids after caesarean section delivery: only 4% reported new haemorrhoids after a section in the study by MacArthur *et al.* (1991). Other studies have also found similar reduced rates after caesarean section (Glazener *et al.*, 1995).

One study has recently documented anal fissure, defined as a split or tear in the skin of the anal canal, as occurring in 9% of the women (Corby *et al.*, 1997). The study included 313 first births and used clinical history and examination to diagnose anal fissures at about 6 weeks postpartum. The authors noted that without such detailed investigation many of these would have been diagnosed (if at all) as acute painful haemorrhoids, with over 90% of cases resolving without treatment. Type of delivery or perineal trauma were not associated with the occurrence of anal fissure, but postnatal constipation was much more common in the symptomatic group.

The occurrence of postpartum faecal incontinence, including frank incontinence, soiling and faecal urgency, is increasingly being documented. It had previously been considered that although obstetric injury was probably the most common cause of faecal incontinence in women, symptoms were unlikely to occur (except after a third-degree tear) until later in life. Several epidemiological studies of unselected obstetric populations have found that between 1–9% of women reported postpartum faecal incontinence, the range depending on how this was defined and the timing of questioning. At 3 months postpartum, Sleep and Grant (1987b) found that 3% reported 'occasional faecal loss', Wilson *et al.* (1996)

documented 4.9% with 'faecal incontinence' and MacArthur *et al.* (2001) found that 9.6% reported 'losing control of bowel motions between visits to the toilet at some time since the birth'. At 10 months postpartum, another study found that 4% had experienced new and 2% recurrent symptoms of frank incontinence, soiling or urgency (described as 'felt the need to go but couldn't hold on') at some time since the birth (MacArthur *et al.*, 1997). This study also showed that less than 15% of the women who reported symptoms had consulted a doctor. Studies using recently developed techniques (endosonography and manometry) to image the anal sphincter muscles have also obtained data on symptoms of faecal and flatus incontinence and have found even higher prevalences (Sultan *et al.*, 1993). These populations, however, are smaller and include women who agree to have the anal investigative techniques, who are therefore likely to have higher symptom rates. Postpartum incontinence of flatus has been shown in all of the studies that have included this to be even more common than incontinence or urgency of faecal matter.

The various pathophysiological studies have shown that childbirth-associated structural damage to the anal sphincter is more likely to be a cause of faecal incontinence than neurological factors affecting the pelvic floor. Sultan *et al.* (1993) examined 202 women with anal endosonography at 34 weeks' gestation and again at 6–8 weeks postpartum. This showed no antenatal sphincter defects among the primiparous women who had a vaginal delivery, but at 6–8 weeks postpartum 35% had defects. Among multiparae, 40% had antenatal defects and 44% had defects at postnatal follow-up, indicating therefore that most anal sphincter damage occurs following a first delivery. Most of the women with this 'occult' sphincter damage do not have symptoms, with about a third experiencing any loss of bowel control (including flatus). Little is known about whether occult damage predisposes to symptoms later in life, although one small study has shown that women who had symptomless anal sphincter defects after a first birth were at higher risk of developing symptoms of faecal incontinence after a second delivery (Fynes *et al.*, 1999).

In addition to third-degree tear, the main risk factor for postpartum faecal incontinence, shown in both the epidemiological and the pathophysiological studies, is instrumental delivery (Assassa *et al.*, 2000; MacArthur *et al.*, 1997; MacArthur *et al.*, 2001; Sultan *et al.*, 1993). Caesarean section delivery is associated with lower symptom rates but faecal incontinence has been documented after emergency procedures. It would be plausible that after elective sections new faecal incontinence

should not occur but there are little data on this. First- or second-degree perineal laceration has not been shown to be associated with an increased risk of faecal incontinence, nor generally has episiotomy.

PERINEAL PROBLEMS

Most women who have a vaginal delivery will have, in the few days afterwards, some degree of perineal pain. It is probably one of the most commonly experienced immediate postpartum symptoms (Sleep, 1995) but it can also be more persistent. Some women experience dyspareunia, defined as pain or discomfort during sexual intercourse, which can be related to perineal problems.

Studies have shown that at least a third of women report experiencing a painful perineum soon after birth. In a study of alternative methods of conducting the second stage of labour, perineal pain was an outcome measure and at 10 days postpartum 33% of the women (no difference between trial arms) reported experiencing this in the previous 24 hours (McCandlish *et al.*, 1998). Glazener *et al.* (1995) found that 42% of the women reported a painful perineum occurring at some time whilst still in hospital. This same study found that between leaving hospital and 8 weeks postpartum, 22% of the women reported experiencing perineal pain, and between 8 weeks and 18 months it was reported by 10% of the sample. Another study found that 21% of women in the sample at 6–7 months postpartum reported that a painful perineum had been a problem for them some time since the birth (Brown and Lumley, 1998).

There is less information on the prevalence of dyspareunia or any other sexual problem, possibly because of the sensitivity of the subject and the reluctance of women to seek medical consultation, although there have been a few recent studies. Brown and Lumley (1998) found that 26% of the women at 6–7 months postpartum reported that they had experienced 'a sexual problem' at some time since the birth, although the types of problems were not specified. At 8 weeks postpartum, Glazener *et al.* (1995) showed that among the women who had attempted sexual intercourse, 28% had found this to be sore or difficult and 9% reported a lack of interest in sex. Between 2 and 18 months, 20% reported sore or difficult intercourse and the proportion reporting a lack of interest in sex had risen to 21%. A recent postal questionnaire study of a range of sexual health problems among almost 800 women 6 months after their first birth, found that 62% recalled experiencing dyspareunia (described as painful penetration and/or pain during intercourse or orgasm) some time in the first 3 months and 31% still had this at 6 months (Barrett *et al.*, 2000). Loss of sexual desire was experienced by 53% of the women in the first 3 months and by 37% at 6 months. Vaginal tightness, looseness, lack of muscle tone and lack of vaginal lubrication was still experienced by at least 20% of the sample. The women were also asked to recall whether they had experienced the same set of sexual health problems in the year before pregnancy and, although this was subject to greater response bias, all of the problems had increased significantly in the first 3 postpartum months and at 6 months were still substantially more common. 32% of the women in the sample recalled that they had resumed sexual intercourse by 6 weeks, 62% by 8 weeks and 81% by 3 months. In the study by Glazener (1997), which included multiparae as well as primiparae, 75% reported having resumed intercourse by the time they responded to their 8-week questionnaire.

The main risk factors of perineal pain and dyspareunia relate to the type of delivery and perineal trauma. Instrumental deliveries are associated with much higher rates of perineal pain, both immediate and longer term, than spontaneous vaginal deliveries, and caesarean sections are associated with the lowest rates (Brown and Lumley, 1998; Glazener *et al.*, 1995). The pattern of association with mode of delivery is similar for dyspareunia, although the differences are less marked (Barrett *et al.*, 2000; Brown and Lumley, 1998).

Perineal trauma is also an important risk factor and is also closely associated with mode of delivery. There has been much discussion since the 1970s concerning the comparative effects of episiotomy compared with spontaneous laceration in relation to subsequent perineal problems. The original rationale for performing episiotomy was to avoid severe lacerations, thus protecting the perineal musculature and preventing subsequent perineal problems. Descriptions from women have suggested that there is more perineal discomfort following an episiotomy than there is after a laceration and several randomized controlled trials have been undertaken to examine this issue. The first of these to provide good evidence was a trial of a 'liberal' compared with a 'restrictive' episiotomy policy. This found that, although there were more intact perinea and more lacerations in the intervention group (restrictive policy), there were no differences in perineal pain experienced at 10 days or at 3 months postpartum; and there was no difference in dyspareunia at 3 months (Sleep *et al.*, 1984). A Cochrane systematic review (Carroli and Belizan, 2001), including six trials on this topic, has

concluded that there is little evidence to justify episiotomy as a means of limiting postpartum perineal pain. The effects on perineal pain and dyspareunia of different materials used for suturing the perineum and of different suture methods are described in Chapter 28.

BACKACHE

Backache is a commonly reported problem within the general population. Backache during pregnancy is even more common, occurring in around half of women and resulting from the hormonal effects of relaxed ligaments, altered posture and extra weight (Östgaard *et al.*, 1991). High rates of backache in the first few days after childbirth have also been reported (Grove, 1973). More recently, numerous studies have documented longer-term backache, with prevalences that still seem to be greater than that among the general population (Breen *et al.*, 1994; Brown and Lumley, 1998; Glazener *et al.*, 1995; MacArthur *et al.*, 1991; Russell *et al.*, 1993; Saurel-Cubizolles *et al.*, 2000).

The range of prevalence estimates of postpartum backache, however, is wide, from 20–50%, and affected by how and when symptom information was obtained. In the Birmingham study of health after childbirth, 14% complained of new backache starting within 3 months of the delivery and lasting for longer than 6 weeks, rising to 23% when women who had also had backache sometime previously were included. Two-thirds of these symptomatic women still had backache at the time of questioning, at least a year later (MacArthur *et al.*, 1991). A similar prevalence (24%) of backache occurring between hospital discharge and 8 weeks postpartum was found in the study by Glazener *et al.* (1995). Between then and 12–18 months 20% experienced backache at some time. A study of backache among all deliveries (*n* = 1042) over a defined period in a Boston hospital showed a prevalence of 44% at 1–2 months (Breen *et al.*, 1994). When followed up at 12–18 months, 49% reported experiencing backache at some time during the preceding 3 months (Groves *et al.*, 1994). The European study of health after birth found even higher rates of backache: 49% in France and 47% in Italy at 5 months and 50% and 65% respectively at 12 months, showing an increase over time in the Italian sample (Saurel-Cubizolles *et al.*, 2000). Russell *et al.* (1993), in a study examining postpartum backache and its risk factors in primiparous women found that 29% had backache that lasted for more than 6 months after delivery, and for 15% this was new backache starting since the birth.

Backache during or before pregnancy is a predisposing factor for postpartum back pain (Breen *et al.*, 1994; Östgaard and Andersson, 1992; Turgut *et al.*, 1998) and some studies have found physically heavy work during pregnancy to be a risk factor (Östgaard and Andersson, 1992). Epidural anaesthesia during labour has been found in some studies to be associated with subsequent longer-term backache (Brown and Lumley, 1998; MacArthur *et al.*, 1990; Russell *et al.*, 1993). Other studies examining this, however, have found no association (Breen *et al.*, 1994; Macarthur *et al.*, 1995). The postulated mechanism to account for a possible association relates to stressed positions, which commonly occur in labour, but are exacerbated by epidural block because of muscular relaxation, the abolition of pain inhibiting the desire to move as well as the inability to move unaided. A woman might remain without immediate discomfort for some time in a potentially damaging position. The observed association with backache, however, may be accounted for by some other factor, for example differences in the types of women who choose to have an epidural. In addition to any antenatal or intrapartum predisposing factor, the physical demands of child care, lifting, bending, carrying and feeding, especially as the child increases in size, are likely to be related to the occurrence of postpartum backache. No specific studies have examined this, but the longitudinal studies have not shown postpartum backache to reduce over time (Glazener *et al.*, 1995; Saurel-Cubizolles *et al.*, 2000), which is a more typical pattern in relation to several other postpartum symptoms.

HEADACHE

The occurrence of short-duration postpartum headaches, in at least a quarter of women, has been reported (Stein *et al.*, 1984) and longer-term headaches have also been documented (Glazener *et al.*, 1993; MacArthur *et al.*, 1991; Russell *et al.*, 1993). Most postpartum headaches are probably tension-type or 'simple' headaches, but the studies, which examined headache among postnatal women, have not generally specified headache type.

MacArthur *et al.* (1991) asked about frequent headaches and migraine (allowing women to define these for themselves), with 4% reporting frequent headaches and 1% migraine as new post-delivery symptoms lasting over 6 weeks; a further 5% and 6% respectively had

also had the same symptoms before. Russell *et al.* (1993) found similar proportions with headache (not specifically frequent headaches) but ones that occurred for more than 6 months after delivery: 4% reported new headaches, with a further 4% for recurrent ones. Glazener *et al.* (1993) found that 22% of the sample reported headaches (new or recurrent) between 1 and 8 weeks; and 15% some time between then and 18 months postpartum. In the European study, headaches increased over the postpartum period, being reported by 22% of Italian and 21% of the French women at 5 months, and 45% and 38% respectively, at 12 months. MacArthur *et al.* (1991, 1993a) found that frequent headaches, in association with backache, were more common in women who had epidural anaesthesia. Headaches without backache, however, were more common in younger, lower social class women with more than one child. Headache is a common complaint, generally related to stress and fatigue, and the additional responsibilities and activities associated with caring for babies and children are likely to be influential factors, irrespective of the childbirth process.

An accidental dural puncture which occurs during epidural insertion in 0.5% to 1% of cases (Stride and Cooper, 1993) often gives rise to a postural type of postdural puncture headache, arising from the loss of CSF and resulting traction on the meninges. The postural nature of this type of headache makes it quite specific. Postdural puncture headache can also occur, although infrequently (1%) after spinal anaesthesia (Hopkinson *et al.*, 1997). A postdural puncture headache is generally considered to be of short duration but there may be persistence of milder headaches (Jeskins *et al.*, 2001; MacArthur *et al.*, 1993a).

DEPRESSION

Depression following childbirth has been well documented in studies and is generally found to occur in about 10–15% of women (O'Hara and Swain, 1996; Romito, 1990). Most studies have been cross-sectional, assessing prevalence at one point in time. In addition to the time after birth that the depression is assessed, variation in prevalence occurs according to the method of assessment. Most studies have assessed depression using standardized psychiatric diagnostic criteria, while the investigations of general postpartum health have been of self-reported depression. The duration of postnatal depression is often relatively short, one longitudinal study showing that two-thirds of the cases lasted for

3 months or less (Cooper *et al.*, 1988), but for some women it is more persistent (Romito, 1990). Even short-lasting depression can be disabling with the demands of caring for a baby, yet many women do not consult health professionals. More recently, validated screening tools, in particular the Edinburgh Postnatal Depression Scale (EPDS) (Cox *et al.*, 1987), are increasingly being used (mainly by health visitors) in the UK to try to ensure that cases of depression are all identified.

The term postnatal depression is commonly used, but given the lack of any evidence of any hormonal association (Romito, 1990), and that the clinical features are the same as depression occurring at other times, whether or not it constitutes a specific entity has been questioned. One longitudinal study of 483 women who completed comprehensive psychiatric assessments antenatally and at 3, 6 and 12 months postpartum compared this with similarly measured psychiatric data from a general-population-based group of non-puerperal women. At 3 and 6 months postpartum the prevalence of depression was 8.7% and 8.8%, which was not significantly different from the 9.9% in the general population sample (Cooper *et al.*, 1988). Another study, however, with controls from the same population and matched with cases for age, marital status and number of children, found a threefold higher rate of depression among the postpartum women within 5 weeks of the birth. But by 6 months the rates in both groups were similar (Cox *et al.*, 1993). These authors concluded that the initial excess is most likely to be the result of the life-event of birth and the new family member, and that postnatal depression remains a useful term.

Risk factors for depression after birth have been extensively examined and associations found with a wide range of characteristics, although few have been consistent across studies (O'Hara and Swain, 1996; Romito, 1990). In general it is now accepted that intrapartum interventions, such as induced labour, operative delivery, or episiotomy, do not have a major effect in relation to an increased risk of depression. The main risk factors are a poor relationship with the partner, history of depression, low social support and socioeconomic deprivation (O'Hara and Swain, 1996; Romito, 1990).

There is accumulating evidence of the adverse effects of postpartum depression on the cognitive and emotional development of the child (Coghill *et al.*, 1986; Cooper and Murray, 1998). A study in Australia has demonstrated a relationship between maternal physical health and recovery, and depression (Brown and Lumley, 2000). It is important, therefore, that health professionals ensure that depression in postpartum women is identified and treated.

FATIGUE

Tiredness in the early postpartum period is well recognized anecdotally, not surprisingly owing to the demands of pregnancy, the delivery, and the additional childcare load and sleeplessness associated with night feeding. However, many women report longer-term exhaustion, which can have a significant effect on their relationships, their social activities and employment and their psychological health. Women rarely consult a doctor about this, possibly because they perceive it as normal at this time, or not a 'medical problem' (Bick and MacArthur, 1995). Glazener *et al.* (1993) found that 59% of the sample reported tiredness between hospital discharge and 8 weeks and 54% between then and 18 months. Brown and Lumley (1998) documented that at 6–7 months 69% of women had experienced tiredness/exhaustion as a problem for them some time since the birth. In an Audit Commission study (Garcia *et al.*, 1998), a representative sample of 2406 women throughout England and Wales at 4 months postpartum were asked to think back to 10 days, 1 month and 3 months; 43%, 31% and 21% said they had experienced fatigue or severe tiredness at these times. In the European study, prevalence of fatigue increased from 46% (France) and 48% (Italy) at 5 months, to 61% and 67% respectively at 12 months postpartum (Saurel-Cubizolles *et al.*, 2000). MacArthur *et al.* (1991) asked about extreme tiredness and found that 17% reported this lasting for more than 6 weeks, with 12% never having had such extreme tiredness before; half of these women said it had lasted for longer than a year.

Various risk factors of postpartum fatigue shown in studies include older maternal age, being unmarried, having twins and breastfeeding (MacArthur *et al.*, 1991; Milligan and Pugh, 1994; Saurel-Cubizolles *et al.*, 2000). No significant relationship has been shown between longer-term fatigue and type of delivery, although caesarean section has been associated with increased short-term fatigue (Glazener *et al.*, 1995; Milligan *et al.*, 1990). MacArthur *et al.* (1991) found that women who had a postpartum haemorrhage reported more tiredness, which could plausibly be related to a low haemoglobin level. Haemoglobin testing is not a routine postnatal practice. In the Grampian study, 7% of women reported anaemia at some time between 2 and 18 months after the birth (Glazener *et al.*, 1993). Paterson and colleagues

(1994), in a study of the effects of low haemoglobin levels in the first 6 weeks after birth, showed a link between low haemoglobin and fatigue. Fatigue is commonly reported in association with depression and anxiety (Glazener *et al.*, 1993; MacArthur *et al.*, 1991), although which problem arises first is not known. Brown and Lumley (2000) have found that tiredness was over three times more likely to be reported by women with high scores on the EPDS.

OTHER PROBLEMS

Pain and weakness in the arms and legs starting after birth and persisting for months or even years were reported four times as often among the Asian compared with the Caucasian women in the study by MacArthur *et al.*, (1991). This could plausibly be accounted for by vitamin D deficiency, commonly found among Asians resident in the UK (Brooke *et al.*, 1980), accentuated by the extra demands and postural stresses of pregnancy and delivery (MacArthur *et al.*, 1993b). Overall, the musculoskeletal system of the parturient woman seems to be more sensitive to various forms of injury, probably because of the laxity of ligaments resulting from the effects of relaxin. Positioning during labour and delivery might be important but this has not been studied.

Paraesthesias in the legs, buttocks and lower back have been reported in a self-selected sample as side-effects of epidural anaesthesia (Kitzinger, 1987). MacArthur *et al.* (1991, 1992) found, in the Birmingham study, that these paraesthesias, as well as those in the fingers and hands, although rare, were more common in women who had had epidural anaesthesia. Dizziness or fainting and visual disturbances, although again rare, were also more common after epidural anaesthesia and after spinal and general anaesthesia (MacArthur *et al.*, 1992). Except for a kind of sensory confusion reported by one or two women as long-term side-effects in a study of problems after epidural in a self-selected sample (Kitzinger, 1987), this relationship has not been documented elsewhere.

KEY POINTS

- Women can experience a range of health problems following childbirth.
- These comprise physical problems as well as psychological problems, including depression.

Reflective Activity 42.1

Use the information in this chapter to devise a symptom checklist to find out about symptoms that women may experience after childbirth.

Have a consultation with a woman in the first month after giving birth and use the checklist. Find out if she had reported any of her symptoms, if not why and how they might be affecting her life.

IMPLICATIONS FOR MIDWIVES

Health problems after childbirth continue well past the routine discharge from maternity services at 6–8 weeks. Many remain unreported to the health services. This has implications for midwives and other members of the primary care team in developing strategies to identify as well as provide for women's postpartum health needs. Community midwives presently have a statutory duty to attend a postpartum woman for a minimum of 10 days to a maximum of 28 days, the former being more common. An extension of the period, routinely to 28 days and with discharge at about 3 months, would allow a more full appraisal of women's health. Since women are often reluctant to initiate consultations about their own health, careful questioning from the midwife and other professionals is needed. Evidence on the nature of common health problems and on their management, including referral criteria is also required. There will be considerable variation in the health needs of individual women and care should be tailored flexibly to take this into account: women with fewer problems will require fewer visits whilst those with several problems may need more visits. A model of postnatal care was redesigned based on these considerations and a randomized controlled trial designed to evaluate it. This has shown a significant improvement in women's psychological well-being at 4 months postpartum, including a reduction in probable depression, in the group who received the redesigned care (MacArthur *et al.*, 2002).

- Some problems are associated with particular birth factors, some with postpartum, maternal or childcare characteristics.

- Many problems currently remain as unmet needs since women often do not report them and

midwives and other health professionals do not always identify them.

REFERENCES

Allen, R.E., Hosker, G.L., Smith, A.R.B. *et al.* (1990) Pelvic floor damage and childbirth: a neurophysiological study. *British Journal of Obstetrics and Gynaecology* 97: 770–779.

Assassa, R.P., Dallosso, S., Perry, C. *et al.* and the Leicestershire MRC Incontinence Study Team (2000) The association between obstetric factors and incontinence: a community survey. *British Journal of Obstetrics and Gynaecology* 107: 822.

Barrett, G., Pendry, E., Peacock, J. *et al.* (2000) Women's sexual health after childbirth. *British Journal of Obstetrics and Gynaecology* 107(2): 186–195.

Bick, D.E. & MacArthur, C. (1995) The extent, severity and effect of health problems after childbirth. *British Journal of Midwifery* 3(i): 27–31.

Breen, T.W., Ransil, J., Groves, P.A. *et al.* (1994) Factors associated with back pain after childbirth. *Anesthesiology* 81: 29–34.

Brooke, O.G., Brown, I.R.F., Bond, C.D.M. *et al.* (1980) Vitamin D supplementation in pregnant Asian women: effects on calcium status and fetal growth. *British Medical Journal* 280(6216): 751–754.

Brown, S. & Lumley, J. (1998) Maternal health after childbirth: results of an Australian population based survey. *British Journal of Obstetrics and Gynaecology* 105: 156–161.

Brown, S. & Lumley, J. (2000) Physical health problems after childbirth and maternal depression at six to seven months postpartum. *British Journal of Obstetrics and Gynaecology* 107: 1194–1201.

Carrolli, F. & Belizan, J. (2001). Episiotomy for vaginal birth (Cochrane Review). *The Cochrane Library*, Issue 4. Oxford: Update Software.

Coghill, S., Caplan, H., Alexandra, H. *et al.* (1986) Impact of maternal postnatal depression on cognitive development of young children. *British Medical Journal* 292: 1165–1167.

Cooper, P. & Murray, L. (1998) Postnatal depression. *British Medical Journal* 316: 1884–1886.

Cooper, P., Campbell, E., Day, A. *et al.* (1988) Non-psychotic disorder after childbirth: a prospective study of prevalence, incidence, course and nature. *British Journal of Psychiatry* 152(799): 806.

Corby, H., Donnelly, V.S., O'Herlihy, C. *et al.* (1997) Anal canal pressures are low in women with postpartum anal fissure. *British Journal of Surgery* 84(1): 86–88.

Cox, J.L., Holden, J.M. & Sagovsky, R. (1987) Detection of postnatal depression: Development of the 10-item Edinburgh Postnatal Depression Scale. *British Journal of Psychiatry* 150: 782–786.

Cox, J., Murray, D. & Chapman, G. (1993) A controlled study of the onset, duration and prevalence of postnatal depression. *British Journal of Psychiatry* 163: 27–31.

Fynes, M., Donnelly, V., Behan, M. *et al.* (1999). Effect of second vaginal delivery on anorectal physiology and faecal continence: a prospective study. *Lancet* 354: 983–986.

Garcia, J., Redshaw, M., Fitzsimons, B. *et al.* (1998) *First Class Delivery. A National Survey of Women's Views of Maternity Care.* Abingdon, Oxford: Audit Commission Publications.

Glazener, C.M.A. (1997) Sexual function after childbirth: women's experiences, persistent morbidity and lack of professional recognition. *British Journal of Obstetrics and Gynaecology* 104: 330–335.

Glazener, C.M.A., Abdalla, M., Russell, I. *et al.* (1993) Postnatal care: a survey of patients' experiences. *British Journal of Midwifery* 1: 67–74.

Glazener, C.M.A., Abdalla, M., Shroud, P. *et al.* (1995) Postnatal maternal morbidity: extent, causes, prevention and treatment. *British Journal of Obstetrics and Gynaecology* 102(4): 282–287.

Glazener, C.M.A., Herbison, G.P., Wilson, P.D. *et al.* (2001) Conservative management of persistent postnatal urinary and faecal incontinence: a randomised controlled trial. *British Medical Journal* 323: 593–596.

Grove, L.H. (1973) Backache, headache and bladder dysfunction after delivery. *British Journal of Anaesthesia* 45: 1147–1149.

Groves, P.A., Breen, T.W., Ransil, B.J. *et al.* (1994) Natural history of post partum back pain and its relationship with epidural anesthesia. *Anesthesiology* 81(3A): A1167.

Hopkinson, J.M., Samaan, A.K., Russell, I.F. *et al.* (1997) A comparative multicentre trial of spinal needles for caesarean section. *Anaesthesia* 52(10): 1005–1011.

Jeskins, G.D., Cooper, C.M. & Lewis, M. (2001) Long-term morbidity following dural puncture in an obstetric population. *International Journal of Obstetric Anaesthesia* 10: 17–24.

Kitzinger, S. (1987) *Some Women's Experiences of Epidurals. A Descriptive Study.* London: National Childbirth Trust.

McCandlish, R., Bowler, U. & van Asten, H. (1998) A randomised controlled trial of care of the perineum during second stage of normal labour. *British Journal of Obstetrics and Gynaecology* 105(2): 1262–1272.

MacArthur, A.J., MacArthur, C. & Weeks, S. (1995) Epidural anaesthesia and low back pain after delivery: a prospective cohort study. *British Medical Journal* **311**: 1336–1339.

MacArthur, C., Lewis, M., Knox, E.G. *et al.* (1990) Epidural anaesthesia and long-term backache following childbirth. *British Medical Journal* **301**: 9–12.

MacArthur, C., Lewis, M. & Knox, E.G. (1991) *Health After Childbirth*. London: HMSO.

MacArthur, C., Lewis, M. & Knox, E.G. (1992) Investigation of long-term problems after obstetric epidural anaesthesia. *British Medical Journal* **304**: 1279–1282.

MacArthur, C., Lewis, M. & Knox, E.G. (1993a) Accidental dural puncture in obstetric patients and long-term symptoms. *British Medical Journal* **306**: 883–885.

MacArthur, C., Lewis, M. & Knox, E.G. (1993b) Comparison of long-term health problems following childbirth in Asian and Caucasian women. *British Journal of General Practice* **43**: 519–522.

MacArthur, C., Lewis, M. & Bick, D. (1993c) Stress incontinence after childbirth: predictors, persistence, impact and medical consultation. *British Journal of Midwifery* **1**(5): 207–215.

MacArthur, C., Bick, D.E. & Keighley, M.R.B. (1997) Faecal incontinence after child birth. *British Journal of Obstetrics and Gynaecology* **104**: 46–50.

MacArthur, C., Glazener, C.M.A., Wilson, P.D. *et al.* (2001) Obstetric practice and faecal incontinence three months after delivery. *British Journal of Obstetrics and Gynaecology* **108**: 678–683.

MacArthur, C., Winter, H.R., Bick, D. *et al.* (2002) *Redesigning Postnatal Care: A Randomised Controlled Trial of Protocol-based Midwifery-led Care Focussed on Individual Women's Physical and Psychological Health Needs.* Health Technology Assessment. Online. Available: http://www.ncchta.org.

Milligan, R.A. & Pugh, L.C. (1994) Fatigue during the childbearing period. *Annual Review of Nursing Research* **12**: 33–49.

Milligan, R.A., Parks, P. & Lenz, E. (1990) An analysis of postpartum fatigue over the first three months of the postpartum period. In: Wang, J., Simoni, P. & Nath, C. (eds). *Vision of Excellence: The Decade of the Nineties.* Charleston WV: West Virginia Nurses' Association Research Conference Group.

Mørkved, S. & Bø, K. (1996) The effect of postnatal exercises to strengthen the pelvic floor muscles. *Acta Obstetricia et Gynecologica Scandinavica* **75**: 382–385.

O'Hara, M. & Swain, A. (1996) Rates and risk of postpartum depression – a meta-analysis. *International Review of Psychology* **8**: 37–54.

Östgaard, H.C. & Andersson, G.B.J. (1992) Postpartum low back pain. *Spine* **17**(1): 53–55.

Östgaard, H.C., Andersson, G.B.J. & Karlsson, K. (1991) Prevalence of back pain in pregnancy. *Spine* **16**: 549–552.

Paterson, J., Davis, J., Gregory, M. *et al.* (1994) A study of the effects of low haemoglobin on postnatal women. *Midwifery* **10**: 77–86.

Romito, P. (1990) Postpartum depression and the experience of motherhood. *Acta Obstetricia et Gynecologica Scandinavica* **69**(Suppl. 154): 7–19.

Russell, R., Grove, P., Taub, N. *et al.* (1993) Assessing long-term backache after childbirth. *British Medical Journal* **306**: 1299–1303.

Saultz, J.W., Toffler, W.L. & Shackles, J.Y. (1991) Postpartum urinary retention. *Journal of the American Board of Family Practitioners* **4**(5): 341–344.

Saurel-Cubizolles, M-J., Romito, P., Lelong, N. *et al.* (2000) Women's health after childbirth: a longitudinal study in France and Italy. *British Journal of Obstetrics and Gynaecology* **107**: 1202–1209.

Sleep, J. (1995) Postnatal perineal care revisited. In: Alexander, J., Levey, V. & Roch, S. (eds) *Aspects of Midwifery Practice. A Research Based Approach,* Ch. 7. London: Macmillan Press.

Sleep, J. & Grant, A. (1987a) West Berkshire perineal management trial: three year follow-up. *British Medical Journal* **295**: 749–751.

Sleep, J. & Grant, A. (1987b) Pelvic floor exercises in postnatal care. *Midwifery* **3**: 158–164.

Sleep, J., Grant, A., Garcia, J. *et al.* (1984) West Berkshire perineal management trial. *British Medical Journal* **298**: 587–590.

Smaill, F. & Hofmeyr, G.J. (2001) Antibiotic prophylaxis for caesarean section. *The Cochrane Library,* Issue 4. Oxford: Update Software.

Stein, G.S., Morton, J., Marsh, A. *et al.* (1984) Headaches after childbirth. *Acta Neurologica Scandinavica* **69**: 74–79.

Stray-Pederson, B., Blakstad, M. & Bergen, T. (1990) Bacteriuria in the puerperium: risk factors, screening procedures and treatment programs. *American Journal of Obstetrics and Gynecology* **162**: 792–797.

Stride, P.C. & Cooper, G.M. (1993) Dural taps revisited. *Anaesthesia* **48**: 247–255.

Sultan, A.H., Kamm, M.A., Hudson, C.N. *et al.* (1993) Anal sphincter disruption during vaginal delivery. *New England Journal of Medicine* **329**(26): 1905–1911.

Turgut, F., Turgut, M. & Cetinsahin, M. (1998) A prospective study of persistent back pain after pregnancy. *European Journal of Obstetrics and Gynecology and Reproductive Biology* **80**: 45–48.

Wilson, P.D., Herbison, R.M. & Herbison, G.P. (1996) Obstetric practice and the prevalence of urinary incontinence three months after delivery. *British Journal of Obstetrics and Gynaecology* **103**: 154–161.

Yarnell, J.W.G., Voyle, G.J., Sweetnam, P.M. *et al.* (1982) Factors associated with urinary incontinence in women. *Journal of Epidemiology and Community Health* **36**: 58–63.

FURTHER READING

Bick, D., MacArthur, C., Knowles, H. *et al.* (2002) Postnatal Care: Evidence and Guidelines for Management. London: Churchill Livingstone.
This book reviews the evidence on the occurrence and risk factors of postnatal health problems and the primary management of these by midwives. It is based on the guidelines that were developed for midwives in the study referred to at the end of this chapter.

Clement, S. (ed) (1998) *Psychological Perspectives on Pregnancy and Childbirth*. Edinburgh: Churchill Livingstone.
This book draws together a range of perspectives relating to the psychological side of pregnancy and childbirth.

Enkin, M., Keirse, M.J.N.C., Neilson, J. *et al.* (2000). *A Guide to Effective Care in Pregnancy and Childbirth,* 3rd edn. Oxford: Oxford University Press.
This book enables midwives to become familiar with and understand the importance of systematic reviews of literature to provide evidence of effectiveness of a wide range of maternity care practices.

MacArthur, C., Winter, H.R., Bick, D. *et al.* (2002) *Redesigning Postnatal Care: A Randomised Controlled Trial of Protocol-based Midwifery-led Care Focussed on Individual Women's Physical and Psychological Health Needs*. Health Technology Assessment.
This report describes a trial in which midwives in the intervention group gave flexible postnatal care tailored to individual needs, and the control group gave standard care. The main effects of the intervention care were a benefit to women's psychological health. Details of the content of the flexible care and how it was tailored to needs are also given. Copies are available from the National Coordinating Centre for Health Technology Assessment (email hta@soton.ac.uk) or can be printed off the web at http://www.ncchta.org.

PART 7

CONDITIONS AND COMPLICATIONS OF CHILDBIRTH

43. Nausea and Vomiting 751

44. Bleeding in Pregnancy 758

45. Hypertensive Disorders of Pregnancy 780

46. Medical Disorders of Pregnancy 793

47. Sexually Transmitted Diseases 815

48. Abnormalities of the Genital Tract 829

49. Multiple Pregnancy 839

50. Preterm Labour 853

51. Induction of Labour and Post-term Pregnancy 862

52. Disordered Uterine Action 876

53. Malpositions and Malpresentations 884

54. Mental Health Problems 918

PART 7

CONDITIONS AND COMPLICATIONS OF CHILDBIRTH

43

Nausea and Vomiting

Patricia Lindsay

LEARNING OUTCOMES

After reading this chapter you will be able to:

- define and differentiate between physiological and pathological vomiting in pregnancy
- plan and implement appropriate midwifery action

- discuss possible treatments, including self-help strategies
- discuss the possible consequences for mother and baby.

Nausea and vomiting is a common 'minor' disorder of pregnancy, affecting up to 90% of normal pregnancies. Vomiting occurs when one of two centres in the brain is stimulated: the emetic centre in the medulla or the chemoreceptor trigger zone, situated on the lateral wall of the fourth ventricle (Billet, 1992). It is often regarded as a normal occurrence and is considered a presumptive sign of pregnancy. Nausea associated with pregnancy may begin before the first period is missed.

It may have a positive effect in enhancing placental development: nausea and vomiting may suppress maternal tissue synthesis in early pregnancy by altering serum levels of insulin and insulin growth factor-1. This optimizes the available nutrients for the developing placenta (Achord, 1995; Huxley 2000).

The causes of nausea and vomiting in pregnancy are poorly understood. Explanations include the following, although the research evidence is equivocal (Tucker Blackburn, 2003; Boyce, 1992; Broussard and Richter, 1998; Hill and Fleming, 1999; Thorp *et al.*, 1991):

- *Rising levels of oestrogen, progesterone and human chorionic gonadotrophin* (hCG) which are thought to stimulate the chemoreceptor trigger zone. hCG levels have been found to be raised in women experiencing nausea and vomiting during pregnancy.
- *Physiological changes* of pregnancy such as reduced gastric motility, reflux oesophagitis.
- *Metabolic changes* such as carbohydrate deficiency, vitamin B deficiency, alteration in serum lipids and lipoproteins.

- *Position of the corpus luteum*: a corpus luteum situated in the right ovary may cause high concentrations of sex steroids in the hepatic portal system, leading to nausea and vomiting.
- *Psychological factors* such as dependent or histrionic personality, rejection of, or ambivalence about, the pregnancy, psychological conflict regarding gender role or maternal role (Lub-Moss and Eurelings-Bontekoe, 1997).

The condition is more common in young and primigravid women and strongly associated with multiple pregnancy, hydatidiform mole and severe pre-eclampsia.

The midwife should remember that vomiting may occur as a result of incidental conditions such as gastroenteritis, hiatus hernia, duodenal ulcer, appendicitis, pyelonephritis or cerebral lesions. Such conditions are more difficult to diagnose in pregnancy but other signs such as pain or pyrexia will be present.

Psychological disturbance should not be assumed to be a cause of vomiting in pregnancy unless pathological causes have been excluded and there are frank signs of psychoneurosis (Beischer *et al.*, 1997).

Tests for underlying pathology include blood tests, such as aspartate aminotransferase (AST), alanine aminotransferase (ALT), urea and electrolytes to assess renal and liver function. A midstream specimen of urine may be sent for culture if urinary tract infection is suspected. An ultrasound scan may also be useful to exclude hydatidiform mole and multiple pregnancy as causes. Early pregnancy nausea, accompanied by pain, is also suspicious of ectopic pregnancy (DoH, 1998). Abdominal X-ray should be avoided.

Vomiting in pregnancy is associated with a decreased risk of spontaneous abortion and seems to have no adverse effect on the length of gestation, birth weight or perinatal morbidity (Broussard and Richter, 1998; Huxley 2000).

MILD VOMITING IN PREGNANCY

Although unpleasant, this is a transient and self-limiting condition. It commonly appears in the fifth week of pregnancy although it may commence in the week of conception. Peak severity is around weeks 11–13, resolving by the 14th week. However, it can persist until the 22nd week and may recur in the third trimester (Lacroix et al., 2000). The woman often feels nauseated on waking, and vomiting occurs on rising from bed. The symptoms usually recede during the day, although nausea may be persistent. The sense of smell is heightened and some women develop aversions to substances such as tea, coffee, alcohol, fatty foods and tobacco. This may be a physiological defence mechanism designed to reduce exposure of the embryo to potential teratogens. On examination, the woman does not appear dehydrated and the urine does not contain ketones. The midwife can reassure her that the condition will improve in time.

Dietary modification may be helpful. Frequent small, light meals and savoury foods are generally well tolerated. Fatty, spicy or strong-smelling food should be avoided. A milky drink at bedtime and dry toast or a biscuit before rising often alleviate early-morning nausea; carbonated drinks such as soda or non-alcoholic dry ginger are useful if nausea persists during the day. *Medication* is not usually required. The woman should be advised to *rest* as much as possible, as tiredness and stress will exacerbate the vomiting.

Reflective Activity 43.1

Contact your local hospital dietician. What dietary modifications does he/she recommend to reduce nausea and vomiting in pregnancy?

Complementary remedies are sometimes used to treat morning sickness. Vitamin B_6 may be useful (Sahakian et al., 1991) but vitamin supplements should be used with caution as overdosage may cause fetal damage. Bananas, avocados, raisins, sunflower seeds and hazelnuts are all rich in vitamin B_6. Ginger is a recognized antiemetic (Fischer-Rasmussen et al., 1990; Langner et al., 1998) and may be taken as powdered ginger root capsules, crystallized stem ginger or in biscuits or drinks. The midwife should be aware that most remedies (complementary or standard pharmaceutical) have not been tested in pregnant women. Some studies have indicated possible antithrombotic and cytotoxic/cytostatic effects of ginger. Thus the potential effects of using ginger in pregnancy are unknown (Backon, 1991; Lee and Surh, 1998; Thatte et al., 2000).

Acupuncture and acupressure using the P6 point have been suggested to relieve vomiting in pregnancy and acupressure wristbands used to prevent motion sickness have been tried (Belluomini et al., 1994; Dundee et al., 1988; Hoo, 1997; Stannard, 1989). However, a clinical trial found no benefit for acupressure (O'Brien et al., 1996).

If medical hypnosis is used, a thorough assessment must be carried out first in order to exclude organic causes for the vomiting (Simon and Schwartz, 1999). Relief may also be obtained through the use of aromatherapy and homeopathic remedies (Tisserand, 1990). The midwife herself may not use any complementary therapy for her clients unless she is properly qualified in that field as some complementary medicines and techniques can be harmful in pregnancy (NMC, 2002). The midwife also has a duty to advise the woman if she believes that any remedy or treatment the woman is using may be harmful to the pregnancy.

Empathic support is an important part of the care of the woman with mild vomiting in pregnancy. Although not clinically ill, the woman often feels miserable and her symptoms should not be regarded as trivial.

MODERATE VOMITING IN PREGNANCY

This is more serious as the woman will be vomiting several times during the day, often after meals. The dietary advice described above may help but often the woman continues to vomit and will begin to show signs of dehydration. There may be some weight loss and ketones will appear in the urine. The woman will usually be feeling anxious about her condition and that of the fetus. The midwife should arrange for the woman to be admitted to hospital. Examinations to exclude any underlying pathology will be carried out.

Medication is used sparingly in pregnancy as many drugs are teratogenic. However, a meta-analysis indicates that antihistamines are safe to use in pregnancy and promethazine hydrochloride (Phenergan, Avomine) may be prescribed to control the vomiting (Seto *et al.*, 1997). The midwife should warn the woman that this drug may cause drowsiness.

Intravenous fluids may be required to correct dehydration and a careful record of fluid balance is kept. The vomiting usually ceases quickly and once the woman is tolerating a normal diet she may be discharged home.

HYPEREMESIS GRAVIDARUM

This is the pathological form of vomiting in pregnancy. It is a serious disorder which may lead to maternal death (DoH, 1996). The vomiting usually begins in the first 10 weeks of pregnancy and is continuous and severe. Ptyalism (excessive salivation) may accompany the symptoms. The woman rapidly shows signs of dehydration such as sunken eyes, loss of skin elasticity, parched mouth and lips, and oliguria. Urinalysis reveals marked ketosis. The woman loses weight and becomes hyponatraemic and hypochloraemic. Any woman with a past history of hyperemesis gravidarum or who has pre-existing liver disease is at an increased risk.

The precise cause is unknown but may be related to the following factors:

- *hormonal activity during pregnancy*
- *psychosocial stress* such as unwanted pregnancy
- *short inter-pregnancy interval*
- *female fetal sex*
- *thyroid activity in pregnancy*: women who are hyperemetic tend also to have significantly higher thyroxin concentrations (Askling *et al.*, 1999; Fantz *et al.*, 1999; James, 2000; Lao *et al.*, 1988)
- *Helicobacter pylori* infection, which may be a cause of intractable vomiting in pregnancy, occasionally complicated by haematemesis.

The diagnosis of *H. pylori* infection is made by serological screening for antibodies and urease (^{13}C urea) breath tests. *H. pylori*-specific IgG antibodies are transferred to the fetus during pregnancy and may afford protection against infection during infancy. The infection responds well to antibiotic therapy such as erythromycin or clarithromycin. Vomiting ceases after treatment and the pregnancy can be expected to proceed normally (Frigo *et al.*, 1998; Jacoby and Porter, 1999; Kocak *et al.*, 1999; Younis *et al.*, 1998).

Despite the severity of this condition there appear to be few adverse fetal effects (Walters, 1999), though there may be an increased risk of intrauterine growth restriction (Gross *et al.*, 1989). However, the woman's condition will deteriorate rapidly unless the disease is treated swiftly. Liver and renal damage may occur and the woman may become jaundiced. Coagulopathy secondary to vitamin K deficiency may develop and vitamin B_1 (thiamine) deficiency will cause neurological symptoms such as polyneuritis. Wernicke's encephalopathy is a rare but serious complication caused by severe thiamine deficiency. Signs include disturbance of consciousness and memory, abnormal eye movements, loss of vision, ataxia, polyneuropathy and temperature instability, particularly hypothermia. Urinary incontinence has been reported. If untreated, Wernicke's encephalopathy may lead to coma and death. The condition responds well to thiamine (Hillbom *et al.*, 1999; Robinson *et al.*, 1998; Sakakibara *et al.*, 1997; Tesfaye *et al.*, 1998).

Oesophageal tears (Mallory–Weiss syndrome) and *haematemesis* may occur in women with severe and persistent vomiting.

> ### Reflective Activity 43.2
>
> Locate and read your local policy for management of severe vomiting in pregnancy.

Care and management

The woman must be referred to an obstetrician and should be admitted to hospital at once. She should be nursed in a single room if possible to avoid undue disturbance. Nothing is given by mouth until the vomiting stops – ice may be given to suck.

A blood sample is taken to estimate urea and electrolyte levels and for liver function tests. The urine is tested for ketones, bile, protein and glucose. A midstream specimen of urine is sent for culture to exclude pyelonephritis. An intravenous infusion is commenced at once to correct the dehydration, using normal saline or Ringer's lactate (Hartmann's) solution, with added potassium if required, to restore the electrolyte balance. Fluids containing dextrose should *not* be used until thiamine replacement has been given (Goodwin, 1998).

Slow-drip enteral feeding and total parenteral nutrition (TPN) have been used in the management of hyperemesis gravidarum (Boyce, 1992; Levine and Esser, 1988; Russo-Stieglitz *et al.*, 1999). Both methods carry risks: persistent vomiting during enteral feeding may cause aspiration pneumonia if vomit is inhaled; TPN used for the management of hyperemesis gravidarum has been associated with cardiac tamponade and maternal and fetal death (Greenspoon *et al.*, 1989).

If parenteral nutritional supplementation is used, the woman must be given thiamine 100 mg daily. Failure to do so may cause an acute depletion of residual thiamine stores, which can precipitate fits (Rees *et al.*, 1997).

An antiemetic drug such as prochlorperazine (Stemetil) or metaclopramide (Maxolon, Primperan) may be effective. Vitamin B injections may also be prescribed. Diazepam has been used in conjunction with parenteral fluids with good results and no apparent adverse effects (Ditto *et al.*, 1999).

Methylprednisolone may be used to treat hyperemesis gravidarum. The drug is given orally as a rapidly tapering course. As prednisolone is largely converted to inactive prednisone within the placenta, there is relatively little fetal transfer of the active compound. It is therefore considered safe for use as a short course during pregnancy (Safari *et al.*, 1998). Most women with hyperemesis gravidarum will experience relief within 2–3 days and the vomiting is less likely to recur than when conventional antiemetics are used.

The midwife should make frequent records of the woman's temperature, pulse, blood pressure and urinalysis. An accurate record of fluid balance is essential. The woman's care will also include attention to personal and oral hygiene. An obstetrician should be called at once if the woman exhibits neurological symptoms such as disorientation, drowsiness, abnormal eye movements or ataxia.

Termination of the pregnancy is only considered if the vomiting is intractable and signs of major organ failure appear, such as persistent pyrexia or hypothermia, persistent tachycardia, jaundice, persistent proteinuria, polyneuritis or encephalopathy.

Once the vomiting ceases, oral fluids and food may be gradually reintroduced. The midwife should provide psychological support for the woman as this condition affects her self-image and also her confidence in her body's ability to bear a child. The partner also needs support as he will be very anxious. The woman may be discharged when she is taking a normal diet and gaining weight. The midwife should be aware that this condition may reappear later in pregnancy. There is a 50% risk of recurrence in future pregnancies (Walters, 1999).

> ### Reflective Activity 43.3
>
> Contact your local hospital pharmacy and find out about total parenteral nutrition. What are the constituents, and how is it made, stored and administered? What special precautions must be taken during administration?

EATING DISORDERS AND VOMITING IN PREGNANCY

Reproductive function is often disturbed in women with eating disorders and consequently pregnancy is relatively uncommon. Amenorrhoea, nausea, vomiting, dizziness and abdominal bloating are often features of conditions such as anorexia nervosa but they are also common early symptoms of pregnancy. A pregnancy may therefore go undetected for some time. Healthcare professionals should consider the possibility of pregnancy if the woman is sexually active; early diagnosis is essential. There is an association between eating disorders and small-for-gestational-age infants. Hyperemesis gravidarum may develop and the eating disorder may worsen during the pregnancy (Bonne *et al.*, 1996; Conti *et al.*, 1998; Lingam and McCluskey, 1996).

Anorexia nervosa

The impaired gonadal function induced by starvation results in amenorrhoea in many cases, and spontaneous pregnancy is therefore unusual. However, fertility treatment has been offered to anorexic women with some success.

Clothing is often baggy to obscure body size and the woman may be evasive about dietary habits. A careful and sensitive history should be taken. A history of subfertility or previous small-for-dates (growth-restricted) babies may indicate problems. The midwife should explain the risks of undernutrition in pregnancy. The woman may be torn between the need to control her size and concern about the impact of poor nutrition on the baby. Eating patterns may improve in pregnancy but weight gain is usually poor. Preterm labour and fetal growth restriction are common.

The course of the pregnancy should be closely monitored by the midwife and obstetrician. This should include assessment of fetal growth and well-being as well as monitoring maternal physical and psychological health. Induction of labour may be necessary if the fetal growth and health are poor.

The health visitor must be informed, as the infant's growth and development may be poor if the maternal eating disorder persists (Treasure and Szmukler, 1995).

Bulimia nervosa

Fertility is not usually impaired with this type of eating disorder, so pregnancy is not uncommon. Fears for the health of the child lead most sufferers to control their symptoms in pregnancy. Weight gain, birth weight and gestation span are therefore usually within normal limits; however, there is a higher than usual miscarriage rate. The secretive nature of the disorder may make it difficult to detect and many women with bulimia may progress through pregnancy without arousing suspicion in the midwife. The eating disorder may recur after the birth and parenting difficulties are not uncommon (Treasure and Szmukler, 1995). Again, the health visitor should be made aware if the midwife suspects that the woman has bulimia.

CONCLUSION

Nausea and vomiting are common in pregnancy. However, the more serious consequences of hyperemesis gravidarum are fortunately rare and some cases may be avoidable if the vomiting is treated promptly and effectively. The midwife should invest time in initial assessment and identification of women who may be at risk, and ensure that support and information is available to them. She should be able to differentiate between normal and pathological vomiting and refer and manage the care accordingly.

Reflective Activity 43.4

Talk to women about their experiences of nausea and vomiting in pregnancy, especially their knowledge and beliefs about its causes, duration and treatment.

KEY POINTS

- Nausea and vomiting are common occurrences in pregnancy, but may, on rare occasions, become pathological.
- Informed and appropriate midwifery care and advice can make the discomfort more tolerable for the woman.
- The midwife must be able to distinguish between physiological and pathological pregnancy vomiting and take appropriate action.
- The woman can be reassured that her baby is unlikely to come to any harm due to the vomiting or the medication which may be used to control it.

REFERENCES

Achord, J. (1995) Nausea and vomiting. In: Hanbrich, W., Shaffner, F. & Berk, J. (eds) *Bockus Gastroenterology*, 5th edn, Vol. 1. London: W.B. Saunders.

Askling, J., Erlandsson, G., Kaijser, M. *et al.* (1999) Sickness in pregnancy and sex of child. *Lancet* 354(9195): 2053.

Backon, J. (1991) Ginger in preventing nausea and vomiting of pregnancy due to its thromboxane synthetase activity and effect on testosterone binding. *European Journal of Obstetrics and Gynecology and Reproductive Biology* 42(2): 163.

Beischer, A., Mackay, E. & Colditz, P. (1997) *Obstetrics and the Newborn*, 3rd edn. London: W.B. Saunders.

Belluomini, J., Litt, R., Lee, K. *et al.* (1994) Acupressure for nausea and vomiting of pregnancy: a randomised, blinded study. *Obstetrics and Gynecology* 84(2): 245–248.

Billet, J. (1992) A closer look at pregnancy sickness. *Professional Care of Mother and Child* Nov–Dec: 310–311.

Bonne, O., Rubinoff, B. & Berry, E. (1996) Delayed detection of pregnancy in patients with anorexia

nervosa: two case reports. *International Journal of Eating Disorders* 20(4): 423–425.

Boyce, R. (1992) Enteral nutrition in hyperemesis gravidarum: a new development. *Journal of the American Dietetic Association* 92(6): 733–736.

Broussard, C. & Richter, J. (1998) Nausea and vomiting of pregnancy. *Gastroenterology Clinics of North America* 27(1): 123–151.

Conti, J., Abraham, S. & Taylor, A. (1998) Eating behavior and pregnancy outcome. *Journal of Psychosomatic Research* 44(3–4): 465–477.

Department of Health (DoH) (1996) *Report on Confidential Enquiries into Maternal Deaths in the United Kingdom, 1991–1993.* HMSO, London.

Department of Health (DoH) (1998) *Why Mothers Die: Report on Confidential Enquiries into Maternal Deaths in the United Kingdom, 1994–1996.* The Stationery Office, London.

Ditto, A., Morgante, G., la Marca, A. *et al.* (1999) Evaluation of treatment of hyperemesis gravidarum using parenteral fluid with or without diazepam: a randomized study. *Gynecologic and Obstetric Investigations* 48(4): 232–236.

Dundee, J., Sourial, F., Ghaly, R. et al. (1988) P6 acupressure reduces morning sickness. *Journal of the Royal Society of Medicine* 81(8): 456–457.

Fantz, C., Dagogo-Jack, S., Ladenson, J. et al. (1999) Thyroid function in pregnancy. *Clinical Chemistry* 45(12): 2250–2258.

Fischer-Rasmussen, W., Kjaer, S., Dahl, C. et al. (1990) Ginger treatment of hyperemesis gravidarum. *European Journal of Obstetrics and Gynecology and Reproductive Biology* 38(1): 19–24.

Frigo, P., Lang, C., Reisenberger, K. et al. (1998) Hyperemesis gravidarum associated with *Helicobacter pylori* seropositivity. *Obstetrics and Gynecology* 91(4): 615–617.

Goodwin, T. (1998) Hyperemesis gravidarum. *Clinical Obstetrics and Gynecology* 41(3): 597–605.

Greenspoon, J., Masak, D. & Kurz, C. (1989) Cardiac tamponade in pregnancy during central hyperalimentation. *Obstetrics and Gynecology* 73 (3 Pt 2): 465–466.

Gross, S., Librach, C. & Cerutti, A. (1989) Maternal weight loss associated with hyperemesis gravidarum: a predictor of fetal outcome. *American Journal of Obstetrics and Gynecology* 160(4): 906–909.

Hill, W. & Fleming, A. (1999) Gastrointestinal disease complicating pregnancy. In: Reece, E. & Hobbins, J. (eds) *Medicine of the Fetus and Mother*. Philadelphia: Lippincott-Raven.

Hillbom, M., Pyhtinen, J., Pylvanen, V. et al. (1999) Pregnant, vomiting and coma. *Lancet* 353(9164): 1584.

Hoo, J.J. (1997) Acupressure for hyperemesis gravidarum. *American Journal of Obstetrics and Gynecology* 176(6): 1395–1397.

Huxley, R. (2000) Nausea and vomiting in early pregnancy: its role in placental development. *Obstetrics and Gynecology* 95(5): 779–782.

Jacoby, E. & Porter, K. (1999) *Helicobacter pylori* infection and persistent hyperemesis gravidarum. *American Journal of Perinatology* 16(2): 85–88.

James, W.H. (2000) Hyperemesis gravidarum and sex of child. *Lancet* 355(9201): 407.

Kocak, I., Akcan, Y., Ustun, C. et al. (1999) *Helicobacter pylori* seropositivity in patients with hyperemesis gravidarum. *International Journal of Gynecology and Obstetrics* 66(3): 251–254.

Lacroix, R., Eason, E. & Melzack, R. (2000) Nausea and vomiting during pregnancy: a prospective study of its frequency, intensity and patterns of change. *American Journal of Obstetrics and Gynecology* 182(4): 931–937.

Langner, E., Greifenberg, S. & Gruenwald, J. (1998) Ginger: history and use. *Advances in Natural Therapy* 15(1): 25–44.

Lao, T., Chin, R., Mak, Y. et al. (1988) Plasma zinc concentration and thyroid function in hyperemetic pregnancies. *Acta Obstetricia et Gynecologica Scandinavica* 67(7): 599–604.

Lee, E. & Surh, Y. (1998) Induction of apoptosis in HL-60 cells by pungent vanilloids (6)-gingerol and (6)-paradol. *Cancer Letters* 134(2): 163–168.

Levine, M. & Esser, D. (1988) Total parenteral nutrition for the treatment of severe hyperemesis gravidarum: maternal nutritional effects and fetal outcome. *Obstetrics and Gynecology* 72(1): 102–107.

Lingam, R. & McCluskey, S. (1996) Eating disorders associated with hyperemesis gravidarum. *Journal of Psychosomatic Research* 40(3): 231–234.

Lub-Moss, M.M. & Eurelings-Bontekoe, E.H. (1997) Clinical experience with patients suffering from hyperemesis gravidarum (severe nausea and vomiting during pregnancy): thoughts about subtyping of patients, treatment and counselling models. *Patient Education and Counselling* 31(1): 65–75.

Nursing and Midwifery Council (NMC) (2002) *Guidelines for the Administration of Medicines*. London: NMC.

O'Brien, B., Relyea, M.J. & Taerum, T. (1996) Efficacy of P6 acupressure in the treatment of nausea and vomiting during pregnancy. *American Journal of Obstetrics and Gynecology* 174(2): 708–715.

Rees, J., Ginsberg, L. & Schapira, A. (1997) Two pregnant women with vomiting and fits. *American Journal of Obstetrics and Gynecology* 177(6): 1539–1540.

Robinson, J., Banerjee, R. & Thiet, M-P. (1998) Coagulopathy secondary to vitamin K deficiency in hyperemesis gravidarum. *Obstetrics and Gynecology* 92(4 Pt 2): 673–675.

Russo-Stieglitz, K.E., Levine, A.B., Wagner, B.A. et al. (1999) Pregnancy outcome in patients requiring parenteral nutrition. *Journal of Maternal–Fetal Medicine* 8(4): 164–167.

Safari, H., Fassett, M., Souter, I. et al. (1998) The efficacy of methylprednisolone in the treatment of hyperemesis gravidarum: a randomised controlled study. *American Journal of Obstetrics and Gynecology* 179(4): 921–924.

Sahakian, V., Rouse, D. & Sipes, S. (1991) Vitamin B6 is effective therapy for nausea and vomiting of pregnancy: a randomised, double-blind, placebo-controlled trial. *Obstetrics and Gynecology* 78(1): 33–36.

Sakakibara, R., Hattori, T., Yasuda, K. et al. (1997) Micturitional disturbance in Wernicke's encephalopathy. *Neurourology and Urodynamics* 16(2): 111–115.

Seto, A., Einarson, T. & Koren, G. (1997) Pregnancy outcome following first trimester exposure to antihistamines: meta-analysis. *American Journal of Perinatology* 14(3): 119–124.

Simon, E.P. & Schwartz, J. (1999) Medical hypnosis for hyperemesis gravidarum. *Birth* 26(4): 248–254.

Stannard, D. (1989) Pressure prevents nausea. *Nursing Times* 85(4): 33–34.

Tesfaye, S., Achari, V., Yang, Y. et al. (1998) Pregnant, vomiting and going blind. *Lancet* 352(9140): 1594.

Tisserand, M. (1990) *Aromatherapy for Women*. London: Thorson's.

Thatte, U., Bagadey, S. & Dahanukar, S. (2000) Modulation of programmed cell death by medicinal plants. *Cellular and Molecular Biology* **46**(1): 199–214.

Thorp, J., Watson, W., & Katz, V. (1991) Effect of corpus luteum positions on hyperemesis gravidarum, a case report. *Journal of Reproductive Medicine* **36**(10): 761–762.

Treasure, J. & Szmukler, G. (1995) Medical complications of chronic anorexia nervosa. In: Szmukler, G., Dare, C. & Treasure, J. (eds) *Handbook of Eating Disorders*. Chichester: John Wiley.

Tucker Blackburn, S. (2003) *Maternal, Fetal and Neonatal Physiology: a Clinical Perspective*, 2nd edn. London: W.B. Saunders.

Walters, B. (1999) Hepatic and gastrointestinal disease. In: James, D., Steer, P., Weiner, C. *et al.* (eds) *High Risk Pregnancy: Management Options*. London: W.B. Saunders.

Younis, E., Abulafia, O. & Scherer, D. (1998) Rapid marked response of severe hyperemesis gravidarum to oral erythromycin. *American Journal of Perinatology* **15**(9): 533–534.

FURTHER READING

Hill, W. & Fleming, A. (1999) Gastrointestinal disease complicating pregnancy. In: Reece, E. & Hobbins, J. (eds) *Medicine of the Fetus and Mother*. Philadelphia: Lippincott-Raven.
This book contains a useful and research-based overview of vomiting in pregnancy.

ADDITIONAL RESOURCES

http://www.sosmorningsickness.com/
Useful resource for women, families and professionals.

http://www.something-fishy.org/pregnancy.htm
Website centred on eating disorders.

http://www.anred.com/pg.html
Website on eating disorders, with information on the impact of pregnancy.

http://rainforest.parentsplace.com/dialog/get/newpregeating disorder1.html
This is a discussion board for women who have had eating disorders and are now pregnant or considering pregnancy.

44

Bleeding in Pregnancy

Patricia Lindsay

LEARNING OUTCOMES

After reading the chapter you will be able to:

- identify the causes of vaginal bleeding in pregnancy
- discuss the midwife's role in bleeding in pregnancy both before and after the 24th week

- describe the possible implications for the health and well-being of the mother and the fetus
- discuss therapeutic termination of a pregnancy.

INTRODUCTION

Vaginal bleeding during pregnancy is always considered to be abnormal, and should always be investigated. It may also be extremely frightening for the woman, and the midwife should manage care with sensitivity, ensuring that the woman is fully informed and involved in her own management. An important part of the management lies within the diagnosis of the cause, and in the accurate assessment and reporting of the woman's previous and present history. It is also important to recognize that medical definitions and terms such as 'abortion' will need to be explained, as this term may have a different meaning for women and their families.

Bleeding from the genital tract is usually considered in two groups, depending on whether it occurs before or after the 24th week of pregnancy (Barron, 1995).

BLEEDING BEFORE THE 24TH WEEK OF PREGNANCY

Bleeding from the genital tract in early pregnancy, that is before the 24th week, may be caused by:

- implantation bleeding
- abortion
- hydatidiform mole
- ectopic pregnancy
- cervical lesions
- vaginitis.

IMPLANTATION BLEEDING

There may be a little bleeding when the trophoblast embeds into the endometrial lining of the uterus. The bleeding is usually bright red and of short duration. As implantation takes place 8–12 days after fertilization, the bleeding usually occurs just before the menstrual period is due. If mistakenly thought to be a menstrual period, this may confuse the expected date of delivery. A careful menstrual history is therefore essential to detect probable implantation bleeding, thereby avoiding miscalculation of dates.

ABORTION

A pregnancy which ends before 24 completed weeks of gestation, and where the fetus is not alive, is termed an abortion. The classification is shown in Figure 44.1.

Spontaneous abortion

15–20% of confirmed pregnancies end in spontaneous abortion, most of these occurring before the 12th week of pregnancy. The true rate of pregnancy loss is much higher as it is not known how many unrecognized pregnancies are lost (Chamberlain, 1995; Rosevear, 1999). Midwives should be aware that the term 'abortion' may cause confusion. Many women who have lost a wanted pregnancy find the word offensive and it

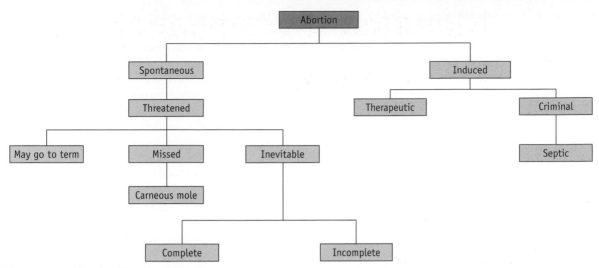

Figure 44.1 The classification of abortion.

should therefore not be used when talking to women about a pregnancy which has ended from natural causes. In these circumstances the use of the word 'miscarriage' is more appropriate.

Causes

- *Maldevelopment of the conceptus.* The most common cause of spontaneous abortion is a defective conceptus. Chromosomal abnormalities account for approximately 70% of defective conceptions, although spontaneous mutations may arise (Beischer *et al.*, 1997; Chamberlain, 1995).
- *Defective implantation* (Beischer *et al.*, 1997).
- *Hydatidiform mole* (Chamberlain, 1995).
- *Maternal infection.* Any acute illness, particularly with a high temperature, may cause abortion. This may be due to the general metabolic effect of a high fever or the result of transplacental passage of viruses. Infections known to be associated include influenza, rubella, pneumonia, toxoplasmosis, cytomegalovirus, listeriosis, syphilis and brucellosis. Appendicitis in pregnancy may also be a cause (Silver and Branch, 1999).
- *Genital tract infection* such as bacterial vaginosis and vaginal mycoplasma infection (Donders *et al.*, 2000; Silver and Branch, 1999).
- *Medical disorders.* These include diabetes, thyroid disease, renal disease and hypertensive disorders (Chamberlain, 1995).
- *Endocrine abnormalities.* These include poor development of the corpus luteum, inadequate secretory endometrium and low serum progesterone levels (Beischer *et al.*, 1997).

- *Uterine abnormalities.* The majority of the female genital tract arises from the two müllerian ducts, which form during embryonic life. Failure of development may cause structural abnormalities such as double uterus, unicornuate, bicornuate, septate or subseptate uterus. Such structural uterine abnormalities are implicated in approximately 15% of early pregnancy losses. Sometimes the uterus fails to develop to the full adult size, remaining infantile. Pregnancy in such a uterus may also end in abortion (Chamberlain, 1995; Silver and Branch, 1999).
- *Fibroids* (Chamberlain, 1995).
- *Retroversion of the uterus.* This does not itself cause abortion. As the uterus enlarges it will usually rise into the abdomen. If it fails to do so, vaginal and abdominal manipulation to correct the retroversion may cause an abortion (Chamberlain, 1995).
- *Cervical weakness* ('incompetent' cervix). Laceration of the cervix or undue stretching of the internal cervical os, produced by a previous abortion or childbirth, may allow the membranes to bulge through the cervical canal and rupture. This condition is often a cause of repeated late pregnancy losses. Cervical cerclage (a nylon tape or suture inserted and tied around the cervix) at about the 14th week may prevent this. The tape must be removed before the onset of labour (Beischer *et al.*, 1997).
- *Environmental factors.* External influences may be a cause. These include environmental teratogens such as lead and radiation, and ingested teratogenic substances such as drugs (especially cocaine) and alcohol (Carr and Coustan, 1999; Silver and Branch, 1999).

- *Smoking.* Exposure to tobacco smoke has been linked with spontaneous abortion but research findings remain inconclusive (Carr and Coustan, 1999).
- *Maternal age.* Women in their late thirties and older have higher rates of pregnancy loss irrespective of obstetric history (Andersen *et al.*, 2000; Silver and Branch, 1999).
- *Stress and anxiety.* Severe emotional upset may cause abortion by disrupting hypothalamic and pituitary functions. However, other factors may be implicated, as women experiencing adverse life events often have higher rates of smoking and alcohol use (Boyles *et al.*, 2000).
- *Paternal causes.* Poor sperm quality may be a factor. The father may also be the source of chromosomal abnormalities, particularly in cases of recurrent abortion (Beischer *et al.*, 1997; Gopalkrishnan *et al.*, 2000).
- *Immunological.* Maternal lymphocytes with natural killer cell activity may affect trophoblast development, disrupting implantation and embryonic growth. Autoimmune diseases such as antiphospholipid syndrome may also cause abortion (Beischer *et al.*, 1997; Silver and Branch, 1999).

Despite detailed investigations no cause can be found in the majority of cases.

Threatened abortion

Slight bleeding may occur, usually during the first 3 months of pregnancy. This may be painless or associated with slight lower abdominal pain or backache, but there is no cervical dilatation.

No aperient or enema should be given and no vaginal examination should be made by the midwife as this may provoke uterine contractions.

There is no evidence that bedrest is effective in preserving an unstable pregnancy and it may put the woman at risk of deep vein thrombosis (Enkin *et al.*, 2000). The woman should be referred for medical attention straight away and may be admitted to hospital or (where available) seen as an outpatient in an early pregnancy unit. A pregnancy test is carried out and an ultrasound scan will be done to assess viability. Heavy or increasing bleeding is an ominous sign and may precede inevitable abortion.

Inevitable abortion

The key feature of inevitable abortion is cervical dilatation. As the name suggests, the outcome is unavoidable pregnancy loss. The bleeding is more severe than in a threatened abortion and the woman may collapse from blood loss. The gestation sac separates from the uterine wall and the uterus contracts to expel the conceptus. This uterine activity causes discomfort similar to that of labour contractions. Speculum examination would reveal a dilating cervix, possibly with products of conception protruding through it. The gestation sac may be expelled complete (*complete abortion*), or part, usually placental tissue, may be retained (*incomplete abortion*).

The midwife who is called by a woman with signs of inevitable abortion should attend at once. The woman's vital signs should be recorded and an estimate of blood loss made. If the fetus has been expelled and the woman is bleeding, an oxytocic drug such as Syntometrine can be given. Any products of conception passed should be saved for inspection. The midwife should contact a medical practitioner who may be the woman's GP or the obstetrician/gynaecologist, and the local hospital unit to arrange transfer into hospital. If the bleeding is severe or the woman is showing signs of shock, a paramedic team from the local ambulance service should be requested. They will resuscitate the woman and stabilize her condition, if necessary giving a blood transfusion. She can then be transferred to hospital. In hospital, *evacuation of retained products of conception* (ERPC) from the uterus may be carried out and a blood transfusion may be given if blood loss has been severe.

Medical management of inevitable or incomplete abortion is possible, using prostaglandin analogues such as *misoprostol* or *gemeprost*.

Once the uterus is empty, vulval hygiene is important for comfort and to reduce the likelihood of infection: the woman should be advised to change her sanitary towels frequently and keep the vulva clean, using a bidet or shower if possible. All women who have required surgical evacuation should be screened for chlamydial infection (RCOG, 2000a).

If the breasts begin to secrete, the woman should be advised to wear a well-fitting brassiere in order to minimize discomfort. *Cabergoline* 1 mg may be prescribed to suppress lactation. The use of *bromocriptine* should be avoided because of its possible association with hypertension, myocardial infarction and mental disorder when used in the puerperium (BMA and RPSGB, 2002). If the woman is rhesus negative, anti-D gammaglobulin 50–100 mg is given within 60 hours of abortion to prevent isoimmunization and potential rhesus problems in subsequent pregnancies. Women who are non-immune to rubella may be given rubella vaccination at this time and advised to avoid the risk of pregnancy for the next 3 months.

Missed abortion (delayed abortion, silent abortion)

This situation occasionally follows threatened abortion. Bleeding occurs between the gestation sac and the uterine wall and the embryo dies. Layers of blood clot are formed, later becoming organized. The uterus ceases to increase in size and as the presence of the retained fetus appears to inhibit menstruation the woman may think that her pregnancy is continuing, although other signs of pregnancy have disappeared. The bleeding from the vagina varies from nothing, to a trickle of brownish discharge. As the signs of pregnancy gradually disappear, some women become aware that all is not well.

The diagnosis is confirmed by ultrasound. The uterus would eventually expel the fetus spontaneously, but this may not occur for some time. Treatment is usually to evacuate the uterus, either surgically or with misoprostol, either alone or in combination with methotrexate (Autry *et al.*, 1999; Ayres-de-Campos *et al.*, 2000).

'Expectant' management is another approach which may be offered: the woman is given the option of returning home for a few days to await spontaneous expulsion of the fetus (Bradley and Hamilton-Fairley, 1998). Some women have found it distressing and disorienting when surgical evacuation rapidly follows the news that the pregnancy is no longer viable. Expectant management gives the woman more time to assimilate the bad news. However, this treatment option is not universally accepted: many women find the idea of going home with a dead fetus in utero very distressing and many who wish to await spontaneous expulsion will eventually require surgical evacuation of the uterus anyway (Jurkovic *et al.*, 1998). Women opting for expectant

management should have 24-hour access to telephone advice (RCOG, 2000a).

If the uterine size is less than that at 12–13 weeks' gestation, the uterus may be evacuated per vaginam with a suction curette. Alternatively, medical abortion may be induced with oral mifepristone 600 mg followed 36–48 hours later with a vaginal prostaglandin analogue. If the uterus is larger than at 13 weeks' gestation, a combination of vaginal prostaglandins and intravenous Syntocinon may be used to empty the uterus. If a well-formed dead fetus is retained in utero it will become flattened and mummified (*fetus papyraceous*; Fig. 44.2) rather than being reabsorbed, though this is more often associated with a multiple pregnancy.

Recurrent abortion

This is a term used when three or more consecutive spontaneous abortions have occurred. Careful investigation should be undertaken to find the cause. Occasionally the causative factors are different for each, with no clear single factor associated. However, some conditions may be implicated in recurrent pregnancy loss (Stirrat and Wardle, 1999):

- *Structural abnormality of the uterus*: these appear in up to 50% of women with recurrent abortion (e.g. bicornuate uterus).
- *Weak ('incompetent') cervix.*
- *Maternal systemic disease*: diabetes and antiphospholipid antibodies.
- *Genetic causes*: the incidence of chromosome disorders is approximately 50% in first trimester abortions. The majority are balanced translocations. In

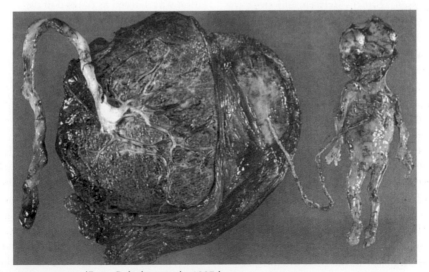

Figure 44.2   Fetus papyraceous. (From Beischer *et al.*, 1997.)

cases of consanguineous or cousin marriage a lethal recessive gene may cause recurrent losses.

- *Uterine infection*, especially toxoplasmosis, *Mycoplasma hominis*, *Ureaplasma urealyticum* and chlamydia.
- *Hormonal deficiency*: luteal phase deficits may be associated, although this theory is not universally accepted.
- *Immunological factors*.

Treatment varies according to the cause. Infections are treated with the appropriate antibiotic. A weak or incompetent cervix may be closed by insertion of a suture (cervical cerclage). The suture is normally removed just before term or earlier if labour commences. Prior to the next pregnancy both partners should attend for karyotyping, and ultrasound examination of the woman's pelvic cavity may be useful. The woman should be investigated for the presence of antiphospholipid antibodies. If these are the suspected cause, treatment with low-dose aspirin and heparin in pregnancy may be helpful (Rai *et al.*, 1997). The use of paternal alloimmunization for suspected immune factors remains controversial, although some studies have indicated that it may be effective (Ramhorst *et al.*, 2000; Scott, 2000).

Psychological effects

Many women experience a marked grief reaction following abortion and may require considerable counselling and support. Psychological distress may be severe and some women become clinically depressed. The grief experienced by the partner may be as intense as that of the woman though he is less likely to receive support (Conway and Russell, 2000). Staff should treat the parents with sensitivity. The couple may wish to see their baby, and staff should take account of their wishes. The guidelines written by the Stillbirth and Neonatal Death Society (Kohner, 1992 and 1995) are useful.

The midwife should remember that the legal age of fetal viability is 24 weeks as defined by the Stillbirth (Definition) Act 1992. After the end of the 24th week of pregnancy the infant must be registered as a stillbirth. Many maternity hospitals offer a funeral or memorial service for pre-viable fetuses and provide a decent burial, and all must offer respectful disposal. In this situation the hospital chaplain may be a valuable source of support and advice. The couple may wish to discuss future pregnancies with the doctor and in some cases may be referred for genetic counselling. The midwife may give the couple the address of the Miscarriage Association (see Additional resources), whose members provide support for those who have undergone a spontaneous abortion.

Reflective Activity 44.1

Talk to the manager of your early pregnancy unit. What are the referral criteria?

If there is no local early pregnancy unit, identify what services are available for women with early pregnancy problems and early fetal loss.

Induced abortion

This term refers to the deliberate termination of a pregnancy. Induced abortions are classified as therapeutic or criminal.

Therapeutic abortion

Therapeutic abortion has been legal in the UK since 1967 when the Abortion Act became law. This Act allows termination of a pregnancy if two registered medical practitioners are of the opinion that continuance of the pregnancy:

1. involves risk to the life of the pregnant woman
2. involves risk of injury to her physical or mental health
3. involves risk to any existing children of her family, greater than if the pregnancy were terminated; or
4. carries a substantial risk that if the child were born it would suffer from such physical or mental abnormalities as to be seriously handicapped.

On 1 April 1991 the Abortion Law was changed as a result of the Human Fertilisation and Embryology Act 1991, and the upper gestation limit for legal termination was defined as the end of the 24th week. The only circumstances in which therapeutic abortion may be carried out after the 24th week are:

1. if there is a risk to the woman's life
2. if there is a risk of grave permanent damage to the woman's physical or mental health; or
3. if there is a substantial risk that the child would be seriously handicapped.

The law also allows for selective fetal reduction in multifetal pregnancy, if continuance of the pregnancy with that number of fetuses would threaten the health or life of the woman, or if one or more of the fetuses were seriously abnormal.

A termination of pregnancy must be carried out in an approved institution and all terminations are notified to the Chief Medical Officer of the Department of Health. Staff are allowed to refuse to advocate or take part in abortions on moral or conscientious grounds.

Abortions after 24 weeks may only be carried out in NHS hospitals.

Pre-procedure tests should include blood sampling for haemoglobin concentration, blood group and rhesus factor and screening for blood-borne or genital tract infection if appropriate. Cervical cytology screening can be offered if required (RCOG, 2000b).

Adequate counselling should be available before a woman undergoes termination of pregnancy so that she is able to make an informed decision, without undue influence of medical opinion or pressure from relatives.

Methods of therapeutic abortion during the first trimester

Medical   Mifepristone (RU 486, Mifegyne) is a drug that blocks the action of progesterone. It is licensed for use in the termination of pregnancy up to 63 days' gestation and effects a complete abortion in 96% of cases. The woman must be under 35 years old and no more than a light smoker.

Oral mifepristone 600 mg is given in the presence of a doctor, and the woman should be observed for 2 hours. 36–48 hours later either gemeprost 1 mg or misoprostol 800 µg is given vaginally and her condition is observed for 6 hours. Abortion may be expected to occur within the next few hours. A follow-up visit should be arranged 8–12 days later to ensure that the products of conception have been completely expelled (BMA and RPSGB, 2002).

Surgical   Suction evacuation is carried out under local or general anaesthesia. Although generally a safe method, complications such as haemorrhage, infection, cervical damage and perforated uterus may still occur. The cervix may be 'primed' or made 'favourable' (softened) by the administration of vaginal prostaglandins 3 hours prior to surgical evacuation. The cervix is dilated and the uterus emptied by suctioning and curettage (Fig. 44.3). Suction evacuation should be avoided in pregnancies of less than 7 weeks' gestation (BMA and RPSGB, 2002; RCOG, 2000b).

Methods of therapeutic abortion during the second trimester

Medical:
- *Oral prostaglandins.* Mifepristone 200 mg or 600 mg is given orally, followed 36–48 hours later by prostaglandins such as gemeprost or misoprostol (BMA and RPSGB, 2002; RCOG, 2000c). Midwives should be aware that misoprostol is a drug licensed for the treatment of gastric or duodenal ulcers. It is also used in medical abortion or induction of labour in the UK.

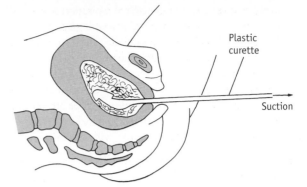

Figure 44.3   Dilatation and vacuum aspiration.

However, it has not yet been licensed for such use and therefore has not undergone the required testing for dose and safety necessary for registration (BMA and RPSGB, 2002; Enkin *et al.*, 2000).
- *Extra-amniotic prostaglandins.* A 16-French gauge self-retaining catheter is passed through the cervical canal into the extra-amniotic space and prostaglandin E_2 is instilled. Abortion can be expected to occur between 12–24 hours later. This method carries a risk of systemic inflammatory response, bacteraemia and infection (Ben-Arie *et al.*, 2000; Rouzi *et al.*, 1999).

Adequate analgesia is essential for women undergoing a second-trimester medical termination of pregnancy.

Surgical:
- *Dilatation and evacuation.* This method may be used in pregnancies of up to 18 weeks' gestation, if the operator is trained in the technique. The cervix is prepared with a prostaglandin pessary prior to the operation (RCOG, 2000c).
- *Hysterotomy.* This is an incision through the muscle wall of the uterus and removal of the fetus and placental tissue. It is rarely performed, as the scar that results is in the upper uterine segment and may rupture in a subsequent pregnancy.

Placental expulsion may be delayed when second trimester abortion is performed and the woman may require a manual removal of the placenta.

Selective fetal reduction   This technique is sometimes employed in higher-order multiple pregnancy in order to reduce the number of fetuses, usually to two. This decreases the risk to the surviving fetuses of preterm birth and impaired growth and reduces the risk to the woman's health. This may also be performed if one of the fetuses is found to be abnormal. It may be undertaken in the first or second trimester.

In the first trimester, transvaginal aspiration of embryonic tissue is performed under ultrasound guidance.

In the second trimester, a needle is inserted, under ultrasound guidance, through the abdominal wall and into the amniotic sac. The needle is then introduced into the fetal chest and a small dose of potassium chloride is injected. The needle is withdrawn after 30 seconds of fetal cardiac asystole. If the procedure is carried out in early pregnancy the tiny fetus will be reabsorbed; if later in pregnancy the fetus may become papyraceous and may be discovered among the membranes at delivery.

Local anaesthesia is used during the procedure for maternal comfort. However recent work has highlighted the possibility of fetal pain and therefore the need for systemic analgesia for fetal reasons. Fetal pain perception is poorly understood and this is a contentious area which urgently requires further research (Glover and Fisk, 1999).

Selective fetal reduction raises some difficult ethical issues and parents require careful counselling prior to the procedure and follow-up after it (Bergh *et al.*, 1999; Shalev *et al.*, 1999).

Follow-up care   After termination of pregnancy at any gestation, contraceptive advice must be given before the woman is discharged, as fertility returns very quickly and an unplanned pregnancy may result if the woman is unaware of this. Rhesus-negative women should receive anti-D gammaglobulin, and women with evidence of genital tract infection should receive antibiotic treatment.

The midwife should remember that termination of pregnancy may have profound psychological effects. Depression and feelings of guilt are not uncommon in the weeks that follow and may be reawakened in future pregnancies. The emotional pain may be particularly severe if the termination was for fetal abnormality, and staff should be sensitive and supportive. The midwife can provide parents with details of the organization ARC (Antenatal Results and Choices), which offers support for those undergoing this painful ordeal (see Additional resources).

Reflective Activity 44.2

Find out what services midwives offer locally to women who have had a spontaneous abortion or second trimester termination of pregnancy

---

Criminal abortion

This is the termination of a pregnancy outside the terms of the Abortion Act, possibly by unauthorized and untrained persons, and is an offence punishable by law. The incidence has fallen sharply since the introduction of the 1967 Abortion Act. However, cases still occur: four such offences were detected in the year 2000–2001 (Home Department, 2001). The abortion may be induced either by the woman herself or by some other person, by use of drugs or instruments. The illegal use of misoprostol preparations has been recorded (Jones and Fraser, 1998). Whether successful or not, the action is illegal. The methods used may cause sudden death from haemorrhage, air embolus or vagal inhibition. Because of lack of asepsis, infection readily occurs and may lead to chronic ill-health or salpingitis and sterility. Since the public are aware that midwives have extensive knowledge of pregnancy and its complications, the midwife's help may be sought if bleeding follows an attempt at criminal abortion. The woman should be immediately referred to a doctor. Any involvement in a case of criminal abortion may render the midwife liable to prosecution.

Septic abortion

Uterine infection may occur after spontaneous or induced abortion. It is more likely to occur following criminal abortion or spontaneous abortion where there are retained products of conception. The incidence of septic abortion has declined in countries which allow legal termination of pregnancy but it is still a cause of maternal death: five maternal deaths from sepsis following spontaneous abortion were recorded in the UK between 1997–1999 (Lewis, 2001). Causative organisms include *Staphylococcus aureus*, *Clostridium welchii*, *Escherichia coli*, group B haemolytic streptococci, *Klebsiella*, *Serratia* and *Bacteroides* species (Rosevear, 1999).

The woman will feel acutely ill with fever, tachycardia, headache, nausea and general malaise. On examination, signs of pregnancy such as breast changes may be evident. The uterus may be tender and the vaginal loss is offensive. The woman should be isolated. A high vaginal swab is sent for microscopy and blood cultures are taken. Antibiotics will be prescribed and are usually commenced before any surgical intervention is undertaken. They may be given intravenously if the woman is very ill.

When her condition allows, the woman is taken to theatre and the uterus is emptied. The midwife must be aware that severe infection may cause septicaemia and endotoxic shock. Other risks include disseminated intravascular coagulation, and liver and renal damage, and the midwife must make careful observations in order to detect signs of organ damage such as oliguria and jaundice. The damage caused by pelvic infection may result in adhesion formation, salpingitis and infertility.

GESTATIONAL TROPHOBLASTIC DISEASE (HYDATIDIFORM MOLE AND CHORIOCARCINOMA)

Hydatidiform mole

This condition occurs as a result of degeneration of the chorionic villi at an early stage of pregnancy (Fig. 44.4). Usually the embryo is absent; occasionally a hydatidiform mole may be found in a twin pregnancy alongside a viable fetus (Kauffman *et al.*, 1999). Molar pregnancy may be complete, with an intrauterine multivesicular mass composed of hydropic chorionic villi, or partial, where vesicular tissue is present, but less well developed, along with a fetus. Vesicle formation may occur within the placenta of an apparently normal pregnancy.

The incidence of complete hydatidiform mole in the UK is approximately 1 in 1000 pregnancies; partial moles occur in 1 in 3000 pregnancies (Seckl *et al.*, 2000).

Molar pregnancy is more common in:

- women under 20 or over 35 years old
- multiparous women
- women with a previous history of hydatidiform mole
- women in Japan, Asia, South-East Asia and Mexico (Beischer *et al.*, 1997; Rosevear, 1999).

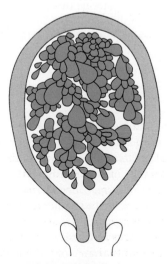

Figure 44.4 Hydatidiform mole.

The appearance of a hydatidiform mole has been likened to grapes or white currants. The villi become distended with fluid and may measure 1 cm in diameter. The outer layer of the villi is trophoblastic tissue and this may later become malignant if it is not completely removed. A complete mole shows degeneration of all villi. The karyotype is almost always 46XX but the chromosomes are of paternal origin. The ovum nucleus has been lost and the full complement (46XX) is achieved by duplication of the chromosomes of the X-bearing haploid sperm which penetrated the ovum. Occasionally an anucleate ovum is penetrated by two haploid sperm (X and Y) to give a chromosome complement of 46XY (Chamberlain, 1995). In partial moles the chromosome complement is triploid (69XXX, 69XXY or 69XYY). This occurs when a normal haploid ovum (23X) is fertilized by a two haploid sperm or one single diploid sperm (Blackburn, 2003; Rosevear, 1999).

Signs and symptoms

Often the minor disorders of pregnancy such as nausea and breast tenderness are more severe. The woman may complain of intermittent bleeding per vaginam from around the 12th week of pregnancy. When the mole begins to abort there may be profuse haemorrhage. Pre-eclampsia may develop even in the early weeks of pregnancy and severe nausea and vomiting may occur. On abdominal examination, the uterus is usually large for the period of gestation and may feel soft and doughy to the fingers. No fetal parts are palpable and the fetal heart is absent. There may be signs of mild thyrotoxicosis due to the thyroid-stimulating hormone (TSH)-like activity of human chorionic gonadotrophin which is secreted in large amounts by the molar vesicles. The diagnosis is suggested by the clinical findings and is confirmed by an ultrasound scan which will reveal no fetal parts but only a speckled or snowstorm appearance (Llewellyn Jones, 1999). Urinary or serum hCG levels are high.

The widespread introduction of early pregnancy dating scans has led to earlier detection of molar pregnancy. Partial moles are harder to recognize but a sonographic finding of cystic spaces within the placenta is suggestive (RCOG, 2000d).

Treatment

Once the diagnosis of molar pregnancy is confirmed, the uterus must be completely evacuated at once. This is achieved by careful suction curettage. Uterine contractions may cause molar tissue to enter the circulation via the sinuses of the placental bed. These emboli may set up metastatic disease in other sites, commonly the lungs. Medical termination should therefore be avoided. Unless the woman is haemorrhaging, oxytocic drugs are withheld until the uterus has been surgically emptied. A Syntocinon infusion may then be used to maintain uterine contraction and haemostasis. The woman should be registered at a specialist follow-up centre in London, Sheffield or Dundee (RCOG, 2000d).

After treatment for hydatidiform mole, careful observation is required as approximately 3% of these women will develop malignant trophoblastic disease (choriocarcinoma). Partial moles are less likely to become malignant but still require follow-up (Seckl *et al.*, 2000). Serum beta-hCG levels are monitored fortnightly until the values fall to within the normal range. Urine samples are then normally tested every 4 weeks until 1 year after evacuation. In the second year of follow-up urinary hCG testing is carried out every 3 months.

If any molar tissue remains in the uterus it will continue to grow and may invade the myometrium. Perforation of the uterine wall is then likely and this will cause major internal haemorrhage. Signs that the mole is continuing to grow are indicated by the persistence of high hCG levels 24 hours after uterine evacuation and high levels 1 month after treatment. If the serum or urinary hCG fails to return to normal levels within 6 months or begins to rise again, the woman is at risk of malignant trophoblastic disease.

The woman must avoid another pregnancy until she has been discharged from the follow-up programme. Use of the oral contraceptive pill increases the risk of the development of invasive disease and should therefore be avoided until hCG levels have been normal for 3 successive months (Rosevear, 1999). The midwife may need to advise the couple on barrier methods of contraception.

Choriocarcinoma

Choriocarcinoma is a malignant disease of trophoblastic tissue. It occurs following approximately 3% of complete moles (Seckl *et al.*, 2000). hCG levels will rise and the pregnancy test will become strongly positive again; bleeding occurs. Choriocarcinoma may occur in the next normal pregnancy following an evacuation of a mole.

As the growth infiltrates the uterus and vagina the pain increases. The condition will be rapidly fatal unless treated. The disease spreads by local invasion and via the bloodstream; metastases may occur in the lungs, liver and brain. Transplacental fetal metastases may occur during a pregnancy but this is very rare. Infantile choriocarcinoma may present with anaemia, endocrine

abnormalities and hepatosplenomegaly (Goldstein, 1999; Szavay *et al.*, 2000).

Choriocarcinoma responds extremely well to chemotherapy. Cytotoxic drugs such as methotrexate, etoposide and actinomycin-D are used singly or as combination therapy, and are nearly always completely successful. The woman should avoid another pregnancy for at least 1 year after the completion of treatment and will require hCG monitoring after any future pregnancy, as there is a risk of disease recurrence (Llewellyn Jones, 1999).

ECTOPIC OR EXTRAUTERINE GESTATION

Ectopic pregnancy occurs when the fertilized ovum implants outside the uterine cavity. In 95% of cases the site of implantation is the uterine tube and these are known as tubal pregnancies. Occasionally the site may be the ovary, the abdominal cavity or the cervical canal but these are rare. The incidence of ectopic pregnancy is 1:150 but is higher in some areas, e.g. in the West Indies where the incidence is 1:28 (Chamberlain, 1995). Ectopic pregnancy is the major cause of maternal death before 20 weeks' gestation in the industrialized world.

Tubal pregnancy

This is the commonest type of ectopic pregnancy and the incidence has increased two- to threefold in the last 30 years (Kadar, 1999). Tubal pregnancy occurs when there is a delay in the transport of the zygote along the fallopian tube. This may be due to a congenital malformation of the uterine tubes or more commonly to tubal scarring following pelvic infection. The ovum implants and begins to develop in the lining of the tube. The ampulla is the commonest site (Fig. 44.5).

Although tubal pregnancy may occur in the absence of any significant history there are certain risk factors (Kadar, 1999; Lemus, 2000):

- *History of previous tubal pregnancy.*
- *Tubal surgery.*
- *Hormonal ovulation induction* – drugs such as clomiphene may interfere with tubal motility.
- *Progesterone-releasing intrauterine contraceptive devices* (this is related to higher-dose devices).
- *Tubal endometriosis.*
- *Pelvic inflammatory disease.*
- *Appendicectomy, pelvic or abdominal surgery* which may cause adhesion formation.
- *Postcoital contraception using diethylstilboestrol.*

- *Contraceptive methods* – the intrauterine contraceptive device and the progesterone-only pill may increase the relative risk because they protect against intrauterine pregnancy but do not prevent ovulation and fertilization. This may make tubal pregnancy more likely in a woman who conceives while using these methods.
- *IVF pregnancy*.

Diagnosis

Diagnosis based on clinical signs alone may be difficult because the clinical picture may appear similar to pelvic inflammatory disease or threatened abortion. Delay in diagnosis and treatment may contribute to maternal mortality and morbidity. The most accurate method currently available is a combination of serum hCG levels and transvaginal ultrasound scanning. hCG levels rise steadily in early pregnancy. Levels lower than normal or falling below the doubling time (the time in which serum levels can be expected to double) are indicative of ectopic gestation (Tin-Chiu *et al.*, 1999). The ultrasound scan may reveal a tubal mass or a fluid collection in the pelvis but is most useful for confirming the *absence* of an intrauterine sac. As the conceptus develops and grows the tube distends to accommodate it.

Initially the woman will experience the usual signs of pregnancy such as nausea and breast changes, although amenorrhoea is not always present. The uterus will soften and enlarge under the influence of the pregnancy hormones. As the tube becomes further distended the woman will experience abdominal pain and some vaginal bleeding. The blood loss is uterine in origin and signifies endometrial degeneration. Gastrointestinal disturbance such as diarrhoea and pain on defecation are also common signs (DoH, 1998).

If the site of implantation is the narrower proximal end of the tube, tubal rupture is likely to occur between the 5th and 7th weeks of pregnancy (Fig. 44.6).

If the pregnancy is located in the wider ampullary section, the gestation may continue until the 10th week. Occasionally the gestation sac is expelled from the fimbriated end (Fig. 44.7).

As the ovum separates from its attachment to the ampullary part of the tube, layers of blood clot may be deposited around the dead ovum to form a mass of blood clot which may remain in the uterine tube or be expelled from the fimbriated end of the tube. When the tube ruptures there will be severe intraperitoneal haemorrhage and the woman will experience intense abdominal pain. There may also be referred shoulder tip pain on lying down as blood tracks up towards the diaphragm. The woman will appear pale, shocked and nauseated and may collapse. The abdomen is tender and may be distended. Pelvic examination is usually exquisitely tender, especially on movement of the cervix. Ruptured ectopic pregnancy is an acute surgical emergency and requires immediate treatment.

Management

If ectopic pregnancy is suspected, a large-bore intravenous cannula (size 14 gauge) should be inserted and blood taken for cross-matching. The woman must be transferred to theatre as soon as possible. Laparoscopic salpingotomy may be performed unless the woman is

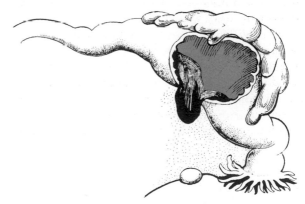

Figure 44.6 Rupture of the uterine tube.

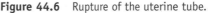

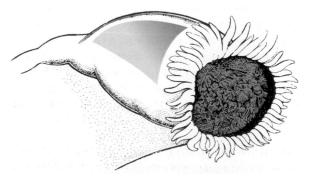

Figure 44.7 Tubal abortion.

Uterine end of tube

Tubal pregnancy

Ampullary end of tube

Ovarian ligament   Ovary

Figure 44.5 Tubal pregnancy.

suffering from haemorrhagic shock, when laparotomy is preferable.

If the condition is detected in the early stages, non-surgical management may be attempted with injections of prostaglandin $F_{2\alpha}$ or systemic prostaglandin E_2. Methotrexate may also be given, either intramuscularly or directly into the gestation sac (RCOG, 2000e; Rosevear, 1999).

Heterotopic or combined pregnancy

Heterotopic pregnancy occurs when a blastocyst from a multiple gestation implants outside the uterine cavity. It is associated with dizygotic twinning, and the extrauterine pregnancy is nearly always tubal. It may follow in vitro fertilization and embryo transfer. The incidence is thought to be approximately 1 : 15 000 and is likely to rise as the incidence of both multiple gestation and ectopic pregnancy rises. Diagnosis can be difficult and management options are limited by the presence of the intrauterine pregnancy. The ectopic sac must be removed but the uterus should be disturbed as little as possible and methotrexate must be avoided if the intrauterine pregnancy is to survive (Kadar, 1999).

Secondary abdominal pregnancy

Very rarely, when rupture of a tubal pregnancy occurs, there may be partial extrusion of the ovum into the peritoneal cavity, but with enough chorionic villi remaining attached to the tube to ensure that the embryo does not die. Chorionic villi on the surface of the ovum then become attached to the neighbouring abdominal organs and the pregnancy continues with the fetus developing free within the abdominal cavity. The fetus is at risk of severe growth restriction because of the relatively poor placentation and may also suffer pressure deformities as there is no protective uterine wall.

This condition is usually detected on ultrasound scanning but may be suggested by a persistently abnormal fetal lie and the fact that fetal parts are unusually easy to palpate. Delivery is by laparotomy. The placenta is usually left in situ to be absorbed, as an attempt to detach it may cause uncontrollable haemorrhage.

Ectopic pregnancy is a significant cause of maternal death and the incidence is rising. There were 13 reported deaths in the UK from this cause between 1997 and 1999 (Lewis, 2001). The midwife must be aware of the associated risk factors and seek an obstetric opinion for any woman with signs or symptoms suggestive of extrauterine gestation without delay.

BLEEDING FROM ASSOCIATED CONDITIONS

The following conditions may cause bleeding, although, strictly speaking, they are not early bleedings of pregnancy since the bleeding is not from the site of the pregnancy.

Cervical polyp

This is a small red gelatinous growth attached by a pedicle to the cervix, close to the external os. It may give rise to slight irregular bleeding.

Ectropion of the cervix

A cervical erosion is formed when the columnar epithelium lining the cervical canal proliferates owing to the action of the pregnancy hormones. The ectropion forms a reddish area on the cervix, extending outwards from the external os. It may give rise to a blood-stained discharge from the vagina. No treatment is necessary and the ectropion will recede during the puerperium.

Carcinoma of the cervix

Invasive cervical carcinoma is rarely seen in pregnancy, although cervical intraepithelial neoplasia (CIN) may occasionally be discovered if a cervical smear is taken. If the cervical cytology report suggests precancerous changes, colposcopy is performed to identify the affected areas and a small cervical biopsy may be carried out. Treatment is deferred until after delivery if the condition is not invasive.

Invasive cervical cancer is very serious as the disease may progress quickly. On vaginal examination the cervix is hard and irregular and bleeds when touched. There may also be a purulent vaginal discharge. If the condition is discovered in the first trimester, the pregnancy may be terminated and treatment initiated. In the third trimester, the fetus is viable and may be delivered by caesarean section. Once the infant is born the obstetrician may carry out a radical hysterectomy (Wertheim's hysterectomy). Vaginal delivery is associated with a poorer prognosis for the mother as cervical dilatation may cause dissemination of tumour cells and metastases have been reported in episiotomy sites (Sood et al., 2000).

A dilemma arises if the condition is discovered in the second trimester because the fetus is unlikely to survive if delivered. The woman may choose to postpone treatment for a time to allow further fetal growth; however, the delay should be no longer than 4 weeks (Chamberlain, 1995).

Bleeding in early pregnancy may occur for a variety of reasons. It is a serious sign and the underlying condition may be life-threatening. Any woman who reports vaginal bleeding during pregnancy must be referred to an obstetrician without delay.

BLEEDING AFTER THE 24TH WEEK – ANTEPARTUM HAEMORRHAGE

Antepartum haemorrhage is defined as bleeding from the genital tract after the 24th week of pregnancy and before the birth of the baby. Bleeding which occurs during labour is sometimes referred to as intrapartum haemorrhage.

Antepartum haemorrhage is a serious complication which may result in the death of the mother or the baby. There are two main varieties of haemorrhage:

- *Placenta praevia* (unavoidable or inevitable haemorrhage) is bleeding from separation of an abnormally situated placenta. (The placenta lies partly or wholly in the lower uterine segment and bleeding is inevitable when labour begins.)
- *Abruptio placentae* (placental abruption) is bleeding from separation of a normally situated placenta.

However, extraplacental bleeding may sometimes occur. This is vaginal bleeding from some other part of the birth canal, e.g. a cervical polyp, as described above.

PLACENTA PRAEVIA

The incidence of placenta praevia at term ranges from 0.5–1%. It is usually detected on ultrasound scanning in early pregnancy and may be seen in as many as one-quarter of all pregnancies in the second trimester. As the lower segment grows and stretches the placental site appears to rise up the uterine wall, away from the internal os uteri, until at term in the majority of cases the placenta no longer occupies the lower segment. Those cases where the placenta overlies the internal os in early pregnancy, are at highest risk of haemorrhage. The classification of placenta praevia is shown in Table 44.1. This is a standard classification and the distinction between types III and IV is purely academic. The types are illustrated in Figure 44.8.

Causes

The cause of placenta praevia is unknown but the following factors are known to be associated (Handler *et al.*, 1994; Konje and Taylor, 1999; Taylor *et al.*, 1994):

- *Multiparity.* The increased size of the uterine cavity following repeated childbearing may predispose to placenta praevia.

- *Multiple pregnancy.* The larger placental site is more likely to encroach on the lower segment of the uterus.
- *Age.* Older mothers are more at risk than younger ones.
- *Scarred uterus.* One previous caesarean section doubles the risk of placenta praevia.
- *Previous myomectomy or hysterotomy.*
- *Smoking.* The exact mechanism is unclear but the relative hypoxia induced by smoking may cause enlargement of the placenta in order to compensate for the reduced oxygen supply.
- *Placental abnormality.* Bipartite and succenturiate placentae may cause placenta praevia. Placenta membranacea (placenta diffusa) may also be a cause. This is a rare developmental abnormality of the placenta where all the chorion is covered with functioning villi. The placenta develops as a thin membranous structure, covering an unusually large surface of the uterus. The condition may be diagnosed on ultrasound. In pregnancy it may cause severe haemorrhage possibly requiring hysterectomy. It may not separate readily in the third stage of labour. Fetal nutrition appears to be relatively undisturbed in cases of placenta membranacea.
- *Fetal sex.* There may be an association between male fetal sex and placenta praevia (Wen *et al.*, 2000).

Associated conditions

A low-lying placenta puts the woman and her fetus at risk of other complications. The most serious of these is placenta accreta. This usually occurs where the previous delivery was by caesarean section. The combination of the relatively thin decidua in the lower segment and the presence of scar tissue increases the likelihood of trophoblastic invasion of the myometrium.

Intrauterine growth restriction may occur, possibly as a result of repeated small haemorrhages (Konje and Taylor, 1999).

Table 44.1	Classification of placenta praevia
Type I	Placenta mainly in the upper segment but encroaching on the lower segment
Type II	Placenta reaches to, but does not cover, the internal os
Type III	Placenta covers the internal os when closed but not completely when it is dilated
Type IV	Placenta completely covers the internal os

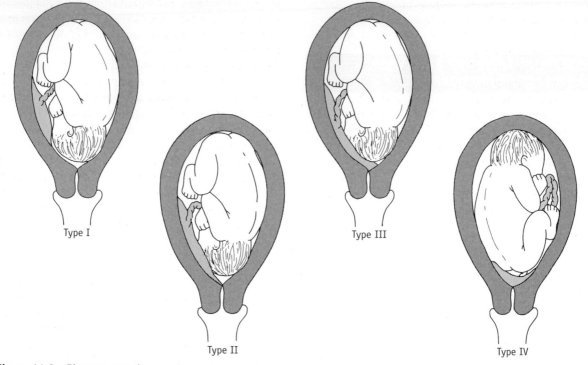

Figure 44.8   Placenta praevia.

Signs and symptoms

As placenta praevia is normally diagnosed on ultrasound scanning in early pregnancy, midwives will usually be aware of any woman in their care who has a low-lying placenta. However, there are women who will not have had an ultrasound scan during pregnancy, such as women who choose not to do so, women who have concealed their pregnancy, women who have not 'booked', or women who may have spent their antenatal period in a country where ultrasound scans are not readily available. Therefore the midwife must be aware of the signs which indicate a possible placenta praevia:

- *Malpresentation of the fetus.* Although the presentation may be cephalic, often it is not. The placenta occupies space in the pelvis and the midwife may find that the breech presents, as there is more room for the head in the fundus, or that the lie is oblique and the fetal shoulder presents.
- *Non-engagement of the presenting part.* This is especially likely with a type III or IV placenta praevia.
- *Difficulty in identifying fetal parts on palpation.* An anterior placenta praevia (especially types I and II) lies between the fetus and the midwife's hand like a cushion. This makes the fetal parts relatively difficult to identify.

- *Loud maternal pulse below the umbilicus.* An anterior placenta praevia (especially types I and II) may often be detected by the presence of loud maternal arterial sounds from the placental bed. This is more easily heard with an electronic fetal heart monitor (Doppler). The fetal heart sounds may be difficult to detect as they are muffled by the placenta, especially in a cephalic presentation.

  An anterior type I or II placenta praevia will cushion some of the fetal movements and the woman may mention that she only feels fetal movement above the umbilicus.

- *Bleeding after sexual intercourse.* Stimulation of the cervix during intercourse may provoke bleeding.

When bleeding occurs it usually begins after the 24th–28th week of pregnancy, although it may occur earlier. In the third trimester of pregnancy the lower segment is completing its development, Braxton Hicks contractions are increasing and, towards the end of pregnancy, the cervix is becoming effaced. Bleeding is caused by detachment of the placenta which cannot stretch to adapt to these changes in uterine structure. As the placenta is in the lower pole of the uterus the blood escapes easily, thus giving rise to the classical unprovoked, fresh, painless bleeding of placenta praevia. 'Warning haemorrhages' are associated with placenta praevia. These are small, recurrent, fresh and painless haemorrhages occurring during the third trimester. Each episode of bleeding indicates further placental detachment. If the placenta is torn, some fetal bleeding will occur and this will further compromise the condition of the fetus. Torrential maternal haemorrhage may occur at any time but is more likely once labour begins as the cervix begins to dilate.

It is impossible to predict the course of events in a case of placenta praevia and even in the absence of bleeding the condition is regarded as a major and life-threatening complication of pregnancy.

Outcome

Conservative treatment When slight to moderate bleeding occurs before the 38th week of pregnancy and the maternal and fetal conditions are satisfactory, conservative treatment aims to maintain the pregnancy until as near the 38th week as possible to avoid prematurity. When the bleeding ceases the obstetrician may carry out a speculum examination to exclude incidental causes of bleeding. The placental site will be identified by ultrasound examination. If the placenta is found to be normally situated the woman may be allowed to go home when the bleeding has ceased, provided her condition, and that of the fetus, is good. If placenta praevia is diagnosed the implications of this condition should be discussed with her. If there is a major degree of placenta praevia the woman should remain in hospital for the rest of her pregnancy as the risk of further and severe haemorrhage is very real. Ultrasound examination should be performed if there is a history of previous caesarean section, in order to rule out placenta accreta. It is essential that the midwife and the senior obstetrician discuss the plan of care with the woman and her partner (RCOG, 2000f).

Delivery If no serious haemorrhage has made it imperative to act before, the woman will be delivered at about 38 weeks' gestation. Delivery at this stage avoids the problems of prematurity for the infant.

If the placental location is unclear, an examination under anaesthetic may be carried out in theatre, by a senior obstetrician, with the woman suitably anaesthetized and the theatre set up in readiness for a caesarean section. An intravenous infusion is commenced and 4 units of cross-matched blood is at hand. With the woman in the lithotomy position, the obstetrician makes a very gentle and cautious vaginal examination, passing a finger through the cervix into the lower pole of the uterus. If the placenta is palpable the obstetrician will immediately perform a caesarean section. If the placenta is not palpable in the lower segment the membranes may be ruptured and the woman allowed to labour. This procedure avoids unnecessary caesarean section for women in whom placenta praevia is not confirmed.

However, nearly all women have access to ultrasound scanning and the diagnosis is usually clear. Vaginal delivery is usually possible in cases of type I placenta praevia, if the fetal head is engaged. However, the presence of placental tissue within 2 cm of the internal os is a contraindication to vaginal birth (Konje and Taylor, 1999; RCOG, 2000f).

Active treatment In cases where bleeding first occurs at 38 weeks or later, conservative treatment is not appropriate, as the fetus is mature. Active treatment is also necessary in cases where labour has started, if bleeding is severe or there are signs of fetal distress. An intravenous infusion is commenced and the woman's condition is stabilized if necessary. A senior obstetrician performs an emergency caesarean section under general anaesthesia. A paediatrician should be present to attend to the baby, who may be asphyxiated at birth. Preterm infants of mothers with placenta praevia have an increased risk of developing respiratory distress syndrome (Lin *et al.*, 2001).

Third stage Postpartum haemorrhage may complicate the third stage of labour since there are few oblique muscle fibres to control bleeding from the placental site in the lower uterine segment.

Placenta accreta may occur in women who have had a previous caesarean section and torrential haemorrhage may result from attempts to separate the placenta. Surgical treatments such as ligation of the internal iliac arteries may be required in order to control the haemorrhage. Hysterectomy is undertaken as a last resort to save the woman's life. The midwife must be familiar with local guidelines for management of massive obstetric haemorrhage, and adequate supplies of cross-matched blood should be available before surgery commences.

It cannot be emphasized too strongly that vaginal examination in placenta praevia is an extremely dangerous procedure and should not be attempted, except with the precautions described above.

ABRUPTIO PLACENTAE

Abruptio placentae is bleeding due to the separation of a normally situated placenta (Fig. 44.9). It is sometimes referred to as placental abruption or accidental bleeding. Placental abruption may occur at any stage of pregnancy, or during labour and may complicate approximately 1% of pregnancies.

Causes

The cause of the placental separation cannot always be satisfactorily explained, and in 40% of cases no cause can be found (Rana *et al.*, 1999). However, the following risk factors have been associated with the condition (Carr and Coustan, 1999; Konje and Taylor, 1999; Ray and Laskin, 1999; Reis *et al.*, 2000):

- *Hypertensive disease*: essential hypertension, PIH or pre-eclampsia

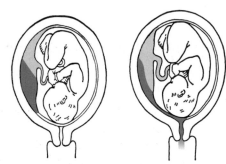

Figure 44.9 Abruptio placentae.

- *Sudden decompression of the uterus* such as may follow spontaneous rupture of the membranes in cases of polyhydramnios
- *Preterm prelabour* rupture of the membranes
- *Previous history* of placental abruption
- *Trauma*, for example following external cephalic version, road traffic accident, a fall or a blow
- *Smoking*
- *Illegal drug abuse*, e.g. cocaine, crack, marijuana
- *Folate and vitamin B_{12} deficiency*; although the evidence for this association is not conclusive.

Maternal hypertension is the most consistent finding in cases of placental abruption.

Types

The bleeding may be revealed, concealed or partially revealed (Fig. 44.10).

Revealed bleeding This occurs when the site of detachment is at the placental margin. The blood thus dissects between the membranes and the decidua and escapes through the os uteri. With revealed placental abruption the degree of shock is in proportion to the visible vaginal blood loss.

Concealed bleeding This occurs when the site of detachment is close to the centre of the placenta. The blood cannot escape and a large retroplacental clot forms. The blood may infiltrate the myometrium, sometimes as far as the peritoneal covering, causing a marbled, petechial pattern of bleeding. This is called a *Couvelaire uterus*. There is no visible blood loss but

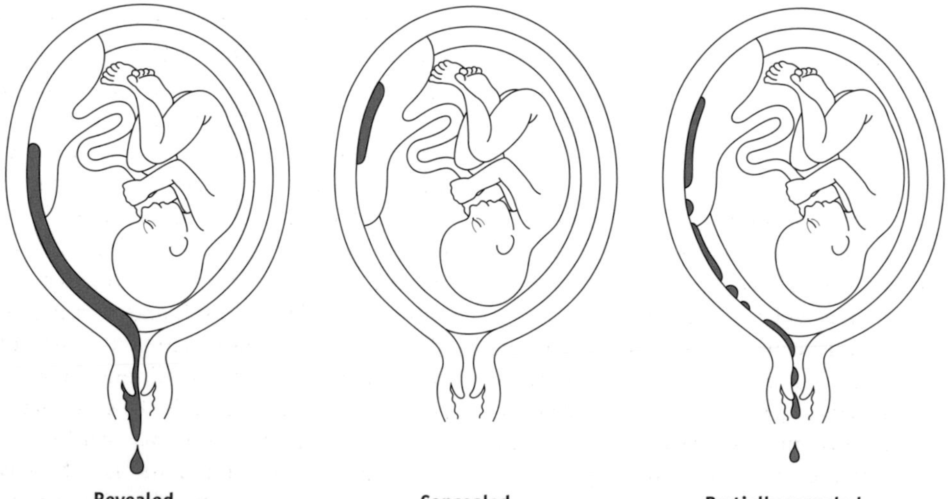

Revealed   **Concealed**   **Partially revealed**

Figure 44.10 Types of abruptio placentae.

the pain and shock may be severe as the intrauterine tension rises. Increasing abdominal girth or rising fundal height are suspicious of concealed haemorrhage. Backache may accompany abruption in a posteriorly sited placenta.

Partially revealed bleeding   This occurs when some of the blood trickles between the membranes and the decidua to become visible as vaginal bleeding. Not all the blood escapes and a variable amount remains concealed. In this situation the bleeding and thus the degree of shock will be much more severe than the visible loss suggests.

The severity of placental abruption may be classified as mild, moderate or severe:

Mild abruptio placentae   The loss is usually slight and the bleeding may be entirely concealed, although often there is a slight trickle per vaginam. The mother may experience no more than mild abdominal pain, the uterus is not tender and the fetus is alive. There is no sign of maternal shock.

Moderate abruptio placentae   The blood loss is heavier, the abdominal pain more severe and, on palpation, the uterus may be tender and firm. The mother may be hypotensive and have a tachycardia and usually there are signs of fetal distress.

Severe abruptio placentae   This is an obstetric emergency. More than half the placenta will have separated, the blood loss will exceed 1 litre and the mother will be very shocked. Abdominal pain will be severe. On palpation the uterus may be hard ('woody') and tender, and on auscultation fetal heart sounds will not be heard. There is an increased risk of coagulation disorders. It is essential to remember that the amount of bleeding per vaginam is no guide to the degree of placental separation.

Outcome

If there is only minor detachment of the placenta and the mother and fetus are in good condition the woman will be advised to stay in hospital for observation. If the bleeding ceases and all is well she may be discharged. The pregnancy will be closely monitored with ultrasound scans and regular cardiotocography to assess fetal growth and well-being. There is an increased risk of poor fetal growth and preterm birth following an episode of placental abruption (Rasmussen *et al.*, 2000).

In a case of moderate or severe abruptio placentae the most important treatment is to empty the uterus. If fetal condition permits, labour is induced by rupturing

the membranes and an oxytocic infusion is commenced. Vaginal delivery may be possible. If the fetus is in poor condition, delivery will be by caesarean section unless the woman is already in the second stage of labour, when a forceps delivery will be performed. Ergometrine 500 µg is given intravenously at delivery to control haemorrhage in the third stage of labour. It is usual to continue the Syntocinon infusion for some hours after delivery in order to maintain uterine contraction.

The best treatment for severe haemorrhage and defective coagulation is the transfusion of fresh blood. If fresh blood is not available, fresh frozen plasma should be given as this contains fibrinogen, platelets and clotting factors III, V and VIII.

> ### Reflective Activity 44.3
> Locate and read your Unit policy for management of bleeding in later pregnancy.

MANAGEMENT OF ANTEPARTUM HAEMORRHAGE AND THE MIDWIFE'S ROLE

At home

If called by a woman with bleeding, the midwife must ascertain the amount of bleeding and, having advised the woman to lie down, attend at once. If the reported bleeding is heavy the midwife should ask a paramedic team from the local ambulance service to attend simultaneously in order to avoid delay in transfer to hospital.

The woman should lie on her side or with a pillow or towel wedged under the right hip to achieve a slight pelvic tilt and avoid supine hypotensive syndrome. Vital signs should be recorded, blood loss noted and a sanitary pad applied. The presence of pain is suggestive of abruptio placentae, while painless bright bleeding may indicate placenta praevia. Soiled pads and clothing should be saved to allow accurate estimation of blood lost. An obstetrician from the local hospital must be contacted, as the woman will need to be admitted. The midwife should inform the obstetrician of the severity of the bleeding, colour (fresh or dark) of the blood, nature and location of pain, if present, and the woman's general condition. If the initial loss is small, the woman's blood pressure and pulse rate will be normal and she will appear well. Should the loss be severe she will present the typical picture of a woman who has had a haemorrhage: pale, sweating, restless, thirsty, with a rising pulse rate and falling blood pressure. In this case emergency assistance is needed and a paramedic team from the ambulance service should be called. An intravenous infusion is started and group O rhesus-negative blood may be given if necessary. Plasma expanders such as *Haemaccel*, *Gelofusine* or *hetastarch* preparations (*Hespan*) may be used. Dextrans should be avoided.

The woman is transferred to hospital. During transfer oxygen can be given at 4 litres/minute via face mask. The midwife should make frequent recordings of pulse and blood pressure until care is handed over to the hospital team.

When attending a woman who is bleeding *no vaginal examination should be made*. If this is a case of placenta praevia, a vaginal examination could precipitate a disastrous haemorrhage. Rectal examinations are similarly dangerous. Abdominal examination should be avoided if possible as this may provoke Braxton Hicks contractions, which may accelerate bleeding.

In hospital

The woman is admitted to the delivery suite and a senior obstetrician is informed. If there are signs of severe haemorrhage a senior anaesthetist and haematologist should also be informed.

Until the diagnosis is clear she must be treated as having a potential placenta praevia, although there may be some features which help in making a diagnosis (see Table 44.2). Often the distinction is not clear; it is particularly difficult if the mother has had a small revealed abruption but no pain, no apparent cause for the bleeding and no signs of pre-eclampsia.

If bleeding has been severe the treatment must be swift, as the woman's condition may deteriorate rapidly. The aim is to restore blood loss and thus improve the mother's general condition, get the baby delivered quickly if necessary, and avoid the dangerous complications of renal failure and blood coagulation disorders. An intravenous cannula (14 gauge) is inserted – in cases of severe haemorrhage two cannulae should be inserted. Blood is taken for grouping and cross-matching and the duty haematologist and blood bank must be informed if large quantities of blood are likely to be needed. Other blood tests include full blood count (essential for haemoglobin estimation and platelet count), urea and electrolytes, clotting studies and fibrin degradation products.

Temperature, pulse, blood pressure, fetal heart and vaginal loss should be observed. The pulse and blood pressure are recorded as frequently as the woman's condition dictates: quarter-hourly if the bleeding is continuing. Maternal oxygen saturation should be observed using a pulse oximeter. Oxygen may be given by face mask if required. The fetal heart should be continuously monitored by external cardiotocography whilst bleeding persists. A Foley urinary catheter is inserted and the urinary output is closely monitored, a marked decrease being a grave sign. The urine is tested for protein. The midwife records an estimate of blood loss.

Analgesia such as morphine may be required if the woman is in pain. An intravenous infusion of normal saline 0.9% or Hartmann's solution (Ringer's lactate) will be commenced. Blood transfusion may be required and several units of blood or packed cells may be

Table 44.2 Differential diagnosis with placenta praevia

Clinical sign	Placenta praevia	Abruptio placentae
Pain	No pain	Uterine pain, may be severe; backache if placenta is posterior
Colour of blood loss	Bright, fresh	May be darker
'Warning' haemorrhages	Yes	No
Onset of bleeding	Possibly following coitus, otherwise unexpected	May follow trauma, exertion
Degree of shock	In proportion to visible loss	May be more severe than visible loss suggests
Consistency of uterus	Soft, non-tender	Increased uterine tone, may be tense, rigid, 'woody'
Palpation	Fetus usually fairly easy to palpate	Tense uterus makes palpation difficult
Presentation	May be a malpresentation	Probably cephalic
Engagement	Not engaged	May be engaged
Fetal heartbeat	Probably present	May be absent
Abdominal girth	Equivalent to gestation	May increase due to concealed haemorrhage

needed if the haemorrhage has been substantial: in such cases central venous pressure should be monitored to avoid the dangers of over- or undertransfusion.

The abdominal girth is sometimes measured and recorded.

Meticulous observation and recording of vital signs, blood loss and fluid balance are essential in order to assess the woman's condition and plan her care. Ongoing management of the situation is governed by the condition of mother and fetus. The midwife may need to involve the social worker if there are other children at home for whom care arrangements need to be made. The needs of the partner should also be addressed, which include support and information.

If the haemorrhage is not severe and urgent delivery is not indicated, the woman may be transferred to the ward once the bleeding settles and her condition is stable. In the absence of pain or active bleeding the woman should not be confined to her bed and can be encouraged to wear her usual clothes during the day. In cases of placenta praevia at least 2 units of cross-matched blood should always be available. If the bleeding is due to placenta praevia she may be advised to remain in hospital until delivery. The midwife must ensure that the woman and her partner are fully informed about her condition and the likely management. Antepartum haemorrhage is a frightening experience for the woman and she must be given the opportunity to ask questions.

Women who find themselves in this situation can very quickly become demoralized by the prospect of having to spend some weeks in hospital. The midwife should make every effort to maintain the woman's morale; the effects of separation from the family may be reduced by allowing unrestricted visiting.

Following antepartum haemorrhage, tests to assess fetal well-being will be carried out because premature separation of the placenta may result in impaired placental function. Fetal growth will be assessed by ultrasound, and periodic continuous fetal heart monitoring will be performed. Women who are rhesus negative should be given anti-D gammaglobulin after each episode of bleeding.

COMPLICATIONS

Blood coagulation disorders When tissue damage occurs there is a release of thromboplastin from the local cells. Thromboplastin activates the clotting mechanism and this results in the conversion of fibrinogen into fibrin. The sticky web of fibrin traps the cellular components of the blood and a clot forms, sealing off the bleeding point. The clot is later dispersed by plasmin which is the active product of the fibrinolytic system. When a clot is broken down fibrin degradation products (FDPs) are formed. Clot dispersal is a protective mechanism to prevent capillary blockage.

The system of initial clot formation followed by fibrinolysis is normally delicately balanced. If the coagulation system fails bleeding will persist, while if the fibrinolytic system fails clotting will persist.

Occasionally tissue damage is so severe or widespread that there is a massive release of thromboplastin into the general circulation. Widespread clotting will then occur throughout the body. This condition is known as *disseminated intravascular coagulation* (DIC). This is extremely dangerous as the microthrombi generated by the thromboplastin will occlude small blood vessels. This results in ischaemic tissue damage within the body organs: the damaged tissue releases thromboplastin, which stimulates further clotting. Thus a vicious circle of tissue damage and uncontrolled clotting occurs. Any body organ may be affected: renal damage will result in oliguria or anuria; liver damage will lead to jaundice. If the lungs are affected dyspnoea and cyanosis will occur; convulsions or coma indicate cerebral involvement. Microthrombi in the retina may cause blindness; if the pituitary gland is affected Sheehan's syndrome may occur.

Eventually the available circulating platelets are depleted. Clotting factors such as prothrombin (factor II), thromboplastin (factor III), proaccelerin (factor V), antihaemophilic factor (factor VIII) and fibrinogen (factor I) are exhausted. No further coagulation can take place: bleeding becomes apparent. This may take the form of oozing from venepuncture sites, mucous membrane bleeding, petechiae and uncontrollable uterine haemorrhage.

DIC is always a secondary event, occurring as a result of massive tissue damage and thromboplastin release. It may complicate conditions such as severe pre-eclampsia, septicaemia or amniotic fluid embolism. It may also occur following abruptio placentae when thromboplastin is released from the damaged placental, decidual and myometrial tissue. Unless DIC is recognized and treated promptly the condition may become uncontrollable and maternal death is almost inevitable. The midwife must be aware of any woman who is at risk of DIC and be alert for the signs of coagulation failure. All maternity units should have an emergency protocol for dealing with such cases. Any woman with an abruptio placentae should have screening tests for coagulation defects. These tests include (Konje and Taylor, 1999):

- partial thromboplastin time (normally 35–45 seconds)
- prothrombin time (normally 10–14 seconds)
- thrombin time (normally 10–15 seconds)
- fibrinogen levels (2.5–4 g/l)
- fibrin degradation products
- whole blood film and platelet count.

Fresh frozen plasma, packed cells and platelets are used in the treatment of DIC. Heparin is rarely used as it may exacerbate the haemorrhage, especially if the uterus is not empty.

Acute renal failure   This may occur following severe shock in cases of antepartum haemorrhage.

Sheehan's syndrome or Simmonds' disease (anterior pituitary necrosis)   This is a rare complication of severe and prolonged shock. The earliest sign is failure to lactate followed by amenorrhoea. The activity of the thyroid and adrenal glands gradually diminishes, hence the woman becomes lethargic and complains of feeling cold, coarsening of hair and skin and loss of libido. The secondary sexual characteristics are affected: the genitalia and the breasts will atrophy (Chamberlain, 1995). Recognition of the condition and treatment is essential if serious ill-health or possible death is to be avoided.

Postpartum haemorrhage   Following severe abruptio placentae, postpartum haemorrhage is most likely to be caused by a blood coagulation disorder, whereas following placenta praevia it is due to the inability of the lower uterine segment to contract effectively. Aortic compression may be necessary to control cases of intractable haemorrhage.

Infection   Sepsis is likely owing to the woman's lowered resistance following a state of severe shock, a large blood transfusion, more interference in labour and anaemia.

Anaemia   The haemoglobin must be checked and anaemia corrected in the puerperium.

Psychological disturbances/psychoses   Psychological disorders after childbirth are more likely following complications of pregnancy and labour, and may be due to the ensuing anaemia or post-traumatic stress (PTS) syndrome (see Ch. 54).

VASA PRAEVIA

This unusual condition may result in vaginal bleeding. It is associated with velamentous insertion of the cord. One of the fetal vessels traverses the membranes in the region of the internal os, in front of the presenting part (see Ch. 30). Occlusion of the vessel may occur as the presenting part compresses the membranes. When the membranes rupture, the vessel is torn and severe fetal bleeding occurs. The perinatal mortality associated with this condition is high. Diagnosis is difficult but a pulsating vessel may be felt on vaginal examination. Velamentous insertion can often be detected on routine ultrasound examination from the second trimester of pregnancy and vasa praevia can be confirmed by transvaginal colour Doppler scanning (Nomiyama *et al.*, 1998).

If vasa praevia is suspected, the midwife should leave the membranes intact and inform the obstetrician.

Vaginal bleeding with sudden severe fetal distress following rupture of the membranes should alert the midwife to the possibility of a ruptured vasa praevia. A sinusoidal fetal heart trace on cardiotocography is also suggestive of fetal bleeding. The blood loss may be tested for the presence of fetal cells using the alkali-denaturation (Apt) test, which will determine whether the blood is fetal or maternal in origin. However, it is unlikely that there will be time for this as delivery must be immediate if there is to be any hope of saving the fetus. Delivery will be by emergency caesarean section if vasa praevia is diagnosed during the first stage of labour. In the second stage of labour, delivery is expedited by an episiotomy and forceps. If born alive, the baby will require expert resuscitation and an appropriately qualified paediatrician, midwife, or neonatal nurse should be present at the delivery. A blood transfusion may be needed to correct hypovolaemia and anaemia. The midwife should be aware that there is a higher risk of vasa praevia in placenta praevia, where there is a succenturiate lobe and in IVF pregnancies (Olayinka *et al.*, 1999).

CONCLUSION

Bleeding in pregnancy remains a major cause of maternal mortality. The midwife must be familiar with local policy for management of bleeding in pregnancy and regular 'fire drills' should be held in maternity units to ensure that the obstetric team can respond to haemorrhage quickly and appropriately (DoH, 1996, 1998; Lewis, 2001). Midwives should be familiar with

Box 44.1 Key points from Guidelines for the Management of Massive Obstetric Haemorrhage (DoH, 1994)

- Immediate involvement of all key staff, including senior obstetrician, anaesthetist, haematologist, blood transfusion service and portering staff.
- Minimum 20 ml sample of blood for cross-matching and coagulation studies.
- 6 units minimum of cross-matched blood, with use of plasma expanders as necessary (not dextrans).
- Blood of the patient's own group to be used for transfusion; uncross-matched O negative blood to be used only if immediate transfusion is required.
- Minimum of two peripheral intravenous lines, using 14 gauge cannulae.
- Immediate commencement of CVP monitoring.
- Facilities for monitoring central venous and intra arterial pressure, ECG, blood gases and acid–base status should be available in consultant units.
- Rapid administration of blood and fluids (blood filtration is not necessary).
- Use of blood-warming equipment.
- Repeated estimation of haemoglobin and coagulation studies.

the recommended Guidelines for the Management of Massive Obstetric Haemorrhage to be found in the *Report on Confidential Enquiries into Maternal Deaths in the United Kingdom* (DoH, 1991, 1994) (Box 44.1) and the subsequent key recommendations (DoH, 1998; RCOG, 2001).

Midwives also need to be able to identify women who might be at risk, and refer appropriately, also ensuring that the woman and her family are informed and supported throughout. Often the midwife will be the continuity during the woman's pregnancy, and can work towards providing holistic, sensitive and appropriate care to the woman, her baby and family.

KEY POINTS

- Vaginal bleeding at any stage of pregnancy is always abnormal and may be indicative of a serious complication.
- Midwives need to educate the woman and her family regarding deviations from normal, and ensure that they are aware of what action should be taken and with whom they should communicate.
- Midwives must be aware of the possible causes of bleeding in pregnancy.
- Prompt and appropriate response may prevent the loss of the fetus and may save the mother's life.
- Midwives must be aware of the possible emotional, social and psychological impact of bleeding or pregnancy loss for the woman and her partner.

REFERENCES

Abortion Act 1967. London: HMSO.

Andersen, N., Wohlfahrt, J., Christens, P. *et al.* (2000) Maternal age and fetal loss: population based register linkage study. *British Medical Journal* 320(7251): 1708–1712.

Autry, A., Jacobson, G., Sandhu, R. *et al.* (1999) Medical management of non-viable early first trimester pregnancy. *International Journal of Gynecology and Obstetrics* 67(1): 9–13.

Ayres-de-Campos, D., Teixeira-da-Silva, I., Campos, B. *et al.* (2000) Vaginal misoprostol in the management of first-trimester missed abortions. *International Journal of Gynecology and Obstetrics* 71(1): 53–57.

Barron, S. (1995) Bleeding in pregnancy. In: Chamberlain, G. (ed) *Turnbull's Obstetrics*. Edinburgh: Churchill Livingstone.

Beischer, N., Mackay, E. & Colditz, P. (1997) *Obstetrics and the Newborn*. London: W.B. Saunders.

Ben-Arie, A., Hazan, Y., Goldchmit, R. & Hagay, Z. (2000) Safety of extraovular catheter insertion for second-trimester abortion. *Obstetrics and Gynecology* 96(4): 529–532.

Bergh, C., Moller, A., Nilsson, L. *et al.* (1999) Obstetric outcome and psychological follow up of pregnancies after embryo reduction. *Human Reproduction* 14(8): 2170–2175.

Blackburn, S.T. (2003) *Maternal Fetal and Neonatal Physiology*, 2nd edn. London: W.B. Saunders.

British Medical Association (BMA) and Royal Pharmaceutical Society of Great Britain (RPSGB) (2003) *British National Formulary*, 46th edn. London: BMA and RPSGB.

Boyles, S., Ness, R., Grisso, J. *et al.* (2000) Life event stress and the association with spontaneous abortion in gravid women at an urban emergency department. *Health Psychology* 19(6): 510–514.

Bradley, E. & Hamilton-Fairley, D. (1998) Managing miscarriage in early pregnancy assessment units. *Hospital Medicine* 59(6): 451–456.

Carr, R. & Coustan, D. (1999) Nonprescription drugs and alcohol: abuse and effects in pregnancy. In: Reece, E. & Hobbins, J. (eds) *Medicine of the Fetus and Mother*. Philadelphia: Lippincott.

Chamberlain, G. (1995) *Obstetrics by Ten Teachers*. London: Arnold.

Conway, K. & Russell, G. (2000) Couples' grief and experience of support in the aftermath of miscarriage. *British Journal of Medical Psychology* 73(4): 531–545.

Department of Health (DoH) (1991) *Report on Confidential Enquiries into Maternal Deaths in the United Kingdom 1985–1987*. London: HMSO.

Department of Health (DoH) (1994) *Report on Confidential Enquiries into Maternal Deaths in the United Kingdom 1988–1990*. London: HMSO.

Department of Health (DoH) (1996) *Report on Confidential Enquiries into Maternal Deaths in the United Kingdom 1991–93*. London: HMSO.

Department of Health (DoH) (1998) *Why Mothers Die: Report on Confidential Enquiries into Maternal Deaths in the United Kingdom 1994–1996*. London: HMSO.

Donders, G., Van Bulck, B., Cauldron, J. et al. (2000) Relationship of bacterial vaginosis and mycoplasmas to the risk of spontaneous abortion. *American Journal of Obstetrics and Gynecology* 183(2): 431–437.

Enkin, M., Keirse, M., Neilson, J. et al. (2000) *A Guide to Effective Care in Pregnancy and Childbirth*. Oxford: Oxford University Press.

Glover, V. & Fisk, N. (1999) Fetal pain: implications for research and practice. *British Journal of Obstetrics and Gynaecology* 106(9): 881–886.

Goldstein, I. (1999) Fetal neoplasm. In: Reece, E. & Hobbins, J. (eds) *Medicine of the Fetus and Mother*. Philadelphia: Lippincott.

Gopalkrishnan, K., Padwal, V., Meherji, P. et al. (2000) Poor quality sperm as it affects repeated early pregnancy loss. *Archives of Andrology* 45(2): 111–117.

Handler, A., Mason, E., Rosenberg, D. et al. (1994) The relationship between exposure during pregnancy to cigarette smoking and cocaine use and placenta praevia. *American Journal of Obstetrics and Gynecology* 170(3): 884–889.

Home Department (2001) *Criminal Statistics England and Wales 2000*. London: The Stationery Office. Online. Available: www.archive.official-documents.co.uk.

Human Fertilisation and Embryology Act 1991. London: HMSO

Jones, M. & Fraser, K. (1998) Misoprostol and attempted self-induction of abortion. *Journal of the Royal Society of Medicine* 91(4): 204–205.

Jurkovic, D., Ross, J. & Nicolaides, K. (1998) Expectant management of missed miscarriage. *British Journal of Obstetrics and Gynaecology* 105(6): 670–671.

Kadar, N. (1999) Ectopic and heterotopic pregnancies. In: Reece, E. & Hobbins, J. (eds) *Medicine of the Fetus and Mother*. Philadelphia: Lippincott.

Kauffman, D., Sutkin, G., Heine, R. et al. (1999) Metastatic complete hydatidiform mole with a surviving co-existent twin. A case report. *Journal of Reproductive Medicine* 44(2): 131–134.

Kohner, N. (1992) *A Dignified Ending*. London: Stillbirth and Neonatal Death Society (SANDS).

Kohner, N. (1995) *Pregnancy Loss and the Death of a Baby: Guidelines for Professionals*. London: SANDS.

Konje, J. & Taylor, D. (1999) Bleeding in late pregnancy. In: James D., Steer P., Weiner, C. et al. (eds) *High Risk Pregnancy: Management Options*. London: W.B. Saunders.

Lemus, J. (2000) Ectopic pregnancy: an update. *Current Opinion in Obstetrics and Gynecology* 12(5): 369–375.

Lewis, G. (ed) (2001) *Why Mothers Die 1997–1999: Fifth Report of the Confidential Enquiries into Maternal Deaths in the United Kingdom*. London: CEMD: associated with NICE, RCOG.

Lin, C., Wang, S., Hsu, Y. et al. (2001) Risk for respiratory distress syndrome in preterm infants born to mothers complicated by placenta previa. *Early Human Development* 60(3): 215–224.

Llewellyn Jones, D. (1999) *Fundamentals of Obstetrics and Gynaecology*, 7th edn. London: Mosby.

Nomiyama, M., Toyota, Y. & Kawano, H. (1998) Antenatal diagnosis of velamentous umbilical cord insertion and vasa previa with color Doppler imaging. *Ultrasound in Obstetrics and Gynecology* 12(6): 426–429.

Olayinka, K., Turner, M., Lees, C. et al. (1999) Vasa previa: an avoidable obstetric tragedy. *Obstetrical and Gynecological Survey* 54(2): 138–145.

Rai, R., Cohen, H., Dave, M. et al. (1997) Randomised controlled trial of aspirin and aspirin plus heparin in pregnant women with recurrent miscarriage associated with phospholipid antibodies (or antiphospholipid antibodies). *British Medical Journal* 314(7076): 253–257.

Ramhorst, R., Agriello, E., Zitterman, S. et al. (2000) Is the paternal mononuclear cells' immunisation a successful treatment for recurrent spontaneous abortion? *American Journal of Reproductive Immunology* 44(3): 129–135.

Rana, A., Sawhney, H., Gopolan, S. et al. (1999) Abruptio placentae and chorioamnionitis – microbiological and histological correlation. *Acta Obstetricia et Gynecologica Scandinavica* 78(5): 363–366.

Rasmussen, S., Irgens, L. & Dalaker, K. (2000) Outcome of pregnancies subsequent to placental abruption: a risk assessment. *Acta Obstetricia et Gynecologica Scandinavica* 79(6): 496–501.

Ray, J. & Laskin, C. (1999) Folic Acid and homocyst(e)ine metabolic defects and the risk of placental abruption, pre-eclampsia and spontaneous pregnancy loss: a systematic review. *Placenta* 20(7): 519–529.

Reis, P., Sander, C. & Pearlman, M. (2000) Abruptio placentae after auto accidents. A case control study *Journal of Reproductive Medicine* **45**(1): 6–10.

Rosevear, S. (1999) Bleeding in early pregnancy, In: James, D., Steer, P., Weiner, C. *et al. High Risk Pregnancy: Management Options*. London: W.B. Saunders.

Rouzi, A., Hawasawi, H. & Abduljabbar, H. (1999) Extra-amniotic prostaglandin E$_2$ for termination in the second and early third trimesters. *International Journal of Gynecology and Obstetrics* **67**(1): 45–46.

Royal College of Obstetricians and Gynaecologists (RCOG) (2000a) *Management of Early Pregnancy Loss*. London: RCOG. Online. Available: http://www.rcog.org.uk/guidelines/guideline25.

Royal College of Obstetricians and Gynaecologists (RCOG) (2000b) *The Care of Women Requesting Induced Abortion*. London: RCOG. Online. Available: http://www.rcog.org.uk/guidelines/induced_abortion.

Royal College of Obstetricians and Gynaecologists (RCOG) (2000c) *Induced Abortion*. London: RCOG. Online. Available: http://www.rcog.org.uk/guidelines/abortion.

Royal College of Obstetricians and Gynaecologists (RCOG) (2000d) *The Management of Gestational Trophoblastic Disease*. London: RCOG. Online. Available: http://www.rcog.org.uk/guidelines/guideline18.

Royal College of Obstetricians and Gynaecologists (RCOG) (2000e) *The Management of Tubal Pregnancies*. London: RCOG. Online. Available: http://www.rcog.org.uk/guidelines/tubal.

Royal College of Obstetricians and Gynaecologists (2000f) *Guidelines for the Diagnosis and Management of Placenta Praevia*. London: RCOG. Online. Available: http://www.rcog.org.uk/guidelines/placentapraevia.

Scott, J. (2000) Immunotherapy for recurrent miscarriage. *Cochrane Database of Systematic Revues* (2): CD000112.

Seckl, M., Fisher, R., Salwerno, G. *et al.* (2000) Choriocarcinoma and partial hydatidiform moles. *Lancet* **356**(9223): 36–39.

Shalev, J., Meizner, I., Mashiach, R. *et al.* (1999) Multifetal pregnancy reduction in cases of threatened abortion of triplets. *Fertility and Sterility* **72**(3): 423–426.

Silver, R. & Branch, D. (1999) Sporadic and recurrent pregnancy loss. In: Reece, E. & Hobbins, J. (eds) *Medicine of the Fetus and Mother*. Philadelphia: Lippincott-Raven.

Sood, A., Sorosky, J., Mayr, N. *et al.* (2000) Cervical cancer diagnosed shortly after pregnancy: prognostic variables and delivery routes. *Obstetrics and Gynecology* **95**(6 Pt 1): 832–838.

Stillbirth (Definition) Act 1992. London: HMSO.

Stirrat, G. & Wardle, P. (1999) Recurrent miscarriage. In: James, D., Steer, P., Weiner, C. *et al.* (eds) *High Risk Pregnancy: Management Options*. London: W.B. Saunders.

Szavay, P., Wermes, C., Fuchs, J. *et al.* (2000) Effective treatment of infantile choriocarcinoma in the liver with chemotherapy and surgical resection: a case report. *Journal of Pediatric Surgery* **35**(7): 1134–1135.

Taylor, V., Kramer, M., Vaughan, T. *et al.* (1994) Placenta praevia and prior caesarean delivery: how strong is the association? *Obstetrics and Gynecology* **84**(1): 55–57.

Tin-Chiu, L., Bates, S. & Pearce, M. (1999) Biochemical tests in complications in early pregnancy. In: O'Brien, P. (ed) *The Yearbook of Obstetrics and Gynaecology*, Vol. 7. London: RCOG Press.

Wen, S., Demissie, K., Liu, S. *et al.* (2000) Placenta praevia and male sex at birth: results from a population-based study. *Paediatric and Perinatal Epidemiology* **14**(4): 300–304.

FURTHER READING

Bonnar, J. (2000) Massive obstetric haemorrhage. *Baillière's Clinical Obstetrics and Gynaecology* **14**(1): 1–18.
A comprehensive and readable guide to the management of major haemorrhage. The tables are clear and very useful. It outlines risks to mother and fetus and also considers other complications associated with this emergency.

Regan, L. & Rai, R. (2000) Epidemiology and the medical causes of miscarriage. *Baillière's Clinical Obstetrics and Gynaecology* **14**(5): 839–854.
This is a useful and well-referenced source which provides an overview of the types of miscarriage and associated causes.

ADDITIONAL RESOURCES

ARC – Antenatal Results and Choices (formerly SATFA)
73 Charlotte Street, London W1P 1LB
Tel: 020 7631 0280
Helpline: 020 7631 0285
Email: arcsatfa@aol.com

Hydatidiform Mole and Choriocarcinoma U.K. Information and Support Service
Website: http://www.hmole-chorio.org.uk

The Miscarriage Association
c/o Clayton Hospital, Northgate, Wakefield, West Yorkshire WF1 3JS

Helpline: Tel. 01924 200799 (Mon–Fri, 9 am–4 pm)
Scottish Helpline (answerphone): 0131 334 8883
Email: miscarriageassociation@care4free.net
Website: http://www.miscarriageassociation.org.uk

SANDS (Stillbirth & Neonatal Death Society)
28 Portland Place, London W1N 4DE
Tel: 020 7436 3715
Email: support@uk-sands.org
Website: http://www.uk-sands.org

45

Hypertensive Disorders of Pregnancy

Chris Bewley

LEARNING OUTCOMES

After reading this chapter you will be able to:

- appreciate the difficulty of defining and classifying disorders which present with maternal hypertension
- be aware that hypertension may be associated with pre-eclampsia, chronic or essential hypertension, or renal disease

- understand the pathophysiology of pre-eclampsia
- recognize the outward signs of pre-eclampsia and relate them to pathophysiology
- be aware of the psychological support needed for women who are diagnosed with pre-eclampsia.

INTRODUCTION

This chapter reviews the available literature on hypertensive disorders in pregnancy to provide an overview of the nature, prevalence, diagnosis and outcomes in women and their babies. A midwifery approach to collaborative care between pregnant women and healthcare professionals is suggested, which maximizes recognition and minimizes adverse pregnancy outcomes for mother and baby, yet retains maternal choice, input and understanding.

Hypertensive disorders in pregnancy accounted for 15 maternal deaths in the UK between 1997 and 1999 (Lewis, 2001), and 20 in the previous triennium (DoH, 1998). The term 'hypertensive disorders' is used to describe conditions in which hypertension is present, and includes essential, chronic and renal hypertensive disorders (see Ch. 46). The term 'pregnancy-induced hypertension' is widely used, but as Roberts (2000) points out, hypertension arising in pregnancy may be only one major characteristic of a multisystem disorder, pre-eclampsia, which should perhaps more properly be called a syndrome. Roberts further suggests that studying the whole pathophysiology has increased knowledge considerably more than limiting study to hypertension only.

TERMINOLOGY

Various terms have been applied to a condition arising in pregnancy which is characterized by a rise in blood pressure, proteinuria, possibly oedema, and convulsions (Chappell *et al.*, 1999). The term pre-eclampsia has been retained in this chapter to denote a condition in which a previously normotensive pregnant woman exhibits hypertension in conjunction with proteinuria, with or without oedema. Chamberlain (1991) observes that the semantics of terminology are less important than the ability of health professionals to recognize the features of a life-threatening disorder of pregnancy.

Classification

A number of authorities have attempted to classify hypertensive disorders which occur in pregnancy (Chappell *et al.*, 1999) but the validity of such classifications is questionable since many conditions are only identified retrospectively, either from post-mortem following maternal death, or from follow-up investigations postnatally. However, greater understanding of the number and forms of hypertensive conditions occurring during pregnancy may be achieved by classification, which provides a common foundation on which research can be based and results assessed.

Most authorities accept the difficulty of defining hypertension, and many use a working definition that a blood pressure of 140/90 mmHg or more and/or an increase in diastolic pressure of 20 mmHg or more from the booking blood pressure after the 20th week of pregnancy constitute grounds for further monitoring.

Reflective Activity 45.1

What does your unit protocol indicate about levels of blood pressure and referral?

What definition of 'hypertensive' is used, and are the protocols evidence-based?

PRE-ECLAMPSIA

The detection and treatment of pre-eclampsia is a vital part of midwifery practice; however, current research and literature suggest that while considerable work is being undertaken into various aspects of pre-eclampsia, little has been discovered to determine its cause. In the absence of such knowledge, midwives, obstetricians and paediatricians work under difficult conditions of second guessing a syndrome whose worst effects are evident only in its advanced stages (Bewley, 2000).

As has already been stated, pre-eclampsia was implicated in 15 maternal deaths between 1997 and 1999 (Lewis, 2001). It may also increase the risk of perinatal mortality and morbidity, since it causes placental dysfunction. Complications such as intrauterine growth restriction (IUGR), intrauterine hypoxia and intrauterine fetal death may occur. Perinatal mortality is raised fivefold (Walker, 2000), not only because of these conditions but also because of prematurity, as early delivery is often necessary for severe pre-eclampsia and eclampsia. Li and Wi (2000) further suggest that maternal pre-eclampsia and eclampsia are associated with subsequent sudden infant death syndrome (SIDS) in the baby of the affected pregnancy.

Pathophysiology

Despite much research, the cause of pre-eclampsia remains uncertain and it has been named the 'disease of theories' (Redman and Walker, 1996). Theories suggest that there may be a basic maladaptation of the maternal circulatory system in response to the trophoblast. It is called a disease of the placenta, because it can also occur in pregnancies where there is trophoblast, but no fetal tissue, such as complete molar pregnancy (Norwitz *et al.*, 1999). Usually there is a physiological dilatation of the spiral arterioles which allows a pooling of maternal blood in the placental bed; this then creates a shunt, which in turn causes the blood pressure to be lowered. In pre-eclampsia and eclampsia this dilatation fails to occur; and the blood pressure is raised as the blood is forced through constricted arterioles. The muscle coating of the vessels is further damaged, leading to arteriosclerosis and local platelet aggregation, causing a further rise in blood pressure (Chamberlain, 1991).

Failure in the reduction of peripheral resistance is further complicated by an increased sensitivity to angiotensin II, leading to vasospasm in the spiral arterioles. Normally, in pregnancy, a delicate balance is maintained between prostacyclin and thromboxane, which prevents this aggravated response to angiotensin II (Chamberlain, 1991). Widespread endothelial damage occurs and this was thought to be caused by hypertensive vascular trauma. However, since the changes in the brain, heart and liver of pre-eclamptic women are similar to those caused by hypovolaemia, hypoperfusion rather than vascular trauma may cause the placenta to produce vasoconstrictors and procoagulant substances (Salas, 1999). Furthermore, changes associated with atherosclerosis are seen in women with pre-eclampsia (Moran and Davison, 1999), and predisposing causes for pre-eclampsia are the same as those for cardiovascular disease (Roberts, 2000).

The effects of hypoperfusion and vasoconstriction are seen in the kidney, liver and the placental bed. Placental abruption may occur due to arteriolar vasoconstriction and spasm resulting in ischaemia and subsequent rupture of arterioles. Disseminated intravascular coagulation (DIC) may also occur (see Chs 44 and 59) and is caused by the release of thromboplastic material into the circulation. In pre-eclampsia and eclampsia the source of thromboplastin is probably the damaged placental tissue, whether or not it is associated with abruptio placentae.

Aetiological factors

Pre-eclampsia is more common in primigravidae than in multigravidae. Even if the first pregnancy results in abortion, especially induced abortion, there is a reduced incidence of pre-eclampsia in the second pregnancy. However, the degree of protection is not as great as that following a first, term pregnancy (Eras *et al.*, 2000). A small study of 1011 pregnant women who delivered consecutively in an obstetric unit in the UK suggested that exposure to partner's semen during intercourse over a period of time prior to conception may also protect against pre-eclampsia (Robillard *et al.*, 1994). Li and Wi (2000) suggest that changing paternity also affects the woman's likelihood of developing pre-eclampsia, while Smith *et al.* (1997) suggest some partner-specific maternal immune response. Racial tendencies and geographical location have been observed (Roberts, 2000) and there is some evidence that eclampsia may be more common in humid rather than dry conditions (Makhseed *et al.*, 1999). Familial tendencies have been described (Kilpatrick *et al.*, 1989) showing a higher rate of pre-eclampsia amongst sisters, suggesting a genetic susceptibility; however, a single-gene hypothesis is disputed by Thornton and Onwude (1991), whose study of identical female parous twins failed to confirm a genetic link, at least on the maternal side. Thornton and Macdonald's (1999) study of female twins suggests that genetic inheritance in pre-eclampsia is multifactorial and may not be as significant as originally believed. Smith *et al.* (1997) suggest that a familial link may arise from the male side. A large-scale study of the genetic contribution to pre-eclampsia is currently underway in the UK (Broughton, 1999).

The condition is more likely to develop in young teenagers and women over 35 years of age; obesity, diabetes mellitus, multiple pregnancy and black race are widely considered to be predisposing factors and women with essential or renal hypertension may develop a superimposed pre-eclampsia (Roberts, 2000). The condition commonly arises, after 32 weeks, but it may occur as early as 20–24 weeks in rare instances, especially when associated with hydatidiform mole.

Dietary aspects have also been considered, and some studies suggest that there is a link between low dietary calcium and pre-eclampsia (Lopez-Jaramillo, 2000). Hypocalciuria appears to be more common in women with pre-eclampsia than in those who are normotensive. Preliminary studies suggest that calcium supplementation may be beneficial and multicentre trials are currently underway (Hojo and August, 2000). Norwitz *et al.* (1999) observe that work is now emerging that suggests that calcium levels are crucial in the production of nitric oxide, which is a potent vasodilator produced in endothelial cells, also capable of inhibiting platelet aggregation. Further work (Chappell *et al.*, 1999) suggests an association with oxidant stress, and a study of antioxidant vitamins administered to pregnant women suggests they may be beneficial.

However, Action on Pre-eclampsia (APEC, 1999) warns pregnant women against self-administration of such vitamins until further trials have taken place.

Diagnosis

It has been customary to describe pre-eclampsia as mild, moderate or severe, but Norwitz *et al.*, (1999) contend that there is no category of moderate pre-eclampsia. They suggest that severe pre-eclampsia should be diagnosed when women with new-onset hypertension and proteinuria (their classification of mild pre-eclampsia) develop one or more of the following: blurred vision, severe headache, confusion, seizures, epigastric pain, oliguria, pulmonary oedema, coagulopathy, or haemolysis elevated liver enzymes low platelets (HELLP) syndrome.

Three major areas for consideration when screening for pre-eclampsia are blood pressure, urinalysis and oedema. These are discussed below.

Blood pressure A reading of 140/90 mmHg is regarded as the upper limit of normal, but a rise in diastolic blood pressure of 15–20 mmHg or more above the level recorded in the early weeks of pregnancy is significant (Moran and Davison, 1999). The diastolic pressure is of more significance than the systolic because it is not affected by posture and other factors such as stress and excitement, although Cartwright *et al.* (1992) suggest that when blood pressure is monitored serially, there is no difference in anxiety levels between women monitored at home and those monitored in hospital. Moran and Davison (1999) suggest that a sustained reading of 140/90 mmHg over 15 minutes warrants further investigation in a relaxed setting. Blood pressure estimations should be made at 30-minute intervals over a 2-hour period, and the mean calculated from this.

Widely differing methods of obtaining blood pressure readings are adopted, leading to gross variability of results (Brown and Simpson, 1992). There is often a lack of consensus about whether the diastolic pressure should be measured at the 'muffling' stage or at the disappearance of sounds. It is recommended that the diastolic measurement is taken at the 'muffling' or IV stage of the Korotkov sounds since, during pregnancy, there may not be complete disappearance of sound. Maternal position should be such that the sphygmomanometer cuff is at the same level as the left atrium. Large-size cuffs should be available for those women who need them; Mahomed and James (1988) suggest a larger cuff size for women weighing more than 85 kg.

Moran and Davison (1999) recommend that blood pressure is recorded from both arms at the initial visit, and thereafter on the right arm. Although automated blood pressure devices may be useful, a small study of 30 women with pre-eclampsia carried out in the USA suggested that automated blood pressure recording machines may underestimate blood pressure by as much as 30 mmHg (Natarajan *et al.*, 1999). This must be taken into account if automatic machines are used. Standardization of techniques within individual institutions will ensure consistency in recordings (Lewis, 2001).

Reflective Activity 45.2

How does *your* technique of taking blood pressure compare with the above?

Does your unit have a clear policy for the standard of measuring blood pressure?

Urinalysis   Proteinuria + or more on dipstick, in an uncontaminated specimen, and in the absence of infection is always serious in conjunction with hypertension. It indicates damage to endothelial tissue with leakage of albumin, the smallest plasma protein, from the blood into the urine. Protein loss changes osmotic pressure within the capillaries and may lead to the development of oedema. The study by North *et al.* (1999) of 1496 nulliparous women suggests that adverse maternal and fetal outcomes increase almost fourfold in the presence of proteinuria. Hypertension and proteinuria occurring prior to 33 weeks' gestation often has a poor prognosis (Mattar and Sibbai, 1999).

Volume and concentration of urine affect random readings and protein excretion is variable according to time of day. 24-hour urine collections remain the 'gold standard' for quantification of protein, and significant proteinuria is said to exist where protein exceeds 300 mg/24 hours.

Urine should also be tested to exclude infection (Moran and Davison, 1999).

Oedema   Although 85% of women with pre-eclampsia will develop oedema, it is no longer considered a cardinal sign of pre-eclampsia, because it is so often a feature of normotensive as well as hypertensive pregnancies. Changes in the cardiovascular system, including increased plasma volume, lead to the development of physiological oedema in pregnancy (Ch. 17). Physiological oedema usually affects only the lower legs, and normally resolves when the woman lies down.

Pathological oedema associated with pre-eclampsia may be present in the pretibial area, hands, face and abdomen, and does not resolve with rest. Excessive weight gain may be due to occult oedema.

During the latter half of pregnancy, normal weight gain should be approximately 0.5 kg per week. Weight gain significantly in excess of this, sometimes defined as exceeding 2 kg in a 1-week period, accompanied by hypertension and proteinuria is likely to be associated with pre-eclampsia (National High Blood Pressure Education Program Working Group, 1990).

Diagnostic tests   Hypertension and proteinuria are not the only signs of pre-eclampsia, or necessarily the most important; they constitute evidence of end organ damage within an ongoing process. Diagnostic tests to assess renal function, cardiovascular changes and liver enzymes are necessary to diagnose the extent to which the maternal system is affected (British Eclampsia Survey Team, 1994; Douglas and Redman, 1994).

The midwife's responsibility

Diagnosis is usually made on physical signs rather than symptoms. This is important, since a woman may have severe pre-eclampsia and yet feel well. Early diagnosis is essential; thus, midwives must begin with an accurate recording of the woman's history to identify risk factors and establish a baseline blood pressure using a standardized technique (Moran and Davison, 1999). Thereafter, regular antenatal screening involves blood pressure readings, testing urine at each visit for protein, and assessing for significant non-dependent oedema.

Although hypertension and proteinuria, with or without oedema, occur in pre-eclampsia, the severity of these signs varies considerably. A small number of women present with symptoms such as headache, visual disturbances, epigastric pain or generally feeling unwell, which may be indicative of serious systemic complications, and may be followed by eclampsia (Barry *et al.*, 1994). If a woman complains of these symptoms, the midwife must take her blood pressure, test the urine for protein, and then refer her to an obstetrician immediately, even if her blood pressure is not significantly raised. It is now known that convulsions may precede hypertension or proteinuria (DoH, 1998; Lewis, 2001). Following referral, women need follow-up care in a multidisciplinary team setting.

Day assessment units (DAUs) or maternity day units (MDUs) offer facilities for ongoing assessment on an outpatient basis, with mothers actively involved in their own screening programmes (Moran and Davison,

1999). All of the following tests can be carried out in this setting.

Assessment of renal functions

- *Uric acid levels* indicate progress and severity of pre-eclampsia with increased levels in cases of hypertension, usually before the development of proteinuria.
- *Blood urea and creatinine* levels are raised, and a high level indicates a late stage of renal involvement.
- *24-hour urinary protein excretion* is >0.3 g.

Assessment of liver functions

Serial measurements of *liver enzymes,* particularly transaminase, and liver function tests should be carried out.

Assessment of coagulation complications

Repeated investigations to detect the development of coagulation complications should also be performed. These investigations include:

- *blood film*
- *platelet count*, which often decreases in pre-eclampsia
- *coagulation studies:* coagulation levels are usually unchanged in pre-eclampsia, unless disseminated intravascular coagulation is present, when thrombin time will be prolonged in the presence of fibrin degradation, heparin or reduced fibrinogen.

The multisystem nature of the condition is reflected in changes which take place in the blood and may give rise to the HELLP syndrome, characterized by <u>h</u>aemolysis, <u>e</u>levated <u>l</u>iver <u>p</u>roteins and <u>l</u>ow <u>p</u>latelets.

Reflective Activity 45.3

Visit a maternity day assessment unit and find out what tests are carried out to assess the progress of pre-eclampsia.

List what the normal test results should be.

Assessment of fetal well-being

Pre-eclampsia is associated with a reduction in maternal placental blood flow which results in IUGR and hypoxia of the fetus. Any deterioration in the fetal condition will influence the management. The following investigations may be used to assess fetal condition:

- *Cardiotocography:* although this can be unreliable at under 30 weeks' gestation, a reactive and variable trace is generally indicative of satisfactory fetal condition. Loss of variability or decelerations suggest

deterioration. Walker (2000) suggests that the tracings can be reassuring for the mother.
- *Measurement of symphyseal–fundal height.*
- *A record of fetal movements* (kick chart).
- *Ultrasound scanning* for:
  - amniotic fluid index
  - fetal growth – as fetal growth restriction may occur prior to any other signs of pre-eclampsia (Lewis, 2001)
  - umbilical artery Doppler analysis.

In case of abnormality in any of the above, Moran and Davison (1999) suggest a biophysical profile is performed, which includes:

- record of fetal breathing movements
- tone
- gross body movements
- heart rate activity
- liquor volume.

Women attending the DAU/MDU will need to be kept fully informed of their situation, and may need considerable support from the midwife. Women who have experienced pre-eclampsia speak of how frightened they were and how they feared for their baby (Redman and Walker, 1996) and reported that compassionate care from the midwife was appreciated.

Reflective Activity 45.4

Review the literature available locally for pregnant women, and the level of information available to women.

Women who develop significant proteinuria, or who experience any of the previously described symptoms of severe pre-eclampsia require admission to hospital. The woman with essential hypertension who develops proteinuria is likely to have superimposed pre-eclampsia rather than a worsening of essential hypertension. During the hospital stay, the monitoring that is undertaken is similar to that in the DAU/MDU, but it will take place more frequently.

Severe pre-eclampsia

Depending on the severity of pre-eclampsia and the gestation, conservative treatment may 'buy time' to bring the fetus to optimum time of delivery, without endangering the mother. Moran and Davison (1999) suggest that, excluding women with diabetes, renal disease, thrombocytopenia and IUGR, pregnancy may be prolonged by up to 15 days without maternal compromise. Antihypertensive drugs control the blood pressure, although they do not improve the underlying effects of the disease. However, controlling the blood pressure reduces the risk of cerebral haemorrhage and eclampsia, and therefore the risk of maternal death (Moran and Davison, 1999). Mattar and Sibai (1999) suggest that outcome is poorest for women who develop pre-eclampsia at or before 32 weeks. However, attempts to secure a more mature fetus must not lead obstetricians to underestimate the dangers of the disease, which may be progressive despite apparent control of the blood pressure by antihypertensive drugs (DoH, 1998).

The dangers to mother and baby are:

- *Maternal:* eclampsia, placental abruption, disseminated intravascular coagulation, pulmonary oedema, cerebral oedema, cerebrovascular accident, renal or hepatic failure, and maternal death.
- *Fetal:* IUGR, fetal hypoxia, preterm delivery, intrauterine death.

Management
The midwife is part of the multidisciplinary team approach in which the aim of management is to deliver the baby before life-threatening complications occur. In addition to ongoing monitoring of blood pressure and urine, the following are significant:

Bedrest Although bedrest is traditionally advised for women with severe pre-eclampsia, Norwitz *et al.* (1999) point out that the course of the disease and the perinatal outcome is unchanged as a result of bedrest, even for women at high risk. Moran and Davison (1999) point out that bedrest itself carries the risk of thromboembolism.

Fluid balance Accurate monitoring of fluid intake and urinary output is essential for the detection of oliguria and the avoidance of overtransfusion. Oliguria (less than 30 ml output per hour) indicates renal involvement. Pulmonary complications due to intravenous overload accounted directly for two maternal deaths in the 1994–1996 triennium (DoH, 1998), and one in the 1997–1999 triennium (Lewis, 2001). Pulmonary oedema was also a factor in some of the six deaths due to adult respiratory distress syndrome (DoH, 1998). Although diuretics are not used to control hypertension in pre-eclampsia, in severe cases where intensive therapy is given, and where a central venous pressure line is in situ, diuretics may be used where pulmonary overload is suspected (Davison and Moran, 1999).

Antihypertensive drugs *Methyldopa* 1–3 mg daily in divided doses given intravenously or orally is commonly used to treat hypertension in pregnancy; it acts centrally by inhibiting sympathetic outflow and the overview of clinical trials on its use suggests that it significantly reduces the risk of developing severe hypertension (Collins and Wallenburg, 1989). One of its side-effects is depression, so it is not suitable for postnatal use (Moran and Davison, 1999).

Labetolol, a combined α- and β-antagonist acts to reduce peripheral resistance and cardiac output, thereby reducing blood pressure, but in common with β-adrenoceptor antagonists such as propanolol and atenolol, may result in severe fetal and neonatal bradycardia (Collins and Wallenburg, 1989). Nevertheless, it is suggested that it is generally as safe and effective as methyldopa, and that its antihypertensive action may be more controlled than that of hydralazine (Collins and Wallenburg, 1989).

Hydralazine is a vasodilator and may be given orally or intravenously. It is an effective antihypertensive drug, but when given intravenously may lead to sudden maternal hypotension.

Calcium antagonists such as *nifedipine* lower blood pressure by the inhibition of calcium ion activity in the smooth muscles of blood vessels, resulting in a decrease in peripheral vascular resistance.

Aspirin has been the subject of clinical trials including the Collaborative Low-dose Aspirin Studies in Pregnancy (CLASP) – to assess its use in the prevention and treatment of pregnancy-induced hypertension. Results of earlier trials (de Swiet and Fryers, 1990) suggest that aspirin is most effective when low doses (60 mg per day) are given to women considered at higher risk of developing pre-eclampsia, rather than for the treatment of those who actually develop these disorders. In addition, low-dose aspirin may be of value in the treatment of IUGR. However, despite hopes for a significant beneficial role, aspirin has not yielded the definite results which were indicated by the initial small trials. In a large multicentre study of 9354 pregnant women, randomly allocated 60 mg aspirin daily or matching placebo, there was no significant reduction in preeclampsia, IUGR, stillbirth or neonatal death (CLASP, 1994). There was a slight, but significant reduction in preterm delivery, and an indication that low-dose aspirin may be beneficial before 20 weeks' gestation for women who have a previous history of early pre-eclampsia.

Debate still continues over dosage and gestation at which aspirin should be given (Duley, 1999).

During the woman's stay in hospital, as well as the need for the monitoring of the physical condition of mother and fetus, it is also important to use the opportunity to ensure that the mother has some parenting education, which should include a visit to the Neonatal Intensive Care Unit, and a chance to talk to the staff there. Women and their families may be extremely anxious, and information and full involvement in decision-making is crucial for them at this time (Hartley, 1998).

Ongoing assessment

The development of any of the following signifies a deterioration in the maternal condition:

1. Severe frontal headache, probably associated with cerebral oedema.
2. Visual disturbances, resulting from oedema of the retina. The vision may be dim or blurred, the woman saying that she cannot see to read; or she may see spots or flashes of light.
3. Vomiting, which may be related to cerebral oedema or associated with (4).
4. Epigastric pain caused by haemorrhages under the liver capsule; this can be a warning that eclampsia is imminent. Barry *et al.* (1994) studied cases where upper abdominal pain was the first indication of pre-eclampsia and this symptom had been variously misdiagnosed as dyspepsia and urinary tract infection. Pain may also be associated with placental abruption.
5. Oliguria, may indicate the onset of eclampsia or renal involvement.

Not all women with severe pre-eclampsia present all these symptoms and signs. Indeed any one symptom, with or without hypertension and proteinuria, is sufficient to indicate that the condition is worsening and that eclampsia may be imminent.

Care at home/in the community

Whilst many women may already be in hospital, having earlier shown some of the signs of pre-eclampsia, the midwife may have to deal with a situation, within the community setting, in which a woman develops eclampsia with little warning. The principles of care which follow will be the same, but will require the midwife to bring medical expertise to the woman, in order to stabilize her condition sufficiently for transfer. A general practitioner may already be present, but a senior obstetrician should be consulted. A plan of management should be made, and practitioners should be aware of the rapidity with which eclampsia can progress, and that delay in adequate treatment following admission to hospital may lead to significant morbidity, or death (DoH, 1998; Lewis, 2001)

> ### Reflective Activity 45.5
>
> Check your unit protocol; how is the development of any of the above assessed and dealt with?

ECLAMPSIA

Eclampsia is the onset of convulsions in a pregnancy usually, but not always, complicated by pre-eclampsia. One in 200 women who have pre-eclampsia will develop eclampsia (Walker, 2000). However, in a national study conducted in the UK in 1992, 38% of cases of eclampsia were not preceded by hypertension and proteinuria (Douglas and Redman, 1994). Eclampsia occurs in the UK once in about 2000 births and carries serious risks for both mother and fetus. Douglas and Redman (1994) found that nearly 1 in 50 women who developed eclampsia died and 1 in 14 of their babies also died. Worldwide, 50 000 women die after suffering an eclamptic convulsion (Duley, 1994).

In severe pre-eclampsia there is likely to be cerebral hypoxia due to intense vasospasm and oedema. Cerebral hypoxia leads to increased cerebral dysrhythmia and this may be the cause of the convulsions. Some women have an underlying cerebral dysrhythmia and therefore convulsions may occur following less severe forms of pre-eclampsia.

The convulsions may occur before, during or after labour. Even if antenatal care and care in labour are of a high standard, postpartum convulsions may still occur. Monitoring of blood pressure and urine for proteinuria should therefore continue during the postpartum period.

There is one sign of eclampsia, namely, the eclamptic convulsion. This is similar to an epileptic seizure, and to aid medical differential diagnosis, it is important to observe carefully the duration and nature of the seizure. Four phases usually occur:

1. *Premonitory stage.* This transient stage may be missed if the woman is not under constant observation. She will roll her eyes, while facial and hand muscles twitch momentarily.
2. *Tonic stage.* Almost immediately muscles go into violent spasm. The fists are clenched and arms and

legs are rigid. The woman will clench her teeth and may bite her tongue. Since respiratory muscles are in spasm, she stops breathing and the colour becomes deeply cyanosed. This spasm continues for perhaps 30 seconds.

3. *Clonic stage.* As the spasm ceases, jerky muscular movements begin and become increasingly violent. The whole body is thrown restlessly from side to side, while frothy, often bloodstained saliva appears at the lips. The breathing is stertorous and mucus or blood may be inhaled from the mouth. Convulsive movements gradually subside. This restless phase lasts up to 2 minutes and is followed by a period of coma.

4. *Comatose stage.* The woman is deeply unconscious and perhaps breathing noisily. The cyanosis fades, but her face may remain swollen and congested. Sometimes she regains consciousness in a few minutes or the coma may persist for hours.

Dangers

Maternal   If hypertension is greatly increased, the woman may have a cerebral haemorrhage. Women with massive oedema and oliguria can develop pulmonary oedema or renal failure. Inhalation of blood or mucus may lead to asphyxia or pneumonia. Any of these complications may be fatal. The number of maternal deaths from eclampsia in the UK in 1997–1999 was 5 (Lewis, 2001), all of which occurred in hospital. It is not unusual for women to die after only one seizure (DoH, 1998; Lewis, 2001).

Fetal   The fetus may already be affected by placental insufficiency. This leads to IUGR and hypoxia. During the seizure when the mother stops breathing, the fetal oxygen supply, already impaired, is further reduced. Intrapartum convulsions are also very hazardous to the fetus because intrauterine hypoxia is already increased owing to the uterine contractions.

Management

During a seizure   The main points are:
- Maintain a clear airway, using position. Use of mouthgags and similar objects is no longer approved.
- Protect the woman from injury.
- The woman should be turned on to her side as gently as possible. The mouth is cleared of mucus and blood with suction apparatus, although vigorous suction should be avoided, as this may induce vomiting.

- Oxygen is given, as it will benefit both mother and fetus.

Subsequent management
- Control of convulsions.
- Control of hypertension.
- Deliver the baby.

Anticonvulsant and antihypertensive drugs are given immediately to try to stabilize eclampsia and to lower the blood pressure. Labour is then induced or caesarean section is performed. The risks of eclampsia, placental insufficiency and abruption, and intrauterine fetal death must be considered against those of prematurity (DoH, 1998; Lewis, 2001).

Magnesium sulphate is an effective anticonvulsant and acts rapidly. The findings of the Eclampsia Collaborative Trial Group (ECTG) conclude that magnesium sulphate is more effective in reducing and preventing eclamptic convulsions than both diazepam and phenytoin (ECTG, 1995). Women in the trial who received magnesium sulphate had a 52% lower risk of convulsions than those given diazepam, and a 67% lower risk than those given phenytoin. The World Health Organization now recommends the use of magnesium sulphate for the treatment of eclampsia (WHO, 1995).

An initial intravenous injection of 4–5 g in a 20% solution may be given, over 5–10 minutes, followed by an infusion of 1–2 g/hour. This should be continued for 24 hours after the last seizure (Lewis, 2001). It is believed to inhibit presynaptic activity but does not have antihypertensive or sedative properties. It is administered intravenously, and blood levels must be monitored regularly to ensure that these remain within the therapeutic range (2–4 mmol/l). Toxicity leads to loss of maternal reflexes and eventually muscle paralysis, respiratory arrest and cardiac arrest. For this reason, midwives must be aware of the signs of toxicity, which are loss of patella reflexes; weakness; nausea; flushes; sleepiness; double vision; and slurred speech. The antidote is intravenous calcium gluconate 10 ml of 10% solution (Moran and Davison, 1999). There are no known long-term adverse fetal or neonatal effects, but a study by Riaz *et al.* (1998) of 26 infants whose mothers received magnesium sulphate, suggests they were hypotonic and had lower Apgar scores immediately after delivery than the control group of 26.

At the consultant's discretion, diazepam may be used if the seizures continue, though it is important to consider other causes of fits if they continue, and a CAT scan may be required.

Blood pressure is controlled by the use of antihypertensive drugs. Diuretic treatment is indicated when the urinary output is less than 20 ml/hour. Antibiotics may be prescribed to prevent pulmonary infection.

Biochemical tests to assess renal function, thrombocytopenia and liver enzymes are performed to give information about the extent to which the maternal system is affected, and early warning of the HELLP syndrome.

Midwifery care   The scope of midwifery care is dependent on the severity of illness, and is similar in severe pre-eclampsia and eclampsia. Women may be extremely ill and may be cared for in a high-dependency unit (HDU) by a multidisciplinary team. An HDU or ICU chart should be used to record all observations and care.

Any stimulus may precipitate convulsions, so external stimuli such as noise, bright lights and handling are reduced to a minimum. The woman is kept in a quiet, single room and, until her condition is stabilized, she must never be left alone. Suction apparatus and oxygen equipment must be available. Although bright sunshine should be excluded, the room should be light enough for the midwife to be able to assess the woman's condition without switching lights on and off. Only essential procedures such as turning 2-hourly to avoid hypostatic pneumonia, mouth care and treatment of pressure areas are carried out initially.

Observations

1. Restlessness or twitching may indicate a convulsion.
2. Continuous oxygen saturation should be measured. Cyanosis is an important sign of cardiorespiratory failure, and therefore the midwife should be able to monitor this visually as well as electronically. Cyanosis is an indication for the administration of oxygen.
3. The temperature is recorded hourly. If there is no obvious sign of infection, a rise in temperature could indicate anoxic damage to the temperature-regulating centres in the midbrain.
4. Pulse and respirations may be recorded as often as every 15 minutes.
5. Blood pressure will be recorded frequently, probably continuously, half-hourly, or hourly. If automatic sphygmomanometers are used, there should be an initial check using a traditional machine to monitor any difference between the two machines (Lewis, 2001; RCOG, 1996). When antihypertensives are used, women should be warned about postural hypotension, and encouraged to get up slowly.

6. Central venous pressure (CVP) readings should be measured every 15–20 minutes.
7. An accurate record of fluid intake and output is essential. Intravenous fluids will be given rather than oral fluids and nourishment and a second infusion may be required for the administration of drugs. The importance of avoiding intravenous overload cannot be overemphasized.

    A self-retaining catheter is inserted into the bladder and released hourly; thus urinary output can be measured accurately and the woman will not have to be disturbed to pass urine. A urinary output of less than 30 ml/hour suggests renal involvement. Urine is tested for protein.
8. The fetal heart is continuously monitored.
9. Monitor for signs of labour, as this may start spontaneously. Any loss per vaginam is noted and the fundus should be gently palpated if the woman appears to be restless at regular intervals because she could be being disturbed by uterine contractions. A comatose woman could progress to an advanced stage of labour unless the signs are recognized by an observant midwife.
10. Blood should be taken every 12–24 hours for full blood count, urea and electrolytes, creatinine and liver function tests.
11. Information and support should be provided to the woman, and to her family, in clear terms that they will understand. This may require the use of a translator if English is not their first language.

CARE DURING LABOUR AND POSTNATALLY

Mode of delivery

Pre-eclampsia will resolve only after delivery. Moran and Davison (1999) contend that fetal maturity can be assumed at 36 weeks, and that if the woman has reached that far she is likely to have a vaginal delivery. The disease usually resolves within 48–72 hours of delivery.

As soon as the woman's condition is stabilized, arrangements are made for delivery. Walker (2000) suggests that rushing the delivery contributes to postpartum risks, but there should be no unnecessary delay. The woman should be transferred to a unit with more specialized facilities, especially those for neonatal intensive care, and discussion between senior medical staff at each institution must occur (Walker, 2000).

Dexamethosone or betamethosone may be given intramuscularly or orally to aid fetal lung maturity, and their effects are beneficial even before 24 hours have elapsed. Walker (2000) suggests that prior to 32 weeks, caesarean section is appropriate, but that after 34 weeks, vaginal delivery should be aimed for.

Care in labour for women with pre-eclampsia or eclampsia

In addition to the midwifery care already described, and the continuation of observations, effective analgesia is essential and can best be achieved by epidural anaesthesia. This has the advantage of lowering the blood pressure, although it is more advantageous in preventing the rise in blood pressure associated with pain in labour. Continuous monitoring of the fetal heart and uterine contractions should be carried out. As long as the woman's condition remains stable there is no need for routine instrumental delivery (Walker, 2000).

Syntocinon should be given for third stage delivery, since ergometrine causes a rise in blood pressure.

A paediatrician, or practitioner skilled in neonatal resuscitation must be present at the birth.

Management after delivery

Following an initial improvement after delivery, 60% of women will worsen within 48 hours, and most maternal deaths occur in the postpartum period (Moran and Davison, 1999; Walker, 2000). Antihypertensive drugs are usually continued for a further 48 hours, and postpartum seizures may occur.

The special midwifery care and observations previously described are continued. Symptoms such as severe headache, vomiting and epigastric pain should alert the midwife to seek help from a senior obstetrician. Unsatisfactory postpartum care accounts for a significant proportion of the mortality from pre-eclampsia and eclampsia (DoH, 1998; Lewis, 2001). Depending on the gestational age, the baby may be cared for in the neonatal intensive care unit or in a postnatal area with the mother. Parents must be appropriately supported to care for their baby, and, given the connection between SIDS and pre-eclampsia, they should be encouraged to follow the protocols for preventing SIDS (Wi and Li, 2000).

Reflective Activity 45.6

Is there a copy of the latest confidential enquiry into maternal deaths available on the maternity unit?

Review the chapter on hypertensive disorders of pregnancy.

Consider:

- Do you think any of these case studies could happen in your unit/locality?
- Does your unit management mirror the recommendations – if not, why not?

Psychological care

Problems which may result from hypertensive disorders may be minor, and be a matter of the woman needing medication to control her blood pressure, or may be major, and result in her having instrumental delivery, and even requiring high-dependency or intensive care. This may be considerably different from the woman's expectations. It can also cause post-traumatic stress syndrome, with debilitating symptoms such as flashbacks, nightmares and depression (Hammett, 1992).

The midwife needs to provide space and an opportunity for the woman, and often her partner, to review and debrief. This will often clarify issues of confusion for the woman, and help her begin to understand and accept events. It also allows the midwife to identify a woman who may require additional support or counselling.

Follow-up investigations of blood pressure or assessment of renal function may be necessary for women who have suffered serious hypertensive disease in pregnancy. They may also be advised to obtain preconception advice and counselling before embarking on a future pregnancy. Eclampsia rarely occurs in a subsequent pregnancy, but pre-eclampsia recurs in up to 1:20 cases where severe pre-eclampsia was present in a first pregnancy, and in up to 1:3 where it occurred in a second pregnancy (Redman and Walker, 1996). It is not associated with a higher incidence of essential hypertension in later life.

The charity Action on Pre-eclampsia (APEC) seeks to inform all pregnant women of the risks of pregnancy-induced hypertension, emphasizing the fact that the disorder is largely asymptomatic and must be diagnosed by active screening. Whilst the charity welcomes the demedicalization of childbirth, it emphasizes the importance of informing women and securing their cooperation in all aspects of antenatal care (APEC, 1992). This is congruent with the midwifery concept of health promotion (Crafter, 2000), and the participation of women in their own antenatal care, by regular antenatal checks, by providing a urine specimen, and by being aware of the significance of headaches, visual disturbances and abdominal pain. It could be argued that some women will be inappropriately stressed by unnecessary tests and investigations, and some will develop pre-eclampsia despite regular antenatal care.

However, pre-eclampsia only reveals itself in its final stages, and until a cause is isolated, midwives and obstet- ricians tread a fine line between over- and underdiagnosis (Bewley, 2000). The Report on Confidential Enquiries into Maternal Deaths (DoH, 1998) notes that recent advances in detection and management of pre-eclampsia mean that few professionals will ever come across severe pre-eclampsia or eclampsia. The report reiterates the need for local specialized teams within regions, who can act either in an advisory capacity, or within suitably equipped and staffed high-dependency units. It also stresses the need for a lead consultant and clear guidelines for the management of severe pre-eclampsia and eclampsia in each maternity unit.

Despite the strong recommendation in recent reports for a regional advisory service, there is no record of help being sought from such a service in any of the deaths from hypertensive disorders in this report (DoH, 1998).

ESSENTIAL/CHRONIC HYPERTENSION

Essential hypertension is a condition of permanently raised blood pressure, often with no apparent cause. It may also be associated with renal disease (see Ch. 48), phaeochromocytoma or coarctation of the aorta. It is familial and complicates 2–5% of all pregnancies (Roberts and Redman, 1993) with 15–20% of women developing a superimposed pre-eclampsia (Sibai, 1991). A woman attending the antenatal clinic is said to have essential hypertension if her blood pressure in early pregnancy is 140/90 mmHg or more, or her 6-week postpartum blood pressure remains high following hypertension in pregnancy. It is distinguished from pre-eclampsia by the fact that it is present in the early weeks of pregnancy, long before pre-eclampsia normally arises, and, in the absence of renal disease, there is no oedema or proteinuria.

Mid trimester, the blood pressure often falls to a normal level, which may mask hypertension if the woman begins antenatal care after the 18th week of pregnancy.

Management

The woman will require antenatal care from a consultant obstetrician, physician and midwife. She is likely to have a normal pregnancy and labour but is advised to avoid excessive weight gain. She should be advised not to smoke, as this contributes to hypertension. Fetal well-being is monitored closely to detect growth restriction. Antihypertensive drugs may be prescribed if the diastolic blood pressure exceeds 100 mmHg (Sibai, 1991). Investigations are carried out as described for pre-eclampsia. In addition, urinary catecholamines or vanillylmandelic acid (VMA) are usually measured because severe hypertension may be caused by phaeochromocytoma, a tumour of the adrenals.

Renal failure, heart failure and cerebral haemorrhage are potential complications if the blood pressure is exceptionally high. The fetus is at risk, because the placental circulation is poor; hence IUGR and hypoxia may occur.

If the blood pressure cannot be controlled or there are signs of fetal growth restriction or hypoxia, labour is induced or, if the danger is more acute or arises earlier, caesarean section may be performed. Women with essential or chronic hypertension require the same midwifery input as women with pre-eclampsia; however, from a psychological point of view, their disease is ongoing and progressive.

CONCLUSION

Hypertension complicates a significant number of pregnancies, causing a number of potential problems. Midwives play a key role in the detection of pre-eclampsia, and the care of women who experience hypertensive disorders during pregnancy. The midwife should work to develop a partnership role, during which she should ensure that the woman is sufficiently informed and prepared, in order that she can report any problems and unusual symptoms early. In addition, within the multidisciplinary team, the midwife may be one of the few constant practitioners, who can provide the element of continuity, and ensure that the care and management of the woman both during and following the pregnancy is holistic and developed to ensure as positive and safe an experience as is possible.

KEY POINTS

- Hypertensive disorders of pregnancy include pre-existing essential or chronic hypertension, hypertension associated with renal disease, pre-eclampsia and eclampsia.
- Pre-eclampsia and eclampsia are major contributors to maternal and perinatal mortality and morbidity.
- Involvement of senior midwifery and medical personnel at an early stage, and throughout the care is essential.

- Women and their partners need information about pre-eclampsia and its effects, given in a sensitive way.
- Effective assessment, monitoring and referral by the midwife will ensure that care is tailored to the woman's needs and that complications are speedily dealt with.
- Follow-up investigations may be necessary to safeguard women's physical and psychological well-being.

REFERENCES

Action on Pre-eclampsia (APEC) (1992) APEC gets the official go-ahead. *APEC Newsletter* **2**: 1.

Action on Pre-eclampsia (APEC) (1999) Don't self treat with megavitamins in pregnancy, warns national charity. Evidence about vitamins C and E for preventing pre-eclampsia needs confirmation and safety checks. *APEC* Sept: 2.

Barry, C., Fox, R. & Stirrat, G. (1994) Upper abdominal pain may indicate pre-eclampsia. *British Medical Journal* **308**(6943): 1562–1563.

Bewley, C. (2000) Abstract writer's comments. *MIDIRS Midwifery Digest* **10**(4): 456.

British Eclampsia Survey Team BEST Report (1994) Eclampsia in the United Kingdom. *British Medical Journal* **309**: 1395–1399.

Broughton, F.B. (1999) Genetics of pre-eclampsia: ideas at the turn of the millennium. *Current Obstetrics and Gynaecology* **9**(4): 179–182.

Brown, M.A. & Simpson, J.M. (1992) Diversity of blood pressure recording during pregnancy: implications for the hypertensive disorders. *Medical Journal of Australia* **156**(5): 306–308.

Cartwright, W., Dalton, K.J., Swindells, H. *et al.* (1992) Objective measurement of anxiety in hypertensive pregnant women managed in hospital and in the community. *British Journal of Obstetrics and Gynaecology* **99**(3): 182–185.

Chamberlain, G. (1991) ABC of antenatal care: Raised blood pressure in pregnancy. *British Medical Journal* **302**(6790): 1454–1458.

Chappell, L., Seed, P.T., Briley, A.L. *et al.* (1999) Effects of antioxidants on the occurrence of pre-eclampsia in women at increased risk: a randomised trial. *Lancet* **354**(9181): 810–816.

Collaborative Low-Dose Aspirin Study in Pregnancy Collaborative Group (CLASP) (1994) CLASP: a randomised trial of low-dose aspirin for the prevention and treatment of pre-eclampsia among 9364 pregnant women. *Lancet* **343**(8898): 619–629.

Collins, R. & Wallenburg, H.C.S. (1989) Pharmacological prevention and treatment of hypertensive disorders in pregnancy. In: Chalmers, I., Enkin, M. & Kierse, M.J.N.C. (eds) *Effective Care in Pregnancy and Childbirth*. Oxford: Oxford University Press.

Crafter, H. (2000) Working with Action on Pre-eclampsia: the role of a childbirth charity advisor and trustee. *MIDIRS Midwifery Digest* **10**(2): 184–186.

De Swiet, M. & Fryers, G. (1990) Review: the use of aspirin in pregnancy. *Journal of Obstetrics and Gynaecology* **10**(6): 467–482.

Department of Health (DoH) (1998) *Why Mothers Die: Report on Confidential Enquiries into Maternal Deaths in the United Kingdom 1994–96*. London: Stationery Office.

Douglas, K.A. & Redman, C.W.G. (1994) Eclampsia in the United Kingdom. *British Medical Journal* **309**(6966): 1395–1400.

Duley, L. (1994) Maternal mortality and eclampsia: the eclampsia trial. *MIDIRS Midwifery Digest* **4**(2): 176–178.

Duley, L. (1999) Aspirin for preventing and treating pre-eclampsia (Editorial). *British Medical Journal* **318**(7186): 751–752.

Eclampsia Collaborative Trial Group (ECTG) (1995) Which anticonvulsant for women with eclampsia? Evidence from the Collaborative Eclampsia Trial. *Lancet* **345**(8963): 1455–1463.

Eras, J.L., Saftlas, A.F. & Triche, E. (2000) Abortion and its effect on risk of pre-eclampsia and transient hypertension. *Epidemiology* **11**(1): 36–43.

Hammett, P.L. (1992) Midwives and debriefing. In: Abbott P. & Sapsford R. (eds) *Research into Practice*, pp. 135–159. Buckingham: Open University Press.

Hartley, J. (1998) Diagnosis, treatment and care of the pre eclamptic woman. *RCM Midwives Journal* **1**(1): 17–20.

Hojo, M. & August, P. (2000) Calcium metabolism in pre-eclampsia: supplementation may help. *Pre-eclampsia Society Newsletter* **39**: 16–18.

Kilpatrick, D.C., Gibson, F. & Liston, W.A. (1989) Association between susceptibility to pre-eclampsia within families and HLA DR4. *Lancet* **11**(8671): 1063–1064.

Lewis, G. (ed) (2001) *Why Mothers Die 1997–99: Fifth Report of the Confidential Enquiries into Maternal*

Deaths in the United Kingdom. London: CEMD: associated with NICE, RCOG.

Li, D. & Wi, S. (2000) Maternal pre-eclampsia/eclampsia and the risk of sudden infant death in offspring. *Paediatric and Perinatal Epidemiology* 14(2): 141–144.

Lopez-Jaramillo, P. (2000) Calcium, nitric oxide, and pre-eclampsia. *Seminars in Perinatology* 24(1): 33–36.

Mahomed, K. & James, D.K. (1988) Hypertension in pregnancy: do we need to admit all mothers to hospital for assessment and management? *Journal of Obstetrics and Gynaecology* 8(4): 314–318.

Makhseed, M., Musini, V.M., Ahmed, M.A. *et al.* (1999) Influence of seasonal variation on pregnancy induced hypertension and/or pre-eclampsia. *Australian and New Zealand Journal of Obstetrics and Gynaecology* 39(2): 196–199.

Mattar, F. & Sibai, B.M. (1999) Eclampsia VIII. Risk factors for maternal morbidity. *American Journal of Obstetrics and Gynecology* 182(2): 307–312.

Moran, P. & Davison, J.M. (1999) Clinical management of established pre-eclampsia. *Baillière's Best Practice: Clinical Obstetrics and Gynaecology* 13(1): 77–93.

Natarajan, P., Shennan, A.H. & Penny, J. (1999) Comparison of auscaltatory and oscillometric automated blood pressure monitors in the setting of pre-eclampsia. *American Journal of Obstetrics and Gynecology* 181 (5 Pt 1): 1203–1210.

National High Blood Pressure Education Program Working Group (1990) National High Blood Pressure Education Program Working Group report on high blood pressure in pregnancy. *American Journal of Obstetrics and Gynecology* 163(5 Pt 1): 1691–1712.

North, R.A., Taylor, R.S. & Schellenberg, J.C. (1999) Evaluation of a definition of pre-eclampsia. *British Journal of Obstetrics and Gynaecology* 106(8): 767–773.

Norwitz, E.R., Robinson, J.N. & Repke, J.T. (1999) Prevention of pre-eclampsia: is it possible? *Clinical Obstetrics and Gynaecology* 42(3): 436–454.

Redman, C. & Walker, I. (1996) *Pre-eclampsia: The Facts.* Harrow: Action on Pre-eclampsia.

Riaz, M., Porat, B., Brodsky, N.L. *et al.* (1998) The effects of maternal magnesium sulfate treatment on newborns: a prospective controlled study. *Journal of Perinatology* 18(6 Pt 1): 449–454.

Roberts, J.M. (2000) Pre-eclampsia: what we know and what we do not know. *Seminars in Perinatology* 24(1): 24–28.

Roberts, J.M. & Redman, C. (1993) Pre-eclampsia: more than pregnancy induced hypertension. *Lancet* 341(8858): 1447–1451.

Robillard, P.Y., Hulsey, T.C. & Perianin, J. (1994) Association of pregnancy induced hypertension with duration of sexual cohabitation before conception. *Lancet* 344(8928): 973–975.

Royal College of Obstetricians and Gynaecologists (RCOG) (1996) *Clinical Green Top Guidelines. Management of Eclampsia.* Online. Available: http://www.rcog.org.uk.

Salas, S.P. (1999) What causes pre-eclampsia? *Baillière's Best Practice: Clinical Obstetrics and Gynaecology* 13(1): 41–57.

Sibai, B.M. (1991) Diagnosis and management of chronic hypertension in pregnancy. *Obstetrics and Gynecology* 78(3 Pt 1): 451–461.

Smith, G.N., Walker, M., Tessier, J.L. *et al.* (1997) Increased incidence of pre-eclampsia in women conceiving by intrauterine insemination with donor versus partner sperm for treatment of primary infertility. *American Journal of Obstetrics and Gynecology* 177(2): 455–458.

Thornton, J.G. & Macdonald, A.M. (1999) Twin mothers, pregnancy hypertension and pre-eclampsia. *British Journal of Obstetrics and Gynaecology* 106(6): 570–575.

Thornton, J.G. & Onwude, J.L. (1991) Pre-eclampsia: discordance among identical twins. *Lancet* 303(6812): 1241–1242.

Walker, J. (2000) Severe pre-eclampsia and eclampsia. *Baillière's Best Practice: Clinical Obstetrics and Gynaecology* 14(1): 57–71.

World Health Organization (WHO) (1995) Magnesium sulphate is the drug of choice for eclampsia. *Safe Motherhood – A Newsletter Of Worldwide Activity.* Issue 18(2), pp. 3, 13. Geneva: WHO.

FURTHER READING

McKay, K. (1999) Biochemical and blood tests in midwifery practice 1. Pre-eclampsia. *Practising Midwife* 2(8): 28–31.
A well set out overview of tests commonly performed in pre-eclampsia, with details of underlying physiology and pathophysiology. Reasons for carrying out tests are explained, and there is a table of normal and pregnancy affected values.

Redman, C.W.G. (2000) Pre-eclampsia. *Yearbook of Obstetrics and Gynaecology* 8: 97–108.
An excellent overview of the recent history of pre-eclampsia. Clear explanations of pathophysiological processes.

Walker, J. (2000) Severe pre-eclampsia and eclampsia. *Baillière's Best Practice: Clinical Obstetrics and Gynaecology* 14(1): 57–71.
A clearly written and practical account of the work of the Department of Obstetrics and Gynaecology, St James University Hospital, Leeds, in relation to pre-eclampsia and eclampsia. Protocols based on available evidence give the rationale for referral, diagnosis, further assessment and management. While written for medical staff, it will be of benefit to midwives.

46

Medical Disorders of Pregnancy

Chris Bewley

LEARNING OUTCOMES

After reading this chapter you will be able to:

- have an overview of some pre-existing medical and other disorders which affect or are affected by pregnancy
- gain insight into the underlying pathophysiology

- be familiar with some of the drugs used in various medical conditions
- realize the importance of the midwife's role in supporting women whose pregnancy is complicated by a medical disorder.

INTRODUCTION

Although pregnancy is a physiological event, it may be complicated by or complicate existing medical disorders. Women with complicated pregnancies report that they feel 'out of control' and experience high levels of anxiety. It is important for midwives to recognize the psychosocial impact on women as well as understand the pathophysiology of medical and other disorders. Women report that when they are ill, the focus of pregnancy tends to be on the developing fetus, and that once the baby is safely delivered, care is not so intense, and they feel isolated in the postnatal period (Thomas, 1999). This chapter highlights some of the existing and pre-existing conditions which women may experience, defines the condition, considers the incidence in pregnancy, outlines the effects on mother and fetus/neonate, describes treatment, and emphasizes specific midwifery care.

ANAEMIA

Anaemia is a deficiency in the quality or quantity of red blood cells, resulting in reduced oxygen-carrying capacity of the blood. It is commonly found during pregnancy, and contributes to maternal mortality and morbidity, particularly in developing countries (Guidotti, 2000). The World Health Organization's view, unchanged since 1979, is that anaemia is present in the pregnant woman when haemoglobin is 11 g/dl

or less (WHO, 1979). More arbitrary levels may be decided locally and usually range between 10–10.5 g/dl. In developing countries, anaemia as defined by WHO is widespread. It may be associated with poor nutrition or may arise as a consequence of intestinal parasites or malaria (van den Broek, 1998).

During pregnancy, total blood volume increases, mainly because of an increase in the volume of plasma. The red cell increase is proportionately less. This results in physiological haemodilution of the blood in pregnancy, leading to a lower level of haemoglobin (see Ch. 17).

To prevent this fall in haemoglobin level, iron was commonly given routinely in pregnancy and some still continue to prescribe it. However, the benefit of iron supplementation is now questioned and some studies show that the routine administration of iron may be superfluous or even harmful (Day, 1998). Oral iron may exacerbate sickness and cause constipation or diarrhoea. Levels of haemoglobin traditionally regarded as pathological in the non-pregnant woman are, in fact, associated with good obstetric outcomes (Steer *et al.*, 1995). The increase in plasma volume is essential to ensure perfusion of the vascular bed and maintenance of blood pressure and it is suggested that an increase in haemoglobin results in a decrease of blood flow through tissues. Mahomed's (1997) review of eight clinical trials revealed that routine supplementation with iron or folates maintained serum iron and ferritin levels, and reduced the number of women with Hb levels of 10 g/dl in late pregnancy. However, there were no significant effects on maternal or fetal outcomes. There is a need, therefore, to differentiate between physiological adaptation and a pathological condition.

Types of anaemia

Anaemias can be classified according to their causes:

1. Iron-deficiency anaemia
2. Folic acid deficiency anaemia
3. Haemoglobinopathies, which include sickle cell disease and thalassaemia
4. Anaemia as a result of blood loss or secondary to infection
5. Aplastic varieties, which are rare in pregnancy.

Effects on pregnancy

During pregnancy, anaemia will have the following effects:

- Undermining of the woman's general health
- Lowering of resistance to infection
- Exacerbation of the minor disorders of pregnancy such as digestive problems
- In severe cases – may cause intrauterine hypoxia
- Perinatal mortality is increased in severe anaemia
- Antepartum and postpartum haemorrhage are more serious
- Higher risk of thromboembolic disorders
- Increased risk of postnatal depression
- Risk of maternal mortality is increased.

Signs and symptoms

- Pallor of mucous membranes
- Tiredness, dizziness and fainting
- Dyspnoea on exertion
- Palpitations
- Oedema
- Digestive upsets and loss of appetite commonly occur and tend to exacerbate the condition.

Iron-deficiency anaemia

Iron deficiency is the commonest cause of anaemia in pregnancy. Anaemia may predate pregnancy and may occur in poorly nourished women, those who have menorrhagia, or those who have repeated pregnancies, especially if close together. Blood loss due to bleeding haemorrhoids or antepartum haemorrhage may also cause anaemia. Chronic infections such as pyelonephritis may also predispose to anaemia.

Malabsorption of iron may be associated with the intake of alkalis to relieve heartburn, or may be due to lack of vitamin C or to gastrointestinal disorders such as vomiting and diarrhoea.

Investigations

After taking a detailed history about general health, diet, infection, blood loss and other relevant information the following investigations may be carried out (McKay, 2000).

- *Haemoglobin measurements*.
- *Packed cell volume* (PCV) is the volume of red cells expressed as a fraction of the total volume of blood. It is normally 35–40% in pregnancy, but is reduced in anaemia.
- *Mean corpuscular volume* (MCV) is the average volume of a single red cell in cubic micrometres. It is normally about $90\,\mu m^3$ but is lower in iron-deficiency anaemia and higher in folic acid deficiency anaemia.
- *Mean corpuscular haemoglobin* (MCH) is the average amount of haemoglobin in each red cell. It is normally about 30 pg and is reduced in anaemia.
- *Serum iron and total iron-binding capacity*: in iron-deficiency anaemia the serum iron will be lower than 60 mg/100 ml (normal 60–120 mg/100 ml) and the total iron-binding capacity over 400 mg/100 ml (normal 325–400 mg/100 ml). This indicates depleted iron stores. Iron is absorbed from the intestines and bound to a protein. Almost two-thirds of the protein is not combined with iron and this is the iron-binding-capacity of the blood. It rises in anaemia. Serum ferritin below 10 mg/l indicates exhausted iron stores. The serum ferritin level falls up to the 28th–30th week of pregnancy. After that time it increases in women receiving iron supplementation but continues to fall in those not receiving iron therapy. Serum B_{12} and serum folate may also be estimated.
- A *midstream specimen of urine* is sent to the laboratory to detect infection.
- *Faecal specimens* are obtained if the anaemia is thought to arise from hookworm infestation.
- *Electrophoresis* may also be carried out to detect abnormal haemoglobins such as sickle cell disease or thalassaemia. This will usually include screening offered to the partner and genetic counselling preconceptually if possible.

Management

Where iron-deficiency anaemia has been diagnosed, oral iron 120–160 mg daily may be given as:

- *ferrous sulphate* – 200 mg tablet twice daily, giving 120 mg iron; or

- *ferrous gluconate* – two 300 mg tablets twice daily, giving 140 mg iron.

Women need to know that iron absorption is enhanced by vitamin C and inhibited by tannin in tea, and that there might be some side-effects such as blackness of stools, nausea, epigastric pain, diarrhoea and constipation. Side-effects are reduced by taking the iron after meals, but the type of iron supplement may need to be changed. This is also a good opportunity for the midwife to provide dietary advice (see Ch. 19).

In more severe cases of anaemia the woman may be given intramuscular injections of iron in the form of iron sorbital citrate complex known as Jectofer. The 2 ml ampoules contain 100 mg of iron, and a dose of 1.5 mg per kilogram body weight is usually given daily for 10–20 days. Special precautions should be taken when administering this, to avoid permanent staining of the skin.

Iron may also be given in an intravenous infusion. An iron–dextran complex (Imferon) is given in a total dose infusion over a few hours, the dose being calculated on body weight and the degree of anaemia. A test dose of 10 drops per minute is given for the first half hour and the woman is closely observed during this time as there is a risk of an anaphylactic reaction. If the woman tolerates the test dose, the infusion rate is then increased, but observations must continue every 15 or 30 minutes throughout the course of the infusion. The haemoglobin should begin to rise 2 or 3 weeks after this treatment.

Blood transfusions to treat anaemia are rarely necessary in pregnancy; though a woman who is very anaemic in late pregnancy may have blood cross-matched when she goes into labour and given if she has a postpartum haemorrhage.

Folic acid deficiency anaemia

Folic acid is necessary for the formation of the nuclei in all the body cells. In pregnancy, when there is proliferation of cells, a deficiency is likely to occur unless the intake of folic acid is increased. In the bone marrow a deficiency of folic acid leads to the formation of *megaloblasts*, which are large red cells (Marieb, 1999).

Megaloblastic anaemia is more common in women who are poorly nourished, in multiparous women and in those with a multiple pregnancy. It may also occur in women being treated with anticoagulant drugs, long-term sulphonamides or anticonvulsants, or in women drinking too much alcohol, as these substances interfere with folic acid metabolism. The anaemia is often fairly severe and fails to respond to iron therapy.

Diagnosis

The diagnosis of megaloblastic anaemia is usually made on examination of the peripheral blood. The red blood cells are large (macrocytic) and in severe cases there is poikilocytosis or irregularity in shape. The polymorphs are large and there may be a low platelet and white cell count. The serum folic acid is lower than 4 µg/ml.

Management

Dietary advice is important for those women considered to be at risk, for example those with a multiple pregnancy. Dietary sources of folic acid are green leafy vegetables such as broccoli and spinach, which must not be overcooked (see Ch. 19). Following the demonstrated link between neural tube defects and intake of folic acid, all pregnant women, and those intending to become pregnant are advised to take 0.4–4 mg folic acid daily (Consumers' Association, 1994; DoH, 1992; HEA, 1996).

Treatment of megaloblastic anaemia is by oral folic acid 5–10 mg daily. Occasionally, when the condition is very severe, folic acid may have to be given parenterally.

Megaloblastic anaemia may continue, or be diagnosed for the first time, during the puerperium. Treatment with iron and folic acid supplements should therefore continue until the haemoglobin has reached a satisfactory level.

Deficiency of vitamin B_{12} also produces a megaloblastic anaemia, but this is extremely rare in pregnancy. Since vitamin B_{12} is found exclusively in products of animal origin, including milk and cheese, women who are vegans are most likely to suffer from this deficiency.

Reflective Activity 46.1

When are blood tests carried out in your unit to determine women's haemoglobin levels, and what tests are done? At what point is action taken? How does this relate to the information given above?

Haemoglobinopathies

Haemoglobin is made up of two components:

- *Haem*: an iron-containing pigment of four pyrrole rings, which are organic molecules joined by bridges. This structure then takes up an iron atom in the ferrous form, which it holds centrally.

- *Globin*: a protein consisting of a long chain of amino acids. In normal haemoglobin, four types of globin molecule exist, which are differentiated by slight changes in the amino acids. These four types are alpha (α) beta (β), delta (δ) and gamma (γ).

Each molecule of haemoglobin contains four globin chains; the globin chains occur in the following combinations, which form the three major normally occurring haemoglobins (Marieb, 1999):

Major adult haemoglobin	HbA	2α plus 2β
Minor adult haemoglobin	HbA	2α plus 2δ
Fetal haemoglobin	HbF	2α plus 2γ

Haemoglobinopathies are inherited conditions in which one or more abnormal types wholly or partly replace the normal adult haemoglobin, HbA. The main haemoglobinopathies which complicate pregnancy are sickle cell disease and thalassaemia. These conditions are complex in terms of genetics and inheritance and are presented here in a relatively simplified form (further information may be obtained from texts included in the list of further reading).

Sickle cell trait and sickle cell disease

Abnormal haemoglobins (HbS) and/or HbC result when valine (HbS) or lysine (HbC) replaces glutamic acid in the sixth position of the beta polypeptide chain (Samuels, 1999). They were formerly associated with those whose ethnic origin lay in countries where malaria was endemic, since the sickle cell gene (in its trait form) is thought to provide some protection against malaria. More recently, however, population movement and the development of sexual relationships between members of different ethnic groups has resulted in a changed pattern of occurrence. In many areas, all women, regardless of ethnic origin are tested routinely, as are their babies. Both haemoglobins S and C are genetically inherited and thus there are heterozygous and homozygous forms of the disease. Heterozygous individuals inherit one normal and one abnormal haemoglobin, and thus have HbAS or HbAC, that is *sickle cell trait*. They are carriers of the disease but sickling does not usually occur. Homozygous individuals inherit abnormal HbS or HbC from both parents, and thus are HbSS or HbCC. Those with HbSS have *sickle cell anaemia* whereas those with HbCC have homozygous CC disease, where sickling does not occur because there is no S haemoglobin. In some cases an individual may inherit two different abnormal haemoglobins, HbS from one parent and HbC from the other,

and thus be HbSC. This is a milder form of the disease than HbSS and there is little anaemia. However, during pregnancy, HbSC can be hazardous, as there is still a possibility of sickling, which doctors and midwives may not anticipate, owing to the absence of anaemia (Nelson-Piercy, 1997) (Tables 46.1 and 46.2).

In sickle cell disease, erythrocytes containing HbS have a short lifespan of 5–10 days, rather than the normal span of 120 days (Samuels, 1999). They become sickle shaped under conditions of low oxygen tension such as hypoxia, dehydration, infection and acidosis and cold (Nelson-Piercy, 1997). They are easily haemolysed, and cause extremely painful vaso-occlusive symptoms in joints, in the abdomen and in the extremities during acute exacerbations, known as crises. This leads to chronic haemolytic anaemia, and an increase in the rate of haemoglobin synthesis in the bone marrow, which may lead to folic acid deficiency. Other complications are thromboembolic disorders, retinopathy, renal papillary necrosis, leg ulcers, and increased

Table 46.1 Haemoglobin combination in sickle cell disorders

HbSS	Homozygous sickle cell disease (sickle cell anaemia)
HbSC	Heterozygous sickle cell disease (sickle cell C disease)
HbCC	Homozygous CC disease (*not* a sickling disorder)
HbS beta/thal	Sickle/beta thalassaemia
HbAS	Sickle cell trait

Table 46.2 Patterns of inheritance in sickle cell anaemia

	Mother		Father	
	Sickle cell anaemia (HbSS)		Normal haemoglobin (HbAA)	
Infants	HbAS	HbAS	HbAS	HbAS
	(All infants will have sickle cell trait)			
	Sickle cell anaemia (HbSS)		Sickle cell trait (HbAS)	
Infants	HbAS	HbAS	HbSS	HbSS
	Sickle cell trait (HbAS)		Sickle cell trait (HbAS)	
Infants	HbAA	HbAS	HbAS	HbSS

risk of infection because of disorders in the function of the spleen (Nelson-Piercy, 1997). Acute chest syndrome may occur, in which there is pyrexia, tachypnoea, leucocytosis and pleuritic chest pain.

Effect on pregnancy The diagnosis is usually made in childhood, once most HbF has been replaced, and all women at risk should be tested. Nelson-Piercy (1997) observes that 35% of pregnancies will be complicated by crises, and perinatal mortality is increased four- to sixfold (Samuels, 1999). Pregnancy may be complicated by increased risk of miscarriage, intrauterine growth restriction (IUGR), preterm labour, and pre-eclampsia.

Management

Pregnancy All women at risk, together with their partners, should be screened for haemoglobinopathies in early pregnancy by means of haemoglobin electrophoresis. Iron therapy should be avoided but folic acid is given routinely throughout pregnancy. Blood transfusions may be required to treat very severe anaemia, and exchange transfusions may be carried out to remove the abnormal HbS and replace it with normal HbA although the advantages of this are debatable (Samuels, 1999).

At each antenatal visit, urinalysis should be carried out because of the increased risk of infection. Any infection should be treated with antibiotics.

Women with sickle cell disease may have poor appetites and should be encouraged to have regular small meals including meat, fish, eggs, cheese, fruit and wholemeal bread. Women and families should be aware of the symptoms of infection, and who to contact if they feel unwell. Since dehydration may lead to crisis, adequate fluids should be taken. Fetal well-being is monitored throughout the pregnancy by serial ultrasound and Doppler assessment.

In the case of crisis, the woman will be admitted to hospital where she should be kept warm, and given pain relief, usually morphine (Nelson-Piercy, 1997). Oxygen levels are monitored by pulse oximetry or arterial blood gases.

Labour Dehydration, acidosis and infection all lead to sickling, so care must be taken to avoid these complications in labour; however, care must also be taken to avoid fluid overload. Unless there is an obstetric indication, caesarean section is not indicated, and general anaesthesia should be avoided. It is important, however, that management involves the haematology department, and colleagues knowledgeable in the care and management of women with sickle cell disease, and that the woman is encouraged to report any problems (Lewis, 2001).

Postnatally Midwives must be aware of sources of specialist help (see p. 814) to which women and their partners may be directed, and of particular screening tests which may be offered during pregnancy and after delivery, to detect the presence of abnormal haemoglobins in the baby.

Thalassaemia

Thalassaemia is a condition in which there is an abnormal amount of HbA_2. It is most common in people of Mediterranean and Asian origin. The condition arises from defects in the alpha or beta globin chains resulting in thin, shortly lived red cells, often misshapen and deficient in haemoglobin, causing profound anaemia. As with sickle cell trait, thalassaemia in its mild forms confers some protection against malaria.

The condition may be mild, moderate or severe, depending on the number of inherited defective genes; in *alpha thalassaemia major*, four defective alpha genes are inherited; this condition produces hydrops fetalis and is incompatible with extrauterine life.

In *beta thalassaemia major*, there are two defective beta genes; the condition usually presents between the ages of 3 and 18 months, when the child becomes pale and fails to thrive. Untreated, these children will die before the age of 8. Treatment is by regular blood transfusions, but excess iron builds up from red cell breakdown, causing damage to the heart and liver. With treatment, patients may survive into their childbearing years (Nelson-Piercy, 1997).

In *thalassaemia minor*, the alpha or beta chains may be affected, resulting in alpha thalassaemia minor (very rare in this country) or beta thalassaemia minor. These minor thalassaemias are often called traits and have significance for women who carry them, in determining what screening tests should be carried out. Ideally, women and their partners should be screened before embarking on a pregnancy, since some thalassaemias are only detectable by blood testing and may coexist with iron deficiency, thereby confusing the diagnosis (Samuels, 1999).

Management As iron stores are likely to be overloaded, rather than depleted, iron supplements are not given unless iron deficiency is proved by measurement of iron stores. Folic acid is given throughout pregnancy, however, because the bone marrow is very active in replacing the short-lived red blood cells.

Other causes of anaemia

Glucose-6-phosphate dehydrogenase (G-6-PD) deficiency

This rare, X-linked inherited enzyme deficiency typically affects people of African, Asian and Mediterranean origin. Haemolytic crises occur if the affected person takes certain drugs, such as antimalarial preparations, sulphonamides, antibiotics (nitrofurantoin, nalidixic acid and possibly chloramphenicol) or eats broad (fava) beans. It may be implicated in cases of prolonged neonatal jaundice.

Secondary causes of anaemia include blood loss and infection, often a urinary tract infection which may be asymptomatic. Hookworm infestation may also cause anaemia because blood is lost in the stools. When the ova of the hookworm are found in the stools, bephenium hydroxynaphthoate (Alcopar) 5 mg is given on an empty stomach and may be repeated if required. Iron therapy will also be necessary.

Reflective Activity 46.2

Where is your nearest specialist centre for haemoglobinopathies? Does this reflect the ethnic mix in your community?

HEART DISEASE

Heart disease is a major cause of maternal mortality, the third most common non-obstetric cause of maternal death in the UK (Lewis, 2001; Oakley, 1999) and is seriously complicated by pregnancy. The cause may be congenital, such as atrial or ventricular septal defect, or acquired, such as mitral stenosis or incompetence, subsequent to rheumatic heart disease. Rheumatic heart disease has declined in developed countries, and accounts for 50% of cardiac disorders in pregnancy, as opposed to a previous level of 80% (Gilbert and Harmon, 1998). More women with congenital heart disease are reaching childbearing age following advances in cardiac surgery, including transplant. The total incidence of cardiac disease in pregnancy is 0.5–2% (Gilbert and Harmon, 1998).

Signs of cardiac disease are:

- dyspnoea
- chest pain

Box 46.1 New York Heart Association classification of cardiac disease

Class I: asymptomatic at all degrees of activity
Class II: symptomatic with increased activity
Class III: symptomatic with ordinary activity
Class IV: symptomatic at rest

- limitation of activity
- palpitations/arrhythmias/dysrhythmias
- cyanosis
- heart sound changes.

Cardiac disease is usually classified according to the limitations in activity it causes (see Box 46.1).

During pregnancy, women with pre-existing heart disease may experience a worsening of symptoms, due to physiological changes of pregnancy (see Ch. 17). Amongst other things, there is an increase in circulating blood volume, increased resting oxygen consumption, profound fall in peripheral vascular resistance, increase in stroke volume and slight increase in resting heart rate (Oakley, 1999). All of these changes influence haemodynamics, and will place a greater strain on an existing heart problem.

Rheumatic heart disease

Rheumatic heart disease is now rare, even in developing countries, and women who have mitral stenosis (narrowing of the mitral valve due to fibrosis following rheumatic fever), may not be diagnosed until they develop signs of dyspnoea, and tachycardia during pregnancy (Oakley, 1999). The major concern is prevention of endocarditis following infection (DoH, 1998).

Congenital heart disease

Atrial septal defects, patent ductus arteriosus and ventricular septal defects are the most commonly seen congenital lesions. Other more serious lesions include Fallot's tetralogy (ventricular septal defect, pulmonary stenosis, overriding aorta and right ventricular hypertrophy), Eisenmenger's syndrome (ventricular septal defect, overriding aorta and right ventricular hypertrophy) and Marfan's syndrome (a genetic condition which includes cardiac anomalies). Outcome of pregnancy is worst where there is pulmonary hypertension, and maternal mortality may be as high as 50% in

Eisenmenger's syndrome and Marfan's syndrome with aortic involvement (Mason and Brobowski, 1998). Early termination of pregnancy may be advised for such women, since the maternal mortality rate is high, although some women will choose to continue with the pregnancy and their choice must be respected (DoH, 1998; Oakley, 1999).

Fetal effects

Where maternal circulation is compromised, intrauterine hypoxia may occur, which may lead to fetal death. The fetus may also be affected by maternal medication, and may be further compromised by an increased risk of congenital heart defect. An echocardiogram may be carried out at 24 weeks, and women need to know the significance of reduced fetal movements (Gilbert and Harmon, 1998).

Antenatal care

The aim of antenatal care is to detect heart failure and disturbances of cardiac rhythm. A multidisciplinary approach involves obstetrician, physician and midwife. Women and their partners need help and support during what may be a particularly anxious time. Practical help may be needed with transport to clinics, household work, and child care.

A high-protein, low-carbohydrate diet, and low-salt diet is recommended, and weight control is important, as excessive weight gain places extra strain on the heart. Women taking diuretics should maintain a good dietary intake of potassium (Gilbert and Harmon, 1998). Prevention of anaemia is important to avoid cardiac compromise and the haemoglobin is estimated frequently.

Infection must be treated with antibiotics to reduce the risk of bacterial endocarditis; therefore dental caries, which may be a potential source of infection, should be treated early in pregnancy.

Cardiac failure   The major antenatal complications are acute pulmonary oedema and congestive cardiac failure. Women and partners should be aware of symptoms which indicate worsening of the condition such as dyspnoea, cough or chest pain, which will need admission immediately for stabilization. Oxygen therapy, digitalization and diuretics such as intravenous furosemide (frusemide) 20 mg may be given. Digoxin in maternal therapeutic levels crosses the placenta but does not harm the fetus. Women who have had valve replacements will be taking anticoagulants, usually

warfarin, to reduce the risk of embolism (de Swiet, 1995; Oakley, 1999). Warfarin is teratogenic in early pregnancy and may lead to fetal haemorrhage at any time. During pregnancy, fetal risks are reduced by changing to subcutaneous, self-administered, or intravenous heparin which does not cross the placenta. The effects of heparin are easily reversed by protamine sulphate.

Labour

Labour may be spontaneous or induced and should take place in a consultant obstetric unit. Prophylactic antibiotics are usually given to reduce the risk of bacterial endocarditis (de Swiet, 1995; Gilbert and Harmon, 1998). Epidural analgesia is recommended, but with caution in regard to hypotension. It is contraindicated in women on anticoagulant therapy. The optimum position for the woman is supported left lateral, or semi-upright (Gilbert and Harmon, 1998). In addition to usual midwifery observations in labour, the following are important:

- colour in case of cyanosis
- respiratory rate – should remain below 24 per minute
- degree of dyspnoea
- radial and apical pulses – should remain below 110 per minute
- ECG may be continuous throughout labour
- fluid balance to prevent overload
- continuous fetal monitoring using CTG.

It is suggested that in the absence of obstetric complications, vaginal delivery is preferable because it causes less haemodynamic fluctuation than caesarean section (Gilbert and Harmon, 1998).

It is sensible to keep the strenuous second stage of labour as short as possible, but there is no reason for elective forceps or vacuum extraction if delivery is proceeding well. Excessive pushing should be avoided since it alters haemodynamics and may compromise cardiac activity. If the woman feels the urge to push, short pushes with the mouth open should be encouraged. Oxytocic drugs are given only with great caution. Sudden strong uterine contraction in the third stage may direct so much of the uterine circulation of blood to the systemic circulation that the impaired heart may become seriously compromised and congestive cardiac failure ensue. Syntocinon should be used with caution, and is contraindicated in cases of heart failure (de Swiet, 1995; Lewis 2001). Serious postpartum haemorrhage is treated in the usual way.

Postnatal care

Continuing close observation is necessary as heart failure may occur in the first few days postnatally. Women require rest, but not complete immobilization. Physiotherapy may help to reduce the risk of thromboembolic disorders.

There is usually no contraindication to breastfeeding.

The risk of congenital heart disease in the baby is increased and ranges from 1 : 4 in Fallot's tetralogy to 1 : 15 with atrial septal defects; therefore, careful examination of the baby is essential.

The woman may need advice on family spacing methods; the intrauterine device with its associated risk of infection may not be appropriate; barrier methods may be used safely, as may the progesterone-only pill.

Careful plans should be made for transfer to the community. Women need practical help to enable them to rest, and cope with the demands of the baby. An appointment should be made with the cardiologist 4–6 weeks postnatally, to assess cardiac function.

Reflective Activity 46.3

Read the section on deaths from cardiac disorders in *Why Mothers Die 1997–9: Fifth Report of the Confidential Enquiries into Maternal Deaths in the United Kingdom* (Lewis, 2001). What influence will the accounts of women in the report have on your practice?

THYROID DISORDERS

Physiological changes to thyroid-binding globulin (tBG) and thyroxine in pregnancy lead to iodine deficiency in pregnancy, as maternal iodine requirements rise to facilitate active iodine transfer to the fetus (see Ch. 17). Iodine excretion in urine increases because of raised glomerular filtration rate (GFR) and decreased renal tubular reabsorption. Plasma iodine levels fall, and there is an increased uptake of iodine from the thyroid gland. Where there is dietary insufficiency, or the woman has thyroid disease, the thyroid will enlarge to increase iodine uptake under the influence of tri-iodothyronine (T_3) and thyroxine (T_4). The signs and symptoms of thyroid disorders may mimic those of pregnancy, and differential diagnosis is important.

Thyrotoxicosis (hyperthyroidism, Graves' disease)

Thyrotoxicosis occurs in about 1 : 500 pregnancies. 95% of cases are familial and associated with an autoimmune disorder in which thyroid-stimulating hormone (TSH) receptor antibodies are produced. Serum levels of free T_4 are high. When untreated, the condition is associated with infertility but conception occurs quite commonly in women who are treated. The condition does not appear to be made worse by pregnancy (Nelson-Piercy, 1997).

Women with thyrotoxicosis experience sensitivity to heat, tachycardia, palpitations, vomiting, palmar erythema and emotional lability, all of which are also features of normal pregnancy. The difference is that women with thyrotoxicosis also experience weight loss, tremor, persistent tachycardia, lid lag and prominent eyes. The disease usually predates pregnancy, but may arise for the first time in the first or early second trimester (Nelson-Piercy, 1997). It may be mistaken for hyperemesis gravidarum (Landon, 1999).

If untreated, there is an increased risk of miscarriage, IUGR, preterm labour, and perinatal mortality. In women who are poorly controlled there is a risk of a thyroid crisis, or 'storm', with hyperpyrexia, palpitations and tachycardia, which may lead to heart failure, especially in labour (Landon, 1999).

Treatment

Treatment is by therapeutic doses of carbimazole or propylthiouracil (PTU), either for 12–18 months following diagnosis, or over a longer period. Both drugs cross the placenta (PTU less so) and may cause fetal hypothyroidism and/or goitre (Nelson-Piercy, 1997), but they are unlikely to cause teratogenic problems at therapeutic levels. In the early management of the disease, beta-blockers may be given to control palpitations, tachycardia and tremor, but these are only usually given for a month.

Fetal effects are unlikely where there is good control, but outcomes are unpredictable. In cases of poor control, there may be fetal tachycardia, IUGR, fetal goitre, and a 50% increase in mortality if the disease is untreated. After delivery, the neonate may develop thyrotoxicosis, with weight loss, tachycardia, jitteriness, and poor feeding. Treatment is by antithyroid drugs. The neonatal condition will resolve once maternal thyroid-stimulating antibodies have cleared from the neonatal system (Gillmer and Hurley, 1999).

Care for women is collaborative, with particular midwifery emphasis on education of women about the effects of pregnancy on their condition, and of the condition on their pregnancy. During the antenatal period, assessment of maternal heart rate, weight gain, experience of nausea and vomiting should be carried out. Clinical assessment of fetal condition will include monitoring for IUGR; listening to the fetal heart; and may include serial ultrasound scans to assess growth and to detect goitre. During labour, careful observation of temperature, heart rate and rhythm are necessary, in addition to usual midwifery care. Minimal amounts of antithyroid drugs are excreted in breast milk, so breast-feeding is not contraindicated (Nelson-Piercy, 1997).

Hypothyroidism

This condition occurs in about 1% of pregnancies and there is usually a family history. It is characterized by weight gain, lethargy, hair loss, dry skin, constipation, fluid retention, carpal tunnel syndrome and possibly goitre. There is also intolerance of cold and a low pulse rate. Like hyperthyroidism, it is thought to be an autoimmune disorder. Untreated, it may lead to infertility, increased risk of miscarriage and fetal loss. Treatment is by thyroxine supplementation, and when well controlled there are no adverse effects on pregnancy. Little thyroxine crosses the placenta, and neonatal hypothyroidism is very rare (Landon, 1999; Nelson-Piercy, 1997).

RENAL CONDITIONS

Three common forms of urinary tract infection occur during pregnancy: *asymptomatic bacteriuria*, *cystitis* and *pyelonephritis*. Infection is particularly liable to arise in pregnancy because of the physiological changes which occur. The ureters and pelvis of the kidney become dilated in response to increased vascular volume, and urinary stasis may occur. The dilatation of the ureters is further accentuated when the enlarging uterus presses on the ureters at the pelvic brim, particularly on the right side since the uterus inclines to the right. Other factors which predispose to infection are vesicoureteric reflux of urine containing bacteria, urinary catheterization even with impeccable technique, and abnormalities of the renal tract (Gilbert and Harmon, 1998).

Causative organisms

The organism usually responsible is *Escherichia coli*, a normal inhabitant of the intestines, which may increase in virulence during pregnancy under the influence of oestrogen. The organisms may gain access to the urinary tract via lymphatics, or from the colon or bladder. Occasionally other organisms such as *Proteus vulgaris*, *Streptococcus faecalis* or *Pseudomonas aeruginosa* are involved.

Asymptomatic bacteriuria

Between 2–10% of all women have asymptomatic bacteriuria, that is, the presence of more than 100 000 colony-forming units of a single organism per millilitre of urine (Nelson-Piercy, 1997). Untreated, it leads to urinary tract infection in 30–40% of women (Gilbert and Harmon, 1998; Robson, 1999), in the form of cystitis and/or pyelonephritis.

Cystitis

Cystitis, or infection of the urinary bladder, occurs in up to 1.5% of pregnancies. Women may experience:

- dysuria
- haematuria
- frequency/urgency
- suprapubic pain.

Diagnosis is by culture from a midstream specimen of urine, and treatment is by antibiotics, typically ampicillin. Follow-up testing of urine should be carried out as the condition may recur. Women should be advised to drink plenty of fluids, preferably not acidic or carbonated, to wipe the perineum from front to back, and to empty the bladder immediately following sexual intercourse. Recent studies indicate that cranberry juice may help in the treatment and prevention of urinary tract infection, specifically that associated with *E. coli* (Lavender, 2000). It is thought that tannins in cranberries prevent p-fimbriated *E. coli* from attaching themselves to uroepithelial cells, thereby inhibiting infection. Cranberry juice is acidic, so may not be well tolerated by some women during pregnancy. Low-sugar versions are as effective and suitable for women with diabetes.

Women also need to know the signs and symptoms of further infection and be encouraged to report these to the midwife or GP (Gilbert and Harmon, 1998), as ascending infection may lead to the more serious condition of pyelonephritis.

Pyelonephritis

Pyelonephritis occurs in 1–2% of all pregnancies and is more common in women who exhibit bacteriuria

(Nelson-Piercy, 1997). The renal tubules become inflamed, and their ability to reabsorb sodium is adversely affected. Normally, sodium and water are excreted in the urine, but where initial reabsorption is affected, sodium and water remain in the body leading to oedema and increased pressure on the cardiovascular system. There is also a decrease in urine output as a consequence. In addition, the ability to produce buffers, such as potassium and ammonia is affected, leading to accumulation of free hydrogen ions and acidaemia.

When glomerular damage occurs, nitrogenous waste cannot be removed from the blood, leading to an increase in serum creatinine, urea and uric acid, and consequent decrease in urinary creatinine, urea and uric acid. Glomerular damage may also lead to loss of plasma proteins into the urine, changing osmotic pressure and leading to further oedema.

Practitioners need to be aware that infection can speedily become overwhelming, and that infections need to be treated quickly and effectively, and the woman's well-being and response to treatment carefully monitored. In the most recent *Confidential Enquiries into Maternal Deaths in the United Kingdom*, two women were reported to have died from such infection, and significant factors were the speed of the deterioration, the risk of overhydration and the need for consultant involvement (Lewis, 2001).

Signs and symptoms
- Pain from the loin to the groin, often on the right side
- Headache
- Nausea and vomiting
- Dysuria
- Frequency
- Pyrexia sometimes accompanied by rigors
- Tachycardia
- The woman may be anaemic and urinary output may be diminished.

Diagnosis
Diagnosis is confirmed by microscopic examination of a midstream specimen of urine. This will reveal pus cells and 100 000 bacteria per millilitre. The urine is usually acid, has an offensive smell and contains some red blood cells and protein.

Blood cultures may also be taken.

Management
The woman is admitted to hospital for rest, observation and treatment. A broad-spectrum antibiotic such as ampicillin (500 mg every 6–8 hours) is usually prescribed but may be changed once sensitivity of the causative organism is established. Initially, intravenous administration is more effective. The woman should drink ample fluids to avoid urinary stasis. An intake and output chart is maintained.

Lying on the unaffected side will help to relieve the pain and assist drainage. Analgesics are prescribed as necessary. The temperature, pulse and respirations are recorded 4-hourly, and a fan may be used if the temperature is very high. Further midstream specimens of urine are obtained for bacteriological examination until the urine is sterile and free of pus. The haemoglobin is checked because risk of anaemia is increased.

A recurrence of the infection is likely during pregnancy or postnatally, so follow-up is necessary. Antibiotic therapy is continued for a month, and in some cases throughout pregnancy. Three months following delivery when the renal tract has returned to normal, an intravenous pyelogram and other renal investigations may be carried out (Gilbert and Harmon, 1998).

Effects on the fetus
The risk of miscarriage and preterm labour is increased, and hyperpyrexia may result in intrauterine fetal death. The pain of uterine contractions associated with preterm labour may not be recognized if the woman is already in severe pain from the illness, and labour may only be detected by cardiotocography. Maternal plasma volume may be reduced, leading to poor placental perfusion. This can result in IUGR. There may also be fetal hypoxia. If the mother has a urinary tract infection at the time of delivery, the infant is at substantial risk of congenital infection.

Chronic renal disease

Chronic renal disease may arise as a result of any of the following:

- glomerulonephritis (acute or chronic)
- polycystic renal disease
- chronic pyelonephritis
- diabetic nephropathy
- systemic lupus erythematosus
- scleroderma
- renal calculi
- congenital abnormality of the lower urinary tract
- solitary kidney
- nephrotic syndrome.

The underlying pathophysiology described for pyelonephritis leads to the same maternal and fetal consequences in chronic renal disease. However, chronic renal disease is further complicated when damage to renal tissue results in reduced blood supply to the kidney. When this occurs, renin is produced to increase blood supply (see Ch. 45), with a consequent rise in blood pressure.

Chronic renal disease is usually classified as mild, moderate or severe, depending on levels of plasma creatinine (Nelson-Piercy, 1997). Women with severe disease may be advised against pregnancy, since 85% of them are likely to experience problems.

The outcome of pregnancy depends on the nature and severity of the disease, and the degree of loss of renal function. Outcome is best in women whose renal function is only moderately compromised, and where there is little or no hypertension. The outlook is worse where renal function is less than 50% (Nelson-Piercy, 1997). The woman is at risk of deterioration of renal function, proteinuria, and worsening of hypertension. There is also an increased risk of miscarriage, superimposed pre-eclampsia, IUGR, preterm delivery and fetal death.

The aim of care during pregnancy is to avoid further deterioration in renal function. In addition to the normal care provided, more frequent antenatal visits are required for maternal and fetal monitoring. The woman may need extra rest and help with childcare and household work. She may need to be admitted to hospital for rest and observation of blood pressure, assessment of renal function, and fetal monitoring. The course of the pregnancy will determine the mode and time of delivery; onset of labour and delivery may be spontaneous or labour may be induced. For some women, an elective caesarean section may be performed, depending on maternal and fetal condition.

Renal transplant

Following a successful renal transplantation, pregnancy will occur in 1 in 20 women transplant patients of childbearing age (Robson, 1999). Pre-pregnancy counselling is essential for these women and, in general, the following advice is given:

- The woman must have been in good health for 2 years after transplantation.
- Her stature should not be one associated with adverse obstetric outcome.
- There should be no proteinuria and no significant hypertension.
- There should be no sign of rejection of the transplanted kidney.

- There should be no sign of distension of the renal pelvis or calyces.
- Plasma creatinine should be 200 mmol/l or less.
- Immunosuppressive drug dosages should be at maintenance levels, e.g. prednisone, 15 mg/day or less and azathioprine 2 mg/kg body weight per day, or less (Davison and Dunlop, 1995).

The woman should be cared for by a nephrologist and an obstetrician; however, she still requires midwifery care and support. Regular monitoring of blood pressure, renal function and fetal condition, including ultrasound assessment of growth, and Doppler studies of umbilical and placental circulation must be carried out.

The predisposition to urinary tract infection associated with pregnancy, coupled with immunosuppressive drugs taken by transplant patients renders the woman more likely to infection. She may also develop hypertension and she may become anaemic.

Labour may occur spontaneously unless there is an obstetric indication for intervention. Steroid therapy is increased and antibiotics must be given prophylactically for any surgical intervention, including episiotomy (Nelson-Piercy, 1997).

Neonatal problems include preterm delivery, IUGR, respiratory distress syndrome, adrenocortical insufficiency, thrombocytopenia, leucopenia, cytomegalovirus and other infections. Theoretically, breastfeeding is possible, but so many uncertainties surround the effects of some of the drugs used that it is not advised (Davison and Dunlop, 1995).

Acute renal failure

A fall in urinary output is the first sign of acute renal failure. An output of less than 500 ml in 24 hours is considered a sign of renal failure.

Causes

Acute renal failure in pregnancy is rare (<0.005%), but mild to moderate renal impairment may occur (1:8000). It may occur in association with severe haemorrhage, pre-eclampsia and eclampsia, infection, including septic abortion. It is rarely associated with pyelonephritis (Nelson-Piercy, 1997). The kidneys are unable to excrete creatinine and urea, and rising serum levels lead to acidosis. Though rare, it is serious and its course is unpredictable. It has been recommended that all women with renal failure should be transferred to a unit where renal dialysis is available.

Management

Management will depend largely on the cause, which may be prerenal, e.g. hypovolaemia, or renal (tubular or cortical necrosis). It is important to be aware that acute renal failure can occur and to prevent its onset by adequate fluid replacement, while avoiding fluid overload, which particularly in cases of pre-eclampsia, can lead to pulmonary oedema (Nelson-Piercy, 1997). Emphasis is on avoiding and/or treating uraemia, acidosis, hyperkalaemia and fluid overload, and renal dialysis may be needed.

Women and their families need support from the multidisciplinary team, since not only is the woman extremely ill, she will also be concerned for her baby. Postnatal care should include full information about the nature of her illness, effects on future pregnancies, and information about appropriate contraception.

Reflective Activity 46.4

This section, and others in this chapter have highlighted the need for women to have practical help with daily activities. How could this be accomplished?

DIABETES MELLITUS

Diabetes mellitus is a medical condition in which there is a total or relative lack of insulin produced by the pancreas for the requirements of the tissues. This means that glycolytic enzymes are inhibited and gluconeogenetic enzymes are activated, resulting in the liberation of additional glucose into the bloodstream. Without insulin, this additional glucose cannot be utilized for energy, since it is unable to cross the cell membrane into muscle and adipose tissue. The body therefore endeavours to utilize energy sources from fat and protein metabolism, breaking down amino acids for gluconeogenesis. Urea, a by-product of amino acid metabolism, is excreted in large quantities in the urine.

Ketogenesis also takes place as fatty acids are liberated from adipose tissue in response to the body's requirements for energy. Ketones can be used by some body tissues as an energy source, but in uncontrolled diabetes, may be produced in excess, resulting in excretion in urine and through the lungs. Ketones are acidic substances and lower the body pH; in an effort to avoid acidosis, the body's buffer pool becomes exhausted, leading to possible shock (Marieb, 1999).

Thus, blood glucose levels are high, and become increasingly higher as gluconeogenesis occurs. This hyperglycaemia means that the transport maximum for reabsorption of glucose in the renal system is exceeded, and glycosuria results. Since glucose is osmotically active, it carries with it a corresponding amount of water as it is excreted in the urine, resulting in polyuria. As more and more water is excreted, so dehydration occurs, and the traditional picture is produced of the hyperglycaemic, dehydrated and ketotic patient with polyuria and polydipsia. Untreated, these symptoms will lead to acidosis, coma and death (Marieb, 1999).

Although the effects of diabetes mellitus are seen principally in relation to glucose metabolism, multiple metabolic pathways are disturbed and the disease exerts its effects on all systems of the body.

Diagnosis and classification

The diagnosis of diabetes is by the glucose tolerance test, which challenges the body's response to a glucose load. The fasting woman is given a drink containing 75 g glucose. Venous blood samples are obtained at regular intervals and compared with results within the normal range. The blood glucose levels rise initially, but should return to normal within 2 hours. Abnormal findings would be a fasting blood glucose of over 7 mmol/l, and a blood glucose level over 10 mmol/l after 2 hours. Where the 2-hour figure is below 10 mmol/l, but greater than 7 mmol/l, glucose tolerance is said to be impaired (WHO, 1980).

The World Health Organization (WHO) classification of diabetes mellitus is as follows:

Type I: insulin-dependent diabetes (IDD) mellitus

The glucose tolerance test is abnormal and patients have signs and symptoms of the disease and require treatment. It is most common in juveniles, and is characterized by an almost complete lack of insulin, possibly because of a decrease in the number of beta cells in the islets of Langerhans. Hyperglycaemia, polyuria and ketosis are present, and this type of diabetes is insulin dependent. It is now thought to be a genetically mediated disorder, involving human leucocyte antigens (HLA) on chromosome 6 (de Swiet, 1995).

Type II: non-insulin-dependent diabetes (NIDD) mellitus

Women have an abnormal glucose tolerance test but no symptoms. In this type of diabetes, there seems to be resistance in the tissues to the action of insulin; it is often diagnosed later in life, and frequently affects those who are overweight. It is not dependent on insulin, and oral hypoglycaemic agents may be used to control it. Some patients may also be controlled by diet alone.

Impaired glucose tolerance (IGT)   The glucose tolerance test is normal except in times of stress when the woman may develop diabetes. When this occurs in pregnancy it is known as *gestational diabetes*. 15–20% of these women go on to develop insulin-dependent diabetes in later life, with the incidence rising to 70% if there is also obesity (Chamberlain, 1997).

Other   This group would include potential IDD and NIDD sufferers, who have certain risk markers, including:

- ethnic origin (Asian, African and Afro-Caribbean)
- glycosuria on two occasions in the antenatal clinic
- history of diabetes in first-degree relatives
- previous baby weighing more than 4.5 kg
- previous unexplained perinatal death
- history of a baby with congenital malformations
- polyhydramnios
- obesity.

Gestational diabetes

This term has traditionally been applied to the condition in women who develop hyperglycaemia with an impaired glucose tolerance test during pregnancy. The supposed association between gestational diabetes and adverse neonatal outcome led to active treatment by diet and insulin therapy for such women. Active screening, including random blood glucose estimation and glucose tolerance testing (in some centres for all pregnant women) aimed to detect and treat the condition in order to improve perinatal outcome. However, Gillmer and Hurley (1999) examine the arguments for and against screening all pregnant women for GDM, concluding that such a policy cannot be justified. De Swiet (1995) points out that although women with GDM produce macrosomic babies, and are more likely to have caesarean section, there is no clear indication that perinatal outcome is improved by aggressive intervention. He further highlights that diagnosis places the woman in an 'abnormal' category, and forces her into a time-consuming and painful regime of dietary restriction, glucose monitoring and insulin. His view is that certain groups are at risk of developing IDD and NIDD (see above), some of whom will be detected for the first time during pregnancy, and these are the groups who

should be targeted for screening, using a glucose load of 50 g with blood glucose estimation 1 hour later.

For midwives, the uncertainty surrounding the diagnosis, or even existence, of gestational diabetes is confusing when it comes to providing care and information for women, since studies are inconclusive.

> ### Reflective Activity 46.5
>
> Does your unit have a policy for routine screening for diabetes?

Midwives need to be aware that women with gestational diabetes and those with pre-existing diabetes mellitus require knowledgeable and skilled care, and a recognition of them as women in their own right rather than a reflection of a medical condition.

Pregnancy and diabetes

A number of hormonal and metabolic changes occur naturally as a result of pregnancy, and these changes, together with their accepted physiological norms have been well-documented (see Ch. 17).

Type I and type II diabetes mellitus are complicated by the physiological changes which take place in glucose metabolism during pregnancy. In the first trimester, fasting blood glucose levels fall from 4 mmol/l until, at term, the level may be as low as 3.6 mmol/l. However, the peak response to food is progressively higher and delayed as pregnancy progresses. In the non-diabetic, rises in insulin production maintain normoglycaemia (Nelson-Piercy, 1997) and there is considerable hypertrophy of the pancreatic islet cells in order to produce additional insulin in response to glucose stimulation. Maternal fat storage takes place in the first trimester, and is followed by fat mobilization in the later months as the fetus accelerates its use of glucose and amino acids. Thus, in non-diabetic pregnancy, the metabolic state is altered to provide preferential perfusion of nutrients across the placenta to the fetus, to ensure embryogenesis, growth, maturation and survival.

Placental hormones exert an influence on the metabolic status both directly and indirectly; progesterones, oestrogens, human placental lactogen and increased free cortisol combine to produce a resistance to insulin. In this sense, pregnancy is said to be diabetogenic.

Glucose carried in plasma passes through the renal system, and is normally reabsorbed in the proximal convoluted tubule of the nephron. The transport system for glucose is linked to the active transfer of sodium ions, in a phenomenon known as co-transfer (Marieb, 1999).

There is a maximum amount of glucose which can be reabsorbed in this way (the transport maximum, or Tm), and, in health, this means that when blood glucose levels are between 4.2–6.7 mmol/l, all glucose will be reabsorbed. However, the maximum rate for glucose reabsorption is 375 mg/min, and when plasma glucose levels exceed 10 mmol/l, the transport maximum is exceeded; therefore all the plasma glucose cannot be reabsorbed. Consequently, glucose is excreted in the urine, producing glycosuria. Normally, the action of insulin would prevent this.

In non-diabetic pregnancy, the glomerular filtration rate is increased, so that even when blood glucose levels are within normal limits, all glucose cannot be reabsorbed, and there may be glycosuria. In diabetic pregnancy, therefore, urinalysis is inadequate as a reflection of blood glucose.

In diabetes, episodes of hyperglycaemia cause haemoglobin to become irreversibly bound to glucose; this glycosylated haemoglobin (HbA_1) normally constitutes 4–8% of the woman's total haemoglobin. This level may rise during hyperglycaemia, and a raised level is associated with fetal abnormalities in pregnancy. Levels of HbA_1 in the blood reflect blood glucose status up to 3 months previously, so that levels of HbA_1 taken at 10 weeks of pregnancy may reveal high blood glucose levels at the time of conception and embryogenesis.

Complications

Although more complications occur in the pregnancies of diabetic mothers, the maternal mortality rate is no higher than 0.5% (Nelson-Piercy, 1997). In the pregnant diabetic woman, insulin requirements will obviously be greatly increased to cope with the relative fasting hypoglycaemia, and up to four times the usual dose of insulin will be required. Women with type II diabetes may also require insulin at this stage, although in both type I and type II diabetes, and gestational diabetes, insulin requirements will return to normal immediately after delivery. Insulin-dependent diabetes becomes more unstable in pregnancy. The renal threshold for glucose is lowered in pregnancy and insulin requirements increase as pregnancy advances, so that diabetic control is more difficult (Marieb, 1999).

Hyperglycaemia leads to glycosuria and ketoacidosis. Monilial vaginitis and urinary tract infections are commonly associated with hyperglycaemia, whereas ketoacidosis may increase the severity of any nausea and vomiting in pregnancy. These metabolic changes can result in a period of instability in diabetic control for the pregnant woman, which may exacerbate existing complications of diabetes.

There are conflicting views as to whether diabetic retinopathy worsens during pregnancy (Lauszus *et al.*, 2000). However, as it is a progressive condition, and is the most frequent cause of blindness in type I diabetes, it is advisable that ophthalmic examinations of the fundi be carried out during each trimester. Lauszus *et al.* (2000) recommend that tight glycaemic control during pregnancy will avoid progression of retinopathy.

Likewise, diabetic nephropathy may be present, or may be detected during pregnancy, and may be complicated by a superimposed pre-eclampsia. Renal disease does not seem to worsen during pregnancy. 25% of pregnant women with diabetes will develop polyhydramnios, and this may be associated with fetal abnormality or may develop as a result of fetal polyuria in response to fetal hyperglycaemia (Gillmer and Hurley, 1999).

There is an increased incidence of pre-eclampsia in diabetic women and it is made worse by poor diabetic control.

Despite good diabetic control, there is still a risk of fetal macrosomia (birthweight over 4000 g), with its attendant maternal and fetal risks. Macrosomia occurs for a number of reasons: maternal hyperglycaemia stimulates the fetus to produce insulin which acts as a growth hormone and results in deposition of fat and protein, particularly around the shoulder girdle of the fetus. Overproduction of the growth hormone from the anterior pituitary gland is also involved in the development of large babies. It is suggested that the fetus in diabetic pregnancy may have an increased potential for growth which is stimulated by relatively small increases in maternal blood glucose (Gillmer and Hurley, 1999). The major risk to the macrosomic fetus is birth trauma, principally brachial plexus injury secondary to shoulder dystocia. Infants need close monitoring to detect any of these conditions.

Intrauterine fetal death occurs frequently in the last 3–4 weeks of pregnancy but the cause is not really understood. Gillmer and Hurley (1999) suggest that long periods of hyperglycaemia in poorly controlled diabetes lead to increased aerobic and anaerobic glucose metabolism which consume oxygen and lead to production of lactate, resulting in lowered pH and fetal acidaemia.

It is particularly likely to occur when:

- the diabetes is not well controlled
- there is marked polyhydramnios

- the baby is very large, or
- the pregnancy is complicated by hypertension.

The incidence of pre-eclampsia is increased in diabetic women and this may be partly responsible for the high perinatal mortality rate. Diabetic vascular disease, hyperglycaemia and ketoacidosis in the mother all increase the risk of fetal death possibly due to chronic fetal hypoxia. Other causes may be related to fetal acidaemia and a compensatory fetal polycythaemia accompanied by thrombocytopenia (de Swiet, 1995; Nelson-Piercy, 1997). In the neonate, the higher haematocrit associated with polycythaemia predisposes the infant to jaundice (Gillmer and Hurley, 1999).

The incidence of malformations in diabetic pregnancy is four times higher than usual, and congenital abnormality is now the commonest cause of perinatal death in diabetic pregnancies. Cardiac anomalies occur four times as often in diabetic pregnancies; other congenital abnormalities include anencephaly and vertebral defects (Landon, 1999). Infants should be examined carefully for signs of congenital abnormality (see Ch. 31). The perinatal mortality rate in diabetic pregnancy has greatly improved in recent years and is now below 5% (de Swiet, 1995) and this is largely due to the improved diabetic management of the pregnant diabetic woman. In cases where diabetic control is poor, the perinatal mortality rate is likely to be higher.

Prematurity is an important factor in perinatal mortality. Early delivery may be necessary because of the severity of the diabetes or the onset of complications. The baby has a sixfold risk of developing respiratory distress syndrome.

Maternal and fetal complications affecting pregnant women with diabetes are summarized in Box 46.2.

Preconception care

Good diabetic control before and at the time of conception as well as throughout the antenatal period greatly improves the outcome of pregnancy. Women with diabetes mellitus should therefore discuss a proposed pregnancy with their doctor so that diabetic control can be improved, if necessary, before conception occurs, particularly given the association between fetal abnormality and hyperglycaemia during the period of fetal organogenesis. Women with diabetes may already be well informed about their condition, and be aware of the importance of pre-pregnancy care. Associations such as Diabetes UK (see Additional resources, p. 814) produce literature specifically related to pregnancy. Clinical nurse specialists in

---

> **Box 46.2 Maternal and fetal complications affecting pregnant diabetic women**
>
> **Maternal complications**
> 1. Unstable diabetic control
> 2. Ketoacidosis
> 3. Polyhydramnios
> 4. Pre-eclampsia
> 5. Preterm labour
> 6. Obstructed labour
>
> **Fetal complications**
> 1. Congenital abnormalities
> 2. Macrosomia
> 3. Intrauterine death
> 4. Respiratory distress syndrome
> 5. Neonatal hypoglycaemia, hypocalcaemia, jaundice, polycythaemia

---

diabetic clinics should also be aware of the importance of periconception care.

Care during pregnancy

Collaborative care is essential for pregnant women who have diabetes; medical, obstetric and midwifery input, together with informed self-care by the woman can help pregnancy to be as fulfilling for the woman with diabetes as for her non-diabetic counterpart. Midwifery input must be knowledgeable and up to date, catering for all aspects of the woman's care during pregnancy, birth and the puerperium.

Regular monitoring of the blood glucose levels at home by the pregnant woman has proved successful in achieving good diabetic control.

Diet The carbohydrate energy content of the diet should be related to the energy requirements of the individual. In most cases it does not exceed 40%, but it can be higher without adverse effects. Fat intake should be restricted because of the increased risk of arterial disease in diabetics. A high fibre intake is recommended because the slower gastric emptying delays the absorption of sugar into the bloodstream. Hypoglycaemia may exacerbate the effects of morning sickness; glucose and sugary foods should be avoided, and hypoglycaemia avoided by taking milk and a light snack. Glucagon should be available to women with diabetes, for use in emergencies.

Diabetes is particularly common in British women of Asian origin. Dietary considerations for such women should avoid sweets such as gulab juman, halwa and jelabi, and, where the woman is also overweight, foods fried in ghee or oil should be reduced.

Insulin   Insulin requirements usually increase in pregnancy owing to the rise in energy requirements and the production of diabetogenic hormones from the placenta (Ch. 17). The dose of insulin is carefully correlated to the glucose levels, which are monitored daily. Better diabetic control is generally achieved if a combination of short- and intermediate-acting insulins are administered twice daily (Gillmer and Hurley, 1999).

Continuous infusion of insulin may be maintained via a subcutaneous syringe pump, although this has not been shown to achieve better control than conventional multidose administration (de Swiet, 1995). Three descriptions have been applied to control of blood glucose in pregnancy complicated by diabetes: *very tight control*, *tight control* and *moderate control*.

1. *Very tight control*: aims for blood glucose below 5.6 mmol/l.
2. *Tight control*: aims for blood glucose 5.6–6.7 mmol/l.
3. *Moderate control*: aims for blood glucose 6.7–8.9 mmol/l.

In normal pregnancy, blood glucose levels rarely exceed 6.6 mmol/l.

The effects of these degrees of control have not been thoroughly researched, but evidence suggests that tight control coupled with a holistic approach to the woman's care results in reduced incidence of macrosomia, urinary tract infection, respiratory distress syndrome, hypertension, preterm labour and perinatal mortality.

Oral hypoglycaemic drugs   The use of oral hypoglycaemic drugs is not recommended in pregnancy as they cross the placenta and may cause severe hypoglycaemia in the baby after birth because of their slow metabolism in the infant's immature liver.

Assessment of blood glucose levels and glycosylated haemoglobin (HbA$_1$)   Blood glucose levels are monitored four or six times on 2 or 3 days a week and the preprandial levels should be below 5.5 mmol/l. The woman can use a glucose monitor to monitor her own blood glucose levels and change her treatment when necessary to remain normoglycaemic (blood glucose between 4–6 mmol/l). She should keep a record of pre-meal and pre-snack blood glucose levels, levels of ketonuria, and hypoglycaemic episodes, which are more common when tight regulation of glucose during pregnancy is required. Family and friends should know how to administer glucagon to reverse the effects of severe hypoglycaemia (Gillmer and Hurley, 1999). Glycosylated haemoglobin (HbA$_1$) can also be measured every 2–4 weeks, and helps to assess diabetic control. It is a type of adult haemoglobin where one part of the beta chain has been combined with glucose. HbA$_1$ has been found to increase in diabetes, especially when the blood glucose control is poor, although as stated earlier, its levels are not indicators of present diabetic status but of blood glucose levels during the preceding 1–3 months. Levels of 10% or lower are considered a sign of good control, while levels of more than 10% indicate poor control (Gillmer and Hurley, 1999).

Fetal well-being   In addition to careful supervision of the diabetes, fetal well-being is monitored closely throughout pregnancy. It may be assessed by 'kick counts' and cardiotocography, and growth is monitored by clinical examination and ultrasonography (see Ch. 18). Biophysical profiles and Doppler blood flow studies may also be performed.

Obstetric care   The frequency of attendance at the antenatal clinic varies but is often every 2 weeks until 32 weeks and then weekly. The incidence of pre-eclampsia is increased in women with diabetes; thus particular care is taken to record the blood pressure and examine the urine for protein. Hospitalization before 38 weeks is necessary only if complications such as pre-eclampsia, polyhydramnios, fetal growth restriction, infection or inadequate diabetic control occur.

Care during labour

The midwife cares for the woman in labour in conjunction with medical and obstetric colleagues; labour onset may be spontaneous or induced, or delivery may be by elective caesarean section if there are obstetric indications.

Dextrose/insulin regimes vary; Gillmer and Hurley (1999) suggest intravenous 10% dextrose 100 ml per hour; it is important that this does not change. Changes in response to blood glucose results should be to the insulin infusion (usually Human Actrapid insulin 6 units in 60 ml normal saline (1 unit in 10 ml) given according to a sliding scale). The aim is to keep blood glucose levels between 4–6 mmol/l. Blood glucose levels are checked hourly and the insulin infusion rate adjusted if necessary. If oxytocin is necessary, it should be infused in normal saline.

Fetal monitoring should be continuous, by external cardiotocography or by fetal scalp electrode, and is essential because of the increased risks of fetal distress and fetal hypoxia during labour.

Satisfactory pain relief may be achieved by epidural anaesthesia.

After labour, insulin requirements usually revert to pre-pregnancy levels and women who began insulin therapy during pregnancy will not normally now require this.

Postnatal care

Maternal insulin requirements fall sharply after delivery, so frequent blood glucose estimations are made to detect hypoglycaemia. The insulin dosage is reduced and the woman is gradually restabilized.

Breastfeeding should be encouraged, and women may need additional carbohydrate to facilitate this. De Swiet (1995) suggests an additional 50 g per day, with less long-acting insulin given at night to prevent nocturnal hypoglycaemia, which may occur during night feeding.

High standards of hygiene are necessary to combat the increased risk of infection in diabetic women (Gilbert and Harmon, 1998).

Diabetic women require careful advice on family spacing, and should be encouraged to have their children early, before vascular complications occur (de Swiet, 1995). The combined oral contraceptive pill may alter carbohydrate metabolism and some women may need a higher dose of insulin, and carries a slight risk of thromboembolism. The intrauterine contraceptive is effective (but unsuitable for nulliparous women) and there is no higher rate of pelvic infection for women with diabetes (de Swiet, 1995). Barrier methods may be used by women for whom further pregnancy would not severely exacerbate diabetic complications.

The baby of the diabetic mother

A paediatrician should normally be present at birth to receive the baby. In the past these babies were invariably large and plethoric (the diabetic 'cherub') but with better diabetic control the baby is more likely to be an appropriate weight for gestational age. Despite being large for gestational age, the baby may be immature and require special care after birth, although routine separation of mother and baby for the simple purpose of observation is not required. These babies are particularly prone to respiratory distress syndrome and hypoglycaemia, so require close observation. In intrauterine life the hypertrophic islets of Langerhans produce more insulin in response to the high maternal blood sugar levels. After birth the pancreas continues to produce excess insulin initially, so the baby becomes hypoglycaemic. To prevent this, early feeding within 2 hours of birth is essential and the infant's blood glucose levels are measured with Dextrostix 2-hourly to detect hypoglycaemia.

Other neonatal complications include skin infections, hyperbilirubinaemia and bleeding from a very thick cord, and the incidence of congenital malformations is increased. Considerable weight loss occurs in the first week or so after birth and initially the baby tends to be lethargic, but then progress should be normal (de Swiet, 1995).

RESPIRATORY PROBLEMS

Tuberculosis

Pulmonary tuberculosis (TB) is responsible for 6% of all deaths worldwide, and available sources suggest that up to half the world's population is infected with the disease in either its latent or active form (Mays, 1993; Nelson-Piercy, 1997). Improvements in housing, nutrition and access to health care, coupled with a mass-screening campaign in the 1950s, resulted in a significant decline in the disease in Great Britain. However, sources suggest that TB is becoming more prevalent, particularly among the homeless, in situations where there is overcrowding, and where there is exposure through contact with people from countries where the disease is widespread. Drug users and those infected with HIV are at increased risk of developing TB (Joint Tuberculosis Committee of the British Thoracic Society, 2000). Women may become pregnant whilst being treated for TB, or may develop the disease during pregnancy.

Classic symptoms are chronic cough and blood-streaked sputum, with fever, weight loss and night sweats occurring late in the disease. The onset is insidious and there is also a feeling of general malaise.

Diagnosis

Diagnosis is made when the causative organism (*Mycobacterium tuberculosis* or tubercle bacillus) is found in sputum, and by chest X-ray.

Pregnancy care

Congenital TB is very rare, so the fetus is not at risk; if chest X-rays are needed, a lead apron is used to protect the woman's abdomen.

Care in pregnancy is by an obstetrician and a respiratory physician. Since social and economic factors

Table 46.3   Drugs used for the treatment of active TB in pregnancy

Drug	Dose	Possible side-effects	
		Maternal	**Fetal**
Isoniazid	5 mg/kg/day Max. 300 mg	Hepatitis Peripheral neuropathy Agranulocytosis	None
Rifampicin	10 mg/kg/day Max. 600 mg	Hepatitis Decreased effectiveness of oral contraceptive	Increase in neural tube defects
Ethambutol	15–25 mg/kg/day Max. 2.5 g	Optic neuritis Visual problems	None
Pyrazinamide	15–30 mg/kg/day	Hepatitis Arthralgias	None

Note: Streptomycin is not given in pregnancy since it causes damage to fetal auditory and vestibular nerves.

feature in the care of women with TB, the midwife must liaise with a social worker where necessary. Help will be needed both during and after pregnancy with housework and childcare, since the woman will be tired. Liaison with other healthcare workers may be necessary, since family members may need to be screened and educated as to the nature of the disease and the steps needed to prevent its spread.

Drugs used to treat TB have side-effects for both mother and fetus (see Table 46.3); courses of treatment are long – 6 to 9 months or longer – but the symptoms of the disease resolve after only 3 weeks, and the woman will be non-infectious after 2 (Nelson-Piercy, 1997). Women must be encouraged to continue treatment, otherwise there is the risk of drug-resistant strains developing.

Infection is spread by airborne transmission of droplet nuclei from a person with active TB. If the woman is infectious, she should be provided with a single room while she is in hospital. Crockery and cutlery are not involved in the transmission of infection and barrier nursing is not required.

In the absence of obstetric indications, labour onset is spontaneous and care is as that of any normal labour.

Where the woman or any close family members have active pulmonary tuberculosis, particularly of a resistant strain, the baby has a 50% risk of developing the disease (Nelson-Piercy, 1997) and may need to be separated from the family. The baby is vaccinated with the BCG (bacille Calmette–Guérin) vaccine and may be given syrup of isoniazid prophylactically. If the disease is not active, the mother and baby are not separated, nor is breastfeeding contraindicated (Nelson-Piercy, 1997; Samuels, 1999).

Advice about family-spacing methods will be needed, as the women with active TB should avoid pregnancy until there are no further signs of the disease, usually for a period of 2 years.

Asthma

Asthma is an obstructive disease of the respiratory system characterized by episodic breathlessness, wheezing, cough and feelings of tightness in the chest. This is caused by decreased expiratory flow rates, hyperinflation and premature airway closure, with some lack of lung compliance. During acute attacks, sufferers experience increased respiratory rate and wheezing, are unable to speak in complete sentences because of breathlessness, and they use their accessory muscles of respiration. These difficulties in breathing are caused by inflammation, narrowing of the airways, and contraction of the smooth muscle of the airway walls. Known factors in asthma attacks are allergens, such as pollen or environmental factors, exercise, and upper respiratory tract infections. Asthma affects approximately 3% of women of childbearing age (Nelson-Piercy, 1997). The effect of pregnancy on asthma appears to be variable. Some women experience fewer asthmatic attacks, possibly owing to the increased production of corticosteroids in pregnancy, but a few may have more, particularly those who have severe asthma. Schatz (1992) suggests that asthmatic women are more likely to develop hyperemesis gravidarum, chronic hypertension, pregnancy-induced hypertension and antepartum haemorrhage. The causes are unknown but the conditions are less likely to arise where asthma is controlled well (Moore-Gillon,

1994). It is also suggested that maternal hypoxia during repeated asthmatic attacks results in IUGR.

The aim in pregnancy is to prevent attacks in order to ensure adequate maternal/fetal oxygenation. This is achieved by maintaining adequate drug therapy with inhaled anti-inflammatory agents, beta agonists or steroids. These are considered safe during pregnancy, and midwives should assure women of this. As Nelson-Piercy (1997) points out, poorly controlled asthma carries greater risks for the fetus than do the drugs used to treat it. Samuels (1999) supports influenza vaccination in the winter, to prevent upper respiratory tract infection, which may lead to attacks. Women should be encouraged to participate in the management of their condition and measure their own peak flow, adjusting their inhaled drug dosage as required. Women should be advised to use spacers when inhaling steroids, to avoid the development of oral thrush (Samuels, 1999), and if they smoke, should be offered help in stopping.

Oral steroids such as prednisolone may be used to control exacerbations; however, these are diabetogenic and women will need regular estimation of blood glucose. Women on oral steroids will need hydrocortisone during labour (Nelson-Piercy, 1997). Entonox, epidural and other forms of pain relief can be used in labour; however, opiates are respiratory depressants, and would not be used if the woman had an attack during labour. Epidural anaesthesia is safer for caesarean section, as it avoids the problems of chest infection and atelectasis associated with general anaesthesia (Samuels, 1999).

Breastfeeding is not contraindicated, and may protect the baby from developing atopic asthma (Nelson-Piercy, 1997).

EPILEPSY

Epilepsy is a condition of abnormal cerebral function in which characteristic, convulsive seizures occur. 1 in 200 people are affected and the incidence in pregnancy is between 0.3–0.5% (Lindsay, 1990). Seizures may be generalized (petit mal and grand mal), partial (temporal lobe epilepsy) or focal (Jacksonian seizure). Seizures frequently result in loss of consciousness for periods of a matter of seconds up to half an hour. In all cases abnormal, paroxysmal electrical discharges, recordable on EEG, occur in the brain. In many cases the cause is unknown (idiopathic), but epilepsy may be due to cerebral trauma, congenital abnormality, the presence of space-occupying lesions in the brain, vascular disorders, degenerative disorders, infection, metabolic disorders such as hypoglycaemia, or following withdrawal from drugs or alcohol.

Epilepsy may be controlled, but not cured, by the use of anticonvulsant drugs such as sodium valproate (Epilim) or phenytoin sodium (Epanutin). Phenobarbitone or benzodiazepines may also be given. Pregnancy has a variable effect on the pattern of seizures, but generally, the more severe the disorder, the greater the effect on the pregnancy. Women aged 25–39 years with treated epilepsy have significantly lower fertility rates than those of the general population (Wallace *et al.*, 1998). However, those who become pregnant achieve successful pregnancy outcome in more than 90% of cases. Successful outcome relates to close monitoring of the epilepsy, cooperation of the woman in taking prescribed medication, and preferably preconception assessment and counselling. There is an increased incidence of congenital abnormalities in infants of women with epilepsy (Consumers' Association, 1994); some sources suggest that this is due to the teratogenic effects of anticonvulsant therapy and some that it is associated with the condition itself. Most common defects are cleft lip and cleft palate, spina bifida and heart disease. Abnormalities occur more often in women who receive combinations of anticonvulsants, so, during pregnancy, treatment with one drug alone is recommended. Prophylactic folic acid for prevention of neural tube defects may reduce serum phenytoin levels, thus affecting control of seizures in some women (Consumers' Association, 1994). Hydantoin syndrome (a condition resembling fetal alcohol syndrome) may occur in infants of women taking hydantoin preparations.

This association between fetal abnormality and drug therapy highlights the importance of counselling for the woman. A balance needs to be maintained between preventing seizures, which in themselves may lead to intrauterine hypoxia and/or maternal injury, and maintenance of drug levels at the lowest maternal therapeutic doses possible. Physiological changes in pregnancy result in lower concentrations of anticonvulsant drugs, which may need to be increased, subject to estimations of plasma levels. These drugs alter the absorption of folic acid and 5 mg/day should be given as a prophylactic precaution. For the same reason, clotting factors may be inhibited in the neonate, who should receive vitamin K. There is no evidence to support the policy of administering vitamin K to women in the last trimester of pregnancy to prevent neonatal vitamin K deficiency (Hey, 1999).

During pregnancy, the woman and her partner need full information about the incidence of congenital abnormalities and the screening tests available to them. They may also need individualized parenting programmes to help them devise strategies for coping safely with their baby. Midwives should be aware of the effects of phenytoin toxicity, which are nystagmus and ataxia in the woman. The confidential enquiry into maternal deaths (Lewis, 2001) records nine deaths related to epilepsy in the 1997–1999 triennium. Two of these deaths were sudden unexpected death in epilepsy (SUDEP), and three from accidental drowning in a bath. Previous reasons for maternal deaths have included aspiration of vomit. The midwife should therefore ensure that partners and families are aware of the importance of using the recovery position to maintain a safe airway, and women should be advised about ensuring that they do not take a bath when alone, to prevent accidental drowning.

Status epilepticus is a serious condition in which myoclonic seizures occur in rapid succession. It arises more commonly in the third trimester or in labour (Licht and Sankar, 1999) and may be associated with failure to take prescribed anticonvulsants or inhibition of their effectiveness during pregnancy because of the effects of oestrogen and progesterone. In the pregnancy of a woman not known to have epilepsy, this could initially be mistaken for eclampsia. It is controlled by increasing anticonvulsant therapy, by administering diazepam and by giving intravenous dextrose to prevent hypoglycaemia.

In the absence of obstetric complications, labour and delivery will be spontaneous.

All anticonvulsants are secreted in breast milk, but as long as the maternal dosage is not excessively high, there is no contraindication to breastfeeding. If the mother has received high doses of phenobarbitone, primidone or benzodiazepines during pregnancy, the baby may be hyperactive, restless, reluctant to suckle and may have vomiting or diarrhoea for up to a month. Parents need extra support postnatally, and the British Epilepsy Association (see Additional resources, p. 814) provides practical written guidance for parents about safety, which includes not bathing the baby when alone, changing the baby on the floor on a changing mat, feeding the baby while sitting on the floor, avoiding having hot drinks or cigarettes near the baby and having safety gates at the top and bottom of stairs.

OBSTETRIC CHOLESTASIS (INTRAHEPATIC CHOLESTASIS OF PREGNANCY

Intrahepatic cholestasis of pregnancy (ICP) is a disease arising in the third trimester, which is characterized by pruritus, dark-coloured urine, anorexia, malabsorption of fat and elevated maternal bile acid levels. It is thought to arise from a genetic hypersensitivity to oestrogen and is associated with increased rates of fetal mortality and morbidity, and with maternal coagulation defects, due to inability to absorb vitamin K, which is fat soluble (Nelson-Piercy, 1997). The condition was once thought to be benign, but it is now recognized that it may be a factor in 'unexplained' fetal deaths. It is thought that bile acids cause placental vasoconstriction, resulting in fetal hypoxia. In up to 40% of pregnancies complicated by ICP, there will be meconium in the amniotic fluid, with the risk of meconium aspiration (Redfearn and Chambers, 1996).

Any woman complaining of severe itching, which often begins on the palms of the hands, should be referred for liver function tests. If ICP is diagnosed, careful monitoring is required to detect and prevent coagulation defects by giving vitamin K. Fetal well-being is monitored, checking growth, liquor volume and blood flow, using Doppler studies. Early delivery may decrease the risk of perinatal mortality (Warwick, 1996).

Antihistamines such as promethazine (Phenergan) may be given to alleviate itching, and women should be encouraged to wear loose cotton clothing.

Although symptoms will disappear following delivery, the risk of recurrence in subsequent pregnancies is as high as 50%. Since the condition is related to oestrogen, women should avoid oral contraceptives containing oestrogen (Nelson-Piercy, 1997).

CONCLUSION

This chapter has reviewed some of the medical disorders midwives may encounter when working with pregnant women. Whilst pathophysiology and practical care are important, emphasis must also be placed on the need to treat women as individuals, and not as a reflection of their condition. The midwife has an important role in identifying women with pre-existing medical conditions, and women who may be at risk of developing such conditions, and in monitoring the well-being of the woman and her baby throughout. The need to educate and support women and involve them in planning and participating in their care will ensure that even should intervention be required, complications and problems should be minimized and the women will feel empowered during the process.

KEY POINTS

● ●

- Women with pre-existing medical disorders may be well informed about their condition and its management and be aware of risks associated with pregnancy.
- The midwife needs to be knowledgeable about medical disorders and contemporary management and care in order that she can interpret and explain this information to women and their families, working towards a partnership model of care.
- Women who develop medical disorders during pregnancy need education and support in relation to their condition.

- Strategies for reducing risk and preventing problems which medical disorders may present, need to be explored with women and their families.
- Women and their families need to be aware of signs and symptoms of deterioration and how to deal with them.
- Women and families may need antenatal education specifically tailored to their needs.
- Collaborative, multidisciplinary care is essential.

REFERENCES

Chamberlain, G. (1997) *ABC of Antenatal Care*. London: BMJ Publishing.

Consumers' Association (1994) Folic acid to prevent neural tube defects. *Drugs and Therapeutics Bulletin* **32**(4): 31–32.

Davison, J.M. & Dunlop, W. (1995) Urinary tract in pregnancy. In: Chamberlain, G. (ed) *Turnbull's Obstetrics*, 2nd edn, Ch. 26. Edinburgh: Churchill Livingstone.

Day, L. (1998) Iron supplementation in pregnancy: can it be justified? *British Journal of Midwifery* **6**(3): 385–390.

Department of Health (DoH) (1992) *Folic Acid and Neural Tube Defects – Guidelines on Prevention*. Circular PL/CMO (92) 18. London: DoH.

Department of Health (DoH) (1998) *Why Mothers Die: Report on Confidential Enquiries into Maternal Death 1994–96*. London: The Stationery Office.

de Swiet, M. (1995) Medical disorders in pregnancy. In: Chamberlain, G. (ed) *Turnbull's Obstetrics*, 2nd edn, Ch. 22. Edinburgh: Churchill Livingstone.

Gilbert, E.S. & Harmon, J.S. (1998) *A Manual of High Risk Pregnancy and Delivery*. New York: Mosby.

Gillmer, M.D.G & Hurley, P.A. (1999) Diabetes and endocrine disorders in pregnancy. In: Edmonds D.K. (ed) *Dewhurst's Textbook of Obstetrics and Gynaecology for Postgraduates*, Ch. 17. Oxford: Blackwell Science.

Guidotti, R.J. (2000) Anaemia in pregnancy in developing countries. *British Journal of Obstetrics and Gynaecology* **107**(4): 437–438.

Health Education Authority (HEA) (1996) *Folic Acid and the Prevention of Neural Tube Defects*. London: HMSO.

Hey, E. (1999) Effect of maternal anticonvulsant treatment on neonatal blood coagulation. *Archives of Disease in Childhood (Fetal and Neonatal Edition)* **81**: F208–F210.

Joint Tuberculosis Committee of the British Thoracic Society (2000) Control and prevention of tuberculosis in the UK: code of practice. *Thorax* **55**(11): 887–901.

Landon, M.B. (1999) Diabetes mellitus and other endocrine diseases. In: Gabbe, S.G., Niebyl, J.R. & Simpson J.L. (eds) *Obstetrics. Normal and Problem Pregnancies*, 4th edn, Ch. 31. New York: Churchill Livingstone.

Lauszus, F., Klebe, J.G. & Bek, T. (2000) Diabetic retinopathy in pregnancy during tight metabolic control. *Acta Obstetricia et Gynecologica Scandinavica* **79**(5), 367–370.

Lavender, R. (2000) Cranberry juice: the facts. *Nursing Times Plus* **96**(40): 11–12.

Lewis, G. (ed) (2001) *Why Mothers Die 1997–99: Fifth Report of the Confidential Enquiries into Maternal Deaths in the United Kingdom*. London: CEMD: associated with NICE, RCOG.

Licht, E.A. & Sankar, R. (1999) Status epilepticus during pregnancy: a case report. *Journal of Reproductive Medicine* **44**(4): 370–372.

Lindsay, P. (1990) Epilepsy in pregnancy *Nursing Times* **86**(24): 36–38.

McKay, K. (2000) Blood tests in pregnancy (2). Iron deficiency anaemia. *Practising Midwife* **3**(4): 25–27.

Mays, M. (1993) Tuberculosis: a comprehensive review for the certified nurse-midwife. *Journal of Nurse-Midwifery* **38**(3): 132–139.

Mahomed, K. (1997) Iron and folate supplementation in pregnancy (Cochrane Review). *The Cochrane Library*, Issue 1, 2002. Oxford: Update Software.

Marieb, E. (1999) *Human Anatomy and Physiology*, 4th edn. California: Benjamin/Cummings Science Publishing.

Mason, B.A. & Brobowski, R.A. (1998) Cardiac disease. In: Queenan, J.T. & Hobbins, J.C. (eds) *Protocols for High-risk Pregnancies*, Ch. 32. Washington: Blackwell Science.

Moore-Gillon, J. (1994) Asthma in pregnancy. *British Journal of Obstetrics and Gynaecology* **101**(8): 658–660.

Nelson-Piercy, C. (1997) *Handbook of Obstetric Medicine*. Cambridge: Isis Medical Media.

Oakley, C.M. (1999) Heart disease in pregnancy. In: Edmonds D.K. (ed) *Dewhurst's Textbook of Obstetrics and Gynaecology for Postgraduates,* Ch. 16. Oxford: Blackwell Science.

Redfearn, J. & Chambers, J. (1996) Obstetric cholestasis: Itching in pregnancy? Midwives must be alert. *Midwives* **109**(1297): 36–37.

Robson, S.C. (1999) Hypertension and renal disease in pregnancy. In: Edmonds D.K. (ed) *Dewhurst's Textbook of Obstetrics and Gynaecology for Postgraduates,* Ch. 15. Oxford: Blackwell Science.

Samuels, P. (1999) Renal disease. In: Gabbe, S.G., Niebyl, J.R. & Simpson J.L. (eds) *Obstetrics. Normal and Problem Pregnancies,* 3rd edn, Ch. 30. New York: Churchill Livingstone.

Schatz, M. (1992) Asthma during pregnancy. *Annals of Allergy* **68**(1): 123–133.

Steer, P., Alam, M.A. & Wadsworth, J. (1995) Relation between maternal Hb concentration and birth weight in different ethnic groups. *British Medical Journal* **310**(6978): 489–491.

Thomas, H. (1999) Women's' experiences of major illness during pregnancy. *MIDIRS Midwifery Digest* **9**(3): 312–316.

Van den Broek, N. (1998) Anaemia in pregnancy in developing countries. *British Journal of Obstetrics and Gynaecology* **105**(4): 385–390.

Wallace, H., Shorvon, S. & Tallis, R. (1998) Age-specific incidence and prevalence rates of treated epilepsy in an unselected population of 2,052,922 and age-specific fertility rates of women with epilepsy. *Lancet* **352**(9145): 1970–1973.

Warwick, K. (1996) Diagnosis and treatment for cholestasis in pregnancy. *Midwives* **109**(1297): 37–38.

World Health Organization (WHO) (1979) *The Prevalence of Nutritional Anaemia in Developing Countries.* WHO. Geneva.

World Health Organization (WHO) (1980) *Expert Committee on Diabetes Mellitus.* WHO Technical Report 646: 1–79.

FURTHER READING

Gilbert, E.S. & Harmon, J.S. (1998) *A Manual of High Risk Pregnancy and Delivery.* New York: Mosby.
An American text with clear emphasis on interventions and support by midwives. Readers must allow for differing provision of healthcare and different units of measurement, but overall, a practical and sensitive approach.

Gillmer, M.D.G. & Hurley, P.A. (1999) Diabetes and endocrine disorders in pregnancy. In: Edmonds D.K. (ed) *Dewhurst's Textbook of Obstetrics and Gynaecology for Postgraduates,* Ch. 17. Oxford: Blackwell Science. Primarily for doctors, but the section on diabetes is well written and explains the complex underlying physiology

and pathophysiology. The rationale behind screening for gestational diabetes is clearly outlined, and regimes for care are suggested.

Nelson-Piercy, C. (1997) *Handbook of Obstetric Medicine.* Cambridge: Isis Medical Media.
A concise and up-to-date handbook in a readable and interesting format. Although intended for medical students and doctors, the background information and pathophysiology is invaluable for student midwives and midwives. In some cases statements are not referenced, but each chapter is followed by suggestions for further reading.

ADDITIONAL RESOURCES

British Epilepsy Association
New Anstey House, Gate Way Drive, Yeadon, Leeds LS19 7XY
Tel: 0113 210 8800
Website: http://www.epilepsy.org.uk

Diabetes UK
PO Box 1, Portishead, Bristol BS20 7EG

Tel: 0800 585 088
Website: http://www.diabetes.org.uk

Sickle Cell Society
Green Lodge, Barretts Green Road, London NW10 7AP

United Kingdom Thalassaemia Society
107 Nightingale Lane, London N8 7QY

47

Sexually Transmitted Diseases

Jane Susan Bott

LEARNING OUTCOMES

This chapter aims to enable the reader to:

- understand the midwife's role in offering and recommending screening for human immuno-deficiency virus (HIV), syphilis and hepatitis B virus (HBV) infection during pregnancy
- be aware of the ethical principles which underpin midwifery practice

- discuss the clinical presentation, where appropriate, pregnancy implications and management of selected sexually transmitted infections (STIs)
- discuss the clinical presentation and management of vaginal candidiasis in pregnancy.

Ideally, sexually transmitted infections are diagnosed in genitourinary medicine (GUM) clinics, where, in addition to testing, facilities exist for contacting, testing and treating sexual partners to prevent reinfection and further spread of infection. Those most at risk are people having unprotected sexual intercourse (i.e. not using a condom), especially those with more than one sexual partner, and those who frequently change partners (PHLS, 2001a).

As all pregnant women have had unprotected sex, midwives should take every opportunity to discuss and promote sexual health, as appropriate. Further discussion of the midwife's role in health promotion is beyond the scope of this chapter. However, suggestions for further reading have been included at the end of the chapter. Routine screening for selected sexually transmitted infections (STIs) during pregnancy is recommended; for example human immunodeficiency virus (HIV), hepatitis B virus (HBV) and syphilis may have adverse effects on pregnancy outcome. If any of these tests are positive, testing for other STIs is recommended (PHLS, 2001a). Midwives should ensure that all women receive information about these blood tests, when offering and recommending screening during the booking visit.

Most STIs, if detected early, are treatable and can be cured with antibiotics, e.g. gonorrhoea and syphilis. However, patients with viral infection, such as herpes simplex virus (HSV) experience recurrences, as the virus remains in the body and reactivates on occasions. HIV is more serious as currently no cure is available, and the effects may be more devastating for a pregnant woman and her family.

This chapter will examine the midwife's role in relation to HIV screening, highlighting the complex issues involved in decision-making. Ethical principles which underpin the midwife's role in relation to offering and recommending HIV testing during pregnancy will be applied (Box 47.1). Midwives should be guided by the principles of *Changing Childbirth* (DoH, 1993), which advocates a woman-centred approach to care. Accurate information based upon the best currently available evidence should be available to enable women to choose for themselves the tests they want. These principles may also be applied to the midwife's role when offering and recommending screening for HBV and syphilis. These STIs, in addition to other relevant STIs, will be discussed, with reference to clinical presentation, pregnancy implications and management. In addition, vaginal candidiasis (moniliasis or thrush) will be discussed. Though not a true STI, an understanding of its clinical presentation and management will enable midwives to meet women's sexual health needs effectively (Young, 2000).

HIV SCREENING DURING PREGNANCY

In 2000, about 1 in 350 pregnant women in London were infected with HIV, according to the unlinked

Box 47.1 Ethical principles

- Beneficence
- Non-maleficence
- Informed consent
- Autonomy
- Confidentiality

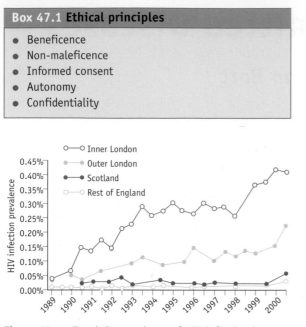

Figure 47.1 Trends in prevalence of HIV infection in pregnant women by area of residence: 1989–2000. (Source of data: DoH, 2001; reproduced by permission of PHLS.)

anonymous prevalence monitoring programme (DoH, 2001). This is the highest ever level since reporting began in 1988, and reflects a ninefold rise. 1 in 240 women were infected in inner London, compared with 1 in 530 living in outer London. HIV prevalence varied according to maternal district of residence within London, ranging from zero to about 1 in 140. The prevalence is less elsewhere in the UK, but has risen since 1998 from about 1 in 6500 to 1 in 3700 in 2000 (Fig. 47.1). The prevalence of HIV infection among pregnant women largely reflects migration of women of black African ethnicity who were probably infected in sub-Saharan Africa.

Better diagnosis rates for HIV infection during pregnancy will enable infected women to make an informed choice regarding interventions, which can almost eliminate the risk of vertical transmission of HIV infection from mother to infant (PHLS, 2001b). These interventions include antiretroviral treatment during pregnancy, at delivery and for the newborn infant, delivery by caesarean section and the avoidance of breastfeeding.

In 2000 there were an estimated 452 births to HIV-infected mothers in the UK. This would have resulted in about 120 HIV-infected infants if none of these maternal infections had been diagnosed (assuming a mother-to-infant transmission rate of about 25% in the absence of interventions; DoH, 2001). However, with a growing proportion of infections diagnosed before delivery

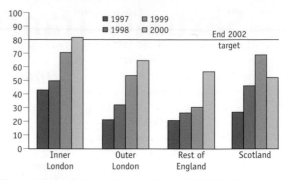

Figure 47.2 Estimated proportion of HIV infections diagnosed before delivery amongst pregnant women. Data are subject to reporting delay, particularly for recent years. (Source of data: CDSC, 2002; reproduced by permission of PHLS.)

(Fig. 47.2), and assuming that 2% of babies will acquire HIV despite the maternal infections being diagnosed prior to delivery, it is estimated that 45 infants were infected with HIV in 2000. National targets have been set by the Department of Health to improve the uptake of HIV testing during pregnancy to 90% by 2002 (DoH, 1999).

Reflective Activity 47.1

What is the incidence of HIV-infected women in your trust, and what services are available?

Disease progression

Different phases of the disease have been identified (Pratt, 1995):

- 2–6 weeks after the initial infection with HIV some people develop acute 'glandular fever-like symptoms'. This is known as the *acute primary infection* (phase A). Symptoms include lethargy and malaise, headache, fever, painful joints, muscular pain, diarrhoea and skin rash. Some people may develop aseptic meningitis, encephalitis, and swollen lymph glands (lymphadenopathy). Other people, however, may have unrecognizable symptoms. Towards the end of this phase, HIV antibodies are produced (seroconversion).
- Phase B is the *antibody-positive phase* following seroconversion. During this phase, which is thought to last 10–15 years, many people remain clinically asymptomatic.
- Phase C is the period of *early symptomatic disease*, during which people usually become chronically ill,

and may be affected by a variety of minor opportunistic infections such as oral candidiasis.

- Phase D is known as the *late symptomatic disease (acquired immunodeficiency syndrome – AIDS) stage*. Patients commonly present with a host of opportunistic infections, as various pathogens are able to take the 'opportunity' of a depressed immune system to establish clinical illness.
- During Phase E, treatment of opportunistic infections results in *periods of remission* and relatively good health.
- Phase F is the *terminal phase*. *Pneumocystis carinii* pneumonia is the commonest cause of death. Patients are frequently blind (due to cytomegalovirus retinitis), incontinent, grossly malnourished and suffer from dementia.

Beneficence

When applying the ethical principle of beneficence, the midwife should ensure that the outcomes of care result in 'good' being done to the woman and her baby. This entails informing women of the advantages of HIV testing during pregnancy. The benefits of HIV testing are as follows:

Reduced rate of vertical transmission   Although the fetus can become infected during the first trimester of pregnancy (Scarlatti, 1996), evidence suggests that at least 65% of infections occur during the final 6 weeks of pregnancy and at delivery (Rouzioux *et al.*, 1993). The following interventions have been found to reduce the risk of vertical transmission:

- *Zidovudine*. In addition to reducing the risk of vertical transmission, zidovudine (Box 47.2) also appears to decrease the risk of stillbirth and deaths after the neonatal period, whilst having no effect on the incidence of premature delivery, birthweight or maternal death (Brocklehurst, 2001a).
- *Bottlefeeding*. Breastfeeding may double the risk of mother-to-child transmission of HIV infection (Newell *et al.*, 1997). Advising the mother to avoid breastfeeding would reduce the risk of transmission by a further 7–22% (Dunn *et al.*, 1992). However, midwives need to be aware of cultural issues when advising and supporting women (see Case scenario 47.1).
- *Elective caesarean section* (i.e., before labour and rupture of membranes). An individual-patient meta-analysis incorporating 8533 mother–infant pairs from 15 prospective cohort studies found that elective caesarean section decreases the risk of transmission by more than 50%, after adjustment for antiretroviral

---

Box 47.2 Zidovudine (AZT) in pregnancy

Action

- Zidovudine is an antiretroviral drug which inhibits HIV replication
- Treatment results in a significant reduction in the risk of vertical transmission from 25.5–8.3% (Connor *et al.*, 1994)

Dosage/route

- Oral zidovudine 100 mg, five times daily started between 14–34 weeks of pregnancy
- Intravenous zidovudine during labour, 2 mg/kg body weight over a 1-hour period, followed by continuous infusion of 1 mg/kg/h until delivery
- Zidovudine syrup given to the baby, 2 mg/kg, four times a day for 6 weeks, beginning 8–12 hours after delivery

---

Case scenario 47.1

Abisola is a 24-year-old African woman who has been living in London for 2 years. She is 14 weeks pregnant and HIV testing has confirmed that she is infected with HIV. Bottlefeeding has been advised in addition to other interventions. The avoidance of breastfeeding will pose problems for Abisola as her cultural background views breastfeeding as the norm. She needs to think about how she will manage to bottlefeed within her social network. Her midwife spends time with Abisola and her partner discussing various strategies for dealing with the potential dilemmas posed when bottlefeeding.

---

therapy, maternal disease stage, and birthweight. Compared with other modes of delivery and no antiretroviral therapy, elective caesarean delivery and the three-part zidovudine regimen combined reduced transmission by more than 85% (International Perinatal HIV Group, 1999). A randomized trial of mode of delivery in Europe found a transmission rate of 1.8% among women randomized to elective caesarean section compared with 10.5% for women randomized to vaginal delivery. Approximately 65% of women were taking prophylactic antiretroviral therapy. There were few postpartum complications and no serious adverse events in either group (European Mode of Delivery Collaboration, 1999). Delivery by caesarean section in women taking the long course of AZT and who do not breastfeed has been shown to reduce the risk of transmission to about 1% (UNAIDS, 1999).

- *Other interventions* that may further reduce the risk of vertical transmission include:
  - the avoidance of invasive procedures, e.g. amniocentesis (Anastos *et al.*, 1997)
  - washing the baby after delivery (Johnstone, 1996)
  - screening and treatment of other sexually transmitted diseases (UNAIDS, 1999)
  - combination antiretroviral therapy: preliminary findings of one study suggest a further decrease in the risk of transmission when a combination of zidovudine and lamivudine is given during pregnancy and labour, or during labour and postnatally (Brocklehurst, 2001a).

Benefits for the mother   Early diagnoses of HIV enables 'optimal control' of HIV infection, improving maternal health and life-expectancy. This is achieved when a woman with a measurable viral burden consistently takes highly active antiretroviral therapy (HAART), has a stable or increasing CD4 lymphocyte count, is receiving appropriate prophylaxis for opportunistic infections, based on the lowest past CD4 count, and has achieved maximum suppression of HIV replication load (Beckerman, 1998).

Combination therapy, using two or more drugs, is associated with prolonged suppression of viral replication, marked reductions in viral load, and a delay in the emergence of viral resistance. In contrast, monotherapy (for example, only using zidovudine) is considered substandard treatment because it is likely to lead to the development of resistant virus which becomes more difficult to treat. Some women who have their infections diagnosed during pregnancy may be advised to commence combination therapy for maternal reasons. Women who become pregnant and are already receiving combination antiretroviral therapy are advised to continue their therapy, as any interruption is likely to be associated with rebound of plasma HIV RNA measurements to pretreatment levels or higher (Beckerman, 1998).

As both HIV disease and pregnancy place major nutritional burdens on a woman's body (Beckerman, 1998), referral to a dietician is beneficial.

Benefits for the baby   It has been estimated that over 1600 children have been born to HIV-infected mothers in the UK (PHLS, 2001b). Of these, 38% have been shown to be infected, 40% are known to be uninfected, and the remainder have not had their infection status established, because all babies initially have

antibodies to HIV as a result of the transfer of maternal antibodies. These antibodies disappear by 18 months in babies who have not become infected. Nevertheless, it is possible to conclusively diagnose most cases of paediatric HIV infection by 1 month of age using sensitive viral tests, while virtually all are diagnosable by 6 months (Josefson, 1997). It is recommended that all infants with confirmed HIV infection under 12 months of age be treated with combination antiretroviral therapy (Josefson, 1997). Thus children would be able to benefit from such treatment in the same way as adults can. Because infants who acquire the infection perinatally are still developing their immune system during the first 6 months of life, they have potentially more to gain from such treatment (Josefson, 1997). Without treatment, approximately 23–26% of HIV-infected babies will develop features characteristic of AIDS within the first year of life, and their health will deteriorate rapidly (Scarlatti, 1996).

About 30–50% of HIV-infected children present with an early onset of opportunistic infections such as *Pneumocystis carinii* pneumonia (PCP), whilst those that do better have no signs or symptoms of disease until 8–10 years of age (Scarlatti, 1996). To reduce the prevalence and severity of infection, the Centers for Disease Control and Prevention (1995) recommend PCP prophylaxis by 4–6 weeks of age for all children born to HIV-positive mothers. A reduction in the frequency of bacterial infections which commonly affect children after the first year of life has been obseved, and it has been suggested that this may be attributable to the use of prophylactic antibiotics, especially co-trimoxazole, and intravenous immunoglobulin (Scarlatti, 1996).

In the UK, prophylactic treatment of most infants born to HIV-infected women from 6 weeks of age has been associated with nearly 60% reduction in progression to AIDS (70% of which was PCP) within the first 6 months of life in infants born after the beginning of 1994 compared with those born before (Duong *et al.*, 1999).

Benefits for the family   Informed decisions can be made regarding the current pregnancy, planning future pregnancies and testing other family members for HIV. Information can also be given in relation to preventing the spread of HIV infection. This is particularly important because in one study 11% of patients were infected with HIV-1 variants harbouring mutations that are associated with resistance to drugs used in the treatment of HIV (Yerly *et al.*, 1999). In such cases, patients may have a poor virological response to combination antiretroviral

---

Box 47.3 Potential 'harm'

- Psychological impact – suicide risk
- Social sequelae – impact on work/family/ relationships
- Stigma/discrimination
- Insurance/mortgage issues (if positive)
- Unnecessary treatment of about 85% of mothers and their uninfected babies (RCOG, 1997)
- Long-term side-effects of zidovudine need to be excluded for children of treated mothers
- Mild neonatal anaemia occurs more frequently (Connor *et al.*, 1994)
- 12–16 caesarean sections would be required to prevent infection in one infant (Scarlatti, 1996)
- Risks associated with sepsis following caesarean section are greater in HIV-infected women (UNAIDS, 1999)
- Transmission to baby via breastfeeding

---

therapy (Cohen and Fauci, 1999). Furthermore, misperception regarding the seriousness of HIV-1 infection in the era of highly active antiretroviral therapy (HAART) has contributed to an increase in high-risk sexual activity among some people (Kelly *et al.*, 1998). These factors, combined with the fact that a safe and effective HIV-1 vaccine has not yet been developed, highlight the crucial need for health promotion/disease prevention.

Non-maleficence

When applying the ethical principle of non-maleficence, the midwife should ensure that any act or omission does not result in harm. An awareness of the potential 'harm' (Box 47.3) will enable midwives to discuss any individual concerns with women, who must decide for themselves whether screening is in their best interests.

Awaiting the results of HIV testing and receiving a positive result can be considerably stressful, and midwives need to be sensitive to an individual's need for support during this time. One piece of research has shown that receiving an HIV diagnosis is a traumatic experience, resulting in reactions of shock, fear, and anguish. For some women, the shadow of death lurked threateningly from the moment they received their diagnosis. The thought of potentially causing death to others was also common. One woman recounted: 'When I found out ... my baby had AIDS, I was thinking, he is going to die. What if he dies? O God, I am a murderer. What have I done?' (Stevens and Tighe, 1997: 527). Women often experience unrelenting misery, escalating drug

use and transmission risks, and destabilization of relationships, income and shelter. Other examples of harm include risk of rejection, isolation, domestic violence (Lester *et al.*, 1995) and suicide (Campbell, 1995). Therefore, it is important that midwives are able to refer women to specialist counsellors and social workers as appropriate, to reduce the potential social and psychological 'harm'. Details of HIV support groups may also be given.

Informing women of the 15–20% risk of vertical transmission is the same as telling them that 80–85% of babies will not be infected, and therefore the majority of mothers who accept the interventions on offer will be exposing themselves and their babies to unnecessary treatment. Zidovudine treatment has been associated with a higher incidence of neonatal anaemia (haemoglobin concentration of less than 9 g/dl), although by 12 weeks of age this effect is no longer apparent (Connor *et al.*, 1994). So far, one study has evaluated the long-term effects of in utero exposure to zidovudine vs placebo among a randomized cohort of uninfected children. No major adverse effects of zidovudine up to the age of 4 years were found (Culnane *et al.*, 1999). However, continued prospective evaluations of children born to HIV-infected women who are exposed to zidovudine are critical to assess the long-term safety, as data from animal studies demonstrate the potential for transplacental carcinogenicity of zidovudine (Olivero *et al.*, 1997).

Research findings support the hypothesis of a link between mitochondrial dysfunction and the perinatal administration of antiretroviral combination therapy (zidovudine and lamivudine). The researchers concluded that zidovudine monotherapy should continue to be recommended, although further assessment of the toxic effects of combination therapy is required (Blanche *et al.*, 1999). Knowledge of the latest research findings will enable midwives to provide accurate information for women regarding treatment implications.

Postoperative complications are significantly more common in HIV-1-positive women compared to HIV-1-negative matches, according to the findings of a randomized controlled trial comparing the clinical outcomes of 62 HIV-infected women who underwent caesarean section between 1987 and 1999 (Grubert *et al.*, 1999). Postpartum pyrexia requiring antibiotics was especially common. HIV-infected women were also more likely to require blood transfusions, as they frequently develop anaemia, a side-effect of antiretroviral therapy. When considering caesarean section, the risk of maternal morbidity and the risk of vertical transmission should be carefully weighed up, particularly for women on HAART.

The advice to avoid breastfeeding is based on relatively few studies of poor quality (Brocklehurst, 2001a). According to the findings of a recent study of 549 HIV-infected women, exclusive breastfeeding carries a significantly lower risk of HIV-1 transmission (almost half the risk) than mixed feeding and a similar risk to no breastfeeding (Coutsoudis *et al.*, 1999). The authors of this study raise the possibility that virus acquired during delivery could have been neutralized by immune factors present in breast milk but not in formula feeds. In addition, breast milk contains growth factors, such as epidermal growth factor and transforming growth factor β, which may enhance maturation of the gut epithelial barrier, thus maintaining its integrity and hindering passage of the virus (Planchon *et al.*, 1994; Udall *et al.*, 1981). In the mixed-feeding group, the beneficial immune factors of breast milk are probably counteracted by damage to the infant's gut by contaminants or allergens in mixed feeds. Further research is urgently required to confirm and elucidate these findings. In the meantime, it is premature to revise infant feeding guidelines on the basis of this one study (Newell, 1999).

If HIV-1-infected women choose to breastfeed, they should be advised to avoid giving any other foods for at least the first 3 months. Early and abrupt weaning should be advised because of the increased risk of late postnatal transmission through breast milk after 3–6 months, (Leroy *et al.*, 1998) and because introduction of other foods becomes more frequent as the infant gets older.

Reflective Activity 47.2

Identify appropriate HIV support groups (voluntary agencies) for women in your area, including contact details and referral information.

Informed consent

Each woman needs to be aware of the implications of receiving an HIV diagnosis in order that she can decide for herself whether testing would be in her best interest and, if necessary, make informed decisions regarding treatment and interventions. According to Gillon (1986) consent is given when an individual makes a voluntary uncoerced decision on the basis of adequate information and deliberation. Midwives have a key role in providing relevant and up-to-date information in an appropriate way (Box 47.4).

Box 47.4 Information for women (Antenatal HIV Testing Working Party, 1998)

- Nature and purpose of test
- Advantages
- Disadvantages
- Insurance/mortgage issues
- Assurances re non-discriminatory service
- Confidentiality policy
- Advice on safer sex
- Unlinked anonymous surveys
- Unit's policy on HIV testing
- Process of testing/informing of results
- Risk assessment

Leaflets can be useful, and if sent to the woman prior to the booking interview, may serve as a basis for further discussion prior to testing. Some women may require more time to consider the implications before making their decision, and midwives should offer a further appointment in such instances. In providing a 'woman-centred' approach to care, midwives need to ensure that all women, including those from different cultural groups, are able to understand the relevant information. Information needs to be targeted more appropriately for such women, e.g. videos or specially designed leaflets. Some hospitals have produced leaflets in different languages, e.g. Somali, French, Bengali, Gujarati, Vietnamese and Turkish.

Reflective Activity 47.3

What care provision exits for women from ethnic minority groups? What cultural factors need to be considered when helping women (and their partners) to make an informed choice in relation to testing and management options?

Autonomy

Autonomy is inextricably linked with consent and entails facilitating a woman's ability to formulate and carry out her own plans so that she is in control of her life, and can act freely within the context of rational decision-making (Downie and Calman, 1987). Midwives should ensure that women do not feel coerced into having the test, as this would cause 'harm' if the woman's rights were infringed, and would undermine women's feelings of being in control. It may also discourage some women from seeking antenatal care.

However, there may be attitudinal barriers to testing and treatment of HIV, which may be overcome as midwives allow time for discussion if necessary. For example, one study found that negative attitudes towards AZT were widely prevalent. Women viewed the drug as highly toxic, prescribed indiscriminately, inadequately tested in women and minorities, promoted for the wrong reasons and inappropriate while they were feeling well (Siegel and Gorey, 1997).

Confidentiality

A breach of confidentiality is particularly serious for women who are HIV positive because of the risk of discrimination, even within the health service. Midwives are required to practice in accordance with the Nursing and Midwifery Council (NMC) standards for professional practice, which are designed to protect the public. Midwives are personally accountable for their practice and must 'protect all confidential information concerning patients and clients obtained in the course of professional practice and make disclosures only with consent, where required by the order of a court or where you can justify disclosure in the wider public interest' (NMC, 2002). At the initial visit, midwives should inform women of the standards of confidentiality that will be maintained. This includes explaining to women that some information, such as an HIV diagnosis, may be made available to other healthcare professionals involved in the delivery of care. They should be informed who this might be, and the woman's explicit consent must be obtained before disclosing specific information. Confidentiality standards can be included in leaflets and posters in the healthcare setting, reinforcing to women what they can expect from the service. Midwives who fail to maintain these standards risk causing personal distress to women in their care, and women may sue through the civil court for alleged breach of confidentiality (NMC, 2002).

HEPATITIS B VIRUS (HBV)

The Department of Health advises that all women should be offered screening for HBV infection during pregnancy. As with HIV, many infected people are asymptomatic and are unaware of their infection. Others experience 'flu-like' symptoms and jaundice (DoH, RCM, 2000). Approximately 10% of infected people become carriers of the virus (Sira, 1998) and 20% of carriers may develop serious liver disease, such as cirrhosis or hepatocellular carcinoma (Wright and Lau, 1993). Vertical transmission may occur at or around the time of birth (DoH, RCM, 2000), and up to 90% of infected infants become chronic carriers (Grosheide and Van Damme, 1996). These infants are at risk of premature death from chronic liver disease. However, immunization can prevent such infants developing carrier status in up to 95% of cases (Hadler and Margolis, 1992).

Screening involves testing a blood specimen for HBV surface antigen (HBsAg). If the screening test is positive, confirmatory testing is undertaken. If infection is confirmed, tests for hepatitis B e-markers are carried out to determine whether the newborn baby should be given hepatitis B specific immunoglobulin (HBIg), in addition to hepatitis B vaccine.

Babies born to carrier mothers should be immunized with hepatitis B vaccine within 24 hours of birth. If the mother carries the hepatitis B e-antigen or has had acute HBV infection during pregnancy, the baby should also receive HBIg. Further doses of vaccine are given at 1 and 2 months of age. At 12 months a booster dose is given, and follow-up testing should also be carried out (DoH, RCM, 2000). As breastfeeding is not contraindicated, mothers should be encouraged and supported to breastfeed during this time. Mothers should also be referred to a specialist with expertise in liver disease.

Reflective Activity 47.4

Refer to your local trust protocol for midwives offering and recommending HIV screening during pregnancy. What guidelines have been included in relation to ensuring that confidentiality is maintained? Are these adequate? If not, what improvements could be made? What support and care would be provided for women who have a positive test result?

Reflective Activity 47.5

Refer to your local trust protocol for midwives offering and recommending HBV screening. What written information is given to infected mothers regarding when injections should be given to their babies, and who is responsible for administering each dose? Who is responsible for ensuring follow-up appointments are made?

The DoH has produced a leaflet in a range of languages for midwives to give to women who have a positive test result (Hepatitis B: how to protect your baby). The leaflet provides information about HBV infection and the health implications for the baby, the mother and close contacts. It emphasizes the importance of a complete course of immunization to protect the baby. Ensure you have these leaflets to give to women as appropriate. They may be obtained by telephoning the NHS Responseline on 0541 555455, by fax from Prolog on 01623 724524, or by email: doh@prologistics.co.uk

SYPHILIS

Syphilis is caused by *Treponema pallidum*, a spirochaete, which is a bacteria-like organism. In the UK, syphilitic infections are relatively uncommon, compared to infections such as chlamydia and gonorrhoea (PHLS, 2001a). Maternal infections have been found in almost every health region but are more prevalent in London and the South East (Hurtig *et al.*, 1998). Being born abroad and belonging to an ethnic minority group are high-risk factors (Hurtig *et al.*, 1998). Nine presumptive cases of children with congenital syphilis were reported during 1994–97.

Symptoms of syphilis are not specific. Indeed, a person may have no symptoms, and transmit the infection unknowingly. Following an incubation period of 3–90 days (Genc and Ledger, 2000), one or more painless but highly infectious sores may appear (primary infection), usually at the site of the infection (PHLS, 2001a). 50% of people also develop lymphadenopathy. The sores resolve spontaneously after 2–6 weeks, although secondary symptoms may develop 6 weeks to 6 months later. These include headache, low-grade fever, generalized lymphadenopathy, rash on the palms and soles, patchy alopecia, mild hepatitis and nephrotic syndrome (Genc and Ledger, 2000). If the infection is undetected or untreated, about 40% of people will develop late symptoms, 4 or more years after the primary infection. Complications may occur in the mucocutaneous tissue, heart, respiratory tract or central nervous system, producing variable symptoms which range from skin lesions (a rash on the palms of the hands or soles of the feet) to dementia (PHLS, 2001a).

During pregnancy, syphilis may cause spontaneous abortion, perinatal or infant death, intrauterine growth restriction and neonatal infection (Genc and Ledger, 2000; Schulz *et al.*, 1987). The risk of vertical transmission diminishes as maternal syphilis advances (Hurtig *et al.*, 1998). Screening during pregnancy enables infected women to benefit from treatment and helps prevent vertical transmission. At least 40 maternal infections are detected annually in the UK (Connor *et al.*, 2000) through routine blood testing using, for example, the Venereal Disease Research Laboratory (VDRL) test and the fluorescent treponemal antibody absorption (FTA-ABS) assay. Women at risk of infection should be retested in the third trimester (Genc and Ledger, 2000).

Penicillin is the treatment of choice during pregnancy. A single intramuscular dose of benzathine penicillin, 2.4 million units, has been shown to prevent fetal infection in 98% of cases (Alexander *et al.*, 1999), although some authorities recommend a second dose a week later (Genc and Ledger, 2000). However, treatment failure has been found to occur in HIV-infected women. Therefore, the HIV status of the mother and the stage of maternal infection should be considered when determining a penicillin regimen. Some authorities recommend that HIV-infected women and women with long-standing syphilis be treated for up to 3 weeks (Donders, 2000; Genc and Ledger, 2000).

Genc and Ledger (2000) state that, despite appropriate treatment, 14% of infected women will have a stillbirth or an infected liveborn infant. Furthermore, treatment may be complicated by the Jarisch–Herxheimer reaction, an allergic response, which can cause fetal distress, premature labour, fever, chills, headache, hypotension, tachycardia and myalgia (Genc and Ledger, 2000). This usually occurs several hours after treatment and resolves within 1–2 days.

Syphilis is not transmitted during breastfeeding, unless an infectious lesion is present on the breast (Genc and Ledger, 2000). Midwives should ensure that women are given this information.

GONORRHOEA

Gonorrhoea, which is the second most common bacterial STI in the UK, is caused by the bacterium *Neisseria gonorrhoeae*. During 1999, the highest rates of female gonorrhoea occurred in women aged between 16–19 years (139/100 000). The recent rise in diagnoses in women suggests that there has been a significant increase in heterosexually transmitted gonorrhoea. Rates of diagnoses were highest in London (PHLS, 2001a).

Many women and some men are unaware of their infection (PHLS, 2001a), as gonorrhoea often causes mild symptoms. Symptoms may appear 2–10 days after becoming infected. Women commonly experience dysuria and yellow or bloodstained vaginal discharge. Men are more likely to experience symptoms, which are typically dysuria and discharge from the penis. Men and women with rectal infections may also experience discharge from the anus, anal discomfort and pain during anal intercourse (PHLS, 2001a). Rarely, untreated gonorrhoea can spread to the bloodstream or the joints.

Gonorrhoea, if untreated, can result in women developing pelvic inflammatory disease (PID), which is difficult to treat. In pregnancy it has been associated with prelabour rupture of the membranes and preterm delivery (Amstey and Steadman, 1976). The infection can be transmitted from the mother's genital tract to the neonate during vaginal delivery. Occasionally, when there is prolonged rupture of the membranes, it can be transmitted to the fetus before birth. The risk of transmission from an infected mother is between 30–47% (Fransen et al., 1986; Galega et al., 1984). Neonatal infection usually manifests itself in the form of gonococcal ophthalmia neonatorum in the first few days of life. Profuse purulent conjunctival discharge, which is frequently bilateral, is apparent. If left untreated, the infection will eventually cause blindness. Occasionally, the neonate may develop gonococcal infection elsewhere, such as gonococcal arthritis (Brocklehurst, 2001b). In the postpartum period, gonorrhoea can cause endometritis and pelvic sepsis in the mother, which may be severe.

Gonorrhoea may be diagnosed by taking a cervical swab, and is usually treated with penicillin during pregnancy. However, for women who are allergic to penicillin or who are infected with penicillinase-producing *Neisseria gonorrhoeae* (PPNG), treatment with ceftriaxone or spectinomycin appears to be as effective in producing microbiological cure (Brocklehurst, 2001b).

HERPES SIMPLEX VIRUS (HSV)

HSV causes genital herpes, which is the commonest ulcerative STI in the UK. Two types have been isolated, HSV-1 and HSV-2. Both types can cause genital infection, although type 1 usually causes lesions of the face, lips and eyes (Adler, 1999). HSV-2 is mostly acquired sexually (Drake et al., 2000). Genital HSV is spread by direct contact via unprotected vaginal or anal sex, genital contact or through oral sex with someone with cold sores. Both genital herpes and cold sores are very infectious when an infected person has either blisters or sores,

although it is possible for the virus to be transmitted when the infected person has no symptoms (PHLS, 2001a).

During 1999 almost 17 500 newly diagnosed primary HSV infections were reported among people attending GUM clinics in the UK, with the highest number of infections occurring in men and women aged between 20–24 years (PHLS, 2001a). However, this is an underrepresentation, as others are diagnosed and managed by general practitioners, gynaecologists or dermatologists (Adler, 1999).

The primary infection is often quite severe, causing multiple painful genital ulcers after an incubation period of less than 7 days. Ulcers may also appear on the buttocks, thighs and anus. The ulcers begin as erythematous areas, which develop into vesicles before becoming ulcers. Finally, they become dry crusts (Adler, 1999). Primary attacks last for 3 weeks, and some people also experience groin pain due to inguinal lymphadenopathy. Patients commonly experience dysuria (PHLS, 2001a), about a third experience fever and malaise, and a few have headaches, photophobia and viral meningitis (Adler, 1999). Seroconversion occurs 4–6 weeks after the primary infection, when type-specific antibodies become detectable (Drake et al., 2000). After the initial infection the virus becomes dormant in the dorsal root ganglion which innervates the affected epithelium (Drake et al., 2000). The virus reactivates from time to time to cause recurrences, which may be preceded by symptoms such as itching, tingling or pain in the genital area. During recurrent phases, the lesions are similar to those occurring in the primary attack, although they are fewer in number and heal more quickly (Adler, 1999). Most people experience mild and infrequent symptoms, although some may experience more frequent and severe recurrent episodes. However, some people may not experience any symptoms during either a primary infection (Drake et al., 2000) or a recurrence (PHLS, 2001a).

Approximately 85% of cases of neonatal herpes result from perinatal transmission of the virus during vaginal delivery because of symptomatic or asymptomatic shedding of the virus from the genital tract. Neonatal infection can cause severe neurological impairment or death. However, neonatal herpes occurs very rarely in the UK (PHLS, 2001a). Approximately 10 cases per year have been reported (Tookey and Peckham, 1997).

Women who have symptoms of primary genital herpes during pregnancy should have the diagnosis confirmed by viral culture, which may take 1 week (Drake *et al.*, 2000). If the diagnosis is made during the first two trimesters of pregnancy, treatment with aciclovir is recommended, and a vaginal delivery may be planned. Women can also be advised to take saline baths, analgesia, and increased fluids to dilute their urine. Local anaesthetics applied topically may relieve pain during micturition or defecation. If lesions are present during labour, many obstetricians consider performing a caesarean section, although there is little evidence to support this approach (Drake *et al.*, 2000). The risk of transmission from a mother to her baby is greatest when the mother presents with primary infection during the last trimester of pregnancy, as the mother will not have had time to produce type-specific neutralizing antibodies (Brown *et al.*, 1997), which may be partially protective when transferred transplacentally. Therefore a caesarean section should be considered. If the baby is delivered vaginally, the baby can be treated with intravenous aciclovir, in addition to treating the mother (Drake *et al.*, 2000).

Women with genital herpes are likely to be tearful and depressed. They require information about the illness, support and ongoing counselling (Drake *et al.*, 2000).

CHLAMYDIA

Genital chlamydial infection, caused by the bacterium *Chlamydia trachomatis*, is the most common bacterial STI in the UK (PHLS, 2001a). Women aged between 16–24 years and men aged 20–24 years are most commonly infected (PHLS, 2001a). During 1999 over 34 000 cases were diagnosed among those aged 16–24 years at GUM clinics in the UK. However, less than 10% of infections are diagnosed in GUM clinics (Renton and Taylor-Robinson, 1994) which, until recently, were the only clinical settings that undertook nation-wide systematic screening (Pimenta *et al.*, 2000). It is estimated that there were another 100 000–200 000 cases among young women aged 16–24 years (PHLS, 2001a), and a large proportion of these cases are undiagnosed. Therefore many women do not receive treatment and are at risk of developing severe complications.

An expert advisory group has recommended that in addition to testing symptomatic patients and those at higher risk (people attending GUM clinics and women seeking termination of pregnancy), opportunistic screening should be offered to sexually active women under 25 and those over 25 with a new sexual partner or who have had two or more partners in the past year

(Chief Medical Officer's Expert Advisory Group, 1998). Accordingly, some GPs, family planning clinics and young people's sexual health clinics now also offer testing (PHLS, 2001a). Urine tests, rather than traditional tests requiring endocervical or endourethral swabs, should greatly increase acceptability and uptake of screening (Pimenta *et al.*, 2000).

Many people are unaware of their infection, as up to 50% of men and 70% of women are asymptomatic (PHLS, 2001a). Women with symptoms may experience unusual vaginal discharge, bleeding between periods, dysuria and pain in the lower abdomen. Men may experience discharge from the penis, burning and itching in the genital area, and pain when passing urine. Symptoms, which appear 1–3 weeks after the infective episode, may persist, or may only last for a few days then disappear (PHLS, 2001a). Men and women can also develop painful arthritis due to inflammation of the joints.

Uncomplicated chlamydial infection is easy to treat and cure (PHLS, 2001a). During pregnancy, clindamycin and azithromycin may be considered if erythromycin and amoxycillin are contraindicated or not tolerated (Brocklehurst and Rooney, 2001). Amoxycillin, when compared with erythromycin, is associated with a lower incidence of side-effects. However, the lack of suitable data on its longer-term effectiveness raises concerns about its routine use (Brocklehurst and Rooney, 2001).

If untreated, approximately 33% of women develop PID, which causes chronic pelvic pain, infertility and ectopic pregnancy. The incidence of ectopic pregnancy in England is 1 in 100 and it accounts for 21% of maternal deaths resulting from complications of pregnancy and childbirth (PHLS, 2001a). One in five women with an episode of PID will become infertile, and may subsequently require in vitro fertilization (IVF) treatment. The consequences of chlamydial infection are therefore immense, bearing in mind all the implications of IVF, for the woman, her partner and a prospective pregnancy.

Complications are rarer in men, but untreated chlamydia can result in epididymitis, which causes pain, testicular swelling and, occasionally, male infertility (PHLS, 2001a).

An infected woman can pass the bacteria on to her baby causing it to be born with conjunctivitis or pneumonia. However, both are treatable.

TRICHOMONAS

Trichomonas vaginalis is one of the most common sexually transmitted organisms (Gülmezoglu, 2001).

Symptoms of infection include green–yellow frothy vaginal discharge, dyspareunia, vulvovaginal soreness, itching and dysuria. It is usually diagnosed on the basis of clinical findings and identification of the parasite in a wet mount smear. Trichomoniasis is known to affect women during pregnancy, although its effect on pregnancy complications is uncertain.

Metronidazole, given as a single dose, is likely to cure the infection, although it is not known whether this will have any effect on pregnancy outcome. It is advisable to commence treatment after the first trimester (Lossick and Kent, 1991; Murphy and Jones, 1994). In early pregnancy a local application of clotrimazole may be recommended (Gülmezoglu, 2001).

VAGINAL CANDIDIASIS

Vaginal candidiasis, a common and frequently distressing infection for many women, is caused by a yeast, *Candida albicans*, which often inhabits warm moist areas of the body such as the mouth, vagina, perineum and groin (Young and Jewell, 2001). Although frequently harmless, causing no symptoms, it can cause vaginal soreness and itching, sometimes with a white curdy discharge and reddening of the labia. Predisposing factors include pregnancy, the use of broad-spectrum antibiotics, diabetes and combined oral contraceptive use (Young, 2001).

Infection can be transmitted between the penis and vagina but recurrent infection is more likely to be a result of reinfection from the bowel (Young and Jewell, 2001). Midwives should inform women of preventive measures, including wiping from front to back and avoiding tight underwear (especially synthetics). In addition, women should be advised to avoid excessive washing, and use of bubble baths and perfumed soaps, which may, like antibiotics, damage the natural protective flora of the vagina.

A variety of antifungal drugs, which may be administered by the oral or local (intravaginal) route, have been used in the treatment of vulvovaginal candidiasis (Royal Pharmaceutical Society of Great Britain, 1999). Although the oral route of administration is the preferred route, no differences exist in terms of the clinical effectiveness (measured as clinical and mycological cure) of antifungals administered by the oral and intravaginal routes (Watson *et al.*, 2001). Topical imidazole appears to be more effective than nystatin for treating symptomatic vaginal candidiasis in pregnancy, and treatment for 7 days may be necessary, rather than the shorter courses more commonly used in non-pregnant women (Young and Jewell, 2001).

Midwives can reassure women that there is no evidence that thrush harms the unborn child (Young and Jewell, 2001).

Reflective Activity 47.6

Identify STIs that occur most frequently in your area of practice.

Design an information leaflet to be given to women for one STI that you have identified. Include details of transmission, clinical presentation, pregnancy implications, management/advice and contact details of useful support groups/sources of further information.

CONCLUSION

There has been a sustained rise in diagnoses of STIs over the last 6 years, probably attributable to the increasing practice of unsafe sexual behaviour, particularly in young heterosexuals and homo/bisexual men (PHLS, 2001c). In view of the severe longer-term complications associated with untreated STIs, as well as their potential role in facilitating HIV transmission, these latest data emphasize the need to improve STI prevention strategies. Midwives, who are in contact with sexually active women, should skilfully elicit details of women's sexual behaviour and health during the booking interview. Individual needs should be identified and health promotion tailored by providing information on disease prevention as necessary. Midwives should also be alert to the possible benefit of additional screening as appropriate, e.g. for chlamydia, and provide further information regarding management of specific STIs during pregnancy for infected women. Specially designed leaflets and details of support groups can be beneficial.

Midwives have an important role to play in screening for HIV, HBV and syphilis during pregnancy. Screening enables infected women to benefit from interventions which are known to improve health outcomes for women and their families, and helps reduce further spread of infection. Women should be given relevant, up-to-date information regarding the issues surrounding testing in order that they can make an informed choice. Midwives should respect women's autonomy by facilitating their ability to make important decisions. The rights of women should be protected in relation to confidentiality, and only those providing care should have access to women's healthcare records. Midwives require appropriate knowledge, skills and attitudes to work effectively within a multidisciplinary context, to ensure maximum benefit and minimum harm for all women.

KEY POINTS

- Midwives need to be aware of the issues surrounding routine testing for HIV, HBV and syphilis when enabling women to make an informed choice regarding testing and treatment.
- Respect for women's autonomy should enable midwives to facilitate the decision-making process, so that women experience maximum 'good' and minimum 'harm'.

- An awareness of the prevention, recognition, pregnancy implications and management of STIs should enable midwives to provide appropriate care.
- Maintaining confidentiality is of paramount importance.

REFERENCES

Adler, M.W. (1999) *ABC of Sexually Transmitted Diseases*, 4th edn. London: BMJ Books.

Alexander, J.M., Sheffield, J.S., Sanchez, P.J. *et al.* (1999) Efficacy of treatment for syphilis in pregnancy. *Obstetrics and Gynecology* 93(1): 5–8.

Amstey, M.S. & Steadman, K.T. (1976) Asymptomatic gonorrhoea and pregnancy. *Journal of the American Venereal Disease Association* 3(1): 14–16.

Anastos, K., Denenberg, R. & Solomon, L. (1997) Human immunodeficiency virus infection in women. *Medical Clinics of North America* 81(2): 533–553.

Antenatal HIV Testing Working Party (1998) *Quality Framework for HIV Testing Services in London.* London: Inner London HIV Health Commissioners Group.

Beckerman, K.P. (1998) Reproduction and HIV disease: pregnancy and perinatal care of HIV-1 infected women. In: Cohen, P.T. (ed) Natural history, clinical spectrum, and general management of HIV disease. Online. Available: http://hivinsite.ucsf.edu/akb/1997/04preg/index.html 4 September 1999.

Blanche, S., Tardieu, M., Rustin, P. *et al.* (1999) Persistent mitochondrial dysfunction and perinatal exposure to antiretroviral nucleoside analogues. *Lancet* 354(9184): 1084–1089.

Brocklehurst, P. (2001a) Interventions aimed at decreasing the risk of mother-to-child transmission of HIV infection (Cochrane Review). *The Cochrane Library,* Issue 1. Oxford: Update Software.

Brocklehurst, P. (2001b) Interventions for treating gonorrhoea in pregnancy (Cochrane Review). *The Cochrane Library,* Issue 1. Oxford: Update Software.

Brocklehurst P, & Rooney G (2001) Interventions for treating genital *Chlamydia trachomatis* infection in pregnancy (Cochrane Review). *The Cochrane Library,* Issue 1. Oxford: Update Software.

Brown, Z.A., Selke, S., Zeh, J. *et al.* (1997) The acquisition of herpes simplex virus during pregnancy. *New England Journal of Medicine* 337(8): 509–515.

Campbell, J. (1995) HIV and suicide: is there a relationship? *AIDS Care* 7(Suppl. 2): S107–S108.

Centers for Disease Control and Prevention (1995) Revised guidelines for prophylaxis against pneumocystis carinii pneumonia for children infected with human immunodeficiency virus. *Morbidity and Mortality Weekly Report* 44(RR-4): 1–11.

Chief Medical Officer's Expert Advisory Group (1998) *Main report of the CMO's Expert Advisory Group on Chlamydia trachomatis.* London: DoH.

Cohen, O.J. & Fauci, A.S. (1999) Transmission of drug-resistant strains of HIV-1: unfortunate, but inevitable. *Lancet* 354(9180): 697.

Communicable Disease Surveillance Centre (CDSC) (2002) HIV infection in women giving birth in the United Kingdom – trends in prevalence and proportions diagnosed to the end of June 2001. *CDR Weekly* [serial on line] 12(17): HIV/STI. Available: www.phls.co.uk/publications/cdr/archive02/News/news17 02.html# antenatal.

Connor, E.M., Sperling, R.S., Gelber, R. *et al.* (1994) Reduction of maternal–infant transmission of human immunodeficiency virus type 1 with Zidovudine treatment. *New England Journal of Medicine* 331(18): 1173–1180.

Connor, N., Roberts, J. & Nicoll, A. (2000) Strategic options for antenatal screening for syphilis in the United Kingdom: a cost effectiveness analysis. *Journal of Medical Screening* 7(1): 7–13.

Coutsoudis, A., Pillay, K., Spooner, E. *et al.* for the South African Vitamin A Study Group (1999) Influence of infant-feeding patterns on early mother-to-child transmission of HIV-1 in Durban,

South Africa: a prospective cohort study. *Lancet* **354**(9177): 471.

Culnane, M., Fowler, M.G., Lee, S., *et al.* (1999) Lack of long-term effects of in utero exposure to zidovudine among uninfected children born to HIV-infected women. *Journal of the American Medical Association* **281**(2): 151–157.

Department of Health (DoH) (1993) *Changing Childbirth*. London: HMSO.

Department of Health (DoH) (1999) Targets to cut numbers of babies born with HIV by 80% by 2002. Online. Available: http://www.nds.coi.gov.uk/coi/coipress.nsf 2 September 1999.

Department of Health (DoH) (2001) Prevalence of HIV and hepatitis infections in the United Kingdom. Annual report of the Unlinked Anonymous Prevalence Monitoring Programme 2000. London: DoH.

Department of Health (DoH) and Royal College of Midwives (RCM) (2000) *Information for Midwives – Hepatitis B Testing in Pregnancy. Helping Women Choose*. London: DoH

Donders, G.G. (2000) Treatment of sexually transmitted bacterial diseases in pregnant women. *Drugs* **59**(3): 477–485.

Downie, R.S. & Calman, K.C. (1987) Health Respect – Ethics in Health Care. London: Faber & Faber.

Drake, S., Taylor, S., Brown, D. *et al.* (2000) Improving the care of patients with genital herpes. *British Medical Journal* **321**(7261): 619–623.

Dunn, D.T., Newell, M.L., Aden, A.E. *et al.* (1992) Risk of human immunodeficiency virus type 1 transmission through breastfeeding. *Lancet* **340**(8819): 585–588.

Duong, T., Ades, A.E., Gibb, D.M. *et al.* (1999) Vertical transmission rates for HIV in the British Isles: estimates based on surveillance data. *British Medical Journal* **319**(7219): 1227–1229.

European Mode of Delivery Collaboration (1999) Elective caesarean section versus vaginal delivery in prevention of vertical HIV-1 transmission: a randomised clinical trial. *Lancet* **353**(9158): 1035–1039.

Fransen, L., Nsaze, H., Klauss, V. *et al.* (1986) Ophthalmia neonatorum in Nairobi, Kenya, the role of *Neisseria gonorrhoeae* and *Chlamydia trachomatis*. *Journal of Infectious Diseases* **153**(5): 862–869.

Galega, F.P., Heymann, D.L. & Nasah, B.T. (1984) Gonococcal ophthalmia neonatorum: the case of prophylaxis in tropical Africa. *Bulletin of the World Health Organization* **61**: 95–98.

Genc, M. & Ledger, W.J. (2000) Syphilis in pregnancy. *Sexually Transmitted Infections* **76**(2): 73–79.

Gillon, R. (1986) *Philosophical Medical Ethics*. Chichester: Wiley.

Grosheide, P.M. & Van Damme, P. (1996) *Prevention and Control of Hepatitis B in the Community*, pp. 1–60. Communicable Diseases Series, No. 1. Antwerp, Belgium: Viral Hepatitis Prevention Board Secretariat.

Grubert, T.A., Reindell, D., Kästner, R. *et al.* (1999) Complications after caesarean section in HIV-1-infected women not taking antiretroviral treatment. *Lancet* **354**(9190): 1612.

Gülmezoglu, A.M. (2001) Interventions for trichomoniasis in pregnancy (Cochrane Review). *The Cochrane Library*, Issue 1. Oxford: Update Software.

Hadler, S. & Margolis, H. (1992) Hepatitis B immunization: vaccine types, efficacy, and indications for immunization. In: Remington, J. & Swart, M. (eds) *Current Clinical Topics in Infectious Diseases*. Boston, Mass: Blackwell Scientific.

Hurtig, A-K., Nicoll, A., Carne, C. *et al.* (1998) Syphilis in pregnant women and their children in the United Kingdom: results from national clinician reporting surveys 1994–7. *British Medical Journal* **317**(7173): 1617–1619.

International Perinatal HIV Group (1999) Mode of delivery and the risk of vertical transmission of human immunodeficiency virus type 1 – a meta-analysis of 15 prospective cohort studies. *New England Journal of Medicine* **340**(13): 977–987.

Johnstone, F.D. (1996) HIV and pregnancy. *British Journal of Obstetrics and Gynaecology* **103**(12): 1184–1190.

Josefson, D. (1997) HIV treatment in children brought into line with that in adults. *British Medical Journal* **315**(7113): 902.

Kelly, J.A., Hoffman, R.G., Rompa, D. *et al.* (1998) Protease inhibitor combination therapies and perceptions of gay men regarding AIDS severity and the need to maintain safer sex. *AIDS* **12**(10): F91–95.

Leroy, V., Newell, M.L., Dabis, F. *et al.* (1998) International multicentre pooled analysis of late postnatal mother-to-child transmission of HIV-1 infection. *Lancet* **352**(9128): 597–600.

Lester, P., Partridge, J.C., Chesney, M.A. *et al.* (1995) The consequences of a positive prenatal HIV antibody test for women. *Journal of Acquired Immunodeficiency Syndrome* **10**(3): 341–349.

Lossick, J.G. & Kent, H.L. (1991) Trichomoniasis: trends in diagnosis and management. *American Journal of Obstetrics and Gynecology* **165**(4 Pt 2): 1217–1222.

Royal Pharmaceutical Society of Great Britain (1999) *Martindale: The Complete Drug Reference*, 32nd edn. London: Pharmaceutical Press.

Murphy, P.A. & Jones, E. (1994) Use of oral metronidazole in pregnancy. *Journal of Nurse-Midwifery* **39**(4): 214–220.

Newell, M.L. (1999) Infant feeding and HIV-1 transmission. *Lancet* **354**(9177): 442–443.

Newell, M.L., Gray, G. & Bryson, T.J. (1997) Prevention of mother to child transmission of HIV-1 infection. *AIDS* **11**(Suppl. A): S165–172.

Nursing and Midwifery Council (2002) *Code of Professional Conduct*. London: NMC.

Olivero, O.A., Anderson, L.M., Diwan, B.A., *et al.* (1997) Transplacental effects of 3'-azido-2', 3'-dideoxythymidine (AZT): tumorigenicity in mice and genotoxicity in mice and monkeys. *Journal of the National Cancer Institute* **89**(21): 1602–1608.

Public Health Laboratory Service (PHLS) (2001a) Sexually transmitted infections. Online. Available: http://www. phls.co.uk/facts/HIV/hiv.htm 23 February 2001.

Public Health Laboratory Service (PHLS) (2001b) *HIV/AIDS* Surveillance in the United Kingdom. Infection probably acquired through: transmission from mother to child. Online. Available: http://www.phls.co.uk/facts/hiv-epi3.htm 17 March 2001.

Public Health Laboratory Service (PHLS) (2001c) Diagnoses of selected sexually transmitted infections (STIs) seen in genitourinary medicine clinics: England and Wales, 1995–2000 (provisional data for 2000). Online. Available: http://www.phls.co.uk/facts/STI/sti_uk_data.html, 20 November 2001.

Pimenta, J., Catchpole, M., Gray, M. *et al.* (2000) Evidence based health policy report: screening for genital chlamydial infection. *British Medical Journal* **321**(7261): 629–631.

Planchon, S.M., Martins, C.A.P., Guerrant, R.L. *et al.* (1994) Regulation of intestinal epithelial barrier function. *Journal of Immunology* **153**(12): 5730–5739.

Pratt, R. (1995) *HIV and AIDS. A Strategy for Nursing Care*, 4th edn. London: Edward Arnold.

Royal College of Obstetricians and Gynaecologists (RCOG) (1997) *HIV Infection in Maternity Care*. Working Party Report. London: RCOG Press.

Renton, A. & Taylor-Robinson, D. (1994) *The Need for an Assessment of Health Technology for Screening for Chlamydia Trachomatis in the Population*. Leeds: NHS Executive.

Rouzioux, C., Costagliola, D., Burgard, M. *et al.* (1993) Timing of mother-to-child transmission depends on maternal status. *AIDS* **7**(Suppl. 2): S49–52.

Scarlatti, G. (1996) Paediatric HIV infection. *Lancet* **348**(9031): 863–868.

Schulz, K.F., Cates, W. Jr. & O'Mara, P.R. (1987) Pregnancy loss, infant death, and suffering: legacy of syphilis and gonorrhoea in Africa. *Genitourinary Medicine* **63**(5): 320.

Siegel, K. & Gorey, E. (1997) HIV-infected women: barriers to AZT use. *Social Science and Medicine* **45**(1): 15–22.

Sira, J. (1998) Hepatitis: exploding the myths. *Primary Health Care* **8**(3): 31–38.

Stevens, P.E. & Tighe Doerr B. (1997) Trauma of discovery: women's narratives of being informed they are HIV infected. *Aids Care* **9**(5): 523–538.

Tookey, P. & Peckham, C.S. (1997) Neonatal herpes simplex virus infection in the British Isles. *Paediatric Perinatal Epidemiology* **10**(4): 432–442.

Udall, J.N., Colony, P., Fritze, L. *et al.* (1981) Development of gastrointestinal mucosal barrier. II. The effect of natural versus artificial feeding on intestinal permeability to macromolecules. *Paediatric Research* **15**(3): 245–249.

UNAIDS (1999) Counselling and voluntary HIV testing for pregnant women in high HIV prevalence countries. Guidance for service providers. Online. Available: http://www.unaids.org/highband/document/mother-to-child/pisani.html, 10 September 1999.

Watson, M.C., Grimshaw, J.M., Bond, C.M. *et al.* (2001) Oral versus intra-vaginal imidazole and triazole antifungal treatment of uncomplicated vulvovaginal candidiasis (thrush) (Cochrane Review). *The Cochrane Library*, Issue 4. Oxford: Update Software.

Wright, T.L. & Lau, J.Y.N. (1993) Clinical aspects of hepatitis B virus infection. *Lancet* **342**(8883): 1340–1344.

Yerly, S., Kaiser, L., Race, E. *et al.* (1999) Transmission of antiretroviral-drug-resistant HIV-1 variants. *Lancet* **354**(9180): 729–733.

Young, F. (2001) Management of genital thrush. *Professional Care of Mother and Child* **11**(1): 12–14.

Young, G.L. & Jewell, D. (2001) Topical treatment for vaginal candidiasis (thrush) in pregnancy (Cochrane Review). *The Cochrane Library*, Issue 4. Oxford: Update Software.

FURTHER READING

Holmes, K. *et al.* (1999) *Sexually Transmitted Diseases*, 3rd edn. New York: McGraw-Hill

This comprehensive textbook provides detailed information on the whole spectrum of sexually transmitted diseases. In addition to providing a useful source of further information generally, it also contains a chapter on 'Sexually transmitted diseases, including HIV in pregnancy'.

Rudd, A., Taylor, D. (eds) (1992) *Positive Women. Voices of Women Living with AIDS*. Toronto: Second Story Press.

This book contains a collection of women's narratives. It is an international anthology, which enables readers to learn more about the lives of women living with HIV/AIDS as they share their stories. It contains a wide variety of

women's experiences, reflecting their responses of tears and courage as they face death and loss.

Stewart-Moore, J. (2000) Sexual health in the postnatal period. In: Alexander, J., Roth, C., Levy, V. (eds) *Midwifery Practice. Core Topics 3*. London: Macmillan.

This chapter examines the implications for midwives when promoting sexual health in the postnatal period.

McNab, M. 1997 Sexual health promotion. In: Crafter, H. (ed) *Health Promotion in Midwifery. Principles and Practice*. London: Arnold.

This chapter discusses various aspects of sexual health, sexual health promotion in midwifery practice and relevant health promotion theory.

48

Abnormalities of the Genital Tract

Patricia Lindsay

LEARNING OUTCOMES

After reading this chapter you will be able to:

- identify the major anomalies of the female genital tract and discuss their origin
- discuss the impact of these anomalies on fertility, pregnancy, labour and the puerperium
- discuss three main types of uterine displacement and discuss their impact on labour
- discuss the clinical and cultural implications of female genital mutilation
- identify the role of the midwife in the care of a woman with genital tract anomaly.

The true incidence of reproductive tract anomalies is unknown and many defects are asymptomatic. Reported rates are often derived from studies which have a selection bias in that they include women who have reproductive difficulties (Goldberg and Falcone, 1999). The true incidence may therefore be higher than was previously thought. While structural abnormalities of the uterus are particularly likely to cause problems, pregnancy and labour may also be affected by other conditions such as fibroids or uterine displacements.

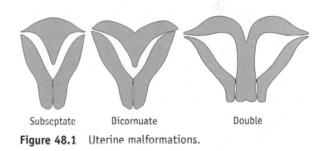

| Subseptate | Bicornuate | Double |

Figure 48.1 Uterine malformations.

DEVELOPMENTAL ANOMALIES

The majority of the female genital tract arises from the müllerian ducts, which form during embryonic life. The ducts fuse and the median septum then breaks down, thus forming a single uterus. Should this process fail, abnormalities such as *double uterus* (with or without a double cervix and vagina), *bicornuate uterus* or *subseptate uterus* will occur (Fig. 48.1). As the müllerian ducts and wolffian ducts develop close together in embryonic life, genital tract anomalies may be accompanied by malformations of the kidney and ureters. Care of the woman with a müllerian duct anomaly should therefore also include assessment of the urinary system (Ross and Kay, 1999).

Provided the cervix and vagina are patent, the woman is usually fertile: the ovaries are almost always present even if the rest of the genital tract is grossly malformed or absent.

Diethylstilboestrol (DES)

This synthetic non-steroidal oestrogen was used for approximately 30 years to treat a variety of conditions, including recurrent pregnancy loss and threatened abortion. It was also used in the 1960s as a form of postcoital contraception (Sundaram, 1995). The drug was withdrawn from use in 1971. Girls who have been exposed to DES in utero have an unusually high incidence of uncommon anomalies, both structural and cellular. These include vaginal adenocarcinoma, vaginal wall cysts, cervical anomalies such as collars and hoods and uterine malformations such as hypoplastic and T-shaped uteri.

Reproductive function in affected women is impaired. Conception may be difficult; spontaneous abortion, ectopic pregnancy and preterm birth appear to be more common. Where pregnancy progresses to term, labour may be prolonged (Goldberg and Falcone, 1999).

Sundaram (1995) estimates that, in the UK, approximately 10 000 girls may have been exposed to DES in utero. The midwife should be aware of the potential problems facing a woman with this history and must be able to advise on appropriate pregnancy and labour care.

Unicornuate uterus

This uncommon abnormality arises from failure of development of one of the müllerian ducts. It is associated with renal tract anomalies on the same side as the missing duct. Occasionally a rudimentary or vestigial horn may be present. There is a higher rate of spontaneous abortion, breech presentation, fetal growth restriction and preterm labour, possibly due to the limited space in the uterine cavity (Goldberg and Falcone, 1999). Incoordinate uterine action may occur in labour and the rudimentary horn may cause an obstruction (Beischer *et al.*, 1997). Caesarean delivery is therefore more likely for women with this type of anomaly. If the pregnancy develops in a rudimentary horn the outcome is usually spontaneous abortion or occasionally rupture of the rudimentary horn, as the myometrium becomes rapidly stretched.

Double uterus (uterus didelphys)

This may be accompanied by a double vagina or a longitudinal vaginal septum (Goldberg and Falcone, 1999). As the pregnancy progresses the midwife will notice that the fundus is abnormal in shape and may feel unusually wide. Breech presentation is common. As the pregnancy continues the non-pregnant uterus will enlarge under the influence of the pregnancy hormones and may occupy space in the pelvis, thus obstructing labour. Twin pregnancy has been recorded, with a fetus in each half of a double uterus (Brown, 1999; Kekkonen *et al.*, 1991).

Reflective Activity 48.1

Think about the potential needs of a woman with a double uterus. What factors would you need to discuss with her, and what would you include in her care plan?

Subseptate and bicornuate uterus

This occurs when complete obliteration of the müllerian septum fails. A subseptate uterus is outwardly normal but the midwife may recognize a bicornuate uterus which has a wide, heart-shaped fundus. This can be detected on abdominal examination and may even be visible under the abdominal wall in a very slim woman, especially after the third stage of labour. These anomalies do not usually cause difficulties in conception or in early pregnancy. However, they are associated with transverse lie and breech presentation, as the abnormal uterine structure hinders the process of spontaneous version which occurs between 30 and 34 weeks' gestation. Attempts at external cephalic version of the fetus will be unsuccessful.

The midwife should be aware of any woman with a history of successive malpresentation as this may indicate the presence of a structural abnormality of the uterus. The progress of the first and second stage of labour is usually normal where there is a subseptate or bicornuate uterus. However, retained placenta may occur in the third stage and the woman with this type of uterine anomaly is more likely to require a manual removal of placenta. The incidence of postpartum haemorrhage is also increased (Beischer *et al.*, 1997).

Vaginal septum

A vaginal septum (Fig. 48.2) may be longitudinal or transverse and may be complete or partial. It may be detected on vaginal examination but as the tissue is usually soft and is easily deflected by the examining fingers the diagnosis is often overlooked. A partial high vaginal septum may prevent cervical dilatation and may obstruct descent of the fetus during labour. Where the breech presents, the fetus may sit astride a longitudinal septum. In the second stage of labour the septum may be visible in front of the advancing

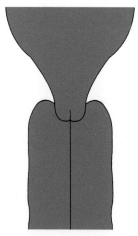

Figure 48.2   Longitudinal vaginal septum.

presenting part and may require division in order to allow delivery of the fetus (Kelsall, 1992).

Associated problems

The presence of a uterine malformation is associated with a fourfold increase in the risk of spontaneous abortion and preterm labour (Llewellyn Jones, 1999). The poorly formed myometrium is unable to stretch and develop to accommodate the rapidly growing fetus. The pregnancy will be unstable and more likely to abort, possibly because of poorer placental perfusion (Leible et al., 1998).

Caesarean delivery is more likely. If vaginal birth is attempted in a subsequent pregnancy there is a greater risk of uterine rupture (Ravasia et al., 1999).

Ultrasound scanning during pregnancy will usually reveal the presence of a uterine abnormality. The midwife should refer the woman to an obstetrician so that appropriate care may be planned as there is a higher likelihood of the need for intervention during labour.

DISPLACEMENTS OF THE UTERUS

Retroversion of the gravid uterus

Retroversion of the uterus, where the pregnant uterus falls back into the hollow of the sacrum (Fig. 48.3), occurs in between 6–19% of women and is normally of little clinical significance (Lettieri et al., 1994). It is not associated with infertility or an increased rate of spontaneous abortion (Llewellyn Jones, 1999). During

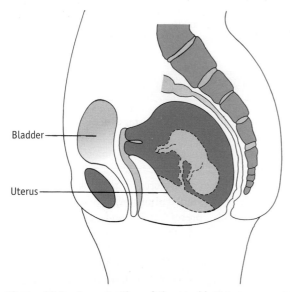

Figure 48.3 Incarceration of the gravid uterus.

pregnancy the condition usually resolves spontaneously as the uterus grows, becomes erect and rises into the abdomen around the 12th week.

However, rarely, the retroversion fails to resolve and the uterus becomes fixed or incarcerated in the pelvis. This is more likely to occur where uterine malformation, endometriosis, pelvic tumours or pelvic adhesions are present (Llewellyn Jones, 1999). By the 14th or 15th week of pregnancy the retroverted pregnant uterus completely fills the pelvis and the cervix is drawn up towards the pelvic brim. The anterior vaginal wall and the urethra become stretched, the urethra narrows and the mother is unable to pass urine.

Diagnosis

The woman will at first complain of pelvic pressure, difficulty in micturition and later of complete inability to pass urine (Lettieri et al., 1994). The bladder becomes more and more distended and, if it is unrelieved, overflow incontinence will occur as small amounts of urine escape.

At this stage the woman will complain of severe abdominal pain. On examination of the abdomen there is a large soft swelling (the bladder) above the pubes, which may extend to the level of the umbilicus or even above it. The fundus is not palpable at the brim of the pelvis.

Treatment

The woman requires hospital treatment. A catheter is passed and the bladder emptied. There is no evidence to support the practice of gradual emptying. However, some degree of hypotension and haematuria may occur (Hanno and Wein, 1994; Nyman et al., 1997). Although this is unlikely to be clinically signifi-cant, the midwife should monitor the woman's condition and seek medical advice if there is marked or persistent haematuria or if hypotension is causing faintness. The bladder is kept empty with a self-retaining catheter draining into a sterile urine collection bag until bladder tone returns. Once the bladder is empty, the uterus usually corrects its malposition spontaneously. This may be assisted if the mother lies in the semi-prone or Sims position. The retroversion will not recur, since the uterus is growing steadily and will, in a few days, be too big to fall back into the pelvis. Occasionally spontaneous correction does not occur and then manipulation under anaesthesia, with ultrasound guidance, is necessary. This may involve the creation of a pneumoperitoneum via a laparoscopy incision to assist in manipulation and correction of the incarceration (Lettieri et al., 1994).

Uterine incarceration which persists into the third trimester has been reported but is very rare (Dietz *et al.*, 1998; Hoenigl, 1999).

Dangers

Urinary tract infection is likely, owing to stasis of urine in the overdistended bladder. The midwife should send a catheter specimen of urine for microscopy, and any infection must be treated promptly. In exceptional cases, sloughing of the bladder and rupture may occur. The pregnancy is at risk, as spontaneous abortion is more likely. Persistent incarceration may cause sacculation of the anterior uterine wall. The pregnancy will then enlarge into the abdomen and this may confuse the diagnosis. Delivery will be by caesarean section. This must be performed by an experienced surgeon as the altered anatomy makes damage to adjacent displaced structures a real risk (Dietz *et al.*, 1998).

Reflective Activity 48.2

What information and advice would you give a woman who (at 8 weeks' gestation) has been told that she has a retroverted uterus?

Anteversion of the gravid uterus (pendulous abdomen) (Fig. 48.4)

This unusual condition is commoner in multiparous women whose abdominal muscles have been weakened by repeated pregnancies. Separation of the recti abdominis allows the uterus to fall forward and in extreme case the fundus may lie below the symphysis pubis. As the uterus becomes heavier, the woman will complain of backache and abdominal pain. The presenting part will not engage and dystocia is likely because the long axis of the uterus is at an angle to the pelvic brim. A well-fitting binder or corset will relieve the mother's discomfort and encourage engagement of the presenting part (Llewellyn Jones, 1999). The binder should be worn during labour to facilitate engagement and descent of the fetus. The 'all-fours' delivery position should be avoided as the combination of gravity and the heavy uterus may exacerbate the abdominal wall weakness and may hinder the woman's own expulsive efforts.

Prolapse of the gravid uterus

Although rarely seen, pregnancy may occur in a partially prolapsed uterus. The condition is much commoner in obese women or multiparae where the uterovaginal

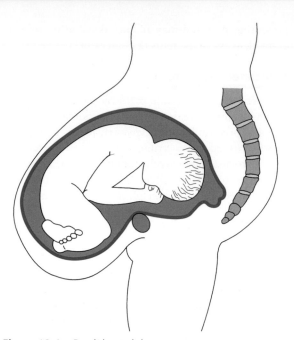

Figure 48.4 Pendulous abdomen.

supports have become lax and allow the uterus to descend so that the cervix is found at or just behind the vaginal introitus. The condition is most troublesome in the first trimester of pregnancy as the uterus increases in size and weight and the ligaments soften and relax. A ring pessary may be inserted to relieve the prolapse. As the uterus grows and becomes an abdominal organ the condition improves although it may recur in late pregnancy. Caesarean section may be recommended to prevent further damage to the uterovaginal supports. Where spontaneous labour occurs it usually proceeds normally and cervical dilatation may be rapid (Beischer *et al.*, 1997; Chamberlain, 1995; Llewellyn Jones, 1999).

FIBROMYOMATA (FIBROIDS)

Fibroids are the most common pelvic tumours, with an incidence possibly as high as 25% (Nowak, 1999). They are commoner in older women and in young West Indian and West African women. The presence of fibroids (leiomyomas) increases the risk of complications such as threatened abortion, antepartum haemorrhage, breech presentation and caesarean birth (Coronado *et al.*, 2000).

On palpation of the uterus one or more smooth rounded swellings may be felt continuous with the wall of the uterus (Fig. 48.5). A large fibroid may be mistaken for the fetal head. In pregnancy, hypertrophy of the

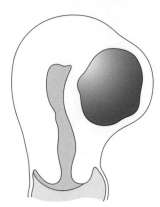

Figure 48.5   Uterine fibroid.

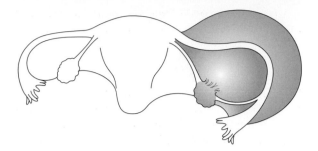

Figure 48.6   A uterus with a simple serous cyst.

myometrial fibres and increased vascularity and oedema cause the fibroid to enlarge and soften. Red degeneration (*necrobiosis*) may occur due to venous obstruction (Chamberlain, 1995). These changes often cause pain and local tenderness. Pyrexia and vomiting may also occur. However, spontaneous recovery is usual and surgical intervention is rarely necessary. Analgesic drugs may be prescribed. Myomectomy during pregnancy is a hazardous procedure carrying a high risk of haemorrhage and abortion (Chamberlain, 1995).

Most fibroids are found in the body of the uterus and do not affect the course of labour. Rarely, one may occur in the lower segment beneath the presenting part. This will prevent descent of the fetus into the pelvis and may obstruct labour. A low-lying fibroid may be felt on vaginal examination.

During the third stage of labour postpartum haemorrhage may occur, especially if the placental site overlies a subendometrial fibroid (Chamberlain, 1995).

Labour and delivery should take place in hospital in case difficulty should arise. During the puerperium, fibroids regress and become smaller as autolysis reduces the myometrial mass.

The midwife should be aware of any woman who has a history of treatment for fibroids prior to pregnancy. Myomectomy involves incisions on the uterus and this may pose a risk of scar rupture in future pregnancy (Hockstein, 2000). Selective embolization of fibroids is often the preferred treatment and successful pregnancy has been documented following this procedure (Pelage *et al.*, 2000).

OVARIAN CYST

With the widespread use of ultrasound scanning in pregnancy it has become apparent that pelvic masses are much more common than was previously supposed. Corpus luteum cysts are common in the first trimester and will usually regress spontaneously. However, other untreated ovarian lesions may cause obstructive complications if they persist (Chan and Reece, 1999). In the second and third trimester approximately 4% of women have sonographically detectable masses (Hill *et al.*, 1998). Ovarian cysts are malignant in about 10% of women under 30, and the incidence of malignancy rises in older women (Chamberlain, 1995).

The cyst may be in the abdomen or in the pelvis and may be discovered on ultrasound scanning or pelvic examination in early pregnancy (Fig. 48.6). It should be removed as soon as possible because of the risk of malignancy or torsion (either before or after delivery). Removal before the 12th week carries a risk of miscarriage if the corpus luteum is removed before the placenta is ready to take over the hormonal support of the pregnancy (Chamberlain, 1995). Simple non-malignant cysts can be successfully aspirated during pregnancy and this may be the only treatment required (Caspi *et al.*, 2000).

If undetected or untreated, an ovarian cyst lying within the pelvic cavity may obstruct labour.

FEMALE GENITAL MUTILATION

The custom of female genital mutilation (FGM, female circumcision) is still relatively common among some groups of women, particularly those from Nigeria, Ethiopia, the Sudan and Egypt. It is a cultural requirement and may be a rite of passage into adult status within the community.

The operation may be performed at any time from shortly after birth to adolescence (Trevelyan, 1994).

The World Health Organization (1998) currently classifies FGM as follows:

- Type 1: excision of the clitoral prepuce with or without excision of all or part of the clitoris (Fig. 48.7).

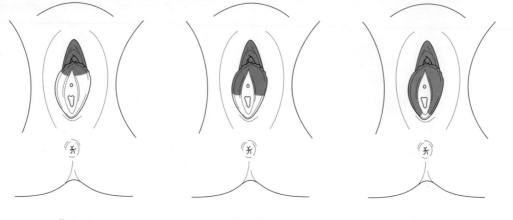

 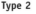

Type 1   **Type 2**   **Type 3**

Figure 48.7   Types of surgery.

- Type 2: excision of the clitoris with partial or total excision of the labia minora (Fig. 48.7).
- Type 3: excision of part or all of the external genitalia and stitching/narrowing of the vaginal opening (*infibulation* or *pharaonic circumcision*) (Figs 48.7 and 48.8). This is the most extensive type and is similar to a simple vulvectomy (Jordan, 1994).
- Type 4: unclassified – includes pricking, piercing, incising or cautery of the clitoris and related structures. It also includes traditional practices such as cutting the vagina (gishiri cuts) or scraping of the vaginal orifice (angurya cuts).

Female genital mutilation is illegal in the UK and many other countries, although there is increasing evidence from some countries of the involvement of doctors, midwives and nurses in the practice (WHO, 1998). Traditionally it is carried out in the family's home village by the local birth attendant or the older women. Fusion of the labial remnants is encouraged by binding the girl's legs together. Infection and acute urinary retention are common. When healing occurs there may be complete fusion of the labia which requires urgent surgical correction. On marriage, penetrative sexual intercourse will be difficult because of the vulval scarring.

Female genital mutilation carries a significant immediate mortality from haemorrhage and sepsis. Lifelong morbidity from urinary infection, pelvic inflammatory disease, endometriosis and renal damage is common. Contraceptive choice is limited by the vulval stenosis and cervical smears are impossible to obtain (Trevelyan, 1994). Psychological trauma and marital disharmony are common (Jordan, 1994).

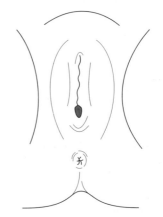

Figure 48.8   Appearance after healing of type 3 (infibulation).

Infibulation presents particular problems in childbearing. In pregnancy, urinary tract infection is likely. Progress during labour is harder to assess owing to the difficulty in performing a vaginal examination (Trevelyan, 1994). The presence of scar tissue may cause delay in the second stage and the fetus is at risk of hypoxia. The midwife must be prepared to perform an anterior episiotomy, separating the labial remnants (see Fig. 48.9). There may be severe damage to the pelvic floor: rupture of the anal sphincter is more likely as the rigidity of the vulval tissue causes undue pressure to be exerted in the posterior part of the birth canal. If the perineum is not meticulously repaired, faecal incontinence will result. This would have disastrous consequences for the woman as divorce and social ostracism often follow such problems. The midwife or obstetrician must be careful not to repair the labia in such a way

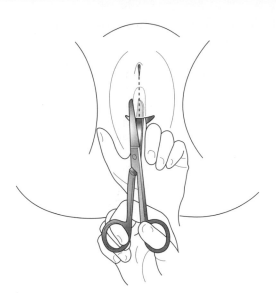

Figure 48.9 Direction of anterior episiotomy for type 3 (infibulation).

as to restore the infibulated state (Jordan, 1994). This would be illegal, although the midwife may face strong pressure to do so from the woman and her relatives.

Uterine prolapse is not uncommon even following a first baby.

If the infant is a girl, the midwife must be aware that the mother may wish to have the child circumcised. The Health Visitor should be informed and this may become a Child Protection issue. The parents can be prevented from taking the child out of the country under the provisions of the Children Act 1989.

In order to avoid adverse consequences, some obstetricians and midwives are offering a targeted Well-Woman service, which includes discussion of the health and legal issues and the option of reversal of infibulation. This is carried out at around 20 weeks' gestation to optimize healing before labour is likely to begin (Momoh and Kaufmann, 1998).

Although the World Health Organization is committed to eradicating the practice (WHO, 1998), there is an argument which suggests that punitive or restrictive approaches are tantamount to cultural imperialism and do not necessarily serve the interests of women who must live in those cultures. A woman who has not conformed to her society's cultural practices may not be marriageable. This is a serious handicap when a woman's status or even survival may depend on being married (Teare, 1998). Scherf (2000) suggests a culturally sensitive and comprehensive approach to women's health issues: strategies which seek to minimize harm

by offering alternative initiation practices are more likely to be effective than rigid prohibitions.

Midwifery care begins at booking, during which the midwife should ascertain whether the woman has undergone genital mutilation. The words used should reflect the midwife's attitude and approach, which must be well-informed, non-judgemental and sensitive. The midwife must remember that to this woman, this may be normal and part of a cultural heritage, and words can be a powerful purveyor of disparagement and disapproval.

> ### Reflective Activity 48.3
>
> Consider how you can add this assessment to your booking interview. How would you phrase the questions, and what sort of information would you give to a woman who has had FGM? You may find it useful to refer to some of the literature on FGM such as the novel *Possessing the Secret of Joy* (Walker, 1993).

Good communication is essential. If the woman and the midwife do not speak the same language, an interpreter must be found – this should *not* be a family member. A careful history must be taken; details of any previous births must be recorded, including any surgical interventions required, the condition of the infant and the woman's health since the birth. A physical examination should be carried out, if the woman consents. Minor degrees of genital mutilation will probably require no special attention, apart from ascertaining the woman's wishes regarding her labour and delivery care.

Infibulation, however, may present problems. Detailed information about previous pregnancies and births will help to inform the current management. The woman's beliefs and knowledge about the impact of her surgery on childbirth must be assessed. Her wishes for this pregnancy and birth should be discussed, but the midwife must make it clear that re-infibulation following the birth is not permitted by law. The possibility of the need for episiotomy should be raised. Advice regarding hygiene in pregnancy is essential, especially the need to reduce the risk of urinary tract infection.

The midwife should refer the woman to an obstetrician. Advice can be sought from centres with specialist knowledge, such as those who run dedicated clinics or African Well-Woman services. De-infibulation during pregnancy can be offered if the woman wishes.

The midwife should be aware of the possible social impact for the woman of her advice and actions. The relationship should be one of respect and acceptance.

Reflective Activity 48.4

Find and read your unit policy for the care of a woman with type 3 genital mutilation. If there is no policy, how would you get one written? What issues would you include?

IMPLICATIONS OF GENITAL TRACT ANOMALIES FOR MIDWIFERY PRACTICE

The true incidence of genital tract anomaly is unknown. The diagnosis may be made only following investigations for reproductive problems such as recurrent pregnancy loss, pain or infertility.

A thorough but tactful history must be taken, with attention to privacy during the consultation. The woman's health status must be assessed and the midwife should enquire about the information and advice which may have been given by other health professionals. The presence of lower abdominal or periumbilical scars is suggestive of gynaecological surgery and the midwife should ask the woman to explain the circumstances of the procedure. If there is a history of reproductive problems or gynaecological surgery the midwife should refer the woman to an obstetrician for an opinion on management of the pregnancy and labour.

Psychological support is essential. The midwife must be especially sensitive in ascertaining the history and giving advice and care during pregnancy. Feelings of womanliness and self-worth may have been damaged and the woman may have been left with a sense of a spoiled identity. A true working partnership can help repair some of the psychological impact by maintaining the focus on the normality of the process, as far as is compatible with safety. Cooperative care, with the woman as an informed and equal partner, will reduce anxiety and enhance feelings of control and satisfaction.

The midwife is often the first healthcare practitioner that the woman may have come into contact with, and may pave the way not just for this pregnancy, but for interactions with the variety of practitioners within the health services. Therefore a sensitive, respectful and caring approach will ensure that the woman's experience of healthcare is positive, and will also contribute to the woman's health, and that of her baby and family.

KEY POINTS

- The true incidence of anomalies is unknown but they may have significant implications for fertility and childbearing.
- Midwives must be able to identify women at potential risk of related problems and implement appropriate care.
- Midwives should be aware of different cultural practices which might be prevalent in their own practice area, and be knowledgeable about the impact of such practices on the reproductive health of the woman and on her baby.
- The legal and ethical difficulties which may present in this area must be considered, but maintaining respect and sensitivity for the views and beliefs of others.

REFERENCES

Beischer, N., Mackay, E. & Colditz, P. (1997) *Obstetrics and the Newborn*. London: Baillière Tindall.

Brown, O. (1999) Twin pregnancy in a uterus didelphys, with unilateral placental abruption and onset of labour. *Australian and New Zealand Journal of Obstetrics and Gynaecology* 39(4): 506–508.

Caspi, B., Ben-Arie, A., Appelman, Z. *et al.* (2000) Aspiration of simple pelvic cysts during pregnancy. *Gynecological and Obstetric Investigations* 49(2): 102–105.

Chamberlain, G. (ed) (1995) *Obstetrics by Ten Teachers*. London: Edward Arnold.

Chan, L. & Reece, E. (1999) Three-dimensional ultrasound and magnetic resonance imaging in obstetrics. In: Reece, E.

& Hobbins, J. (eds) *Medicine of the Fetus and Mother*. Philadelphia: Lippincott-Raven.

Children Act 1989. London: HMSO.

Coronado, G., Marshall, L. & Schwartz, S.M. (2000) Complications in pregnancy, labor and delivery with uterine leiomyomas: a population-based study. *Obstetrics and Gynecology* 95(5): 764–769.

Dietz, H., Teare, A. & Wilson, P. (1998) Sacculation and retroversion of the gravid uterus in the third trimester. *Australian and New Zealand Journal of Obstetrics and Gynaecology* 38(3): 343–345.

Goldberg, J. & Falcone, T. (1999) Müllerian anomalies: reproduction, diagnosis and treatment. In: Gidwani, G. &

Falcone, T. (eds) *Congenital Malformations of the Female Genital Tract*. London: Lippincott Williams & Wilkins.

Hanno, P. & Wein, A. (1994) *Clinical Manual of Urology*, 2nd edn. London: McGraw-Hill.

Hill, L., Connors-Beatty, M., Nowak, A. *et al.* (1998) The role of ultrasonography in the detection and management of adnexal masses during the second and third trimesters of pregnancy. *American Journal of Obstetrics and Gynecology* 179(3 Pt 1): 703–707.

Hockstein, S. (2000) Spontaneous uterine rupture in the early third trimester after laparoscopically assisted myomectomy. *Journal of Reproductive Medicine* 45(2): 139–141.

Hoenigl, W. (1999) Asymptomatic uterine retroversion at 32 weeks gestation. *Journal of Ultrasound in Medicine* 18(11): 795–798.

Jordan, J. (1994) Female genital mutilation (female circumcision). *British Journal of Obstetrics and Gynaecology* 101(9): 94–95.

Kekkonen, R., Nuutila, M. & Laatikainen, T. (1991) Twin pregnancy with a fetus in each half of a uterus didelphys. *Acta Obstetricia et Gynecologica Scandinavica* 70(4–5): 373–374.

Kelsall, J. (1992) Unusual delay in the second stage. *Midwifery Matters* 52(Spring): 21, 30.

Leible, S., Munoz, H., Walto, R. *et al.* (1998) Uterine artery blood flow velocity waveforms in pregnant women with müllerian duct anomaly: a biologic model for uteroplacental insufficiency. *American Journal of Obstetrics and Gynecology* 178(5): 1048–1053.

Lettieri, L., Rodis, J., McLean, D. *et al.* (1994) Incarceration of the gravid uterus. *Obstetrics and Gynaecology Survey* 49(9): 642–646.

Llewellyn Jones D (1999) *Fundamentals of Obstetrics and Gynaecology*, 7th edn. London: Mosby.

Momoh, C. & Kaufmann, T. (1998) Female genital mutilation (female circumcision). *RCM Midwives Journal* 1(7): 216–217.

Nowak, R. (1999) Fibroids: pathophysiology and current medical treatment. *Baillière's Clinical Obstetrics and Gynaecology* 13(2): 223–238.

Nyman, M., Schwenk, N. & Silverstein, M. (1997) Management of urinary retention: rapid versus gradual decompression and risk of complications. *Mayo Clinic Proceedings* 72(10): 951–956.

Pelage, J-P., Le Dref, O., Soyer, P. *et al.* (2000) Fibroid-related menorrhagia; treatment with superselective embolization of the uterine arteries and midterm follow-up. *Radiology* 215(2): 428–431.

Ravasia, D., Brain, P. & Pollard, J. (1999) Incidence of uterine rupture among women with müllerian duct anomalies who attempt vaginal birth after cesarean delivery. *American Journal of Obstetrics and Gynecology* 181(4): 877–881.

Ross, J., & Kay, R. (1999) Management of associated renal anomalies. In: Gidwani, G. & Falcone, T. (eds) *Congenital Malformations of the Female Genital Tract*. London: Lippincott Williams & Wilkins.

Scherf, C. (2000) Ending genital mutilation. *British Medical Journal* 321(7260): 570–571.

Sundaram, B. (1995) Tackling the aftermath faced by daughters of DES. *Nursing Times* 91(33): 34–35.

Teare, P. (1998) Culture shocks. *Nursing Times* 94(27): 34–35.

Trevelyan, J. (1994) Women's health: discrimination, tradition. *Nursing Times* 90(15): 49–50.

World Health Organization (WHO) (1998) *Female Genital Mutilation: an Overview*. Geneva: World Health Organization.

FURTHER READING

Gibeau, A. (1998) Female genital mutilation: when a cultural practice generates clinical and ethical dilemmas. *Journal of Obstetric, Gynecologic and Neonatal Nursing* 27(1): 85–91.
This is an overview of the practice and health implications of FGM. It includes considerations of ethical and professional issues for nurse/midwives.

Gidwani, G. & Falcone, T. (eds) (1999) *Congenital Malformations of the Female Genital Tract*. London: Lippincott Williams & Wilkins.
This is an up-to-date and comprehensive text discussing most aspects of this topic, including genetics, presentation, implications for reproduction and management.

Toubia, N. (1999) *Caring for Women with Circumcision*. New York: Rainb♀.
This book, subtitled 'A technical manual for health care providers' is written by an African-American female physician. It gives a clear overview of the clinical and cultural issues including care of children and communication issues. Case studies are included to highlight specific areas of care. UK readers should be aware that Section 4 (Legal Considerations) relates to American law.

Walker, A (1993) *Possessing the Secret of Joy*. New York: Pocket Books.
This is an excellent and compelling novel which deals with FGM from the perspective of a woman who has this performed on her, and deals with her transition to womanhood.

OTHER RESOURCES

Channel 4 (2003) *The Day I Will Never Forget*, broadcast
18 August 2003. A film by Longinolto K (2002) available
from Women Make Movies, 462 Broadway, Suite 500 WS
New York, USA.

A detailed documentary about FGM in Kenya, including
pioneering work in reversing this tradition, and personal
experiences of FGM.

49

Multiple Pregnancy

Jane Denton and Margie Davies

LEARNING OUTCOMES

After reading this chapter you should be aware of the following:

- the incidence of multiple births
- how twins arise and the importance of determination of chorionicity and zygosity
- the additional information and support required in preparing women for caring for two or more babies
- the risks and potential complications associated with delivering twins and how to support and care for bereaved parents, particularly if one baby survives.

INTRODUCTION

The incidence of multiple births is rising in many countries, mainly because of the increased availability of treatments for infertility (Imaizumi, 1997). A decline in the 1970s was followed by a rise from the early 1980s onwards (MacFarlane and Mugford, 2000) (Fig. 49.1). In the UK, the multiple birth rate in 2001 was 14.8 per thousand maternities (Table 49.1). The most dramatic change has been the threefold increase in the rate of triplet and higher-order births and this has considerable consequences for families, health services and society (Mugford and Henderson, 1995) (Fig. 49.2).

Not only do multiple pregnancies carry higher risks for the mothers and babies, they also impose a greater burden practically, financially and emotionally on the parents (Botting *et al.*, 1990) and also on the neonatal services (Collins and Graves, 2000).

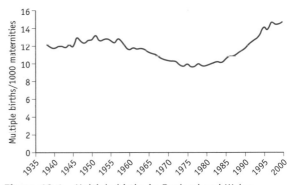

Figure 49.1 Multiple births in England and Wales, 1938–2000. (Source: Office for National Statistics, Birth Statistics, Series FM1.) (Graph by Alison Macfarlane, National Perinatal Epidemiology Unit.)

Table 49.1 Multiple birth rates per 1000 maternities 1989–2000

	1989	1990	1991	1992	1993	1994	1995	1996	1997	1998	1999	2000	2001
England and Wales	11.4	11.6	12.1	12.5	12.8	13.2	14.1	13.8	14.5	14.4	14.46	14.68	14.77
Northern Ireland	10.9	10.3	12.3	10.5	11.7	13.0	14.1	13.3	13.7	13.3	14.95	14.98	15.65
Scotland	11.0	11.4	11.0	12.6	12.5	13.0	14.2	14.1	13.8	14.6	13.72	14.39	15.22
Whole of UK	11.3	11.6	12.0	12.4	12.7	13.2	14.1	13.8	14.4	14.4	14.42	14.67	14.83

Source: Office for National Statistics London, General Register Office Northern Ireland, General Register Office Scotland
NB: Figures include live births and stillbirths

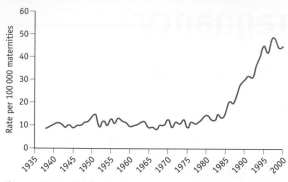

Figure 49.2   Triplet and higher-order births in England and Wales, 1938–2000. (Source: Office for National Statistics.)

THE INCIDENCE OF MULTIPLE BIRTHS

The rate of conception of multiple pregnancies is almost certainly higher than the recorded data suggest. Early ultrasound scans have shown that although there may be two or more fetal sacs in the first few weeks, some of the fetuses may die during the first trimester. This is often described as 'the vanishing twin syndrome' (Landy and Neis, 1995). If a multiple birth occurs before 24 weeks' gestation and includes both live births and dead fetuses, the fetal deaths are not registerable.

If after 24 weeks' gestation a dead fetus is delivered with a live birth, it should be registered as a stillbirth even if death occurred much earlier in the pregnancy (MacFarlane and Mugford, 2000).

The triplet rate in the UK used to be about 1 in 10 000 maternities. Since the early 1980s there has been a threefold increase in triplet and higher-order births and this is attributed to ovarian stimulation and assisted conception (Dunn and MacFarlane, 1996). In 1998/99, 1756 twin births and 235 triplets resulted from IVF (HFEA, 2000).

FACTS ABOUT MULTIPLES

How twins arise

There are two types of twins: monozygotic and dizygotic.

- Monozygotic ('identical', MZ, monozygous, uniovular) twins arise when a fertilized egg (zygote) divides into two identical halves during the first 14 days after fertilization. They will have the same genetic make-up and will therefore be of the same sex apart from the rare case of an XO/XY chromosomal anomaly (Perlman *et al.*, 1990).

- Dizygotic ('non-identical', DZ, dizygous, fraternal or binovular) twins result from the fertilization of two separate ova (eggs) by two separate sperm. They may be the same or of different sex and are no more genetically alike than any other siblings.

Causes of twinning

The cause of monozygotic twinning is unknown but recent reports suggest that slightly more are born after the use of drugs to stimulate ovulation. The incidence of MZ twins throughout the world has been constant at 3.5 per 1000 until the recent slight rise which may be associated with ovulation induction (Derom *et al.*, 2001). Occasional cases have been reported where there are several sets of monozygotic twins in one family but this is very rare and there is no general genetic predisposition.

Dizygotic twinning is different as there are several known associated factors (Harvey *et al.*, 1977):

- *Race:* black races have the highest rates (45 per 1000 maternities in Nigeria) and Orientals the lowest (5.6 per 1000 in parts of Japan). Caucasians and Indians are in between.
- *Maternal age:* the multiple birth rates rise until women reach their mid-30s.
- *Parity:* the higher the parity, the greater the likelihood of having twins or more.
- *Maternal height and weight:* taller and heavier women have a greater chance of conceiving twins.
- *Infertility treatment:* the use of drugs to stimulate the ovaries or replacement of multiple embryos or oocytes (eggs) increases the risk of twins and higher-order births.

DETERMINATION OF ZYGOSITY AND CHORIONICITY

Zygosity determination means finding out whether or not twins, triplets or more are monozygotic (identical). Midwives should understand the importance of this and be able to provide accurate information about zygosity and how it can be determined, as soon as a multiple pregnancy is diagnosed.

Placentation

The placenta can be single (monochorionic) separate or fused (dichorionic) (Fig. 49.3). All dizygous twins

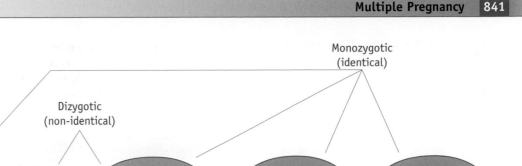

Figure 49.3   The relationship between zygosity and chorionicity.

have dichorionic (two chorions) and diamniotic (two amnions) placentae. About one-third of monozygous twins also have dichorionic placentae; this arises if the embryo divides within the first 3 or 4 days after fertilization. In about two-thirds of cases, the division occurs up to approximately the middle of the second week, and placentae will be monochorionic and diamniotic. Monoamniotic twins occur in about 1% of cases and arise when the embryo divides later in the second week.

Despite the now well-established facts about placentation and zygosity, many parents are still told that if same-sex twins are dichorionic they must be non-identical, which is of course incorrect.

Chorionicity

When two or more gestational sacs or fetal hearts are seen on an ultrasound scan, an assessment should be made of the chorionicity by measuring the thickness of the membranes (Fisk and Bryan, 1993). Blood vessels linking the two sides of the placenta are present in nearly all monochorionic placentae. Changes in the haemodynamics between the twins can have profound effects on the developing fetuses. Careful monitoring is needed to detect this condition, which is referred to as twin-to-twin transfusion syndrome.

Zygosity determination after birth

DNA testing

The most accurate method of zygosity determination currently is to compare DNA.

Physical features

About one-third of twins are of different sex and therefore non-identical. However, if they are the same sex it can be more difficult. Dizygotic twins can look remarkably similar, often until they are about 2 years old or even older. The colour of the hair and eyes, shape of the ears, hands and feet, teeth eruption and formation and pattern of growth are good indicators of zygosity. Nevertheless, parents often require confirmation, and they should be offered the opportunity for DNA testing.

> ### Reflective Activity 49.1
>
> Find out what information is available in your unit about zygosity determination and DNA tests.

DIAGNOSIS OF A MULTIPLE PREGNANCY

Ultrasound examination

It is now very uncommon for multiple pregnancy to remain undiagnosed, as most maternity centres routinely scan all pregnant women. Some units report nearly 100% detection rates of multiple pregnancies (Patel *et al.*, 1984). Ultrasound screening may be carried out as early as 6 weeks into the pregnancy and most women are aware of the multiple conception by the 18th week (Spillman, 1993a). When the diagnosis is made in the first trimester of the pregnancy, the risk of the 'vanishing twin syndrome' should be explained (Landy and Neis, 1995). Chorionicity should be determined in the first trimester.

Although in the UK, multiple pregnancy is most likely to be diagnosed by the sonographer, there may be situations, particularly in the developing world, where such technology is not available. A skilled midwife can apply other methods of detection.

Inspection

A midwife should always be alert to the possibility of twins if, on inspection, the uterus looks larger than expected for the gestation, especially after 20 weeks, and fetal movements are seen over a wide area, although the diagnosis need not always be of twins. A history of twins in the family should also be taken into account.

Palpation

On palpation, the fundal height may be greater than expected for the period of gestation.

If two fetal poles (head or breech) are felt in the fundus of the uterus, and multiple fetal limbs are palpable, this may be indicative of a multiple pregnancy. A smaller than expected head for the size of the uterus may suggest that the fetus is small and there may be more than one present. Location of three poles is diagnostic of at least two fetuses.

Auscultation

Hearing two fetal heart rates is not diagnostic of a twin pregnancy, as one heart rate can be heard over a wide area. The use of 'Sonicaid' machines in monitoring fetal heartbeats has improved detection of more than one fetal heart rate, but heartbeats must be listened too simultaneously for at least 1 minute. If the two heartbeats have a variation of more than 10 beats per minute, almost certainly twin infants are present.

ANTENATAL SCREENING

Serum screening is not usually performed in multiple pregnancies, as results are complex to interpret. Nuchal translucency (NT) refers to ultrasound measurement of the depth of fluid between the skin and the tissue underlying it at the back of the neck of the fetus. Increased nuchal translucency can be associated with an increased risk of the baby having Down's syndrome. The test should be performed between the 11th and 13th weeks of pregnancy.

Chorionic villus sampling (CVS) is not usually recommended in a multiple pregnancy because of the increased risk of miscarriage.

Amniocentesis can be performed in twin pregnancies, usually between 15–20 weeks. It should be performed in a specialist fetal medicine centre; most obstetricians do a dual needle insertion to avoid any contamination between the two fetuses.

ANTENATAL PREPARATION

Early diagnosis of a multiple pregnancy and chorionicity is extremely important so that parents can have the additional specialist support and advice they need.

At whatever stage parents are told, it is essential that whoever shares the news is aware of the effect the revelation may have (Spillman, 1985). Although some mothers and fathers are delighted to know that more than one baby is expected, in many cases there are reactions of shock and disbelief (Spillman, 1986). It is important that an obstetrician or midwife is available to answer questions and give appropriate counselling at this time. It is also helpful if the mother can be put in touch with someone who has twin children, who can understand and give reassurance. Contact numbers for a local twins group and information about other relevant support organizations can be a great source of reassurance (see Additional resources, p. 852).

Parent education

As soon as a multiple pregnancy is diagnosed, written information should be given containing contact numbers of the local twins club, parentcraft department at the hospital, and the national twin organizations such as the Multiple Births Foundation (MBF), and the Twins and Multiple Births Association (TAMBA). The news that two babies are expected can come as a considerable shock to some families and the midwife should give them the opportunity to discuss any concerns and check whether they need to be referred to a social worker.

Routine parentcraft classes need to be booked as early as possible; the mother should start them at around 24 weeks' gestation, which is earlier than for a singleton pregnancy when classes usually begin at 32 weeks. Specialist multiple pregnancy classes begin at 28 weeks. Some hospitals will run their specialist classes on a regular monthly basis, whilst others may choose to run a short course of two or three classes every couple of months (Davies, 1995). When planning these classes, contact with the local twins club can provide a very useful source of practical information. Mothers from the clubs are usually delighted to participate and offer practical information on equipment and clothes as well as on breastfeeding (Denton and Bryan, 1995).

Although the aim, as for all pregnant women, should be continuity of care throughout the pregnancy, this is often difficult to achieve. Broadbent (1985) reported that most of the mothers in her study who expected twins received all their antenatal care in consultant units and were seen by a variety of different midwives and doctors, thereby missing the one-to-one care they would have liked. As has been done for other medical problems occurring in pregnancy, specialist antenatal clinics are now being established for multiple pregnancies. Multiples are considered high-risk pregnancies, so dedicated 'twin clinics' should be held with midwives specializing in the care of women with multiple pregnancies to offer these mothers the specific care and support they need.

Midwives should be aware of the enhanced role of fathers in the care of multiples, and their cooperation in the mother's care should be sought from the start.

> ### Reflective Activity 49.2
>
> Plan a parentcraft session with information specific to multiple births.

Preparation for breastfeeding

Mothers expecting twins or triplets will inevitably give a lot of thought to how they are going to feed their babies, not only from the nutritional aspect but from the practical one as well, because it will take up a large part of the first months. Mothers should be encouraged that breastfeeding is not only possible for two babies, and in some cases three (Fuducia, 1995), but can be a very rewarding experience for the mother. Breast milk is ideal for babies and this is especially important because twins, and more so triplets, tend to be born prematurely and of low birthweight.

Early in the pregnancy the mother should be given as much information on breastfeeding as possible, with contact numbers of local breastfeeding organizations. Both parents should have the chance to talk through any concerns they may have; it is a good idea to suggest they meet with another mother who is successfully breastfeeding twins.

COMPLICATIONS ASSOCIATED WITH A MULTIPLE PREGNANCY

When the pregnancy is a multiple one, minor disturbances are likely to be exaggerated. Morning sickness is often severe and prolonged. Heartburn is also often persistent. Increased pressure may cause oedema of the ankles and varicose veins of the legs and vulva. As the pregnancy progresses, dyspnoea, backache and exhaustion are common.

More serious complications

- *Pre-eclampsia* is reported to be more frequent in multiple pregnancies (Bryan *et al.*, 1997) with the incidence higher in monozygotic than in dizygotic primigravid twin pregnancies (McMullan *et al.*, 1984). The woman who has pre-eclampsia in her first pregnancy is usually less likely to have it in subsequent pregnancies, unless of course she has changed her partner. Then the risk is the same as in the first pregnancy, but the midwife must be aware of confidentiality in dealing with this (Salha *et al.*, 1999).
- *Anaemia* is a risk. Two or more fetuses make much greater demands on the mother's stores of iron and folic acid. However, recent research suggests that iron and folic acid supplements prescribed to prevent the development of anaemia are unnecessary in most cases, as the condition is transient and resolves. Only mothers with evidence of significant anaemia should be treated (MacGillivray, 1991).
- *Acute polyhydramnios* can occur as early as 18–20 weeks. It may be associated with fetal abnormalities, but with monochorionic twin pregnancies it is more likely to be due to twin-to-twin transfusion syndrome (TTTS) (see below).

  The midwife should always be alert for the mother who complains of a rapid increase in her abdominal girth in the second trimester, as well as a uterus that is continuously hard. This is due to the rapid increase in amniotic fluid (polyhydramnios). Urgent obstetric intervention is required to prevent premature labour and fetal death.
- *Twin-to-twin transfusion syndrome* can be acute or chronic. TTTS complicates 4–35% of diamniotic monochorionic twin pregnancies (Fisk, 1995) and accounts for 15–17% of perinatal mortality in twins (Steinberg *et al.*, 1990). The placenta in TTTS transfuse blood from one twin fetus to the other. The donor twin transfuses blood via arteriovenous anastomoses of the placenta to the recipient twin. This results in growth restriction, oligohydramnios and anaemia in the donor twin ('stuck twin') and polycythaemia with circulatory overload in the recipient twin (hydrops). The fetal and neonatal mortality is high; early intervention with serial

amnioreduction, laser coagulation of connecting placental vessels or amniotic septostomy may prolong the pregnancy until the fetuses are viable. Amnioreduction may have to be repeated regularly as fluid can re-accumulate rapidly.

- *Preterm labour* is a major risk, not just because of monochorionicity, but low or very high parity, low maternal age, and monozygosity have been shown to predispose to the onset of early labour (Weekes *et al.*, 1977). The same study showed that cervical cerclage had no effect in reducing the incidence of preterm delivery.

- *Antepartum haemorrhage* is significantly increased in multiple pregnancy (MacGillivray and Campbell, 1988). Placenta praevia is also more common because of the large placental site encroaching on the lower uterine segment, and placental abruption may occur following rupture of the membranes and subsequent diminution in uterine size, or be associated with pregnancy-induced hypertension.

FETAL ABNORMALITIES ASSOCIATED WITH MONOZYGOTIC TWINS

Conjoined twins   These result from the incomplete monozygotic division of the fertilized ovum. This is extremely rare, occurring in approximately 1.3 per 100 000 births. Delivery has to be by caesarean section; separation of the babies is sometimes possible depending on which internal organs are involved.

Acardiac twins (twin reversed arterial perfusion: TRAP)   In acardia, one twin presents without a well-defined cardiac structure and is only kept alive through placental anastomoses to the circulatory system of the healthy co-twin (Moore *et al.*, 1990).

Fetus-in-fetu (endoparasite)   In fetus-in-fetu, parts of a fetus become lodged within the other usually healthy twin. This can only happen in monozygotic twins and is seen equally in both sexes (Baldwin, 1994).

INTRAPARTUM CARE

It is advisable that all mothers expecting a multiple birth be booked for delivery in a consultant unit. Ideally, in the case of triplets and higher-order births, this should be a hospital that can offer neonatal intensive care facilities, i.e. a regional referral unit.

Complications

The risk during labour to mother and babies is much greater in multiple pregnancy. As well as preterm delivery, other complications are more common.

Malpresentation   Although malpresentations can occur more frequently than with singleton births, in about half of twin pregnancies both babies are cephalic presentations and in three-quarters of cases the first baby presents as a vertex (Campbell and MacGillivray, 1988a).

Cord prolapse   This is a particular risk in cases of malpresentation, polyhydramnios and in the interval between the births of the first and second twin. Premature rupture of the membranes, malpresentation and polyhydramnios may predispose to this.

Prolonged labour   The length of the first stage of labour is usually similar to that of a singleton birth. However, because of the overdistension of the uterus and abdominal muscles there may be uterine inertia in some mothers.

Monoamniotic twins   This occurs in approximately 1% of twin pregnancies, and because monoamniotic twins share the same sac there is the risk of cord entanglement. Delivery is usually at around 32–34 weeks' gestation and by caesarean section.

Locking of twins

This is an extremely rare phenomenon. However, the condition is potentially disastrous and therefore midwives should be aware of the possibility, particularly when the labour is preterm and the babies small. Primigravidae are also more at risk (Khunda, 1972).

If locked twins are suspected during the first stage of labour, a caesarean section is performed to prevent obstruction occurring. The second stage of labour may be underway before it is realized that, during the breech delivery of the first infant, progress has halted. The descending second baby's head engages in the pelvis ahead of the first twin's head and interlocking of the chins occurs. The first twin will die of asphyxia unless delivered quickly. The mother is anaesthetized without delay and the doctor may attempt to push the head of the second twin out of the way. The first twin can then be delivered followed by the second. Even if caesarean section is attempted, results are poor. A high fatality rate of the first twin is reported in such cases (Khunda, 1972).

Deferred delivery of the second twin

In the last few years there have been cases when the first twin has been born, often very prematurely, and then labour has stopped. Labour in some cases has not started again for a period of time; cases have been recorded of the gap being 30 days or more. This can be beneficial to the second twin, as a course of betamethasone can be administered to help mature the lungs. Throughout this period, the mother will need an enormous amount of support as she will be concerned about the twin who has been delivered as well as still being pregnant and having concerns for that baby. She will need to be closely monitored for signs of infection.

Onset of labour

The average durations of multiple pregnancies with two, three and four babies are as follows.

- twins: 37 weeks
- triplets: 34 weeks
- quadruplets: 32 weeks.

Approximately 30% of twins and 80–95% of triplets are born spontaneously before 37 weeks (Clarke and Roman, 1994). If labour does begin very early, the chances of survival are not good and the mother may be given drugs to inhibit uterine activity. Intravenous salbutamol and sulindac tablets are the drugs most commonly used. The cause of the premature labour must be determined quickly, so that it can be treated if possible; for example a urinary tract infection should be treated with antibiotics. Most twin pregnancies are induced at 38 weeks, and it is only in very rare cases that they go beyond to 40 weeks.

Care in labour

When a mother expecting a multiple birth is admitted in labour, the team who will be present at the delivery should be alerted. As well as midwives and obstetric medical staff, an anaesthetist and paediatricians should be available (Bryan et al., 1997). All those in attendance should be introduced to the parents and their presence and role explained. If students and other observers are included, the mother's permission should be sought; ideally this should have been done before labour begins.

First stage

The first stage of labour is conducted as for a singleton labour, though a multiple pregnancy is considered high risk. Regular monitoring of each baby must be observed – two external transducers can achieve this, once the membranes are ruptured, with a scalp electrode on the presenting twin and the external monitor on the second twin. Uterine activity should also be monitored. Epidural anaesthesia is now the pain relief of choice offered to mothers giving birth to multiples (Crawford, 1978). This form of pain relief has the added advantage that if manoeuvres such as internal version, forceps delivery, ventouse extraction and emergency caesarean section are needed, adequate pain relief is in situ. The use of analgesia such as pethidine is usually avoided as this may cause respiratory depression, particularly in the case of the second baby who may already be experiencing reduced oxygen levels (Bryan et al., 1997). It is widely accepted that the risk to the second-born infant is significantly higher (Campbell and MacGillivray, 1988b). Thompson et al. (1983) in a Scottish study report a death rate for first twins of 47.6 per 1000 compared with 64.6 for second twins. Mortality is also higher for boys than girls (Campbell and MacGillivray, 1988b).

If there are any signs of fetal distress at any time during the first stage of labour to either baby, then an emergency caesarean section must be performed.

Second stage

The obstetrician, anaesthetist and paediatrician should be present together with the midwife because of the risk of complications. Continuous monitoring of contractions and both infants' heartbeats should be in progress.

The delivery room should be suitable for an emergency caesarean section or in close proximity to an operating theatre. Two sets of resuscitation equipment and incubators should be prepared. The delivery trolley should include the requirements for episiotomy, amniotomy, instrumental delivery and extra cord clamps. Equipment for local and general anaesthesia should be available if epidural anaesthetic is not already established and effective.

The second stage is conducted as usual for the birth of the first baby. When the labour is preterm, forceps may be used to protect the infant's head during delivery. The cord should be firmly clamped in two places and cut between the clamps. If the maternal side is not secure, the second baby in the case of monochorionic twins may suffer exsanguination. When the first twin is born, the time of delivery must be noted. The first infant and the cord should be clearly labelled 'Twin 1' or with the parents' chosen name if that is known.

The baby should be shown to the mother if the condition is satisfactory, or the parents constantly informed of progress if resuscitation is required. The baby may be put to the breast if its condition is satisfactory, as its sucking will stimulate uterine activity.

The lie, presentation and position of the second baby should be ascertained by abdominal palpation and confirmed by vaginal examination. If transverse or oblique, this must be corrected by external version to longitudinal. If this is not possible, an emergency caesarean section is performed. The fetal heart rate and the mother's blood pressure and pulse rate must be checked after each procedure. The alternative of a doctor performing an internal version, grasping a foot and delivering the baby by breech extraction, is seldom carried out nowadays. Such manoeuvres carry high mortality rates.

When it has been confirmed that there is no cord presentation, the second sac of membranes is ruptured and a scalp electrode applied. Once again a check is made to make sure that the cord has not prolapsed. If contractions do not resume very soon after delivery of the first twin, then an infusion of Syntocinon may be used. The delivery is now conducted in the normal way, taking care to note the time and label the baby 'Twin 2', and the same for the cord. The interval between the births varies considerably. It has been suggested that 30 minutes should be the maximum time. Campbell and MacGillivray (1988a) conclude that avoidance of undue haste or undue delay would seem to be the safest policy.

If more than two babies are expected, the delivery is usually by caesarean section (see below).

Undiagnosed twins   It is unusual nowadays for a multiple pregnancy to remain undiagnosed at the time of delivery. However, where ultrasonography is not available or not used routinely for all expectant mothers, or in the case of an unbooked woman, this can still occur. In this situation, ergometrine or Syntometrine should not be administered until after the birth of the baby, so there is no risk to a possible twin from severe anoxia, which may lead to death, or precipitate delivery of a possibly brain-damaged infant. Rupture of the uterus is also a risk. If drugs have been administered, the second baby requires immediate delivery. A general anaesthetic may be required and a muscle relaxant given. Caesarean section may be indicated.

It should be appreciated that both parents in this situation are likely to be in a state of shock (Theroux, 1989). Suddenly there are two babies to whom they must relate. They may already have formed a bond with the first infant and find it difficult to accept the unexpected baby (Bryan et al., 1997). Midwives, if aware of the possible problem, can give extra support to allow expression of negative feelings and help acceptance of the new situation.

Third stage

Management may vary in different hospitals. It is usual to give an injection of ergometrine maleate 250–500 mg intravenously or Syntometrine 1 ml intramuscularly with the birth of the anterior shoulder of the last baby. When the uterus is felt to contract, controlled cord traction is applied to both/all cords at the same time.

Following delivery, there is an increased risk of haemorrhage from the large placental site and overdistended uterine muscles, which may also contribute, as the abdominal muscles are more relaxed.

Examination of placenta and membranes

The midwife must make the usual examination to ensure completeness and detect any deviation from normal. If the babies are of different sex then they must be dizygotic twins, with either two separate placentae or one that has fused together, but each will have its own set of membranes, i.e. amnion and chorion. When the babies are of the same sex, they may be monozygotic or dizygotic. It used to be thought that there was always a single chorion in the case of monozygotic twins. However, research has revealed that one-third of monozygotic twins have dichorionic placentae (Corney, 1975; Strong and Corney, 1967). It is important that the placentae and membranes are sent for histological examination to help establish the zygosity. This is particularly important if one twin has an abnormality, is stillborn or dies.

Delivery of triplets and higher-order births

The greatest problem for triplet and higher-order births is preterm delivery. A study in the UK over a 5-year period revealed that a quarter of triplets were born before 32 weeks' gestation and just over three-quarters before 36 weeks (Botting et al., 1990).

The most likely method of delivery is by caesarean section and in many series of data this rate is greater than 90% for triplets (Lipitz et al., 1994). The higher the order, the more likely this becomes (Pons et al., 1988). The method of delivery for triplets is much debated and practice varies between units, with some obstetricians favouring vaginal delivery (Thiery *et al.*, 1988).

The delivery of triplets or more is a major event for all staff as well as parents. As much information as possible should be given to the parents about the procedure, and the roles of the many personnel in the delivery room should be explained (Bryan *et al.*, 1997). It is crucial that the resuscitation teams are briefed well in advance of the delivery and that each baby has its own paediatric team.

However many infants are involved, the parents should be shown their babies as soon as possible after delivery.

If it is necessary to transfer some or all of the infants to the neonatal unit, photographs should be taken and brought to the mother as soon as possible. Ideally, the babies should be photographed together so that the realities of the multiple birth are established. However, if this is not possible, the pictures should be clearly labelled with the birth order of the babies.

POSTNATAL CARE

The immediate postnatal care for a mother who has given birth to twins or more is the same as for a singleton mother, but with special attention to her blood loss and the involution of the uterus. As the babies are likely to be smaller and preterm, it is more difficult for them to maintain their body temperature so they must be kept warm.

Following delivery, the mother is likely to be very tired. She has probably suffered from a sleep deficit over several months and a more complicated delivery or caesarean section may compound her exhaustion. The lochia in the first few days is often heavier than after a singleton delivery and the mother is more likely to complain of afterpains.

In addition, the mother has two or more babies to whom she must relate and give care. Her anxieties may be increased if her babies are preterm. One, both, or in the case of triplets or more, all, may be nursed in the neonatal unit. The mother will need additional support and help if she has one baby on the postnatal ward with her and one in the NICU. She may feel more inclined to stay with the healthy baby on the ward than the sick one, especially if the long-term outcome is uncertain.

Some units have established transitional care wards where small, well babies can remain with their mothers with the aid of specially trained midwives or nurses who are available to support, assist and advise them on the care and specialized feeding the babies need.

Sadly, it is not uncommon for very sick babies to be transferred, sometimes without their mother, from the delivery hospital to a regional referral unit where intensive neonatal nursing care can be offered. The distances involved can be great and extremely costly to the parents and the neonatal services (Papiernik, 1991). This situation is traumatic for all the family. Midwifery staff must strive to reunite the family as soon as the condition of the babies allows. Regular communication during the separation is vital. The splitting up of the family group is often avoided if the babies are transferred to the regional referral unit in utero. Bowman *et al.* (1988) demonstrated that such babies had a better prognosis than those who needed to be transferred after birth.

Feeding multiples

Twins can breastfeed separately or together; if fed together the feeds will only take a little longer than with a single baby.

The mother can have more quality time with her babies, as she has no bottles to sterilize or feeds to make up.

During the first few weeks, the mother is going to need a lot of support and advice in order to get her breastfeeding established. She should allow herself 4–6 weeks to get into a routine and to establish breastfeeding.

Whilst in hospital, help should be available at every feed until the mother feels confident. It is advisable in the first few days for her to feed her babies separately, this gives her a chance to get to know each baby as an individual and to feel confident handling and putting the baby to the breast. If it is her first pregnancy, it can be overwhelming for the mother to try to perfect feeding two babies together right from the start. Once breastfeeding is established, some mothers prefer to feed both infants together, thus saving time; others prefer to feed separately but wake the second to feed immediately after the first so the routine is maintained. There is no one right way (Davies and Denton, 1999); it has to be the mother's preference and what fits in with her family. The important thing is that the mother should be confident and able to cope. One of the main causes of nipple soreness and backache is incorrect positioning of both babies at the nipple and the mother's sitting position whilst feeding. It is very important that

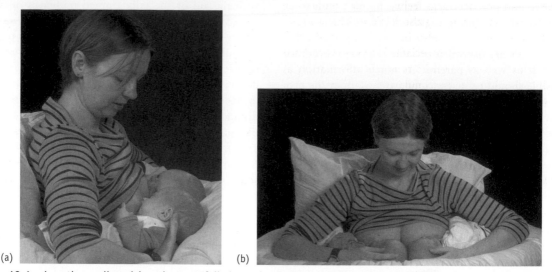

(a)   (b)

Figure 49.4   A mother well positioned successfully breastfeeding twins using the football hold.

the mother is taught right from the start to use plenty of pillows to support her back, and also to take the weight of the babies for feeding. A V-shaped pillow can be a great asset. The pillows should bring the babies up to nipple level so the mother can sit with her back straight and not be leaning over the babies. The weight of the babies is taken by the pillows, leaving the mother's hands free to reposition a baby should either of them come off the nipple and to lift one baby up for winding purposes. There are a variety of positions in which the mother can hold her babies for feeding. The most usual one for newborns is the football hold (Fig. 49.4).

Some mothers will choose to wholly or partially bottlefeed their babies. Partners, family and friends are then able to share in feeding routines. Whatever the mother's choice of feeding method, the midwife should support her in that choice.

Coming home

If the babies have been born preterm, the mother may be discharged several days or weeks before her babies. It is very unusual for the babies to be discharged home at different times, but there are occasions when this happens. In these cases great strains are put on the parents, who have to care for one baby at home whilst finding time to visit the sick one in hospital. Criticism of parents who are unable to visit frequently should be avoided. It may be necessary to arrange for a mother to room in for a few days before both the infants are discharged, to be sure that she has confidence in caring

for them. This transition will be smoother if the mother has adequate help. She should be advised to try to arrange help for the first few weeks after discharge.

Sources of help

There is no statutory help routinely available for mothers of twins, triplets or more in the UK. If there are concerns about the family circumstances and the parents' ability to cope, then social services should be contacted before the babies are born. Further Education Colleges running the Council for Awards in Children's Care and Education (CACHE) Diploma in Child Care and Education often welcome the opportunity to place their students with families for work experience. Anecdotal feedback indicates that this is very valuable for both parents and students and it is well worth contacting the local colleges for further information. Home Start is another organization which may be able to assist.

Family relationships

A mother may find it more difficult to relate to both/all of her babies at the beginning. This is very common and the mother should be reassured that these feeling will pass.

A strong preference may develop for one of the babies in the early days. Research has shown that this is usually for the baby who was heavier at birth (Spillman, 1984). The mother should be reassured that this is normal and in time her relationship with the other baby or babies will improve.

Becoming overtired and feeling overwhelmed with the immensity of their task is also a risk for both mothers and fathers. There may also be problems with other children in the family, especially toddlers. It is hard enough for a 2-year-old child to accept one new baby. When two or more arrive simultaneously there may be real difficulties. Single older children may see their parents as a pair and the twins as a pair, and themselves on their own, and it is helpful for the parents to arrange for a special friend to spend time with the older child. It is usual for the new babies to give a present to their older sibling, but it can be very helpful if the older child is taken out to choose a small different gift for each twin. Cuddly toys are a good idea, and being the first gifts the twins receive can make them very special.

Individuality and identity

Most parents of twins these days appreciate the importance of their children developing their own identities, and the importance of this should be discussed in the antenatal period. Parents of twins should always be encouraged to treat their children as individuals, giving them the same opportunities as a single-born child. Ways in which they can emphasize their individuality should be discussed in parentcraft classes. These include choosing names that do not sound the same or rhyme, and start with a different first letter, and dressing the children in different-coloured clothes (Bryan and Hallett, 2001).

Postnatal depression

In view of all the possible complications, increased risk of surgical intervention and other stresses involved in having a multiple birth, it is perhaps not surprising that there is an increased risk of depression (Spillman, 1993; Thorpe *et al.*, 1991).

The health professionals caring for the mother should recognize the signs that such depression is developing. It is helpful if there is continuity of care by a known midwife and a health visitor who has been introduced to the family before the babies are born. If the babies are still in hospital, it is still important for the mother to receive visits from her midwife and health visitor.

Bereavement

Mortality rates for multiple births have long been established as significantly higher than those of singletons,

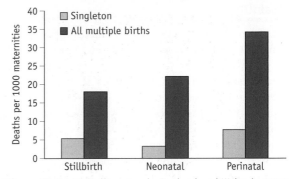

Figure 49.5 Mortality rates in England and Wales in 1998.

with twins about 5 times, and triplets about 10 times, more likely to die within the first year of life (MacFarlane and Mugford, 2000) (Fig. 49.5).

The higher incidence of preterm delivery and the associated complications are the main reason for the increased death rates (Dunn and MacFarlane, 1996). The loss of all the babies in a multiple pregnancy is tragic and the grief of the parents is usually fully recognized, but the situation may be more complex when one twin or triplet dies. Parents then have to cope with grieving for the dead baby (or babies if two triplets die) at the same time as caring for the survivor. Professionals as well as family and friends can fail to realize that the grief is just as great when one baby dies, and the joy of having a healthy child will not diminish the depth of the emotions or compensate for the loss. Parents may be regarded as ungrateful for the survivor, particularly if one twin dies during pregnancy or delivery or shortly after birth. They may need help to fully acknowledge their feelings and should be given information and support and offered counselling, which should be ongoing, as soon as the death is confirmed. The loss of status of being parents of twins, triplets or more should not be underestimated. They will continue to be parents of however many children are born and this should always be acknowledged (Bryan, 1986).

Encouragement should be given to the parents to talk about the confusing, contradictory feelings they may have and to think about their dead baby, as this will allow the mourning process to take place (Lewis, 1979).

Each case must be treated individually, and the information and care required will vary in some ways depending upon when the baby died. The different situations and recommendations for the care of these families is given in detail in the section on bereavement in the Multiple Births Foundation *Guidelines for Professionals* (Bryan and Hallett, 1997).

Disability

The risk of disability is greater with multiple births. The chance of a triplet pregnancy resulting in a baby with cerebral palsy is 47 times, and for a twin pregnancy 8 times, that of a singleton pregnancy (Petterson *et al.*, 1990). Caring for one child with a disability and another who is healthy brings many challenges, especially with twins. Often the healthy child has just as many problems, and may imagine that he or she caused the problem or resent the attention paid to the other child. Many potential emotional and behavioural problems may be avoided if the family are supported and advised appropriately as early as possible.

Multifetal pregnancy reduction

Multifetal pregnancy reduction may be offered to parents who conceive triplets or more on the basis that reduction to two or even one fetus provides a better chance of the healthy survival of each baby. The procedure is usually carried out between the 10th and 12th weeks of gestation and the most common method is to inject potassium chloride into the fetal thorax. When parents are presented with this immensely difficult decision, they must be provided with information about the risks and consequences of the procedure and offered counselling so that they consider the implications fully before making a final choice.

Selective feticide

If one of the babies in a multiple pregnancy has a serious abnormality, the same clinical procedure as that described for multifetal pregnancy reduction may be used. Again the parents will need very detailed information about the risks and counselling before making the final decision. As the dead baby will remain in the uterus until the delivery, the midwife has an important role to play in acknowledging the bereavement and supporting the mother through this very emotional time before and after the birth.

> **Reflective Activity 49.3**
>
> Find out what services are available nationally and locally to support bereaved parents.

Planning ahead

It is important that good family planning advice is offered to the parents following a multiple birth. Genetic counselling may be needed for those who have lost a baby. Follow-up of survivors should be arranged, especially when the infants are monozygous or have experienced neonatal complications. Multiple birth families have special needs. Midwives should be prepared for the additional and different management, information and support needed to ensure the best outcomes for the whole family.

KEY POINTS

- The incidence of multiple births is increasing because of the wider availability of infertility treatments.
- It is important to determine chorionicity and zygosity accurately.

- Risk management is an important part of care.
- Obtaining adequate support throughout childbirth and beyond is essential.
- Established voluntary networks are an important source of support.

REFERENCES

Baldwin, V.J. (1994) *Pathology of Multiple Pregnancy.* New York: Springer-Verlag.

Botting, B., MacFarlane, A.J. & Price, F.V. (1990) *Three Four and More: A Study of Triplet and Higher Order Births.* London: HMSO.

Bowman, E., Doyle, L.W., Murton, L.J. *et al.* (1988) Increased mortality of preterm infants transferred between tertiary perinatal centres. *British Medical Journal* 297: 1098–1100.

Broadbent, B.A. (1985) Multiple births – women's needs. *Midwife, Health Visitor and Community Nurse* 21: 425–430.

Bryan, E.M. (1986) The death of a newborn twin. How can support for the parents be improved? *Acta Geneticae Medicae et Gemellologiae* 5: 166–170.

Bryan, E.M. & Hallett, F. (1997) *Guidelines for Professionals: Bereavement.* London: The Multiple Births Foundation.

Bryan, E.M. & Hallett, F. (2001) *Guidelines for Professionals: Twins and Triplets: The First Five Years and Beyond.* London: The Multiple Births Foundation.

Bryan, E.M., Denton. J. & Hallett, F. (1997) *Guidelines for Professionals: Multiple Pregnancy.* London: The Multiple Births Foundation.

Campbell, D.M. & MacGillivray, I. (1988a) Management of labour and delivery. In: MacGillivray, I., Campbell, D.M. & Thompson, B. (eds) *Twinning and Twins*, pp. 143–160. Chichester: John Wiley.

Campbell, D.M. & MacGillivray, I. (1988b) Outcome of twin pregnancies. In: MacGillivray, I., Campbell, D.M. & Thompson, B. (eds) *Twinning and Twins*, pp. 179–205. Chichester: John Wiley.

Clarke, J.P. & Roman, J.D. (1984) A review of 19 sets of triplets. *Australian and New Zealand Journal of Obstetrics and Gynaecology* **134**: 50–53.

Collins, J. & Graves, G. (2000) The economic consequences of multiple gestation pregnancy in assisted conception cycles. *Human Fertility* **3**: 275–283.

Corney, G. (1975) Placentation. In: MacGillivray, I., Nylander, P.P.S. & Corney, G. (eds) *Human Multiple Reproduction*, pp. 40–76. London: W.B. Saunders.

Crawford, J.S. (1978) *Principles and Practice of Obstetric Anaesthesia*, 4th edn, p. 218. Oxford: Blackwell.

Davies, M.E. (1995) Managing multiple births, supporting parents. *Modern Midwife* **5**(11): 10–14.

Davies, M.E. & Denton, J. (1999) *Feeding Twins Triplets and More*. London: The Multiple Births Foundation.

Denton, J. & Bryan, E.M. (1995) Prenatal preparation for parenting twins, triplets or more: the social aspect. In: Whittle, M. & Ward, R.H. (eds.) *Multiple Pregnancy*, Ch. 12, p. 119. London: RCOG Press.

Derom, R., Derom, C. & Vlietnick, R. (2001) The risk of monozygotic twinning. *Lancet* **i**: 1236–1238.

Dunn, A. & MacFarlane, A.J. (1996) Recent trends in the incidence of multiple births and associated mortality in England and Wales. *Archives of Disease in Childhood* **75**(1): F10–F19.

Fisk, N.M. (1995) The scientific basis of feto-fetal transfusion syndrome and its treatment. In: Humphrey Ward, R. & Whittle, M. (eds.) (1995) *Multiple Pregnancy*, Ch. 24, pp. 235–250. London: RCOG Press.

Fisk, N.M. & Bryan, E.M. (1993) Routine prenatal determination of chorionicity in multiple gestation: a plea to the obstetrician. *British Journal of Obstetrics and Gynaecology* **100**: 975–977.

Fuducia, A. (1995) Breastfeeding three babies at once. *Twins, Triplets and More* **6**(3): 10–11.

Harvey, M.A.S., Huntley R.M.C. & Smith, D.W. (1977) Familial monozygotic twinning. *Journal of Pediatrics* **90**: 246–247.

Human Fertilisation and Embryology Authority (HFEA) (2000) *Human Fertilisation and Embryology Authority Annual Report*. London: HFEA.

Imaizumi, Y. (1997) Trends of twinning rates in ten countries, 1972–1996. *Acta Geneticae Medicae et Gemellologiae* **46**: 209–218.

Khunda, S. (1972) Locked twins. *Obstetrics and Gynecology* **39**: 453–459.

Landy, H.J. & Nies, B.M. (1995) The vanishing twin. In: Keith, L., Papiernik, E., Keith, D. & Luke, B. (eds) *Multiple Pregnancy, Epidemiology, Gestation, and Perinatal Outcome*, Ch. 6, p. 59. New York: Parthenon.

Lewis, E. (1979) Mourning by the family after a still birth or neonatal death. *Archives of Disease in Childhood* **54**: 303–306.

Lipitz, S., Reichman, B. & Uval, J. (1994) A prospective comparison of the outcome of triplet pregnancies managed expectantly of by multifetal reduction to twins. *American Journal of Obstetrics and Gynecology* **170**: 874–879.

MacFarlane, A.J. & Mugford, M. (2000) Characteristics of babies. In: *Birth Counts Statistics of Pregnancy and Childbirth*. Norwich: The Stationery Office.

MacGillivray, I. (1991) Obstetrical aspects of multiple births. In: Harvey, D. & Bryan, E.M. (eds) *The Stress of Multiple Births*, pp. 11–21. London: The Multiple Births Foundation.

MacGillivray, I. & Campbell, D.M. (1988) Management of twin pregnancies. In: MacGillivray, I., Campbell, D.M. & Thompson, B. (eds) *Twinning and Twins*, pp. 111–139. Chichester: John Wiley.

McMullan, P.F., Norman, R.J. & Marivate, M. (1984) Pregnancy-induced hypertension in twin pregnancy. *British Journal of Obstetrics and Gynaecology* **91**: 240–243.

Moore, T.R., Gale, S. & Benirschke, K. (1990) Perinatal outcome of forty nine pregnancies complicated by acardiac twinning. *American Journal of Obstetrics and Gynecology* **163**: 907–912.

Mugford, M. & Henderson, J. (1995) Resource implications of multiple births. In: Humphrey Ward, R., & Whittle, M. (eds.) *Multiple Pregnancy*, pp. 334–345. London: RCOG Press.

Papiernik, E. (1991) Costs of multiple pregnancies. In: Harvey, D. & Bryan, E.M. (eds) *The Stress of Multiple Births*, pp. 22–34. London: The Multiple Births Foundation.

Patel, N., Bowie, W. & Campbell, D.M. (1984) *Scottish Twin Study 1983 Report*. Glasgow: Social Paediatric and Obstetric Research Unit, University of Glasgow & Greater Glasgow Health Board.

Perlman, E.J., Stetton, G., Tuckmuller, C.M. *et al.* (1990) Sexual discordance in monozygotic twins. *American Journal of Medical Genetics* **3**: 551–557.

Petterson, B., Stanley, F. & Henderson, D. (1990) Cerebral palsy in multiple births in Western Australia. *American Journal of Medical Genetics* **37**: 346–351.

Pons, J.C., Mayenga, J.M., Plu, G. *et al.* (1988) Management of triplet pregnancy. *Acta Geneticae Medicae et Gemellologiae* **37**: 99–103.

Salha, O., Sharma, V., Dada, T. *et al.* (1999) The influence of donated gametes on the incidence of hypertensive disorders of pregnancy. *Human Reproduction* **14**(9): 2268–2273.

Spillman, J.R. (1984) *The Role of Birthweight in Maternal–Twin Relationships*. MSc Thesis, Cranfield Institute of Technology.

Spillman, J.R. (1985) 'You have a little bonus my dear': the effect on mothers of the diagnosis of multiple pregnancy. *British Medical Ultrasound Society Bulletin* **39**: 6–9.

Spillman, J.R. (1986) Expecting a multiple birth: some emotional aspects. *British Journal for Nurses in Child Health* **10**: 298–299.

Spillman, J.R. (1993a) Midwives responding to the needs of multiples. In: *Proceedings: 23rd International Congress of Midwives,* Vancouver, Canada, Vol. IV, pp. 1752–1765.

Spillman, J.R. (1993b) Perinatal loss in multiple pregnancy. In: *Proceedings: 23rd International Congress of Midwives,* Vancouver, Canada, Vol. IV, pp. 1776–1785.

Steinberg, L.H., Hurley, V.A., Desmedt, E. *et al.* (1990) Acute polyhydramnios in twin pregnancies. *Australian and New Zealand Journal of Obstetrics and Gynaecology* **30**: 196–200.

Strong, S.J. & Corney, G. (1967) *The Placenta in Twin Pregnancy.* Oxford: Pergamon Press.

Theroux, R. (1989) Multiple birth: a unique parenting experience. *Journal of Perinatal and Neonatal Nursing* **3**(1): 35–45.

Thiery, M., Kermans, G. & Derom, R. (1988) Triplet and higher order births. What is the optimal delivery route? *Acta Geneticae Medicae et Gemellologiae* **37**: 89–98.

Thompson, B., Pritchard, C. & Corney, G. (1983) Perinatal mortality in twins by zygosity and placentation. Paper given at the 4th Congress of International Society of Twin Studies, London.

Thorpe, K., Golding, J., MacGillivray, I. *et al.* (1991) Comparison of prevalence of depression in mothers of twins and mothers of singletons. *British Medical Journal* **302**: 875–878.

Weekes, A.R.L., Menzies, D.N. & de Boer, C.H. (1977) The relative efficacy of bed rest, cervical suture and no treatment in the management of twin pregnancy. *British Journal of Obstetrics and Gynaecology* **84**: 161–164.

FURTHER READING

Bryan, E., Denton, J. & Hallett, F. (2001) *Multiple Births and their Impact on Families: Guidelines for Professionals.* London: The Multiple Births Foundation.
A series of five booklets, available individually or in a pack, covering multiple births from preconception up to the first 5 years.

Davies, M. & Denton, J. (1999) *Feeding Twins, Triplets and More.* London: The Multiple Births Foundation.
A booklet for parents and professionals with advice and information on all aspects of feeding.

Bryan, E. (1995) *Twins, Triplets and More: Their Nature, Development and Care.* London: The Multiple Births Foundation.
Written by an internationally acknowledged expert on twins, this book answers many questions that arise about multiple births. Useful for parents, relatives and all professional disciplines.

Cooper, C. (1997) *Twins and Multiple Births.* London: Vermilion.
A mother of twins and practising GP gives professional and practical advice to help parents cope with the development and rearing of multiple birth children.

ADDITIONAL RESOURCES

The Multiple Births Foundation (MBF)
Hammersmith House, Level 4, Queen Charlottes Hospital, Du Cane Road, London
W12 0HS
Tel: 020 8383 3519
Fax: 020 8383 3041
E-mail: mbf@hhnt.nhs.uk
http://www.multiplebirths.org.uk

Twins and Multiple Births Association (TAMBA)
2 The Willows, Gardner Road, Guildford, Surrey GU1 4PG
Tel: 0870 770 3305
Fax: 0870 770 3303
E-mail: enquiries@tamba.org.uk
http://www.tamba.org.uk
Tamba Twinline tel: 0800 138 0509

Council for Awards in Children's Care and Education (CACHE)
8 Chequer Street, St Albans, Hertfordshire AL1 3XZ
Tel: 01727 847 636
Fax: 01727 867 609
http://www.cache.org.uk

HOME START UK
2 Salisbury Road, Leicester LE1 7QR
Tel: 0116 233 9955
Fax: 0116 233 0232
E-mail: info@home-start.org.uk
http://www.home-start.org.uk

50

Preterm Labour

Patricia Lindsay

LEARNING OUTCOMES

After reading this chapter you will be able to:

- identify the factors associated with preterm labour and birth
- highlight the implications of risk factors and the value of risk assessment
- discuss the available tocolytic drugs, including associated risks
- critically explore midwifery management of preterm labour and birth
- discuss the implications of preterm birth for the baby, and the family.

INTRODUCTION

Labour is defined as preterm when it occurs before the end of the 37th week of pregnancy. Babies are described in terms of either birthweight or gestational age. Infants delivered less than 37 completed weeks from the first day of the last menstrual period are referred to as preterm, irrespective of weight, while infants weighing less than 2500 g are classified as of low birthweight. Babies may be both preterm and of low birthweight.

Recent advances in neonatal care have resulted in the survival of very small and immature infants and these classifications have been expanded: *very low birthweight infants* (VLBW) are defined as those weighing less than 1500 g at birth and *extremely low birthweight infants* (ELBW) as less than 1000 g at birth. Some authorities add a further category which describes infants weighing 750 g or less: these may be referred to as *incredibly low birthweight* (ILBW) (Amon, 1999).

It is important to differentiate between the low birthweight preterm infant and the baby whose birthweight is low because of intrauterine growth restriction, as each group has different needs and problems after birth.

The incidence of preterm delivery as a proportion of all births, ranges from 6 to 10% in developed countries and this has changed little over the past 20 years. Rates of preterm delivery increase with increasing gestational age, up to 37 weeks, with less than a quarter occurring before 32 weeks. Preterm birth is directly responsible for 75–90% of all neonatal deaths not due to lethal congenital malformations and is a major cause of both short- and long-term neonatal morbidity (Amon, 1999).

AETIOLOGY

Preterm birth may occur as a result of any of the following situations:

- *Elective preterm delivery:* this may be undertaken as a result of severe pre-eclampsia, maternal renal disease or severe intrauterine growth restriction.
- *Premature rupture of the membranes:* this is an antecedent in about 20% of cases of preterm birth.
- *Complicated emergency delivery:* the complications include placental abruption, eclampsia, rhesus isoimmunization, maternal infection or prolapsed cord. This group accounts for about 25% of preterm births.
- *Uncomplicated spontaneous preterm labour of unknown cause:* this is the largest group, accounting for up to 40% of preterm births.

Risk factors

A number of risk factors have been associated with preterm labour and these may be related to maternal or fetal circumstances. It is important to remember that many of these factors are not causative agents but only markers which may indicate the woman who is at increased risk of preterm labour. Identification of the higher-risk woman may, in theory, make intervention and prevention easier. However, many of the factors are interlinked and it is difficult to disentangle the effects of discrete risks such as drug abuse from the pattern of deprivation which often accompanies it (Amon, 1999; El Bastawissi *et al.*, 2000; French *et al.*, 1999a; Minakami *et al.*, 2000; Schieve *et al.*, 2000; Shah and Bracken, 2000; Shumway *et al.*, 1999; Walkinshaw, 1995).

Biological/medical factors

- Age less than 16 or more than 35 years.
- Low weight for height.
- Chronic medical conditions such as diabetes or renal disorders.
- Generalized infections, especially viral.

Reproductive history

- History of previous preterm birth, i.e. a history of more than two preterm deliveries increases the risk by 70%.
- Bleeding in previous pregnancy.
- Uterine abnormality such as bicornuate, unicornuate or didelphic uterus, which increase the risk of preterm birth to 19%.

Current pregnancy

- Poor nutrition – especially if the pre-pregnancy body mass index (BMI) is low, i.e. less than 19.8.
- Bleeding.
- Retained intrauterine contraceptive device.
- Abdominal surgery.
- Infections, especially pyelonephritis.
- Genital tract infection, especially non-specific vaginitis, bacterial vaginosis, *Chlamydia*, *Ureaplasma urealyticum* and group B haemolytic *Streptococcus*. This latter organism is carried by 5% of women and is associated with preterm prelabour rupture of the membranes. Amnionitis resulting from genital tract infection may stimulate cytokine production and the local release of prostaglandin E_2 and $F_{2\alpha}$: this may cause labour to begin. Evidence of infection is common in preterm labour occurring before 30 weeks' gestation. This association seems to weaken with advancing gestation (Goldenberg *et al.*, 2000).
- Multiple pregnancy: the risk of preterm birth is nine times higher for a multifetal pregnancy compared to a singleton pregnancy.

- Polyhydramnios.
- Fetal malformation.
- Rhesus disease.
- Fetal death.
- Violence – including verbal abuse – may cause a fourfold increase in preterm labour.
- Hypertensive disease.

Socioeconomic

- Poverty and social deprivation.
- Employment which involves hard physical work.
- Psychological – psychological distress is associated with preterm delivery.

Cultural/behavioural

- Cigarette, alcohol or drug use.
- Short inter-pregnancy interval.
- Late antenatal booking.
- Poor attendance for antenatal care.

The pathophysiology of spontaneous preterm labour is poorly understood. It seems most likely that uterine contractions begin as a result of the interplay of several factors which result in an increase in myometrial oxytocin receptors, gap junction formation and changes in cervical structure. Infection appears to be a factor in about 30% of preterm labours (Amon, 1999)

PREDICTION AND PREVENTION OF PRETERM LABOUR

Several methods have been used to try to identify women at risk of preterm labour. However, prediction is difficult and may not be effective in preventing preterm birth. Formal *risk-scoring* systems have been used, based on the factors described above. This method has relatively poor predictive value for spontaneous preterm labour, especially for primigravid women; a low score may induce a false sense of security (Amon, 1999). However, it may be more useful where it is possible to identify factors relating to past obstetric history and current events.

Home monitoring of uterine activity has also been used, though evaluation of effectiveness has produced inconclusive results. Where rates of preterm labour appear to be reduced, it is difficult to determine whether it is the intervention which is beneficial or whether increased support and education are also factors (Amon, 1999; Iams *et al.*, 1987).

Regular pelvic examination will reveal signs of cervical changes which may herald the onset of labour. However, this procedure may of itself introduce infection and has a low predictive value for women at risk of preterm birth (Enkin *et al.*, 2000).

Ultrasonographic measurement of cervical length may be an accurate predictive tool in high-risk women. Funnelling of the internal cervical os may indicate impending preterm labour and this sign cannot be elicited on digital examination alone (Amon, 1999; Cook and Ellwood, 2000).

Fetal fibronectin tests may predict the onset of preterm labour (Lockwood *et al.*, 1991; Mast Diagnostics Ltd, 1993). Fetal fibronectin is a component of the extracellular matrix, secreted by the anchoring trophoblastic villi. Although its presence in vaginal secretions is a normal finding in the first half of pregnancy, concentrations greater than 50 ng per ml after 22 weeks' gestation are indicative of chorio-decidual disruption (Amon, 1999).

If preterm labour is imminent there is separation of maternal and fetal tissue at the chorio-decidual junction, leading to leakage of fibronectin. However, false positive results can occur which means that some women may be subjected to unnecessary interventions. A false positive result can arise if the test is carried out after vaginal examination, following sexual intercourse, when the uterus is contracting or where there is vaginal bleeding. There is also a higher false-positive rate in multiparous women (Amon, 1999). However, a review conducted by Lopez *et al.* (2000) revealed a positive predictive value significantly greater than reported in previous studies. Those women with negative test results received less intervention and delivered at later gestations. This test may therefore help clinical decision-making and concentrate activity on those women most likely to actually deliver, while releasing those unlikely to deliver from unnecessary intervention.

The test should be carried out every 2 weeks from 24 weeks' gestation and cannot be used in the presence of vaginal bleeding or rupture of the membranes as both blood and amniotic fluid contain fibronectin.

Vaginal pH monitoring may be useful, as a rise in pH often indicates the presence of infection which may precipitate labour. Monitoring can be carried out by the woman herself, using a disposable glove which carries an indicator strip (Pelican Health Care, 2001).

Fetal breathing movements cease before preterm labour commences and, although this may not occur in every case, it is a reasonably reliable indicator of imminent preterm delivery (Amon, 1999; Castle and Turnbull, 1983). However, the time and resources required to screen large populations of at-risk women may also make this unattractive as a screening procedure. Indometacin may be used as a tocolytic agent but can cause an increase in fetal breathing movements, which may confuse the interpretation of the examination findings (Amon, 1999).

Prevention of preterm birth is dependent upon preventing uterine activity and/or cervical dilatation. In the past, *bedrest* was advocated as a preventive measure though now has been shown to be ineffective, and it may actually increase the risk for deep vein thrombosis (Enkin *et al.*, 2000; Kovacevich *et al.*, 2000). Increased antenatal care and education about preterm labour may reduce the incidence of birth before 34 weeks' gestation (Papiernik *et al.*, 1985). *Antibiotic therapy* has been used in the management of women at risk of preterm labour, though there is no powerful evidence to support the routine use of antibiotics where the membranes are intact. A large randomized study of metronidazole treatment for asymptomatic bacterial vaginosis also failed to demonstrate any reduction in the incidence of preterm labour (Carey *et al.*, 2000; Enkin *et al.*, 2000; King and Flenardy, 2000).

Prophylactic *cervical cerclage* may be helpful where there is a recognized cervical weakness such as may follow previous second trimester abortions or cone biopsy, or where there is a diethylstilboestrol-related abnormality of uterine structure. It is also sometimes employed in the management of multifetal pregnancy (Silver and Ware Branch, 1999; Smith-Levitin *et al.*, 1999). The technique involves the insertion of a strong, non-absorbable suture such as Mersilene tape or Mersilk 4 around the cervix at the level of the internal os. This keeps the cervical canal closed (Llewellyn Jones, 1999). The procedure is carried out under general anaesthesia and carries the attendant risks of surgery in pregnancy. The suture is removed at 39 weeks' gestation or when labour commences.

The role of *social support* in preventing preterm birth has been examined and does not appear to have any influence on physical outcomes, although it may improve psychological well-being (Enkin, 2000; Oakley, 1989).

Reflective Activity 50.2

Consider a care plan for a woman who has a history of three preterm births, at 36, 30 and 28 weeks' gestation respectively. What advice and support might this woman need for her pregnancy? How would you develop a plan of care that would adequately meet her needs and reduce the risk of preterm birth?

PRETERM PRELABOUR RUPTURE OF THE MEMBRANES

Spontaneous rupture of the membranes before 37 weeks' gestation and before labour commences is termed preterm prelabour rupture. The cause may be unclear but it is associated with maternal smoking, vaginal bleeding in the second trimester, cervical incompetence and genital tract infection, especially group B haemolytic *Streptococcus, Chlamydia trachomatis* and bacterial vaginosis (Walkinshaw, 1995).

If preterm rupture of the membranes occurs at home, the midwife must contact the doctor and arrange for the woman to be admitted to a hospital with a neonatal unit. On admission of the woman to hospital, the midwife should assess the maternal and fetal condition, noting any uterine activity. A speculum examination is carried out to visualize the cervix. A pool of amniotic fluid may be seen in the posterior fornix. A cervical swab is taken and sent for microscopy and culture. Digital vaginal examination should be avoided in order to reduce the risk of ascending infection.

Steroids, such as dexamethasone 12 mg, or betamethasone 12 mg may be prescribed, and will be administered intramuscularly in two doses 12 hours apart. This accelerates surfactant production in the fetal lungs and reduces the risk of respiratory distress syndrome (hyaline membrane disease) to the neonate. These drugs are effective after 24 hours and for up to 7 days, and of most benefit between 24 and 32 weeks' gestation.

The woman's temperature and pulse should be recorded at least twice daily as chorioamnionitis occurs in at least 20% of cases of preterm rupture of the membranes. Blood may be taken to estimate the white cell count and for serum screening for C-reactive protein. This is a globulin of hepatic origin which rises in the acute phase of any infection. A single measurement of more than 30–40 mg/l or consecutive values of more than 20 mg/l indicate infection (Walkinshaw, 1995). If there is evidence of infection or vaginal colonization, antibiotic therapy may improve perinatal outcome.

The midwife should monitor the fetal condition and observe the state of any liquor draining from the vagina. Abnormal maternal signs such as pyrexia, tachycardia, uterine tenderness or offensive liquor, or fetal signs such as abnormal fetal heart patterns or alterations in fetal activity should be reported to the obstetrician. The midwife must observe for any signs of bleeding, as a sudden reduction in liquor volume may cause some placental detachment. If the membranes have been ruptured for more than 3 weeks, the fetal lungs may fail to develop properly because of the reduced liquor volume. This is a particular problem if rupture of the membranes occurs before 24 weeks' gestation.

MANAGEMENT OF PRETERM LABOUR

Preterm labour may be difficult to recognize but documented uterine contractions (2 in 10), documented cervical changes, cervical effacement of 80% or cervical dilatation of 2 cm or more are accepted as diagnostic (Amon, 1999). The midwife should be aware of the likelihood of preterm labour in any woman who complains of:

- menstrual-like cramps
- backache
- urinary frequency
- pink vaginal secretions
- diarrhoea
- pelvic pressure or increased vaginal discharge (Amon, 1999).

If labour begins at home, the midwife must arrange for the woman to be admitted to a hospital with an appropriate level of neonatal unit. On admission, she should be made comfortable and the fetus should be continuously monitored. The plans for the management of labour and its implications should be discussed with the couple in language that they understand, with time for questions to be asked, and the information to be assimilated. The neonatal unit should be informed and a member of the neonatal unit staff should visit the parents to discuss the proposed management of the baby at delivery. It is essential that accurate information is available regarding number of fetuses, estimated gestation, estimated fetal weight and presentation.

If the gestation is 35 weeks or more, labour will probably be allowed to continue as most babies of this age make good progress if given appropriate care after birth. Below 35 weeks, tocolytic drugs may be used if both mother and fetus are in good condition, with no signs of current vaginal bleeding or rupture of the membranes.

Tocolytic drugs

Tocolytic agents are used to suppress uterine activity in an attempt to buy the fetus more 'growing time' in utero or allow steroid-induced lung maturation to take place. Although it may be possible to prolong the pregnancy, no medication has been found to be universally effective and all have adverse side-effects (Gyetvai *et al.*, 1999). It is important that midwives are familiar with the use and likely effects of the drugs: close monitoring is essential.

The group of drugs most commonly used are the beta-adrenergic agonists such as ritodrine hydrochloride (Yutopar), salbutamol (Ventolin, Salbuvent) and terbutaline (Bricanyl). These compounds stimulate the beta-receptors of the autonomic nervous system and thus relax smooth muscle. They are used for the suppression of preterm labour occurring between 20 and 35 weeks' gestation (RCOG, 2000).

Ritodrine hydrochloride is administered by intravenous infusion, commencing at 50 µg/min and gradually increasing to 300–350 µg/min or until uterine contractions are suppressed, provided the maternal pulse does not exceed 130–140 beats per minute. The infusion is continued for 12–48 hours after cessation of contractions. There is no evidence that oral maintenance therapy is of benefit (RCOG, 2000). As ritodrine crosses the placenta there will be fetal effects such as tachycardia, hyperglycaemia and hyperinsulinaemia.

Salbutamol is another beta-receptor stimulant drug which reduces uterine activity. The dose is usually 10 µg/min by intravenous infusion but may be increased up to 45 µg/min if required to suppress uterine contractions, providing the maternal pulse rate does not exceed 130–140 beats per minute. The infusion is maintained until contractions are controlled.

Terbutaline is administered by intravenous infusion, 5 µg/min for 20 minutes, increasing in increments of 2.5 µg/min every 20 minutes until uterine activity ceases. Dosage should not exceed 20 µg/min (BMA, 2003).

Maternal *side-effects* include nausea, flushing, tremors, hypotension and palpitations. More serious effects are cardiac arrhythmias, myocardial ischaemia and pulmonary oedema which may develop in up to 5% of women. These drugs should therefore not be used in women with cardiac disease.

It is thought that beta-adrenergic agonists activate the renin – angiotensin system, thus causing sodium and water retention, which increases pulmonary capillary pressure. *Pulmonary oedema* is particularly likely to occur in multiple pregnancies, or where there is evidence of maternal infection (Lamont, 2000). Symptoms include retrosternal chest pain, cough and dyspnoea. Other signs of fluid retention will be present such as a positive fluid balance and haemodilution with a decrease in haematocrit. Chest X-ray will confirm the diagnosis. The midwife should inform the doctor of any woman complaining of chest pain or dyspnoea whilst being treated with these drugs. The oedema disperses once the treatment is stopped.

A new approach is *Atosiban* (Tractocile), a synthetic peptide which acts as an oxytocin competitor (Ferring Pharmaceuticals, 2000). This has a specific action which inhibits uterine contractions by blocking myometrial oxytocin receptors. Clinical trials indicate that it seems to be an effective tocolytic which is well tolerated by women and produces fewer adverse maternal or fetal effects (Moutquin *et al.*, 2000; Romero *et al.*, 2000). Atosiban is used mainly for women in uncomplicated preterm labour: it is not suitable where there is active vaginal bleeding, in severe pre-eclampsia, where there is premature rupture of the membranes or evidence of intrauterine infection. The manufacturers do not recommend its use at gestations below 24 or above 33 weeks. The drug is given as an initial intravenous bolus of 6.75 mg, followed by a high-dose 'loading infusion' of 18 mg/h for 3 hours. This is followed by a low-dose intravenous infusion of 6 mg/h for up to 45 hours (Ferring Pharmaceuticals, 2000). Valenzuela *et al.* (2000) found a subcutaneous maintenance regime of atosiban to be effective in preventing recurrence of contractions. There is no oral form of this preparation as yet.

As with any other tocolytic, the midwife must monitor maternal and fetal condition closely. Any apparent adverse reaction must be reported to the doctor and the hospital pharmacist. The Medicines Control Agency should be notified.

Magnesium sulphate has been used as a tocolytic agent in the United States but is not commonly used for this purpose in Britain. Evidence for its effectiveness in preventing preterm birth appears to be weak (Crowther and Moore, 2000). A major hazard is maternal hypermagnesaemia, which produces respiratory depression and loss of deep tendon reflexes. The antidote is calcium gluconate by intravenous injection. When this drug is used, for whatever purpose, the midwife should be aware that, should labour persist and progress, residual depression of myometrial activity may cause an atonic haemorrhage in the third stage of labour.

Prostaglandin synthesis inhibitors such as *indometacin* may be used to arrest preterm labour. Prostaglandin endoperoxide synthase converts free arachidonic acid to prostaglandin, which induces changes in the cervical collagen and facilitates cervical dilatation. Indometacin acts by inhibiting production of this enzyme. Maternal side-effects include nausea, vomiting, diarrhoea, dizziness and headaches. Long-term use may cause fetal effects such as constriction of the ductus arteriosus, right-sided heart failure and fetal death. Ductal constriction seems to be enhanced when corticosteroids are also administered, although the effects may be transient. Fetal exposure to this drug may also be associated with an increased incidence of necrotizing enterocolitis in low birthweight infants (Levy *et al.*, 1999; Major *et al.*, 1994). Contraindications are maternal infection, bleeding disorders, renal disease or peptic ulcers (Amon, 1999).

Calcium channel blockers such as *nifedipine* may be used. These are drugs which reduce muscle contraction by controlling the influx of calcium across the plasma membrane. Nifedipine seems to have fewer cardiovascular and metabolic effects than ritodrine. A recent small randomized study indicated that it is not only a more effective tocolytic than ritodrine but also produces better neonatal outcomes. *Nifedipine* is given orally, with a loading dose of 10–40 mg in the first hour, then 60–160 mg (slow release) daily until 34 weeks (Papatsonis *et al.*, 2000).

Glyceryl trinitrate (GTN) skin patches have been used as a method of suppressing preterm labour (Lees *et al.*, 1994). Although this drug does not seem to be commonly used, it appears to be a relatively safe and effective means of tocolysis (Smith *et al.*, 1999).

Corticosteroids

Dexamethasone or *betamethasone* may be given as described earlier to accelerate fetal production of pulmonary surfactant. Although a single course may be helpful in preventing neonatal respiratory disease there is some doubt about the value of repeated courses (Crowley, 2000).

There is also some evidence that repeated exposure to corticosteroids has deleterious effects. Measurable adrenal suppression has been found in women. Infants tend to be of lower than expected birthweight and

(where corticosteroid therapy is continued after birth) there is an increased incidence of cerebral palsy. Corticosteroids should not be used where there is evidence of chorioamnionitis or tuberculosis. Their use in women with diabetes mellitus has not been researched (Banks *et al.*, 1999; French *et al.*, 1999b; Helal *et al.*, 2000; Penney, 2000; Shinwell *et al.*, 2000).

Monitoring

In all cases where drugs are used to suppress uterine activity, the maternal and fetal condition must be closely observed. Continuous monitoring of uterine contractions should be carried out and recordings of maternal pulse and blood pressure made every 15 minutes. If the maternal pulse exceeds 130–140/min the tocolytic infusion should be stopped and the obstetrician informed. A strict record of fluid balance is essential. Women with diabetes mellitus in pregnancy should have their blood glucose levels monitored (RCOG, 2000). Continuous external monitoring of the fetal heart is preferable to intermittent recordings every 15 minutes. Side-effects of the drugs must also be recorded. If the dilatation of the os uteri reaches 4 cm or more or the membranes rupture, it is unlikely that the attempt to prevent labour progressing will be successful.

Labour and delivery

If the labour progresses despite attempts to control it, the midwife must inform both an obstetrician and a paediatrician. Continuous monitoring of the uterine contractions and fetal heart are carried out and all tocolytic drugs are stopped. Fetal hypoxia due to cord compression may occur, particularly if the membranes have ruptured before the onset of labour. Amnio-infusion has been used to reduce cord compression following oligohydramnios but this remains a contentious and relatively unevaluated technique (Enkin *et al.*, 2000).

It is essential that an accurate assessment of fetal presentation is made; many fetuses present by the breech prior to 34 weeks' gestation. An ultrasound scan may be helpful if the presentation is difficult to define.

There is little evidence that elective caesarean section produces better long-term outcomes for the baby (Grant, 2000). A retrospective cohort study by Wolf *et al.* (1999) also concluded that caesarean section is of no proven benefit even when the presentation is breech.

Care must be exercised in the choice and timing of drugs given for pain relief. Epidural anaesthesia or the inhalation of nitrous oxide and oxygen are the preferred methods of pain relief as they have no adverse effect on the fetus. Analgesic drugs, especially morphine and its derivatives, should be given as sparingly as possible and avoided altogether within 3–4 hours of delivery, as they may severely depress the fetal respiratory centre. The midwife should be aware that recent use of tocolytic drugs may increase the risk of uterine atony during and following the third stage of labour.

A paediatrician should be present at delivery. Because of the poor ossification of the fetal skull, the infant is at risk of intracranial injury. However, there is no evidence in favour of routine elective episiotomy for the delivery of a preterm infant. The midwife should be guided by the circumstances of each particular birth. Equally, there is no evidence that elective forceps delivery reduces trauma (Enkin *et al.*, 2000). Ventouse delivery should be avoided because of the risk of vascular rupture and subsequent haemorrhage in an immature infant (Edebiri, 1999).

The paediatrician will resuscitate the baby should it be necessary. The child should be given an injection of phytomenadione (Konakion) 0.5–1 mg IM to lessen any risk of haemorrhage. Antenatal administration of vitamin K to the mother has been attempted but has little effect on the subsequent development of periventricular haemorrhage in the preterm baby (Crowther and Henderson-Smart, 2000).

When the mother has seen and held her baby, the baby is transferred to the neonatal unit.

The midwife has a multifaceted role in caring for the woman, her baby and family in the situation of preterm labour and delivery. The first is the educative role in ensuring that the woman is in optimum health during pregnancy, and that any deviations from the norm can be identified and reported by the woman. The midwife provides the continuity and support through the stress of admission and preterm labour, and can ensure that the woman and her family are fully informed and as prepared as possible for the birth.

Preterm delivery is extremely stressful for the parents. The birth often comes as a shock and they may be psychologically unprepared for the baby's arrival. Any feelings of joy are quickly submerged by fears for the child's health. Both parents need time to discuss the event and its implications with the midwife. This will include fears about immediate events and also about long-term prospects: there is significant morbidity, mortality and developmental delay in infants born weighing less than 750 g (Agustines *et al.*, 2000). The parents may also experience the grief of dashed expectations, both of the expected birth experience and of the healthy term baby. Again the midwife can prepare the mother and her family for the normality of these feelings and assist them in coming to terms with the reality of preterm birth, and help them to develop their relationship with this new baby.

Breastfeeding confers benefits to the preterm infant, and the mother should be encouraged to express her milk if the baby is too small or ill to suckle. She will need a great deal of support from the midwife in establishing and maintaining lactation while her baby is in the neonatal unit.

The financial burden may be considerable if the infant is transferred to another hospital and the parents have to travel long distances to visit. In addition to this there may be the needs of older children to consider, and the midwife should not underestimate the stress which preterm birth causes to all the family. Viewing the preterm neonate and the family in context will assist the midwife in understanding and supporting the family appropriately.

Reflective Activity 50.4

Consider the management of preterm labour and birth in your unit. Identify one midwifery strategy which could be implemented to improve either the experience or outcome of preterm birth.

KEY POINTS

- Preterm birth continues to be a major cause of perinatal death and morbidity.
- The pathophysiology of preterm birth is unclear and individual aetiology may include a range of interrelated factors.
- Antenatal education may be helpful in preventing some cases by allowing earlier intervention and providing women and their families with sufficient information to be properly prepared for birth.
- The midwife must be aware of the associated factors in order to provide optimum care for women at higher risk.

REFERENCES

Agustines, L., Lin, Y., Rumney, P. *et al.* (2000) Outcomes of extremely low birth-weight infants between 500 and 750 g. *American Journal of Obstetrics and Gynecology* **182**(5): 1113–1116.

Amon, E. (1999) Premature labour. In: Reece, E. & Hobbins, J. (eds) *Medicine of the Fetus and Mother.* Philadelphia: Lippincott-Raven.

Banks, B., Cnaan, A., Morgan, M. *et al.* (1999) Multiple courses of antenatal corticosteroids and outcome of premature neonates. *American Journal of Obstetrics and Gynecology* **181**(3): 709–717.

British Medical Association (BMA) and Royal Pharmaceutical Society of Great Britain (RPSGB) (2003) *British National Formulary,* 46th edn. London: BMA and RPSGB.

Carey, J., Klebanoff, M., Hauth, J. *et al.* (2000) Metronidazole to prevent preterm delivery in pregnant women with asymptomatic bacterial vaginosis. *New England Journal of Medicine* **342**(8): 534–540.

Castle, B. & Turnbull, A. (1983) The presence or absence of fetal breathing movements predicts the outcome of preterm labour. *Lancet* **ii**(8348): 471–472.

Cook, C. & Ellwood, D. (2000) The cervix as a predictor of preterm delivery in 'at risk' women. *Ultrasound in Obstetrics and Gynecology* **15**(2): 109–113.

Crowley, P. (2000) Prophylactic corticosteroids for preterm birth. *Cochrane Database of Systematic Reviews* (2): CD000065. Oxford: Update Software.

Crowther, C. & Henderson-Smart, D. (2000) Vitamin K prior to preterm birth for preventing neonatal periventricular haemorrhage (Cochrane Review). *The Cochrane Library,* Issue 3. Oxford: Update Software.

Crowther, C. & Moore, V. (2000) Magnesium for preventing preterm birth after threatened preterm labour. *Cochrane Database of Systematic Reviews* (2): CD000940. Oxford: Update Software.

Edebiri, A. (1999) Is the vacuum safe for preterm vaginal delivery? *Journal of Maternal–Fetal Medicine* **8**: 234.

El Bastawissi, A., Williams, M., Riley, D. *et al.* (2000) Amniotic fluid interleukin-6 and preterm delivery: a review. *Obstetrics and Gynecology* **95**(6 Pt 2): 1056–1064.

Enkin, M., Keirse, M.J.N.C., Neilson, J. *et al.* (2000) *A Guide to Effective Care in Pregnancy and Childbirth.* Oxford: Oxford University Press.

Ferring Pharmaceuticals (2000) *Tractocile Resource Pack.* Langley, Berkshire: Ferring Pharmaceuticals.

French, J., McGregor, J., Draper, D. *et al.* (1999a) Gestational bleeding, bacterial vaginosis and common reproductive tract infections: risk for preterm birth and benefit of treatment. *Obstetrics and Gynecology* **93** (5 Pt 1): 715–724.

French, N., Hagan, R., Evans, S. *et al.* (1999b) Repeated antenatal corticosteroids; size at birth and subsequent development. *American Journal of Obstetrics and Gynecology* **180**(1 Pt 1): 114–121.

Goldenberg, R., Hauth, J. & Andrews, W. (2000) Intrauterine infection and preterm delivery. *New England Journal of Medicine* **342**(20): 1500–1507.

Grant, A. (2000) Elective versus selective caesarean section for delivery of the small baby. *Cochrane Database of Systematic Reviews* (2): CD000078. Oxford: Update Software.

Gyetvai, K., Hannah, M., Hodnett, E. *et al.* (1999) Tocolytics for preterm labor: a systematic review. *Obstetrics and Gynecology* **94**(5 Pt 2): 869–877.

Helal, K., Gordon, M., Lightener, C. *et al.* (2000) Adrenal suppression induced by betamethasone in women at risk of premature delivery. *Obstetrics and Gynecology* **96**(2): 287–290.

Iams, J., Johnson, F., O'Shaughnessy, R. *et al.* (1987) A prospective random trial of home uterine activity monitoring in pregnancies at increased risk of preterm labour. *American Journal of Obstetrics and Gynecology* **157**: 638–643.

King, J. & Flenardy, V. (2000) Antibiotics for preterm labour with intact membranes. *Cochrane Database of Systematic Reviews* (2): CD000246. Oxford: Update Software.

Kovacevich, G., Gaich, S., Lavin, J. *et al.* (2000) The prevalence of thromboembolic events among women with extended bed rest prescribed as part of the treatment for premature labor or preterm premature rupture of membranes. *American Journal of Obstetrics and Gynecology* **182**(5): 1089–1092.

Lamont, R. (2000) The pathophysiology of pulmonary oedema with the use of beta-agonists. *British Journal of Obstetrics and Gynaecology* **107**: 439–444.

Lees, C., Campbell, S., Jauniaux, E. *et al.* (1994) Arrest of preterm labour and prolongation of gestation with glyceryl trinitrate, a nitric oxide donor. *Lancet* **343**(8909): 1325–1326.

Levy, R., Matitiau, A., Ben Arie, A. *et al.* (1999) Indomethacin and corticosteroids: an additive constrictive effect on the fetal ductus arteriosus. *American Journal of Perinatology* **16**(8): 379–383.

Llewellyn Jones, D. (1999) *Fundamentals of Obstetrics and Gynaecology,* 7th edn. London: Mosby.

Lockwood, C., Senyei, A., Dishe, M. *et al.* (1991) Fetal fibronectin in cervical and vaginal secretions as a predictor of preterm delivery. *New England Journal of Medicine* **325**(10): 669–674.

Lopez, R., Francis, J., Garite, T. *et al.* (2000) Fetal fibronectin as a predictor of preterm birth in actual clinical practice. *American Journal of Obstetrics and Gynecology* **182**(5): 1103–1106.

Major, C., Lewis, D., Harding, J. *et al.* (1994) Tocolysis with indomethacin increases the incidence of necrotizing enterocolitis in the low birth weight neonate. *American Journal of Obstetrics and Gynecology* **170**(1 Pt 1): 102–106.

Mast Diagnostics UK Ltd (1993) *Fetal Fibronectin Membrane Assay Kit*. Bootle, Merseyside: Mast Diagnostics.

Minakami, H., Kosuge, S., Fujiwara, H. *et al.* (2000) Risk of premature birth in multifetal pregnancy. *Twin Research* 3(1): 2–6.

Moutquin, J-M., Sherman, D., Cohen, H. *et al.* (2000) Double-blind, randomized, controlled trial of atosiban and ritodrine in the treatment of preterm labor: a multicenter effectiveness and safety study. *American Journal of Obstetrics and Gynecology* 182(5): 1191–1199.

Oakley, A. (1989) Can social support influence pregnancy outcome? *British Journal of Obstetrics and Gynaecology* 96(3): 260–262.

Papatsonis, D., Kok, J., Van Geijn, H. *et al.* (2000) Neonatal effects of nifedipine and ritodrine for preterm labor. *Obstetrics and Gynecology* 95(4): 477–481.

Papiernik, E., Bouyer, J. & Dreyfus, J. (1985) Risk factors for preterm births and results of a prevention policy. The Haguenau Perinatal Study, 1971–1982. In: Beard, R. & Sharp, F. (eds) *Preterm Labour and its Consequences. Proceedings of the Thirteenth Study Group of the Royal College of Obstetricians and Gynaecologists*, pp. 15–20. London: RCOG.

Pelican Health Care (2001) *Careplan VpH*. Cardiff, Pelican Health Care.

Penney, G. (2000) *Antenatal Corticosteroids to Prevent Respiratory Distress Syndrome: RCOG Guidelines*. London: Royal College of Obstetricians and Gynaecologists. Online: Available http://www.rcog.org.uk/guidelines/corticosteroids.html.

RCOG (Royal College of Obstetricians and Gynaecologists) (2000) *Beta-agonists for the Care of Women in Preterm Labour (Guidelines)*. London: Royal College of Obstetricians and Gynaecologists. Online. Available: http://www.rcog.org.uk/guidelines/beta_agonists.htm

Romero, R., Sibai, B., Sanchez-Ramos, L. *et al.* (2000) An oxytocin receptor antagonist (atosiban) in the treatment of preterm labor: a randomized, double-blind, placebo-controlled trial with tocolytic rescue. *American Journal of Obstetrics and Gynecology* 182(5): 1173–1183.

Schieve, L., Cogswell, M., Scanlon, K. *et al.* (2000) Prepregnancy body mass index and pregnancy weight gain: associations with preterm delivery. *Obstetrics and Gynecology* 96(2): 194–200.

Shah, N. & Bracken, M. (2000) A systematic review and meta-analysis of prospective studies on the association between maternal cigarette smoking and preterm delivery. *American Journal of Obstetrics and Gynecology* 182(2): 465–472.

Shinwell, E., Karplus, M., Reich, D. *et al.* (2000) Early postnatal dexamethasone treatment and increased incidence of cerebral palsy. *Archives of Disease in Childhood Fetal and Neonatal Edition* 83: F177–181.

Shumway, J., O'Campo, P., Gielen, A. *et al.* (1999) Preterm labor, placental abruption and premature rupture of membranes in relation to maternal violence or verbal abuse. *Journal of Maternal–Fetal Medicine* 8(3): 76–80.

Silver, R. & Ware Branch, D. (1999) Sporadic and recurrent pregnancy loss. In: Reece, E. & Hobbins, J. (eds) *Medicine of the Fetus and Mother*. Philadelphia: Lippincott-Raven.

Smith, G., Walker, M. & McGrath, M. (1999) Randomized double-blind, placebo controlled pilot study assessing nitroglycerin as a tocolytic. *British Journal of Obstetrics and Gynaecology* 106(7): 736–739.

Smith-Levitin, M., Skupski, D. & Chervenak, F. (1999) Multifetal pregnancies: epidemiology, clinical characteristics and management. In: Reece, E. & Hobbins, J. (eds) *Medicine of the Fetus and Mother*. Philadelphia: Lippincott-Raven.

Valenzuela, G., Sanchez Ramos, J., Romero, R. *et al.* (2000) Maintenance treatment of preterm labor with the oxytocin antagonist atosiban. *American Journal of Obstetrics and Gynecology* 182(5): 1184–1190.

Walkinshaw, S. (1995) Preterm labour and delivery of the preterm infant. In: Chamberlain, G. (ed) *Turnbull's Obstetrics*. London: Churchill Livingstone.

Wolf, H., Schaap, A., Bruinse, H. *et al.* (1999) Vaginal delivery compared with caesarean section in early preterm breech delivery: a comparison of long term outcome. *British Journal of Obstetrics and Gynaecology* 106: 486–491.

FURTHER READING

Elder, M., Romero, R. & Lamont, R. (1997) *Preterm Labor*. Churchill Livingstone, London.
This book provides a broad and readable overview of the mechanisms, prevention and management of preterm birth.

Lopez Bernal, A. & TambyRaja, R. (2000) Preterm labour. *Baillière's Clinical Obstetrics and Gynaecology* 14(1): 133–153.
This is a useful overview of the biological and chemical mechanisms which influence myometrial activity, with reference to preterm labour.

51

Induction of Labour and Post-term Pregnancy

Pat McGeown

INDUCTION OF LABOUR

Labour is induced when an artificial intervention is used to initiate labour and delivery before spontaneous onset occurs. It has been described as being 'one of the most drastic ways of intervening in the natural process of pregnancy and childbirth' (Enkin *et al.*, 2000: 375). Despite this, it is routine practice in modern maternity units in the UK. In NHS units in England the incidence was 21.3% in 1997–98 (Government Statistical Service, 2001) in comparison to a rate of 41% in the mid-1970s (DHSS, 1976). The decline is due to the widespread public criticism in the early 1970s and a greater understanding of the adverse effects of unwarranted induction (Chalmers *et al.*, 1978).

The recent Royal College of Obstetricians and Gynaecologists' (RCOG) guidelines on induction of labour state:

> Induction of labour should only follow informed consent by the woman. For consent to be fully informed it should include the reasons for induction, the choice of method to be used, and the potential risks and consequences for accepting or refusing an offer of induction of labour.
>
> (RCOG, 2001: 33)

Indications for induction of labour mainly relate to increased risk of fetal and maternal compromise if delivery is delayed. However, there are other circumstances where the decision is less clear as to whether induction confers benefit or harm. In these situations careful assessment of each individual woman and fetus is needed to select those in whom the risk of continuing the pregnancy is greater than the potential risk of intervention. But induction should only be considered when vaginal birth is felt to be the appropriate route (RCOG, 2001).

Reflective Activity 51.1

Find out the induction rate in your local maternity unit and compare it with other regional and national rates. Analyse and reflect upon the rationale for any variability between the rates.

Maternal indications

Hypertension   Hypertensive disorders are one of the principal indications for induction, and timely intervention may become necessary to avoid serious maternal morbidity and perinatal compromise (see Ch. 45).

Diabetes   Diabetes is associated with increased risk of maternal and perinatal mortality and morbidity. Specific risks include the increased rate of late fetal death (Casson *et al.*, 1997; Hawthorne *et al.*, 1997) and the potential for macrosomia and its attendant risks of brachial plexus injury (Acker *et al.*, 1998). Induction or elective delivery prior to term has been proposed as a means of improving maternal and perinatal outcomes (RCOG, 2001). However, the potential benefits of induction need to be balanced against the potential risk of respiratory complications in the neonate.

Other medical conditions   Pre-existing renal, cardiac or other medical disease can deteriorate as pregnancy progresses and induction may be indicated in some of these pregnancies.

Prelabour rupture of the membranes

Definitions   Preterm, prelabour rupture of the membranes (PPROM) occurs before the onset of regular uterine contractions and before 37 weeks. At 37 weeks or after it is known as prelabour rupture at term (PROM).

The two main risks of PPROM are preterm birth and infectious morbidity due to ascending intrauterine infection. PROM occurs in 6–19% of all term pregnancies (Hannah *et al.*, 1996; Tan and Hannah, 2003a) and results in 86% of these women going into labour within 23 hours and 91% within 47 hours (Savitz *et al.*, 1997). Complications include: maternal and neonatal infection, prolapsed cord, increased risk of caesarean section and a low 5 minute Apgar score. Induction of labour may reduce the risks of infective sequelae for the woman and baby (Tan and Hannah, 2003b).

Current guidelines recommend offering women with PROM either immediate induction or expectant management not exceeding 96 hours following membrane rupture (RCOG, 2001).

Maternal request   Induction of labour may be requested by women for social or psychological reasons; for example, difficulties may arise in arranging social support or they may become anxious or stressed as pregnancy progresses. Each individual case should be considered on the potential benefits and risks for both mother and baby. In these circumstances, induction is preferably performed when the woman has a favourable cervix at term and where resources allow. Reasons given for requesting induction include increased feelings of safety and a desire to shorten the length of pregnancy (Out *et al.*, 1986).

Reflective Activity 51.2

You may have cared for a woman requesting induction of labour for no obvious medical indication. Reflect upon the advice and/or information given to her. Consider the reasons why some women request induction of labour. How do healthcare professionals respond to such requests? How do you feel about (a) the woman and (b) the caregivers? Discuss this issue with a colleague(s).

Poor obstetric history   Induction is sometimes undertaken to alleviate the anxiety and stress associated with subsequent pregnancies following previous adverse outcome, although it may have no clinical relevance to the current pregnancy, e.g. previous explained stillbirth or neonatal death associated with labour and delivery.

Unstable lie   Induction may be offered to women at term with an unstable lie once underlying abnormalities such as placenta praevia have been excluded. The lie is corrected to longitudinal by external version followed by controlled rupture of the membranes with an assistant stabilizing the presenting part. However, the risk of cord prolapse may lead the obstetrician to decide on caesarean section as the safest option.

Fetal indications

Abnormal fetal growth   Induction is indicated if there is evidence of diminished fetal well-being caused by uteroplacental insufficiency, which is often characterized by intrauterine growth restriction, abnormal fetal movements or abnormal fetal umbilical blood flow detected by Doppler ultrasound. However, if the fetus is severely compromised, caesarean section will be performed.

Macrosomia not associated with diabetes may be an indication to induce labour in order to avoid difficult delivery, shoulder dystocia and their consequences. The management is dependent upon accurate estimation of fetal size and other factors such as maternal choice, size and parity. However, current evidence is inconclusive as to whether induction of labour for suspected idiopathic fetal macrosomia can reduce maternal or neonatal morbidity (RCOG, 2001).

Fetal death   When fetal death has occurred there are no overwhelming benefits or risks of induction of labour over expectant care and the woman should be allowed to choose the best option for her and her family. The main medical complication is the possible increase in the risk of blood coagulation disorders whilst awaiting spontaneous labour; this is usually when the death has been associated with placental abruption (Enkin *et al.*, 2000).

Rhesus isoimmunization   Induction of labour is an optional management for established isoimmunization when the fetus is considered sufficiently mature, is not too severely affected and can be effectively treated after birth (Enkin *et al.*, 2000).

Fetal anomaly   Labour may be induced to terminate pregnancy if the fetus has a lethal abnormality or a malformation likely to result in handicap. It may also be useful when the baby would benefit from planned early surgery.

Contraindications

Contraindications for induction of labour are the same as those for a vaginal delivery. If the woman cannot have a safe vaginal delivery, induction of labour should not be considered.

Placenta praevia   Even with marginal placenta praevia there is almost no indication for vaginal birth when the fetus has reached a viable age because of the risks of maternal and fetal haemorrhage, cord accidents and malpresentations (Enkin *et al.*, 2000).

Cephalopelvic disproportion   Proven cephalopelvic disproportion may be a contraindication for induction of labour. Although it is rarely possible to make this diagnosis except in cases of known altered anatomy, e.g. severe contracture or pelvic fractures. The literature shows that successful vaginal birth occurs over 50% of the time following a caesarean section for disproportion, dystocia or failure to progress (Paterson and Saunders, 1991; Rosen and Dickinson, 1990; Rosen *et al.*, 1991).

Oblique or transverse lie   These are absolute contraindications because of the risks of cord prolapse and obstruction.

Severe fetal compromise   In this situation the fetus is unlikely to tolerate the stress of labour, and caesarean section is the safest option.

Timing of induction

Induction is usually timed for when it will be most successful, that is, near to the onset of spontaneous labour. But there are situations when it will be necessary to intervene before term in order to reduce the risk of fetal and/or maternal compromise. Corticosteroids should be administered to a woman who will deliver before 36 weeks to promote fetal pulmonary maturity and thereby reduce the risk of mortality, respiratory distress syndrome and intraventricular haemorrhage in preterm infants (Crowley, 2003a).

Methods

Methods used to induce labour mainly aim to replicate the physiological processes that naturally occur in spontaneous labour. However, the mechanisms that control this complex process are not clearly understood and therefore limit the methods available for the purpose. Current methods available attempt to stimulate cervical ripening and uterine contractions.

Cervical ripening

The success of induction and subsequent length of labour are primarily determined by the state of the cervix at the time of induction. An 'unripe' or unfavourable cervix fails to dilate adequately and results in high failure rates (Enkin *et al.*, 2000). Prior to induction the state of the cervix is assessed using a score based on that originally proposed by Bishop (1964). Five qualities are rated (see Table 51.1):

- cervical dilatation
- cervical consistency
- length of cervix
- position of the cervix
- station of the presenting part.

When the total score is greater than eight the cervix is said to be favourable (RCOG, 2001).

Table 51.1   Modified Bishop's scoring system

Features for assessment	Score			
	0	**1**	**2**	**3**
Dilatation of cervix (cm)	<1	1–2	2–4	>4
Consistency of cervix	Firm	Medium	Soft	–
Length of cervix (cm)	>4	2–4	1–2	<1
Position of cervix	Posterior	Mid	Anterior	–
Station in cm above (−) ischial spines	−3	−2	−1/0	+1/+2

Risks of cervical ripening   Cervical ripening is the first step to inducing labour; it should not be attempted unless the aim is to bring pregnancy to an end. The complications that can arise include:

- intrauterine infection
- uterine hyperstimulation
- fetal heart rate abnormalities
- maternal discomfort and inconvenience.

Intrauterine infection is mainly associated with invasive techniques, such as mechanical devices and extra-amniotic procedures. Iatrogenic uterine hyperstimulation and fetal heart rate abnormalities during the cervical ripening period can lead to emergency caesarean section with its associated morbidity. Failure to produce any significant change in cervical favourability may lead to delivery by caesarean. The consequences of initiating any procedure that may have such significant sequelae should always be considered by the clinician and discussed in full with the woman prior to its commencement.

Sweeping the membranes

Sweeping or stripping the membranes from the lower uterine segment at term has frequently been used to induce labour in the hope that amniotomy or oxytocic drugs may be avoided. It involves placing a finger inside the cervix and making a circular, sweeping action to separate the membranes from the cervix. The theory behind this method is that localized prostaglandin production is increased (Mitchell *et al.*, 1977).

Boulvain and colleagues (2003a) found that membrane sweeping reduced the time from intervention to spontaneous onset of labour or birth by a mean of 3 days. It also reduced the incidence of prolonged pregnancy if performed from 38–40 weeks and thereby reduced the need for formal induction of labour. Interestingly, the reviewers felt there was little justification to undertake the procedure routinely prior to 40 weeks' gestation.

Sweeping the membranes was not associated with an increase in maternal or neonatal infection but one trial (Boulvain *et al.*, 1998) reported increased maternal discomfort during and after the procedure with both vaginal bleeding and painful contractions not leading to the onset of labour during the 24 hours following the intervention.

The RCOG induction of labour guideline (2001) recommends that all women with uncomplicated pregnancies at 40 or more weeks should be offered sweeping of the membranes prior to formal methods of induction. This offer should also include evidence-based information to allow women to make an informed choice.

Prostaglandin

Prostaglandin (PG) has been used since the late 1960s for cervical ripening and induction of labour in a variety of different forms and rates of administration. In the UK, vaginal prostaglandin is one of the most commonly used induction agents. It is more likely than either placebo or no treatment to start labour and to avoid the need for induction with oxytocin (Enkin *et al.*, 2000).

A series of systematic reviews has recently been undertaken that compare the various preparations and the methods of administration. Table 51.2 contains the main results.

One of the reviews (Kelly *et al.*, 2003a) that compared vaginal PGE_2 gel, tablet, pessary, suppository and sustained-release formulations concluded that vaginal PGE_2 tablets seem to be as cost-effective as gel preparations. Although PGE_2 gel does reduce the need for oxytocin augmentation, the significance of a reduction in the use of oxytocin is uncertain.

The associated complications of prostaglandin administration include (Enkin *et al.*, 2000):

- maternal gastrointestinal side-effects
- maternal pyrexia from the effect on the thermo-regulating centre in the brain
- uterine hyperstimulation with or without fetal heart rate abnormalities.

There is also the risk of an 'unjustified' induction of labour because of the ready availability of prostaglandin.

Prostaglandin is associated with an increased successful vaginal delivery rate within 24 hours, a reduced caesarean section rate and a reduced risk of the cervix remaining unchanged at 24–48 hours when compared to oxytocin (RCOG, 2001). There was also a reduction in the use of epidural analgesia and more women were satisfied with the method of induction. The relative safety of these drugs for the baby has yet to be determined.

Vaginal prostaglandin E_2 should be considered for formal induction of labour irrespective of cervical favourability or membrane status (RCOG, 2001).

Amniotomy

Amniotomy is the deliberate artificial rupture of the amniotic membranes. During a vaginal examination

Table 51.2 Current evidence from Cochrane Systematic Reviews on prostaglandin as an induction of labour agent

Preparation	Technique	Results	Review comments	Reference
PGF$_{2\alpha}$	Vaginal	Cervical changes likely. Caesarean section rate unchanged. Oxytocin augmentation reduced	Effective induction agent	Kelly *et al.*, 2003a
Prostaglandin	Oral v other methods	Less likely to have delivered in 24 h. Increased maternal side-effects	No advantage over other methods. Frequent side-effects	French, 2003
PGE$_2$	Vaginal	Reduced number undelivered in 24 h. Caesarean section rate unchanged. Oxytocin reduced. Increased hyperstimulation with fetal heart rate changes	Effective induction agent	Kelly *et al.*, 2003a
PGE$_2$	Vaginal tablet, pessary and gel	As efficacious as each other. Lower doses as effective as higher doses. Tablet is most cost-effective	Tablet to be recommended	Kelly *et al.*, 2003a
PGE$_2$ v PGF$_{2\alpha}$	Vaginal		Insufficient data to make conclusions	Kelly *et al.*, 2003a
Prostaglandin	Extra-amniotic	Reduced use of oxytocin	Little clinical evidence. Rarely used in modern obstetrics	Hutton and Mozurkewich, 2003
Prostaglandin v oxytocin	Intravenous	High incidence of hyperstimulation with fetal heart rate changes. Increased maternal side-effects. Equal delivery rates	No difference in effectiveness but more hyperstimulation and side-effects	Luckas and Bricker, 2003
Misoprostol (prostaglandin E$_1$ analogue)	Oral v vaginal	Oral less effective than vaginal. Caesarean section rate lower	Oral effective but safety issues	Alfirevic, 2003
Prostaglandin	For PROM	Decreased chorioamnionitis and admission to neonatal unit. No difference in caesarean section rate. More pain relief and maternal diarrhoea	As results	Tan and Hannah, 2003c
Prostaglandin v oxytocin	For PROM at or near term	PGE$_2$ = Increased chorioamnionitis and maternal side-effects. Reduced epidurals and internal fetal heart rate monitoring	As results	Tan and Hannah, 2003a
Prostaglandin v oxytocin	For PROM at term	PGE$_2$ = Increased chorioamnionitis and neonatal infection. Reduced epidurals and internal fetal heart rate monitoring	As results	Tan and Hannah, 2003d
Misoprostol (prostaglandin E$_1$ analogue)	Vaginal	Increased cervical ripening 12–24 h and delivery in 24 h. Reduced oxytocin. Increased uterine hyperstimulation without fetal heart rate changes	Appears to be more effective than other methods but concerns over hyperstimulation and anecdotal reports of ruptured uterus. Warrants further trials	Hofmeyr and Gulmezoglu, 2003

the clinician digitally identifies the cervical os and membranes and pierces the forewaters using a specially designed plastic 'Amnihook' (EMS Medical Group). Less commonly, surgical steel forceps are used. Artificial rupture of the hindwaters used to be done with an S-shaped metal Drew Smythe catheter. This procedure is rare in the UK but may have a place in countries where resources are limited.

More than any other method of induction, amniotomy implies a firm commitment to delivery (Enkin et al., 2000).

Amniotomy can be used alone if the membranes are accessible, although the time interval from amniotomy to established labour and thus delivery is unpredictable. This may or may not be acceptable to clinicians and women, and in a number of cases induction by amniotomy alone may fail (Bricker and Luckas, 2003).

It may be used with oxytocic drugs either at the time of membrane rupture or after an interval of a few hours if uterine contractions have not commenced. Evidence from clinical trials (Saleh, 1975, cited in Bricker and Luckas, 2003) shows that women who receive oxytocin at the time of amniotomy are more likely to be delivered within 12 hours, less likely to have a caesarean section or forceps delivery, require less analgesia and sustain lower rates of postpartum haemorrhage than those who do not receive oxytocin. Less depressed Apgar scores are also found. However, this method is not without certain risks. Potential hazards of amniotomy include:

- ascending intrauterine infection: including mother-to-child vertical transmission of HIV infection
- early decelerations of the fetal heart rate
- umbilical cord prolapse
- bleeding from the cervix, fetal vessels in the membranes (vasa praevia) or the placental site.

Oxytocin

Oxytocin is the commonest induction agent used worldwide. Intravenous infusion is the licensed method of administration. It is used to augment labour as well as being a method of induction. The RCOG guideline on induction of labour (2001) recommends that oxytocin should be delivered via an infusion pump or a syringe driver with the dosage expressed in milliunits per minute, commencing at a starting dose of 1–2 milliunits per minute and increased at intervals of no less than 30 minutes.

The dose of oxytocin is regulated by the intensity of uterine contractions, aiming for a maximum of three to four contractions every 10 minutes. The maximum licensed dose is 20 milliunits per minute.

Concerns over achieving a minimal effective dose are related to the serious complication of excessive uterine contractions. Excessively frequent (hyperstimulation/tachysystole) or prolonged contractions (hypertonus) may cause fetal hypoxia due to compromised

placental circulation. Uterine rupture is a rare but life-threatening consequence of uterine hypercontractility. The suggested management for uterine hyperstimulation is to stop the oxytocin, as the short half-life of the drug will reduce the degree of fetal compromise, dependent upon fetal reserve. Tocolytics may be needed to halt labour: subcutaneous terbutaline 0.25 mg is the suggested drug of choice (RCOG, 2001: 20).

The antidiuretic effect of oxytocin can lead to water retention and hyponatraemia with serious associated maternal sequelae, although this is preventable with strict fluid management and minimal infusion volume.

There is also evidence that the incidence of neonatal hyperbilirubinaemia is increased with the use of oxytocin (Enkin et al., 2000).

Other methods

Medical   Table 51.3 includes reviews of other medical methods that have been used for cervical ripening or induction of labour but are not currently recommended for routine clinical use. Although it is acknowledged that certain agents, i.e. misoprostol and mifepristone, are effective, they require further rigorous evaluation.

Non-medical   Castor oil combined with a bath and enema has traditionally been used for initiating labour but has been shown to be ineffective and causes uncomfortable gastrointestinal side-effects (Kelly et al., 2003c). Its use has mainly been abandoned in modern maternity practice.

Breast stimulation has historically been used to induce and augment labour in many different cultures. A meta-analysis of six trials of breast stimulation showed that more women progress to labour and that there is a reduced incidence of postpartum haemorrhage but it is associated with hyperstimulation (Kavanagh et al., 2003c).

Regular sexual intercourse has been found to be ineffective as a method of inducing labour (Kavanagh et al., 2003d).

The use of acupuncture and homeopathic remedies, such as raspberry leaf tea, have not been adequately studied to assess their usefulness for induction of labour, although observational studies suggest they may be effective (Smith, 2003; Smith and Crowther, 2003) and may warrant further evaluation.

More natural methods of cervical ripening and induction of labour allow women to have greater control over the induction process, are inexpensive and

Table 51.3 Reviews of other medical methods to effect cervical ripening or induction of labour

Method	Review findings	Reference
Oestrogen	Ineffective for cervical ripening	Thomas *et al.*, 2003
Oxytocin (cervical ripening)	Ineffective for cervical ripening	Kelly and Tan, 2003
Mechanical devices, e.g. Laminara tents, cervical, or extra-amniotic catheters	Appear effective but uncomfortable and not commonly used in UK	Boulvain *et al.*, 2003b
Mifepristone	Insufficient evidence but data suggest it is more effective and reduces caesarean section rate. Warrants further evaluation	Neilson, 2003
Relaxin	Insufficient evidence. Not commonly used. Not licensed in UK	Kelly *et al.*, 2003b
Corticosteroids	Insufficient evidence. Not commonly used. Not licensed in UK	Kavanagh *et al.*, 2003a
Hyaluronidase	Insufficient evidence. Not commonly used. Not licensed in UK	Kavanagh *et al.*, 2003b
Misoprostol	Appears cost-effective. Associated with uterine hyperstimulation and meconium-stained liquor. Not licensed. Warrants further evaluation	Alfirevic, 2003; Hofmeyr and Gulmezoglu, 2003

are perceived as being less medicalized. However, further research is required to establish the safety and efficacy of certain methods. They should not be used when induction of labour is considered necessary for the safety of the mother or baby.

POST-TERM PREGNANCY

Post-term pregnancy is classified as a pregnancy continuing for more than 42 weeks or greater than 294 days (International Federation of Gynecology and Obstetrics (FIGO), 1980). The reported incidence of post-term pregnancy is between 4 and 14% (Enkin *et al.*, 2000). A previous prolonged pregnancy increases the incidence of subsequent prolonged pregnancy two- to threefold and daughters of mothers who have had prolonged pregnancy have increased risk (Mogren *et al.*, 1999).

Population studies indicate that perinatal mortality and morbidity are increased in pregnancies of more than 42 weeks (RCOG, 2001), although the incidence is much reduced from that previously cited (Campbell, 1997). In addition, the incidence of congenital malformation in babies born post-term is higher and data should be adjusted to account for life-threatening anomalies (Enkin *et al.*, 2000). Perinatal death occurs mainly during the intrapartum and neonatal periods and not during the pregnancy (Enkin *et al.*, 2000). Asphyxia associated with meconium-staining of the amniotic fluid is a common feature of these deaths. The incidence of neonatal seizures is increased two to five times in babies born after 41 weeks (Enkin *et al.*, 2000).

Accurate dating

Post-term pregnancy and social factors account for approximately 70% of inductions (Thomason, 1999). The common method of establishing the due date is by the last menstrual period (LMP) following Naegele's rule. However, inaccuracies in maternal recollection of LMP (Geirsson and Busby-Earle, 1991) and the wide variance in the distribution of ovulation and conception dates (Guerrero and Florez, 1969) introduce substantial error when using LMP as the principal tool for dating. In developed countries ultrasound scanning is also routinely used to check the LMP-derived date. Dating by ultrasound scan alone has been shown to be a more accurate predictor of the birth date than dating by LMP alone or with a 14-, 10- or 7-day adjustment 'rule' (Mongelli *et al.*, 1996). A recent systematic review (Crowley, 2003b) concluded that an early ultrasound scan to assess gestational age more accurately predicts the birth date and thus reduces the number of inductions of labour for perceived post-term pregnancy.

Associated features of post-term pregnancy

Uteroplacental insufficiency A tenaciously held but mistaken belief is that the placenta ages as pregnancy progresses. No morphological feature of the term placenta can be considered as a manifestation of ageing (Fox, 1979; Larsen *et al.*, 1995); indeed, fresh villous growth and continuing DNA synthesis have been demonstrated in the placenta at term (Fox, 1978; Sands and Dobbing, 1985). However, the fetoplacental circulation decreases after 35 weeks of pregnancy (Lingman and Marsel, 1986) and Doppler studies show varied and numerous fetal circulatory modifications in the post-term fetus (Vetter, 1998). Calcification in the term and especially the post-term placenta is a frequent clinical observation in normal pregnancy; it is also seen on ultrasound scanning (Gudmundsson and Laurini, 1998).

Some studies have shown a gradual deterioration in placental function in the post-term pregnancy associated with chronic progressive uteroplacental insufficiency which is thought by some to 'mimic a mild fetal growth restriction' (Battaglia *et al.*, 1995).

Fetal behaviour also changes in normal post-term pregnancy. Van de Pas and colleagues (1994) found that the increasingly 'wakeful' fetal heart rate (FHR) pattern could imitate an abnormal pattern that might lead to intervention. However, further studies are required to evaluate the usefulness of assessment of fetal behavioural states in differentiating the at-risk fetus from normal.

Oligohydramnios Amniotic fluid volume diminishes in post-term pregnancies, thereby limiting the cushioning effect on the umbilical cord and fetus. Cord compression during uterine contractions may lead to fetal heart rate abnormalities. Meconium-staining of the amniotic fluid is also associated with a decreased volume (Crowley *et al.*, 1984) which in turn may lead to meconium aspiration syndrome in the baby (Katz and Bowes, 1992). This often has a significant influence on the care and management of labour and the newborn.

Fetal macrosomia In the absence of uteroplacental insufficiency, fetal growth continues, though at a reduced rate after 38 weeks' gestation (Boyd *et al.*, 1988; Gruenwald, 1967). Babies born at 42 completed weeks are three to seven times more likely to weigh over 4000 g than those delivered before 41 completed weeks (Fabre *et al.*, 1998). Macrosomia increases the risk of dysfunctional labour, shoulder dystocia, brachial plexus injury and clavicular fracture in the baby and subsequent morbidity to the woman as a result of intervention.

At and beyond term, some unpredictable and random changes occur within a few days. Interpreting the significance of these variable findings continues to be controversial and remains a challenge to modern obstetrics.

Post-maturity syndrome This condition affects babies born post-dates. Gibb (1985) first described the features of the postmature infant. Such infants are alert and appear mature but have a decreased amount of soft tissue mass, particularly subcutaneous fat; their body length is increased in relation to body weight; and the skin may hang loosely on the extremities and is often dry and peeling. There is an absence of vernix and lanugo, although they often have abundant scalp hair. The fingernails and toenails are long. The nails and umbilical cord may be stained with meconium passed in utero.

It is also associated with oligohydramnios (Clement *et al.*, 1987), with similar features to those seen in the growth-restricted infant. Knox Ritchie (1992) describes this syndrome as an expression of chronic fetal malnutrition which is not confined to post-term pregnancy. However, as few as 10% of post-term pregnancies are complicated by this syndrome (Resnik, 1994).

Management of post-term pregnancy

The recommended alternatives available to clinicians when caring for women with confirmed post-term pregnancy are either membrane sweeping from 40+ weeks, expectant management with increased antenatal surveillance of fetal well-being from 42 weeks or active induction of labour from 41+ weeks (Crowley, 2003b; RCOG, 2001). Thus interventionalist methods are to be offered before the pregnancy is strictly post-term, i.e. 42 completed weeks or more.

Membrane sweeping This has been discussed earlier in the chapter (see p. 865).

Expectant management with increased surveillance Women who decide not to be induced and await spontaneous labour are offered tests that aim to assess fetal well-being. Tests that are commonly used include:

- *Cardiotocography* (CTG), also referred to as the non-stress test, has become the primary method of assessment of fetal well-being during the antenatal period. The antenatal cardiotocograph is thought to be reassuring if fetal heart rate and variability are normal, accelerations are present and there are no decelerations. However, a recent systematic review of the use of CTG for antenatal assessment (Pattison and McCowan, 2003) concluded that there was inadequate evidence to evaluate its usefulness, it has poor predictive value and is susceptible to inter-observer interpretation errors. Midwives and obstetricians should be conscious of the limitations of this commonly used tool for assessing fetal well-being.

- *Biophysical profile* (BPP) *scoring* was first described by Manning *et al.* (1980). Minor refinements have been made but it usually involves the scoring of five biophysical variables: fetal breathing movements, gross body movements, fetal tone, fetal heart rate reactivity, and amniotic fluid volume. The BPP is based on physiological and pathophysiological features that are affected by fetal compromise. This and the extensive observational data accumulated over the years suggest a link between low biophysical profile scores and poor pregnancy outcome.

  More recently, a meta-analysis of the efficacy of BPP in high-risk pregnancies states that at present there are insufficient trial data to be able to make meaningful conclusions about the benefits or otherwise of this widely used fetal surveillance method (Alfirevic and Neilson, 2003).

- *Measurement of amniotic fluid volume by ultrasound alone* is commonly used as a method of fetal surveillance. Amniotic fluid volume is measured using a variety of ultrasound techniques that have been developed to improve the accuracy of the measurement. There has been an ongoing debate about which of the techniques is the most efficacious and there is a dearth of research studies undertaken to evaluate the accuracy of each technique and its predictive value. The predictive value of amniotic fluid volume estimation has been questioned (Williams *et al.*, 1993) and certain techniques may increase obstetric intervention (Alfirevic *et al.*, 1997).

- *The use of Doppler ultrasound* in high-risk pregnancies, e.g. hypertensive disorders and intrauterine growth restriction, has been shown to be beneficial in predicting those babies at risk of adverse peri-natal outcome (Neilson and Alfirevic, 2003). However, the technique has been found to confer no benefit in low-risk pregnancy and there are concerns over the safety of higher-intensity techniques (Bricker and Neilson, 2003).

Hannah and colleagues (1992) found that there was no difference in outcomes between complex antenatal fetal monitoring techniques (computerized CTG and BPP) when compared to more simple tests (standard CTG and maximum pool depth of amniotic fluid) in post-term pregnancies. The RCOG (2001: 26) currently recommend twice-weekly CTG and estimation of maximum amniotic pool depth in pregnancies that continue after 42 weeks. However, women and clinicians who influence their decision-making should be aware of the limitations of the efficacy of current methods of antenatal surveillance (Crowley, 2003b). Indeed, some suggest that antepartum surveillance in pregnancies where the risk of adverse outcome is very low, may actually cause rather than prevent morbidity (Alfirevic *et al.*, 1997).

Active induction of labour from 41+ weeks   This is the third option available in managing post-term pregnancy. Crowley (2003b) concludes that a policy of routine induction of labour after 41 weeks reduces the risk of perinatal death in normally formed babies and does not affect the rate of caesarean section. It is considered, however, that over 500 inductions would need to be performed to prevent one perinatal death. Women should be advised of the evidence and also have the opportunity to discuss the efficacy of the various methods available.

Management of otherwise uncomplicated prolonged pregnancy remains controversial with varied maternity unit policies and individual clinician's and women's preferences affecting the decision-making process. It does appear from the evidence that both induction of labour and expectant management are valid options and ultimately the woman should choose whichever pathway is best suited to her and her family.

Economic considerations

Cost-effectiveness and clinical governance now dominate the processes that evaluate financial calculations about patient management. The cost–benefit analysis of induction of labour versus expectant management and the cost-effectiveness of the various methods of induction have only recently been calculated (RCOG, 2001). Comparisons of the efficacy and cost of the various preparations and cost of length of stay can be achieved more simply than estimating the cost of individual tests, midwifery and obstetric resources and time. The cost of an induction depends on how it is managed and the outcome achieved (MacKenzie, 1998).

The Canadian Post-term Pregnancy Trial (Goeree et al., 1995) found that routine induction of labour was less expensive than serial monitoring of post-term pregnancy. A second study comparing expectant management with induction found that there was no difference in cost (Gafni et al., 1997).

The RCOG (2001: 41) analysed the available evidence of the cost-effectiveness of different prostaglandin preparations and conclude that overall, prostaglandin vaginal tablets are the most cost-effective. Another study concludes that prostaglandin is cost-neutral or cost-saving when compared to oxytocin once operative deliveries and postpartum complications are considered (Davies and Drummond, 1991). Available evidence and analysis are limited and further local and national analysis of the cost-effectiveness of these policies is required in order to make the findings representative.

WOMEN'S VIEWS

Studies of women's experiences of induction of labour show that women who have had their labour induced would prefer not to have the same experience repeated (Boland et al., 1990, cited in MacKenzie, 1998; Cartwright, 1977).

Available research suggests that women prefer induction of labour to expectant management when pregnancy is prolonged (Out et al., 1986; Roberts and Young, 1991), and Sarkar (1997) has confirmed that women have significantly high levels of anxiety when pregnancy goes beyond the expected date.

Garcia and colleagues (1998) sought women's views of maternity care and found that 61% of women did not feel they had a say in their labour being induced; whilst another survey established that 48% of women wanted more information about induction (Singh and Newburn, 2000). These data suggest that women receiving maternity care in the UK were unable to make informed choices or give informed consent regarding induction of labour.

MIDWIFERY CARE

The decision to pre-empt the spontaneous onset of labour needs to be made in a climate of honest interchange of information, with the benefits and risks of induction explained by the obstetrician and midwife, so that an informed choice may be made. It is the responsibility of the clinicians involved to ensure women are given evidence-based information, where it is available, to make the most appropriate decision for them.

Women and their partners are likely to experience a range of emotions when faced with induction of labour. However, involving the woman and her partner in decision-making is likely to increase their feelings of control over what happens. An individual plan of care can then be made and documented in the woman's notes.

Planning for induction

For women with complicated pregnancies and clear indications for induction, thought needs to be given to the timing of the procedure. Liaison with the antenatal ward, delivery suite, neonatal unit and any other specialist services, if appropriate, may be required to communicate any relevant details, and ensure the availability of a bed and appropriate staff.

The midwife providing care for a woman with a normal pregnancy will need to consider the appropriate time for referral to an obstetrician in the event of the pregnancy becoming post-term. Adjustment of expected date of delivery should not occur on the day a woman presents to discuss management options for supposed prolonged pregnancy.

Place of induction

Women who decide to have membrane sweeping from 40+ weeks to reduce the risk of post-term pregnancy may be cared for in the community. However, it is important that they have access to advice and assessment if required.

Induction protocols have differed between maternity units. With the publication of the RCOG national guideline (2001) it is likely that a more standardized approach to induction of labour will develop. It recommends that:

- Formal methods of induction should take place in the hospital setting
- In the absence of specific risk factors, prostaglandin induction may be initiated on the antenatal ward
- Women with recognized risk factors (including suspected fetal growth compromise, previous caesarean section and high parity) should be induced on the delivery suite
- Following insertion of prostaglandin the woman should lie down for 30–60 minutes to ensure absorption
- CTG should be undertaken to establish fetal well-being

- The administration of oxytocin should occur on the delivery suite
- Women receiving oxytocin should receive one-to-one midwifery care
- Clinical discussions, regarding induction of high-risk cases, should be undertaken at consultant level
- Wherever induction of labour occurs, facilities should be available for continuous uterine and fetal heart rate monitoring.

(Adapted from RCOG, 2001: 18–23)

These guidelines provide basic requirements for the safety of mother and baby. However, they do not consider the woman's physical, cultural, emotional or psychological needs that remain to be addressed. These topics are considered in previous chapters.

> **Reflective Activity 51.3**
>
> Review your unit's guidelines for induction of labour and assess if it reflects the principles of the RCOG guideline. Where there are any inconsistencies, evaluate whether they are supported with valid evidence.

KEY POINTS

- Prostaglandin is currently the most efficacious induction agent.
- Accurate dating of pregnancy is essential to avoid unnecessary induction of labour.
- Expectant management and induction of labour are both valid options for management of post-term pregnancy.

REFERENCES

Acker, D.B., Gregory, K.D., Sachs, B.P. *et al.* (1998) Risk factors for Erb–Duchenne palsy. *Obstetrician and Gynaecologist* **71**: 389–392.

Alfirevic, Z. (2003) Oral misoprostol for induction of labour. *Cochrane Database of Systematic Revues*, Issue 3. Oxford: Update Software.

Alfirevic, Z. & Neilson, J.P. (2003) Biophysical profile for fetal assessment in high risk pregnancies (Cochrane Review). *The Cochrane Library*, Issue 3. Oxford: Update Software.

Alfirevic, Z., Luckas, M., Walkinshaw, S.A. *et al.* (1997) A randomised comparison between amniotic fluid index and maximum pool depth in the monitoring of post-term pregnancy. *British Journal of Obstetrics and Gynaecology* **104**(2): 207–211.

Battaglia, C., Artini, P.G., Ballestri, M. *et al.* (1995) Hemodynamic, hematological and hemorrhological evaluation of post-term pregnancy. *Acta Obstetricia et Gynecologica Scandinavica* **74**(5): 336–340.

Bishop, E.H. (1964) Pelvic scoring for elective induction. *Obstetrics and Gynecology* **24**: 266–268.

Boulvain, M., Fraser, W., Marcoux, S. *et al.* (1988) Obstetric consequences of postmaturity. *American Journal of Obstetrics and Gynecology* **158**: 343–348.

Boulvain, M., Stan, C. & Irion, O. (2003a) Membrane sweeping for induction of labour. *Cochrane Database of Systematic Reviews*, Issue 3. Oxford: Update Software.

Boulvain, M., Kelly, A.J., Stan, C. *et al.* (2003b) Mechanical methods for induction of labour. *Cochrane Database of Systematic Reviews*, Issue 3. Oxford: Update Software.

Boyd, M.E., Usher, R.H., McClean, F.H. *et al.* (1988) Obstetric consequences of postmaturity. *American Journal of Obstetrics and Gynecology* **158**: 343–348.

Bricker, L. & Luckas, M. (2003) Amniotomy alone for induction of labour (Cochrane Review). *The Cochrane Library*, Issue 3. Oxford: Update Software.

Bricker, L. & Neilson, J.P. (2003) Routine Doppler ultrasound in pregnancy (Cochrane Review). *The Cochrane Library*, Issue 3. Oxford: Update Software.

Campbell, M.K. (1997) Factors affecting outcome in post-term birth. *Current Opinion in Obstetrics and Gynecology* **9**(6): 356–360.

Cartwright, A. (1977) Mothers' experiences of induction. *British Medical Journal* **2**: 745–749.

Casson, I.F., Clarke, C.A., Howard, C.V. *et al.* (1997) Outcomes of pregnancy in insulin dependent diabetic women: results of a five year population cohort study. *British Medical Journal* **315**: 275–278.

Chalmers, I., Dauncey, M.E., Verrier-Jones, E.R. *et al.* (1978) Respiratory distress syndrome in infants of Cardiff residents 1965–1975. *British Medical Journal* **ii**: 1119–1121.

Clement, D., Schifrin, B.S. & Kates, R.B. (1987) Acute oligohydramnios in postdate pregnancy. *American Journal of Obstetrics and Gynecology* **157**: 884–886.

Crowley, P. (2003a) Prophylactic corticosteroids for preterm birth. *Cochrane Database of Systematic Reviews*, Issue 3. Oxford: Update Software.

Crowley, P. (2003b) Interventions for preventing or improving the outcome of delivery at or beyond term

(Cochrane Review). *The Cochrane Library*, Issue 3. Oxford: Update Software.

Crowley, P., O'Herlihy, C. & Boylan, P. (1984) The value of ultrasound measurement of amniotic fluid volume in the management of prolonged pregnancies. *British Journal of Obstetrics and Gynaecology* 91: 444–448.

Davies, L.M., Drummond, M.F. (1991) Management of labour: consumer choice and cost implications. *Journal of Obstetrics and Gynaecology* 11: S23–33.

Department of Health and Social Security (DHSS) (1976) *On the State of the Public Health for the Year 1975.* London: HMSO.

Enkin, M., Keirse, M.J.N.C., Neilson, J. *et al.* (2000) *A Guide to Effective Care in Pregnancy and Childbirth*, 3rd edn. Oxford: Oxford University Press.

Fabre, E., Gonzalez de Aguero, R., de Augustin, J.L. *et al.* (1998) Macrosomia: concept and epidemiology. In: Kurjak, A. (ed) *Textbook of Perinatal Medicine*, Vol. 2, pp. 1273–1289. London: Parthenon Publishing Group.

International Federation of Gynecology and Obstetrics (FIGO) (1980) International classification of disease: update. *International Journal of Gynecology and Obstetrics* 17: 634–640.

Fox, H. (1978) *Pathology of the Placenta.* London: W.H. Saunders.

Fox, H. (1979) The placenta as a model for organ ageing. In: Beaconsfield, P. & Villee, C. (eds) *Placenta – A Neglected Experimental Animal.* Oxford: Pergamon.

French, L. (2003) Oral prostaglandin E$_2$ for induction of labour (Cochrane Review). *The Cochrane Library*, Issue 3. Oxford: Update Software.

Gafni, A., Goeree, R., Myhr, T.L. *et al.* (1997) Induction of labour versus expectant management for prelabour rupture of the membranes at term: an economic evaluation. *Canadian Medical Association Journal* 157: 1519–1525.

Garcia, J., Redshaw, M., Fitzsimons, B. *et al.* (1998) *First Class Delivery: A National Survey of Women's Views of Maternity Care.* Abingdon: Audit Commission Publications.

Geirsson, R.T. & Busby-Earle, R.M.C. (1991) Certain dates may not provide a reliable estimate of gestational age. *British Journal of Obstetrics and Gynaecology* 98: 108–109.

Gibb, D. (1985) Prolonged pregnancy. In: Studd, J. (ed) *The Management of Labour.* London: Blackwell Scientific Publications.

Goeree, R., Hannah, M. & Hewson, S. for the Canadian Post-term Pregnancy Trial Group (1995) Cost-effectiveness of induction of labour versus serial antenatal monitoring in the Canadian Multicenter Postterm Pregnancy Trial. *Canadian Medical Association Journal* 152: 1445–1450.

Government Statistical Service (2001) *NHS Maternity Statistics, England: 1995–96 to 1997–98.* London: DoH.

Gruenwald, P. (1967) Growth of the human fetus. In: McLaren, A. (ed) *Advances in Reproductive Physiology*, Vol. 2, pp. 279–309. London: Logos Press.

Gudmundsson, S. & Laurini, R.N. (1998) Placental haemodynamics and morphological evaluation. In: Kurjak, A. (ed) *Textbook of Perinatal Medicine*, Vol. 2, pp. 1273–1289. London: Parthenon Publishing Group.

Guerrero, R. & Florez, P.E. (1969) The duration of pregnancy. *Lancet* 2(7614): 268–269.

Hannah, M.E., Hannah, W.J., Hellman, J. *et al.* (1992) Canadian Multicenter Post-Term Pregnancy Trial Group. Induction of Labour as compared with serial antenatal monitoring in post-term pregnancy. A randomized controlled trial. *New England Journal of Medicine* 326: 1587–1592.

Hannah, M.E., Huh, C., Hewson, S.A. *et al.* (1996) Postterm pregnancy: putting the merits of a policy of induction of labor into perspective. *Birth* 23: 13–19.

Hawthorne, G., Robson, S., Ryall, E.A. *et al.* (1997) Prospective population based survey of outcome of pregnancy in diabetic women: results of the Northern Diabetic Pregnancy Audit, 1994. *British Medical Journal* 315: 279–281.

Hofmeyr, G.J. & Gulmezoglu, A.M. (2003) Vaginal misoprostol for cervical ripening and induction of labour. *Cochrane Database of Systematic Reviews*, Issue 3. Oxford: Update Software.

Hutton, E. & Mozurkewich, E. (2003) Extra-amniotic prostaglandin induction of labour (Cochrane Review). *The Cochrane Library*, Issue 3. Oxford: Update Software.

Katz, V.L. & Bowes, W.A. (1992) Meconium aspiration syndrome: reflections on a murky subject. *American Journal of Obstetrics and Gynecology* 166: 171–183.

Kavanagh, J., Kelly, A.J. & Thomas, J. (2003a) Corticosteroids for induction of labour (Cochrane Review). *The Cochrane Library*, Issue 3. Oxford: Update Software.

Kavanagh, J., Kelly, A.J. & Thomas, J. (2003b) Hyaluronidase for induction of labour. *Cochrane Database of Systematic Revues*, Issue 3. Oxford: Update Software.

Kavanagh, J., Kelly, A.J. & Thomas, J. (2003c) Breast stimulation for cervical ripening and induction of labour (Cochrane Review). *The Cochrane Library*, Issue 3. Oxford: Update Software.

Kavanagh, J., Kelly, A.J. & Thomas, J. (2003d) Sexual intercourse for induction of labour. *Cochrane Database of Systematic Revues*, Issue 3. Oxford: Update Software.

Kelly, A.J. & Tan, B. (2003) Intravenous oxytocin alone for cervical ripening and induction of labour (Cochrane Review). *The Cochrane Library*, Issue 3. Oxford: Update Software.

Kelly, A.J., Kavanagh, J. & Thomas, J. (2003a) Vaginal prostaglandin (PGE$_2$ and PGF$_{2a}$) for induction of labour at term (Cochrane Review). *The Cochrane Library,* Issue 3. Oxford: Update Software.

Kelly, A.J., Kavanagh, J. & Thomas, J. (2003b) Relaxin for cervical ripening and induction of labour (Cochrane

Review). *The Cochrane Library*, Issue 3. Oxford: Update Software.

Kelly, A.J., Kavanagh, J. & Thomas, J. (2003c) Castor oil, bath and/or enema for cervical priming and induction of labour (Cochrane Review). *The Cochrane Library*, Issue 3. Oxford: Update Software.

Knox Ritchie, J.W. (1992) Obstetrics for the neonatologist. In: Roberton, N.R.C. (ed) *Textbook of Neonatology*, 2nd edn, pp. 83–119. London: Churchill Livingstone.

Larsen, L.G., Clausen, H.V., Anderson, B. *et al.* (1995) A stereologic study of postmature placentas fixed by dual perfusion. *American Journal of Obstetrics and Gynecology* 172: 500–507.

Lingman, G. & Marsel, K. (1986) Fetal central blood circulation in the third trimester of normal pregnancy. Longitudinal study. 1 Aortic and umbilical blood flow. *Early Human Development* 13: 137–150.

Luckas, M. & Bricker, L. (2003) Intravenous prostaglandin for induction of labour (Cochrane Review). *The Cochrane Library*, Issue 3. Oxford: Update Software.

MacKenzie, I.Z. (1998) Induction and augmentation of labour. In: Kurjak, A. (ed) *Textbook of Perinatal Medicine*, Vol. 2, pp. 1732–1748. London: Parthenon Publishing Group.

Manning, F.A., Platt, L.D. & Sipos, L. (1980) Antepartum fetal evaluation: development of a fetal biophysical profile. *American Journal of Obstetrics and Gynecology* 136: 787–795.

Mitchell, M.D., Klint, A.P.F., Bibby, J. *et al.* (1977) Rapid increases in plasma prostaglandin concentrations after vaginal examination and amniotomy. *British Medical Journal* 2: 1183–1185.

Mogren, I., Stenlund, H. & Hogberg, U. (1999) Recurrence of prolonged pregnancy. *International Journal of Epidemiology* 28(2): 253–257.

Mongelli, M., Wilcox, M. & Gardosi, J. (1996) Estimating the date of confinement: ultrasonographic biometry versus certain menstrual dates. *American Journal of Obstetrics and Gynecology* 174(1): 278–281.

Neilson, J.P. (2003) Mifepristone for induction of labour (Cochrane Review). *The Cochrane Library*, Issue 3. Oxford: Update Software.

Neilson, J.P. & Alfirevic, Z. (2003) Doppler ultrasound for fetal assessment in high risk pregnancies (Cochrane Review). *The Cochrane Library*, Issue 3. Oxford: Update Software.

Out, J.J., Vierhout, M.E., Verhage, F. *et al.* (1986) Characteristics and motives of women choosing elective induction of labour. *Journal of Psychosomatic Research* 30(3): 375–380.

Paterson, C.M. & Saunders, A.J. (1991) Mode of delivery after one caesarean section: audit of current practice in a health region. *British Medical Journal* 303: 818–821.

Pattison, N. & McCowan, L. (2003) Cardiotocography for antepartum fetal assessment (Cochrane Review). *The Cochrane Library*, Issue 3. Oxford: Update Software.

Resnik, R. (1994) Post-term pregnancy. In: Creasy, R.K. & Resnik, R. (eds) *Maternal Fetal Medicine Principles and Practice*, 3rd edn, pp. 521–526. London: W.B. Saunders.

Roberts, L.J. & Young, K.R. (1991) The management of prolonged pregnancy – an analysis of women's attitudes before and after term. *British Journal of Obstetrics and Gynaecology* 98: 1102–1106.

Rosen, M.G. & Dickinson, J.C. (1990) Vaginal birth after cesarean: a meta-analysis of indicators for success. *Obstetrics and Gynecology* 76: 865–869.

Rosen, M.G., Dickinson, J.C. & Westhoff, C.L. (1991) Vaginal birth after cesarean: a meta-analysis of morbidity and mortality. *Obstetrics and Gynecology* 77: 465–470.

Royal College of Obstetricians and Gynaecologists (RCOG) (2001) *Induction of Labour*. Evidence-based Clinical Guideline No. 9. London: RCOG Press.

Saleh, Y.Z. (1975) Surgical induction of labour with and without oxytocin infusion: a prospective study. *Australian and New Zealand Journal of Obstetrics and Gynaecology* 15: 80–83.

Sands, J. & Dobbing, J. (1985) Continuing growth and development of the third-trimester human placenta. *Placenta* 6: 13–22.

Sarkar, P.K. (1997) Anxiety in women who go postdates. *Contemporary Reviews in Obstetrics and Gynecology* 9(2): 107–111.

Savitz, D.A., Ananth, C.V., Luther, E.R. *et al.* (1997) Influence of gestational age on the time from spontaneous rupture of the chorio amniotic membranes to the onset of labor. *American Journal of Perinatology* 14: 129–133.

Singh, D. & Newburn, M. (2000) *Access to Maternity Information and Support*. London: NCT Publications.

Smith, C.A. (2003) Homeopathy for induction of labour. *Cochrane Database of Systematic Reviews*, Issue 1. Oxford: Update Software.

Smith, C.A. & Crowther, C. (2003) Acupuncture for induction of labour. *Cochrane Database of Systematic Reviews*, Issue 3. Oxford: Update Software.

Tan, B.P. & Hannah, M.E. (2003a) Prostaglandins versus oxytocin for prelabour rupture of membranes at or near term. *Cochrane Database of Systematic Reviews*, Issue 1. Oxford: Update Software.

Tan, B.P. & Hannah, M.E. (2003b) Oxytocin for prelabour rupture of membranes at or near term. *Cochrane Database of Systematic Reviews*, Issue 2. Oxford: Update Software.

Tan, B.P. & Hannah, M.E. (2003c) Prostaglandins for prelabour rupture of membranes at or near term (Cochrane Review). *The Cochrane Library*, Issue 2. Oxford: Update Software.

Tan, B.P. & Hannah, M.E. (2003d) Prostaglandins versus oxytocin for prelabour rupture of membranes at term (Cochrane Review). *The Cochrane Library*, Issue 2. Oxford: Update Software.

Thomas, J., Kelly, A.J. & Kavanagh, J. (2003) Oestrogens alone or with amniotomy for cervical ripening or induction of labour (Cochrane Review). *The Cochrane Library*, Issue 3. Oxford: Update Software.

Thomason, J.S. (1999) Elective induction of labour. Why, when and how? *Obstetrician and Gynaecologist* **1**(1): 20–25.

Van de Pas, M., Nijhuis, J.G. & Jongsma, H.W. (1994) Fetal behaviour in uncomplicated pregnancies after 41 weeks of gestation. *Early Human Development* **40**(1): 29–38.

Vetter, K. (1998) Doppler velocimetry in late normal pregnancy: fetal arterial circulation. In: Kurjak, A. (ed) *Textbook of Perinatal Medicine*, Vol. 1, pp. 427–432. London: Parthenon Publishing Group.

Williams, K., Wittmann, B. & Dansereau, J. (1993) Intraobserver reliability of amniotic fluid volume estimation by two techniques: amniotic fluid index vs. maximum vertical pocket. *Ultrasound in Obstetrics and Gynecology* **3**(5): 346–349.

FURTHER READING

Enkin, M., Keirse, M.J.N.C., Neilson, J. *et al.* (2000) *A Guide to Effective Care in Pregnancy and Childbirth*, 3rd edn. Oxford: Oxford University Press.

Royal College of Obstetricians and Gynaecologists (2001) *Induction of Labour*. Evidence-based Clinical Guideline No. 9. London: RCOG Press. Online. Available: http://www.rcog.org.uk/guidelines/eb_guidelines.html.

52

Disordered Uterine Action

Sarah Church and Tracey Hodgson

LEARNING OUTCOMES

After reading this chapter you will be able to:

- identify the factors that contribute to prolonged labour
- recognize disordered uterine action and understand how this may contribute to a prolonged or precipitate labour

- discuss the midwife's role in the prevention, care and management of disordered uterine action.

INTRODUCTION

This chapter looks at prolonged labour and explores the issues that surround disordered uterine action: prevention, diagnosis, management and associated problems. To maximize learning it is anticipated that the reader has a working knowledge of the care and management of normal labour.

In normal labour the uterine contractions are progressively longer, stronger and increase in frequency, causing completion of effacement and progressive dilatation of the os uteri in the first stage, steady delivery of the baby in the second stage, expulsion of the placenta and membranes and the control of haemorrhage to complete the third stage of labour. Disordered uterine action can occur at any stage of labour and is often attributed to an abnormal pattern of uterine contractility, resulting in slow or rapid progress. Vigilant observation and assessment of a woman in labour is therefore paramount in the prevention, detection and diagnosis of disordered uterine action. Unfortunately there is no way to predict the kind of labour progression (in terms of dilatation and descent) that a given contractile pattern will produce, i.e. the quality of contractions can tell little about the course of labour. In this context, the value of antenatal education in preparing the woman and her partner for labour and the possibility of a non-perfect labour is paramount. Since abnormal uterine action may be inefficient or overefficient, a useful tool to assess progress of labour is the partogram.

The partogram

The partogram is a chart used to facilitate assessment of the progress of labour, including maternal and fetal well-being. A glance at the partogram will indicate if progress is satisfactory, since progress is measured by linear progression along a prescribed time scale, whereby a curve of cervical dilatation is measured in centimetres plotted against time in hours (Friedman, 1955), and descent of the head abdominally. Modifications to the partogram have occurred resulting in the introduction of alert and action lines. The action line is 2 hours to the right of the alert line, and augmentation is instituted at this time (Fig. 52.1). Once labour is confirmed, cervical dilatation is expected to progress at a rate of 1 cm/h, and augmentation is employed in primigravidae at any deviation to the right of a simple diagonal line drawn at 1 cm/h from the diagnosis of labour. However, recent data from the USA (Albers, 2001) suggest that this is an unrealistic expectation and a rate of 0.5 cm/h was proposed as being more realistic. This illustrates the international variation in the assessment of normal labour.

PROLONGED LABOUR

The term 'prolonged labour' is difficult to define, since it is dependent upon the actual time at which labour is presumed to have begun. Defining the onset of labour is complicated, since differentiating between a prolonged

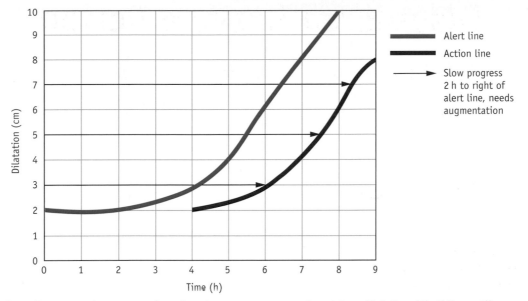

Figure 52.1   Normogram/partogram of cervimetric progress commencing at 2 cm dilatation. 'Alert' line outlines normal progress. 'Action' line indicates when augmentation should be instituted. (After Studd, 1973.)

latent phase and false labour is often difficult. Enkin *et al.* (2000) suggest that the most frequently used marker for the onset of labour for women choosing to deliver in hospital is the time of admission. Since this is an arbitrary measurement, it can lead to an inaccurate diagnosis of the onset of labour. The presumed failure of the cervix to dilate within a given time limit based on the inaccurate diagnosis of labour, can result in inappropriate intervention, preventing the woman from following her own labour pattern.

Labour used to be termed 'prolonged' when it exceeded 24 hours (Baird, 1952). Nowadays O'Driscoll *et al.* (1993) espouse the 12-hour period as the generally accepted limit. The rationale behind such an arbitrary time is the belief that the longer labour continues, the greater the hazard to both mother and fetus. To try to prevent this, the National Maternity Hospital Dublin (O'Driscoll *et al.*, 1993) define 'active labour', as painful uterine contractions, accompanied by either complete effacement of the cervix or partial effacement of the cervix with a show and/or ruptured membranes. If the women do not meet this criteria they are discharged from the labour ward; however, it is interesting to note that 40% return in established labour within 24 hours.

The following factors can contribute to the development of prolonged labour:

- Substandard midwifery care can compromise maternal well being.

- Maternal dehydration, resulting in ketosis and excessive tiredness (Keirse, 1989), can lead to maternal distress, a condition of psychological and physical exhaustion. In this condition the temperature, pulse and blood pressure rise, dehydration, oliguria and ketosis develop and may be accompanied by vomiting. Psychologically the woman becomes demoralized and restless and her pain threshold is lowered.
- A full bladder and/or rectum can impede progress by delaying descent and cause potential damage to maternal structures.

All these factors can create potential hazards to the mother and fetus.

Dangers to the mother and fetus

Owing to the early rupture of membranes and increased intervention, there is a greater risk of intrauterine infection, which can be transmitted to the fetus. An obstructed labour caused by undetected cephalopelvic disproportion may lead to a ruptured uterus. The risk of operative intervention, anaesthesia and postpartum haemorrhage is increased owing to the inability of the uterus to contract strongly. The risk of psychological trauma associated with the cumulative effects of interventions in labour and at delivery cannot be ignored. Prolonged labour is associated with fetal acidosis and intrauterine hypoxia, which can result in meconium aspiration and may lead to perinatal death (MCHRC, 2000).

Causes of prolonged labour

1. Inefficient uterine action.
2. Cephalopelvic disproportion.
3. Posterior position of the occiput.
4. Malpresentation of the fetus.
5. Macrosomia – infants who are above 90th weight centile for gestational age (Lissauer and Clayden, 2001).
6. Very rarely the cause is cervical dystocia.

Any one of these factors or a combination of them may cause prolonged labour, which remains a major cause of maternal death and infant morbidity in developing countries (Berhane & Hogberg, 1999).

Inefficient uterine action

The majority of women whose labours are prolonged are primigravidae, with inefficient uterine action the most common cause (O'Driscoll *et al.*, 1993). The birth of the first child alters the birth canal, and subsequent deliveries are usually easier, since the mother has the potential benefit of experience and belief in herself.

The active management of labour

Active management was first implemented by a group of obstetricians in Dublin during 1968 (O'Driscoll *et al.* 1969). They emphasized the importance of:

1. accurate diagnosis of the onset of labour, especially the need for complete effacement of the cervix
2. early use of amniotomy once labour was diagnosed
3. use of oxytocin within 1 hour of amniotomy if minimal progress
4. one-to-one support from a midwife or medical student who walks with the woman, promoting upright posture and mobility throughout the whole course of labour
5. rectal examinations for assessment of progress (in order to reduce the incidence of infection, unless there are specific reasons for vaginal examination, e.g. to apply a fetal scalp electrode)
6. supportive and thorough peer review to evaluate standards.

A high spontaneous vaginal delivery rate is achieved with this type of management. There is a low number of operative deliveries with impressively low mortality and morbidity rates. In order to achieve such outcomes, the labours of 45% of primigravidae are augmented with oxytocin (O'Driscoll *et al.*, 1993). However, an overview of trials evaluating the outcomes of active management, concludes that although the operative delivery rate is reduced, the presence of a constant companion for the woman in labour is the effective ingredient, not the use of amniotomy and oxytocin (Thornton and Lilford, 1994).

Active management of labour is not normally applied to women in labour with twins or malpresentations. Augmentation should be used with extreme caution in multigravidae and women with uterine scars because of the risk of uterine rupture (DoH, 1998). To appreciate the implications of active management, an understanding of amniotomy and use of oxytocin is required.

Amniotomy

Amniotomy is when the membranes are ruptured to accelerate labour; it may also reveal the presence of meconium. The underlying physiology that instigates contractions is the increase in prostaglandin release and the pressure from the fetal head upon the cervix, which is associated with the increase in pain and the use of epidural anaesthesia (Barrett *et al.*, 1992). Although the UK Amniotomy Group (1994) demonstrated that the average length of labour was only reduced by 30 minutes, Fraser *et al.* (1993) reported that labour was reduced by 136 minutes, but commented that the caesarean section rate had increased. If amniotomy is performed too early in labour it results in reduced amniotic fluid which predicts increased fetal risk and subsequent obstetric intervention (Menard, 1998; Wingfield *et al.*, 1993).

Henderson (1990) points out that the benefits of intact membranes are the maintenance of an even hydrostatic pressure to the whole fetal surface during labour and a reduced likelihood of infection. Fetal hypoxia is therefore less likely because retraction of the placental site, and thus impairment of the uteroplacental circulation will not occur. Accurate assessment of established labour and justification of amniotomy must be carefully addressed. The woman needs to retain control and make informed choices even when deviation from normal progress occurs (DoH, 1993). The most important views of amniotomy are those of women who experience this intervention. A large trial conducted by the National Childbirth Trust (1989) found that the great majority of women found labour harder to cope with following amniotomy and felt their physiology had been disturbed. A discussion with the mother regarding the need and the implications should take place and her consent should be obtained (DoH, 1993; Moran-Ellis, 1991). Following amniotomy, it may be necessary to augment labour with oxytocin.

Augmentation with oxytocin

The use of oxytocin in the active management of labour varies. Keirse (1989) recommends that, while there is a place for oxytocic augmentation in slow labour, other measures such as enabling women to mobilize, and to eat and drink (Baker, 1996), should be considered in the first instance, rather than medical intervention, to treat non-existent dystocia (Crowther *et al.*, 1989). The relationship between anxiety and the need for oxytocin to augment uterine contractions has been documented (Haddad & Morris, 1985).

Whilst it is thought that high maternal anxiety interferes with normal uterine activity (Lederman *et al.*, 1978), the value of providing sufficient information to meet women's individual needs during preparation for childbirth has been recognized (Lee, 2001). O'Driscoll *et al.* (1969) placed an importance on educating women for the childbirth process, by the provision of information during the antenatal period in order to 'train' women how to achieve a spontaneous delivery.

Alternative approaches such as the use of water during labour to ease pain, reduce anxiety and induce relaxation have also been suggested (Garland, 2000) as a means of encouraging the woman to return to her normal labour pattern.

If augmentation with oxytocin is required, vigilant midwifery care is essential. Although it is rare for a primigravid uterus to rupture, in a multigravida, oxytocin should be used with extreme caution after obstructed labour has been excluded (DoH, 1998). In these situations, a multidisciplinary approach to care is required.

Reflective Activity 52.1

To complete this activity you will need access to your local database.

What is the normal delivery rate in your unit?

How long is the average length of labour for primigravid and multigravid women?

How many women had their labours augmented with: (a) amniotomy; (b) amniotomy with intravenous oxytocin?

Of these, how many women had: (a) normal deliveries; (b) instrumental deliveries; (c) caesarean section?

The role of the midwife in prolonged labour

If the principles in management of labour care are followed, it should alert the midwife to the development of a prolonged labour and, therefore, the subsequent action necessary. The following points are particularly relevant:

- The midwife should continue to carefully assess the woman's condition, both physically and psychologically, reporting any deviations from normal to an obstetrician. Continuous fetal heart monitoring will be required (NICE, 2001), although intermittent auscultation may be appropriate to encourage mobility if only an amniotomy has been performed.
- One-to-one support is very important for the woman and her partner to facilitate assessment of progress, aid good communication and enhance informed consent (Hunt & Symonds, 1995).
- Accurate contemporaneous records should be maintained (UKCC, 1998).
- The midwife should act as an advocate for the woman as required and work collaboratively with members of the multidisciplinary team (UKCC, 1998).
- Adequate management of pain may help reduce the anxiety and give opportunity for the body to return to natural rhythms. Water is a medium which might meet these needs (Garland, 2000). Research is currently being undertaken to find out whether water can be an alternative method in the management of prolonged labour (E. Cluett, personal communication, 2001; Cluett *et al.*, 2001).

Use of oxytocin

- Oxytocin is administered intravenously using an infusion pump and titrated according to local policies.
- The midwife carefully observes uterine action, ensuring that the uterus relaxes adequately between contractions and there are no signs of hyperstimulation and fetal distress. As labour progresses the infusion rate may need to be decreased.
- If uterine hyperstimulation or fetal distress occurs, the oxytocin infusion should be turned off immediately. In addition to being referred to an obstetrician (UKCC, 1998), the woman should be encouraged to adopt the left lateral position and oxygen should be administered via a face mask. NB: Oxygen should not be administered for long periods as it is thought it may be detrimental to the fetus. This is an area requiring further research (NICE, 2001).
- If intravenous fluids are necessary, oral fluids may be restricted and a drug to reduce gastric aspiration

syndrome (e.g. ranitidine) should be administered in case of the need for a general anaesthetic (DoH, 1998).

- After delivery the infusion is usually continued for 1 hour to reduce the risk of postpartum haemorrhage.

Reflective Activity 52.2

Consider the information given in Case scenario 52.1:

- Does Ruth require obstetric intervention to augment her labour?
- How do you justify your decision?
- Discuss your plan of care.

Discussion of case scenario

It is recommended that the midwife in conjunction with Ruth and Dave, re-evaluate the plan of care based on a full assessment of labour progress. The two key issues here are the management of pain and the development of efficient uterine action. Pain management needs to be addressed first, as this might facilitate an increase in uterine efficiency. As Ruth has had intramuscular pain relief, options available may be limited depending on the drug used, time of administration and the local policies. Alternative positions, increased mobilization, the use of a water pool and the provision of high-calorie isotonic drinks may be restricted.

It is evident that contractions are inefficient and to assist progress, contractions must be sufficient to facilitate pressure on the cervix to assist dilatation, accompanied by rotation and flexion of the baby. Possible options include a second intramuscular injection, which may inhibit uterine contractions further and provide limited pain relief, which Ruth might not find acceptable. Alternatively, an epidural may provide sufficient pain relief to allow rest and reduce anxiety, giving opportunity for the uterus to regain efficiency, thus enabling avoidance of the use of augmentation.

Management of a prolonged second stage of labour

It is important to consider that prolonged labour can occur at any stage and the progress of the first stage may influence the management of the second and third stages. Historically, time limits have been imposed on the length of the second stage; however, it is now considered good practice to assess each woman on an individual basis, ensuring that maternal and fetal observations remain within normal limits (McCandlish, 1997).

Case scenario 52.1

Ruth, a 22-year-old primigravida at term, has been in labour for 8 hours. Since her admission she has been contracting 3 : 10 fair to moderate, lasting 35–45 seconds and has been progressing slowly. On abdominal palpation, the fetus is a long lie, cephalic presentation, 3/5th palpable and in the right occipitoposterior position. On vaginal examination, the cervix is thick and 6 cm dilated, and poorly applied to the presenting part. Liquor is clear. The fetal heart rate is within normal limits and is being intermittently auscultated. Ruth feels tired and exhausted, and has had intramuscular analgesia and Entonox for pain relief. She is well supported by her husband Dave who is now also very tired.

The main causes of delay in the second stage of labour are inefficient uterine action, full bladder or rectum, a rigid perineum and, rarely, a contracted pelvic outlet.

Fetal causes include a persistent occipitoposterior position, deep transverse arrest, malpresentations, fetal macrosomia and fetal abnormality such as hydrocephaly.

If progress is slow and the woman is able and wishes to adopt an upright position, the midwife should support this as it is believed that the direct pressure of the presenting part against the posterior wall of the vagina stimulates the release of oxytocin (Ferguson's reflex), and thereby enhances the urge to bear down (Burns, 1992). Meticulous observations continue during the second stage, as in the first. The obstetrician must be informed if there appears to be lack of progress or if fetal or maternal distress develops. In this instance an assisted vaginal delivery or occasionally a caesarean section may be necessary.

Midwifery management of the third stage of labour following a prolonged first and/or second stage

Invariably, if the first and second stage of labour have progressed normally the third stage will too. However, the midwife must remain observant and if problems have occurred during the labour, active management will be the method of choice because of the associated risks. Women at greater risk of complications of prolonged third stage are those who have had inadequate contractions, or developed a constriction ring, full bladder or morbidly adhered placenta.

In addition to the active management of the third stage with oxytocic drugs, the midwife should be vigilant, avoid 'fiddling' with the uterus and ensure that the bladder is empty, since a full bladder can interfere with uterine activity. Alternative strategies may be used, which include the encouragement of skin-to-skin contact between mother and infant (Ashmore, 2001), change of maternal position, and breastfeeding, which may stimulate the uterus to contract by the release of oxytocin (Stuart-Macadam and Dettwyler, 1995). In some instances oxytocin may have to be administered intravenously by infusion, if contractions are inadequate or absent and the above management has failed. If this is the case, the obstetrician must be informed whilst the midwife remains with the woman (UKCC, 1998). Continuous monitoring of maternal condition is paramount, with adequate and appropriate explanation of events and potential subsequent management.

The psychological aspects of prolonged labour

Throughout a prolonged and augmented labour the woman and her partner should be cared for and supported by a midwife with whom they have developed a trusting relationship. Good communications are essential to allay unnecessary anxiety and to enable the woman and her partner to understand what is happening and to be involved in all discussions and decisions regarding care.

It is most important for the woman's psychological well-being, that she is consulted about all interventions and retains a sense of control (Weaver, 1998). A debriefing discussion (Smith and Mitchell, 1996), between the woman and the midwife who cared for her in labour, should take place at a suitable time after delivery. This can help the woman to come to terms with the events of her labour and raise her self-esteem. Some women experience a sense of failure and become depressed after a prolonged and difficult labour (Cartwright, 1979), which is further complicated by postnatal ill-health.

OVEREFFICIENT UTERINE ACTION (PRECIPITATE LABOUR)

Labour is sometimes very rapid with intense frequent contractions, and delivery occurs within an hour (Stables, 1999). This is more common in the multiparous woman and is usually caused by the minimal resistance of the maternal soft tissues. The first stage of labour may occur almost without pain and only when the head is about to be born does the woman become aware of it. The mother may sustain lacerations of the cervix and perineum and is at risk of postpartum haemorrhage. Fetal complications include hypoxia as a result of intense frequent contractions and intracranial haemorrhage that may occur as a result of rapid descent through the birth canal. Other dangers include injuries sustained as a result of being delivered in an unsuitable place or falling to the ground. If the woman has a history of precipitate births, it is advisable for her to have a delivery pack at home and for local midwives to be made aware of her history and address. Some obstetricians advocate admission to the maternity unit from 38 weeks' gestation for controlled induction. In a small study of 11 women, it was reported that whilst a shorter labour was preferable, several women were frightened they would not reach hospital in time and frustrated that midwives did not believe them when they said they wanted to push (Rippin-Sisler, 1996).

TONIC UTERINE ACTION

Definition

This is a rare condition in which the uterus increases powerful contractions to overcome an obstruction; eventually one long contraction is maintained. It is synonymous with severe acute pain accompanied by rapid deterioration in maternal condition and intrauterine death due to cessation of delivery of oxygen to the fetus.

Midwifery management

The midwife's role is to administer oxygen while summoning emergency medical and midwifery aid to resuscitate the mother, as immediate delivery is required to prevent a ruptured uterus. The management is usually by caesarean section.

Caution must be taken not to confuse tonic uterine action with tetanic uterine action, which occurs as a result of uterine hyperstimulation, caused usually by injudicious use of oxytocics. If oxytocin is being administered intravenously the infusion should be stopped. Encourage the woman to adopt the left lateral position to enhance uteroplacental blood flow, and inform the obstetrician.

CERVICAL DYSTOCIA

This is when the uterus contracts normally but the cervix fails to dilate. Its occurrence is rare but diagnosis is important to prevent maternal and fetal distress. The cervix might efface but fails to dilate; the woman may have a history of cervical surgery or congenital abnormality of the cervix. It is important that this condition is excluded prior to the use of oxytocin because of the associated risk of uterine rupture. Vaginal delivery is therefore impossible and a caesarean section is performed.

SUMMARY

Good midwifery care, including the accurate diagnosis of establishment of labour, prevention of maternal dehydration, and good communication skills, may prevent the development of prolonged labour. However, if prolonged labour occurs, the midwife needs to remember the importance of vigilance and accurate record-keeping. Working in partnership with the woman and liaising with relevant healthcare professionals is essential. Sensitive and empathetic midwifery care is also required to support women experiencing precipitate delivery, and in the careful planning of future births. In either situation the midwife should recognize the potential need for an opportunity for the woman to discuss her labour experiences.

KEY POINTS

- An accurate assessment of the onset of labour should be made, to minimize the introduction of unnecessary intervention.
- Collaboration and cooperation between the woman, midwife and obstetrician are essential.

- The midwife should remain vigilant throughout labour and recognize that prolonged labour can occur at any stage and the progress of the first stage may influence the management of the second and third stages.

REFERENCES

Albers, L. (2001) Rethinking dystocia: patience please. *MIDIRS Midwifery Digest* **11**(3): 351–353.

Ashmore, S. (2001) Implementing skin to skin contact in the immediate postnatal period. *MIDIRS Midwifery Digest* **11**(2): 247–250.

Baird, D. (1952) The cause and prevention of difficult labour. *American Journal of Obstetrics and Gynecology* 63: 1200–1212.

Baker, C. (1996) Nutrition and hydration in labour. *British Journal of Midwifery* 4(11): 568–572.

Barrett, J.F.R., Savage, J., Phillips, K. *et al.* (1992) Randomized trial of amniotomy versus the intention to leave membranes intact until the second stage. *British Journal of Obstetrics and Gynaecology* **99**: 5–10.

Berhane, Y. & Hogberg, U. (1999) Prolonged labour in rural Ethiopia: a community based study. *African Journal of Reproductive Health* 3(2): 33–39.

Burns, K.M.L. (1992) The second stage of labour – a battle against tradition. *Midwives Chronicle* 105: 92–94.

Cartwright, A. (1979) *The Dignity of Labour*. London: Tavistock.

Cluett, E.R., Pickering, R.M. & Brooking, J.I. (2001) An investigation into the feasibility of comparing three management options (augmentation, conservative and water) for nulliparae with dystocia in the first stage of labour. *Midwifery* **17**(1): 35–43.

Crowther, C., Enkin, M., Keirse, M.J.N.C. *et al.* (1989) Monitoring the progress of labour. In: Chalmers, I., Enkin, M. & Keirse, M.J.N.C. (eds) *Effective Care in Pregnancy and Childbirth*, pp. 833–845. Oxford: Oxford University Press.

Department of Health (DoH) (1993) *Changing Childbirth: Report of the Expert Maternity Group*, Part one. London: HMSO.

Department of Health (DoH) (1998) *Why mothers die? Report on Confidential Enquiries into Maternal Deaths in the UK 1994–1996*. London: HMSO.

Enkin, M., Keirse, M.J.N.C., Neilson, J. *et al.* (eds) (2000) Prolonged labour. In: *A Guide to Effective Care in Pregnancy and Childbirth*, Ch. 35, pp. 332–340. Oxford: Oxford University Press.

Fraser, W.D., Marcoux, S. & Moutquin, J.M. (1993) Effect of early amniotomy on the risk of dystocia in nulliparous women. *New England Journal of Medicine* 328(16): 1145–1149.

Friedman, E.A. (1955) Primigravid labor – a graphicostatistical analysis. *Obstetrics and Gynecology* 6: 567–589.

Haddad, P.F. & Morris, N.F. (1985) Anxiety in pregnancy and its relation to use of oxytocin and analgesia in labour. *Journal of Obstetrics and Gynaecology* 6: 77–81.

Henderson, C. (1990) Artificial rupture of the membranes. In: Alexander, J., Levy, V. & Roch, S. (eds) *Intrapartum Care – A research Based Approach*. Hampshire: Macmillan Education.

Garland, D. (2000) *Waterbirth: An Attitude to Care*, 2nd edn. Oxford: Books for Midwives.

Hunt, S. & Symonds, A. (1995) *The Social Meaning of Midwifery*. Basingstoke: Macmillan.

Keirse, M.J.N.C. (1989) Augmentation of labour. In: Chalmers, I., Enkin, M. & Keirse, M.J.N.C. (eds) *Effective Care in Pregnancy and Childbirth*. Oxford: Oxford University Press.

Lederman, R.P., Lederman, E., Work, B.A. *et al.* (1978) The relationship of maternal anxiety, plasma catecholamines and plasma cortisol to progress in labor. *American Journal of Obstetrics and Gynecology* **132**: 495–500.

Lee, B. (2001) Royal Society of Medicine forum: active birth, active management. *RCM Midwives Journal* **4**(7): 228–230.

Lissauer, T. & Clayden, G. (2001) *Illustrated Textbook of Paediatrics,* 2nd edn. London: Mosby Wolfe.

McCandlish, R. (1997) Care during the second stage of labour. In: Alexander, J., Levy, V. & Roth, C. (eds) *Midwifery Practice Core Topics 2*, Ch. 7, pp. 98–112. Hampshire: Macmillan Press.

Maternal and Child Health Research Consortium (MCHRC) (2000) *Confidential Enquiry into Stillbirths and Deaths in Infancy: 7th Annual Report*. London: MCHRC.

Menard, M.K. (1998) Early amniotomy increased the rate of fetal heart decelerations. *Evidence-based Medicine* **3**(1): 18.

Moran-Ellis, J. (1991) Rupture of the membranes in labour. *Journal of Obstetrics and Gynaecology* **11**(Suppl. 1): S6–S10.

National Childbirth Trust (1989) *Rupture of the Membranes in Labour: Women's Views*. London: National Childbirth Trust.

National Institute for Clinical Excellence (NICE) (2001) *The Use of Electronic Fetal Monitoring*. London: NICE.

National Midwifery Council (NMC) (2002) *Code of Professional Conduct*. London: NMC.

O'Driscoll, K., Jackson, R. & Gallagher, J. (1969) Prevention of prolonged labour. *British Medical Journal* **2**: 477–480.

O'Driscoll, K., Meagher, D. & Boylan, P. (1993) *Active Management of Labour: The Dublin Experience*. London: Mosby.

Rippin-Sisler, C.S. (1996) The experience of precipitate labour. *Birth* **23**(4): 224–228.

Smith, J.A. & Mitchell, S. (1996) Debriefing after childbirth: a tool for effective risk management. *British Journal of Midwifery* **4**(11): 581–586.

Stables, D. (1999) Abnormalities of uterine action and onset of labour. In: *Physiology in Childbearing with Anatomy and Related Biosciences,* Ch. 41, pp. 495–503. London: Baillière Tindall.

Stuart-Macadam, P. & Dettwyler, K.A. (1995) *Breastfeeding: Biocultural Perspective*. New York: Adline-de Gruyter.

Studd, J. (1973) Partograms and normograms of cervical dilatation in mangement of primigravid labour. *British Medical Journal* **4**: 451–455.

Thornton, J.G. & Lilford, R.J. (1994) Active management of labour: current knowledge and research issues. *British Medical Journal* **309**: 366–369.

UK Amniotomy group (1994) A multicentre randomised trial of amniotomy in spontaneous first labour at term. *British Journal of Obstetrics and Gynaecology* **101**: 307–309.

United Kingdom Central Council for Nursing, Midwifery and Health Visiting (UKCC) (1998) *Midwives Rules and Code Of Practice*. London: UKCC.

Weaver, J. (1998) Choice, control and decision-making in labour. In: Clement, S (ed) *Psychological Perspectives on Pregnancy and Childbirth,* Ch. 5, pp. 81–99. Edinburgh: Churchill Livingstone.

Wingfield, M., Turner, M.J. & Stronge, J.M. (1993) Significance of absent amniotic fluid in labour following spontaneous or artificial rupture of the membranes. *Journal of Obstetrics and Gynaecology* **13**(5, Pt 2): 891–896.

FURTHER READING

Hammett, P.L. (1997) Midwives and debriefing. In: Kirkham, M.J. & Perkins, E.R. (eds) *Reflections on Midwifery,* Ch. 7, pp. 135–159. London: Baillière Tindall.
A thought-provoking chapter, which highlights a number of pertinent midwifery issues in relation to the psychological trauma that may be experienced by women during labour.

McDonald, S. (1997) Active management of labour. In: Alexander, J., Levy, V. & Roth, C. (eds) *Midwifery Practice Core Topics 2*, Ch. 4, pp. 51–62. Hampshire: Macmillan Press.
An excellent critical review of the policy of active management.

O'Driscoll, K. & Meagher, D. (1993) *Active Management of Labour*, 3rd edn. London: W.B. Saunders.
This is a classic text, which underpins the active management of labour and provides a historical perspective for practices still advocated today.

ADDITIONAL RESOURCE

Cluett, E. (1998) Waterbirth study hopes to bring more choice and less pain to mothers in prolonged labour. University of Southampton. Online. Available: http://www.soton.ac.uk/~pubaffrs/1998/98172.htm.

53

Malpositions and Malpresentations

Paul Lewis

LEARNING OUTCOMES

After reading this chapter you will be able to:

- have an understanding of the factors which predispose to malpositions and malpresentations of the fetus
- recognize features of malposition and malpresentation and take the appropriate action
- consider the management and care that may facilitate normality, and ensure a safe and positive experience for the woman and her baby
- use appropriate sources of evidence and research to underpin and support effective and caring practice
- be aware of current practice controversies relevant to the identification, care, and management of malposition and malpresentation.

INTRODUCTION

This chapter considers the recognition, management and care of the fetus when it presents in an occipitoposterior position, by the breech, face or brow and when an oblique or transverse lie results in a shoulder presentation. Compound presentation is also discussed.

Malpositions and malpresentations of the fetus can occur in both pregnancy and labour. The midwife has a key role in identifying these, using best evidence to inform and support the mother and effective skills to undertake her management and care. With associated higher rates of maternal and perinatal morbidity and mortality it is essential that careful attention be given to the diagnosis of malpositions and malpresentations in order to maximize fetal outcomes (Baxley, 2001).

While primarily a practitioner of the 'normal', the midwife needs to be fully conversant with the problems and practicalities that both malpositions and malpresentations can give rise to. Indeed, it is in such circumstances that skills are often tested to the limit and the midwife's ability to gain the confidence of the woman and to work effectively with the wider healthcare team will be paramount in achieving a safe and successful outcome for both mother and baby (ALSO, 2000). In dealing with malpositions and malpresentations of the fetus, the midwife needs to be knowledgeable about the latest evidence that will help to inform a woman's decisions in relation to her care and provide her with the options available.

This may be difficult and, in spite of the evidence, some women may choose for personal, cultural and religious reasons, a path that is not in keeping with the recommended evidence. Nevertheless, it is a woman's right to choose for herself and the midwife needs to ensure that in such circumstances, the woman continues to receive the relevant information, advice and support that is available. In achieving this, the midwife should consult with her supervisor of midwives and, with the woman's permission, share the proposed plan of care with her and the lead obstetrician. All discussions with the woman must be clearly documented in her maternity notes and accurately reflect the advice given, the options available and choices she has made.

IDENTIFYING MALPOSITIONS AND MALPRESENTATIONS OF THE FETUS

Midwives must be able to employ a range of skills to assist them in identifying the fetus that is lying in a deflexed attitude such as an occipitoposterior position, or where the fetus presents in an extended attitude, by the face or brow. In addition to these malpresentations, they must also be able to identify those of breech and shoulder presentation.

These all require midwives to be able to take a detailed history, to keenly observe the woman's body and behaviours and to carry out a considered and careful clinical examination. Above all, they must be able to draw the findings together in order to analyse and make sense of them. From this the midwife can then make a diagnosis, upon which discussions with the woman, clinical decisions and further professional judgements will be based.

INCIDENCE

The incidence of malpositions and malpresentations varies according to lifestyle, gestation and parity as well as the condition of the mother and fetus. The midwife needs to consider the likelihood of such presentations and the reasons why they might occur as part of the assessment, diagnosis and plan of the woman's care.

Malposition of the occiput

Occipitoposterior positions occur in approximately 10% of all labours, most of which end normally. However, it has been suggested that the modern lifestyle of less physical activity and poorer posture has led to an increase in the number of babies presenting in posterior positions. Although most may be persuaded to change their position before labour begins, midwives need to be conversant with ways that will help the mother and fetus if the baby remains in an occipitoposterior position (Sutton, 2000).

Malpositions may also be more common with the use of epidural anaesthesia (Saunders et al., 1989; Thorp et al., 1993). It is postulated that the use of epidural anaesthesia reduces the tone of the muscles of the pelvic floor and consequently, the resistance to the presenting part. This may result in a failure of the vertex to rotate and therefore increases the chance of persistent occipitoposterior positions, asynclitism and transverse arrest of the fetal head. In a study by Gardberg et al. (1998), persistent OP position at birth, primarily resulted from a malrotation rather than the absence of rotation.

It is essential that the midwife recognize that a malposition is the commonest cause of non-engagement of the fetal head at term in a primigravida. In addition,

it is the commonest cause of prolonged labour and mechanical difficulties associated with the birth.

Although the cause of occipitoposterior position is not satisfactorily explained, it is often associated with an android pelvis whose narrow forepelvis forces the fetal head to adjust and take up a posterior position in order to enter the pelvic brim. The anthropoid pelvis may also lead to a persistent occipitoposterior position. Other causes may be a pendulous abdomen or a flat sacrum. An anterior placenta is also associated with an OP position towards term (Gardberg and Tuppurainen, 1994).

Breech presentation

Malpresentation of the breech will alter significantly as gestation increases. The MIDIRS informed choice leaflet (2003) identifies the incidence of singleton breech presentation as 20% at 28 weeks. However, most of these babies will turn spontaneously before delivery and by term the incidence falls to 3–4% (approximately 1 in 25–33 pregnancies at term) (ALSO, 2000). It is suggested that in association with low birth order and high maternal age, the occurrence of breech presentation at term appears to be rising (Albrechtsen et al., 1998).

The fetus adopts this position for a variety of reasons. Most common is a 'benign error of orientation'. That is, the fetus sits in the breech for no known cause and without any obvious abnormalities. Some breech presentations occur because of the size and shape of the pelvis and that of the uterus. A breech presentation may also result when the placenta or fibroids occupy the lower uterine segment or when there is abnormal liquor volume. Significantly, multiple pregnancy, fetal abnormalities or maternal conditions that result in poor postural tone can also result in breech presentation, and midwives needs to exclude these as they seek to identify the possible cause of the malpresentation.

Shoulder presentation

The shoulder presents when the fetus is in a transverse or an oblique lie and the long axis is perpendicular to that of the mother. At term, an unstable or transverse lie presents a considerable risk to both mother and fetus with cord prolapse being 20 times more common than with a flexed vertex presentation (Baxley, 2001). Unless the lie is corrected, a caesarean section is the only mode of delivery.

The incidence of transverse lie and shoulder presentation is about 0.3–0.4% of all births and according to Baxter (2000) is 10 times higher in grand multiparous women than in nulliparous women. Other causes include conditions that obstruct the lower uterine segment such as placenta praevia, fibroids, uterine anomalies and abnormalities of the fetus.

Face presentation

Deflection, extension and hyperextension of the fetal head can lead to both brow and face presentations. The reported incidence of face presentation varies widely from 0.2% to 0.8%, which is 1 in 500 to 1 in 1200 pregnancies at term (ALSO, 2000). The causative factors are those leading to general malpresentations and those that prevent flexion of the fetal head (Napolitano and Parker, 2002).

Brow presentation

The brow presentation is the least common of all fetal presentations with a reported incidence of less than 0.02%; this is approximately 1 in 4500 pregnancies at term (ALSO, 2000).

The causes of brow presentation are generally similar to those causing face presentation and include cephalopelvic disproportion, fetal prematurity and increasing parity (Parker and Napolitano, 2002). These account for more than 60% of cases in which there is persistent brow presentation.

Reflective Activity 53.1

Whenever a malposition or malpresentation is identified at term or in labour and the woman chooses to proceed with a vaginal birth, it is imperative that the midwife is familiar with the alternative mechanisms as the fetus seeks to negotiate the birth canal.

Review Chapters 5 and 15, looking at the landmarks of the pelvis and fetal skull. Use a doll and pelvis to practise the normal mechanisms of labour.

CLINICAL ASSESSMENT

In identifying malpositions and malpresentations the midwife should take into account the gestational age of the fetus, the woman's parity and any history that might suggest the likelihood of such anomalies or abnormalities. The clinical skills of abdominal and vaginal assessment that the midwife may perform as part of a woman's antenatal and intrapartum care are central to the recognition of the presentation, engagement, attitude, lie and position of the fetus (see Ch. 16).

Underlying this is the need to be fully conversant with the anatomy of the maternal pelvis, the engaging diameter of the fetal presentations and the implications of these for the birthing process.

MALPOSITION OF THE OCCIPUT

The fetus is in an occipitoposterior position when the fetal occiput lies adjacent to the sacroiliac joint and occupies either the left or right posterior quadrants of the mother's pelvis with the brow directed anteriorly.

Sutton and Scott (1996) suggest that the position of a baby in a woman's pelvis at the end of her pregnancy will have a major influence on the kind of labour she will experience and will affect the way in which her baby is born. They have been strong advocates for midwives to work with women during pregnancy to facilitate and correct any malposition before labour begins, to encourage the fetus to adopt an occipitoanterior position.

While not based on research evidence, their seminal text on optimal fetal positioning is derived from a wealth of observational experience over many years and has enabled midwives and childbirth educators to learn ways that may help women to increase their chances of normal childbirth. A recent study by Kariminia et al. (2004) suggests otherwise and concludes that 'hands and knees' exercise with pelvic rocking from 37 weeks gestation to the onset of labour did not reduce the incidence of persistent occipitoposterior position at birth.

Reflective Activity 53.2

What do you understand by the term 'optimal fetal positioning'? What exercises in pregnancy or labour might facilitate the fetus to adopt an occipitoanterior position?

Although occipitoposterior positions (Fig. 53.1) throw a heavy responsibility on the midwife, being overly pessimistic does little to help the mother. Where the labour is progressing satisfactorily the outcome is likely to be spontaneous rotation to an anterior position followed by a normal vertex delivery.

While the case history described in Case scenario 53.1 indicates that malpositions can and do resolve, the midwife should be aware of the potential for delay and the possibility of adverse outcomes that may arise when the labour is prolonged or the occipitoposterior position persists.

Slow progress should alert midwives to the possibility of abnormal labour and they must be vigilant to

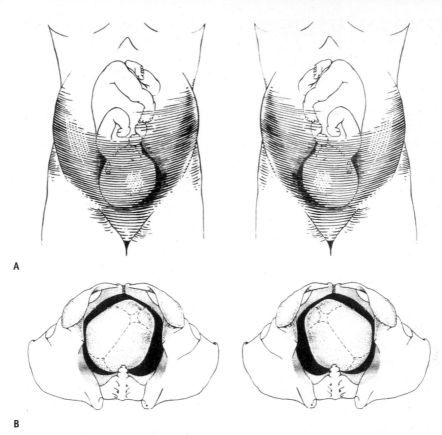

A

B

Figure 53.1 Occipitoposterior positions. **A.** Abdominal findings – the anterior shoulders are well out from the midline or fetal limbs are easily palpable. This may cause a misdiagnosis of multiple pregnancy. **B.** Vaginal findings – on vaginal examination, the anterior fontanelle is easily felt and recognized by its shape and size.

promptly recognize any complications that may arise and to call for assistance. They should be ready to act and make decisive professional judgements when indicated by either the maternal or fetal condition, poor progress of labour, the mother's psychological state and frame of mind. In the presence of an obstetric urgency or emergency, such as deep transverse arrest or cord prolapse, the midwife should seek immediate medical assistance.

In caring for a woman in prolonged labour, the midwife has the exacting task of maintaining a close watch on the progress she is making, attending to her physical care and at the same time, providing the encouragement, reassurance and emotional support that the woman needs.

The midwife also needs to be aware of the altered mechanism of a fetus in a posterior position, during which the fetus tends to be in a deflexed attitude, with the anterior fontanelle immediately over the internal cervical os. The fetal spine is towards the forward curve of the maternal lumbar spine, so that the fetus finds it

difficult or impossible to adopt a flexed position. As the fetal spine straightens, the fetus tends to 'square' the shoulders and raise the chin from the chest, resulting in a deflexed, erect 'military' attitude of the fetal head as shown in Figure 53.2.

Such movements bring the fetal head into a more difficult relationship with the inlet of the maternal pelvis. Misaligned above the pelvic brim, the fetal head is slow to engage as its larger diameters present. This ill-fitting presentation may also result in early rupture of the membranes and the danger of cord prolapse.

There is also a loss of fetal axis pressure, contractions are not effectively stimulated and descent is delayed. This can lead to slow, uneven cervical dilatation and prolonged labour. In the process of birth, the engaging diameter of the fetal head is reduced with that at right angles being elongated. In an occipitoposterior position, the fetal head is compressed in unfavourable diameters, resulting in 'sugar loaf' moulding creating a greater risk of damage to the tentorium cerebelli and the likelihood

Case scenario 53.1

Angela was a 29-year-old woman who, in her second pregnancy, chose to stay at home when she went into labour. On abdominal palpation her symphysis–fundal height was equivalent to term and the baby was a good size with an estimated fetal weight of approximately 4.0 kg. However, on assessment, the abdominal contour was slightly flattened and there was a slight depression below Angela's umbilicus. The presentation was cephalic and both the occiput and cephalic prominence could be palpated at the same level. The head was not engaged and while the lie was clearly longitudinal, the fetal parts were easily felt on the maternal right.

The position was suggestive of left occipitoposterior and the fetal heart was auscultated in the midline and in an extreme left lateral position. On vaginal examination the head remained high.

Angela remained at home, continued to labour and was mobile throughout, undertaking small tasks about the house as well as caring for her 2-year-old daughter. As labour progressed, the presenting part descended and with engagement, the cephalic prominence could be felt on the maternal right, on the opposite side to the fetal back. This indicated that the occiput had entered the pelvic inlet and that flexion had begun to occur.

On vaginal examination, the anterior fontanelle was easily felt as the fetus remained in an occipitoposterior position, but luckily, the membranes had remained intact. This was important, as it is believed that the presence of the amniotic fluid lubricates and facilitates the fetus to rotate from an occipitoposterior to the occipitoanterior position.

Angela continued to mobilize and during contractions moved her pelvis forward with her weight in front of her sitting bones (the ischial tuberosities). Although she was experiencing back pain, this was easier when she knelt down. Back massage and encouragement were also supportive. Occasionally Angela would try to raise her left leg as if trying to create more space in her pelvis to help the baby move down and within a few hours, it was obvious that Angela had entered the second stage of labour.

The presenting part advanced well and after a labour of 8 hours, Angela gave birth to a healthy and robust baby boy weighing 4.2 kg. He was born in an occipitoanterior position and Angela sustained no vaginal or perineal tears.

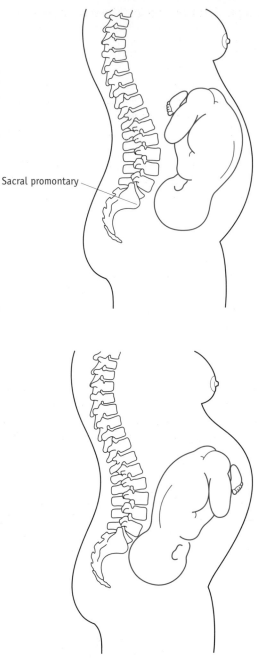

A

B

Figure 53.2   The 'military' posture of the fetus in an occipitoposterior position. **A.** Well-flexed fetus. **B.** OP position. Deflexed with straight spine and wider engaging diameter.

of intracranial haemorrhage. With a persistent occipitoposterior position, these wider diameters may also result in increased trauma to the woman's vagina and perineum.

Diagnosis of the occipitoposterior position

During pregnancy

The diagnosis is often made by abdominal examination. On inspection, the abdomen appears flattened, or slightly depressed, below the umbilicus (see Fig. 53.3). On palpation, the fetal head is commonly high. If the fetus is almost occipitolateral, the deflexed head may feel large because the occipitofrontal diameter is palpated.

The occiput and brow may be felt at the same level at the pelvic inlet, while the fetal back can be palpated out in the flank. If the occiput is markedly posterior, the high head feels small, as the bitemporal diameter is palpated; movements of the fetal limbs can often be seen or easily felt and it may be impossible to feel the back (see Fig. 53.1A and B). The fetal heart sounds can be heard in the midline just below the umbilicus. If the heart sounds are audible in one flank, it suggests that the fetal back is directed towards that side.

During labour

As described above, the diagnosis may be made by abdominal examination, though as labour advances, the head may become flexed and engaged. In this case, the cephalic prominence of the sinciput can be felt above the pubic bone and on the opposite side to the fetal back. The midwife should be alert whenever the cephalic prominence is felt on the same side as the fetal back and should consider the possibility of a face or brow presentation and seek to exclude these. A deflexed head prior to or in the process of engagement in the maternal pelvis can become extended to a brow, or hyperextended to a face, presentation. The coupling of contractions is associated with occipitoposterior positions. The midwife may identify this phenomenon when she palpates the mother's abdomen. Coupling of contractions might also be seen on the tocograph tracing if electronic fetal monitoring is in progress.

On vaginal examination the findings will depend on the degree of flexion of the fetal head. Palpation of the anterior fontanelle is usually diagnostic of an occipitoposterior position (Fig. 53.1A and B). When the head is partially or well flexed, the anterior fontanelle is felt towards the front of the pelvis, while occasionally the posterior fontanelle is just within reach at the back. With a deflexed head, the anterior fontanelle is almost central and, unless obscured by caput, it is easily recognizable by its size and shape.

Progress in labour

The progress of labour will depend upon the regularity and strength of uterine contractions and the degree of flexion of the fetal head. In addition, the shape of the maternal pelvis and the maternal position may be significant in determining how the fetus negotiates the pelvic inlet, cavity and outlet.

Reflective Activity 53.3

Review the characteristics and variation of the different types of pelvis. Consider how the difference in diameters and shape of the inlet, a flattened sacrum, prominent ischial spines and a narrow forepelvis might affect the management of care and outcomes of labour.

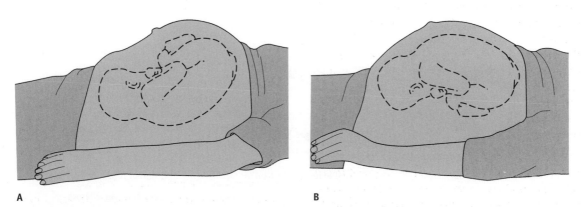

A   B

Figure 53.3 Abdominal contour. **A.** When the fetus is in the occipitoposterior position, compared to **B.** the more rounded contour of the occipitoanterior position.

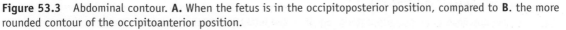

Flexion of the fetal head

If the head is flexed, labour will probably be completely normal. The engaging diameter is the suboccipitofrontal (10 cm). The occiput reaches the pelvic floor and rotates anteriorly through three-eighths of a circle (135 degrees) and the baby is born with the occiput anteriorly (Fig. 53.4).

When the head remains deflexed it tends to remain high or to take some time to engage. Labour is slow to become established with hypotonic and irregular uterine contractions. However, flexion may improve and, once the head becomes flexed, labour usually speeds up and continues normally, with a long internal rotation and an occipitoanterior birth (Fig. 53.4A).

Deflexion of the fetal head

The midwife needs to be fully conversant with the mechanism of the persistent occipitoposterior position and how this translates into what the woman experiences. If the head remains deflexed, labour is likely to be prolonged and painful, backache being a prominent characteristic. The outcome is then dependent on the size, shape and dimensions of the pelvis in relation to those of the fetal skull.

Persistent occipitoposterior position

The mechanism is that the lie is longitudinal, presentation vertex and attitude deflexed, so that the engaging diameter is the occipitofrontal and measures 11.5 cm. The position may be either right or left occipitoposterior and the presenting part is the anterior aspect of either the right (ROP) or left (LOP) parietal bone. Descent takes place with deficient flexion and the biparietal diameter of the fetal head is held up on the sacrocotyloid diameter of the maternal pelvis, so that the sinciput becomes the leading part. When the sinciput

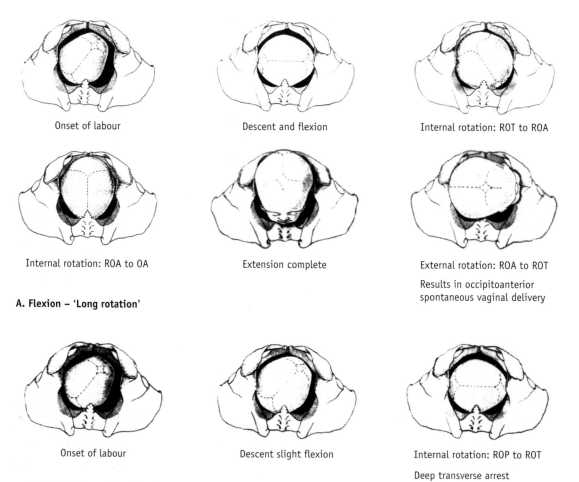

Onset of labour   Descent and flexion   Internal rotation: ROT to ROA

Internal rotation: ROA to OA   Extension complete   External rotation: ROA to ROT

Results in occipitoanterior
spontaneous vaginal delivery

A. Flexion – 'Long rotation'

Onset of labour   Descent slight flexion   Internal rotation: ROP to ROT

Deep transverse arrest

B. Slight flexion – Arrest in the transverse

Figure 53.4   Possible outcomes of an occipitoposterior position. The fetal head enters the pelvis with the occiput posteriorly.

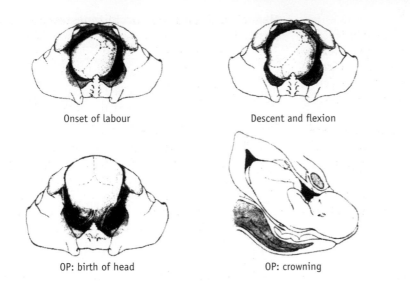

Onset of labour

Descent and flexion

Internal rotation: ROP to OP

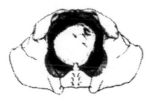

OP: birth of head

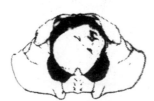

OP: crowning

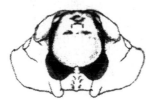

OP: flexion complete

Persistent occipitoposterior position – 'face to pubes'

C. No flexion, 'military position' – 'short rotation'

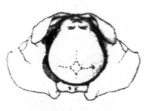

No mechanism for delivery

D. Slight flexion – Brow presentation

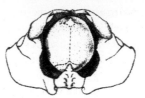

LMA: onset of labour

Extension and descent

Internal rotation: LMA to MA

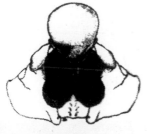

Flexion

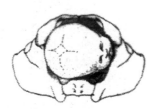

Extension

External rotation: LMA to LMT

E. Extension – face presentation

Figure 53.4 *(continued)*.

meets the resistance of the pelvic floor, it rotates forward one-eighth of a circle (Fig. 53.4C). The sinciput passes under the pubic arch and the occiput into the hollow of the sacrum. With good contractions, spontaneous delivery ensues and, with flexion, the occiput sweeps the maternal perineum and, once the glabellar is visible, the brow and face are delivered by extension. The rest of the mechanism follows that of a normal, vertex presentation (see Ch. 29). This is called *persistent occipitoposterior position* or 'face-to-pubes' delivery and is often associated with an anthropoid pelvis (Fig. 53.4C).

Deep transverse arrest (DTA)

Deep transverse arrest (Fig. 53.4B) may occur if the head remains deflexed. In this condition the fetal head may attempt a long rotation, but because of the wider diameters and the prominence of the ischial spines, it can become caught in the transverse diameter of the obstetric outlet, between the ischial spines.

This should be suspected if there is delay in the second stage of labour. On vaginal examination, the sagittal suture is found in the transverse diameter of the pelvis with a fontanelle at each end, close to the ischial spines. In the past, Kielland's forceps were used to rotate the fetal head but concern about safety has led to a decrease in their use. Today, in such circumstances, appropriately skilled midwifery or medical assistance should be obtained and, with the use of vacuum extraction (ventouse), the fetal head may be rotated to an anterior position and delivered. Manual rotation of the occiput may also be considered if the circumstances are favourable, the midwife understands the manoeuvre and the mother gives her consent. However, this should not delay summoning additional support.

Occasionally, caesarean section is necessary to deliver the fetus in an occipitoposterior position. This is likely when complications such as cord prolapse and fetal distress occur, or when true cephalopelvic disproportion is diagnosed.

Extension of the fetal head

It is possible that the fetal head may either be in a slightly extended position, or may adopt this as labour progresses, resulting in a *brow* presentation (see p. 913) (Fig. 53.4D). Unless the fetus is particularly small or preterm then it is unlikely that it will be born vaginally. Full extension of the fetal head may lead to a face presentation, which, if mento-anterior, may deliver vaginally under medical supervision (Fig. 53.4E).

Manual rotation of the occipitoposterior position

Faced with the fetus in a persistent occipitoposterior position, a prolonged second stage and a failure to deliver, the midwife, as suggested above, may also consider manual rotation to assist the birth of the baby. This requires the procedure to be fully explained to the woman and her consent obtained.

This is no more invasive than vacuum extraction and carries less risk than rotational forceps. According to ALSO (2000), this becomes an attractive alternative during a long second stage of labour because it can be attempted during a vaginal examination. If successful, delivery can be expedited and if unsuccessful, no harm has been done. The midwife seeks to enhance the normal forces of rotation, which result when the fetal head is flexed and meets the resistance of the muscles of the pelvic floor.

The midwife introduces a hand into the mother's vagina. The hand used should be opposite to that of the fetal position, i.e. when the fetus is LOP, the right hand is introduced and when the fetus is ROP, the left hand is used. The midwife's hand attempts to reach up behind the fetal occiput and cup it; the thumb is placed close to but not over the anterior fontanelle and pressure is applied to flex the fetal head. The hand essentially replicates and enhances the action of the pelvic floor (ALSO, 2000). After the fetal head has been flexed, and with the next contraction, the mother is encouraged to push. The midwife rotates her hand according to the fetal position; where this is LOP the rotation used is counterclockwise, and when ROP it is clockwise. At the same time, the midwife or an assistant can apply suprapubic pressure to the mother's abdomen in the same direction as the rotation. Although this procedure is taught on ALSO courses throughout the UK and it is believed that with time and practice, confidence and skill improve, there have been no trials to evaluate this procedure. The mother needs to be aware of this and midwives need to ensure that their practice is consistent with the requirements and standards of the Nursing and Midwifery Council's Code Of Professional Conduct (NMC, 2002).

Reflective Activity 53.4

Using a doll and mannequin, rehearse the manoeuvres of manual rotation of the posterior fetal occiput.

Complications

Midwives need to carefully consider complications that might arise (Table 53.1) and should be fully aware of what action should be taken to prevent or minimize these occurring in their management and care of a woman whose baby is in an occipitoposterior position.

Care in labour

When caring for a woman in labour whose baby is in an occipitoposterior position, the following aspects of care are paramount:

- communications and support
- one-to-one care
- general comfort and pain relief
- ambulation and position
- assessment of progress
- assessment of maternal and fetal well-being
- appropriate and decisive clinical decisions
- appropriate referral when necessary
- accurate and detailed record-keeping
- careful debriefing following the birth of the baby.

MALPRESENTATIONS OF THE FETUS

Malpresentation refers to the orientation of the fetus and may be diagnosed during pregnancy or in labour.

Table 53.1 Complications of occipitoposterior positions

Complication	Reason
Early rupture of the membranes	Poorly fitting presenting part and uneven pressure on the forewaters
Cord prolapse	As with any ill-fitting presenting part the membranes tend to rupture early and the cord may prolapse
Prolonged labour	This is associated with a deflexed head, poorly fitting presenting part and misaligned fetal axis pressure. A slightly contracted pelvis may compound this. Hypotonic and inefficient or over-efficient uterine contractions may result. In such circumstances, the development of either fetal or maternal distress is more likely and operative intervention and anaesthesia are often necessary. Postpartum haemorrhage is therefore an added risk
Retention of urine	This may occur with prolonged labour and the pressure on the urethra that results from the wider diameters of the OP position
Premature expulsive effort	The wider diameter of the OP position results in pressure on the sacral nerves and the woman may feel the need to push before full dilatation of the cervix. Early distension of the perineum and dilatation of the anus can also occur while the head is still high
Infection	This is more likely because of early rupture of the membranes, especially if labour is prolonged and can be compounded by an increased number of vaginal assessments
Trauma to the mother's soft tissues	The risk of trauma is increased with the wider diameter of the OP position. When this is persistent, the biparietal diameter and large occiput distend the maternal perineum. Instrumental delivery may also increase the risk of maternal trauma
Post-traumatic stress disorder or postnatal depression	Prolonged, difficult, painful and traumatic labour might result in mental ill-health. This can be exacerbated when the mother has no control over events and is not involved in decision-making. This, together with maternal exhaustion and an unsettled baby, may lead to difficulty in maternal–infant bonding
Maternal exhaustion	In prolonged labour maternal exhaustion may follow the birth
Unsettled or difficult-to-feed infant	In an OP position and a prolonged labour the baby's head will have been compressed in an unnatural angle resulting in discomfort and pain
Fetal intracranial haemorrhage	Upward moulding of the fetal skull may lead to stretching and damage of the tentorium cerebelli and consequent tearing of the great vein of Galen resulting in haemorrhage and intracranial damage
Increased perinatal mortality and morbidity	This might result from cord prolapse, prolonged labour, instrumental delivery, infection and intracranial haemorrhage and is increased because of hypoxia and birth trauma

Any presentation other than vertex is termed a malpresentation and therefore includes *breech*, *face*, *brow* and *shoulder*. When midwives encounter a malpresentation of the fetus, they will draw upon similar knowledge and many of the skills they used in the care and management of women whose babies were in an occipitoposterior position.

In all malpresentations, as in malpositions, there is commonly an ill-fitting presenting part. This is often associated with early rupture of the membranes because of uneven pressure on the bag of forewaters and results in an increased risk of cord prolapse. An ill-fitting presenting part is also associated with poor uterine action and slower cervical dilatation, and therefore labour may be prolonged with the concomitant risk of infection and operative intervention.

Breech presentation

A breech presentation occurs when the fetal buttocks lie lowermost in the maternal uterus and the fetal head occupies the fundus. The lie is longitudinal, the denominator is the sacrum and the presenting diameter is the bitrochanteric, which measures 10 cm.

Types

Four types of breech presentation are described (Fig. 53.5). They are determined by the way in which the fetal legs are flexed or extended, and these have implications for the birth.

- *Flexed* or *complete* breech is when the fetus sits with the thighs and knees flexed with the feet close

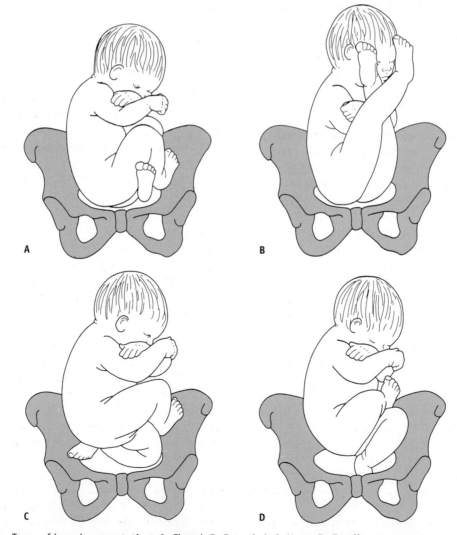

Figure 53.5   Types of breech presentation. **A.** Flexed. **B.** Extended. **C.** Knee. **D.** Footling.

to the buttocks. The flexed breech occurs more commonly in multigravidae.

- *Extended* or *frank* breech is when the fetal thighs are flexed, but the legs are extended at the knees and lie alongside the trunk, the feet being near the fetal head. This is the commonest type of breech presentation and occurs most frequently in primigravidae towards term. This is because their usually firm uterine and abdominal muscles allow only limited fetal movement and the fetus is therefore unable to flex its legs and turn to a cephalic presentation.

- *Footling presentation* is when one or both feet present below the fetal buttocks, with hips and knees extended. This type of breech presentation is more likely to occur when the fetus is preterm, but is relatively rare. A foot may occasionally be felt at the level of the buttocks and might be confused with a footling presentation. Usually, as labour advances, it slips behind the buttocks returning to an obvious flexed breech position.

- *Knee presentation* occurs when one or both knees present below the fetal buttocks, with one or both hips extended and the knees flexed. This is the least common of all types of breech presentation.

It is widely acknowledged that there is a higher perinatal mortality and morbidity with breech presentation, which is largely due to prematurity and congenital abnormalities of the fetus as well as birth asphyxia and birth trauma (Cheng and Hannah, 1993).

In providing care to women with a breech presentation, the midwife needs to be conversant with the latest developments surrounding the management and optimal mode of delivery. Although the 'Term Breech Trial' did not consider breech births at home or under the care of midwives, it did demonstrate a significant increase in perinatal mortality and morbidity with planned vaginal breech birth (Hannah *et al.*, 2000) and women need to be made aware of this information, which may inform their decisions about both mode and place of birth.

However, as Shennan and Bewley (2001) point out, the need to provide expertise in vaginal breech delivery will not disappear, as the Term Breech Trial showed that nearly 6% of women with breech presentation still have a vaginal breech delivery. This is because some women present too late, even when a policy of planned caesarean section is in place. Moreover, in spite of the evidence, some women will reject the choice of a planned caesarean section and choose to have a vaginal breech birth in either the hospital or

home setting because of personal, cultural or religious reasons.

Although the Term Breech Trial did not implicate the level of experience of the obstetrician as a factor in determining fetal outcomes, there is strong evidence that the number of vaginal breech births in the UK is limited (Thornton and Hayman, 2002). In these circumstances, it is unlikely that midwives or even obstetricians are well prepared to manage unexpected or planned vaginal breech births, and alternative training methods need to be developed.

Thornton and Hayman (2002) advocate that vaginal breech drills should be added to the teaching syllabus. ALSO (UK) along with many higher education institutes, already teach this as part of their programmes. While midwives need to be familiar with the theoretical knowledge that underpins breech presentation and birth, they must also acquire the skills necessary to manage the vaginal breech and optimize the safety of the birth.

> ### Reflective Activity 53.5
>
> Identify the guidelines for the management of breech presentation that exist in your unit or university. Explore what skills and drills training is available for unexpected or planned vaginal breech birth and if any differences exist between how midwives and obstetricians would conduct the delivery.

Causes

One fetus in four will present by the breech at some stage in pregnancy. In preterm labour it is not surprising to find the breech presenting and these infants comprise a quarter of all babies born by the breech. However, by the 34th week of pregnancy, the majority will have turned to a vertex presentation.

The commonest reason for the breech to present is a benign error of orientation for which no cause may be identified. Nevertheless, many of the probable causes of breech presentation are associated with conditions that either restrict the freedom of the fetus to turn in the uterus, or because excessive space within the uterus allows the fetus to frequently change its presentation (Table 53.2).

Breech presentation may also result from the presence of congenital anomalies, the incidence of which is known to be two to three times higher in those fetuses that present by the breech (Lauszus *et al.*, 1992). Examples of these are listed in Table 53.3.

Table 53.2   Causes of breech presentation

Primigravidae	Firm abdominal and uterine muscles may prevent flexion of the fetal legs, especially when they are already extended
Uterine anomalies	Bicornuate uterus may restrict fetal movement Previous breech birth may also be strongly associated with a uterine anomaly
Oligohydramnios	Reduced liquor volume restricts the ability of the fetus to turn in the uterus. The condition may also be associated with fetal anomalies and fetal compromise
Placental location	Placenta praevia may prevent the fetal head from fitting into the lower uterine segment and entering the pelvis. A placenta situated in one or other cornua of the uterus reduces the breadth of space in the upper segment and can lead to a breech presentation
Uterine fibroids	These can interfere with fetal activity or when situated in the lower uterine segment can prevent the fetal head from entering the lower pole of the uterus
A contracted pelvis	The fetal head is unable to enter the pelvic brim
Fetal anomalies such as trisomy 21 and hydrocephalus	These can lead to fetal hypotonia in which the lack of movement, reduced or restricted fetal activity makes it difficult for the fetus to turn Hydrocephalus can prevent the fetal head engaging in the pelvis
Multiple pregnancy	There is usually insufficient space to turn. Twins may present vertex and breech and as such, spontaneous version is unlikely
Maternal alcohol or drug abuse	May lead to fetal hypotonia in which the lack of movement, reduced or restricted fetal activity makes it difficult for the fetus to turn
Grande multiparity	Lax abdominal and uterine muscles allow movement and may lead to an unstable lie
Polyhydramnios	Overdistension of the uterus enables the fetus to be more mobile
Prematurity	Increased incidence at earlier gestation Smaller fetus with greater space within the uterus to adopt a breech position
Impaired fetal growth, short umbilical cord and fetal death	Compromised fetus may result in decreased fetal activity May be associated with fetal or maternal conditions having an adverse effect on the fetus, which results in reduced or restricted fetal mobility

Table 53.3   Congenital abnormalities in breech presentation (ALSO, 2000)

Anomaly	Breech (%)	Non-breech (%)
Hydrocephalus	0.5	0.1
Anencephaly	0.2	0.0
Urinary system	0.8	0.6
Cardiovascular system	1.0	0.5
Respiratory and GI systems	1.5	0.4
Trisomy 21 – Down's syndrome	0.2	0.1
Skeletal system	0.9	0.5
Multiple abnormalities	1.1	0.1
Total congenital abnormalities	6.2	2.3

Diagnosis during pregnancy

The midwife needs to be alert to the gestational age of the fetus and should not be unduly concerned prior to 36 weeks' gestation. A history of a previous breech presentation may be significant, as the cause could be a uterine anomaly. If the breech persists, then referral to an obstetrician should be made and the likely cause identified.

The woman may give a history of discomfort under the ribs due to the presence of the hard fetal head or describe fetal movements in the lower pole of the uterus.

Abdominal examination   The clinical skills of abdominal and vaginal examination are central to the midwife's ability to detect a breech presentation or indeed, any other malpresentation or malposition. It may be difficult to distinguish between a breech and a vertex presentation but a high index of suspicion is an asset for diagnosis (ALSO, 2000).

The diagnosis is usually made by abdominal examination. However, the method of conducting the abdominal examination may have consequences for detecting a breech presentation or finding a ballottable fetal head in the uterine fundus.

Although inspection of the maternal abdomen usually reveals nothing that indicates a breech presentation, occasionally fetal movements can be seen in the lower pole. On palpation the presenting part feels firm but less hard and less rounded than the head. The diagnosis is usually made by feeling the hard, round and ballottable head in the fundus of the uterus, which may be very easy and obvious.

Over time, the sequence in which Leopold manoeuvres have been applied during abdominal palpation have changed, with identification of the lie often taking place before palpation of the presenting part (see Ch. 16). In such circumstances, especially at term, the uterus might be stimulated, with an increase in tone or even the onset of a contraction. This results in the presenting part feeling hard and the fetal head, which is in the uterine fundus, becoming fixed and more difficult to ballot. As a consequence, breech presentations can be missed.

A primigravida with an extended breech may simulate a cephalic presentation. The woman's firm abdominal muscles brace the extended legs and compress the breech, allowing it to enter deep into the pelvis. The presenting part may be out of reach of the midwife's palpating fingers and can be mistaken for the deeply engaged head. In addition, the baby's feet, lying under the chin, also immobilize the fetal head making ballottement difficult. The placenta may lie on the anterior uterine wall and further obscure identification of the fetal head.

The fetal heart sounds, classically heard above the umbilicus in breech presentations, may well be heard at maximum intensity in an extended breech where the heart sounds are commonly heard in a vertex presentation; that is, halfway between the superior anterior iliac spine and the maternal umbilicus.

Ultrasound imaging may be helpful in confirming the presentation and can identify fetal attitude, estimate fetal weight and liquor volume and may confirm or rule out possible abnormalities. It might also be used to confirm those women with breech presentation after 36 weeks' gestation, for which external cephalic version (ECV) should be offered (Vause *et al.*, 1997).

Vaginal examination A vaginal examination may be carried out by the midwife or obstetrician, to exclude a deeply engaged head and confirm a breech presentation. If the head is deeply engaged, the shoulders palpate just above the pelvic brim and are sometimes difficult to distinguish from the breech. On vaginal examination, an extended breech has a hard, compressed presenting part similar to a cephalic presentation and the cleft of the buttocks may imitate the line of the sagittal suture.

Midwives should be aware of these deceptive findings and unless they are certain that the presentation is vertex, should be cautious. If in doubt or convinced that the presentation is breech after 36 weeks' gestation, they should inform the woman of the findings, discuss the evidence and implications and, with the woman's permission, refer her to a senior obstetric colleague.

Diagnosis during labour

In labour the presenting part may initially be high. On vaginal examination the breech feels soft and irregular and no sutures or fontanelles are palpable. The hard sacrum and the anus should be felt and it is important to distinguish the breech from a face presentation.

The midwife will note that in a breech presentation, the landmarks of the fetal ischial tuberosities are on either side of the fetal anus and form a straight line. This differs from a face presentation in which the fetal mouth and malar prominences form a triangle (ALSO, 2000).

Fresh, 'toothpaste like', thick meconium may be found on the examining finger and is diagnostic of a breech presentation. The fetal genitalia are soft and not easily recognized because they become oedematous.

In a flexed breech the feet may be palpable alongside the buttocks but these usually fall back behind the presenting part as labour advances. On vaginal examination, the features of the foot that distinguish it from a hand are; shorter digits, larger size but limited range of movements of the big toe, and the presence of a heel.

Associated risks

Breech presentation places a healthy mother and fetus at increased risk from either a complicated vaginal delivery or caesarean section (Cheng and Hannah, 1993; Hofmeyr, 1991). Regardless of the mode of delivery, a breech presentation carries four times the risk of perinatal morbidity and mortality than the fetus presenting by the vertex (Rovinsky *et al.*, 1973).

A high incidence of childhood handicap following breech presentation has also been identified and found to be similar in those infants delivered after a trial of labour and following an elective caesarean section (Danielian *et al.*, 1996). It is likely therefore that poor outcomes following vaginal breech delivery might result from some underlying condition causing breech presentation rather than damage during delivery (Hofmeyr and Hannah, 2002) and breech presentation, per se, appears to be a marker for poor perinatal outcome.

Nevertheless, caesarean section for breech presentation was seen as a way of reducing some of the risk, and the Royal College of Obstetricians and Gynaecologists'

Clinical Green Top guidelines (RCOG, 2002) identify that 'in many countries in Northern Europe and North America, caesarean section is the normal mode of delivery for breech presentation'. However, prior to the Term Breech Trial, the evidence was at best, equivocal, and therefore some mothers, midwives and obstetricians continued to show a strong preference for vaginal breech birth.

In 1993, Cheng and Hannah carried out a review of the management of breech pregnancy at term. The two studies that compared elective caesarean section with planned vaginal delivery of the breech showed no differences in mortality between the groups, but a short-term morbidity was noted in those babies who were born vaginally (Hofmeyr and Hannah, 2002). In a meta-analysis of infant outcomes after breech delivery, a higher risk of fetal injury or death was found in selected term breech infants allowed a trial of labour than in those electively delivered by caesarean section. The authors concluded that methodological problems and a lack of systematic evaluation of maternal and fetal outcomes made clinical application of the results difficult (Gifford et al., 1995).

Other evidence that supported elective caesarean section for the term breech came from hospital audits (Thorpe-Beaston et al., 1992). However, these failed to compare a policy of intended caesarean section with a policy of intended vaginal birth.

The Term Breech Trial was funded to conduct a randomized controlled trial (RCT) comparing planned vaginal delivery with planned elective caesarean section for the uncomplicated term breech (Hannah et al., 2000). This study confirmed that vaginal delivery is more hazardous than elective caesarean section for the term breech and that planned caesarean section reduced the overall risk of perinatal death for the extended or flexed breech fetus at term by 75% (relative risk 0.23; confidence interval 0.07–0.8). While the trial did not evaluate the long-term outcomes for the mother or child, the Hannah study did make the definitive recommendation that the best method of delivering a term extended or flexed singleton breech is by planned caesarean section.

The Term Breech Trial has been criticized for reflecting a medical model of birth that sanctioned the conventional dorsal lithotomy position for delivery. It has been argued that this missed an opportunity to evaluate labour and delivery in upright positions, which are considered by some to be physiologically and anatomically more sound (Gyte and Frohlich, 2001). The RCOG guidelines acknowledge that this remains an area that requires further research by those clinicians and women who remain undecided (RCOG, 2002).

Reflective Activity 53.6

Obtain a copy of the 'Term Breech Trial' paper and critically review the findings. Explore the sub-analysis and consider the implication this has for mothers, midwives and obstetricians.

In a study that revisited undiagnosed breech in labour, it was found that vaginal breech birth was more common in undiagnosed than diagnosed breech presentation (Leung et al., 1999). They concluded that their findings were 'useful in advising women concerning the mode of delivery when the breech presentation is diagnosed only after the onset of labour' and that with careful monitoring, safe vaginal delivery can certainly be achieved.

The Term Breech Trial has therefore not ended the disagreement about vaginal delivery of breech infants at term. In a well-argued commentary, van Roosmalen and Rosendaal (2002: 969) suggest that 'a policy of planned vaginal birth for selected breeches with a low threshold to proceed to caesarean section when problems arise may still be in the best interests of the mother and child'. Importantly they argue that the perinatal mortality in the Term Breech Trial was not necessarily related to the mode of delivery. In fact there were three perinatal deaths in the caesarean section group, one of which was a direct consequence of this mode of delivery. This compared to 13 perinatal deaths in the planned vaginal birth group, and of these, only four, not 13, were directly related to the mode of delivery (van Roosmalen and Rosendaal, 2002).

Similar criticisms were made in relation to maternal morbidity. Since follow-up was only carried out to 6 weeks postpartum, it was unlikely to identify problems associated with caesarean section and flies in the face of the accumulating knowledge that highlights the risks of this mode of birth. In their discussions with women, midwives should be clear about the risks of caesarean section and its implications for poorer outcomes in subsequent pregnancies.

In a breech delivery, the fetal head does not approach the maternal pelvis until after the thorax and arms are born. Once this has occurred the fetal head is usually delivered within 5 minutes. Previously, it was thought that the traumatic stresses undergone by the aftercoming head as it passed quickly through the birth canal, caused rapid compression and an equally sudden decompression as it emerged from the birth canal. It was postulated that this resulted in abnormal pressure on the tentorium cerebelli leading to rupture of the blood vessels and intracranial haemorrhage. It is now known that fetal anoxia is the major cause of intracranial haemorrhage following vaginal breech birth.

The midwife should note that placental separation may also occur in the second stage of labour and may be more likely when an upright, standing birthing position is adopted. Equally, as the aftercoming head enters the pelvis, it inevitably compresses the cord; this lack of oxygen continues and while the fetal head is still in the vagina, this hypoxia can stimulate breathing. As a result liquor, blood and mucus may be inhaled, so that after birth it is difficult or impossible to clear the airway and initiate normal breathing. Additional dangers to the baby that may result from the delivery are fractures, rupture of abdominal organs and damage to muscles and nerves.

Care and management during pregnancy

The midwife who diagnoses or suspects a breech presentation at 36 weeks should, with the mother's consent, refer her to a senior obstetrician. Having reviewed the woman's obstetric and medical history and assessed the condition of the fetus, with reference to available evidence, both midwife and obstetrician should be able to inform the woman as to her options of care. These, together with the mother's choices, should be clearly documented in her notes.

Spontaneous cephalic version of the breech   While the vast majority of breech presentations will have turned to the vertex by term, spontaneous version occurs with diminishing frequency as pregnancy advances. It happens in around 57% of pregnancies after 32 weeks' gestation and in 25% after 36 weeks' gestation (Westgren et al., 1985). It is more likely to occur in multigravidae, especially in those who have not had a previous breech presentation. It is least likely when the fetus has extended legs or a short umbilical cord.

The use of alternative approaches and techniques to promote spontaneous cephalic version has been widely reported, though the effectiveness of these has yet to be confirmed. In four RCTs, postural management using the knee–chest position showed no significant benefits in converting breech to cephalic presentations (Hofmeyr and Kulier, 2000).

One technique that may have a positive effect and play a part in reducing the number of breech presentations at term is that of moxibustion. This is used in traditional Chinese medicine to encourage fetal activity and version of the fetus in breech presentations. Budd (2000) describes 11 years' experience of this technique within an NHS hospital and while the case studies reported are interesting, the evidence is not strong. However, a small RCT investigating the use of moxibustion for correction of breech presentation, found that among primigravidae with breech presentation during the 33rd week of gestation, moxibustion for 1–2 weeks increased fetal activity during the treatment period and cephalic presentation after the treatment period and at delivery. At term, 75.4% (98/130) of the fetuses in the intervention group were cephalic at birth against 62.3% (81/130) in the control group (Cardini and Weixin, 1998).

Although further research is required to support these findings, the value of this treatment is that it can be self-administered, is simple to perform, does not involve needles and enables the woman to be fully involved and empowered in her care (Budd, 2000). If successful, it is also likely to be cost-effective.

External cephalic version (ECV)   The use of external cephalic version (ECV) has been well evaluated (Hofmeyr and Kulier, 2001) and the results are consistent and clear: ECV should be offered to all women with an uncomplicated breech presentation at term.

The procedure is considered both safe and effective and, if successful, its use avoids the associated risks of vaginal breech delivery and caesarean section. In spite of the recommendations of the RCOG that a skilled service for ECV should be available and offered, this is not the case in the majority of consultant units within the British Isles (Coltart et al., 1997). This challenges midwives and obstetricians to ensure that evidence-based practice is implemented in the best interests of women and the service (Lewis, 1997).

ECV is best carried out where facilities for emergency delivery are readily available. Cardiotocography should be performed both prior to and following the procedure and ultrasound guidance has been found to be helpful. Tocolysis is also associated with fewer failures of ECV (Hofmeyr, 2002). However, the most significant factor in providing an ECV service is the availability of suitably trained personnel. This extended role could be undertaken by some midwives and together with obstetric colleagues, a service delivered in which the incidence of breech presentation at term could be effectively reduced (Taylor and Robson, 2003).

Reflective Activity 53.7

What facilities exist in your place of practice to offer ECV? Examine the guidelines for ECV and explore the feasibility of this procedure being offered by midwives.

Mechanism of vaginal breech delivery

Although caesarean section is increasingly considered as the optimal mode of delivery for the breech presentation (Hannah *et al.*, 2000), women may still choose to have a vaginal breech birth or may present in advanced labour with an undiagnosed breech. Midwives must be fully conversant with the management and mechanism of breech presentation and be able to orientate themselves to the position that the mother adopts in labour.

There are six positions in breech presentation. The denominator is the sacrum, and its relationship to the maternal pelvis determines the position. The positions are the same as the vertex presentations, substituting the sacrum for the occiput (Fig. 53.6):

1. *Left sacroanterior position (LSA).* The sacrum points to the left iliopectineal eminence and the abdomen and legs are directed towards the right sacroiliac joint. The left buttock is anterior and the bitrochanteric diameter is in the left oblique diameter. The natal cleft is in the right oblique diameter. A caput may form on the left buttock and on the genitals.

2. *Left sacrolateral (LSL).* The sacrum is towards the left side of the pelvis.

3. *Left sacroposterior (LSP).* The sacrum points to the left sacroiliac joint, and the abdomen towards the right iliopectineal eminence.

4. *Right sacroanterior position (RSA).* The sacrum points to the right iliopectineal eminence, and the abdomen is directed towards the left sacroiliac joint. The right buttock is anterior and the bitrochanteric diameter is in the right oblique diameter. The natal cleft is in the left oblique diameter. A caput may form on the right buttock and on the genitals.

5. *Right sacrolateral (RSL).* The sacrum is towards the right side of the pelvis.

6. *Right sacroposterior (RSP).* The sacrum points to the right sacroiliac joint, and the abdomen towards the left iliopectineal eminence.

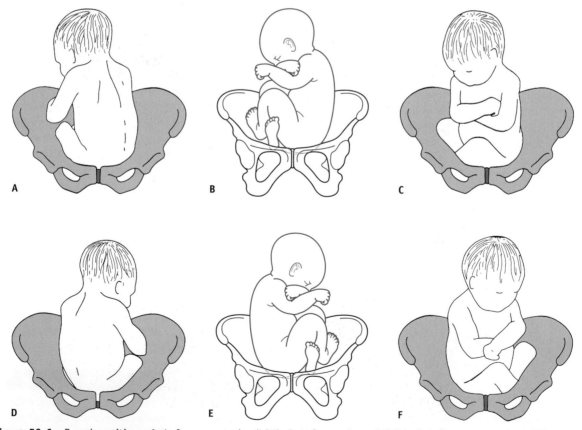

Figure 53.6   Breech positions. **A.** Left sacroanterior (LSA). **B.** Left sacrolateral (LSL). **C.** Left sacroposterior (LSP). **D.** Right sacroanterior (RSA). **E.** Right sacrolateral (RSL). **F.** Right sacroposterior (RSP).

The fetus may also be positioned in a direct anterior or posterior position.

With the breech in either the right or left sacroanterior position and good contractions, there is descent. The mechanism of the right sacroanterior position is illustrated in Figure 53.7. The fetus engages with the bitrochanteric diameter (10 cm) in the right oblique diameter of the pelvic brim and descends into the pelvic cavity.

With further contractions, the anterior buttock meets the resistance of the pelvic floor and rotates forwards through one-eighth of a circle (45 degrees) and comes to lie behind the symphysis pubis. The bitrochanteric diameter now lies in the anteroposterior diameter of the outlet. Lateral flexion of the trunk allows the continued descent of the buttocks along the curve of the birth canal (Fig. 53.8). The anterior buttock normally passes

under the symphysis pubis and is born, followed by the posterior buttock, which passes over the perineum.

With the birth of the buttocks the shoulders descend into the pelvis with the bisacromial diameter (11 cm) in the left oblique diameter of the brim. Internal rotation of the shoulders through one-eighth of a circle brings the anterior shoulder behind the symphysis. The left (anterior) shoulder and arm escape under the symphysis and the right (posterior) shoulder and arm pass over the perineum (Fig. 53.9).

The flexed head engages with the suboccipitobregmatic (9.5 cm) or suboccipitofrontal diameter (10 cm) lying in the right oblique or transverse diameter of the brim. Internal rotation of the head carries the occiput behind the symphysis. The face now lies in the hollow of the sacrum. External rotation of the buttocks and shoulders is produced by the internal rotation of the

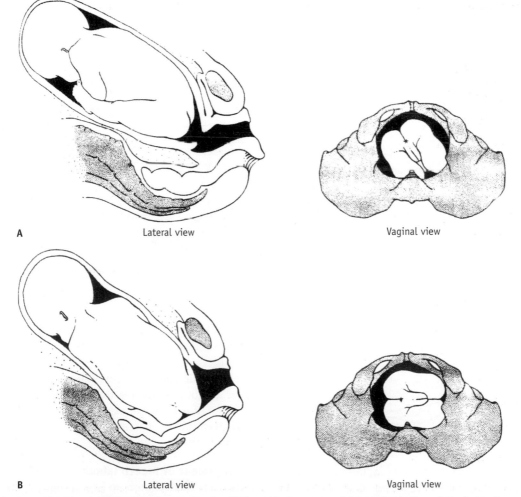

A   Lateral view   Vaginal view

B   Lateral view   Vaginal view

Figure 53.7   Right sacroanterior position. **A.** Onset of labour. **B.** Descent and internal rotation of the buttocks.

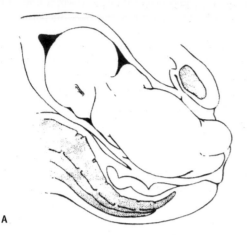

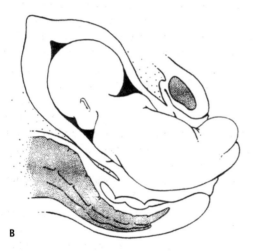

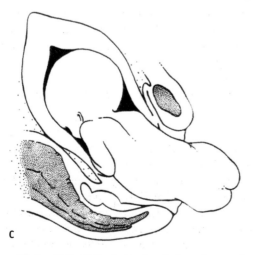

Figure 53.8 Birth of the buttocks. **A.** Breech crowning or 'rumping'. **B.** Birth of posterior buttock. **C.** Birth of anterior buttock.

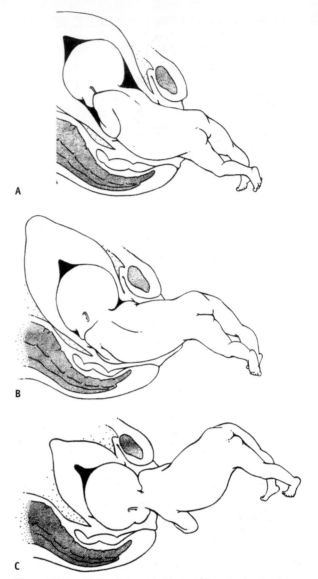

Figure 53.9 Birth of the shoulders. **A.** Feet born, shoulders engaging. **B.** Descent and internal rotation of shoulders. **C.** Posterior shoulder born; head has entered the pelvis.

head. The back of the baby's head and body now face in the same direction as the mother's abdomen.

It is essential that the back of the fetus orientates in the same direction as the mother's abdomen, and if it does not, it is gently assisted to do so. The chin, face, vertex and occiput are expelled over the perineum by a movement of flexion to complete the delivery (Fig. 53.10).

Management of breech labour

When a woman chooses to have a vaginal breech birth the midwife needs to ensure that she does so from an

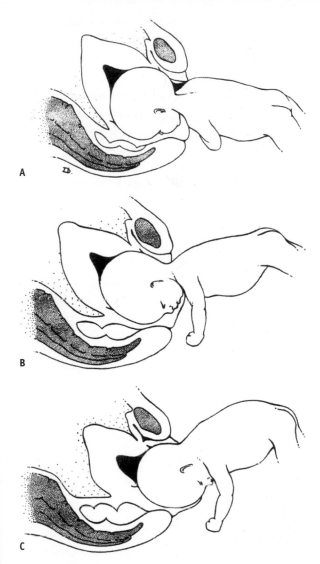

Figure 53.10 Birth of the head. **A.** Anterior shoulder born; descent of the head. **B.** Internal rotation and beginning flexion of the head. **C.** Flexion of the head complete.

informed position. Consultation with an experienced obstetrician, midwife and supervisor of midwives is important and a 'checklist' of investigations and issues should be considered and completed. A careful history should be taken to ensure that there are no medical or obstetric contraindications for vaginal breech birth and that both woman and baby are in good health.

If possible, a detailed ultrasound scan should be carried out to:

- confirm a singleton pregnancy
- exclude obvious fetal abnormality
- estimate fetal weight and attitude

- determine placental position
- assess liquor volume.

In the past, pelvimetry was advocated as a means of ensuring adequate maternal pelvic diameters for safe delivery in vaginal breech birth, though it did not significantly lower the overall caesarean section rate (Walkinshaw, 1997) and its value remains debatable (Van Loon *et al.*, 1997). A thorough clinical assessment of pelvic capacity should be performed.

Even when labour is established, consideration should be given to performing an ECV in an attempt to alter the presentation of the fetus to cephalic. While it is preferable for a vaginal breech labour to be conducted in hospital and under the supervision of an experienced obstetrician, this may not always be possible; maternal choice, as well as unexpected and rapid delivery, sometimes prevent transfer to hospital. Supervisors of midwives also have a role in facilitating the woman's admission to hospital and in supporting those midwives with the relevant skill to accompany her if requested to do so by the mother.

Given the known risks associated with breech presentation, hospital birth is preferable as it provides ready access to emergency facilities and the assistance of additional midwifery, obstetric, paediatric and anaesthetic personnel.

The process and protocol for vaginal breech delivery should be fully explained to the woman. This should involve identifying, if possible, the midwife or obstetrician who will be conducting the care and letting the woman know who, with her permission, would be in attendance at the birth.

The issues of induction of labour with a breech presentation are less likely to be encountered following the recommendations of the Term Breech Trial, because fewer breech presentations are delivered vaginally, and induction of labour will need to be carefully considered for women at term who have chosen vaginal birth.

First stage of labour This differs little from that of normal labour. If the breech is not engaged, as is probable in a flexed breech, there is a risk of early rupture of the membranes and prolapse of the umbilical cord. The midwife should be vigilant and immediately exclude the possibility of cord prolapse when the membranes rupture in such circumstances. Where the breech is engaged, the legs are probably extended and the risk of cord prolapse reduced.

The value of upright positions, ambulation and support in labour is equally pertinent to women labouring with a breech presentation. The midwife needs to provide continued support and continuity, carefully monitoring the progress of labour and the condition of the woman and fetus. A close working relationship with the wider maternity care team is also essential and while the experienced midwife may conduct the breech delivery, the support of a senior obstetrician should be readily available if necessary.

Because of the associated risk in breech presentation, continuous monitoring of the fetal heart should be offered and recommended in breech labour (NICE, 2001). Nevertheless, having been apprised of this evidence, the woman may still opt for intermittent monitoring. In such circumstance, observations on the maternal condition and progress in labour should be carried out in keeping with the recommended guidelines for intermittent monitoring (NICE, 2001).

Fetal blood sampling from the buttocks also provides an accurate assessment of the acid–base status, when the fetal heart rate trace is not reassuring (Brady *et al.*, 1989).

In most cases, the first stage of labour progresses normally. Augmentation may be required should uterine action be hypotonic. This should be done with extreme caution, and breech presentation in some units may be considered a contraindication for augmentation. There is no evidence that epidural anaesthesia is essential and its use will depend upon the wishes and needs of the woman.

Occasionally, the breech may begin to descend through the cervix before the cervical os is fully dilated and this gives the woman a desire to push. Although uncommon, the buttocks may then descend easily, but the larger head cannot pass through the incompletely dilated cervix and dangerous delay results. The use of epidural anaesthesia makes this less likely as the woman does not experience the premature urge to push; however, a large retrospective study on breech presentation found that epidurals were associated with a longer duration of labour, increased need for augmentation and a significantly higher caesarean section rate in the second stage (Chadha *et al.*, 1992).

When a women does not use epidural analgesia with a breech presentation in labour, it is important that when she first shows signs of 'bearing down' the midwife offers inhalation analgesia and discourages her from pushing until full dilatation of the cervical os is confirmed by vaginal examination.

Second stage of labour When full dilatation of the cervical os has been confirmed, the mother may adopt a semi-recumbent, all-fours, upright or supported squatting position that will aid her expulsive efforts and the descent of the fetus.

Case scenario 53.2

An audit of midwifery practice

Between August 1993 and September 1994, a number of women approached a London hospital asking for a 'standing breech birth' supported by a midwife rather than undergoing a medically managed vaginal breech delivery or a caesarean section. The hospital had a firm policy of supporting a woman's right to choose, especially if the evidence was equivocal, and during this time, 20 women with breech presentations sought midwife care.

All of the women were seen by a supervisor of midwives and the majority were referred to and seen by a consultant obstetrician. The meeting between the woman, supervisor and consultant obstetrician provided a forum in which questions could be asked and informed choices made. At that time, the research evidence as to the optimal method of delivery for breech presentation was limited and equivocal.

Maternal complications which might have affected a vaginal breech were excluded and ECV was offered after confirming gestation, fetal weight, placental location, liquor volume and fetal attitude.

Out of the 20 women in the audit, six did not have an ECV, three because of obstetric reasons and three because of maternal choice. From the 14 women who received ECV only four had the breech converted to a cephalic presentation, a success rate of approximately 28%. Three of these women went on to have spontaneous vaginal births and one had a ventouse delivery.

Given the options of a caesarean section, a medically managed breech birth or a standing breech birth conducted by the midwife, all the remaining 16 women initially chose a standing breech birth. Four women had caesarean sections; two prior to labour for reduced liquor volume and an oblique lie and two in labour for failure to progress and a footling presentation.

The remaining 12 women achieved their wish to have a standing breech birth conducted by the midwife (a vaginal delivery rate of 75%). It should be noted that two babies required admission to the neonatal unit and in both cases, placental separation occurred during the birth of the fetal trunk.

Standing position for the birth should be treated with caution, as in a small, unpublished series of standing breech deliveries known to this author, premature separation of the placenta has occurred with significant consequence for all those involved. In conducting vaginal breech births, experienced independent midwives advocate women adopting an all-fours or a forward-leaning 'prayer position' for the birth (Evans and Cronk, personal communication, 2002).

Where an obstetrician is conducting the delivery, the woman is usually in the lithotomy position. The woman can mobilize prior to the onset of the second stage and lithotomy may be delayed until the breech is visible.

The midwife should ensure that appropriate and experienced help is at hand and that a paediatrician and senior obstetrician are present or readily available and that an anaesthetist can be quickly in attendance in case operative intervention suddenly becomes necessary.

If the fetal breech and body descend well, then it is likely that spontaneous breech delivery will occur with little assistance from the midwife or obstetrician. This is more common in multigravidae or when the fetus is small and preterm.

Assisted breech delivery

A medically managed vaginal breech birth employs techniques to assist the delivery of the fetus. The woman is predominantly in the lithotomy position. The bladder is emptied prior to delivery. When the posterior buttock distends the perineum, the perineum is infiltrated with local anaesthetic (unless the mother has had an epidural anaesthetic or a pudendal block) and an episiotomy is performed. The posterior buttock then emerges and the breech advances more quickly.

As the trunk descends, the back will rotate anteriorly allowing the fetal shoulder to enter the maternal pelvis in the transverse of oblique diameter of the inlet. Traction on the fetus is not a part of British practice as this can give rise to extension of the head and nuchal displacement of the arms. There should be no interference and, increasingly, obstetricians, like midwives, apply the rule of 'hands off the breech' and will try to avoid unnecessary manipulations.

Once the umbilicus is visible, previous practice dictated that a loop of the umbilical cord should be gently pulled down to relieve any tension. This is no longer advocated. At this stage compression of the cord is likely and time is an imperative.

From the complete delivery of the buttocks, some authorities advocate that the baby should be delivered within 15 minutes. It has been argued that in vaginal breech birth, there may be benefits from rapid delivery of the baby to prevent progressive acidosis. This needs to be weighed against the potential trauma of a quick delivery and to date there is not enough evidence to evaluate the effects of expedited vaginal breech birth (Hofmeyr and Kulier, 2002).

If the fetal legs do not deliver spontaneously, inserting the index finger behind the thigh to flex the knee and abduct the leg may gently disengage them. However, if the practitioner is prepared to wait, they will deliver as the trunk descends.

With the next contraction the shoulder blades appear; the arms, which are normally flexed across the chest, will usually slip out on their own and the shoulders are born in the anteroposterior diameter of the pelvic outlet. The head at this stage is entering the transverse or oblique diameter of the pelvic inlet. Some authorities advocate that from complete delivery of the baby's body until full delivery of the head, no more than 5 minutes should elapse.

At this stage, a number of manoeuvres may be used to facilitate the delivery of the head. If all is proceeding well, spontaneous, but controlled, delivery may be used when the head is at the pelvic outlet. Some independent midwives who assist women to give birth using a forward-leaning position, use the analogy of 'getting the woman to move from a Christian prayer position to a Muslim prayer position' as this aids release of the head and facilitates its delivery. It has been observed that when the fetus begins to draw up its knees, the fetal head also flexes. If the woman then moves forward as described above, her pelvis rotates over the fetal head causing its spontaneous release (Evans and Cronk, personal communication, 2002).

Alternatively the Mauriceau–Smellie–Veit manoeuvre may be used, using flexion and traction to deliver the fetal head. The Burns–Marshall manoeuvre with or without forceps to the aftercoming head may be used to avoid rapid compression and decompression of the fetal skull and to maximize control in delivering the head.

Mauriceau–Smellie–Veit manoeuvre This manoeuvre is an effective method of delivering the fetal head, and the underlying principle is that of 'flexion before traction' (Fig. 53.11). This method is more often employed by the midwife and should ensure good control of the head and may also be used when there is delay in the descent of the head.

This manoeuvre is a combination of jaw flexion and shoulder traction and can be used for any breech delivery, but is of particular value when the fetal head is extended and forceps may be difficult to apply.

The practitioner supports the baby on the left hand, with the baby's legs straddling the arm (Fig. 53.11), and slides three fingers into the vagina feeling for the baby's cheekbones, also known as the malar bones. Originally, the middle finger was inserted into the baby's mouth in order to maximize traction but this is not recommended as it can result in dislocation of the jaw (ALSO, 2000). Instead, the ring and index fingers

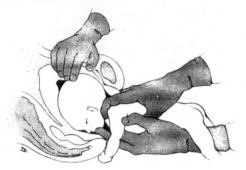

Figure 53.11 Mauriceau–Smellie–Veit manoeuvre.

rest on the cheekbones while the middle finger applies pressure to the chin.

The index and ring fingers of the practitioner's right hand are hooked over the baby's shoulders, to apply traction, while the middle finger presses on the occiput to aid flexion. An assistant may apply suprapubic pressure if needed.

As gently as possible the baby's head is flexed and aided through the pelvic cavity to the outlet, after which the trunk is raised to bring the mouth into view. The air passages are then cleared and the birth of the head completed in the usual way. The midwife can, in an emergency, perform this manoeuvre, though it is rarely required.

Burns–Marshall manoeuvre Once the body is born, the baby is allowed to hang by his own weight for a few moments to facilitate descent and flexion of the head. When the nape of the neck and hairline come into view, the head is ready to be delivered (Fig. 53.12).

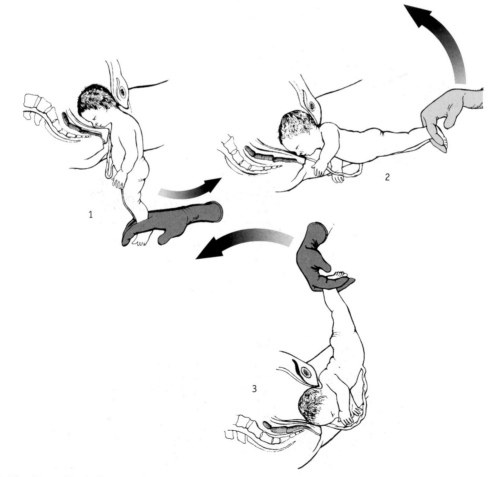

Figure 53.12 Burns–Marshall manoeuvre.

Grasping the baby by the ankles and using slight traction, the practitioner directs the trunk upwards in a wide arc over the woman's abdomen.

The perineum should then be depressed with the fingers to expose the mouth of the fetus and allow it to be cleared of any blood or mucus. The baby should then be able to breathe freely.

The birth of the head then proceeds very slowly to avoid any sudden release of pressure that might give rise to an intracranial haemorrhage. To avoid this danger Wrigley's or Neville–Barnes forceps may be applied to the aftercoming head, which allows careful control of the speed with which the head is born.

Complications of vaginal breech delivery

Extended arms If the baby's arms are not flexed across the chest, they are likely to be stretched up alongside the head. It is not possible for head and arms

to enter the pelvis together, so the arms must come first and then the head. This is best achieved by Lövset's manoeuvre, shown in Figure 53.13. With the baby in a right sacrolateral position, the manoeuvre depends on the fact that the posterior shoulder is below the sacral promontory while the anterior shoulder is above the symphysis pubis.

The practitioner grasps the baby's thighs with thumbs over the sacrum and being careful to avoid pressure above the pelvic girdle, which could cause abdominal injury, pulls the baby gently downwards at the same time turning him, back upwards, through a half circle (180 degrees). The former posterior shoulder now becomes anterior and is released under the symphysis pubis, while at the same time, the other shoulder is brought into the pelvic cavity. The baby is then turned back through a half circle in the opposite direction and the other arm is released in the same way. This procedure

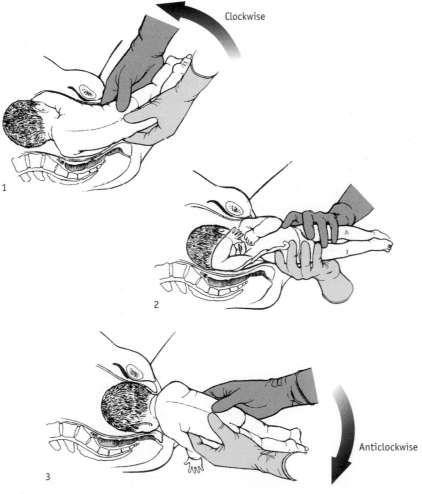

Figure 53.13 Lövset's manoeuvre.

does not require an anaesthetic, can be carried out by a midwife and, correctly performed, is safe and successful, even in cases where the baby has one arm at the back of the neck (nuchal displacement).

Reflective Activity 53.8

Using a manikin or doll and pelvis, rehearse the mechanisms of a breech presentation, and the different manoeuvres that can be used (Mauriceau–Smellie–Veit; Lövset's manoeuvres).

Extended head   After the birth of the shoulders the baby is allowed to hang from the vagina to facilitate descent and flexion of the head. If the neck and hairline are not visible within a few seconds, the most likely reason is extension of the head. The head may be delivered by the Mauriceau–Smellie–Veit manoeuvre, described above. Alternatively, forceps delivery may be required.

Entrapment of the fetal head   Although extremely rare in the term breech, this is an extremely dangerous situation. It occurs when the breech is delivered, but an incompletely dilated cervix traps the head. In this situation the midwife must call for urgent medical assistance and try to create a channel for air to reach the fetal airways by placing her fingers or a Simm's speculum into the vagina and holding the maternal tissues away from the baby's nose and mouth (see Fig. 53.14). If possible, secretions from the air passages should be aspirated. The obstetrician will try to release the head from the cervix, but mortality and morbidity rates are high. Although more commonly used in shoulder dystocia, McRobert's manoeuvre (see Ch. 55) has been used as a means to facilitate release of the fetal head (Shushan and Younis, 1992).

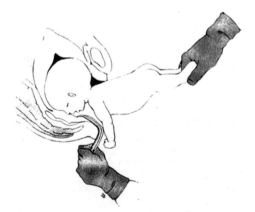

Figure 53.14   Vaginal retractor providing airway to baby's mouth and nose.

It is possible, for a variety of reasons, for a midwife to be faced with an unexpected and emergency breech delivery. In community practice, the midwife should, with the mother's consent, make every effort to transfer her into hospital. When labour is not advancing very quickly this is usually possible.

If the labour is progressing rapidly, however, delivery may be imminent and it may be deemed that the risks of transfer might be too great. If the contractions are strong and effective, there is every chance that the breech will deliver easily, though the midwife should call for skilled help as unexpected complications may still occur. Meanwhile the midwife's management of the breech birth is as described above.

Face presentation

Face presentation is uncommon, and occurs when the head and neck are hyperextended but the limbs flexed, so that the fetus lies in the uterus in a curious S-shaped attitude with the occiput against its shoulder blades and the face directly over the internal os (Fig. 53.15). The presenting portion is between the orbital ridges and the chin, with the latter being the denominator (Napolitano and Parker, 2002).

In primary face presentation, which is present before the onset of labour, the fetus is often abnormal. In *anencephaly*, there is no vertex to present and where tumours of the fetal neck occur the head is unable to flex. Occasionally excessive tone in the fetal extensor muscles may result in an extended attitude and face presentation, and this might persist for a few days after birth.

Secondary face presentations develop in labour for no obvious reason. In a deflexed occipitoposterior position the biparietal diameter may have difficulty in passing the sacrocotyloid diameter of the maternal pelvis. The bitemporal diameter descends more quickly, the head extends and the face presents.

Where the uterus is tilted sideways (uterine obliquity) the force of the uterine contractions may be directed towards the front of the head, so that the head extends as it enters the pelvis. Face presentation is also more likely to occur in a flat pelvis, where the uterus is lax, in prematurity and where there is polyhydramnios or a multiple pregnancy.

The presenting diameters of the face presentation are to some degree favourable (i.e. 9.5 cm); however, the initial reason for the fetus adopting this position, the risk of the fetus being in a mentoposterior position, and the reduced ability of the facial bones to mould, carry additional risks to the fetus (see Table 53.4).

Identification in pregnancy

Face presentation is not easily diagnosed in pregnancy. It should be suspected if a deep groove is felt between the fetal head and back and when the cephalic prominence and the fetal back are palpated on the same side.

If heart sounds are heard through the anterior chest wall on the side where the limbs are palpated, these may seem unusually loud and clear when the position is mentoanterior (MA). In mentoposterior (MP) positions the fetal heart sounds are more difficult to hear because the chest is posterior.

When face presentation is suspected, ultrasound should be used to confirm the clinical diagnosis.

During labour the high presenting part may give rise to suspicion. The diagnosis can be made on vaginal examination, when gentle palpation will reveal the orbital ridges and the gums within the mouth. The presence of the gums distinguishes the face presentation from the breech presentation in which the anus would be identified. Occasionally the fetus will further help the diagnosis by sucking the examining finger.

Once a face presentation is diagnosed it is essential to determine the position of the chin, whether it is anterior or posterior. A posterior face presentation, unless it rotates to an anterior position, will lead to obstructed labour. When the midwife diagnoses a face presentation a senior obstetrician should be informed as soon as possible. If the chin is lateral or posterior the urgency of the situation should be stressed.

As labour progresses it becomes increasingly difficult to distinguish facial landmarks on vaginal examination because the face becomes very oedematous. Vaginal examinations must be carried out with great care to avoid trauma to the eyes.

Mechanisms

The lie is longitudinal, the presentation is the face, the denominator is the chin and the attitude is hyperextended. The engaging diameter is submentobregmatic,

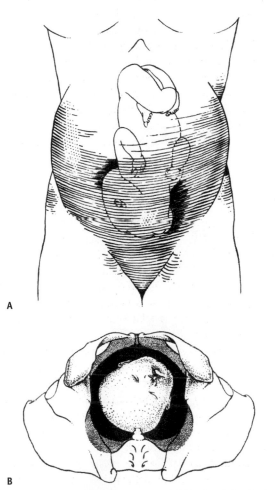

Figure 53.15   Anterior face presentation. **A.** Abdominal view. **B.** Vaginal view.

Table 53.4   Complications that may occur with a face presentation

Complication	Reason
Cord prolapse	Ill-fitting presenting part and early rupture of the membranes
Obstructed labour	The face does not mould and therefore cannot overcome minor degrees of cephalopelvic disproportion
	A persistent posterior face presentation leads to obstructed labour
Emergency operative delivery	As a result of obstructive labour or fetal distress
Severe perineal trauma	Wider diameters. Although the presenting diameter is the submentobregmatic at 9.5 cm, it is the submentovertical of 11.5 cm that distends the vagina and perineum. Risk of operative delivery
Intracranial haemorrhage	Anoxia and abnormal moulding of the fetal skull
Facial bruising and oedema	The inability of the face to mould and injury to the soft tissue

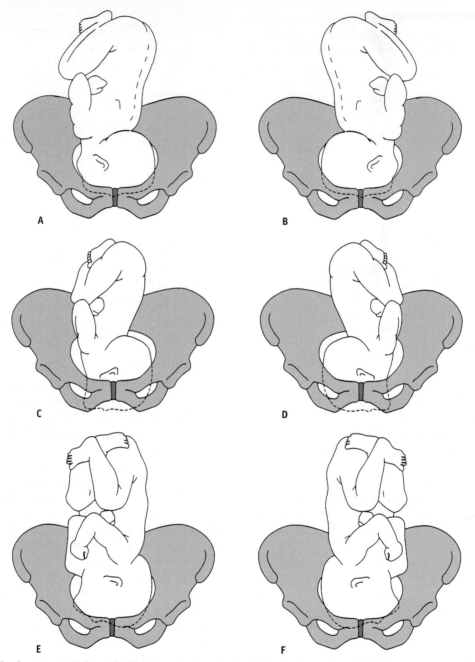

Figure 53.16   Face presentations. **A.** Right mentoposterior. **B.** Left mentoposterior. **C.** Right mentolateral.
D. Left mentolateral. **E.** Right mentoanterior. **F.** Left mentoanterior.

which is 9.5 cm. There are six positions in which the
face may present (Fig. 53.16).

1. *Right mentoposterior* (RMP) is an extension of an
   LOA. The chin points to the right sacroiliac joint.
2. *Left mentoposterior* (LMP) is an extension of an
   ROA. The chin points to the left sacroiliac joint.

3. *Right mentolateral* (RML) is an extension of an
   LOL. The chin is directed towards the right side of
   the pelvis.
4. *Left mentolateral* (LML) is an extension of an
   ROL. The chin is directed towards the left side of
   the pelvis.

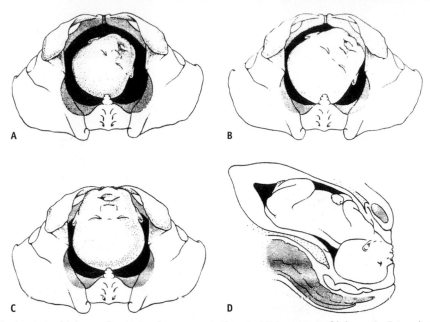

Figure 53.17 Mechanism of labour of anterior face presentation. **A.** LMA – onset of labour. **B.** Extension and descent. **C.** Vaginal view. **D.** Lateral view.

5. *Right mentoanterior* (RMA) is an extension of an LOP. The chin points to the right iliopectineal eminence.
6. *Left mentoanterior* (LMA) is an extension of an ROP. The chin points to the left iliopectineal eminence.

Face presentation develops before the head is engaged in the pelvis. The left mentoanterior position is the most common, occurring in 60–80% of cases. The mentum is transverse in 10–12% of cases and posterior in 20–25% (Napolitano and Parker, 2002).

In a mentoanterior position, the extended head enters the brim of the pelvis with the face presenting. The chin points to the iliopectineal eminence and the sinciput to the opposite sacroiliac joint (Fig. 53.17). The submentobregmatic diameter (9.5 cm) engages and the face descends into the pelvis. The chin, being the lowest part, meets the resistance of the pelvic floor and rotates through one-eighth of a circle (45 degrees), to escape under the pubic arch. The face appears at the vulval outlet (Fig. 53.18). Further uterine contractions drive the vertex and occiput over the perineum and thus, by a movement of flexion, the head is born. Restitution and external rotation take place.

A face presentation can only be born spontaneously if the chin is anterior. There is no mechanism by which the chin can be born when it lies at the back of the pelvis. This is because the neck is too short to span the length of the sacrum and is already at the point of maximum extension. For birth to occur in a mentoposterior position, the head and chest of the fetus would have to enter the pelvis together. This is normally impossible and obstructed labour will occur (see Fig. 53.19). However, spontaneous rotation of the head from the mentolateral or mentoposterior to the mentoanterior position can, and occasionally does, take place. Also, a small fetus may be able to traverse the pelvis, should the pelvic diameters permit. Spontaneous delivery may then occur.

In a face presentation with the chin to the front, an adequate pelvis, a healthy fetus and good contractions, the labour will usually progress normally, with a vaginal delivery rate of 60–70%. However, in spite of this, in developed countries in the 21st century there is a lower threshold to move to caesarean section when face presentation is identified.

Reflective Activity 53.9

Using a manikin and doll that presents by the face, explore how the contours feel on vaginal examination. Alter the position from anterior to posterior and examine again. Attempt to feel and describe the difference.

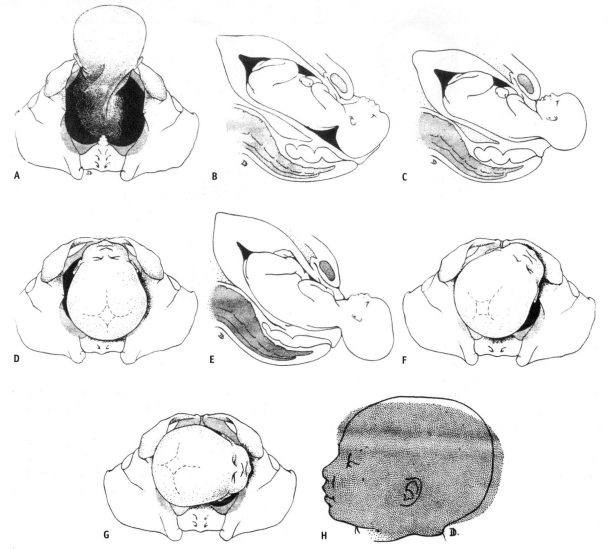

Figure 53.18 Mechanism of labour of anterior face presentation – birth of the face. **A.** Flexion; **B.** Flexion beginning; **C.** Flexion complete; **D.** Vaginal view; **E.** lateral view; **F.** Restitution – MA to LMA; **G.** External rotation – LMA to LMT; **H.** Moulding.

Management

In a mentoanterior position labour often proceeds normally, though, as in any malpresentation, the membranes may rupture early, prolapse of the cord is possible, and labour is sometimes prolonged. In the second stage normal delivery is anticipated, aided by an episiotomy, since, although the submentobregmatic diameter is only 9.5 cm, it is the submentovertical of 11.5 cm which distends the perineum at the time of delivery.

If there is delay in the second stage the obstetrician will apply forceps. If normal delivery occurs, extension

is maintained by applying pressure on the sinciput until the chin has escaped under the symphysis pubis; the head is then flexed to allow the vertex and occiput to sweep the perineum.

Mentolateral and mentoposterior positions are much more hazardous. Spontaneous delivery is unlikely, obstructed labour is possible and immediate treatment is thus essential.

The obstetrician may attempt to manually convert the face to a vertex presentation or to rotate the head to a more favourable mentoanterior position and carry out a forceps delivery (see Fig. 53.20). These manoeuvres

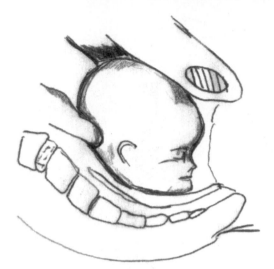

Figure 53.19 Obstructed labour, with fetus in the mentoposterior position.

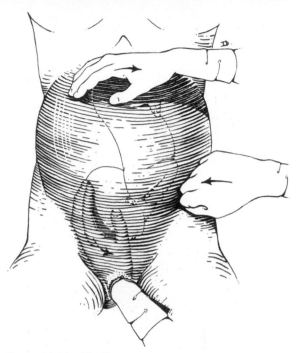

Figure 53.20 The Thorn manoeuvre.

are rarely successful and are associated with high perinatal mortality and maternal morbidity. Because of this, a caesarean section is preferable and is more commonly the treatment of choice.

At birth, the baby is usually in good condition, although the eyelids and lips will be grossly oedematous and the face congested. The bruising and unsightly appearance can cause the mother considerable alarm and anxiety. The midwife should warn her what to expect and describe how the baby might look. The mother should be reassured that the bruising and oedema will subside within a few days and suckling, which at first may be difficult, is usually normal in 48 hours.

Brow presentation

Brow presentation (Fig. 53.21) is the least common presentation and the causes are, with the exception of anencephaly, the same as in face presentation.

The head is midway between flexion and extension, with the mentovertical diameter of 13.5 cm attempting unsuccessfully to enter the 13 cm transverse diameter of the pelvic brim. A small head might enter a large pelvis only to be arrested in the cavity. Brow presentation, undiscovered and untreated, will lead to obstructed labour, uterine rupture, and raised perinatal and maternal mortality and morbidity.

Identification

On abdominal examination the head is high and the presenting diameter unusually large. As with face presentation, a groove may be felt between the occiput and the back, and the cephalic prominence will be on the same side as the fetal back.

On vaginal examination the presenting part may be too high to identify. If the brow is within reach, the orbital ridges may be felt on one side and the anterior fontanelle on the other. The diagnosis should be confirmed by ultrasound.

Management

In brow presentation, three possible outcomes are possible. The brow may:

- convert to a vertex presentation
- convert to a face presentation, or
- remain as a persistent brow presentation.

The midwife must immediately call an obstetrician if a brow presentation is suspected or diagnosed in labour, and a woman at home should be alerted to the situation and its dangers and transferred into hospital.

As in all malpresentations, the membranes are likely to rupture early and there is a risk of cord prolapse; thus a vaginal examination should be made as soon as the membranes rupture to exclude this.

If brow presentation is diagnosed early in labour it may convert to a face presentation becoming fully extended or it may flex to a vertex presentation.

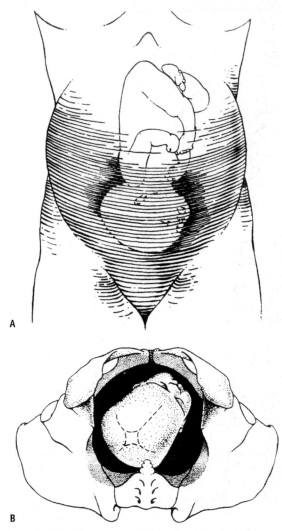

A

B

Figure 53.21 Brow presentation. **A.** Abdominal view. **B.** Vaginal view.

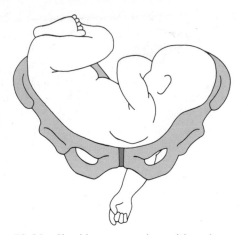

Figure 53.22 Shoulder presentation, with prolapse of one arm.

If the brow presentation persists, however, and the fetus is a normal size, it will be impossible to deliver vaginally and a caesarean section will be performed.

Oblique and transverse lie leading to shoulder presentation

A shoulder presentation occurs as a result of a transverse or an oblique lie (Fig. 53.22). Shoulder presentation is not uncommon and is only problematic if the fetus is not cephalic by 36 weeks' gestation. If uncorrected, shoulder presentation will result in obstructed labour and must be readily identified.

The commonest cause of an unstable lie and shoulder presentation is laxity of the uterine and abdominal muscles. Thus transverse and oblique lie are seen most frequently in women of high parity. Among the other likely causes, placenta praevia is one of the most serious. If a woman has a persistent oblique lie, even without sentinel bleeding, placenta praevia should be considered as a possible cause. Other contributory factors are multiple pregnancy, polyhydramnios, uterine abnormality, a contracted pelvis and occasionally a large uterine fibroid. An overdistended bladder may displace the presenting part and cause a transient oblique lie.

Identification

Abdominal examination and continuity are key to making the diagnosis of an oblique, transverse or unstable lie and therefore the presence of a shoulder presentation. The abnormal lie is easily diagnosed in pregnancy from the shape of the uterus, which appears too broad, with the fetal poles felt on either side of the abdomen, while the fundus is unusually low. Palpation will reveal the fetal head on one side and the breech on the other and no presenting part within the pelvis.

In an oblique lie the fetal head, or breech, is found in one or other iliac fossa. If a non-longitudinal lie is found after the 36–37th week of pregnancy, an obstetrician should be informed. Ultrasound may be used to confirm the diagnosis, identify the presentation and detect the possible cause.

Management

As pregnancy advances a non-longitudinal lie tends to revert to longitudinal and stabilize; however, if this does not occur, after 36 weeks' gestation, the obstetrician will attempt to correct the lie by external version to a longitudinal lie and cephalic presentation. At term, labour may then be induced while the lie remains longitudinal and the presentation cephalic.

The likelihood of reversion to an oblique or transverse lie is high. The attendant risk that the membranes may rupture and the cord or even the arm prolapse, or labour start before the lie is corrected, often leads to the woman being admitted to hospital for observation.

Ultrasound examination should exclude placenta praevia, and fetal or uterine abnormalities. A vaginal examination may be made to detect any pelvic abnormality such as a contracted pelvis. In labour, the lie is closely monitored and, if necessary, gentle lateral pressure may be applied to the uterus to help maintain a longitudinal lie. External cephalic version is normally contraindicated when labour has started, as high uterine tone may result in uterine rupture or fetal damage.

If a longitudinal lie is maintained, once labour is established and the fetal head enters the pelvis, the membranes can be ruptured. Labour should then progress normally. In cases where the woman has a poor obstetric history, or if complications occur in labour, there is likely to be early recourse to caesarean section as the safest mode of delivery.

If undetected or inadequately monitored, an unstable lie in labour is a serious obstetric emergency. With contractions the fetal shoulder will be forced down into the pelvis, the membranes are likely to rupture and the cord and/or the fetal arm may prolapse.

The midwife should recognize shoulder presentation during abdominal examination, as described above. Once placenta praevia has been excluded, vaginal examination can be carried out, and the fetal ribs or the hand may be felt.

On detecting an unstable lie or shoulder presentation, the midwife should immediately send for an obstetrician. If in independent or community practice, the emergency services should be contacted, to rapidly transfer the woman to hospital. Turning the woman onto all fours is of value in displacing the shoulder and reducing the mother's urge to push. Where an arm or cord prolapses, this manoeuvre is essential. If the lie is uncorrected, caesarean section will be necessary and it may well be the safest mode of delivery even when the fetus has died.

In a twin delivery, the midwife may identify, after the birth of a first twin, that the second child is lying transversely, and this requires urgent action. If no obstetrician is available, the midwife will need to correct the lie by external version and rupture the second bag of membranes, thus stabilizing the longitudinal lie and hastening the birth of the child.

Compound presentation

This term is used to describe a presentation in which a hand or foot lies alongside the head. Very rarely both a hand and a foot come down. This tends to occur when the fetus is small and the pelvis large or when there is any condition preventing the descent of the head into the pelvis. Lower abdominal pain and a lack of fundal dominance is often noted in compound presentations. The pain experienced by the mother is best dealt with through effleurage, where the midwife applies light circular stroking movements to massage the mother's lower abdomen. Compound presentation is only of significance in advanced labour when the membranes have ruptured. Usually the presenting limb will recede as the presenting part descends. Replacement of an arm or leg is hardly ever necessary. Labour usually ends in a normal or a low instrumental delivery but where the compound presentation persists, there is an increased risk to the mother of vaginal and perineal trauma.

CONCLUSION

It is important that the midwife is knowledgeable about contemporary care and management of malpositions and malpresentations, and is able to impart this information to the woman in a realistic and accessible manner. Good preparation for the birth, and different strategies which might be required, should be discussed prior to labour if possible, and a plan agreed and documented, involving the whole maternity care team.

The midwife's primary role is to monitor, support and enhance the experience of the pregnancy and birth, and where there are deviations from normal, make quick and appropriate referral. Midwives should be familiar with the mechanisms of deviations from normal, and the manoeuvres which they may use in facilitating delivery. Not only must midwives be able to inspire confidence in the mother, they must have confidence in themselves and in their ability to support the woman in her choice of birth and to manage this effectively when a malposition or malpresentation occurs.

The midwife should provide continuity of care, through to the puerperium, and should provide an opportunity for debriefing for the woman and her partner following the birth.

KEY POINTS

- Malpositions and malpresentations of the fetus may increase the risks of fetal and neonatal morbidity and mortality.
- The midwife should be able to identify women and babies at risk of malpositions and malpresentations through effective clinical assessment, and then take appropriate and timely action.
- The midwife should ensure that the woman and her partner feel prepared and supported for

birth and have an opportunity for informed discussion.
- Effective communication and teamwork are crucial in the provision of safe and appropriate care to women and their babies.
- Manoeuvres and other skills based on physiological and evidence-based principles should be practised by those providing care to women and their babies, on a regular basis.

REFERENCES

Albrechtsen, S., Rasmussen, S., Dalaker, K. *et al.* (1998) The occurrence of breech presentation in Norway 1967–1994. *Acta Obstetricia et Gynecologica Scandinavica* 77(4): 410–415.

Advanced Life Support in Obstetrics (ALSO) (2000) *Advanced Support in Obstetrics Manual*, 4th edn. Kansas City, USA: American Academy of Family Physicians.

Baxley, E.G. (2001) Malpresentations and malpositions. In: Ratcliffe, S.D., Baxley, E.G., Byrd, J.E. *et al.* (eds) *Family Practice Obstetrics*, 2nd edn, Ch. 16, pp. 477–502. Philadelphia: Hanley & Belfus.

Brady, K., Duff, P., Read, J.A. *et al.* (1989) Reliability of fetal buttock sampling in assessing the acid–base balance of the breech fetus. *Obstetrics and Gynecology* 74(6): 886–888.

Budd, S. (2000) Moxibustion for breech presentation. *Complementary Therapies in Nursing and Midwifery* 6(4): 176–179.

Cardini, F. & Weixin, H. (1998) Moxibustion for correction of breech presentation; a randomised control trial. *Journal of the American Medical Association* 280(18): 1580–1584.

Chadha, Y.C., Mahmood, T.A., Dick, M.J. *et al.* (1992) Breech delivery and epidural anaesthesia. *British Journal of Obstetrics and Gynaecology* 99(2): 96–100.

Cheng, M. & Hannah, M. (1993) Breech delivery at term: a critical review of the literature. *Obstetrics and Gynecology* 82(4 Pt 1): 605–618.

Coltart, T., Edmonds, D.K. & Al-Mufti, R. (1997) External cephalic version at term: a survey of consultant obstetric practice in the United Kingdom and Republic of Ireland. *British Journal of Obstetrics and Gynaecology* 104(5): 544–547.

Danielian, P.J., Wang, J. & Hall, M.H. (1996) Long term outcome by method of delivery of fetuses in breech presentation at term: population based follow up. *British Medical Journal* 312(7044): 1451–1453.

Gardberg, M. & Tuppurainen, M. (1994) Anterior placental location predisposes for occiput posterior presentation near term. *Acta Obstetrica Gynecolgica Scandinavia* 73(2): 151–152.

Gardberg, M., Laakkonen, E. & Salevaara, M. (1998) Intrapartum sonography and persistent occiput posterior position: a study of 408 deliveries. *Obstetrics and Gynecology* 91(5 Pt 1): 746–749.

Gifford, D.S., Morton, S.C. & Kahn, K. (1995) A meta-analysis of infant outcomes after breech delivery. *Obstetrics and Gynecology* 85(6): 1047–1054.

Gyte, G. & Frohlich, J. (2001) Planned caesarean section versus planned vaginal birth for breech presentation at term: a randomised multicentred trial (Commentary). *MIDIRS Midwifery Digest* 11: 80–83.

Hannah, M.E., Hannah, W.J., Hewson, S.A. *et al.* (2000) Term Breech Trial Collaborative Group. Planned caesarean section versus planned vaginal birth for breech presentation at term: a randomised multicentre trial. *Lancet* 356(9239): 1375–1383.

Hofmeyr, G.J. (1991) External cephalic version at term: how high are the stakes? *British Journal of Obstetrics and Gynaecology* 98(1): 1–3.

Hofmeyr, G.J. (2002) External cephalic version facilitation for breech presentation at term. *The Cochrane Library*, Issue 1. Oxford: Update Software.

Hofmeyr, G.J. & Hannah, M.E. (2002) Planned caesarean section for term breech delivery. *The Cochrane Library*, Issue 4. Oxford: Update Software.

Hofmeyr, G.J. & Kulier, R. (2000) Cephalic version by postural management for the breech presentation. *Cochrane Database of Systematic Revues,* Issue 4. Oxford: Update Software.

Hofmeyr, G.J. & Kulier, R. (2001) External cephalic version for breech presentation at term. *The Cochrane Library*, Issue 2. Oxford: Update Software.

Hofmeyr, G.J. & Kulier, R. (2002) Expedited versus conservative approaches for vaginal delivery in breech presentation. *The Cochrane Library*, Issue 1. Oxford: Update Software.

Kariminia, A., Chamberlain, M.E., Keogh, J. *et al.* (2004) Randomised controlled trial of effect of hands and knees posturing on incidence of occiput posterior position at birth. *British Medical Journal* 328(7438):490. Epub 2004 Jan 26.

Lauszus, F.F., Petersen, A. & Praest, J. (1992) Strategy for delivery in breech presentation. A retrospective study. *Ugeskrift for Laeger* **154**(3): 123–126.

Lewis, P. (1997) This breech is not for turning – professional ideology or evidenced based practice. *MIDIRS Midwifery Digest* **7**(3): 318–319.

Leung, W.C., Pu, T.C. & Wong, W.M. (1999) Undiagnosed breech revisited. *British Journal of Obstetrics and Gynaecology* **106**(7): 638–641.

MIDIRS (Midwives Information and Resource Service) (2003) *Breech Presentation Options for Care.* Informed Choice Leaflet No. 9. Bristol: MIDIRS in collaboration with the NHS Centre for Reviews and Dissemination. Online. Available: http://www.infochoice.org.

Napolitano, P.G. & Parker, J. (2002) Face Presentation. *eMedicine Journal* **3**(3) (March 11), http://www.emedicine.com/med/topic3273.htm (accessed June 2002).

National Institute of Clinical Excellence (NICE) (2001) *The Use of Electronic Fetal Monitoring.* London. NICE. Online. Available: http://www.nice.org.uk.

Nursing and Midwifery Council (NMC) (2002) *Code of Professional Conduct.* London: NMC. Online. Available: http://www.nmc-uk.org.

Parker, J. & Napolitano, P.G. (2002) Brow Presentation. *eMedicine Journal* **3**(3) (March 8), http://www.emedicine.com/med/topic3274/htm (accessed June 2002).

Royal College of Obstetricians and Gynaecologists (RCOG) (2002) *The Management of Breech Presentation (20), Clinical Green Top Guidelines.* Online. Available: http://www.rcog.org.uk/guidelines.asp?PageID=106 &GuidelineID-19 (accessed August 2002).

Rovinsky, J.J., Miller, J.A. & Kaplan, S. (1973) Management of breech presentation at term. *American Journal of Obstetrics and Gynaecology* **115**(4): 497–513.

Saunders, N.J., Spiby, H., Gilbert, L. *et al.* (1989) Oxytocin infusion during second stage of labour in primiparous women using epidural analgesia. *British Medical Journal* **299**(6713): 1423–1426.

Shennan, A. & Bewley, S. (2001) How to manage term breech deliveries (Editorial). *British Medical Journal* **323**(7307): 244–245.

Shushan, A. & Younis, J.S. (1992) McRoberts manoeuvre for the management of the aftercoming head in breech delivery. *Gynecologic and Obstetric Investigation* **34**(3): 188–189.

Sutton, J. (2000) Occipito-posterior positioning and some ideas about how to change it. *Practising Midwife* **3**(6): 20–22.

Sutton, J. & Scott, P. (1996) *Understanding and Teaching Optimal Foetal Positioning.* New Zealand: Tauranga.

Taylor, P. & Robson, S. (2003) External cephalic version – a new midwifery role. *British Journal of Midwifery* **11**(4): 207–210.

Thornton, J. & Hayman, R. (2002) Staff experience in vaginal breech delivery (Editorial). *British Journal of Midwifery* **10**(7): 408–410.

Thorp, J.A., Hu, D.H., Albin, R.M. *et al.* (1993) The effects of intrapartum epidural analgesia on nulliparous labour: a randomised, controlled prospective trial. *American Journal of Obstetrics and Gynaecology* **169**(4): 851–858.

Thorpe-Beaston, J.G., Banfield, P.J & Saunders, N.J. (1992) Outcome of breech delivery at term. *British Medical Journal* **305**(6586): 746–747.

Van Loon, A.J., Mantingh, A., Serlier, E.K. *et al.* (1997) Randomised controlled trial of magnetic-resonance pelvimetry in breech presentation at term. *Lancet* **350**(9094): 1799–1804.

Van Roosmalen, J. & Rosendaal, F. (2002) There is still room for disagreement about vaginal delivery of breech infant at term. *British Journal of Obstetrics and Gynaecology* **109**: 967–969.

Vause, S., Hornbuckle, J. & Thornton, J.G. (1997) Palpation or ultrasound for detecting breech babies? (Editorial). *British Journal of Midwifery* **5**(6): 318–319.

Walkinshaw, S. (1997) Pelvimetry and breech delivery at term. *Lancet* **350**(9094): 1791–1792.

Westgren, M., Edvall, H., Nordstrom, E. *et al.* (1985) Spontaneous cephalic version of breech presentation in the last trimester. *British Journal of Obstetrics and Gynaecology* **92**(1): 19–22.

FURTHER READING

Advanced Life Support in Obstetrics (ALSO) (2000) *Advanced Support in Obstetrics Manual,* 4th edn. Kansas City, USA: American Academy of Family Physicians.
A useful text which deals with complications and their management, and includes a good section on dealing with malpresentations and malpositions.

Enkin, M.E., Keirse, M.J.N.C., Neilson, J. et al. (2000) *A Guide to Effective Care in Pregnancy and Childbirth,* 3rd edn. Oxford: Oxford University Press.
A useful text overarching evidence-based practice.

54

Mental Health Problems

Mary Sidebotham

LEARNING OUTCOMES

After reading this chapter you will be able to:

- have an understanding of the wider factors influencing women's mental health
- appreciate the impact of pregnancy, childbirth and transition to parenting on mental health
- understand the importance of early detection of mental illness, and know how to contribute effectively to treatment and management of minor and major disorders
- appreciate the value of working collaboratively within the wider multidisciplinary team

- understand the importance of maintaining professional boundaries whilst working as a member of the wider multidisciplinary team
- contribute to care models designed to prevent the primary occurrence of mental illness or prevent exacerbation of existing symptoms
- confidently offer advice and support to women and be aware of the sources of help and support available locally and nationally
- recognize your own emotional needs and feel able to access appropriate levels of personal support.

INTRODUCTION

Pregnancy is a time that is associated with joy and happiness. The reality, however, is that for many women, pregnancy will in fact cause a recurrence of impaired mental health or will be the precursor of a primary illness. There is a recognition that despite improvements in the understanding, detection and treatment of pregnancy-related mental health disorders, many women will not seek help and try to cope with their illness, hiding their unhappiness from their care-givers and family. Women still fear discrimination and long-term repercussions if they reveal a previous emotional disturbance or psychiatric illness (MIND, 2001; Oates, 2001; Robinson, 2002).

> I feel reluctant to admit I've got mental health problems: the stigma and rejection are too hard to face.

This quotation taken from the home page of the website of MIND, the mental health charity, shows there is still a stigma attached to mental illness within British society. This remains the case despite the fact that one in four people will experience mental health problems at some time during their life. Up to 50% of all women

are thought to have suffered some form of emotional disturbance during their lives and the risk is much higher amongst women who are socially excluded (MIND, 2001).

There is an increased risk of mental illness associated with childbirth, mostly in the postpartum period, but problems may also be present before or during pregnancy. Many of the factors associated with postnatal mental illness, such as lack of a confiding relationship and support, marital tension, socioeconomic problems and a previous psychiatric history, are present before and during pregnancy (O'Hara and Zekowski, 1988; Romito, 1989) and so depression may occur both in pregnancy and the postpartum period (Evans *et al.*, 2001; Clement *et al.*, unpublished data, 1994; Green and Murray, 1994; Watson *et al.*, 1984). Whilst there is a growing understanding of the factors associated with depression and psychotic illness following childbirth, there is relatively little published work on the incidence of, and morbidity associated with, *antenatal* depression. This is despite the fact that depressed mood in pregnancy has been associated with poor attendance at antenatal clinics, substance misuse, low birthweight and preterm labour (Hedegaard *et al.*, 1993; Pagel *et al.*,

1990). Whereas it was once thought that pregnancy was a protective factor against depression, Watson *et al.* (1984) found that in 24% of cases of detected postnatal depression, symptoms were present in pregnancy.

There is now clear evidence that psychopathological symptoms in pregnancy have physiological consequences for the fetus (Teixeira *et al.*, 1999). A cohort study of depressed mood during pregnancy and after childbirth concluded that research and clinical efforts towards recognizing and treating antenatal depression must be improved (Evans *et al.*, 2001). The Confidential Enquiry into Maternal Deaths (Lewis, 2001) recommended better detection and management of psychiatric disorders antenatally to reduce the mortality rate. Services must be designed to meet the needs of all women, and a crucial part of the service should address the mental health needs of women.

WHO IS AT RISK

Many women may experience mixed reactions to their pregnancy with transient feelings of anxiety, and fear. Women should be reassured that this is normal and be encouraged to discuss these feelings openly. The incidence of detected mental illness in the first trimester of pregnancy is thought to be as high as 15%. Only about 5% of these women will have suffered from previous episodes of mental illness. In the second and third trimesters of pregnancy the incidence of new episodes of mental illness is less, only about 5%.

The majority of episodes of new mental illness during pregnancy are minor conditions or neuroses. The commonest condition is the depressive neurosis with anxiety, but phobic anxiety states and obsessional compulsive disorders may also occur. In most cases these neurotic mental illnesses resolve by the second trimester of pregnancy and there seems to be no added risk of these women developing postnatal depression.

The outlook is different for those women who begin their pregnancies with chronic neurotic conditions. Their illness is likely to continue throughout pregnancy and may be exacerbated during the puerperium.

Minor mental illness is more likely to occur in the first trimester of pregnancy in women who have marked neurotic traits in the premorbid personality. It also tends to occur in women who have a history of neurotic disorders and in those with social problems such as marital tension. Other predisposing factors include a history of previous abortion and the possibility of the present pregnancy being terminated. Women with a poor obstetric history or those who have undergone extensive infertility treatment may exhibit signs of increased anxiety in early pregnancy.

The onset of minor mental illness later in pregnancy, usually during the third trimester, is less common than in the first trimester. When it occurs at this stage in pregnancy, however, the risk of the woman developing postnatal depression is increased (Clement *et al.*, unpublished data, 1994; Oates, 1989).

Major mental illnesses include *manic depression, severe depression* and *schizophrenia*. The risk of a woman developing a new episode of one of these conditions in pregnancy is lower than at other times in her life. When women with a history of major mental illness become pregnant, there is no particular increase in the risk of a relapse during pregnancy if they are well stabilized and their illness is in remission. Although the risk of major mental illness is reduced in pregnancy, it is greatly increased in the first 3 months after delivery.

THE MIDWIFE'S ROLE IN THE ANTENATAL PERIOD

Case histories from an innovative midwifery project developed to provide one-to-one caseload midwifery care for women with mental health problems are used throughout for illustrative purposes (Ferguson and Thomson, 1999).

There is a growing emphasis on the development of the public health role of the midwife, and promotion of mental well-being is an area where the midwife can make a valuable contribution (DoH, 1999). The midwife has a responsibility to provide holistic care, meeting the physical, psychological and emotional needs of all women. There should be an emphasis on promoting emotional and psychological well-being for all women, not just those perceived to be at risk. Ideally all women should be treated with sensitivity during pregnancy and enabled during meetings with the midwife to reveal and discuss any issues that may predispose them to impaired mental health. Women should be provided with an opportunity to discuss how they feel about the current pregnancy, explore their expectations, and reflect upon their previous birth experiences. Some women will approach a new pregnancy with unresolved issues from previous pregnancies, causing high levels of anxiety to be evident. Midwives should be aware of the social and cultural barriers that may prevent a woman from being open in discussions, ensuring that every effort is made to make the woman feel safe and supported. Some

Case scenario 54.1

Nina

Nina was a 20-year-old woman who with her child had recently arrived in England from Somalia. She was seeking refugee status and was referred to the midwives by the link worker who had been selected by the community to provide support and translation services for the women. Nina had one small child and was living in crowded conditions with another family. Her child was very demanding and she was obviously finding things difficult to cope with.

She denied feeling 'depressed' though this was difficult to assess, as there is no word within her language to describe depression. She did, however, report frequent distressing physical symptoms including hyperemesis, backache, dizziness, toothache, reduced fetal movements and others. She described her toddler as very naughty.

The midwives worked directly with all members of the primary care team. They ensured that Nina saw the welfare rights officer regularly, supported by the link worker to help her with benefits claims and sorting out her immigration status. She was seen by the dentist. The link worker introduced her to other families living within the community and she attended the preparation for parenthood sessions held in the health resource centre. She used the crèche facilities to enable her to have a break from her toddler whom she found to be very demanding. The health visitor was alerted to the problems Nina was having in coping and made more regular contact with Nina, offering support. She was referred to the therapeutic massage service to alleviate her back pain, which reminded her of being at home in Somalia where it was normal practice for women to be massaged with aromatic oils during pregnancy by female relatives.

Nina became happier as the pregnancy progressed. Her confidence grew as did her coping abilities. She began to interact well with her peers and her care-givers, and the relationship with her child improved. Her physical complaints diminished and referral to the physiotherapist for back pain was cancelled as she felt 'cured' by the massage. She had a normal delivery and coped well postnatally. She had developed her own support network that was culturally acceptable to her. She was well on discharge to the care of the health visitor.

women will live within a culture where there is no recognition of minor depressive illness or anxiety states (Clifford *et al.*, 1999). Any attempt to enquire whether the woman is symptomatic may be restricted by other family members who associate impaired mental health only with major psychotic illness to which there is shame and stigma attached (Oates, 2001). The midwife should recognize that descriptions of ongoing minor physical disorders and concerns about the pregnancy may be the only way the woman can express her feelings (Case scenario 54.1). To ensure that all women receive adequate support and help, independent, trained interpreters should be available for women whose first language is not English and every attempt must be made to see the woman at least once on her own.

Reflective Activity 54.1

Consider Nina's experience of maternity care in Case scenario 54.1, and think about whether your maternity service could have managed the care as described. Do you consider there were any aspects of care which could have been provided in a better way?

Important lessons to be learned from Case scenario 54.1

- Where a woman's first language is not English, the person translating must be a true advocate, putting the woman's needs first.
- Physical signs can sometimes mask emotional distress.
- Within some cultures there is greater stigma attached to emotional distress, and it is therefore not recognized or acknowledged.
- Social circumstances can greatly affect a woman's mental health status.
- Women fleeing from war-torn countries may be suffering from post-traumatic stress disorder.
- Depression in a mother will be reflected in her child's well-being and development.

The midwife should be alerted to the socioeconomic factors that predispose a woman to depression and anxiety, and a careful history must be taken to ensure that warning signs of significant mental illness do not go undetected. The association between drug and alcohol misuse, and depressive illness is well documented (Oates, 2001), so, should a woman reveal a problem in this area, an appropriate referral for support must be made (Case scenario 54.2).

Case scenario 54.2

Ella

Ella was an 18-year-old girl referred to the midwifery project by the community alcohol team. She was 12 weeks' pregnant at first referral and was accompanied by her mother. She had been treated for alcoholism and depression. She had not been drinking for the last few months and had taken herself off her antidepressant medication on discovering she was pregnant.

She appeared to be very aggressive and defensive to questioning, and expressed quite a marked fear of the pain of labour. She said she hoped for a caesarean section as she thought it would be easier. She continued attending the alcohol support unit and saw her psychiatric social worker regularly. She wanted to remain off antidepressant medication so was referred to the community psychiatric nurse (CPN) for assessment and support. She attended the parent education and aquanatal sessions and became more open and trusting of the midwives as the pregnancy progressed. As the relationship with the midwife developed, she became less defensive.

She was proud of her preparations for the baby and enjoyed showing the midwife during home visits what she had done to prepare at home. It was during one of these visits that the midwife approached the subject of the birth again. Ella told the midwife she was afraid of giving birth because she thought it would be too painful to bear. She went on to tell the midwife she had been sexually abused by her uncle at the age of 12. She had told her mother and aunt at the time, but they did not believe her and warned her not to ever tell anybody else. They told her she was bad and wicked for saying such things and it was never discussed again. She said that was why she started drinking and in her words 'became bad'. She hadn't told anybody during her treatment for alcoholism as she thought nobody would believe her, but that was why she was afraid of the birth.

Ella began specialist counselling. She attended an active birth workshop and began preparing for the birth experience fully informed and with an open mind. She was supported by her named midwife throughout labour and she had a normal delivery of a daughter. She was strong and confident and coping well on discharge to the health visitor.

There is a clear association between victims of domestic violence, sexual and physical abuse being predisposed to mental illness, so midwives should use and develop their communication skills to allow them to establish a trusting relationship with the woman, making the likelihood of disclosure more possible (Bloom, 2002).

Important lessons to be learned from Case scenario 54.2

- Women need to be given time to disclose their feelings.
- Midwives should be aware that the presence of other family members may alter women's reactions and responses. They must be given privacy and assured confidentiality.
- They need to feel in control and trust their care-giver.
- Alcohol and substance abuse can sometimes mask other major problems.
- Irrational fears of birth may indicate previous sexual abuse.
- Women need the opportunity to be seen alone where they can talk openly and honestly without fear or reprisal.
- An aggressive and confrontational attitude may be masking insecurity and fear.
- Midwives need to recognize their boundaries and refer for specialist help where required.

It is essential that an accurate history is taken and any reported current or past mental illness is adequately investigated and assessed. This should be done with extreme sensitivity to eradicate any fears the woman may have of discrimination (Robinson, 2002). Where necessary, the GP should be involved and asked to contribute to the woman's care in pregnancy. If the woman is under the care of a psychiatrist, community psychiatric nurse or psychologist, attempts should be made to work collaboratively to ensure the woman's needs are met.

Reflective Activity 54.2

Do you know the practitioners that you can refer to for specialist assistance in this sort of case? Find out about the specialist services in your area which may be useful to childbearing women, i.e. specialist counsellors, drugs and alcohol support, community psychiatric nursing services. Make sure that you have the contact details of these services in your resource file/work diary.

The majority of minor illnesses will resolve spontaneously by the second trimester of pregnancy. The woman will require support, counselling, reassurance and information communicated in a caring, intelligible way. Psychotropic drugs are rarely necessary or prescribed at this stage of pregnancy. Instead, therapy to help the woman relax and reduce her anxiety may be employed and seems to be effective. Midwives may be involved in counselling and supporting these women and teaching relaxation techniques. Sometimes a social worker is also required to help tackle social problems which may be the cause of the problem.

Social support in pregnancy can have a beneficial effect on women with obstetric and social problems (Hodnett, 1994a,b), and strategies to diagnose depression and the institution of appropriate psychological interventions to treat the condition in pregnancy may prevent it becoming a long-term postnatal problem. Clement (1995) suggests the use of the Edinburgh Postnatal Depression Scale (EPDS) for the detection of depression in pregnancy for high-risk groups, followed by 'listening visits' in pregnancy and continued in the postpartum period.

Women who have had single episodes of major mental illness in the past but who have been well for some time are usually advised by their psychiatrist to stop their medication before conception and throughout their pregnancy (Case scenario 54.3). There is no substantial risk of relapse during pregnancy, but there is a marked risk of developing a puerperal psychosis during the first 3 months after delivery (Cox, 1986).

Case scenario 54.3

Carol

Carol was a 30-year-old woman who was pregnant for the fourth time.

She had two daughters and had terminated her last pregnancy 'because I couldn't cope'. She booked with a conventional maternity service model of care, and a hospital-based midwife took a routine history at her original hospital-booking visit. She reported experiencing 'bad' postnatal depression, requiring medication in the past and said she felt anxious this time in case it happened again. She had been on antidepressant medication following the termination of pregnancy but had stopped on discovering the current pregnancy. Her plan of care was to attend a satellite hospital midwife-led clinic, based in the community, for antenatal care and deliver at hospital.

She met a project midwife at the community-based clinic who told her about a midwifery project offering one-to-one care and extra support. Carol was invited to join the project because of her history of depression and she readily accepted. Carol was physically and emotionally well during her pregnancy, but had social and relationship problems. She was referred to the counselling service and accessed help from the welfare rights officer.

She was very anxious about the birth, as she felt her depression last time was due to her sense of being out of control of her labour, and disappointment because she did not have an epidural. It was very important to

her that she would know her midwife, and that her wishes be respected. She also wanted to know she would not be abandoned after the baby was born, as she was afraid she would become depressed again and not know where to turn.

Carol had an uncomplicated labour. Both project midwives were present and her wishes were respected. She walked around the park and the art gallery until established in labour and requesting pain relief. She had an epidural sited, which was effective as she entered the second stage of labour. Her delivery was pain free and she remained in control.

She needed lots of reassurance and listening time when she went home, and was well supported by her GP, midwives and health visitor. The midwives visited until Carol felt she no longer needed the reassurance of the midwives' 'listening time'. She was encouraged to attend a baby massage group and access other sources of social support. Although she did experience a period of despondency and weepiness within the first week, she also felt euphoric when reflecting on how much she had 'enjoyed the birthing experience'. She used her newly found coping strategies to get through, and her carefully planned support systems came into place. She recovered quickly and felt strong. She did find it hard saying goodbye to her midwives, as many women do, but was well and happy 1 year later when she came back to say hello.

Important lessons to be learned from Case scenario 54.3

- Women who give a history of 'postnatal depression' at booking must be encouraged to discuss what that illness meant to them then and how they feel about it in the current pregnancy.
- Previous birth experiences should be discussed.
- Carol viewed the midwife as a friend and found saying goodbye difficult. Midwives must avoid allowing long-term dependency in vulnerable women by helping them to identify ongoing sources of support.
- Some women require very simple measures to avoid distressing postpartum illness, namely time, empathy, respect and support.

- Whilst this woman was part of an innovative project, this care could have been delivered by any midwife in any setting, with the same positive results.

The problem is more complex in the woman who has had several episodes of major mental illness (Case scenario 54.4).

The Confidential Enquiry into Maternal Deaths using the Office for National Statistics (ONS) linkage data indicated that suicide is the current leading cause of maternal death. In the report's recommendations, it is suggested that women with a history of severe depression or psychotic disorder be referred to a specialist perinatal mental health team and an appropriate care

Case scenario 54.4

Jenny

Jenny was 24 years old when referred to the midwifery project by her mental health social worker. She had a major personality disorder and acute anxiety state. She had a history of self-harm and had made a previous attempt at suicide. She was under the care of the psychiatric team and supported on a daily basis by a home-visiting service. She was taking prescribed antipsychotic medication. She was married to an asylum seeker and was experiencing financial and social problems at the time of her referral.

She came to the midwifery project for extra support to help her cope with the pregnancy. The perinatal care team, including Jenny and her partner, met regularly to discuss her total progress and ensure that suitable plans were in place to support her through the delivery and postnatal period. Jenny had been a psychiatric inpatient for in excess of 1 year prior to meeting her husband, and was living in a supported house when the relationship developed. At the time of her referral she was living in a privately rented house with her husband. It was felt that Jenny would experience major difficulties at and around the time of the birth and the anticipated plan was that she would require admission to the mother and baby unit for a prolonged period of time after the birth to learn parenting skills and develop confidence. As she was self-harming, delusional and psychotic, there were grave concerns expressed about her ability to care for herself and the child on a long-term basis.

Jenny cooperated at all times with her treatment plan. There was extensive collaboration and cooperation

within the wider healthcare team. All of Jenny's social, emotional, physical and practical needs were met and she visibly gained confidence in her own ability to cope, gradually gaining more control over her own future throughout the process. Jenny expressed a desire to breastfeed, so under the guidance of her psychiatrist, her medication was adjusted and monitored accordingly. With the support of the team Jenny re-established contact with her family, who became an important source of support.

She had a normal delivery assisted by her two named midwives. The psychiatrist assessed her and her postnatal progress was carefully monitored on a daily basis both in hospital and on her discharge home at day 4. Her level of home support was increased in the early postnatal period, and the midwives visited regularly, assisting with childcare and feeding, and monitored Jenny's ability to care for the baby. The health visitor was invited to join the team planning meetings in the antenatal period and became well known to Jenny and therefore trusted, ensuring that the handover from the midwives to the health visitor would be smooth and efficient. Jenny's mental health status improved considerably during the course of the pregnancy but particularly in the long-term postnatal period. She successfully breastfed the baby for in excess of 1 year. Her required level of home support reduced and her ability to care for the baby was unquestioned. She maintained her relationship with her family and felt she had regained control of her life. She complied with her medication regime and was well and happy.

plan be developed, aiming to support the woman through pregnancy and minimize the risk of severe postnatal disorder (Lewis, 2001).

Where a woman is under the care of a psychiatrist when pregnancy is diagnosed, then there should be careful liaison between the obstetrician, midwife and mental health team to ensure that the woman's care is seamless, and that appropriate management plans are made to maximize the outcome for mother and baby. This is especially relevant when deciding upon the woman's ongoing and future drug regime.

Important lessons to be learned from Case scenario 54.4

- The recognition of professional boundaries.
- The importance of working collaboratively, and respecting each person's contribution.
- The value of early and thorough care-planning.
- The need to involve the woman and her family in the care-planning process in order to develop a trusting relationship.
- The value to the assessment process of continuity of carer.
- The importance of avoiding attachment to one caregiver, by phased introduction of new carers, i.e. staged handover from midwife to health visitor.

LABOUR AND DELIVERY

Some women find childbirth to be a fulfilling experience, but for others it is the most traumatic experience of their life (Niven, 1992). There is an increasing awareness that events around the time of birth can seriously affect a woman's mental well-being (Laing, 2001; Pantlen and Rohde, 2001). Women have reported experiencing intense fear, helplessness and a loss of control when recalling their birth experiences. One study found that women who suffered an adverse birth experience were likely to develop trauma symptoms analogous to those associated with post-traumatic stress disorder (Creedy et al., 2000), described as 'extreme psychological distress following exposure to a traumatic and threatening experience' (Lyons, 1998). There is evidence that women who have undergone an emergency caesarean section delivery are less likely to have another child than those women who had a normal vaginal delivery, because of the fear of recurrence of the bad memories associated with the experience. Women often do not understand the sequence of events that led to the delivery, but feel traumatized by the

experience many years later. Women contact support groups such as Maternity Alliance or The National Childbirth Trust (NCT) for help in coming to terms with their birth experience, having in some cases suffered the symptoms of depression for many years.

The midwife's role

Midwives have a responsibility to ensure that the women in their care retain control over their childbirth experiences and understand what is happening to them, and may act as a woman's advocate when required. This is particularly important for woman with a history of mental illness (Robinson, 2002). Where possible, the delivery should have been discussed beforehand and any potential issues such as former sexual abuse should be addressed, as these may later distress the woman (Gutteridge, 2001). Where a woman has a history of an acute disorder, the midwife should liaise with the psychiatrist or primary mental health worker to ensure that appropriate medication is prescribed. If necessary, a trusted mental health worker should accompany the woman in labour. The aim should at all times be to empower the woman and help her to retain control (Robinson, 2002).

Problems may arise where there is doubt about a woman's capacity to consent to, or refuse treatment. Where a woman's capacity is questioned, a supervisor of midwives should be involved and appropriate legal advice should be sought (North West LSA, 2002). The primary aim should always be to act in the woman's best interests and as her advocate.

All women should be given the opportunity to discuss the birth and be offered the opportunity to ask questions and discuss their feelings freely. They should be offered support and most importantly, listening time. To date there is very little published research into the effectiveness of postnatal debriefing but there is a growing body of opinion that women would benefit from a form of postnatal debriefing to help reduce the psychological morbidity experienced by many women following pregnancy and childbirth (Lavender and Walkinshaw, 1998; Pantlen and Rohde, 2001). However, some studies have concluded that for some women, debriefing could have contributed to their emotional health problems. This is an area in need of further research.

THE POSTNATAL PERIOD

The risk of becoming mentally ill during the puerperium is greater than at other times in the woman's

Table 54.1   ICD-10 classification of puerperal disorders

F53	**Mental and behavioural disorders associated with the puerperium, not elsewhere classified** This classification should be used only for mental disorders associated with the puerperium (commencing within 6 weeks of delivery) that do not meet the criteria for disorders classified elsewhere in this book, either *because insufficient information is available*, or because it is considered that *special additional clinical features are present which make classification elsewhere inappropriate*. It will usually be possible to classify mental disorders associated with the puerperium by using two other codes: the first is from elsewhere in chapter V (F) and indicates the specific type of mental disorder (usually affective (F30–F–39)), and the second is 099.3 (mental diseases and diseases of the nervous system complicating the puerperium) of ICD-10
F53.0	***Mild* mental and behavioural disorders associated with the puerperium, not elsewhere classified** Includes: postnatal depression NOS postpartum depression NOS
F53.1	***Severe* mental and behavioural disorders associated with the puerperium, not elsewhere classified** Includes: puerperal psychosis NOS
F53.8	**Other mental and behavioural disorders associated with the puerperium, not elsewhere classified**
F53.9	**Puerperal mental disorders, unspecified**

Source: Reproduced by permission of WHO, from *The ICD Classification of Mental and Behavioural Disorders: Clinical Descriptions and Diagnostic Guidelines*. Geneva, World Health Organization, 1992.

reproductive life. In 1992 the World Health Organization included puerperal mental disorders in their International Classification of Diseases (Table 54.1).

Postnatal blues

Between 50–80% of women will experience a transient period of weepiness and mood instability known as *postpartum blues* (George and Sandler, 1988; Kendall *et al.*, 1981; Romito, 1990; Stein *et al.*, 1981). The condition typically presents between 2 and 4 days after birth and symptoms include tearfulness, irritability, mood instability, headache, tiredness and oversensitivity (Hannah *et al.*, 1992; O'Hara *et al.*, 1991). The woman needs the opportunity to talk about her feelings, and her physical discomfort should be reduced as the condition frequently coincides with breast discomfort. The woman should be helped to rest and be offered extra support if possible. In most cases the condition is self-limiting but studies have found that women who suffer from this condition are more likely to go on to develop postnatal depression (Beck *et al.*, 1992; O'Hara *et al.*, 1991).

Postnatal depression

The reported incidence of depression after childbirth is between 10–15% of women (Cox *et al.*, 1993; Kumar and Robson, 1984), but when questioned, many midwives and women report a higher incidence.

Postnatal depression is a non-psychotic depressive disorder of variable severity, which occurs in the first year after childbirth. In many cases it is not detected by professionals, and only a few women seek or receive the medical help which is available.

> Everybody kept saying to me 'Oh how well you're coping' And yet behind the closed walls, you think, 'Why can't I tell them what's going on.'
> (MIND, 2001)

Postnatal depression can have enduring consequences for both the woman and her family. Although some women may recover spontaneously in time, in a significant number of cases the illness becomes chronic and may persist for the first year or more after the birth of the child (Taylor *et al.*, 1994). This chronic illness is particularly evident amongst women of low socioeconomic status (Seguin *et al.*, 1999). Long-standing untreated depressive illness is distressing not only for the mother, but also for her partner and her children. It may result in marital problems, or exacerbate existing problems, and have an adverse effect on the children's intellectual and emotional development (Coghill *et al.*, 1986; Murray and Cooper, 1997; Sinclair and Murray, 1998; Uddenberg and Englesson, 1978). Early diagnosis and effective treatment are therefore important for the health of the whole family.

Some researchers have questioned whether postnatal depression is any different from depression which may occur at other times in a woman's life. A controlled study by Cox *et al.* (1993) compared depression in parturient and non-parturient women, and found a marked increase in the onset of depression in parturient women within 1 month of delivery. They therefore concluded that postnatal depression is a direct consequence of the physical and psychological stresses of childbirth. Others consider postnatal depression unique because it follows childbirth and has atypical signs and symptoms (Dalton, 1980; Pitt, 1968).

Aetiology

The actual cause of depressive illness following childbirth is unknown but is thought to be multifactorial, a combination of biological, psychological and social factors.

Biological reasons include genetic make-up, gynaecological and obstetric problems (Stein *et al.*, 1989), parity and maternal age, the hormonal changes which occur in the early puerperium and the appearance and behaviour of the baby. The mother may experience a reactive depression if her baby dies or is born with a congenital abnormality, particularly if it was previously undiagnosed. Psychological factors may include the woman's early relationship with her parents, personality development, acceptance of her sexuality and the ability to accept dependence (Cox, 1986). Women who display anxious or obsessional traits in their personality, or appear too controlled and compliant have a greater risk of developing postnatal depression. The previous psychiatric history of the woman (and her family) has been found to be a risk factor in many cases (Wolkind *et al.*, 1988). The consistent finding of epidemiological studies carried out to date is that the major factors of aetiological importance are psychosocial in nature (Cooper and Murray, 1998). The occurrence of stressful life events and lack of personal support from family, partner or friends have all consistently been found to raise the risk of postnatal depression (Levy and Kline, 1994; Paykel *et al.*, 1980; Playfair and Gowers, 1981; Stein *et al.*, 1989).

The midwife's role

The midwife's role is primarily one of prevention. Where signs of illness are present, early detection and treatment are essential. It is important that women are adequately prepared for the surge in emotions they will feel following the birth of their baby. They should be aware that they are likely to experience extreme emotions following the birth, possibly feeling weepy for no reason. Parent education programmes should be designed to prepare women and their partners for the realities of parenting. Programmes should be designed to meet the needs of all women, and women should feel able to attend whatever their social circumstances without feeling stigmatized or disadvantaged. Women should be prepared realistically for the birth experience, emphasizing the importance of being informed and in control whatever the outcome. This needs to avoid the implication of 'failure' if the normal vaginal delivery is not achieved. Success should be gauged by the degree of control and ability to contribute to the decision-making process achieved and the perception of having her wishes respected at all times.

Women and their partners should be given the opportunity to discuss their fears, in a safe supportive way. Women should be helped to develop strategies to avoid family conflicts, through empowerment and development of self-confidence, to enable them to stand up to anybody who may be controlling and making decisions for them. The realities of disturbed sleeping patterns, crying babies and the commitment in time and emotion required in the early weeks to achieve successful breast-feeding need to be fully discussed and strategies for dealing with them explored. Women need to know where to go for help, and that they will not be alone.

Midwives have a major role in recognizing women at high risk of developing postnatal depression, and of detecting the early signs of this distressing condition when it does occur. It is sometimes difficult at first to distinguish between the tiredness and emotional instability that are common features of the puerperium, and the onset of a depressive illness. Careful assessment of the woman's emotional state is an essential part of the midwife's role in postnatal care. To achieve this the midwife must encourage the woman to express her feelings and anxieties, not only about her baby but also about herself, and listen carefully both to what she says and to what she may not be able to express openly. Many women are embarrassed by what they see as their inability to cope and are sometimes reticent about admitting it. An empathic, non-directive, empowering approach by the midwife can enable the mother to voice her anxieties and true feelings. This process is more likely to be successful in detecting depressive illness if the midwife has known the woman throughout pregnancy. If depression is suspected, help can then be offered. The midwife should be trained appropriately and have access to adequate resources and time to offer appropriate levels of help and support to those women showing signs of depressive illness (Bick *et al.*, 2002). Where midwives have been trained to deliver evidence-based postnatal advice and support, based upon the woman's description of

Box 54.1 Early signs and symptoms of postnatal depression

- Tearfulness, despondency.
- Feelings of inadequacy.
- Inability to cope, anxiety.
- Ruminative worry, often about the baby, and guilt about her perceived poor mothering skills, yet the baby is usually well cared for and thriving.
- Sleep disturbance is a common symptom and may be early-morning waking or difficulty in getting off to sleep. Because so many postnatal women are disturbed at night by their baby, this symptom is often missed.
- During the day the mother will feel constantly tired and will often go to bed to rest and avoid the company of others.

symptoms, rates of postnatal depression have been shown to be reduced (MacArthur *et al.*, 2002).

Women at risk of postnatal depression will require particularly close observation in the postnatal period. Early signs and symptoms of the condition are listed in Box 54.1.

Profound and consistent lowering of the mood, depressive ideation, slowing of psychomotor functions and biological symptoms such as early-morning waking are features of severe depression. Another symptom is *anomie*, which is a painful feeling of inability to experience love or pleasure. These mothers often feel that they do not or cannot love their babies, but their baby is obviously lovingly handled and cared for by the mother. This dissonance between the mother's comments and behaviour is an important diagnostic point and one that the midwife, if still in attendance, should recognize.

Detection

The Edinburgh Postnatal Depression Scale has been developed for the diagnosis of postnatal depression (Cox and Holden, 1994) (see Figs 54.1 and 54.2). It is a simple, self-rating, 10-item scale which was designed to be used at about 6 weeks postpartum, but can also be used at other times, including the antenatal period, for high-risk women (Clement, 1995). Scores for individual items range from 0 to 3 according to severity, and the total score is the sum of the scores for the individual items.

Because of the difficulties associated with detecting postnatal depression within other cultures, a Punjabi version of the EPDS scale has been developed which has proved to be successful in trials to date (Clifford *et al.*, 1999).

Reflective Activity 54.3

Is the Edinburgh Postnatal Scale in use in your maternity service? If not, why not? Consider when this tool is and could be used.

Treatment

Women who score 12 or more on the scale are likely to be suffering from depressive illness. Referral for further assessment and treatment should then be offered. Initially the midwife's responsibility is to detect the symptoms, and refer the woman for specialist support. The general practitioner should be informed and the midwife should liaise with the health visitor, developing effective communication channels, and thus ensure that the woman will receive increased levels of support following discharge from the midwife. Postnatal depression may be treated by counselling, cognitive therapy or medication. Non-directive counselling has proved to be a very useful method of managing postnatal depression in many cases. The Cochrane review on the subject shows this form of therapy to be as effective as a course of antidepressant medication (Hoffbrand *et al.*, 2001).

Postnatal support groups may be very helpful to women who feel isolated and lonely after childbirth, and can offer the support which a woman needs from those who are experiencing similar problems. The Association for Postnatal Illness and The National Childbirth Trust provide peer support and information about postnatal depression. In some cases, support groups are linked to healthcare workers who can identify those who are in need of treatment or a review of their treatment.

Antidepressant drugs may be required for the treatment of some mothers suffering from postnatal depression. Good supervision and support are also required. Referral to a psychiatrist is necessary if the woman fails to respond to antidepressant drugs, or has suicidal tendencies.

> late one afternoon, I stood washing up at the kitchen sink. The water was hot. The next thing I remember is that the water was cold and it was dark outside. I was glad that we lived near Kings Cross Station because there were lots of trains and I could walk under one.
>
> (MIND, 2001)

HOW ARE YOU FEELING

As you have recently had a baby, we would like to know how you are feeling now. Please underline the answer which comes closest to how you have felt in the past 7 days, not just how you feel today.
Here is an example, already completed:

I have felt happy:
Yes, most of the time   No, not very often
Yes, some of the time   No, not at all

This would mean: 'I have felt happy some of the time' during the past week. Please complete the other questions in the same way.

IN THE PAST SEVEN DAYS

1. I have been able to laugh and see the funny side of things:
As much as I always could
Not quite so much now
Definitely not so much now
Not at all

2. I have looked forward with enjoyment to things:
As much as I ever did
Rather less than I used to
Definitely less than I used to
Hardly at all

3. I have blamed myself unnecessarily when things went wrong:
Yes, most of the time
Yes, some of the time
Not very often
No, never

4. I have felt worried and anxious for no very good reason:
No, not at all
Hardly ever
Yes, sometimes
Yes, very often

5. I have felt scared or panicky for no very good reason:
Yes, quite a lot
Yes, sometimes
No, not much
No, not at all

6. Things have been getting on top of me:
Yes, most of the time I haven't been able to cope at all
Yes, sometimes I haven't been coping as well as usual
No, most of the time I have coped quite well
No, I have been coping as well as ever

7. I have been so unhappy that I have had difficulty sleeping:
Yes, most of the time
Yes, sometimes
Not very often
No, not at all

8. I have felt sad or miserable:
Yes, most of the time
Yes quite often
Not very often
No, not at all

9. I have been so unhappy that I have been crying
Yes, most of the time
Yes, quite often
Only occasionally
No, never

10. The thought of harming myself has occurred to me:
Yes, quite often
Sometimes
Hardly ever
Never

Edinburgh Postnatal Depression Scale: Scoring Sheet

1. I have been able to laugh and see the funny side of things:

As much as I always could	0
Not quite so much now	1
Definitely not so much now	2
Not at all	3

2. I have looked forward with enjoyment to things:

As much as I ever did	0
Rather less than I used to	1
Definitely less than I used to	2
Hardly at all	3

3. I have blamed myself unnecessarily when things go wrong:

Yes, most of the time	3
Yes, some of the time	2
Not very often	1
No, never	0

4. I have felt worried and anxious for no very good reason:

No, not at all	0
Hardly, ever	1
Yes, sometimes	2
Yes, very often	3

5. I have felt scared or panicky for no very good reason:

Yes, quite a lot	3
Yes, sometimes	2
No, not much	1
No, not at all	0

6. Things have been getting on top of me:

Yes, most of the time I haven't been able to cope at all	3
Yes, sometimes I haven't been coping as well as usual	2
No, most of the time I have coped quite well	1
No, I have been coping as well as ever	0

7. I have been so unhappy that I have had difficulty sleeping:

Yes, most of the time	3
Yes, sometimes	2
Not very often	1
No, not at all	0

8. I have felt sad or miserable:

Yes, most of the time	3
Yes, quite often	2
Not very often	1
No, not at all	0

9. I have been so unhappy that I have been crying:

Yes, most of the time	3
Yes, quite often	2
Only occasionally	1
No, never	0

10. The thought of harming myself has occurred to me:

Yes, quite often	3
Sometimes	2
Hardly ever	1
Never	0

Figure 54.1 Edinburgh Postnatal Depression Scale. (*Source*: Cox, J. and Holden, J. (eds) (1994) *Perinatal Psychiatry*, pp. 139–143. Reproduced with permission from Gaskell and Royal College of Psychiatrists, London.)

Health professional .... District ....

Name	Baby's D.O.B	5–8 wk EPDS		10–14 wk EPDS		20–26 wk EPDS		Counselling support		Referred?
		Date	Score	Date	Score	Date	Score	Start	End	Date

Fig. 54.2 Edinburgh Postnatal Depression Scale record sheet. (*Source*: Cox, J. and Holden, J. (eds) (1994) *Perinatal Psychiatry*, pp. 139–143. Reproduced with permission from Gaskell and Royal College of Psychiatrists, London.)

The Confidential Enquiry into Maternal Deaths shows suicide to be the leading cause of maternal death (Lewis, 2001). There has been a growing emphasis on studying the factors associated with deaths in women with mental illness, and recommendations made within this report will be discussed later.

Mothers with severe depressive illness should be admitted to a psychiatric unit, preferably a special mother and baby unit with their baby. Admission is to enable the woman to receive adequate assessment and support and to ensure her treatment and recovery in the initial stages are appropriately supervised. Treatment with ECT may be required, together with antidepressant drugs, which should be continued for 6 months. Most mothers with postnatal depression respond very well to treatment, usually within 4–6 weeks.

Puerperal psychosis

The most severe form of mental illness following childbirth is *puerperal psychosis*. The term is used to describe a group of illnesses that occur following childbirth and are characterized by delusions, hallucinations and impaired perception of reality. The majority of puerperal psychoses are affective (manic or depressive) conditions. A minority are schizophrenia-like conditions. True, chronic schizophrenia arising for the first time in the puerperium is very uncommon.

The incidence of puerperal psychosis is 2–3 per 1000 live births (Cox, 1986).

A sudden onset of illness at 2 weeks following a period of relative well-being is common (Riley, 1995; Thurtle, 1995). This should be borne in mind by those midwives working within a model where women are discharged early from postnatal care. The signs and symptoms of puerperal psychosis are listed in Box 54.2.

The symptoms are generally very severe in women suffering from puerperal psychosis; more severe than in non-puerperal patients suffering from a major mental illness. This can be a very frightening and distressing time for other family members, who may try to hide the behaviour from the midwife because of the perceived shame and stigma attached to mental illness (Lewis, 2001) and this places the mother and baby at greater risk.

Aetiology

It is now thought that biological factors, including genetic factors, are likely to be as important, or perhaps even more important, than possible psychosocial and obstetric factors (Cox and Holden, 1994). A family or personal history of affective psychosis is therefore a major risk factor and should always be elicited when the history is taken in early pregnancy. The risk for a woman with a previous history of affective psychosis

Box 54.2 Signs and symptoms of puerperal psychosis

- The woman will present with symptoms of extreme irritability, often expressing grandiose ideas and possibly becoming violent if these are thwarted (Piper, 1992).
- She looks physically unwell and is in a state of perplexity, confusion, fear and distress.
- She is restless, suffers from insomnia and may also be disoriented about time and place. *Insomnia is one of the most important symptoms and any woman who has a sleep disturbance not explained by a crying baby, noise, or other legitimate reasons should be closely observed by the midwife.*
- The woman will often talk very rapidly, sometimes weaving normal aspects of activity within her words, but may be delusional, and bizarre in meaning.
- From the primary onset of symptoms the woman's mental state changes rapidly, with the emergence of prominent delusions, hallucinations and disturbances of behaviour.
- The symptoms often focus on the baby or the recent delivery.
- The mother may have delusions that the baby has died, or that something dreadful is going to happen to it.

is estimated to be as high as 1 in 3 and 1 in 2 (Kendell *et al.*, 1987; Wieck *et al.*, 1991). Cox and Holden (1994) recommend that a woman with a history of affective psychosis should be referred to a specialist psychiatrist during her pregnancy. Prophylactic treatment, started usually soon after delivery, can then be considered.

Another recent explanation for the development of puerperal psychosis is the major change which occurs in the levels of the steroid hormones at this time, especially the drop in oestrogen (Wieck, 1989). It is thought that high-risk patients develop a hypersensitivity of the central D_2 receptors and that this may be related to the effect of the drop in the oestrogen level on the dopamine system. Another theory is that the condition is related to the fall in progesterone levels which occurs after delivery (Dalton, 1985).

Psychosocial and obstetric factors are also thought to be possible causes of puerperal psychosis. Those who appear to be at higher risk include:

- primiparae who have had major obstetric problems, including caesarean section

- those from the higher socioeconomic groups
- those who are older than average at the birth of their first child, are married, and have a relatively long interval from marriage to the birth of their first child, and
- those who have had a major life event shortly before or after the birth of their child.

Severe episodes of the blues may lead to postnatal depression, and untreated depression may develop into a major depressive psychosis (Cox, 1986).

The midwife's role

Most midwives will come across this condition at some time in their career, and the priority is that of recognition, appropriate referral, and support for the woman and her family. The midwife will potentially be the healthcare professional who detects the behavioural changes associated with this condition, and it is essential that once it is suspected, the woman is referred to specialist medical support for immediate assessment and treatment. These women are profoundly disturbed and require admission to hospital together with their babies, where possible. Psychiatric units with specialized mother and baby sections where such mothers can be skilfully nursed and treated should be available (Oates, 1994). Whilst some women can be cared for on an outpatient basis the majority will require inpatient care. It is a sad reflection, though, that despite the recommendations of two Confidential Enquiry reports that a perinatal mental health service should be available for all women, less that 50% of women will have access to this level of help (RCPSYCH, 2002).

Once admitted, the immediate priority is to sedate the mother sufficiently to reduce symptoms, yet allow for adequate hydration and nutrition. If the mother is in a postnatal ward when puerperal psychosis first presents, she may be sedated there for about 48 hours and closely observed. In a significant minority of cases the illness will resolve quickly and admission to a psychiatric unit will then be unnecessary. This is particularly likely if a psychotic episode arises following a caesarean section. The majority of mothers, however, will eventually require admission to a psychiatric unit.

The short- and long-term prognosis is good, despite the initial severity of the illness. Manic patients usually respond to treatment within 2 weeks, often in a few days. Most of the severe depressive puerperal psychoses will resolve within 6–8 weeks. By 6 months after the onset of the illness, most mothers will have made a full recovery, though a few have a more protracted recovery.

There is a danger of relapse occurring, however, particularly in the early weeks after delivery. Accurate documentation particularly related to first onset of symptoms is essential in order to plan appropriately for future pregnancies. Up to half of all women who have had a puerperal psychosis will be at risk of developing a further episode of mental illness following the birth of their next child. The illness is likely to follow a similar pattern with symptoms developing at the same time, and will have the same prognosis (Lewis, 2001). The risks are lower for those who developed a psychosis following a caesarean section or a major life event. Nearly one-third of all women who suffer from puerperal psychosis will develop a manic depressive illness not related to childbearing at a later stage in life. It therefore seems that women who are susceptible to manic depressive illness are especially vulnerable in the puerperium.

DRUGS AND BREASTFEEDING

Psychotropic drugs are invariably prescribed for women who develop severe mental illness following childbirth. It is when the mother is breastfeeding that particular care must be taken to ensure that drugs are prescribed that are not only effective for the mother but also safe for the baby. The continuation of breastfeeding is often very important to the mother and, indeed, should be encouraged, as it will aid the recovery of her self-esteem and promote her relationship with her baby. Discontinuing breastfeeding only adds to the burden of guilt the mother often feels later.

The *tricyclic antidepressants* appear to be safe in full dosage for breastfeeding mothers. The *phenothiazines* are also probably safe in moderate dosages, although the baby should be closely observed and breastfeeding may have to be suspended if the baby becomes too drowsy and does not feed well. In this case the breast milk must be expressed and discarded. It is important to try to maintain lactation by regular expression of the breasts until it is considered safe for the baby to resume breastfeeding. *Lithium* is not considered a safe drug to give to breastfeeding women. With close consultation and cooperation between the professionals caring for the woman it is usually possible to enable the mother to maintain her lactation and breastfeed successfully in due course. If a midwife is in doubt as to whether breastfeeding can continue in the presence of prescribed medication, advice should be obtained from the local pharmacist, who may also be in a position to suggest alternatives. There is an increasing amount of information available about drug safety and breastfeeding and the midwife should be aware that the woman herself may have already accessed this via the World Wide Web (Gardiner, 2001).

> **Reflective Activity 54.4**
>
> Using Chapter 71, and the British National Formulary, review drugs and medications which are in use for treating and managing postnatal depression. You should be familiar with dosage, route administration and possible side-effects and interactions.

CONFIDENTIAL ENQUIRIES INTO MATERNAL DEATHS (CEMD)

As medical treatment has improved, and deaths from direct causes have reduced, there has been a growing emphasis on the public health aspects of maternal deaths. There is now a clear association between social exclusion, poverty, substance misuse, domestic violence and maternal death. As the main aetiology of depressive illness is psychosocial in origin it is not surprising that an emerging major theme within the ongoing enquiry is the association of mental illness with maternal deaths. Psychiatric disorders are now known to have caused or contributed to 12% of all maternal deaths, 10% of which were due to suicide, all of which were characterized by their violent nature; suicide is now the leading cause of maternal death. In many of these cases, clear psychiatric risk factors were present but not ascertained, and staff caring for the women who died, failed to appreciate and act on symptoms of depression or psychosis.

The midwife's role

All professionals working within the National Health Service are obliged to contribute to and act on the findings of the four national Confidential Enquiries (DoH, 1998). From April 2003 there has been a closer association between the enquiries, and where possible links will be made. The Confidential Enquiry into Suicides and Homicides (CISH) by People with Mental Illness works closely with the newly formed Confidential Enquiry into Maternal and Child Health (CEMACH) to further raise awareness amongst all healthcare professionals and the public of the need for early recognition, appropriate treatment and adequate resources to support women with these distressing conditions.

Midwives should now, however, be aware of the recommendations made by the former Confidential Enquiry into Maternal Deaths (CEMD) pertaining to mental health:

- Protocols for the management of women at risk of relapse or recurrence of a serious mental illness should be in place in every trust providing maternity services.
- Enquiries about previous psychiatric history, severity, care received and clinical presentation should be routinely made in a systematic and sensitive way at the booking clinic.
- The term postnatal depression or 'PND' should not be used as a generic term for all types of psychiatric disorder. Details of previous illness should be sought and recorded in line with the recommendations made above.
- Women who have a past history of serious psychiatric disorder, whether postpartum or non-postpartum, should be assessed by a psychiatrist in the antenatal period and a management plan instituted with regard to the high risk of recurrence following delivery.
- Women who have suffered from serious mental illness after childbirth or at other times should be counselled about possible recurrence of that illness after further pregnancies.

CONCLUSION

All women should be cared for with sensitivity, and encouraged to explore their own feelings in a safe and supported way. They should be confident that their care will be non-prejudiced and that there will be no stigma associated with disclosure of previous mental illness. When there is a need for extra support, or the services of other professionals are required, then adequate resources must be made available to ensure the woman receives the care appropriate to her needs. There is a growing recognition amongst midwives of the value of self-reflection, and in some cases midwives caring for women with profound emotional disturbances may reflect on their own life experiences, identifying a personal need for support.

Initially midwives should be encouraged to discuss any areas of difficulty with their supervisor of midwives, but ultimately they will only be able to offer holistic woman-centred care if they are emotionally well themselves. It is essential that employers recognize the potential stress midwives may be under when caring for women with profound problems and ensure that an adequate level of non-judgemental support exists for staff as well as for women using the service (Hammett, 1997).

KEY POINTS

- It is important that midwives assess and monitor women's mental health during pregnancy and childbirth.
- Mental health problems may be experienced prior to, during or after the physiological and socio-psychological impact of pregnancy and childbirth.
- Midwives can support and prepare women should they experience minor or major mental health problems.

- Collaborative working and effective referral are crucial in supporting and managing women who experience mental health difficulties, and their families.
- Midwives need to be aware of the potential impact of mental health problems on the family and wider society.

REFERENCES

Beck, C., Reynolds, M.A. & Rutowski, P. (1992) Maternity blues and postpartum depression. *Journal of Obstetric, Gynecologic and Neonatal Nursing* 21(4): 287–293.

Bick, D., MacArthur, C., Knowles, H. *et al.* (2002) *Postnatal Care: Evidence and Guidelines for Management*, pp. 129–146. Edinburgh: Harcourt.

Bloom, J. (2002) Midwifery and perinatal mental health care provision. *British Journal of Midwifery* 9(6): 385–388.

Clement, S. (1995) 'Listening visits' in pregnancy: a strategy for preventing postnatal depression? *Midwifery* 11: 75–80.

Clifford, C., Day, A., Cox, J. *et al.* (1999) A cross-cultural analysis of the use of the Edinburgh Post-Natal depression scale (EPDS) in health visiting practice. *Journal of Advanced Nursing* 30(3): 655–664.

Coghill, S.R., Caplan, H.L., Alexandra, H. *et al.* (1986) Impact of maternal postnatal depression on cognitive development of young children. *British Medical Journal* 292: 1165–1167.

Cooper, P.J. & Murray, L. (1998) Postnatal depression. *British Journal of Midwifery* 316: 1884–1886.

Cox, J. (1986) *Postnatal Depression. A Guide for Health Professionals.* Edinburgh: Churchill Livingstone.

Cox, J. & Holden, J. (eds) (1994) *Perinatal Psychiatry.* London: Gaskell.

Cox, J., Murray, D. & Chapman, G. (1993) A controlled study of the onset, duration and prevalence of postnatal depression. *British Journal of Psychiatry* 150: 27–31.

Creedy, D.K., Shochet, I.M., & Horsfall, J. (2000) Childbirth and the development of acute trauma symptoms: incidence and contributing factors. *Birth* 27(2): 104–108.

Dalton, K. (1980) *Depression after Childbirth.* Oxford: Oxford University Press.

Dalton, K. (1985) Progesterone prophylaxis used successfully in postnatal depression. *Practitioner* 229: 507–508.

Department of Health (DoH) (1998) *A First Class Service – Quality in the New NHS.* London: DoH.

Department of Health (DoH) (1999) *Making a Difference.* London: HMSO.

Evans, J., Francomb, H., Oke, S. *et al.* (2001) Cohort study of depressed mood during pregnancy and after childbirth. *British Medical Journal* 323: 257–260.

Ferguson, K. & Thomson, A.M. (1999) *An Evaluation Of The Kath Locke Maternity Project.* Report To Manchester Health Authority And Central Manchester Health Care Trust. Manchester: University Of Manchester.

Gardiner, S. (2001) *Prescriber Update Articles. Drug Safety in Lactation.* Online. Available: http://www.medsafe. govt.nz/prof s/PU articles/lactation.htm.

George, A. & Sandler, M. (1988) Endocrine and biochemical studies in puerperal mental disorders. In: Kumar, R. & Brockington R.F. (eds) *Motherhood and Mental Illness,* Vol. 2, pp. 78–81. Cambridge: Wright (Butterworths).

Green, J.M. & Murray, D. (1994) The use of the Edinburgh Postnatal Depression Scale in research to explore the relationship between antenatal and postnatal dysphoria. In: Cox, J.L. & Holden, J.M. (eds) *Perinatal Psychiatry: Use and Misuse of the Edinburgh Postnatal Depression Scale.* London: Gaskell.

Gutteridge, K.E.A. (2001) Failing women: the impact of sexual abuse on childbirth. *British Journal of Midwifery* 9(5): 312–315.

Hammett, P.L. (1997) Midwives and debriefing. In: Kirkham, M.J. & Perkins, E.R. *Reflections on Midwifery,* pp. 135–159. London: Baillière Tindall.

Hannah, P., Adams, D., Lee, A. *et al.* (1992) Links between early post-partum mood and post-natal depression. *British Journal of Psychiatry* 160: 777–780.

Hodnett, E.D. (1994a) Support from caregivers during at-risk pregnancy. In: Enkin, M.W., Keirse, M.J.N.C., Renfrew, M.J. *et al.* (eds) *Pregnancy and Childbirth Module. Cochrane Database of Systematic Reviews:* Revue No. 04169, Issue 1. Oxford: Update Software.

Hodnett, E.D. (1994b) Support from caregivers for socially disadvantaged mothers. In: Enkin, M.W., Keirse, M.J.N.C., Renfrew, M.J. *et al.* (eds) *Pregnancy and Childbirth Module. Cochrane Database of Systematic Reviews:* Revue No. 07674, Issue 1. Oxford: Update Software.

Hedegaard, M., Henriksen, T.B., Sabroe, S. *et al.* (1993) Psychological distress in pregnancy and preterm delivery. *British Medical Journal* 307: 234–239.

Hoffbrand, S., Howard, L. & Crawley, H. (2001) Antidepressant drug treatment for postnatal depression. *Pregnancy and Childbirth Module. Cochrane Database of Systematic Reviews* (2): CD002018. PMID: 11406023. Oxford: Update Software.

Kendall, R.E., McGuire, R.J., Connor, Y. *et al.* (1981) Mood changes in the first three weeks after childbirth. *Journal of Affective Disorders* 3: 317–320.

Kendell, R.E., Chalmers, L. & Platz, C. (1987) The epidemiology of puerperal psychoses. *British Journal of Psychiatry* 151: 662–673.

Kumar, R. & Robson, K. (1984) A prospective study of emotional disorders in childbearing women. *British Journal of Psychiatry* 144: 35–47.

Laing, K.G. (2001) Post-traumatic stress disorder; myth or reality. *British Journal of Midwifery* 9(7): 447–451.

Lavender, T. & Walkinshaw, S.A. (1998) Can midwives reduce postpartum psychological morbidity? A randomized trial. *Birth* 25(4): 215–219.

Levy, V. & Kline, P. (1994) Perinatal depression: a factor analysis. *British Journal of Midwifery* 2(4): 154–159.

Lewis, G. (ed) (2001) *Why Mothers Die 1997–99: Fifth Report of the Confidential Enquiries into Maternal Deaths in the United Kingdom.* London: CEMD: associated with NICE, RCOG.

Lyons, S. (1998) A prospective study of post traumatic stress symptoms one month following child birth in a group of 42 first-time mothers. *Journal of Infant and Reproductive Psychology* 16(2/3): 91–105.

MacArthur, C., Winter, H.R., Bick, D.E. *et al.* (2002) Effects of redesigned community postnatal care on women's health 4 months after birth: a cluster randomised controlled trial. *Lancet* 359(9304): 378–385.

MIND (2001) *Understanding Postnatal Depression.* London: Mind Publications.

Murray, L. & Cooper, P. (1997) Effects of postnatal depression on infant development. *Archives of Disease in Childhood* 77(2): 99–101.

Niven, C. (1992) *Psychological Care for Families: Before During and After Birth.* Oxford: Butterworth-Heinmann.

North West Local Supervising Authorities (LSA) (2002) Guidelines for supervisors of midwives supporting midwives caring for women with mental health problems. In: *LSA Guidance for Supervisors of Midwives*. North West Local Supervising Authorities, Morecambe Bay Health Authority.

Oates, M.R. (1989) Management of major mental illness in pregnancy and the puerperium. In: Oates, M.R. (ed) *Psychological Aspects of Obstetrics and Gynaecology. Clinical Obstetrics and Gynaecology*, Vol. 3, pp. 839–856. London: Baillière Tindall.

Oates, M.R. (1994) Postnatal mental illness: organisation and function of services. In: Cox, J. & Holden, J. *Perinatal Psychiatry*, pp. 18–19. London: Gaskell.

Oates, M. (2001) Deaths from psychiatric causes. In: Lewis, G. (ed) *Why Mothers Die 1997–99: Fifth Report of the Confidential Enquiries into Maternal Deaths in the United Kingdom*, pp. 165–187. London: CEMD: associated with NICE, RCOG.

O'Hara, M.W. & Zekowski, E.M. (1988) Postpartum depression: a comprehensive review. In: Kumar, R. & Brockington, I.F. (eds) *Motherhood and Mental Illness*. London: John Wright.

O'Hara, M.W., Schlechte, J.A. & Lewis, D.A. (1991) Prospective study of post partum blues. *Archives of General Psychiatry* **48**(9): 801–806.

Pagel, M.D., Smilkstein, G., Regen, H. *et al.* (1990) Psychological influences on newborn outcome; a controlled prospective study. *Social Science and Medicine* **30**(5): 597–604.

Pantlen, A. & Rohde, A. (2001) Psychological effects of traumatic deliveries. *Zentralblatt fur Gynakologie* **123**(1): 42–47.

Paykel, E.S., Emms, E.M., Fletcher, J. *et al.* (1980) Life events and social support in puerperal depression. *British Journal of Psychiat*ry **136**: 339–346.

Piper, M. (1992) Emotional and mental disturbances of the puerperium. *Midwives Chronicle* **105**(1255): 228–235.

Pitt, B. (1968) Atypical depression following childbirth. *British Journal of Psychiatry* **114**: 1325–1335.

Playfair, H.R. & Gowers, J.I. (1981) Depression following childbirth – a search for predictive signs. *Journal of the Royal College of General Practi*ce **31**: 201–208.

Riley, D. (1995) *Perinatal Mental Health: A Source Book for Health Professionals*. Oxford: Radcliffe Medical Press.

Robinson, J. (2002) The perils of psychiatric records. *British Journal of Midwifery* **10**(3): 173.

Romito, P. (1989) Unhappiness after childbirth. In: Chalmers, I., Enkin, M. & Keirse, M.J.N.C. (eds) *Effective Care in Pregnancy and Childbirth*. Oxford: Oxford University Press.

Romito, P. (1990) Postpartum depression and the experience of motherhood *Acta Obstetricia et Gynecologica Scandinavica* **69**(Suppl. 154): 7–19.

Royal College of Psychiatrists (RCPSYCH) (2002) Maternity services failing women with severe mental illnesses. *Press Release,* 24 June.

Seguin, L. Potvin, L., St-denis, M. *et al.* (1999) Depressive symptoms in the late postpartum among low socioeconomic status women. *Birth* **26**(3): 157–160.

Sinclair, D. & Murray, L. (1998) Effects of postnatal depression on children's adjustment to school. Teachers' reports. *British Journal of Psychiatry* **172**: 58–63.

Stein, G., Marsh, A. & Morton, J. (1981) Mental symptoms, weight change and electrolyte excretion during the first postpartum week. *Journal of Psychosomatic Research* **25**: 395–408.

Stein, A., Cooper, P.J. & Campbell, E.A. (1989) Social adversity and perinatal complications: their relation to postnatal depression. *British Medical Journal* **171**: 1073–1074.

Taylor, A., Adams, D. & Glover, V. (1994) Postnatal depression: identification, risk factors and effects. *British Journal of Midwifery* **2**: 253–257.

Thurtle, V. (1995) Post natal depression: the relevance of sociological approaches. *Journal of Advanced Nursing* **22**: 416–422.

Teixeira, J.M.A., Fisk, N.M. & Glover, V. (1999) Association between maternal anxiety in pregnancy and increased uterine artery resistance index: cohort based study. *British Medical Journal* **318**: 153–157.

Uddenberg, N. & Englesson, X. (1978) Prognosis of postpartum mental disturbances. *Acta Psychiatrica Scandinavica* **58**(3): 201–212.

Watson, J.P., Elliot, S.A., Rugg, A.J. *et al.* (1984) Psychiatric disorder in pregnancy and the first postnatal year. *British Journal of Psychiatry* **144**: 453–462.

World Health Organization (WHO) (1992) *The ICD-10 Classification of Mental and Behavioural Disorders.* Geneva: WHO.

Wieck, J.P. (1989) Endocrine aspects of postnatal depression. *Baillière's Clinical Obstetrics and Gynaecology* **3**(4): 857–877.

Wieck, A., Kumar, R., Hirst, A.D. *et al.* (1991) Increased sensitivity of dopamine receptors and recurrences of affective psychoses after childbirth. *British Medical Journal* **303**: 613–616.

Wolkind, S., Zajicek-Coleman, E. & Ghodsian, M. (1988) Continuities in maternal depression. *International Journal of Family Psycho*logy **1**: 167–181.

ADDITIONAL RESOURCES

Depression Central
Website: http://www.psycom.net/depression

MAMA (Meet a Mum Association)
Tel: 01761 433598
Website: http://www.mama.org.uk

Maternity Alliance
Tel: 020 7588 8583
Website: http://www.maternityalliance.org.uk

Mind (National Association for Mental Health)
Tel: 020 8519 2122
Website: http://www.mind.org.uk

The Association For Post Natal Illness
Tel: 020 7386 0868
Website: http://www.apni.org.uk

The Mental Health Foundation
Tel: 020 7802 0300
Website: http://www.mentalhealth.org.uk

The National Childbirth Trust
Tel: 0870 444 8707
Website: http://www.Nctpregnancyandbabycare.com

The Royal College of Psychiatrists
Tel: 020 7235 2351
Website: http://www.rcpsych.ac.uk

Sane
Tel: 0845 767 8000
Website: http://www.sane.org.uk

PART 8

OBSTETRIC EMERGENCIES

55. Shoulder Dystocia 939

56. Presentation and Prolapse of the Umbilical Cord 954

57. Disproportion, Obstructed Labour and Uterine Rupture 960

58. Procedure in Obstetrics 970

59. Complications of the Third Stage of Labour 987

Shoulder Dystocia

Terri Coates

LEARNING OUTCOMES

After reading this chapter you will be able to:

- identify risk factors for shoulder dystocia
- describe shoulder dystocia and be able to recognize the signs which suggest it
- demonstrate a series of manoeuvres that are likely to be effective in resolving shoulder dystocia
- identify which manoeuvres are not likely to be effective in this emergency situation
- state which manoeuvres are likely to cause harm if undertaken

- anticipate the consequences of shoulder dystocia for the mother and the infant
- perform or participate in a locally agreed drill or procedure for shoulder dystocia
- provide support and information to women and their families during and after a case of shoulder dystocia.

Shoulder dystocia is an obstetric emergency with a potentially catastrophic outcome. It refers to deliveries where manoeuvres other than gentle downward traction are needed to complete the delivery of the anterior shoulder (Resnik, 1980). One of the difficulties of shoulder dystocia lies within the subjectivity that may be applied to the definition, which may range from a situation in which the shoulders have not properly rotated to the anteroposterior diameter, through wedging of the shoulder girdle within the maternal pelvis, to one or both shoulders being trapped above the brim of the pelvis.

MECHANISM

In a normal labour the shoulders enter the pelvic brim in the oblique or transverse diameter. The anterior shoulder then passes behind the superior pubic ramus and above the obturator foramen. (For a complete description of the normal mechanism of labour, see Ch. 29.)

In shoulder dystocia there is an arrest of the normal mechanism of labour as the shoulders attempt to enter the pelvis in the anteroposterior diameter of the pelvic brim. The diameter of the fetal shoulders or bisacromial diameter is 12.4 cm and should fit comfortably through the widest diameter of the pelvic brim.

Shoulders are sufficiently flexible to allow those of even a large baby to negotiate the pelvis, as they adduct to reduce the bisacromial diameter. With shoulder dystocia the shoulders may not have had a chance to adduct and are trapped, abducted, at the pelvic brim.

There is no current agreement on a definition for shoulder dystocia. Smeltzer (1986) suggests that shoulder dystocia is a failure of the shoulders to spontaneously traverse the pelvis after the fetal head has been delivered.

Gibb (1995) has described three degrees of shoulder dystocia, in order of seriousness:

- A tight squeeze when delivering a big baby; the mechanism of labour is normal
- A unilateral dystocia, where the anterior shoulder has become stuck above the symphysis pubis and the posterior shoulder has entered the pelvis
- A bilateral dystocia where both shoulders have arrested above the pelvic brim.

A sign that shoulder dystocia may have occurred, is that the infant's chin burrows into the mother's perineum, and the head looks as though it is trying to return into the vagina. This is the *turtle sign* and is caused by reverse traction from the anterior shoulder, which is wedged on to the symphysis pubis, and the posterior

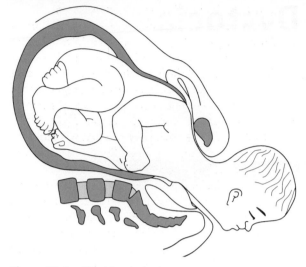

Figure 55.1 Shoulder dystocia.

shoulder, which may not have negotiated the pelvic inlet (Fig. 55.1).

Instinct may suggest pulling to deliver the anterior shoulder, but pulling on the infant's head is likely to further impede delivery by wedging the infant's anterior shoulder more firmly on to the symphysis pubis and can cause damage to the brachial plexus (Fig. 55.10).

The midwife must recognize shoulder dystocia and summon help immediately from midwifery, obstetric, paediatric and anaesthetist colleagues, as the outcome for both mother and infant is potentially very serious. She must then institute proven effective manoeuvres to release the shoulders and complete delivery.

The midwife's anxiety is likely to be communicated to the mother even if little is said. The midwife should remain calm and in control of the situation, and maintain communication with the mother and her partner. The parents must be kept informed in simple and understandable terms.

INCIDENCE AND RISK

It is generally agreed that the incidence of shoulder dystocia is around 2 or 3 per 1000 deliveries (0.2–0.3%) at term, but the risk increases to 1.3% by 42 weeks' gestation (Eden *et al.*, 1987; Johnstone and Meyerscough, 1998). However, a lack of agreement over the definition affects the number of cases reported (Johnstone and Myerscough, 1998).

The risk of shoulder dystocia rises with increasing birthweight and length of gestation, birth order and maternal age (Acker *et al.*, 1986; Al-Najashi *et al.*, 1989; Gross *et al.*, 1987; Johnstone and Myerscough, 1998). Johnstone and Myerscough (1998) point out that half of all babies with shoulder dystocia weigh less than 4 kg and are not considered to be large, and only 4% of large babies suffer shoulder dystocia.

The work of Mortimore and McNabb (1998) suggested that some practitioners may use the term to describe any general difficulty with the delivery of the shoulders, and that the option of including a category of 'difficulty with delivery of the shoulders' may identify the true and false shoulder dystocia cases.

Identification of risk factors

Ideally all potential cases of shoulder dystocia would be identified antenatally; the associated maternal and neonatal morbidity and mortality could then be prevented. The sensitivity of single predictive risk factors is poor. At present, midwives and obstetricians can do no more than anticipate the problem by identifying those factors which give a strong index of suspicion.

The antenatal booking history should alert the midwife to certain risk factors:

Maternal age   The definition of advanced maternal age is over 35 years. O'Leary (1992: 13) suggests that the significance of advanced maternal age in this context is its relationship to increased birthweight and therefore shoulder dystocia.

Maternal obesity   A frequently occurring factor associated with shoulder dystocia is maternal obesity (maternal weight at delivery over 90 kg). The greater the maternal weight the higher the risk (Acker *et al.*, 1986; Boyd *et al.*, 1983; Modanlou *et al.*, 1982; Sack, 1969; Spellacy *et al.*, 1985).

Maternal birthweight   It has been demonstrated by Klebanoff *et al.* (1985) that a mother's own birthweight has a strong influence upon her infant's birthweight. This study looked at 1335 women and concluded that maternal birthweight was an accurate predictor of macrosomia (birthweight over 4000 g). These results were verified by a larger study (16 320 mothers, 17 092 infants) undertaken by Seidman *et al.* (1988). O'Leary (1992) suggests that on the strength of these studies the mother's birthweight should be recorded at the antenatal booking to help to predict macrosomia and thus prevent some cases of shoulder dystocia.

Maternal diabetes and gestational diabetes   Spellacy *et al.* (1985) studied the data from 33 545 deliveries and concluded that women with either insulin-dependent or gestational diabetes are more likely to deliver a macrosomic infant and are therefore at a higher risk of a delivery complicated by shoulder dystocia. Maternal diabetes is also a risk factor as it is associated with asymmetrical fetal growth acceleration with relatively limited head growth (Acker *et al.*, 1985). The body and particularly the shoulders are larger than in babies of mothers who are not diabetic.

Fetal size   The risk of shoulder dystocia increases with increased birthweight. Infants of non-diabetic mothers who have birthweights of 4000–4449 g have a 10% risk of shoulder dystocia, while infants of the same weight born to diabetic mothers have a 31% risk of developing shoulder dystocia because of their asymmetrical growth (Acker *et al.*, 1985; Spellacy *et al.*, 1985).

Pelvic abnormality   Those women who have a platypelloid type of pelvis have an increased risk of developing shoulder dystocia (O'Leary, 1992: 65).

Previous shoulder dystocia   A previous delivery complicated by shoulder dystocia is a predictive risk factor with a recurrence rate of around 10% for subsequent deliveries (Olugbile and Mascarenhas, 2000; Smith *et al.*, 1994).

Use of ultrasound to predict the macrosomic fetus
Ultrasonic estimation of fetal weight is widely used, as it is objective and can be reproduced (Combs *et al.*, 1993). However, Chauhan *et al.* (1992) suggest that ultrasonic diagnosis of the large infant is generally no more accurate than clinical estimation and that if a woman has had a baby before, her own estimate is likely to be as good as an ultrasound measurement. Elective induction for infants diagnosed as macrosomic on ultrasound scan increases the risk of caesarean section and does not prevent shoulder dystocia (Combs *et al.*, 1993; Hall, 1996).

In spite of the inadequacy of ultrasound estimation of fetal weight, it is currently used along with clinical judgement to assess the safest method of delivery, especially for the postmature, large for gestational age or suspected macrosomic fetus. Magnetic resonance imaging may be used to measure shoulder width, but this has not yet been demonstrated on a large population (Johnstone and Myerscough, 1998).

Prediction of impending shoulder dystocia
Most labours preceding shoulder dystocia are normal (McFarland *et al.*, 1995). In some cases the first hint of trouble the midwife may experience during a delivery is the slow extension of the baby's head and then the chin remaining tight against the mother's perineum (Coates, 1995). In spite of current technology, shoulder dystocia usually occurs unexpectedly (Al-Najashi *et al.*, 1989).

Unfortunately, the absence of risk factors cannot be relied upon to exclude the possibility of shoulder dystocia. It is therefore important that the midwife has a sound knowledge of the interaction between the physiology and mechanism of labour and the manoeuvres that may be used to complete the delivery in the shortest time possible, thus ensuring the best outcome for the mother and her infant. All members of the labour ward team should be familiar with the agreed protocol, and 'drills' should be practised on a regular basis by all grades of staff (MCHRC, 1998).

MANOEUVRES FOR MANAGEMENT OF SHOULDER DYSTOCIA

The following descriptions of manoeuvres are arranged from the simple, requiring only movement of the mother, to the complex, where direct manipulation of the baby is required. These manoeuvres cannot really be learned or fully understood by reading alone and it is suggested that the reader works through the manoeuvres using a doll and pelvis or phantom.

McRoberts' manoeuvre

This is the first choice of manoeuvre in most circumstances as it has been proven to be safe and effective. The manoeuvre is named after William A. McRoberts Jr MD, who taught the method in Houston, Texas (Gonik, 1983) but it was first described in 1899 (Johnstone and Myerscough, 1998). The manoeuvre (Fig. 55.2) requires the mother to lie flat on her back (or with a slight lateral tilt to prevent supine hypotension). The mother is then assisted into an exaggerated knee–chest position.

Once the mother has adopted this position, the midwife should be able to proceed with a normal delivery of the shoulders. Smeltzer (1986) suggests that this manoeuvre:

1. rotates the symphysis pubis superiorly by approximately 8 cm
2. elevates the anterior shoulder

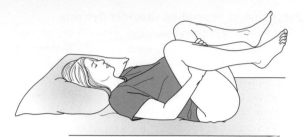

Figure 55.2   McRoberts' manoeuvre.

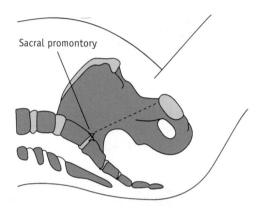

Sacral promontory

Figure 55.3   Diagram to show brim of pelvis in dorsal position.

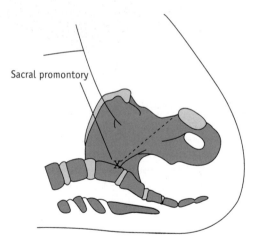

Sacral promontory

Figure 55.4   Diagram to show brim of pelvis in McRoberts' position.

3. pushes the posterior shoulder over the sacrum
4. flexes the fetal spine
5. straightens maternal lordosis
6. opens the pelvic inlet to its maximum
7. brings the inlet perpendicular to the maximum expulsive force
8. removes weight-bearing forces from the sacrum, and
9. removes the sacral promontory as a point of obstruction (Figs 55.3 and 55.4).

This was supported by later radiological studies (Gherman *et al.*, 2000).

Maternal and fetal models were used by Gonik *et al.* (1989) to assess the forces used to extract the fetal shoulders. The McRoberts' manoeuvre was compared with the lithotomy position and consistently required less force to remove the shoulders.

Gonik *et al.* (1983), Smeltzer (1986), O'Leary and Leonetti (1990), Gherman *et al.* (1997), and Johnstone and Myerscough (1998) advocate the use of the McRoberts' manoeuvre as a first step if shoulder dystocia is diagnosed, and most suggest that if the manoeuvre is unsuccessful at the first attempt to try it a second time before attempting other manoeuvres. McRoberts' position is comparatively safe, though spontaneous symphysiotomy has been described in a case where shoulder dystocia was expected in which the manoeuvre was used prophylactically (Heath and Gherman, 1999). It is therefore important to ensure that excessive force is not used, and that the woman's legs are not hyperflexed for longer than required.

All-fours position

When there is a minor degree of shoulder dystocia, movement of the mother can dislodge the obstruction so the shoulders can negotiate the pelvis normally; assisting the mother into an *all-fours position* can work in this way. The all-fours position (Fig. 55.5) also can be used to optimize the space in the sacral curve for the midwife to undertake the direct or rotational manoeuvres as described below. Generally, this position, which acts as an 'upside-down McRoberts' position' carries the same positive effects as above, and will allow the posterior shoulder to deliver first (Macdonald and Day-Stirk, 1995).

If a mother has already adopted this position for delivery and shoulder dystocia is encountered, then the midwife should assist her to move into the McRoberts' position. If this is not possible, then direct manoeuvres can be undertaken whilst the all-fours position is maintained.

The all-fours position can only be used if the woman is willing and able to manoeuvre onto her knees, and is not suitable for women who have a dense epidural block. Whilst the woman is in the all-fours position it is difficult to maintain eye contact and the midwife must ensure that good clear verbal contact is maintained. It is a useful position for a larger or overweight woman, who may find the McRoberts' position overly difficult. A retrospective study of this manoeuvre

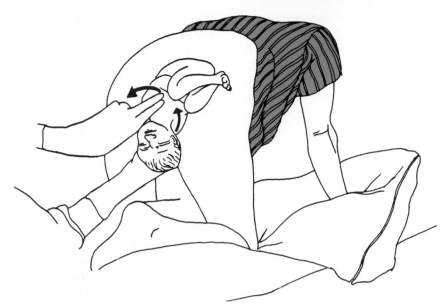

Figure 55.5 Wood's manoeuvre with the woman in the all-fours position.

used for 82 consecutive cases, indicated an incidence of 1.8% shoulder dystocia. 83% of the women delivered with no other manoeuvres required, with a delivery interval of between 1–6 minutes between head and shoulders, and a morbidity rate of 4.9% (Bruner *et al.*, 1998).

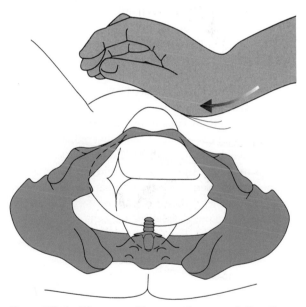

Figure 55.6 Diagram to illustrate the use and direction of suprapubic pressure when the back is on the woman's left.

Reflective Activity 55.1

Using role play, with one of you 'playing' the woman and one the midwife, work with a colleague and try:

- assisting a woman from the lithotomy position into:
  - the McRoberts position
  - the all-fours position
- assisting a woman from a semi recumbent position into:
  - the McRoberts position
  - the all-fours position.

Practise the instructions that you might have to give to a mother moving from one position to another.

Consider how easy/difficult it was getting into these different positions, and how you could prepare women antenatally for such an emergency.

Suprapubic pressure

The application of suprapubic pressure is intended to adduct and then displace the anterior shoulder away from the symphysis pubis and so allow it to enter the pelvis in an oblique diameter (Fig. 55.6). Pressure is applied either by the midwife or assistant using the flat of the hand against the baby's back in the direction that the baby is facing. Steady, gentle, downward traction can be utilized at the same time to effect delivery (Johnstone and Myerscough, 1998).

Suprapubic pressure can be used on its own or with other non-invasive manoeuvres such as the McRoberts or all-fours manoeuvre; it may also be used with the Rubin manoeuvre or the Woods manoeuvre (see below).

Non-invasive procedures have been shown to be effective in up 69/76 (91%) of cases of shoulder dystocia (Luria *et al.*, 1994). However, if the non-invasive manoeuvres described have been unsuccessful, then direct rotational manoeuvres are required. It is at this stage that extra analgesia or anaesthesia may be required. Meanwhile, the midwife should not delay attempting to complete the delivery.

Episiotomy

Shoulder dystocia is a bony dystocia and as such is not greatly affected by soft tissue. However, all the authors mentioned thus far have recommended the use of an episiotomy to try to prevent any further injury to the mother's pelvic floor and perineum during any direct manipulation of the fetus and/or to accommodate the midwife's or obstetrician's hand whilst undertaking direct rotational manoeuvres.

The timing of the episiotomy is controversial, with some advocating it as first-line management and others suggesting that it should be undertaken only if non-invasive manoeuvres have been unsuccessful.

Administering local anaesthesia for the procedure and performing an episiotomy will be very difficult when the head has already been delivered, as the head and chin will be in the way of the scissors and the perineum is no longer stretched. The midwife must secure the best pain control for the mother possible before undertaking the procedure and protect the baby's tissue against damage from the incision.

Woods' manoeuvre and Rubin manoeuvre

Woods' manoeuvre

The laws of physics were applied by Woods (1943) to overcome the problem of shoulder dystocia. Using a wooden manikin he demonstrated that after the head has been delivered, the shoulders of the baby resemble a longitudinal section of a screw engaged in three threads' (Woods, 1943: 797). These 'threads' are the sacral promontory, the symphysis pubis and the coccyx. As a screw offers the greatest resistance to its release by pull, Woods points out that pulling on the baby's head or neck would be inappropriate as it contravenes the laws of physics.

To undertake the Woods' or the Rubin manoeuvre, the midwife should assist the woman into the lithotomy position with her buttocks well over the edge of the bed so that there is no restriction to the sacrum or coccyx during the manoeuvre. If this is not possible, in a home confinement for instance, then the McRoberts' manoeuvre should be used, as it provides a useful and practical position for undertaking further manoeuvres. Alternatively, the woman could be assisted into an all-fours position. These positions will remove restrictions to the sacrum and coccyx, which are present when the mother is in the dorsal or semi-recumbent position. These positions will facilitate manoeuvres to rotate the fetal shoulders off the symphysis pubis and complete the delivery.

The method Woods used to relieve shoulder dystocia involves applying one hand to the mother's abdomen, putting firm but gentle pressure on to the fetal buttocks, and inserting as much of the hand as is necessary into the vagina to locate the anterior surface of the posterior shoulder (clavicle). The shoulder is then rotated through 180 degrees in the direction of the fetal back (Fig. 55.5), which actually causes an abduction of the fetal shoulders.

This rotation may dislodge the anterior shoulder and enable the posterior shoulder to enter the pelvic brim. The posterior shoulder becomes the anterior following the rotation, and may be delivered by normal downward traction and the delivery completed.

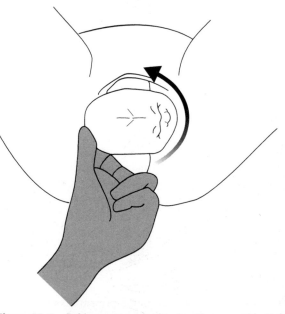

Figure 55.7   Rubin manoeuvre: the shoulders are adducted as the shoulder is rotated anteriorly.

Rubin manoeuvre

Rubin (1964) emphasized the importance of having both of the infant's shoulders adducted, and presented measurements to demonstrate that in this position the circumference of the baby's body is less than if the shoulders were abducted. To achieve the Rubin manoeuvre, a hand must be inserted into the vagina as far as is necessary to locate a shoulder. Then, working from behind the fetus, the shoulders are pushed into the oblique diameter. Once the shoulders are in the oblique diameter and free of the symphysis pubis, then delivery can be completed (see Fig. 55. 7).

O'Leary (1992) suggests that both the Woods and Rubin manoeuvres may be more successful if they are used in conjunction with gentle but firm suprapubic pressure in the direction that facilitates the vaginal rotation (Fig. 55.6).

Delivery of the posterior arm

Schwartz and McClelland Dixon (1958) advocate this manoeuvre to relieve shoulder dystocia as they found it caused less fetal injury when compared with traction and pressure (50 cases). The technique is to insert a hand into the vagina along the curve of the sacrum and locate the posterior arm or hand. The fetal arm should then be swept over the chest and delivered (see Fig. 55.8).

If this manoeuvre fails once the posterior arm has been delivered, the fetus may be rotated using either the Woods or Rubin manoeuvre so that the shoulder and arm that have been delivered are rotated to the anterior position, thus unlocking the obstruction (this is similar to the Burns–Marshall manoeuvre as described in Ch. 53).

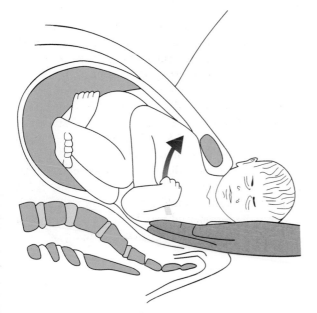

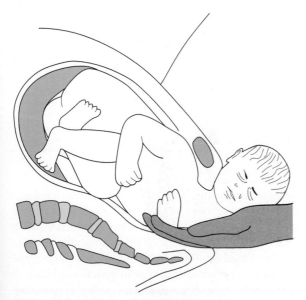

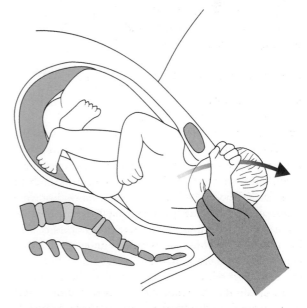

Figure 55.8 Delivery of the posterior arm.

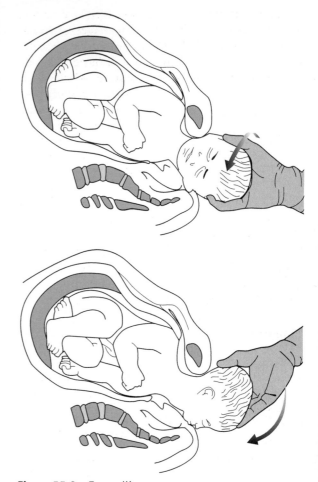

Figure 55.9   Zavanelli manoeuvre.

Zavanelli manoeuvre

The Zavanelli manoeuvre is a revolutionary concept (Sandberg, 1985). Unlike the other manoeuvres described, it reverses the whole mechanism of delivery. Cephalic replacement is followed by a caesarean section. Whist it is unlikely that a midwife would ever need to undertake this manoeuvre it may be a last resort if practising in a remote area away from immediate obstetric support.

To carry out the manoeuvre, the fetal head is returned to the pre-restitution position of either direct occipitoanterior or direct occipitoposterior position. The head is then manually flexed and returned to the vagina (Sandberg, 1985) (Fig. 55.9). Delivery is then completed by caesarean section.

The role of the midwife in such circumstances would normally be to support the mother, monitor and record the condition of both the mother and the fetus, and ensure that all the personnel necessary are available to deal with this obstetric emergency.

O'Leary (1992) and Sandberg (1999) reviewed the available data for cases where the Zavanelli manoeuvre had been used and concluded that the procedure seemed simple and successful, even when operators had no prior experience. Maternal and infant morbidity were discussed; neither cited the Zavanelli manoeuvre as the cause of fetal injury and maternal morbidity was reported as similar to that in women undergoing emergency caesarean sections.

Sandberg (1985: 482) suggests that the Zavanelli manoeuvre 'must occupy the bottom priority until its virtue and applicability ... can be confirmed'. The

Zavanelli manoeuvre must remain the last resort; however, it has proved to be a life-saving procedure. Midwives should understand the mechanisms of the Zavanelli manoeuvre and hope that they will never need to use it.

OTHER PROCEDURES

Symphysiotomy

Surgical separation of the symphysis pubis to enlarge the pelvis for delivery has been proven clinically useful for cephalopelvic disproportion but is associated with high maternal morbidity. Although symphysiotomy has been used for the relief of shoulder dystocia, the few cases reported reveal high maternal morbidity. It is therefore difficult to assess the value or potential value of this technique (Broekman *et al.*, 1994). A case report described three cases in which symphysiotomy was 'the last resort'. All three babies were injured and later died. Maternal morbidity was reported as 'significant', though this was considered to have been influenced by operator inexperience (Goodwin *et al.*, 1997).

Cleidotomy

A clavicle can fracture spontaneously during a normal delivery of a normal-weight infant or a delivery complicated by shoulder dystocia. Deliberate fracture of the clavicle has also been considered by some authors to be necessary to accomplish delivery. This is a difficult procedure, especially in a large, mature fetus. O'Leary (1992: 78) points out that although clavicular fracture is often mentioned 'its use has never been substantiated'. In the past, cutting of the clavicle has also been advocated but is considered to be dangerous and potentially mutilating for both mother and fetus.

Fundal pressure

Fundal pressure together with traction provides the worst outcome for brachial plexus injury (Gross *et al.*, 1987). Fundal pressure will further impact the shoulder or shoulders and impede progress, can damage the brachial plexus and has also been associated with uterine rupture and maternal death (O'Leary, 1992). Fundal pressure has also been implicated in uterine rupture, and thus maternal morbidity and mortality. It is a practice which *should not* be used.

MATERNAL OUTCOME

Shoulder dystocia is associated with a higher risk of physical and psychological morbidity and mortality for mother and baby:

- potential for physical and psychological trauma to mother
- possibility of uterine rupture from fundal pressure
- postpartum haemorrhage (PPH) and/or shock
- soft tissue damage – cervix and vagina
- infection
- postnatal depression
- the loss of the perfect birth and the perfect baby
- possible problems with maternal–infant interaction.

Uterine rupture

Maternal deaths associated with shoulder dystocia have been caused by the use of fundal pressure causing uterine rupture (Seigworth, 1966), and from haemorrhage during delivery or immediately postpartum (O'Leary, 1992: 155).

Postpartum haemorrhage and/or shock

Benedetti and Gabbe (1978) described maternal morbidity from shoulder dystocia as considerable: in their study 68% of cases had an estimated blood loss of more than 1000 ml. Others have recorded extensive vaginal, cervical and perineal lacerations, uterine rupture and vaginal haematoma as sequelae to shoulder dystocia (Gross *et al.*, 1987).

It is wise for the midwife to anticipate postpartum haemorrhage if shoulder dystocia is encountered, and to have prepared equipment, personnel, and the woman and her partner, for such an eventuality.

Soft tissue damage – cervix and vagina

Soft tissue damage may include vulval haematoma and minor and major lacerations. As these may cause a significant degree of blood loss, the midwife should examine the cervix, vagina and labia very carefully following delivery to diagnose any lacerations and take appropriate action (see Chs 28 and 44).

Infection

Increased vaginal examinations, and manoeuvres are likely to increase the risk of infection for the woman. This may be exacerbated by soft tissue damage and blood loss.

The loss of the perfect birth and the perfect baby

Women will have had plans and expectations for the birth of the baby, and the reality of a shoulder dystocia birth and its sequelae may be difficult for the woman to come to terms with. As with any traumatic experience, the mother and her partner may wish to discuss the events surrounding the delivery with their midwife.

It is useful to undertake this review soon after the birth, and also provide an opportunity for discussion at a later date, perhaps after 3 or 4 weeks, when the woman and her partner may have further questions about what happened. (This is discussed further in Ch. 54.)

Post-traumatic stress syndrome

Studies have highlighted post-traumatic stress syndrome as being a risk following normal birth (Ayers and Pickering, 2001; Czarnocka and Slade, 2000) and that the risk is raised in women with high expectations, lack of control and previous negative childbirth experiences (Charles, 1997).

BIRTH INJURY AND FETAL OUTCOMES

The most obvious and immediate consequence for the infant whose birth has been complicated by shoulder dystocia is asphyxia. Meconium aspiration is also frequently associated with these deliveries (Benedetti and Gabbe, 1978; Boyd *et al.*, 1983; MCHRC, 1998; Gordon *et al.*, 1973).

Meconium may not have been seen prior to the second stage of labour. However, the asphyxia caused by the delay in completion of the delivery is likely to cause the fetus to expel meconium prior to delivery. Airway protective reflexes are reduced by asphyxia. Midwives should therefore prepare for the reception of an asphyxiated baby, and must call for a paediatrician to attend the delivery (Box 55.1). (Resuscitation of the newborn is described in Ch. 35.)

Careful examination of the newborn is always important but is imperative following a traumatic delivery. The most commonly reported injuries following deliveries complicated by shoulder dystocia involve the brachial plexus (see also Ch. 36).

Brachial plexus injury

The prevalence of congenital brachial palsy (CBP) is 1:2300 of all live births, 64% of CBP is associated with shoulder dystocia compared to the normal population risk of 0.2–1% (RCPCH, 2000). Whilst many brachial plexus injuries are associated with shoulder dystocia, high birthweight and assisted delivery, around 7.5% of cases have no associated risks reported (RCPCH, 2000). There is no reliable method of predicting risk of either shoulder dystocia or brachial plexus injuries, and diagnosis can be complex as there may be a combination of injuries.

Erb's palsy is the most commonly reported brachial plexus injury following shoulder dystocia. This is the result of damage to the nerve roots C5–6 (Fig. 55.10). The arm on the affected side lies in the classical 'waiter's tip' position (Fig. 55.11).

Box 55.1 Calling for help (hospital)
• Senior midwifery colleagues
• Senior obstetrician
• Senior paediatrician/neonatologist
• Anaesthetist

Following delivery, if the baby has a flaccid arm or an unequal Moro reflex, then the midwife must suspect a brachial plexus injury and inform a senior paediatrician. Serious conditions are associated with congenital brachial plexus injury such as cervical cord injury, cerebral injury or fractures, and these may require urgent treatment.

Some lesions of the brachial plexus are less common. C4 injury causes a phrenic nerve palsy and the potentially serious paralysed hemidiaphragm. C8–T1

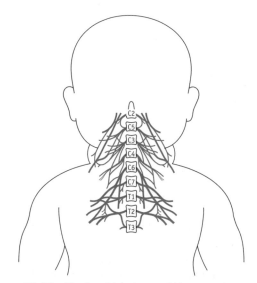

Figure 55.10   The brachial plexus of the neonate.

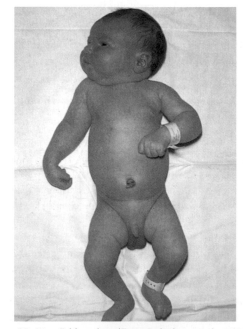

Figure 55.11   Erb's palsy. (From Beischer *et al.*, 1997.)

involvement will result in Klumpke's paralysis: the Moro reflex may be present, but there is no palmar grip, a claw hand and a flail arm. The skin of the affected arm may have a marbled appearance, which is due to vasomotor disturbance. This level of injury is sometimes associated with Horner's syndrome (ipsilateral ptosis) where pigmentation of the eye on the affected side will fade (RCPCH, 2000). The midwife should therefore examine the baby carefully following delivery, including an observation of the face and eyes; a review of the baby's limb movements, assessing appropriate flexion and muscle tone; the baby's respiration rate, observing that the chest is moving equally; and the baby's colour.

A large proportion of brachial plexus injuries will resolve with physiotherapy within 6 months, with no sequelae. However, around 30% of Erb's palsies may be permanent.

There are four degrees of injury to the brachial plexus:

1. *Stretch injury.* Injury depends on the degree of stretch. Further damage is caused by compression due to swelling and bruising. This is the least severe injury; recovery may be complete within 6–18 months.
2. *Rupture.* The nerve is torn, perhaps in several places and may require surgery to restore function.
3. *Neuroma.* Scar tissue that develops following injury.
4. *Avulsion.* Nerves are pulled or torn from the spinal cord. This is the most severe injury and is likely to require several stages of surgery to restore nerves, and may require muscle graft and tendon transfer.

Diagnosis may be complex as there may be a combination of injuries. Parents should be referred to support groups (contact addresses can be found at the end of this chapter).

Treatment for congenital brachial plexus injury

The baby will be referred to a physiotherapist and the parents will be taught how to maintain the affected arm in a natural position until any bruising or swelling resolves. The physiotherapist will then teach the parents a series of exercises for the affected arm.

Physiotherapy is used to maximize the use of the arm to prevent muscle contracture. Motion exercises develop strength and flexibility, and tactile stimulation is used to improve sensory awareness and feeling. It is important to keep the joints supple for the best outcome. However, these exercises are time consuming,

and parents will require support and encouragement, as well as as much information as is available concerning their baby and his condition.

Most congenital brachial plexus injuries resolve within 6–12 months; those that have not resolved may need surgery to improve function.

Bony injury

Shoulder dystocia and high birthweight are considered risk factors for clavicular fractures (Roberts *et al.*, 1995). Clavicular fractures can also be unpredictable and unavoidable, and may occur in 2–4% of normal births (Roberts *et al.*, 1995). The baby may be in considerable pain and on examination an irregularity may be felt over the site of the fracture. However, if the fracture is not displaced an irregularity may only be felt over the site of the fracture several days after birth as a callus forms as part of the healing process. The callus will resolve within a couple of months. If a midwife suspects that a clavicle has been fractured then a paediatrician must examine the baby. The paediatrician may order X-rays to confirm the diagnosis and to rule out other bony injury: an analgesic such as paracetamol may be prescribed if the baby appears to be suffering any discomfort.

The humerus may have also been damaged following shoulder dystocia, especially if the posterior arm has to be delivered to release the impaction. Both arms should be examined carefully after delivery, and in the first weeks following delivery, to exclude bony injury and monitor CBP.

Careful examination of the newborn must be undertaken following any delivery and special attention taken following a traumatic delivery to exclude any injury not immediately apparent (Box 55.2).

Box 55.2 Injuries associated with shoulder dystocia

- Sternomastoid tumour
- Congenital brachial palsy (CBP)
- Horner's syndrome
- Paralysed hemidiaphragm
- Facial palsy
- Phrenic nerve palsy
- Fractured clavicle
- Fractured humerus
- Shoulder dislocation
- Bruising
- Cerebral palsy

NOTES AND RECORD-KEEPING

There are many events in midwifery that happen with alarming rapidity (NMC, 2002) and as such are difficult to record contemporaneously. Accurate records are vital for all deliveries and especially following any emergency situation. The midwife must take care to record all events in chronological order. The important or main events in a case of shoulder dystocia are:

- time of delivery of the head
- position of the woman before and during birth
- time assistance was summoned
- time of each manoeuvre
- time and duration of traction
- episiotomy and when this was performed
- effect of each manoeuvre used
- time assistance arrived
- time of delivery of the body
- Apgar score and condition of the baby
- results of the examination following birth
- information provided to parents at and after the birth (RCM, 2001).

EDUCATION, TRAINING AND DEVELOPMENT

Regular scenario training or 'drills' and thorough knowledge of local procedure for shoulder dystocia are recommended by the Confidential Enquiry into Stillbirth and Deaths in Infancy (CESDI) (MCHRC, 1998). Most maternity units have instituted such educational and development strategies, and these are especially useful when the 'skills drill' is preceded by a review of the theoretical issues, i.e. risk identification, mechanisms of the delivery, etc. Some units have regular drills which include all staff, and which as closely as possible mimic a real situation. It is also a fundamental part of the 'drill' that the whole group then reflects on the drill, identifying where colleagues may have made an error, or where there might be a local difficulty in the communication or management of the emergency.

The Advanced Life Support in Obstetrics (ALSO) training has been a useful means of gathering multidisciplinary groups together to practise emergency skills in a safe environment, and for the emergency of shoulder dystocia has promoted the HELPERR mnemonic (see Box 55.3). Other mnemonics are in use (see Box 55.4).

Whatever mnemonic is in use, it should be underpinned by a clear evidence-based rationale and should be clear and known to the whole team.

Box 55.3 The HELPERR mnemonic (ALSO, 1992)

H   Help – call for help
E   Episiotomy
L   Legs hyperflexed (McRoberts' position)
P   Pressure suprapubically
E   Enter the vagina
R   Remove the posterior arm
R   Roll the woman on to her hands and knees

Box 55.4 The SLEEP mnemonic (Etches and Klein, 1995)

S   Shout for help
L   Legs hyperflexed
E   External suprapubic pressure
E   Enter vagina to perform Woods' screw manoeuvre
P   Posterior arm removal

The nature of shoulder dystocia as a comparatively rare, but serious emergency means that some practitioners may never have the experience of dealing with it, or may never observe a case before they have to deal with it as lead practitioner. It is therefore vital that following an incident of shoulder dystocia (and any other emergency) there is a forum to discuss the individual case and its management in a systematic and critically reflective way, highlighting elements of good practice, and communication, and identifying areas which require additional attention. This forum should be multidisciplinary, and should at its heart have a non-blame and development principle (DoH, 2000). Individual midwives may feel that they would wish to discuss the case with their supervisor of midwives prior to this more open forum, and the supervisor of midwives should attend the forum partly as support to the midwife, but also to be aware of issues which may emerge from the discussion.

Reflective Activity 55.3

Review your local protocols and clinical guidelines. Are these up to date and evidence-based? Is there a regular shoulder dystocia drill carried out locally? You may wish to work with colleagues to plan a regular drill as recommended by CESDI (MCHRC, 1998), involving a range of colleagues, to practise the manoeuvres and management. Ensure that there is an opportunity to reflect together after the sessions.

CONCLUSION

Shoulder dystocia is a rare but serious complication of labour. The midwife should commit to memory a series of manoeuvres that have been proven to be effective and be aware of those manoeuvres that have been proven ineffective or dangerous. This should be supported by appropriate evidence and by a clear rationale. Current knowledge of labour ward protocol or procedure is necessary for all members of the labour ward staff. All members of staff who would be involved in such an emergency should take part in practice 'drills' on the labour ward (MCHRC, 1998). Developments such as the Commission for Health Improvement (CHI), National Institute for Clinical Excellence (NICE) and Clinical Negligence Scheme for Trusts (CNST) have encouraged the development of evidence-based policies and protocols, and this has included the multi-disciplinary approach to emergencies such as shoulder dystocia.

Permanent damage is a rare complication of shoulder dystocia but can be disabling, and the risk of this may be minimized by rapid detection, diagnosis and management of dystocia. The main problem of shoulder dystocia is in fact its apparent unpredictability, and practitioners should be alert to its possibility and be ready to act accordingly. Babies who do suffer more permanent damage should be swiftly referred to a specialist centre, and parents provided with appropriate support and information to help them care for their child. The psychological impact of such a traumatic birth should be considered by the care team, and opportunities provided for debriefing and for further counselling, should this be necessary.

KEY POINTS

- Shoulder dystocia is an emergency and midwives should prepare for the unexpected, be involved in 'drills' and ensure that local procedures are manageable.
- If shoulder dystocia occurs, help should be summoned immediately.
- The most simple and non-invasive manoeuvres should be attempted, progressing to the direct and rotational manoeuvres as needed.
- The midwife should be prepared for a complicated delivery in which the mother and baby are at higher risk, and have taken appropriate measures in preparing equipment and personnel.
- Careful examination of the newborn must be carried out to exclude injuries not immediately obvious at birth. Any deviations from the normal should be investigated and specialist referral organized, ensuring parents are fully informed throughout.
- Full and accurate records should be maintained.
- Reflection and discussion with the mother and partner and all those involved in the delivery is essential.

REFERENCES

Acker, D.B., Sachs, B.P. & Friedman, E.A. (1985) Risk factors for shoulder dystocia. *Obstetrics and Gynecology* **66**(6): 762–768.

Acker, D.B., Sachs, B.P. & Friedman, E.A. (1986) Risk factors for shoulder dystocia in the average weight infant. *Obstetrics and Gynecology* **67**(5): 614–618.

Advanced Life Support in Obstetrics (ALSO) (1992) *Advanced Life Support in Obstetrics*. Kansas: America Academy of Family Physicians.

Al-Najashi, S., Al-Suleiman, S.A., El-Yahia, A. *et al.* (1989) Shoulder dystocia – a study of 56 cases. *Australian and New Zealand Journal of Obstetrics and Gynaecology* **29**(2): 129–131.

Ayers, S. & Pickering, A.D. (2001) Do women get posttraumatic stress disorder as a result of childbirth? A prospective study of incidence. *Birth* **28**(2): 111–118.

Beischer, N., Mackay, E. & Colditz, P. (1997) *Obstetrics and the Newborn*. London: W.B. Saunders.

Benedetti, T.J. & Gabbe, S.G. (1978) Shoulder dystocia a complication of fetal macrosomia and prolonged second stage of labour with mid pelvic operative delivery. *Obstetrics and Gynecology* **52**(5): 526–529.

Boyd, M.E., Usher, R.H. & McLean, F.H. (1983) Fetal macrosomia, prediction risks and proposed management. *American Journal of Obstetrics and Gynecology* **61**(6): 715–722.

Broekman, A.M.W., Smith, Y.G. & van Dessel, T. (1994) Shoulder dystocia and symphysiotomy: a case report. *European Journal of Obstetrics and Gynecology and Reproductive Biology* **53**(2): 142–143.

Bruner, J.P., Drummond, S.B., Meenan, A.L. *et al.* (1998) All-fours manoeuvre for reducing shoulder dystocia during labor. *Journal of Reproductive Medicine* **43**(5): 439–443.

Charles, C. (1997) When the dream goes wrong – post traumatic stress disorder. *Midwives* **110**(1317): 250–252.

Chauhan, S.P., Lutton, P.M., Bailey, K.J. *et al.* (1992) Intrapartum clinical, sonographic, and parous patients' estimates of newborn birth weight. *Obstetrics and Gynecology* **79**(6): 956–958.

Coates, T. (1995) Shoulder dystocia. In: Alexander, J., Levy, V. & Roch, S. (eds) *Midwifery Practice*, Vol. 5. London: Macmillan.

Combs, A.C., Singh, N.B. & Khoury, J.S. (1993) Elective induction versus spontaneous labour after sonographic diagnosis of fetal macrosomia. *Obstetrics and Gynecology* **81**(4): 492–496.

Czarnocka, J. & Slade, P. (2000) Prevalence and predictors of post-traumatic stress symptoms following childbirth. *British Journal of Clinical Psychology* **39**(1): 35–51.

Department of Health (DoH) (2000) *An Organisation with a Memory: Report of an Expert Group on Learning from Adverse Events in the NHS*. London: Department of Health.

Eden, R., Seifert, L., Winegar, A. *et al.* 1987 Perinatal characteristics of uncomplicated postdate pregnancy. *Obstetrics and Gynecology* **69**(3 Pt 1): 296–299.

Etches, D. & Klein, M. (1995) 'SLEEP' a mnemonic to use in shoulder dystocia. *Accoucheur* **2**(2): 1–2.

Gherman, R.B., Goodwin, T.M. & Souter, I. (1997) The McRoberts' manoeuvre for the alleviation of shoulder dystocia: how successful is it? *American Journal of Obstetrics and Gynecology* **176**(3): 656–661.

Gherman, R.B., Tramont, J., Muffley, P. *et al.* (2000) Analysis of McRoberts' manoeuvre by X-ray pelvimetry. *Obstetrics and Gynecology* **95**(1): 43–47.

Gibb, D. (1995) Clinical focus: shoulder dystocia. The obstetrics. *Clinical Risk* **1**(2): 49–54.

Gonik, B., Allen, R. & Sorab, J. (1989) Objective evaluation of the shoulder dystocia phenomenon: effect of maternal pelvic orientation on force reduction. *Obstetrics and Gynecology* **74**(1): 44–48.

Gonik, B., Stringer, C.A. & Held, B. (1983) An alternate manoeuvre for management of shoulder dystocia. *American Journal of Obstetrics and Gynecology* **145**(7): 882–883.

Goodwin, T.M., Banks, E., Millar, L.K. *et al.* (1997) Catastrophic shoulder dystocia and emergency syphysiotomy. *American Journal of Obstetrics and Gynecology* **177**(2): 463–464.

Gordon, M., Rich, H., Deutschberger, J. *et al.* (1973) The immediate and long-term outcome of obstetric birth trauma. I. Brachial plexus paralysis. *American Journal of Obstetrics and Gynecology* **117**(1): 51–56.

Gross, S.J., Shime, J. & Forrine, D. (1987) Shoulder dystocia: predictors and outcome. A five year review. *American Journal of Obstetrics and Gynecology* **56**(2): 336–344.

Hall, M.H. (1996) Guessing the weight of the baby. *British Journal of Obstetrics and Gynaecology* **103**(8): 734–736.

Heath, T. & Gherman, R.B. (1999) Symphyseal separation, sacro iliac dislocation and transient femoral cutaneous neuropathy associated with McRoberts manoeuvre. A Case report. *Journal of Reproductive Medicine* **44**(10): 902–904.

Johnstone, F.D. & Myerscough, P.R. (1998) Shoulder dystocia. *British Journal of Obstetrics and Gynaecology* **105**(8): 811–815.

Klebanoff, M.A., Mills, J.L. & Berendes, H.W. (1985) Mother's birthweight as a predictor of macrosomia. *American Journal of Obstetrics and Gynecology* **153**(3): 253–256.

Luria, S., BenArie, A. & Hagay, Z. (1994) The ABC of shoulder dystocia management. *Asia-Oceania Journal of Obstetrics and Gynaecology* **20**(2): 195–197.

Macdonald, S.E. & Day-Stirk, F. (1995) A midwife's perspective (shoulder dystocia). *Clinical Risk* **1**(2): 61–65.

McFarland, M., Hod, M., Piper, J.M. *et al.* (1995) Are labor abnormalities more common in shoulder dystocia? *American Journal of Obstetrics and Gynecology* **173**(4): 1211–1214.

Maternal and Child Health Research Consortium (MCHRC) (1998) *Confidential Enquiry into Stillbirth and Deaths in Infancy: 5th Annual Report*. London: MCHRC.

Modanlou, H.D., Komatsu, G., Dorchester, W. *et al.* (1982) Large-for-gestational-age neonates: anthropometric reasons for shoulder dystocia. *Obstetrics and Gynecology* **60**(4): 417–423.

Mortimore, V.R. & McNabb, M. (1998) A six year retrospective analysis of shoulder dystocia and delivery of the shoulders. *Midwifery* **14**(3): 162–173.

Nursing and Midwifery Council (NMC) (2002) *Guidelines for Records and Record Keeping*. (Reprint replacing UKCC 1998 publication.) London: NMC.

O'Leary, J.A. (ed) (1992) *Shoulder Dystocia and Birth Injury: Prevention and Treatment*. New York: McGraw-Hill.

O'Leary, A. & Leonetti, H.B. (1990) Shoulder dystocia: prevention and treatment. *American Journal of Obstetrics and Gynecology* **162**(1): 5–9.

Olugbile, A. & Mascarenhas, L. (2000) Review of shoulder dystocia at the Birmingham Women's Hospital. *Journal of Obstetrics and Gynaecology* **20**(3): 267–270.

Resnik, R. (1980) Management of shoulder girdle dystocia. *Clinical Obstetrics and Gynecology* **23**(2): 559–564.

Roberts, S.W., Hernandez, C., Maberry, M.C. *et al.* (1995) Obstetric clavicular fracture: the enigma of normal birth. *Obstetrics and Gynecology* **86**(6): 978–981.

Royal College of Midwives (RCM) (2000) Clinical risk management Paper 2: Shoulder dystocia. *RCM Midwives Journal* **3**(11): 348–351.

Royal College of Paediatrics and Child Health (RCPCH) (2000) *British Paediatric Surveillance Unit 14th Annual Report 1999–2000*. London: BPSU.

Rubin, A. (1964) Management of shoulder dystocia. *Journal of the American Medical Association* 189(11): 835–837.

Sack, R.A. (1969) The large infant. *American Journal of Obstetrics and Gynecology* 104(2): 195–203.

Sandberg, E.C. (1985) The Zavanelli maneuver: a potentially revolutionary method for the resolution of shoulder dystocia. *American Journal of Obstetrics and Gynecology* 152(4): 479–484.

Sandberg, E.C. (1999) The Zavanelli maneuver: 12 years recorded experience. *Obstetrics and Gynecology* 93(2): 312–317.

Schwartz, B.C. & McClelland Dixon, D. (1958) Shoulder dystocia. *Obstetrics and Gynecology* 11: 468–471.

Seidman, D.S., Ever-Hadani, P., Stevenson, D.K. *et al.* (1988) Birth order and birth weight re-examined. *Obstetrics and Gynecology* 72(2): 158–162.

Seigworth, G.R. (1966) Shoulder dystocia a review of five years experience. *Obstetrics and Gynecology* 28(6): 764–767.

Smeltzer, J.S. (1986) Prevention and management of shoulder dystocia. *Clinical Obstetrics and Gynecology* 29(2): 299–308.

Spellacy, W.N., Miller, S., Winegar, A. *et al.* (1985) Macrosomia, maternal characteristics and infant complications. *Obstetrics and Gynecology* 66(2): 158–161.

Smith, R.B., Lane, C. & Pearson, J.F. (1994) Shoulder dystocia: what happens at the next delivery? *British Journal of Obstetrics and Gynaecology* 101(8): 713–715.

Woods, C.E. (1943) A principle of physics as applicable to shoulder delivery. *American Journal of Obstetrics and Gynecology* 45: 796–805.

FURTHER READING

Maternal and Child Health Research Consortium (MCHRC) (1998) *Confidential Enquiry into Stillbirth and Deaths in Infancy: 5th Annual Report*. London: MCHRC. Includes a focus group/central review of shoulder dystocia.

Royal Collage of Midwives (RCM) (2000) Clinical risk management paper 2: shoulder dystocia. *RCM Midwives Journal* 3(11): 348–351.

This provides a good overview of the management of shoulder dystocia, and provides some useful references and a management algorithm.

Rennie, J. & Roberton, N.R.C. (eds) (1999) *Textbook of Neonatology*. Edinburgh: Churchill Livingstone. Useful text to refer to in the context of problems for the neonate following a difficult delivery.

ADDITIONAL RESOURCES

Addresses

Brachial Plexus Foundation
c/o 210 Spring Haven Circle, Royersford, PA 19468, USA

Erb's Palsy Support Group
50 Bassetts Way, Farnborough, Kent BR6 7AF

Websites

http://www.shoulderdystocia.com
Gives a broad overview of the problem from both the practitioner's and the parents' view. It also gives some interesting (American) medico-legal insights. Whilst there are many other shoulder dystocia sites available, many are based on personal practice and experience and should be used with extreme caution.

http://www.calebsjourney.anderson-clan.org/
This site has links to several different sources. It has been designed by a mother of a baby with Erb's palsy, and gives some useful information for parents; it is a very positive site.

http://www.erbs-palsy-help.com
This American site gives a broad overview of the problem, treatment and potential outcome, and also has some useful links to sites with help for parents. For both shoulder dystocia and Erb's palsy, parents' stories make interesting reading and all clinicians could learn from the case histories from the parents' perspective.

http://www.gentlebirth.org/
This site is a useful springboard with hotlinks to shoulder dystocia and other midwifery and obstetric sites. It is American, but has some useful discussions.

56

Presentation and Prolapse of the Umbilical Cord

Patricia Lindsay

LEARNING OUTCOMES

After reading this chapter you will be able to:

- differentiate between presentation and prolapse of the umbilical cord
- identify situations when this emergency might occur
- discuss the midwife's management of cord presentation and prolapse
- discuss the possible consequences to the woman and the infant.

In approximately 1 in 300 births the umbilical cord descends below the presenting part (Llewellyn Jones, 1999). The vessels in the cord may become occluded by pressure of the descending presenting part. Such a profound hypoxic insult will result in irreversible brain damage, stillbirth or neonatal death.

Presentation of the cord occurs when a loop of cord lies below the presenting part of the fetus (Fig. 56.1), the membranes being intact. When the membranes rupture the cord is said to be *prolapsed* (Fig. 56.2).

Occult cord presentation occurs when a loop of cord lies beside, rather than before, the presenting part (Beischer *et al.*, 1997). This will not be felt on vaginal examination but may be the cause of unexplained fetal distress in labour, characterized in the early stages by deep early decelerations of the fetal heart. When confronted with a case of unexplained fetal distress the midwife should consider the possibility of cord compression.

CAUSES

Presentation and prolapse of the umbilical cord may occur in any situation which results in a poorly fitting

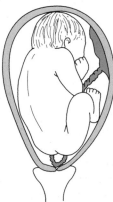

Figure 56.1 Cord presentation.

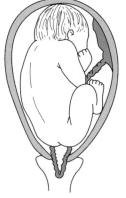

Figure 56.2 Cord prolapse.

presenting part: under normal circumstances the well-flexed fetal head enters the pelvis in late pregnancy or in early labour and thus prevents the descent of the cord.

An unusually *long umbilical cord* may also constitute a risk for this condition. Cord presentation and prolapse is common in malpresentations such as *shoulder presentation* and *breech presentation*, especially a flexed or footling breech: the available space around the fetal legs in the lower pole of the uterus favours descent of the cord (Beischer *et al.*, 1997; Llewellyn Jones, 1999).

Preterm fetuses are at increased risk because there is a higher incidence of malpresentation, especially before 34 weeks' gestation, owing to the relatively large quantity of amniotic fluid compared to the fetal size, which permits increased mobility of the fetus. The small and immature parts of the preterm fetus do not fit into the lower pole of the uterus as snugly as those of a term fetus and this adds to the risk. Cord prolapse may occur as a result of preterm prelabour rupture of the membranes (Romero *et al.*, 1999).

Malpositions such as *occipitoposterior positions*, where the presenting part tends to remain high, may also favour cord presentation and prolapse. *Polyhydramnios* encourages fetal mobility and often results in a high presenting part. When the membranes rupture, the gush of amniotic fluid may bring down the cord. Similarly, the cord may prolapse during *artificial rupture of the membranes* if the presenting part is ill-fitting or high. The fetal heart should always be auscultated before and after artificial rupture of the membranes and if any unexplained fetal distress occurs after this procedure the possibility of cord compression should be considered.

Multiple births are associated with cord presentation and prolapse, as malpresentation is not unusual. The second fetus in a twin delivery may take advantage of the extra available space in the uterus and turn to become a malpresentation after the birth of the first child. This predisposes to cord presentation and the person conducting the delivery must be mindful of this when rupturing the second amniotic sac.

Multiparous women are at an increased risk because their relatively lax abdominal musculature favours non-engagement of the fetal head until labour begins. *Malformation or contracture of the pelvis* and *cephalopelvic disproportion* are associated with a high presenting part and therefore constitute a risk for cord presentation and prolapse, as do conditions such as *fibroids* or *placenta praevia* because they occupy space in the pelvis and prevent the fetal head from becoming engaged. The midwife should remember that obstetric manipulations such as *external cephalic version* of the fetus also promote cord presentation (Llewellyn Jones, 1999).

A 5-year review suggested that, while many cases are unavoidable, obstetric interventions contribute to 47% of umbilical cord prolapses (Usta *et al.*, 1999).

DIAGNOSIS

Cord presentation may be diagnosed in pregnancy by ultrasound scanning (Pelosi, 1990). In 1985 the reliability of this method was demonstrated in a study of 1471 high-risk-women (Lange *et al.*, 1985). In nine of these women cord presentation was suggested on ultrasound examination and this was later confirmed in eight of the nine. There were no cases of cord prolapse among the remaining women whose cord position was normal on ultrasonography. These authors suggest that women with a malpresentation or poorly fitting presenting part at term should have an ultrasound scan to exclude cord presentation, in order to identify the fetus at risk and so plan the appropriate place and mode of delivery.

Vaginal examination may occasionally reveal a cord presentation, the soft, irregular, rope like cord being palpated through the fetal membranes. Pulsation will be evident and will be synchronous with the fetal heart. If the presenting part is very high, the cord may float away from the examining fingers. Pulsation caused by the uterine arteries will be felt in the vaginal fornices and will be synchronous with the maternal pulse. Therefore the midwife should auscultate the fetal heart and simultaneously take the maternal pulse if she is unsure of the source of pulsation. If a cord presentation is suspected, the midwife must aim to keep the membranes intact and should attempt to reduce any cord compression by placing the mother in an exaggerated Sims' position with the hips and buttocks elevated by a wedge or pillows (Fig. 56.3). Medical assistance should be called at once and the midwife should stay with the woman. Elevating the maternal pelvis may encourage the umbilical cord to move, but if the cord presentation persists, the fetus will be delivered by caesarean section.

When the membranes rupture it is essential to auscultate the fetal heart and to make a vaginal examination in order to diagnose cord prolapse. The risk of cord prolapse should be borne in mind whenever there is a high head, malpresentation or malposition, polyhydramnios or multiple pregnancy. The prolapsed cord may be palpated in the cervical canal or in the vagina or may be visible in the vulva. The midwife should quickly assess cervical dilatation and the descent of the presenting,

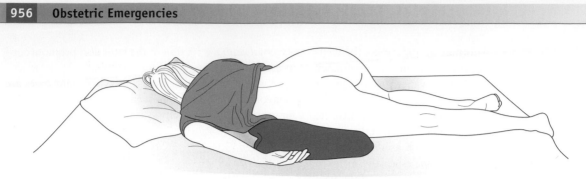

Figure 56.3   Exaggerated Sims' position. (After Farrer, 1985.)

part as management of this condition depends upon the stage of labour.

DANGERS

The fetus is at risk of having its oxygen supply cut off when the cord is compressed between the presenting part and the maternal pelvis. In addition, cooling, drying or handling the cord may cause the umbilical vessels to go into spasm, which will also affect blood supply to the fetus. The prognosis for the fetus depends on where the mother is when the emergency occurs. If she is in hospital where delivery can be immediately effected, the perinatal mortality may be 15–20%, whereas in isolated centres or at home it may be more than 50% (Beischer *et al.*, 1997). The outcome for the fetus may be worse where the presentation is cephalic as the hard head is more likely to compress the cord than the breech or shoulder (Lewis and Chamberlain, 1990).

The dangers for the mother are those associated with operative delivery and anaesthesia and include the risk of Mendelson's syndrome, haemorrhage and sepsis. The midwife should remember that, unless sensitively handled, the psychological trauma inflicted by the emergency and the need for a rapid and often operative delivery may cause distress and may affect the woman's ability to form a nurturing relationship with the child.

Reflective Activity 56.1

Locate and read your local policy for management of umbilical cord presentation and prolapse. What instructions does it give with regard to midwifery management of such incidents at home and in the community?

MANAGEMENT OF CORD PROLAPSE

Key points in management:
- Call medical assistance urgently
- Relieve pressure on the cord
- Improve fetal oxygenation
- Expedite delivery
- Keep a clear, accurate and contemporaneous record.

The management will depend upon the stage of labour and whether the fetus is alive or dead. If there are no pulsations in the cord and the fetal heart is not heard, then the fetus is probably dead. However, this should be confirmed by ultrasound scan: sonographic evidence of fetal cardiac activity has been reported even in the absence of cord pulsation and an audible fetal heartbeat (Cruikshank, 1999). If fetal death is confirmed, labour is allowed to proceed without further intervention and may culminate in the normal delivery of a stillborn infant. If the fetus is known or suspected to be alive, the treatment is immediate delivery, which may be instrumental or by caesarean section. The midwife must attempt to keep the fetus in good condition until delivery is effected.

Reflective Activity 56.2

Write out your own emergency 'Action Plan' for dealing with cord prolapse at home or in hospital.

Prelabour and first stage

Obstetric medical assistance is summoned urgently and the time that the prolapse was detected is noted. (Anaesthetic and paediatric assistance will also be required.)

If the emergency occurs at home, the midwife should call the paramedic ambulance service at once.

Meanwhile, the midwife must attempt to relieve pressure on the cord by moving the woman into the knee–chest position or the exaggerated Sims' position.

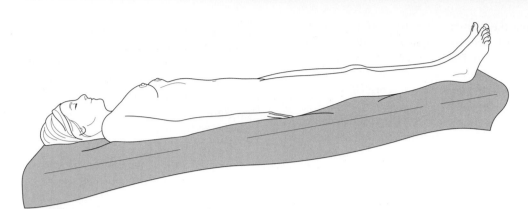

Figure 56.4 The Trendelenburg position. (After Taylor and Campbell, 1998.)

The foot of the bed is elevated if possible. In addition, the midwife should introduce two fingers into the vagina and push up the presenting part during contractions to further relieve cord compression. This must be maintained until the obstetrician is ready to deliver the baby. If the cord is protruding from the vulva, the midwife may attempt to replace it gently within the vagina in order to prevent chilling and spasm of the umbilical vessels. Care should be taken to avoid excessive handling, and if the cord cannot be replaced easily at the first attempt it may be preferable to leave it alone.

Should this emergency arise while labour is being induced or augmented, the midwife should stop the Syntocinon infusion. Oxygen may be administered by facemask at a rate of 4 l/min. Maternal oxygen therapy has been shown to increase PO_2 levels in the hypoxic fetus. It does not appear to cause constriction in the placental bed (Battaglia, 1999; McClure and James, 1960; Nicolaides *et al.*, 1987). However, this treatment can only be of benefit if there is still some fetoplacental circulation; the midwife must make every effort to ensure that cord compression is relieved and the fetoplacental circulation maintained.

Manual replacement of the umbilical cord within the *uterine* cavity (*funic reduction*) has been shown to have some success in selected parous women (Barrett, 1991). However, the midwife should not attempt this manoeuvre, as successful replacement is unlikely and this degree of cord manipulation may cause vasospasm which will exacerbate fetal hypoxia. The obstetrician may prescribe an intravenous infusion of a tocolytic drug such as ritodrine (Yutopar) to arrest uterine contractions. The use of tocolytic intravenous infusions combined with filling the maternal urinary bladder with 500–700 ml of normal sterile saline to elevate the presenting part has been successful in maintaining good fetal condition while preparations are made for delivery by caesarean section.

Bladder filling

The woman should be placed in the Trendelenburg position (see Fig. 56.4) while a self-retaining (Foley) catheter is passed. Sterile saline is then rapidly instilled using a bag of normal saline for intravenous infusion and an administration set connected to the catheter. The fluid should not be cold, that is, it should be at least at room temperature. This procedure has been shown to dislodge the fetal head to 2 cm above the ischial spines and should relieve pressure on the umbilical cord. The amount of fluid required is assessed by the degree of elevation of the presenting part but would probably be a *minimum* of 500 ml. The fetal condition should be continuously monitored and response to this intervention assessed (Katz *et al.*, 1988; Runnebaum and Katz, 1999). Once the bladder has been filled, the woman's position should be altered to achieve a lateral tilt and avoid supine hypotension, which would exacerbate the fetal hypoxia.

Bladder filling may be useful if there is likely to be a delay of more than a few minutes before caesarean section can be performed, such as in a community setting. The urinary catheter is secured by filling the self-retaining balloon and remains in situ until the woman is in theatre and the obstetric surgeon requests that the bladder is drained.

Second stage

If the cervix is fully dilated and there is no evidence of cephalopelvic disproportion or malpresentation, an immediate forceps delivery is performed. Late in second stage the midwife should make an episiotomy and encourage the woman's expulsive efforts in order to effect a quick delivery. Caesarean section may be the preferred mode of delivery even in second stage if there is evidence of malpresentation which would require correction or if the presentation is breech with the buttocks high in the pelvis.

The midwife should remember that the woman and her partner are likely to be confused and frightened by the sudden nature of the emergency and the speed with which delivery is effected. This has implications for informed consent in this situation.

Careful explanations should be given as soon as the midwife is aware of the possibility of cord presentation or prolapse. Even if the outcome is good, the feelings of powerlessness engendered by the situation may cause the couple to feel resentful or angry. The midwife should ensure that she makes the opportunity for time to discuss the events with them and reflect on their reactions and feelings.

Reflective Activity 56.3

What are the possible emotional/psychological consequences for the woman and her family following

---

prolapse of the umbilical cord? If you have cared for a woman who has experienced this, reflect on what you observed in her, and her interaction with the baby. What were her perceptions of what happened and how did these match with the 'professional' perceptions of events? If there are radical differences, why would this be?

Prolapse of the umbilical cord threatens the life of the fetus. The midwife must be aware of potential high-risk situations and be able to take the appropriate action when this emergency is suspected or detected. The psychological and support needs of the woman and her partner must not be forgotten in the haste to save the life of the baby. The safe management of this emergency demands a high level of clinical and interpersonal skills from the midwife.

Reflective Activity 56.4

Consider what you have read and the previous activities you have done. Has your understanding of this emergency changed? What are the key points of management for you as a practitioner?

KEY POINTS

- Umbilical cord presentation and prolapse happen relatively infrequently.
- They are often unexpected occurrences but there is an association with particular conditions.
- The midwife is often the professional who makes the diagnosis.
- The outcome is likely to be poor for the baby if action is not swift and effective.

- The midwife must be aware of those women who are at higher risk and know what emergency action to take in the event of cord presentation or prolapse.
- Accurate record-keeping is vital, particularly with regard to times and action taken.
- Psychological care and 'debriefing' after the event are essential for the woman and her family.

REFERENCES

Barrett, J.M. (1991) Funic reduction for the management of umbilical cord prolapse. *American Journal of Obstetrics and Gynecology* 165(3): 654–657.

Battaglia, F. (1999) Fetoplacental perfusion and transfer of nutrients. In: Reece, E. & Hobbins, J. (eds) *Medicine of the Fetus and Mother*. Philadelphia: Lippincott-Raven.

Beischer, N., Mackay, E. & Colditz, P. (1997) *Obstetrics and the Newborn*, 3rd edn. London: W.B. Saunders.

Cruikshank, D. (1999) Malpresentations and umbilical cord complications. In: Scott, J., Di Saia, P., Hammond, C. *et al.* (eds) *Danforth's Obstetrics and*

Gynecology. Philadelphia: Lippincott Williams & Wilkins.

Farrer, H. (1985) *Gynaecological Care*. London: Churchill Livingstone.

Katz, Z., Shohan, Z., Lancet, M. *et al.* (1988) Management of labor with umbilical cord prolapse: a 5 year study. *Obstetrics and Gynecology* 72(2): 278–281.

Lange, I.R., Manning, F.A., Morrison, I. *et al.* (1985) Cord prolapse: is antenatal diagnosis possible? *American Journal of Obstetrics and Gynecology* 151(8): 1083–1085.

Lewis, T. & Chamberlain, G. (eds) (1990) *Obstetrics by Ten Teachers*. London: Edward Arnold.

Llewellyn Jones. D, (1999) *Fundamentals of Obstetrics and Gynaecology*, 7th edn. London: Mosby.

McClure, J. & James, B. (1960) Oxygen administration to the mother and its relation to blood oxygen in the newborn infant. *American Journal of Obstetrics* 80: 554–557.

Nicolaides, K., Bradley, R., Soothill, P. *et al.* (1987) Maternal oxygen therapy for intrauterine growth retardation. *Lancet* 1(8539): 942–945.

Pelosi, M.A. (1990) Antepartum ultrasonic diagnosis of cord presentation. *American Journal of Obstetrics and Gynecology* 162(2): 599–601.

Romero, R., Athayde, N., Maymon, E. *et al.* (1999) Premature rupture of the membranes.

In: Reece, E. & Hobbins, J. (eds) *Medicine of the Fetus and Mother*. Philadelphia: Lippincott-Raven.

Runnebaum, I. & Katz, M. (1999) Intrauterine resuscitation by rapid urinary bladder instillation in a case of occult prolapse of an excessively long umbilical cord. *European Journal of Obstetrics and Gynecology and Reproductive Biology* 84(1): 101–102.

Taylor, M., & Campbell, C. (1998) Surgical practice. In: Clarke, P., Jones, J. *Brigden's Operating Department Practice*. London: Churchill Livingstone.

Usta, I., Mercer, B. & Sibai, B. (1999) Current obstetrical practice and umbilical cord prolapse. *American Journal of Perinatology* 16(9): 479–484.

FURTHER READING

Calder, A. (2000) Emergencies in operative obstetrics. *Baillière's Clinical Obstetrics and Gynaecology* 14(1): 43–55.

This provides a readable overview of the aetiology, diagnosis and management of umbilical cord prolapse.

Prabulos, A-M. & Philipson, E. (1998) Umbilical cord prolapse. Is the time from diagnosis to delivery critical? *Journal of Reproductive Medicine* 43(2): 129–132.

This 7-year case review compares neonatal outcome with management and concludes that time from diagnosis to delivery is not the only determinant of outcome.

Roberts, W., Martin, R., Roach, H. *et al.* (1997) Are obstetric interventions such as cervical ripening, induction of labor, amnioinfusion or amniotomy associated with umbilical cord prolapse? *American Journal of Obstetrics and Gynecology* 176(6): 1181–1185.

This is a review of 37 cases of umbilical cord prolapse in a 5-year period at one American medical centre. Interventions in labour such as amniotomy are now commonplace but there is little evidence regarding any association with complications such as cord prolapse. Although an association was not found, this article will help midwives to maintain a critical awareness that any intervention, however minor, may have adverse consequences.

57

Disproportion, Obstructed Labour and Uterine Rupture

Margaret Brock

LEARNING OUTCOMES

By the end of the chapter the reader should:

- be aware of the principles of antenatal pelvic assessment
- be able to recognize CPD (cephalopelvic disproportion)
- be able to recognize signs of obstructed labour

- be aware of the hazards of obstructed labour
- be able to recognize predisposing factors for ruptured uterus
- be aware of sites of occurrence of ruptured uterus.

CEPHALOPELVIC DISPROPORTION

Cephalopelvic disproportion is failure of the fetal head to descend through the pelvis in the presence of efficient uterine contractions and moulding of the head. It is caused by a misfit between the fetal head and the maternal pelvis, because the presenting diameter of the fetal head is larger than the diameters of the maternal pelvis through which it has to pass. Malpresentations, malpositions, pelvic tumours and fetal abnormalities which prevent the head descending through the pelvis are viewed as constituting *obstruction* rather than as causes of cephalopelvic disproportion.

The head is the largest part of the fetus and if it has passed through the brim of the pelvis the rest of the fetus should pass through without difficulty. The probability is that the cavity and outlet are also of adequate dimensions to accommodate the passage of a normal fetus. However, in practice, there can be cephalopelvic disproportion at the cavity or outlet of the pelvis too. The reader is reminded of the different types of pelves and how these may influence the way the fetal head negotiates its passage through the bony canal (see Ch. 5).

During the last 2 or 3 weeks of pregnancy it will sometimes be found that the head is not engaged and, in some cases, cannot be made to engage. Reasons for non-engagement of the fetal head have been discussed in Chapter 16. The most common reason for non-engagement is an occipitoposterior position of the fetal head, because of the larger presenting diameter of the deflexed head, the occipitofrontal diameter of which is 11.5 cm. In labour, however, the head usually flexes, and descends into the pelvis.

Diagnosis

The possibility of disproportion should be considered if there is a history of:

- medical conditions such as rickets or osteomalacia which could adversely affect the size and shape of the pelvis
- spinal deformities such as scoliosis
- pelvic fractures or injuries which may have altered the normal shape and dimensions of the pelvis
- obstetric complications such as previous prolonged labour, difficult birth, caesarean section or perinatal death.

On examination of the woman, the possibility of cephalopelvic disproportion should be considered if:

- the woman is of short stature, less than 150 cm, or
- the fetus seems unduly large.

Maternal height continues to be used as a predictor for cephalopelvic disproportion. McGuiness and Trevidi

(1999) noted a 30% incidence of caesarean section with a height of less than 140 cm. They point out, however, that short stature *alone* does not greatly predispose to cephalopelvic disproportion, and as Barnhard *et al.* (1997) conclude, predicting cephalopelvic disproportion rests with the collective assessment of:

- symphyseal–fundal height
- maternal height of <150 cm
- estimate of fetal weight by abdominal palpation and/or ultrasonography.

The possibility that disproportion is present is much greater in a primigravida than in a multigravida with a history of previous normal deliveries, but it can never be ruled out since the size of the fetus may have been smaller in previous pregnancies. Worthy of mention is that excessive fetal size can be controlled by good management of maternal diabetes, a predisposing factor in macrosomia.

It is difficult to assess the size of the fetus accurately by palpation, but with experience it is possible to determine whether the fetus is unduly large for the duration of pregnancy. As ultrasound technology and expertise become increasingly more sophisticated, more accurate estimation of fetal size is possible. Technology, however, is no substitute for the expert midwifery skills required to obtain an accurate medical and obstetric history from the woman, or for midwives developing the clinical expertise to assess fetal and pelvic size and interpret the idiosyncratic combinations of all the above findings and take appropriate action.

If the head is not engaged by the 38th week of pregnancy in a primigravida, the mother is normally referred to an obstetrician for an opinion, primarily to exclude the possibility of cephalopelvic disproportion. When clinical examination reveals no evidence of pelvic contraction or cephalopelvic disproportion, no further action is taken and a vaginal birth is anticipated.

Reflective Activity 57.1

Consider what midwifery skills and strategies could be employed that may enhance/encourage flexion and descent of the fetal head through the pelvis.

X-ray pelvimetry

In recent years the benefit of X-ray pelvimetry has been questioned. Ikhena *et al.* (1999) point out that there are no agreed measurements considered satisfactory to allow vaginal birth, and in addition, X-ray pelvimetry may serve to increase the caesarean section rate (Thubisi *et al.*, 1993). Furthermore, Pattinson (1998) and the RCOG Guidelines (2001) conclude that even in situations of anticipated cephalopelvic disproportion, women do better if allowed to labour. A serious consideration is the risk of exposing women and their babies to radiation if the investigation does not assist clinical management or decision-making. The evaluation of the progress of labour is considered a far more accurate indicator of cephalopelvic disproportion (Chhabra *et al.*, 2000; Impey and O'Herlihy, 1998). Hence, there are only rare situations where pelvimetry is indicated (e.g. history of fractured pelvis).

Management

From these examinations and investigations the clinician is able to place the mother into one of three categories:

1. No disproportion is present and spontaneous labour and vaginal birth can be awaited.
2. There is a slight degree of disproportion which may well be overcome successfully in labour. Provided there are no other complications, the woman is admitted to hospital for trial of labour. Careful monitoring and surveillance of both mother and fetus are conducted and the facilities and personnel required for any emergency intervention are readily available.
3. There is definite disproportion, either because the pelvis is small or abnormal in shape or because the fetus is unusually large. Vaginal birth is out of the question and caesarean section is necessary.

Dangers

If cephalopelvic disproportion is not detected it will lead to obstructed labour which may result in a ruptured uterus and in maternal and fetal death.

Trial of labour

Trial of labour is an ordinary labour conducted in hospital with the special object of ascertaining if the contractions of labour will flex and mould the fetal head sufficiently to make it engage and descend through the pelvis when there is a minor degree of cephalopelvic disproportion. If the head engages, labour is likely to continue normally. The purpose is to give maximum opportunity for the woman to benefit from a vaginal birth within the parameters of fetal and maternal safety. A successful trial of labour prevents unnecessary operative intervention and the associated risks of increased morbidity and mortality, including psychological problems. It also influences the management of future labours, in that if the woman delivers safely vaginally, this is likely to be the pattern in the future.

It is considered that all primigravidae with a non-engaged head are undergoing a trial of labour and, with careful selection in the antenatal period and an upright position in labour, or the active management of labour which ensures effective uterine action, most experience a normal birth. A hands–knees posture may be of benefit to encourage anterior rotation of the lateral or posterior head positions in the pelvis (Hofmeyr and Kulier, 2000).

Conditions necessary in labour when a minor degree of cephalopelvic disproportion is suspected

The presentation must be *cephalic*. A trial of labour is never carried out in breech presentations. There should be no major degree of cephalopelvic disproportion. The woman should be *young* and *healthy* with an uncomplicated medical and obstetric history. There should be *no complications* of pregnancy such as hypertension or antepartum haemorrhage and the pregnancy must not be postmature, otherwise the fetal head will not mould satisfactorily. There is strong evidence to suggest that it is safe to conduct a trial of labour with a transverse lower segment uterine scar, provided there is careful management and monitoring in labour (Flamm *et al.*, 1994; Impey and O'Herlihy 1998). The probability is that there will be a successful vaginal birth with minimal risks of morbidity associated with scar dehiscence or uterine rupture (Flamm *et al.*, 1994). The midwife caring for a woman with a uterine scar in labour will be constantly on the alert for the signs and symptoms of impending rupture of the uterus, which are described later in this chapter.

Management

Labour will take place in a major obstetric unit where there are both the facilities and the personnel available for electronic monitoring and any interventions which may be required to achieve a safe outcome to the labour for both mother and baby. Although midwifery care is given as in normal labour, the obstetrician will be the lead professional in a trial of labour. The midwife may find that the couple require a high level of support and will need to be kept very well-informed of progress, or the lack of it. Good preparation of the woman and her partner before the onset of labour is essential to gain their understanding of the situation and their cooperation in labour. When faced with obstetric emergencies and the need to minimize morbidity and mortality, available options/choices may be diminished. However, women and their partners can still experience a sense of control through the sharing of information and in the decision-making process (Weaver, 1998).

During labour the mother is encouraged to be ambulant because an upright position promotes flexion and descent of the head, cervical dilatation and the maintenance of contractions (Enkin *et al.*, 1993).

Continuous monitoring of the fetal heart and uterine contractions is preferable to intermittent recordings and may be carried out by telemetry in order to encourage ambulation. Progress is assessed by:

- the efficiency of the uterine contractions
- abdominal palpation to determine descent of the fetal head
- vaginal examination to note descent and position of the head, effacement of the cervix and dilatation of the os uteri.

All observations and findings of examinations are plotted on a partogram (see Ch. 26). This facilitates rapid recognition of any delay in cervical dilatation and descent of the head and indicates when action should be taken to aid progress. Once labour is established, cervical dilatation of less than 1 cm per hour over a 2-hour period is regarded as delayed progress (O'Driscoll and Meagher, 1993).

If progress is found to be slow due to inefficient uterine action, active management of labour may be undertaken, after the mother has been carefully assessed by an obstetrician. Oxytocic drugs are used to overcome active phase arrest which is unrelated to cephalopelvic disproportion (Satin, 1996; Warenski, 1997). Otherwise a diagnosis of cephalopelvic disproportion may be made in cases when the real problem is inefficient uterine action. The use of oxytocin in trial of labour may be viewed as controversial because of the risk of uterine rupture. However, there is support for its use, provided electronic cardiotocography is carried out and facilities for the management of any emergencies are readily available (Leung *et al.*, 1993). Having said that, Sweeten *et al.* (1995) confirm that an increase in the incidence of ruptured uterus was caused by the overuse of Syntocinon. It should be stressed that active management would never be undertaken if more than a minor degree of cephalopelvic disproportion was suspected. Selective and judicious use of oxytocin is necessary when it is used to improve uterine efficiency in cases of minor cephalopelvic disproportion.

Conditions necessary for the use of oxytocin in a trial of labour can be summarised thus:

- expert midwifery care to monitor uterine activity both by abdominal palpation and by skilled interpretation of the cardiotocograph trace
- continuous electronic cardiotocography
- close surveillance of fetal and maternal well-being
- avoidance of hyperstimulation of uterine activity by oxytocin and, in the absence of significant progress, a limited period of use.

If uterine hyperstimulation or fetal distress occurs, the oxytocin is immediately stopped and the obstetrician informed. If progress in labour does not improve with the use of oxytocin for a limited period, caesarean section is indicated.

It is never possible to forecast exactly how labour will progress, as so many factors are uncertain. However, if the uterine contractions are effective, the fetal head moulds, the pelvic joints relax and the maternal and fetal condition remains satisfactory, vaginal birth is likely.

If contractions are ineffective, no 'trial' is possible. Oxytocic drugs may therefore be used to augment labour, as described above. If with effective contractions the head fails to engage, a caesarean section will be performed. Studies by Impey and O'Herlihy (1998) and Perveen and Shah (1997) show a 64–68% success rate for vaginal birth following previous caesarean section for cephalopelvic disproportion or failure to progress in labour. In these studies the incidence of morbidity in the mothers was no higher than that found in women undergoing trial of labour following previous caesarean section for non-recurrent conditions. This leaves open to question how absolute are the diagnoses of cephalopelvic disproportion.

Engelkes and van Roosmalen (1992) suggest that symphysiotomy is worthy of consideration in the management of cephalopelvic disproportion in selected cases. Such cases may include the following:

- to facilitate a ventouse extraction when the os uteri is fully dilated – forceps delivery is contraindicated following a symphysiotomy because of the risk of injury to the bladder and to the thinned lower segment of the uterus
- when operative intervention is best avoided, perhaps due to lack of facilities, particular hazards or cultural preferences
- in cases of entrapment of the after-coming head of the breech (Pust *et al.*, 1992).

According to Engelkes and van Roosmalen (1992) symphysiotomy is associated with minimal morbidity in expert hands and so is another form of management to be considered in cases of cephalopelvic disproportion. Equally, it should be contrasted with the risks of caesarean section performed in less than optimal circumstances and the future risk of scar rupture (Bergstromm *et al.*, 1994). Symphysiotomy is rarely carried out in the UK because caesarean section is considered safe and is more culturally acceptable. (See Ch. 55 for more on symphysiotomy.)

OBSTRUCTED LABOUR

Obstructed labour will occur in any case in which there is an insuperable barrier to the passage of the fetus through the birth canal, in spite of good uterine contractions.

Causes

Obstructed labour may occur in the following circumstances:

- if the maternal pelvis is grossly contracted, probably due to rickets, osteomalacia or severe injury
- if the available space in the pelvis is occupied by a large tumour, e.g. a fibroid or an ovarian cyst
- if the fetus is unusually large or abnormal with a condition such as hydrocephalus
- if malpositions or malpresentations such as shoulder, brow and persistent mentoposterior face presentations occur
- if cephalopelvic disproportion is unrecognized.

It is important to distinguish clearly between *delay in labour*, known as *active phase arrest*, when progress is slow, probably because the uterine contractions are not sufficiently strong, but delivery is possible, and *obstruction*, when there is no progress in spite of good uterine contractions, because vaginal birth is mechanically impossible.

Signs and symptoms

Obstructed labour should be suspected if there is little or no progress in labour, including no descent of the fetus, despite good uterine contractions. On examination, the presenting part remains high and the cervix dilates slowly, and because the presenting part remains high, the cervix is therefore not well applied to it. The membranes can rupture early and so there is a risk of prolapsed cord. Recognition of the condition at this stage will prevent serious complications.

If the condition is allowed to continue the contractions become longer, stronger and more frequent in an effort to overcome the obstruction, until eventually tonic contractions occur. Uterine exhaustion may occur, especially in primigravidae, when the contractions cease for a while and then restart with renewed vigour. The mother is in severe and continuous pain, greatly distressed and looks very anxious and ill. The temperature is raised, the pulse is rapid; she may be vomiting and showing signs of dehydration with reduced urinary output. When the abdomen is inspected, the uterus appears closely moulded around the fetus, the liquor amnii having drained away. On palpation, the presentation remains high and the uterus is continuously hard instead of contracting intermittently. In advanced obstructed labour an oblique ridge may actually be seen running across the abdomen. This is *Bandl's retraction ring*, which denotes a marked difference in thickness between the tonically retracted upper uterine segment and the dangerously thinned lower segment, which is now in imminent danger of rupturing. The continuous retraction soon cuts off the fetal oxygen supply, resulting in fetal demise. The woman herself is in grave danger of dying from exhaustion or from rupture of the uterus. On vaginal examination the vagina may feel hot and dry and the presenting part remains high. A large caput succedaneum will be present and, if the presentation is cephalic, there will be excessive moulding.

Morbidity and mortality associated with obstructed labour

Morbidity and mortality associated with obstructed labour are greatly increased in cases where the condition is not recognized at an early stage, and where there is delay in referral and perhaps inadequate facilities and trained personnel to cope with such an emergency. When obstructed labour is prolonged, the presenting part is impacted against the soft tissues of the pelvis causing ischaemic vascular injury and ensuing tissue necrosis resulting in either vesico- or rectovaginal fistula formation. Arrowsmith *et al.* (1996) report that such fistulae can be up to 2 cm long and 2.5 cm wide and carry with them a wide spectrum of both physical and social trauma (Muleta, 1997).

According to Chhabra *et al.,* (2000), obstructed labour and its sequelae is mainly a problem in certain well-defined geographical regions in Africa and the Indian subcontinent. These authors emphasize the value of the use of a partogram to aid early recognition of delay in labour and to initiate prompt referral. This view is supported by the WHO (1994). Where there is provision for good ante- and intrapartum care by well-qualified professionals, obstructed labour should not occur.

Management

Prevention

By good antenatal care and close observation in early labour, the causes of obstructed labour can be recognized and treatment instituted before obstruction occurs. Thus, an ovarian cyst is removed during pregnancy, a caesarean section is planned in late pregnancy for conditions such as cephalopelvic disproportion, a transverse lie is corrected at the onset of labour, or earlier, and safe birth is achieved. If obstruction occurs later in labour, for instance when the fetal head extends to a brow presentation or to a posterior face presentation, immediate caesarean section is performed. In the second stage of labour, early recognition of deep transverse arrest is essential so that the woman can be safely delivered with ventouse or forceps once the fetal head has been rotated.

A midwife attending a mother at home and finding her in obstructed labour should immediately arrange for ambulance paramedics to transfer the woman to hospital. The midwife may give the woman an injection of meptazinol or pethidine hydrochloride to relieve her pain, blood is taken for cross-matching and an intravenous infusion of Hartmann's solution will be set up before the woman is transferred to hospital. Nothing is given by mouth as the woman will need to be prepared for anaesthesia, and careful observations of the maternal and fetal condition are made and recorded.

In hospital the treatment is immediate caesarean section to deliver the fetus, whether alive or dead. Once the baby is delivered, the obstetrician will closely examine the uterus for signs of rupture.

There is rarely a place in modern obstetrics for destructive operations such as craniotomy and cleidotomy in cases of obstructed labour, because of the risk of trauma to the overstretched and thinned lower uterine segment and to other parts of the birth canal. There is also the profound psychological trauma to the parents to be considered when such procedures are undertaken. Gupta and Chitra (1994), however, suggest that there remains a limited place for destructive operations in developing countries in carefully selected cases which present late with obstructed labour, an intrauterine death and advanced intrauterine sepsis.

Reflective Activity 57.2

Outline the factors that would alert you to the possibility of obstructed labour.

UTERINE RUPTURE

Rupture of the uterus is a serious obstetric emergency which can result in fetal and/or maternal death. In the *Report on Confidential Enquiries into Maternal Deaths in the United Kingdom 1994–1996* (DoH, 1998), five cases of ruptured uterus are reported.

The true incidence of ruptured uterus is difficult to determine from the medical literature because authors have different interpretations of what constitutes a ruptured uterus. Some only include a complete rupture, whereas others do not distinguish between complete and incomplete ruptures. The incidence of ruptured uterus is higher in parts of the world where ante- and intrapartum care are deficient and obstructed labour is a more frequent occurrence. Mesleh (1999a) suggests this occurs up to 10 times more often in developing countries than in developed countries.

Causes

Ziadeh *et al.* (1996) conclude that the most common contributing factor to uterine rupture in developing countries is obstructed labour, whereas rupture of previous uterine scars is the most common cause in developed countries (possibly constituting 70% of reported uterine ruptures (MCHRC, 1998; Mesleh, 1999a)). The latter is undoubtedly influenced by the rising caesarean section rates and the corresponding increase in vaginal birth after caesarean (VBAC) with its 80–85% success rate and its high degree of maternal and neonatal safety (Flamm *et al.*, 1994). The VBAC success rate, in turn, is possibly influenced by improved intrapartum care, assisted by established guidelines and policies.

Reflective Activity 57.3

Consider how a midwife could present the evidence to enable a woman to make her decision to plan a home birth after a previous caesarean section.

How might a supervisor of midwives contribute constructively to support the woman and the midwife in the above scenario?

Scar rupture

This can result from previous uterine surgery, usually a caesarean section. A classical scar (that is a longitudinal scar in the body of the uterus) is particularly likely to rupture (Caughey *et al.*, 1999). The most likely time for rupture to occur is in late pregnancy or in labour. Because of the high risk of uterine rupture following a classical uterine incision, an elective caesarean section is usually planned in a subsequent pregnancy at about 38 weeks' gestation.

The incidence of uterine rupture following a lower segment caesarean section is 0.8% (Caughey *et al.*, 1999). In these cases the rupture is more likely to occur when the woman is in labour.

Other causes of scarring of the uterus include surgery for conditions such as evacuation of the uterus or fibroids, and some investigations, for example hysteroscopy. During these procedures trauma or perforation which is not always recognized may lead to a scarred uterus, which results in rupture, usually at the fundus, in a subsequent pregnancy (Pelosi and Pelosi, 1997; Ripley, 1999).

Traumatic rupture

Traumatic (and often iatrogenic) rupture is caused by:

- the misuse of oxytocic drugs and prostaglandins
- the use of instruments
- intrauterine manipulations.

Because of the increased maternal and fetal morbidity and mortality associated with high or mid-cavity forceps deliveries, caesarean section is now considered a preferable mode of birth. Similarly, intrauterine manipulations to correct unstable lie or malpresentation, such as a shoulder presentation, are considered hazardous procedures for both mother and fetus because of the high risk of uterine rupture. The risks are increased when manipulations are attempted in cases of prolonged or obstructed labour, because of the excessive thinning of the lower uterine segment, and also when the integrity of the uterus is suspect, as in grande multigravidae and when there is scarring.

A dominating predisposing risk factor to ruptured uterus in the literature is the misuse of oxytocic drugs and uterine stimulants such as prostaglandins (Caughey *et al.*, 1999; Mesleh, 1999a; Raskin *et al.*, 1999; Ripley, 1999). Great care must be exercised in the use of oxytocic drugs for inducing or augmenting labour, especially in multiparous women because hypertonic contractions are more easily stimulated. The DoH (1998) and CESDI (MCHRC, 1998) reports specifically recommend only one prostaglandin administration to women with previous uterine scars unless great vigilance is exercised. There is also an increased risk of uterine rupture in those with an intrauterine fetal death if high levels of oxytocic drugs are administered because the effects on the fetus do not have to be considered. A cervical tear may extend into the lower uterine segment and cause serious haemorrhage because of the poor retraction there.

Spontaneous rupture

This may occur as a result of very strong uterine contractions (not induced or augmented by the use of oxytocic drugs). The cause of spontaneous rupture is not always clear. It may be due to unrecognized trauma to the uterus which occurred in a previous pregnancy. Another cause is neglected obstructed labour which results in tonic uterine contractions; this will lead to a ruptured uterus if the condition is not diagnosed and delivery effected quickly. In this case the rupture is usually in the lower uterine segment. Abruptio placentae increases the risk of uterine rupture, because of disruption and distension of the uterine wall. The risk is further increased when oxytocic drugs are used to stimulate uterine action. Although spontaneous rupture of the primigravid uterus is rare, several authors cite examples of this occurrence (Churchill and Bloomfield, 1992; DoH, 1998; Mesleh, 1999b).

Types of uterine rupture

Complete or true rupture   This involves the full thickness of the uterine wall and pelvic peritoneum. Ripley (1999) describes it as a sudden, acute event associated with pain and blood loss and a raised maternal and fetal morbidity. It is most commonly associated with spontaneous or traumatic rupture of an unscarred uterus.

Incomplete rupture   This involves the myometrium but not the pelvic peritoneum, which remains intact. It may also be called *occult* or *silent rupture*, or sometimes *dehiscence* or *uterine window*. Incomplete rupture is more frequently associated with a previous lower segment caesarean section scar and tends to present with less violent and dramatic signs and symptoms, possibly owing to the avascular nature of the scar tissue.

Sites of uterine rupture

The unscarred uterus   Longitudinal tears appear to be more common in ruptures in the unscarred uterus.

Many cases in the literature describe a cervical tear which extends longitudinally into the lower uterine segment, either anteriorly or posteriorly (Eden *et al.*, 1986; Golan *et al.*, 1980). It may further extend into the vascular upper uterine segment, thereby increasing morbidity and mortality (Mahomed, 1987). In some cases a rupture may occur in the upper uterine segment only. Ruptures in the unscarred uterus are usually complete and tend to be more extensive and therefore associated with higher maternal and fetal morbidity and mortality rates (Mesleh, 1999a; Sweeten *et al.*, 1995).

The scarred uterus   In these cases the rupture is usually through the scar. The risk of scar rupture in a subsequent pregnancy following a longitudinal incision in the upper uterine segment (i.e. a classical caesarean section) is estimated to be 4–12% (Caughey *et al.*, 1999). In a pregnancy following a previous lower segment caesarean section the risk of rupture is 0.8%.

Although the rupture usually follows the line of the scar, there are cases documented when this does not happen, for example transverse rupture into the posterior lower uterine segment, or vertical lower segment ruptures (Golan *et al.*, 1980).

Signs and symptoms

Complete rupture of the uterus often presents as an acute event with dramatic maternal collapse. The mother usually complains of severe and constant abdominal pain, followed by a marked reduction or cessation of uterine contractions, and vaginal bleeding. The fetus may be palpated in the abdomen separate from the uterus and fetal distress followed by intrauterine death is usual.

An incomplete rupture is far less dramatic. It may be called a silent rupture as the onset of signs and symptoms is gradual and it is often difficult to diagnose. Sometimes it is diagnosed after the birth or at caesarean section, especially in cases where there are no signs and symptoms before the birth (Ripley, 1999). The mother may complain of constant abdominal pain and her contractions may slow or cease. Although abdominal pain and/or scar tenderness are regarded as classical signs, Rachagan *et al.* (1991) found that these symptoms presented in only 35.3% of cases. A rise in maternal pulse rate and the cessation of fetal heart sounds or significant change (variable/late decelerations or bradycardia) were identified by Menihan (1998), Sakka *et al.* (1998) and Sweeten *et al.* (1995)

as the most common clinical features of impending rupture. Vaginal bleeding may also occur. There is a gradual deterioration in the mother's condition. If the rupture is diagnosed early and delivery is expedited, the fetus might survive.

Management

All obstetric units should have a written protocol for this emergency and staff familiar with the management of sudden unexpected haemorrhage. The initial management will depend on the maternal and fetal condition. If the mother is in a state of shock she is urgently resuscitated and prepared for immediate surgery, either caesarean section or, if the rupture is suspected after delivery, laparotomy. A blood transfusion will be necessary for severe haemorrhage and/or shock. Once the baby is delivered and the obstetrician has identified the type, location and extent of the rupture, the appropriate treatment can be instituted.

The surgical options are:

- simple repair of the rupture; this is the treatment of choice whenever possible (Mesleh, 1999a)
- uterine and internal hypogastric artery ligation to control haemorrhage
- hysterectomy; the uterus should always be sent for histological examination.

Aftercare

It is essential that mothers and their partners who have experienced such traumatic complications in childbirth receive adequate support and a clear explanation of the events from their obstetrician and midwife during the postnatal period. Some mothers suffer long-term psychological problems after a traumatic birth experience. Lyons (1998) likens it to post-traumatic stress disorder. The opportunity to debrief and the provision of good support from midwife, doctor and family may help to prevent these additional problems. The circumstances may be even more complex if the baby has died and the parents require an approach which facilitates the grieving process. On occasions the midwife will realize that the mother needs specialist help which is beyond her capabilities and referral for appropriate professional counselling or treatment may be required. Midwives themselves often benefit from the opportunity to debrief after caring for a woman who has experienced such traumatic complications in childbirth. Reflecting on the events with colleagues not only helps midwives to learn from the experience (Taylor, 2000), but also helps them to work through their own feelings and obtain support.

> ### Reflective Activity 57.4
>
> From your own clinical experience, what features would indicate that a woman/family's emotion and psychological needs, following childbirth, had advanced beyond your supportive and listening skills and would benefit from referral for professional counselling/psychiatric assessment?

CONCLUSION

The advent of risk management strategies in most maternity units has resulted in a system of follow-up on situations of less than optimal clinical outcomes. This encourages a structured examination of critical events aimed *not* to apportion blame, but rather to identify aspects of care that went well, along with things that have been learnt and areas for improvement and change (RCM, 2000), thereby improving standards of care.

KEY POINTS

- The use of a partogram aids recognition of obstructed labour.
- There is a 68% chance of successful vaginal birth with VBAC (vaginal birth after caesarean) for previous CPD.
- Look for the 'big picture' when assessing for CPD, obstructed labour and uterine rupture.
- *Any* scars on the uterus may rupture during labour, and the likelihood increases when oxytocin and prostaglandins are used. Midwives need to be aware of this and should monitor progress carefully.
- Sharing information and decisions made with parents is of crucial importance.

REFERENCES

Arrowsmith, S., Hamlin, C. & Wall, L. (1996) Obstructed labor injury complex: obstetric fistula formation and the multifaceted morbidity of maternal birth trauma in the developing world. *Obstetrical and Gynecological Survey* 51(9): 568–574.

Barnhard, Y.B., Divon, M.Y. & Pollack, R.N. (1997) Efficacy of the maternal height to fundal height ratio in predicting arrest of labour disorders. *Journal of Maternal–Fetal Medicine* 6: 103–107.

Bergstrom, S., Henrik, L. & Molin, A. (1994) Value of symphysiotomy in obstructed labour: management and follow-up of 31 cases. *Gynecological and Obstetric Investigations* 38: 31–35.

Caughey, A., Shipp, T., Repke, J. *et al.* (1999) Rate of uterine rupture during a trial of labor in women with one or two prior caesarian deliveries. *American Journal of Obstetrics and Gynecology* 181(4): 872–876.

Chhabra, S., Gandhi, D. & Jaiswal, M. (2000) Obstructed labour – a preventable entity. *Journal of Obstetrics and Gynaecology* 20(2): 151–153.

Churchill, D. & Bloomfield, P.I. (1992) Uterine rupture in the primigravida. *Journal of Obstetrics and Gynaecology* 12(5): 314.

Department of Health (DoH) (1998) *Why Mothers Die – Report on Confidential Enquiries into Maternal Deaths in the United Kingdom 1994–96.* London: HMSO.

Eden, R.D., Parker, R.T. & Gall, S.A. (1986) Rupture of the pregnant uterus: a 53 year review. *Obstetrics and Gynecology* 68(5): 671–674.

Engelkes, E. & van Roosmalen, J. (1992) The value of symphysiotomy compared with caesarian section in cases of obstructed labour. *Social Science & Medicine* 35(6): 789–793.

Enkin, M.W., Keirse, M.J.N.C., Renfrew, M.J. *et al.* (1993) Upright versus recumbent position during first stage of labour. In: *Pregnancy and Childbirth Module. Cochrane Database of Systematic Revues*: Review No. 03334. Cochrane Updates on Disk. Oxford: Update Software.

Flamm, B.L., Goings, J.R., Liu, Y. *et al.* (1994) Elective repeat caesarean delivery versus trial of labour: a prospective multi-centre study. *Obstetrics and Gynecology* 83(6): 927–932.

Golan, A., Sandbank, O. & Rubin, A. (1980) Rupture of the pregnant uterus. *Obstetrics and Gynecology* 56(5): 549–554.

Gupta, U. & Chitra, R. (1994) Destructive operations still have a place in developing countries. *International Journal of Gynecology and Obstetrics* 44(1): 15–19.

Hofmeyr, G.J. & Kulier, R. (2000) Hands/knees posture in late pregnancy or labour for fetal malposition (lateral or posterior) (Cochrane Review). *The Cochrane Library,* Issue 4. Oxford: Update Software.

Ikhena, S.E., Halligan, A.W.F. & Naftalin, N.J. (1999) Has pelivimetry a role in current obstetric practice? *Journal of Obstetrics and Gynaecology* 9(5): 463–466.

Impey, L. & O'Herlihy, C. (1998) First delivery after caesarean delivery for strictly defined cephalopelvic disproportion. *Obstetrics and Gynecology* 92(5): 799–802.

Leung, A.S., Farmer, R.M., Leung, E.K. *et al.* (1993) Risk factors associated with uterine rupture during trial of labour after caesarean delivery: a case-study control. *American Journal of Obstetrics and Gynecology* 168(5): 1358–1363.

Lyons, S. (1998) Post traumatic stress disorder following childbirth: causes, prevention and treatment. In: Clement, S. & Page, L. (eds) *Psychological Perspectives on Pregnancy and Childbirth.* London: Churchill Livingstone.

McGuiness, B.J. & Trivedi, A.N. (1999) Maternal height as a risk factor for caesarean section due to failure to progress in labour. *Australian and New Zealand Journal of Obstetrics and Gynaecology* 39(2): 152–154.

Mahomed, K. (1987) A five year review of rupture of the pregnant uterus in Harare, Zimbabwe. *Journal of Obstetrics and Gynecology* 7: 192–196.

Maternal and Child Health Research Consortium (MCHRC) (1998) *Confidential Enquiry into Stillbirths and Deaths in Infancy: 5th Annual Report.* London: MCHRC.

Menihan, C. (1998) Uterine rupture in women attempting a vaginal birth following prior caesarean birth. *Journal of Perinatology* 18(6, Pt 1): 440–443.

Mesleh, R., Kurdi, A., Algwiser, A. *et al.* (1999a) Intrapartum rupture of the gravid uterus. *Saudi Medical Journal* 20(7): 531–535.

Mesleh, R., Kurdi, A. & Algwiser, A. (1999b) Brief communication. Intrapartum rupture of the uterus – 19 years' experience. *International Journal of Gynecology and Obstetrics* 64: 311–312.

Muleta, M. (1997) Obstetric fistulae : a retrospective study of 1210 cases at the Addis Ababa Fistula Hospital. *Journal of Obstetrics and Gynaecology* 17(1): 68–70.

O'Driscoll, K. & Meagher, D. (1993) *Active Management of Labour,* 3rd edn. Eastbourne: Saunders.

Pattinson, R.C. (1998) Pelvimetry for cephalic presentations (Cochrane Review). *The Cochrane Library,* Issue 3. Oxford: Update Software.

Pelosi, M.A. III, Pelosi, M.A. (1997) Spontaneous uterine rupture at thirty three weeks subsequent to previous superficial laparoscopic myomectomy. *American Journal of Obstetrics and Gynecology* 177: 1547–1549.

Perveen, F. & Shah, Q. (1997) Obstetric outcome after one previous caesarean section. *Journal of Obstetrics and Gynaecology Research* 23(4): 341–346.

Pust, R.E., Hirschler, R.A. & Lennox, C.E. (1992) Emergency symphysiotomy for the trapped head in breach delivery: indication, limitation and method. *Tropical Doctor* 22(2): 71–75.

Rachagan, S.P., Raman, S., Balasundram, G. *et al.* (1991) Rupture of the uterus – a 21 year review. *Australian and New Zealand Journal of Obstetrics and Gynaecology* 31(1): 37–40.

Raskin, K., Dachauer, J., Doeden, A. *et al.* (1999) Uterine rupture after use of prostaglandin E_2 vaginal insert during vaginal birth after caesarean. *Journal of Reproductive Medicine* 44(6): 571–574.

Royal College of Midwives (RCM) (2000) *Reassessing Risk: A Midwifery Perspective*. London: RCM.

Royal College of Obstetricians and Gynaecologists (RCOG) (2001) *Pelvimetry – Clinical Indications*. Green Top Guidelines (14). London: RCOG.

Ripley, D. (1999) Uterine emergencies – atony, inversion and rupture. *Obstetrics and Gynecology Clinics of North America* 26(3): 419–433.

Sakka, M., Hamsho, A. & Khan, L. (1998) Rupture of the pregnant uterus – a 21 year review. *International Journal of Gynecology and Obstetrics* 63: 105–108.

Satin, A.J. (1996) ACOG technical bulletin. Dystocia and the augmentation of labor. *International Journal of Gynecology and Obstetrics* 53: 73–80.

Sweeten, K.M., Graves, W.K. & Athanassiou, A. (1995) Spontaneous rupture of the unscarred uterus. *American Journal of Obstetrics and Gynecology* 172(6): 1851–1856.

Taylor, B.J. (2000) Reflective Practice: *A Guide for Nurses and Midwives*. Buckingham: Open University Press.

Thubisi, M., Ebrahim, A., Moodley, J. *et al.* (1993) Vaginal delivery after previous caesarean section: is X-ray pelvimetry necessary? *British Journal of Obstetrics and Gynaecology* 100: 421–424.

Warenski, J.C. (1997) Managing difficult labor: avoiding common pitfalls. *Clinical Obstetrics and Gynecology* 40(3): 525–532.

Weaver, J. (1998) Choice, control and decision-making in labour. In: Clement S. (ed) *Psychological Perspectives on Pregnancy and Childbirth*. London: Churchill Livingstone.

World Health Organization (WHO) (1994) *Partograph Reduces Complications of Labour and Childbirth*, 7 June. Geneva: WHO.

Ziadeh, S., Zakaria, M. & Sunna, E. (1996) Obstetric uterine rupture in North Jordan. *Journal of Obstetrics and Gynaecology Research* 22(3): 209–213.

FURTHER READING

Kohn, I., Moffitt, P-L., with Wilkins, I.A. (2000) *A Silent Sorrow*. London: Routledge.
This text is primarily written from the perspective of the parents/families and the experiences pertaining to the loss of a baby, and has enormous relevance for professionals as well.

Stainsby, D., MacLennan, S. & Hamilton, P.J. (2000) Management of massive blood loss: a template guideline. *British Journal of Anaesthesia* 85(3): 487–491.
This paper outlines the collaborative efforts that are required by surgeons, anaesthetists and haematologists in situations of massive blood loss to achieve haemostasis, restoration of circulatory blood volume and blood component replacement. The template is a particularly useful guide.

Vincent, C. (ed) (2001) *Clinical Risk Management*. London: BMJ Publishing Group.
Whilst this text does not specifically focus on obstetrics, the chapters pertaining to risk management in obstetrics are valuable. The rest of the book is useful in putting risk management into the context of the health service as a whole and how it relates to clinical governance.

58

Procedures in Obstetrics

Stephanie Meakin

LEARNING OUTCOMES

After reading this chapter you will be able to:

- reflect upon your own practice to assess what is considered normal and any aspects of it that may influence operative delivery rates
- explore local protocols, policies and guidelines that may have the potential to impact on the increasing operative delivery rates
- examine the information given to women regarding choices in their labour and delivery

- ensure that appropriate and effective care is provided for women experiencing instrumental and operative deliveries
- ensure that the most appropriate and relevant postdelivery care is provided for both mother and baby.

INTRODUCTION

A baby may enter the world spontaneously through the mother's vagina, with only the occasional need for guidance from attendants, or by operative means with the use of forceps, vacuum extraction, or by caesarean section. At the beginning of the 21st century, the spontaneous vaginal delivery route is becoming less common. This was highlighted in the ENB midwifery audit (1999) undertaken in 178 units in 1998–1999, the results of which showed that in some units, the rate for normal deliveries undertaken by midwives was down to as low as 52%. Instrumental delivery rates were increasing annually along with caesarean sections. Recent statistics presented to Government suggest the rate is even lower – 44.4% (Birth Choice, 2001). It might be considered that, soon, spontaneous vaginal delivery will no longer be the accepted normal route.

The following chapter will explore some of the issues for midwives within the trends of increasing operative deliveries, including the impact that this can have on women's and children's health. The sections on instrumental and caesarean style deliveries will begin with the morbidity associated with them. Indications for each type of delivery will be listed followed by an exploration of aspects of care given to the woman in labour that may have the potential to increase the need for an instrumental or an operative delivery. The techniques involved in each of these styles of delivery will then be briefly explained and the midwife's role in providing the most effective and appropriate care for each will be discussed. Cervical cerclage will be introduced to complete the chapter.

OPERATIVE VAGINAL DELIVERIES

Up until three centuries ago, choices in the means of childbirth were severely restricted and the maternal and infant morbidity associated with operative delivery was appalling. Operative intervention was undertaken as a measure of desperation when all other means failed. The roots of modern high-technology western birth can be traced to the 17th century when men began to use both surgery and forceps to extract babies from women (Wagner, 1994). These men were not physicians but barbers, tailors and butchers, who called themselves barber-surgeons. Their first priority was the woman's life. In obstructed labour, their job was to save the life of the woman even if this meant, as it sometimes did, the destruction of the fetus.

Forceps and ventouse have the potential to safely remove the infant and mother from a hazardous situation (Dennen and Hayashi, 1999), and even to save lives. Taking this into consideration, however, the increase in their use has an impact on the health of women and infants. The consensus of opinion from an international forum held in Brazil looking at technology for birth, concluded that forceps and ventouse are often performed without medical need, carry serious risks to both women and babies and have real social and economic costs to the family and the nation (Wagner, 1994). Highest rates of trauma are consistently observed with operative procedures with short- and long-term morbidity.

Neonatal complications

After any instrumental vaginal delivery, the baby may suffer hypoxia, have lower Apgar scores and need appropriate resuscitation. Facial or scalp abrasions or bruising are common. Alopecia has occurred in infancy following ventouse delivery (Teng *et al.*, 1997). A cephalhaematoma may develop because of friction between the fetal head and pelvis or forceps blade, as well as from the suction of the ventouse cup. There may be an increase in jaundice due to reabsorption of haemoglobin associated with this bruising (Dennen and Hayashi, 1999). Facial palsy, which is usually temporary, may occur because of the forceps blade compressing the facial nerve, which runs anteriorly to the ear. Intracranial trauma and haemorrhage is higher among infants delivered by vacuum extraction, forceps or caesarean section (Towner *et al.*, 1999). In more rare circumstances, tentorial tears and rupture of the great vein of Galen may occur, leading to bleeding and compression of the brainstem (Hibbard, 1989). Skull fractures are usually linear but occasionally a depressed fracture can result in a subarachnoid haemorrhage. Kielland's forceps can cause unexplained convulsions. Retinal haemorrhages are more common in vacuum extraction deliveries (Vacca, 1996). The most serious complication to occur is that of subgaleal haemorrhage. This potentially life-threatening condition is reported to have increased since the introduction of the vacuum extractor (Chadwick *et al.*, 1996).

Maternal complications

The most common injuries to the genital tract are cervical, vaginal and perineal tears, haematomas and rectal lacerations. Bladder or urethral injury may occur, causing urinary retention and even the formation of a fistula. Perineal pain due to bruising, oedema, trauma and episiotomy can impair sexual function and infant feeding. Faecal incontinence as an immediate consequence of childbirth is more common following instrumental deliveries (Bick *et al.*, 1997). There is an increased risk of haemorrhage (Walsh, 2000). A rare complication is that the cervix and lower segment of the uterus may be damaged. The psychological effects of instrumental delivery may include fear and anxiety in relation to subsequent pregnancy, and feelings of failure, inadequacy and disappointment. Both forceps and ventouse-assisted deliveries were found to be predictive factors of acute trauma symptoms and post-traumatic stress disorder as a result of women's birth experiences (Creedy *et al.*, 2000). Jolly *et al.* (1999) conclude that caesarean section or vaginal instrumental birth is associated with voluntary and involuntary infertility as it can leave many mothers frightened about future childbirth. 13% more of women who had a caesarean section and 6% more of those who had instrumental births had not had a second child compared with those following normal birth.

Reflective Activity 58.1

Owing to the maternal and neonatal morbidity associated with instrumental deliveries, it appears appropriate for all midwives to reflect in and on their own practice to ensure that aspects of care for women in normal labour are not increasing the possibility of operative deliveries. Take time to explore your beliefs regarding the points for midwifery practice below. Each time you care for a woman who requires an instrumental delivery or an emergency caesarean section, reflect upon the course of her labour to assess whether there were any aspects of her care that may have contributed to the outcome. Record your thoughts for future reference.

Key aspects of midwifery practice

Some critical consideration of aspects of care may enable the midwife to plan care not just to ensure the woman's comfort and safety, but also to reduce the need for intervention and augmentation. This has wide-ranging implications for the quality of care and for effective use of both human and other resources within the service.

One of the most important issues for the midwife and the consultant team to consider is that of ensuring that the woman is informed and prepared for the labour and birth of her baby. It is imperative that her expectations and experiences are considered early during the pregnancy, usually at booking. Exploring the process of birth allows the midwife to then provide information about possible management and care which may be required should there be any minor or major deviations from normal, and this ensures that the woman should feel more confident and prepared.

Policies

Blanket policies to treat prolonged labour and 'failure to progress' should be examined as there is much literature available to explore long-held beliefs of the definition of the duration and progress of labour. Even in 1973, when medicalization was really taking control of childbirth, Studd questioned the arbitrary application of time limits on labour considering the confusion over the diagnosis of the onset of active labour. Yet this confusion remains and time limits for stages of labour remain in place.

Position for labour and delivery

An upright position, preferably mobile, assists the woman to feel in control, can reduce her distress and help her to adopt comfortable positions more easily. During a review of the trials for The Cochrane Library, Gupta *et al.* (2001) highlighted that adopting upright positions in labour appeared to reduce the number of assisted deliveries and fewer abnormal fetal heart rate patterns were noted.

Diet, fasting and nutrition

Fasting women throughout a normal labour can add to exhaustion, as labour is a time of great energy demand and it is estimated that a labouring woman may require 800–1100 kcal/h (Ludka and Roberts, 1993). Whilst women adapt to a small rise of ketones in labour, blood pH can be reduced in starving women and result in ketoacidosis. Mark (1961) discovered that uterine activity was influenced by environmental pH and that myometrial cells spontaneously contract with increased alkalinity, preferably between 7.8–7.1. Ketones that build up may also cross the placenta and if there is an accumulation in the fetus this can affect fetal well-being and fetal activity (Swift, 1991).

Supportive presence during labour

Cochrane reviews highlight that the presence of an appropriate support person throughout labour is associated with a decreased incidence of epidural anaesthesia, dystocia and instrumental deliveries (Hodnett, 2001).

Amniotomy and Syntocinon

Amniotomy can increase the requirement for instrumental delivery and caesarean section (Johnson *et al.*, 1997). It is recognized that amniotomy causes fetal heart abnormalities due to cord and head compression, which then increases the risk of interventions. It can inhibit the rotation of some malpresentations, for example occipitoposterior, which may predispose to delay. There is an increase in pain during contractions which may in turn increase the demand for epidural analgesia.

Syntocinon reduces the oxygen supply to the baby's brain. The fetus may then display signs of fetal distress, increasing the need to dramatically shorten the labour (O'Regan, 1998).

Pain relief

Epidurals are associated with a substantially increased use of assisted vaginal delivery (Mander, 1994). Epidurals increase the length of first and second stages, often affecting the efficacy of contractions, increasing the need for Syntocinon (Page, 2000).

Indications for the use of assisted vaginal delivery

The following short list is not absolute but meant to give a general idea of the most common indications for the use of forceps or vacuum extraction during the second stage of labour:

- When a shortening of the second stage of labour is required, most frequently due to maternal distress/exhaustion.
- Fetal jeopardy.
- To spare the mother muscular effort, as is necessary in medically significant indications including cardiopulmonary or vascular conditions.

Contraindications to instrumental delivery

- Unengaged head.
- Malpresentation (face/brow).
- Inability to define position.
- Fetal macrosomia (>4–4.5 kg estimated weight, especially in maternal diabetes).
- Inexperienced operator.

If an instrumental delivery is necessary

The woman and her companion are likely to be extremely apprehensive once the need for an instrumental delivery is recommended. When the midwife has summoned the appropriate personnel, who will preferably include a senior obstetrician, a paediatrician and another person who can assist with assembling equipment, there will be several strangers in the room. Midwives then have to prioritize the care they give and, where possible, involve other members of the team to assist the doctors rather than leave the woman's side. They must remember that they remain the woman's advocate and must be present to explain all the procedures, support, encourage and ensure that there is a respectful environment within the delivery room. There should be little discussion in the room that does not include the woman.

Procedure

- Prior to the procedure, consent should be obtained from the woman. This will require full, but simple explanation and rationale of the procedures being provided to the woman, which may require the presence of a translator.
- An abdominal examination is performed to check lie, presentation and descent and that uterine contractions are satisfactory.
- Adequate analgesia/anaesthesia must be considered.
- Prior to the delivery, the mother is placed in the lithotomy position. The midwife must ensure that the woman is covered with a sheet as much as, and for as long as possible to protect her dignity. Both legs are flexed simultaneously and gently on to the abdomen, and the feet moved to the outer sides of the supports and placed in the leg rests or stirrups together to avoid sacroiliac strain. To prevent obstruction of venous return and possible thrombosis by pressure, care is taken to ensure that the legs are fully abducted. Once the mother is correctly positioned, the foot part of the bed is lowered and the mother's buttocks lifted to the edge of the bed. The operator can now proceed.
- The bladder is emptied by means of a catheter.
- A vaginal examination is performed to ensure that the cervix is fully dilated and that the membranes are ruptured, the position and station of the fetal head is defined, the degree of moulding is ascertained and there is a final check that there is no cephalopelvic disproportion present.
- Checks are made that necessary equipment is present, correct and in good working condition.
- A paediatrician should be in attendance for the delivery (where possible).
- Checks are made that neonatal resuscitation equipment is available and in good working order (see Ch. 31). The resuscitaire, including the overhead heater should be switched on.

Ventouse vs forceps

Debate exists over the preferred instrument for vaginal delivery once it is believed to be necessary. There are two methods for instrumental delivery: forceps and vacuum (ventouse) extraction. A Cochrane systematic review of nine randomized controlled studies involving 2849 primiparous and multiparous women compared vacuum extractions with forceps. Ventouse appears to be significantly more likely to fail at achieving a vaginal delivery, but is less likely to produce maternal trauma and is less likely to be associated with severe perineal pain. However, it does produce increased rates of cephalhaematoma, retinal haemorrhages and low Apgar scores at 5 minutes. There appeared no difference in long-term outcome between the two instruments (Johanson and Menon, 2000).

Forceps (Fig. 58.1)

Forceps were first described in 400 BC by Hippocrates to extract dead fetuses. From a birth room scene on a marble relief, it would appear that forceps were also used in Roman times, but in modern history the use of forceps as an aid to vaginal delivery has been known only since their invention by the Chamberlen family in the 1600s (Pearson, 1981). The family tried to keep the nature of their instruments a secret, as these forceps offered a practical possibility of live births from obstructed labours and were a source of fame and money to those who used them.

Since the introduction of forceps, many attempts have been made to improve the efficacy and safety of the instrument for specific obstetrical situations, and the shortcomings of current forceps design is acknowledged. In fact the blades of some designs were designed for delivery of the long ovoid moulded head which was a common shape adapted from the prolonged labour. As a result of present-day care, this shape is less frequently seen and the head is less moulded and more spherical (Hibbard, 1989).

The basic instrument consists of two interlocking parts, one right and one left, and this is according to the side of the mothers pelvis in which they lie when applied. They each have a handle which leads into the shank where the lock is situated stabilizing the forceps during delivery. The blades of the forceps have a heel and a toe, the heel positioned nearest the shank. The blades are curved on the inner medial side producing the cephalic curve to conform to the fetal head. The superior and inferior edges produce the pelvic curve which conforms to the mother's pelvis. In addition

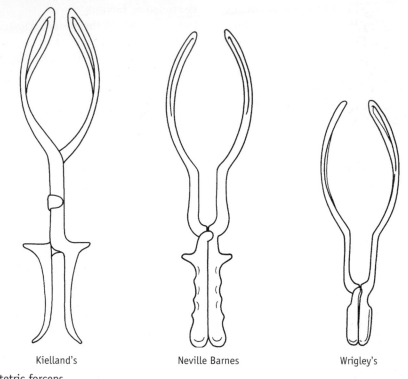

Kielland's   Neville Barnes   Wrigley's

Figure 58.1 Obstetric forceps.

there may be a locking or traction device (ALSO, 1996).

Forceps may be used in two ways: to exert traction without rotation; and to correct malposition, e.g. occipitoposterior position, by rotation prior to traction. Rotation is rarely performed now owing to the trauma to the mother and the baby. There are definitive texts available which outline the procedures for forceps delivery but here, it would appear more pertinent to discuss certain principles for all types of the delivery.

The operation may be performed at the pelvic outlet or controversially at the mid-pelvic level where rotation remains incomplete. High forceps should now never be contemplated because of the high morbidity associated with them.

There are three phases to the operation, *application* of the blades, *adjustment and articulation* and *traction*.

Application

Correct application is of great importance to the safe control of the head, allowing the operator to know the exact attitude of the head (Dennen and Hayashi, 1999). The left blade is usually applied first, avoiding having to cross the handles to engage the lock. Both are inserted holding the handle with finger and thumb

grip and cupping the blade with fingers of the other hand to protect maternal tissue and to guide the blade into position (ALSO, 1996) (Fig. 58.2).

Adjustment and articulation

If anything more than minimal force is necessary, then there is something wrong. Blades should come together and lock easily and if they do not, there is a problem which may require undue manipulation and cause trauma. They should be removed and reapplied (Hibbard, 1989). Forceps are correctly applied to the sides of the fetal head when the blades are located symmetrically between the orbits and the ears, reaching from the parietal eminences to the malar area and cheeks.

Traction

Traction is used to reproduce the normal mechanism of labour and there should be descent throughout the contraction. Assuming the clinical situation permits, traction should be timed to coincide with contractions and the direction should be in the axis of the pelvic curve (Fig. 58.3). A steady pull should be maintained and delivery should be effected within three contractions (Dennen and Hayashi, 1999).

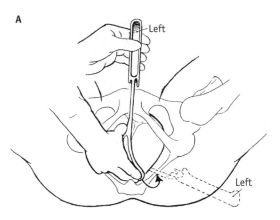

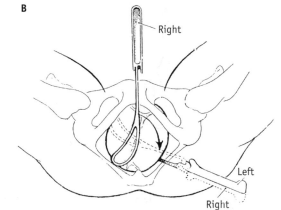

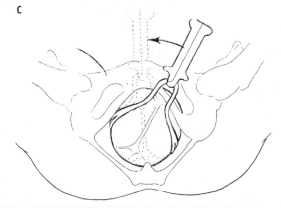

Figure 58.2 Forceps application. (From Dennen and Hayashi, 1999.)

Vacuum extraction

Vacuum extraction is a method of instrumental delivery which involves the use of a vacuum device as a traction instrument to assist delivery. The technique was developed from early work by Young, a Royal Navy surgeon in 1705, and Simpson in the 1840s (Chamberlain, 1989). The modern version was developed by Malmstrom in the 1950s.

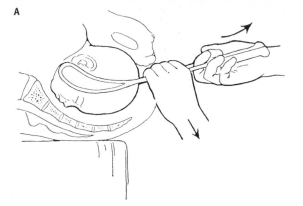

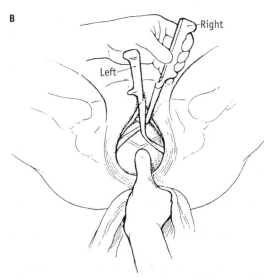

Figure 58.3 **A.** Traction. **B.** Removal of forceps. (From Dennen and Hayashi, 1999.)

The vacuum extractor or ventouse consists of a cup made of metal or soft material such as silicone rubber, a traction device and a vacuum system which provides negative pressure, by which the cup is attached to the fetal scalp. The cups were originally metal but the softer caps which have been available since the early 1980s are proving more popular. Previously, the metal cup formed a 'chignon', but now the soft cup relies on covering a larger surface area in order to develop sufficient traction, and this has led to less scalp trauma.

Contraindications specific to ventouse and in addition to those listed above for all instrumental deliveries are:

- malpresentations, e.g. face, brow, breech
- preterm labour at less than 36 weeks' gestation
- suspected fetal coagulopathy.

A

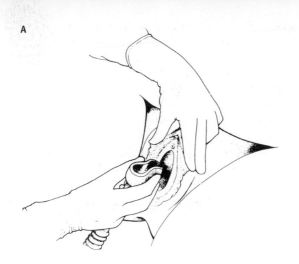

B

C

D

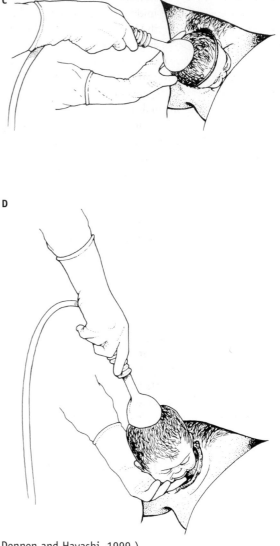

Figure 58.4   Application and delivery with ventouse. (From Dennen and Hayashi, 1999.)

Equipment and procedure (Fig. 58.4)

The cup is applied to the fetal head and, using suction, a vacuum is created applying a negative pressure of 0.2 kg/cm. The cup is checked for position and to exclude any entrapment of maternal tissue, and the vacuum is increased either in stages or rapidly to a maximum of 0.8 kg/cm. The artificial 'caput', is drawn into the cup, which is thus firmly fixed. Traction is then applied to coincide with the uterine contractions. The ventouse procedure should be abandoned if the cap falls off three times or if there is no progress after three pulls (ALSO, 1996). Once the delivery is completed, the vacuum is released and the cup is detached. The large caput succedaneum, described from its shape as a 'chignon', may give the baby a bizarre appearance. This subsides quickly, becoming a circular bruised area which clears more slowly.

> **Reflective Activity 58.2**
>
> Reflect on the last instrumental delivery that you attended. Consider whether you felt that you adequately prepared:
>
> - the woman
> - her partner
> - the equipment.
>
> Looking through the information here, what would you have done differently?

Midwife ventouse practitioners

The first course to prepare midwife ventouse practitioners was run by Bournemouth University in 1997. Whilst there is an ever-increasing number of midwives successfully completing the course and undertaking ventouse deliveries in clinical practice, concerns have been expressed that this expansion of their role will be to the detriment of normal midwifery (Rampersad, 1997). A survey undertaken in 2000 to seek information concerning the experiences of the midwife ventouse practitioners (MVP) interestingly found that from a total of 505 women to whom these midwives had been called because a ventouse delivery was thought to be needed, 129 (26%) achieved a normal birth facilitated by the MVP (Alexander *et al.*, unpublished work, 2000). The importance placed on maintaining the centrality of normality appears to be very evident, thereby reducing the medicalized influence.

Reflective Activity 58.3

Do you believe that midwives should perform forceps deliveries or undertake caesarean sections? Talk to colleagues and reflect on your beliefs of what constitutes midwifery practice and its boundaries. Read the available literature on the subjects and then write a list of what you feel is complementary to woman-centred midwifery practice and what is obstetric practice that might soon be provided by midwives only because of financial savings to trusts or convenience to obstetricians.

Postnatal care

At delivery, if the baby's condition permits, he or she should be given to the mother immediately. If resuscitation is required, then as soon as the condition is satisfactory, the baby should be given to the mother with relevant explanation for any necessary procedures that were undertaken. If the baby is transferred to the neonatal intensive care unit, then the parents must be kept informed of the baby's condition and taken to visit as soon as possible. Once the doctors have left, then the midwife should ensure that the parents have a quiet and protected time to recover and develop a relationship with their baby.

Postnatal observations will be as for any delivery, but particular attention should be paid to pain from perineal trauma, urinary output in case any damage has occurred to the bladder, and signs of postpartum haemorrhage due to uterine atony and trauma. Particular requirements may include analgesia and assistance with feeding owing to discomfort. It is also important to observe the neonate for any sign of trauma, and ensure that a thorough, careful examination is carried out with appropriate referral should any deviations from the normal be noted. Owing to the possible link discussed earlier with acute trauma symptoms and post-traumatic stress disorder, there must be an opportunity for the midwife to review with the woman, her experience, and discuss any concerns regarding the intervention and the procedure with the parents. It is also an appropriate time to ensure that the woman is assured that she did not 'fail'.

CAESAREAN SECTION

Caesarean section is the delivery of the fetus, placenta and membranes through a surgical incision in the abdominal wall and uterus. There are two types of caesarean section:

- *Lower segment caesarean section* (LSCS) is most frequently performed through a suprapubic (Pfannenstiel) transverse incision. This is the method of choice as there is a low incidence of wound dehiscence with an excellent cosmetic appearance (Dickinson, 1999). Occasionally a midline vertical incision proves necessary as it allows rapid access and can be enlarged without difficulty.

- *Classical upper segment caesarean section* involves a longitudinal incision in the upper uterine segment and is rarely performed because of the higher risk of scar rupture in a subsequent pregnancy (incidence 2.2%). It may be used in the case of a major degree of placenta praevia, cervical carcinoma, lower segment uterine myomas, or for the delivery of preterm infants prior to the 28th week when the lower uterine segment has not fully formed (Crichton *et al.*, 1991).

There is a public health concern associated with the well-publicized rise in the caesarean section rate and therefore, in 2000, an audit began to evaluate the role of caesarean sections in maternity care. The National Sentinel Caesarean Section Audit involved a collaboration between the Royal Colleges (RCOG, RCM, RCA) and the National Childbirth Trust, funded by the Department of Health through the National Institute for Clinical Excellence. The full report was published in October 2001. The audit found that 21.5% of births were by caesarean section, though there was a regional variation where the rate was 19.3% in the Northeast and 24.2% in London and Wales.

Other peripheral findings were that, though in most units a midwife was likely to be providing care to one woman at a time, there were a small number of units where a midwife would be responsible for three women at a time.

The increasing caesarean section rate in the UK is attributed to a variety of causes in varying sources of literature. These include delivery of preterm infants now likely to survive with good neonatal care, avoidance of litigation, lack of staff on maternity units, maternal request, increased medicalization of childbirth, increased induction rate and individual obstetrician's preferences in their practice. The Sentinel study also illustrates that the caesarean rate is raised in older women, black African or Caribbean women, previous caesarean section, and breech presentation and multiple pregnancy (Thomas and Parenjothy, 2001) (Table 58.1). It was suggested that in all of these categories, there may be an increased risk of complications requiring such intervention.

Caesarean section is a major surgical procedure and, in a small number of cases, it can save both neonatal and maternal lives, improve outcome for some babies who may have undergone extended labour, and reduce the potential risks of infection associated with some vaginal deliveries (Duff, 2000). Nevertheless, though the caesarean section rates have significantly increased, maternal and neonatal mortality does not appear to be decreasing, and indeed neonatal and maternal morbidity is increasing. Hillan (2000) realized

from available figures that 9–15% of women delivered by caesarean section suffer serious maternal morbidity, whilst another 65% did not feel fully recovered 3 months after caesarean section.

There is a plethora of literature highlighting the morbidity and the increased risk of mortality associated with caesarean section. Physical effects range from tiredness, backache, sleeping difficulties and depression, to wound and urinary tract infection (Hillan, 2000). There is an increased risk of haemorrhage, thromboembolism, peripartum hysterectomy, future miscarriages, ectopic pregnancies, placenta abruptio and praevia and reduced fertility (Wagner, 2000). Some mothers experience a sense of loss or failure because they have been unable to deliver their baby vaginally. Psychological effects of caesarean section include extreme disappointment, intense anxiety and a sense of inadequacy and failure, and may include acute trauma symptoms and post-traumatic stress disorder as previously associated with instrumental delivery (Creedy et al., 2000). There appears little difference between emergency or elective surgery.

Risks of caesarean section to the fetus

Owing to maternal cardiovascular changes, especially with spinal anaesthesia, low Apgar scores and relative fetal acidosis may occur. Later, respiratory distress may develop, which is usually due to transient tachypnoea of the newborn (see Chs 31, 35), the incidence being four times greater in babies delivered by elective caesarean section than in those who are delivered vaginally. This is thought to be due to the lack of catecholamines being produced by the mother, which would normally cross the placenta and 'switch off' the production of lung fluid by the fetal lung pneumocytes. It was thought that at birth there was an excess of up to 30 ml of fluid which may not have been absorbed by the lymphocytes, or by 'vaginal squeezing' as would happen during a vaginal birth, and therefore the neonate needs to cry lustily at birth to assist the absorption of this excess lung fluid (Strang, 1991). However, it is now thought that there is only about 35% of this fluid at term, and that it is absorbed, through the lymphatics, and changes in the pulmonary blood flow (Blackburn, 2003), and that the vaginal squeeze has a minor effect on fluid clearance.

Annibale et al. (1995) concluded in their study that abdominal delivery following an uncomplicated pregnancy remains a risk factor for adverse neonatal outcome. During a conference in 1999 entitled *The Rising Caesarean Section Rate: A Public Health Issue*, a

Table 58.1 Indications for caesarean section (Thomas and Parenjothy, 2001)

Indications	Caesarean section rate
Fetal distress/abnormal CTG	22%
Failure to progress/induction	20.4%
Previous caesarean section	13.8%
Breech position	10.8%
Maternal request	7.3%
Malpresentations	3.4%
Placenta praevia/bleeding	2.2%
Pre-eclampsia/eclampsia/HELLP	2.3%
Multiple pregnancy	1.2%

neonatologist came to the conclusion that babies should only be born by caesarean section if they are very large, in a difficult position or known to have a mother with a serious viral condition such as HIV (Duff, 2000).

Costs of caesarean section

The UK Audit Commission (1997) found that a caesarean section delivery cost approximately £760 more than a spontaneous delivery, not taking into account all the postoperative hospital and community support. It could be argued that there is no other major surgery undertaken in the NHS for a predominantly physiological event. It seems an inappropriate expenditure when there is a wealth of evidence available highlighting that 'one-to-one midwifery care' reduces intervention and morbidity and costs far less than expensive surgery and a surgical team. Investing in midwives would seem to prove a more valuable investment.

Indications for caesarean section

Examples of some indications for caesarean section include the following:

- hypertensive disorders, e.g. pre-eclampsia and eclampsia
- fetal distress
- failure or delay to progress in labour
- malpresentations such as breech, brow or shoulder presentations, but a breech presentation may be delivered vaginally if there is no suspected cephalopelvic disproportion or other complications
- previous or predicted shoulder dystocia
- prolapse of the umbilical cord in the first stage of labour
- antepartum haemorrhage due to severe abruption or placenta praevia
- major cephalopelvic disproportion
- severe intrauterine growth restriction
- severe rhesus isoimmunization
- active herpes genitalis
- maternal HIV infection
- previous vaginal reconstruction surgery
- pelvic tumours, e.g. cervical myomas (fibroids)
- fetal abnormality, e.g. hydrocephalus, gastroschisis.

Implications for midwifery practice

Whilst the majority of the list above appears appropriate for caesarean section, there is an increase of caesarean section due to 'failure to progress' and fetal distress. It would be advantageous now to revisit the areas discussed earlier in relation to instrumental delivery as they are also relevant to caesarean section. Additional points to be considered include:

- Early amniotomy is associated with an increased risk of caesarean section (Segal *et al.*, 1999).
- The use of continuous electronic fetal monitoring during labour can lead to an increase in caesarean sections and instrumental delivery. Thacker and Stroup (2000) reviewed the effects of routine electronic fetal monitoring during labour compared with intermittent auscultation. The review included 58855 women in 10 clinical trials. The results showed that there was no change in perinatal deaths or neonatal unit admissions and there was no evidence that cerebral palsy was reduced.

Reflective Activity 58.4

How do you normally gauge whether a woman is in the active stage of labour? Is this normally by examination or by maternal behaviour? If you were unable to examine the woman, how would you measure her progress?

Midwife's role

Whether surgery is an emergency or elective procedure, the midwife should ensure that the woman understands the reasons for surgery and that a written consent form is obtained for the operation.

A sample of venous blood must be collected for full blood count, haemoglobin level and cross-matching. The woman should be dressed in a theatre gown and wearing identification labels. Antiembolic (TED) stockings should be applied. It is preferable that the woman is not wearing any make-up to ensure that the anaesthetist can observe her colour, that jewellery is taped or removed for safety reasons because of the use of diathermy during the procedure and that her pubic area has been shaved, removing as little as absolutely necessary for the incision.

In theatre Along with the usual theatre staff, a paediatrician will be present for each case and the midwife will usually assist at the resuscitaire after receiving the baby at delivery. It is preferable that the anaesthetist can meet, examine and discuss any procedures with the woman prior to the surgery, although this may not be possible in emergency circumstances. The anaesthetist will be fully involved with the woman once in theatre but the midwife should remain with her and her partner as support for both of them. Operating theatres can be quite frightening areas to be in.

The fetal heart will still require frequent auscultation, and this should be recorded.

Anaesthesia

General anaesthesia in obstetric patients is fraught with difficulties. In the last Confidential Enquiries into Maternal Deaths (Lewis, 2001), three women died as a direct consequence of anaesthetic problems, though there were also a number of deaths in which anaesthetic care was substandard.

The problems include raised maternal intragastric pressure; acidity of gastric contents; aortocaval occlusion if the supine position is employed; the adverse effects on the fetus of the drugs used, or of maternal hypoxia or hypotension; placental insufficiency; and intrapartum fetal hypoxia. These problems are exacerbated in the case of preterm infants, or in the woman whose condition is poor, i.e. if she is eclamptic.

Intubation in the pregnant woman may be difficult because of the posture of the neck in pregnancy or laryngeal oedema in cases of pregnancy-induced hypertension.

To minimize the risk of supine hypotensive syndrome, the operating table is tilted laterally, or the woman is wedged at a lateral tilt until the infant is delivered. A foot cushion is usually employed to elevate the legs from the table to avoid venous stasis in the calf muscles; other means, such as TED stockings, should be used to avoid the risk of venous thrombosis. The bladder will be emptied and a catheter inserted which will remain in place during the procedure. The fetal heart will be listened to prior to surgery.

Acid aspiration syndrome (Mendelson's syndrome)

One of the complications that may occur is acid aspiration syndrome, a life-threatening condition which should not occur if adequate precautions are taken. It arises as a result of aspiration of acidic stomach contents into the lungs (Sharp, 1997).

Available evidence states that for acid aspiration to be severe, the minimum amount of gastric juice would be 0.4 ml/kg, approximately 28 ml for a 70 kg woman, at a pH level 2.5 or less (Sharp, 1997). Yet it has been observed that whatever the time of the last oral intake and the onset of the anaesthetic, there is never usually less than 100 ml in the stomach, as the secretory activity of the stomach is increased in the absence of oral intake.

Obstetric anaesthesia requires prevention of acid aspiration syndrome, which is characterized by wheezing, cyanosis and tachycardia and gives rise to adult respiratory distress syndrome (ARDS) due to aspiration pneumonitis. Because of the risk of this potentially life-threatening syndrome, Mendelson, who recognized the syndrome in 1946, suggested that all women should be prohibited from eating and drinking in labour. The pregnant woman is at risk because of delayed gastric emptying arising from gastric hypotonia, altered relationship between the oesophagus, stomach and diaphragm, pressure of the enlarged uterus, gastric hypersecretion in labour and compromised lower oesophageal tone (Tsen and Datta, 1999). Unfortunately, though Mendelson's research was carried out more than 50 years ago, it continues to influence care provided, and many women in normal labour are still restricted to little or no food and restricted fluids.

Sellick's manoeuvre (cricoid pressure) during the passage of an endotracheal tube is essential in all cases to protect the airway from regurgitated stomach contents (see Fig. 58.5).

The cricoid cartilage is compressed with the fingers towards the cervical spine to occlude the oesophagus (Vanner, 1993). The assistant, who may be the midwife, maintains the pressure until the endotracheal tube is in place. One woman in the last triennium, 1997–1999, died through aspiration pneumonia following anaesthetic, during which it was not clear whether cricoid pressure was used (Lewis, 2001).

There must be protocols to follow in the case of 'failed or difficult induction' to prevent fatalities and it is recommended that administration of obstetric anaesthesia should only be performed by an experienced anaesthetist. Prevention is the significant feature and a number of measures are employed to prevent the occurrence of acid aspiration syndrome. These include the administration of antacid preparations such as sodium citrate 30 ml given orally 30 minutes prior to the induction of the anaesthetic (Ostheimer, 1992). A histamine-2 receptor antagonist such as ranitidine 150 mg may be given, usually prior to surgery. It is recommended that it is administered to all women suffering from pre-eclampsia because of the high incidence of mortalities from acid aspiration syndrome in this group of women. Metoclopramide may be given by intramuscular injection preoperatively as it is an antiemetic and increases gastric emptying.

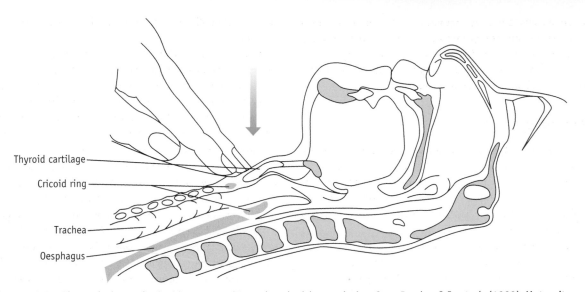

Thyroid cartilage

Cricoid ring

Trachea

Oesphagus

Figure 58.5 The technique of cricoid pressure. (Reproduced with permission from Reeder, S.J. *et al.* (1983) *Maternity Nursing,* 15th edn, p. 585. Philadelphia: Lippincott.)

Spinal (subarachnoid) and epidural anaesthesia

Many caesarean sections are now performed under epidural or spinal, rather than general, anaesthesia (see Ch. 27). This removes the risks associated with general anaesthesia and enables the mother to see and hold her baby at birth. It is reported that this method is superior in facilitating the mother–baby relationship. The partner may be present so that he can be supportive to the mother and share in the experience.

However, even this technique carries its own risk, as illustrated by one of the women who died in the 1997–1999 triennium (Lewis, 2001) following a high sensory and motor block, through an epidural 'top-up'.

This text is inappropriate for discussion of either epidural or spinal anaesthesia in depth and the reader is recommended to visit anaesthesia text books to explore the technicalities further.

Immediate postoperative care

If the woman is awake, the midwife should ensure that the baby is shown to her as soon as possible. If the baby does not require resuscitation following delivery, opportunity for the mother to hold and touch her baby as soon as possible should be actively encouraged (see below).

In the immediate postoperative recovery period, regardless of the method of anaesthesia, pulse, blood pressure, respirations, colour, state of consciousness, vaginal loss, wound dressing, catheter and wound drainage are observed, as appropriate. If the woman

has had a general anaesthetic, extubation is performed. This involves removal of the endotracheal tube once reflexes have returned, suction is carried out and the operating table is tilted head down. Vigilance at this stage is important as the woman may not be fully conscious and inhalation of gastric contents may still occur. The woman is placed on her side to maintain the airway, assist drainage of secretions and prevent airway obstruction by the tongue.

Infusion of intravenous fluids is monitored and recorded on the anaesthetic sheet. An analgesic may be administered for pain relief. When the woman's postoperative condition is satisfactory, the anaesthetist will give permission for her to be discharged to the care of the ward staff. Instructions and details of the surgery and anaesthetic are recorded in the notes and given to the receiving midwife.

Maternal–infant attachment

The baby is received by the midwife and any resuscitative measures are carried out by a paediatrician, or by a midwife skilled in neonatal resuscitation. However, if the mother is conscious and the baby appears well at birth, the baby should be given to the mother immediately. There are many maternity units now that actively encourage breastfeeding in the theatre if the mother wishes it, and skin-to-skin contact if it is safe and convenient to do so. A preterm or ill baby will be admitted to the neonatal unit for special or intensive care. The parents will naturally be very anxious if their baby requires such care and should be encouraged to visit as soon as possible. The neonatal unit staff often take photographs of the baby to give to the parents whilst visiting is difficult.

Record-keeping

Accurate and contemporaneous records are made of all observations and treatments. The midwife responsible for the care of mother and baby will give a detailed handover report to the ward midwife. This report will include the condition of the mother and the baby at birth, and the care and any treatment given before transfer to the ward or, in the case of a sick or preterm baby, to the neonatal unit. This information will enable all staff involved with the mother and baby during the early postnatal period to give appropriate care and support.

Subsequent postnatal care

Postnatal observations

There is a high risk of postpartum haemorrhage, adding to the amount of blood lost during the operation. The uterus may not contract effectively and there is also the very serious complication of the unsuspected continuation of intraperitoneal bleeding after the operation. The following observation and care routines are guidelines only, but denote safe and best practice:

- Pulse and blood pressure should be checked every 15 minutes for the first 2 hours, then every 30 minutes for the next 2 hours, reducing to hourly for 2 hours, 2-hourly for 2 days then 4-hourly for 3 days.
- Temperature, should be recorded twice daily for the first 3 days then daily, because of the frequency of infection following caesarean section. Other symptoms of infection vary according to the virulence of the organisms involved. A mild uterine infection would present on about the third postnatal day with a raised temperature and pulse rate, subinvolution of the uterus and profuse red, offensive lochia. If untreated, it may cause peritonitis, and the danger signs, for which the midwife should be constantly alert, include a rising pulse rate, pyrexia, vomiting, and abdominal pain and distension.
- Ensure that the intravenous line is patent and effective whilst it is in situ to assist with fluid administration until the woman maintains her own fluid balance and provide an emergency line should there be a haemorrhage.
- Check vaginal loss for excessive bleeding and wound loss on the dressing at each observation.

- Adequate pain relief should be offered frequently, acknowledging that the woman has undergone major abdominal surgery. Initially, pain relief may be administered in the form of intramuscular opiates, e.g. morphia, but later suppositories or oral analgesics will be given, as required, within prescribed limits.
- Oral fluids are offered soon after the operation. A light diet can be started when the woman feels ready to eat, unless the surgeon requests that food is withheld until bowel sounds are heard, usually if the bowel has been handled excessively during surgery. Intravenous fluids are then maintained until bowel sounds are heard and the woman has started to eat. *Paralytic ileus* frequently accompanies peritonitis and is recognized by an inability to pass flatus or have the bowels open because the bowel has become paralysed. This is a very serious complication. Antibiotic drugs are given to overcome the infection. Because the absorption of fluids and nutrients from the paralysed intestinal tract is disrupted, fluids, electrolytes and glucose are given intravenously until the condition is resolved. Aspiration of the stomach with a Ryle's tube is necessary until the paralytic ileus recovers and the mother is able to take fluids by mouth without vomiting.
- The urinary catheter if in situ is removed as per the surgeon's recommendations. However, even without a catheter, fluid balance should be observed for the first 3 days as the woman may be actually passing urine but not in significant amounts leaving a residual amount in the bladder.
- Antiembolic stockings, early ambulation, active and passive leg exercises are encouraged to help reduce the incidence of deep vein thrombosis. There is always a possibility of pulmonary embolism whenever a laparotomy has been performed. Collapse and even sudden death may occur from this serious complication, often between the 10th and 14th postoperative days.
- A bed bath and a vulval toilet are still enjoyed by women following a caesarean section. They should have an opportunity to clean their teeth and put on fresh and light clothing. The dressing is usually removed on the following day and the woman is assisted with a shower and afterwards shown how to dry the wound. She will be encouraged to shower daily when she can manage safely alone.
- Wound care includes inspection and, if a drain is present, it is shortened and removed according to the doctor's instructions. If clips or non-absorbable

skin sutures have been used, they too will be removed at a time directed by the surgeon, usually about the fifth postoperative day. If possible, the woman should be encouraged to expose the wound to the fresh air to dry the wound and assist with healing when she is resting.

- The mother with a painful abdominal wound will require help in finding a comfortable position in which to breastfeed her baby. The midwife can suggest that she tries lying on her side in bed with her baby alongside her, or on a pillow tucked under her arm, with the baby's trunk and feet under her arm, rather than lying across her abdomen. Although early contact and involvement in the care of her baby is encouraged, a caesarean section is a major abdominal operation and the mother will require more help and support during the first few postoperative days, and again when she is transferred home.

- Following caesarean section, most women are transferred home on the fifth postoperative day to the care of their midwife in the community. An earlier discharge may not always be appropriate, as some women may not have any support at home and may have other children to care for, and are sometimes in inadequate housing.

- Contraception will be discussed before discharge and advice given, if required, about the provision of services and appropriate methods.

- Once again, psychological support may be necessary because of the findings discussed earlier of acute trauma symptoms and post-traumatic stress disorder. Discussion regarding the reasons for the operation and the procedures is necessary.

Trial of scar – vaginal birth after caesarean section (VBAC)

There are many different rates of successful vaginal birth reported after caesarean section. Dickinson (1999) gave the results of two studies undertaken in the last decade: one, by Flamm, included 5022 women and revealed a 75% vaginal birth rate; the other was by Miller who reviewed 12 707 trials of labour and reported an 82% successful vaginal birth rate. The indication for the previous caesarean section should, of course, come into consideration.

There is no evidence to support the policy of some trusts that these women should have an intravenous cannula sited and continuous electronic fetal monitoring once labour has commenced. There is also debate

regarding place of birth, some opting for home birth and others in hospital. This has to be considered individually with each woman. As in all labours, close observations of maternal and fetal condition are made, especially noting any tenderness or pain over the caesarean scar. The other signs that may occur include signs of abnormal uterine action, signs of maternal haemorrhage and acute fetal bradycardia.

CERVICAL CERCLAGE

Cervical cerclage is a surgical intervention performed usually under general anaesthetic in the second trimester of pregnancy, whereby a suture is placed around the cervix to prevent it from dilating where there is cervical incompetence (Fig. 58.6). The aim of the procedure is to prolong pregnancy and thus improve the fetal and neonatal outcome. 'Cervical incompetence', a term first used by Gream in 1865, is a condition where there is laxity of the cervix which causes the cervical os to dilate very easily (Jackson and Garite, 1992). It may be the cause of mid-trimester miscarriage, or preterm labour and delivery.

Causes
Cervical incompetence may be congenital, for example uterine abnormality, or it may be caused by intrauterine

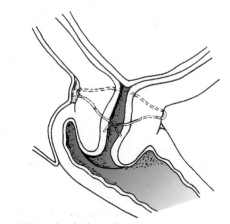

Figure 58.6 Cervical cerclage.

exposure to diethylstilbestrol, or it may be the result of previous cervical surgery; for example, excessive dilatation for curettage, cone biopsy, Manchester repair or cervical amputation. Other causes include hormonal and biochemical influences (Jackson and Garite, 1992).

Diagnosis

Typically the history is one of successive mid-trimester abortions, characterized by rupture of the membranes in the absence of painful uterine contractions and a short, relatively painless labour with a live fetus (Ware Branch, 1986). It may also be diagnosed by serial vaginal examinations to assess the dilatation of the cervix. Ultrasound scans show changes in the length of the cervix, with the internal os more than 3 cm dilated and funnelling of the membranes.

Recent evidence indicates that cervical cerclage should be offered to women who have had two previous mid-trimester abortions or preterm labours, and that it is beneficial in these cases despite the risks associated with increased medical intervention and infection.

Techniques

Cervical cerclage may be performed by the technique described by Shirodkar in 1960, or by McDonald in 1957, the latter being simpler and more commonly used. The Shirodkar suture involves making an incision in the supravaginal portion of the cervix so that a non-absorbable tape or silk can be placed higher around the cervix, whereas the McDonald suture is inserted into the actual cervix, rather like the purse-string suture in an appendicectomy (Stirrat and Wardle, 1999). This holds the cervix closed and therefore prevents spontaneous abortion. The suture is removed just before term, or earlier if labour commences.

The treatment is successful in many cases, but is not without risk and involves a general anaesthetic for insertion of the suture. Obstetric interventions such as induction of labour and caesarean section may be necessary and there is a higher risk of puerperal sepsis (Stirrat and Wardle, 1999).

Contraindications

These include:

- significant uterine contractions
- ruptured membranes
- proven or suspected intrauterine infection
- uterine bleeding
- fetal abnormality.

Complications

Complications that may occur following cerclage include:

- cervical laceration
- premature rupture of the membranes
- stimulation of myometrial activity
- sepsis
- endotoxic shock
- cervical dystocia or cervical stenosis
- vesicovaginal fistula
- uterine rupture
- anaesthetic complications.

CONCLUSION

The number of normal physiological births appears to be decreasing in the UK, whilst figures for caesarean section and instrumental deliveries are rising, with increasing neonatal and maternal morbidity and static mortality (ENB, 1999; Thomas and Parenjothy, 2001). This rise may cause an eroding of the midwife's role, skills and knowledge with an associated lack of confidence in the ability of midwives to care for physiological birth. In this climate, midwives should reflect upon their own practice and make continuous professional and practice development part of their work. Nevertheless, there are still a significant number of women who will require an operative-style delivery, and they require the midwife's unique skills and understanding in addition to 'normal' postnatal care. Midwives must ensure that they provide appropriate and relevant care tailored to each individual woman to minimize the associated morbidity.

KEY POINTS

- The potential morbidity and mortality risk to woman and neonate of any operative delivery must be balanced by the value of these procedures in bringing the woman and baby at risk to safety.

- There are several aspects of the care provided by midwives and their colleagues which may reduce the need for intervention and augmentation, such as positioning, nutrition and the presence of a supportive person.

- It is important that midwives are familiar with the principles of anaesthesia and caring for women who may require anaesthesia or instrumental delivery.
- The midwife must consider strategies for ensuring adequate preparation for the woman and her partner for all possibilities, and work to ensure that whatever intervention may be needed they will feel positive, empowered and supported throughout.

REFERENCES

Advanced Life Support in Obstetrics (ALSO) (1996) *Advanced Life Support in Obstetrics Training Manual.* Missouri: American Academy of Family Physicians.

Annibale, D., Hulsey, T. & Wagner, C. (1995) Comparative neonatal morbidity of abdominal and vaginal deliveries after uncomplicated pregnancies. *Archives of Pediatrics and Adolescent Medicine* 149(8): 862–867.

Audit Commission (1997) *First Class Delivery: A National Survey of Women's Views of Maternity Care.* Oxford: Audit Commission.

Bick, D., MacArthur, C. & Keighley, M. (1997) Faecal incontinence after childbirth. *British Journal of Obstetrics and Gynaecology* 104(1): 46–50.

Birth Choice UK (2001) Accessible on www.BirthchoiceUK.com

Blackburn, S.T. (2003) *Maternal, Fetal and Neonatal Physiology – A Clinical Perspective*, 2nd edn. Philadelphia: W.B. Saunders.

Chadwick, L., Pemberton, P. & Kurinczuk, J. (1996) Neonatal subgaleal haematoma: associated risk factors, complications and outcome. *Journal of Paediatrics and Child Health* 32(3): 228–232.

Chamberlain, G. (1989) The vacuum extractor. In: Turnbull, A. & Chamberlain, G. (eds) *Obstetrics.* London: Churchill Livingstone.

Creedy, D., Shochet, I. & Horsfall, J. (2000) Childbirth and the development of acute trauma symptoms: incidence and contributing factors. *Birth* 27(2): 104–111.

Crichton, S.M., Pierce, J.M. & Stanton, S.L. (1991) Complications of caesarean section. In: Studd, J.W.W. (ed) *Progress in Obstetrics and Gynaecology*, Vol. 9. Edinburgh: Churchill Livingstone.

Dennen, P.C. & Hayashi, R. (1999) Assisted vaginal delivery. In: James, D.K., Steer, P.J., Weiner, C.P. & Gonik, B. (eds) *High Risk Pregnancy Management Options.* London: W.B. Saunders.

Dickinson, J.E. (1999) Cesarean section. In: James, D.K., Steer, P.J., Weiner, C.P. et al. (eds) *High Risk Pregnancy Management Options.* London: W.B. Saunders.

Duff, E. (2000) Risks of caesarean section: who is sneezing, who is catching the cold? *MIDIRS Midwifery Digest* 10(1): 73–74.

English National Board for Nursing, Midwifery and Health Visiting (ENB) 1999 *Midwifery Practice: Identifying the Developments and the Difference.* London: ENB.

Gupta, J.K. & Nikodem, V.C. (2001) Women's position during the second stage of labour. *The Cochrane Library*, Issue 1. Oxford: Update Software.

Hibbard, B.M. (1989) Forceps delivery. In: Turnbull, A. & Chamberlain, G. (eds) *Obstetrics.* London: Churchill Livingstone.

Hillan, E. (2000) The aftermath of caesarean delivery. *MIDIRS Midwifery Digest* 10(1): 70–72.

Hodnett, E.D. (2001) Caregiver support for women during childbirth (Cochrane Review). *The Cochrane Library*, Issue 1. Oxford: Update Software.

Jackson, D.J. & Garite, T.J. (1992) Surgical correction of uterine abnormalities. In: Plauche, W.C., Morrison, J.C. & O'Sullivan, M.J. (eds) *Surgical Obstetrics.* Philadelphia: W.B. Saunders.

Johanson, R. & Menon, B. (2000) Vacuum extraction versus forceps for assisted vaginal delivery (Cochrane Review). *The Cochrane Library*, Issue 1. Oxford: Update Software.

Johnson, N., Lilford, R., Guthrie, K. et al. (1997) Randomised trial comparing a policy of early with selective amniotomy in uncomplicated labour at term. *British Journal of Obstetrics and Gynaecology* 104(3): 340–346.

Jolly, J., Walker, J. & Bhabra, K. (1999) Subsequent obstetric performance related to primary mode of delivery. *British Journal of Obstetrics and Gynaecology* 106(3): 227–232.

Lewis, G. (ed) (2001) *Why Mothers Die 1997–99: Fifth Report of the Confidential Enquiries into Maternal Deaths in the United Kingdom.* London: CEMD: associated with NICE, RCOG.

Ludka, L.M. & Roberts, C. (1993) Eating and drinking in labour: a literature review. *Journal of Nurse–Midwifery* 38(4): 199–207.

Mander, R. (1994) Epidural analgesia 2: research basis. *British Journal of Midwifery* 2(1): 12–16.

Mark, R. (1961) Dependence of uterine muscle contractions on pH with reference to prolonged labour. *Journal of Obstetrics and Gynaecology* 68: 584.

O'Regan, M. (1998) Active management of labour. *AIMS Journal* 10(2): 1–7.

Ostheimer, G.W. (1992) *Manual of Obstetric Anaesthesia.* New York: Churchill Livingstone.

Page, L. (2000) *The New Midwifery: Science and Sensitivity.* London: Churchill Livingstone.

Pearson, J.F. (1981) A short history of the obstetric forceps. *Maternal and Child Health* 6(May): 198–204.

Rampersad, K. (1997) Letter to the editor. *British Journal of Midwifery* 5(11): 704.

Segal, D., Sheiner, E., Yohai, D. *et al.* (1999) Early amniotomy – high risk factor for cesarean section. *European Journal of Obstetrics and Gynecology and Reproductive Biology* 86(2): 145–149.

Sharp, D. (1997) Restriction of oral intake for women in labour. *British Journal of Midwifery* 5(7): 409–412.

Stirrat, G.M. & Wardle, P.G. (1999) Recurrent miscarriage. In: James, D.K., Steer, P.J., Weiner, C.P. *et al.* (eds) *High Risk Pregnancy Management Options*, 2nd edn. London: W.B. Saunders.

Strang, L.B. (1991) Fetal lung fluid secretion and reabsorption. *Physiological Reviews* 71: 991–1016.

Studd, J. (1973) Partograms and nomograms of cervical dilatation in management of primigravid labour. *British Medical Journal* 4(5890): 451–455.

Swift, L. (1991) Labour and fasting. *Nursing Times* 87(48): 64–65.

Teng, F.Y. & Sayre, J.W. (1997) Vacuum extraction: does duration predict scalp injury? *Obstetrics and Gynecology* 89(2): 281–285.

Thacker, S. & Stroup, D. (2000) Continuous electronic heart rate monitoring for fetal assessment during labour.

The Cochrane Library, Issue 3. Oxford: Update Software.

Thomas, J. & Parenjothy, S. (CESU) (2001) *The National Sentinel Caesarean Section Audit.* London: RCOG Press.

Towner, D., Castro, M., Eby-Wilkens, E. *et al.* (1999) Effects of mode of delivery in nulliparous women on neonatal intracranial injury. *New England Journal of Medicine* 342(23): 1709–1714.

Tsen, L.C. & Datta, S. (1999) Anaesthesia for high risk parturients. In: James, D.K., Steer, P.J., Weiner, C.P. *et al.* (eds) *High Risk Pregnancy Management Options.* London: W.B. Saunders.

Vacca, A. (1996) Birth by vacuum extraction: neonatal outcome. *Journal of Paediatrics and Child Health* 32(3): 204–206.

Vanner, R.G. (1993) Mechanisms of regurgitation and its prevention with cricoid pressure. *International Journal of Obstetric Anesthesia* 2(4): 207–215.

Wagner, M. (1994) *Pursuing The Birth Machine.* Australia: ACE Graphics.

Wagner, M. (2000) Choosing caesarean section. *Lancet* 356(9242): 1677–1680.

Walsh, D. (2000) Evidence based practice Part 4: Fetal monitoring should be controlled. *British Journal of Midwifery* 8(8): 511–516.

Ware Branch, D. 1986 Operations for cervical incompetence. *Clinical Obstetrics and Gynecology* 29(2): 240–254.

FURTHER READING

Berg, M., Lundren, I., Hermansson, E. *et al.* (1996) Women's experience of the encounter with the midwife during childbirth. *Midwifery* 12(1): 11–15.
The study examines the uniqueness and the importance of the relationship between midwife and woman and provides an opportunity for midwives to reflect upon their communication and behaviour towards the women that they care for.

Dickinson, J.E. (1999) Previous cesarean section. In: James, D.K., Steer, P.J., Weiner, C.P. *et al.* (eds) *High Risk Pregnancy Management Options.* London: W.B. Saunders.
With the increase in caesarean section, there is a risk of setting a precedent for the future. However, there is a reluctance by some women and clinicians to accept vaginal birth as a viable option after caesarean section. This chapter is highly recommended to those offering truly informed choice to women because of its unbiased analysis and comprehensive list of references.

Jordan, L. (2001) Reducing obstetric risk. Why do women sue? *MIDIRS Midwifery Digest* 11(1): 117–119.
One of the reasons given for the increase in instrumental and caesarean deliveries is fear of litigation. This article written by a solicitor, investigates reasons for claims against maternity services, and is of great importance to all who work within them in these litigious days.

Wagner, M. (2000) Choosing caesarean section. *Lancet* 356(9242): 1677–1680.
This paper debates the issues around caesarean section, skilfully handling the most controversial issues such as its convenience to both women and obstetricians, arguing the ethical dilemma, resource implications, effect on public health, with an honest approach to safety. Useful for midwives, obstetricians and women.

59

Complications of the Third Stage of Labour

Patricia Lindsay

LEARNING OUTCOMES

After reading this chapter you will be able to:

- discuss the types and causes of complications of the third stage of labour
- describe the midwife's management of the emergency situation
- outline further treatments which may be necessary
- discuss the implications of complications in the third stage for the woman and her partner.

POSTPARTUM HAEMORRHAGE

Postpartum haemorrhage is one of the most serious of all the complications of midwifery. It may happen without warning after any delivery and, as there is a placental circulation of approximately 600 ml/min at term, the mother can lose blood with alarming rapidity (Blackburn, 2003). Postpartum haemorrhage is still a significant cause of maternal mortality and morbidity in the UK. Often there is no doctor present and in this situation the prompt and intelligent action of the midwife may spare the mother dangerous blood loss and perhaps even save her life. It is therefore essential that the midwife has a thorough understanding of this subject. All maternity units should have a policy for management of postpartum haemorrhage and regular 'fire drills' should be organized to ensure that all staff respond quickly and appropriately (DoH, 1998; Lewis, 2001).

Reflective Activity 59.1

Locate and read your local policies for management of third stage emergencies. Are they in line with the recommendations of the CEMD (Confidential Enquiries into Maternal Deaths; DoH, 1998; Lewis, 2001)?

Definition

Postpartum haemorrhage is defined as excessive bleeding from the genital tract occurring any time from the birth of the child to the end of the puerperium.

Primary haemorrhage refers to the first 24 hours. This is the commonest and most dangerous type, complicating approximately 6% of all deliveries (including caesarean sections).

Secondary or puerperal haemorrhage occurs after 24 hours and before the end of the puerperium, that is, the sixth postnatal week. This is apparently uncommon, affecting 1–3% of all deliveries; however, this may be an underestimation (Pelage *et al.*, 1999a).

The word 'excessive' requires careful interpretation. Traditionally a loss of 500 ml or more at delivery has been regarded as a postpartum haemorrhage. However, definitions may vary between maternity units according to the general health profile of their particular client group. Smaller losses later in the puerperium would be considered excessive.

Estimating blood loss

Blood lost at the end of labour is extremely difficult to measure. It stains sheets, towels and gowns; it mixes with liquor; it trickles to the floor and is mopped up; it clots and the clot is conscientiously collected and measured in a jug, but it is not always appreciated that the 360 ml clot is only the solid part of more than

600 ml of blood. Visual estimation is at best approximate and is often unreliable. Prasertcharoensuk *et al.* (2000) demonstrated an average underestimation of 100 ml, with greater inaccuracies in measurement of higher losses. This echoed earlier findings that blood loss can be underestimated by 30–50% (Levy, 1990; Levy and Moore, 1985).

Thus, definitions of the amount which constitutes postpartum haemorrhage are of little clinical usefulness. It is much more important to assess the effect of the blood loss on the mother. In this context 'excessive' means any amount, however small, which adversely affects the mother.

Causes of postpartum haemorrhage

Postpartum haemorrhage arises from two sources:

- the placental site – usually due to myometrial atony
- genital tract laceration – so-called 'traumatic' haemorrhage.

Primary postpartum haemorrhage from the placental site

The immediate cause of primary placental site postpartum haemorrhage is failure of the uterus to contract and retract adequately. If the many uterine blood vessels are not squeezed or ligated by compression from the muscle fibres surrounding them, blood loss can be rapid and dangerous. This may occur because the myometrium is flaccid or atonic, or because retained placental tissue is preventing effective uterine contraction. These two causes account for 80% of all cases of postpartum haemorrhage (Lewellyn Jones, 1999).

Prediction and risk factors

It is not possible to predict accurately that any particular woman will have a postpartum haemorrhage, but the risk is increased in certain circumstances:

- *A history of previous postpartum haemorrhage or retained placenta.* This may recur.
- *Multiple pregnancy, polyhydramnios and fetal macrosomia.* In these circumstances the overdistended uterus may not retract well. In multiple pregnancy there is a larger placental site, which is also more likely to encroach upon the poorly retractile lower uterine segment, thus increasing the risk of haemorrhage.
- *Anaemia.* An anaemic woman is less able to withstand haemorrhage and may collapse after even a small loss.

- *Antepartum haemorrhage.* A woman who has suffered either placenta praevia or abruptio placentae may subsequently have a postpartum haemorrhage. In the case of placenta praevia this is because the retractile ability of the lower uterine segment is deficient and therefore control of bleeding from the placental site is poor. A Couvelaire uterus may occur in severe, concealed placental abruption and the damaged muscle fibres fail to contract and retract effectively to control haemorrhage (Fig. 59.1). The midwife should remember that a woman who has had an antepartum haemorrhage may be somewhat anaemic and this further increases the threat from postpartum haemorrhage.
- *Prolonged labour.* If contractions have been weak or uncoordinated during the first and second stages of labour, this may be expected to continue in the third stage and the uterus will fail to contract and retract effectively. Occasionally prolonged labour because of mechanical difficulty may lead to uterine exhaustion, atony and thus postpartum haemorrhage.
- *Pre-eclampsia/hypertensive disease in pregnancy.* This association may be a reflection of the fact that these women are more likely to have induced labours and an operative delivery. Coagulopathy is also a potential complication of hypertensive disease and

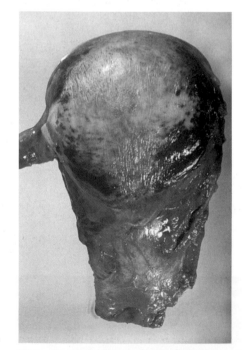

Figure 59.1   Couvelaire uterus. (From Beischer *et al.*, 1997, with permission of Harcourt Publishers Ltd.)

some drugs used to prevent seizures may contribute to uterine atony.

- *General anaesthesia.* Uterine atony may occur if anaesthesia is prolonged. It is especially likely if halogenated anaesthetic agents are used.
- *Fibroids.* The presence of uterine fibroids may interfere with efficient contraction and retraction.
- *Mismanagement of the third stage of labour.* Massaging, squeezing or otherwise 'fiddling' with the uterus can disrupt the rhythm of myometrial activity, causing only partial separation of the placenta.
- *Retained placenta.* Unless the uterus is empty it cannot retract completely, so a partially separated retained placenta (whether or not the result of mismanagement) or retained blood clot can itself diminish the contractions and worsen the bleeding.
- *Tocolytic drugs.* Drugs given to suppress uterine activity in preterm labour may cause atony in the third stage should labour progress. This will contribute to postpartum haemorrhage.
- *Induced or augmented labours.* The uterine inefficiency which necessitates the use of oxytocics may contribute to postpartum haemorrhage.
- *Inversion of the uterus.* Any degree of uterine inversion will interfere with efficient contraction and retraction and will precipitate postpartum haemorrhage.
- *Infection.* Chorioamnionitis is associated with primary postpartum haemorrhage.

There is little evidence that postpartum haemorrhage is commoner in grande multiparae. High parity is no longer considered to be a risk per se. However, the woman who has borne several children, particularly with short inter-pregnancy intervals, may have depleted iron stores. In this case, a comparatively small blood loss may produce signs of hypoxaemia and underperfusion. The midwife should assess each woman's history and current health status on an individual basis.

The midwife must remember that postpartum haemorrhage may occur as a complication of otherwise completely normal labours when even the most careful retrospective assessment fails to explain it (ACOG Technical Bulletin Number 243, 1998; Park and Sachs, 1999).

Other causes

Disseminated intravascular coagulation (DIC) is a coagulopathy which results in a steady, persistent oozing of blood even though there is adequate uterine contraction and retraction. No clot forms and the blood remains liquid. Venepuncture sites may ooze and petechiae may appear. It can occur as a result of severe primary postpartum haemorrhage. In this case it arises when supplies of circulating fibrinogen and other blood clotting factors become depleted and the coagulation system fails. The hypoxia which accompanies major haemorrhage may cause the local release of thromboplastin from the damaged tissue, triggering the formation of microthrombi all round the body. This further exhausts the circulating coagulation factors. The thrombi will block capillary vessels, thus causing more tissue damage and release of thromboplastin. Disseminated intravascular coagulation may also occur as a secondary effect of other major problems such as concealed abruptio placentae, amniotic fluid embolus, severe pre-eclampsia and eclampsia. It can also follow prolonged retention in the uterus of a dead fetus.

As the condition worsens, blood levels of fibrin degradation products (FDPs) rise. These are toxic to the myometrium and will interfere with efficient uterine contraction and retraction, thus exacerbating the haemorrhage.

At every delivery the midwife should note whether the blood is clotting and whether the clot is firm or friable. Absent or unstable clot formation is an indication of coagulopathy: this must be treated promptly and the midwife should call for medical assistance without delay. If DIC is allowed to progress, the condition will become uncontrollable and maternal death may ensue.

Medical disorders such as idiopathic thrombocytopenia and inherited coagulopathies such as von Willebrand's disease also increase the risk of both primary and secondary postpartum haemorrhage (Economides and Kadir, 1999).

Prophylaxis

Pregnancy Prevention of postpartum haemorrhage begins at the initial booking interview when the midwife will identify those women at higher risk. Any woman whose history suggests that she is at risk of postpartum haemorrhage should be booked for delivery in hospital where, should haemorrhage occur, immediate and effective treatment can be given. Conditions such as anaemia should be treated with iron and folic acid supplements. In severe cases intramuscular iron or even blood transfusion may be required to raise the haemoglobin level to 11 g/dl before delivery.

Labour During labour, careful management will reduce the likelihood of postpartum haemorrhage for those women at risk. When labour starts, an intravenous cannula is inserted and a blood sample is taken: the haemoglobin level is estimated and the blood group confirmed. The serum is saved: this speeds up the process of cross-matching donor blood should it become necessary. The midwife will monitor the progress of labour; it is important to avoid dehydration and exhaustion and an obstetrician should be called if there are any signs of prolonged labour. A Syntocinon infusion may be required and this should be maintained for at least 1 hour after the end of the third stage of labour. The bladder should also be kept empty, as a full bladder may impede efficient uterine action.

Correct management of the third stage of labour is crucial. Syntometrine 1 ml (containing ergometrine maleate 500 μg and Syntocinon 5 units) is given by intramuscular injection with the birth of the anterior shoulder. Ergometrine maleate 500 μg should be available for intravenous injection if required. The midwife should discuss the management of the third stage of labour with the woman, preferably before the onset of labour. Some women would prefer not to have Syntometrine, but physiological management is considered unsafe for the woman at risk of postpartum haemorrhage.

Treatment of postpartum haemorrhage

The basic principles of management are to:

- arrest bleeding
- resuscitate the mother
- replace fluids.

Before delivery of the placenta   The midwife must call for skilled medical assistance at once. She must stay with the mother and treat her while waiting for help to arrive. In the community or in a hospital without resident obstetricians this will be a paramedic team from the ambulance service, or (less commonly now) the emergency obstetric service from the local maternity hospital. The midwife should always be aware of what assistance is available in the area. In the case of postpartum haemorrhage at home, a blood transfusion should be started and the placenta removed if possible before transferring the woman to hospital.

When haemorrhage is first noted, the midwife must quickly determine the likely cause by locating the fundus and assessing the degree of uterine contraction. In primary postpartum haemorrhage due to uterine atony the fundus will feel soft and flaccid. The first consideration is to make the uterus contract. The

Reflective Activity 59.2

Find out how emergency transfer of a woman from her home to hospital is managed in your area.

If there is a local emergency obstetric unit ('flying squad') find out what equipment is used and where it is kept.

If the local ambulance service provides a paramedic team, find out what equipment they carry and what they are able to do in an obstetric emergency.

quickest way to do this is by massaging the uterus. The midwife should therefore take the following actions:

1. *'Rub up' a contraction* by massaging the uterus, (see Fig. 59.2) when, within a few minutes, it will become hard.
2. *Give an oxytocic drug*, either an intramuscular injection of Syntometrine 1 ml which will make the uterus contract within 2.5 minutes or an intravenous injection of either Syntometrine 1 ml or ergometrine maleate 500 μg, which will act in 45 seconds. The midwife should not, on her own authority, administer more than two 500 μg doses of ergometrine maleate, as this drug may cause severe peripheral vasoconstriction and a sharp rise in blood pressure (BMA and RPSGB, 2003).
3. *Deliver the placenta*; if possible, when the uterus contracts.

If the bladder seems full, a catheter can be passed and, having ensured again that the uterus is well contracted, another attempt made to deliver the placenta by controlled cord traction.

If the placenta is still unable to be delivered, prepare for the doctor to perform a manual removal of the

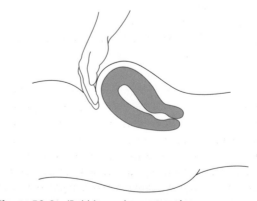

Figure 59.2   'Rubbing up' a contraction.

placenta and membranes. Before this procedure is carried out it is essential to set up an intravenous infusion, if not already in progress, and to take blood for cross-matching.

When dealing with a case of postpartum haemorrhage the midwife should not elevate the foot of the bed as this encourages blood to pool within the uterine cavity and would hinder uterine contraction and retraction. Instead, the woman's legs may be elevated on pillows, taking care to avoid undue pressure on the calves which would predispose to venous thrombosis.

After delivery of the placenta   The above principles still apply:

- 'rub up' a contraction
- give an oxytocic drug
- if necessary, empty the bladder.

Firm massage or 'rubbing' of the uterus will usually stimulate a contraction and expel any blood clot (Fig. 59.2). The administration of an intravenous injection of ergometrine maleate 500 μg or an intramuscular injection of Syntometrine 1 ml are usually sufficient to control the bleeding. Passing a catheter to ensure that the bladder is empty may be useful as a full bladder can impede uterine contraction and retraction. In most cases these actions are effective if used in good time.

It is essential that these steps are taken as soon as the midwife suspects that the uterus is failing to contract and bleeding is unusually heavy. Delay will result in further blood loss and the woman's condition can deteriorate with frightening rapidity.

The placenta and membranes are examined to ensure that they are complete. If the placenta is incomplete, an exploration and evacuation of the uterus is carried out by an obstetrician under general or epidural anaesthesia.

Further measures
If bleeding continues despite the above treatment, compression of the uterus or main abdominal vessels may be carried out.

External bimanual compression   The left hand dips down as far as possible behind the uterus; the right hand is pressed flat on the abdominal wall; the uterus is compressed and, at the same time, pulled upwards in the abdomen. The bleeding area is thus compressed while the pulling up of the uterus straightens the kinked uterine veins and, by allowing free drainage from them, relieves the congestion and decreases the bleeding.

Internal bimanual compression (Fig. 59.3)   This may be carried out when the mother is anaesthetized if bleeding persists after a manual removal of the placenta and membranes or following evacuation of the uterus. The right hand is introduced into the vagina, closed to form a fist, and pushed up in the direction of the anterior vaginal fornix. The left hand, on the abdominal wall, dips down behind the uterus and pulls it forwards and towards the symphysis. The two hands are pressed firmly together, thus compressing the uterus and therefore the placental site. The pressure is maintained until the uterus contracts and remains retracted.

Both of these manoeuvres are extremely tiring to perform and cannot be maintained for long periods.

Abdominal aortic compression   This has been used as a short-term emergency measure to control severe haemorrhage while awaiting emergency assistance. The midwife places a fist on the mother's abdomen, above the fundus and below the level of the renal arteries, which arise from the aorta at the level of L1/L2 (Marieb, 1995). Strong pressure is directed towards the vertebral column in order to compress the aorta against the spine and reduce blood flow to the uterus (Fig. 59.4). Adequacy of compression can be assessed by checking for the absence of femoral pulses (Keogh and Tsokos, 1997).

Once bleeding is controlled, uterine contraction is maintained by an intravenous infusion of Hartmann's

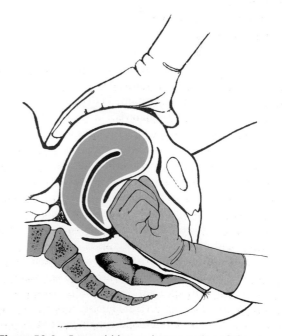

Figure 59.3   Internal bimanual compression of the uterus.

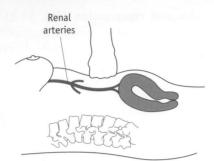

Figure 59.4 Abdominal aortic compression.

(compound sodium lactate; Ringer's lactate) solution to which oxytocin is added. The usual dose is 20–40 units of Syntocinon in 500 ml of Hartmann's solution. The concentration of the drug and the rate of infusion are determined by the obstetrician. This will help prevent further bleeding when the effect of the bolus oxytocics used begins to wear off. Blood transfusion may be required. If the bleeding persists or recurs, an exploration of the genital tract under general anaesthesia may be required.

Reflective Activity 59.3

Visit your local delivery unit and obstetric theatres and find out where the drugs and intravenous fluids required for management of haemorrhage and shock are kept.

Massive obstetric haemorrhage

The definition of 'massive' is somewhat arbitrary as blood loss is so often underestimated. However, most midwives and obstetricians would probably accept that a haemorrhage of 1.5 litres or more, or any lesser amount which causes a sustained fall in systolic blood pressure to less than 80 mmHg, is a life-threatening event and constitutes a massive bleed (Maresh *et al.*, 1999).

In cases of massive obstetric haemorrhage, the protocol or 'drill' for managing severe haemorrhage should be initiated at once. The team should consist of the midwife caring for the woman and key senior staff including midwives, obstetricians, haematologists and anaesthetists. Portering staff should be available to ensure rapid transfer of specimens for laboratory analysis. One member of staff should take responsibility for documenting all care given during the emergency.

Two large-bore (at least 16 gauge) intravenous cannulae and a central venous pressure line are inserted. Blood samples are taken for full blood count, cross-matching and clotting studies. At least six units of cross-matched

blood are requested; plasma expanders such as Gelofusine, Haemaccel or Hespan may be used. The use of dextrans should be avoided as they may interfere with typing and cross-matching of blood and can also cause transient prolongation of the bleeding time (BMA and RPSGB, 2003). All maternity units should keep at least two units of emergency group O rhesus-negative blood in the blood fridge and this may be used while awaiting cross-matched supplies. The blood should be passed through a warming device and infused as rapidly as possible using a compression cuff. Martin's pumps should not be used as they do not provide a sufficiently rapid infusion rate (DoH, 1994).

Other oxytocic agents

- *Hemabate.* If the uterus remains flaccid in spite of conventional oxytocics the doctor may order Hemabate (carboprost) 250 µg. This is given as a deep intramuscular injection and may be repeated at intervals of 15–90 minutes, up to eight doses (maximum dosage of 2 mg) and depending on the unit protocol.
- $PGF_{2\alpha}$. Continuous intrauterine irrigation with small doses of $PGF_{2\alpha}$ has been successful in controlling severe postpartum haemorrhage (Kupferminc *et al.*, 1998).

Surgical procedures

- *Selective uterine artery embolization*, using absorbable gelatin sponge as embolic material, has been effective in controlling haemorrhage and averting the need for hysterectomy (Pelage *et al.*, 1999b).
- *The use of a brace suture* (B-Lynch suture) to maintain uterine compression following either vaginal or caesarean birth (B-Lynch *et al.*, 1997; Ferguson *et al.*, 2000). The woman is placed in the lithotomy position and any clots evacuated from the vagina. If delivery has been vaginal, the abdomen is opened by a low transverse (Pfannenstiel) incision, the uterus is exteriorized and manual compression applied. If this controls bleeding, then the use of the suture is likely to be successful. Compression must be maintained by the surgical assistant until the procedure is complete. A tight suture is inserted along the long axis of the uterus, from one side of the lower segment and incorporating that edge of the wound if the procedure follows caesarean section. The suture is then carried up over the outside of the uterine fundus, down the posterior wall where it is passed back through the uterine wall, returned over the outside of the fundus and secured (Fig. 59.5). This technique has successfully controlled haemorrhage on more

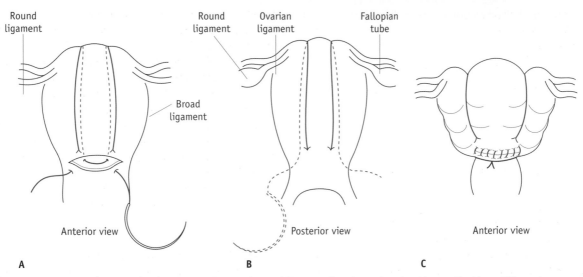

Figure 59.5   B-Lynch suture in the uterus: **A.** anterior and **B.** posterior views showing the application of the suture; **C.** the anatomical appearance after competent application. (Reprinted from the *British Journal of Obstetrics and Gynaecology*, 104, B-Lynch, C., Coker, A., Lawal, A. *et al.*, The B-Lynch surgical technique for the control of massive postpartum haemorrhage: an alternative to hysterectomy?, pp. 372–375, copyright 1997, with permission of Elsevier Science. Illustrations by Mr Philip Wilson FMAA, RMIP.)

than 900 applications worldwide (C. B-Lynch, personal communication, 2002).

- *Internal iliac artery ligation.* If measures such as the injection of oxytocic drugs directly into the uterus and direct compression of the aorta fail to stop the bleeding, internal iliac artery ligation will be necessary. The obstetrician will make every attempt to conserve the uterus but if these measures fail to control the bleeding, hysterectomy may be necessary to save the woman's life.

Observations

The amount of blood loss is measured and assessed and, once bleeding is controlled, the total loss is estimated. The greater the blood loss the more difficult it is to estimate it accurately (Prasertcharoensuk *et al.*, 2000).

A fluid balance chart is maintained to record the fluid intake and urinary output. A self-retaining catheter is inserted, attached to a urometer, and urine output is measured and recorded hourly. Central venous pressure must be measured when it is necessary to give large volumes of fluid intravenously, in order to avoid overtransfusion. The mother's general condition is assessed and her pulse and blood pressure are recorded every 15 minutes until her condition is satisfactory.

It is important to palpate the fundus repeatedly to ensure that it remains well contracted and to observe the lochia.

The best treatment for hypovolaemic shock is to replace the circulating blood volume. Elevating the woman's legs may help to maintain the core circulation. Sedation may be required and oxygen can be given by face mask. All wet bed linen is removed and the mother is kept dry and comfortable.

If it is noted that the blood does not clot or the clotting studies indicate incipient coagulation failure the haematologist should be called. Fresh blood is usually the best treatment as this will contain platelets and coagulation factors V (pro-accelerin) and VIII (anti-haemophilic factor). Fresh frozen plasma also contains factors V and VIII as well as fibrinogen (factor I).

Traumatic postpartum haemorrhage

Approximately 20% of cases of postpartum haemorrhage arise from a laceration of some part of the genital tract (Lewellyn Jones, 1999). Occasionally these are perineal tears or episiotomies. Lacerations involving the labia or clitoris also often bleed freely. Deep lacerations of the vaginal walls, cervix and, exceptionally, lower uterine segment will produce severe haemorrhage. This is much more likely to complicate a difficult, instrumental delivery than a normal one for which the midwife would be taking responsibility, though it sometimes follows a very rapid labour. Uterine rupture may also occur in obstructed labour or if a scar ruptures.

Superficial bleeding points are easily seen and treated by direct pressure. A laceration of the cervix is suspected if the bleeding begins the moment the child is born and continues steadily though the uterus is well contracted. It may be temporarily controlled by digital pressure or by the application of a sponge or arterial pressure forceps. An obstetrician must be summoned and the laceration sutured. Tears of the upper part of the vagina, the cervix or the uterus are sutured under general or regional anaesthesia. In cases of severe haemorrhage from a ruptured uterus, it may be necessary to perform a hysterectomy.

A *vulval haematoma* may be a cause of postpartum haemorrhage. These may occur following perineal repair with inadequate haemostasis, where there has been damage to a vulval varicosity or (occasionally) where the perineum is intact (Beischer *et al.*, 1997). The appearance is of a localized vulval swelling, usually on one side, which will be tense and shiny in appearance. The pain may be severe and there may be signs of shock. A surprisingly large amount of blood may be present. Morgans *et al.* (1999) record a case in which 2 litres of blood were evacuated from a vulval haematoma. The midwife must call for medical assistance. Intravenous access must be secured, as replacement fluids may be needed. The haematoma should be drained under anaesthesia. Attention to perineal hygiene and pain relief is essential.

Following postpartum haemorrhage

Following postpartum haemorrhage, the mother is liable to suffer from chronic iron-deficiency anaemia unless adequate treatment is instituted during the puerperium. She is more likely to develop puerperal sepsis, and lactation may be poor. In cases of severe and prolonged shock the woman may develop anuria due to tubular necrosis. Another serious complication is anterior pituitary necrosis. If the mother survives, she will suffer from Sheehan's syndrome. Lactation will not occur, owing to deficient prolactin secretion. Atrophy of the breasts and genital organs will follow.

The midwife should make the opportunity to discuss the events which have occurred with the couple. They will both wish to know the reason for the haemorrhage and whether it is likely to happen again. The partner, in particular, is very vulnerable in the emergency situation and is likely to have been very frightened. The sudden nature of the emergency often means that explanations given at the time are brief, hurried and poorly assimilated by the couple. The midwife should give them time to ask questions and can advise

them about the likely management of future deliveries. The woman should avoid another pregnancy until she has completely recovered.

Postpartum haemorrhage is still an important cause of maternal death in the UK, although with improving social conditions, including better nutrition and better obstetric care, the number of deaths attributed to this cause is decreasing. It should be noted that previous confidential enquiries have highlighted that the main dangers to the woman lie in poor intra-professional communication, delay in appropriate referral, and a lack of realization of the speed with which a woman's condition may deteriorate (DoH, 1998; Lewis, 2001).

Subsequent pregnancies

All mothers who have had a postpartum haemorrhage should be booked for subsequent deliveries in hospital under the care of an obstetrician. An intravenous cannula is sited when labour begins and Syntometrine 1 ml or ergometrine 500 µg is administered by injection with the birth of the anterior shoulder to reduce the risk of a further postpartum haemorrhage.

Reflective Activity 59.4

Find out if 'fire drills' (practice sessions for management of emergencies) are in place on your delivery unit. If they are, make sure you attend; if not, talk to the manager about starting them.

PROLONGED THIRD STAGE

The third stage of labour lasts, on average, 6–7 minutes (Beischer *et al.*, 1997). With active management it is considered prolonged when the time exceeds 30 minutes, though the doctor should be summoned after 20 minutes or earlier if there is excessive bleeding or if the midwife is in any way concerned about the mother's condition. With physiological management of the third stage a longer time may be allowed, up to 1 hour, provided the maternal condition is good, with no signs of undue bleeding.

The retained placenta may be partially or completely separated but trapped in the cervix or lower uterine segment, so bleeding will occur from the placental site. If the retained placenta is completely adherent to the uterine wall there may be no bleeding from the placental site.

The incidence of retained placenta is approximately 2%. If the woman has a history of previous prolonged third stage her risk is two to four times higher. It is the second most common indication for blood transfusion in the third stage of labour (Adelusi *et al.*, 1997).

Causes

Causes of a prolonged third stage include the following:

- *Inadequate uterine contraction and retraction.* This may follow prolonged or (occasionally) very rapid labour (Loeffler, 1995).
- *Uterine abnormality.* Retained placenta may be more likely if the uterus contains a fibroid (Berck and Baxi, 1999). A bicornuate or subseptate uterus may also be a cause, as the uterine contour is irregular.
- *Preterm birth*, especially if there is an associated chorio-amnionitis (Adelusi *et al.*, 1997).
- *Induced labour* (Adelusi *et al.*, 1997).
- *High parity* – more than five previous births (Adelusi *et al.*, 1997).
- *History of retained placenta* (Adelusi *et al.*, 1997).
- *History of uterine surgery* such as D&C and caesarean section (Adelusi *et al.*, 1997).

Morbid adherence of the placenta

This occurs when the placental villi penetrate deeper than the decidua basalis. It is commoner in multiparous women, particularly those with a history of previous caesarean section or other uterine surgery. A combination of previous caesarean section and current placenta praevia are high-risk factors for abnormal trophoblastic penetration.

There are three types of abnormally adherent placenta:

1. *Placenta accreta.* The decidua basalis is deficient and the chorionic villi are attached to the myometrium.
2. *Placenta increta.* The villi deeply invade the myometrium.
3. *Placenta percreta.* The villi have penetrated the myometrium as far as the serous coat of the uterus. Involvement of the bladder and adjacent structures may occur. This type is very rare.

The area of adherence may be focal, partial or total. Cases of focal or partial adhesion may be successfully treated by manual removal of the placenta, possibly followed by curettage. Attempts to remove a placenta percreta are likely to result in uterine perforation and haemorrhage. The obstetrician may carry out a hysterectomy or may leave the placenta in situ to be reabsorbed. In the latter situation, methotrexate has been used to achieve destruction of the trophoblastic tissue and thus accelerate reabsorption. However, use of this drug is not successful in all cases (Dildy *et al.*, 1999).

The following may cause delay in the third stage by interfering with the descent and expulsion of a separated placenta:

- *full bladder*
- *constriction ring* – a localized spasm of uterine muscle just above the lower segment – this is unusual.

Management

An attempt is made to deliver the placenta and membranes following catheterization to empty the bladder, and, if this fails, the woman is prepared for manual removal of the placenta and membranes.

Oxytocin injected via the umbilical vein has been used in an attempt to shorten the third stage of labour and reduce blood loss. However, randomized controlled trials have produced conflicting evidence for the clinical usefulness of this intervention and it is not considered part of routine management of prolonged third stage (Carroli *et al.*, 1998; Gazvani *et al.*, 1998).

Manual removal of the placenta may be carried out under regional or general anaesthesia. First, however, blood is taken for cross-matching, and an intravenous infusion is commenced because there is a risk of severe haemorrhage occurring during the procedure.

Once a satisfactory anaesthetic has been administered, the woman is put into the lithotomy position. Strict aseptic precautions are essential; the vulva is cleaned with antiseptic solution and chlorhexidine (Hibitane) obstetric cream 1% is used for lubrication of the tissues. Special sterile elbow-length gloves are sometimes worn during this procedure. The obstetrician forms the right hand into a cone shape and inserts it into the vagina. With the left hand on the abdomen (a sterile towel intervening) he or she steadies the uterus from above. It is helpful if an assistant holds the cord taut. The cord is followed up to its placental insertion and the separated area or the edge of the placenta is located. With a gentle sawing motion the remainder of the placenta is stripped off the uterine wall. The obstetrician removes the placenta and then explores the uterine cavity to ensure that no placental fragments have been missed (Fig. 59.6).

Following manual removal of the placenta, uterine contraction is achieved by intravenous Syntometrine or ergometrine maleate 500 µg. An intravenous infusion of Hartmann's solution with Syntocinon is commenced.

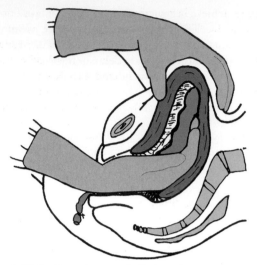

Figure 59.6 Manual removal of placenta.

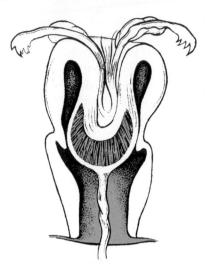

Figure 59.7 Inversion of the gravid uterus.

The dose and rate of administration is prescribed by the doctor: 20 units of Syntocinon in 500 ml of infusion solution is the usual amount. This will maintain uterine contraction. If bleeding recurs or continues, bimanual compression may be required. Antibiotics are given, as manual removal of the placenta is a highly invasive procedure and there is a risk of puerperal sepsis.

If the placenta is retained in community practice the midwife should call for emergency obstetric help without delay. An intravenous infusion is commenced at home and blood is taken for cross-matching. If attempts to deliver the placenta fail, the mother should be transferred to hospital for a manual removal of placenta and membranes under general anaesthesia.

Though the activities of a midwife include the manual removal of placenta in an emergency (UKCC, 1998), in the developed world it is unlikely that the midwife would be required to undertake this role. However, it is useful for the midwife to understand the principles of manual removal, and some practitioners may wish to learn this skill under supervision of an obstetrician.

The midwife should carefully monitor the woman's condition in the postnatal period and refer her for medical attention if signs of uterine infection appear. The woman should be advised to have future births in hospital as there is a high risk of recurrence.

ACUTE INVERSION OF THE UTERUS

This is a rare but most serious complication of the third stage of labour, and occurs in approximately

1 : 20 000 births (Calder, 2000). The uterus is partly or completely turned inside out (Fig. 59.7). It is classified according to severity or degree (Ripley, 1999):

- *First degree inversion.* The fundus is inverted but does not pass through the cervix.
- *Second degree inversion.* The inverted fundus protrudes through the cervix and lies in the vagina.
- *Third degree inversion.* The uterus is completely inverted and the fundus appears outside the vulva.

Causes

Inversion of the uterus may be due to various causes, including the following:

- *Mismanagement of the third stage of labour.* This is the commonest cause of uterine inversion and results either from pressure on the fundus or from traction on the cord when the uterus is relaxed. It is particularly likely to occur when the placenta is situated in the uterine fundus.
- *Short cord.*
- *Manual removal of placenta.* Inversion of the uterus may occur if the operator's hand is quickly withdrawn from the uterus while the other hand is still applying some degree of fundal pressure.
- *Precipitate delivery.* Especially if the woman is in an upright position.
- *Spontaneous inversion.* Occasionally spontaneous inversion occurs and the cause is unknown. It may result from uterine atony and a sudden increase in the intra-abdominal pressure such as occurs during coughing, sneezing or a straining effort.

Dangers

The condition is associated with profound shock and possibly haemorrhage, if the placenta has partly or wholly separated from the uterus. If the mother survives, she may suffer from anuria and Sheehan's syndrome as a result of shock, and the risk of puerperal sepsis is high.

Diagnosis

Minor degrees of uterine inversion may not be recognized if there is only a slight indentation of the fundus. The woman may complain of pain and the lochia will probably be heavy.

If the inversion is more serious, the woman will complain of severe pain and on palpation of the abdomen a hollow will be felt in the fundus of the uterus. Haemorrhage will occur if the placenta has separated.

If there is a complete inversion, the uterus will not be palpable in the abdomen and the inverted fundus will be visible at the vulva. If the uterus cannot be palpated in the abdomen or seen at the vulva, a vaginal examination should be made, as it is likely to be in the vagina. The woman will complain of severe lower abdominal pain and may report a sensation of prolapse or 'something coming down'. Haemorrhage and neurogenic shock occur owing to traction on the infundibulopelvic and round ligaments and compression of the ovaries (Calder, 2000).

Management

Where possible, the uterus should be replaced immediately, as maternal shock will increase and may become irreversible. Vascular congestion and oedema of the uterus will also occur, making replacement more difficult the longer it is delayed. If immediate replacement is not possible and the uterus is outside the vulva, it should be gently replaced inside the vagina, if possible. Rough or prolonged digital manipulation will increase the accompanying vasovagal shock and must be avoided. The foot of the bed should be raised in order to reduce traction on the infundibulopelvic ligaments and to alleviate shock. An intravenous infusion is commenced: plasma expanders such as Gelofusine or Haemaccel may be given. Blood is taken for crossmatching as blood transfusion will probably be required. The woman can be given an injection of morphine 15 mg intramuscularly. If the placenta is still attached to the inner uterine wall, the midwife must make no attempt to detach it as torrential haemorrhage may result.

Once shock is treated the uterus must be replaced without any delay. The mother is anaesthetized and the uterus is replaced either manually or by the hydrostatic method. By manual manipulation the part of the uterus which inverted last, that is the lower segment, is replaced first and the fundus last. The other hand should be placed on the abdomen to give counterpressure, otherwise the uterus may be pushed up too high.

Some obstetricians prefer the hydrostatic method as described by O'Sullivan (1945). Opinion varies as to whether the placenta should be removed just prior to replacement of the uterus: removal of the placenta reduces the mass which must be replaced but may precipitate haemorrhage. The woman is usually given an anaesthetic. The lithotomy position may be required but a better vaginal seal can be obtained if the woman lies flat with her legs together when the obstetrician begins to instil the fluid. A head-down tilt may be useful to relieve shock and assist reduction of the inversion. The obstetrician replaces the uterus in the vagina. Warm normal saline (0.9%) is then infused into the vagina via a large bore (20 G) Foley catheter attached to an infusion bag suspended approximately 1 m above the uterus. At least 2–3 litres of fluid will be required. The catheter is held in the vagina and the introitus sealed around the forearm by the other hand while an assistant compresses the infusion bag. The use of a Silastic ventouse cup in the vagina also produces a good seal (Ogueh and Ayida, 1997; Ward, 1998). The pressure exerted by the fluid distends the vagina and effects replacement of the uterus without aggravating the shock. Surgical correction via a laparotomy incision may be preferred by some surgeons. Following replacement of the uterus, an intravenous injection of ergometrine maleate 250–500 µg is given to ensure that the uterus contracts and bleeding is controlled. Further treatment for shock may then be required. The woman should be seen by the obstetrician 6–8 weeks after delivery in order to exclude chronic uterine inversion. The midwife should encourage the woman to carry out her postnatal exercises; referral to an obstetric physiotherapist may be helpful if the abdominal and pelvic floor muscle tone is particularly poor. This condition may recur in future births and a woman who has suffered an acute inversion of the uterus should be advised to deliver in hospital if she becomes pregnant again (Calder, 2000).

SHOCK

Shock is a condition in which the circulation cannot meet cellular nutritional requirements or remove metabolic waste. The ensuing hypotension and reduced tissue perfusion may result in irreversible organ damage or death. Shock is usually classified according to its cause (Campbell, 1993; Dildy *et al.*, 1999):

- *Cardiogenic shock*. This is reduced cardiac output because of heart failure. In midwifery it may occur as a result of pulmonary embolism, congenital cardiac defects, acquired valvular disease or severe anaemia.
- *Hypovolaemic shock*. This occurs when the circulating blood volume is too low to meet tissue requirements. It is associated with severe obstetric haemorrhage, such as antepartum or postpartum haemorrhage, ruptured ectopic pregnancy and genital tract trauma. It may follow coagulopathy such as that associated with amniotic fluid embolism.
- *Neurogenic shock*. This occurs as a result of an insult to the central nervous system. It is associated with uterine inversion, regional anaesthesia and aspiration of gastric contents.
- *Toxic shock* (septic shock, bacterial shock). This occurs as a result of a severe generalized infection. This topic will be considered separately.
- *Anaphylactic shock*. This may occur as a result of an adverse drug reaction.

The effects of shock may be exacerbated by pain, dehydration and exhaustion.

The term 'obstetric shock' has been used to describe collapse. This rather catch-all term, which generally signifies hypovolaemic shock, should no longer be used.

Signs of deterioration

Midwives should be alert for changes in the condition of any woman in their care. The following signs indicate deepening shock which will affect all the body organs and systems:

1. *Pulse.* A pulse rate of over 90 is not normal. As it continues to rise, the volume grows weaker until the rapid thready pulse of severe haemorrhage is noted.
2. *Blood pressure.* Though the mother is losing blood, for some time the compensatory mechanisms in her body will keep her blood pressure at a normal level. Peripheral, splanchnic and renal vasoconstriction ensure that vital organs such as the heart and brain continue to be perfused. If the systolic pressure falls below 100 mmHg there is cause for anxiety. Readings of 90 and 80 mmHg indicate seriously deepening shock.

3. *Increasing pallor of the skin.* The skin is covered with a cold sweat. The lips are bluish and the mucous membranes blanched.
4. *Temperature.* This falls to a subnormal level.
5. *Respiration.* Breathing becomes deep and sighing. The mother is sometimes restless and may complain of thirst, nausea or faintness. She may lose consciousness.

Most childbearing women are healthy, and a woman who enters labour in good general condition is unlikely to suffer harm provided that blood loss does not exceed the physiological volume expansion which occurs in pregnancy. Up to 1 litre may be lost without signs of physiological compromise. A loss of more than 35% of the total circulating volume will generally have occurred before clinical signs of hypovolaemia appear.

The pulse and blood pressure will remain normal in the early stages of shock. The woman may appear pale but the vital signs will be deceptively reassuring. An increasing tachycardia reflects cardiac response to underperfusion of the vital organs. Hypotension is a late sign, indicative of deepening central hypoperfusion. Cellular metabolism becomes deranged and a metabolic acidosis develops. The woman is now close to death (Bobrowski, 1999; Dildy *et al.*, 1999; Loeffler, 1995).

The midwife *must* closely observe the woman's condition and call for obstetric assistance at once at the first sign of a rising pulse rate.

Whether the cause is clearly postpartum haemorrhage or whether some less obvious condition is present is immaterial. In either case the mother is in urgent need of resuscitative treatment.

Treatment

The principles underlying treatment are as follows (Dildy *et al.*, 1999):

- *Administration of fluid.* Two large-bore (at least 16 gauge) intravenous cannulae are sited. Blood is taken and cross-matching requested: at least six units of donor blood will be required. In the meantime, the circulation can be maintained by plasma expanders such as Gelofusine, Haemaccel or Hespan.
- *Other means of maintaining the circulation.* Inotropic drugs such as dopamine increase myocardial contractility and may be effective in maintaining cardiac output. Vasopressor agents such as noradrenaline (norepinephrine) may be useful, especially in cases of septic shock where fluid volume replacement alone is insufficient to maintain

blood pressure. These types of drug are used with caution as pulmonary and renal vasoconstriction may occur. They should also be used with caution in the treatment of shock which is due to hypovolaemia following haemorrhage. Volume replacement is essential (BMA and RPSGB, 2003).

In an emergency situation, raising the woman's legs may assist in maintaining the core circulation.

- *Monitoring*. A central venous pressure (CVP) line is inserted to monitor maternal response to fluid therapy. There should be no delay in inserting a CVP line: accurate volume replacement is essential to save the woman's life and this cannot be safely managed without central venous monitoring.

The heart rate should be monitored continuously by electrocardiograph (ECG) if possible and a pulse oximeter applied. Blood is taken for estimation of plasma gases, haemoglobin, clotting studies, urea and electrolytes. The patency of the airway must be monitored and the woman's position should be adjusted so as to allow adequate ventilation and lung expansion. The midwife must watch carefully for any signs of cyanosis. Frequent records of pulse, blood pressure, respiratory rate, blood loss, urine output and level of consciousness are maintained.

- *Oxygen* should be administered by nasal prongs or face mask at an initial rate of 6 l/min. The rate may be adjusted according to the results of blood gas estimation or pulse oximetry.
- *Pain relief*, such as an intramuscular injection of morphine, may be given to relieve pain and allay anxiety. The mother should be kept as quiet and undisturbed as possible.

No attempt should be made to warm the skin: the cold, pale skin is evidence that the body's compensatory mechanism is at work. The superficial capillaries and arterioles are constricted and blood is being diverted to the parts of the body where the need is greatest, that is the heart and brain. To warm the skin until it is flushed may well undo this important compensatory mechanism and even deepen the shock to an irreversible degree.

The woman should be transferred to a high-dependency or intensive care unit as soon as possible.

Bacterial shock

This is cardiovascular collapse due to septicaemia. In up to 80% of cases the causative organisms are Gram-negative bacteria, particularly the Enterobacteriaceae.

Escherichia coli, *Klebsiella*, *Serratia* and *Clostridium welchii* may all cause septic shock. Occasionally Gram-positive aerobic organisms such as staphylococci and streptococci may be implicated. Endotoxins released by organisms such as *Escherichia coli* or *Clostridium welchii* enter the bloodstream and cause intense vasoconstriction of the postcapillary vessels. Blood therefore collects in the capillary bed rather than returning to the heart, the cardiac output is reduced and peripheral failure ensues. This results in tissue destruction, especially in the kidneys.

Signs

- Temperature instability – temperature >38°C (possibly with rigors) or <35°C.
- Tachycardia – >90 beats/min.
- Tachypnoea – >20 breaths/min.
- Oliguria – <0.5 ml/kg body weight/h.
- Hypoxaemia (Roseveai, 1999)

The skin is usually hot and dry and the woman looks acutely ill. Uterine infection may be accompanied by acute abdominal tenderness and scanty lochia. Hypoxaemia may cause a confusional state. Multiple organ failure, adult respiratory distress syndrome and disseminated intravascular coagulation may develop. Mortality can be high unless appropriate measures are instituted rapidly (DoH, 1998; Lewis, 2001).

Septic shock may follow puerperal uterine infection, septic abortion, intra-amniotic infection and urinary tract infection.

Management

The midwife must call for medical assistance if there is any evidence of infection. The woman should be admitted to a hospital which has high-dependency or intensive care facilities.

A midstream specimen of urine, high vaginal swab, wound swab (if appropriate) and blood cultures are sent for bacterial investigation. Serum electrolytes and blood urea are measured and screening tests for clotting disorders performed.

Treatment may include:

- Intravenous fluids including blood transfusion if required.
- Monitoring of vital signs – blood pressure, pulse, temperature, pulse oximetry, cardiac monitoring, level of consciousness. Intensive monitoring if required – central venous pressure.
- Intravenous antibiotics.

- Correction of acidosis.
- Accurate assessment of urinary output.
- Inotropic agents may be used. Steroids may be given to decrease peripheral resistance and improve pulmonary circulation.

Any infected products of conception must be removed from the uterus. The midwife should pay attention to the woman's personal hygiene and general comfort.

AMNIOTIC FLUID EMBOLISM

Amniotic fluid embolism occurs when amniotic fluid is forced into the maternal circulation via the uterine sinuses of the placental bed. It may occur at or close to term, during labour or immediately after delivery. Most deaths occur within 1 hour of the event and the diagnosis is usually made post-mortem when fetal squames or debris are found in the lungs (Thomson and Greer, 2000). The mortality rate associated with this condition is very high, approaching 80%. It may occur in older, multiparous women and where labour has been tumultuous or hypertonic. This includes cases where oxytocic drugs have been used to induce or accelerate labour. However, amniotic fluid embolism has occurred during elective caesarean section (DoH, 1998). It may also complicate multiple pregnancy or follow polyhydramnios.

In all these cases the intra-amniotic pressure is increased and when the membranes rupture, either spontaneously or artificially, amniotic fluid may be forced into the maternal circulation. The incidence of amniotic fluid embolism seems to be rising and there may be an association with increased maternal age in childbearing (DoH, 1998). Signs of fetal hypoxia ('fetal distress') commonly precede or accompany amniotic fluid embolus (Thomson and Greer, 2000).

Symptoms
- Respiratory:
  - cyanosis
  - chest pain
  - dyspnoea
  - bloodstained frothy sputum
  - respiratory arrest.
- Cardiovascular:
  - hypotension
  - cardiac arrest.
- Haematological:
  - disseminated intravascular coagulation.

- Neurological:
  - fits (Park and Sachs, 1999).

The respiratory difficulties may be due, in part, to the effect of amniotic fluid endothelin, which causes pulmonary vasoconstriction and bronchoconstriction (Khong, 1998).

If the woman survives the initial embolus, the thromboplastin-like effects of amniotic fluid may cause a coagulopathy and she may subsequently die from coagulation failure. As the presence of intravascular amniotic fluid depresses myometrial activity, the uterus may become atonic and this will compound the haemorrhage due to coagulopathy (Clark, 1990).

The midwife must call for medical assistance at once and should commence cardiopulmonary resuscitation. High concentrations of oxygen should be administered. An intravenous infusion and a central venous pressure line are inserted. The woman may be intubated and mechanically ventilated. Delivery is effected by caesarean section as quickly as possible: the aim here is not simply to salvage the fetus but also because adequate and effective resuscitation of the mother is better achieved when the uterus is empty. Signs of amniotic fluid embolus may also appear in the first few hours after childbirth, although this is rare.

Amniotic fluid embolus is an uncommon event but often fatal, and midwives must remember that care of the partner forms a large part of their role in this situation.

Known or suspected cases of amniotic fluid embolism should be notified to the UK Amniotic Fluid Embolism Register in Bradford, West Yorkshire; telephone 01274 364520 (DoH, 1998; Tuffnell and Johnson, 2000).

The third stage is the most dangerous part of labour for the woman. Complications can arise without warning and an apparently normal birth can rapidly become a life-threatening event. As the senior professional present at the majority of births in the UK, it is usually the midwife who has the responsibility for identifying the problem and beginning emergency treatment. It is essential that midwives are aware of the potential dangers and, while supporting the physiological process, unobtrusively watch for signs of impending problems and know how to respond appropriately. The emotional needs of the parents must be addressed once the emergency is over and they will probably need to talk through the events with the midwife. The long-term consequences may be physical, such as infection or anaemia, or psychological such as postnatal depression. The emergency often results in separation from the baby for some hours or even days, which may cause distress. Breastfeeding may be more difficult to establish and the woman's long-term relationships both with her baby and her partner may suffer.

Accurate records are essential and a discussion with the Supervisor of Midwives may be helpful.

Adequate emotional support should be available for the midwife.

KEY POINTS

- The third stage is the most dangerous part of labour for the woman.
- Postpartum haemorrhage is still a major cause of maternal death in the UK.
- Complications may arise without warning and the woman's condition can deteriorate rapidly.
- Effective management of blood loss and shock is crucial.

- Accurate assessment and rapid response to emergencies may save the woman's life.
- The midwife is the most senior professional present at the majority of births in the UK and needs to be able to monitor the woman's condition, refer appropriately and work collaboratively to ensure safe and effective care at this time.

REFERENCES

ACOG Technical Bulletin No. 243 (1998) Postpartum haemorrhage. *International Journal of Gynecology and Obstetrics* **61**(1): 79–86.

Adelusi, B., Soltan, M., Chowdhury, N. *et al.* (1997) Risk of retained placenta: multivariate approach. *Acta Obstetricia et Gynecologica Scandinavica* **76**(5): 414–418.

Beischer, N., Mackay, E. & Colditz, P. (1997) *Obstetrics and the Newborn*. London: Baillière Tindall.

Berck, D. & Baxi, L. (1999) Benign tumours in pregnancy. In: Reece, E. & Hobbins, J. (eds) *Medicine of the Fetus and Mother*. Philadelphia: Lippincott-Raven.

B-Lynch, C., Coker, A., Lawal, A. *et al.* (1997) The B-Lynch surgical technique for the control of massive postpartum haemorrhage: an alternative to hysterectomy? Five cases reported. *British Journal of Obstetrics and Gynaecology* **104**(3): 372–375.

Blackburn, S.T. (2003) *Maternal, Fetal & Neonatal Physiology*, 2nd edn. Philadelphia: W.B. Saunders.

British Medical Association (BMA) and Royal Pharmaceutical Society of Great Britain (RPSGB) (2003) *British National Formulary*, 46th edn. London: BMA and RPSGB.

Bobrowski, R. (1999) Trauma in pregnancy. In: James, D., Steer, P., Weiner, C. *et al.* (eds) *High Risk Pregnancy: Management Options*. London: W.B. Saunders.

Calder, A. (2000) Emergencies in operative obstetrics. *Baillière's Clinical Obstetrics and Gynaecology* **14**(1): 43–55.

Campbell, J. (1993) Making sense of shock. *Nursing Times* **89**(5): 34–36.

Carroli, G., Belizan, J., Grant, A. *et al.* (1998) Intra-umbilical vein injection and retained placenta: evidence from a collaborative large randomised controlled trial.

British Journal of Obstetrics and Gynaecology **105**(2): 179–185.

Clark, S. (1990) New concepts of amniotic fluid embolism: a review. *Obstetrical and Gynecological Survey* **45**(6): 360–368.

Dildy, G., Mason, B. & Cotton, D. (1999) Trauma, shock and critical care obstetrics. In: Reece, E. & Hobbins, J. (eds) *Medicine of the Fetus and Mother*. Philadelphia: J.B. Lippincott.

Department of Health (DoH) (1994) *Report on Confidential Enquiries into Maternal Deaths in the United Kingdom, 1988–1990*. London: HMSO.

Department of Health (DoH) (1998) *Why Mothers Die: Report on Confidential Enquiries into Maternal Deaths in the United Kingdom, 1994–1996*. London: HMSO.

Economides, D. & Kadir, R. (1999) Inherited bleeding disorders in obstetrics and gynaecology. *British Journal of Obstetrics and Gynaecology* **106**(1): 5–13.

Ferguson, J., Bourgeois, J. & Underwood, P. (2000) B-Lynch suture for postpartum hemorrhage. *Obstetrics and Gynecology* **95**(6 Pt 2): 1020–1022.

Gazvani, M., Luckas, M., Drakeley, A. *et al.* (1998) Intra-umbilical oxytocin for the management of retained placenta: a randomized controlled trial. *Obstetrics and Gynecology* **91**(2): 203–207.

Keogh, J. & Tsokos, N. (1997) Aortic compression in massive postpartum haemorrhage – an old but lifesaving technique. *Australian and New Zealand Journal of Obstetrics and Gynaecology* **37**(2): 237–238.

Khong, T. (1998) Expression of endothelin-1 in amniotic fluid embolism and possible pathophysiological mechanism. *British Journal of Obstetrics and Gynaecology* **105**(7): 802–804.

Kuperminc, M., Gull, I., Bar-Am, A. *et al.* (1998) Intra-uterine irrigation with prostaglandin F$_{2\alpha}$ for management of severe postpartum haemorrhage. *Acta Obstetricia et Gynecologica Scandinavica* **77**(5): 548–550.

Levy, V. (1990) The midwife's management of the third stage of labour. In: Alexander, J., Levy, V. & Roch, S. (eds) *Midwifery Practice: Intrapartum care – a Research-Based Approach*. London: Macmillan.

Levy, V. & Moore, J. (1985) The midwife's management of the third stage of labour. *Nursing Times* **1**(5): 47–50.

Lewellyn Jones, D. (1999) *Fundamentals of Obstetrics & Gynaecology*, 7th edn. London: Mosby.

Lewis, G. (ed) (2001) *Why Mothers Die 1997–1999*. The fifth report of the Confidential Enquiries into Maternal Death in the United Kingdom. London: CEMD.

Loeffler, F. (1995) Postpartum haemorrhage and abnormalities of the third stage of labour. In: Chamberlain, G. (ed) *Turnbull's Obstetrics*. London: Churchill Livingstone.

Marieb, E. (1995) *Human Anatomy and Physiology*. Wokingham: Benjamin/Cummings.

Maresh, M., James, D. & Neales, K. (1999) Critical care of the obstetric patient. In: James, D., Steer, P., Weiner, C. *et al.* (eds) *High Risk Pregnancy: Management Options*. London: W.B. Saunders.

Morgans, D., Chan, N. & Clark, C. (1999) Vulval perineal haematomas in the immediate postpartum period and their management. *Australian and New Zealand Journal of Obstetrics and Gynaecology* **39**(2): 223–226.

Ogueh, O. & Ayida, G. (1997) Acute uterine inversion: a new technique of hydrostatic replacement. *British Journal of Obstetrics and Gynaecology* **104**(8): 951–952.

O'Sullivan, J.V. (1945) Acute inversion of the uterus. *British Medical Journal* **2**(Sept 1): 282–283.

Park, E. & Sachs, B. (1999) Postpartum haemorrhage and other problems of the third stage. In: James, D., Steer, P., Weiner, C. *et al.* (eds) *High Risk Pregnancy – Management Options*. London: W.B. Saunders.

Pelage, J-P., Soyer, P., Repiquet, D. *et al.* (1999a) Secondary postpartum hemorrhage: treatment with selective arterial embolization. *Radiology* **212**(2): 385–389.

Pelage, J-P., Le Dref, O., Jacob, D. *et al.* (1999b) Selective arterial embolization of the uterine arteries in the management of intractable post-partum hemorrhage. *Acta Obstetricia et Gynecologica Scandinavica* **78**(8): 698–703.

Prasertcharoensuk, W., Swadpanich, U. & Lumbiganon, P. (2000) Accuracy of the blood loss estimation in the third stage of labour. *International Journal of Gynecology and Obstetrics* **71**(1): 69–70.

Ripley, D. (1999) Uterine emergencies. *Obstetric and Gynecology Clinics of North America* **26**(3): 419–434.

Rosevear, S. (1999) Bleeding in early pregnancy. In: James, D., Steer, P., Weiner, C. *et al.* (eds) *High Risk Pregnancy – Management Options*. London: W.B. Saunders.

Thomson, A. & Greer, I. (2000) Non-haemorrhagic obstetric shock. *Baillière's Clinical Obstetrics and Gynaecology* **14**(1): 19–41.

Tuffnell, D. & Johnson, H. (2000) Amniotic fluid embolism: the UK register. *Hospital Medicine* **61**(8): 532–534.

United Kingdom Central Council for Nursing, Midwifery and Health Visiting (UKCC) (1998) *Midwives Rules and Code of Practice*. London: UKCC.

Ward, H. (1998) O'Sullivan's hydrostatic reduction of an inverted uterus: sonar sequence recorded. *Ultrasound in Obstetrics and Gynecology* **12**: 283–286.

FURTHER READING

Bonnar, J. (2000) Massive obstetric haemorrhage. *Baillière's Clinical Obstetrics and Gynaecology* **14**(1): 1–18.
An up-to-date overview of the topic, which addresses causes and management. The tables are particularly useful.

Drife, J. (1997) Management of primary postpartum haemorrhage. *British Journal of Obstetrics and Gynaecology* **104**(3): 275–277.
This is a clear and concise commentary on management. The text takes a step-by-step approach, starting with basic measures. The aim of management is to eliminate substandard care.

Ekeroma, A., Ansari, A. & Stirrat, G. (1997) Blood transfusion in obstetrics and gynaecology. *British Journal of Obstetrics and Gynaecology* **104**(3): 278–284.
This is a useful and readable review of blood transfusion. It addresses rates, trends, indications for transfusion and complication rates. It also considers how the use of blood transfusion can be reduced, an important issue as many women are concerned about the safety of blood products and would prefer to avoid them.

PART 9

HEALTH, SOCIAL SERVICES AND PUBLIC HEALTH

60. The Changing National Health Service 1005

61. Quality in Midwifery 1021

62. Epidemiology 1034

63. Children Act and Social Services 1050

The Changing National Health Service

Tara Kaufmann

LEARNING OUTCOMES

After reading this chapter you will be able to:

- identify key developments in National Health Service (NHS) policy and practice
- be aware of the key reforms in the changing NHS, and understand how these reforms impact on the role of the midwife

- appreciate the implications of changes in the NHS for midwives and for the maternity services
- view the potential opportunities which reforms may offer midwives and women and babies.

INTRODUCTION

Why is it important to understand the wider NHS and its policy drivers? There are many health professionals who do a very good job while paying little attention to the world outside their own practice. But getting to grips with the bigger picture makes the practitioner more effective and able to work as an advocate for women and families. Without that understanding, it is difficult to respond effectively to change and to proactively use the opportunities that change provides; and unlocking funding streams and policy initiatives that can transform the service that is offered are lost opportunities. Just as importantly, understanding the environment and context of midwives' practice allows more control to be exerted, and helps prevent staff alienation and burnout (Sandall, 1999).

It is particularly important that midwives engage with NHS reform. Too often, midwives feel oppressed rather than supported by the system within which they work. Some see midwives' gradual loss of autonomy – as they came under NHS control, and then into the hospital system – as the loss of a golden age, and believe that the only way to rejuvenate midwifery and improve care for women is to 'liberate' midwives from external control – and, in particular, from control by doctors. Much has been written about the historic battle for

control between (male) medicine and (female) midwifery (Donnison, 1988), and this polarization is still evident in maternity services today (a battle in which midwives usually fare badly and child-bearing women fare worse). While gender is an important factor in this dynamic, there are others: the balance of power and resources between primary and secondary healthcare, between the needs of the ill few and the healthy majority, between regulating quality and allowing local flexibility, between the advancement of knowledge and the strengthening of basic healthcare provision. In other words, midwives are facing similar challenges to those experienced by many others in the NHS, and midwives – as much as anyone else in the health service – can work to influence and benefit from NHS reform.

Midwives are proud to be an 'autonomous' profession, but the reality is that no health worker is truly autonomous in today's NHS. We are all as effective as the partnerships we create, the opportunities we seize and the resources we identify and use. That means that the current wave of NHS reform is of crucial interest to all those concerned about the future of maternity services.

As devolution increases the diversity of policy and practice across the UK, it is becoming increasingly difficult to provide accurate and comprehensive detail on all four countries without resorting to long and unwieldy lists. The escalating pace of reform means that any chapter of this kind is liable to become out of date almost before it is published. Therefore, the focus is on the main policy drivers and trends that are consistent across the UK, as NHS reforms in each of the four UK countries share common themes and philosophies. While this may change in the years to come, as devolution begins to make a real difference, for now most of what is written here will be applicable nationally.

BACKGROUND

The creation of the National Health Service, over 50 years ago, is rightly remembered as among our nation's finest expressions of collective will. One of the central planks of the post-war reforms that sought to tackle social inequalities, build public health, and create a society which provided its most vulnerable with a safety net 'from the cradle to the grave', the health service still commands great loyalty and affection in the public psyche. Yet preoccupation over the accessibility and effectiveness of the NHS's services is equally a national pastime, and the future of the NHS has become highly contested – between political parties, in the media, and in public discourse.

Before the NHS was established, there was not a single maternity care system: women chose, according to their means, from a plethora of competing providers, including midwives, family doctors, obstetricians and hospitals (private and charitable). The 1946 National Health Service Act, which became operational in 1948, established a comprehensive if fragmented model of care, comprising hospital maternity services, community midwifery services (which were under the control of local authorities), and general practitioners. This fragmentation caused duplication and poor continuity, and many midwives were frustrated by what they saw as the encroachment of doctors on the provision of midwifery care. This was exacerbated by the expansion of hospital maternity beds resulting from the 1962 Hospital Plan, and by the Peel Report of 1970 (DHSS, 1970), which recommended that all women give birth in hospital, cared for by multidisciplinary teams of midwives, obstetricians and GPs. In 1973, the National Health Service Reorganisation Act brought all midwives under the responsibility of the NHS.

These reforms, along with the opportunities offered by evolving obstetric expertise, exacerbated the erosion of community-based midwifery. Childbirth became increasingly medicalized, with hospital delivery and many obstetric interventions becoming routine. The

development of general management during the early 1980s meant that midwives reported up through general or nursing management, making them feel even more isolated from decision-making power.

Meanwhile, the wider NHS was experiencing repeated restructuring and reform in order to reduce its complex, multi-layered bureaucracy. At the end of the 1980s, it also underwent ideological revolution as the Government aimed to introduce 'market forces' to public services. A competitive internal market was established within the NHS, within which the functions of purchasing and providing were separated. Hospitals, community and ambulance services were encouraged to become self-governing trusts. GPs were encouraged to become fundholders, with power over their own resources and responsibility for purchasing care for their patients. The aim of this was to increase choice and efficiency, but both aims were frustrated: efficiency was undermined by the unavoidable management costs of implementing and running the system, while choice was subverted by the system of block contracts and restrictions on extra-contractual referrals.

By the time the Labour Party assumed government in 1997, after 18 years of uninterrupted Conservative administration, it appeared that the NHS was feeling sick and tired itself. Those who worked within it were fatigued and demoralized by continued structural reform and the implicit (often explicit) message that they could not run their own affairs efficiently. Conflict over wages, differentials, professional territories and management influence were widespread. Long waiting lists and poor customer care were alienating NHS users and supporters. The NHS had become a political football, and its future management was one of the key reasons why the country felt ready for change.

> During the past 30 years, attitudes to public services have evolved from a paternalistic assumption that the state will provide, through stringent public spending restraint and wholesale privatisation, to the current philosophy that accepts an underlying societal responsibility for good public services but increasingly expects empowered individuals to take responsibility for themselves. This reality is full of contradictions: between local autonomy and central control, between consumer expectations and the capacity of services that have been starved of investment, between what people say they want and what they are prepared to pay for.
>
> (Audit Commission, 2001)

THE CURRENT CHALLENGE

The election of the Labour Government in 1997 was perceived by many as an opportunity to halt the gradual erosion of the NHS. The state of the NHS had been a significant election issue and the incoming administration's credibility was to a great degree pinned to its ability to meet its pledge to restore public pride in the health service. Nevertheless, the subsequent relationship between the Government and the NHS has not always been easy. Undoubtedly, many welcomed the philosophical underpinning of new policy, and few demurred at the impressive investment produced in 2001. But the Government also signalled its determination to produce improved results for this money, and has shown itself as willing as its predecessors to break up the entrenched power cabals within the NHS. As a result, it has continued the same cycle of structural reform and centralized micro-management that has so wearied NHS personnel over the years.

One of the most significant reforms has been in the constitutional arena, with devolution to a Scottish Parliament and Welsh Assembly. 'Local solutions to local problems' was the guiding principle for the handover of health responsibilities to these assemblies – indeed, health was the biggest single issue to be devolved. The result has been a comprehensive 'rebranding' of health service reform, with each country determined to show that it does things its way and in response to particular local circumstances. A significant divergence in health service policy or practice is yet to be seen, but it is starting and it is probable that in the future, midwives will work in markedly different ways across the UK.

There are, undoubtedly, significant and persistent problems in the NHS. Its inflexibility, lack of responsiveness and perceived indifference to patients' wishes have shown it to be out of step with our modern consumer society. As a monopoly provider, it has been too quick to prioritize its own interests over patients' needs. The services that are provided are not always of high quality: too often, users face excessive delays, fragmentation, poor coordination, and conflicting advice. Quality is variable, and clinicians are sometimes slow to adopt best practice or apply research evidence to their practice. Above all, patients often feel that services are not geared to their needs; rather, they are expected to fit into the service's requirements, and sometimes treated with less than full respect.

The causes of these problems are multifactorial. Some are structural; the sheer size of the NHS, and many of its constituent institutions, lead to impersonality and inflexibility. The complexity of the system defies attempts to reform and throws up unexpected effects of the most carefully planned change programme. Persistent over-centralization deadens local initiative and ownership. The barriers between services confuse and alienate patients and disrupt effective, seamless treatment. Hospital and community services are not sufficiently integrated; the gaps between health and social care are even more marked. The volume and pressure of work never seem to allow for adequate communication or relationship-building across these barriers, and the development of information technology (IT) and communication systems to help bridge the gap has not been given sufficient priority. Paradoxically, given the problems arising from NHS structures, it is also clear that successive governments' addiction to structural change has caused and is causing real damage – lowering morale, diverting priorities, consuming resources, and inhibiting the development of expertise and partnerships.

The general public and some clinicians are fond of blaming managers for all the health service's woes, and certainly poor management has played its part in the slow pace of service improvement. Performance management – while necessary and important – has often been badly executed: lack of incentives, targets that are seen as meaningless or perverse, and a culture of blame have all been evident. The very definition of quality is contested between different professions, organizations and sectors. The management of information and knowledge systems is particularly poor, and is significantly delaying the development of efficient care systems, and of effective performance management.

Reflective Activity 60.1

'The values that produce high quality clinicians are not always compatible with either conventional approaches to management or other characteristics of high performance organisations such as team working and effective resource management' (NHS Confederation, 2002a).

Do you agree with this? What are the qualities that make a leader in midwifery? What can the profession do to identify, develop and sustain its leaders?

However, important though it undoubtedly is to ensure that structure serves purpose, and that leadership and management are of the highest quality, culture is the trump card that so often defeats attempts to create change. Ham and Alberti (2002) have written convincingly of the breakdown of the compact between the NHS and its doctors. They point out that the implicit contract, agreed at the founding of the NHS, was based on the Government providing resources and the medical profession taking care of clinical standards. Prior to 1948, British doctors were private practitioners and their freedom to practise as they wished was curtailed less by the State than by the strong moral and ethical context in which they worked. Although many were not enthusiastic about the establishment of the NHS, they ceded to government the right to determine the budget and the national policy framework for their work, in return for continued medical control over regulation and clinical decision-making. In these early years of the NHS, managers were administrators and saw their job as facilitating doctors, rather than managing them. Patients, too, accepted that 'doctor knows best', and were happy to acquiesce to medical authority.

This implicit contract was undermined by the growing consumer movement in the 1960s, the increased publicity given to poor standards, and the medical profession itself becoming more vocal and lobbying for higher budgets to keep pace with growing technological opportunities. Over the next 30 years, the implicit compact was further undermined by growing regulation, clinical audit and patient involvement. Public spending constraints led governments to seek efficiency improvements in the NHS, and increased management power led to strained relationships between managers and doctors. The rise in litigation and challenges to self-regulation further undermined doctors' sense of professionalism. Doctors, along with other health professionals and managers, have become increasingly frustrated by their workloads and by the growing gap between what it is possible to do for patients and what can be done with available resources.

Midwives, meanwhile, have experienced the breaching of their own implicit compact. In the first half of this century, midwives worked very hard and their pay was poor. Compared to other working women, however, their lot was not so bad. Although their social status never rivalled that of doctors, they worked with a significant degree of autonomy and often enjoyed high status in the communities where they worked. The level of continuity of care they were able to offer provided them with job satisfaction that was some compensation for their long hours. It should also be remembered that they were often unmarried and childless, wedded to the job in a way that today's midwives – many of

whom have children, and most of whom believe in a life outside work – could not countenance.

50 years of NHS reform have not been altogether negative for midwifery, but they have altered this original agreement out of recognition. NHS midwives generally work shorter hours with lighter caseloads than their predecessors. They have the support of medical back-up, technological and other resources, and employment benefits. Yet the highly risk-averse nature of modern healthcare does not allow for the full flourishing of essential midwifery skills, and as midwives have been drawn into the traditional doctor–nurse dyad that characterizes our system of healthcare they have lost status and pride. Many midwives would go so far as to argue that the modern hospital environment – fast-moving, technological, strongly directive – is intrinsically oppositional to birthing and to the midwifery philosophy of care.

In addition, the last century's drive to professionalize midwifery has had ambivalent results. While it may have saved midwifery from near-extinction, as happened in other countries, it did so at the cost of autonomy from medical direction (and of the livelihoods of many working-class midwives). 100 years on from the establishment of legal regulation of midwifery in England (followed rapidly by the other UK countries), midwifery is not fully a profession, and midwives continue to feel devalued by their role and status within the health service.

Reflective Activity 60.2

Some feel it is vital that midwives continue to behave as full professionals, to control their own education and body of knowledge, and continually strive to improve their practice and status. Others feel that midwives should give the NHS only what it pays for, and resist the imposition of unrewarded responsibility.

How can these two viewpoints be brought together to create forward movement for the midwifery workforce?

With the expansion of alternative – and more lucrative – occupations for educated women, this lack of consensus on the relationship between midwifery and its paymaster is finding expression in chronic staff shortages and a growing sense of crisis. The future for midwifery is uncertain, and it is in this area, as much as any other, that the necessity for effective NHS reform is most marked.

That is at least partly why the NHS is currently undergoing one of the most ambitious and relentless programmes of reform since its establishment. Many analysts and commentators feel that this is the NHS's last chance to prove that it is possible to provide a publicly funded health system that is clinically effective, free at the point of use and good value for the taxpayer. The size of the challenge is reflected in the scope of the reforms. The Government wants to produce demonstrable and sustainable improvements in all areas of the health service. It wants to shift emphasis and investment to the primary sector while also producing ambitious improvements in acute sector care; it wants to provide more and better hospitals and community facilities, bring down death rates from the 'big killer' diseases, close health inequalities, ensure better access and shorter waiting times, empower frontline staff and service users, and develop imaginative new ways of working. And it aims to do all this while becoming more cost-efficient and avoiding explicit rationing.

THE CURRENT WAVE OF REFORM

Improving performance and outcomes

In the early years of the NHS it was generally expected, and accepted, that doctors should define for themselves what constituted a quality service, and work towards it. Fellow doctors had little influence over the standard of a doctor's clinical practice, even if it fell below the norm. The encroachment of management into clinical quality was strongly contested, and clinical autonomy has often been understood (and not only by clinicians) as a vital defence of the doctor–patient relationship against the forces of penny-pinching bureaucracy.

Medicine itself created the seeds of change by developing the technology of evidence-based practice – audit, controlled trials, meta-analyses, guidelines, and organizations such as the Cochrane Collaboration. No longer is it enough to have clinical experience; doctors accept that their practice must be guided by demonstrable evidence. Midwives and nurses have similarly come to know that experience and instinct are not in themselves sufficient arbiters of best practice. In addition, as knowledge has grown, new technologies have been developed, and the threat of litigation has expanded, the potential and the price for negligent practice have become increasingly evident.

The new era of quality improvement is not just about clinicians guiding and monitoring each other; or indeed about management monitoring clinicians. Increasingly, the NHS is characterized by central control of local clinical management. The previous Government introduced market forces, competition and contracting to exert their own regulatory drivers, though it is worth noting that they created a host of new regulatory authorities to manage the performance of the public sector (Walshe, 2002). The current Government has preferred to explicitly build on the significant expansion, over the last two decades, of external regulation.

Now, tight and centralized performance management holds NHS organizations to account against a range of exacting targets and standards. In England, those that fail to meet these standards are subject to closer monitoring and less autonomy; those that fail badly may have new senior managers imposed on them. They will also suffer poorer public esteem and find it harder to attract and retain staff. In contrast, those who 'succeed' enjoy increased autonomy from central control, better access to funding, and lighter-touch performance management from the strategic health authority. They may also be able to apply to become *foundation trusts* (DoH, 2002), with greater financial and regulatory freedoms.

The main elements of the new quality improvement agenda are:

1. *National targets.* These commonly address access (waiting times and waiting lists), reduced mortality from major killer diseases, the introduction of more patient-centred systems such as booked admissions, and financial balance. These targets have been contested, because they can divert from other priorities, be inflexible to local needs, create perverse incentives, and place great stress on staff and resources. Nevertheless, they address some of the issues that matter most to patients, and given the political importance to the Government of achieving tangible improvements in the short term, they are likely to continue to be accorded high priority.
2. *National standards and service models.* In England, National Service Frameworks (NSFs) set national standards and define service models for specific services or care groups, and establish programmes to support implementation and performance measures against which progress will be measured. The National Institute for Clinical Excellence (NICE) is the main standard-setting body for England, Wales and Northern Ireland. Scotland has established its own Clinical Standards Board.
3. *Clinical governance.* All NHS organizations must now have systems and structures in place to ensure

a consistent and institutionalized approach to improving clinical quality. These must include strategies for quality improvement, monitoring care, audit, risk management, poor performance and continuing professional development.

A number of new regulatory agencies have been created to monitor and encourage best practice. In England alone, there are five:

- *The National Institute for Clinical Excellence* (NICE), a special health authority that provides formal advice for clinicians and managers on the clinical and cost-effectiveness of new and existing technologies, develops clinical guidelines, and promotes clinical audit and confidential inquiries.
- *The Commission for Health Improvement* (CHI) (soon to be the Commission for Healthcare Audit and Inspection (CHAI)) monitors clinical standards, conducting local and national reviews on the implementation of NSFs and NICE guidelines, and provides national leadership to develop clinical governance.
- *The Modernisation Agency* works to spread best practice through a range of service improvement and leadership development programmes. It also provides a rapid response unit that can offer intensive intervention to improve services in trouble.
- *The National Patient Safety Agency* runs a mandatory reporting system for logging failures, errors and near-misses across the NHS, with the aim of creating a learning, blame-free NHS.
- *The National Clinical Assessment Authority* has the role of streamlining procedures for dealing with poorly performing doctors.

In addition, the Government is planning to introduce an overarching Council for the Regulation of Healthcare Professionals, which will coordinate and harmonize the operation of the different regulatory bodies. These will include the new Nursing and Midwifery Council (NMC) and its associated Boards in each of the four UK countries.

These agencies are funded by, and accountable to, the Department of Health and tighten central political control over clinical quality in the NHS. They signify how far we have come from the status quo throughout the early years of the NHS, in which clinicians expected to be accountable to themselves and their vocational calling, but rarely to other clinicians and only very exceptionally to non-clinicians. Rightly or wrongly, professional self-regulation is no longer trusted to effectively guard against poor practice.

> ### Reflective Activity 60.3
>
> What is happening to improve your service? What plans exist for modernization within your workplace that will affect the service you provide? If you were planning a change programme, what would you put in it?

Strengthening primary care

For many years, primary care has been the 'poor sister' of the acute sector. It has suffered from low political priority and relative lack of investment. Yet there is increasing recognition that this imbalance must be put right; not just because the vast majority of NHS consultations take place in the primary sector, but because primary care is vital for improving public health, for managing demand on the acute sector, and for reducing health inequalities.

The recognition that primary care services are often better placed to understand the complexity of individuals' and communities' health needs, and to work with the range of local service providers, led to a belief that it should be the primary sector, and not a remote health authority, that should plan local services. In England, primary care trusts (PCTs) were established from April 2000, and assumed full powers from April 2002. Revenue allocations are made directly to them, rather than via health authorities, and they are responsible for commissioning the bulk of secondary care services (some specialist services are still commissioned at sectoral level, with strong PCT input). In addition, they are responsible for developing primary and community health services, managing family health services contractors (GPs, dentists, pharmacists and optometrists), assessing and addressing the health needs of local populations, and working with other organizations to deliver care. Similar, though not identical provision has been made in the rest of the UK; in Wales, local health groups are developing into local health boards with commissioning powers. Local health councils in Scotland, and local health and social care groups in Northern Ireland will provide similar functions.

It is not yet clear what scale and speed of impact this will have on patterns and content of service provision. Primary care organizations are facing an enormous organizational development agenda in order to master their extensive responsibilities. As well as mastering secondary care commissioning, they must develop new and robust relationships with local authorities and the voluntary sector, expand access to primary care services, develop clinical and sectoral networks, and negotiate access arrangements with GPs. To compound this, they are experiencing chronic problems with recruitment and retention, and mounting pressures from evolving health needs. There are growing tensions between expectation and capacity (National Primary Care Research and Development Centre, 2001).

Reflective Activity 60.4

Are you involved with your local commissioning body? Do you know where it is and what it is doing? Who represents midwives on it and how can you influence its decision-making?

Promoting public health and tackling health inequalities

Public health aims to address the health and healthcare needs of populations, bringing together all the factors that shape and influence the health of individuals and communities. Its activities include epidemiology, health education, immunization and vaccination programmes, health-promoting service provision (such as clean water supplies), and social policy measures to address the wider determinants of health. In recent years, the 'new public health' has embraced the growing evidence that social inequality is a key determinant of public health, having a negative impact not just on those living in poverty, but on the whole of society. This perspective has been strongly influential on public health policies in all four UK countries.

In 1998, Sir Donald Acheson's *Independent Inquiry into Inequalities in Health* encapsulated this new approach, summarizing the evidence that health inequalities negatively affect the health and well-being of individuals and communities at all levels of society, and arguing that effective action must encompass wider social change, individual empowerment and community development, as well as clinical interventions. It recommended that high priority be given to the health of families with children, and particularly to improving health and reducing inequalities in women of childbearing age, expectant mothers and young children.

Each of the four UK countries has a national strategy for public health, which sets national targets to improve health and reduce health inequalities. There are also UK and country strategies to tackle specific public health issues, such as teenage pregnancy and smoking. National strategies for nursing, midwifery and health visiting have called for an enhanced midwifery role in

maximizing women's health and in contributing to public health targets. The Sure Start programme is now running across the UK, targeting support to pregnant women and pre-school-age children in areas of deprivation.

Midwifery contribution to public health could be further enhanced. The shift of midwifery management and service delivery into the acute sector has obscured midwifery's community focus and inhibited its partnership with other primary and social care practitioners. But there is plenty of potential to enhance the midwife's contribution to, for example:

- Assessing the health needs of local populations through needs assessment and community profiling
- Designing, managing and evaluating maternity services with the aim of improving health outcomes and reducing health inequalities
- Building healthy alliances and a supportive infrastructure for community development initiatives
- Engaging with local statutory and voluntary groups to work towards health-related policies and activities
- Contributing midwifery expertise and information to health strategy
- Identifying groups that have particular needs, or are missing out on maternity care – such as women who are refugees, or homeless, or misusing drugs, or from minority ethnic communities – and developing services that are appropriate, culturally sensitive and accessible to them
- Developing family-centred care, through strategies for improved parenting education, father/partner involvement, and help with domestic violence and other family problems.

If they are to make an effective contribution to public health, midwives need to examine their priorities and make hard choices. A recent review of the contribution of nurses, midwives and health visitors to public health in Scotland found much good practice, but also lack of clear leadership and direction, contributions that were often ad hoc and uncoordinated, little involvement with strategy, little or no use of evidence to support and inform practice, a focus on individuals and families rather than communities, poor preparation from education, and professionals often working in isolation, with little sharing of good practice or opportunity to be challenged on their own practice. In addition, there was little structured contact either between nurses, midwives and health visitors, or with other key partners in the public health effort (Scottish Executive, 2001).

Reflective Activity 60.5

'There is almost no convincing evidence anywhere in the world that spending money on health services has any impact on population health – as measured by life expectancy. Investment in education, improving 'health conditions', increasing the income of the poor, and promoting rights and status of women may all be better social investments to improve health. Government expenditure on tertiary facilities, specialist training and interventions that provide little health gain for the money spent should be abandoned in favour of increased public health interventions and decentralisation of government health services. Most people are kept healthy or made ill long before they have contact with the health services. Health is not a 'commodity' that can be bought through the purchase of ameliorative clinical service interventions. It is a 'social product' arising from the cumulative impact on individuals of what happens in families, workplaces, schools, on transport systems and so on' (World Bank, 1993).

What do you make of these arguments? What are their implications for midwifery? Can you envisage a future in which midwives worked to improve the 'social product' of health?

Empowering patients and the public

Many health professionals, including midwives, are committed to the concept of patient-centredness in service provision. But the NHS as a whole has not matched commitment with reality, and institutional or professional convenience is still commonly prioritized over patients' own needs and wishes. The need to involve patients has been a key feature of NHS policy and recommendations over recent years (Modernisation Agency, 2002), and was given a major impetus with the publication on the Kennedy Report on the Bristol Royal Infirmary (BRI) enquiry (BRI, 2001).

Too often, 'patient involvement' is limited to tokenistic consultation on minor areas of service provision – for example, cosmetic improvements to the environment. Even in midwifery, which has a stronger history of partnership with service users, the content of 'woman-centred care' is often assumed rather than negotiated, and 'choice' usually equates to a very limited menu of carer-defined options.

The new NHS will need to do better. All parts of the health service have been asked to develop new and meaningful systems for engaging with patients, their carers and the general public. This engagement should go beyond the tokenism, and should encompass information exchange, consultation and partnership in strategic and operational development.

In England, the National Commission for Patient and Public Involvement in Health has been established to guide this work. Every trust is now required to set up a patient advice and liaison service (PALS) to provide information to patients, their carers and families and help them resolve problems quickly. In addition, every trust must establish a patient forum, to consult patients and represent their views. These will be able to inspect all areas of work, and will have a representative on the trust board. Controversially, community health councils – set up in 1974 to represent the public's interest in the health service – are to be abolished in England. In Wales, they will be retained and reinforced with a new complaints system and a network of '*expert patients*' to support individuals with specific conditions.

Nobody should underestimate the challenges inherent in this work. Given that no patient is truly representative of any other, it is difficult to identify and develop a group of patient representatives that is small enough to be coherent and effective, and large enough to carry the diversity and the support of the local community. Patient representatives often find it hard to hold their own in negotiating with NHS personnel; they lack knowledge of the system and are too easily 'fobbed off' or patronized. Indeed, this is often taken advantage of: NHS trusts are, in a very real sense, coalitions of competing interest groups, and the addition of a new lobby – whose perspective and priorities may sit far outside any consensus that has been built between the others – is bound to be resisted, even at a subliminal level.

NHS organizations, and individual staff, will need to work hard and courageously to ensure patient involvement receives the investment and support it needs. The rewards for doing so are many: better communication, better-quality services, more patient-centredness, greater local ownership and fewer complaints.

Supporting and developing NHS staff

NHS trusts spend between 60–70% of their revenue on staff costs and so it is vital to ensure that the workforce is up to strength, appropriately skilled, and working effectively (NHS Confederation, 2002b). The chronic difficulties in attracting and retaining staff to many parts of the NHS over recent years have paid testament to the difficulties faced by the NHS in managing its human resources effectively. The reform agenda must ensure strategic investment in recruiting and retaining staff, improving the quality of their working lives, and providing the management capacity and capability to deliver this agenda.

There are shortages of staff in many areas. Medical shortages have been exacerbated by the Calman Report (DoH, 1993), which has decreased junior doctors' hours, meaning that work has had to be picked up by other staff. The European Working Time Directive will also have a significant impact on service delivery (European Union, 1996). In midwifery, staff shortages have been chronic over many years, and these show no signs of abating (RCM, 2002a). The Government is tackling this in a number of ways:

Modernising pay   The *Agenda for Change* structure is likely to produce a restructured and simplified NHS pay system for non-medical staff, matched by greater flexibility in roles and responsibilities.

Enhancing and extending roles   Recruitment and retention problems, plus the escalating rate of change in working practices, point to the need for much greater flexibility in workforce planning and deployment. This new flexibility has been most evident with nurses, with the extension of prescribing rights and the rapid expansion of nurse-led clinical initiatives. Midwives, too, are in some places undertaking tasks that were once outside of the scope of their role – ultrasonography, ventouse deliveries and examination of the newborn, for example. Clearly this offers opportunities for improving continuity of carer, providing midwife-led care in new settings, and reducing unnecessary delays or distances in accessing care. It also raises the risk that midwives' core role will be pulled off-centre, and unduly medicalized, by NHS needs that have little to do with improving the quality or continuity of midwifery care (RCM, 2002b).

Meanwhile, there is a strong move across all disciplines to develop the contribution of healthcare assistants and other support workers. Many maternity units are extending the roles of maternity care assistants (often called by other titles) in order to free up midwives to concentrate on essential midwifery. While traditionally these staff have been ward-based and task-oriented, there is great potential to develop their contribution to ante- and postnatal care in community settings, working under midwifery supervision and as an integral part of the maternity care team (RCM, 1999, 2003a).

A positive development has been the creation of 'consultant midwife' posts, which aim to provide strong clinical leadership alongside the managerial leadership of Heads of Midwifery. Consultant midwives commonly focus on key priority areas – such as labour ward, or public health, or midwife-led care – and lead clinical and service developments while also carrying a teaching and research function. The challenge now is to develop career ladders that lead into these posts, and so encourage the brightest and best to stay within midwifery.

Training and development   Significant investment in training and development is being provided, in order to tackle recruitment and retention problems, and increase role flexibility. Extra training places have been provided for midwifery and nursing, and work is under way to broaden access to them – for example, to healthcare assistants. In addition, the *Agenda for Change* (NHS, 2003) programme aims to introduce a 'skills escalator' into NHS training and employment, which will allow every employee to develop competencies and proceed – with associated remuneration – to the next stage of the career ladder. This should allow for more opportunity, career progression, flexibility and skill. It could also have benefits for local regeneration, by encouraging more socially excluded people into first-time employment. This has been further developed by the RCM to illustrate possibilities for those entering midwifery, and pathways for those within the profession (RCM, 2003b).

Improving working conditions   A significant programme of investment and reform is under way to improve the often substandard working conditions of NHS staff. These programmes include work on violence against staff, improving the working environment, more family-friendly working practices and improved childcare provision.

Reflective Activity 60.6

NHS reform plans for all four UK countries promise more decision-making power for frontline staff. In your experience, is this likely to be real or rhetoric? How would different groups of staff use any increased powers? What are the opportunities, and threats, in this for midwives? What should be done to maximize the potential benefits?

Developing partnerships

In years past, NHS organizations have been characterized by their 'silo' mentality. District general hospitals provided a reasonably comprehensive range of services to their local population, and did not need to worry overmuch about what their neighbours were doing. Individual clinicians provided the best care they could as they saw fit, and did not need to concern themselves with what other clinicians in other institutions were up to. Within hospitals, clinical departments and directorates have been characterized by their territorialism and the strict boundaries fenced around their roles and responsibilities.

This isolationism was only encouraged by the NHS reforms of the 1980s and 1990s, which introduced the competition of 'market forces' into the health service. But today it is clear that the old culture must be transformed into a new ethos of partnership, if the NHS is to thrive and develop. Demand to provide a wider range of specialist services, the need to drive quality through sharing innovation and resources, and the urgency of improving continuity of care throughout the 'helping agencies' all point to the need to break down traditional boundaries and develop new models of partnership working.

The drive for partnership is evident in the following areas:

Multidisciplinary practice   Multidisciplinary teamworking is not new, but the need to move from rhetoric to full implementation has been made particularly urgent by NHS reform. The increasingly complex needs of many communities, and of many clinical conditions, require a team problem-solving approach that moves far beyond the traditional doctor–nurse dyad. Teams, and the individuals within them, need to be flexible, multiskilled, and able to work with others from a wide range of disciplines and agencies.

Clinical networks   The development of clinical networks is designed to ensure that people receive seamless continuity of care, however complex their condition, and that they are able to access the services they need even where these are not provided by their local NHS trust. Networks usually operate on a sector-wide basis, ensuring that referrals are rapid and appropriate, and unnecessary and expensive duplication of specialist services in neighbouring trusts is avoided. Their potential is not so immediately obvious in maternity services – where most women need a relatively simple care pathway – but the growth of tertiary maternal–fetal medicine technologies will undoubtedly lever their early development.

Health and social care   The structural and operational gap between health and social care agencies has been a major problem in the provision of seamless support. Midwives know this from their own work with pregnant teenagers, women who are homeless or refugees, women with substance use difficulties or families with child protection issues. NHS reform throughout the UK has placed new responsibilities on both health and social care providers to work in closer partnerships, and flexibilities have been put in place to enable joint or pooled budgeting, commissioning and management. The 2001 Health and Social Care Act also allows for the creation of care trusts, which will provide health and social care services for defined population groups – likely to be those who need continuing and complex support, such as older people and people with mental health problems.

The UK health reform strategies also envisage closer working between health agencies and those addressing the environment, transport and investment. Local strategic partnerships will bring together local government, public health, housing, social care, voluntary, independent sector and other agencies to formulate and implement strategies for health and well-being, and ensure joint planning of interface services.

Public–private partnerships   More controversially, the Government has expressed its commitment to expanding and diversifying a 'mixed economy' of providers, working within an NHS regulatory framework to provide a publicly funded, universally available service. There is considerable debate about whether these represent value for money for the NHS, and whether they herald the introduction of creeping privatization. Currently, the private sector has four main roles within the NHS:

- Spare capacity within the private sector is used where it will be more efficient or convenient, and most commonly when NHS trusts are attempting to clear backlogs of waiting lists.
- Private sector management of some selected services such as the planned 'Surgi-centres'.
- The private finance initiative (PFI) aims to reduce public expenditure by the use of private funds to renovate and build. For example, the private sector partner may build a new hospital, then lease it and

many of its support systems to the NHS partner for a defined period.

- Public–private partnerships (PPP) are increasingly being used to achieve improvements and additions to the NHS estate, such as diagnostic and treatment centres.

Restructuring the NHS

Across the UK, the NHS has ambitious plans to:

- devolve power to frontline staff
- further involve patients and the public within the NHS
- change the NHS structure and culture, in order to support devolved responsibility, user involvement and the development of cross-sectoral, multidisciplinary working.

In order to achieve this, the NHS is being restructured – again. The aim is to streamline the hierarchy so that there is clearer scrutiny and accountability between local organizations and the centre.

- In *England*, regional offices have been abolished. The previous 95 health authorities have been replaced by 28 strategic health authorities, whose core function is to performance manage PCTs and NHS trusts, and drive reform throughout the health economy. They will do this through supporting local strategic partnerships and clinical networks, brokering strategic solutions, creating capacity through planned capital investment, workforce planning and information management, and ensuring public consultation takes place on major service configurations.
- In *Wales*, health authorities will be abolished altogether. Local health boards and NHS trusts will report to the Welsh Assembly NHS Directorate through three local regional offices.
- In *Scotland*, boards and trusts are being regrouped into 15 new unified NHS boards, with responsibility for strategic planning, resource allocation and performance management.
- In *Northern Ireland*, there will be 15 new local health and social care groups. There will be further concentration of acute services for patients with more complex conditions, but the Assembly has promised that no hospitals will be closed and clinical networks will be developed. Everyone will be within 1 hour of emergency care and consultant-led maternity services, the development of midwife-led maternity units alongside consultant-led units will

be encouraged, and two stand-alone midwife-led units will be piloted.

What is expected of and for midwives?

NHS reform strategies have had little to say explicitly or directly about the future direction of maternity care. But although a blueprint for the development of maternity services is lacking, there is little doubt about what is expected of and for midwives over the next 10 years.

Across the UK, government plans for maternity services aim to combine the best of all worlds, with:

- more community-based care, alongside improved secondary and tertiary care
- greater choice and user involvement
- skilled and empowered staff working in innovative partnerships
- stronger links to social care and to the primary sector
- the development of existing and new career paths for midwives and support staff
- a greater focus on public health, and especially on breastfeeding, smoking cessation and family well-being
- the development of midwife-led services (Welsh Assembly, 2002).

Scotland has led the way with its *Framework for Maternity Services in Scotland* (Scottish NHS Executive, 2001), which favours a community-based maternity service with a woman-centred approach, underpinned by a philosophy of normality and generally provided within midwife-led services. Midwives will have a wider role in health promotion and supporting women with the effects of pregnancy and birth on their wider lives and relationships. One-to-one midwifery care is promised throughout labour and childbirth, preferably with continuity of carer. Women are promised a right to choose how and where to give birth. These progressive ideals are currently being translated into implementation plans. Wales and Northern Ireland have produced policy statements that are broadly in line with this philosophy. In England, a national service framework (NSF) is being developed for children's and maternity services.

For a busy midwife in an overstretched maternity unit, the promised results of reform may seem very distant. Nonetheless, significant reform is underway and its impact on maternity services will be marked, though not necessarily immediate. It will pose the midwifery profession with a number of key challenges and choices about the direction of maternity care in the

21st century. Among these are the following questions and considerations:

What is a midwife?   Midwives have been encouraged to maintain expertise across the breadth of their role, but increasing specialization and role enhancement offers new opportunities and challenges. Can a midwife be an expert community-focused practitioner, working in partnership with a range of partners across health and social care and the primary and secondary sectors, while also providing increasingly technological intrapartum care? Should there be a return to the days when midwives worked either in hospital or the community? Should the profession embrace more specialization – high-dependency care midwives, public health midwives, community support midwives?

Who is in the maternity care team?   Given the increasing scope of the midwife's role, coupled with chronic staffing problems, should midwives embrace new entrants into the maternity care team? What would be the potential benefits, and risks, of developing new roles for non-midwives specializing in, for example, breastfeeding support, counselling for antenatal testing, additional support for women with particular needs, antenatal health education?

Redefining partnerships   Who are midwives' natural partners? If the answer is 'women', or 'obstetricians', then extra attention may also be needed for other health and social care partners, whose contribution can be utilized to improve the effectiveness of maternity care. Most midwives are employed by and managed within the acute sector, and this can distort the focus of the partnerships they create and sustain. There is no justification for a claim of providing 'woman-centred' or 'holistic' care if that care is solely framed by acute sector inputs and processes. This does not mean that relationships with obstetricians are obsolete; there is an urgent need to improve them and make them more equal and constructive. But with the transfer of planning and commissioning powers to the primary care sector, midwives should ensure that their communication and influence is appropriately placed and effective.

Defining priorities, making best use of resources
As more and more tasks and responsibilities are loaded onto an already overburdened workforce, midwives will need to identify and agree the priorities for their working time – the things that must be done and that only midwives can do – and find ways of dropping or reallocating the other tasks. This will involve process-mapping,

analysis and redesign. In many areas this is long overdue; for example, who can say that if asked to design antenatal and postnatal care from scratch they would come up with the present structure and content? Similarly, hard choices may need to be made about how best to tailor resources to need in order to produce best outcomes for particular population groups. For example, if continuity of carer or one-to-one care in labour cannot be provided to all women, should it be targeted to those who need it most?

Positioning the profession   In common with some other professional groups within the NHS, midwifery stands at a defining moment in its development. If the profession is serious about achieving full professional status, significantly increasing its remuneration and assuming greater power in decision-making and management, it will need to embrace responsibility (and therefore shoulder blame), develop its own support staff, accept further specialization, actively develop its own evidence-based body of knowledge, develop its management capacity and capability, get slicker at understanding and using the wider NHS agenda, and agree a new compact with its medical colleagues.

The investment needed to do this will be significant and may not be rewarded. It may feel like too high a price to pay to a workforce that is relatively low-paid, has been demoralized by its recent history, is largely female and often has caring responsibilities. There is no right or wrong answer to this question; a number of different pathways are possible and plausible. But midwifery will need to develop greater consensus over its own future, and find the energy and will to drive that consensus forward, if it is to avoid having its fate decided for it by others.

Whatever the answers to these questions, it is evident that the status quo is not an option. The NHS reform agenda is gathering scope and speed, and the midwifery profession cannot choose to opt out of it. Some midwives may feel that an inordinate amount is being demanded of them in return for their remuneration and reward. Nevertheless, change always creates opportunities, and the opportunities currently on offer to midwives are the most significant since *Changing Childbirth*, back in the early 1990s.

THE FUTURE OF THE NHS

Successive governments have sought to reform the NHS, and they have all discovered the strength of its resistance. Although the present Government's reforms have been largely welcomed by the NHS, their implementation has been fraught and highly criticized. Despite significant new investment, guidance and support, the health service has struggled to respond to the ambitious agenda imposed on it. Pessimistic voices suggest that this just demonstrates the impossibility of running a vast, complex and unwieldy organization with efficiency, and that the NHS of the future will have to be pared down and contracted out to external providers. Others still believe that the NHS can continue to be the jewel in Britain's crown. Whatever the view, it is instructive to examine the causes of this resistance to change. They include:

The right people in the right place Workforce capacity and capability continues to be one of the main enemies of creating effective change. The NHS performs daily miracles in simply providing basic services, given the scale of staffing shortages in many areas. Creating change requires intensive human resources: to learn and implement changes while carrying out their usual tasks; to manage, monitor and evaluate those changes; and to provide clinical and managerial leadership to inspire and sustain change. The NHS needs to revitalize its workforce and make the health service an attractive career option for the rising generation. But the size of its workforce makes that an extraordinarily expensive programme of work, and the Government is insistent that its new investment should not be 'swallowed up' in the NHS wages bill, without delivering manifest improvements in care.

Sustaining improvement over the longer term It is relatively easy to demonstrate improvement in the short term, but far harder to sustain improvement over the longer term. To create and sustain change in an organization as complex as the health service takes a long time, but time is precisely what governments – whose deadline is always the next general election – never have. Hence the plethora of short-term reform initiatives, often competing, which focus on 'quick wins' and neglect the importance of sustainability and replication. These initiatives often drink up the available funding, leaving little to strengthen core services and infrastructure.

The balance of power between the centre and the frontline Governments that are focused on quick wins before the next election cannot risk devolving power, however much they espouse doing just that.

Centralization ensures stronger control over maverick or under-performing NHS organizations; it keeps accountability clear and makes sure that everybody works to the same end. But it stifles local initiative, and undermines the development of leadership and management. It also means that health service managers are over-occupied with managing upwards, and the creation of a range of external agencies has exacerbated this over-accountability. Central management may lead to the creation of excessive targets, as the Government attempts to micro-manage every part of the health service. The more targets are created, the less real priority will be given to anything and the less staff will understand what is required of them.

The need to create cultural change At the heart of much of the resistance to NHS reform lies a fundamental dissonance between the cultural values of clinicians, management and government. The original compact between the state and the medical establishment – autonomy with very little accountability (Klein, 1983) – has been superseded by the needs to contain costs, respond to patients' demands for empowerment, ensure standardization in quality and impose management on a complex system. Clinicians' autonomy is being reined in, and this causes alienation and suspicion that management demands for productivity are given precedence over patient needs. In addition, there is little team culture with the NHS. The health service socializes its clinicians to be individualistic and hierarchical, and undermines team working through its training, its response to problems and accidents, and its competitive approach to funding allocations. Although this is changing, it still requires far greater investment and support in order to ensure that clinicians feel confident and supported within the new NHS.

Meanwhile, managers may also resist change. The scale and the scope of the reform agenda may overwhelm them, creating managers who are overly focused on detail, fearful, short-term, upward-facing, and neglectful of internal relationships. The high management turnover within the NHS, and the macho ethic of much health service management, suggests that cultural change is needed here, too. Instead, because of the difficulty of creating cultural change, governments have preferred to rely on structural change – which usually fails to remedy the root causes of dysfunction.

Working smarter, not harder The stringency of NHS reform targets and standards has forced the health service to run faster and work harder in order to achieve them (and therefore avoid penalties including loss of management freedoms). Intensified effort is no bad thing, but it cannot be sustained year-on-year. Incremental, piecemeal change simply cannot deliver the step change in efficiency and strategic focus that the NHS needs in order to meet the challenges of the coming years. Unfortunately, the intensity and the multiplicity of government reform targets mean there is little resource left over for analysing underlying processes and redesigning service delivery. In addition, the reform agenda creates perverse incentives and distorts priorities. The creation of high performance depends on pulling the objectives of clinicians, management and government into line, and ensuring this direction of travel is supported by systems, structures, staffing, leadership and culture. Although some of this work is being resourced and supported by organizations like the Modernisation Agency, it needs to be brought centre-stage to the reform agenda, not relegated to secondary status.

The future of the NHS is crucially dependent on its ability to tackle these challenges. The health service is a complex adaptive system – an interconnection of parts sharing an environment, with each part having some freedom to act independently (NHS Confederation, 2001). This means that change cannot be delivered by simply issuing instructions and expecting that implementation will just happen; policy pronouncements may have completely unexpected effects when put into practice, and anything that discourages creativity and innovation will act as treacle in the system. Instead, the Government needs to abandon micro-management, and resource the NHS to work towards a very limited set of high-level targets. It would need to help create an environment in which NHS staff had permission to be innovative, while understanding risks and boundaries. It would need to pull back the net of performance management to allow experimentation – and sometimes failure. This would be high risk in a country where governments are held accountable for every failure of individual patient care, and so will require a more mature public discourse on the NHS than we are used to. Nevertheless, the government that will truly save the NHS will be the one that will steer forward on this path.

CONCLUSION

For now, the health service is continuing to struggle with continuing questions over its very existence. There is an increasing divide between those who believe that

the dream of a system of universal provision of healthcare, funded by universal taxation, is redundant and doomed to failure, and those who see the NHS as the foundation block of a society that is committed to fairness and equality. Most of the general public does not seem to actively want a market in healthcare, but wonder if a European-style insurance system is inevitable in the future.

This Government, meanwhile, grows ever more committed to developing a health service that provides services not just by line-managed NHS organizations, but by a range of agencies working within a national framework of standards and inspection. It is eyeing the potential for new forms of organization such as mutual or public interest companies working within a public ethos, and will shortly be creating the first tranche of 'Foundation Trusts' – former three-star trusts that will be run by their local communities and enjoy greater financial freedoms. Even more fundamentally, its 'Patient Choice' programme aims to reintroduce competitiveness and selection into the NHS; to its supporters, this promises consumer empowerment; to its detractors, the growing inevitability of a two-tier NHS.

> Our reforms are about redefining what we mean by the National Health Service. Changing it from a monolithic, centrally-run, monopoly provider of services to a values-based system where different health care providers – in the public, private and voluntary sectors – provide comprehensive services to NHS patients within a common ethos: care free at the point of use, based on patient need and their informed choice and not their ability to pay. Who provides the service becomes less important than the service that is provided. Within a framework of clear national standards, subject to common independent inspection, power will be devolved to locally run services so they have the freedom to innovate and improve care for NHS patients.
>
> (Tony Blair, speech to New Health Network, 15 January, 2002)

The future of individual NHS organizations, and indeed of the NHS as a whole, will largely be determined by the ability of health service staff to pull rabbits out of hats – to demonstrate that, despite chronic shortages, growing pressures, and systemic disincentives, they can deliver a step change in performance capable of transforming the pride of 20th century Britain into the pride of the 21st.

KEY POINTS

- Since its inception in 1948, the NHS has been undergoing a process of constant change.
- Midwives need to be conversant with the structures and systems within the NHS, and their place within it, and be able to visualize opportunities in policy documents, modernization proposals and changing patterns of care.
- The midwife's focus is on the woman, her baby and family, and any changes to the NHS and its service provision must be seen in this context, and translated to the midwife's practice appropriately.
- Some of the modernization proposals fundamentally change the way acute and primary services will be controlled, and it is crucial that midwives place themselves in a position to influence, contribute and shape services and workforce planning.

REFERENCES

Acheson, Sir D., Chair (1998) *Independent Inquiry into Inequalities in Health.* London: The Stationery Office.

Audit Commission (2001) *Change Here! Managing Change to Improve Local Services.* London: Audit Commission.

Bristol Royal Infirmary (BRI) (2001) *Learning from Bristol: the Report of the Public Enquiry into Children's Heart Surgery at the Bristol Royal Infirmary 1984–1995.* Command Paper CM 5207 July 2001. London: The Stationery Office.

Department of Health (DoH) (1993) *Hospital Doctors: Training for the Future, the Report of the Working Group on Specialist Medical Training* (The Calman Report). London: DoH.

Department of Health (DoH) (2002) *A Guide to NHS Foundation Trusts.* London: DOH.

Department of Health and Social Security (DHSS) (1970) *Report of the Sub-Committee on Domiciliary and Maternity Bed Needs* (Chair: Sir John Peel). London: HMSO.

Donnison, J. (1988) *Midwives and Medical Men.* London: Heinemann.

European Union (EU) (1996) *Working Time Directive* (93/104/EC). Brussels: European Union.

Ham, C. & Alberti, K.G.M.M. (2002) The medical profession, the public and the government. *British Medical Journal* 324: 838–842.

Health and Social Care Act 2001 London: HMSO.

Klein, R. (1983) *The Politics of the National Health Service.* London: Longman.

Modernisation Agency (2002) *Improvement Leaders' Guide to Involving Patients and Carers.* London: Modernisation Agency.

National Health Service Act 1946 London: HMSO.

National Health Service Reorganisation Act 1973 London: HMSO.

National Health Service (NHS) (2003) *Agenda For Change 2003.* London: DoH. Online. Available: http://www.doh.gov.uk/agendaforchange/proposedagreement.htm.

National Primary Care Research and Development Centre (2001) *The National Tracker Survey of Primary Care Groups and Trusts 2000/2001: Modernising the NHS.* Online. Available: www.npcrdc.man.ac.uk.

NHS Confederation (2001) *Why Won't the NHS Do as it is Told – and What Might We Do About it?* Leading Edge Briefing No. 1. London: NHS Confederation.

NHS Confederation (2002a) Creating high performance: why is it so hard? *Leading Edge* No. 4, May.

NHS Confederation (2002b) *The Pocket Guide to the NHS in England.* London: NHS Confederation.

Royal College of Midwives (RCM) (1999) *Support Workers in the Maternity Services.* Position Paper No. 5a. London: RCM.

Royal College of Midwives (RCM) (2002a) *Evidence to the Review Body for Nursing Staff, Midwives, Health Visitors and Professions Allied to Medicine for 2003.* London: RCM.

Royal College of Midwives (RCM) (2002b) *Refocusing the Role of the Midwife.* Position Paper No. 26. London: RCM.

Royal College of Midwives (RCM) (2003a) *The Use of Non Midwifery Staff in the Maternity Services.* Position Paper. London: RCM.

Royal College of Midwives (RCM) (2003b) *Valuing Practice: a Springboard for Midwifery Education: The RCM Strategy for Education.* London: RCM.

Sandall, J. (1999) Team midwifery and burnout in midwives in the UK: practical lessons from a national study. *MIDIRS Midwifery Digest* 9(2): 147–152.

Scottish Executive (2001) *Nursing for Health: a Review of the Contribution of Nurses, Midwives and Health Visitors to Improving the Public's Health in Scotland.* Edinburgh: The Stationery Office.

Scottish NHS Executive (2001) *The Framework for Maternity Services in Scotland.* Online. Available: http://www.scotland.gov.uk/library3/ffms.

Walshe K (2002) The rise of regulation in the NHS. *British Medical Journal* 324: 967–970.

Welsh Assembly (2002) *Delivering the Future in Wales: a Framework for Realising the Potential of Midwives in Wales.* Cardiff: Welsh Assembly.

World Bank (1993) *World Development Report: Investing in Health. World Development Indicators.* New York: Oxford University Press.

FURTHER READING

Rivett, G. (1998) *From Cradle to Grave: Fifty Years of the NHS*. London: King's Fund.
This book tells the extraordinary story of the NHS, and was published on the 50th anniversary of the King's Fund. It describes the major achievements and events in medicine, nursing, hospital development, primary health care and health management, and has been described as a unique review of the NHS.

This is mirrored by Rivett's innovative website, which provides dynamic and up-to-date information of NHS developments (http://www.nhshistory.net/).

ADDITIONAL RESOURCES

Department of Health
Website: http://www.doh.gov.uk

Health Development Agency
Website: http://www.had-online.org.uk

National Clinical Assessment Authority
Website: http://www.ncaa.nhs.uk

National Institute for Clinical Excellence
Website: http://www.nice.org.uk

NHS Direct
Website: http://www.nhsdirect.nhs.uk

NHS Modernisation Agency
Website: http://www.modernnhs.nhs.uk

NHS Plan
Website: http://www.nhs.uk/nationalplan

NHSPlus
Website: http://www.nhsplus.nhs.uk

Sure Start
Website: http://www.surestart.gov.uk

Commission for Health Improvement
Website: http://www.chi.nhs.uk

National Service Frameworks
Website: http://www.doh.gov.uk/nsf/nsfhome

National Patient Safety Agency
Website: http://www.npsa.org.uk

NHS University
Website: http://www.doh.gov.uk/nhsuniversity/index.htm

National Electronic Library for Health
Website: http://www.nelh.nhs.uk

61

Quality in Midwifery

E. Rosemary Buckley

LEARNING OUTCOMES

After reading this chapter you will be able to:

- put quality in midwifery practice in the context of the NHS agenda
- discuss the relevance of clinical governance to healthcare and in particular midwifery care
- highlight issues that need to be addressed in midwifery in order to improve care
- describe ways of improving quality in midwifery.

The success of a maternity service is to be measured by the saving of life, by the improvement in the standard of health of mothers and babies and also by the extent to which it can diminish the fears, difficulties and discomforts which, in some measure, have to be faced by every woman who embarks on motherhood.

(MoH, 1959)

A BRIEF HISTORY OF QUALITY ISSUES IN THE NHS

Midwives have always aspired to give quality care. The aim of their first professional organization The Midwives Institute (which later became the Royal College of Midwives (RCM)) was 'to encourage the training of midwives so as to lead to a better standard of care for mothers and babies' (Cowell and Wainwright, 1981). It is only comparatively recently, however, that midwives, along with other health professionals, have been required both to place their care on an evidence base and to quantify the quality of their care.

Working for Patients (DoH, 1989) first introduced the concept of quality in healthcare by formulating its vision to 'bring all parts of the Health Service up to the very high standard of the best'. Medical audit was introduced as the 'systematic, critical analysis of the quality of medical care, including the procedures used for diagnosis and treatment, the use of resources, and the resulting outcome and quality of life for the patient'.

Audit in the paramedical professions was to be addressed by local managers in consultation with their professional colleagues.

This apparent need for non-medical professionals to be directed by local managers was corrected in *Framework of Audit for Nursing Services* (DoH, 1991a) when the concept of nursing audit was introduced and nurses and midwives were given the lead in auditing and implementing improvements in their clinical practice.

In the 1980s and 1990s, quality circles (or standard-setting groups) were introduced in many hospitals. This was a 'bottom-up' approach to implementing quality. Groups composed of health professionals met regularly to discuss and produce standards and audit them at a local level. The setting of standards was commonly based on Donabedian's (1966) structure, process, outcome model which required a standard statement to be produced, which was then broken down into components (structure and process) which, together, produce the outcome to achieve the standard.

Maxwell's (1984) dimensions for quality care (accessibility, equity, relevance to need, social acceptability, efficiency, effectiveness) were also used, albeit less commonly, as an alternative model for assuring quality – another example of the 'bottom-up' approach. Whichever method was used, the aim was to implement the standards after ratification by the appropriate manager. The standards would then be audited and change implemented, based on the results of audit.

In 1993, *Clinical Audit* (DoH, 1993b) proposed that audit should remain clinically led but should develop links with resource management, risk management, quality assurance and total quality management (TQM). Clinicians were to be encouraged to be involved in multidisciplinary audit as part of a wider quality management programme and it was recommended that audit become part of basic, undergraduate and postgraduate education.

Several government documents relating to clinical audit, guidelines and effectiveness (DoH, 1996a,b,c) followed. However, it became increasingly clear that local groups, and the standards they produced, were only as effective as the support they received from managers, and that the concept needed to become embedded into the culture rather than remain an issue for enthusiasts.

Total quality management, also known as continuous quality improvement, a 'top-down' initiative used in factories to improve quality throughout the organization, was implemented in some hospitals in the 1990s. TQM seeks to ensure quality at every interface, involving every person working at every level in the organization from the top down. Some hospitals used it successfully (Forsberg, 1997); others found it did not work (Porter, 1993).

The time was ripe for a top-down approach based around clinical care, not borrowed from industry. The term 'clinical governance' first appeared in *The New NHS: Modern, Dependable* (DoH, 1997). This describes a framework, the aim of which is to 'provide an NHS that continually improves the overall standard of clinical care, whilst reducing variations in outcomes of, and access to services as well as ensuring that clinical decisions are based on the most up-to-date evidence of what is known to be effective' (DoH, 1999a). Clinical governance was an idea which not only provided a framework for the 'bottom-up' work produced over previous years, but for the first time, made quality central to all aspects of clinical care.

PUTTING QUALITY INTO MIDWIFERY PRACTICE

The aim of midwifery care is to provide safe, effective and satisfactory care for all mothers and their babies. Clinical governance provides the frame-work for this to happen. How can this be achieved in practice?

The 'quality cycle' was first described by Lang (1976) and is sometimes known as the quality 'spiral' (Bucknall *et al.*, 1992). Delivering quality midwifery is about implementing the cycle of quality (Fig. 61.1).

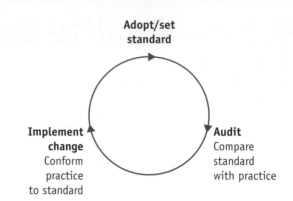

Figure 61.1   Cycle of quality.

Standards

Standards are the starting point of quality midwifery. Midwifery practice is regulated by standards which have been defined as 'professionally agreed levels of performance appropriate to the population addressed which are achievable, observable and measurable' (Sale, 1991). These have been produced by the United Kingdom Central Council for Nursing, Midwifery and Health Visiting (UKCC) (now the Nursing and Midwifery Council, NMC), the Government, trusts and local professional groups and should be based on the most up-to-date, best-quality evidence. The Royal Colleges (RCM and Royal College of Obstetricians and Gynaecologists (RCOG)) also produce standards for midwifery and obstetric care with guidelines based on best evidence in order to standardize practice and improve outcomes.

Clinical audit

'Nothing shall be called good practice until there is evidence that it achieved and continues to achieve the desired outcome' (DoH, 1993a).

Good standards, unfortunately, do not guarantee good practice. Standards need to be audited in order to demonstrate whether they have been achieved and to inform the need for change. Audit is also used to provide baseline data for future audits, to identify trends and to gather information for national audits, health authorities, professional bodies and other agencies.

Clinical audit is 'a clinically led initiative which seeks to improve the quality and outcome of patient care through structured peer review whereby clinicians examine their practices and results against agreed standards and modify their practice where indicated' (DoH, 1996a). Audit in midwifery measures practice against standards, providing information about how far practice falls short, with the aim of informing the need for change to improve care for women, babies

Table 61.1 Audit methods

Method	Strengths	Weaknesses
Surveys		
Questionnaires	Easy to administer Cheap Can be analysed by a computer program Suitable for large numbers	Low response rate Unsuitable for those who cannot read or write English Questions may be missed or misunderstood Susceptible to bias as lower-motivated people less likely to complete and/or return
Interview schedules	High response rate Suitable for those unable to read or write Extra comments can be noted Can be analysed by a computer program	Time-consuming Intra-interviewer variation Inter-interviewer variation Unsuitable for those who cannot understand English
Observation	Direct view of what actually happens Qualitative information gained Contemporaneous data	Resource intensive Time-consuming/suitable only for small-scale studies Observer bias Can be difficult to interpret data 'Hawthorne' effect Ethical issues Sample may not be representative
Examination of records		
Hand written	Direct record of care Possible to identify who gave care Does not rely on client's memory	Inaccessible records Incomplete/illegible records Time-consuming Dependent on access to database
Computer	Quick Can analyse large quantities of data easily	Training of personnel to access data Incomplete records/unusable data

and their families. Audit which is divorced from this process becomes merely 'orphan data' (Shaw, 1992).

The difference between audit and research is sometimes confused. Though there are areas of considerable overlap, particularly in methodologies, they have different functions. Research provides the evidence for standards against which audit measures practice. 'Research is concerned with finding out the right thing to do: audit in ensuring it is done right' (Smith, 1992). Nixon (1992) observed that '(audit) is designed to influence "me" rather than "you"'.

There are four main ways to audit practice against standards (Table 61.1). Each method has advantages and disadvantages and is limited by time and resources, human and monetary. Some methods lend themselves more to one kind of audit than another.

Surveys (questionnaires and interview schedules) are useful for audits of patient satisfaction, information and support. Observation may be used to monitor staff attitudes or information giving to women. Examining records directly is an ideal way of auditing standards of record-keeping and clinical care, observations, etc.

Auditing computer records is being used increasingly as units employ clinical computing systems. It is a quick and easy way to handle large amounts of data to produce, for example, rates of method of delivery, breastfeeding, smoking, transfusion, low haemoglobins (Hb).

'It must never be lost sight of what observation is for. It is not for the sake of piling up miscellaneous information or curious facts, but for the sake of saving life and increasing health and comfort' (Nightingale, 1860).

Audit is pointless without evaluation. Audit data need to be evaluated with a view to being incorporated into the cycle of quality leading to implementation of change. Making sense of the data involves looking at the larger picture to see what is really going on and how practice can be improved. Questions need to be asked about audit data. What do the results mean? How well do they conform to the standard? Are the results acceptable or unacceptable? In whose view? Are they improving or getting worse? Is the change real? Is like being compared with like? How well do the results compare with those of other units or with national benchmarks?

For example, a falling postnatal transfusion rate may at first seem to be a positive outcome of good care which in turn will lead to reduced maternal morbidity with less risk of adverse reactions, shorter hospital stays and lower cost to the NHS. However, there may be other reasons. An apparent fall in the transfusion rate needs to be supplemented with other information – the data quality (how much missing/unusable data was there?), sample size (was it representative?), the number of postnatal women going home with low Hb levels, the threshold for giving transfusions and the number of women declining transfusion. The fall in the transfusion rate may have occurred because more women are discharged with low Hb levels – either because the threshold for transfusions has dropped or because of client refusal.

'Averages seduce us away from minute observation' (Nightingale, 1860).

Although averages and percentages give a feel for what is going on, it is invariably necessary to look further to get a fuller picture in order to evaluate data. Why did these women lose so much blood in the first place? Were their antenatal haemoglobins within normal limits? Were they at a high risk of haemorrhage and if so, what measures were put in place to minimize blood loss? If they were low risk, was there a deficiency in care which caused excessive blood loss? Clinical audit does not stand on its own. It interacts with risk management, which is concerned with identifying risks and reducing them. A need for education may be highlighted. Audit can also identify substandard practice which should be addressed through midwifery supervision or management pathways.

Ideally, all standards regulating midwifery practice should be audited for compliance. In the real world this is not possible and professional bodies, government, local units and professionals themselves decide which are the most important standards to audit. Standard outcome data such as delivery rates, smoking in pregnancy rates, stillbirth rates and breastfeeding are commonly requested but are almost meaningless unless the data are evaluated and meaningful comparisons are made over a period of time and with other units or benchmark data.

Reflective Activity 61.1

Review the results of the last two clinical audits in your unit and determine how they have influenced practice. Discuss other areas where audit would be helpful in changing practice.

Implementing change

Effective audit may be regarded as a three point circle of setting standards, evaluating care and modifying practice in the light of evaluation. Many audits fail in the last stages because there is no formal feedback of information and no formal decision to remedy the deficiencies. Without feedback and remedy, 'orphan data' merely accumulate.

(Shaw, 1992)

Implementing change is the most difficult part of the quality cycle. The setting or choosing of standards and their audit is relatively easy, particularly when there are dedicated personnel to coordinate the process. Implementing change which improves care and can be demonstrated to do so is a considerable challenge involving, as it usually does, the 'shop floor' clinician. Change does not happen automatically just because it is indicated.

People respond to change in different ways and at different paces. Rogers (1983) found that in a population required to implement change, innovators (2.5%) and early adopters (around 13.5%) take on change earliest. Innovators are venturesome and enthusiastic and influence the 'early adopters' who tend to be senior opinion leaders in the organization. They in turn are able to influence the 'early majority' (around 34%) to implement the change, which creates the momentum for the 'late majority' (also around 34%) to take on the change. The change is thus established and embedded. Only the laggards (the remaining 16%) remain to take on the change. They tend to be traditional in outlook and adopt change very late, if at all.

Taking personalities into account when introducing change is important. But *how* the change is introduced is also important. Several principles make implementation of change more likely to be successful (see Box 61.1). The key is good communication.

Quality midwifery and clinical governance

A First Class Service (DoH, 1998a) put clinical governance at the heart of the NHS: 'a framework through which NHS organisations are accountable for *continuously improving* the quality of their services and safeguarding *standards* of care by creating an environment in which excellence can flourish'.

Clinical governance is an umbrella under which evidence-based practice, clinical audit, risk management, education, clinical or midwifery supervision, research and partnership with users work together to continuously

- *Evaluation* – systematic analysis and communication of data, in verbal and written reports
- *Dissemination* – wide discussion of audit results leading to a plan of action
- *Education* – update of clinicians as appropriate
- *Communication* – what and how changes will be made and by whom
- *Setting a date* – communication of a specific start date
- *Facilitation* – making change as easy as possible, e.g. giving support, using posters, stickers, tick lists, computer 'pop-up' prompts
- *Delegation* – giving people clear roles in implementing change
- *Re-evaluation* – re-audit and analysis of results to see if there is improvement, then *Dissemination* ...

improve care. As part of implementing clinical governance, two government-appointed bodies have been established to produce standards and guidelines to provide a national framework for standardizing and improving clinical practice.

The *National Institute for Clinical Excellence* (NICE) provides patients, health professionals and the public with authoritative, robust and reliable guidance on current best practice. It has produced guidelines for electronic fetal monitoring interpretation (RCOG, 2001a) and induction of labour (RCOG, 2001b). *National Service Frameworks* (NSF) are being introduced in which national standards are set for specific service or care groups. These act as performance indicators against which progress is measured within an agreed time scale. In 2001 a NSF for children was announced. This includes maternity services, and an external group is working on standards for maternity care, which will form part of the framework. This is due to be completed by 2003. Progress of this work can be found via the Department of Health website.

Clinical benchmarks

Clinical benchmarks are 'agreed standards of best practice which can be used by practitioners to compare and share practices, to ensure that quality care is delivered in a fair and consistent way' (NHS Executive Trent, 2000). Clinical practice benchmarking is another way of standardizing and improving care, with the goal of reducing unacceptable variations in care and raising the average mean to 'universalize the best'.

The Government has produced eight national benchmarks: nutrition, hygiene and mouth care, tissue viability, continence, safety of clients with mental health needs, record-keeping, privacy and dignity, and principles of self-care (DoH, 2001).

With the exception of record-keeping and privacy and dignity, the benchmarks seem somewhat unrelated to midwifery practice. However, each benchmark is fundamental to midwifery practice. For example, issues around mental health have been identified in the confidential enquiry into maternal deaths (DoH, 1998b) with suicide being a significant cause of maternal deaths. Midwives have a key role in identifying women at risk of developing psychiatric problems, i.e. postnatal depression and psychosis. With the increasing use of epidural anaesthesia, pressure ulcers have been reported in the literature (Malone, 2000). Midwives have an established role in advising on dietary matters and the importance of a balanced diet to assist in maintaining healthy iron levels in pregnancy and for helping to maintain breastfeeding. Eating disorders have been identified in pregnancy and in the puerperium (Franko and Spurrell, 2000). Issues around self-care need to be considered for women with disabilities. Urinary and faecal incontinence are uncommon but extremely distressing complications of childbirth which need to be identified and managed appropriately (Dandy, 1999; Wells, 1996).

Clinical benchmarking standards present a challenge for midwifery care. As specific midwifery benchmarks are developed, there is the potential to further universalize good practice in areas such as breastfeeding, low-risk care, normal childbirth, reducing anaemia and smoking in pregnancy.

At the local level, the essence of clinical governance is a partnership between patient and professional. High-quality care is delivered through clinical effectiveness, risk management, research, effective communication, lifelong learning, supervision and effective leadership, strategic planning and use of resources.

Risk management

Risk management is a fundamental element of clinical governance. It is 'the process of planning and organising to minimise the impact of risk to patients, staff, Trust finance and reputation and to increase the chance of success' (Nottingham City Hospital, 1999). *A First Class Service* (DoH, 1998a) stated that hospitals should have controls assurance in place to identify and control risks, and clinical risk should be systematically assessed with programmes to reduce risk.

Compared with other specialities, obstetrics is a risky business with large claims making up a major part of every trust's annual litigation (Symon, 1998). In no other speciality is the old adage 'prevention is better than cure' more relevant. Risk management aims to improve the quality of care, prevent occurrences which may harm clients or staff, reduce the risks of adverse events and reduce costs to healthcare providers. This process begins by identifying and assessing risks, e.g. poor outcomes and 'near misses', through critical incident reporting which is followed by prompt, open investigation. Why something went (or nearly went) wrong is established, not to apportion blame but so that processes can be put into place to prevent recurrence. Poor performance is addressed and other lessons learned, with the overall aim of improving care and reducing complaints and litigation.

Reflective Activity 61.2

Discuss how clinical governance works in your unit and what happens about adverse incidents particularly.

Measuring outcomes

Measuring outcomes is another important component of clinical governance, much of which takes place at the local level through clinical audit. At a national level the *Commission for Health Improvement* (CHI) is an independent body which assesses how trusts are implementing standards and the guidelines laid down by NICE and NSF. It visits trusts on a rolling programme to assess and monitor, with the aim of improving patient care. It is a collection point for good practice and will investigate serious service failures. Details of its activities can be found at: http://www.chi.nhs.uk/.

Clinical indicators   These are quantitative measures, which are used to evaluate and compare important aspects of patient care. National clinical indicators such as death rates and readmission rates are not a sensitive measure of midwifery and obstetric care. However, specific clinical indicators can be used in midwifery and obstetric practice to reflect the quality of care and to compare with other units so that best practice can be shared to improve outcomes.

Indicators should be easily and objectively measurable, able to be improved and drawn from government or professional recommendations, confidential enquiries,

national initiatives or in some other way to be a measure of safe, effective care.

Like clinical benchmarks, clinical indicators can be developed and used by midwives to compare outcomes over a period of time, to highlight weaknesses and strengths and to compare with other units. Normal delivery and caesarean section (CS) rates have been used for years as 'clinical indicators'. Although there is at present no national consensus on optimum rates, they are already being used as units of comparison both regionally and nationally. Stillbirth rates are another standard measure, a clinical indicator with a national average published for units to compare themselves against. Two measures of perinatal morbidity are the admission rate to neonatal units of non-dysmorphic term babies and the rate of occurrence of hypoxic ischaemic encephalopathy (HIE). Other useful indicators are breastfeeding rates, low postnatal Hb rates and transfusion rates. The percentage of women who smoke the day before delivery is a measure of clinicians' input and advice throughout pregnancy, related to the government document *Smoking Kills* (DoH, 1999b), working towards the government's target of only 15% of women smoking by the end of pregnancy by 2010. 'Standard primipara' data (a subset of the obstetric population) can also be used to make inter-unit comparisons of the process and outcomes of midwifery and obstetric care.

Supervision

Since its inception in 1902, midwifery supervision has played an important part in improving midwifery care. Its purpose is to 'safeguard and enhance the quality of care for the childbearing mother and her family' (ENB, 1996). The roles and responsibilities of supervisors are, amongst others, to monitor standards of midwifery practice, contribute towards risk management and clinical audit, investigate critical incidents and provide leadership which supports and empowers good practice through evidence-based decision-making (ENB, 1997). Working effectively, supervision contributes significantly towards clinical governance and producing a first class maternity service.

Quality care starts with evidence-based standards and guidelines. Care, based on those standards and guidelines, is delivered by competent, confident clinicians who are well supported by supervision and work in partnership with women and their families. Their practice is regularly and rigorously audited and shortcomings identified and corrected so that lessons are learned and care is continuously improved.

REDUCING MATERNAL MORTALITY AND MORBIDITY (BOX 61.2)

Providing safe and effective care for women starts pre-conceptually. Encouraging women to stop smoking and eat a healthy, well-balanced diet will help to promote healthy pregnancies.

Though most women have perfectly normal preg-nancies, deliveries and babies, a small number do not. Women at risk should be identified early: diabetics, women with thromboembolic disease, HIV-positive women, drug abusers and women with other major medical, psychiatric or social problems. Audit of the management of high-risk women needs to be carried out and evaluated to ensure that those women who need spe-cific interventions and care get them. Other research-based recommendations should be carried out, among them: prompt treatment of asymptomatic bacteriuria (RCOG, 1997) and offering external cephalic version to women with breech presentation after 36 weeks' gesta-tion (RCOG, 1997). Just as important is to identify low-risk women who become high risk during preg-nancy or labour.

In the intrapartum period, the recommendations of the confidential enquiries (DoH, 1998b) on managing obstetric haemorrhage and other emergencies, infec-tion and thromboembolic disease (RCOG, 1995) should not only be in place but regularly audited to ensure that policies are complied with. A research-based standard recommends the use of routine antibi-otics at caesarean section to reduce the risk of infection (RCOG, 1997).

Common complications of the postpartum period are anaemia, wound and perineal infection, depression and sequelae of perineal damage – all causing consid-erable morbidity and occasional deaths. Again, safe and effective care means that practitioners base their practice on evidence-based guidelines which are regularly audited and acted upon. Midwives should develop innovative ways of preventing problems hap-pening in the first place; for example, reducing blood loss at delivery, early identification of those at risk of psychiatric problems, being aware of those at risk of third- and fourth-degree tears.

The last confidential enquiry into maternal deaths (RCOG, 2001c) offers guidance for good practice. Dennett (2002) identifies three things that midwives need to consider in maximizing their effectiveness: improving accessibility, effective midwifery practice and collaborative working.

Box 61.2 Reducing maternal morbidity and mortality: main points

Preconception
- Encouragement and support of women to stop smoking
- Encouragement of healthy, well-balanced diet

Antepartum
- Early identification and management of high-risk women
- Early identification and management of complications of pregnancy
- Prompt treatment of asymptomatic bacteriuria
- Offer of external cephalic version (ECV) to women with breech presentation over 36 weeks' gestation

Intrapartum
- Early and effective management of complications and obstetric emergencies
- Routine antibiotics at emergency caesarean section
- Reduction of blood loss at delivery
- Early identification and management of third- and fourth-degree tears

Postpartum
- Early identification and management of infection
- Early identification and management of psychiatric problems

Reflective Activity 61.3

Identify three areas, from the latest confidential enquiry (http://www.cemd.org.uk) where practice might be improved in your unit. Discuss these with other midwives and your supervisor of midwives.

REDUCING PERINATAL MORTALITY AND MORBIDITY (BOX 61.3)

Improving perinatal outcomes also starts preconceptu-ally. Research has shown that taking 400 mg of folic acid daily before pregnancy and up to the 12th week of gestation reduces the incidence of open neural tube defects (RCOG, 1997). In the antepartum period, early identification and management of intrauterine growth

Box 61.3 Reducing perinatal mortality and morbidity: main points

Preconception
- Folic acid before conception and up to 12 weeks' gestation
- Encouraging and supporting women to stop smoking

Antepartum
- Encouraging and supporting women to stop smoking
- Early identification of IUGR and reduced fetal movements
- Administration of steroids to women at risk of preterm labour/delivery

Intrapartum
- Early identification and management of abnormal CTGs
- Administration of antibiotics in labour to women with GBS
- Appropriate treatment of women with HIV

Postpartum
- Encouraging and supporting women to breastfeed
- Advice on how to reduce the risk of cot death, especially providing a 'smoke-free zone' for babies
- Early identification of deviations from norm
- Timely education, advice and support

restriction (IUGR) and reduced fetal movements, encouraging and supporting mothers to stop smoking, and administration of steroids to mothers at risk of preterm delivery are some evidence-based ways of reducing risks and improving outcomes.

Although it is well known that much of the damage to babies who develop hypoxic ischaemic encephelopathy occurs antenatally, CESDI reports (DoH, 1995; MCHRC, 2000) have highlighted deficiencies in cardiotocograph (CTG) interpretation and action on abnormal CTGs, leading to avoidable perinatal mortality and morbidity. A national guideline (RCOG, 2001a) has now been produced with the aim of standardizing CTG interpretation and leading to a reduction in avoidable intrapartum deaths. Evidence indicates that administration of antibiotics in labour to women infected with group B haemolytic streptococcus (GBS) is an effective way of reducing perinatal

mortality and morbidity. HIV-positive women should be given appropriate treatment to help prevent transmission of HIV to their infants.

Postnatally, encouraging and supporting mothers to breastfeed, advising them about how to reduce the risk of cot death (especially by advice to stop smoking) and giving timely education, advice and support all contribute towards reducing perinatal morbidity and mortality.

Defective practice, lack of knowledge and poor communication are commonly found to be causes of avoidable maternal and perinatal mortality and morbidity. Whilst these problems may never be completely eliminated, much can be done to improve care by evidence-based practice which is regularly and rigorously audited and acted upon by addressing deficiencies and 'near misses' through management or supervision.

INCREASING SATISFACTION WITH CARE (BOX 61.4)

Though the majority of women are satisfied with their maternity care, a small proportion are not. Causes of dissatisfaction have been found to be lack of continuity of care, poor-quality information and advice and long waiting times (Williamson and Thomson, 1996). Symon (1998) found that poor and insensitive communication increases dissatisfaction and is a factor in litigation. On the other hand, open communication, a nurturing and caring environment and a democratic management structure were felt by Too (1996) to empower women. The unsurprising conclusions of a study by Morgan *et al.* (1998) were that friendliness, support, consistency of care, good communication and participation in decisions were important determinants of satisfaction.

The NMC lays down strict standards for professional conduct and practice (UKCC, 1992, 1996) regarding the care of clients. *The Patient's Charter* (DoH, 1991b) set important standards for privacy, dignity and respect for religious and cultural backgrounds. *Changing Childbirth* (DoH, 1993c) did much to place the woman at the centre of maternity care, making recommendations designed to give more choice, continuity and control. Women have the right to be supported in their choices, and to be given high-quality, timely information, privacy and dignity. Midwives have a key role in ensuring that women are involved in decisions about their care as much as they want to be and in being facilitators of normal childbirth.

Box 61.4 Increasing satisfaction with care

- Caring, supportive and competent care
- Open, friendly communication
- Timely, appropriate information-giving
- Participation in decision-making
- Facilitation of women's choice
- Consistency and continuity of care
- Respect for privacy and dignity, religious and cultural backgrounds
- High standards of confidentiality
- Appropriate management of pain in labour and the postpartum period
- Prompt attention to complaints

The Government aims to address patient satisfaction through a national patient and users' survey. Involvement of the users in the planning of services is an important part of implementing the NHS plan (DoH, 2000). Local surveys of satisfaction with care should be carried out regularly and acted upon. Complaints tend to be about staff attitude, lack of confidentiality, poor management of pain in labour and lack of support in the postnatal period. They should be dealt with promptly and fairly, in accordance with local policy.

THE WAY FORWARD

What are the challenges that face midwives in the future in their quest to give quality care? Midwives should continue in their role doing what they do best – facilitating normality. The gains of recent decades should not be lost.

Changing Childbirth (DoH, 1993c) empowered midwives to organize their practice around giving continuity, choice and individualized care to women in both hospital and community settings. Choice, however, raises difficulties of its own. How far should choice extend? For example, should women be able to request caesarean section? Caesarean sections for non-clinical reasons carry significantly more risks for both mothers and babies than vaginal deliveries and are more costly in terms of resources, both human and financial (Wagner, 2000). Respecting women's choices need to be balanced with the need to enable women to make safe, informed choices by giving confident, evidence-based advice and care which optimizes outcomes, reducing maternal and perinatal morbidity and mortality.

Ethical issues will continue to challenge midwives. As screening tests continue to become ever-more sophisticated, it will be possible to screen for more conditions, with accompanying ethical dilemmas for both midwives and mothers.

Computers will be used increasingly to store clinical data on databases. Midwives need to seize opportunities to use these systems to improve care. Midwives also need to be innovative, to build on existing structures and processes and develop new ones in order to standardize excellent practice. It is vital to have midwifery representation in the decision-making processes involving procurement of systems and to ensure that systems are flexible enough to introduce developments which can improve care and be audited easily (preferably by a clinician) to monitor standards of care (see Box 61.5). Flexible clinical computer systems lend themselves extremely well to incorporating prompts and audit tools which appear on screen under specific conditions, taking little time to complete and, with appropriate software, being easy to audit. Successful innovations in this and other areas should be shared through publication, conferences and other local and national forums.

Midwives will need to become familiar with accessing the latest research evidence, e.g. Cochrane database, MEDLINE, National electronic Library for Health (NeLH) to inform and develop their practice.

Changing Childbirth (DoH, 1993c) gave midwives an ideal opportunity to focus care on women. However, midwives should not fall into the trap of focusing only on the narrow issues of giving individualized, quality care to women, babies and their families. Midwives do not practise in a vacuum but in a local context, with their peers, obstetricians, paediatricians, anaesthetists, GPs and paramedical staff. Over the last few years, midwives have at times retreated into a midwifery ghetto and have sometimes minimized or even dismissed the contribution of their professional colleagues. Midwives need to contribute meaningfully to multidisciplinary policies, protocols and guidelines in order to improve standards of care and universalize good practice, whilst retaining their unique and distinctive role.

A further challenge for midwives is to be aware not only of their role as individual and local practitioners but also of their wider contribution to public health. Midwives have an important part to play and their impact should not be underestimated. Smoking in pregnancy, reducing cot death, promoting breastfeeding, healthy diet, parentcraft education and reducing teenage pregnancies are just some of the issues on which midwives can and do have enormous influence,

---

Box 61.5 Smoking and pregnancy

It has long been recognized that smoking is harmful in pregnancy (Royal College of Physicians, 1992) and poses considerable risks to babies. *The Health of the Nation* (DoH, 1992) aimed to reduce by a third the number of women who smoke at the start of their pregnancy. In 1999, *Smoking Kills* (DoH, 1999b) set targets of reducing smoking in pregnancy to 18% by 2005, and 15% by 2010.

It is well known that advice given by health professionals influences quitting rates and, based on grade A strength of evidence, Raw *et al.* (1998) stated that 'pregnant smokers should be given firm and clear advice to stop smoking throughout pregnancy, and given assistance when it is requested'. These recommendations were updated (West *et al.*, 2000) with the addition that pregnant smokers should be offered specialist support with stopping smoking and that nicotine replacement therapy be offered to women who could not quit on their own.

In 1994, a standard was set at Nottingham City Hospital that 'All mothers who smoke will be advised about the risks of smoking and encouraged to stop' (Buckley, 2000). To fulfil the standard, interactive software 'SmokeScreen' was developed which was integrated into the computerized booking process. The programme generates questions in response to previous answers, to establish whether the woman smokes, for how long, and where she is on the 'cycle of change' (Prochaska and DiClemente, 1983). On the basis of this information, the midwife is prompted to advise the woman about the risks of smoking and the benefits of stopping, and give relevant leaflets and contact phone numbers. Referral to a specialist advisor is offered to pregnant smokers. The midwife then records on computer whether advice and leaflets were given.

Postnatal mothers are asked about smoking on hospital discharge, using a questionnaire. This is to ascertain how many mothers were still smoking the day prior to delivery, providing statistical data and prompting the midwife to give advice about the risks of neonatal exposure to smoke and how to reduce the risks, particularly of cot death.

Compliance with the standard is monitored regularly. The results of one audit indicated that the percentage of smokers being given advice at booking had decreased to 89% from the previous year's level of 97%. On investigation it was found that several midwives were not giving advice. The midwives were seen by their supervisors who discussed with them the reasons for not giving advice. The importance of complying with the evidence-based standard was reiterated and for one midwife the need for updating was highlighted. Audit of the standard for the following year demonstrated an improvement and it was found that 97% of smokers were given advice at booking.

Audit of postnatal advice consistently demonstrates that around 91% of women are given advice on hospital discharge. Audit results are discussed at unit meetings to try to improve rates of compliance.

Around 24% of women are smokers at booking. About 21% of women are still smoking the day before delivery, a 12.5% reduction and an indication of health professionals' input. The rate of smoking the day before delivery is one of the unit's clinical indicators and is a continuing measure of the progress being made towards the national target.

Helping pregnant smokers to quit is a good example of how midwives can influence the health of mothers and babies through practice based on a research-based standard. Audit of compliance with the standard identified deficiencies in care which were acted upon. Re-audit demonstrated an improvement in practice, thus 'closing the audit loop'. Standards, evidence-based practice, risk management, clinical audit, clinical indicators, ongoing education and midwifery supervision all have a role in improving practice and outcomes for mothers and babies as part of the clinical governance programme.

---

not only on women, but also their partners, families and beyond.

Nationally, midwives need to be at the forefront of policy-making processes around maternity care. *The NHS Plan* (DoH, 2000) articulated the need to examine leadership throughout the NHS in order to take the NHS forward into the new millennium. At a national level, midwives should grasp opportunities to work more closely on policy, research and education with their medical and nursing colleagues to further improve the health of the nation.

CONCLUSION

Quality midwifery care is both competent and caring. It aims to involve the woman and her family so that she experiences as positive and safe and normal a pregnancy, delivery and puerperium as possible. The midwife whose practice is woman centred and evidence based, working cooperatively with her peers in her local situation and being aware of her unique role and contribution in the wider context of society, is ideally placed to have an impact on both the short-term and long-term health and well-being of mothers, babies and their families.

KEY POINTS

- To achieve 'quality midwifery', midwives should base their practice on evidence-based standards and guidelines, and audit and evaluate their practice against those standards, taking action where necessary to further improve care.
- Clinical governance is a framework which midwives can use to continuously improve the quality of their care through clinical audit and other processes such as risk management, professional regulation, education, research and supervision.
- Midwives should work collaboratively with their medical and nursing colleagues to improve care and outcomes.

- Midwifery benchmarks should be developed in order that practice between units can be compared and best practice shared.
- Clinical indicators are a useful way of quantifying aspects of midwifery practice in order to evaluate outcomes over a period of time, raise awareness of positive results and identify areas of suboptimal practice.
- Midwives have a unique role and impact in their practice as individuals, in the local context and in society as a whole.

REFERENCES

Buckley, E.R. (2000) Helping pregnant women to stop smoking. *British Journal of Midwifery* 8(10): 101–105.

Bucknall, C., Robertson, C., Moran, F. *et al.* (1992) Improving management of asthma: closing the loop or progressing along the spiral? *Health Care* 1: 15.

Cowell, B. & Wainwright, D. (1981) *Behind the Blue Door*, p. 99. London: Baillière Tindall.

Dandy, D. (1999) Assessment tool promotes continence after childbirth. *Nursing Times* 95(28): 42–43.

Dennett, S. (2002) Maternal deaths: still a concern for midwives. *British Journal of Midwifery* 10(2): 68–70.

Department of Health (DoH) (1989) *Working for Patients*. London: Department of Health.

Department of Health (DoH) (1991a) *Framework of audit for nursing services*, p. 3. London: Department of Health.

Department of Health (DoH) (1991b) *The Patient's Charter*. London: HMSO.

Department of Health (DoH) (1992) *The Health of the Nation*, p. 18. London: HMSO.

Department of Health (DoH) (1993a) *Targeting practice: the contribution of nurses, midwives and health visitors*. London: Department of Health.

Department of Health (DoH) (1993b) *Clinical Audit: Meeting and Improving Standards in Healthcare*. London: DoH.

Department of Health (DoH) (1993c) *Changing Childbirth: Report of the Expert Maternity Group*. London: HMSO.

Department of Health (DoH) (1995) *Confidential Enquiry into Stillbirths and Deaths in Infancy: Annual Report from 1 January–31st December 1994*. London: HMSO.

Department of Health (DoH) (1996a) *Clinical Audit in the NHS: Using Clinical Audit in the NHS: a Position Paper*, p. 3. London: Department of Health.

Department of Health (DoH) (1996b) *Promoting Clinical Effectiveness: A Framework for Action in and through the NHS*. London: Department of Health.

Department of Health (DoH) (1996c) *Clinical Guidelines*. London: Department of Health.

Department of Health (DoH) (1997) *The New NHS: Modern, Dependable*. London: Department of Health.

Department of Health (DoH) (1998a) *A First Class Service*. London: Department of Health.

Department of Health (DoH) (1998b) *Why Mothers Die. Report on Confidential Enquiries into Maternal Deaths in the United Kingdom 1994–1996*, pp. 140–153. London: Department of Health.

Department of Health (DoH) (1999a) *Clinical Governance*. London: Department of Health.

Department of Health (DoH) (1999b) *Smoking Kills*. London: Department of Health.

Department of Health (DoH) (2000) *The NHS Plan*. London: Department of Health.

Department of Health (DoH) (2001) *Essence of Care*. London: Department of Health.

Donabedian, A. (1966) Evaluating the quality of medical care. *Millbank Memorial Fund Quarterly* 44(2): 166–206.

English National Board for Nursing, Midwifery and Health Visiting (ENB) (1996) *Supervision of Midwives: the*

English National Board's Advice and Guidance to Local Supervising Authorities and Supervisors of Midwives, p. 13. London: ENB.

English National Board for Nursing, Midwifery and Health Visiting (ENB) (1997) Preparation of Supervisors of Midwives. Module 1, p. 12. London: ENB.

Forsberg, S.A. (1997) Infant metabolic screening: a total quality management approach. *Journal of Obstetric, Gynecologic and Neonatal Nursing* 26(3): 257–261.

Franko, D.L. & Spurrell, E.B. (2000) Detection and management of eating disorders during pregnancy. *Obstetrics and Gynecology* 95(6 Pt 1): 942–946.

Lang, N. (1976) Quality assurance – the idea and its development in the United States. In: Willis, M. & Linwood, M. (eds) *Measuring the Quality of Care.* Edinburgh: Churchill Livingstone.

Maxwell, R. (1984) Quality assessment in health. *British Medical Journal* 288: 1470–1472.

Malone, C. (2000) Pressure sores in the labour ward. *RCM Midwives Journal* 3(1): 20–23.

Maternal and Child Health Research Consortium (MCHRC) (2000) *Confidential Enquiry into Stillbirths and Deaths in Infancy: 7th Annual Report.* London: MCHRC.

Ministry of Health (MoH) (1959) *Report of the Maternity Service Committee*, p. 15. London: HMSO.

Morgan, M., Fenwick, N., McKenzie, C. *et al.* (1998) Quality of midwifery led care: assessing the effects of different models of continuity for women's satisfaction. *Quality in Health Care* 7(2): 77–82.

NHS Executive Trent (2000) *Supporting Clinical Governance.* Leicester: Clinical Governance Support Team.

Nightingale, F. (1860) *Notes on Nursing.* Reprinted 1969. New York: Dover Publications.

Nixon, S.J. (1992) Defining essential hospital data. In: Smith, R. (ed) *Audit in Action*, p. 113. London: BMJ.

Nottingham City Hospital (NHS) Trust (1999) *Risk Management Manual.* Nottingham: NCHT.

Porter, J.L. (1993) Commentary on ten reasons why TQM doesn't work. *Nursing Scan in Administration* 8(4): 5.

Prochaska, J. & DiClemente, C. (1983) Stages and processes of self-change of smoking towards an integrative model of change. *Journal of Consulting and Clinical Psychology* 51: 390–395.

Raw, M., McNeil, A. & West, R. (1998) Smoking cessation guidelines for health professionals. *Thorax* 53(5): S1–S19.

Rogers, E.M. (1983) *Diffusion of Innovations*, 3rd edn, pp. 246–251. New York: Free press.

Royal College of Physicians (1992) *Smoking and the Young.* London: Royal College of Physicians.

Royal College of Obstetricians and Gynaecologists (RCOG) (1995) *Report of the RCOG Working Party on Prophylaxis against Thromboembolism in Gynaecology and Obstetrics.* London: RCOG.

Royal College of Obstetricians and Gynaecologists (RCOG) (1997) *Effective Procedures in Maternity Care Suitable for Audit*, pp. 30–35. London: RCOG.

Royal College of Obstetricians and Gynaecologists (RCOG) (2001a) *The Use of Electronic Fetal Monitoring. Evidence Based Clinical Guideline No. 8.* London: RCOG.

Royal College of Obstetricians and Gynaecologists (RCOG) (2001b) *Induction of Labour. Evidence Based Guideline No. 9.* London: RCOG.

Royal College of Obstetricians and Gynaecologists (RCOG) (2001c) *Why Mothers Die 1997–1999. The Fifth Report of CEMD in the UK.* London: RCOG Press.

Sale, D. (1991) *Quality Assurance*, p. 54. Hampshire: Macmillan.

Shaw, C.D. (1992) Acceptability of audit. In: Smith, R. (ed) *Audit in Action*, p. 27. London: BMJ.

Smith, R. (1992) Audit and research. *British Medical Journal* 305: 905–906.

Symon, A. (1998) *Litigation. The Views of Midwives and Obstetricians*, p. 6. Cheshire: Hochland and Hochland.

Too, S. (1996) Do birthplans empower women? A study of midwives' views. *Nursing Standard* 10(32): 44–48.

United Kingdom Central Council for Nursing, Midwifery and Health Visiting (UKCC) (1992) *Code of Professional Conduct.* London: UKCC.

United Kingdom Central Council for Nursing, Midwifery and Health Visiting (UKCC) (1996) *Guidelines for Professional Practice.* London: UKCC.

Wells, M. (1996) Continence following childbirth. *British Journal of Nursing* 5(6) (British Journal of Continence Suppl.): 353–354, 356, 358 passim.

West, R., McNeil, A. & Raw, M. (2000) Smoking cessation guidelines for health professionals: an update. *Thorax* 55: 987–999.

Williamson, S. & Thomson, A.M. (1996) Women's satisfaction with antenatal care in a changing maternity service. *Midwifery* 12(4): 198–204.

Wagner, M. (2000) Choosing caesarean section. *Lancet* 356(9242): 1677–1680.

FURTHER READING

Buckley, E.R. (1997) *Delivering Quality in Midwifery.* London: Baillière Tindall.

A practical book about quality in midwifery, offering step-by-step guidelines for setting standards, carrying out audits and implementing change. Examples of midwifery audits are given throughout the book.

Morris, M. (1998) *Midwifery Audit: Good Practice Guide.* London: Royal College of Midwives.

A guide to assist midwives to participate effectively in the audit process, to work with other disciplines in order to deliver effective, quality services to women.

Royal College of Obstetricians and Gynaecologists (1997) *Effective Procedures in Maternity Care Suitable for Audit*. London: RCOG.
A guide containing standard statements with supporting evidence covering important aspects of maternity care. A framework for the audit process is provided which encourages a collaborative approach to the process of improving care.

Royal College of Nursing, Clinical Governance Research and Development Unit (2002) *Principles of Best Practice in Clinical Audit*. London: Heinemann.
This book was funded by NICE and CHI in response to demands of professionals, and encourages staff to follow examples of best practice.

Epidemiology

Mary Sidebotham

INTRODUCTION

The constantly changing patterns of fertility and child-bearing in England and Wales are monitored by the Office for National Statistics (ONS). This information plays an important part in future planning for health, education and social welfare needs. Within this country there is a legal duty imposed to notify and register all live births, stillbirths and deaths. It is from these data that trends and patterns may be identified, and services planned accordingly to meet the needs of the current and emerging population. It is important that midwives recognize the processes for gathering these data, and are able to utilize this information in their day-to-day practice.

NOTIFICATION AND REGISTRATION OF BIRTHS

The National Health Service Act (1977) requires that that the father, or any person in attendance at the birth or within 6 hours after, notify the birth to the Director of Public Health within 36 hours. In practice this duty is commonly undertaken by the midwife, who is supplied with printed cards and stamped envelopes by the health authority, or completes a computerized notification.

All live births (even before the 24th week) and stillbirths must be notified.

The purpose of notification is to communicate information about the birth to the health visitor, including in particular any babies who may appear to be at risk. The information is then computerized, and this ensures recall at appropriate times for screening, vaccination and immunization, and provides data to be used for statistical and epidemiological purposes.

Registration of births

The Registration of Births and Deaths Act (1953) requires all live births and stillbirths to be registered with the Registrar of Births and Deaths within 42 days of the birth of the baby. The baby is usually registered with the registrar of the district in which the child was born, but arrangements can be made to register the child in the mother's district of residence.

All stillborn babies, including those born following termination of pregnancy, and those babies who died in early pregnancy but are born after 24 weeks (*fetus papyraceous*) must be registered. This will understandably be difficult for the parents to accept, and the midwife must show tact and understanding in these difficult circumstances. A stillbirth must be registered before burial and for this a certificate must be produced, signed by a medical practitioner or the midwife who was present at birth or examined the body afterwards.

Registration is the responsibility of the child's parents. If the parents fail to register the birth, the duty falls on the occupier of the premises in which the birth took place, usually the midwife or some other person of authority. A short certificate giving the full name and sex of the child and the date and place of birth is issued free. A fee is charged for a more detailed certificate which includes information about the parents of the child.

An increasing number of children (40.3%) are born to parents who are unmarried (ONS, 2002) and in these circumstances the mother registers the birth. The father's name can be entered on the birth certificate only if he accompanies the mother and requests that his name be entered; or it may be entered without his consent on production of an order made under the Affiliation Proceedings Act 1957.

FERTILITY RATE

The general fertility rate is described as the number of births per 1000 women aged 15–44 years. There was increasing fertility in the UK between 1952 and 1964 when it peaked at 94 births per 1000 women (DoH, 1994) In the last decade there has been a shift downwards in the general fertility rate which in 1999 was 57.7 (ONS, 2000a).

The total fertility rate (TFR) is the average number of children who would be born per woman if they experienced the age-specific fertility rates of the given year throughout their childbearing years. There has been a steady decline since the mid-60s 'baby boom'. The recorded TFR of 2000 was 1.64 – the lowest ever recorded rate. There has been a corresponding rise in the reported infertility rate with an increasing demand being made upon health authorities to provide services for assisted conception with a frequently quoted rate of 1 in 6 couples (Kon, 1993) trying and failing to conceive within 2 years of trying.

BIRTH RATE

The birth rate is the number of registered live births per 1000 population, and has been in decline in England and Wales since 1990 (Fig. 62.1). The live birth rate for England and Wales in 2000 was down to 11.4 per 1000 population (ONS, 2002) and this will have an impact

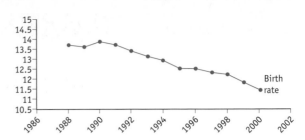

Figure 62.1   Crude birth rate 1988–2000 (source ONS).

upon the planned provision of maternity services in the future.

Women are delaying childbirth for many reasons, with the mean age at birth of the first child now 26.9 years and the mean age for all births 29.1 (ONS, 2002). This factor could explain in part the increasing number of women seeking treatment for infertility, as general fertility decreases with age. Women of 35 are known to be on average half as fertile as those of 31 (Challoner, 1999). Other factors influencing the birth rate are the availability, safety and reliability of methods of contraception, with a noted increase in conception rates being observed when the safety of the contraceptive pill was in doubt. Environmental factors are also thought to play a part in the general downward trend in fertility and have been linked with decreasing sperm counts (Balen et al., 1997) and exposure to sexually transmitted disease.

Despite the reduction in births in the general population, England and Wales has the highest teenage conception rate in Europe (64.9) with a teenage birth rate of 30.6 per 1000 births. The reported mortality and morbidity in young mothers is higher than average and there are concerted attempts by Government to improve sex education and make family planning services more accessible to young people in an attempt to reduce the teenage conception rate. The Government have supported this strategy with the introduction of Sure Start Plus (SEU, 1999). Maternity services are being planned and delivered to monitor pregnant teenagers in a supportive environment in an attempt to reduce the perceived risk of higher morbidity and mortality.

Reflective Activity 62.1

Review your unit's birth register and other sources of statistical information (as in the reference list).

What are the following in your unit:

- birth rate?
- teenage pregnancy rate?

- maternal mortality rate?
- perinatal mortality rate?

Have these rates changed during the last few years? If so, why do you think this has happened? How has this information been used to design services?

FETAL AND INFANT DEATHS

Reduction in fetal and infant deaths has been a major factor in health policy throughout the 20th, and into the 21st century. In 1958 and again in 1970, nationwide perinatal surveys provided increased knowledge of perinatal deaths. These highlighted valuable information, and allowed an analysis of the factors which might influence the survival rates. The Report of the Committee on Child Health Services made unfavourable comparisons between perinatal and infant mortality in Great Britain and in other developed countries (DHSS, 1976) which were reiterated by *The Way Forward* report (DHSS, 1977).

Since then the perinatal mortality rate in the UK has fallen considerably. The Social Services Committee's second report (Social Services Committee, 1984) welcomed the improvements in perinatal and neonatal mortality since the publication of its earlier report in 1980 (Social Services Committee, 1980). The highest perinatal and infant mortality rates continued to be mainly associated with the lower socioeconomic groups. This was echoed by the Black report (DHSS, 1980).

A further report (DHSS, 1988) addressed the persisting concerns of marked geographical and socioeconomic variations in infant mortality rates, along with the high prevalence of deaths amongst babies of low birthweight and those deaths attributed to sudden infant death syndrome. The group recommended that a system of confidential enquiry into stillbirths and deaths in infancy be implemented and this resulted in the establishment of the Confidential Enquiry into Stillbirths and Deaths in Infancy (CESDI) in 1992.

CONFIDENTIAL ENQUIRY INTO STILLBIRTHS AND DEATHS IN INFANCY (CESDI)

On 1 April 2003 CESDI amalgamated with the Confidential Enquiry into Maternal Deaths (CEMD) to form the new organization the Confidential Enquiry into Maternal and Child Health (CEMACH).

The overall aim of CESDI was 'to improve understanding of how the risks of death in late fetal life and infancy, from 20 weeks of pregnancy to one year after birth may be reduced' (MCHRC, 1999). CESDI aimed to identify risks, which can be attributed to suboptimal clinical care (MCHRC, 1999).

CESDI was organized on a regional basis with each regional coordinator contributing data to the National Secretariat. All fetal and infant losses from 20 weeks' gestation up to 1 year after birth were reported to CESDI using the Rapid Report form. From the total number of fetal and infant losses, relevant subsets were identified, and areas of practice critically examined by means of panel or focus group work, using the confidential enquiry process. Since 1993 annual reports of activity have used this approach, highlighting avoidable factors and making recommendations to improve the care offered to women and babies. This function has remained an integral part of the newly formed organization CEMACH and a major part of the role of the Regional CEMACH Coordinator is local dissemination of this information. This obligation is focused centrally upon the Secretariat, guided by professional consortia of advisors.

In 1999 the introduction of the government paper *A First Class Service* (DoH, 1998a) saw the creation of the National Institute of Clinical Excellence (NICE), which is now responsible for all of the national Confidential Enquiries. Within the same paper the Government acknowledged the value of the enquiries and placed an obligation on all professionals to contribute to them.

CESDI have examined factors surrounding intrapartum deaths and the subsequent impact on stillbirth and perinatal mortality rates (MCHRC, 1995, 1997); sudden expected and unexpected deaths in infancy (MCHRC, 1999): and antepartum stillbirths at term (MCHRC, 1998). Intrapartum-related deaths amongst home births have been examined and recommendations have been made to ensure that birth at home is as safe as possible. Focus groups have looked at the influence that events such as shoulder dystocia, induction of labour, and breech presentation may have had on mortality rates. Recommendations based on analysis of these events have been published (MCHRC, 1998, 2000), and the more recent report includes audit and uptake of those recommendations (MCHRC, 2000). The focus of enquiry for 1998–2000 was premature birth and the findings from this large gestational age-based study are published within the 8th (MCHRC, 2001) and 9th CESDI reports (MCHRC, 2002).

FACTORS INFLUENCING DEATH RATES

Fetal and infant deaths are divided into defined categories. Whilst there may be similarities between these groups, it is important to look at them individually in order to identify areas for future research, and potential improvement in outcome.

Stillbirths

A baby who has issued forth from its mother after the 24th week of pregnancy and has not at any time after being completely expelled from its mother breathed or shown any sign of life is a stillborn baby.

(UKCC, 1998)

The stillbirth rate is the number of stillbirths registered during the year per 1000 registered total (live and still) births. In 1999 the stillbirth rate for England and Wales was 5.3 (ONS, 2000b).

Certain duties are imposed by statute regarding stillbirths. These include completion of the following:

1. *Notification of stillbirth.*
2. *Certification of stillbirth.* This may be completed by the medical practitioner or midwife who was present at a stillbirth or examined the body. This certificate is then given to the woman or partner. Whenever possible the cause of death and the estimated duration of pregnancy should be recorded on this certificate to the best of the practitioner's knowledge and belief.
3. *Registration.* On receipt of the stillbirth certificate the Registrar of Births and Deaths issues a certificate for burial or cremation. The parents should be advised that the stillbirth certificate issued to them by the Registrar of Births and Deaths can, on request, include the chosen name of their stillborn baby. It is usual for the hospital or health authority to make

arrangements for the baby's burial or cremation, although some parents prefer to do this personally.

Sometimes the Coroner issues an Order for Burial and then a certificate is not required. The hospital or health authority meets the cost of the burial or cremation.

Following a stillbirth the midwife must be prepared to provide much help and support to the mother and her family during the postnatal period. Her understanding of the family's grief and her skill as a counsellor can do much to comfort and support them (see Ch. 3).

Perinatal deaths

The perinatal mortality rate comprises all stillbirths and deaths in the first week of life per 1000 registered total births (Fig. 62.2). The group includes all babies who have died 'around' the time of birth.

The perinatal mortality rate in England and Wales fell from 19.3 per 1000 in 1975 to 8.1 per 1000 in 2000 (ONS, 2002).

The main causes remain unchanged:

- anoxia
- congenital abnormalities
- immaturity
- cerebral birth injury (MCHRC, 2002).

Predisposing causes of perinatal death

Social factors The perinatal mortality rate is very much higher in socioeconomic groups IV and V and the gap between the social classes is widening rather than decreasing (DHSS, 1980; DoH, 2000; ONS, 2002; Social Services Committee, 1980, 1984; Whitehead, 1987). Social class differences in access to social and medical care also continue, with women from lower socioeconomic and minority groups not fully utilizing the services available. Several researchers have found that the decline in perinatal mortality may be attributed to an increase in birthweight, and this is regarded as an indicator of improved environmental and social factors rather than medical care (Editorial, 1986). Low birthweight remains more prevalent in lower socioeconomic and certain ethnic groups. Even if a low birthweight baby survives the perinatal period, recent studies indicate that those who are small or disproportionate at birth, or who have altered placental growth, are at an increased risk of developing coronary heart disease, hypertension and diabetes during adult life (Godrey and Barker, 1995). The perinatal mortality rate for babies of unsupported mothers is nearly double that of their married (or supported) counterparts. Biological factors such

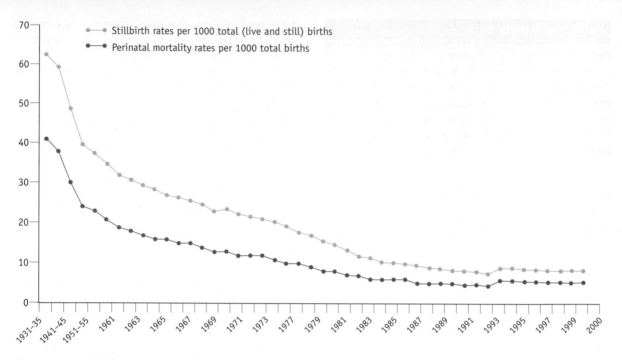

Figure 62.2 Stillbirth and perinatal death rates in England and Wales.

as short stature, maternal age under 20 or over 35 years and first pregnancies or high parity all increase the risk. Similarly, the risk is higher in most immigrant groups.

Obstetric factors Conditions such as bleeding in pregnancy, hypertensive disorders, malpresentations, malposition, multiple pregnancy, cephalopelvic disproportion, prolonged labour, preterm and postmature labours, prolapsed cord and rhesus haemolytic disease all increase the perinatal risk.

Medical conditions The risk of perinatal death is increased when the mother suffers from conditions such as diabetes mellitus, autoimmune disorders, haemoglobinopathies, renal conditions, anaemia, respiratory conditions, epilepsy, infections such as rubella, cytomegalovirus, toxoplasmosis, listeria, chlamydia, haemolytic group B streptococcus, syphilis and hyperpyrexia, whatever the cause.

Teratogenic factors Some drugs taken by the mother, alcohol and smoking all increase the risk to the fetus. Tobacco smoking has been positively linked with prematurity, low birthweight and stillbirth, and there is growing evidence showing that maternal and passive smoking during pregnancy can have a direct influence on the child in utero. The harmful effects remain after

birth and the link between tobacco exposure and subsequent increased risk of sudden infant death syndrome, along with an increased tendency towards respiratory and infective illness in the child have been published widely. Likewise regular or 'binge' intake of alcohol has been linked to increased risk of miscarriage, growth restriction and fetal alcohol syndrome. Drug abuse is linked to fetal abnormality, growth restriction and an increased risk of sudden infant death (see Chs 71 and 36).

Dietary deficiencies Folic acid deficiency preconceptually and in early pregnancy has been shown to be a cause of neural tube defects (MRC, 1991; Smithels *et al.*, 1980; Wald and Bower, 1995). Periconceptional vitamin supplementation is therefore advised, especially when there is a history of these malformations. Poor intrauterine nutrition may also affect the long-term health of the individual into adult life (Godrey and Barker, 1995).

Reducing the perinatal mortality rate

There are marked geographical differences in mortality rates, and improvements will only be seen when efforts to improve the whole aspect of the nation's health, through improvements in healthcare provision, housing, education, employment prospects and general social welfare are effective. The detrimental effect of socioeconomic deprivation is recognized universally and there are innovative government-led schemes established to tackle the inequalities. The creation of *Health Action Zones* (HAZ) and *Centres for Health Improvements* provide opportunities for agencies to work together to eliminate the worst health inequalities. Midwives should be in a position to influence policy at PCT level to encourage investment in maternal and child health services.

The *Sure Start* and *Sure Start Plus* programmes are becoming well established throughout the country to improve the health of young children, especially those living in socially deprived areas, and innovative midwifery posts are supporting the scheme in a variety of ways.

Reflective Activity 62.3

Is your area a designated health action zone? What maternity and paediatric innovations are supported within the zone, and who is the Sure Start coordinator in your area?

Maternity services

The Changing Childbirth initiative quickly became associated with 'choice, continuity and control' (DoH, 1993). Concerted efforts have been made around the country to develop maternity services which meet all 10 changing childbirth recommendations (DoH, 1999). Whilst advances and improvements have been made, inequalities still exist.

In order to have a measurable impact on improvements in perinatal mortality, maternity services need to be designed to meet the specific needs of the clients they are serving, and should be evidence based, accessible and non-judgemental. Care should be provided by appropriate personnel, with the skills of the midwife utilized accordingly, and no duplication of effort or resources. Evidence of collaborative working among all relevant members of the health and social welfare team across primary and secondary services and encompassing both statutory and voluntary services should be sought. Outcomes should be accurately audited, and changes implemented efficiently where necessary. Models and systems of care should be flexible and individualized, providing extra social support where needed (DoH, 1993; Oakley *et al.*, 1990). There should be a heightened emphasis on the health education and public health role of the midwife and this is reflected in areas where consultant midwife roles are developing in the speciality of public health (DoH, 2001). A woman is receptive to lifestyle change during pregnancy, and this window of opportunity should be capitalized upon.

Other essential components that should be reflected within any model of care are:

- early booking;
- appropriate selection of place of confinement
- identification of, and close supervision of all 'at-risk' mothers
- effective screening tests to detect abnormalities
- genetic counselling
- early detection and treatment of complications.

Intrapartum events have a major impact on perinatal mortality rates and there are positive measures that can be taken to reduce intrapartum deaths:

- referral to fetal medicine units for monitoring of high-risk pregnancies where appropriate, with planned induction of labour to avoid an unfavourable intra-uterine environment
- stringent guidelines to support the practice of induction of labour (RCOG, 2001a) and the management of shoulder dystocia
- active management of labour, where necessary, to avoid prolonged labour
- appropriate use of cardiotocography, with all staff responsible for the care of women in labour regularly trained in the interpretation of CTGs (RCOG, 2001b)
- prompt and skilful management of intra- and extra-uterine hypoxia
- adequate neonatal special and intensive care facilities throughout the country
- further improvements in the staffing levels and training of midwives and doctors involved in obstetrics and neonatal paediatrics; neonatal resuscitation training should be made available to all disciplines that may be responsible for delivery or immediate aftercare of the neonate, including student midwives, paramedics and general practitioners.

Perinatal mortality rates are considered a good indicator of the standards of obstetric and neonatal care, although, as previously discussed, there are factors in addition to the health service that have an important influence. Nowadays there is concern not only about mortality, but also about the quality of life of the survivors. Some babies who survive perinatal complications may be left with a permanent handicap. There is a growing trend towards aiming to measure morbidity, with many regions producing data relating to outcomes of all babies born below a certain birthweight. The EPI-CURE study (Wood *et al.*, 2000) focuses particularly on the mortality and morbidity of babies born between 24–26 weeks' gestation and will provide important information to those planning ongoing services for these children.

Neonatal mortality

The neonatal mortality rate (Fig. 62.3) is the number of deaths of babies within 4 weeks of birth per 1000 registered live births. The neonatal mortality rate, like the other mortality rates, is declining and fell from 11.0 in 1975 to 3.9 in 2000 (ONS, 2002).

The majority of neonatal deaths occur in the first day or two after birth, which closely relates the death of the baby to gestational age, labour and delivery. The causes of perinatal and neonatal deaths occurring in the first week of life are obviously related and may also be responsible for later neonatal deaths; however, other factors such as infection may be more strongly implicated in later deaths. The reasons for reduction in the neonatal mortality rate are similar to those responsible for the decline in perinatal mortality.

Infant mortality

The infant mortality rate is the number of deaths of infants during the first year of life (including those occurring during the first 4 weeks) per 1000 registered live births in the year. There has been a remarkable decline in infant deaths from 140 per 1000 live births in 1900, to 5.6 per 1000 in 2000 (ONS, 2002) (see Fig. 62.3).

Although the infant mortality rate has declined greatly in the last 50 years, of the total number of deaths in the first year, most still occur in the first 4 weeks of life. The majority of these neonatal deaths occur within a day or two of delivery.

Causes

The main causes of death include:

- infection, mainly acute respiratory and gastro-intestinal infection
- congenital malformations
- sudden infant death syndrome (SIDS)
- accidents
- child abuse
- consequences of prematurity.

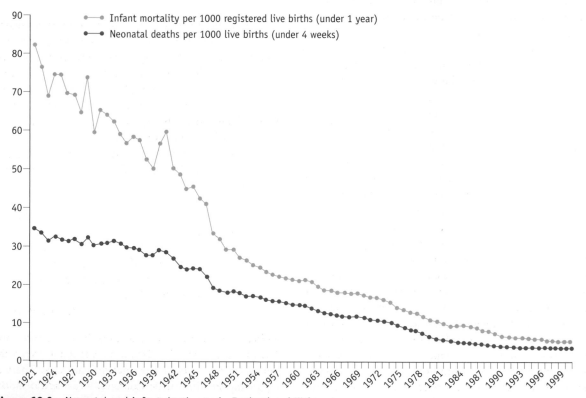

Figure 62.3   Neonatal and infant death rate in England and Wales.

The social factors discussed under perinatal mortality are predisposing causes of infant death. Children born into families in socioeconomic groups IV and V are twice as likely to die between the end of the first month and the end of the first year of life, since it is during this time that environment and other related factors have the most impact. Infant mortality is also increased in children born to young mothers and to those who have inadequate antenatal care, smoke heavily, have low birthweight babies and live in inner city areas.

Reducing the infant mortality rate

One of the major factors influencing the reduction in infant mortality in the last decade has been the reduction in deaths attributed to SIDS. The 'reducing the risk' information leaflet (DoH, 2001) is widely distributed to all expectant and new mothers, and the message is taken up well. The Foundation for the Study of Infant Deaths (FSID) and Cot Death Research Association strive to find answers through research as to why this distressing condition is still responsible for unexpected infant deaths. Special leaflets for grandparents and teenagers who may be caring for babies and young children are produced and available free of charge from the Foundation. The Care of the Next Infant (CONI) scheme provides support and resources to families where there is an increased risk of cot death where one sibling has already died from this condition.

Midwives must be aware of their responsibilities in child protection issues, and appropriate training in managing these issues should be widely encouraged. Many families are living in extreme conditions and stress levels are high. There is a growing awareness of the condition *shaken baby syndrome*, illustrated by highly publicized cases where babies, originally thought to have died from cot death syndrome, have been rediagnosed as having been victims of child abuse. This has caused great strain for families and professionals involved, and has highlighted the need for good collaboration and effective communication systems between professionals.

Scarce resources should be appropriately targeted to ensure that those families in need of extra support are detected and receive the help that they need. This includes referral to voluntary sector services and agencies such as the NSPCC, who provide positive parenting support. Parenting skills are being highlighted as an important theme within education, and midwives can support this initiative by supporting schemes locally by going into the schools and contributing to the programme. The detrimental effect of domestic violence within families on maternal and infant welfare is also well known, and services should be designed to recognize and support women who are victims of domestic violence (DoH, 2000; Lewis, 2001; RCM, 1997).

Measures to reduce infant and perinatal mortality rates are similar, and the introduction of Sure Start programmes should have a measurable impact over the coming years. In parts of the country, services have changed their approach and go out and seek those in need (Davies, 1988; McKee, 1980; Reid *et al.*, 1983; Thomas *et al.*, 1987; Zander *et al.*, 1987).

Reflective Activity 62.4

What initiatives could be developed to reduce stress levels in families with new babies?

What strategies are in place to reduce or minimize the harm caused by:

- maternal drug abuse?
- domestic violence?

Who is your local child protection midwife, and how do you report suspicion of child abuse in your area?

MATERNAL MORTALITY (FIG. 62.4)

The maternal mortality rate for any year, is expressed as the number of deaths attributed to pregnancy and childbearing per 1000 registered total births, or more commonly as the number of deaths per 100 000 maternities (Fig. 62.5). Maternal deaths occurring more than 42 days after pregnancy or childbirth are no longer included in the figures, in line with the international definition of maternal deaths.

The International Classification of Diseases, Injuries and Causes of Death (ICD9) defines a maternal death as:

> the death of a woman while pregnant or within 42 days of termination of pregnancy, irrespective of the duration and the site of the pregnancy, from any cause related to or aggravated by the pregnancy or its management but not from accidental or incidental causes.
>
> (Lewis, 2001)

Maternal deaths are divided into *direct*, *indirect* and *fortuitous deaths*. This definition is in accord with the definition adopted by the International Federation of Gynaecology and Obstetrics (FIGO). In addition, the latest revision, ICD10, recognizes that some women

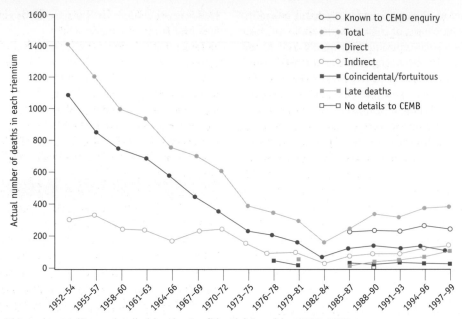

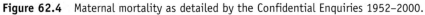

Figure 62.4 Maternal mortality as detailed by the Confidential Enquiries 1952–2000.

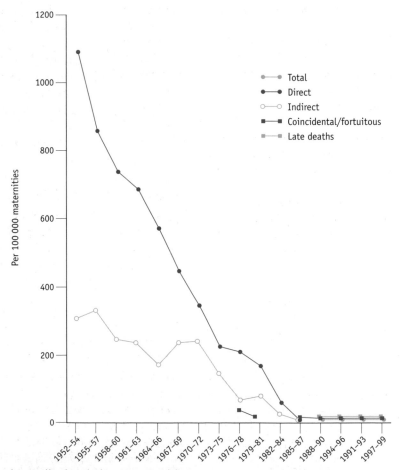

Figure 62.5 Maternal mortality in relation to maternities.

die as a consequence of direct or indirect obstetric causes after this period and has introduced the category of *late maternal deaths* (Lewis, 2001).

The World Health Organization (WHO) Safe Motherhood initiative was launched in 1987 and maintains its aim to reduce mortality and morbidity significantly among mothers and infants. Most of the annual total of 500 000 maternal deaths occur in developing countries, but women still die, albeit in small numbers, in the more affluent nations of the world. The maternal mortality rate is 11.4 per 100 000 births in the UK (see Fig. 62.5), with a direct rate of 5.0 per 100 000, and an indirect rate of 6.4 per 100 000. In some parts of Europe it is lower, for example in Belgium 3.42 and in Sweden 4.78, whereas in some developing countries it is over 600 per 100 000 births (DoH, 1994; WHO, 1996). The relative risks are described in Table 62.1.

Confidential Enquiries into Maternal Deaths

In the UK a confidential enquiry into every maternal death is undertaken to look for factors which may have influenced the outcome, in an attempt to make recommendations and guide future practice. A detailed report is published at 3-yearly intervals on all maternal deaths reported. Ascertainment has improved over the last decade as better computer software at ONS is assisting in the recognition of maternal deaths. Reporting has improved owing to the introduction of standards surrounding maternal deaths by local supervising authority (LSA) officers, so what could appear to be an increase in deaths is actually attributed to improved ascertainment (Lewis, 2001).

Information surrounding the care of the woman is gathered by the regional coordinating body and is then sent to regional obstetric and, where appropriate, midwifery and anaesthetic assessors for comment.

The assessors then send the completed form to the Chief Medical Officer at the Department of Health. In Scotland and Northern Ireland, the system of enquiry is similar, but one panel of assessors deals with all cases.

At the Department of Health, only advisors in obstetrics, gynaecology, midwifery and anaesthetics see the forms. An analysis of the cases is undertaken and recommendations are made, highlighting areas of concern and seeking to ensure improvements in coming years. A report on Confidential Enquiries into Maternal Deaths in England and Wales was published for each successive 3-year period from the 1952–54 report until the 1982–84 report, and since 1985 reports have included all four countries of the UK.

In the latest report for the 3-year period 1997–99 (Lewis, 2001) maternal deaths are divided into *direct deaths*, which result from obstetric complications of pregnancy, labour and the puerperium, and *indirect deaths*, which are caused by either a previously existing disease or by a disease which developed during pregnancy, or was worsened by pregnancy. *Coincidental* (formerly known as fortuitous) deaths may also occur and are the result of causes which are not at all related to pregnancy, for example, road traffic accidents.

In the 1997–99 enquiry there were a total of 378 maternal deaths. Of these, there were 106 (28%) direct deaths, 136 (36%) indirect deaths, 29 coincidental deaths (8%) and 107 (36%) late deaths.

The main causes of maternal death are shown in Table 62.2.

Table 62.1 Women's risk of dying from pregnancy and childbirth (WHO, 1996)

Region	Risk of dying
All developing countries	**1 in 48**
Africa	1 in 16
Asia	1 in 65
Latin America and Caribbean	1 in 130
All developed countries	**1 in 1800**
Europe	1 in 1400
North America	1 in 3700
Country-level differences are even more dramatic.	

Table 62.2 Main causes of maternal death in the UK 1997–99

Cause	No. of deaths	Rate per million maternities
Thrombosis and thromboembolism	35	16.5
Hypertensive disease of pregnancy	15	7.1
Early pregnancy deaths (including abortions)	17	8.0
Haemorrhage	7	3.3
Amniotic fluid embolism	8	3.3
Genital tract sepsis (excluding abortions)	14	6.6
Anaesthesia	3	1.4
Genital tract trauma	2	1.0
Total	**101**	**5.9**

Thrombosis and thromboembolism

This remains the commonest cause of maternal deaths in the UK, with 35 deaths reported in 1997–99 (Lewis, 2001). There were 13 antepartum deaths (8 of which occurred in the first trimester), 7 deaths following caesarean section and 10 deaths following vaginal delivery.

Key recommendations from the CEMD report (Lewis, 2001) were:

- There should be wider use of prophylaxis and better investigation of classic symptoms.
- First trimester pregnancy carries a risk and prophylaxis is indicated in situations where there is an increased risk, i.e. prolonged bedrest, dehydration, or familial history.
- Close attention should be paid to any pregnant woman with chest or leg symptoms, which should be investigated using duplex ultrasound or ventilation–perfusion scanning.
- All women undergoing caesarean section should be assessed for prophylaxis.
- Midwives should pay attention to women in the puerperium complaining of chest or leg symptoms and exclude the possibility of deep vein thrombosis (DVT) or pulmonary embolism (PE).

Whilst pulmonary embolism is a leading cause of maternal death in the UK, the total of 31 deaths following PE in 1997–99 represents a substantial reduction from the 46 cases in 1996–98. This may be due to the implementation of the RCOG guidelines on thromboprophylaxis at caesarean section (RCOG, 1995). There is a need to address the issue of detection and treatment of classic symptoms, especially in women perceived to be at low risk, as there was a significant rise in deaths where diagnosis was delayed or missed, particularly within primary care or accident and emergency settings. There were also a number of women with recognized risk factors who were not offered thromboprophylaxis, emphasizing the continuing need for widespread education in this area.

Hypertensive disorders of pregnancy

This remains a major cause, with 15 deaths due to this condition during 1997–99 representing a reduction from 20 deaths in 1994–96. Cerebral complications, mainly intracerebral haemorrhage, were the commonest cause of death. There were 5 deaths from HELLP syndrome (haemolysis, elevated liver enzymes, low platelets). Despite recommendations made in previous reports, there were still substandard aspects of care

associated with these deaths, with criticisms made by panels for failure to react quickly enough to impending signs of eclampsia and lack of seniority and experience in the teams caring for these women. There were also examples where healthcare professionals misdiagnosed and failed to make standard routine measurements of blood pressure and urinalysis. Midwives must be vigilant in their approach to early detection and management of any women presenting with risk factors and ensure appropriate management and referral.

The key recommendations for the management of pregnancy-induced hypertension (PIH) include:

- Each unit should have an obstetric-led team to coordinate policy and training programmes in the management of pre-eclampsia and eclampsia.
- Junior staff should not be exposed to potentially dangerous clinical situations of which they have little experience.
- A single clinician should have overall responsibility for the management of these potentially difficult cases, and communication should be clear and concise to other team members.
- All women should receive antenatal information on the signs of pre-eclampsia and should have direct access to immediate professional advice.
- There is an immediate need for ongoing professional education, particularly for those staff who work in the community, with regard to the implications of pre-eclampsia and the need for accurate assessment, diagnosis and referral when required.

Haemorrhage

There were 7 direct deaths from haemorrhage, both ante- and postpartum, in 1997–99, representing a reduction from 15 deaths in 1994–96 in the UK. Haemorrhage remains a major cause of maternal death throughout the world, and it is estimated that a quarter of all direct obstetric deaths are due to haemorrhage (WHO, 1994, 1996). Whilst not the direct cause of death, haemorrhage played a significant role in a further 7 deaths in the 1997–99 report. Of the 7 direct deaths, 3 were associated with placental abruption, 3 with placenta praevia and 1 was following delivery (PPH). In 11 cases, care was assessed to be substandard, with failures in communication and failure to take appropriate action cited.

The midwife is often the first person to see the woman who may present with acute pain or bleeding. The midwife should always refer a woman who complains of abdominal pain in early pregnancy to a doctor.

Ectopic pregnancy is often a difficult condition to diagnose, especially as it may present with or without bleeding before the woman realizes that she is pregnant. Early investigations and appropriate treatment may be life saving. Similarly, a woman presenting with pain and tender abdomen may have a concealed haemorrhage.

Postpartum haemorrhage will always remain a risk, and midwives must be trained appropriately to manage the situation whilst awaiting medical aid. The woman's haemodynamic status should be checked in pregnancy and when anaemia is detected it should be appropriately treated. Midwives caring for women at home or in birth centres should have access to immediate resuscitation facilities until medical assistance can be summoned.

The key recommendations made by the Confidential Enquiries encompass many of these points and can be summarized as:

- Placenta praevia presents a risk and an experienced operator and a consultant should be available.
- Minor signs and symptoms may have a considerable significance in pregnancy and all those who may come into contact with pregnant women should assess whether there may be an obstetric element to the symptoms, e.g. abdominal pain without bleeding could indicate concealed haemorrhage or ectopic pregnancy. Accident and emergency department staff should be especially vigilant in this area and should be advised accordingly when seeking a midwifery or obstetric opinion.
- Every unit should have a major haemorrhage policy.
- Every unit should regularly practice the management of major haemorrhage using 'fire drills'.
- Good communication and speed of access particularly to blood supplies are essential.

Other causes of maternal deaths

There were 8 deaths from amniotic embolism in 1997–99, representing a reduction from 17 in 1994–96. None of the cases assessed was felt to have received suboptimal obstetric/midwifery care. Whilst the condition is rare it carries a high mortality. Risk factors associated with this condition include higher maternal age, and as the average age of childbearing is increasing this may influence future statistics. The use of oxytocic drugs to induce or augment labour (DoH, 1994) has been linked to an increased risk of amniotic embolism, though in the last report 3 of the women did not receive any oxytocic or prostaglandin drugs. Sudden collapse in labour is a common feature in this condition, which should be suspected in any woman regardless of type of labour or delivery. Despite prompt treatment and good intensive care, death remained unavoidable in all cases. There is little evidence guiding practice towards prevention or treatment, and further research would increase understanding and provide information on best practice in its management.

Genital tract sepsis

There were 14 deaths in 1997–99 due directly to genital tract sepsis, and a further 4 others in which it may have played a significant part (8.4 per million maternities). This represents an increase from 7 direct deaths (7.3 per million maternities) in 1994–96.

Deaths from puerperal sepsis remain a risk to all women and midwives must be vigilant in the detection and management of any signs of infection. The growing trend towards early discharge from hospital, especially following operative delivery, and reduced postnatal visiting may adversely affect puerperal sepsis rates. The spread of disease can be rapid and devastating, and early detection and treatment are essential.

Whilst numbers are small, cases of substandard care are identified throughout the report, highlighting that care fell short of generally accepted standards.

Indirect causes of maternal death

Social and environmental factors are now recognized as having an effect on a woman's risk of mortality or long-term morbidity in pregnancy. Mortality rates amongst the socially excluded, including women from lower socioeconomic groups, the very young and women from certain ethnic communities are higher than amongst the population as a whole.

Analysis of the data within the 1997–99 report on maternal mortality shows that women were more likely to die during pregnancy or childbirth if they were:

- from the most disadvantaged groups in society and lower socioeconomic groups (risk increased by about 20 times)
- from ethnic groups other than white and those who speak little English (risk increased by 2)
- from the travelling community
- women who had reported that they were subjected to violence in the home
- those who were late to book or had missed four antenatal visits
- those with known mental health problems (Lewis, 2001).

Results of an ONS/CEMD linkage study show when all deaths up to 1 year after delivery are taken into account, that suicide is not only the leading cause of indirect death, but is also the leading cause of maternal death overall (Lewis, 2001).

Midwives should ensure that services are planned to meet the needs of the most vulnerable women in our society. There should be safeguards built into monitoring systems to ensure that women shown to be at higher risk do not 'slip through the net'.

Midwives should be aware of their professional accountability when caring for women with psychiatric and psychological problems during pregnancy and the puerperium, should be vigilant in identifying women at risk, and should have access to an appropriate source of referral should a problem arise. Midwives should work within the remit of their professional boundaries at all times, and therefore access to an appropriate mental health practitioner is essential.

Reflective Activity 62.5

Is there a Confidential Enquiry document available in your area? Are the recommendations implemented and audited?

Are all policies and guidelines in use in your unit evidence based and subjected to annual review?

Attend the next perinatal meeting in your unit, and consider the structure of the meeting, who attends, and the type of discussion which emerges. Do clear recommendations emerge from this forum?

CONCLUSION

Recommendations made by the Confidential Enquiries are endorsed by the Royal Colleges within *Towards Safer Childbirth* (RCOG, 1999) and by the Clinical negligence schemes for trusts auditable standards (CNST, 1997; NHS Litigation Authority, 2002).

Midwives are accountable for their own professional development and should ensure that they take full advantage of any training opportunity to enable them to cope with unexpected obstetric and paediatric emergencies.

With the restructuring of the four national Confidential Enquiries there is a growing opportunity for midwives to become involved in the monitoring of maternal and infant care through the formation of a new organization, the Confidential Enquiry into Maternal and Child Health (CEMACH). In April 2003 CEMACH was created by the amalgamation of CESDI and CEMD with a renewed and widened remit to report extensively on many aspects of maternal and child health. There will be increasing opportunities for joint working with the remaining two Confidential Enquiries (Confidential Enquiry into Perioperative Deaths (CEPOD) and, significantly in view of the findings from the maternal enquiries, Confidential Enquiry into Suicides and Homicides (CISH)).

Midwives should be aware of their role as the woman's advocate. It is vital to give evidence-based, clear information, but it is also imperative that the woman's understanding of the information should be assessed. When discussing how to summon help in an emergency, local knowledge of communication or travel links is invaluable. Language remains a barrier to effective communication for many women, and adequate and accessible interpreter services should be available for all women.

Midwives must develop their public health role as reflected in the proposed expansion of the role of the midwife highlighted in *Making a Difference* (DoH 1999) and further confirmed by the growing number of public-health-related consultant midwife posts. Collection of statistics is meaningless unless the information gathered is put to good use.

Midwives should be aware of how local regional and national statistics can be used in the provision and development of services, as a means of improving clinical practice and as a means of supporting bids for service innovations in all areas, particularly when aimed at reducing inequalities.

KEY POINTS

- Statistics are an important part of measuring quality and quantity of service, of highlighting shortcomings in practice and supporting the development of appropriate protocols and guidelines to prevent and manage high-risk situations in obstetrics and neonatal care.
- Confidential Enquiries into maternal and perinatal mortality have been an important strategy in

improving clinical practice and reducing risks for mothers and their babies.

- Midwives play a key role in the gathering of statistical data, and in translating the ensuing reports into practice outcomes. They therefore must be knowledgeable about the whole process and be familiar with the most recently available information.

REFERENCES

Affiliation Proceedings Act 1957 London: HMSO.

Balen, H.A., Jacobs, H. & de Cherney, A. (1997) *Infertility in Practice*. London: Churchill Livingstone.

Challoner, J. (1999) *The Baby Makers: The History of Artificial Conception*. London: Macmillan.

Clinical Negligence Scheme for Trusts (CNST) (1997) Clinical Negligence Scheme for Trusts Manual Of Risk Management Standards. London: CNST.

Davies, J. (1988) Cowgate Neighbourhood Centre – a preventative health care venture shared by midwives and social workers. *Midwives Chronicle* 101(1200): 4–7.

Department of Health (DoH) (1993) *Changing Childbirth. Report of the Expert Maternity Group*, Part 1. London: HMSO.

Department of Health (DoH) (1994) *Report on Confidential Enquiries into Maternal Deaths in the United Kingdom 1988–1990*. London: HMSO.

Department of Health (DoH) (1998a) *A First Class Service – Quality in the New NHS*. London: The Stationery Office.

Department of Health (DoH) (1998b) *Report on Confidential Enquiries into Maternal Deaths in the United Kingdom 1994–1996*. London: HMSO.

Department of Health (DoH) (1999) *Making a Difference*. London: The Stationery Office.

Department of Health (DoH) (2000) *Domestic Violence: A Resource Manual for Health Care Professionals*. London: DoH.

Department of Health (DoH) (2001) *Reduce the Risk of Cot Death: An Easy Guide*. London: DoH. Online. Available: http://www.doh.gov.uk/pub/docs/doh/ cotdeath.

Department of Health and Social Security (DHSS) (1976) *Fit for the Future. Report of the Committee on Child Health Services*. (Chairman: Professor S.D.M. Court) London: HMSO.

Department of Health and Social Security (DHSS) (1977) *The Way Forward*. London: HMSO.

Department of Health and Social Security (DHSS) (1980) *Inequalities in Health*. (Chairman: Sir Douglas Black) London: HMSO.

Department of Health and Social Security (DHSS) (1988) *Infant mortality in England. A report to the Chief Medical Officer by an Expert Working Group*. London: HMSO.

Editorial (1986) Perinatal care: organisation and outcome. *Lancet* 1(8484): 777–778.

Godrey, K.M. & Barker, D.J.P. (1995) Maternal nutrition in relation to fetal and placental growth. *European Journal of Obstetrics and Gynecology and Reproductive Biology* 61(1): 15–22.

Kon, A. (1993) *Infertility: The Real Costs*. London: ISSUE and CHILD.

Lewis, G. (ed) (2001) *Why Mothers Die 1997–99: Fifth Report of the Confidential Enquiries into Maternal Deaths in the United Kingdom*. London: CEMD: associated with NICE, RCOG.

Maternal and Child Health Research Consortium (MCHRC) (1995) *Confidential Enquiry into Stillbirths and Deaths in Infancy: 2nd Annual Report*. London: DoH.

Maternal and Child Health Research Consortium (MCHRC) (1997) *Confidential Enquiry into Stillbirths and Deaths in Infancy: 4th Annual Report*. London: MCHRC.

Maternal and Child Health Research Consortium (MCHRC) (1998) *Confidential Enquiry into Stillbirths and Deaths in Infancy: 5th Annual Report*. London: MCHRC.

Maternal and Child Health Research Consortium (MCHRC) (1999) *Confidential Enquiry into Stillbirths and Deaths in Infancy: 6th Annual Report*. London: MCHRC.

Maternal and Child Health Research Consortium (MCHRC) (2000) *Confidential Enquiry into Stillbirths and Deaths in Infancy: 7th Annual Report*. London: MCHRC.

Maternal and Child Health Research Consortium (MCHRC) (2001) *Confidential Enquiry into Stillbirths and Deaths in Infancy: 8th Annual Report*. London: MCHRC.

Maternal and Child Health Research Consortium (MCHRC) (2002) *Confidential Enquiry into Stillbirths and Deaths in Infancy: 9th Annual Report*. London: MCHRC.

McKee, I. (1980) Community antenatal care: the Sighthill Community Antenatal Care Scheme. In: Zander, L.I. & Chamberlain, G. (eds) *Pregnancy Care for the 80s*. London: Royal Society of Medicine/ Macmillan Press.

Medical Research Council (MRC) (1991) Vitamin Study Research Group. Prevention of neural tube defects: results of the MRC vitamin study. *Lancet* **338**(8760): 132–137.

National Health Service Act 1977 London: HMSO.

NHS Litigation Authority (2002) Clinical Risk Management Standards for Maternity Services. Bristol: Willis.

Oakley, A., Rajan, L. & Grant, A. (1990) Social support and pregnancy outcome. *British Journal of Obstetrics and Gynaecology* **97**(2): 152–162.

Office for National Statistics (ONS) (2000a) *Population Trends,* Winter 2000. London: The Stationery Office.

Office for National Statistics (ONS) (2000b) *Health Statistics Quarterly,* Aug. 2000. London: The Stationery Office.

Office for National Statistics (ONS) (2002) *Health Statistics Quarterly,* Spring 2002. London: The Stationery Office.

Registration of Births and Deaths Act 1953 London: HMSO

Reid, M.E., Gutteridge, S. & McIlwaine, G.M. (1983) *A Comparison of the Delivery of Antenatal Care between a Hospital and a Peripheral Clinic.* Glasgow: Social Paediatrics and Obstetric Research Unit, University of Glasgow.

Royal College of Midwives (RCM) (1997) *Domestic Abuse in Pregnancy.* Position Paper 19. London: RCM.

Royal College of Obstetricians and Gynaecologists (RCOG) (1995) *Report of a Working Party on Prophylaxis against Thromboembolism in Gynaecology and Obstetrics.* London: RCOG.

RCOG Clinical Effectiveness Support Unit (2001a) *Induction of Labour.* Evidence Based Guideline No. 9. London: RCOG.

RCOG Clinical Effectiveness Support Unit (2001b) *The Use of Electronic Fetal Monitoring.* Evidence Based Guideline No. 8. London: RCOG.

Royal College of Obstetricians and Gynaecologists (RCOG) & Royal College of Midwives (RCM) (1999) *Towards Safer Childbirth.* London: RCOG.

Smithels, R.W., Sheppard, S., Schorah, L.J. *et al.* (1980) Possible prevention of neural tube defects by periconceptual vitamin supplementation. *Lancet* 1(8164): 339–340.

Social Exclusion Unit (SEU) (1999) Teenage pregnancy. In: *Preventing Social Exclusion.* London: SEU. Online. Available: http://www.socialexclusionunit.gov.uk/publications/reports/html/pse/pse_html/contents.htm.

Social Services Committee (1980) *Perinatal and Neonatal Mortality.* (Chairman: Renee Short) London: HMSO.

Social Services Committee (1984) *Perinatal and Neonatal Mortality: Follow-up.* (Chairman: Renee Short) London: HMSO.

Thomas, H., Draper, J., Field, S. *et al.* (1987) Evaluation of an integrated antenatal clinic. *Journal of the Royal College of General Practitioners* **37**(305): 544–547.

United Kingdom Central Council for Nursing, Midwifery and Health Visiting (UKCC) (1998) *Midwives Rules and Code of Practice.* London: UKCC.

Wald, N.J. & Bower, C. (1995) Folic acid and the prevention of neural tube defects. *British Medical Journal* **310**(6986): 1019–1020.

Whitehead, M. (1987) *The Health Divide: Inequalities in Health in the 1980s.* London: Health Education Council.

Wood, N.S., Marlow, N., Costeloe, K. *et al.* (2000) Neurologic and developmental disability after extremely preterm birth. *New England Journal of Medicine* **343**(6): 378–384.

World Health Organization (WHO) (1994) Mother–Baby Package: Implementing Safe Motherhood in Countries. Geneva: WHO.

World Health Organization (WHO) (1996) *WHO revised 1990 Estimates of Maternal Mortality: A New Approach by WHO and UNICEF.* Geneva: WHO.

Zander, L., Lee-Jones, M. & Fisher, C. (1987) The role of the primary health care team in the management of pregnancy. In: Kitzinger, S. & Davis, J. (eds) *The Place of Birth.* Oxford: Oxford Medical Publications.

FURTHER READING

Department of Health (DoH) (1990) *Confidential Enquiry into Stillbirths and deaths in Infancy: Report of a Working Group Set up by The Chief Medical Officer.* London: DOH.

Department of Health (DoH) (1996) *Report on Confidential Enquiries into Maternal Deaths in the United Kingdom 1991–1993.* HMSO: London.

Department of Health and Social Security (DHSS) (1986) *Report on Confidential Enquiries into Maternal Deaths in England and Wales 1979–1981.* HMSO: London.

Maternal and Child Health Research Consortium (MCHRC) (1996) *Confidential Enquiry into Stillbirths and Deaths in Infancy: 3rd Annual Report.* London: DoH.

Office for National Statistics (ONS) (2001) *Health Statistics Quarterly,* Autumn 2001. London: The Stationery Office.

ADDITIONAL RESOURCES

CEMACH (Confidential Enquiry into Maternal and Child Health)
Chiltern Court, 188 Baker Street, London NW1 5SD
Tel: 020 7486 0091
Website: http://www.cemach.org.uk

FSID (The Foundation for the Study of Infant Deaths)
14 Halkin Street, London SW1X 7DP
Tel: 020 7235 0965
Website: http://www.sids.org.uk/fsid/

Office for National Statistics
1 Drummand Gate, London SW1V 2QQ
Tel: 0845 601 3034
Website: http://www.Statistics.gov.uk

SANDS (Stillbirth and Neonatal Death Society)
28 Portland Place, London W1B 1LY

Sure Start
Website: http://www.surestart.gov.uk
Links to: What is Sure Start; Sure Start programmes; Common questions; History planning pack; Sure Start Plus; and Sure Start: a guide to planning and running your programme

63

Children Act and Social Services

Barbara Burden and Helen Wenman

LEARNING OUTCOMES

By the end of this chapter you will have been able to:

- develop an understanding of the legislative basis and key principles within the Children Act 1989
- appreciate the range of resources available to support families in caring for their children
- assess the role and responsibilities of local authority and voluntary sector organizations in providing and monitoring services for children and families

- evaluate the role and responsibilities of the midwife in assisting social services departments to promote and safeguard the welfare of children in need and at risk
- realize the midwife's contribution to the assessment of children and families
- identify the particular needs of children with disability and those from different racial and cultural backgrounds.

INTRODUCTION

Decisions about children's welfare and safety are complex, and continuing high-profile deaths of children such as Victoria Climbié raise criticisms and anxieties about professional decision-making (DoH, 2003a). Government documents highlight the requirement for professionals to work together to safeguard and promote the well-being of children and young people (DoH, 1999a; 2000a). These guidelines reflect the outcomes of research and reports from child protection inquiries during the 1980s and 1990s.

This chapter seeks to enable midwives to understand the legislative framework and related policies, procedures and resources, to carry out their role effectively in working together with parents and other professionals to ensure the well-being and safety of the child. Please note that those working outside England and Wales need to access legislation and policy guidelines relevant to that country.

Discussion is linked to three scenarios that may be encountered by midwives (Case scenarios 63.1, 63.2 and 63.3), and a range of activities are suggested which enable the reader to consolidate learning.

Reflective Activity 63.1

Consider the role and responsibilities of the midwife in situations like those of Case scenarios 63.1–63.3:

- What might be your concerns?
- Who would you report your concerns to?
- What can you contribute to a pre-birth assessment?
- What would you be looking for in your contact with the parents?
- How do you think parents could be supported to care for their baby whilst not putting the child at risk?

BACKGROUND TO THE CHILDREN ACT

The Children Act was implemented in 1991 and brought about a fundamental change in childcare law. It pulled together previously fragmented legislation to cover almost all aspects of the care, upbringing and protection of children (Allen, 1998; White *et al.*, 1995). This includes the welfare and protection of children in disputed divorce proceedings, children in need, children

Case scenario 63.1

Gill aged 28 has just given birth to a baby boy. A previous child was removed from her at 6 months because care was found to be inadequate. Gill has learning difficulties.

A pre-birth assessment, in which Gill cooperated, commenced when she notified her general practitioner (GP) of her pregnancy at 28 weeks' gestation.

Initially Gill maintained that she was raped at a party and did not know the baby's father. She claimed that she had separated from Jack, the father of her first baby, a year ago. Jack has spent the last 4 months in prison for grievous bodily harm and has a reputation for violent behaviour. He was released from prison 2 days ago. Gill now states that Jack is the father of this baby. She is no longer willing to cooperate with the hospital or social services and is threatening to discharge herself. Jack is encouraging her in this.

The paediatric consultant would like the baby to stay in hospital for observation because antenatal care was poor and the baby has low birthweight. Gill's health also requires monitoring. She suffers from epilepsy and is extremely obese.

Case scenario 63.2

Susan is aged 16 and is 16 weeks pregnant. She was previously in care, but has left her foster home and is living rough in a local squat. There is concern that Susan is abusing drugs and alcohol and that she may be involved in prostitution.

Case scenario 63.3

Yasmin came to this country from Pakistan at the age of 27, is married and has one child aged 3 years. Following her last pregnancy she suffered with postnatal depression and her baby was provided with respite care until she recovered. Yasmin is attending regularly for antenatal care and was recently diagnosed with intrauterine growth retardation.

Social services have stated they will be undertaking a pre-birth assessment because of Yasmin's fragile mental health.

Box 63.1 Legal definition of a child

The Children Act defines a child as a person under the age of 18. This accords with the current age of majority in Britain. It is important to note that in current British law, an individual has no legal entity until the moment of birth. Similarly, a person does not become a parent until his or her child is born.

at risk, children with disability or special educational needs, and those who need to live away from home (either short or long term) including children in hospital, boarding schools, residential homes and foster homes.

Guidelines and regulations produced by the Department of Health provide detailed information about how the legislation should be implemented. Two published examples of these are *Working Together to Safeguard Children* (DoH, 1999a) and *Framework for the Assessment of Children in Need and their Families* (DoH, 2000a), which provide blueprints for agencies to work together with children (Box 63.1) and families in the future.

Midwives are in an effective position to comment on all aspects of the health and care of newborn babies and on preparations made by mothers and other family members for this. In contrast to some other professionals, for example social workers and police, who tend to only get involved with families when there is a problem, the midwife has a universal and accepted role in working with pregnant mothers, newborn babies and their parents. As such, families easily accept them since their involvement does not label or stigmatize. Whilst midwives have been involved with all children, (12 million in England), intervention by social services departments only affects a small proportion of families, estimated to be about 5% (DoH, 1999b).

KEY FEATURES OF THE CHILDREN ACT

The Children Act was formulated on key beliefs about children, young people, parents and the role of the state, which are given statutory recognition in the Act.

These include the following:

- There is a universal duty to promote and safeguard the welfare of the child.
- Children are best brought up within their family, and local authorities have a duty to give support to children and families to facilitate this.

- Even where children are separated from their families they should maintain contact with them, except where this puts them at risk.
- The state should only intervene where it is in the child's best interests and legal measures are only taken as a last resort.
- Professionals should work in partnership with parents, involving them in care and decisions made about their children where possible.
- The wishes and feelings of children and young people should be sought (depending on their age and level of understanding), and taken into account when making decisions about their lives.
- The child's welfare should be the paramount consideration in the majority of court decisions.
- The race, religion, culture and language of a child should be taken into account in provision of any services.

The Act underpins the responsibility of everybody to safeguard and promote the welfare of children as the primary and universal duty. Whilst other objectives such as working in partnership with parents are also important principles it is important to recognize that the concept of partnership does not eliminate the prevailing duty of the local authority to safeguard and promote the welfare of children (Brayne and Martin, 1999).

Reflective Activity 63.2

Consider how these principles would affect your work with Gill, Susan and Yasmin.

CONTENT AND STRUCTURE OF THE CHILDREN ACT

The Act comprises 108 sections organized into 12 parts and followed by 15 schedules which give more detail about specific areas of the Act. In addition there are 10 volumes of guidance and regulation (DoH, 1991). Of particular interest to midwives are the parts of the Act that deal with the responsibilities of the local authority (LA) in providing support for children and families (Part III) and the protection of children (Part V).

The child's welfare

It is significant that the Children Act begins with a statement that the child's welfare is the paramount issue to be taken into account in the majority of decisions made by a court in respect of children and young people

under the Act. The court is required to take account of the following factors, outlined in the *'welfare checklist'* (Section 3):

- the ascertainable wishes and feelings of the child (subject to age, understanding and maturity)
- the child's physical, emotional and educational needs
- the likely effect on him of having any changes in his circumstances
- sex, age, background and any characteristics the court considers relevant
- any harm which the child has suffered or is at risk of suffering
- how capable each of the parents and any other relevant party are in meeting the child's needs
- the range of powers available to the court.

Whilst this is not applicable in every case, and relates specifically to decisions of the court, the impact of the list is that these are important factors that professionals are expected to take into account when making decisions about a child.

Avoidance of delay

The Act seeks to avoid delay in making decisions about a child's upbringing. Research had shown that children were suffering through a lack of planning and certainty about, for example, whom they should live with (DHSS, 1985; Law Commission, 1998). Children were often left to 'drift', moving from foster home to foster home or back and forward between different carers and their parent(s). The lack of security and difficulties for these children due to a lack of opportunities to experience stability and make secure attachments was shown to have a damaging effect on their development.

Non-intervention

Section 1(5) of the Act states that courts can only make an order in respect of a child if this would be better for the child than not making an order. This is based on the principle that the state should intervene in private family life only as a last resort. This conforms to Article 8 of the European Convention on Human Rights and the Human Rights Act 1998 (Dimond, 2000a).

Parents and parental responsibility

The concept of *parental responsibility* was introduced in the Children Act and is described in Sections 2, 3, and 4. Parental responsibility is defined as: 'the collection of rights, duties and authority, which by law a parent has in respect of a child' (Children Act 1989: S.3(1)).

This includes the responsibility to care for a child and promote and protect the child's moral, physical and emotional health. Although not specifically defined in the Act, this is generally considered to include decisions in respect of the name, religion and education of the child, the right to consent or not to medical treatment, to have contact and to arrange for the burial or cremation of a child (Hardy and Hannibal, 1997).

Who has parental responsibility?

Having parental responsibility does not automatically equate with being the legal or biological parent of the child. For example, the natural (birth) mother automatically acquires parental responsibility at the moment of birth. However, the father does not have parental responsibility as a right unless he was married to the mother at the time of birth. The unmarried father has parenthood if he is registered as the father on the child's birth certificate or if DNA testing has proved paternity. In these cases he has succession rights and can agree or refuse consent for adoption. The Children Act was amended in 2002 following the implementation of the Adoption and Children Act 2002 enabling fathers to have parental responsibility if registered as the child's father, if it was mutually agreed by the parents or if ordered by the court. Other people may also acquire parental responsibility through decisions of the court, for example grandparents, a guardian, foster carer or the local authority. In these circumstances parental responsibility can be shared among several people. The only circumstance in which a birth mother and married father would lose parental rights is when their child is adopted or freed for adoption. In divorce, both parents retain parental rights, even if it is decided that the child should live with one of the parents.

Having parental responsibility does not have the same meaning in law as being the parent; for example, it does not convey the right to give or refuse consent to adoption, it does not make the person or body with parental rights a relative of the child, for example in respect of succession or inheritance, and in some cases the right to change the child's name is restricted (Bainham, 1998).

The issue of parenting and parental responsibility is becoming increasingly complicated with the advent of surrogacy and IVF (in vitro fertilization). In respect of surrogacy, the woman who gives birth is the legal mother and has parental rights. The natural parent(s) need to adopt the child in order to become the legal parents and gain parental rights. In cases of IVF the situation is even more complex.

> **Reflective Activity 63.3**
>
> In considering the case scenarios:
>
> - Who has or will have parental responsibility in the case of Susan's, Gill's and Yasmin's babies?
> - What difference will this make to any plans or decisions which need to be made in respect of the child?

STRATEGIES FOR PROMOTING THE WELFARE OF CHILDREN SINCE THE CHILDREN ACT

The Government is encouraging a task-focused response across different departments of government and local authorities to address particular issues in society. This is reflected in cross-departmental strategies to address social exclusion (SEU, 2001), including strategies to reduce poverty, neighbourhood renewal (SEU, 2000) and teenage pregnancies (SEU, 1999). These strategies include the implementation of Health Action Zones (HAZnet, 2001), Sure Start (Sure Start, 2001), the Children's Taskforce (DoH, 2001a) and Connexions (DfEE, 2000). The strategies encourage the involvement of voluntary and private sectors, local communities and parents in their development and implementation.

> **Reflective Activity 63.4**
>
> Find out where your local social services department is. How has it organized its responsibilities to children?
>
> What initiatives do you have in your area for helping vulnerable children and their families?
>
> See if you can obtain a copy of the Children's Services Plan for your area? What are the key aims and objectives for your area?

THE CHILDREN ACT AND THE HUMAN RIGHTS ACT

There was concern that the implementation of the Human Rights Act 1998 would create conflicts for the role of the state in intervening in family life in order to protect children. Article 8 of the Act states that:

> Everyone has the right to respect for his private and family life … [and] that there shall be

no interference by a public authority with the exercise of this right except such as is in accordance with the law and is necessary in a democratic society ... For the protection of health or morals or for the protection of the rights and freedoms of others.

This article is known as a *qualified right*, in that the rights are limited and qualified by particular constraints. It is thought that the 'interference by a public authority', for example a local authority social services department, to protect children does not contravene this right providing that the strict criteria of the Children Act have been followed and that interference only went as far as necessary to meet the aim.

SUPPORT FOR CHILDREN AND FAMILIES

The changing nature of family

Any consideration of support for children and families needs to take account of the changing nature of family life in Britain (Utting, 1995). Britain has become an increasingly multicultural society, and these factors taken together have brought a diversity of ideas in respect of different family structures and ways of life. This diversity has been recognized both within the Children Act and within Department of Health publications in two ways. Firstly the Act widened the concept of people who are important to children by allowing absent parents and other relatives to be consulted and involved in decisions about the care of children. Secondly, for the first time in English law, the diversity and multicultural context of families have been recognized and it is required that these be taken account of and respected.

Poverty and social exclusion

Sources of stress and disadvantage for children and families include poverty and accompanying social exclusion. Research has estimated that a considerable proportion of children (between 3–4 million) are living in poverty (defined as below half the national average income) (Gregg *et al.*, 1999; Utting, 1995). Two-thirds of children with lone parents fall into this category, compared with only one-quarter of children who have two parents. In 1999, 2 million children were living in households where there was no adult in paid work. Babies born in social classes IV and V are 20% more likely to be born underweight than those in higher

social classes. The impact of poverty on children and their families has been recognized as having a major effect on life chances, health and education (Utting, 1995).

It is important to note here that households comprising families from black and Asian origins are significantly more likely to experience poverty (Butt and Box, 1998); over four-fifths of Pakistani and Bangladeshi households receive an income below half the national average, compared with only one-quarter of white families.

Reflective Activity 63.5

Access the Social Exclusion Unit (SEU) website or contact them direct to obtain a copy of their report *Preventing Social Exclusion*: http://www.socialexclusionunit.gov.uk.

Review the document in relation to your practice as a midwife and the support required by Gill, Susan and Yasmin.

Pregnant women can access a range of benefits to help combat social inequality caused by poverty. Under the Employment Rights Act 1996 women retain employment rights whilst pregnant and should not be discriminated against (Dimond, 2000b). This includes the right to attend antenatal appointments, protection from suspension, the right to maternity leave, maternity pay, redundancy payment, and return to work following pregnancy. This is supported by the Employment Relations Act 1999 which addresses the right to maternity leave, protection against detrimental treatment during pregnancy and parental leave (Dimond, 2000b). These are basic rights for employees, which may be enhanced by the employer.

Reflective Activity 63.6

Because of the changing nature of maternity benefits it is important that you are able to access current and relevant information for the families in your care. Gaining experience of accessing the Department of Work and Pensions website will enable you to keep your practice informed by new initiatives.

Access the Department of Work and Pensions website at http://dwp.gov.uk and review the sections on:

- Statutory maternity pay
- Maternity allowance
- Incapacity benefit

- Time off for maternity leave
- Council tax benefit
- Income support
- Social Fund
- Sure Start maternity grants.

Which of these benefits do you think Gill, Susan and Yasmin could be entitled to?

Paternity leave Every working father is entitled to 2 weeks' paid paternity leave, paid at the same rate as statutory maternity pay.

Reflective Activity 63.7

The Inland Revenue offers support for families through the Working Families Tax Credit. This is awarded to families who have one or more children, where the parents work at least 16 hours per week and are entitled to work in this country as UK residents.

Access the Inland Revenue website on http://www.inlandrevenue.gov.uk.

Review the current information relating to Working Families Tax Credit and Childcare Tax Credit.

Sure Start programme (Sure Start, 2001) This aims to provide universal services for children under 4 and their families within some of the most disadvantaged communities, addressing the health and well-being of children and families before and after birth. The aim is to improve the health of children before entry to school to enhance their achievements at school. Sure Start programmes are run by local partnerships, including parents. The programmes provide access to family support, advice on nurturing, health services and early learning, through outreach and home visiting, support, provision of play and learning experiences, information about child health and diet and support for children and families with special needs.

Reflective Activity 63.8

Obtain a copy of 'Good News for Babies: Sure Start Maternity Grant' from the Department for Work and Pensions or from http://www.dwp.gov.uk.

Review the content of this document.

How relevant is this to Gill, Susan and Yasmin?

Family support and the Children Act

Whilst there are central and local government strategies designed to aid vulnerable children, such as Sure Start programmes, the Children Act places a duty on local authorities to target particular services to children defined as being *in need*.

Local authorities have a general duty to:

- safeguard and promote the welfare of children 'in need' and
- promote the upbringing of such children by their families

by providing a range and level of services appropriate to those children's need (Children Act 1989: S.17(1)).

The aim of the duty to children in need within the Children Act is to target services to the most vulnerable, including those children thought to be at risk, providing positive support to avoid the need for the state to have to seek statutory control, or for a child to have to live away from home.

Child welfare had become preoccupied with the investigation of child abuse, leading to an imbalance between provision of support services and child abuse investigation (DoH, 1995). Gibbons *et al.* (1995) found that too many children were being dealt with through a child protection process, which alienated families and led to a concentration of resources on child protection to the extent that there was little time and money for anything else. It is now recognized that helpful intervention at an early stage by provision of support services enables parents to look after their children differently and may prevent abuse (Fraser, 1997).

ASSESSING CHILDREN 'IN NEED' AND THEIR FAMILIES

The new *Framework for the Assessment of Children in Need and their Families* (DoH, 2000a) and *Working Together to Safeguard Children* (DoH, 1999a) guidelines emphasize that promoting the welfare of children and safeguarding their needs are not separate activities. They aim to refocus attention on preventive work, together with producing a more holistic and interagency assessment focusing on strengths as well as needs (Calder, 2000). Assessment begins from the point of referral and emphasizes the corporate responsibility of local authority departments and voluntary organizations in contributing to both the assessment and the provision of services to children in need. The assessment seeks to discriminate between different types and levels of need and is crucial to improving the success of services for children (DoH, 2000a).

Focus on an interagency approach starts as soon as there are concerns about a child's welfare, not just when there is concern about the child being at risk of significant harm.

Midwives should identify vulnerable children and decide whether to refer them to social services for assessment. They contribute to the assessment, planning and intervention required. In this context they may attend a range of meetings. The most common situations where midwives are involved in working with social service departments in respect of children in need or at risk are pre-birth assessments and post-birth concerns.

The new assessment framework takes account of recent research to produce a framework that retains the child at the centre of three domains which interact to affect the well-being and development of a child within the family. These are (a) the child's developmental needs, (b) parenting capacity, and (c) family and environmental factors (see Fig. 63.1). Midwives are well placed to comment on all of these, given their close and frequent contact with newborn babies and their parents and their knowledge and understanding of early childhood development and needs. In visiting the home, midwives may become aware of the care,

not only of newborn babies, but also of older children in the family, injuries, conditions in the home, parenting and lifestyles.

Reflective Activity 63.9

Have a look at the categories included in the triangle in Figure 63.1 and consider what information you could contribute from contact with parents during the antenatal and postnatal periods both in hospital and through home visits.

What factors across these three domains would give cause for concern in respect of the child being in need?

When you are next out visiting a family think about how you assess parenting capacity, what criteria you use to decide whether a child is developing 'normally', and what you observe about family resources, networks and support systems.

What circumstances would alert you to the need to make a referral to the Social Services Department (SSD)?

Making a referral

Working Together to Safeguard Children states that:

> all PCHT members should know when it is appropriate to refer a child to SSD as a 'child in need' and how to act on concerns that a child may be at risk of significant harm through abuse or neglect.
>
> (DoH, 1999a: 19)

Before referring to social services the midwife should discuss concerns with a senior member of staff or supervisor of midwives and, unless this would place the child at increased risk, discuss concerns with the family and gain their agreement to the referral. The GP should also be informed. In making the referral it is important to be clear about the nature of the concerns and document these, referring only to known facts.

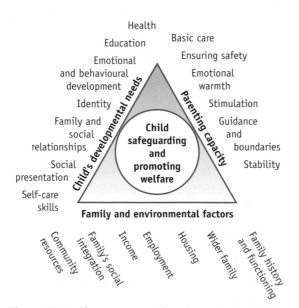

Figure 63.1   The asssessment framework (DoH, 2000a).

Reflective Activity 63.10

How would you present your concerns about Susan to the Social Service Department if making a referral?

Reflective Activity 63.11

Obtain a copy of *What to do if You're Worried a Child is Being Abused – Summary* (DoH, 2003b).

Familiarize yourself with Flow Charts 1–5 concerning referral, initial assessment, emergency action and actions necessary after the Strategy Discussion and Child Protection Conference.

Consent and confidentiality

Personal information about children and families is subject to a duty of confidence and should not normally be shared without consent (DoH, 2000a). However, the law permits disclosure of confidential information if it is necessary to safeguard a child. In all cases consent should be sought from parents before sharing information. Trusts have local policies regarding this. Under the Data Protection Act 1998 it is important that explanations are given to the family as to why it is necessary to disclose information or seek information from other agencies.

In circumstances where there are concerns about the child being at risk or suffering significant harm the overriding duty is to safeguard the child. This appears to be in accord with Article 8 of the Human Rights Act, which states there should be no interference by a public authority *unless* it is in accordance with the law (in this case the Children Act) and is for the protection of health and morals, the rights and freedoms of others or prevention of disorder or crime. If in any doubt it is important to seek legal advice. Midwives are required to be open and honest with families when child protection becomes an issue to ensure this relationship is not compromised and care for both the mother and the child can continue (Calder, 2000).

The midwife's role in assessment

The midwife may be asked to contribute to an assessment of whether a child is in need and, if so, the services which may be appropriate to promote the child's welfare and upbringing within the family. The midwife in respect of both Gill and Yasmin would be contacted for information about previous pregnancies, attitudes towards antenatal and self-care, or home conditions, as part of the *initial assessment* phase. This is a brief assessment of each child referred to SSD and should be undertaken within a maximum of 7 working days. This includes gathering information from other agencies and interviewing the child and family.

In circumstances requiring a more in-depth exploration, a *core assessment* is undertaken, and completed within 35 days. Again, depending on the degree of involvement, the midwife may be invited to provide information, specialist knowledge and advice and in some cases undertake specific assessments. The midwife is expected to contribute to the *plan* for providing support – *The Child in Need Plan*. However, it is important to note that it is not necessary to wait until the outcome of the assessment to begin to provide services.

FAMILY SUPPORT SERVICES

Once the local authority has decided that a child is in need under the criteria of the Children Act, they have a duty to provide a range of services, either directly to the child or to any member of the child's family. Effective assessment determines which services would best meet the needs of the child.

The services and range of placements should reflect the racial, cultural, linguistic and religious needs of the child. These services are provided by a range of local authority agencies, together with the voluntary and private sector. Such services include family centres, day nurseries, fees for childminding or playgroups, and support within the home, such as family aides. Different local authorities organize the provision of these services in different ways depending on the identified needs of the community and resources. Some offer basic services, whilst others, particularly within the voluntary sector, offer specialized, creative and innovative projects. Examples of voluntary organizations providing family support and other specialized projects for vulnerable children and their families include NCH Action for Children, Barnardo's, Children's Society, Home-Start, Gingerbread, Family Service Units and the NSPCC. The services may be means tested and liable to repayment, although any person in receipt of income support or family credit is exempt from this.

Reflective Activity 63.12

Find out what family support services exist in your area. How are these publicized?

Give some examples of how family centres and day nurseries take account of the different racial groups of children in their area when providing services.

Which of these services would be helpful to Gill, Susan or Yasmin?

Accessing services

Whilst there is a duty to provide services to children in need, it has been found that more families gained relevant help where there was a range of broadly based neighbourhood services (Gibbons, 1994). It is important that parents do not feel stigmatized in accessing services and this is improved by open access. For example, local authorities enable access to play groups, day care provision (DfEE, 1998), and family centres (Armstrong, 1996), which are open to all children, by payment of fees and provision of transport. Research in respect of open access parenting support found the establishment of networks, friendships and support from other parents reduced isolation and raised self-esteem (Grimshaw and McGuire, 1998). Services include provision of family support workers, family aides or home helps who go to parents' homes to provide direct care, help or assistance.

Child minding and day care

For babies and younger children, child minding can provide appropriate support. Childminders are paid for caring for a child under 8 for more than 2 hours a day, in their own home. In cases of children in need the Social Service Department may pay fees for either childminding or day care. The Early Years Directorate arm of OFSTED undertakes the regulation and delivery of these services (Care Standards Act, 2000).

Everyone providing day care or child minding must be registered. To do so without registration is an offence.

The local authority imposes requirements on childminders and day care providers in respect of:

- number and age of children to be looked after
- safety of their premises and equipment
- quality of care and learning provided
- health needs
- number of staff (day care).

Children living away from home

Whilst the aim of the Act is to promote the upbringing of children within their family, there may be occasions when it is necessary for the child to be cared for by others, if only for a limited period of time (Aldgate *et al.*, 1996). In this context the Act has broadened the concept of family to include parents and other close relatives. The local authority has a duty to provide accommodation in a range of situations, including when children are *in need* and there is no person who

has parental responsibility for them or they are lost or abandoned, or the person who has been caring for them is prevented from providing them with suitable accommodation or care (Children Act: S.20). When the local authority accommodates children they become *looked after* children.

Children may be accommodated in a variety of placements; however, there has been an increase in the number of children cared for in foster homes in comparison to residential care during the last 20 years, and younger children will predominately be placed with foster carers (Berridge, 1996).

Foster carers   These are suitable people selected and approved by the local authority or registered foster-care agency to provide care for children. Foster carers are subject to inspection and registration under the Foster Placement (Children) Regulations 1991. Foster carers may be approved to care for particular groups of children, for example in respect of age, disability, number of children, for emergency, respite or in short- or long-term situations (Steele, 2000).

Accommodation for young babies

Where there are concerns about a young baby it is likely that the local authority would, unless there is very good reason, try to maintain the mother and child in their own home by provision of a family aide and/or home help. If this is not possible, efforts would be made to try to place mother and child together. For example, there may be particular foster carers within a local authority who work with mothers to help them to care for their babies. There are still some residential mother and baby homes, predominantly managed by the private and voluntary sector, which provide care, support and training for mothers, including some specialist services for very young mothers, or those with drug or alcohol dependency. If none of these options were feasible, it would still be important to facilitate frequent contact between mother and child unless this was felt to put the baby at risk.

TEENAGE MOTHERS

The national agenda for teenage mothers and parenting has been established following the presentation of the report on *Teenage Pregnancy* to Parliament (SEU, 1999) and incorporated aspects of the Children Act (1989). The political agenda is aimed at reducing the incidence of teenage pregnancy, helping prevent adverse outcomes of teenage pregnancy and parenting (by tackling health inequalities (DoH, 2001b), eradication of child poverty and reduction of infant mortality), and reducing long-term social exclusion of young parents (Connexions Service *et al.*, 2001; SEU, 2001: Annexe D: Teenage Pregnancy). The theme of reducing and preventing social exclusion of teenage parents is supported at strategic level through a range of initiatives. These include the National Strategy for Neighbourhood Renewal, which outlines the need to tackle teenage pregnancy among minority groups (SEU, 2000), and *Preventing Social Exclusion*, which addresses the special risks associated with teenage pregnancy, particularly in black and minority ethnic groups (SEU, 2001). A key theme is the education of young parents by returning to education (DoH, 2000d).

Young mothers, if under the age of 18, may be defined as children 'in need' in their own right. Both they and their babies may be entitled to an assessment of need and provided with services, including the provision of accommodation. However, the mother also has parental responsibility for her baby, regardless of her age. Teenage mothers may be eligible for 'after care' by virtue of the Children Leaving Care Act 2000 if they have been *looked after* or accommodated in a health authority, residential care home, or nursing home, and are between the ages of 16–21. This requires the local authority to advise, assist and befriend them by providing suitable accommodation and a personal adviser.

ADOPTION

Adoption is the dissolution of parental rights and duties, which are subsequently transferred to the new adoptive parent(s).

Adopted children have legal status in relation to their adoptive parents as do any other children to their parents, except that they cannot inherit titles. The Adoption and Children Act 2002 outlines the adoption service, placement and adoption orders, status of adopted children, adoption registers and overseas adoption. The Act ensures that the welfare of the children is central to any decisions made about them. Council adoption rates vary between 0.5–10.5% of *looked after* children being adopted each year. The average time between being placed for adoption and actual placement is 1 year 11 months. At present in this country there are approximately 4000 adoptions each year (including step-parent adoptions), of which 2700 were 'looked after' children in 1999/2000 (DoH, 2001c; 2001d).

In some cases, midwives become involved with a mother who has decided to give up her child for adoption. In rare circumstances the mother may decide that she does not want to care for the baby after birth. If this is the case, then midwives will be involved in planning with the SSD or adoption agency to manage this process.

CHILDREN WITH DISABILITIES

The Children Act 1989 recognizes children with disabilities as children first and includes them in the definition of children *in need* enabling them to benefit from the same services as other children. The Act imposes a duty on local authorities to provide services for children with disabilities to minimize the effect of their disabilities and to give them the opportunity to lead lives that are as normal as possible. The term 'child with disability' covers children affected by physical disability, chronic sickness, mental disability, sensory disability, communication impairment and mental illness (White *et al.*, 1995). Approximately 3–5% of children are classified as disabled in this country (DoH, 1998).

The child with disability is entitled to assessment and provision of services under the Children Act, but also under the Chronically Sick and Disabled Persons Act 1970, Education Act 1996, the Disability Discrimination Act 1995 and the Carers and Disabled Children Act 2000. At the same time as the assessment of need of the child, the carers are entitled to an assessment of their needs under the Carers (Recognition of Services) Act 1995 (Section 2). This includes young carers who may be caring for a disabled parent.

Midwives are at the front line of working with parents who are expecting a child with disability or where a disability is diagnosed at birth. They need to be sensitive to how information is conveyed to parents and ensure openness and honesty. In many cases, this involves referral to paediatric specialists. It is useful for the midwife to be aware of support groups and resources available to parents locally. Information can be obtained from social service departments who have specialist teams working with children with disabilities.

Reflective Activity 63.13

Find out what resources are available in your locality to help children with disabilities.

An important principle in working with children with disabilities is to ensure that the views and wishes of the child are sought and not to make the assumption that this is not possible.

Disabled children have been found to be particularly vulnerable and face an increased risk of abuse in many settings (Westcott and Jones, 1999). This may arise in part from social attitudes and special treatment resulting in disabled children being more isolated, more dependent, having less control over their lives and bodies and being less able to communicate their abuse. Special attention should be given to the needs of disabled children who receive multiple care-givers as part of their regular routine, and to their needs for reasonable continuity of care-givers.

THE PROTECTION OF CHILDREN

The impact of domestic violence on children and adolescents is becoming increasingly recognized and has been well researched (Cleaver, 2000). A network of women's refuges has been established to provide a safe haven and advice for women and their children, accessed through the Samaritans, the police or social services.

In some circumstances, alcohol and drugs misuse and mental illness may also adversely affect parents' abilities to care for their children (Cleaver *et al.*, 1999; Falkov, 1998). Careful assessment of the child and family's needs is required in any of these situations.

Along with all other professionals and voluntary sector workers involved with children, midwives have a responsibility to be alert to the possibility of child abuse and to take appropriate action where indicated (DoH, 1999a, 2000b) This involves discussion with a supervisor of midwives, senior colleague or doctor (see Box 63.2). *Working Together to Safeguard Children* (DoH, 1999a) addresses the entire area of cooperation and responsibilities of different agencies and professionals to work together to promote children's welfare and to protect them from abuse and neglect. Section 47 of the Children Act places a duty on any health authority or NHS trust to help a local authority in its inquiries in cases where there is reasonable cause to suspect that a child is suffering or is likely to suffer

---

Box 63.2 Responsibilities of the senior midwife (DoH, 1997: 9–10)

Those who manage midwifery should ensure that:

- There are agreed arrangements to give the name and telephone number of the health visitor to the mother the first week after the birth.
- They provide professional advice and guidance to any midwife who is concerned about a child or who is involved where a child is suspected of being at risk or has been abused or neglected.
- There is an early response to information of a pregnancy in a family where there has been an identified concern. The concern should be shared with other professionals as appropriate but particularly the health visitor.
- Where the mother is known to have abused drugs or alcohol during pregnancy, the risk factors are taken into account for the unborn child and any other children. Where a baby is born with fetal alcohol syndrome or has signs or symptoms of addiction to narcotics, a referral to social services should be made.
- Midwives and nurses in neonatal units are aware that infants separated from their mother at birth may be at greater risk of child abuse later in childhood. Their observations may be the first crucial step in alerting others to an 'at risk' situation.
- Midwives and nurses have an important part to play in promoting parent and child contact that forms the foundation of a strong parent/child relationship and the development of good parenting skills. This is particularly important where there are problems, e.g. mental or physical illness, physical or learning disability.
- Where the midwife is notified of a child or young person under 18 who is pregnant, she should consider whether there is a child protection concern.
- The special needs of the mother and father are met, e.g. a parent(s) with a disability including a learning disability and referring them to the appropriate source of support.

---

significant harm. It is important for midwives to recognize the roles and responsibilities of other professionals in working with children and where possible access joint multidisciplinary training in respect of assessment and child protection (DoH, 1997). With respect to child protection, the midwife is required to *refer* to social services departments if there are concerns that a child's welfare or safety may be at risk (DoH, 2003b). Social services or the NSPCC may contact the midwife to provide information in respect of knowledge about a child and family to assist their enquiries. Where it is agreed, following a *strategy decision*, that a *Section 47 enquiry* should be instigated and the child may be at risk of significant harm, the midwife may become involved in a *child protection conference*. If the child is placed on the *Child Protection Register*, involvement in a *child protection plan*, *core group meetings* and *review conferences* may be necessary.

Health authorities

Each health authority is required to identify a senior nurse with a health visiting qualification as designated senior professional to the Area Child Protection Committee (ACPC). Each NHS trust must also identify a named nurse or midwife to lead on child protection matters (DoH, 1997).

The Area Child Protection Committee (ACPC)

The overall management of the cooperation between various agencies in respect of child protection in any local authority is the responsibility of the Area Child Protection Committee (http://www.acpc.gov.uk). Each committee has a representative at a senior management level from each of the relevant agencies. They have responsibility to develop local policies and procedures for interagency work to protect children and evaluate these through setting objectives and performance indicators, to specify training needs and raise awareness within the wider community. They also conduct a review of any particularly difficult cases that arise, or where a child dies as a result of abuse or neglect in their area.

Reflective Activity 63.14

Find out who is the designated senior professional and the named doctor and midwife in your area.

Obtain a copy of the Area Child Protection Committee procedures in your area of practice.

Significant harm

Important in the assessment of risk is the concept of *significant harm*. If there is reasonable cause to suspect

---

Box 63.3 Categories of abuse and neglect

Abuse and neglect are generally considered under the following categories:

- physical abuse
- emotional abuse
- sexual abuse
- neglect.

These are generally used as the basis for registration of children on the Child Protection Register.

---

that a child who lives or is found in their area, is suffering or is likely to suffer significant harm, the local authority has a duty to make such enquiries as they consider necessary to enable them to decide whether they should take any action to safeguard or promote the child's welfare (Children Act 1989: S.47). This enquiry is commonly known as a *Section 47 investigation*.

Significant harm is defined in Section 31(9) and (10) of the Children Act as follows: 'Harm means ill treatment or impairment of health or development.'

Ill-treatment includes sexual abuse and other forms of ill-treatment that are not physical (see Box 63.3). The decision as to whether the harm is *significant* is measured on a comparison with the health and development reasonably expected of a similar child. The lack of a specific definition or of accompanying guidelines about how it should be applied in practice means that decisions about significant harm take into account a range of factors, and legal advice is usually sought. Assessments under the new framework aim to cover the range of factors and are child centred so that the impact of parenting capacity, family and environment on the child can be clearly identified and understood (DoH, 2000a). Ayre (1998) in analysing the factors taken into account by professionals in determining significant harm found that of 400+ factors cited, only one-quarter related to observations concerning the child, whereas more than half related to factors in respect of the parent.

Working Together to Safeguard Children (DoH, 1999a) advises that abuse or neglect is caused by inflicting harm. Abuse may occur in the family or in an institution.

Whilst it is not within the remit of this chapter to provide detail of signs and symptoms of abuse, there are well-documented warning signs which may alert the midwife (DoH, 1999a; Owen and Pritchard, 1993; Simpson, 1999a, 1999b). Physical abuse includes hitting, shaking, throwing, poisoning, burning, scalding, or suffocating. Midwives should be concerned about any bruising on a baby, particularly bruising around the face or on any soft tissues, bruising consistent with an implement being used to hit a child, fingertip bruising or slap marks, black eyes or ears, bites, scald and burn marks anywhere on the body, or a torn frenulum. Suspicion may be particularly raised if parents delay seeking advice about injuries or if there are discrepancies between the parents' explanation and the actual injuries found.

Emotional abuse may be observed by the midwife in terms of poor emotional bonding and possible rejection of the pregnancy and child, unrealistic expectations and/or demands of the child, constant criticism, unequal treatment, or a child being made to feel worthless and unloved. Failing to meet a child's basic physical or psychological needs in respect of food, clothes and safety, failing to protect the child from harm and failing to ensure access to appropriate medical care or treatment may be examples of neglect. Failure to follow medical advice through pregnancy and postnatal care, the mental state of the mother, rough handling or a history of drug or alcohol abuse also give cause for concern.

Munchausen syndrome by proxy   This condition is where a parent or carer fabricates the symptoms of injury or ill-health or deliberately causes this. For example, a mother may put blood into a baby's nappy or give drugs which make the child ill (DoH, 1997).

The time immediately after birth is important in establishing a positive relationship between parent and baby. Prematurity, illness of either mother or child, or other factors sometimes hinder this relationship. The midwife is a key figure in fostering a positive relationship, recognizing what is likely to support this and what may hinder it.

Reflective Activity 63.15

Make a list of the factors which you consider would encourage a positive and affectionate relationship between a baby and its parents.

Whilst stress does not automatically lead to child abuse it may make it more likely. Sources of stress for families include issues relating to social exclusion (Calder, 1999; DoH, 2000a; SEU, 2001), domestic violence (DoH, 2000c; Haggerty *et al.*, 2001), mental

illness of parent (Cleaver *et al.*, 1999), drug or alcohol abuse (Cleaver, 2000).

Whilst acknowledging that these factors do not necessarily lead to abuse or neglect, the potential or actual impact of these on a child need to be assessed and action taken to support the child and family as well as ensuring the child's safety.

A midwife who is involved with a child where there is concern may be involved in a *strategy discussion* with other professionals to share information, determine a plan for *Section 47 enquiries*, and consider how to immediately safeguard the child and provide interim services and support. This includes consideration of how to take race and ethnicity into account, including use of interpreters, the needs of other children, decisions about what information should be shared with the family, and the role of the police where an offence may have been committed.

Pre-birth assessment

Pre-birth assessments are undertaken when the local authority is concerned that the baby when born is in need or at risk of significant harm. The safety of the child is paramount, with the pre-birth assessment assessing the needs of the child and the support necessary to enable the family to succeed (Fraser, 1997). Assessments include consideration of parenting skills, preparation for the baby, use of medical advice and guidance, and consideration of the family and environment. In these situations the identified midwife works with social workers and other professionals in contributing to the assessment (Calder, 2000).

Particular issues, which may trigger a referral to a social services department or a pre-birth assessment, are:

- a mother who has learning disability or physical disability which makes it difficult for her to care for her baby
- consistent use of illegal drugs or alcohol by the mother or within the environment (Cleaver *et al.*, 1999)
- a mother living with or having frequent contact with a violent partner or Schedule 1 offender (a Schedule 1 offender is someone who has been convicted of an offence against children)
- young and vulnerable mothers with no support mechanisms – for example, this may be a girl who is herself 'in need', accommodated by the local authority or subject to a Care Order
- concerns about the mental health of the mother (or anyone else likely to have care of the child) and the

impact of her ill-health on the baby (Cleaver *et al.*, 1999)

- extreme poverty or inadequate housing
- families where a child has previously been placed on the Child Protection Register or removed from the home
- where pregnancy is the result of rape.

The unborn baby can be placed on the *Child Protection Register* but no further action can be taken until the child is born.

> It has been held that where a Local Authority wish to take early action to protect a newly born baby from potentially inadequate parents, they cannot intervene before birth. (The fetus cannot be made a ward of court.) However, they can intervene immediately after the birth and base this intervention on the mother's behaviour whilst pregnant and the presumption that this would lead to the child being at risk of significant harm.
>
> (Bainham, 1998: 70)

In rare cases where there is serious concern about the welfare of the child, the child may be made subject to an *Emergency Protection Order* or a ward of court and removed from the mother after birth. This should be planned ahead through the core group, to enable removal to take place as sensitively as possible. It can be a very traumatic time for all concerned, including professionals, and it is essential that all involved be supported throughout.

Reflective Activity 63.16

Consider the situations in Case scenarios 63.1–63.3. What would be the role of the midwife?

What evidence could the midwife contribute to a pre-birth assessment?

The Emergency Protection Order

In general the plans to protect a child proceed in agreement with parents; however, some cases may require emergency action. The Children Act (Section 44) allows for an Emergency Protection Order (EPO) to be made if there is reasonable cause to believe that a child is likely to suffer significant harm if:

- the child is not removed to accommodation; or
- the child does not remain in the place in which he or she is then being accommodated.

An EPO can be made if access to a child is being denied as part of a Section 47 enquiry. It gives the authority to remove a child or cause the child to remain in the protection of the local authority or NSPCC for a maximum of 8 days. Police also have powers to remove children to suitable accommodation or to prevent their removal from hospital or safe accommodation (Section 46).

In situations where parents are refusing to cooperate with Section 47 but there is not sufficient concern to justify an EPO, the local authority can apply for a Child Assessment Order (Section 45). This order directs the parents or carer to cooperate with an assessment of the child.

In respect of young babies an EPO may be applied for at birth if there are concerns that the parent will remove the child. Other examples may include a child who has been seriously injured by a parent who is refusing to allow access to the child or threatening to remove the child from hospital. In line with the best interests of the child, the Family Law Act 1996 allows for a perpetrator to be removed from the home instead of the child being removed, through an *exclusion order* attached to an EPO or Interim Care Order.

Female genital mutilation

In *Working Together to Safeguard Children* (DoH, 1999a) the possibility or reality of female genital mutilation has been identified as a legitimate reason for a Section 47 investigation and can constitute physical injury and abuse. In certain circumstances it provides evidence for an Emergency Protection Order or Care Order. Female genital mutilation can take place any time from 1 week after birth to 12 years (Owen and Brown, 1993). Female genital mutilation is against the law in this country by virtue of the Prohibition of Female Circumcision Act 1985.

The Child Protection Conference

The Child Protection Conference is the first meeting at which representatives of all the agencies which have dealings with the child or the child's family get together to share and evaluate information and consider the level of risk to a child or children. The conference decides whether the child should be placed on the Child Protection Register and makes plans for the future (DoH, 1999a). Social services departments or in some areas, the NSPCC, have responsibility for calling and arranging the conference.

The midwife may be required to attend a case conference to present and share information about the child and family, and will be one of many professionals in attendance. Generally there is a manager representing each agency that attends regularly, including a representative from health, education and the police. Other professionals include the social worker and his or her manager, the local authority solicitor, paediatrician, general practitioner, health visitor, housing officer, police, teachers, foster carers and any one who may have a significant contribution to make to the assessment. Parents and/or carers should be invited to attend (Cleaver and Freeman, 1995). This someimes places professionals in a situation where they feel unwilling to speak frankly in front of the parents for fear of jeopardizing their relationship with them.

All discussions which take place within child protection conferences, are confidential. Professionals involved in child protection have their duty of confidentiality to their client overridden by their duty to contribute to the protection of a child at risk. It is important for midwives to be adequately prepared for attendance at a conference. Box 63.4 provides a checklist of things to consider.

The Child Protection Register

The Child Protection Register records that a child has been, is at risk of, or is suspected of being abused. Children's names are put on the register under different categories of abuse, as described in Box 63.3. A designated officer within either the Social Services Department or NSPCC maintains the register, and access to it is restricted to those professionals offering direct services to the child. It can be checked in situations where abuse is suspected, to provide information of previous incidents.

Child Protection Plan   If a child is placed on the Child Protection Register a *key worker* is appointed. The key worker is a social worker from either the Social Services Department or NSPCC. They have responsibility for making sure the Child Protection Plan is developed into a more detailed interagency plan, ensuring completion of the core assessment, putting the plan into effect and monitoring it.

A *core group* of professionals, composed of those who have direct contact with the family or child, is established to develop and implement the Child Protection Plan in conjunction with the family. Members of the core group are jointly responsible for developing, implementing and monitoring the plan. A meeting of

> **Box 63.4 Checklist of preparation for a child protection conference**
>
> Who is the health representative who is attending?
> Where and at what time is the meeting to be held?
> Will the parents be present?
> Do I need a written report?
> Am I clear about the information to be presented? – Is my opinion based on facts?
> What is my view of the child's developmental needs? – What is my evidence?
> What is my view of the parents' capacity to parent? – What is my evidence?
> What is my view of family support systems and resources? – What is my evidence?
> Have I taken into account the needs of the child as being the primary concern?
> What do I think needs to happen to promote the welfare of this child/children?
> Is there anything I can contribute to this directly?
> Do I know of other resources/aids/assistance, which may be helpful?

the core group should take place within 10 working days of the initial conference.

The Child Protection Plan identifies how the child can be protected, including completion of a core assessment, short- and long-term aims to reduce risk to the child and promote the child's welfare, clarity about who will do what and when, and ways of monitoring progress.

If the child is not placed on the Register, this does not mean that all work with the child and family ceases. Whether children are placed on the Register or not, they may still be eligible to be considered as children 'in need' for whom a range of services may be provided.

CONCLUSION

The Children Act protects the rights of children promoting their status within society. Midwives must be aware of the implications of the Act and apply them to their practice. Midwives are uniquely situated to identify risk factors and act as advocates for newborn babies and other children during their professional practice. Detailed and contemporaneous records should be maintained throughout, as these may be required in assessments and child protection conferences. Key amendments are constantly made to the Children Act and so it is important to keep up to date and access relevant websites and support organizations so that knowledge is current. Using the three case scenarios identified at the start of this chapter will have helped you explore aspects of the Children Act in relation to midwifery practice, through exploration of supporting concepts, on-line materials and professional and statutory documents. In all cases it is important that the midwife liaises with the Supervisor of Midwives and other professionals, thus perpetuating a team approach to child support.

KEY POINTS

- The key features of the Children Act 1989 include paramountcy, parental responsibility, promotion of upbringing within the family, provision of services and support to enable this, and protection of children at risk.
- Midwives need to know the context of working with vulnerable families and how this impacts on their practice.

- The role of the midwife is significant to interprofessional working promoting the welfare of children defined by the Children Act as being *in need*, including those at risk of significant harm.
- The midwife plays a vital role in both pre-birth and post-birth assessments.

REFERENCES

Aldgate, J., Bradley, M. & Hawley, D. (1996) Respite accommodation: a case study of partnership under the Children Act 1989. In: Hill, M. & Aldgate, J. (eds) *Child Welfare Services: Developments in Law, Policy, Practice and Research*, Ch. 10, pp. 147–159. London: Jessica Kingsley.

Allen, N. (1998) *Making Sense of the Children Act*, 3rd edn. London: John Wiley.

Armstrong, H. (1996) *Annual Reports of the Area Child Protection Committees 1994–95*. London: DoH.

Ayre, P. (1998) Significant harm: making professional judgement. *Child Abuse Review* 7: 330–342.

Bainham, A. (1998) *Children: the Modern Law*, 2nd edn. Bristol: Family Law/Jordan.

Berridge, D. (1996) *Foster Care: A Research Review*. London: HMSO.

Brayne, H. & Martin, G. (eds) (1999) *Law for Social Workers*, 6th edn. London: Blackstone Press.

Butt, J. & Box, C. (1998) *Family Centred: A study of the Use of Family Centres by Black Families*. London: REU.

Calder, M. (1999) Towards an anti-oppressive practice with ethnic minority groups. In: Calder, M. & Howarth, J. (eds) *Working for the Child on the Child Protection Register*. Aldershot: Arena.

Calder, M. (2000) Towards a framework for conducting pre-birth risk assessments. *Child Care in Practice* 6(1): 53–72.

Cleaver, H. (2000) *Fostering Family Contact*. London: The Stationery Office.

Cleaver, H. & Freeman, P. (1995) *Parental Perspectives in Cases of Suspected Child Abuse*. London: Stationery Office Books.

Cleaver, H., Unell, I. & Aldgate, J. (1999) *Children's Needs – Parenting Capacity: The Impact of Parental Mental Illness, Problem Alcohol and Drug Use and Domestic Violence on Children's Development*. London: The Stationery Office.

Connexions Service, Teenage Pregnancy Unit & Sure Start (2001) Working Together: Connexions And Teenage Pregnancy. London: DfES Publications. Online. Available: http://www.connexions.gov.uk/pdf/teenagepregnancy.pdf.

Department of Health (DoH) (1991) *The Children Act (1989) Guidance and Regulations*, Vols 1–10. London: HMSO.

Department of Health (DoH) (1995) *Child Protection: Messages from Research*. London: HMSO.

Department of Health (DoH) (1997) *Child Protection Guidance for Senior Nurses, Health Visitors, Midwives and their Managers*, 3rd edn. London: The Stationery Office.

Department of Health (DoH) (1998) *Disabled Children Directions for their Future Care*. London: DoH.

Department of Health (DoH) (1999a) *Working Together to Safeguard Children: A Guide to Inter-agency Working to Safeguard and Promote the Welfare of Children*. London: HMSO.

Department of Health (DoH) (1999b) *Children Looked After by the Local Authority*. London: Government Statistics Services.

Department of Health (DoH) (2000a) *Framework for the Assessment of Children in Need and their Families*. London: HMSO. Online. Available: http://www.open.gov.uk/doh/quality.htm.

Department of Health (DoH) (2000b) *The Protection of Children Act 1999: A Practical Guide to the Act for all*

Organisations Working with Children. London: DoH. (Available free from the Department of Health.)

Department of Health (DoH) (2000c) *Domestic Violence: A Resource Manual for Health Care Professionals*. London: DoH. Online. Available: http://www.doh.gov.uk/domestic.htm. (Also obtainable free from the NHS Response line: 0541 555 455.)

Department of Health (DoH) (2000d) *Teenagers to Work Initiative: Information Pack for Local Authorities*. London: DoH.

Department of Health (DoH) (2001a) *Children's Taskforce: An Introduction*. Online. Available: http://www.doh.gov.uk/childrenstaskforce.

Department of Health (DoH) (2001b) *Tackling Health Inequalities: Consultation a Plan for Delivery*. Online. Available: http://www.doh.gov.uk/healthinequalities.

Department of Health (DoH) (2001c) *Adoption*. London: Department of Health. Online. Available: http://www.doh.gov.uk/adoption.

Department of Health (DoH) (2001d) *New Adoption Bill – a Fresh Start for Children*. Online. Available: http://www.nds.coi.gov.uk/coi/coipress.nsf/.

Department of Health (DoH) (2003a) *The Victoria Climbié Inquiry: Report of an Inquiry by Lord Laming*. London: Stationery Office.

Department of Health (DoH) (2003b) *What to do if You're Worried a Child is Being Abused – Summary*. London: DoH.

Department of Health and Social Security (DHSS) (1985) *Review of Child Care Law*. London: HMSO.

Department for Education and Employment (DfEE) (1998) National Child Care Strategy, Green Paper: Meeting the childcare challenge. Online. Available: www.dfes.gov.uk/eydcp/.

Department for Education and Employment (DfEE) (2000) *Connexions: The Best Start in Life for Every Young Person*. Online. Available: http://connexions.gov.uk.

Dimond B (2000a) The Human Rights Act 1998: Implications for practice. *British Journal of Midwifery* 8(10): 616–618.

Dimond B (2000b) Maternity rights for the employee. *British Journal of Midwifery* 8(4): 201–205.

Falkov, A. (ed) (1998) *Crossing Bridges: Training Resources for Working with Mentally Ill Parents and their Children*. Brighton: Pavilion Publishing.

Fraser, J. (1997) *Child Protection: A Guide for Midwives*. Cheshire: Books for Midwives Press, Hockland and Hockland.

Gibbons, J. (ed) (1994) *Family Support and The Children Act 1989*. London: HMSO.

Gibbons, J., Conroy, S. & Bell, C. (1995) *Operating the Child Protection System*. London: HMSO.

Gregg, D., Harkness, H. & Machin, S. (1999) *Child Poverty and its Consequences*. York: Joseph Rowntree Foundation.

Grimshaw, R. & McGuire, C. (1998) *Evaluating Parenting Programmes: A Study of Stakeholder's Views*. London: National Children's Bureau/Joseph Rowntree Foundation. Online. Available: http://www.jrf.org.uk/knowledge/findings/socialpolicy/SPR978.asp#top.

Haggerty, L., Kelly, U., Hawkins, J. *et al.* (2001) Pregnant women's perceptions of abuse. *Journal of Obstetrics, Gynaecology and Neonatal Nursing* 30: 283–290.

Hardy, S. & Hannibal, M. (1997) *Law for Social Workers*. London: Cavendish.

HAZnet (2001) What are health action zones? Online. Available: http://www.haznet.org.uk.

Law Commission (1998) *Family Law: Review of Child Care Law*. Law Commission No. 172. London: HMSO.

Owen, H. & Brown, L. (1993) Preventing female genital mutilation. In: Owen, H. & Pritchard, J. (eds) *Good Practice in Child Protection – A Manual for Professionals*, Ch. 6, pp. 88–89. London: Jessica Kingsley.

Owen, H. & Pritchard, J. (1993) *Good Practice in Child Protection – A Manual for Professionals*. London: Jessica Kingsley.

Simpson, D. (1999a) The midwife's role in child protection, Part 1: The legal framework. *Practising Midwife* 2(3): 28–31.

Simpson, D. (1999b) The midwife's role in child protection, Part 2: Practical matters. *Practising Midwife* 2(4): 32–35.

Social Exclusion Unit (SEU) (1999) *Teenage Pregnancy* (Cm 4342). London: The Stationery Office.

Social Exclusion Unit (SEU) (2000) *National Strategy for Neighbourhood, Minority Ethnic Issues in Social Exclusion and Neighbourhood Renewal*. Online. Available: http://www.socialexclusionunit.gov.uk.

Social Exclusion Unit (SEU) (2001) *Preventing Social Exclusion*. Online. Available: http://www.socialexclusionunit.gov.uk.

Steele, L. (2000) The day fostering scheme: a service for children in need and their parents. *Child and Family Social Work* 5(4): 317–325.

Sure Start (2001) *What is Sure Start?* Online. Available: http://www.surestart.gov.uk.

Utting, D. (1995) *Family and Parenthood: Supporting Families; Preventing Breakdown*. York: Joseph Rowntree Foundation.

Westcott, H. & Jones, D. (1999) The abuse of disabled children. *Journal of Child Psychology and Psychiatry* 40(4): 497–506.

White, R., Carr, P. & Lowe, N. (1995) *The Children Act in Practice*, 2nd edn. London: Butterworth.

STATUTES

Adoption and Children Act 2002 London: HMSO.
Care Standards Act 2000 London: HMSO.
Carers (Recognition of Services) Act 1995
    London: HMSO.
Carers and Disabled Children Act 2000 London: HMSO.
Children Act 1989 London: HMSO.
Children Leaving Care Act 2000 London: HMSO.
Chronically Sick and Disabled Persons Act 1970
    London: HMSO.
Data Protection Act 1998 London: HMSO.
Disability Discrimination Act 1995 London: HMSO.

Education Act 1996 London: HMSO.
Employment Relations Act 1999 London: HMSO.
Employment Rights Act 1996 London: HMSO.
Family Law Act 1996 London: HMSO.
Foster Placement (Children) Regulations 1991
    London: HMSO.
Human Rights Act 1998 London: HMSO. Online.
    Available: http://www.hmso.gov.uk/acts.htm.
Prohibition of Female Circumcision Act 1985
    London: HMSO.
Protection of Children Act 1999 London: HMSO.

FURTHER READING

Clarke, E. (1993) The Children Act 1989: implications for
midwifery. *British Journal of Midwifery* **1**(1): 26–30.
This article provides midwives with a concise outline of the
Children Act and how it impacts on midwifery practice. Of
particular importance is Table 2, which outlines the practice
implications in the form of a checklist for midwives.

Dimond, B. (2000) Maternity rights for the employee.
British Journal of Midwifery **8**(4): 201–205.
The arrangements for maternity leave and pay often appear
complex and confusing for the practitioner. In this article
Bridgit Dimond clearly presents the key components of the
Employment Rights Act 1996 and the Employment

Relations Act 1999, both of which impinge on rights of
women as employees.

Simpson, D. (1999) The midwife's role in child protection
Part 2: Practical matters. *Practising Midwife* **2**(4). 32–35.
This is the second part of two articles addressing concepts
of child protection (the first discusses legal issues). The
article is divided into important points to include, physical
abuse, sexual abuse, emotional abuse, referrals to social
services, child protection conferences, action plans,
outcomes, concerns about a baby's welfare, records
and reports, confidentiality, allegations of abuse by
staff and liaison with other professionals.

ADDITIONAL RESOURCES

Helplines

Childline
Tel: 020 7239 1000
Childline: 0800 1111
Website: http://www.childline.org.uk

NSPCC
Weston House, 42 Curtain Road, London, EC2A 3NH
Tel: 020 7825 2500
Child Protection Helpline: 0808 800 5000
Website: http://www.nspcc.org.uk/

Parent Line Plus
Tel: 0808 800 2222
Website: http://www.parentlineplus.org.uk/

Samaritans
Tel: 08457909090
Website: http://www.samaritans.org.uk/

The Maternity Alliance
Tel: 020 7588 8582
Website: http://www.maternityalliance.org.uk/

Websites

Acts of Parliament
http://www.hmso.gov.uk/acts.htm

Adoption
http://www.doh.gov.uk/adoption/

Area Child Protection Committees
http://www.acpc.gov.uk/

Children and Young People's Unit
http://www.dfee.gov.uk/cypu/

Connexions
http://www.connexions.gov.uk

Department for Work and Pensions
http://www.dwp.gov.uk

Department of Trade and Industry
http://www.dti.gov.uk

National Family and Parenting Institute
http://www.nfpi.org/

NCH Action for Children
http://www.nchafc.org.uk

Neighbourhood Renewal Unit
http://www.neighbourhood.dtlr.gov.uk/

Social Exclusion Unit
http://socialexclusionunit.gov.uk

Sure Start
http://www.surestart.gov.uk

Teenage Pregnancy Unit
http://www.teenagepregnancyunit.gov.uk

PART 10

THE MIDWIFE

64. A History of the Profession in the UK 1071

65. International Perspectives 1100

66. Statutory Framework for Practice 1116

67. Ethics and the Midwife 1133

68. Law and the Midwife 1142

69. Management and Leadership in Midwifery 1167

70. The Midwife as a Lifelong Learner 1185

71. Drugs and the Midwife 1209

A History of the Profession in the UK*

Jean Donnison

LEARNING OUTCOMES

After reading this chapter you will be able to appreciate:

- the significance of socioeconomic factors in the development of an occupation
- the extent to which ruling ideas about women's abilities and social status have affected the occupation of midwives in the UK
- the innate power of healthy women, except in a small minority of cases, to give birth safely without intervention

- the importance of clarity and rigour in the use of concepts like 'normality' and 'risk'
- the necessity for persistence, patience, pugnacity and organization among midwives to the continuance of the midwifery profession as guardians of normal childbirth.

THE OFFICE OF MIDWIFE: A FEMALE DOMAIN

The office of midwife is an ancient calling, and is represented universally in the art and literature of antiquity (Fig. 64.1). Sculptures of midwives attending birth date back at least 8000 years, and in the temples of ancient Egypt, Hat-hor, goddess of fertility and childbirth, is frequently portrayed in this role. Midwives appear, too, in the Old Testament; the quick-witted Shiprah and Puah outmanoeuvre Pharaoh, and the birth of Tamar's twins testifies to the midwife's resourcefulness and skill.

Until early modern times childbirth was considered 'women's business' – a matter of which women alone had special understanding. Certainly, no word existed in any language to signify a *male* birth attendant, and when, in the early 17th century, such appeared, new terms had to be created. The word 'obstetrician' came even later, being a 19th century invention constructed from '*obstetrix*', the Latin for 'midwife'.

---

*Unless otherwise referenced, material in this chapter is taken from Donnison, J. (1988) *Midwives and Medical Men: A History of the Struggle for the Control of Childbirth.* London: Historical Publications.

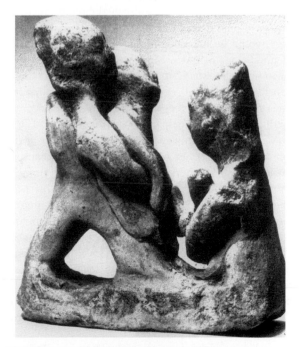

Figure 64.1   Sixth century BC terracotta group from Cyprus. The mother sits on a woman's lap (a traditional position for giving birth) while the midwife holds the newborn infant (Louvre, Paris).

Literally, 'she who stands before', 'obstetrix', like the Anglo-Saxon 'midwife' or 'with-woman', denotes the midwife's office, to be with the labouring woman. Other designations derive from her function of receiving the child and include the old French 'leveuse'; the Italian 'levatrice' and the German 'Hebamme'. The later French usage, 'sage-femme' (wise-woman), implies wider concerns and, indeed, midwives were commonly consulted on the care of the newborn, on matters of fertility, and on female ailments.

Occasionally, when the child could not be delivered normally, a man might be called in. Traditionally the use of instruments belonged to surgeons who, with the increasing exclusion of women from medicine and surgery from the 1300s, were overwhelmingly men. Yet the surgeon's scope was limited. Using hooks and scissors, he might extract piecemeal an infant presumed dead, or swiftly perform a caesarean section on the newly dead mother in the hope of saving the infant. Hence a man's advent into the birth chamber usually presaged the death of mother or child, or both. Where surgeons were not available, however, midwives themselves might undertake such operations.

What manner of women were midwives?

Little is known about the individual circumstances of European midwives before the 16th century. As later, they would be married women or widows, generally of middle age or older. Most would have given birth, since until the late 1700s this experience was usually considered essential, except for daughters following their mothers into the work. The case of the great German midwife Justina Siegemundin (1636–1705) illustrates this principle. Having suffered greatly at the hands of midwives in what proved to be a phantom pregnancy, she set herself to study midwifery, though, as a parson's daughter with a comfortably-off husband, she had no intention of practising for money. Learning through reading and through accompanying a local midwife to the labours of poor peasant women, she gradually acquired a reputation for skill in difficult births, eventually being called in to such cases among the nobility. Despite her renown, a physician-backed proposal in 1670 that she become a City Midwife for Liegnitz was nearly lost on account of standard regulations requiring appointees to have borne children. Later Siegemundin became midwife to the Prussian Court and author of an outstanding book on abnormal births, the 'child' she left to the world (Siegemundin, 1690: preface).

Before the 16th century most midwifery knowledge, like knowledge in other fields, would be transmitted by example and by word of mouth. Few women, even if literate, would have had the Latin necessary to read medical works, in which, even after the advent of printing in Europe in the mid-1400s, most were written. The first midwifery text printed in English was Richard Jonas' Byrth of Mankynde (1540), translated via the Latin from a 1513 German work addressed to pregnant women and midwives. Though containing nothing new, being largely drawn from ancient and mediaeval authors, the Byrth's huge popularity demonstrated the enormous hunger for such information in the vernacular (Hagelin, 1990: 12). Nevertheless, it would mainly benefit the literate minority who could afford its price. Significantly, the 1545 edition claimed that 'many honorable ladies and worshypfull gentyl wemen' took the book with them when visiting birthing neighbours. There they had appropriate parts read out for the education of the midwife and of the 'gossips' (the wife's friends and relations, themselves mothers, who by general custom were invited to witness the event).

What formally educated midwives there were came generally from the artisan class or from the lower gentry, and by the 17th century most of these would be literate. Such women invested time and possibly money in several years' apprenticeship to a senior midwife, while daughters commonly followed mothers into the work. These professional midwives would be found mostly in towns, where there was sufficient prosperity to make their outlay worthwhile. Even so, most would start by practising among the poor, acquiring a more affluent clientele in town and countryside as their reputation grew. Town midwives engaged by country nobility would arrive well beforehand, and stay several days afterwards, being recompensed accordingly.

These midwives occupied a respected position within the community, enjoying the title 'Mistress', indicating the propertied status borne out by wills and inventories they left behind (Ashcroft, 2002: 58–62; Evenden, 2000: 132–137). Such was the Kendal widow 'Mistress' Elizabeth Thompson (d. 1675), whose clientele included wives of solid citizens and of country gentry. However, Mrs Thompson clearly attended many poorer women, probably charging according to their means, or sometimes not at all. Her peak earnings (in 1673) were £27 9s 2d from 89 cases (Ashcroft, 2002), her average remuneration per case, including any attended gratis, being just over 6s.

Her London counterparts, with more prosperous clients, could do much better. In 1699 one such, although attending only 21 women, including two gratis, received over £28, her receipts ranging from 5s to nearly £5 and her average of approximately £1 6s 6d per case attended being over four times Mrs Thompson's. In her peak year of 1717, with four out of 30 deliveries unremunerated, she nonetheless received over £51, a sum representing a comfortable annual income for a London middle-class family keeping a servant (Anon, 1694–1723; Earle, 1989: 14). Attendance on royalty, however, was the most rewarding. Madame Peronne, who in 1630 came over from France to attend Charles I's French queen, received £300, with £100 for 'diet and entertainment', and in 1688 Mrs Labany and Mrs Wilkins, the midwives who delivered James II's heir, each received 500 guineas (Aveling, 1872: 60, 62).

However, such professional midwives were probably a minority compared with the numerous untrained, possibly illiterate women who might turn their hands to midwifery. Deriving their knowledge from their own birthing experiences and from watching neighbours' deliveries, these women were by custom considered qualified for the work by virtue of their advanced years or the large number of children they had borne (McMath, 1694: preface; Siegemundin, 1690: preface). They would serve the very poor, especially in rural areas, for perhaps a few pence or a small payment in kind, eking out a poor living with sick nursing, laying out the dead, and any other work they could find, as did their successors until the early 20th century.

'In the Straw'

Generally birth took place at home, poor women delivering in the communal room, before the hearth, the floor covered with straw that would later be burnt. In all classes the birth chamber would be darkened, its windows and doors sealed, and a fire kept burning for several days. These precautions were taken lest the woman took 'cold', a constant concern, as midwifery texts were to demonstrate. Also at work were ancient superstitions that malevolent spirits might gain entrance, harming the mother, or stealing away the infant and leaving behind a 'changeling', a puny thing, to grow up retarded or misshapen (Gélis, 1996: 97; Thomas, 1973: 728–732). Care was taken, too, that the afterbirth and its attachments, all credited with potent magical properties, should be disposed of safely, lest they be used in spells to harm the family. Such beliefs still persisted in remote parts of Europe in the early 20th century.

To hasten matters in early labour the parturient would from time to time be encouraged to walk, as the *Byrth* advised, supported by two sturdy women, her strength sustained by warm broth or spicy drinks. The midwife, inspired by the ancient and universal belief sanctioned by medical authority that the *child* provided the motive power for its birth, would follow time-honoured practice in greasing and stretching the woman's genitalia, also dilating the mouth of the womb, to 'help' the infant emerge. In recommending these procedures, the Graeco-Roman physician Soranus of Ephesus (late first to early second century AD), required his 'ideal' midwife to possess, along with appropriate qualities of character, small hands with long tapering fingers (Temkin, 1956: 5, 72–73).

The second stage of labour usually took place, as it had for millennia (Kuntner, 1988: Ch. 3), with the woman in upright or semi-upright position, known to provide the advantages of easier breathing and gravity. In rich households a birth chair might be used (Fig. 64.2), but more commonly the parturient sat on a woman's lap. Some women knelt or stood, leaning against a support; some adopted a half-sitting, half-lying posture, with a solid object to push their feet against during contractions, while others delivered on all fours (Blenkinsop, 1863: 8, 10, 73; Gélis, 1996: 21–36). As labour progressed, the woman would

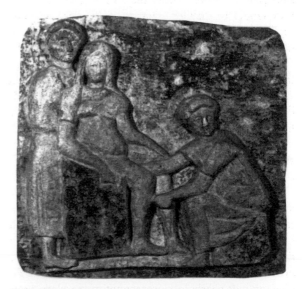

Figure 64.2 First century tablet from Ostia from the tomb of Scribonia Attice, midwife, commissioned by her for herself, her mother and her doctor husband. It shows the parturient seated on a birth chair, while the woman helper behind her presses the fundus with both hands and the midwife prepares to receive the child (Rome Museum).

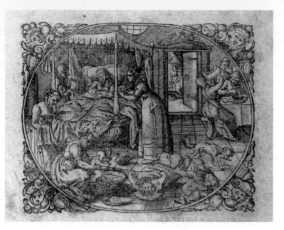

Figure 64.3 After the birth in a wealthy 16th century German household. The Midwife (centre) hands the mother a bowl of broth, while the monthly nurse bathes the newborn preparatory to its swaddling for the cradle. On the extreme right, the 'gossips' celebrate the new arrival. (Jacobus Rueff, *De conceptu et generatione hominis*, 1580, Frankfurt-am-Main (Wellcome Library, London).)

instinctively change her position, 'as shall seeme commodious and necessarye to the partie', as the *Byrth* put it. The midwife, it urged, should comfort her with refreshments and with 'swete wurdes', encouraging her to 'pacience and tolleraunce' with the hope of a 'spedefull deliveraunce'. Not all births were straightforward, however, and the *Byrth* gave directions for dealing with abnormal cases, including instrumental removal of the dead fetus and caesarean section on the dead mother. Following delivery, the mother would be put to bed to 'lie in' – rich women for up to a month, the poor for days at most. The first few hours, however, were considered critical and the mother was denied sleep until her attendants were sure all was well. The infant would be washed, then swaddled to 'straighten' its limbs, and an all-woman celebration of this female life event would ensue, the spread varying with the means of the household (Fig. 64.3).

THE MIDWIFE, THE CHURCH AND THE LAW

The midwife's duties did not end with the birth, however, and she carried heavy responsibilities concerning baptism. This rite was considered vital by the Church lest the child should remain in the state of 'original sin' in which it was born and its soul be lost. Hence the midwife was required to take weak infants directly to

the priest for baptism, but if time did not permit, to perform the ceremony herself, taking care, on pain of severe punishment, to use only the Church's prescribed words. When the woman died undelivered, the midwife's responsibility if no surgeon had been called was immediately to open the body in hope of finding a living infant for baptism. Stillbirths and unbaptized infants, in their unhallowed state unfit for Christian burial, she was to bury in unconsecrated ground, safely and secretly, where neither man nor beast would find them.

Otherwise baptism would generally take place within a week of the birth, and it was the midwife, infant in arms, who headed the procession to the church, carrying the child to the font. After the christening, the midwife enjoyed an honoured place at the ensuing celebration, and in prosperous households would be liberally tipped by family and friends. Later, after the lying-in was over, she would accompany the mother to her churching. Under Catholicism, this was a ritual of 'purification' from the 'defilement' of carrying an unchristian creature. Taking place at the church door, the woman kneeling with white veil and candle, it was a condition, physically and metaphorically (together with the priest's fee), of the mother's readmission to the Church. With the advent of Protestantism, however, the ceremony took place within the church, becoming merely one of maternal thanksgiving for safe deliverance.

The midwife also had an important role in legal matters. Where a woman condemned to death pleaded pregnancy in the hope of mitigating or postponing punishment, a panel of midwives would be summoned to examine her, though the discovery of a fetus in some post-execution dissections showed such examinations were not always reliable (Pechey, 1696: 55–56). Midwife panels were also called in to examine unmarried women alleging rape, women accused of aborting themselves or of concealing the birth (and possible murder) of an unwanted infant, or the prematurity or otherwise of infants born within less than 9 months of marriage. They could also be asked to certify virginity in prospective brides or impotence in prospective or actual husbands. Midwives attending an unmarried woman were also expected to make her name the father, lest he escape his responsibility to the parish for the child's upkeep.

Governing the midwife

Inevitably, in view of these religious and social functions, and the prevalence of old magical beliefs, the midwife's character and religious orthodoxy were of grave concern to the Church. In 1481 Agnes Marshall of Emeswell, Yorkshire, was 'presented' at the Bishop's Court, not merely because she lacked skill in midwifery, but also because she used (pagan) 'incantations' to 'help' the labour. Midwives were suspect, too, because of their access to stillbirths, and in 1415 a successful Parisian midwife, Perette, was turned in the pillory and banned from practice for supplying a tiny fetus subsequently used, unbeknownst to her, in witchcraft.

Fear of witchcraft was stronger on the Continent, as indicated by the popularity there of the witch-finder's manual, the viciously misogynist *Malleus Maleficarum* (*Hammer of the Witches*) (1484–1486). The work of two German members of the Inquisition, it singled out 'witch-midwives', who 'surpass all other witches in their crimes'. These women, it claimed, secretly killed infants, either in the womb or at the birth, dedicating their souls to the devil and using their bodies in satanic rites. All midwives should therefore be sworn in as good Catholics before the magistrates. Although it does not appear that midwives were especially persecuted during the episodic witch-crazes of the next two centuries, they were among women executed for witchcraft in France, Germany and post-Reformation Scotland. Charges included the use of 'sorcery' to relieve labour pain, or more lurid accusations drawn from the *Malleus*, confessions commonly being extracted by torture (Harley, 1996: 103–115). Church condemnation of artificial birth control also threatened midwives, likely to be consulted on such matters, and in 1477 a Hamburg woman was burned for advising on abortion (Heinsohn and Steiger, 1985: 120).

Probably the first system of compulsory midwife licensing in Europe was instituted in the Bavarian city of Regensberg in 1452, a system gradually followed in other European cities. Applicants for a licence were commonly examined by a panel of physicians who, innocent of practical midwifery, would base their examination on classical texts. Questions dealt with signs of pregnancy, detection of the dead fetus, correction of malpresentations, management of the umbilical cord, expulsion of the afterbirth, and care of mother and newborn. Generally such licensing imposed limits on midwives, requiring them to send for a doctor or surgeon in difficult cases, Strasbourg midwives being prohibited from using hooks or sharp instruments on pain of corporal punishment. Many cities appointed midwives to serve the poor, supplementing their remuneration with payment in kind and providing from the town coffers for their relief in old age or disability (Gélis, 1988: 25; Marland, 1993: Ch. 4).

In England the first formal arrangements for controlling midwives were made under the 1512 Act for regulating physicians and surgeons. The Act's aim was to limit unskilled practice and the use of sorcery and witchcraft in medicine, not just in towns as on the Continent but throughout the land. It therefore provided for Church Courts to license those practitioners producing testimony to their skill and religious orthodoxy and to prosecute the rest. A midwife applicant for a licence would normally bring to the ceremony references to her character and religious conformity, together with 'six honest matrons' whom she had delivered and who were willing to testify to her competence. There was, however, no *formal* examination on this point as existed under Continental schemes, an omission that in 1547 drew unfavourable comparisons from the much-travelled physician, Andrew Boorde, in his *Breviary of Helthe*, and, indeed, the system was never completely enforced.

Successful applicants swore a long and detailed oath, promising 'faithfully and diligently' to help childbearing women, to serve 'as well poor as rich', not to charge more than the family could afford, nor to divulge private matters. They swore not to use witchcraft or sorcery to shorten labour; to use only appointed words when christening infants; and to personally bury stillborn infants in the prescribed manner. They undertook not to procure abortion nor connive at child destruction, false attribution of paternity or substitution of infants. Neither were they to allow any woman to be delivered secretly but always see that 'two or three honest women' were present, a requirement clearly aimed at preventing the speedy disposal of an unwanted child.

ADVENT OF THE MAN-MIDWIFE

Around the mid-16th century came other changes laden with import for midwives, as the new Renaissance spirit of enquiry in anatomy was applied by surgeons to the process of childbirth. Outstanding among pioneers in this field was Ambroise Paré (1510–1590), surgeon to four French Kings, chiefly remembered here for his introduction of podalic version in certain malpresentations. The success of men like Paré was to encourage the extension of male attendance in childbirth, first to 'extraordinary' cases, then to ordinary ones. This development gradually spread throughout Europe, gaining recognition in Britain with the coining in the early 1600s of the term 'Man-Midwife', just as the new construct 'accoucheur' had been adopted in France.

Leading practitioners, male and female, recognized the centrality of anatomy to good midwifery practice. Louise Bourgeois (midwife to the Queen of France) emphasized this in her 1609 *Observations* (the first midwifery text published by a midwife and soon translated into several languages). Later, the London midwife Jane Sharp began her *Midwives Book* by deploring:

> the many Miseries Women endure in the Hands of unskilful Midwives; many professing the Art (without any skill in Anatomy, which is the Principal part effectually necessary for a Midwife) meerly for Lucres sake.
>
> (Sharp, 1671: preface)

The man-midwife Percivall Willughby (1596–1685) concurred, reporting that many country midwives could not manage malpresentations. Also attracting his censure, however, were inexperienced young surgeons, but, more particularly, apothecaries trying their hand at midwifery, whose fatal ignorance Willughby considered deserving of the branding-iron or the hangman's noose.

Maternal mortality

Given the general lack of statistics, the extent of contemporary maternal mortality (calculated as death at or within the month after the birth) is difficult to discover. In his 1662 study of the London Bills of Mortality, John Graunt estimated the maternal death rate at about 15 per 1000 births. Those dying from the 'hardness' of their labour (anaemia and rachitic pelves were probably implicated here) as distinct from other causes, he put at less than 1 in 200. However, along with many authorities, Graunt believed that poor hard-working countrywomen did best in childbirth, a widely held view dating far back into antiquity.

Dr William Harvey (discoverer of the circulation of the blood) indicated a possible factor in this apparent disparity. Condemning 'officious' midwives who hurried the birth by dilating the genitalia and cervix for bringing women 'in danger of their lives', Harvey pointed to 'much happier' obstetrical outcomes in cases 'where the midwife's help is never required', namely, cases of poor women, and of women who, for fear of society's penalties for illicit sexual relations, concealed both pregnancy and birth. Harvey's friend

Willughby, who admitted having earlier recommended such intervention, now insisted that such 'haling, pulling and stretching' did great harm and never any good, and condemned interference in all but abnormal births.

Significantly, Willughby links such interference with the woman's 'taking cold' (Blenkinsop, 1863: 6), a likely reference to 'puerperal' fever, not then so named, but recognized under 'fevers' and 'agues' occurring after childbearing. Following ancient humoral theory, the condition was ascribed to an imbalance of the bodily 'humours' (Jonas, 1540; Sharp, 1671) and was probably then as later the principal cause of maternal death. Not until the late 18th century was it publicly proposed that this deadly malady might be carried to the woman on the attendants' clothing or unwashed hands (Gordon, 1795: 98–99), a view not completely accepted, even in medical circles, until the 1940s.

However, snobbery may also have played a part in this reported differential mortality. Traditionally, wealthier mothers employed wet-nurses to suckle their infants, thus forgoing the potentially contraceptive effects of the customary protracted breastfeeding. They therefore risked another pregnancy soon after the birth, with increased possibility of adverse consequences for mother and fetus (Conde-Agudelo and Belizan, 2000; Smith and Pell, 2003).

Midwives under threat

When urging midwives to study anatomy, Jane Sharp had recognized that women's exclusion from the Universities and 'Schools of learning', where this was taught, disadvantaged them compared with men. Girls were also barred from grammar schools and hence from knowledge of Latin, which was the mark of an educated person and which was still used for many medical texts. Men-midwives, therefore, enjoyed higher status than midwives, irrespective of the skill of either, and the distinction of the great 18th-century practitioners like Smellie, Manningham, Ould and Hunter, was to reflect credit on every man-midwife, deserved or not.

However, it was probably the general introduction in the 1720s of the midwifery forceps that precipitated the rapid acceleration of the existing trend. The forceps enabled its user in certain circumstances to deliver live infants where previously child or mother would have been lost, and to shorten tedious labour. Since custom discouraged the use of instruments by midwives,

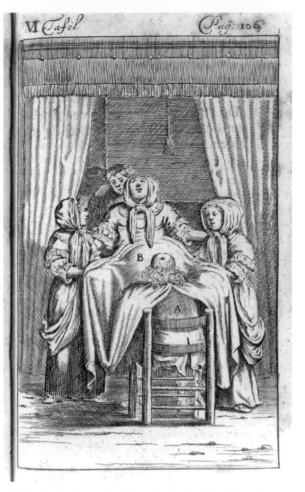

Figure 64.4   Man-midwife attending a birth. To protect the woman's modesty the corners of a sheet are pinned around his neck so that he must work 'blind', increasing the risk of error. The woman holds on to her attendants' shoulders while they push against her feet to provide purchase for her expulsive efforts. (Janson S, *Korte en Bonding verhandeling, van de voortteelingen't Kinderbaren*, 1711, Amsterdam (Wellcome Library, London).)

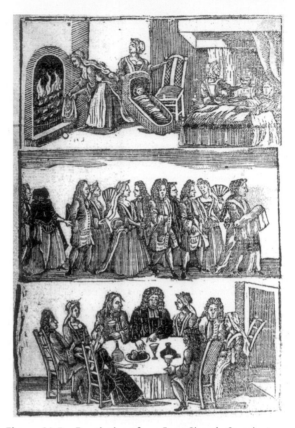

Figure 64.5   Frontispiece from Jane Sharp's *Compleat Midwife's Companion* (1724). (1) The midwife hands the mother a bowl of broth after the birth. (2) Infant in arms, she heads the christening procession to the church. (3) A guest at the christening party, she will receive substantial tips from the company (Wellcome Library, London).

this development further enhanced the position of men and many surgeon-apothecaries, taking up midwifery, became general practitioners in fact if not yet in name. Some men, too, saw childbirth as a *mechanical* process and men, with their right to use instruments, as better suited to preside over it. Indeed, many saw the educated male practitioner as representing the new enlightened age, while the midwife, in whose ranks were many hampered by illiteracy and superstition, remained a relic of a benighted past.

Midwives, keenly aware of the threat to their livelihood, fought back, supported in books and pamphlets by both medical and lay sympathizers. Many women for reasons of modesty would not send for a man, these argued, nor would their husbands allow it. More could not afford men's fees, and in any case male assistance, especially in the country, was commonly unavailable. Furthermore, many men-midwives resorted to unnecessary and damaging use of instruments to save their time and to demand extra fees; consequently more mothers and infants were lost than formerly. Men also exaggerated the dangers of childbirth, frightening women into believing that extraordinary measures, and therefore male attendance, were more generally necessary than they were. Moreover, by insisting on being called to every trifling difficulty, men were reducing midwives to mere nurses, also taking every opportunity to denigrate their competence and to blame them, however unjustly, for any mishap, including their own mistakes.

Lying-in hospitals and 'out-door' charities

One champion of the midwives' cause was John Douglas, a well-known London surgeon. In rebutting male claims that difficult births were beyond female capacities, Douglas instanced Mme du Tetre, formerly Head Midwife at the great religious foundation in Paris, the Hôtel-Dieu, whose midwives' manual demonstrated her standing in the field. English midwives, Douglas maintained, could reach equally high standards if they had the same educational opportunities as Frenchwomen. (Indeed, midwives had been trained in the Hôtel-Dieu's lying-in wards since 1631; in Britain however, most hospital provision had disappeared with the demise of the monasteries 200 years before.) Seeing hospital instruction as vital for improved midwife education, Douglas therefore demanded the establishment of lying-in hospitals in all the principal cities in England. The first such permanent foundation in the British Isles, however, was the Dublin 'Rotunda', founded in 1745. In London, two lying-in wards were created in the Middlesex Hospital in 1747, followed by the British Lying-in Hospital (1749), the City of London (1750) and the General Lying-in Hospital (later Queen Charlotte's) in 1752. Similar institutions appeared in other major cities in the UK as the century progressed.

Lying-in hospitals, like other hospitals founded at the time, were initially very small philanthropic institutions, funded by subscriptions from the wealthy and run by a voluntary (largely lay) board. Although officially for the benefit of the poor (generally 'respectable' married women), these hospitals were in fact a mixed blessing for those attended there. Outbreaks of puerperal fever, a regular feature until the inception of antiseptic practice in the late 19th century (and still occurring in the 1930s) boosted death rates and necessitated closure for weeks on end. Safer, and cheaper, were 'out-door' charities such as London's Royal Maternity Charity, founded in 1757, which provided poor women with midwife attendance at home, with designated medical assistance where necessary.

Hospitals certainly benefited the medical staff. These men gave their services free, but apart from receiving pupils' fees, their status as public appointees guaranteed them lucrative private practice, while the 'objects of the charity' provided readily available

training material. Some hospitals took midwife pupils, others only men. Midwife instruction lasted 3–4 months, being limited, however, to what was 'necessary for Women to know'. Pupils generally came from the artisan class and had to be married women or widows. Numbers trained were small, probably because of the cost. Instruction by the medical staff cost about £20 per head and this, together with board and lodging, probably came to over £30. Some of the larger outdoor charities also took midwife pupils and pos-sibly made a greater contribution to midwife training. There was, however, no move in England from government, central or local, on this matter; and by the 1720s Bishops' licensing, though no great guarantee of skill, and never properly enforced, had generally ceased.

Continental comparisons

Meanwhile on the Continent, notably in Holland, Germany and France, government involvement in matters perceived to be in the public interest, such as provision of midwife schools and services, grew ever stronger. In France in 1759 the eminent midwife, Mme Ducoudray, was commissioned by the King to travel around the country to lecture to midwives *and* surgeons, and to found lying-in hospitals, a task she discharged for over 20 years. Moreover, in 1770 a government-endorsed midwifery manual was issued free (Marland, 1993: Chs 4, 5, 7–10). Yet in the UK, central government, materially weakened by the curtailment of monarchical power following the execution of Charles I in 1649 and the expulsion of James II in 1688, showed no interest in such questions. Educated midwives, realizing that the lack of instruction and regulation was contributing to the occupation's decline, pointed, like Boorde 200 years before, to Continental regulatory systems, calling, though vainly, for similar measures at home.

Scotland, where Continental influence was stronger, was a different case. In 1726 Edinburgh Town Council had created an (honorary) Chair in Midwifery, the first in the British Isles. Its professor, Joseph Gibson was to teach midwives, but probably also took male pupils. Edinburgh also tightened up its 1694 regulation of midwives. Further, in 1740 the Glasgow Faculty of Physicians and Surgeons instituted a system for the examination and licensing of midwives in the city and surrounding counties, which, like Edinburgh's, appears to have operated throughout the century.

'Towards a new system of midwifery'

By the mid-18th century male practitioners, disdaining the familiar 'man-midwife', began to adopt the French term 'accoucheur', as conveying greater status. Their approach to labour and delivery varied greatly, however. Some still dilated the cervix and the labia vulvae, practices continuing among the more ignorant at the century's close (Clarke, 1793: 21). Some extracted the afterbirth immediately after delivery by introducing the hand into the womb and detaching it with their finger nails (in the absence of asepsis, a highly dangerous manoeuvre), while others roundly condemned this (Smellie, 1752: 238–239). The trend in normal births, however, was towards non-intervention. This stemmed from the new, but not yet general, realization that it was uterine action rather than fetal exertion that provided the expulsive force for the birth, as explained by the Scot, William Smellie in his 1752 *Treatise on the Theory and Practice of Midwifery*. Significantly, Smellie (since regarded as the 'father of British obstetrics') concluded from his vast experience that, out of 1000 parturients, 990 would be safely delivered 'without any other than common assistance' (ibid: 195–196).

Differences existed, too, on care in the puerperium. Some accoucheurs encouraged the mother to sit up in bed after delivery, as depicted in 16th century manuals, to facilitate drainage of the lochia (White, 1773: 115–116). Others prescribed a supine position for several days, a practice still followed in the 1940s (Strachan, 1947: 265–266). The low diet traditionally recommended for fear that solid food, especially meat, would engender fever, became poorer, and repeated 'prophylactic' purging was routine (Anon, 1803: 248–251). All this, together with enforced recumbency, contributed to the increasing invalidization of lying-in women, which continued until the mid-20th century. Salutary changes, however, were the encouragement of sleep following delivery, hitherto considered dangerous, and the admission of light and air to the lying-in chamber (Clarke, 1793: 289; White, 1773: 112–113).

Though ambulation in the first stage was still encouraged, women's freedom to choose their delivery position was gradually being curtailed. Earlier authorities, male and female, had encouraged women to adopt the position most comfortable to them as facilitating the best outcome for mother and infant. Smellie, too, underlined the advantages of upright positions in furthering labour through gravity and the equalization of the uterine force, recommending them for tedious labours (Smellie, 1752: 202). Despite this, many accoucheurs, including Smellie, generally insisted on delivery in bed, for fear that otherwise the woman might take 'cold' (ibid: 204), or the delivery be too precipitate (White, 1773: 103–104). Equally important to the accoucheur, however, seems to have been his own convenience (Burton, 1751: 106–107) and sense of control. Sitting by the edge of the bed, with his hand concealed by a sheet was less tiring and less undignified for the accoucheur aspiring for recognition of his art as part of medicine proper than crouching before the seated parturient on the midwife's low stool.

So it was that recumbent delivery positions (left lateral in Britain, dorsal in France) gradually became the norm for 'civilized' practice. Although delivery out of bed persisted in some rural areas into the 20th century, it was generally considered low-class, if not inhumane. Significantly, the parturient's transfer to bed, together with her increasing designation as a 'patient' (a word traditionally used only of the sick), indicated her transition from an active to a passive role in this important female life-event, and, implicitly, the incipient medicalization of childbirth itself.

THE DECLINE OF THE MIDWIFE

By the early decades of the 19th century the midwife's situation had deteriorated further. Growing prudery, largely the result of the Evangelical movement, had rendered reference to childbirth, and even the word 'midwife', taboo in polite society. Together with the male capture of the better-paid private practice and the growing reluctance of the middle classes to allow their women to work, this prudery meant that fewer educated women entered midwifery, leaving many who wanted skilled assistance in childbirth forced to send for a man. Midwife supporters argued that midwives' instruction (where it existed) had not kept pace with men's and increasingly demands arose for the instruction of female practitioners to the highest professional standards, not only in midwifery but also in women's diseases, demands which foreshadowed the coming battle for the re-entry of women into medicine.

The medical response was predictable. The academic distinction of midwives like Lachapelle and Boivin at the Paris Maternité, and of Charlotte von Siebold, the German midwife who delivered both the future Queen Victoria and her consort Prince Albert, was ignored. Women were unfitted by nature for 'scientific mechanical employment' (which midwifery was), and could never use obstetrical instruments with 'advantage or precision' even if they had 'presumption' enough to try. Such remarks, together with allegations that midwives were necessarily abortionists, prompted one midwife supporter to remark that 'the greatest slanders against the moral and intellectual characters of women have been uttered by practitioners of man-midwifery'.

This animosity towards midwives arose partly from men-midwives' own low status within the medical profession in England and Wales. Their speciality was not officially recognized as part of medicine and there was no official qualification to distinguish men with midwifery training from those with none, like the Rochdale mill worker recorded in 1823 who left the mill to turn man-midwife. Hence men seeking officially recognized midwifery qualifications were forced to go to Scotland or the Continent. Leading accoucheurs had repeatedly requested the English chartered medical corporations to establish such a qualification but had always been rebuffed. Many prominent medical figures viewed attendance on childbirth as 'women's work' and hence below the dignity of professional men. Thus in 1827 Sir Anthony Carlisle, later President of the English College of Surgeons, denounced man-midwifery as a 'dishonorable vocation', accusing men-midwives of seeking, from financial motives, to turn a natural process into a 'surgical operation'. It was 1852 before the College established a Midwifery Licence and 1888 before similar qualifications were required by the General Medical Council, the doctors' regulatory body established under the 1858 Medical Act, for admission to its Medical Register. Thenceforth midwifery was formally recognized in the UK as part of medicine.

Maternal mortality and the Registrar-General's Office

Hitherto there had been no national maternal mortality figures, these only becoming available from 1839 from the newly created Registrar-General's Office for Births, Marriages and Deaths. The estimated maternal death rate for 1841 of nearly 6 per 1000 live births (stillbirths were not registered until 1929) caused the Office's Statistical Superintendent, Dr W Farr, to look wistfully at Continental legislation for midwife instruction and regulation. However, British suspicion of state direction, together with national 'delicacy' (prudery) in such matters, he regretfully concluded, ruled out the

establishment of comparable arrangements at home. Yet with properly instructed midwives, Farr believed, the annual 3000 maternal deaths could be reduced by a third. That some grossly incompetent midwives existed was demonstrated by press reports of women who had pulled out the womb or torn the child's body from its head. Such disasters were paralleled, however, in accounts of ignorant male practitioners cutting out the womb or part of the intestines with scissors or knife. Some of these men (graphically described in the *London Medical Gazette* as 'disembowelling accoucheurs') were regularly qualified medical men; others were chemists, but in neither case was instruction in midwifery required by law.

The end of the midwife?

Meanwhile the midwife's image had not been helped by Charles Dickens' caricature in his 1844 novel *Martin Chuzzlewit* of the unsavoury 'Mrs Gamp', a poor widow who, like so many over the centuries, earned her living by practising midwifery, sick and 'monthly' nursing, and laying out the dead (Fig. 64.6).

A blowsy, tippling, unscrupulous character, Mrs Gamp soon became the midwife stereotype. But although with Dr Farr some medical men advocated the replacement of such midwives by respectable, trained women, certain accoucheurs, seeking a male monopoly of midwifery (actually achieved in North America by the 1950s), were fiercely advocating the midwife's total abolition. 'All midwives are a

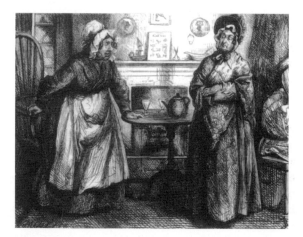

Figure 64.6 Dickens' Mrs Gamp quarrels with her friend and colleague Betsy Prig, a nurse from St Bartholomew's Hospital, London, both being the worse for drink (Dickens 1844, *Martin Chuzzlewit*).

mistake', Tyler Smith, Midwifery Lecturer at the Hunterian School of Medicine, told his students in 1847, 'and it should be the aim of every obstetric practitioner to discourage their employment'. Furthermore, because of its origin, the word 'midwifery' should no longer be used to describe male attendance on childbirth but be superseded by the new construct 'obstetrics'. Here Smith well understood that a Latin-sounding name, though derived from the Latin for 'midwife' (a fact known only to a classically educated élite), had a snob value which would further elevate men above their female competitors. This substitution of 'obstetrics' for 'midwifery' in male practice was, however, not fully achieved until after World War II.

The Royal Maternity Charity and maternal mortality

Directly in Smith's line of fire was the century-old Royal Maternity Charity. The Charity's employment of midwives, however well instructed, Smith contended, was 'degrading' to 'obstetrics' and harmful to its clients, who instead should be attended by 'educated' practitioners. Yet the Charity's statistics, published annually by the eminent practitioners supervising its work, repeatedly disproved his allegations. Although serving only poor women, many undernourished and living in unhealthy conditions, the Charity (and other similar foundations) consistently demonstrated mortality rates considerably lower (in the Charity's case less than half) than the Registrar-General's recorded rate for England and Wales of over 5 per 1000 live births.

Another onslaught in this continuing controversy came in 1870 from the distinguished obstetrician Mathews Duncan. In his *Mortality of Childbed*, Duncan dismissed the charities' results as 'Munchausen' successes which 'educated accoucheurs', who in their private practice generally lost five times as many women, could not accept. Otherwise it followed that poor women delivered by 'imperfectly educated' midwives in filthy slums fared better than wealthy patients attended in salubrious conditions by experienced practitioners, clearly an absurd conclusion. Questioning the Registrar-General's estimate of 5 deaths per 1000, Duncan postulated an irreducible minimum of at least eight. Duncan's stance was challenged by equally respected obstetricians, while Florence Nightingale acidly concluded that his figures created a 'very painful impression' of the practice of his 'educated accoucheurs' themselves.

Despite this contrast between the relative safety of poor women attended by the charities' trained midwives and the admitted high mortality among Duncan's affluent cases the anti-midwife faction had an answer. The cause of higher mortality among the rich lay not with their medical attendants, but with the 'artificial state of society', which disabled wealthier women for parturition. Increased (medical) vigilance (and hence higher fees) was therefore necessary in attending them, not less. The degree to which childbirth among the prosperous classes was progressively seen as pathology was evident in Dr P Chavasse's 1842 handbook *Advice to a Wife*. While describing childbirth as a natural event, Chavasse required the 'pregnant female' to rest for 2–3 hours a day while the post-parturient should keep to a meagre diet and lie flat on her back for 10–14 days lest she faint, haemorrhage, or suffer a prolapsed womb. Such a regimen was only possible for women with servants and, for the puerperium, is now considered positively dangerous. This invalidization of childbirth naturally implied more medical attention and higher fees. Furthermore, women were now caught in a double bind. Not only were they regarded as incapable of competent attendance on this uniquely female function but were increasingly seen as requiring male assistance even to perform it.

The advent of artificial pain relief

Another factor working to enhance the prestige of the male practitioner was the use from the 1840s of chloroform to produce analgesia or anaesthesia in childbirth, a practice not open to midwives. This was not greeted with universal acclaim, however. Quoting Genesis, certain churchmen viewed labour pain as women's divinely ordained punishment for Eve's disobedience in the Garden of Eden in tasting the fruit of the Tree of Knowledge, while medical opponents argued that, being natural, it should not be interfered with. Among these was the eminent American obstetrician Charles Meigs, who contended that women sustained by cheering counsel and 'carefully' freed from terror could endure this pain without much complaint. 'The sick need a physician', he declared, 'not they that are well'. In the event the practice received royal sanction in 1853 when Dr John Snow administered chloroform as an analgesic to Queen Victoria at the birth of her eighth child. Yet such analgesia was only available to the better-off. Indeed, it was not until the second half of the 20th century that artificial pain relief (though no longer chloroform, which proved dangerous) became general. However, as we shall see, some modern methods also attract criticism.

Return of the woman doctor

By the 1850s it seemed that eventually women would lose their time-honoured occupation of midwifery while remaining excluded from professionalized medicine. Answering demands from those who considered women the most appropriate attendants in childbirth and in the diseases of women and children, the medical weekly, *The Lancet*, countered that these were the very departments of medicine for which 'weak and tender women' were 'morally, psychologically and physically' least fitted. Furthermore, although it was unthinkable that men should be attended by female doctors, it was nonsense to suggest that women's modesty suffered if they had to consult men (Anon, 1874; 1877).

Nevertheless by 1877, after a long and bitter battle that formed part of a wider struggle for equal political and civil status with men, women won the right to qualify as medical practitioners. Woman doctors, driven out centuries before, and facing many obstacles in future years, were again available for women desiring female attendance.

The female doctor's medical opponents had alleged women's 'unfitness', not only for medicine, but also for midwifery. However, in 1892 when Parliament enquired into the midwife situation in England, the midwife's medical adversaries claimed that women doctors could provide female attendance on childbirth for all those desiring it. There was consequently no need for midwives, who could find employment as monthly nurses, carrying out those duties more appropriate for a 'mere woman'. This stance ignored the reality that midwives still attended probably over half the births throughout the country, while only a fifth of the 150 or so medical women on the Register (in any event unlikely to content themselves with the midwife's low fee) practised at home, the rest working in India. What was certain, however, was that the arrival of women qualified in midwifery *and* medicine meant that henceforward midwives, improved or not, would perforce occupy a position subordinate to the medical profession.

THE MIDWIVES' INSTITUTE, MIDWIFE REGISTRATION AND MATERNAL MORTALITY

Accepting this reality, in 1880 a tiny group of educated midwives, supported by a wealthy pioneer in women's employment, Louisa Hubbard, formed the Matrons' Aid Society, later to become the Midwives' Institute and ultimately the Royal College of Midwives (RCM). The Institute's avowed aim was the philanthropic one of improving the practice of midwives to benefit the poor women they attended, and, by implication, to reduce maternal mortality, to be achieved through a registration Act similar to other professional legislation. Also attainable through registration, the Institute hoped, was the eradication of the 'Gamp' (the term employed to disparage midwives lacking formal training), and the rehabilitation of midwifery as a respectable profession for educated women. Realizing that general practitioners might view registered midwives as competitors, the Institute stressed that these would attend only women too poor to pay doctors' fees and would not encroach on medical ground by acting in abnormal labour.

Yet what proportion of annual maternal mortality (still around 5 per 1000 live births in England and Wales) could be laid at the midwife's door? Testifying in favour of registration to the 1892 Commons' Select Committee, the obstetrician JH Aveling implied that most of this was attributable to untrained midwives. However, since there was as yet no notification of births, nor any system of identifying the birth attendant, this could only be guesswork. Indeed, WC Grigg, Physician to Queen Charlotte's Hospital, concluded in 1891 that more cases of 'injury and disaster' resulted from imprudent use of forceps and turning by doctors than from the negligence and ignorance of midwives.

The Midwives Act 1902

But how was a Midwives Act to be obtained? Despite continued strengthening of Continental midwife legislation, Government at home, still heavily imbued with 'laissez-faire' ideology, declined to intervene. The Midwives' Institute therefore began seeking friendly medical and parliamentary support for the promotion of a Private Member's Bill, a difficult task when childbirth was a taboo subject in genteel society, and one not achieved until 1890. For 12 long years thereafter the Institute and its allies struggled against indifference and ridicule from an all-male parliament and, latterly, the bitter opposition of many general practitioners, the British Medical Association and the General Medical Council. Finally, in 1902, probably consequent on growing parliamentary concern about the falling birth rate and the nation's health, the first State registration measure for an all-female occupation became law,

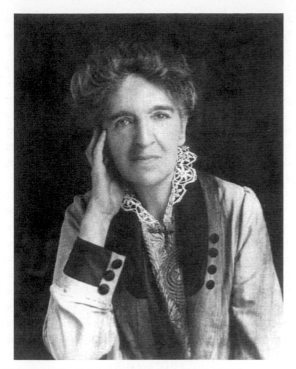

Figure 64.7   Dame Rosalind Paget (1855–1948). (Courtesy of the Royal College of Midwives.)

the fruit, as Miss Rosalind Paget (Fig. 64.7) for the Midwives' Institute pointed out, of that body's 20 years' unflagging dedication to the cause. Similar legislation for Scotland and Ireland (though there midwife pupils had first to be qualified nurses) followed respectively in 1915 and 1918.

However, the late arrival of secular regulation at home meant that by 1902 midwives' status had greatly deteriorated relative to their Continental counterparts, while that of their medical competitors, now part of a highly organized and increasingly respected profession, was much strengthened. It followed therefore that the Act (the result of a private, rather than a Government initiative) would establish the new registered midwife at a level unlikely to threaten the medical profession. Inevitably, this would be greatly inferior to that of midwives in leading Continental countries, where systematic regulation and instruction at a higher level had long since safeguarded the midwife's position.

The Central Midwives Board

The Act established a midwives' regulatory authority, the Central Midwives Board (CMB). Unlike other professional regulatory bodies, the Board, in recognition of the extreme poverty of many midwives, would be financed largely out of public funds, rather than by its registrants (an arrangement repeated with the 1919 Nurses Act). Moreover, midwives, unlike doctors and chemists, were not to be self-regulating. To keep their vital medical alliances intact, the Bill's promoters had conceded total medical membership of the Board, even the Institute's representative being a doctor. There was, at Privy Council insistence, to be a woman member, this being a symbolic break with tradition, not only on account of her sex, but also of her function, as a laywoman and a mother, of representing the user interests of childbearing women. Belatedly, however, midwives gained a spokeswoman when the Queen's Nursing Institute, which employed many rural midwives, was awarded representation, choosing Miss Paget as its member.

The justice of appointing midwife members as such was recognized in 1920, with, however, the proviso that they should never constitute a majority, and not until 1973 did a midwife become Chairman. Significantly, in 1928 the Privy Council's appointment of a member to represent childbearing women was discontinued, in favour of one of its medical officials, by the new Ministry of Health (1919), to which the Board's oversight (together with that of the new Nursing Council) had been transferred.

The Board had responsibility for keeping a 'Roll' of 'certified' midwives, determining conditions of entry, approving training and exercising discipline. Allowed on the Roll were over 22 000 existing practitioners, less than half of whom held certificates of formal training. Some, indeed, proved illiterate and had to seek help with record-keeping and reading a thermometer. Before taking the Board's examination, new entrants to the occupation were required to have 3 months' approved training (doubled to 6 months in 1916 for non-nurse-trained applicants, in 1926 to 1 year, and in 1938 to 2 years). However, despite the Act's ban on unregistered midwives after 1910, it was to be 30 years or so before these were stamped out.

The Board's rules limited midwives to attendance on natural labour (which included twin and breech deliveries), requiring them to send for a doctor in difficult cases, and forbade them to lay out the dead, traditionally a significant part of poorer midwives' work. Detailed directions also governed their daily practice, extending to their clothing, equipment and record-keeping. Breaches of the rules could be punished by erasure from the Roll, as could also 'misconduct' (undefined) in daily life, a penalty not applying in any male profession. The Act also provided for local supervision of midwives to be exercised by County Councils through the agency of (possibly hostile) Medical Officers of Health. Thus not only were midwives subjected to stricter control than obtained under other professional regulation but at both national and local level were placed under the governance of a rival profession.

'Certified Midwife'

Despite these restrictions on midwives' independence, the Act worked gradually to raise the occupation's status, consequently preventing the disappearance from this country (as virtually happened in North America) of this ancient female calling. Following the requirement of hospital training and examination for new entrants, however, came changes in the occupation's social composition. Gradually more younger, single women entered its ranks, while the poor local working-class women who had for centuries served their poorer neighbours were excluded by the cost of training, uniform, books and examination fees (Leap and Hunter, 1993: 44–47).

Other changes taking place in the organization of midwife services were equally fundamental. In 1910 few women gave birth in institutions, either in voluntary hospitals or Poor Law infirmaries. Of the rest, about half were attended by doctors, mainly general practitioners, the others by midwives. Some midwives worked in hospitals, some for out-door maternity charities, others for voluntary district nursing associations, but most practised privately. In the years preceding World War I, however, concern to breed a healthier race capable of defending home and Empire persuaded Government to subsidise midwifery care for the poor through local government, separately from services for paupers under the stigmatizing Poor Law. By the 1920s competition from such subsidized services and from expanding charitable hospital provision, together with the falling birth rate, meant that many midwives practising privately could hardly make a living.

As always, the midwife's life could be very arduous, especially in the country, where long distances would be travelled in all weathers, possibly over difficult terrain, by bicycle or on foot. Urban practice could also be taxing and one Portsmouth midwife recorded how she once went without sleep for 4 days while single-handedly conducting seven deliveries, one of a 12½lb baby, finally going home to sleep the clock round twice (Leap and Hunter, 1993: 50–56, 63–68). Fees were low (possibly 30s–£2, generally paid in instalments beforehand), and bad debts were common. Though in 1929 a few midwives with extensive practices were found to be earning over £275 annually, many working full time earned only £90–£100. Nursing association salaries in rural areas could be as low as £84 p.a., the life very lonely and the hours worked very long, some midwives delivering 90–100 women a year (Leap and Hunter, 1993: 50–56, 63–68).

Yet despite these hardships, midwives remembered with pride and pleasure the work that for many single women had been a vocation filling their whole lives. Some formed strong social ties with families, sending regular gifts to 'their' babies and being invited to family occasions. Nevertheless, they kept a certain distance, conscious of their professional status as certified midwives. This status was recognized by the public with its bestowal on them (whether officially due or not) of the 'respectable' title of 'Nurse', to distinguish them from the old untrained woman – still, significantly, referred to as 'the midwife' (Leap and Hunter, 1993: 8–9, 50–56, 63–68).

Domiciliary midwife practice, which included twin and breech births, appears to have followed guidelines laid down in contemporary obstetricians' textbooks. Midwives were allowed by the CMB to give mild analgesics, but many employed warm baths and back-rubbing to ease pain, and only in the 1940s did the self-operated Minnit inhalation analgesic apparatus become available in portable form for carriage on the midwife's bicycle. Ambulation in the first stage was encouraged but (left lateral) delivery in bed insisted on to allow manual protection of the perineum. Perineal tears, midwives considered, resulted largely from the attendant's impatience. As one retired midwife concluded, 'It's all patience in midwifery', while another, horrified at the 1970s hospital practice of routine episiotomy, stressed that the whole thrust of her midwifery training had been to protect the perineum, 'not to split it' (Leap and Hunter, 1993: 170–171).

Sometimes the medical help sent for in difficult cases was delayed and midwives might have to manage alone. In any case many GPs were inexperienced in midwifery, and midwives might have to apply the forceps for them. Midwife–doctor relations varied but, as in earlier centuries, some doctors sought to blame midwives for their own incompetence. After delivery, the mother was to lie flat for at least a day, remaining entirely in bed for 10–14 days, for fear of uterine prolapse (Leap and Hunter, 1993: 57–58, 164–171, 175–179). She was also kept on the low diet originally prescribed as a prophylactic against puerperal fever (long after this was known to result from bacterial infection) and which, as contemporary midwifery textbooks show, only began to change in the 1950s.

The continuing problem of maternal mortality

When the 1902 Act was passed, the maternal mortality rate had been expected to fall, as untrained midwives, known to be reluctant to send for medical help in difficult cases, were gradually replaced by trained women mindful of the CMB's requirement. Instead, the rate remained puzzlingly stable. Worse still, from 1928 it had shown a significant increase, rising to exceed 4 per 1000 live births in 1930. Indeed, analysis of the records of Queen's Institute midwives (all trained women) for the years 1905–1925 by JS Fairbairn, obstetrician Chairman of the CMB, produced interesting results. As expected, the proportion of midwives' cases to which GPs were called had risen; yet the maternal death rate, instead of falling, had climbed in step with this increase, suggesting a possible causal connection. Supporting evidence came from the 1930 Ministry enquiry, which found that many GPs lacked appropriate expertise in complicated cases. Many also neglected aseptic and antiseptic precautions, unsurprisingly when that same year at London's prestigious Queen Charlotte's Hospital, the director of its new puerperal fever research unit, Leonard Colebrook, discovered that staff did not customarily wear gloves or masks or even sterilize instruments (Loudon, 2000: 178).

By this time allegations of fatal overuse of instruments had followed male practitioners for two centuries. Yet *The Lancet* could still report that many GPs openly admitted routinely using instruments to save their time, maintaining they could not afford to do otherwise (Anon, 1929). Significantly, 'premature application of forceps' (the cervix being insufficiently dilated) was found to be a common cause of death (Munro Kerr, 1933: 51–52). Another factor in the high MMR, contended Eardley Holland, President of the recently formed British (later Royal) College of Obstetricians and Gynaecologists, was the increasing tendency among GPs to view childbirth as a pathological rather than a physiological process, interfering upon insufficient indications and without appreciating the risks involved (Holland, 1935). Significantly, Ministry enquiries showed that charitable and municipal outdoor midwife services for the poor (many of whom were in poor health and living in insanitary conditions) consistently returned a maternal death rate of half the national figure, and lower than rates in more affluent areas where medical attendance was the norm.

State midwifery

Parliament's response to continuing worries about high maternal mortality and the falling birth rate, was the 1936 Midwives Act which required County and County Borough Councils to provide for a whole-time midwife service for poor women, adequate to local needs and free or at reduced cost. Thenceforward, the great majority of midwives would be salaried, uniformed, pensioned professionals (Fig. 64.8), with time off and annual leave, offering a more complete service and receiving official acknowledgement of their contribution to national well-being. In recognition of the superfluity of midwives and the competition presented by the new subsidised service, many not selected for this were bought out of their practices and those considered unfit compulsorily retired. The Act passed without adverse comment from the medical press, probably as a result of the improvement in general practitioners' financial security largely consequent on

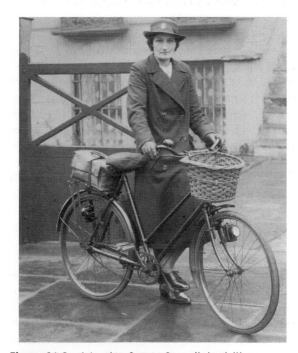

Figure 64.8 A London County Council domiciliary midwife prepares to go out on a call (London Metropolitan Archives, Corporation of London).

the 1911 National Insurance panel system. GPs were now content to leave 'cheap midwifery' to the midwife. But although municipal midwives were better off, broken nights followed by a full working day remained a feature of domiciliary practice.

Further official appreciation of the midwife's work was the honouring in 1935 of Rosalind Paget as a Dame of the British Empire. Moreover, in 1941 the Midwives Institute was elevated to a College, its Charter proclaiming its purpose as 'promoting the art and science of midwifery'. The prefix 'Royal' was granted in 1947, but unlike the medical Royal Colleges, the RCM (like the RCN) is not permitted to set qualifying examinations.

THE NATIONAL HEALTH SERVICE, MATERNITY CARE AND THE MIDWIFE

In 1948, under the free and comprehensive National Health Service (NHS) established by the 1945 Labour government as part of the new Welfare State, midwife, general practitioner and hospital services were provided free to all women, irrespective of income. A great expansion of professional education also took place and, at last, midwife training was free. Yet persistent prejudice was directed against non-nurse midwives. The upper-middle-class ladies who had led the Midwives' Institute to victory had come into midwifery from the already 'respectable' occupation of nursing, thus establishing an enduring ethos which labelled as 'second class' midwives lacking the sanitizing badge of 'nurse'. The Scottish and Irish registration Acts had required all midwife pupils to be qualified nurses, and in England nurse-qualified midwives tended to be preferred for hospital midwifery promotion despite possibly inferior midwifery experience (Radford and Thompson, unpublished work, 1988). Gradually English 'direct-entry' midwifery courses were officially discouraged until by 1980 only one such school remained. Yet many nurses qualifying in midwifery at the taxpayer's expense never practised it, whereas most direct-entry midwives stayed in the work.

Place of birth

By the 1950s the long-sought fall in maternal mortality had arrived. Sulphonamide drugs had appeared in 1936, followed a decade later by antibiotics. Together with stricter attention to asepsis and antisepsis in delivery and puerperium, these drugs had virtually eliminated puerperal sepsis, in 1930 still responsible for around 40% of maternal deaths. By 1945 the 1931–1935 figure of 4 deaths per 1000 live births had been halved, and by 1950 halved again. A crucial factor in this continued decline, however, as McKeown noted in relation to other health problems (McKeown, 1976), has been the generally improved standard of living, resulting, in particular, in a dramatic reduction in rachitic pelves and anaemia (Worth, 2002).

Despite these advances and the excellent results consistently achieved by domiciliary midwives, the trend to (more expensive) hospital delivery was officially encouraged, on obstetricians' advice, as being safer for mother and baby in *all* cases, a view subsequently challenged by independent statistical analysis (Tew, 1978). By 1958, 64% of births took place in hospital, many in general practitioner units (GPUs), smaller and more local than consultant-led units (CUs). With estimated maternal mortality rates (now more widely defined as deaths from causes attributed to pregnancy and childbirth per 1000 total live and still-births) as low as 0.18 per 1000 for 1968 for England and Wales and 0.14 per 1000 for 1969 in Scotland (Macfarlane *et al.*, 2000: II, Tables 1.3A 3.3.2, A 10.2.1), attention had turned increasingly to perinatal mortality. Defined as stillbirth and infant death within the first week, and standing at over 23 per 1000 births, this was higher in England and Wales than in comparable Continental countries. Significantly, also, it was higher in low-income groups (where maternal health was poorer) than among the better-off.

In 1970, the Health Department's Maternity Advisory Committee, chaired by Sir John Peel, President of the Royal College of Obstetricians and Gynaecologists (RCOG), presented its recommendations for remedial measures. These were based (unscientifically, in the absence of impartial statistical analysis) on the facile but erroneous equation between the falling perinatal mortality rate (PMR) and increasing hospitalization. Ignoring substantial general practitioner and midwife opinion to the contrary, the Committee recommended the transfer of home midwifery services to hospital control, effected in 1974 with their removal from elected local councils to the new unelected, hospital-dominated area health authorities. Hospital delivery was now over 80% and, expecting this soon to reach 100%, the Committee pronounced 'academic' any discussion of their scheme's advantages or disadvantages. The consultant-led 'obstetric team' (to include general practitioners and midwives) should therefore undertake the 'education' of the community on the 'benefits' of the reorganization.

Most obvious were the benefits to obstetricians' status and career prospects, with increased resources directed to CUs at the expense of home midwifery and GPUs. Equally clear were the drawbacks for midwives and mothers. Midwives who had successfully looked after women throughout pregnancy, labour and the puerperium, enjoying independence and variety in their duties, and receiving recognition and respect in their localities, were forced into the impersonal hospital ward to work under the direction of the obstetrician, or restricted to community postnatal care. Women's choice of place of delivery under the NHS was also disappearing. Many had preferred the familiarity of home, with the attention of a known midwife; others had chosen the local GPU, again with attendants known to them. Increasingly, however, they were to be compelled, possibly with children in tow, to make time-consuming visits to the large central district hospital for antenatal care, and to deliver in its stark, impersonal surroundings among strangers. In many areas women insisting on home birth or other non-interventionist care made private arrangements with a midwife or doctor at their own expense.

The 'New Obstetrics'

Perinatal mortality was considered further by the 1980 Commons' Social Services Committee (the Short Committee). Although hospital births now stood at 98%, and despite preferential allocation of medical resources to less favoured regions, the gap between perinatal mortality rates in the wealthier and the poorer classes had widened. While admitting that some procedures employed in intrapartum care had never been scientifically evaluated, the Committee nevertheless accepted its medical advisers' view that it was 'reasonable' to believe that 'professional' intervention could substantially lower the PMR. It therefore recommended a further increase in consultant obstetrician posts with even greater concentration of births in large CUs and further restriction of home birth. Furthermore, wholly accepting the view of childbirth as pathology, its report demanded its routine management on a par with acute illness, in conditions of 'intensive care'.

This was already the case in many CUs. Here older obstetricians' 'watchful expectancy' in normal birth had been superseded by the current North American doctrine of 'active management'. With the arrival in the late 1950s of Syntocinon, a synthetic version of oxytocin (the hormone governing uterine contractions) had come a more reliable means of inducing labour.

Hitherto induction had generally been employed only in instances of fetal post-maturity and maternal pre-eclampsia: thenceforth its use escalated, cases rising from 13% in 1958 to nearly 40% in 1974 (75% with particular consultants). Significantly, fewer births took place on weekends or Bank Holidays, indicating that many inductions were undertaken for the convenience of obstetricians. Syntocinon could also be used to accelerate labour already ongoing and to shorten it to conform to new restricted definitions of 'normality' derived from the averages of the new 'partogram' rather than the limits of healthy experience.

Yet neither of these procedures was wholly benign but led, observed critics, to a 'cascade of interventions', as obstetricians persuaded themselves that techniques helpful in abnormal labours would assuredly benefit *all* cases, and that no birth was normal except in retrospect. The syntocinon 'drip', together with electronic fetal monitoring (which carries a high false-positive rate and is associated with higher caesarean section rates) inhibited mobility, hitherto valued as facilitating labour. Contractions were more violent and more painful than in natural labour, with greater danger of uterine rupture. Enhanced pain required stronger pain relief, progressively supplied with new drugs and lumbar epidural analgesia. Since epidurals diminish uterine activity, tending to hinder the natural rotation and descent of the fetus and inhibiting the urge to push, they prolong labour, with the risk also of maternal circulatory collapse. More malpresentations and forceps deliveries resulted, with attendant risk to the child, and the discomfort of episiotomy, with possible lasting adverse sequelae, for the mother (Wagner, 2002). Persistent headache and backache are also associated with its use, and if the procedure is mismanaged, permanent paralysis, coma or even death can ensue (May, 1994, Ch. 9). Episiotomy was now used routinely, mistakenly justified as preventing serious perineal tears and pelvic floor damage, and by 1980 employed in 52% of deliveries in England and Wales (Tew, 1995: 165). Dorsal delivery (the legs possibly raised in stirrups), replaced left lateral delivery, becoming the standard delivery position. Though it was known to be more painful for the woman and problematic for the fetus, it was praised in a leading midwives' manual as more 'comfortable', and as facilitating pushing (Myles, 1981: 309). Recently condemned by leading authorities (Steer and Flint, 1999), it has still not completely disappeared, and many believe that the now popular semi-recumbent position is only marginally better.

Moreover, as 'failure to progress' (defined by the strict timetables routinely governing labour), increasingly resulted in caesarean section (CS), rates for this major operation rose rapidly. This fact alone led to further intervention – the prohibition or restriction of nutrition to *every* parturient to fit her for general anaesthesia in case a caesarean section should be performed. Clearly such debilitating deprivation at a time when women needed all their physical and mental strength – a deprivation still imposed in many UK hospitals (Speak, 2002) – was itself likely to contribute to 'failure to progress'. The growing use of analgesic drugs, too, had consequences for the baby. These pass across the placenta and have a depressing effect on the fetus, which may result in protracted difficulties in breathing and suckling, necessitating time in the (expensive) special care baby unit.

Responses of the midwifery profession

Although the Peel and Short Committees had both recommended that full use should be made of midwives' expertise, their recommendations pointed in the opposite direction. The disappearance of home midwifery and increased medicalization of hospital birth meant that midwives, officially excluded by the 1902 Act from attending abnormal labour, were now losing their role as guardians of normal birth. Midwifery skills were devalued in favour of interventionist methods, which midwives themselves, many unwillingly, and against their professional judgement, were required to adopt (Reid, 2002). Moreover, experienced midwives were increasingly required to defer to senior house officers (SHOs) who, despite their designation, were merely junior doctors doing their 6 months' obstetric training. Further, hospital midwives' work was increasingly compartmentalized into antenatal, intrapartum or postnatal care, some midwives seldom delivering a baby and practically none following a pregnancy through to delivery. Only the few midwives allowed to undertake home delivery, and those operating a 'DOMINO' system (where the midwife supervises the pregnancy, accompanies the labouring woman to hospital, conducts the labour, and brings her home a few hours afterwards), could be said to be acting as midwives proper within the NHS.

For domiciliary midwives whose long years of low pay and broken nights had nonetheless given them the immense satisfaction of delivering women successfully in their own homes, the condemnation of home midwifery, despite excellent safety records, as 'unsafe' was

tantamount to the negation of their life's work. For many the experience was traumatic and retirement could not come too soon (Allison, 1996: ix–x). Others tolerated the transfer to hospital as bringing shorter, more convenient hours, less responsibility and improved career opportunities. Nor did the RCM seriously oppose this transformation of the midwife's work. Overcome by the confidence with which obstetricians, generally male, and of higher social status, put their case to government, the College merely acquiesced as the ancient office of midwife was increasingly eroded, and its own avowed purpose, 'the advancement of the art and science of midwifery', effectively abandoned. Signalling its acceptance of the total hospitalization of birth, in 1974 it abolished its longstanding Domiciliary Midwives Council. Some leading midwives expressed regret at these changes; others espoused them wholeheartedly, seeing reliance on technology as increasing midwives' status, rather than, in fact, reducing it. Here was no sympathy for midwives seeking to undertake home delivery; and women desiring this, or intervention-free hospital care, were constrained into acceptance of what was now NHS policy.

Especially striking was the turnabout demonstrated in the 1975, 1981 and 1987 editions of Margaret Myles' *Textbook for Midwives*, a standard work used in many midwifery schools since 1953. Hitherto Myles, herself a midwife, had spoken of home as the 'ideal' place of delivery, affirming Nature's power in the vast majority of cases to complete childbirth successfully unaided, and warning against the dangers of 'meddlesome midwifery'. Yet these later editions dismissed the older philosophy of 'watchful expectancy' in labour as 'negative', applauding instead the 'modern concept' of 'active management', with its 'planned positive approach'. The management of 'normal' labour now included routine interventions, justified as ensuring greater maternal and fetal safety, while psychophysical methods of pain management were dismissed in favour of drugs. Midwives must accept 'modern ideas', working to secure the compliance of the 'misinformed' minority of expectant mothers who demanded intervention-free birth and 'outmoded' continuity of carer. Hospital delivery was strongly advocated: indeed, for a midwife to take sole charge of a woman, depriving her of the 'scientific expert care' of the 'obstetric team', would be a retrograde step. Midwives should relish their new, more fulfilling role as technically qualified members of the medically controlled 'team' (as 'mini-obstetricians' is implied) rather than seeing themselves as clinically independent practitioners as sanctioned by the Midwives Acts.

Not all midwives approved of these developments. Some left the NHS in order to practise privately as independent practitioners, offering home delivery and choice of birth positions. Others, however, decided to fight the trend from within the NHS. In 1976 a group of student midwives formed the Association of Radical Midwives (ARM), which aimed to challenge what it saw as the RCM's connivance at the destruction of the midwife. The use of the word 'radical' signified members' desire to return to the 'roots' of midwifery, namely, attendance on normal, physiological birth, rather than practise as maternity nurses in interventionist obstetrics. Over the years ARM was to grow in strength, its members gaining positions of responsibility in practice, in education and in the College.

User protest and the 'Active Childbirth' Movement

Protests came, too, from among childbearing women themselves, their complaints supported by healthcare user organizations forming part of the post-war consumer movement. Among these were the National Childbirth Trust (NCT) and the increasingly assertive Association for Improvements in the Maternity Services (AIMS). AIMS demanded more sympathetic maternity care, including choice of home birth, of intervention-free care and of birthing positions, ideas generally dismissed in medical circles as fads of a misguided middle-class minority. Such women, wrote one obstetrician, were too ignorant or selfish to accept their role as 'patients', even for their infants' safety. Clearly viewing the womb as a railway engine, he censured complainants for 'dictating their treatment', thus relegating professionals *from the signal-box to the footplate*, presumably from their imagined rightful position of routinely controlling labour to one of merely observing it. Moreover, despite radiological evidence that squatting enlarged the pelvic outlet by almost 30% compared with the generally used supine position (Russell, 1982), upright delivery was condemned as too 'primitive' (outdated) or too 'innovative' (untested). Furthermore, the 'bizarre' positions 'professionals' would have to adopt would adversely affect their 'sense of security' in their work.

Evidence was mounting, however, that women's objections to the 'new obstetrics' were more widespread than had been supposed. In 1982, 5000 women demonstrated outside London's Royal Free Hospital, demanding choice of birthing positions, and a BBC survey of 6000 women showed that most were dissatisfied with restrictions imposed by hospital obstetricians. Public interest was further aroused by the BBC TV programme featuring the clinic of the French obstetrician Michel Odent, and showing women giving birth upright or in water. For Odent, birth is an *involuntary* process, which can be hindered by *any* interference, however well-intentioned. Women should therefore be encouraged to relax so that the body can do its work, which in all but a few cases it will complete successfully. Formidable scientific evidence supporting Odent's views came from the research of Mendez-Bauer, which demonstrated the positive effects of upright posture on uterine contractions. Likewise, that of the eminent obstetric physiologist Caldeyro-Barcia indicated similar benefits to the fetal oxygen supply, known to be compromised by the supine position. Significantly, women in both these comprehensive studies reported much less pain when remaining upright. A convert to active birth in normal labour, Caldeyro-Barcia concluded that the supine position was the worst for parturition 'short of being hanged by the feet', and that 'Nature will provide if we do not interfere' (Inch, 1982: 49–51).

Indicative of the impact of consumer protest on hospital practice during the 1980s were certain concessions, some of which, like cheerfully decorated 'birth rooms', were largely palliative in nature. Some centres installed birth chairs and birthing pools, but their use was not always actively encouraged. Compromises were made on labour positions, though generally only as far as a semi-recumbent posture in bed, which, though conferring some benefit from gravity, still restricts maximum opening of the pelvic outlet (Gardosi *et al.*, 1989). Rates for induction, forceps delivery and episiotomy declined markedly, though not enough to challenge the ruling concept of medicalized management. Moreover, statistics for amniotomy and labour augmentation were not collected, while rates for the ultimate intervention, caesarean section, rose steadily, reaching a 14% average by 1993 (Tew, 1995: 187–188).

NURSES, MIDWIVES AND HEALTH VISITORS ACT 1979

Meanwhile midwives faced other problems following the implementation in 1983 of the government-sponsored Nurses, Midwives and Health Visitors Act

1979. This replaced the different regulatory machinery for these three professions in England, Scotland and Northern Ireland with one umbrella organization, the United Kingdom Central Council (UKCC). Following representations to Government by a re-invigorated RCM, the midwife's distinctive nature was recognized with the establishment of a statutory Standing Midwifery Committee to consider 'matters relating to midwifery'. However, since the Committee was subordinate to the nurse-dominated UKCC, midwives were no more a self-regulating profession than under the CMB.

Nurses' lack of empathy for midwifery matters was especially manifest in *Project 2000*, the UKCC's 1986 proposal for combining the basic education of the three professions in one 18-month nursing programme followed by another 18 months specialization, with midwifery as one of the specialities. Midwifery education for students taking such courses would thus be reduced by 18 months, although 18-month courses for qualified nurses would remain. Opposing strongly, the RCM argued that midwives' clinical responsibilities clearly distinguished them from nurses, and that to cut midwife education would demote midwifery to a branch of nursing (RCM, 1986). Moreover, the proposal contravened the 1980 European Community requirements for UK midwives wishing to practise in EC countries, where midwives, as in former times, had longer midwifery training and generally were not nurses. Faced with this reality, the Council yielded. An interesting turnabout then took place. Direct entry midwifery courses, instead of being phased out, were to be extended to 3 years, thus reversing a century-old trend towards the elimination of the midwife pure and simple, and preventing official downgrading of midwifery to obstetric nursing. (More recently, such courses have been instituted in Scotland.) However, the struggle to defend midwifery education from nursing control in the higher education institutions, where nursing and midwifery are now jointly placed, continues.

Finding a new voice

A further sign of a more vigorous, enterprising outlook among midwives was the 1989 edition of Myles' *Textbook for Midwives*, now under new authorship and with an approach contrasting sharply with the celebration of authoritarian interventionist obstetrics characteristic of the previous three editions. In a new departure for midwifery manuals, it emphasized the midwife's duty to accommodate, where feasible, women's choice of labour and delivery positions, forms

of pain relief and so on. Midwives should also strive to make this normal but critical life event as happy as possible for mother, partner and family. Another 'first' was the referencing of the text, along with suggestions for further reading, indications of a new vision among midwife educators, who now held up the ideal of the midwife as a lifelong learner in a 'research-based' profession. Significantly, similar emphases characterized the corresponding edition of *Mayes' Midwifery*, the other standard textbook in the field. Further noteworthy professional developments originating in the ranks were the foundation in 1986 of MIDIRS, a midwife-run quarterly critical digest of recent literature and research in maternity care. This, together with the arrival in 1993 of the *British Journal of Midwifery*, soon followed by other midwife-led publications, was to present a serious challenge to the staid *Midwives Chronicle*, official journal of the RCM, ultimately for-cing it also to adopt a more proactive stance.

'Choice in Childbirth'

In 1991, on the initiative of Audrey Wise MP, maternity services were again studied by MPs, this time by the House of Commons' Health Committee (the 'Winterton Committee'), which reported the following year. Unlike its predecessors, the Committee started not from the negative standpoint of childbirth as an inevitably hazardous event needing medical management, but saw it as a normal physiological function that healthy women could generally perform successfully without intervention. For the first time, too, midwives were included among the advisers, and submissions, written and oral, invited from service users as well as providers.

Again unlike previous committees, Winterton placed more credence on impartial statistical analyses than on the unproven assertions of obstetricians, concluding that without compelling evidence a medical model was inappropriate for the care of low-risk women. Taking maternal satisfaction with maternity services as its criterion of success, the Committee argued that no one professional group had a greater claim to control over maternity care than any other, such control belonging properly to mothers and mothers-to-be (House of Commons Health Committee, 1992: 1, xii). Moreover, since evidence on safety did not support the policy of 100% CU delivery, wider choice of place of birth should be made available (ibid: xlviii). GPUs, whether rural or urban, offered a compromise between home birth and delivery in a CU, and their closure on presumptive grounds of safety or cost should be abandoned forthwith (ibid: lxvii).

The Committee also condemned the failure of the medical and midwifery professions, in their concentration on perinatal mortality as the sole yardstick of performance, to audit their care in terms of maternal morbidity. Like other medical specialities, obstetrics had been subject to fashion, procedures being introduced merely because they were available, and used routinely without consideration of possible adverse maternal consequences (ibid: xlviii–xlix). Women should therefore be given the option of refusing interventions such as induction, electronic fetal monitoring, epidurals and episiotomies rather than having to undergo them as routine (ibid: xxiii). Furthermore, hospital delivery units should as far as practicable reproduce home conditions, with privacy, a relaxing atmosphere, refreshments, and continuity of carer by a known midwife. Women would thus be enabled to feel in control of their labours and to adopt positions of choice (ibid: lxix). The Committee summed up its philosophy under the heads, '*Choice, Continuity and Control*'.

Essential to the development of more user-friendly maternity services, the Committee concluded, was a reassessment of the midwife's role. Condemning current use of midwives as '*a scandalous waste of money*' (ibid: lxxxi), it recommended what was in fact a restoration of former responsibilities. In CUs, midwives should have principal charge over normal labour, no longer being subject to SHOs, who should have trainee status only. They should have their own caseloads, taking full responsibility for the women in their care, their professional status recognized in their terms and conditions of employment. Antenatal care should be community based and midwife managed, with ready access to specialist assessment, midwives themselves referring as necessary to appropriate specialists (ibid: xlv). Further, to allow more women the choice of non-medicalized care, the Health Department should pursue the development of midwife-managed units, near enough to CUs for transfer should this be required (ibid: lxviii–lxix, lxxii). Finally, since midwives working independently but in close cooperation with their medical colleagues provided the best route to excellence in maternity care, they should be granted the same rights over all aspects of their education as were enjoyed by all other professions in the NHS or elsewhere (ibid: lxxxvi).

The Government's response, *Changing Childbirth* (DoH, 1993), accepted Winterton's philosophy of 'woman-centred' care, suggesting 5-year targets towards the implementation of its recommendations. However, this document was merely consultative and lacked the teeth necessary to enforce any widespread change. Women seeking home birth still reported GPs threatening to strike them off their NHS lists, while many health authorities refused on the ground of midwife shortages. Where they existed, midwife-run units, despite their recorded low intervention rates and increased maternal satisfaction, remained on sufferance, health authorities resenting the expense of maintaining these 'experiments' in addition to their ordinary hospital establishments. Yet, argue reformers, if these centres became general, with midwives (with appropriate medical back-up) attending women with normal pregnancies (the vast majority), obstetricians would be freed to concentrate on abnormal cases, the ensuing reduction in highly paid CU staff and expensive technology bringing overall savings to the taxpayer.

Whose choice in childbirth?

Responding to *Changing Childbirth*, the RCOG qualified its acceptance of the ideal of 'woman-oriented care', invoking considerations of 'safety', a veiled justification of current practice. It also argued, significantly, for 'equal attention' to be paid to the welfare of the fetus, 'the other important person' in the case (RCOG, 1993). For centuries, however, English law had not recognized the unborn child as a 'person' (the principle underlying current abortion law). Yet in 1992, displaying to an extreme degree the paternalism condemned by Winterton, obstetricians from a London hospital obtained a court order for a forced caesarean on a mother refusing her consent on religious grounds. Similar orders followed, all granted without maternal representation in court, until in May 1998 the Appeal Court ruled illegal the forcible invasion of a competent adult's body, even if a woman's life *or* that of her fetus depended on it. The fetus was *not* a separate person from its mother and its medical needs could not override her rights to self-determination. Notwithstanding this definitive judgement, many obstetricians persist in a curious doublethink. This allows them, while accepting abortion of the (non-person) fetus (up to term in the case of handicap), illogically and incorrectly to endow it with full person status, by implication on a par with the mother, by describing it as a 'patient' (RSM, 2002).

Apart from the Appeal Court's clear-cut confirmation of the parturient's legal autonomy, how has user choice fared in general? In a recent study undertaken to assess the effectiveness in promoting choice of the widely used evidence-based MIDIRS *Informed Choice* leaflets (dealing with home birth, labour and delivery positions, etc.) researchers found that in some units, choice was not on the agenda. The leaflets might not be distributed at all, either because of time constraints or professional disapproval of the content. Where they *were* distributed, generally midwives did not offer to discuss them, and such was women's trust in, and deference to health professionals, that they rarely asked questions or requested alternatives to what was being offered. Indeed, some of the choices mentioned in the leaflets were unavailable in the unit. However, interventions such as ultrasound scanning and electronic fetal monitoring, driven by fear of suits for damages relating to intrapartum injury to the infant, had become so routine that some health professionals did not even perceive them as optional. In effect, women were steered towards acceptance of technological intervention through information-giving which minimized its risks and exaggerated the potential harm of doing without. Based on deficient information, women's 'choice' was illusory rather than real, being in fact merely *compliance* with the unit's obstetrician-determined regimen (Stapleton *et al.*, 2002).

Childbirth 'A Surgical Operation'?

However, obstetricians may accede to user choice when this fits with the medical model of childbirth. Indeed, the 2001 Government-sponsored National Sentinel CS Audit showed that nearly 75% of obstetricians responding to the enquiry were willing to grant requests for CS from 25-year-olds with no medical indications for intervention. Critics of this practice argue that increasing numbers of women, frightened by previous bad experiences and by medical overemphasis on complications in childbirth, see CS as a safe and relatively painless, stress-free procedure. Yet it is a major invasive operation, with increased maternal mortality and morbidity, and with potential complications in future births which may terminate in emergency hysterectomy (Gould *et al.*, 1999; Langdana *et al.*, 2001). It is therefore questionable how many women, if given all the facts, would freely choose this procedure. Observers also contrast medical compliance with women's requests for CS, which can be scheduled to suit obstetricians' convenience, with the resistance frequently encountered by women wanting intervention-free birth, which cannot (Robinson, 1999). Another powerful factor in the increasing caesarean section rate (CSR) may be obstetricians' fear of litigation,

damages in childbirth cases now comprising almost two-thirds of NHS compensation payments (RCOG and RCM, 1999).

It was therefore no surprise when the 2001 report of the Scottish Expert Advisory Group on CS found that Scotland's rate approached 20%, while the National Sentinel Audit revealed even higher rates in England, Wales and Northern Ireland. Remarkable variations existed between regions and between hospitals, inexplicable by reference to case-mix, as were variations in CS percentages ascribed to different primary indications. Disturbingly, while half the obstetricians responding to the enquiry considered current rates too high, 21% did not. Furthermore, in private hospitals, where obstetricians are paid not by salary, as in the NHS, but by item-of-service, receiving more for performing this invasive procedure than for the oversight of vaginal delivery, the caesarean section rate (CSR) averages around 50% (BBC, 2002). Yet the World Health Organization's 1985 Consensus Conference had concluded that no improvement in outcomes could be expected from a CSR exceeding 10–15%, a rate maintained by the Scandinavian countries. Moreover, together with Holland, which has about 30% home births and a CSR of just over 11% (CBS, 1999), these countries have some of the world's lowest maternal and perinatal mortality rates (Wagner, 2000).

Given, then, the Hippocratic injunction to all doctors, '*First (and foremost), do no harm*', it is to be hoped that the RCOG will actively discourage the performance, in the absence of well-defined, evidence-based medical indications, of this fashionable but problematic and costly operation. Furthermore, since every attempt to show a positive correlation between increasing CSRs and lower perinatal mortality rates has failed (Wagner, 2002), and every 1% increase in CS costs the NHS £5 million a year (NCT *et al.*, 1999: 9), it is remarkable that successive governments, always anxious for best value for taxpayers' money, have not enquired into this phenomenon earlier. Indeed, private healthcare insurers are also concerned about the rising CSR in private hospitals, this averaging around 2½ times the NHS figure, and the operation, even without complications, costing around £7000. Significantly, one major insurer is now refusing to finance caesareans, the company finding it 'increasingly difficult' to distinguish between those performed out of medical necessity and those determined by patient 'personal or life-style choice' (BBC, 2002; Brown, 2002).

A pressing question now presents itself. Women are healthier and taller than ever before, and estimated maternal mortality from direct causes has fallen to around 5 per 100 000 registrable live births and still-births (Lewis, 2001: Table 1.1). Why then has intervention in childbirth increased to the point where, in Anthony Carlisle's prescient words of 1827, this natural function has increasingly become a 'surgical operation'? One factor may be the nature of medical education, which in general is oriented to the study of the body as a structure, and to the 'mechanisms' of disease, rather than to their underlying causes. This has resulted in failure critically to assess the effectiveness of medical intervention, the beneficence of which tends to be over-estimated, while patients' needs additional to, but possibly more important than, medical ministrations are ignored (McKeown, 1976: 127–128, 158–159).

Nowhere has this approach been more evident than in obstetrics, where training has long been gynaecology oriented and directed to the abnormal. It may therefore be difficult for obstetricians to accept incontrovertible evidence that old-fashioned 'watchful expectancy', with appropriate emotional support, can in most cases produce better results than modern interventionist management (Tew, 1995: 297–298; Wagner, 2001). Yet such is the addiction to technology that, as the experience of the Viennese obstetrician Rockenschaub demonstrates, it can be practically impossible for reputable accounts of highly successful 'low-tech' maternity care to find publication in medical journals, which, indeed, dismiss such results as 'unbelievable' (Beech, 1996). Worse still, when the adverse consequences of any one intervention necessitate more drastic procedures, the reaction may be not to reassess the need for the first intervention, but to demand more resources be devoted to the second. Thus obstetricians at a London hospital, recently finding that CS was the most significant risk factor in the need for emergency hysterectomy in the hospital, recommended, not a reduction in the caesarean sections that had rendered this catastrophic mutilation necessary, but further obstetrician training in major pelvic surgery (Gould et al., 1999). The problem of perinatal mortality is equally interesting in this connection. Although a high PMR is clearly associated with social deprivation, and in particular with poor maternal health, obstetricians consistently demand more resources for interventionist technology, rather than material aid for poor mothers to help *prevent* its underlying causes.

WHAT IS 'NORMAL' BIRTH?

Another puzzle facing researchers into maternity care is the current use of the term 'normal' concerning childbirth. In the early 1950s, as before, 'normal' birth meant a birth in which no instruments were used and no special measures taken. Generally such births, except for initial doses of castor oil and the requirement of delivery in bed, would be intervention-free. However, since 'active management' brought intervention in the absence of medical indications, inducing and shortening labours in conformity with the arithmetical averages of the Procrustean partogram, no clear dividing line has existed. Consequently today's doctors and midwives may never have seen a completely intervention-free birth, and along with childbearing women themselves, may not believe it possible.

Indeed, a recent study in the Trent region discovered that in over 60% of the 956 deliveries recorded as 'normal' or 'spontaneous' (i.e. excluding instrumental or CS deliveries), interventions had occurred. These included amniotomy, induction, augmentation of labour, episiotomy and epidural anaesthesia. In about a third, induction or augmentation of labour had taken place, while 89% of amniotomies were performed before the cervix was fully dilated (Downe et al., 2001). In reality, rather than having a spontaneous labour and delivery, which in the vast majority of cases (i.e. *normally*), Nature has equipped healthy women for, these women have been subjected to what is now 'usual' or 'normal' *obstetric practice*. Complaints to user organizations from women traumatized by such 'normal' birth suggest that in future they may seek CS, seeing this as a lesser evil (ibid). Confusion on what constitutes 'normal' birth is worse confounded by the recent pronouncement from two leading obstetricians that only *two-thirds* of births are 'normal' (Chamberlain and Steer, 1999). This is not only a contradiction in terms, but also a wilful misuse of English, since in no other field do we admit a definition of 'normality' which designates *one-third* of any group as deviant. Clearly, this definition of 'normal' does not imply, as in the past, intervention-free birth, but birth with *less intervention*, compared to 'abnormal' birth (where instruments or CS are employed), with *more intervention*. Obviously, official statistics based on such bogus definitions are worthless.

Can we measure 'risk'?

Accompanying this redefinition of normality is the now ubiquitous concept of 'risk'. That certain risks exist in pregnancy and childbirth has always been known. The most serious are generally readily recognizable by expert clinicians; however, to assess *every* risk for *every* parturient, given individual differences in health and physique, and to use such assessment as a basis for 'prophylactic' intervention, is indeed a tall order. Antenatal screening tests are known to be far from infallible, while electronic fetal monitoring, in common use in labour, has a high false-positive rate. Moreover, difficulties in 'risk factor' definition and quantification render risk-scoring 'systems' highly suspect, and their predictive values, positive and negative, have proved poor (Enkin *et al.*, 2000: 49–51; Tew, 1995: 110–111, 256–268, 330–338). Yet the risk 'bogey' is increasingly paraded to secure women's compliance with interventions which may be unnecessary and which bring their own hazards.

Furthermore, as the 1997 Audit Commission noted, definitions of commonly used indications for intervention, such as 'failure to progress' and 'fetal distress', lack consistency, and thresholds used in the making of such diagnoses vary. Further, the incidence of these 'prophylactic' interventions differs from unit to unit (Audit Commission, 1997). Clearly many of these procedures are driven by considerations other than women's objective need, with immediate professional convenience and 'defensive obstetrics' probably both playing a part. Moreover, labelling women 'at risk' or intervening 'just in case' can engender a disabling anxiety. The resulting adrenaline secretions inhibit the flow of oxytocin and endorphins and contract the circular muscle fibres of the womb, thus hindering labour and producing the very problems it was intended to avoid (Clement, 2001; Enkin *et al.*, 2000: 51–52; Tew, 1995: 337–338). This power of the mind over the body in childbirth has long been recognized. Nearly 200 years ago, Soranus of Ephesus warned against creating anxiety in the parturient (Temkin, 1956: 73–74), advice repeated down the centuries. 'Fear and want of confidence', wrote Dr John Clarke in 1793, 'will disturb and retard, just as confidence and hope will facilitate, labour' (Clarke, 1793: 15–16). The lesson is clear. While remaining aware of the *possibility* of adverse developments, birth attendants should follow the positive advice of the *Byrth of Mankynde*, making it their first care to strengthen women's faith in their bodies' natural power to give birth, rather than, through words, demeanour or actions, to undermine it.

REGULATION, RECRUITMENT AND RETENTION

So what is now the midwife's statutory position, a century after the first Act to regulate the occupation in modern times? On the new regulatory body instituted under the 1999 Health Act, the Nursing and Midwifery Council (NMC), nurses still predominate, with eight places to the midwives' four. However, they are not, as under the UKCC, in the majority, there now being eleven lay members, evidence of the Government resolve to enhance representation of the public interest in professional regulation. Midwives have also retained their Statutory Midwives Committee for the consideration of midwifery matters', a re-endorsement of their legal status as clinical practitioners in their own right, distinct from nursing. An important change is the location of the nurses' and midwives' regulatory body under the supervision of the Privy Council, rather than as before under the Department of Health (DoH), whose interests as the main employer might conflict with the necessary impartial oversight of registrants' rights. The change also puts the regulation of these two predominantly female professions on a par with other State-regulated occupations.

Interestingly, also, in the light of the UKCC's 1986 *Project 2000* proposal to amalgamate midwifery and nurse education, 3-year 'direct-entry' midwifery students in England now outnumber nurses taking 18-month post-registration courses. Direct-entry numbers in Scotland are rising and courses are planned in Northern Ireland. Problems of recruitment and retention remain, stemming partly from low pay, low status, poor career structure and family responsibilities. Recently the remuneration issue has been partly addressed in England by the Health Department's agreement that qualified midwives, by virtue of their clinical responsibilities, should commence practice on the second rung of the pay scale, rather than, as nurses do, on the first. The Government is also expanding training, encouraging family-friendly employment practices and extending the clinical career structure by creating consultant midwife posts. Such posts (also planned in Scotland) are intended to provide promotion for expert midwives in the practice field (Cooper, 2000), as happens in medicine, rather than, as heretofore, mainly in administration. These posts, supposedly on a level with medical consultant posts, are linked to academic institutions, and it is hoped that postholders will foster research initiatives and provide clinical leadership in the promotion of midwifery skills and of childbirth as a normal physiological event. Though there are some hopeful signs from this venture, there is a danger that some appointees may be diverted into public health roles; in any case, unless their numbers are substantially increased, consultant midwives will not be strong enough to withstand, let alone influence, today's medical regime (Barber, 2002).

The most important cause of midwives' dissatisfaction, however, appears to be the disparity between new midwives' expectations of their role, derived from their professional education, and the much more limited one they experience in practice, especially in the larger CUs (Ball *et al.*, 2002). It is here that shortages are most acute, especially in the London, Southeast and Eastern regions. These have the highest rate of heavy midwife workloads, the lowest rates of one-to-one care of labouring women and of midwife deliveries, and, correspondingly, the highest rate of units with high CSRs (ENB, 2001; Lee, 2001). Rising CSRs, midwife critics conclude, stem from there being too few midwives but too many obstetricians (NCT *et al.*, 1999: 9). An increase in midwife-led units, perceived as a way of attracting more midwives and of increasing user choice, has been promised by the Government (Cooper, 2000), and is envisaged elsewhere in the UK. Many such units however, have been lost in repeated organizational amalgamations.

New skills – new opportunities?

In line with the Audit Commission's call for more cost-effective care, the English Health Department's 1999 paper, *Making a Difference*, declared its intention of making better use of midwives and nurses. Yet 11 years after the Winterton Report drew attention to the matter, the ENB's 2001 *Audit of Midwifery Practice* confirmed that midwives' skills were still being wasted. Whereas 20 years ago the midwife was the senior person present at over 75% of births, now only 36% of maternity units had midwife delivery rates of over 70%, while some (generally, larger units) had midwife deliveries of only 52%, a concomitant of higher intervention rates and especially of the rising CSR. However, home-births have increased to around 2% in England, being higher in the south (ENB, 2001), but remaining under 1% in Scotland and Northern Ireland.

One consequence of this DoH initiative is the 'training up' of midwives to perform tasks lately confined to doctors. Midwives may now qualify to undertake the examination of the newborn; and also to deliver breech births (ENB, 2001) as they did before the post-war medical takeover. A further new feature on the ward is the scheduled reduction of SHOs to trainee status only, as Winterton recommended. Hitherto SHOs, despite being only trainees on a 6-month 'rotation' in obstetrics, which they might never practise again, had taken precedence in decision-making over experienced

midwives, and had also undertaken instrumental deliveries. Now midwives themselves may qualify to perform forceps or ventouse deliveries, and also ultrasonography. While all these cost-saving changes are to be welcomed, fears are expressed that midwives performing instrumental delivery may adopt the current medical ethos, perceiving such intervention as conferring higher status than do midwifery skills proper.

There are concerns too, about DoH plans for a wider public health role for midwives. Although the use of maternity care assistants is planned, midwife critics point not only to the midwife shortage, but also to the need to re-establish midwives as the custodians of normal physiological birth. Efforts in this direction, they fear, will be nullified if the midwife's role becomes diluted and diffused. Another challenge is the downward shift in the balance of financial power to the primary care trusts as part of the Government's policy of devolution in resource control to local areas. The question now arises as to whether this development will give midwives more, or less, influence over the organization of maternity services and the nature of their work. At the same time, will the proposed increase in user involvement in decision-making finally produce *real* choice for childbearing women?

WHAT OF THE FUTURE?

Attendance on childbirth in the UK, as in the rest of the western world, has changed in many ways since the appearance 460 years ago of the *Byrth of Mankynde*. It is no longer, as it was once, a solely female domain. In the institutions where most midwives now work, they do so under restrictions laid down by (mostly male) obstetricians. Midwives now include not only women who have not borne children, but also, since the implementation of the 1975 Sex Discrimination Act, a small number of men. Fathers, too, are no longer excluded from the birth, but encouraged to be present to support their partners. A tiny (though now growing) minority of midwives still attend women at home, some working for the NHS, some independently, keeping alive the concept of childbirth as a normal domestic event (Fig. 64.9). Demonstrating the power of Nature, also, are those who now, as in Willughby's day, deliver alone, concealing their infants' birth from family, friends and State authorities.

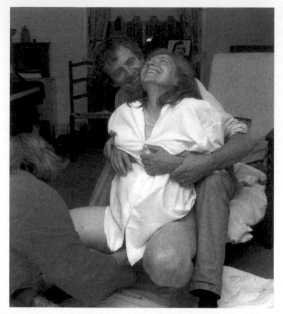

Figure 64.9 A modern homebirth (Sally and Richard Greenhill Photo Library).

More confident than their post-war predecessors, midwives' leaders today argue for a return to a physiological model of birth, whether in hospital or at home, a theme recently re-emphasized by the RCM (Davis, 2002; Downe, 2001). These midwives, along with their 17th century foremother Jane Sharp, do not deny 'due honour to able Physicians and Chyrurgions, when occasion is' (Sharp, 1671: 3). However, they wish to free women from the industrialized medical production line which is the current CU, where childbearing women are, in effect, treated as baby-making machines to be manipulated and speeded up at the operator's behest, and where midwives are prevented from practising the 'gentle art' of true midwifery. In this culture of childbirth-as-pathology, they maintain, scant regard is paid to the potential adverse physical and psychological sequelae to the *mother*, whose general welfare is too often considered of secondary importance to the smooth running of the system. Repudiating this pathogenic ethos, with its frequently iatrogenic procedures, these critics urge a concentration, not on 'risk factors', but on 'health factors'. In the resultant climate of what Antonowski calls 'salutogenesis' (Antonowski, 1993: 111–122), it is argued, childbirth can, in the vast majority of cases, be not only safe, but also joyous (Davis, 2002). Yet it is only too easy in this technological age to jettison 'old-fashioned' knowledge and methods in favour of the latest 'scientific' intervention, and equally difficult to

resist powerful pressures from the self-interested groups driving this on. Here we should take a lesson from William Smellie, who was humble enough to recognize among the ignorance and superstition of the ancients 'valuable jewels' of wisdom, which, even in the 21st century, we would do well not to disregard (Smellie, 1752: lxxi). Today's genuinely reflective practitioners, whether midwives or obstetricians, will not stand by as old skills are lost, but adopt the *truly* scientific approach of seeking the evidence-base of *all* methods, old and new.

So what must the RCM do to succeed in its declared enterprise? In 2002, the College celebrated the centenary of the passing of the first Midwives Act, the fruit of 20 years' gruelling endeavour by the RCM's forerunner, the Midwives' Institute. Certainly the RCM undertakes its mission in more favourable circumstances than those which faced its predecessor. The Institute's membership comprised a tiny fraction of the number of women practising as midwives, many of whom were elderly, isolated and uneducated. No support came from Government, personal health services for the majority being considered a private matter. Childbirth was deemed an unfit topic for polite conversation, and hence assistance from members of the (all-male) Parliament had to be sought through an approach to their wives.

Now, however, childbirth is shown on television, Government has responsibility for the universal provision of health services, there are women MPs, and in recent years the Health Minister overseeing maternity care has been a young woman and a mother. The College, through the NCT and AIMS, has a more broadly based female backing than had the Institute, though its most outspoken medical support probably comes through the medium of the World Health Organization. A crucial change in recent years, however, has been the increasing preoccupation of Government with the need for evidence-based practice in the NHS, and hence for the achievement of best value for money for users and taxpayers. In this connection, urge midwife campaigners, the cheapest option, midwife-led care, is, for most women, also the safest and most satisfying option. All in all, it appears that the signs are more auspicious for a reversal of the technological tide than at any period since the creation of the NHS.

However, with its female leadership and largely female allies, the RCM will need all the tenacity and political skill of its Victorian counterparts in this battle against the male-dominated, technology-driven management of our maternity services if it is to achieve *true* choice for women in what is still essentially 'women's business'. Nonetheless leaders need foot soldiers. It hence behoves all midwives who value their art to recognize the lessons of the past, using these to shape their future – a future which, if sought with the passion and patience of earlier campaigners, can ensure, not merely the survival, but essentially the regeneration, of that most ancient of all offices – the office of midwife.

Reflective Activity 64.1

How many continuing themes can you detect in this history?

How do you think society's perceptions of women have influenced their roles as birth givers and birth attendants?

Which 'valuable jewels' can you find in the midwifery practice of former times that you could use in your own practice?

REFERENCES

Allison, J. (1996) *Delivered at Home*. London: Chapman and Hall.

[Anonymous] *A London Midwife's Diary 1694–1723*. Bod. Rawl Mss. D1141.

[Anonymous] (1803) *The London Practice of Midwifery*. London.

[Anonymous] (1874) Editorial. *Lancet* 2: 561.

[Anonymous] (1877) Editorial. *Lancet* 1: 618.

[Anonymous] (1929) Editorial. *Lancet* 1: 507.

Antonowski, A. (1993) The implications of salutogenesis: an outsider's view. In: Turnbull, A.P., Patterson, J., Behr, S.K et al. (eds) *Cognitive Coping: Families and Disability*. Baltimore: Brookes.

Ashcroft, E.L. (ed) (2002) *The Diary of a Kendal Midwife: Elizabeth Thompson*. Kendal: Curwen Archives Trust.

Audit Commission (1997) *First Class Delivery: Improving Maternity Services in England and Wales*. Abingdon: Audit Commission Publications.

Aveling, E.H. (1872) *English Midwives: Their History and Prospects*. London.

Ball, L., Curtis, P. & Kirkham, M. (2002) *Why do Midwives Leave*. London: RCM.

Barber, T. (2002) Consultant midwives: cameos from clinical practice. *RCM Midwives Journal* 5(5): 166–169.

Beech, B. (1996) A visit to Vienna. *AIMS Journal* 8(1): 6–10.

Blenkinsop, H. (ed) (1863) *Observations in Midwifery by Percival Willughby*. Warwick.

Bourgeois, L. (1609) *Observations Diverses sur la Stérilité, Perte de Fruict, Foecundité, Accouchements, Maladies des Femmes et des Enfants Nouveaux Naiz*. Paris.

British Broadcasting Corporation (BBC) (2002) *Health News*, 2 November. Online. Available: http//news.bbc.co.uk/1/hi/health/2391843.stm.

Brown, D. (2002) Insurers to halt caesarean payouts. *The Independent*, 2 November.

Burton, J. (1751) *An Essay Towards a Complete New System of Midwifery*. London.

Centraal Bureau voor de Statistiek (CBS) (1999) *Vademecum Health Statistics*. Rijswijk: CBS.

Chamberlain, G. & Steer, P. (1999) The ABC of labour care: labour in special circumstances. *British Medical Journal* 318(7191): 1124–1127.

Clarke, J. (1793) *Practical Essays on the Management of Pregnancy and Labour*. London.

Clement, C. (2001) Amniotomy in spontaneous, uncomplicated labour at term. *British Journal of Midwifery* 9(10): 629–634.

Cooper, Y. (2000) *Hansard*, April 19, Cols 225–226 WH.

Conde-Agudelo, A. & Belizan, J.M. (2000) Maternal morbidity associated with interpregnancy interval: cross sectional study. *British Medical Journal* 321(7291): 1255–1259.

Davis, K. (2002) General Secretary's address to the RCM Annual Conference, Bournemouth. *RCM Midwives Journal* 5(6): 210–214.

Department of Health (DoH) (1993) *Changing Childbirth, the Report of the Expert Maternity Group*. London: HMSO.

Downe, S. (2001) In: Lee, B. (ed) Active birth, active management. *RCM Midwives Journal* 4(7): 228–230.

Downe, S., McCormick, C. & Beech, B.L. (2001) Labour interventions associated with normal birth. *British Journal of Midwifery* 9(10): 602–606.

Earle, P. (1989) *The Making of the English Middle Class*. London: Methuen.

English National Board (ENB) (2001) *Audit of Midwifery Practice*. London: ENB.

Enkin, M., Keirse, M.J.N.C., Neilson, J. et al. (2000) *A Guide to Effective Care in Pregnancy and Childbirth*. Oxford: Oxford University Press.

Evenden, D. (2000) *The Midwives of Seventeenth-Century London*. Cambridge: Cambridge University Press.

Gardosi, J., Sylvester, S. & B-Lynch, C. (1989) Alternative positions in the second stage of labour. *British Journal of Obstetrics and Gynaecology* 96(11): 1290–1296.

Gélis, J. (1988) *La Sage-Femme ou le Mèdecin: une Nouvelle Conception de la Vie*. Paris: Fayard.

Gélis, J. (1996) *History of Childbirth* (trans. Morris R). Cambridge: Polity Press.

Gordon, A. (1795) *A Treatise on the Epidemic Puerperal Fever of Aberdeen*. London.

Gould, D.A., Butler-Manuel, S.A. & Turner, M.J. (1999) Emergency obstetric hysterectomy. *Journal of Obstetrics and Gynaecology* **19**: 580–583.

Hagelin, O. (1990) *The Byrth of Mankynde, Otherwyse Named the Womans Booke: Embryology, Obstetrics, Gynaecology through Four Centuries*. Stockholm: Svenska Lakaresallekapet.

Harley, D. (1996) Historians as demonologists: the myth of the midwife-witch. In: Wilson, P.K. (ed) *Midwifery Theory and Practice*. London: Garland Publishing.

Heinsohn, G. & Steiger, O. (1985) *Die Vernichtung der Weisen Frauen*. Hemsbach über Weinheim: Verlag Marz.

Holland E. (1935) *Lancet* **1**: 936.

House of Commons Health Committee (1992) *Second Report: Maternity Services*, Vol. 1. London: HMSO.

Inch, S. (1982) *Birthrights*. London: Hutchinson.

Jonas, R. (1540) *Byrth of Mankynde*. London.

Kuntner, L. (1988) *Die Gebährung der Frau: Schwangerschaft und Geburt aus geschichtlicher, völkerkundlicher und medizinischer Sicht*. Munich: Marseille Verlag.

Langdana, M., Geary, W., Haw, D. *et al.* (2001) Peripartum hysterectomy in the 1990s: any new lessons? *Journal of Obstetrics and Gynaecology* **21**(2): 121–123.

Leap, N. & Hunter, B. (1993) *The Midwife's Tale: An Oral History from Handywoman to Professional Midwife*. London: Scarlet Press.

Lee, B. (ed) (2001) Active birth, active management. *RCM Midwives Journal* **4**(7): 225–230.

Lewis, G.D. (ed) (2001) *Why Mothers Die 1997–9: fifth report of the Confidential Enquiries into Maternal Deaths in the United Kingdom*. London: CEMD: associated with NICE RCOG.

Loudon, I. (2000) *The Tragedy of Childbed Fever*. Oxford: Oxford University Press.

Macfarlane, A., Mugford, M. & Henderson, J. (2000) *Birth Counts: Statistics of Pregnancy and Childbirth*. London: HMSO.

McKeown, T. (1976) *The Role of Medicine: Dream, Mirage or Nemesis?* Oxford: Blackwell.

McMath, J. (1694) *The Expert Mid-Wife: A Treatise of the Diseases of Women with Child and in Childbed*. Edinburgh.

Marland, H. (ed) (1993) *The Art of Midwifery: Early Modern Midwives in Europe*. London: Routledge.

May, A. (1994) *Epidurals for Childbirth*, Ch. 9. Oxford: Oxford University Press.

Munro Kerr, J.M. (1933) *Maternal Mortality and Morbidity*. Edinburgh: E&S Livingstone.

Myles, M. (1981) *Textbook for Midwives*, 9th edn. London: Churchill Livingstone.

National Childbirth Trust (NCT), Royal College of Midwives (RCM) & Royal College of Obstetricians and Gynaecologists (RCOG) (1999) *The Rising Tide*. London: Profile Publications.

Pechey, J. (1696) *A General Treatise of the Diseases of Maids, Big-Bellied Women, Child-Bed Women, and Widows*. London.

Reid, L. (2002) Turning tradition into progress: moving midwifery forward. *RCM Midwives Journal* **5**(8): 250–254.

Robinson, J. (1999) The demand for caesareans: fact or fiction? *British Journal of Midwifery* **7**(5): 306.

Royal College of Midwives (RCM) (1986) *Project 2000: Comments of the Royal College of Midwives*. London: RCM.

Royal College of Obstetricians and Gynaecologists (RCOG) (1993) *Response to the Report of the Expert Maternity Group: Changing Childbirth*. London: RCOG.

Royal College of Obstetricians and Gynaecologists (RCOG) & Royal College of Midwives (RCM) (1999) *Towards Safer Childbirth: Minimum Standards for the Organisation of Labour Wards*. London: RCOG.

Royal Society of Medicine (RSM) (2002) 'The Fetus as a Patient'. Meeting of Obstetrics and Gynaecology Section Programme, 11 November. London: RSM.

Russell, J.G.B. (1982) The rationale of primitive delivery positions. *British Journal of Obstetrics and Gynaecology* **89**: 712–715.

Sharp, J. (1671) *The Midwives Book*. London.

Siegemundin, J. (1690) *Die königliche Preussische und Chur = Brandenburgische Hof = Wehe = Mutter, Das ist, Ein höchstnötiger Unterricht von schweren und unrechtstehenden Geburthen*. Coln an der Spree.

Smellie, W. (1752) *A Treatise on the Theory and Practice of Midwifery*. London.

Speak, S. (2002) Food intake in labour: the benefits and drawbacks. *Nursing Times* **98**(21): 42–43, reprinted *MIDIRS Midwifery Digest* September: 357–358.

Stapleton, H., Kirkham, M. & Thomas, G. (2002) Qualitative study of evidence based leaflets in maternity care. *British Medical Journal* **324**(7338): 639–643.

Steer, P. & Flint, C. (1999) ABC of labour care: physiology and management of normal labour. *British Medical Journal* **318**: 793–796.

Strachan, G. (1947) *Textbook of Obstetrics*. London: H.K. Lewis.

Temkin, O. (ed) (1956) *Soranus' Gynecology*. Baltimore: Johns Hopkins University Press.

Tew, M. (1978) The case against hospital deliveries: the statistical evidence. In: Kitzinger, S. & Davis, J. (eds) *The Place of Birth*. Oxford: Oxford University Press.

Tew, M. (1995) *Safer Childbirth? A Critical History of Maternity Care*. London: Chapman and Hall.

Thomas, K. (1973) *Religion and the Decline of Magic*. London: Penguin.

United Kingdom Central Council for Nursing, Midwifery and Health Visiting (UKCC) (1986) *Project 2000: A New Preparation for Practice*. London: UKCC.

Wagner, M. (2000) Choosing caesarean section. *Lancet* **356**(9242): 1677–1680.

Wagner, M. (2001) Fish can't see water: the need to humanize birth. *International Journal of Gynecology and Obstetrics* 75(Suppl.): S25–37, reprinted *MIDIRS, Midwifery Digest*, June 2002, 213–220.

Wagner, M. (2002) Critique of the British RCOG National Sentinel Caesarean Section Audit Report of Oct 2001. *MIDIRS Midwifery Digest* September: 366–370.

White, C. (1773) *The Management of Pregnant and Lying-in Women*. London

Wiesener, M. (1993) The midwives of South Germany. In: Marland, H. (ed) *The Art of Midwifery: Early Modern Midwives in Europe*. London: Routledge.

Worth, J. (2002) District midwifery in the 1950s. *MIDIRS Midwifery Digest* June: 174–175.

FURTHER READING

Donnison, J. (1988) *Midwives and Medical Men: a History of the Struggle for the Control of Childbirth*. London: Historical Publications.
Told in fascinating detail, this definitive account of the development of the midwifery profession in the UK presents an acute analysis of the socioeconomic factors and interprofessional rivalries influencing this from the 17th century to the present.

Mathers, H. & McIntosh, T. (2000) *Born in Sheffield: a History of the Women's Health Services 1864–2000*. Barnsley: Wharncliffe Books.

A valuable social history of Sheffield's women's health service, vividly bringing to life the development of hospital and home maternity care and the lives of childbearing women during this period.

Worth, J. (2002) *Call the Midwife*. Twickenham: Merton Books.
A compelling account of the troubles, trials and joys of a young domiciliary midwife practising in 1950s London docklands, and of the women she served.

65

International Perspectives

Gaynor D Maclean

LEARNING OUTCOMES

The chapter aims to enable readers to:

- gain insight into critical issues affecting midwifery practice worldwide
- identify the major causes of maternal death historically and geographically, exploring predisposing factors
- examine epidemiological factors associated with MMR reduction internationally
- contemplate activities engendered by the Safe Motherhood Initiative and current

- efforts to 'ensure skilled attendance during childbirth'
- consider the role of international organizations
- reflect on issues raised through studying international perspectives and how these may impact on personal midwifery practice at home and in countries other than their own.

CHALLENGES IN INTERNATIONAL MIDWIFERY FOR THE 21ST CENTURY

Midwives originating from the West will hold very different perspectives of childbirth and midwifery practice by comparison with colleagues from the 'developing world'. Midwives worldwide aspire to meet the needs of their clients, providing a safe environment in which to give birth. However, countless women in today's world are forced to experience childbirth, not as a fulfilling experience, but as one fraught with fear and danger. At the beginning of the 21st century, a majority of women still cannot dissociate birth from death. Consequently, midwives are challenged to play a leading part in making childbirth safer. Little wonder that the focus of international perspectives in midwifery centres on this aspect of sexual and reproductive health and upon the Safe Motherhood Initiative (SMI, 1987). A slogan promoted by the World Health Organization (WHO) clearly expresses sentiment needing to become reality: 'Pregnancy is special, let's make it safe' (WHO, 1997a). Making pregnancy safe challenges not only health professionals, but also technical experts, including water engineers, road builders, telecommunication experts and vehicle mechanics. Community mobilization

even in the farthest reaches of the globe needs to find resonance in political will at the highest levels.

CONTRASTS AND INEQUALITIES

It has been stressed that one of the most striking measurable contrasts between industrialized and developing countries becomes evident in examining *maternal mortality ratios*. The maternal mortality ratio (MMR) represents the risk associated with each pregnancy or 'the obstetric risk'. It is calculated as the number of maternal deaths during a given year per 100 000 live births during the same period. Although this measure has traditionally been referred to as a 'rate', it is actually a 'ratio'. The *maternal mortality ratio* is described as:

> The estimated number of maternal deaths per 100 000 live births
>
> (WHO, 1998)

The most appropriate denominator for such a calculation would be the total number of pregnancies including live births, stillbirths, induced and spontaneous abortions, ectopic and molar pregnancies. But this total is

Table 65.1 Estimates of maternal mortality by United Nations regions

UN region	Number of maternal deaths (rounded figures)	Maternal mortality ratio
World	515 000	400
'More developed countries'	2800	21
'Less developed regions'	512 000	440
'Least developed countries'	230 000	1000
Africa	273 000	1000
Eastern Africa	122 000	1300
Middle Africa	39 000	1000
Northern Africa	20 000	450
Southern Africa	4500	360
Western Africa	87 000	1100
Asia	217 000	280
Eastern Asia*	13 000	55
South-central Asia	158 000	410
South-eastern Asia	35 000	300
Western Asia	11 000	230
Europe	2200	28
Latin America/Caribbean	22 000	190
Caribbean	3100	400
Central America	3800	110
South America	15 000	200
Northern America	490	11
Oceania	560	260

* Japan, Australia and New Zealand have been excluded from the regional figures. They are included under the section 'More developed countries'.
Source: WHO/UNICEF/UNFPA estimates in 1995 (WHO, 2001)

seldom available in either low income or industrialized countries; therefore the number of live births is used in this calculation (WHO, 1999).

The *maternal mortality rate* measures both the obstetric risk and the frequency with which women are exposed to this risk. It is calculated as:

The number of maternal deaths in a given period per 100 000 women of reproductive age (usually 15–49 years).

(WHO, 1998)

The terms 'ratio' and 'rate' are sometimes used interchangeably, but it is essential to clarify which denominator has been used. Researchers now prefer the term 'maternal mortality ratio' and this is the interpretation of MMR that has been used in this chapter.

On a global scale, it is estimated that every minute of every day, a woman dies of pregnancy-related complications; the massive death toll exceeds half a million each year (WHO, 1997a). 99% of these deaths occur in developing countries, figures varying considerably (Table 65.1).

Causes of maternal death

Major causes of maternal death worldwide have been identified as haemorrhage, infection, eclampsia, obstructed labour and abortion (Fig. 65.1). Maternal death is influenced by numerous factors. The reasons why women die have been described as 'many layered' (AbouZahr and Royston, 1991). These layers include social, cultural and political factors that determine crucial issues including the status of women, women's health and fertility, and their 'health seeking behaviour'. Other factors, further increasing the chance of a woman dying, relate to failures in healthcare systems and transportation problems.

The global problem of AIDS and HIV-related illness further compounds the situation, adding to the horrendous slaughter of young women and their babies. Africa currently demonstrates highest infection rates,

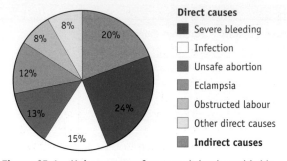

8%   8%   20%

8%

12%

13%   24%

15%

Direct causes

■ Severe bleeding

☐ Infection

■ Unsafe abortion

■ Eclampsia

▨ Obstructed labour

☐ Other direct causes

■ **Indirect causes**

Figure 65.1   Major causes of maternal death worldwide. Other direct causes include ectopic pregnancy, embolism and anaesthesia-related deaths. Indirect causes include anaemia, malaria and heart disease. (*Source*: WHO, 1997b.)

Table 65.2   Lifetime risks of dying in pregnancy: regional contrasts

'More developed regions'	1 in 2500
'Less developed regions'	1 in 60
'Least developed regions'	1 in 16
Europe	1 in 2000
Western Europe	1 in 4000
North America	1 in 3500
Latin America and Caribbean	1 in 160
Asia excluding Japan	1 in 110
Africa	1 in 16
Oceania excluding Australia and New Zealand	1 in 260

Source: WHO/UNICEF/UNFPA estimates in 1995 (WHO, 2001)

Table 65.3   Lifetime risks of dying in pregnancy: some contrasts between selected countries

Finland	1 in 7700
United Kingdom	1 in 4600
United States of America	1 in 3500
Thailand	1 in 1100
China	1 in 710
Solomon Islands	1 in 280
India	1 in 55
Nepal	1 in 21
Angola	1 in 9
Ethiopia	1 in 7

Source: WHO/UNICEF/UNFPA estimates in 1995 (WHO, 2001)

and in Botswana one in two pregnant women are reported HIV positive (Kroeger, 2000).

In addition to the maternal death toll, every year nearly 3.4 million babies die within the first week of life. For every baby that dies another is stillborn (WHO, 1997a).

Risk of dying

A woman's 'lifetime risk of maternal death' is regarded as a reproductive health indicator and defined as: 'The estimated risk of an individual woman dying from pregnancy or childbirth during her lifetime, based on maternal mortality and the fertility rate in the country.' (WHO, 1998).

This average lifetime risk of dying is also influenced by where a woman lives (Tables 65.2 and 65.3).

These represent average figures. The actual lifetime risk can be much higher. Women with high fertility rates living in rural areas are particularly vulnerable. Amongst the most vulnerable are teenagers, older women and those of higher parity (AbouZahr and Royston, 1991).

Previous studies in Bangladesh and Nigeria demonstrated that mothers under 15 years of age have MMRs five to seven times higher than women aged 20–24 years (Chen *et al.*, 1974; Harrison, 1985). More recently it has been shown that sexually active adolescent women experience higher levels of reproductive mortality and morbidity than women in their 20s and early 30s (Senderowitz, 1995). Women aged 35–39 years were between 85% and 460% more likely to die than women aged 20–23 years (Rochat, 1981). These vulnerable groups still feature high in the maternal mortality league tables throughout the world. Indeed a recent Indian study demonstrates increased figures. In women aged 18 years or less, it was found that 12% of

maternal deaths occurred in this group during 1994–1996 by comparison with 7% between 1983 and 1985. Almost a quarter of the deaths occurred in women over 30 years. Women of gravida 5 or above accounted for 21% in the earlier study and 24% in the latter. The death of older women echoes trends in states across India (Pendse, 1999). Danel *et al.* (1998) report that two of the most important characteristics associated with pregnancy-related death in the USA are age and race. Increased risk is associated with increased age, but whilst this is true for all races it is increased for black and Hispanic women with black women over 40 years facing a risk six times more than white women in the same age group.

Survival of women at risk is extremely precarious in countries where health services are inaccessible, inadequate or non-existent. Risk is not eliminated in the West; vulnerable women still face enormous challenges to achieving safe motherhood wherever they struggle to exist. The birth of children to so many of the world's women may still be aptly described: 'Too many, too early, too late and too close together' (Royston and Armstrong, 1989).

WHO emphasizes that recently published figures are intended to draw attention to the existence and likely dimensions of the problem of maternal mortality. They indicate orders of magnitude and are not intended to portray precise estimates (WHO, 2001). In reviewing the most recent MMR statistics (Tables 65.1–65.3), WHO sounds a note of caution in respect of monitoring trends over the short term and also in making cross-country comparisons. This is because of the very large 'margins of uncertainty' associated with the estimates. Having said this, it is acknowledged that there are substantial regional differences between the 1990 MMR estimates (WHO, 1996) and the 1995 figures issued in 2001.

The following statement summarizes the situation:

In general, the 1995 estimates for Asia and Central America are lower compared with 1990 whereas the 1995 estimates for Africa are substantially higher. Whereas in 1990 Africa accounted for 40% of the global total of maternal deaths, the 1995 estimates indicate that Africa accounts for some 53% of the total. By contrast whereas in 1990, Asia contributed 55% of total maternal deaths, in 1995 it contributes 42%.

(WHO, 2001)

Maternal morbidity

Morbidity is less easily measurable. It is estimated that for every woman who dies, at least 30 develop 'chronic, debilitating problems' (WHO, 1997a). These include horrific injuries such as vesicovaginal fistulae. There may be secondary infertility. In industrialized countries, morbidity is also associated with debilitating conditions (Ch. 42). However, estimates of maternal morbidity anywhere in the world indicate merely the tip of an iceberg. It becomes apparent that, regardless of geographical location, childbirth can result in an enormous health deficit. Opportunities to receive appropriate treatment will, however, be significantly reduced for women living in impoverished countries constituting home for the majority of the world's population.

THE SAFE MOTHERHOOD INITIATIVE

It has been estimated that 88–98% of all maternal deaths could 'probably have been avoided' (WHO,

> **Box 65.1 The Safe Motherhood Initiative (WHO, 1990–1994; FCI, 1998)**
>
> The Safe Motherhood Initiative, launched in 1987, is a global effort to reduce maternal mortality and morbidity. It is led by a unique partnership of international organizations that work together to raise awareness, set priorities, stimulate research, mobilize resources, provide technical assistance and share information according to each organization's mandate. Their cooperation and commitment have enabled governments and non-governmental partners from more than 100 countries to take action and make motherhood safer.
>
> The Initiative aims to enhance the quality and safety of the lives of girls and women through the adoption of a combination of health and non-health strategies.
>
> The Initiative places special emphasis on the need for better and more widely available maternal health services, the extension of family planning education and services, and effective measures aimed at improving the status of women.

1986). This implies that maternity services have an important function preventing maternal death and disease. Midwives can make significant contributions to this goal.

In order to address this enormous death toll and health deficit, an international and interdisciplinary effort was inaugurated in 1987. The Safe Motherhood Initiative (Box 65.1) was launched with the expressed aim of reducing maternal mortality by at least 50% by the year 2000 (SMI, 1987).

Co-sponsors of the Safe Motherhood Initiative include major international organizations (Box 65.2).

The co-sponsors form an 'interagency group' (IAG) for safe motherhood with the Secretariat based at Family Care International, New York.

The initial 16-year period of the Initiative cannot be regarded as a success, since mortality figures remain high. Yet it has succeeded to a variable extent in raising awareness at national and international levels and there is evidence of reduced MMRs in some low income countries over the past, 20–30 years. Sri Lanka has shown one of the most dramatic declines in MMR during the latter half of the 20th century (Table 65.4).

Box 65.2 Co-sponsors of the Safe Motherhood Initiative

United Nations Development Programme (UNDP)

United Nations Children's Fund (UNICEF)

United Nations Population Fund (UNFPA)

The World Bank

World Health Organization (WHO)

International Planned Parenthood Federation (IPPF)

The Population Council

Box 65.3 Action messages for the next decade of the Safe Motherhood Initiative (FCI, 1997)

1. Advance safe motherhood through human rights.
2. Empower women; ensure choices.
3. Perceive safe motherhood as a vital social and economic investment.
4. Delay marriage and first birth.
5. Acknowledge that every pregnancy faces risks.
6. Ensure skilled attendance at delivery.
7. Improve access to quality maternal health services.
8. Prevent unwanted pregnancy; address unsafe abortion.
9. Measure progress.
10. Utilize the power of partnership.

'Action message 6' (Box 65.3) is of particular interest to midwives. Safe Motherhood Partners are currently leading efforts to ensure skilled attendance during childbirth. This is outlined below. Between conferences and face-to-face meetings, international debate between technical experts continues through electronic mail. Thus lessons learned are constantly shared and the route ahead reviewed.

THE IMPACT OF MODERNIZATION AND DEVELOPMENT

The process of modernization and development is inextricably linked with numerous health issues. Undoubtedly, as countries develop, childbirth becomes safer. This is a complex issue and the reader would do well to explore the manifold matters that contribute to maternal health and safe motherhood, piecing together the jigsaw that makes life for women what it is in the 21st century (Fig. 65.2). Inevitably, progress of modernity is inversely related to the lifetime risk of dying in childbirth.

Table 65.4 Countries demonstrating reduced MMRs

Country	Earlier MMR (year)	Recent MMR (year)
Cuba	118 (1962)	22 (1997)
Malaysia	148 (1970)	53 (1996)
Sri Lanka	1530 (1941)	62 (1996)
	100 (1975)	
Thailand	110 (1981)	44 (1995–1996)

Nationally reported figures cited
Source: WHO (1998)

THE SIGNIFICANCE OF HISTORICAL ISSUES

Periodically, progress of the Safe Motherhood Initiative is formally reviewed in international arenas. In 1992 a meeting of 'Partners for Safe Motherhood' was held in Washington DC, comprising participants from 33 countries in the 'developed' and the 'developing' world. Programme priorities for the years ahead were discussed and necessary resources identified and mobilized. In 1997, at a meeting hosted in Sri Lanka, Safe Motherhood Partners set priorities for the next decade (Box 65.3).

In a literature survey undertaken for Family Care International (Maclean, 2000a), historical data were utilized in examining the relationship between skilled

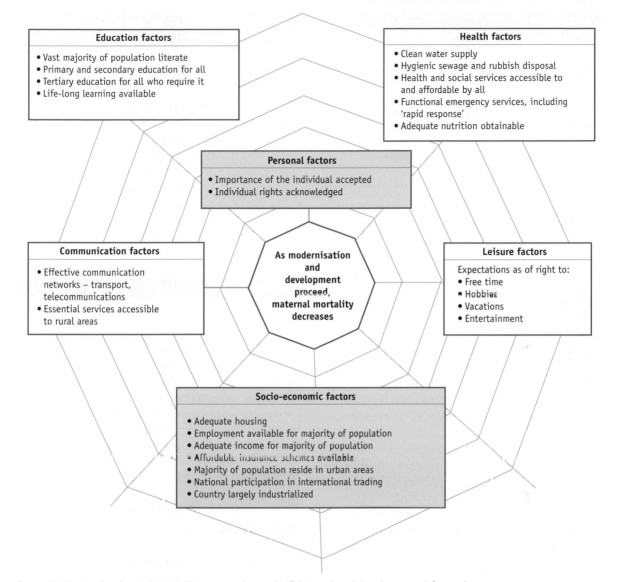

Figure 65.2 Modernity and mortality: a complex web of 'interrelated developmental factors'.

attendance at delivery and reduced maternal mortality. Because it would be impossible to conduct a randomized controlled trial, history is used to provide data about factors associated with reduced death rates in western countries at stages of development comparable with the situation in much of the developing world today. Hence, the influence of advances in pharmacology, surgery and technology can be eliminated from the enquiry.

Historically, high maternal mortality has been associated with poor standards of maternity care, inappropriate interventions and incompetent practice (De Brouwere *et al.*, 1998). Loudon (1992) identified two distinct phases in the history of MMR reduction in Scandinavia, Western Europe and the USA. These phases were separated by 'a plateau', when significantly reduced MMRs remained static. The first phase of improvement was associated with the development of good basic midwifery practice, especially the use of aseptic technique and skilled labour management. This phase was characterized by the recognition of obstetrics as a medical speciality and the development of midwifery as a profession. Legislation made skilled attendance at delivery mandatory. The second phase of improvement was associated with the advent of antibiotics, the use of ergometrine, blood transfusion,

Table 65.5   Examples from historical experiences of promoting safe motherhood

Primary approach	Secondary approach
Accumulation of reliable vital statistics	Investigation into the cause of every maternal death. Confidential enquiry
Diligent use of aseptic techniques	Use of sulphonamides, antibiotics
Skilled management of labour	Use of ergometrine
Adapted from Maclean (2000b)	

caesarean section and improved anaesthesia. During the latter phase, the establishment of systematic enquiry into every maternal death built a recognized vehicle to learn from experience and identify avoidable factors that would make childbirth significantly safer in modernized society.

Sweden led the way in ensuring skilled attendance at delivery during the 19th century at a time when 90% of the population resided in rural areas and poverty was rife. There was emphasis on using aseptic technique, evacuating a full bladder, managing the third stage skilfully, providing pain relief and preparing 'instrumentally competent' midwives (Hogberg, personal communication, 1999). This contrasted with early attempts in the USA, epitomized in the obstetric practice promoted by Dr Joseph B De Lee. He advocated that every woman should be anaesthetized for 'prophylactic forceps delivery' and manual removal of the placenta (De Lee, 1920–1921).

However, a steady decline in maternal mortality in the USA later occurred and this was maintained during the severe economic depression of the 1930s. This, along with further extensive research, prompted the conclusion that maternal mortality is: 'remarkably resistant to the ill-effects of social and economic deprivation' whilst it is 'remarkably sensitive to the good and bad effects of medical intervention' (Loudon, 1986).

Considering the attempts that have been made to address maternal mortality, it appears that some activities have been associated with the first phase of MMR reduction and some with the second phase described by Loudon and cited above. These have been termed primary and secondary approaches respectively (Maclean, 2000a,b,c). Whilst some of these approaches may appropriately originate during the first or second phase of MMR reduction, it is prudent that some secondary approaches are built upon primary approaches if safe motherhood is to be achieved. Examples of these are summarized in Table 65.5.

Belgian researchers considering what may be learned from the historical experience of the industrialized West and reasonably transferred to the developing world caution that: 'The combination of circumstances and conditions that allowed for early reduction in some countries and paved the way for technological developments in the late 1940s has not been present in many developing countries.' (De Brouwere *et al.*, 1998).

There is an obvious need to build upon a sure foundation, with logical selectivity. Using antibiotics without first emphasizing the need for basic aseptic technique, using oxytocics without understanding the physiology of labour and utilizing that knowledge in care provision, is a potential recipe for disaster (Maclean, 2000b,c).

Reflective Activity 65.1

Consider the influences of 'primary and secondary approaches' in promoting safe motherhood. What may be the consequences of utilizing secondary approaches without due attention to the primary approaches:

- in your own practice?
- in a developing country?

'ENSURING SKILLED ATTENDANCE DURING CHILDBIRTH'

During the second decade of the Safe Motherhood Initiative, focus moves towards a new era in promoting the concept of skilled attendance at every delivery. The term 'skilled attendant' refers exclusively to people with midwifery skills who have been 'trained to proficiency' in the necessary skills to enable them to 'manage normal deliveries and diagnose, manage or refer complications'. These may be doctors, midwives or nurses but do not include traditional birth attendants (WHO, 1999, 2000a). The skilled attendant at delivery is regarded as a 'reproductive health indicator' (WHO, 1998) and as such is considered a proxy for a healthcare provider who can provide skilled care throughout pregnancy, labour and the postnatal period.

During the year 2000 there was extensive investigation and debate about the importance and implications of promoting the use of skilled attendants. International efforts to promote this concept are already afoot and likely to continue. Political commitment has been historically and contemporarily associated with successful MMR reduction. Countries that have demonstrated a dramatic improvement in maternal mortality statistics include Sri Lanka and Cuba (Table 65.4). Political commitment in Sri Lanka has resulted in the promotion of a policy ensuring skilled attendance at delivery with coverage reaching 96% (Seneviratne and Peiris, 1997). MMR reduction has been dramatic in the past 50 years. In Cuba, maternal and child healthcare has been a priority since the national health system was established in 1961 with an impressive fall in MMR (Cardoso, 1986; WHO, 1998).

Box 65.4 Definitions of some socioeconomic and demographic indicators (WHO, 1998)

Female literacy rate. 'The percentage of women aged 15 years and over who can both read and write with understanding a short simple statement on her everyday life.'

Total fertility rate (TFR). 'The number of children a woman would have if she experienced the prevailing age-specific fertility rates throughout her childbearing life.'

Urban population. 'Percentage of the total population residing in urban areas.'

Reflective Activity 65.2

Think about the concept of 'skilled attendance during childbirth'.

- How would you define 'skilled'?
- What influence has this policy had in your area of practice?
- What helps to ensure the availability of a 'skilled attendant' for every woman?

---

childbirth is safer in an institutional setting is set to continue.

Reflective Activity 65.3

What factors do you think influence whether women are likely to achieve safe motherhood in your area of practice? What could interfere with these?

EPIDEMIOLOGICAL FACTORS

If skilled attendance during childbirth were the only issue claiming association with significant MMR reduction, cause and effect, process and outcome may be easier to define and declare. However, certain socioeconomic and demographic indicators have been associated with safer motherhood internationally. These include female literacy rate, total fertility rate and urban population. The terms are defined in Box 65.4.

Statistical analyses reveal higher MMRs amongst illiterate women who have a high total fertility rate (TFR) and reside in rural areas. Those who live in rural areas are least likely to have access to skilled attendance during labour, since the majority of the health services are habitually situated in urban areas. This issue is compounded by problems of transport and communication. With notable exceptions, countries with high MMRs frequently demonstrate low female literacy rates, high TFRs and low urban population percentages. Frequently there is also a low incidence of skilled attendance during childbirth (Fig. 65.3A–E).

Since skilled attendants without access to essential equipment and a functional referral chain will be limited in their ability to save life, debate concerning whether

INTERNATIONAL ORGANIZATIONS

Numerous organizations provide both human and fiscal assistance. The Safe Motherhood Initiative and its 'Partners' have been described above and are excellent examples of international cooperation. International organizations may comprise governmental, intergovernmental or non-governmental organizations. There are also voluntary organizations both religious and secular that may offer support. Currently, there is an explosion of international aid sweeping into a volatile world economy, with an apparent movement of wealth from rich to poor nations. However, the reality is much more complex. Issues surrounding aid and trade between governments and the role of such giant organizations as the World Bank have raised ethical queries concerning who really benefits from some aid schemes (Juva, 1994; Madeley *et al.*, 1994). This is not the place to debate the matter, but the reader may find it instructive to consider the role of governments as well as international organizations in the context of poverty relief and debt repayment. These topics have received much media publicity in recent years. In this climate of international cooperation, there are increasing opportunities and demands for midwives to share

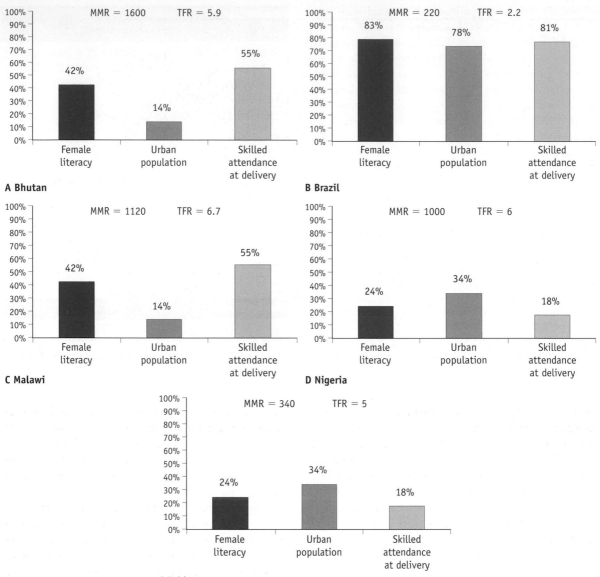

Figure 65.3 Some country profiles: **A.** Bhutan; **B.** Brazil; **C.** Malawi; **D.** Nigeria; **E.** Pakistan.

professional expertise. Without underestimating the valuable contribution of numerous others, brief descriptions of a few organizations are provided.

World Health Organization

The World Health Organization (WHO) has the objective of the attainment by all peoples of the best possible level of health. WHO has two main constitutional functions:

1. To act as the directing and coordinating authority on international health work

2. To encourage technical cooperation for health with member states.

WHO performs its functions through three principal bodies:

- World Health Assembly
- Executive Board
- Secretariat.

The global headquarters is in Geneva, Switzerland. Each of the six world regions has a regional office and committee (Fig. 65.4). Increasingly, decentralization is practised in relation to policy formation, implementation

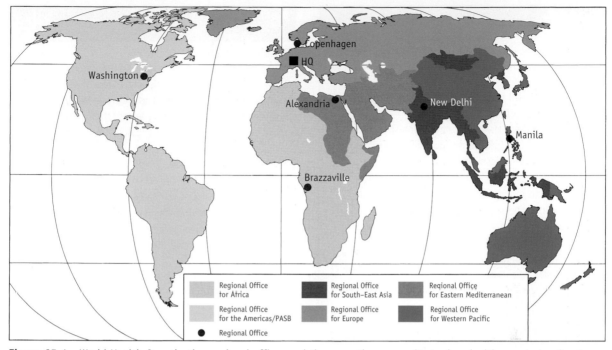

Figure 65.4 World Health Organization regional offices and the areas they serve. (Reproduced with permission from WHO *Biennial Report* 1988–1989.)

and monitoring of regional activities. WHO officially designates leading health-related institutions around the world as WHO Collaborating Centres (WHO, 1990). WHO works closely with other organizations within the United Nations system. It is a constitutional requirement that WHO should 'establish and maintain effective collaboration with the United Nations ... and provide health services and facilities' (WHO, 1990). WHO provides technical, professional and educational health information.

Published documents of particular interest to midwives include the Safe Motherhood Midwifery Modules comprising five teaching manuals designed to help midwifery teachers in developing countries teach prevention and management of major causes of maternal death (WHO, 1996). Currently, manuals are being prepared to provide guidance on essential care provision by healthcare workers to pregnant or parturient women and their babies, with specific direction for those trained to conduct deliveries (WHO, 2000b). The South East Asia Regional Office (SEARO) has led the way in designing and field testing 'standards' for midwifery practice (WHO SEARO, 1998). WHO has been instrumental in promoting traditional birth attendant (TBA) training, though currently there is heated debate about the value of this cadre of worker. Global initiatives to

address major health problems, such as HIV/AIDS, malaria and tetanus, fall within the remit of WHO. New health dilemmas continue to challenge technical expertise, professional will power and national and international commitment from the outset of the 21st century.

At the second WHO Ministerial Conference in Munich in June 2000, the new policy document 'Health 21' was endorsed by all 51 European member states. The document affirms 21 targets and offers a framework for the European region to tackle major health problems. This is complemented by a further document identifying the important contributions that nurses and midwives can make to achieving these targets (Spernbauer, 2000).

UNICEF

The United Nations Children's Fund (UNICEF) aims to raise public awareness of the needs of children, promoting strategies to meet those needs and raising funds for UNICEF-sponsored programmes in more than 130 countries. The organization provides help and care for women and children, and emergency relief and health education in war-torn countries as well as in situations

Box 65.5 10 steps to successful breastfeeding

1. Have a written breastfeeding policy.
2. Train all health staff to implement this policy.
3. Inform all pregnant women about the benefits of breastfeeding.
4. Help mothers initiate breastfeeding within half an hour of birth.
5. Show mothers the best way to breastfeed.
6. Give newborn infants no food or drink other than breast milk, unless medically indicated.
7. Practice 'rooming in' by allowing mothers and babies to remain together for 24 hours a day.
8. Encourage breastfeeding on demand.
9. Give no artificial teats, pacifiers, dummies or soothers.
10. Help start breastfeeding support groups and refer mothers to them.

Source: 'Take the Baby Friendly Initiative' leaflet (UNICEF)

Box 65.6 'World Breastfeeding Week' themes

1993	Women, work and breastfeeding: Everybody benefits
1994	Protect breastfeeding: Make the code work
1995	Breastfeeding: Empowering women
1996	Breastfeeding: A community responsibility
1997	Breastfeeding: Nature's way
1998	Breastfeeding: The best investment
1999	Breastfeeding: Education for life
2000	Breastfeeding – It's your right!

Source: WABA

of poverty in industrialized and non-industrialized countries. UNICEF has a four-part strategy for the protection of children, designated 'GOBI':

G Growth monitoring
O Oral rehydration
B Breastfeeding
I Immunization.

UNICEF, in collaboration with WHO, defined a global standard for maternity services described as 'baby friendly care' in 1989. The emerging 'Baby Friendly Initiative' involves a global effort with hospitals, health services and parents, encouraging them to focus on the needs of mothers and their newborn. It strives to implement 10 steps to successful breastfeeding (Box 65.5).

In order to help promote breastfeeding globally, the World Alliance for Breastfeeding (WABA) was formed

Box 65.7 The International Confederation of Midwives

Mission Statement
'The International Confederation of Midwives will advance worldwide the aims and aspirations of midwives in the attainment of improved outcomes for women in their childbearing years, their newborn and their families wherever they reside.' (May, 1996)

Statement of Purpose
'In looking forward to the 21st century, midwives and women share many of the same concerns and will work toward achieving the vision that empowers both women and midwives to be fully respected as persons who are also productive members of all societies.' (May, 1996)

Source: ICM, 2000

at UNICEF headquarters in New York in 1991 and encourages active participation of individuals and organizations in this effort to protect, promote and support breastfeeding. More than 120 countries designate a 'World Breastfeeding Week' every August. A different theme helps to provide focus on specific aspects of breastfeeding each year (Box 65.6).

The International Confederation of Midwives

The International Confederation of Midwives (ICM) is a unique midwifery professional organization. ICM's ideology is expressed in Box 65.7.

There are four regions of the confederation: Africa, the Americas, Asia Pacific and Europe. An International Council governs ICM, normally meeting every 3 years, when an international congress is also held. A Board of Management oversees management and financial obligations, and Executive and Finance Subcommittees act as advisory bodies to the Board of Management and the Council. The Secretary General is the chief executive officer of ICM and is appointed by the Council. ICM headquarters is in The Hague, Netherlands.

ICM has played a leading role promoting the Safe Motherhood Initiative since its inception in 1987 and currently makes a significant contribution to the inter-agency group (IAG) described above. ICM was instrumental in establishing an 'international day of the midwife'. This takes place at the beginning of May each year when there are efforts to raise awareness of the role and function of midwives and their invaluable contribution to promoting safe motherhood.

European Community Committees

There are some committees within the European Union (EU) of particular interest to the midwife.

The Midwives Liaison Committee is composed of representatives of midwives' organizations within the European Community. It was established in 1968 by ICM in order to give consideration to the EC Midwives Directives and advise governments of the professional views of midwives. The committee looks at the provision of maternity care and midwifery practice issues in all the countries of the European Economic Community.

The EU Advisory Committee on training midwives was established in accordance with EU Midwives Directives in 1980, becoming effective from 1983. It was set up in order to facilitate freedom of movement of midwives across the Community and advises the European Commission on matters concerning their education and practice. The Committee is made up of six members per Member State (EEC, 1977, 1980). Midwives as well as other professions are currently opposing a recent initiative proposing to eliminate the seven specialist directives and replace them with a general directive. This would affect midwifery and nursing amongst a total of seven healthcare professions currently controlled by the specialist directives.

The 'EU round table'. Recently, the EU opted to make maternal health a new priority on its health agenda. A forum has been set up in order to increase dialogue on safe motherhood issues and develop thinking within the EU on most appropriate policies and strategy directions for its projects in developing countries. The EU experts' round table is designed to facilitate discussion between researchers, technical experts, EU member state representatives and others (De Brouwere, personal communication, 2000).

The White Ribbon Alliance for Safe Motherhood

The goals of this alliance incorporate raising awareness about safe motherhood, building alliances and acting as a catalyst for action. The Alliance urges supporters to wear the symbolic white ribbon dedicated to the memory of women who have died in childbirth, uniting individuals, organizations and communities working on MMR reduction (NGO Networks for Health, 2000).

IMPORTANT CONSIDERATIONS FOR MIDWIVES INTENDING TO WORK OVERSEAS

The 21st century is already characterized by increasing international exchange. Midwives from the West provide technical assistance in the developing world. Opportunities for professional education and experience continue to attract midwives into industrialized countries. Clearly, midwives practising in any country other than that in which they were educated must adapt to vastly differing situations.

Midwives who have been educated in an industrialized country intending to work in a low income country need considerable experience. It can be helpful to learn some advanced clinical skills where practicable; for example, vacuum extraction, suturing cervical and vaginal tears, manual removal of placenta, neonatal intubation, inserting intrauterine contraceptive devices. Regulations may restrict midwives from acquiring some of these skills in the UK, but policy and tradition can sometimes be overcome in consultation with obstetricians and supervisors of midwives willing to arrange suitable learning opportunities. Short courses in tropical medicine and health can be most valuable. Discussions with persons experienced in the intended country of practice can be invaluable.

National authorities will specify their own country's priorities in health. Increasingly, needs are expressed for midwives with expertise in education or management, but all midwives must be clinically skilled, able and willing to adapt to local needs. Ability to speak another language or a willingness to learn is an asset, and respect for different cultures and religions crucial. It is important for any expatriate workers to appreciate that they will never know nor understand many things in another country and that change must come from within a country. They must appreciate that 'experts' from another country can best help colleagues by demonstrating appropriate knowledge, skills and attitudes with sensitivity. Midwives practising in cross-cultural situations need an acute sense of awareness, and an attitude of humility and willingness to learn. In a developing country, they need to be able to empathize with colleagues working in very different situations, exercise patience and cope using limited resources.

Midwives who have been educated in low income countries intending working or studying in industrialized countries will find more advanced technology in use than experienced at home. There may also be more emphasis on informed choice for women and partnership in care. These midwives therefore need a good understanding of current issues and popular demands. They must constantly update their knowledge and practice by critically evaluating research. There are benefits and hazards associated with both technology and freedom of choice demanding consideration. In returning to developing countries, indigenous midwives, as expatriates, need to evaluate new practices in the light of local situations, available resources and national priorities, before attempting to transfer them from one country to another.

Midwives who have practised in countries where resources are scarce may be skilled at improvising and can sometimes share innovations with colleagues who face different, though significant resource limitations. Midwives, who have practised in regions remote from medical services, can share with colleagues their experience of complications rarely seen in the West. It is salutary for all midwives to appreciate the consequences of delayed referral and intervention; the reality of, for example, obstructed labour and ruptured uterus as inevitable consequences of cephalopelvic disproportion, and the frightening speed with which septicaemia can occur. Such complications will, of course, result in maternal death anywhere in the world unless there is appropriate and skilled intervention.

CONCLUSION

During the past decade, international perspectives have evolved from being an 'optional extra' to becoming an essential component of the body of knowledge owned by midwives working in the West. International studies now form part of pre-registration and post-registration programmes in the UK. In low income countries, safe motherhood is beginning to establish its rightful place. The attainment of safe motherhood is at the heart of every midwife's practice and whilst tragedies associated with childbirth are not observed on such a great scale in the West, experiences from the rest of the world can provide salutary lessons about fundamentals of midwifery care. Assertions that 'that could never happen here' must find evidence in reality. Safe motherhood should be

> ### Reflective Activity 65.4
>
> **For midwives originating from low income countries**
> Think about one new approach you have observed:
>
> - What may be the benefits in your country?
> - What may be the hazards?
> - Do you suggest any adaptations?
> - Is further research advisable before transferring the practice? If so, what do you propose?
>
> **For midwives educated in industrialized countries**
> Think about a complication identified during your practice:
>
> - What may have been the outcome if you were in a remote area?
> - What could you do to minimize such dangers?
> - What further skills do you need if you intend to practice in remote areas of the developing world? Make an action plan to prepare yourself.

a priority in every country, including the UK. Historically, midwives have played a critical part and the concept of promoting maternal and neonatal health and safe motherhood still falls naturally into the midwife's domain. It is the midwife who makes her profession what it is today and what it will be tomorrow. This warrants critical evaluation and constant reappraisal of essential professional issues including midwifery curricula, standards of practice, professional politics and practice ethics. These must reflect safety as a priority. Other issues, whilst important, will always be secondary.

May 21st century midwifery practice help render a statement made early in the experience of the Safe Motherhood Initiative no longer ring true: 'In practically every society, celebration of life is the dominant theme, while the grimmer side of childbearing is often, shrouded in silence, known only to those who suffer it and those who attend them.' (Royston and Armstrong, 1989).

The shroud has been removed. It is high time that the monumental maternal mortality figures beneath that shroud are removed too, so that unjust suffering gives way to a vibrant celebration of life and health. This provides perspective for an international challenge during the century ahead.

KEY POINTS

- MMRs vary enormously across the globe, with large discrepancies between industrialized and 'low income' countries. Hence the rationale for activities directed at promoting maternal and neonatal health. Midwives play a key role in promoting these basic human rights.

- There are five major causes of maternal death worldwide, predisposed to by numerous and complex factors. The World Health Organization estimates that most of these deaths are avoidable. Promoting safe motherhood embraces health, education, socioeconomic and political issues. The importance of skilled attendance during childbirth motivates current

- endeavours to promote maternal and neonatal health.

- Historical experience of MMR reduction in the West offers some inspiration in world regions where risks associated with childbirth remain as high in the 21st century as they were in the West more than a century ago.

- Internationally, high female literacy rates, low total fertility rates and large urban population ratios have been associated with MMR reduction.

- A midwife intending to work internationally needs special preparation, but studying international perspectives should enrich personal professional development wherever she chooses to practice.

REFERENCES

AbouZahr, C. & Royston, E. (eds) (1991) *Maternal Mortality: A Global Factbook*. WHO/MCH/MSM91.3. Geneva: WHO.

Cardoso, U.F. (1986) Giving birth is safer now. *World Health Forum* 7: 348–352.

Chen, L.C. *et al.* (1974) Maternal mortality in rural Bangladesh. *Studies in Family Planning* 5(11): 334–341.

Danel, I., Berg, C. & Atrash, H. (1998) pregnancy in the USA: risks are higher for some women. *World Health* 1(Jan–Feb): 20–21.

De Brouwere, V. *et al.* (1998) Strategies for reducing maternal mortality in developing countries: what can we learn from the history of the industrialized West? *Tropical Medicine and International Health* 3(10): 771–782.

De Lee, J.B. (1920–21) The prophylactic forceps operation. *American Journal of Obstetrics and Gynecology* 1: 34–44, 77–78.

European Economic Community (EEC) (1977) The EEC Directives on the activities responsible for general care. *Official Journal of the European Communities* 20(176) July.

European Economic Community (EEC) (1980) The EEC Midwives Directives. *Official Journal of the European Communities* 23(33) February. Obtainable from HMSO.

Family Care International (FCI) (1997) *The Safe Motherhood Action Agenda: Priorities for the Next Decade. Report of the Safe Motherhood Technical Consultation, Sri Lanka, October*. New York: FCI.

Family Care International (FCI) (1998) *Safe Motherhood: Critical Issues for Policy-makers*. New York: FCI.

Harrison, K.A. (1985) Childbearing, health and social priorities: a survey of 22,774 consecutive births in Zaria, Northern Nigeria. *British Journal of Obstetrics and Gynaecology* 92(Suppl. 5).

ICM (2000) *Journal of the International Confederation of Midwives*, Vol. 13, 4(2). The Netherlands: ICM.

Juva, M. (1994) The roots of development co-operation. In: Lankinen, K.S. *et al. Health and Disease in Developing Countries*, Ch. 3. London: Macmillan.

Kroeger, M. (2000) *Breastfeeding and HIV/AIDS*. Keynote address presented at NGO Networks for Health Workshop, Chiang Mai, Thailand, November. Conference Proceedings of NGO Networks for Health Chiang Mai Workshop.

Loudon, I. (1986) Obstetric care, social class and maternal mortality. *British Medical Journal* 293: 606–608.

Loudon, I. (1992) *Death in Childbirth. An International Study of Maternal Care and Maternal Mortality 1800–1950*, Vol. 30, pp. 1–41. London: Oxford University Press.

Maclean, G.D. (2000a) In: *Skilled Attendance at Delivery: A Review of the Evidence*. Paper prepared for the Safe Motherhood Technical Consultation, WHO, Geneva, April 2000.

Maclean, G.D. (2000b) *Skilled Attendance at Delivery, Reviewing the Evidence*. Paper presented at 'Improving Provider Performance' workshop, MotherCare, May 2000, Washington DC.

Maclean, G.D. (2000c) *Lessons Learned about the Impact Of Skilled Attendance at Delivery*. Keynote address presented at NGO Networks for Health Workshop, Chiang Mai, Thailand, November.

Madeley, J., Sullivan, D. & Woodroffe, J. (1994) *Who Runs the World*? London: Christian Aid.

NGO Networks for Health (2000) *The White Ribbon Alliance for Safe Motherhood, Information Card*. Washington DC: NGO Networks for Health.

Pendse, V. (1999) Maternal deaths in an Indian hospital: A decade of (no) change? In: Berer, M. & Ravindaran, T.K.S. (eds) (1999) *Safe Motherhood Initiatives: Critical*

Issues, pp. 119–126. Reproductive Health Matters. Oxford: Blackwell Science.

Rochat, R.W. (1981) Maternal mortality in the United States of America. *World Health Statistics Quarterly* 34(1): 2–13.

Royston, E. & Armstrong, S. (1989) *Preventing Maternal Deaths*. Geneva: WHO.

Senderowitz, J. (1995) *Adolescent Health: Reassessing the Passage to Adulthood. World Bank Discussion Papers* No. 72. Washington DC: The World Bank.

Seneviratne, H. & Peiris, G.L. (1997) In: *The New Challenge: Safe Motherhood at Ten*. Presented at the Safe Motherhood Technical Consultation, Sri Lanka, October. New York: Family Care International.

Safe Motherhood Initiative (SMI) (1987) *Preventing the Tragedy of Maternal Deaths. A Report of the International Safe Motherhood Conference, Nairobi, Kenya, February*. Geneva: WHO.

Spernbauer, M. (2000) The 2nd WHO Ministerial Conference on Nursing & Midwifery, 15–17 June 2000, Munich. *Journal of the International Confederation of Midwives* 13(4): 4–5.

World Health Organization (WHO) (1986) Maternal mortality: helping women off the road to death. *WHO Chronicle* 40(5): 175–183.

World Health Organization (WHO) (1990) *Facts about WHO*. Geneva: WHO.

World Health Organization (WHO) (1990–1994) *Safe Motherhood Newsletter, Various Issues*. Geneva: WHO.

World Health Organization (WHO) (1996) *Safe Motherhood Midwifery Education: Materials for Teachers of Midwifery*. Modules 1–5. Geneva: WHO.

World Health Organization (WHO) (1997a) *Maternal Health around the World. Summary Chart of Available Statistics*. Geneva: WHO.

World Health Organization (WHO) (1997b) *Coverage of Maternity Care. A Listing of Available Information*, 4th edn. Geneva: WHO.

World Health Organization (WHO) (1998) *Country Profiles of Reproductive Health Indicators*. Updated November 1998. Geneva: WHO.

World Health Organization (WHO) (1999) *Reduction of Maternal Mortality. A Joint Statement WHO/UNFPA/UNICEF/World Bank*. Geneva: WHO.

World Health Organization (WHO) (2000a) *Update of Statement on the 'Skilled attendant at delivery' in WHO (1999) Reduction of Maternal Mortality. A Joint Statement WHO/UNFPA/UNICEF/World Bank*. Geneva: WHO.

World Health Organization (WHO) (2000b) *Essential Care Series: (1) Essential Care Practice Guide for Pregnancy and Childbirth (2) Managing Complications in Pregnancy and Childbirth: A Guide for Midwives and Doctors*. (Draft document) Geneva: WHO.

World Health Organization (WHO) (2001) *Maternal Mortality in 1995: Estimates Developed by WHO, UNICEF, UNFPA*. Department of Reproductive Health & Research. Geneva: WHO.

World Health Organization South East Asia Regional Office (WHO SEARO) (1998) *Standards of Midwifery Practice for Safe Motherhood in SEAR Countries*. New Delhi: WHO SEARO.

FURTHER READING

Berer, M. & Ravindaran, T.K.S. (eds) (1999) *Safe Motherhood Initiatives: Critical Issues*. Reproductive Health Matters. Oxford: Blackwell Science.
The book provides valuable and extensive up-to-date information on maternal mortality and morbidity measurement. Case studies examine aetiological issues and the debates surrounding effective policies and programmes. When supplies are no longer available, the text will be obtainable on the World Wide Web: RHMjournal@compuserve.com

World Health Organization *Safe Motherhood: A Newsletter of Worldwide Activity*. Geneva: WHO
Published three times a year in English, French and Arabic. Providing news, reviews, special features. Resources and events relevant to Safe Motherhood activities worldwide are listed. Available free from WHO, Geneva (contact details below).

ADDITIONAL RESOURCES

Addresses
The British Council
10 Spring Gardens, London SW1A 2BN, UK

Center for Population & Family Health (Prevention of Maternal Mortality)

Columbia University, 60 Haven Avenue, Level B-3, New York, NY 10032, USA

Family Care International (FCI)
588 Broadway, Suite 503, New York, NY 10012, USA
Website: http://www.familycareintl.org

International Confederation of Midwives (ICM)
Eisenhowerlaan 138, 2517 KN The Hague, The Netherlands
Email: intlmidwives@compuserve.com

Program for Appropriate Technology
1990 M Street, NW, Suite 700, Washington, DC 20036, USA

The Royal College of Midwives (WHO Collaborating Centre)
15 Mansfield Street, London W1M OBE
The RCM library is situated at: 35 Portland Street, London W1F 1QB

White Ribbon Alliance for Safe Motherhood
c/o NGO Networks for Health, 1620 1 Street, NW, Suite 900, Washington, DC 20006, USA
Email: whiteribbonalliance@hotmail.com

World Alliance for Breastfeeding Action (WABA)
Email: secr@waba.po.my

World Health Organization Global Headquarters
CH-1211 Geneva 27, Switzerland
Regional Offices:
  Africa: PO Box 6, Brazzaville, Congo
  Americas: Pan American Sanitary Bureau, 525 23rd Street, NW, Washington, DC 20037, USA
  Eastern Mediterranean: PO Box 1517, Alexandria-21511, Egypt
  Europe: 8 Scherfigsvej, DK-2100, Copenhagen, Denmark
  South East Asia: World Health House, Indraprastha Estate, Mahatma Gandhi Road, New Delhi-110002, India
  Western Pacific: PO Box 2392, 1099 Manila, Philippines

Websites

Aga Khan Foundation
http://www.interaction.org/mb/akf_usa.html

Co-operative for Assistance & Relief Everywhere
http://www.care.org

Centre for Development & Population Activities
http://www.cedpa.org

Family Health International
http://www.fhi.org

Healthlink Worldwide
http://www.ahrtag.org/mission.html

International Confederation of Midwives (ICM)
www.intlmidwives.org

NGO Networks for Health
www.ngonetworks.org

Pathfinder International
www.pathfind.org

Prevention of Maternal Mortality Network
http://cpmcnet.columbia.edu/dept/sph/popfam/papers/PMM.html

World Alliance for Breastfeeding Action
http://www.waba.org.br

World Health Organization
http://www.who.int

66

Statutory Framework for Practice

Belinda Ackerman

LEARNING OUTCOMES

After reading this chapter you will be able to:

- understand the legislation surrounding midwifery practice
- appreciate the role and functions of the Nursing and Midwifery Council (NMC)
- be conversant with the Midwives Rules and Code of Practice and the midwife's statutory responsibilities for clinical practice

- be familiar with the role of the Local Supervising Authority Midwife
- have a working knowledge of the role of the Supervisor of Midwives
- understand the importance of the practitioner in maintaining individual PREP and portfolio requirements.

INTRODUCTION

This chapter provides an overview of the history of midwifery regulation, the profession's drive to remain in control of its legislation for the protection of the public, and the rules and codes by which midwives are supported. The role of midwifery supervision is discussed, and how this differs from but works in conjunction with midwifery management and is an integral component of clinical governance.

It is vital that midwives grasp the fundamentals of the unique professional support provided by midwifery supervision and use it to improve the quality of care given to women and their babies.

LEGISLATION REGULATING THE MIDWIFERY PROFESSION

Historical background

The first Midwives Act in 1902 sanctioned the establishment of a statutory body, the Central Midwives' Board for England and Wales (CMB), prescribed its constitution and laid down statutory powers. This came at a time when there was enormous opposition from the medical profession, who felt their livelihood was threatened and that the legal status of midwives

(who would charge a lower fee than doctors) would deprive them of some of their income (Jowitt and Kargar, 1997: 82). Opposition also came from the nursing profession (see Ch. 60). This Act was amended in 1918, 1926, 1934, 1936 and 1950. The Midwives Act of 1951 consolidated all previous Acts.

The Nurses, Midwives and Health Visitors Act of 1979 established a combined statutory structure for nursing, midwifery and health visiting in the UK. This consisted of the United Kingdom Central Council (UKCC) and four national boards (see Fig. 66.1). It established a register of the three professions, containing 15 parts to include all the different specialities of nursing. Midwives registered on Part 10. This was the first time midwives were amalgamated in law with other professional groups.

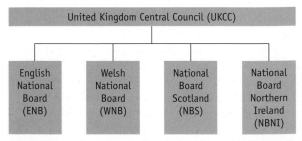

Figure 66.1 Statutory bodies for nursing, midwifery and health visiting.

This created particular concern within the profession that midwifery issues would be overruled by nurses who were in the majority on the Central Council. The Royal College of Midwives (RCM), alongside other midwifery groups including the Association of Radical Midwives (ARM), fought to ensure that a Midwifery Committee was set up in Statute (Jowitt and Kargar, 1997). This was finally accepted and agreed and all matters related to midwifery were to be delegated to the Midwifery Committee prior to review by the UK Central Council. Initial membership of the UKCC and four National Boards was approved and appointments made by the Secretary of State.

Changes to the management structure of the four National Boards in 1987 removed professional-specific Board education officers and replaced them with *generic* education officers. This resulted in midwifery education matters being dealt with by generic education officers, as education was no longer deemed to be specific to one particular profession. Despite protest from members at the time, the Midwifery Committee was overruled on this matter.

An external review of the functioning of the 1979 Act was commissioned by the Health Department in 1989, carried out by Peat Marwick McClintock (1989). The review recommended that the UKCC should become a directly elected body and membership of the National Boards should be smaller and appointed rather than elected. It suggested removing responsibility for the management and funding of education from the National Boards and placing it with regional health authorities, thus removing the professional accountability. National Boards were to be relegated to course validation and accreditation only.

Government proposals that followed in Working Paper 10 (DoH, 1989) suggested setting up the purchaser–provider model – hospitals would contract with education providers for the requisite number of places to fulfil local workforce planning. The future of midwifery education was moving towards greater integration with universities that would eventually reduce the Board's role and functions even further.

These recommendations were accepted by the Government (DoH, 1991; Northern Ireland Office, 1991; Scottish Office, 1991) and were incorporated into the 1992 Nurses Midwives and Health Visitors Act including the revised structure of the UKCC and National Boards. Consolidation of the 1979 and 1992 Acts incorporating all the reforms was made in the 1997 Nurses, Midwives and Health Visitors Act.

Recent changes to legislation

A further review of nursing and midwifery legislation was commissioned by the four UK health departments in 1997 and carried out by JM Consulting. This followed a change of government and its plans for modernization of the health service, including reforms of all professional regulation. The review caused uproar amongst the midwifery professional groups and lay women's groups such as the Association for Improvements in the Maternity Services (AIMS) and the National Childbirth Trust (NCT) as it appeared to diminish the role of the midwife.

Complete reform of the UKCC and four National Boards was required to deal with the four main issues that had arisen (JM Consulting, 1998):

- weakness in the powers to protect the public from unsafe practice
- changes in the healthcare environment and in the education, structure and roles of the professions
- changed public expectations of the accountability of health professionals
- devolution within the UK.

The drive to strengthen control of the healthcare professions followed several scandals involving nursing (Clothier *et al.*, 1994) and the medical profession (DoH, 2002a). The nurses, midwives and health visitors may have appeared to be the easiest and largest group of professionals to target. The majority are women and historically they have never held 'power' with governments in the same way as the medical profession. The next largest group of healthcare professionals are the professions allied to medicine (e.g. physiotherapists, dieticians, occupational therapists and chiropodists). It gave the Government the chance to use the same statutory template as that used for the nurses, midwives and health visitors.

The JM Consulting report recommended the setting up of a new Nurses and Midwives Act with its main purpose:

> to protect the public through setting and monitoring standards of professional practice, education, and conduct for nurses and midwives; and to influence the development of these professions in the public interest.
>
> (JM Consulting, 1998)

The Review recommended that the UKCC and the four National Boards be replaced by a smaller, more strategic Nursing and Midwifery Council with the ultimate responsibility for setting and monitoring standards of training and conduct.

The proposed changes gave nurses a $2:1$ majority for voting, thus setting midwives (and their care of women) back a century. Midwifery professional groups such as the RCM, ARM, the Association of Supervisors of Midwives (ASM) and the Independent Midwives Association (IMA) linked with lay maternity groups protested and meetings took place with JM Consulting following public consultation. The professional and lay groups all agreed that the only way forward was for midwives to return to separate legislation rather than succumb to being overruled by nurses.

As far as protection of the public was concerned, the midwifery profession had the lowest ever number of its members brought in front of the Professional Conduct Committee – possibly owing to the quality control conferred by statutory supervision of midwives.

In February 1999 the government response to the recommendations made in the Review accepted the need for new regulation of the 'various health professions' and proposed an amendment to the new Health Bill in progress at the time 'to make provision to repeal the Nurses, Midwives and Health Visitors Act 1997' (NHS Executive, 1999). Replacement legislation, by Order, regulating the professions was to be made subject to full consultation and publication of the Order in Draft. The third reading of the Health Bill took place in April 1999. The Regulation of Health Care and Associated Professions under Clause 47(2) and Schedule 3.1 of the Health Bill clearly stated the scope of the Secretary of State's powers of regulation via an 'Order' following a period of 3 months' consultation.

This haste to replace primary legislation and substitute it with a Statutory Instrument by 'Order' for Nursing and Midwifery was a departure from the normal practice of parliamentary procedure customary during the previous century. Nursing and midwifery legislation had previously been subject to professional scrutiny throughout all the earlier stages including a Green and White Paper. The midwifery protests to the restrictions of the legislation went unheeded.

Current legislation regulating midwifery

Health Act 1999 (Section 60)

The current legislation for midwives has been drawn up under the Health Act 1999 (DoH, 1999) which set out the Order for the changes from the previous UKCC to the new regulatory body now known as the Nursing and Midwifery Council.

Modernising Regulation – The New Nursing and Midwifery Council – A Consultation Document (NHS Executive, 2000)

This consultation document proposed the new structure of the UK body: the Nursing and Midwifery Council (NMC), to replace the United Kingdom Central Council (UKCC) set up in 1979. It proposed a smaller, more transparent Council that would not only have equal representation of elected nurses, midwives and health visitors from each country but also an emphasis on lay membership. The lay membership would be almost equal numerically to the professional membership with a lay chair. Partnership with the public was important to reduce concern about safety issues with self-regulation.

Establishing the new Nursing and Midwifery Council (DoH, 2001a)

The Government set out their plans for the new regulatory body, the NMC, in the form of draft legislation. It accepted that the NMC should be answerable to a more independent body and chose the Privy Council rather than the Secretary of State who may have been potentially biased as the main employer.

A 'shadow' Council was set up in May 2001 to ensure the seamless takeover from the UKCC. The shadow President was appointed alongside 24 nurses, midwives and health visitors (two from each country) and 11 lay members, totalling 35 members. Completion of work by the UKCC continued during this time with the revision of the Code of Professional Conduct, new processes for consulting the public and consumer organizations and development of guidance for local supervising authorities.

Modernising Regulation in the Health Professions – NHS Consultation document (DoH, 2001b)

The NHS Plan (DoH, 2000) set out the need to strengthen professional regulation and proposed the establishment of a *UK Council of Health Regulators* to act as a forum and coordinate complaints from all the professions and their regulatory bodies. The spotlight was on nurses and midwives to ensure that they put 'patients first' in their revised legislation, following the weaknesses identified in medical regulation.

This framework was also suggested in the Kennedy report on the Bristol Royal Infirmary Inquiry (DoH, 2002a). This Council would be independent of the State and accountable to Parliament, as would all the professional regulatory bodies, through the new Council. This in turn would have the power to require changes to the regulatory framework. It would not have the power to take over or intervene in individual fitness to practise cases.

Nursing and Midwifery Order 2001 Statutory Instrument 2002 No. 253 (DoH, 2002b)

The Orders to establish the Nursing and Midwifery Council were set out in Draft and laid before Parliament in October 2001 for approval under Section 62(9) of the Health Act 1999. Royal Assent was given in February 2002, and the Nursing and Midwifery Council were appointed and commenced office in April 2002.

Reflective Activity 66.1

Look on the Department of Health website and find the legislation that currently regulates your practice.

THE NURSING AND MIDWIFERY COUNCIL (NMC)

The Nursing and Midwifery Council (NMC) was established under the Nursing and Midwifery Order

2001 and came into force on 1 April 2002, succeeding the UKCC and four National Boards (Fig. 66.2). The ratio of nurses to midwives on the Council remains at 2 : 1. However, the concession to include a Midwifery Committee affords protection to the profession on all matters relating to midwifery, including midwifery education.

Function

The primary function of the NMC is protection of the public. This is maintained by:

1. establishment and maintenance of a register of all nurses, midwives and health visitors
2. setting standards for the education and training of all nurses, midwives and health visitors (including appointment of 'Visitors' to oversee education institutions)
3. establishment and review of the standards of conduct and performance of registrants to ensure fitness to practise.

The Midwives Rules are legally binding and the Midwives Code of Conduct and the Code of Professional

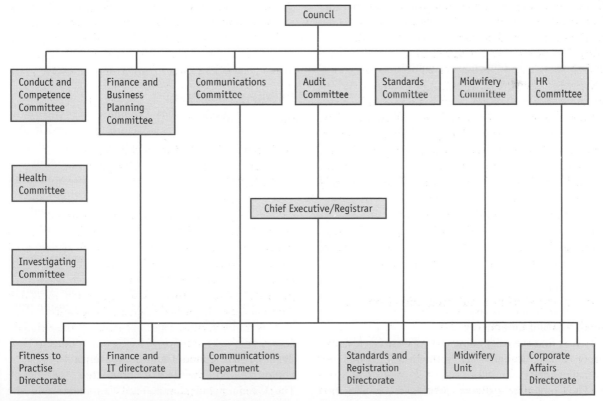

Figure 66.2 Nursing and Midwifery Council structure (from 2004).

Conduct (for all registrants) set standards and guide-lines for professional behaviour and accountability.

The Council has the power to remove a person from the Register, thus preventing the individual from practising as a nurse, midwife or health visitor. It also has a statutory duty to inform and educate registrants and to inform the public about its work.

Membership

The first Registrar was appointed by the Secretary of State. A transitional NMC membership was appointed by the Privy Council. This included an appointed President, Chairperson and a membership of 23 : 12 elected practitioners (four nurses, four midwives and four health visitors) and 11 appointed lay members. In addition 12 'alternate' members were to be elected, who could attend if the elected practitioner was unable to do so. Each member will serve a 4-year term of office and no more than three consecutive terms of office.

Statutory committees

The standards of conduct and performance of regis-trants set by the NMC are monitored by four statutory committees:

1. Investigating Committee
2. Conduct and Competence Committee
3. Health Committee
4. Midwifery Committee.

The first three committees have a strategic and oper-ational role. The role of the Midwifery Committee is to advise the Council on all matters that affect mid-wifery. The concept of a separate committee for mid-wifery was not laid down in the initial plans for the NMC. However, the RCM, ARM and other midwives made it abundantly clear that the profession needed to be in control of its own rules and standards. Midwives argued for and achieved the establishment of a Mid-wifery Committee on the UKCC and, with history repeating itself, did the same for the new NMC.

Investigating Committee

At this first level, preliminary screeners, lay and professionals, initially sift through the complaints and allegations.

The Committee's role is to investigate any allegation referred to it and to notify the registrant immediately

and invite written representations within a specific period of time. It decides whether there is a case to answer. If there is, it undertakes mediation via the Screeners, or refers on to the Health Committee or the Conduct and Competence Committee (DoH, 2002b).

Screeners are appointed by the NMC to 'consider the allegation and consider whether it is well-founded or whether the case should be closed'. The number of screeners on the panel must not be greater than the lay representation.

Conduct and Competence Committee

Its role is to consult: 'other Practice committees as it thinks appropriate and advise the Council on the standards of conduct, performance and ethics expected of registrants; requirements as to good character and good health to be met by registrants; protection of the public from registrants whose fitness to practise is impaired and consider any allegation referred to it by the Council, Screeners, the Investigating Committee or the Health Committee and application for restoration referred to it by the Registrar' (DoH, 2002b).

Health Committee

Its role is to consider: 'any allegation referred to it by the Council, Screeners, the Investigating Committee or the Conduct and Competence Committee and any application for restoration referred by the Registrar' (DoH, 2002b).

Midwifery Committee

The role of the Midwifery Committee is to advise the Council on any matters affecting midwifery. It also advises Council on the regulation of midwifery practice through rules. The rules include the procedure for sus-pension of a midwife from practice, the requirement for midwives to notify their annual 'intention to prac-tise' to the local supervising authority (LSA) midwife and the requirement of midwives to attend courses of instruction.

It advises Council on LSA midwives and establishes standards for the exercise of their function. The Council delegates the power of general supervision of all midwives practising in its area and suspension from practice to the LSAs.

Orders of the Conduct and Competence Committee and the Health Committee

The Conduct and Competence Committee and the Health Committee have to establish in cases referred

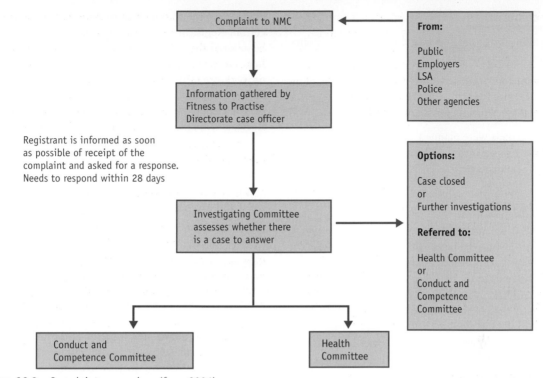

Figure 66.3   Complaints procedure (from 2004).

to them (see Fig. 66.3) whether fitness to practice is impaired. This is determined in Section 22(1) of the Order. They may decide on no further action; refer to the Screeners for mediation; or make one of the following orders to the Registrar:

a. a 'striking-off' order – this is for a minimum of 5 years and will probably be implemented for cases of misconduct

b. a 'suspension' order – not exceeding 1 year; this is more in respect of lack of competence (LOC) and health

c. a 'conditions of practice' order – not exceeding 3 years; this also is more in respect of LOC and health

d. a 'caution' order – not less than 1 year and not more than 5 years; the practitioner works normally and the caution remains on the register entry for the prescribed period.

An appeal may be made by the Registrant within 28 days of a committee's decision.

Restoration to the Register of persons who have been struck off

An application may be made before the end of 5 years, or in any period of 12 months in which an application

for restoration to the Register has already been made by the person who has been struck off. The application for restoration to the Register is made via the Registrar and is forwarded to the relevant Committee that made the 'striking-off' order. If the Committee is satisfied that the registrant has achieved the additional education or training or experience required, then the registration fee is paid and the practitioner is restored to the Register.

If an application is unsuccessful an appeal may be made within 28 days of the decision date. If a second or subsequent application is made while a striking-off order is in force and is rendered unsuccessful, the Committee may direct that the person be suspended indefinitely (DoH, 2001a).

Legal assessors and medical assessors

Legal assessors and medical practitioners (who may be appointed to be medical assessors) are employed to advise the Screeners, the Practice Committees, the Registrar and the Council if required.

Registrant assessors

Registered professionals may be appointed to give advice to the Council, committees of Council, Screeners or the Registrar.

Other committees

In addition, two joint (nursing and midwifery) policy committees were set up:

1. Registration Standards and Professional Development Committee
2. Strategic Resources and Planning Committee.

Advisory panels were planned, consisting of consumers and a professional from each profession across a wide range of practice areas.

Other requirements

The NMC are required to appoint legal assessors, medical assessors and registrant assessors to advise the Council or its committees as appropriate.

The current term of office for Council members expires in 2006. It is planned to create a new internal structure at the NMC to increase efficiency and effectiveness and to hold elections in 2004. 12 registrant members and 12 alternate members will stand for election and the lay members will continue to be appointed by the Privy Council. The Council elects its own president and vice-president.

FUNCTIONS OF THE NMC

The Register (Function 1)

The Council establishes and maintains the Register of qualified nurses and midwives. It ensures the Register is available for inspection by members of the public, though there is currently a debate concerning issues of confidentiality and anxieties about professionals' privacy if the Register is available to be viewed by members of the public.

The Register is divided into parts determined by the Privy Council. Following consultation in September 2002, it was agreed that in future it would only consist of three parts: Nursing, Midwifery and Specialist Community Public Health Nursing. The midwifery groups registered a negative response to the maintenance of three parts that includes *two* sections for nurses on the Register as it does not reflect the simplified legislation title in the 'Nursing and Midwifery' Order 2001.

Further consultation took place in May 2003 (via the NMC website and direct mailing to the professional midwifery groups and other stakeholders) as to what information from the Register should appear in the public domain. In the spirit of openness it has to offer certain Registrant information so that the public can be assured they can check whether a midwife is bona fide. However, if personal details of address and area of work are published, this could cause security problems in midwives' personal lives and would encroach on their right to privacy. It is planned that the new Register will come into effect in April 2004.

The Council determines the fee to be charged and coordinates initial registration or renewal to the Register.

Visiting EEA nurses or midwives are deemed registered and can practise in the UK subject to knowledge of English and comparable qualifications.

Setting standards for education and training (Function 2)

Pre-registration midwifery

The NMC is charged with establishing the pre-registration standards of education and training including requirements for good health and good character.

It appoints 'Visitors' to visit institutions and report back on the 'nature and quality of the instruction given, including facilities provided. The NMC Visitors are trained for their role and are midwives drawn from the profession. Visitors are not allowed to be NMC employees or employees of the universities being visited or anyone who has a close connection with the university through, for example, lecturing. Visitors are required to complete a report summarizing the information gained and are reimbursed by the NMC for expenses incurred. If the Council is of the opinion that the standards established under Article 15(1) are not met it may refuse to approve, or withdraw approval from the particular institution (DoH, 2002b).

Institutions are required to provide information to the Council about all the programmes they offer for registration to the different parts of the Register.

The *Requirements for Pre-registration Midwifery Programmes* (UKCC, 2000) were developed following the Peach Committee's report (UKCC, 1999). The midwifery competencies set out guiding principles to be followed by all pre-registration midwifery students during their education and training (UKCC, 2000). These competencies include: effective midwifery practice; professional and ethical practice; developing the individual midwife and others; and achieving quality care through evaluation and research. Universities are required by the NMC to have incorporated these competencies, in order to ensure the student has been tested against the standard required for professional 'fitness to practise' prior to registration as a midwife.

Fitness for practice

Changing public expectations and new patterns of health and maternity care led to the review of regulation of healthcare practitioners. In addition, concern had been expressed about the practical skills of newly qualified midwives (as well as nurses) and whether the learning environments were adequate for provision of women-centred care and autonomous practice. In response to this, the UKCC established a Commission for Education charged with providing 'an authoritative stance on pre-registration nursing and midwifery education'. The report *Fitness for Practice* (UKCC, 1999) produced 33 recommendations to ensure fitness for practice based on healthcare need including:

- Subject bench-marking of specific standards addressing outcomes consistent with the Quality Assurance Agency's (QAA) threshold for degrees and diplomas
- Consideration of pre-registration midwifery moving to an outcomes-based competency approach
- Charging service-providers with the responsibility to provide good-quality practice placements for students on pre-registration programmes and employment opportunities for newly qualified midwives
- The use of portfolios for practice and assessment through rigorous practice assessment tools
- 3 months' supervised practice towards the end of the pre-registration programme
- An expansion of graduate preparation for midwifery.

This final point linked to the NHS guidance and the requirement of higher education institutions (HEI) and trusts to increase the overall number of pre-registration nursing and midwifery degree commissions following extra funding from the DfEE (NHS Executive, 1998). The phasing out of rostered service was planned for all students beginning from September 1999. The increase in the number of midwifery students has to be carefully thought through and is dependent on the size of the maternity unit and number of midwifery staff that can provide mentorship to students. The numbers are carefully planned in line with the local Workforce Development Confederations (WDCs) so that students can be observed and mentored in a safe environment.

The Royal College of Midwives has set out recommendations for student learning environments in its recent strategy for education (RCM, 2003).

Quality Assurance Agency (QAA) benchmarks for midwifery

The QAA benchmarking statements for pre-registration midwifery education set out both Diploma and Honours Degree standards and incorporated a teaching, learning and assessment strategy (QAA, 2001).

These statements were developed in collaboration with other healthcare professions so that a common structure could be used. The section on teaching, learning and assessment highlights the importance of the central role of practice in the design of learning opportunities for students, and the importance of integrating theory and practice for professional competence.

HEIs are expected to set the QAA standards as a minimum for the award offered at the end of the programme. Thus, universities offering pre-registration midwifery programmes are required to comply with the professional standards set out by the NMC (UKCC, 2000) and the midwifery benchmark statements set out by the QAA (QAA, 2001). HEIs are subject to audit of both by two different bodies, though in reality the two have always worked together to prevent duplication.

Midwives Rules relating to pre-registration midwifery education

The Education rules are found in Section A of the *Midwives Rules and Code of Practice*, and span Rule 28 to 35 (UKCC, 1998). The Rules are currently undergoing review by the NMC and publication of the new Rules is expected in the spring of 2004.

Rule 28

- This states that the 'standard, kind and content of the programme of education' and the conditions of the person being admitted to a midwifery programme leading to registration as a midwife shall be in accordance with these sections of the Rules.

Rule 29

- Sets the minimum age of entry for midwifery education – 17 years and 6 months.

Rule 30

- Sets out the educational requirements for entry to an approved institution leading to registration as a midwife.

The proposal for greater flexibility in the proposed new rules (see above) in leaving the HEI to set the entry requirements, may lead to inequity across the UK as entry requirements may vary from city to city and may be lowered in some institutions in order to fill empty places.

Rule 31

- Sets the length of the long pre-registration midwifery programme (for non-nurses):
  - 3 years, with each year containing 45 'programmed weeks'; these students are protected by supernumerary status
  - 18 months – 'shortened' programme for nurses already registered with the NMC.

The 'shortened' programme has been the same length since 1981 (and has moved from certificate to degree level), and has been criticized for its shortness in preparing the midwife adequately for practice (see Ch. 70).

Rule 32

- Spells out conditions for students who have an 'interruption' to their training.

Greater flexibility is proposed in the new rules, which do not give a specific period of time for completion, but will require the student to complete the outstanding period of the training programme and meet the competencies set out by the NMC.

The bursary is only paid for a period of 3 years, which leaves no 'slack' in the system for students to reorientate back into clinical practice if, for instance, they have had maternity leave (there is no payment for maternity leave for bursaried students). Students may transfer between higher educational institutions subject to local arrangements.

Rule 33

- The outcomes of the education programme required by the NMC.

Instead of spelling out its requirements it will be worded to allow updating from the NMC when necessary.

The RCM has proposed a national curriculum for pre-registration midwifery in its strategy for education (RCM, 2003) in order to prevent major discrepancies of content nationally. This will require further discussion within the profession.

Rule 34

- Outlines the student indexing process.

Under the previous statutory framework, students were indexed with the National Board, and interruptions in training and completion were tracked. Students will no longer be indexed, and this rule will be deleted. This means that there will no longer be a national record of how many times a student has attempted different midwifery programmes nationally

and failed or been required to withdraw for poor professional practice. It will also be problematic in gathering national data on entry and attrition rates.

Rule 35

- Sets out the requirement of a student to have passed the assessment strategy approved by the NMC in order to qualify.

Post-registration education

Under the Nursing and Midwifery Order 2001 the NMC Council 'may make rules requiring registrants to undertake such continuing professional development as it shall specify in standards' (DoH, 2001b). Nurses and midwives who do not keep up their post-registration education and practice (PREP) requirements would then find their registration would 'cease to have effect' (DoH, 2001b).

Post-registration education and practice (PREP)

PREP is a set of standards and guidance developed originally by the UKCC in 1995 and carried forward by the NMC. It enables practitioners to demonstrate that they are keeping up to date with developments in professional practice and expanding knowledge and competence within their own field (UKCC, 2001b).

Every registrant is required to complete a minimum of 100 days (750 hours) during the 5 years prior to renewal of registration. Those practitioners who hold dual qualifications must demonstrate 100 days of practice in both nursing and midwifery (i.e. 200 days total).

The PREP continuing professional development (CPD) standard requires every registrant to undertake at least 5 days or 35 hours of learning activity within each 3-year registration period. A personal profile must be kept up to date to demonstrate this activity. For midwives, this will usually be discussed and agreed with the Supervisor of Midwives at the annual interview.

All practitioners are required to declare compliance with PREP requirements when they renew their registration every 3 years. Audit of compliance with PREP standards commenced in April 2001 and has been continued by the NMC (UKCC, 2001a).

Though universities provide quality control locally for post-registration programmes, Council may establish standards of training and education in respect to additional qualifications which may be recorded on the Register, and certain standards in relation to continuing professional development (DoH, 2001a).

For further information on midwifery education, see Chapter 70.

Midwives Rules relating to post-registration midwifery education
See practice rules below.

Establishment and review of the standards of conduct and performance of registrants to ensure fitness to practise (Function 3)

The Council is required to keep under review 'the standards of conduct, performance and ethics expected of registrants and prospective registrants and give them such guidance on these matters as it sees fit'. In addition, it must 'establish and keep under review effective arrangements to protect the public from persons whose fitness to practise is impaired' (DoH 2001a).

If any misconduct or lack of competence is reported about a registrant to the NMC, it is immediately referred to the Investigating Committee, then on to either the Health Committee or Conduct and Competence Committee.

The over-arching structure of the committees is laid down in the Nursing and Midwifery Order 2001 but the detail of the procedures to be followed is to be agreed and laid down by the Council. Such details are still under discussion at the time of writing, e.g. fitness to practise (see below).

Fitness to practise consultation
In preparation for establishing the new rules processes and procedures, the NMC sent out a consultation document to all the relevant stakeholders to elicit information on such issues as: the constitution of the new Practice Committees; the definition of fitness to practise; the definition of misconduct; lack of competence; standards of proof and other detailed questions. Publication of these will provide more detailed guidance to midwives, their supervisors and employers. The following definitions are proposed:

Fitness to practise A practitioner's suitability to be on the Register without restrictions (NMC, 2003a).

Misconduct Conduct which falls short of that which can reasonably be expected of a registrant (NMC, 2003a).

Lack of competence Lack of knowledge, skill, or judgement which may be accompanied by a negative attitude. This is of such a nature or extent that the nurse, midwife or health visitor is unfit to practise,

and that such concerns having been drawn to their attention, they have either:

- undergone training and supervision but have failed to make the required improvements to their practice, or
- refused to undergo further training or supervision (NMC, 2003a).

In dealing with lack of competence it is proposed to consider and process allegations in the same way as those currently alleging misconduct. The panel of the Conduct and Competence Committee will consider whether or not the facts are proved to the required standard. The present standard of proof used in professional conduct hearings is the criminal standard (facts must be proven 'beyond reasonable doubt'). It is proposed by the NMC that this is changed to the civil standard of proof (facts must be proven on a 'balance of probabilities') (NMC, 2003a).

Midwives Rules and Code of Practice (UKCC, 1998)
The NMC publishes rules and a code of practice for midwives, codes of practice for nurses and midwives, and general guidelines. These provide support to midwives in their practice and can be used to underpin practice development and problem-solving.

The *Midwives Rules* are part of the law and are therefore legally binding (Dimond, 2003). They are divided into regulation of education (discussed earlier), and practice and supervision (discussed below). For example, in Rule 40, midwives must call a doctor or relevant practitioner if a deviation from the norm occurs which is outside their sphere of practice. In other words, if a situation outside of 'normal midwifery' occurs and a midwife does not call for assistance from a suitably qualified practitioner, she or he will be found to be acting outside the law.

The NMC completed a consultation period in January 2003 on changes to the Rules in line with the new Statutory Framework and a revised edition is currently awaited.

The *Midwives Code of Practice* is a matter of guidance on the rules and can be used as the basis for determining whether there is evidence of professional misconduct (Dimond, 2003). An example is the use of homoeopathic medicines. A midwife must be familiar with the requirements of Rule 41 in relation to the administration of medicines. The midwife is reminded to comply with locally agreed policies and procedures. If self-medication has occurred and there are side-effects, the midwife has a responsibility to discuss this with the woman first then contact the relevant practitioner and seek advice (UKCC, 1998).

The NMC re-published some codes immediately following their inception such as:

The Code of Professional Conduct (NMC, 2002b)

This sets standards and guidelines for professional behaviour and accountability for all registrants. It incorporates gaining informed consent prior to treatment or care, maintenance of confidentiality, team working and good communications, maintenance of knowledge and competence, being trustworthy and minimizing risk to the clients.

Following publication of the Code of Professional Conduct, the NMC created a further 3-month period of consultation on the subject of professional indemnity insurance. The Council received legal advice suggesting its responsibility for protecting the public extended to proposing a requirement for all practitioners to take out such indemnity insurance if they were not already covered by their employer (Reyes-Hughes, 2002). The wide-ranging consultation resulted in the NMC ruling out making it a requirement and merely recommended it 'in principle' for independent practitioners. The RCM, RCN, Community Practitioners and Health Visitors Association jointly responded and raised concerns that a mandate for personal injury would allow insurance companies to dictate standards and shift the responsibility for ensuring safe practice away from employers (NMC, 2002c).

Guidelines for the Administration of Medicines (NMC, 2002d)

Principles in relation to the prescription, patient group directions, self-administration of medicines, complementary and alternative therapies and the various drugs Acts are listed and discussed.

Guidelines for Records and Record Keeping (NMC, 2002e)

The principles and purpose of record-keeping are discussed including the promotion of clinical care by improving communications, care plans, treatment, audit and evaluation of care given. The Acts related to documentation are listed.

Other codes published by the previous UKCC remain extant until new publications are made available. These can be accessed on the website: www. nmc-uk.org

Midwives Rules relating to midwifery practice (currently under revision)

Section B of the *Midwives Rules and Code of Practice 1998* sets out the practice rules and spans Rule 36 to 43.

Rule 36

- Requires midwives to notify their intention to practise annually to each LSA within each area of their practice.
- The notification is sent from the LSA to the NMC.
- A form is sent annually to all practising midwives by the NMC and must be completed and returned by March 31 to the midwife's individual supervisor of midwives who can update the NMC records electronically.
- Information about every midwife is forwarded by the supervisor to the LSA midwife who keeps a tally of all midwives practising within her jurisdiction.

Rule 37

- Related to refresher courses for midwives every 5 years and is now obsolete as it has been superseded by the NMC PREP rules (see above).

Rule 38

- Sets out the powers of the LSA to suspend a midwife from practice when necessary:
  - to prevent the spread of infection
  - in any case that has been reported to the NMC pending an investigation or proceedings referred via the Conduct and Competence Committee or Health Committee.
- A midwife would only warrant suspension from practice if considered a danger to the public pending the investigation, such as being under the influence of drugs or alcohol while caring for a mother or baby.

Rule 39

- Gives the LSA the powers to refer a midwife for a medical examination to prevent the spread of infection, such as a midwife who has contracted chickenpox or any other communicable disease.

Rule 40

- Sets out the midwife's responsibility and sphere of practice.
- Requires that midwives must be properly trained in an area of practice before they can undertake care or treatment, unless in an emergency.

- It also requires them to refer any cases outside their area of practice to the most appropriate professional. An example would be referring a women in delayed second stage to an obstetrician unless the midwife was a trained ventouse practitioner and able to carry out the procedure safely. (In the case of a woman experiencing a massive intrapartum haemorrhage, a midwife is trained to carry out a manual removal of a placenta as a life-saving measure pending transfer to obstetric care and theatres.)

Rule 41

- Sets out the requirement for midwives to administer medicines only if they have been trained in their use, dosage and side-effects.
- Midwives can give drugs locally under standing orders as well as individually charted prescriptions. An example would be giving a woman anti-D in either the antenatal or postnatal period. The midwife must be aware of the fact that this is derived from a blood product and discuss the exact purpose and actions of the drug and gain informed consent from the woman prior to administration.

Rule 42

- Requires a midwife to keep contemporaneous records and sets out details of their storage once a midwife ceases to practise.
- Following discharge, both mother and baby records will be stored by the health authority (or other suitable arrangement if a private case) for up to 25 years for legal purposes.

The value of such records is paramount as a form of communication about the plan of care for a woman and baby, especially in a midwifery group practice where a team of six midwives may be providing the total care. The records are usually kept with the woman until both mother and baby have been discharged from the care of the midwife.

Rule 43

- Requires midwives to allow access to the NMC for the purposes of inspection of their practice and premises.
- Inspection of NHS premises traditionally took place every 3 years by the English National Board. Since the inception of the NMC, the inspection of premises will now be undertaken by the LSA and reported back to the NMC. Independent midwives and private practice premises come under the same arrangements.

Supervision of midwives

Midwives Rules and Code of Practice 1998 relating to supervisors of midwives and local supervising authority midwives (currently under review)

Section B of the *Midwives Rules and Code of Practice 1998* set out the rules relating to supervisors and LSAs in Rules 44 and 45.

Rule 44

- Sets out the requirements for the appointment of a supervisor of midwives.
- It includes a minimum of 3 years' experience as a practising midwife and successful completion of an approved course of no less than 100 hours. Once appointed, the supervisor must complete at least 15 hours' study relating to supervision every 3 years.

Rule 45

- Sets out the functions of the LSA midwife.
- It includes the requirement of LSA midwives to publish information about how they will support supervisors of midwives and investigate prima facie cases of misconduct.

The new rules propose a change for the LSA role to 'discharge the statutory functions of the role in accordance with the standards which the Council shall from time to time require' (NMC, 2002a).

Proposed LSA standards (NMC, 2002a, 2003b)

The NMC is responsible for standards of midwifery practice and supervision and it sets the standards for how the LSAs perform their supervisory functions (NMC, 2003b). The draft standards proposed in the two NMC consultation documents propose the first-ever UK-wide framework for supervision (NMC, 2002a, 2003b).

The overall standards are expected to include the following: reporting to the NMC Midwifery Committee; compliance with Rule 44 of the Midwives Rules and Code of Practice; equity of access to a supervisor of midwives; communication; record-keeping systems; supervisory systems and investigation of misconduct allegations; and supporting and developing future leaders (NMC, 2002a).

Consultation issues in the second document cover the following areas: the appointment process of the LSA officer; investigation of poor performance of LSA midwifery officers and supervisors of midwives; LSA support for the supervision of midwives; public engagement with the supervision of midwives; midwifery access to supervision; and the leadership of LSA midwives (NMC, 2003b).

History of supervision

Statutory supervision of midwives began with the 1902 Midwives Act and the setting up of the CMB. The Board had a medical majority and was required to discipline midwives who disobeyed or ignored the Rules or who were guilty of negligence, malpractice or misconduct (personal or professional). The CMB delegated supervision and monitoring to local supervising authorities which were then under the control of county councils and county borough councils until 1973 when they came within the NHS.

The main function of the LSA was negative and punitive towards midwives, and supervision gained a bad reputation in the first half of the 20th century for over-investigating charges of misconduct, negligence or malpractice and reporting these to the CMB.

The 1936 Midwives Act empowered the CMB to make rules relating to the qualifications of medical and non-medical supervisors of midwives. It required the non-medical supervisors to be practising midwives. In 1937, a Ministry of Health letter was released which changed the approach of supervision to a more positive role, expanding on the detail of the 1936 Act, and said that inspectors of midwives were now to be known as supervisors of midwives; and most importantly it stated that the supervisor should act as a 'counsellor and friend'. It was still marred by the inclusion of the desirability of appointing a medical supervisor of midwives.

The 1973 NHS Reorganisation Act abolished LSAs under borough councils and nominated regional health authorities as LSAs. The delegation of duties to supervisors of midwives was nominated by district health authorities. The 1977 Statutory Instrument (SI) No. 1850 eradicated the role of 'medical supervisor' and removed the words 'non-medical' from the title of supervisor.

Since 1996, employment of LSA officers has been devolved to health authorities, many of which went into consortia arrangements. For the first time in history, LSA officers in England were required to be practising midwives. The 1999 reorganization of regional boundaries has meant LSAs work together more closely in some areas to provide a seamless service to supervisors and midwives.

Education and training for supervisors of midwives

In 1978 the CMB introduced courses of instruction for supervisors, initially only for those in post since 1974.

These courses later became mandatory before or immediately after appointment as a supervisor (Rule 44(2) Midwives Rules: UKCC, 1986). A formal open learning programme and training package 'Preparation for Supervisors of Midwives' was developed at diploma level in 1992 by the English National Board (ENB, 1992) and successful completion of the programme was required prior to being nominated to become a supervisor. It was updated by the ENB in 1997 and an NMC update is currently awaited.

The local supervising authority midwife

The Local Supervising Authority (LSA) is responsible for the provision of statutory midwifery supervision on behalf of the NMC (DoH, 2002b). The provision of the LSA became the responsibility of the new English health authorities under the Health Authorities Act 1995 which became effective in April 1996.

'Responsible Midwifery Officers' were appointed by the health authority to carry out the LSA function. Many health authorities have formed consortia and employ an LSA midwife to carry out the role across the consortium (ENB, 1999b).

The LSA officer was required to be a practising midwife in line with the DoH document *Managing the New NHS* (DoH, 1994).

The role of the LSA midwife is to provide leadership and support for supervisors of midwives in order to develop and improve professional practice. The ultimate goal is protection of the public. LSA midwives receive the annual notifications of intention to practise from the supervisors within their consortium. They appoint supervisors of midwives and develop standards that are audited annually. They ensure access to continuing education for midwives and meet regularly with the supervisors to agree strategies and guidelines (ENB, 1999b). They must ensure that systems are in place for investigating substandard care and any prima facie case of misconduct. The LSA midwife determines whether to suspend a midwife from practice in accordance with Rule 38 of the *Midwives Rules and Code of Practice* (UKCC, 1998).

Responsibilities of the Supervisor of Midwives

The role of the Supervisor of Midwives is a unique service of protection of the public and support of midwives in providing a high standard of care to women and their babies. It combines *professional* and *practice* responsibilities for challenging inferior practice and setting required standards as well as carrying out clinical audit, acting as a guide to midwives and ensuring the provision of a 24-hour service. Supervisors ensure that midwives have access to the statutory Rules and Codes and access to local clinical guidelines.

Supervision involves administrative and education tasks, including receipt of a midwife's Notification of Intention to Practise annually and ensuring adequate in-service education sessions to support midwives' practice. Supervisors audit records, arrange regular meetings with individual midwives, at least annually, and work with them to identify areas of practice that need development (ENB, 1999a). They monitor staffing levels and skill-mix in relation to safe practice, and notify senior management when there is a shortfall. They contribute to risk management and clinical governance within the NHS, investigate any allegations of professional misconduct and report upwards to the LSA (ENB, 1997).

Every midwife should have a named supervisor of her or his choosing. The ratio of supervisors to midwives should be 1:15 but locally may be reduced to 1:10 if there are adequate numbers of supervisors.

Reflective Activity 66.2

Have you been allocated a named supervisor? What is the ratio of midwives to supervisors in your locality?

Supervision in action

Statutory supervision has been found to enhance and empower midwives' practice where strategies are in place (Stapleton *et al.*, 1998). It offers a confidential, 24-hour support service to midwives working across the spectrum, both independently and within the NHS. Midwives can change their named supervisor if they feel the relationship has been compromised. In situations where midwives need more in-depth support than they have received from their supervisor, they can contact another supervisor or the LSA midwife directly for advice. There is no hierarchy in supervision and it is not trust-specific, though for practical purposes, most midwives will choose a supervisor employed within their trust. There are a number of supervisors who are employed in institutes of higher education and in the private sector.

Supervision ensures that education opportunities are accessible to support practice as the supervisor liaises with management and education to plan workforce development needs (ENB, 1997). This leads to well-educated and clinically confident and competent midwives who will provide a safe service to women and their babies.

Supervisors provide individual support to midwives who may have been involved in a critical incident and this can help with problem-solving, reflection and professional development. This support is separate from any management and risk management investigations (ENB, 1999a). Group supervision to reflect on clinical practice in a supportive and safe environment has been found to be effective and less time-consuming than individual supervision (Derbyshire, 2000), and is becoming a popular method of statutory supervision.

Allocation of a named supervisor to student midwives was recommended by the ENB in order to assist in the students' understanding and use of supervision at qualification and registration. Though it is a positive and proactive way of promoting the use of supervisors, it has not been readily taken up across England in areas where the supervisor : midwife ratios are high.

Supervision and management

> Supervision and management roles could be clarified by ensuring that, in every case, the distinction between suspension from practice and suspension from duty is made clear to all concerned.
> (Stapleton *et al.*, 1998)

Supervision and management are distinct and separate from each other, and midwives should be appraised of the difference. Midwives should be given access to a named supervisor who is not their manager so that the roles are not confused.

The differences that have been identified are shown in Table 66.1.

Supervision and clinical governance

Supervision is a vital component of clinical governance within the maternity services, supporting clinical risk management by its system of 'quality assurance' (Gorzanski, 1997). It provides a proactive service and can limit the volume of *serious adverse incidents* within an organization by the very nature of its practice and education support to every individual midwife in the UK. Specifically, supervisors can work with midwives and risk management to carry out the recommendations of the most recent reports on the Confidential Enquiry into Stillbirths and Deaths in Infancy (MCHRC, 2001) and Confidential Enquiry into Maternal Deaths (Lewis, 2001).

The Clinical Negligence Scheme for Trusts (CNST) Standards for Maternity Services has incorporated statutory supervision within its standards for the first time (NHS Litigation Authority, 2003). This publicly

Table 66.1   Management and supervision (ENB, 1996; North Thames RHA, 1995)

Manager	Supervisor
NHS trust/private company employee	Appointed by the LSA
Accountable to the employer	Accountable to the LSA and NMC
Has a job description and terms and conditions of service	Undertakes a statutory programme before taking up the role defined by the NMC
Holds a budget	Is not a budget holder
Must fulfil duties and responsibilities defined by the job description and updated in individual performance review	Must ensure midwives are safe and competent practitioners for the protection of women and their babies
Ensures a safe environment under the Health and Safety at Work Act, Employment Act and local trust/employment policies	Ensures safety through audit and monitoring of individual midwives' practice
Implements policies of employer	Promotes midwifery skills and competence through education and training, PREP and supervised practice according to the Midwives Rules and Code of Practice (UKCC, 1998) and Nursing and Midwifery Order 2001
Deals with poor performance and standards in accordance with the local employment policy	Handles incompetent practitioners through the statutory supervision process and education
Deals with complaints and takes disciplinary action if required	Deals with issues of professional misconduct and negligence and reports to the LSA if required
Can suspend from duty	Recommends suspension from practice to the LSA
Must be conversant with trust policies	Must be conversant with NMC Midwives Rules and Codes

confirms the importance of supervision working alongside risk management within a clinical governance framework.

Like risk management, supervision promotes the quality of care provided to women and their babies. The supervisors' involvement in the development of standards and clinical guidelines and their regular audit can be carried out jointly with risk managers. Potential problems and trends can be identified and acted upon to support midwives and protect the public (ENB, 1997).

The supervisor must ensure there is a system of record-keeping that is appropriate for child protection issues (Fowler, 1999) and ensure that midwives are aware of the local child protection policy and supported in their practice during any involvement in child protection cases. Multidisciplinary training can be arranged jointly by the supervisor and risk manager.

CONCLUSION

Midwifery legislation has provided over 100 years of statutory supervision, and protection of the public has been upheld through its quality and standards. The number of midwifery registrants referred to the regulating body for professional misconduct has remained insignificant, demonstrating a mature forward-thinking approach to continuing professional development.

The *Midwives Rules and Code of Practice* have been updated and changed as midwifery practice encompasses different challenges. The legislation has helped to promote the midwife's role as an expert in normal midwifery care through the use of evidence-based practice.

Previous and current government directives and legislation encourage transparency and partnership with the users of the service (DoH, 1993, 1999, 2000, 2001a). Midwives have always worked closely with the users of the service throughout their history and continue to do so through the NMC and RCM.

The *Nursing and Midwifery Order 2001* provides a challenge to midwives with regard to the protection of the midwife and therefore protection of the public. It remains to be seen whether midwives will need to campaign for a new Midwives Act, as despite the inclusion of a Midwifery Committee, a two-thirds majority of nurses on the Council could mean midwives losing control of their own profession.

KEY POINTS

- Midwives should be knowledgeable about the statutory framework within which they practise, which includes familiarity with the rules and codes of practice.
- The statutory framework provides safety of practice for women and their families.

- Midwifery supervision is a key part of clinical risk management and improving care for mothers and babies, and supporting and developing midwifery practice.

REFERENCES

Clothier, C., Macdonald, C.A. & Shaw, D.A. (1994) *The Allitt Enquiry*. London: The Stationery Office.

Department of Health (DoH) (1989) *Working for Patients: Education and Training*. Working Paper 10. London: HMSO.

Department of Health (DoH) (1991) *Statement by the Secretary of State for Health on Nursing, Midwifery and Health Visiting Education and the Future Role and Structure of the Statutory Bodies*. London: HMSO.

Department of Health (DoH) (1993) *Changing Childbirth. Report of the Expert Maternity Group*. London: HMSO.

Department of Health (DoH) (1994) *Managing the New NHS*. London: HMSO.

Department of Health (DoH) (1999) *Health Act 1999*. London: The Stationery Office.

Department of Health (DoH) (1999) *Making a Difference*. London: DoH.

Department of Health (DoH) (2000) *The NHS Plan; A Plan for Investment, A Plan for Reform*. London: DoH. Online. Available: http://www.nhs.uk/nhsplan

Department of Health (DoH) (2001a) *Establishing the New Nursing and Midwifery Council*. London: DoH.

Department of Health (DoH) (2001b) *Modernising Regulation in the Health Professions – NHS Consultation Document*. London: DoH. Online. Available: http://www.doh.gov.uk/modernisingregulation

Department of Health (DoH) (2002a) *Learning from Bristol: The Department of Health's Response to the Report of the Public Inquiry into Children's Heart Surgery at the Bristol Royal Infirmary 1984–1995. Executive Summary*. London: DoH.

Department of Health (DoH) (2002b) *Nursing and Midwifery Order 2001 Statutory Instrument 2002 No. 253*. London: The Stationery Office.

Derbyshire, F. (2000) Clinical supervision within midwifery. In: Kirkham, M. *Developments in the Supervision of Midwives*. Oxford: Books for Midwives Press.

Dimond, B. (2003) Midwifery Rules and Supervision. *British Journal of Midwifery* 11(2): 108–120.

English National Board (ENB) (1992) *Preparation of Supervisors of Midwives*, Module 1–4. London: ENB.

English National Board (ENB) (1996) *Advice and Guidance to Local Supervising Authorities and Supervisors of Midwives*. London: ENB.

English National Board (ENB) (1997) *Preparation of Supervisors of Midwives*, Module 1–4. London: ENB.

English National Board (ENB) (1999a) *Supervision in Action – A Practical Guide for Midwives*. London: ENB.

English National Board (ENB) (1999b) *Advice and Guidance – for Local Supervising Authorities and Supervisors of Midwives*. London: ENB.

Fowler, J. (1999) The role of the supervisor of midwives in child protection. *Maternity Matters* 80(Spring): 4–5.

Gorzanski, C. (1997) Raising the standards through supervision. *Modern Midwife* 7(2): 11–14.

JM Consulting (1998) *Regulation of Nurses, Midwives and Health-Visitors. Report on a review of the Nurses, Midwives and Health-Visitors Act 1997*. Bristol: JM Consulting.

Jowitt, M. & Kargar, I. (1997) *Radical Midwifery. Celebrating 21 Years of ARM*. Lancashire: Association of Radical Midwives.

Lewis, G. (ed) (2001) *Why Mothers Die 1997–99: Fifth Report of the Confidential Enquiries into Maternal Deaths in the United Kingdom*. London: CEMD: associated with NICE, RCOG.

Maternal and Child Health Research Consortium (MCHRC) (2001) *Confidential Enquiry into Stillbirths and Deaths in Infancy 8th Annual Report*. London: MCHRC.

NHS Executive (1998) *Changes in Pre-registration Nursing and Midwifery Degree Commissions. Extension of Practice Placements to all Pre-registration Nursing and Midwifery Students*. Health Service Circular 1998/149, 2 September. London: DoH.

NHS Executive (1999) *Review of the Nurses, Midwives and Health Visitors Act*. Health Service Circular HSC 1999/030 9th February. Leeds: DoH.

NHS Executive (2000) *Modernising Regulation – The New Nursing and Midwifery Council: A Consultation Document*. DoH. Online. Available: www.doh.gov.uk/nmcconsult

NHS Litigation Authority (2003) *Clinical Negligence Scheme for Trusts – Clinical Risk Management Standards for Maternity Services*. London: NHSLA.

North Thames RHA (1995) *Local Supervising Authorities for Midwives: Guidance for Midwives, Managers, Health Professionals and Consumers.* London: North Thames RHA.

Northern Ireland Office (1991) *Statement by the Secretary of State for Northern Ireland on Peat Marwick McClintock Review of Statutory Nursing Bodies.* London: HMSO.

Nursing and Midwifery Council (NMC) (2002a) *Consultation on Revised Midwives Rules and Proposed Standards for Local Supervising Authorities.* London: NMC.

Nursing and Midwifery Council (NMC) (2002b) *Code of Professional Conduct.* London: NMC.

Nursing and Midwifery Council (NMC) (2002c) *Regulator Listens on Indemnity Insurance Issue.* Press Statement, Nov 8th. London: NMC.

Nursing and Midwifery Council (NMC) (2002d) *Guidelines for the Administration of Medicines.* London: NMC.

Nursing and Midwifery Council (NMC) (2002e) *Guidelines for Records and Record Keeping.* London: NMC.

Nursing and Midwifery Council (NMC) (2003a) *Fitness to Practise. Consultation Background Information.* London: NMC.

Nursing and Midwifery Council (NMC) (2003b) *LSA Standards. Proposed Standards for Local Supervising Authorities and LSA Midwifery Officers.* London: NMC.

Peat Marwick McClintock (1989) Review of the United Kingdom Council and the Four National Boards for Nursing, Midwifery and Health Visiting. London: Peat Marwick McClintock.

Quality Assurance Agency for Higher Education (QAA) (2001) *Subject Benchmark Statements: Health care programmes: Midwifery.* 16th August. London: QAA.

Reyes-Hughes, A. (2002) *NMC News,* June 10th. Online. Available: www.nmc-uk.org/cms/content/news

Royal College of Midwives (RCM) (2003) *Valuing Practice: A Springboard for Midwifery Education.* London: RCM.

Scottish Office (1991) *Statement by the Secretary of State for Scotland on Policy Review of the Statutory Nursing Bodies and the Future Funding and Management of Nursing, Midwifery and Health-Visiting Education.* London: HMSO.

Stapleton, H., Duerden, J. & Kirkham, M. (1998) *Evaluation of the Impact of Supervision of Midwives on Professional Practice and the Quality of Midwifery Care.* London: ENB.

United Kingdom Central Council for Nursing, Midwifery and Health Visiting (UKCC) (1986) *Midwives Rules.* London: UKCC.

United Kingdom Central Council for Nursing, Midwifery and Health Visiting (UKCC) (1998) *Midwives Rules and Code of Practice.* London: UKCC.

United Kingdom Central Council for Nursing, Midwifery and Health Visiting (UKCC) (1999) *Fitness for Practice. The UKCC Commission for Nursing and Midwifery Education.* (Chair: Sir Leonard Peach) London: UKCC.

United Kingdom Central Council for Nursing, Midwifery and Health Visiting (UKCC) (2000) *Requirements for Pre-registration Midwifery Programmes.* London: UKCC.

United Kingdom Central Council for Nursing, Midwifery and Health Visiting (UKCC) (2001a) *The PREP Handbook.* London: UKCC.

United Kingdom Central Council for Nursing, Midwifery and Health Visiting (UKCC) (2001b) *Supporting Nurses, Midwives and Health Visitors Through Lifelong Learning.* London: UKCC.

ADDITIONAL RESOURCES

Nursing and Midwifery Council
Website: http://www.nmc-uk.org

Royal College of Midwives
Website: http://www.rcm.org.uk

67

Ethics and the Midwife

Shirley R. Jones

LEARNING OUTCOMES

After reading this chapter, you should be:

- aware of the difference between morality and ethics
- aware of the three areas of ethics and which of them is most applicable to practice
- able to recognize the importance of ethics in midwifery practice
- familiar with the difference between moral conflicts and dilemmas
- able to distinguish between the various normative ethical theories and their tenets

- able to apply certain pluralist duties within the duty of care
- able to recognize the need to uphold the principle of client autonomy in practice
- able to reflect on the ethical aspects of your practice
- able to follow up principles and issues raised in the chapter by further reading.

Ethics is now recognized as a major part of both midwifery education and practice; it permeates all professional relationships. Many childbearing women are no longer willing to be passive recipients of care; they expect to be fully informed of all aspects of their care so that they, rather than the professionals, make informed decisions, thereby retaining their autonomy and control. A knowledge of ethics will enable midwives to have a clear understanding of issues related to their practice and, in particular, of their role in empowering women to achieve a pleasurable, fulfilling experience of childbirth.

WHAT IS ETHICS?

Ethics is basically moral philosophy, or at least the vehicle by which we transport moral philosophy into practical, everyday situations. There is a tendency to consider 'moral' to be related to matters of sexuality; however, here it relates to the 'rights and wrongs' or the 'oughts and ought nots' of any situation. There are three levels to ethics:

1. *Meta-ethics* involves the deeper philosophy of examining everything in abstract; for instance, what we mean by 'right' and 'wrong'. In everyday situations we do not have time for this level of consideration.
2. *Ethical theory* aims to create mechanisms for problem solving, much as mathematicians created formulae for solving problems related to their field. Whether such theories are of use to midwives will be discussed later.
3. *Practical ethics*, as the term suggests, is the active part where the work of the moral philosophers is put into practice. It is also the area on which this chapter will generally concentrate.

For readers who wish to know more about some of the philosophers, a specific book is included in the list of annotated reading at the end of this chapter.

In everyday life, morality underpins our actions; particularly those which involve other people and their possessions. It is translated into our thoughts and actions by principles and concepts that we have learned since early childhood, such as truth-telling. This obviously should start within the family but there are outside influences: educational and religious institutions, the media and peer groups. This is not to say that all adults will behave within a given moral code. As is all too obvious, there are those who never receive the principles and concepts in the first place and others who choose to take a different path. However, these individuals will still be judged according to the code which is generally accepted by society at the time of the incident, and which underpins our civil law. Everyone has the right to expect that moral principles will be upheld; these, therefore, become 'moral rights'. As professionals in healthcare, it is important that midwives have a deeper understanding of morality than members of the general public. This depth of understanding is achieved by education regarding relevant moral principles, concepts and theories; by analysing real-life situations and posed dilemmas; by evaluation of the actions of ourselves and others. In this way we move from morality into ethics.

There are numerous principles, concepts and doctrines, some of which are listed below:

- Accountability
- Beneficence
- Non-maleficence
- Confidentiality
- Justice
- Autonomy
- Paternalism
- Consent
- Value of life
- Quality of life
- Sanctity of life
- Status of the fetus
- Acts and omissions
- Killing or letting die
- Ordinary or extraordinary means
- Double effect
- Truth-telling.

Further reading in relation to these principles, concepts and doctrines is suggested, sources for which are included at the end of this chapter, as these cannot all be discussed in depth here. However, autonomy will be discussed later in the chapter.

WHY IS ETHICS IMPORTANT IN MIDWIFERY?

Clients do not surrender their moral rights once they seek care; these rights have to be observed within their new experience, in any setting. In midwifery, care is very intimate – from the handling of personal information through the spectrum of physical, psychological, social and educational care. Added to this there is another dimension: there is no other field of human care where there is one person at the first point of contact and more than one at the end (obstetrics is considered with

midwifery here). This transition itself is the source of great complexity when decisions have to be made. An understanding of ethics will not only assist the carer to make decisions, it will also help with the empowerment of the clients to make informed decisions and assist the carer in understanding the basis of those decisions. There are ethical issues (i.e. debate or concern regarding the right and wrong actions) in all areas of midwifery. It is fairly easy to construct a list of the various areas from preconception care, through fertility and screening issues, to the end of the puerperium. Most people's lists would consist mainly of the highly emotive areas, which gain media coverage, but there are many issues involved in the care of 'normal' pregnancy, labour, puerperium and the neonatal period. Where there are ethical issues there is the potential for conflicts and dilemmas to occur.

Moral conflict

A moral conflict could be considered to be a show of strength within a moral principle, for instance the autonomy of the client versus that of the midwife or, more commonly, the autonomy of two or more professionals (Castledine, 1994). Both of these situations were seen with regard to *Changing Childbirth* (DoH, 1993). The recommendations were intended to create choice and flexibility, among other things, for those clients who wanted such a service. However, many midwives became anxious because the flexibility required was not compatible with their own family commitments. In some areas there was also tension between midwives, general practitioners and obstetricians. It could be argued that there had been this tension for many years, but it became more acute once the balance of power had to be seen to change.

A conflict could also arise between two or more different principles. On closer examination of the conflict one side becomes a clear winner. Consider the case outlined in Reflective Activity 67.1.

Reflective Activity 67.1

On immediate visual examination, a neonate is thought to have Down's syndrome and the mother's first question is: 'Is he alright?' Should the midwife protect the mother (non-maleficence) by answering 'yes', on the grounds that the Apgar scores were good and chromosome studies need to be performed for confirmation? Alternatively, should the midwife tell the truth and explain that tests are required to confirm the suspicion?

Ethically, telling the truth wins. The mother has the right to know, especially as a positive test will indicate to her that she was initially deceived and this could affect her ability to trust the midwives, or other healthcare professionals, in future encounters. Added to which, the mother's permission should be sought regarding tests to be performed on her baby; and she cannot consent unless she has the information. It is hoped that the reader can see, from this example, that a conflict is logical in resolution, once thought through properly. It is also acknowledged that in some units, in circumstances similar to this example, not all practitioners take this particular action; they obviously find that their clear solution is to protect the mother. Beauchamp and Childress (2001) feel that it is often this initial conflict which goes on to create the dilemma.

Moral dilemma

This starts as an apparent conflict between principles but, on further examination, there is no obvious solution, because the options are equally weighted but neither is satisfactory (Purtilo, 1999). One such dilemma is outlined in Case scenario 67.1.

The Code of Professional Conduct (UKCC, 1992), states that we must '…promote the interests of the patients and clients'.

What the client feels is in her best interests may not correspond with the midwife's view; it could be detrimental to the woman's condition, or that of her fetus. However, where at one time paternalism was virtually encouraged, the code now states:

> You must respect patients' and clients' autonomy, their right to decide whether or not to undergo any healthcare intervention – even where a refusal may result in harm or death to themselves or a [fetus], unless a court of law orders to the contrary.
> (NMC 2002: 3.2)

HOW ARE DILEMMAS SOLVED?

This is where level two of ethics is required – ethical theory. There are possibly nearly as many theories as there are philosophers, as they will all have their own particular stance, but generally speaking their views fit broadly into major theories. Two such theories of normative ethics, at either end of the spectrum, are utilitarianism and deontology.

Case scenario 67.1

A primiparous woman is admitted in established labour. She has a birth plan which states that under no circumstances will she give consent to an episiotomy. During the second stage of labour, progress is slow but positive; however, the perineum remains thick and rigid. The situation is explained to the woman but she maintains her position regarding episiotomy. As time progresses the fetal heart shows signs of slight distress, to the point where most midwives would consider episiotomy to be the action of choice, but still the woman withholds consent. The midwife could either continue and hope that the fetus will survive (obviously notifying appropriate personnel), or she could perform the procedure without consent, in order to protect the fetus. If she carries out the episiotomy without consent she could face a claim of battery against the woman. Neither is the ideal solution (Jones, 2000).

Utilitarianism

Utilitarianism is a consequentialist theory, where possible actions are considered in terms of their probable consequences. The original aim was for all actions to create the greatest happiness for the greatest number of people. Current thinking would probably use the term benefit rather than happiness, which would describe the essential outlook of those managing the National Health Service (NHS). It would also describe the intentions of Hitler in the Second World War, with his views of improving the human race, because, unfortunately, a belief within this theory is 'the end justifies the means'.

There are two forms of the theory: act-utilitarianism and rule-utilitarianism. The first is the purer form, developed in the 18th and 19th centuries by Bentham, Mill and Sidgwick (Norman, 1988), which expects every potential action to be assessed according to its predicted outcomes in terms of benefit. The second form does not look directly at the actual benefit of each act, rather it considers moral rules which are intended to ensure the greatest benefit, and each act is assessed as to its conformity to the rules.

Using in vitro fertilization (IVF) as an example, a technique initially researched in the concentration camps of the Second World War, it can be shown how these two schools of thought differ. Act-utilitarians would view the actions taken in light of the anticipated outcomes: many people today benefit from IVF, therefore, they may believe that this beneficial consequence justifies the research methods used. Rule-utilitarians, however, would want the benefit but would consider whether society would accept the means by which it was achieved. It is likely that they would want to find a more acceptable method of achieving the outcome.

Deontology

Deontology is a duty-based theory. Consequences are not considered, as deontologists believe that what is good in the world is brought about by people doing their duty. This theory divides into three schools of thought, each competing with the others as well as with utilitarianism. A well-known name in philosophy is Immanuel Kant (Norman, 1988). He developed *rational monism* which he believed was how people already thought – that one's actions should be rational and stem from 'good will'; he believed in duty for its own sake – the 'categorical imperative'. He used two tests for the moral value of an action. The first was whether it would be suitable if universalized, i.e. if everyone were to do it. The second test involved whether the act would use someone as a means to an end, which would not be acceptable, or as an end in himself, which would be acceptable as this is the basis of autonomy (Palmer, 1999). For instance, in a healthcare research project, is the research to benefit the individual (treating him as an end in himself), or to benefit others: treatment of future patients, achievement of academic acclaim for the researcher, or making a profit for a company (a means to someone else's end)?

The second school is *traditional deontology* (Jones, 2000); this is firmly seated in a belief in God and the sanctity of life. Each religion has its own model for behaviour, for instance Christians have the Ten Commandments. With this system there is little room for conflict, as it is possible to carry out all the commands at one time.

The third form is *intuitionistic pluralism*, where it is believed that there are a number of moral rules which are of equal importance; unfortunately the possibility of rule conflict exists. To minimize this, Ross considered seven *prima facie* duties which he felt were reasonable for people to abide by:

1. Duty of fidelity – this duty involves keeping promises, being loyal and not deceiving.
2. Duty of beneficence – the obligation to help others.
3. Duty of non-maleficence – not harming others; which is more stringent than the previous duty.
4. Duty of justice – to ensure fair play.
5. Duty of reparation – an obligation to make amends.
6. Duty of gratitude – to repay in some way those who have helped us (owed to special people such as parents); this also includes loyalty.
7. Duty of self-improvement.

(Jones, 2000: 22)

As these duties are equal in importance, it is still possible for conflict to arise between them. However, there is a system which can assist in such a conflict – *casuistry*; this system allows for the duties to be prioritized according to the circumstances.

Readers have probably already identified that, although the NHS is generally essentially utilitarian, midwifery, medicine and other similar disciplines tend towards a deontological approach. In fact, the duty with which we are most familiar – the duty of care – would appear to encompass at least the first four of the above duties. This deontological approach is certainly apparent in the Code of Professional Conduct (NMC, 2002).

To assist understanding of the different focus of utilitarianism and deontology when faced with a dilemma, Reflective Activity 67.2 offers a non-midwifery story; readers are invited to determine the end.

Reflective Activity 67.2

Jim is a botanist on expedition in South America. He finds himself in a small town where 20 Indians are lined up ready for execution, following acts of protest against the government. The captain, Pedro, having explained the situation, offers Jim a guest's privilege of killing one of the Indians himself. If he accepts, as a special mark of the occasion, the other Indians will be freed. If he refuses, then there is no special occasion and Pedro will have them all killed as previously planned (Smart and Williams 1988: 98–99).

You are Jim – what will you do?

If you are utilitarian then your decision would be to shoot one (which one is another problem), thus saving the other 19 as a consequence. As a deontologist, however, you would feel a duty 'not to harm' each man; nor would you don a mantle of responsibility and guilt for Pedro's actions.

As midwives, whatever our personal learnings may be, we may be professionally 'schizophrenic' with regard to our ethical actions. Consider the midwife in Case scenario 67.2.

On the first day Anita was carrying out her 'duty of care' for each client in line with her 'activities of a

Case scenario 67.2

Anita is an experienced F grade midwife. On Friday she was one of a team of on-duty midwives, students and healthcare assistants. She was allocated to a six-bedded postnatal bay, along with a student midwife, where they cared for six mothers and their babies. Although she was kept busy throughout her shift, Anita felt able to fulfil her specific duties to each individual in her care.

On Saturday, in the absence of a G grade midwife, Anita was in charge of the whole ward. There were 27 women, 12 of whom were antenatal, plus 14 babies, which included one set of twins – the babies of two of the women were in the neonatal unit. Having allocated staff to clients, Anita adopted a supervisory role, generally overseeing the care given, ensuring that staff were able to fulfil their duties.

Reflective Activity 67.3

Consider the tragic situation of the conjoined twins known as Mary and Jody (Walsh, 2000); there surely could be no greater professional dilemma for medical and legal practitioners than presented in this case. Analyse the situation through the different philosophical (not legal) viewpoints and determine the decisions which each school might have made.

If you had been a student or qualified midwife assisting in the care of Mary and Jodie, you might have been involved in a case conference. What view would you have put forward and what ethical justification would you have given?

midwife' (UKCC, 1998): this approach would be basically deontological, fulfilling duties to each individual. However, on the second day her remit was to ensure the greatest benefit for the greatest number – both clients and staff – by making decisions for the good of the ward as a whole. While clinicians at the bedside, or in people's homes, can be deontological in their approach, the further up the management line that is considered, the more it becomes obvious that a utilitarian approach is essential. It would not be acceptable to society, for instance, if the NHS purse were to be emptied by caring for a few; the limited resources are expected to do as much as possible for as many as possible.

It must be remembered, however, that most people have to deal with conflicts and dilemmas in their lives without knowledge of these theories. There are some philosophers in fact who suggest that it would be sufficient to teach rights and principles while omitting the formal theories. This idea is not supported by Hanford (1993: 979–982) who feels that teaching principles in place of theories (principlism) is 'reinforcing a sense of professional superiority among health care professionals', rather than creating 'a learning environment that promotes and enhances caring'. Whether we wish to embrace the formal or the informal approaches, it is important for healthcare professionals to know something about each of them, if only to understand how and why some decisions are made. It is also useful to have some idea of the approach which managers or clinicians might take when proposals for implementing schemes or changes are being made.

THE DUTY OF CARE

As health professionals, midwives have a duty of care to those persons who could be affected by their actions or omissions. In midwifery it is important to note that 'persons' relates directly to the mother and neonate. (Legally the fetus is not yet a 'person': readers may wish to pursue the subjects of 'personhood' and 'potential' in texts marked with an asterisk in the Further reading list.) This duty of care would include at least the first four deontological duties listed earlier; failure in the duty of care would result in a civil law case for negligence.

The duty of fidelity

The duty of fidelity requires us to avoid deceiving our clients and their families; this suggests, therefore, that promises should not be made if they cannot be kept and that truth-telling is paramount. An example used earlier, to illustrate a moral conflict, involved a baby with suspected Down's syndrome. If the practitioners involved were to withhold the truth from the mother, then they would be failing in their duty of fidelity, however good their motives might be. Verbal reports by students and qualified midwives suggest that this deception does occur sometimes, in the paternalistic belief that the mother is being protected.

The duty of beneficence

The duty of beneficence creates the obligation to help our clients. This is a positive duty which covers numerous activities, ranging from the various ways of helping to make them comfortable, to the educational aspects of caring for their babies. What this duty does not include is the paternalistic attitude so often experienced within the health service, where practitioners feel that they 'know what is best'. This attitude, although generally well meant, deprives the client of her right to self-determination (autonomy).

The duty of non-maleficence

The duty of non-maleficence is a negative duty – to do no harm. On the surface this would suggest that conducting unpleasant or painful procedures may breach this duty; this would be the case if the intention was to hurt the client. If the intention is to eventually benefit her and, knowing that she might experience pain or discomfort, she is in agreement, then there is no breach in duty. Administration of analgesic injections, the siting of an epidural analgesic or urinary catheterization would come into this category. This duty, although negative in its statement, can have a positive aspect; that of safety and protection from harm. This includes, among other things, consideration of the environment, observance of drug policies and adequate education and training of practitioners.

The duty of justice

The duty of justice requires us to treat our clients equally, without discrimination. For many people, the word 'discrimination' is immediately associated with terms such as race, skin colour or ethnic origin. While it is essential that we consider these areas, it is also important that we are aware of the other forms of discrimination which can occur, such as between articulate and less articulate clients. It is often easier to spend more time with the articulate clients, giving as much information and as much choice as possible, than it is with those who require greater explanations or who ask fewer questions. It could be argued that, to consider equality, we should aim to get all clients to the same endpoint; this would then necessitate that more time be spent with the less articulate clients.

PRINCIPLES

Contrary to Hanford's opinion (1993), the view being taken here is that knowledge of the underlying moral principles is important, if only to ensure that practitioners are 'talking the same language'. It is not possible, in one short chapter, to consider each of the major principles. However, in the author's opinion, one of the most basic moral principles is that of autonomy, since an understanding and observance of this principle should automatically lead professionals into the understanding and observance of many other principles.

Autonomy

> To be an autonomous person is to have the ability to be able to choose for oneself or more extensively to be able to formulate and carry out one's own plans and policies.
>
> (Downie and Calman, 1994: 52)

This definition suggests that autonomy involves self-control of one's actions and destiny. It could be argued that it is impossible to be totally autonomous, as society imposes certain rules, often sitting in judgement on the actions of individuals. However, there is a broad band of acceptability in most areas of life, at least in democratic societies, which gives individuals varying degrees of freedom of choice. What is expected of individuals is that their actions and decisions should be rational, i.e. based on sound reasoning. These decisions should then be accepted, whether or not they match the views of others, such as midwives and doctors.

For midwifery clients to make rational decisions about their care, the carers must ensure that sufficient information is given at the level and pace required by the individual. Many factors need to be considered. The *environment* should be conducive to the giving and receiving of information. The *language* that is being used should be in the 'mother tongue' of the client, with the avoidance of jargon and abbreviations. The *circumstances* in which a decision is required may vary, depending on whether there is time for contemplation or a fairly urgent situation is faced. Having given the information, it is also important for professionals to assess the client's understanding of it.

Having determined that a client has made an informed decision based on what she thinks is sound reasoning, i.e. an autonomous decision, health professionals have no right to overrule that decision (ICM, 1999). This principle is inextricably bound to informed consent: if the client is autonomous then nothing should be done to her without her prior consent; to do so would be to commit a trespass against the person, i.e. battery (Jones, 2000). If her consent is being sought, then she is being considered to be autonomous; therefore a situation should not arise where, on her refusal to consent to a procedure, professionals attempt to overrule her. There are two groups of people who might be deemed to be not autonomous, therefore unable to give consent. One group includes children, but there is no longer a set age, it depends on the circumstances and degree of rationality of the child (DoH, 1989). The other group includes those who are mentally incapacitated, either by disability or by severe mental illness. With both groups, consent by proxy would be sought. There is also the possibility of temporary mental incompetence, in cases of unconsciousness or possibly the effects of drugs (including alcohol). In such cases the professionals would be expected to act out of necessity, in the best interest of the client, unless there was sound evidence that the client would refuse consent if aware of the situation, such as a Jehovah's Witness carrying a card refusing blood products.

It is the author's firm belief that, if client autonomy were truly considered, then it would be unlikely that the varying aspects of the duty of care would be breached. This would not remove situations of conflict and dilemma, but it would make decision-making more straightforward, with all practitioners working to the same ground rules. The use of reflective practice would assist in this area, by midwives analyzing and reflecting upon their actions, particularly with regard to their observance of autonomy, then using this experience to formulate their plans for future decision-making.

Reflective Activity 67.4

Client autonomy

At the end of a shift, consider the clients for whom you cared. In each case consider:

- Which aspects of her care did you discuss with her?
- Which aspects of her care did you not discuss with her?
- What information did you give her?
- What decisions did she make?
- What decisions did you make?
- Did you accept her decisions or did you try to change then?
- What did you write in the records?
- Did you enable her to be autonomous?
- In light of this exercise, what will you do in similar circumstances in the future?

Client autonomy is a relatively new concept. The autonomy of the midwife, however, is not new. Midwives have used the term 'autonomous practitioner' for many years, particularly when trying to explain to the uninitiated the difference between nurses and midwives. Unfortunately, however, this autonomy is not always evident in practice, particularly in the hospital setting. Midwives often plead that they are constrained by the policies within which

they are expected to work. This pleading suggests that, either the policies are too constrictive for both the midwife and the woman, and should be addressed, or that the midwives are comfortably hiding behind them.

Reflective Activity 67.5

Midwife autonomy

Consider your last working week. How many times did you do the following:

- Inform a client that the proposed course of action was 'policy'?
- Discuss the relevant policy with the client but include the alternatives?
- Politely challenge a colleague's (any discipline) decision or course of action because it was not evidence based?
- Notify your manager or supervisor of midwives that a policy needs to be reviewed?
- Make a decision based on the circumstances, not on the policy, then *inform* the appropriate person (midwife-in-charge, registrar, consultant) rather than *ask* him or her?
- Assertively justify a decision in relevant documentation, as opposed to wording suggestive of 'covering your back'?

On reflection, given the same circumstances in the future, which of these actions would you change?

CONCLUSION

This chapter is intended to help readers to accept the need for awareness of moral rights along with the will of individual practitioners to uphold them. An understanding of ethics will help midwives to make decisions in difficult circumstances, even if they do not choose to directly follow the theories outlined. The author firmly believes that observance of ethical principles, in particular autonomy, is the most direct route to assisting childbearing women to have the degree of choice and control which each individual feels is right for her. It is possible that the woman who achieves control in childbearing is better placed to do so in the parenting years ahead of her. By practising in this way, the midwife will also be fulfilling personal, professional accountability.

KEY POINTS

- Ethics is essential to professional midwifery practice.
- There are numerous ethical principles with which midwives and their students should be familiar.
- Moral conflicts and dilemmas cannot be avoided in some cases; they can be disconcerting but must be resolved. Theories and principles are available to help resolve the dilemmas.

- Professional practice in the NHS requires both deontological and utilitarian consideration.
- The duty of care has an ethical basis and is not only a legal principle.
- Client autonomy is an essential basis for good midwifery practice – it also enables midwife autonomy.

REFERENCES

Beauchamp, T.L. & Childress, J.F. (2001) *Principles of Biomedical Ethics*, 5th edn. Oxford: Oxford University Press.

Castledine, G. (1994) Is respect for patient autonomy declining? *British Journal of Nursing* 3(16): 847.

Department of Health (DoH) (1989) *The Children Act*. London: HMSO.

Department of Health (DoH) (1993) *Changing Childbirth*. Report of the Expert Maternity Group. London: HMSO.

Dimond, B. (1994) The duty of care. *Modern Midwife* **4**(8): 17–18.

Downie, R.S. & Calman, K.C. (1994) *Healthy Respect – Ethics in Health Care*, 2nd edn. Oxford: Oxford Medical Publications.

Hanford, L. (1993) Ethics and disability. *British Journal of Nursing* 2(19): 979–982.

International Confederation of Midwives (ICM) (1999) *International Code of Ethics for Midwives*. The Hague, Netherlands: ICM.

Jones, S.R. (2000) *Ethics in Midwifery*, 2nd edn. London: Mosby.

Norman, R. (1988) *The Moral Philosophers*. Oxford: Blackwell.

Nursing and Midwifery Council (NMC) (2002) *Code of Professional Conduct*. London: UKCC.

Palmer, M. (1999) *Moral Problems in Medicine*. Cambridge: Lutterworth Press.

Purtilo, R. (1999) *Ethical Dimensions in the Health Professions*, 3rd edn. Philadelphia: W.B. Saunders.

Smart, J.J.C. & Williams, B. (1988) *Utilitarianism For and Against*. Cambridge: Cambridge University Press.

United Kingdom Central Council for Nursing, Midwifery and Health Visiting (UKCC) (1998) *Midwives Rules and Code of Practice*. London: UKCC.

Walsh, A. (2000) Can a life ever not be worth living? *British Journal of Midwifery* 8(9): 536–538.

FURTHER READING

Ashcroft, B. (1998) Court-ordered caesarean sections: a midwife's dilemma. *British Journal of Midwifery* 6(4): 259–261.
This is just one of a number of articles dealing with the facts and issues inherent in these cases.

Beauchamp, T.L. & Childress, J.F. (2001) *Principles of Biomedical Ethics*, 5th edn. Oxford: Oxford University Press.
This book is a good starting point for gaining depth of understanding of ethical theory beyond the narrow application to midwifery.

Bowden, P. (1997) *Caring, Gender-sensitive Ethics*. London: Routledge.
As midwives deal mainly with adult women, reference to this book which deals with ethics through gender sensitivity might be enlightening to some readers.

Frith, L. (ed) (2003) *Ethics and Midwifery*, 2nd edn. Oxford: Butterworth-Heinemann.
This book contains chapters by different authors on different contemporary issues. It would be natural to progress to this book having grasped the fundamentals of ethical theory and its relationship to and usage in midwifery.

Harris, J. (ed) (2001) *Bioethics*. Oxford: Oxford University Press.
This book has chapters related to beginning and end of life issues, the value and quality of life and professional ethics; all of which are important in midwifery.

House of Commons Health Committee (2003) *Inequalities in Access to Maternity Services*: Eighth Report of Session 2002–3. The Stationery Office.
This report was produced along with the Ninth Report, identified below, when the 'Drown Committee' was appointed 'to examine the expenditure, administration, and policy of the Department of Health and its associate bodies'.

House of Commons Health Committee (2003) *Choices in Maternity Services*. Ninth Report of Session 2002–3. The Stationery Office.

This report was produced by the 'Drown Committee', in addition to the one above, and supersedes *Changing Childbirth*. Every practising midwife should become familiar with it and with the Government's response.

Jones, H. (1996) Autonomy and paternalism: partners or rivals? *British Journal of Nursing* 5(6): 378–381.

Jones, S.R. (2000) *Ethics in Midwifery*, 2nd edn. London: Mosby.
This book outlines major theories and principles, applying them to midwifery and obstetric practice. Analysis of case studies is used for the purpose of assisting readers in the application of theory to practice.

Jones, S.R. (2001) *Ethico-legal Issues in Women's Health*. In: Andrews, G. (ed) *Women's Sexual Health*, 2nd edn. London: Baillière Tindall.
Childbearing is just one aspect of women's lives (and not all women). It is important for midwives to study more broadly into women's health in order to enrich their knowledge of those for whom they provide a service.

Norman, R. (1988) *The Moral Philosophers*. Oxford: Blackwell.
This book is very useful to 'dip into' to discover something about the philosophers who we find referenced in the various texts. It enables a certain amount of understanding of where their views come from.

68

Law and the Midwife

Bridgit Dimond

LEARNING OUTCOMES

After reading this chapter you will be able to:

- understand the language and sources of the law
- have an understanding of the legal framework within which you work
- make judgements as to when expert help needs to be brought in
- ensure that your practice is within the law
- advise your patients and families.

INTRODUCTION TO THE LAW: THE COURTS AND HOW LAWS ARE MADE

The courts (Fig. 68.1)

The main courts dealing with criminal proceedings are the Crown Courts and the Magistrates Courts. Those dealing with civil proceedings are the High Court, the County Courts and the Small Claims Courts. The Court of Appeal and the House of Lords will hear both criminal and civil cases.

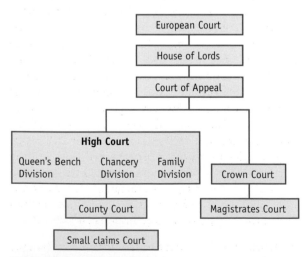

Figure 68.1   The court hierarchy.

In addition to the court system outlined above, there are Coroners Courts and various administrative tribunals which also administer the law, for example Employment Tribunals.

Whilst Northern Ireland and Scotland share the main legislative provisions of England and Wales, they also have their own statutes in particular areas. Since devolution, Wales is able to enact its own statutory instruments.

Classification of the law

The most common distinction made is between criminal and civil law. A criminal offence is where the law (statute or common law – see below) forbids a particular activity which can then be followed by criminal proceedings against the accused. The prosecution must establish beyond reasonable doubt the guilt of the accused. In the Crown Courts, if the accused pleads not guilty, a jury will hear the case and determine guilt or innocence.

Civil proceedings take place between individuals and organizations in order that one party can obtain a remedy (e.g. an injunction forbidding the other party to act in a particular way) or compensation. In civil courts, the standard of proof is 'on the balance of probabilities'.

Some actions may give rise to both civil and criminal proceedings. Thus touching a person without the person's consent may be both a trespass to the person (which is a civil matter) and also constitute the criminal offence of assault or battery.

Another distinction in law is that between private and public law:

- *Private law* is concerned with matters between private individuals and others or between organizations. It comes within the ambit of civil law.
- *Public law* is concerned with matters affecting the public. This comprises constitutional law, administrative law and the criminal law.

Some statutes may cover both areas: thus the Children Act 1989 has some sections which deal with matters of a private nature; others deal with public issues such as the role of local authorities in child protection.

Sources of the law

The law recognized in this country derives from two main sources:

- legislation – Acts of Parliament statutory instruments and Regulations and Directives of the European Union
- common law, which is formed from decisions made by courts in particular cases – this is also sometimes known as *judge-made law* or *case law*.

Legislation

Since Britain joined the European Union (EU) it is obliged as a member state to ensure that EU Directives and Regulations are enforced in this country, and appeals can be made to the European Court of Justice.

In this country, when legislation is proposed, the usual practice is for a consultation paper to be issued (known as a *Green Paper*). Following consideration of the feedback, a *White Paper* is then issued setting out the Government's intentions. The contents of this White Paper are incorporated into a Bill which is then passed through the various stages of Parliament and, when agreed by both House of Commons and House of Lords, is signed by the Queen. The Bill then becomes an Act and comes into force on a date set either in the Act itself or at a later date set out in a Statutory Instrument. The Act of Parliament may provide for the delegation to Ministers and others of powers enabling detailed rules to supplement the Statute to be enacted. These are known as *Statutory Instruments* or *secondary legislation*. They must be placed before Parliament before coming into effect.

Common law

Decisions by judges in courts create what is variously known as the common law, case law or judge-made law. The decisions of the courts create precedents which may be binding on courts below them in the court hierarchy. This is called the Doctrine of Precedent. Thus decisions of the House of Lords are binding on those courts below it, but not itself; and decisions of the Court of Appeal are binding on itself and those courts below it.

The Doctrine of Precedent relies on a recognized system of reporting of judges' decisions, which ensures certainty over what was stated and the facts of the cases. The decisions are recorded in law books such as the *All England Law Reports* or the *Weekly Law Reports*. Every case is identified by the year it was heard, the volume number and page number. For example the case of *Bolam v. Friern Hospital Management Committee* is cited as [1957] 1 WLR 582. This means that it was reported in 1957, in the first volume of the *Weekly Law Reports* at page 582. It is also reported in other series such as the *All England Law Reports*.

The main principles which are set out in a case are known as the *ratio decidendi* (reasons for the decision). Other parts of a judge's speech which are not considered to be part of the ratio decidendi are known as *obiter dicta* (things said by the way). Only the *ratio decidendi* are directly binding on lower courts, but the *obiter dicta* are said to be 'persuasive' because they may influence the decision of judges in later court cases. It may be possible for judges to 'distinguish' the current case under consideration from previous cases and not follow them on the grounds that the facts are significantly different.

The Human Rights Act 1998

The European Convention for the Protection of Human Rights and Fundamental Freedoms (1951) provides protection for the fundamental rights and freedoms of all people. The UK is a signatory, as are many European countries which are not members of the European Union. Thus Norway is a signatory to the European Convention on Human Rights but not a member of the European Union. The Convention is enforced through the European Commission and the European Court on Human Rights, which meets in Strasbourg. However, following the passing of the Human Rights Act 1998, since 2 October 2000 most of the articles are directly enforceable in the UK courts in relation to public authorities or those exercising functions of a public nature. (In Scotland, the Act came into force on devolution of power to the Scottish Parliament.) Of particular significance in healthcare are:

- Article 2 and the right to life, which may be used to justify the allocation of more resources, and has already been used (unsuccessfully) to press for the continuation of treatment for a severely disabled baby (*A National Health Service Trust v. D*, 2000).

- Article 3 and the right not to be tortured or subjected to inhuman or degrading treatment or punishment. (It has been argued that chaining a pregnant prisoner to a bed during her confinement is a breach of Article 3.)
- Article 5 and the right to liberty and security.
- Article 6 and the right to a fair trial (this includes civil hearings and tribunals as well as criminal proceedings).
- Article 8 and the right to respect of privacy and family life.

Other articles may also be relevant to the rights of patients and employees.

Under the Human Rights Act 1998, judges have a duty to refer back to parliament for its consideration, legislation which they consider is incompatible with the rights set out in the European Convention. Parliament can then decide if that Act should be changed. The existence of a right to take a case for violation of rights to the courts of this country does not prevent a person taking a case to the European Court in Strasbourg.

Reflective Activity 68.1

Read through and consider Article 3 of the European Convention on Human Rights and analyse the extent to which any woman could claim that her rights under this Article are infringed.

Midwives Rules and the Code of Professional Conduct

Under the Nurses, Midwives and Health Visitors Act 1997, the regulation of nursing and midwifery was undertaken by the United Kingdom Central Council for Nursing, Midwifery and Health Visiting (UKCC) supported by country boards. This included the development of rules regulating the practice of midwives, codes of practice and practice guidelines. Box 68.1 indicates the purpose of these rules, which are set out under Statutory Instruments, and Box 68.2 sets out the midwife's responsibility and sphere of practice.

The statutory system of the regulation of nursing, midwifery and health visiting set out in the Nurses, Midwives and Health Visitors Act 1979 (as amended by the 1992 Act) went through radical changes following a review of the statutory bodies (JM Consulting 1998) and the revised Health Act (1999) and Orders

---

Box 68.1 Aims of the Midwives Rules

1. Determine the circumstances in which and the procedure by means of which midwives may be suspended from practice.
2. Require midwives to give notice of their intention to practise to the local supervising authority in the area in which they intend to practise (in addition if midwives practise in an emergency outside their normal authority they have to notify the new health authority within 48 hours).
3. Require registered midwives to attend courses of instruction in accordance with the rules.

Box 68.2 Rule 40: Responsibility and sphere of practice

1. A practising midwife is responsible for providing midwifery care to a mother and baby during the antenatal, intranatal and postnatal periods.
2. Except in an emergency, a practising midwife shall not provide any midwifery care, or undertake any treatment which she has not, either before or after registration as a midwife, been trained to give or which is outside her current sphere of practice.
3. In an emergency, or where a deviation from the norm which is outside her current sphere of practice becomes apparent in the mother or baby during the antenatal, intranatal or postnatal periods, a practising midwife shall call a registered medical practitioner or such other qualified health professional who may reasonably be expected to have the requisite skills and experience to assist her.

(UKCC, 1998a: 17/8)

(2002). In April 2002 the UKCC and the National Boards were replaced by a streamlined Nursing and Midwifery Council (NMC). All publications of the former UKCC are now under the NMC remit, though some documents (currently under revision) are in original UKCC format.

The UKCC produced the Midwives rules and code of practice (UKCC 1998), formerly two documents. Codes of practice are complementary to the rules but, unlike the practice rules, do not have the force of law. Of course, the midwives would also be expected to comply with the NMC Code of Professional Conduct (NMC 2002a) and other guidance from the NMC. Every midwife should ensure that they have copies of all the relevant UKCC/NMC guidance.

Supervision

Midwives are the only group of health professionals to have a statutory system of supervision. Appointed by the local supervising authority, the supervisor of midwives has clear statutory responsibilities in relation to the positive promotion of a high standard of midwifery practice, and the protection of the public.

LITIGATION AND CLINICAL NEGLIGENCE

The scale of the problem

In 2001, the National Audit Office (NAO) carried out a study on the handling of clinical negligence claims in England. The NAO noted that the majority of cases were against acute trusts, particularly those with obstetric and gynaecology services. Money spent on legal claims cannot be spent on patient care, therefore the NAO emphasized the importance of effective claims management so that:

- claims with merit are settled quickly and cost-effectively
- disputed claims are defended robustly
- claims with no merit are not pursued.

Box 68.3 highlights some key facts from the NAO study.

The NAO recommended action to reduce the time taken to conclude cases, provide patients and relatives with more information when things go wrong so that they do not feel that legal action is the only way to obtain the answers they need, and find alternatives to legal action so that small and medium claims can be resolved – for example identifying non-financial remedies and offering mediation. The NAO also recommended providing trusts with incentives to reduce the incidents that lead to claims (i.e. improve risk-management arrangements) and ensuring that performance measures are developed for the solicitors working for the NHS so that they can be closely monitored.

NEGLIGENCE

What is negligence?

Negligence is the most common civil action, brought in situations when the claimant alleges that there has been personal injury, death or damage or loss of property. Compensation is sought for the loss which has occurred. To succeed in the action, the claimant has to

> **Box 68.3 Clinical negligence claims in England: key facts from the NAO study**
>
> - Around 10 000 new claims were received in 1999/2000.
> - At 31 March 2000, provisions to meet likely settlements for up to 23 000 outstanding claims were £2.6 billion. In addition, it was estimated that a further £1.3 billion would be required to meet likely settlements for claims expected to arise from incidents that have occurred but not been reported.
> - Only 24% of claims funded by the Legal Services Commission (formerly Legal Aid) are successful.
> - The total annual charge to NHS income and expenditure accounts for provisions for settling claims has risen sevenfold since 1995/96.
> - Cerebral palsy and brain damage cases account for 80% of outstanding claims by value and 26% of claims by number in the Existing Liabilities Scheme.
> - For claims closed in 1999/2000 with settlement costs in excess of £10 000, the average time from claim to payment of damages was 5½ years.
> - In 65% of settlements in 1999/2000 below £50 000, the legal and other costs of settling claims exceeded damages awarded.

show the following elements:

1. that the defendant owed to the person harmed a duty of care
2. that the defendant was in breach of that duty
3. that the breach of duty caused reasonably foreseeable harm
4. that the claimant has suffered harm.

Duty of care

The law recognizes that a duty of care will exist where one person can reasonably foresee that his or her actions and omissions could cause reasonably foreseeable harm to another person. A duty of care will always exist between the health professional and the patient, but it might not always be easy to identify what it includes. Where there is no pre-existing duty to a person (e.g. an existing professional and patient relationship), the usual legal principle is that there is no duty to volunteer services (i.e. perform a 'good Samaritan' act). The NMC recognizes that there may be a professional duty to volunteer help in certain circumstances (NMC, 2002a).

In one case the House of Lords defined the duty of care owed at common law (i.e. judge-made law) as being:

> You must take reasonable care to avoid acts or omissions which you can reasonably foresee would be likely to injure your neighbour. Who then in law is my neighbour? The answer seems to be persons who are so closely and directly affected by my act that I ought reasonably to have them in contemplation as being so affected when I am directing my mind to the acts or omissions which are called in question.
>
> (*Donoghue* v. *Stevenson*, 1932)

Reflective Activity 68.2

Consider any incident of which you are aware, when harm (nearly) occurred to a woman or baby. What potential hearings could take place as a result of this harm and what would have to be shown to secure a conviction/guilt/liability?

Breach of duty

Determining the standard of care In order to determine whether there has been a breach of the duty of care, it will first be necessary to establish the required standard of care. The courts have used what has become known as the 'Bolam Test' to determine the standard of care required by a professional. In the case from which the test took its name the court laid down the following principle to determine the standard of care which should be followed: the standard of care expected is 'the standard of the ordinary skilled man exercising and professing to have that special skill' (*Bolam* v. *Friern Hospital Management Committee*, 1957).

The Bolam Test was applied by the House of Lords in a case where negligence by an obstetrician in delivering a child by forceps was alleged:

> When you get a situation which involves the use of some special skill or competence, then the test as to whether there has been negligence or not ... is the standard of the ordinary skilled man exercising and professing to have that special skill. If a surgeon failed to measure up to that in any respect (clinical judgement or otherwise) he had been negligent and should be so adjudged.
>
> (*Whitehouse* v. *Jordan*, 1981)

In this particular case, the House of Lords found that the surgeon was not liable in negligence and held that an error of judgement may or may not be negligence. It depends upon the circumstances.

This standard of the reasonable professional man following the accepted approved standard of care can be used to apply to any professional person: architect, lawyer, accountant as well as those working in health. The standard of care which a practitioner should have provided would be judged in this way. Expert witnesses would give evidence to the court on the standard of care they would expect to have found in the circumstances before the court. These experts would be respected members of the profession of obstetrics and midwifery, possibly a head of a department or training college, and lawyers would look to the leading organizations of individual professional groups to obtain recommended names.

In a civil action, the judge would decide in the light of the evidence that has been given to the court, what standard should have been followed.

The standards at the time of the alleged negligence apply; not the standards at the time of the court hearing. This is significant, since many cases take several years to come to court, in which time, standards may have changed. Reference is made to literature and procedures which applied at the time of the alleged negligence to establish if a reasonable standard of care was followed.

Experts can of course differ. A case may arise where the expert giving evidence for the claimant states that the accepted approved standard of care was not followed by the defendant or its employees. In contrast, the expert evidence for the defendant might state that the defendant or its employees followed the reasonable standard of care. Where such a conflict arises the House of Lords has laid down the following principle:

> It was not sufficient to establish negligence for the plaintiff (i.e. claimant) to show that there was a body of competent professional opinion that considered the decision was wrong, if there was also a body of equally competent professional opinion that supported the decision as having been reasonable in the circumstances.
>
> (*Maynard* v. *W Midlands Regional Health Authority*, 1985)

The determination of the reasonable standard of care has been more recently considered by the House of Lords in the case of *Bolitho* v. *City and Hackney Health*

Authority, when it was stated that:

> The court had to be satisfied that the exponents of the body of opinion relied on can demonstrate the such opinion has a logical basis. In particular in cases involving, as they often do, the weighing of risks against benefits, the judge, before accepting a body of opinion as being responsible, reasonable or respectable, will need to be satisfied that, in forming their views, the experts had directed their minds to the question of comparative risks and benefits and had reached a defensible conclusion on the matter.
>
> The use of the adjectives 'responsible, reasonable and respectable' (in the Bolam case) all showed that the court had to be satisfied that the exponents of the body of opinion relied upon could demonstrate that such opinion had a logical basis.
>
> It would seldom be right for a judge to reach the conclusion that views held by a competent medical expert were unreasonable.
>
> (*Bolitho* v. *City and Hackney Health Authority*, 1997)

Recent government documents (DoH, 1997, 1998, 1999, 2000) have placed increasing emphasis on standard setting, clinical governance and effective risk management. The National Institute of Clinical Excellence (NICE), the Commission for Health Improvement (CHI), from April 2004 the Commission for Health Care Audit and Inspection (CHAI), and the National Service Frameworks (NSF) are leading to more guidance on standards to be achieved in all departments of a hospital and in community care. They are described in more detail later in this chapter and in Chapters 61 and 66. It is anticipated that these standards will be incorporated into the Bolam Test of reasonable professional practice. Practitioners will be expected to follow the results of clinical effectiveness research in their treatment and care of patients. Patients will be able to use these national guidelines to argue that inadequate care has been provided in their case, as a result of which they have suffered harm.

Midwives who decide that in the light of the specific circumstances of a case, a procedure or protocol or guideline is not entirely appropriate should ensure that clear documentation is completed of all the circumstances and the reasons for the inappropriateness of the guideline, so that their practice can be seen to be justifiable against the standard of the reasonable practitioner.

Communication – between professionals, departments and with patients – is crucial to a reasonable standard of care. This is particularly important where one person is designated as the key worker on behalf of the multidisciplinary team. However, the Court of Appeal has stated that the courts do not recognize a concept of team liability and it is therefore for each individual professional to ensure that his or her practice is according to the approved standard of care (*Wilsher* v. *Essex Area Health Authority*, 1986). Professionals should not take instructions from another professional which they know would be contrary to the standard of care that their profession would require. Failure to follow up a cytology report led to compensation being paid to the dead patient's husband (*Taylor* v. *West Kent Health Authority*, 1997). This is supported by the Code of Conduct for nurses, midwives and health visitors which states that *when facing professional dilemmas, your first consideration in all activities must be the interests and safety of patients and clients* (NMC, 2002:9)

Has there been a breach of the duty of care?   Once it has been established in court what the reasonable standard of care should have been, the next stage is to decide whether or not what took place was in accordance with the reasonable standard, i.e. whether there has been a breach of the duty of care or not. Evidence will be given by witnesses of fact as to what actually took place. Clear comprehensive documentation will be an important element in determining the facts of what took place.

Causation

The claimant must show that not only was there a breach of the duty of care, but that this breach of duty caused actual and reasonably foreseeable harm to the claimant. This requires:

- factual causation to be shown, and also
- evidence that the type of harm that occurred was reasonably foreseeable
- there to have been no intervening cause which breaks the chain of causation.

Factual causation   There may be a breach of the duty of care and harm, but no link between them. In the case of *Barnett* v. *Chelsea Hospital Management Committee* (1968), a casualty officer failed to examine patients who came to the A&E department, when they were vomiting very badly. However, the widow of one was unable to obtain compensation, since it was established on the facts that because the man was suffering from arsenic poisoning, he would have died even if reasonable care had been provided. The breach of duty by the doctor did not therefore cause the man's death.

The onus is on the claimant to establish that there is this causative link between the breach of the duty of care and the harm which occurred. In the case of *Wilsher* v. *Essex Area Health Authority* (1988), the claimants failed to establish that excess oxygen (resulting from the placing of a catheter to monitor oxygen in the vein, rather than in the artery) had caused the retrolental fibroplasia suffered by the baby. The House of Lords ordered a new hearing on the issue of causation, because excess oxygen was only one of five factors which might have caused the blindness. The parties then agreed to a settlement.

Reasonably foreseeable harm   The harm which might arise may not be within the reasonable contemplation of the defendant so that even though there is a breach of duty and there is harm, the defendant is not liable. This is because a negligent act may set off a 'chain reaction' of consequences and the courts have decided that there should be some limit on the liability of the defendant. For example, a practitioner may have delivered the wrong dose of a drug, and therefore be in breach of the duty of care, but the client may have become more ill because of an underlying medical condition, not because of the wrong dose.

No intervening cause which breaks the chain of causation   It may happen that any causal link between the claimant's breach of duty and the harm suffered by the client is interrupted by an intervening event.

Harm

The final requirement to succeed in an action for negligence is that claimants or their representatives must establish that the claimant has suffered harm which the court recognizes as being subject to compensation. Personal injury, death, loss or damage to property are the main areas of recognizable harm. In addition the courts have ruled that nervous shock where an identifiable medical condition exists (now known as post-traumatic stress syndrome) can be the subject of compensation within strict limits of liability. A test of proximity to the defendant's negligent action or omission has been set by the House of Lords.

Vicarious and personal liability

As stated above, it is unlikely that employees will be sued personally, since the employer will usually be vicariously liable for their actions. The NHS's responsibility for the actions of employees (which in certain circumstances includes students, trainees and volunteers) was clarified by guidance issued in 1996 (NHSME, 1996) – referred to as 'NHS indemnity'.

To establish the vicarious liability of the employer the claimant must show the *employee* was *negligent* or was guilty of another wrong whilst acting in the *course of employment*.

Independent practitioners would have to accept personal and professional liability for their actions but they may also be vicariously liable for the harm, caused during the course of employment, by anyone they employ. Each of the elements shown above must be established so that employers are not liable for the acts of their independent contractors (i.e. self-employed persons who are working for them on a contract for services) unless they are at fault in selecting or instructing them.

The employer may challenge whether the actions were performed in the course of employment. For example, a midwife may have undertaken training in a complementary therapy such as acupuncture. If she used these new skills whilst at work, without the express or implied agreement of the employer, and through use of this therapy caused harm to the client, the employer might refuse to accept vicarious liability on the grounds that the employee was not acting in the course of employment.

Liability for student, unqualified assistant: supervision and delegation

Exactly the same principles apply to the delegation and supervision of tasks as to the carrying out of professional activities. Midwives delegating a task, should only do so if they are reasonably sure that the person to whom the task is delegated is reasonably competent and experienced to undertake that activity safely. They must also ensure that the person undertaking that activity has a sufficient level of supervision to ensure that the delegated activity can be carried out reasonably safely. Should harm befall a client because an activity was carried out by a junior member of staff, student or assistant, it is no defence to the legal action to argue that the harm occurred because that person did not have the ability, competence or experience to carry out that task reasonably safely (*Wilsher* v. *Essex Area Health Authority*, 1986). There will be some midwifery tasks, such as attendance at a birth, which can never be delegated. Other activities may be delegated if the delegatee is assessed as competent and the requisite level of supervision is provided.

Defences to an action

The main defences to an action for negligence are listed below:

- Dispute allegations
- Deny that all the elements of negligence are established
- Contributory negligence
- Exemption from liability
- Limitation of time
- Voluntary assumption of risk.

Dispute allegations

Many cases will be resolved entirely on what facts can be shown to exist. Thus the effectiveness of the witnesses for both parties in establishing the facts of what did or did not occur will be the determining factor in who wins the case. Clearly, record-keeping and the witnesses in court will play a significant role in determining the facts of what took place. It might appear before the court hearing that one party has a particularly strong case, but unless the facts on which its case rests can be proved in court or are admitted by the other party, the actual outcome of the case might be that the opponent wins.

Deny that all the elements of negligence are established

The claimant must establish that all elements required to prove negligence are present, i.e. duty, breach, causation and harm. If one or more of these cannot be established, then the defendant will win the case. In some situations, the claimant may be able to claim that 'the thing speaks for itself' (i.e. a *res ipsa loquitur* situation). This means that the claimant will say that there is no explanation for the damage other than a negligent act having taken place. If this claim is made, the defendant is then required to explain how what has happened could have occurred without negligence on his or her part.

Contributory negligence

If the claimant is partly to blame for the harm which has occurred, then there may still be liability on the part of the professional but the compensation payable might be reduced in proportion to the claimant's fault. In extreme cases, if 100% contributory negligence is claimed, such a claim may be a complete defence. In determining the level of contributory negligence, the physical and mental health and the age of the claimant would be taken into account.

The Law Reform (Contributory Negligence) Act 1945, enables an apportionment of responsibility for the harm that has been caused, which may result in a reduction of damages payable. The Court can reduce the damages 'to such extent as it thinks just and equitable having regard to the claimant's share in the responsibility for the damage.' (Section 1(1)).

One of the most frequent examples of contributory negligence being taken into account is in road traffic accidents where the injuries sustained by the claimant are greater because the claimant was not wearing a seat belt.

Exemption from liability

It is possible for people to exempt themselves from liability for harm arising from their negligence, but the effects of the Unfair Contract Terms Act 1977 mean that this exemption only applies to loss or damage to property. A defendant cannot exclude liability from negligence which results in personal damage or death either by contract or by a notice. A midwife could not therefore agree with a woman that she would provide her with a waterbirth on the understanding that the mother would not hold the midwife (or the midwife's employer) liable for any negligence.

Where exemption from liability for loss or damage to property is claimed by the defendant, it must be shown by the defendant that it is reasonable to rely upon the term or notice which purported to exclude liability. The provisions of the Unfair Contract Terms Act 1977 are shown in Box 68.4.

Reasonableness in relation to a notice not having contractual effect, means that: 'it should be fair and reasonable to allow reliance on it, having regard to all the circumstances obtaining when the liability arose or (but for the notice) would have arisen.' (Unfair Contract Terms Act 1977: S.11 (3)).

Under Section 11(5) it is for those claiming that a contract term or notice satisfies the requirements of reasonableness, to show that it does.

> **Box 68.4 Unfair Contract Terms Act 1977**
>
> S.2 (1) A person cannot by reference to any contract term or to a notice given to persons generally or to particular persons exclude or restrict his liability for death or personal injury resulting from negligence.
> S.2 (2) In the case of other loss or damage, a person cannot so exclude or restrict his liability for negligence except in so far as the term or notice satisfies the requirement of reasonableness.

The effect of this legislation, is that notices which purport to exempt a department from liability for negligence are invalid if that negligence leads to personal injury or death. However, a notice which excludes liability for loss or damage to property may be valid if it is reasonable for the negligent person or organization to rely upon it.

Limitation of time

Actions for personal injury or death should normally be commenced within 3 years of the date of the event which gave rise to the harm, or 3 years from the date on which the person had the necessary knowledge of the harm and the fact that it arose from the defendant's actions or omissions. There are, however, some major qualifications to this general principle and these are shown in Box 68.5.

The implication of the rules relating to limitation of time is that, in those cases which might come under one of the exceptions to the 3-year time limit, records should be kept and not destroyed. This is particularly important in the case of children and those with learning disabilities. For example, one case was brought 18 years after the birth (*Bull and Wakeham* v. *Devon HA* (1989)). In a news item report in 1995, a man now aged 33 obtained compensation of £1.25 million because of a failure to diagnose severe dehydration a few weeks after birth (Laurance, 1995).

The definition of knowledge for the purposes of the limitation of time is that a person must have knowledge of the following facts:

- that the injury in question was significant
- that the injury was attributable in whole or in part to the act or omission which is alleged to constitute the negligence, nuisance or breach of duty

Box 68.5 Situations where the limitation of time can be extended

- Those suffering from a disability:
  - children under 18 years – the time does not start to run until the child is 18 years
  - those suffering from a mental disability – time does not start to run until the disability ends. In the case of those who are suffering from severe learning disabilities or brain damage this may not be until death.
- Discretion of the judge. The judge has a statutory power to extend the time within which a claimant can bring an action for personal injuries or death, if it is just and equitable to do so.

- the identity of the defendant
- if it is alleged that the act or omission was that of a person other than the defendant, the identity of that person and the additional facts supporting the bringing of an action against the defendant.

Knowledge that any acts or omissions did or did not, as a matter of law, involve negligence, nuisance or breach of duty is irrelevant. A person is not fixed with knowledge of a fact ascertainable only with the help of expert advice so long as he has taken all reasonable steps to obtain and, where appropriate, to act on, that advice.

Voluntary assumption of risk

Volente non fit injuria is the Latin term for the defence that a person willingly undertook the risk of being harmed. It is unlikely to succeed as a defence in an action for professional negligence since professionals cannot contract out of liability where harm occurs as a result of their negligence (see Box 68.4). The defence of *volenti non fit injuria* would not be available to an employer as a defence against a midwife who argued that she had been exposed to HIV/AIDS as a result of negligence by her employer. The employers have a duty to take reasonable care of the health and safety of employees and it cannot be argued successfully that an employee accepts a risk of being harmed as an occupational hazard, where the employer has failed in its duty of care.

Compensation

The legal term for the amount of compensation to be paid is *quantum* (literally how much?). The general rule governing the award of damages is that they should compensate the claimant for the loss he has suffered. This means that the claimant should be restored to the position he would have been in but for the negligent act. The following is an example of a case where following negligence at birth, the baby suffered from cerebral palsy of a spastic quadriplegic type. Liability was admitted and compensation of £1 849 890 was awarded, including the amounts shown below. The damages awarded reflect the additional costs of caring for the claimant for the rest of his life and thus it is necessary to calculate the claimant's life expectation. A calculation is made of the annual cost of looking after the claimant. The idea of the award is that it will pay for the cost of looking after the claimant until his death, and thus damages are calculated on the basis that the income and part of the capital will be spent each year. In order to work out the damages that should be paid, the annual cost of care is multiplied by the 'multiplier'. In this particular case, it was agreed that the claimant's expectation of life was reduced by 10 years to 64, that the appropriate lifetime multiplier for the purposes of the agreed damages was 17 with a multiplier of 12 for loss of earnings.

General damages	£115 000
Past care	85 000
Other special damages	37 320
Future care	937 783
Future loss of earnings	121 586
Other future expenses	277 065

(including physiotherapy, computer aids, occupational therapy, chiropody, mobility, personal care, seating, bed, clothing, transport, security and leisure)

(*Dyer (A Minor)* v. *Lambeth, Southwark and Lewisham Health Authority*, 1999)

There are two kinds of damages: *general* and *special* damages. *Special damages* refer to the actual financial losses between the negligent act and the trial (or settlement if there is no trial), for example loss of earnings, purchase of special equipment or adaptations to the home and the costs of medical and nursing care. *General damages* basically reflect compensation for pain and suffering from the injury and loss of amenity (reduced enjoyment of life) plus future financial losses, for example loss of earnings and future expenses.

In some cases of negligence, liability might be accepted by the defendant, but there might be disagreement between the parties over the amount of compensation. In others, both liability and quantum might be in dispute.

CONSENT

It is a general legal and ethical principle that valid consent must be obtained before starting treatment or physical investigation, or providing personal care, to a patient. This principle reflects the right of patients to determine what happens to their own bodies, and is a fundamental tenet of good practice. Health professionals who do not respect this principle may be liable both to legal action by the patient and to action by their professional body.

There are two distinct aspects of the law relating to consent to treatment. One is the actual giving of consent by the patient, which acts as a defence to an action for trespass to the person. The other is the duty on the practitioner to give information to the patient prior to the giving of consent. The absence of consent could result in the patient suing for trespass to the person. The failure to provide sufficient relevant information could result in an action for negligence. These two different legal actions will be considered separately.

Trespass to the person

There are two types of trespass to the person. An assault is when an individual perceives a threat that she may be touched without her consent. If she is actually touched without her consent then this is known as a battery. Thus threatening behaviour, but without any physical contact would be assault, while a vaginal examination carried out without the woman's consent could be battery.

The person who has suffered the trespass can sue for compensation in the civil courts (and in criminal cases a prosecution could also be brought). In the civil cases, the victim has to prove:

- the touching or the apprehension of the touching, and
- that it was a (potentially) direct interference with her person.

The victim does not have to show that harm has occurred. This is in contrast with an action for negligence in which the victim must show that harm has resulted from the breach of duty of care.

Defences to an action for trespass to the person

The main defence to an action for trespass to the person is that consent was given by a mentally competent person. In addition there are two other defences in law, which are:

1. statutory authorization, e.g. Mental Health Act 1983
2. common law power to act out of necessity.

Consent and negligence

As part of the duty of care owed in the law of negligence the professional has a duty to inform the patient about the significant risks of substantial harm which could occur if treatment were to proceed.

If the harm has not been explained to the patient, and the harm then occurs, the patient can claim that had she known of this possibility she would not have agreed to undergo the treatment. She could then bring an action in negligence. To succeed the patient would have to show that:

- there was a duty of care to give specific information
- the defendant failed to give this information and in so doing was therefore in breach of the

reasonable standard of care which should have been provided

- as a result of this failure to inform, the patient agreed to the treatment, and
- the patient subsequently suffered the harm.

The Department of Health has issued new guidance on consent which incorporates recent case law on the subject (DoH, 2001a). This includes an aide-memoire for health professionals (DoH, 2001b) with the key points as illustrated by Box 68.6.

Box 68.6 **12 key points on consent: the law in England (DoH, 2001b)**

When do health professionals need consent from patients?

1. Before you examine, treat or care for competent adult patients you must obtain their consent.
2. Adults are always assumed to be competent unless demonstrated otherwise. If you have doubts about their competence, the question to ask is: 'can this patient understand and weigh up the information needed to make this decision?' Unexpected decisions do not prove the patient is incompetent, but may indicate a need for further information or explanation.
3. Patients may be competent to make some healthcare decisions, even if they are not competent to make others.
4. Giving and obtaining consent is usually a process, not a one-off event. Patients can change their minds and withdraw consent at any time. If there is any doubt, you should always check that patients still consent to your caring for or treating them.

Can children consent for themselves?

5. Before examining, treating or caring for a child, you must also seek consent. Young people aged 16 and 17 are presumed to have the competence to give consent for themselves. Younger children who understand fully what is involved in the proposed procedure can also give consent (although their parents will ideally be involved). In other cases, someone with parental responsibility must give consent on the child's behalf, unless such a person cannot be reached in an emergency. If a competent child consents to treatment, a parent *cannot* override that consent. Legally, a parent can consent if a competent child refuses, but it is likely that taking such a serious step will be rare.

Who is the right person to seek consent?

6. It is always best for the person actually treating the patient to seek the patient's consent. However, you may seek consent on behalf of colleagues if you are capable of performing the procedure in question, or if you have been specially trained to seek consent for that procedure.

What information should be provided?

7. Patients need sufficient information before they can decide whether to give their consent: for example information about the benefits and risks of the proposed treatment, and alternative treatments. If patients are not offered as much information as they reasonably need to make their decision, and in a form they can understand, their consent may not be valid.

Is the patient's consent voluntary?

8. Consent must be given voluntarily: not under any form of duress or undue influence from health professionals, family or friends.

Does it matter *how* the patient gives consent?

9. No: consent can be written, oral or non-verbal. A signature on a consent form does not itself prove the consent is valid – the point of the form is to record the patient's decision, and also increasingly the discussions that have taken place. Your trust or organization may have a policy setting out when you need to obtain written consent.

Refusals of treatment

10. Competent adult patients are entitled to refuse treatment, even where it would clearly benefit their health. The only exception to this rule is where the treatment is for a mental disorder and the patient is detained under the *Mental Health Act 1983*. A competent pregnant woman may refuse any treatment, even if this would be detrimental to the fetus.

Adults who are not competent to give consent

11. *No-one* can give consent on behalf of an incompetent adult. However, you may still treat

such a patient if the treatment would be in the patient's best interests. 'Best interests' go wider than best medical interests, to include factors such as the wishes and beliefs of the patient when competent, the patient's current wishes, general well-being and spiritual and religious welfare. People close to the patient may be able to give you information on some of these factors. Where the patient has never been competent, relatives, carers and friends may be best placed to advise on the patient's needs and preferences.

12. If an incompetent patient has clearly indicated in the past, while competent, that he or she would refuse treatment in certain circumstances (an 'advance refusal'), and those circumstances arise, you must abide by that refusal.

Box 68.7 Refusal of blood transfusion (*Re T*, 1992)

A woman had made it clear that she would not wish to have a blood transfusion. She was very much under the influence of her mother, a Jehovah's Witness. When it became evident that she would need blood to stay alive, the court allowed the cohabitee's and father's application for the blood to be given on the grounds that her refusal was not valid. This decision was confirmed by the Court of Appeal.

Elements of consent

For consent to treatment to be valid, it must be given *voluntarily* by an appropriately *informed* person (the patient or where relevant someone with parental responsibility for a patient under the age of 18) who has *capacity* to consent to the intervention in question.

Voluntarily

To be valid, consent must be given voluntarily and freely, without pressure or undue influence being exerted on the patient by partners, family members or health professionals (Box 68.7).

Informed

To give valid consent, the patient needs to understand in broad terms the nature and purpose of the procedure, together with risks of the procedure.

The leading case is that of Sidaway where the House of Lords stated that the professional was required in law to provide information to the patient according to the Bolam Test (*Sidaway* v. *Bethlem Royal Hospital Governors*, 1985). It is advisable to advise the patient of any material or significant risks in the proposed treatment and any alternatives to it, and the risks of doing nothing. A recent Court of Appeal judgement (*Pearce* v. *United Bristol Healthcare NHS Trust*, 1999) stated that it will normally be the responsibility of the doctor to inform a patient of 'a significant risk which would affect the judgement of a reasonable patient'.

To ensure that the patient understands the information which is given, there are considerable advantages in a leaflet being provided (checking of course that the patient can understand it). This would also assist if there was any dispute over the information having been given.

Reflective Activity 68.3

Good communication is an essential part of professional practice. How do you communicate with the women you care for, and record this? Could any of these communications be supported by leaflets? Are they?

Capacity

The person giving consent must be mentally competent. A child of 16 and 17 has a statutory right to give consent and a child below 16 may, if 'Gillick competent', also give consent. This means that the child, although below 16, has sufficient understanding and intelligence to enable him or her to understand fully what is involved in a proposed intervention.

For a person to have capacity, he or she must be able to comprehend and retain information relevant to the decision, especially as to the consequences of having or not having the intervention in question, and must be able to use and weigh this information in the decision-making process.

The existence of a mental illness will not automatically mean that a person is incapable of giving a valid refusal of treatment in her or his best interests, as in the case of *Re C*, where a Broadmoor patient was considered to have the capacity to refuse an amputation of the leg which doctors had advised him was indicated as a life-saving measure. An injunction was ordered against any doctors carrying out an amputation on him without his consent (*Re C*, 1994).

The principles established by the court for consent to be seen as competent were:

* comprehending and retaining treatment information
* believing it to be true, and
* weighing it in the balance to arrive at a choice.

In applying this test to C, the Judge was completely satisfied that the presumption that C had the right of self-determination had not been replaced. Although his general capacity had been impaired by schizophrenia, he had understood and retained the treatment information, and believed it and had arrived at a clear choice.

The right of the adult mentally competent person to refuse food was upheld in the case of a prisoner who had gone on hunger strike. Although the prisoner was diagnosed as suffering from a personality disorder, he was held to be of sound mind so that the law required the Home Office, prison officers and doctors to accept his refusal to take food or drink (*Secretary of State for the Home Department* v. *Orb*, 1995). This case overruled a case where suffragettes who went on hunger strike were force fed (*Leigh* v. *Gladstone*, 1909), where the defence of acting out of necessity was applied. It is now clear that this defence is only available when the adult is mentally incompetent (see below).

Refusal to consent

The principle of the right of self-determination if the adult is mentally competent has been applied and extended by the Court of Appeal in two cases where a compulsory caesarean section had been carried out. In the first case (*Re MB*, 1997), the pregnant woman suffered from needle phobia and would not agree to an injection preceding the caesarean. The court held the needle phobia to render her mentally incapable and therefore it declared that doctors performing a caesarean, acting in her best interests would not be acting illegally. (For the common law power to act in the best interests out of necessity, see below.)

The facts of the second case (*St George's Healthcare National Health Service Trust* v. *S*, 1998) are as follows. S was diagnosed with pre-eclampsia and advised that she needed urgent attention, bedrest and admission to hospital for an induced delivery. Without that treatment, the health and life of both herself and the unborn child were in real danger. She fully understood the potential risks but rejected the advice. She wanted her baby to be born naturally.

She was then seen by an approved social worker and two doctors in relation to compulsory admission to hospital under the Mental Health Act 1983 Section 2 for assessment. They repeated the advice which she had been given and she refused to accept it. On the basis of the written medical recommendations of the two doctors, the approved social worker applied for her admission to hospital for assessment under Section 2 of the Mental Health Act 1983. Later that day, again against her will, she was transferred to St George's Hospital. In view of her continuing adamant refusal to consent to treatment, an application was made ex parte on behalf of the hospital authority to Mrs Justice Hogg who made a declaration that the caesarean section could proceed, dispensing with S's consent to treatment. The operation was carried out and a baby girl delivered. She was then returned to Springfield Hospital and 2 days later her detention under Section 2 of the Mental Health Act was ended.

The woman then sought judicial review of her detention, the High Court judgement and the caesarean operation. The Court of Appeal held that the Mental Health Act 1983 could not be deployed to achieve the detention of an individual against her will merely because her thinking process was unusual, even apparently bizarre and irrational, and contrary to the view of the overwhelming majority of the community at large. A woman detained under the Act for mental disorder could not be forced into medical procedures unconnected with her mental condition unless her capacity to consent to such treatment was diminished. The Court of Appeal was not satisfied that she was lawfully detained under Section 2 of the Mental Health Act 1983 because she was not suffering from mental disorder of a nature or degree which warranted her detention in hospital for assessment. Although on the face of the documents her admission would appear to have been legal, her transfer to St George's Hospital was unlawful and at any time she would have been justified in applying for a *habeas corpus* which would have led to her immediate release. The declaration made by the High Court Judge should not have been made on an ex parte basis (i.e. without representation of the woman) and was unlawful.

The difference between the two cases is that in the first case the woman was held, as a result of the needle phobia to be mentally incompetent, and therefore the caesarean section could be carried out in her best interests without her consent. However, in the second case S was not held to be mentally incompetent and therefore the compulsory caesarean was a trespass to her person. In neither case did the court consider the rights of the fetus to influence the decision-making. The fetus is not regarded in law as a legal personality until birth. Until then, the wishes of a mentally competent pregnant woman will prevail whatever the effect on the fetus.

Following these cases, the Court of Appeal set out principles to be followed regarding applications to the court when the patient's capacity to consent is in doubt. This advice applies to any cases involving capacity when surgical or invasive treatment may be needed by a patient. This advice is summarized in Box 68.8.

Common law power to act out of necessity

Where the patient lacks the capacity to give consent to treatment, treatment can proceed on the basis that it is in the best interests of that individual and is given according to the reasonable standard of the profession. This is known as the right at common law (i.e. judge-made law) to act out of necessity in the best interests of the mentally incompetent person. In such circumstances, the health professional would not be committing a trespass to the person. For example, if a woman who had delivered at home, unattended, had a postpartum haemorrhage and was admitted to hospital in a state of collapse, with no information available

---

Box 68.8 Summary of principles laid down by the Court of Appeal to be followed regarding applications to the court when the patient's capacity to consent is in doubt

1. The principles have no application when the patient is competent to accept or refuse treatment. In principle a patient may remain competent notwithstanding detention under the Mental Health Act.
2. If a patient is competent and refuses to consent to the treatment, an application to the High Court for a declaration would be pointless. However, the information given to the patient should be documented and patients should be asked to sign a written indication of their refusal, including that they understand the nature and reasons for the proposed treatment and the likely results of refusing or accepting it. If they refuse to sign, then this should be documented.
3. If patients are incapable of giving or refusing consent, either permanently or temporarily, then they must be cared for according to their best interests. However, any advance directive must be complied with, unless it does not apply to the particular circumstances. In this case an application for a direction may be made.
4. The hospital should identify as soon as possible whether there is a concern about a patient's competence to consent to or refuse treatment.
5. If the capacity of a patient is seriously in doubt, then it should be assessed as a matter of priority. In many cases the patient's GP or other responsible doctor may be able to make this assessment, but in serious or complex cases, the issue of capacity should be examined by an independent psychiatrist. If competence is in

serious doubt, then legal advice should be sought and, if patients are not able to manage their property or affairs and thus instruct their own solicitor, then they will require a guardian ad litem to act on their behalf.
6. If the patient is incapable of instructing solicitors, then the hospital must notify the Official Solicitor and invite him to act as guardian ad litem.
7. The hearing before the judge should be inter partes (i.e. both the patient and the hospital should be legally represented).
8. The judge must be provided with all relevant information, including the reasons for the proposed treatment, risks involved of proceeding or not proceeding with the treatment, what the alternatives are, and the patient's reasons for refusing consent. The judge will need sufficient information to reach an informed conclusion about the patient's capacity and the issue of best interest.
9. The precise terms of any order should be recorded and approved before being transmitted to the hospital, and the patient should be advised of the precise terms.
10. There may be occasions when, assuming a serious question arises about the competence of a patient, the situation facing the hospital is so urgent and the consequences so desperate that it is impracticable to comply with these guidelines. Where delay may itself cause serious damage to the patient's health or put the patient's life at risk, then compliance with these guidelines would be inappropriate.

as to her preferences, it would be lawful to examine her and undertake any necessary procedures to preserve her life, including surgery and the administration of blood products, without obtaining prior consent.

However, the defence of necessity cannot be used to do something to which people did not give their consent when they were able to do so. For example, if a mentally competent woman refuses blood or blood products, these cannot be given to save her life should her condition become critical.

Relatives do not have the power to consent on behalf of the mentally incompetent adult. At present there is a vacuum in the law. If mentally incapacitated adults are unable to make their own decisions, no relative can give or withhold consent on their behalf. The Law Commission has made recommendations on how this vacuum should be filled (Law Commission, 1995) and this was followed by the consultation document: *Who Cares* (Lord Chancellor's Office, 1997). *Making Decisions* (Lord Chancellor's Office, 1999) was the Government's response to the consultation. A draft bill was published in June 2003, and commented upon by a Joint Committee of the Houses of Parliament. A revised bill is now awaited.

Forms of consent and consent forms

Consent can be given by word of mouth, in writing or can be implied, i.e. the non-verbal conduct of the person may indicate that consent is being given, for example offering an arm for an injection. All these ways of giving consent are valid, but where procedures entail risk and/or where there are likely to be disputes over whether consent was given, it is advisable to obtain consent in writing, since it is then easier to establish in a court of law that consent was given.

New consent forms were issued in April 2002. These contained more emphasis on the patient's right to give or withhold consent and the need for health professionals to provide comprehensive information about the intervention that is proposed, and to answer all the patient's questions.

There are clear advantages in obtaining the patient's consent in writing if there are any risks inherent in the treatment or investigation or if there is likely to be a dispute later as to whether consent was actually given.

What if someone wishes to leave hospital?

It is a principle of consent, that a person who has given consent can withdraw it at any time. This means that if people wish to leave hospital contrary to their best

interests, unless they lack the capacity to make a valid decision, they are free to go. Clearly there are advantages in obtaining the signature of the patient that the self-discharge or refusal to accept treatment was contrary to clinical advice. If patients refuse to sign a form that they are taking discharge contrary to clinical advice, that refusal must be accepted. It would in such a case be advisable to ensure that there is another professional who is a witness to this and that a careful record is made by both professionals.

Reflective Activity 68.4

Analyse the activities which you undertake in relation to women in your care and note the extent to which you obtain consent by word of mouth, consent in writing or consent by non-verbal communication. What changes, if any, do you consider should be made to your practice?

LAWS REGULATING PREGNANCY, BIRTH AND CHILDREN

Abortion Act 1967 as amended (Box 68.9)

The provisions set out in Box 68.9, including the requirement to have two registered medical practitioners, do not apply in an emergency when a registered medical practitioner is of the opinion, formed in good faith, that the termination is immediately necessary to save the life, or to prevent grave permanent injury to the physical or mental health, of the pregnant woman.

Registration of births and stillbirths; births under 24 weeks

The law requires that every birth is registered. When there is a stillbirth, this is registerable if it occurred after 24 weeks or more of gestation. Miscarriages of less than 24 weeks do not have to be registered, but the body must be disposed of with public decency and the wishes and feelings of the parents taken into consideration. Where a live birth is followed by a death (whatever the length of gestation) there must be a registration of both the birth and the death. In other words, if the baby is born alive, even if only for a brief time, and even where the gestation is less than 24 weeks, a birth must be registered and if the baby subsequently dies, then a death must be registered.

Box 68.9 Abortion Act 1967 Section 1(1) as amended by the Human Fertilisation and Embryology Act 1990

A person shall not be guilty of an offence under the law relating to abortion when a pregnancy is terminated by a registered medical practitioner if two registered medical practitioners are of the opinion, formed in good faith:

(a) that the pregnancy has not exceeded its 24th week and that the continuance of the pregnancy would involve risk, greater than if the pregnancy were terminated, of injury to the physical or mental health of the pregnant woman or any existing children of her family; or

(b) that the termination is necessary to prevent grave permanent injury to the physical or mental health of the pregnant woman; or

(c) that the continuance of the pregnancy would involve risk to the life of the pregnant woman, greater than if the pregnancy were terminated; or

(d) that there is a substantial risk that if the child were born it would suffer from such physical or mental abnormalities as to be seriously handicapped.

Human Fertilisation and Embryology Act 1990 and 1992

These Acts provide a legal framework within which infertility treatment and embryo growth and implanting can take place. The Human Fertilisation and Embryology Authority is responsible for licensing centres and issuing a code of practice, and has general responsibility for ensuring that the law is followed.

Criminal law and attendance at birth

A midwife could face criminal proceedings in respect of her work if she offends against the criminal laws, such as health and safety laws or road traffic Acts. If she acts with gross recklessness or negligence in her professional practice, then she could face criminal proceedings. For example, an anaesthetist was held guilty of the death of a patient in theatre where he acted with such gross recklessness as to amount to a criminal offence of manslaughter (R v. *Adomako*, 1995).

Section 16 of the 1997 Nurses, Midwives and Health Visitors Act made it a criminal offence for a person other than a registered midwife or a registered medical practitioner (or student of either) to attend a woman in childbirth except in an emergency or undergoing professional training as doctor or midwife. This is re-enacted in Article 45 of the Nursing and Midwifery Order 2001. There have been some prosecutions under this section and its predecessor. For example, Rupert Baines from Bristol was found guilty of delivering a baby without assistance and Brian Radley from Wolverhampton was charged with attending a woman in childbirth otherwise than under the direction and personal supervision of a duly qualified practitioner and was fined £100 (August 1983).

If the midwife is obstructed by an aggressive partner during a home confinement, she would be able to call upon police powers to assist her.

Children Act 1989

This Act set up a framework for the protection and care of children and established clear principles to guide decision-making in relation to their care. The principles which the court should take into account are shown in Box 68.10. The overriding principle is that 'The child's welfare shall be the court's paramount consideration.'

The involvement of the child in the decision-making is also a major principle and Box 68.11 sets out the considerations which the court should take into account in making certain orders.

Finally in deciding whether or not to make an order, the court 'shall not make the order or any of the orders unless it considers that doing so would be better for the child than making no order at all.'

Where practitioners are concerned that a child, or the sibling or child of one of their patients, is being abused, whether physically, sexually or mentally, they should take immediate action to ensure that this is drawn to the attention of the appropriate persons. This means that they must be familiar with the provisions for child protection and the persons to be contacted. It is not always easy to decide if action is necessary, but practitioners should see as their main priority the safety of the child. As Paragraph 1.13 of the guidelines on interagency cooperation states: 'The difficulties of assessing the risk of harm to a child should not be underestimated. It is imperative that everyone who deals with allegations and suspicions of abuse maintains an open and inquiring mind.' (Home Office *et al.*, 1991).

Should the practitioner's fears prove to be wrong, and it appears that there is no abuse, the name of the practitioner should not be divulged to the parents

Box 68.10 Principles of the Children Act 1989

1. The welfare of the child is the paramount consideration in court proceedings.
2. Wherever possible, children should be brought up and cared for in their own families.
3. Courts should ensure that delay is avoided, and may only make an order if to do so is better than making no order at all.
4. Children should be kept informed about what happens to them, and should participate when decisions are made about their future.
5. Parents continue to have parental responsibility for their children, even when their children are no longer living with them. They should be kept informed about their children and participate when decisions are made about their children's future.
6. Parents with children in need should be helped to bring up their children themselves.
7. This help should be provided as a service to the child and the family, and should:
   a. be provided in partnership with parents
   b. meet each child's identified needs
   c. be appropriate to the child's race, culture, religion, and language
   d. be open to effective independent representations and complaints procedures, and
   e. draw upon effective partnership between the local authority and other agencies including voluntary agencies.

Box 68.11 Circumstances to be taken into account by the court under the Children Act 1989

1. The ascertainable wishes and feelings of the child concerned (considered in the light of the child's age and understanding).
2. The child's physical, emotional and educational needs.
3. The likely effect on the child of any change in his or her circumstances.
4. The child's age, sex, background and any characteristics of the child which the court considers relevant.
5. Any harm which the child has suffered or is at risk of suffering.
6. How capable each of the child's parents, and any other person in relation to whom the court considers the question to be relevant, is of meeting the child's needs.
7. The range of powers available to the court under this Act in the proceedings in question.

(*D. v. National Society for the Prevention of Cruelty to Children*, 1977).

Procedure for the management of child abuse

There should be in existence a locally developed and agreed procedure for the management of child abuse cases and the midwife should be familiar with this. The procedure should require any professional staff working in the service who suspect that there is a possibility of ill-treatment, serious neglect, sexual or emotional abuse of a child, to inform the senior practitioner in charge of the department, who should contact a consultant paediatrician. If the consultant confirms the possibility of abuse, then he or she should inform the Social Services Department immediately.

Interagency cooperation and future development

Each local authority should have an Area Child Protection Committee (ACPC) to ensure interagency cooperation towards children at risk, the tasks of which are set out in Box 68.12. This committee should include senior medical and nursing representation, and a designated lead professional for child protection within the hospital or community service.

Following the death of Victoria Climbie, an enquiry was conducted by Lord Laming, which made significant recommendations for the reform of child protection procedures. The Department of Health published a detailed response *Keeping children safe* (DfES, 2003) and this was followed by a single source document for safeguarding children. A Green Paper, *Every Child Matters*, was published in 2003. Changes will include the appointment of a Children's Commissioner, and a Minister for Children, Young People and Families.

Child protection register

Each local authority must maintain a child protection register, the purposes of which are set out in Box 68.13.

Access to this register is limited to an agreed list of personnel which includes senior medical staff or paediatric social workers in the local hospital departments. Difficulties can sometimes arise if the register is kept within the social services department and there is not 24-hour access to it. This should be brought up at the ACPC and arrangements could be made for the

Box 68.12 Tasks of the Area Child Protection Committee

1. Establishing, maintaining and reviewing interagency guidelines on procedures to be followed in individual cases
2. Monitoring the implementation of legal procedures
3. Identifying significant issues arising from the handling of cases and reports from inquiries
4. Scrutinizing arrangements to provide treatment, expert advice and interagency liaison and make recommendations to the responsible agencies
5. Scrutinizing progress on work to prevent child abuse and making recommendations to the responsible agencies
6. Scrutinizing the work related to interagency training and making recommendations to the responsible agencies
7. Conducting reviews required under Part 8 of the Guide
8. Publishing an annual report about local child protection matters

Box 68.13 Purpose of the Child Protection Register

1. To provide a record of all children in the area who are currently the subject of a Child Protection Plan and to ensure that the plans are formally reviewed at least every 6 months
2. To provide a central point of speedy inquiry for professional staff who are worried about a child and want to know whether the child is the subject of a Child Protection Plan
3. To provide statistical information about current trends in the area

register to be kept by the paediatric department or by the police.

Further information will be found in Ch. 63.

HEALTH AND SAFETY LAWS

The basic health and safety duties are placed upon employers by the Health and Safety at Work Act 1974. This Act has been supplemented by many statutory instruments defining more specific duties in relation to manual handling, protective clothing, and the management of health and safety in the workplace. These statutory duties are enforceable by the Health and Safety Executive in the criminal courts. In addition they are paralleled by duties placed on the employer under the common law. As a result of an implied term in the employment contract recognized by the courts, every employer must take reasonable care of the physical and mental health and safety of the employee. Therefore employers may be liable to pay compensation to an employee where (a) the employee is known to be suffering from unacceptable stress, and (b) there is reasonable action which the employer could take but fails to take to relieve the situation and (c) as a consequence the employee suffers from mental harm. Duties laid down under the manual handling regulations are also paralleled by the employer's responsibility for ensuring that reasonable action (including that of implementing the regulations) is taken to prevent the employee being harmed through manual handling. Every employer has a responsibility to carry out a risk assessment of dangers and hazards in the workplace, including an assessment for substances hazardous to health under the Control of Substances Hazardous to Health Regulations (1999). Regulations also require any incident involving injuries to be reported (RIDDOR; HSE, 1995) and the Medical Devices Regulations (1995) require incidents involving medical devices to be reported to the Medical Devices Agency, and for any warnings from the Agency to be acted upon.

LEGAL ASPECTS OF RECORD-KEEPING

Midwives have clear responsibilities under the Rules to ensure that their documentation of their midwifery care is kept properly (UKCC, 1998). In addition, if they leave their post, then there are specified duties for the transfer of their records. Their supervisor of midwives is also entitled to inspect their records and record-keeping standards. Guidance is provided by the UKCC on standards in record-keeping (NMC, 2002b). It is recommended that records should be kept for at least 25 years. However, where the midwife is aware that a child has been born with serious mental disabilities it would be wise for those records to be retained until at least 3 years after that person's death, since in the case of those under a mental disability, there is no time limit for bringing a legal action for compensation as long as they are alive.

The Data Protection Act 1998 covers both computerized and manual-held records and requires those who deal with personal records to register their storage and use of those records. The duties laid down in the Act are enforced by criminal proceedings. Rights of subject access to personal health records are given by the Act subject to specified exceptions where serious harm would be caused to the physical or mental health of the applicant or another, or where a third party (not being a health professional caring for the patient) who would be identified by the disclosure, has requested not to be identified.

Reflective Activity 68.5

How do your records get audited in your maternity service? Do you have your own personal strategy for auditing your own records? Review the UKCC and NMC guidelines, consider how you could develop a simple checklist tool to check your records, and consider how often you would do this.

MEDICINES

Midwives have statutory powers in relation to the prescribing of medication. These are set out in the Rules, and guidance is provided in the code of practice (UKCC, 1998a). Refer to Ch. 71 for specific laws and rules governing drugs and medicines.

COMPLAINTS

The complaints procedure is of relevance in this chapter, firstly because a comprehensive and detailed complaints investigation may provide the family with the information they need, avoiding the need for them to pursue their concerns through the legal process. An essential part of the complaints procedure is that lessons are learnt to prevent a recurrence. Some complainants will progress from the complaints procedure to taking legal proceedings and any documentation in the complaints file will be disclosable as part of the legal process. It is therefore important that statements and other documents created during the investigation of the complaint are accurate and free of subjective opinions.

The Hospital Complaints Act 1985 required every hospital to establish a complaints procedure. In 1996 a new complaints procedure was introduced following the Wilson Report (DoH, 1994). This identified three levels in dealing with complaints: the first level is called local resolution (NHSE, 1996a,b). During this stage, the complaint is investigated and responded to locally, with the Chief Executive Officer responsible for the reply to the complainant. If the complainant remains aggrieved, then an application can be made to the non-executive director known as the Complaints Convenor who can decide if there should be an independent review (the second stage) panel to consider the complaint. The panel is chaired by an independent lay person and the non-executive director, and an independent health professional would also sit on the panel. If the complainant is dissatisfied with the findings of the panel or the convenor has refused to agree to a panel being set up, then the complainant can appeal to the Health Service Commissioner or Ombudsman. This is the third and final stage.

A review of the complaints procedure has been commissioned by the health departments across the UK and is likely to lead to significant recommendations in terms of its independence and its efficiency in processing complaints. Draft regulations for the reform of the NHS complaints procedure were published in December 2003.

MISCELLANEOUS LEGAL ISSUES OF RELEVANCE TO THE MIDWIFE

Care of property

Failure to look after another person's property could lead to criminal prosecution, e.g. theft, civil action for trespass to the person, or negligence in causing harm to property. In an action for negligence, the person who has suffered the loss or damage of property must establish the same four elements that must be shown in a claim for compensation for personal injury, i.e. duty, breach, causation and harm.

Where, however, property is left by a person (known as the bailor) in the care of another person (the bailee), then, should the property be lost or damaged, the burden would be on the bailee to establish how that occurred without fault on his or her part. This is the situation when a client hands over money or valuables for safekeeping in the ward safe. It should be noted that liability for loss or damage to property can be excluded if such an exclusion is reasonable (see the Unfair Contract Terms Act above).

Vaccine damage

A statutory scheme for compensation was introduced under the Vaccine Damage Payments Act 1979 to compensate those who have suffered harm as a consequence of receiving vaccines. Public health requires a high level of herd immunity to ensure that major infectious diseases are eradicated, and therefore a high level of vaccination in the community is required. Since it is recognized that there is a tiny risk of harm from these vaccinations, it was accepted that as a consequence, there should be compensation for those few who suffered such harm as a result of being vaccinated. The amount available has recently been increased from £40 000 to £100 000. Any applicant must establish that he or she has been severely disabled as a result of a vaccination against the specified diseases of diphtheria, tetanus, whooping cough, poliomyelitis, measles, rubella, tuberculosis, smallpox, and any other disease specified by the Secretary of State for Health. The severe disability must be at least 60% (this was formerly 80%). Whether the disability has been caused by the vaccination shall be established on a balance of probabilities. There was a 6-year time limit on making claims but this is being raised to any time up to the age of 18 years. This will enable more persons disabled by vaccines to claim the payment, including those who have already been rejected, who can reapply under the new rules. An applicant under the statutory scheme is not barred from pursuing a claim in negligence where, if successful, the level of compensation may be far higher. However, an award under the statutory scheme would be taken into account in a negligence payment and vice versa.

Congenital Disabilities (Civil Liability) Act 1976

This Act enables a child who is born disabled as a result of pre-birth negligence to obtain compensation from the person responsible for the negligent act. The mother can only be sued if she was negligent when driving a motor car (in this case the child would be suing the mother's insurance company). A recent amendment enables those whose children have been disabled during IVF treatment to obtain compensation.

Negligent advice

There can be liability for negligence in giving advice, but the claimant would have to show that it was clear to the defendant that he or she would rely upon the advice and in so doing had suffered reasonably foreseeable loss or harm. For example, providing a reference for a student or colleague can lead to liability both to the recipient of the reference, if in reliance

upon that reference the recipient has suffered harm, and also to the person who is the subject of the reference (*Hedley Byrne & Co Ltd* v. *Heller & Partners Ltd*, 1963) and also to the person on whose behalf the reference is given. The latter would have to show that the reference was written without reasonable care, and harm occurred to the subject of the reference as a result of potential employers relying upon the reference (*Spring* v. *Guardian Assurance*, 1994) Every care should therefore be taken to ensure that a reference is written accurately in the light of the facts available.

THE CLINICAL NEGLIGENCE SCHEME FOR TRUSTS

In 1995, the Clinical Negligence Scheme for Trusts (CNST) was initiated. This scheme requires member trusts to pay an annual amount into a central pool, from which justified claims over an agreed amount will be paid. This means that NHS trusts do not have to set aside large amounts of money 'just in case' they have to pay out on a major negligence claim. Instead the risk, and costs, are spread across the NHS and the maximum amount that will have to be paid out by a single NHS trust on a single claim is capped.

The CNST lays great emphasis on the importance of clinical risk management, as good risk-management policies and practices should reduce the number and cost of legal claims. It has therefore developed a system of risk-management standards for trusts participating in the scheme (CNST, 2000), and payments into the pool are based upon assessments of the individual organizations carried out by the CNST. There are three levels of attainment:

Level 1 The trust must have a basic structure of policies and procedures. For maternity services this includes clear lines of accountability throughout the client's care, handover between professionals, a labour ward forum and a comprehensive set of multidisciplinary policies.

Level 2 Standards are more challenging, and require that:

- there must be a lead consultant obstetrician and clinical midwife for labour ward matters (in midwife-led units this role can be fulfilled by a midwife alone)
- minimum levels of consultant and specialist registrar input to the labour ward must be laid down (i.e. a minimum of 40 hours a week of consultant cover and a specialist registrar to be resident or on the ward within 5 minutes).

Level 3 It is required that emergency caesarean sections are undertaken quickly and that, when the decision is made that a section is necessary, the urgency with which it is required has to be documented (e.g. within 30 minutes) together with the time the decision was made. In addition, level 3 requires that there is a personal handover to and from obstetric locums, either by the post holder or senior members of the team.

There is a clear financial incentive for NHS trusts to attain the higher levels of participation but this also reflects more rigorous practices and thus better care for women and their babies.

The NHS Litigation Authority (NHSLA) oversees the CNST and also administers the scheme for meeting liabilities of health service bodies to third parties for loss, damage or injury arising out of the exercise of their functions. In practice this means claims by employees for accidents at work, or by visitors for accidents taking place in NHS premises.

In 2000 the NHSLA announced that it was taking over responsibility for making all existing liability scheme payments (i.e. those liabilities where the incident occurred before April 1995) for clinical negligence schemes. From April 2002, the NHSLA took over responsibility for managing claims (other than very minor ones) arising from incidents after April 1995. Thus, from 1 April 2002, all significant clinical negligence claims are managed centrally, by the NHS Litigation Authority.

Reflective Activity 68.6

Find the CNST standard relating to policies and protocols – do your labour ward policies comply with this standard?

THE NEW STANDARD-SETTING ORGANIZATIONS (NICE AND CHI) AND NATIONAL SERVICE FRAMEWORKS (NSF)

Statutory duties are placed upon the Secretary of State for Health to provide a comprehensive service to meet all reasonable needs, and these duties are in turn delegated to the NHS organizations. In each area a strategic health authority arranges for the commissioning of health services by NHS trusts and others and is responsible for the provision of primary care services through independent contractors such as family practitioners, pharmacists and dentists. Following the Health Act 1999, these responsibilities have mainly transferred to primary care trusts (in Wales, local health groups), and most recently health authorities have been reorganized into a smaller number of strategic health authorities which focus on strategic planning for the area they cover.

The Primary Care Act 1997 and the Health Act 1999 have enabled a variety of different organizational systems to be set up and, over the coming years, there are likely to be changes as community health staff and social services staff are transferred to new organizations.

Clinical governance and the duty of quality

A statutory duty under Section 18 of the Health Act 1999 requires each health authority (HA), primary care trust and NHS trust to put and keep in place arrangements for the purpose of monitoring and improving the quality of healthcare which it provides to individuals. Failures in fulfilling this statutory duty could result in the removal of a board or the dismissal of its chief executive and chairman.

The National Institute of Clinical Excellence (NICE) was established in April 1999 to promote clinical and cost effectiveness across the country. It investigates medicines, and other treatments, and in the light of its research makes recommendations to the Department of Health on the clinical and cost effectiveness of such treatments. For example, in October 2000 it issued guidelines on the use of the drug Ritalin within the NHS to treat children suffering from attention deficit/hyperactivity disorder. It also recommended that *ribavirin*, a drug used to treat hepatitis C (that many health authorities had said was too expensive) should be made available in the NHS in combination with *interferon alpha*. It is estimated that the cost of this drug to the NHS could be £18 million a year.

The 2001 programme for NICE included the following up of a survey carried out by the National Sentinel Audit on the reasons behind caesarean sections, induction of labour and fetal monitoring so that national and widely tested evidence-based guidelines can be produced. Guidelines and recommendations made by NICE can be used by midwives to press for additional resources if they are aware that the standards of care and services provided in their units are lower than those nationally recommended.

The Commission for Health Improvement (CHI) was established under Sections 19 to 24 of the Health Act 1999 as a body corporate (i.e. it can sue and be sued on its own account), with significant powers:

● to provide advice or information with respect to arrangements for monitoring and improving the quality of healthcare by primary care trusts and NHS trusts

- to conduct reviews of, and make reports on, arrangements by primary care trusts or NHS trusts for the purpose of monitoring and improving the quality of healthcare for which they have responsibility
- to carry out investigations into, and make reports on, the management, provision or quality of healthcare
- to conduct reviews of, and make reports on, the management, provision or quality of, or access to or availability of, particular types of healthcare for which NHS bodies or service providers have responsibility, and
- other functions as may be prescribed relating to the management, provision or quality of, or access to or availability of, healthcare for which prescribed NHS bodies or prescribed service providers have responsibility.

CHI can also work with the Audit Commission in carrying out these functions. Effectively these powers make it a 'watchdog' for the NHS, and immediately after its appointment, it was asked by the Secretary of State for Health to visit Garlands Hospital in Carlisle run by the North Lakeland Healthcare NHS Trust in Cumbria. An independent investigation had found that staff had physically and mentally abused patients. The Chairman of the NHS Trust was dismissed by the Secretary of State, who then asked CHI to visit the hospital and report on its findings.

From April 2004, CHI will become the Commission for Health Care Audit and Inspection (CHAI) with wider duties including audit.

National service frameworks (NSF)

It is the intention of the Government to publish national standard frameworks in most clinical areas so that there are identifiable quality standards which should be provided across the country. At the time of writing, NSFs had been provided for mental health and coronary heart disease. A national cancer plan was published in the autumn of 2000 and the NSF for diabetes at the end of 2001 (specific strategy: 2003). Midwifery and obstetric care is a module in the children's national service framework (publication 2004). This will assist midwives in establishing minimum levels of care and services for the women and babies they care for.

CURRENT DEVELOPMENTS IN CIVIL LAW

Many commentators suggest that the system of obtaining compensation for personal injuries is extremely unsatisfactory – it is slow, expensive, uncertain and by no means ensures that justice is done or seen to be done. However, the Royal Commission which reported in 1978 recommended that the current system of liability by establishing fault should be retained, except in some specific circumstances (e.g. vaccine damage, those harmed by BSE, volunteers in medical research).

More recently, Lord Woolf undertook a review of the civil justice system, the results of which were contained in his report *Access to Justice* (1996). The resultant reforms to civil litigation were introduced in April 1999. These were designed to address some of the weaknesses identified above – to speed up the process and reduce costs. The Civil Procedure Rules, resulting from recommended improvements to the civil justice proceedings, are a new procedural code with the overriding objective of enabling the court to deal with cases justly. Dealing with a case justly includes, so far as is practicable:

- ensuring that the parties are on an equal footing
- saving expense
- dealing with the case in ways which are proportionate:
  - to the amount of money involved
  - to the importance of the case
  - to the complexity of the issues, and
  - to the financial position of each party
- ensuring that it is dealt with expeditiously and fairly, and
- allotting to it an appropriate share of the court's resources, while taking into account the need to allot resources to other cases.

The Woolf reforms aim to make the present system work better, but the system is still based on establishing that negligence has occurred, i.e. based on fault. There are calls for a much more radical reorganization of the process, to introduce a system of no fault liability. In a scheme for 'no fault liability', following an arrangement (usually) between insurance companies, employers and the state, a compensation fund is set up from which payment is made to the person who was injured. Countries such as Sweden, Finland and New Zealand have adopted no-fault liability systems. In such schemes, it is not necessary to prove that the defendant (or its employees) has been at fault, but that something which had not been anticipated has occurred which has caused harm to an individual. The

Pearson Report (1978) did not recommend no fault liability in the case of medical negligence (though it did recommend statutory payments for vaccine damage) but there are strong calls for its introduction.

In 2001 the Department of Health issued a consultation document on a new clinical negligence scheme for the NHS. A Consultation paper on a new scheme for obtaining compensation for clinical negligence was published in 2003.

Conditional fees

Legal aid is being phased out from personal injury litigation. The Government has approved the system of conditional fees being introduced into this country. The claimant is able to negotiate, with a solicitor, payment on a 'no win – no fees' basis, i.e. if the claimant loses, the solicitor does not charge any fees. However, a claimant who does not succeed will have to pay the costs of the successful defendant, and this possibility is covered by taking out insurance to meet these and other costs not covered by the agreement with the solicitor. Recent statutory changes enable a successful party to claim the enhanced fees agreed with lawyers under the conditional fee agreement, from the unsuccessful party. The impact of these changes on personal injury cases involving claims against NHS organizations is not yet clear.

CONCLUSION

This chapter covers a large area of law of considerable importance to midwifery practice. It is suggested that the reader should follow up this chapter by referring to some of the recommended texts to obtain a more detailed knowledge of the law. The current emphasis on human rights, the growth of litigation, the requirement that there must be sound professional practice, all show the importance of midwives having an understanding of the laws which apply to their practice and how essential it is, as in all other areas of their competence, that they keep up to date.

KEY POINTS

- It is important that the midwife is aware of how laws, statutes and regulations are developed.
- An understanding of the rules and laws governing practice and healthcare can assist the practitioner in developing strategies and approaches which can improve care, and prevent situations which might lead to litigation.

- It is crucial that midwives keep abreast of development and changes within the law.
- The principles of good communication and informed consent are key to quality of care and experience for clients and their relatives.

REFERENCES

Clinical Negligence Scheme for Trusts (CNST) (2000) *Risk Management Standards and Procedures Manual of Guidance*. London: NHS Litigation Authority.

Department of Education and Skills (DeES) (2003) *Every Child Matters*. London: Stationery Office.

Department of Health (DoH) (1994) *Being Heard: the Report of a Review Committee on NHS Complaints Procedures*. (Chair: Professor Alan Wilson) London: HMSO.

Department of Health (DoH) (1997) *The New NHS – Modern – Dependable*. London: The Stationery Office.

Department of Health (DoH) (1998) *A First Class Service*. London: DoH.

Department of Health (DoH) (1999) *Clinical Governance*. London: DoH.

Department of Health (DoH) (2000) *The NHS Plan*. London: DoH.

Department of Health (DoH) (2001a) *Reference Guide to Consent for Examination or Treatment*. London: HMSO.

Department of Health (DoH) (2001b) *12 Key Points on Consent: the Law in England*. London: Stationery Office. Online. Available: http://www.doh.gov.uk/consent/twelvekeypts.htm January 2002.

Health and Safety Executive (HSE) 1995 *Reporting of Injuries, Diseases and Dangerous Occurrences Regulations (RIDDOR)*. Online. Available: htttp://www.allriskmgmt.co.uk/hse/accidents/guide.htm#1 January 2002.

Home Office, Department of Health, Department of Education and Science, Welsh Office (1991) *Working Together Under the Children Act 1989: a Guide to Arrangements for Inter-Agency Co-Operation for the Protection of Children from Abuse*. London: HMSO.

JM Consulting (1998) *Independent Review Report of the Nurses, Midwives and Health Visitors Act. Report to the Department of Health*. Bristol: JM Consulting.

Laurance, J. (1995) Man handicapped as a baby 33 years ago wins £1.25 m. *The Times* 15 November, p. 5.

Law Commission (1995) *Report No 231 Mental Incapacity*. London: HMSO.

Law Commission (1996) *Damages for Personal Injury: Medical, Nursing and Other Expenses*. London: The Stationery Office.

Lord Chancellor's Office (1997) *Who Cares?* London: The Stationery Office.

Lord Chancellor's Office (1999) *Making Decisions*. London: Lord Chancellor's Office.

Murray, I. (1998) NHS faces £2.3 bn bill for negligence payouts. *The Times,* 21 July.

National Audit Office (NAO) (2001) *Handling Clinical Negligence Claims in England*. London: The Stationery Office.

NHS Executive (NHSE) (1996a) *Complaints: Listening, Acting, Improving Guidance on Implementation of the NHS Complaints Procedure*, London: DoH.

NHS Executive (NHSE) (1996b) *Implementation of New Complaints Procedure: Final Guidance*. EL(96)19. London: DoH.

NHS Management Executive (NHSME) (1996) *NHS Indemnity: Arrangements for Clinical Negligence Claims in the NHS*. (HSG 96) 48. London: DoH.

North Lakeland Healthcare NHS Trust (2000) *Report of Independent Inquiry into Garlands Hospital*. North Lakeland Healthcare NHS Trust and North Cumbria HA London: DoH.

Nursing and Midwifery Council (NMC) (2002a) *Code of Professional Conduct*. London: NMC.

Nursing and Midwifery Council (NMC) (2002b) *Guidelines for Records and Record Keeping*. London: NMC (NMC reprint of UKCC Guidelines of 2000).

Nursing and Midwifery Council (NMC) (2002c) *Guidelines for the Administration of Medicines*. London: NMC (NMC version of UKCC Guidelines of 2000).

Pearson, Lord (Chairman) (1978) *Royal Commission on Civil Liability and Compensation for Personal Injury*. Cmnd 7054. London: HMSO.

UKCC (United Kingdom Central Council for Nursing, Midwifery and Health Visiting) (1998) *Midwives Rules and Code of Practice*. London: UKCC.

Woolf, Lord (1996) *Access to Justice. Final Report by the Right Honourable the Lord Woolf, Master of the Rolls to the Lord Chancellor on the Civil Justice System in England and Wales*. London: HMSO.

STATUTES

Children Act 1989 London: HMSO.

Hospital Complaints Act 1985 London: HMSO.

Congenital Disabilities (Civil Liability) Act 1976 London: HMSO.

Control of Substances Hazardous to Health Regulations 1999 London: HMSO.

European Convention for the Protection of Human Rights and Fundamental Freedoms (1951) London: HMSO.

Health Act 1999 London: HMSO.

Hospital Complaints Act 1985 London: HMSO.

Human Fertilisation and Embryology Act 1990 London: HMSO.

Human Fertilisation and Embryology (Disclosure of Information) Act 1992 London: HMSO

Human Rights Act 1998 London: HMSO.

Law Reform (Contributory Negligence) Act 1945 London: HMSO.

Mental Health Act 1983 London: HMSO.

National Health Service Litigation Authority (Establishment and Constitution) Order 1995 SI No. 2800. London: HMSO.

Nurses, Midwives and Health Visitors Act 1997 London: HMSO.

Nursing and Midwifery Order 2001 London: HMSO.

Primary Care Act 1997 London: HMSO.

Reporting of Injuries, Diseases and Dangerous Occurrences Regulations (RIDDOR) 1995 London: HMSO.

Statutory Instruments 1986 No. 786, 1990 No. 1624, 1993 No. 1901 and 1993 No. 2106 and the Nurses, Midwives and Health Visitors (Midwives Amendment) Rules 1998 SI 2649 London: HMSO.

Stillbirth Definition Act 1992 London: HMSO.

Unfair Contract Terms Act 1977 London: HMSO.

Vaccine Damage Payments Act 1979 London: HMSO.

CASES

A National Health Service Trust v. *D Lloyd, Rep Med* [2000] 411.

Barnett v. *Chelsea Hospital Management Committee* (HMC) [1968] 1 All ER 1068.

Bolam v. *Friern Hospital Management Committee* (HMC) [1957] 1 WLR 582.

Bolitho v. *City and Hackney Health Authority* (HA) [1997] 3 WLR 1151.

Bull and Wakeham v. *Devon Health Authority* [1993] 4 Med LR 117. CA [1989] 2 February 1989 Transcript.

D. v. *National Society for the Prevention of Cruelty to Children* [1977] 1 All ER 589.

Donoghue v. *Stevenson* [1932] AC 562.

Dyer (A Minor) v. *Lambeth, Southwark and Lewisham Health Authority* [1999] reported in Kemp and Kemp, March.

Hedley Byrne & Co Ltd v. *Heller & Partners Ltd* House of Lords [1963] 2 All ER 575.

In re MB (Caesarean Section) [1997] TLR 18 April; *Re MB (Adult Medical Treatment)* [1997] 2 FLR 426

Leigh v. *Gladstone* [1909] 26 TLR 139.

Maynard v. *W Midlands Regional Health Authority* HL [1985] 1 All ER 635.

Pearce v. *United Bristol Healthcare NHS Trust* [1999] 48 BMLR 118.

R. v. *Adomako* House of Lords [1995] 1 AC 171.

Re C (Adult: Refusal of Medical Treatment) [1994] 1 All ER 819.

Re T (Adult) Refusal of Medical Treatment [1992] 4 All ER 649.

Secretary of State for the Home Department v. *Orb* [1995] 1 All ER 677.

Sidaway v. *Bethlem Royal Hospital Governors* [1985] 1 All ER 643.

Spring v. *Guardian Assurance plc and others* [1994] TLR 8 July.

St George's Healthcare National Health Service Trust v. *S* [1998] TLR August 3 CA: 3 All ER 673.

Taylor v. *West Kent Health Authority* [1997] 8 Med LR 251.

Walker v. *Northumberland County Council* [1995] 1 All ER 737.

Whitehouse v. *Jordan* [1981] 1 All ER 267.

Wilsher v. *Essex Area Health Authority* [1986] 3 All ER 801 CA.

Wilsher v. *Essex Area Health Authority* [1988] AC 1074 HL.

FURTHER READING

Dimond, B. (2002) *Legal Aspects of Midwifery,* 2nd edn. Oxford: Butterworth Heinemann.
This text covers main areas of law relating to midwifery practice.

Dimond, B. & Walters, D. (1997) *Legal Aspects of Midwifery: Workbook.* Hale: Books for Midwives Press.
This text can be used as a partner text to *Legal Aspects of Midwifery* (see above) and provides practical exercises for understanding the legal principles.

Symon, A. (2001) *Obstetric Litigation from A to Z.* Salisbury: Quay Books, Mark Allen Publishing.
This is a useful text which clarifies the key concepts within obstetric litigation, and is clearly presented in A–Z format, making it a useful ward/unit resource.

Kennedy, I. & Grubb, A. (2001) *Medical Law.* London, Butterworths.
This is a more specialized and in-depth presentation of the main cases and statutes and commentaries.

69

Management and Leadership in Midwifery

Frances Day-Stirk

LEARNING OUTCOMES

At the end of the chapter readers will be able to:

- understand leadership and management theories and be able to apply them to midwifery practice
- identify their own leadership/management style and potential

- determine their development needs
- understand some of the issues in career planning.

INTRODUCTION

This chapter explores the theories on leadership and management, and provides practical application and parallels to midwifery. The reflective exercises and outcomes are to assist the reader to develop further awareness of self, personal attributes and qualities of leadership and management.

Leadership and management are essential to support the development and direction of midwifery education, practice and service. Whether at entry level, newly qualified or as experienced practitioner, individual self-management as well as wider leadership and management are important in underpinning autonomous practice. Junior students or maternity care assistants also benefit greatly from working with midwives with these transferable skills. The principles can also be applied to practice and in midwives' engagement with childbearing women in planning the management of their care. Key elements of leadership and management such as anticipation, reflection, thinking ahead, forward planning are valuable adjuncts in the pathway from student to qualified practitioner and beyond to the development of the expert practitioner (Benner, 1984). The understanding and development of these skills and their application determine success, innovation and progress in both practice and career.

ORGANIZATIONS AND THE NHS CONTEXT

It is impossible to look at leadership and management without considering the organization, as this is the context in which both take place. Organization is the generic term for any entity such as a company, a free-standing directorate of a company or a unit in the public sector, for example a hospital, which provides products or services. The term structure – hierarchical, matrix, horizontal – is used to indicate the internal organization of such a unit and is often graphically illustrated by an organizational chart or organogram (Fig. 69.1).

Organizations that bring together the skills and effort of large numbers of people, to achieve specific objectives, vary widely depending on the scale and nature of the activities in which they are engaged and are a distinguishing feature of an industrialized society and modern life. However, the appropriateness of their structure to the type of business is important to their effectiveness.

Hierarchy is based on a vertical, pyramidal multi-layered structure of central decision-making, power and control. Within this structure a single head and other key managerial positions are defined, and decisions are made in a linear vertical sequence at the top, and implemented lower down the structure.

A

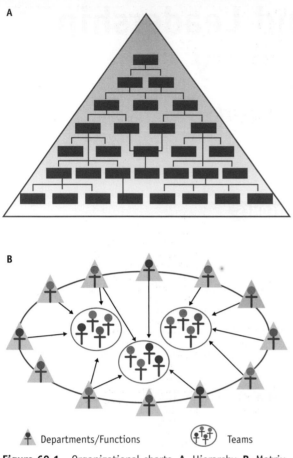

B

Departments/Functions   Teams

Figure 69.1   Organizational charts. **A.** Hierarchy. **B.** Matrix.

A matrix organization is a horizontal and vertical combined structure, which results in more teams within a flatter structure that offers scope for involvement and decision-making by more than a few key people (Handy, 1988).

The key features of a pure bureaucracy are specialization, formalization, clear hierarchy, promotion by merit, impersonal rewards and sanctions, career tenure and separation of careers and private lives (Handy, 1988). There are two other forms of bureaucracy: machine bureaucracy and standardized and professional bureaucracy, within which professionals' power base of expertise affords a high degree of autonomy and local control over professional standards (Hunt, 1992). The NHS exhibits many features of the latter, and the negative consequences of the hierarchical structure within the health service and institutionalization in reducing midwives' autonomy have been articulated (McAnulty, 1993; Page, 2001).

Organizational structures can be empowering or disempowering, and reliant on the people in them: 'organization charts and titles count for next to nothing as endeavours succeed or fail because of the people involved' (Powell, 1996).

The media often portray the NHS as 'top heavy' but in reality good management is crucial in ensuring effective organization. The NHS, the largest organization in Europe, employing over 1.25 million people, is an example of a hierarchical organization and has a reputation as bureaucratic, centralized, inflexible and unwieldy (Wedderburn Tate, 2001). In parallel with other organizations of this type, a key accusation is that there are fundamental problems with the NHS being 'under-led and over managed' (Bennis, 1999: 82) and fostering management over leadership (Wedderburn Tate, 2001: 82). This is associated with problems with the NHS's well-being (Wedderburn Tate, 2001), an over-reliance on 'policies, practices, procedures and rule book' and a lack of concern for important issues like empowerment, trust, mission and vision (Bennis, 1999; DePree, 1989).

It is argued that organizations like the NHS need decentralized models 'to replace hierarchical bureaucracies' (Bennis, 1999). Examples of this are group practices, clinical areas and such services that have autonomy and responsibility for a delegated budget, staff and organization of care. Midwives complain about their inability to practice autonomously because they feel bound by rigid procedures and policies, yet there is sometimes limited take-up of opportunities to work within structures such as group practices, caseload and other similar systems. This can be problematic, and confusing for a DoMS working to achieve autonomous systems of practice, when there are recruitment and retention problems. Many midwives, irrespective of their level within the organization, express dissatisfaction with managers without appreciating the wider picture (Curtis et al., 2003).

Management and leadership are a shared responsibility of many at all levels, not merely the 'person at the top', and therefore whatever the level of the practitioner, it is crucial to invest energy and commitment in the service. This requires an active interest in theories

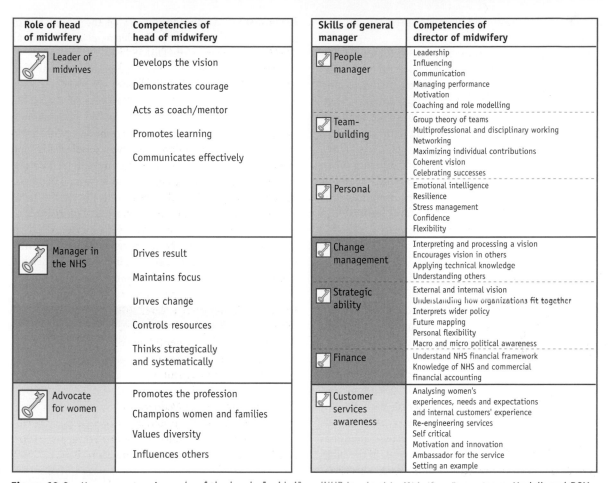

Role of head of midwifery	Competencies of head of midwifery	Skills of general manager	Competencies of director of midwifery
Leader of midwives	Develops the vision Demonstrates courage Acts as coach/mentor Promotes learning Communicates effectively	People manager	Leadership Influencing Communication Managing performance Motivation Coaching and role modelling
		Team-building	Group theory of teams Multiprofessional and disciplinary working Networking Maximizing individual contributions Coherent vision Celebrating successes
		Personal	Emotional intelligence Resilience Stress management Confidence Flexibility
Manager in the NHS	Drives result Maintains focus Drives change Controls resources Thinks strategically and systematically	Change management	Interpreting and processing a vision Encourages vision in others Applying technical knowledge Understanding others
		Strategic ability	External and internal vision Understanding how organizations fit together Interprets wider policy Future mapping Personal flexibility Macro and micro political awareness
		Finance	Understand NHS financial framework Knowledge of NHS and commercial financial accounting
Advocate for women	Promotes the profession Champions women and families Values diversity Influences others	Customer services awareness	Analysing women's experiences, needs and expectations and internal customers' experience Re-engineering services Self critical Motivation and innovation Ambassador for the service Setting an example

Figure 69.2 Key competencies: role of the head of midwifery (NHS Leadership Midwifery Competency Model) and RCM role of director of midwifery.

of leadership and of organizations, as failure to do so will be the continual repetition of mistakes with predictably familiar results (Wedderburn Tate, 2001; DoH, 2000a). There are indicators that the NHS is beginning a new stream of consciousness and planning, with the establishment of NHS Modernisation Agency Leadership, National Nursing Leadership Programme and other UK government initiatives (CNAC, 1996; DoH, 2000b; Scottish NHS Executive, 2001; Welsh Assembly, 2002).

As part of a national leadership initiative, a Midwifery Leadership Competency Model (NHS, 2002) was devised. This identified three broad roles:

- leader of midwives
- manager in the NHS
- advocate for women and families.

and 14 competencies (see Fig. 69.2). These competencies were required to ensure a superior performance;

develop a model to support succession planning and leadership development programmes; and to enhance skill and knowledge required to widen the circle of control and influence of Heads of Midwifery Services (HoMS). The model also provides a pathway for practitioners interested in becoming managers.

Subsequent to the NHS reforms of the 1990s, there is concern within the profession at the demise of midwives at senior level within midwifery management, with recommendations that HoMS should be appointed at an appropriate decision-making level within the senior management structure (Curtis *et al.*, 2003; Henderson, 1997). This has culminated in a strategy document clarifying the roles of Heads of Midwifery Services (HoMS) and Directors of Midwifery Services (DoMS) and the competencies required for both (RCM, 2003). This is not merely a change of words from 'Head' to 'Director,' as both would be the most senior practising midwife within the service. The word *director* signals visibility and a combined strategic, professional and operational remit.

Widespread disenchantment with midwifery management and the prevalence of bullying and horizontal violence were factors reported as adversely influencing retention of midwives (Ball *et al.*, 2002). Managers were perceived as unapproachable, but themselves reported feelings of powerlessness whilst being denied access to decision-making bodies within their trusts (Curtis *et al.*, 2003). The most effective environment emerges when a supportive DoMS enjoys the support and loyalty of staff in return. Successful partnerships are analogous to marriage – both need nurturing – and leaders who are able to sustain such relationships give a valuable 'collective advantage' to the organization (Moss Kanter, 1994, cited in Kippenberger, 2002). This partnership concept is also fundamental to midwives and their relationships with women.

The insularity of the NHS, prevalence of macho management styles and the common command-and-control leadership style leaves it particularly vulnerable to large-scale failures of leadership (Wedderburn Tate, 2001). A proposed change of mind-set, aligning human resources and creating a culture which encourages ideas and empowers, would be helpful. This along with organizational structures which resemble networks or modules, flattened hierarchies and more cross-functional linkages (Bennis, 1999) would be beneficial. In the NHS this will mean decentralization and more multidisciplinary working, which may go some way to avoiding such failure.

THE ORGANIZATION–LEADER INTERFACE

Leaders are essential to organizations in providing strategic vision and direction, and need to be concerned with the value systems that underpin the principles and standards that guide practices within the organization (DePree, 1989; Drucker, 1977). Leadership is the key determinant in the success or failure of any human institution (Bennis, 1999), in creating a human community held together by the work bond for a common purpose (Drucker, 1977).

In many organizations there are two kinds of leaders: hierarchical leaders, those in designated managerial positions, e.g. DoMS; and roving leaders, e.g. F and G grade midwives, who take charge in varying degrees (DePree, 1989). Midwifery leadership is crucial to facilitating new models of care, for professional development and high-quality care (Kirkham and Stapleton, 2000;

RCM, 2000). Midwives also value the leadership of supervisors of midwives (Stapleton *et al.*, 1998) as distinct from that of the DoMS.

German composer Gustav Mahler insisted that each principal musician in the orchestra sit in the audience at least once a week to get some sense of the whole (Stone Zander and Zander, 2000). DoMS who maintain a small 'hands-on' role enjoy credibility with grass roots midwives and, similarly, midwives with shadowing or secondment experience, or who have been patients, have a different perspective of the service. The measure of an organization can be seen in the way it 'facilitate[s] and accelerate[s] the competency of its leaders' (Bennis, 1999: 135), yet the NHS is described as deficient in 'the leadership and vision needed at many levels', and as imposing barriers which inhibit leadership potential (DoH, 2002; Wedderburn Tate, 2001).

Reflective Activity 69.2

Use the 'six things a leader creates' criteria (Bennis, 1999) to gauge your organization. Is there:

1. a compelling vision
2. a climate of trust
3. clear meaning
4. success: feedback on mistake – another way of doing things
5. a healthy empowering environment
6. a flat, flexible, adaptive, decentralized system?

Trust and reliability are essential to all organizations – effective leaders are fair and trust people to do a good job (Wedderburn Tate, 2001). Bennis argues that people would much rather follow individuals they can count on, even when they disagree with their viewpoint, than people they agree with but who shift positions frequently. Midwives need to know that their manager will support them. Trust is a huge issue for midwives – though unfortunately some do not feel that they can trust their supervisors, managers and colleagues (Kirkham and Stapleton, 2000). Before one generates trust, this mutual exchange is important between the DoMS and midwives, and between team leaders and members, and midwives and women. Trust is constantly observed, hard earned and easily dissipated. It is valuable social capital and not to be squandered (O'Neill, 2002).

The management of resources and maintenance of the financial integrity of organizations also rests with managers, and decisions around service provision, pay, costs and staffing levels have traditionally been the responsibility of those at the most senior level (Wedderburn Tate, 2001). Today, management responsibility permeates every level, and all practitioners need to understand issues and deal with the impact of 'finite financial resources' or staff selection, recruitment and retention, working patterns and creative decision-making.

NHS trusts tend to follow a rigid pattern of seeing full-time work as the norm, with few alternatives being offered, though part-time midwifery posts now outnumber full-time posts. This inflexibility within the NHS makes managing work–life balance difficult and therefore does not make it an employer of choice; this challenges DoMS to find a way of accommodating midwives, injecting flexibility – job-share, part time, etc. – which many midwives desire (Ball *et al.*, 2003).

Another concern is customer satisfaction, originating from a combination of quality products and service and capable contented employees. This often involves change – the ultimate leadership challenge. This is highly relevant in the maternity services, when responsiveness to women's needs is determined by a changing society. DoMS have a responsibility for the development of midwifery, and midwives in providing a responsive woman-centred care service. Wedderburn Tate (2001) urges 'alternative ways of thinking about what we do, who we do it with and why we do it and how we do it'.

DEFINITIONS AND DIFFERENCES

> Leaders are people who do the right thing; managers are people who do things right. Both roles are crucial yet differ profoundly.
>
> (Bennis, 1999: 82)

In every sphere of life there is a need for leadership and organization, whether in an orchestra (Stone Zander and Zander, 2000), in politics or in the NHS. There is broad consensus that a leader may not always be a manager and a manager may not always be a leader; therefore, the two roles are not synonymous, but both are important, albeit in different ways and in different circumstances (Bennis, 1999; Hunt, 1992). Midwives are exposed daily to leadership and management in different guises, and often function within their personal and family lives as leader, manager, or as the managed. It can be difficult to disentangle the two; therefore it is important to have a clear understanding

of definitions in order to recognize and understand the differences between and the distinguishing features of the terms, and how each is interpreted and applied in practice and the potential impact.

Leaders and leadership

There are many definitions of leadership; words used to describe it are 'art', 'process' or 'attitude' (DePree, 1989; Kippenberger, 2002; Kouzes and Posner, 1995, cited in Wedderburn Tate, 2001; Ulrich, 1996). It also involves the interdependent engagement of leader, followers, the task and situation (Hunt, 1992: 242).

Whilst there is no commonly agreed definition, there is general agreement that leaders are made, that leadership can be learnt and that leaders exist at every level or emerge from circumstances or situations (Wedderburn Tate, 2001). Leaders do not always occupy senior posts, often not realizing that they are 'everyday leaders', the person that everyone goes to for advice and is listened to (Myerson, 2001, cited in Kippenberger, 2002; Shamir, 1995; Tichy and Cohen, 2000, cited in Wedderburn Tate, 2001).

Leaders impart an intelligence of vision, purpose, strategic intent (Bennis, 1999), define reality, say 'thank you', are servants and debtors (DePree, 1989). In the midwifery context the DoMS' role is to analyse and interpret policy documents, to clarify and translate the meaning for staff, to make available resources needed for implementation and acknowledge each staff member's contribution, however small. Leaders need to have a balanced portfolio of skills and experience (Fig. 69.3), encourage and reward contrary opinions, and recognize the importance of 'effective talk-back' in the decision-making process as increasing their ability to make good decisions (Bennis, 1999; DePree, 1989). This is illustrated in the use of forums such as unit meetings, group meetings or user focus groups, during which there is discussion, debate and an openness to criticism. Another noticeable trait in leaders is an ability to draw others to them by communicating 'an extraordinary focus of commitment' (Bennis, 1999). In terms of midwifery, a good DoMS who invests personal involvement is able to generate excitement and creativity in others, and will often attract staff from other units.

Effective leaders recognize the benefits of diversity, and welcome a varied team. Leaders create an adaptive learning environment that encourages the development of intellectual capital and realizes the creative powers of individuals (Bennis, 1999). They spend considerable

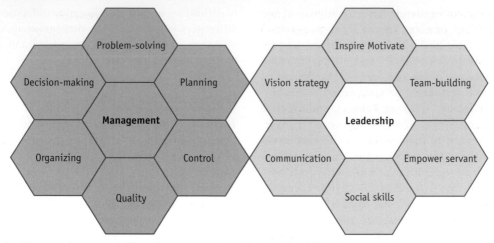

Figure 69.3   Hexagonal representation of management and leadership. (After Cross, 1996.)

time in the field, looking at their own operations and talking with both employees and customers (Peters and Waterman, 1995). Anyone in charge of an organization must be accessible to its members and its constituents, i.e. be connected (Bennis, 1999). This can be achieved by the DoMS who 'walks the talk', i.e. is accessible and approachable, visible in the clinical area and participates in clinical practice. Midwives themselves have some responsibility in developing a relationship based on integrity, honesty, openness and support (Curtis *et al.*, 2003).

The collective effect of good leadership is empowerment that can be felt throughout an organization: in midwifery there is evidence that empowered midwives empower women (Kirkham and Stapleton, 2000). Midwives can gauge their own effectiveness by adapting the following three questions used to gauge a leader's effectiveness (Bennis, 1999):

- Do workers (women) feel significant?
- Is the work felt to be exciting? (job satisfaction)
- Does the leader embody the organization's ethics and values? (philosophy).

Reflective Activity 69.3

What perception do you think the women in your practice have of their importance?

Does your organization have a midwifery philosophy and does this embody the centrality of women?

How would you make the woman feel significant? Reflect on your own role, the purpose of your team, ward or unit.

Managers and management

Management is perceived as getting people to do what needs to be done (Bennis, 1999). It is associated with efficiency, maintaining the status quo, control and command mechanisms, systems, procedures, policies and structures (Bennis, 1999).

It is a highly complex process that encompasses a wide range of tasks that make definition difficult. Managers are often on the receiving end of 'bad press' with the person being lost and replaced by the term 'management' (Cross, 1996). Good managers are 'the dynamic, life-giving force in every business' (Drucker, 1955), enabling innovative practice developments. Being in charge of 'bringing it all together' demands proactivity and entails a range of attributes, activities and actions that have been applied to maternity services by Cross (1996). They can be summarized as follows:

- *Planning and development.* Being future-focused, developing the maternity services though short- and long-term objective-setting and the implementation of systems of continuous quality improvement.
- *Coordination.* Harmonizing the responsibilities and activities of employees for realizing successful care.
- *Control.* Ensuring plans are effected, and evaluating progress and outcomes. This includes clinical reviews, quality audit, user satisfaction surveys and feedback and monitoring maternity service statistics as well as recognizing, rewarding and celebrating successes.
- *Communication.* Much of a manager's time is spent listening, a key managerial skill, a function which denotes 'responsiveness' and which people value most (Hunt, 1992). It involves being accessible,

e.g. having an open door policy to staff, sharing and understanding, steering, influencing, talking to and with individuals and groups of individuals, internal and external professional and user groups and the public. It is also a key midwifery skill as midwives learn to listen to what women say and do not say.

- *Information management.* Reading, interpreting, disseminating, reports, documents, special information and converting data relevant to the service, self and others. It includes vertical and horizontal transfer of information (plans, policies, actions and outcomes) to the NHS trust board, commissioners and to external audiences.
- *Human resource management.* Responsibility for recruitment and retention, direction, motivation, delegation, empowerment, education, training and development of midwives and support staff in keeping with the corporate strategy and culture of the maternity service and the NHS trust.
- *Policy formulation.* Developing policies through which maternity service objectives will be achieved. This entails agreeing goals and targets through consultation and objective setting for maternity service provision.
- *Budget management and organization.* Ensuring the provision and integration of primary (human) and secondary (non-human, e.g. finances, equipment, buildings, time) resources to deliver an effective, productive and safe service.
- *Problem-solving and decision-making.* Anticipating, identifying and investigating problems, collaborative decision-making and action planning to solve problems, initiate improvements and bring about change to shape the future maternity services. This includes representing maternity services within organizational negotiations, dealing with problems and implementing remedial action.

Managers need to have acute political antennae in order to operate effectively within different environments. One way of viewing how managers work politically was described by Baddley and James (1987) using animals as a metaphor (Fig. 69.4). The traits associated with these animals provide good illustrations. The clever foxes are politically astute and will manoeuvre people and situations to their own advantage; whereas the politically naïve sheep will often find *themselves* being manipulated, though acting honourably.

Politics and power and the capacity to influence are all closely connected and exist within individuals or within functions. Hunt (1992) describes politics as

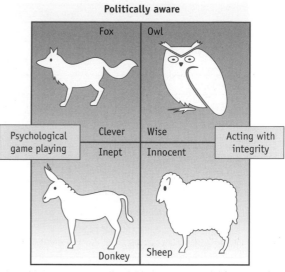

Figure 69.4   Distinguishing features of 'political animals'.

power in action and deems it necessary to get things done. There are main sources of power – interpersonal (social), structural, cultural and external – and several legitimized power bases (Table 69.1).

Midwives need to develop skills of political awareness in their dealings with other professionals and in grasping the bigger national picture. An awareness and understanding of their use in organizations is a distinct advantage.

Reflective Activity 69.4

In which quadrant of Figure 69.4 do you fit? What political animal best describes your peers and other colleagues – are you amongst sheep or foxes? Can you identify the powers being used in your team or organization?

Management is both a micro and a macro function – not simply vested in the most senior post-holder but occurring at several levels, in ward or team managers as well as in the individual manager of self, junior colleagues, and the woman and her family.

Manager or leader?

Just as there is often uncertainty between management and supervision, there can be a similar confusion with leadership and management. Leaders are distinguished from day-to-day managers by what they do, their

Table 69.1 Legitimized power bases (adapted from Hunt, 1992: 67)

Power bases	Effect
Authority – positional power (DoMS)	The right to control resources – financial, human, information and access to decision-making processes
Function	Importance within the organization, e.g. neonatal services
Access	To powerful people, e.g. the DoMS to the Chief Executive
Intellect	Capacity to diagnose, solve problems and provide solutions for uncertain situations
Interpersonal skills	Empathy, sensitivity, intuition, social skills, articulate, listening, observing
Expertise – Consultant Midwife	Based on experience, knowledge and skill
Performance – Team Leader	Super, outperforming others
Referent power – midwife and DoMS; DoMS and Chief Executive	Use of others' power, i.e. link to a powerful internal person or external body, e.g. the Health Authority

actions and behaviours (Hunt, 1992), in getting people to *want* to do what needs to be done (Bennis, 1999; Kippenberger, 2002) and in creating the appropriate culture (Schein, 1985) (see Table 69.2). Although some functions are specific to role, there is a degree of tension and overlap, making communication essential.

Unlike the long-term perspective associated with leadership, management appears aligned with a short-term approach. Ostensibly leadership as a concept appears to be favoured over the mundane management; however, management is needed to make it happen (Kotter, 1990). In the NHS this view is polarized with the leadership focus lacking and management often associated with negative press and media connotations. However, the features distinguishing leaders from managers are the identical ones that can damage leaders and their organization.

Both groups usually have an understanding of their respective and complementary roles. One useful description of leadership emerged from a group of managers (Jones, 1999) and reflects the four leader competencies – 'managements' – identified by Bennis (1999) (Fig. 69.5).

The ability to create and *manage meaning* is critical, the more decentralized and complex the organization. In bringing devolved responsibility to clinical midwives the DoMS is critical; imagining possibilities and translating ideas into realities, whilst always ensuring everyone 'sings from the same hymn sheet'. This applies equally to all of the team, from maternity care assistant to midwives and medical colleagues. It also has parallel application for midwives in their interactions with women.

Cautionary warnings that 'leaders who cannot manage and managers who cannot lead create the worst of both worlds' and that incompetent managers can make life worse, make people sicker and less vital, with profound effects on long-term health, are offered by Ball *et al.* (2003), Bennis (1999) and Kotter (1990). When considering management and leadership it should be noted that it cascades from the highest level, i.e. from the Chief Executive through all levels of staff to clients, patients and the family.

Reflective Activity 69.5

Reflect on the people in leadership and management positions (within and outside midwifery): Think about units you have worked in: who are the leaders and who are the managers?

Think about the skills that you have observed in leaders and managers. Are they the same?

Which do you prefer? Why? Which are you?

THEORIES UNDERPINNING LEADERSHIP AND MANAGEMENT

Organization theory can be categorized into two main schools of thought:

- Classic – focusing on organizational structure and function

Table 69.2 Distinguishing features of leaders and managers

Distinguishing features	Leaders	Managers	References
Traits	Innovate Original Questioning and challenging Focus on people Inspire control Long-range perspective Originate Ask what and why Create a tapestry of intentions Pull Communicate Align, create, empower Servants	Administer Copy Accept the status quo Focus on systems and structures Rely on control Short-range view Imitate Ask how and when Push Command	Bennis, 1999 DePree, 1989 Alimo-Metcalf, 1996
Skills and attributes	Ability to articulate a vision Embrace error Encourage 'reflective backtalk' Competencies: management of attention, meaning, trust and self	Relevant professional knowledge Command of basic facts Proactivity Emotional resilience Social skills and abilities Analytical, problem-solving, decision/judgement-making skills Continuing sensitivity to events Self-knowledge Balanced learning habits and skills Mental agility Creativity	Pedler *et al.*, 1997 Bennis, 1999
Personal qualities	Self-knowledge Open to feedback Eager to learn and improve Curious, risk takers Concentrate at work Learn from adversity Balance tradition and change Open style Work well with systems Serve as models and mentors Politically aware Emotional intelligence 'Crap detectors'	First child or first son, i.e. 'special' High achievers: motivated to succeed, competitive, take careers seriously High energy levels: required to persist, be disappointed and to fight back in the hierarchy-climbing stakes Longer time span: think 3–5 years Goal directed: endless pursuit of goals Politically active, loners content and confident with their own company Field-independent: psychologically capable of differentiating the important from the unimportant; the central from the peripheral	Bennis, 1999 Hunt, 1992 Wedderburn Tate, 2001
Functions	Leadership Align people into teams and coalitions Set direction Focus on change Motivate, inspire	Management Staff and structure, policies and procedures Plans and budgets Predictability and order Problem-solving and control Energize	Kotter, 1990

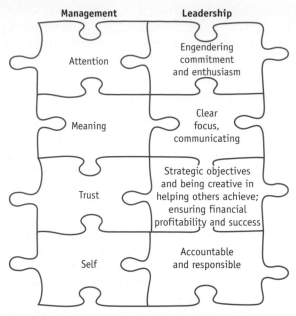

Figure 69.5 Management–leadership jigsaw.

- Human relations – focusing on people in organizations and how they view and accept their work.

Scientific management, the only Classic theory considered here, concentrated on the division of work between workers and managers but ignored leadership (Kippenberger, 2002). The principal object of management was seen to be to secure mutual benefit and satisfaction, and maximum prosperity for the employer and the employee (Pugh and Hickson, 1989, cited in Wedderburn Tate, 2001). Fayol identified five elements of management – namely forecast and plan; organize; command; coordinate; and control – and 14 general principles of management which included kindliness and justice to ensure equity and each employee must have one boss for unity of command (Burnes, 1996).

Human Relations School

The Human Relations School of management theory put people first. It focused on the limitations of the scientific theories and task-focused approaches, concluding that feeling important and valued was more important than the actual physical work conditions. This model stresses three core elements: leadership and communication; intrinsic job motivation and rewards; and organizational structures and practices that facilitate flexibility and involvement (Burnes, 1996). Midwives have cited all three factors as contributing to their decision to leave midwifery where there was 'no

specific sense or belonging', whilst expressing frustration at not being able work in systems which enable the development of effective midwife–woman relationships (Ball et al., 2002).

Motivational theories

Motivational theories argue that the effective manager is responsible for increasing productivity by creating a supportive environment for each employee, encouraging satisfaction and removing obstacles. A significant finding was the different manager and employee perspectives, with employees being motivated by recognition, security and a sense of belonging and managers by the 'logic of cost and efficiency' (Mayo, 1993, cited in Wedderburn Tate, 2002).

Theory X–Y model

This model constructed by McGregor proposed that managers assumed two types of workers (X and Y) and, over time, had the ability to change the psychology of their employees. X–Y theory application may seem to have parallels within the obstetric philosophy of normal in retrospect and the midwifery philosophy of presumed normal unless it becomes complicated.

Theory X manager style is based on a negative assumption that most people do not want to work and that employees:

- must be supervised to maintain quality and production
- only respect authority
- are motivated solely by money
- do not want the responsibility of decision-making
- are not ambitious and wish to remain distanced from management, which results in low productivity and a demotivated workforce.

Theory Y managers, whose assumptions are based on trust and a positive belief that employees naturally enjoy work and will be efficient if trusted with responsibility, hold an opposite view; though employees do need:

- to be committed to the job
- recognition for their contribution
- to be allowed to retain their dignity and self-respect
- to be given maximum freedom to get on with the job as they see fit (Wilson, 2000).

Theory Y managers are facilitators and are more likely to create an open structure, with formal and informal communication channels. In terms of midwifery service organization this approach can be seen in decentralization of caseload practices; self-managed teams or units with delegated budgets; and management models which encourage freedom to arrange own workload, patterns or sphere of work. The benefits of occupational autonomy and the development of meaningful relationships with women and strong relationships with peers and partners within midwifery are well evidenced (Sandall, 1997: 2001) as positive triggers to improved recruitment and retention of midwives (Ball *et al.*, 2002).

Trait theory approach

This approach to leadership attempts to understand the leadership phenomenon by seeking to identify individual personality traits that can be attributed to effective leaders, i.e. ambition, decisiveness, charisma (Hunt, 1992), in accordance with Fielder's 'Great Man' theory (Wedderburn Tate, 2001). Although no special traits have been proven, and some believe the all-knowing individual to be 'anachronistic' (Kippenberger, 2002), 10 traits of dynamic leaders have been identified (Bennis, 1999). Others suggest that leaders possess a unique combination of cognitive skills and competencies, which have been shown in studies of strategic thinking (Hunt, 1992) and which Kotter (1990) describes as needed in 'creating an agenda for change' (Table 69.3).

Situational/contingency theory

This theory argues that the scientific and motivational theories omitted a significant factor – the environment. Path–goal theory is based on the assumption that an individual's motivation to undertake a task is related to achieving the desired outcome; personal satisfaction and reward (Cross, 1996). These leaders emerge from and epitomize two aspects of leadership behaviour – relationship-based and task-completion – simultaneously apparent in the same person.

Leader–member exchange (LMX) theory, or the relationship-based leader, focuses on the relationship and communication established between the leader and each member of the team. The existence of two subgroups, an in-group and out-group, that may become divisive is recognized. Research on LMX theory suggests that the high-quality relationships enjoyed lead to 'lower stress levels, better job appraisals, more commitment with beneficial spin offs for the organization' (Northhouse, 1997, cited in Wedderburn Tate, 2001).

Researchers have separated leadership into two further categories, transformational and transactional, although Hunt (1992) believes this separation is not particularly helpful.

Transformational leadership

This is often cited as the ideal leadership style, yielding many positive outcomes: lower levels of staff stress; more collaboration, innovation and shared responsibilities; better financial performance, job satisfaction, motivation and performance of followers. Despite psychological questionnaires to identify such leaders, cynics argue that there is little experiential evidence to support their predicted success (Kippenberger, 2002). However, Schein (1985) argues that transformational leaders must change the culture of the organization by their own behaviours in harmony with organization structure, systems, physical space, new philosophy or values. The UK model of transformational leadership that highlights leading others, personal qualities and organizational skills (Alimo-Metcalf and Alban-Metcalf, 2000) contrasts with the US models which emphasize charisma, inspiration and vision, and the leader as change agent and a role model for followers (Wedderburn Tate, 2001). Transformational leaders are confident to lead from a distance, delegating responsibility and allowing decisions to be made by those closest to the service or users. Decentralized models of care such as community-based services – antenatal clinics, home assessments in labour, one-stop shops and midwife accommodation – are demonstrations of this.

Transactional leadership

Transactional leaders engage by offering a deal or a transaction to followers, such as opportunities for further study or development (Hunt, 1992). Such leadership has a strong association with management, including immediate results, and structures and process for control. It focuses on the current situation, protects the culture, and derives power from position and authority in the organization (Jones, 1999).

Style theory

This theory, which is addressed below, has superseded the trait and situational theories of leadership and concentrates on the manner in which a leader exercises control and motivates staff to achieve organizational goals.

Table 69.3 Spectrum of current thoughts on leadership (adapted from Kippenberger, 2002: 47)

	School of thought											
	Charismatic	Transformational	Adaptive	F's of leadership	Leader as builder	Nearby leaders	Learning	Co-leadership	'Quiet'	Creative	Swedish	Leadership for greatness
Main ingredient	Inspirational charisma	Self-confident Powerful vision Charisma passionate, values-based Intellectual stimulation, encouraging people Challenge systems in organizations Questioning self, lateral thinking, challenge me as leader Individualized consideration – openness not status, value people, proactive UK model: 14 dimensions; 3 clusters	Fresh eye and fast reaction	Fast Flexible Fun Focused Friendly	Embeds organizational ability	Dynamic, active, sociable, open, considerate, expert, intelligent, physically impressive, original, unconventional Set high standards	Leaders released at all levels	Complementary partnership	Thoughtfulness rooted in experience	Innovating, initiating Creative, adaptive, agile Looks at the horizon, not just at the bottom line Effectiveness What and why Trust in people	Discuss, analyse then decide Calm, patient, composure Trust and empower staff (high-trust cultures) Build commitment Learning organization Incremental development of staff Respect and praise – facilitative confidence-building Respect for individuals	Humility and steely determination
Time frame	Early 1980s	Mid-1980s	1990s		Mid-1990s	Mid-1990s	1990s	Late 1990s	Late 1990s			2001
Author	Continuing research and promotion	Bass and Avolio, 1994 Alimo-Metcalf, 1996	Growing research and literature	Moss Kanter, 1994	Continuing influence	Shamir, 1995	Diverse, research continues	Needs more work and research	Beginnings of anti-hero investigation	Bennis, 1999	Scase, 2001	Brand new research

GENDER AND RACE

There was little evidence of the impact of gender and race on leadership until the 1990s. Rosener's (1990) study found fundamental differences in how women and men described leadership with women characterized as transformational and men as transactional. Wedderburn Tate (2001) suggested that women were more likely to structure flatter organizations and to emphasize frequent contact and sharing of information in 'webs of inclusion'. Most of the prior research comparing male and female leaders has been restricted to a very narrow range of leadership styles. An interesting survey by Bass and Avolio in 1994 showed that women rated higher on three of the following four 'I' criteria:

- Idealized influence (charisma)
- Inspirational motivation
- Intellectual stimulation
- Individualized consideration.

This study confirmed Rosener's (1990) findings which characterized women as transformational, i.e. being more democratic and participative, adopting an interactive, consensus-building style sharing power and information, but disappointingly this appears to change as they move up the ladder. This is pertinent to DoMS as managers of a workforce primarily of women delivering a service to women receiving the service. How they use their personal power can have negative or positive influence in enhancing the self-worth of women in their care.

There is little written on leadership and race; however, there appears to be a concrete ceiling, with women and black people experiencing a reinforced concrete ceiling (Alimo-Metcalf and Alban-Metcalf, 2000; Booysen, 1995). Nowhere is this more evident than in the NHS with its primarily female workforce and large black and ethnic minority workforce that is invisible in top management posts. It has been revealed that black and minority ethnic (BME) staff are blocked or deterred from progressing to senior positions within the NHS (DoH, 2002). Leaders in a culturally diverse world will have to develop 'mindfulness', the ability to be attentive to what is actually happening, to view it in new ways and respond appropriately, not from habit (Kippenberger, 2002). Leaders have to be increasingly cosmopolitan in their outlook to avoid stereotyping and in developing services that meet the needs of the local population and staff. Similarly, midwives need to respect the different value systems, cultural norms and accepted behaviours of childbearing women.

LEADERSHIP AND MANAGEMENT STYLES

In this section the styles of leadership and management, their differences and how and when their use is beneficial or inappropriate will be considered.

Leadership and management styles come in many forms, are dependent on several factors and are often determined by the organization's culture. Leadership style is defined as the manner and approach used to provide direction, implement plans and motivate people; and management style as a blend of personal qualities, attitudes, perception and intuition which makes each person's approach to a given situation unique (DePree, 1989; Wilson, 2000).

Of the three distinct leadership styles recognized (Table 69.4) there is no one that is ideal; each technique has its own set of advantages and disadvantages and uses leadership differently. Although most leaders commonly use all three styles, and develop an eclectic approach, one style usually becomes dominant. A particular style of leadership or management cannot be totally explained by the behavioural models described (see Table 69.3); it cannot be given or imitated: 'it has to be discovered and developed by detailed and diligent self-analysis and experiment' (Wilson, 2000). The situation and prevailing culture will also influence and determine which style is adopted. Determining the approach to a problem is influenced by several factors including; the situation, the leader's personality, attitudes of the people involved, recent events, the urgency and importance of the task, organization culture, long-term strategy and the cost of failure (Wilson, 2000).

It is also important that the person managing or leading is seen in the context of the time and the level of organization. During times of change, the whole organization or service needs a leader to provide vision, and suggest creative solutions to problems. In the same organization, there is also a need for good management. All organization needs a balance of managers and leaders. An example would be the DoMS as an effective leader and the senior midwife managers as good managers. This framework is, however, fluid, in that a leader may have elements of a good manager, and a manager may have elements of leadership – and this may be in varying weights. Each characteristic may actually be a continuum (Bennis, 1999). The style continuum describes the spectrum of approaches which

Table 69.4 Leadership/management styles

Style and characterization	Advantages	Disadvantages
The autocrat Directive style: dictates what to do, and how to do it without involving staff or seeking advice No room for questions with this unilateral approach Leader dominates team members Expects orders to be carried out Associated with a Theory X manager (gives little consideration to Maslow's theory of needs (Fig. 69.6) or motivating theories) Depends on a hierarchical structure to function effectively Often leads to demotivation	Effective when urgent action is needed, i.e. in a clinical emergency or combat situation	Staff become dependent May be passive resistance from staff Need for constant pressure and direction from the leader to maintain control
Laissez-faire Allow staff to make decisions May be seen by subordinates as being left to get on with the job Minimum interference or direction Success or failure is dependent on employees' own energies Inappropriate for some organizations, i.e. the armed forces	Employees are fully involved in decision-making Autonomy and creativity may be enhanced	Employees may feel unfairly delegated to or unsupported There may be a lack of direction
Democratic or participative An inclusive approach Consultation with employees in decision-making The leader maintains final authority but encourages participation and delegates sensibly Most closely associated with a Theory Y manager	Employees are involved in designing their jobs and tasks and in decisions about how the job will be done and by whom	Decisions may take longer to be reached

can be plotted between the two poles of authoritarianism at one end and acquiescence at the other. There is no one best style; success lies in the skill in being able to locate the correct point on the spectrum for each situation and level of management.

SELF AND CAREER DEVELOPMENT

Leadership is a journey not a destination …
There are more opportunities than ever for midwifery career development within the NHS, with clear pathways, competencies and functions. These are demonstrated in service management (DoMS), education (Head of School) and clinical practice (Consultant Midwife) (NHS, 1999), where leadership is demanded and these skills and competencies are imperatives and provide direction for aspiring midwifery leaders. Historically, few practitioners actually plan out their career pathway.

Personal growth development inevitably involves personal transformation – becoming yourself and being responsible for it (Bennis, 1999). The term self-development is used to describe a range of personal and interpersonal skills: leadership, team working,

time management, communication and presentation, conflict handling, appraisal, mentoring, creativity, managing stress, etc. (Reeves, 1997: 114). An important first step on the personal development pathway is self-awareness. This involves the ability to examine one's own thinking, motives, habits and paradigms and how to make a 'paradigm shift' (Covey, 1989: 23). It involves knowing one's skills and deploying them effectively (Bennis, 1999). It entails taking primary responsibility for your learning and deciding how to attain it. It requires career development and advancement and embraces improving performance in an existing job which ultimately leads to the achievement of full potential and self-actualization (Pedler *et al.*, 1997; Wedderburn Tate, 2001).

Self-actualization is the apex of Maslow's hierarchy of needs. Only when the basic needs at the base have been satisfied can higher-order needs be achieved. This is a continuously evolving process, and differs from person to person throughout a person's lifetime. It often results in a change of attitudes, an awareness and altered preferred way of behaviour, a self re-appraisal and altering of values (Alimo-Metcalf, 1996; Reeves, 1997).

Midwifery is seen as a coping profession and midwives often have difficulty in saying 'no'. An individual's basic nature is to *act and not be acted upon* (Covey, 1989), therefore understanding autonomy and responsibility; the ability to choose is fundamental to being autonomous. Behaviour, interpersonal skills, being assertive, honest and dealing with complexity, are important both in our relationship with women and in our daily work.

Reflective Activity 69.6

At your next perinatal meeting, case presentations or multidisciplinary meetings, observe the interactions and contributions of the members. Who sits at the back? Who speaks and who doesn't?

In order to develop, it is important to know what skills and competencies are required (Fig. 69.6) and how leaders are identified and chosen (Fig. 69.7). 'Powell's Rules for Picking People' recommends looking for intelligence and judgment, capacity to anticipate, to see around corners, loyalty, integrity, a high energy drive, a balanced ego and the drive to get things done' (http://www.blaisdell.com/powell).

Career development is an iterative process requiring different skills and competencies at different levels; some increase and others decrease according to the stage of progression.

Career development opportunities

Opportunities in leadership or management will vary from developing skills from a single study to diploma,

degree or mentorship programme, shadowing, coaching or networks. Possibly the most effective way of learning the skills and finer nuances of leadership and management is through working alongside a good role model who might be a team leader, DoMS or teacher.

In thinking about the future there are a wide range of developmental situations useful to career development (DoH, 2002). In the future you may have an opportunity to lead a project or task group that consists of a wide range of people, and experience various aspects of the service or a variety of roles and jobs throughout your career. Overseas experience expands an individual's perspective and is one of the best precursors of effective leadership. Many students now

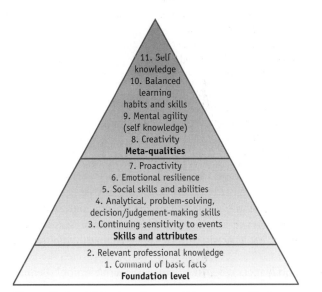

Figure 69.6 Attributes of successful managers (Pedler *et al.*, 1997).

Leaders' skills and competencies	
Cognitive	Information search Concept formation Concept flexibility
Interpersonal	Interpersonal search Managing interaction Developmental orientation
Presentational	Self-confidence Presentation impact
Motivational	Proactive orientation Achievement oriented

Attributes to choose leaders *Most important	
Technical competence	Business of midwifery literacy and knowledge of the the field
Conceptual skills	Facility of abstract or strategic thinking
People skills*	Ability to communicate, motivate and delegate
Taste*	Ability to identify and cultivate talent
Judgment*	Making difficult decisions in a short time-frame with imperfect data
Character*	Defining qualities: trust a key attribute which depend on four Cs: caring, constancy, competence and congruity
Track record	A history of achieving results

Figure 69.7 How leaders are identified (Hunt, 1992) and chosen (Bennis, 1999).

take the opportunity of an elective placement outside their practice placement.

There are steps that can be taken to help your development of decision-making, including judging the context and timeliness of decisions and assessing your own style of decision-making (Wilson, 2000). Several useful self-development exercises on negotiation, collaboration, looking after yourself, relaxation and proactivity are offered (Pedler *et al.*, 1997; Wedderburn Tate, 2001; Wilson, 2000) specifically for BME midwives (DoH, 2002).

Students and newly qualified midwives usually play an important follower role. The essential importance of good followers is unappreciated despite their making good leaders (Bennis, 1999). Effective followers are easy to identify; they challenge and provide constructive criticism, but may find themselves at odds with their colleagues/leader for speaking the truth, despite this being precisely the kind of initiative that leadership entails (Bennis, 1999: 112). In some organizations, staff who follow the status quo are rewarded while those who are critical, have innovative ideas and are independent all too soon find their position untenable (Wedderburn Tate, 2001). The process is interdependent; leaders elicit follower goals, give meaning to possibilities and improve performance without manipulation (Hunt, 1992: 242). Leaders are only as good as their followers. Parallel examples are maternity care assistants and midwives; group practice leaders and ward leaders; 'shop floor' midwives and empowering DoMS. The combination of 'followers who tell the truth and leaders who listen is an unbeatable union' (Bennis, 1999: 112).

Reflective Activity 69.7

Examine the context of a situation and decide what your leadership has to offer and whether you are ready to lead. Identify what skills would be helpful in this role, and how these could be developed.

Then read about the importance of 'homework' and personal space in Wedderburn Tate (2001: 74).

Covey described how incredibly easy it is to get caught up in an activity trap, in the business of life, to work harder and harder at climbing the ladder of success only to discover, upon reaching the top rung, that the ladder is leaning against the wrong wall. If the ladder is not leaning against the right wall, every step we take just gets us to the wrong place faster (Covey, 1989).

If midwives are to thrive we have to recognize and accept our potential as leaders. This means having a clearer idea about leadership behaviour (Wedderburn Tate, 2001) when planning our career pathway and development.

CONCLUSION

There is a wealth of information and theory surrounding leadership and management, which underpins our knowledge and understanding of individual and organizational development. The midwife needs to appreciate this underpinning knowledge and the theories which allow leadership and management to be effective and well supported from bottom up and from top down. All midwives need to see themselves as both a leader and a manager of their particular team, caring for other midwives and the women and babies for whom they are responsible.

In today's health service and in the maternity services particularly, good leadership and management are crucial to providing a midwifery voice and to ensuring that the needs of mothers and babies are met, whilst the professional development needs of the midwives are harnessed and enhanced. The impact of poor leadership and management is negatively evident in the recruitment and retention of midwives, which is in stark contrast to the vision and pioneering spirit of those who campaigned for the 1902 Midwives Act. A service which has an effective midwifery leader will have 'added value' in that there is a shared and dynamic philosophy which respects women both as professionals and as consumers of the service, and which has a vision that will allow the service to develop and grow.

Good clinical leadership is central to the delivery of government policies for the National Health Service. Its future is dependent on future-focused managers with a helicopter view, and leaders who are willing to embrace and drive through the radical transformation in services that the NHS requires. West (2002) suggested that the best prospect for the NHS is that well-selected teams of professionals and sufficient non-professionals will ensure that their local communities get the best value for money. Without leaders able to attract and retain talent, manage knowledge, and release people's capacity to adapt and innovate, an organization's future is in jeopardy (http://westy.itwn.k12.pa.us/users/sja/Bennis/html).

KEY POINTS

- Leadership is essential to innovation and progress.
- It is vital that midwives are able to manage themselves and others effectively to ensure high-quality care and optimal outcomes.
- Nurturing leadership means identifying potential and actual leaders and investing in their development.

- Management skills can be developed; leadership can be learnt.
- Leadership and management theories and concepts can be utilized to understand and enhance everyday practice and are useful in career progression.
- Empowered employees are the result of good leadership and management.

REFERENCES

Alimo-Metcalf, B. (1996) Leaders or managers? *Nursing Management* 3(1): 22–24.

Alimo-Metcalf, B. & Alban-Metcalf, R. (2000) Heaven can wait. *Health Service Journal* 12 October: 26–29.

Baddley, S. & James, K. (1987) Political skills for managers. *Management Education and Development* 18(1): 3–19.

Ball, L., Curtis, P. & Kirkham, M. (2000) *Why do Midwives Leave?* London: RCM.

Bass, B.M. & Avolio, B.J. (1994) Shatter the glass ceiling: women make better managers. *Human Resource Management* 33(4): 549–560.

Benner, P. (1984) *From Novice to Expert*. California: Addison-Wesley Publishing.

Bennis, W. (1999) *Managing People is Like Herding Cats*. London: Kogan Page.

Booysen, A.E. (1995) *An Examination of Race and Gender Influences on the Leadership Attributes of South African Managers*. DBL dissertation. Pretoria: University of South Africa. Online. Available: http://unisa.ac.za/contents/faculties/sbl/Pdfdocs.2.4.1pdf.

Burnes, B. (1996) *Managing Change*, 2nd edn. London: Pitman Publishing.

Central Nursing Advisory Committee (CNAC) (1996) *Working Together: a Focus on Health and Social Well-being. An Action Plan for Community Nurses, Midwives and Health Visitors*. Belfast: HMSO.

Covey, S. (1989) *The Seven Habits of Highly Effective People*. New York: Simon and Schuster.

Cross, R. (1996) *Midwives and Management – A Handbook*. Hale: Books for Midwives Press.

Curtis, P., Ball, L. & Kirkham, M. (2003) *Why do Midwives Leave? Talking to Managers*. London: Royal College of Midwives.

Department of Health (DoH) (2000a) *An Organisation with a Memory*. London: DoH. Online. Available: www.doh.gov.uk/orgmemreport/.

Department of Health (DoH) (2000b) *The NHS Plan: A Plan for Investment, a Plan for Reform*. London: The Stationery Office.

Department of Health (DoH) (2002) *Getting on Against the Odds. National Nursing Leadership Programme – How Black and Ethnic Minority Nurses Can Progress into Leadership – A Resource for Health and Social Care Professionals and Managers*. London: NHS Leadership Centre.

DePree, M. (1989) *Leadership is an Art*. New York: Dell Publishing.

Drucker (1955) *The Practice of Management*. London: Heinemann.

Drucker (1977) *People and Performance*. New York: Harpers College.

Handy, C. (1988) *Understanding Organizations*. England: Penguin Books.

Henderson, C. (1997) Changing structures, status of heads of midwifery. In: *Changing Childbirth and the West Midlands Region 1995–6*, Section 4.1–4.4. Cardiff: RCM.

Hunt, J. (1992) *Managing People at Work. A Manager's Guide to Behaviour in Organisations*, 3rd edn. London: McGraw Hill.

Jones, P. (1999) *The Performance Management Pocketbook*. Hampshire: Management Pocketbooks.

Kippenberger, T. (2002) *Leadership Express*. Oxford: Capstone Publishing.

Kirkham, M. & Stapleton, H. (2000) Midwives' support needs as childbirth changes. *Journal of Advanced Nursing* 32(2): 465–472.

Kotter, J. (1990) *A Force for Change: How Leadership Differs from Management*. London: Free Press.

Kouzes, J.M. & Posner, B.M. (1995) *The Leadership Challenge: How to Keep Getting Extraordinary Things Done in Organizations*. San Francisco: Jossey-Bass.

McAnulty, L. (1993) *Midwifery Professionalism and Professionalisation*. London: Distance Learning Centre, South Bank University.

Moss Kanter, R. (1994) Collaborative Advantage. *Harvard Business Review* July–August.

Myerson, D. (2001) *Tempered Radicals: How People use Differences to Inspire Change at Work*. Cambridge, Mass: Harvard Business School Press.

National Health Service (NHS) (1999) *Nurse, Midwife and Health Visitor Consultants 1999/2000*. Advance Letter NM 2/1999. Online. Available: http://www.nursingleadership.co.uk/pubs/consultant.htm

National Health Service (NHS) (2002) *Midwifery Leadership Competency Model. The National Nursing*

Leadership Programme. Manchester: NHS Modernisation Agency, Leadership Centre.

O'Neill, O. (2002) *A Question of Trust. The BBC Reith Lectures 2002.* Cambridge: Cambridge University Press.

Page, L. (2001) Keeping birth normal. In: Page, L. (ed) *The New Midwifery: Science and Sensitivity in Practice.* London: Churchill Livingstone.

Pedler, M., Burgoyne, J. & Boydell, T. (1997) *A Manager's Guide to Self-development,* 3rd edn. Maidenhead. McGraw-Hill.

Peters, T. & Waterman, R. (1995) *In Search of Excellence.* London: Harper Collins.

Powell, C. (1996) A Leadership Primer. Online. Available: http://www.blaisdell.com/powell (accessed 2002 and Feb 2004).

Pugh, D.S. & Hickson, D.J. (1989) *Writers on Organisations.* 4th edn. London: Penguin.

Reeves, T. (1997) *Alchemy for Managers: Turning Experience into Achievement.* Oxford: Butterworth-Heinemann.

Rosener, J. (1990) Ways women lead. *Harvard Business Review* Nov/Dec: 119–125.

Royal College of Midwives (RCM) (2000) *Vision 2000.* London: RCM.

Royal College of Midwives (RCM) (2003) *Directors of Midwifery in the Modern NHS – Contributing to More than Maternity Services.* London: RCM.

Sandall, J. (1997) Midwives' burnout and continuity of care. *British Journal of Midwifery* 3(2): 106–111.

Scase, R. (2001) Swede smell of success. London: *The Observer,* 14 October.

Schein, E. (1985) *Organisational Culture and Leadership: A Dynamic View.* San Francisco: Jossey-Bass.

Scottish NHS Executive (2001) *Caring for Scotland: The Strategy for Nursing and Midwifery in Scotland.* Edinburgh: Scottish NHS Executive.

Shamir, B. (1995) Social distance and charisma. *Leadership Quarterly* 6(1): 19–47.

Stone Zander, R. & Zander, B. (2000) *The Art of Possibility: Transforming Professional and Personal Life.* Boston: Harvard Business School Press.

Stapleton, H., Duerden, J. & Kirkham, M. (1998) *Evaluation of the Impact of the Supervisor of Midwives on Professional Practice and the Quality of Midwifery care.* London: ENB.

Tichy, N. & Cohen, E. (2000) *The Leadership Engine: How Winning Companies Build Leaders at Every Level.* London: HarperCollins.

Ulrich, D. (1996) The leader of the future: credibility × capability. In: Hesselbein, F. Goldsmith, M. & Beckhard, D. (eds) *The Leader of the Future.* San Francisco: Jossey-Bass.

Walters, H., Mackie, P., Mackie, R. *et al.* (1997) *Global Challenge: Leadership Lessons from the World's Toughest Yacht Race.* Book Guild.

Wedderburn Tate, C. (2001*) Leadership in Nursing.* London: Churchill Livingstone.

Welsh Assembly (2002) *Delivering the Future in Wales: A Framework for Realising the Potential of Midwives in Wales.* Cardiff: Welsh Assembly.

Wilson, J. (2000) *Institute of Management Test: Your Management Style.* London: Hodder & Stoughton.

FURTHER READING

Cross, R. (1996) *Midwives and Management – A Handbook.* Cheshire: Books for Midwives. Written by a midwife with specific translations and application of leadership and management theories to midwifery.

Wedderburn Tate, C. (2001) *Leadership in Nursing.* London: Churchill Livingstone. An easily accessible comprehensive text covering all aspects of leadership and management theory. Personal development exercises with application to the National Health Service.

ADDITIONAL RESOURCES

Bennis, Warren
http://westy.jtwn.k12.pa.us/users/sja/Bennis/html

Drucker Foundation
http://www.pfdf.org
http://www.druckerfoundation.net/leaderbooks

INSEAD
http//www.insead.edu/tilde/vires/fullcv.htm

Kotter, John
http://www.eitforum.com/Experts/john-kotter.htm

Leadership Trust Foundation
http://www.leadership.org.uk

National Health Service
http://www.nursingleadership.co.uk

Powell, Colin
http://www.blaisdell.com/powell

70

The Midwife as a Lifelong Learner

Sue Macdonald

LEARNING OUTCOMES

After reading this chapter, you will:

- have an understanding of the development of pre- and post-registration education for midwives in the UK
- be familiar with educational and academic structures
- be conversant with your own learning style and be able to consider your education and development needs and how these might best be met
- have a framework within which to effectively reflect on practice, and use this knowledge to guide future practice

- be able to develop a dynamic and appropriate curriculum vitae
- have commenced a portfolio which demonstrates your achievements so far, and utilizes your learning needs
- be able to utilize the clinical area fully, whether community or hospital based, as a learning environment, and facilitate the learning and development of those with whom you work.

INTRODUCTION

Chapter 64 explored the history of midwifery within the UK. In this chapter, the more recent history of midwifery education will be discussed, together with some of the policy and practice issues which have shaped and influenced the provision of pre- and post-registration education. To understand midwifery education in the UK now, and to think about the future direction it will take, it is helpful to appreciate some of the influencing factors and history of midwifery. Education and learning will also be explored in a broader sense and how they can be utilized by midwives in their present and future practice.

LIFELONG LEARNING

Lifelong learning has become an everyday term espoused by the Government, and is included in several policy and guidance documents which have informed curriculum development at both pre-registration and post-registration levels (DoH, 1998; ENB, 1995; Tuckett, 1997). This does not mean subscribing to a lifetime of academic courses, and a tranche of qualifications and

certificates, but a view that the pre-registration education is a springboard for future practice and the clinical area a place of learning and development. This allows midwives to think and reflect on their practice, and to learn from each experience, refining and improving their knowledge and skills and imparting this philosophy to their clients and students. This encourages a more creative and positive approach, in which the health service is a learning organization, able to learn and develop from positive events and mistakes, and provide a high quality of service to women and their babies.

In reality, this must be more than paying lip service. The pace of change and of the development of knowledge means that midwives must continually be updating their knowledge and skills in order to provide a safe level of care.

MIDWIFERY EDUCATION

Midwifery has traditionally emerged from an apprenticeship model of education (Leap and Hunter, 1993). Generally, women would have had personal experience of pregnancy and childbirth and would literally 'learn by Nellie' by accompanying a midwife in her daily work. The 'education' of midwives was therefore variable as regards the quality of experience that learner midwives could be exposed to, and was limited by the difficulty of accessing scientific information which would have been available to their male counterparts (Donnison, 1988) (see Ch. 64). Education and practice reflected the society of the time, and were often guided by superstition, custom and practice.

The Midwives Act was passed in 1902, after many years of campaigning by the Midwives Institute (later to become the Royal College of Midwives) and its redoubtable members, including Rosalind Paget and Louisa Hubbard, supported by a small number of powerful politicians. Midwives were amongst the first to achieve professional regulation and were set on the pathway to standardized education, training and practice. Other parts of the UK attained registration of midwifery practice at a later date: Scotland in 1915 and Ireland in 1918. The Nurses Registration Act was passed in 1919, setting up the General Nursing Council, and bringing nursing training and standards into similar lines to those of midwives.

The primary purpose of the legislation was to *safeguard the public* from the practices of uneducated and untrained women, who assisted those who were too poor to pay for medical care during childbirth. The most obvious beneficiaries of the Act were women and their babies, though the loss of the lay midwives or non-professional midwives has been criticized as a loss to working-class women, as many of these midwives were from comparatively humble backgrounds (Leap and Hunter, 1993).

The Central Midwives' Board (CMB), established by the 1902 Act, was charged by Government with responsibility for training midwives and conducting their examinations. The educational programmes developed accordingly, as shown in Table 70.1 and Figure 70.1.

Nurses in maternity care

The increase in the length and content of midwifery training mirrors the reduction in the time student nurses spent learning about maternal and child care. A 12-week compulsory obstetric course introduced into general nurse training in the early 1960s, was steadily reduced to 4 weeks as it became more difficult to accommodate large numbers of nursing students in maternity areas. Today, student nurses may have as little as 4 days in actual practice to gain a perspective on midwifery care.

In the late 1980s there was increasing concern within the profession about both the direction midwifery

education was taking and reduced recruitment into the profession. By 1988 only one school in England provided a direct entry programme, though it was believed that the 'direct entry' route would be more cost-effective and a more health-focused way of training midwives.

Acting on the findings of an ENB/DoH-funded study (Radford and Thompson, 1988), the Department of Health provided pump priming funds for seven pilot schools to develop direct entry programmes, generally at DipHE level, linked to a higher education institution (HEI).

The success of these programmes has been such that by 2000, three-quarters of midwives had been trained through the direct entry route (UKCC, 2001). There continues to be some debate about whether the shortened course for nurses should be retained, but this route is still supported by midwives, and its retention was recommended by the UKCC Commission for Education (1999).

The EC Directives mean that midwives trained through the direct entry route can work in Europe as midwives at the point of qualification, though midwives who have completed the 18-month programme need to practise in midwifery for a further 18 months.

A women's profession?

Historically, midwifery has been the domain of women, and it has previously been argued that this in itself has led to midwifery being sometimes seen as subservient to more male dominated professions, and even prevented midwives campaigning for better pay and conditions (McKenna, 1991). Restrictions on men practising midwifery were lifted in 1983 in response to the Sex Discrimination Act (1975) and the EC Midwives Directives (EEC, 1980) based on the non-discriminatory Treaty of Rome. Male midwives have become an accepted part of the maternity service landscape, though they remain a minority group. In nursing men comprise 10% of the workforce – in midwifery around 0.2% (NMC, 2002). As in the nursing profession, men appear to be disproportionately represented in more senior positions, though they may not be any better qualified than their female counterparts (Finlayson and Nazroo, 1998). One study quoted a rate of 56% of male managers as opposed to 31% female at G grade, and 11% of male to 6% of female managers at I grade level.

Moving into higher education

The last 20 years have been a time of tremendous change, from a scenario where midwifery education

Table 70.1   The progress of education courses

Year	Course	Length of course	Comments	Examination	Award
Late 19th century	London Obstetrical Society	3 months	Small number of students meant impact on practice negligible		Certificate of proficiency
1902–1915	Central Midwives Board (CMB)	3 months	Focus on labour and postnatal care	3-hour written examination 15-minute viva conducted by an obstetrician	Certificate
1916	CMB	6 months (2-month exemption for nurses)			Certificate
1926	CMB	1 year for non-nurses			
1938	CMB	Part 1: 12 months for non-nurses; 6 months for nurses	Midwifery and obstetric theory and hospital-based practice	Practical assessment and submission of set number of case histories	Certificate
		Part 2: 6 months for all	Clinical experience based in community and some lectures from the local Medical Officer of Health		
1968	CMB	1 year for nurses 2 years for direct entrants	Normal midwifery and complicated obstetrics and neonatal care	Two 3-hour written examinations Viva voce	Certificate
1980	CMB	18 months for nurses 3 years for direct entrants	Normal midwifery and complicated obstetrics and neonatal care + new technologies (i.e. CTGs, inductions, etc.) – some doctors' lectures	Two 3-hour written examinations Viva voce	Certificate
1990s	UKCC/National Boards	18 months for nurses 3 years for direct entrants	Increased focus on psychology, sociology, physiology and social policy	Development of continuous assessment and devolvement of assessment processes	Diploma of Higher Education (DipHE) Degrees in Midwifery

was provided locally, closely supervised and supported by the head of midwifery in the hospital, and funded from the maternity care budget, through to midwifery being absorbed into schools of nursing and midwifery, through colleges of health and/or nursing, through to the final move into universities, and the more complex funding streams controlled by workforce development confederations and strategic health authorities.

The Committee on Nursing (DHSS, 1972) also had major implications for nursing and midwifery education,

recommending that 'nursing (including midwifery) become a research based profession' – at a time when research in midwifery (and in the curriculum) was almost unheard of.

Project 2000 (UKCC, 1986) then recommended that nursing and midwifery education have an 18-month shared core, followed by an 18-month 'branch' in midwifery, children's nursing, mental health, acute care or learning disabilities; that students be supernumerary, and courses be offered in higher education (HE) at

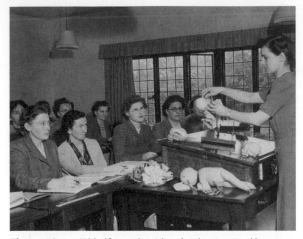

Figure 70.1   Midwifery education in the 1950s. (Courtesy of the Royal College of Midwives.)

diploma or degree level. Midwives overwhelmingly rejected this model for midwifery education, choosing to retain the direct entry route or 18-month programme, generally keeping control over their curriculum, though midwifery education moved, like nursing, into higher education. It is possible that this rejection avoided some of the problems experienced in nursing as described in the Peach Report (UKCC Commission for Education, 1999).

It has been suggested that the move into higher education, which coincided with Project 2000 development, impacted on the student experience and the development of clinical expertise and confidence. Contributory factors were the larger class sizes and geographical move from hospitals and clinical areas (Bower, 2002). Though some worked closely with their nursing colleagues to the extent of sharing elements of their programmes, others retained their midwifery identity, preferring to develop shared learning between the direct entry and 18-month route (Eraut *et al.*, 1995).

The RCM Education Strategy (RCM, 2003) highlights what could be done to redress the balance and align education more closely with clinical practice. Some recommendations, such as the development of a national midwifery curriculum, are straightforward, especially given the development of a national curriculum in children's education. Others are more challenging, e.g. that students undertake at least five home births; two births within a birth centre setting; complete at least two experiences of physiological third stage, and have experience in a variety of settings. Operationalizing the strategy may assist students and

midwives to move clinical practice towards normality and community settings.

This strategy also focused on midwifery educationalists' roles, recommending that educationalists spend a minimum of 20% of their time within the clinical area; that clinical managers seek to find a space for educators, and work to mitigate the negative effects of the geographical move away from practice. Undoubtedly this would require commitment from clinical colleagues, universities and most importantly the educationalists themselves.

> There may be midwives who seek the academic ivory towers, but there are also a significant number of midwives locked in the turret!
>
> (RCM, 2003: 9)

The regional shortages of midwives mirrors a corresponding shortage of educationalists. The proliferation of different roles, such as practice facilitator, clinical facilitator and practice development midwives, may in part replace the traditional role of the midwife teacher, but this may remove a potentially valuable resource from students and qualified staff. Midwifery teachers were usually highly experienced in clinical practice and thoroughly grounded in the theory of advanced midwifery, enhanced by a knowledge of the principles and practice of the education of adults. This level of knowledge and skills is a significant investment, and makes the educationalist a useful member of the maternity services, if fully involved and utilized.

Diplomas, degrees and scholarship

There are a variety of programmes available to the person wishing to enter midwifery, including DipHE and BSc programmes, from 18 months (usually BSc Hons level for nurses), to 3 or 4 years. Presently this is heavily influenced by the funding from the Department of Health: students on DipHE programmes are entitled to a non-means-tested bursary, currently worth around £6000, in comparison to those entering a degree programme who are only entitled to a student grant. The anomaly is that students who are already nurses, completing the 18-month 'top-up' to midwifery continue to be salaried, at present generally on a staff nurse or equivalent grade. In Scotland, all students receive a non-means tested bursury.

Courses are provided within university settings, with linkages to the NHS – usually the acute sector. Most courses allow students to take holidays around Christmas, Easter and the August holiday, and aim to provide a 'university experience'. Courses are designed around the key competencies and clinical experience as laid down by the EC Midwives Directives, and the clinical component is a crucial part of the programme. Students are generally expected to work some shifts and weekends, though mostly this is not supported by extra duty payments. Students are provided with 'self-directed study time', have supernumerary status, and can focus on their studies with comparative exclusivity. Today's students are often mature people who might be on their second or third career, and may be the family breadwinner; therefore students have a different set of stressors from those of traditional university students.

Applicants to midwifery are usually expected to have a minimum educational qualification of five 'GCSEs', and two 'A' levels. Mature students may be accepted with five 'O' levels or a pass at the DC test. Figure 70.2 illustrates the educational system in the UK.

Practitioners who have completed midwifery programmes in the past, or who have completed a diploma, can apply to 'top up' to BSc (Hons) level. As in Figure 70.3, most universities stipulate a total of 360 credits to gain an honours degree – usually consisting of 120 credits at each of levels 1, 2 and 3. Most universities require individuals to complete a significant part of their programme at that university and, even though midwives may only need 120 credits to 'top up' from DipHE to degree level, this may mean they complete more credits. The midwife can then move into advanced 'higher' degree study towards either Postgraduate Certificate and Diploma, Masters or Doctorate qualification.

There is a debate about whether qualifications make the practitioner a better midwife (Bower, 2002). By moving into HE and reducing the clinical practice time, the neophyte practitioner has less accumulated experience and therefore less confidence with which to practice. Research into graduate practitioners in nursing, demonstrates that 6 months after qualification, given appropriate support, practitioners were at a similar point to those who had followed a less academic path. Graduate practitioners tend to remain in practice (Bircumshaw, 1988), demonstrate the ability to problem-solve and have a similar level of competence to their diplomate colleagues (Bartlett *et al.*, 2000; While *et al.*, 1998). One study found that graduate nurses were more likely to be motivated to undertake continuing professional education (CPE) than their diplomate colleagues (Dolphin, 1983).

Midwifery is moving towards being a graduate profession (RCM, 2003), and this should result in practitioners equipped with analytical thinking and reflective skills, in addition to practical skills. Though this may discourage some people from pursuing midwifery, it is likely to raise the status of the profession; therefore, strategies will need to be employed to provide academic and pastoral support.

The RCM strategy proposed a continuum of midwifery, from a 'pre-midwifery' programme, through pre-registration training to the different pathways of consultant midwife, educationalist or manager, always with a firm foundation of clinical practice. The process of moving along the continuum of midwifery establishes a belief that though practitioners may not start at the same point, there is potential for professional and personal growth and reiterates the commitment to continuing professional education (see Fig. 70.4).

Continuing professional development/education (CPD/E) forms a crucial and enduring part of the midwife's continuing development, and has been part of midwifery practice since the 1936 Midwives Act, requiring midwives to undertake periodic refreshment in order to be able to continue practising. This developed from a formal and inflexible week-long programme of residential study, to more flexible provision, either a week's residential course, 7 separate study days, practice placement or other formal study (ENB, 1988).

The Post-registration Education and Practice Project (PREP) (UKCC, 1990) brought these principles to nursing and health visiting, increasing the study days to 5 days every 3 years, and requiring that the practitioner keep a professional portfolio illustrating self-assessment, development plan and reflective activities.

The PREP standard requires that practitioners complete a minimum of 100 days (750 hours) during the 5 years prior to renewal of registration, and practitioners holding dual qualifications must demonstrate 100 days of practice in nursing *and* midwifery (i.e. 200 days total).

'PREP', portfolios and practice

A Profile is a record of career progress and professional development … It is based on a regular process of reflection and recording what you learn from everyday experiences, as well as planned learning activity.

Your profile is your personal document. It does not belong to the UKCC or your employer and its contents are private and confidential to you. Your employer or manager does not have the right to look at it.

(UKCC, 1997: 13)

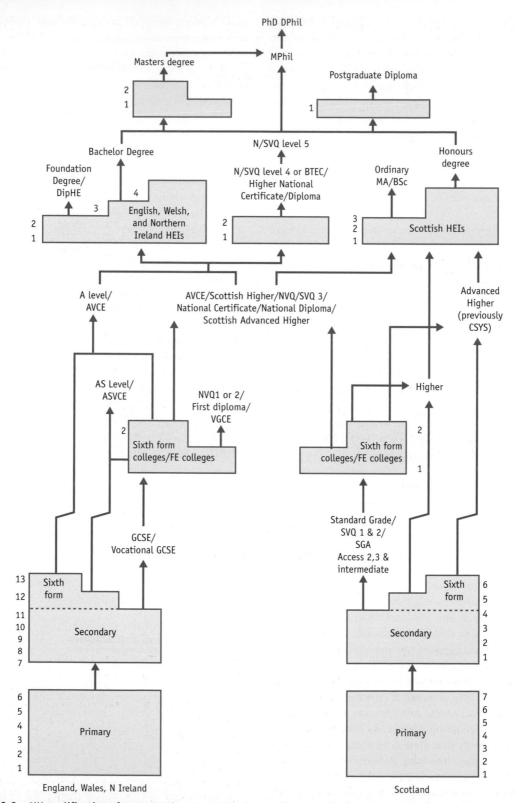

Figure 70.2 UK qualifications from secondary to postgraduate education. (National Academic Recognition Information Centre for the United Kingdom, 2003.)

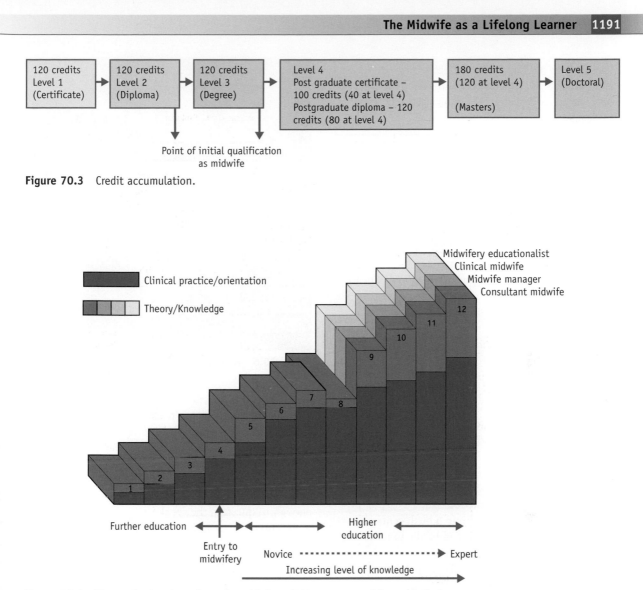

Figure 70.3   Credit accumulation.

Figure 70.4   The professional escalator for midwives (RCM, 2003: 4, with permission).

The PREP (UKCC, 1990) requirement to keep a professional portfolio has led to practitioners having a more formal approach to recording their learning and development. It is important to consider the 'shape' of the portfolio – and whether it is viewed simply as a collection of certificates from different study days, or whether it is a dynamic tool which allows the practitioner to record activities, reflect on practice, and consider learning and development in the past, present and future, as a development plan. The latter approach will include a curriculum vitae (CV), and indeed one way of seeing the portfolio is to think of it as a dynamic CV.

Reflective Activity 70.1

Is your CV up to date? Do you have one? If not, look at the headings provided (see below) and begin to fill in the gaps. Start with the easy information: your school; your qualifications; what professional roles you have had; and then consider what things you do in your role which may not appear in a job description – such as that you take a lead in mentoring junior midwives in your unit; or that you have developed a leaflet with information about waterbirth in your unit; or you are the person that people come to for help in accessing that computer!

> Your CV does not have to be perfect – it is dynamic, and you need to review it every time you apply for a new job or course, or achieve another landmark.

The UKCC published a number of papers and a handbook on keeping a portfolio (UKCC, 1997: 2001). The practitioner can use a commercially produced portfolio, a loose leaf binder, computer or even a personal digital assistant (PDA) unit (see Fig. 70.5). The portfolio should include the following sections:

- Short and concise curriculum vitae
- Personal details – schooling, professional education and career details
- All certificates
- Professional life:
  - a current job description
  - appraisal records
  - minutes or notes from meetings
  - working groups or committees that the midwife has been a member of
- Continuing education and development records
- Practice section – include birth register
- Academic section
- Previous essays, assignments or projects
- Particular achievements:
  - implementing new practice – such as group practice midwifery or setting up a birth centre
  - leaflets or material designed by the practitioner
  - completion of a challenging role – for example, examination of the newborn programme and practice
- References
- Reflective section for critical incidents
- Personal professional plan and objectives – short and long term.

These sections can be added to according to the practitioner's main work area and can be adapted to suit personal styles and workload, and in response to changes in either. For example, a midwife working in parenting education may have a section on health promotion and education.

The portfolio should be under the midwife's control and therefore, if it is shared with another practitioner or supervisor of midwives, sections which are personal to that practitioner (i.e. appraisal records, or some of the reflective accounts) can be taken out.

Updating can be through study days, conferences, working in different practice areas or private study.

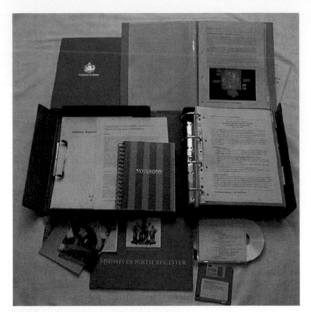

Figure 70.5 A midwifery portfolio.

The important element is identifying the learning in the activity, and maximizing its effect. Prior to attending a study day, for example, practitioners should take some time to read around the subject of the study day, and reflect on this in relation to their own practice. This ensures that the midwife is prepared and can participate fully in the study day, and may feel confident enough to question the speakers.

If a literature search is used as an updating activity, this must include considering a topic, with a rationale in mind, refining the area so that the literature search is focused and effective, resulting in the generation of a list of articles or books to be read and digested, and then considered for application to practice.

It is useful to read actively and to take notes from what is read. This may seem rather onerous, but it saves time and effort later and, more importantly, ensures that any reading is recorded, considered, and a summary made in the practitioner's own words. This is also a good way to aid memory. Box 70.1 illustrates how this can be recorded. These notes include the full reference details, abstract and the reader's notes, which include quotations (with page numbers). This is very helpful as a means of ensuring that any quotations are accurate if they are used in an assignment or project. It can also be helpful to include the place where the book or journal has been accessed, as this may assist if the reference needs to be found in the future. This recording system has the advantage of making any reading active, and of summarizing the key points; therefore

Box 70.1 Taking notes

The culture of midwifery in the National Health Service in England
Kirkham, M

Abstract: The culture of midwifery in the National Health Service was examined in order to foster understanding of the context of midwifery practice. In-depth interviews were conducted with midwives in five very different sites across England. The culture which emerged was one of service and sacrifice where midwives lacked the rights as women which they were required to offer to their clients. There was a lack of mutual support and of positive role models of support, with considerable pressure to conform. Guilt and self-blame were common, as were learned helplessness and muting. The dilemmas of this culture are considered and the resistance which it offered to change in relationships. Change was either resisted, brought about by stealth or strategically planned to equip midwives to change their culture.

Notes: This was part of a multi-site study (5 sites) – grounded theory.
Ethnographic approach – semi-structured interviews. Midwives are working within a male-dominated culture (hospital itself). Midwives as an oppressed group. Midwives make statements which reflect their feeling of sacrifice. Midwives need to be empowered in order to support and empower women.

Quotes:
'This was seen as essentially a culture of women which emphasizes, and internalizes, the values of caring and commitment, irrespective of personal sacrifice' (p. 734).
'Midwives take on far more than they should ...' (p. 734).
'We don't support each other ... we don't even stand up for each other ...' (p. 735).

(1999) *Journal of Advanced Nursing* **30**(3): 732–739.

NB: If this were a review of a book, instead of a journal article, the name of the publisher, and place of publication would be included.

there is no need to store vast numbers of photocopied articles, or whole journals. Instead notes can be kept in a notebook, on index cards in an index box, as files within a computer, or even by using a formal database.

There are a number of commercial bibliographical packages such as *Endnote* and *RefWorks* which offer the ability to record the details of what is read, search functions and the ability to generate bibliographies for essays and other work. These computer-based packages are certainly useful (see Additional resources, p.1208), but require time in setting up and becoming familiar with the software, and still require energy in reading and recording.

After the study day ...

An important part of the portfolio is the recording of all study activities. A certificate of attendance can be placed in the portfolio, but must be supported with a critical reflection of the key learning, and what can be implemented in practice. Some practitioners jot down these reflections on the back of their certificate, or on a separate sheet – this is probably more important than the certificate itself, as it focuses on what was actually learned.

Reflective Activity 70.2

After your next study day, spend half an hour in the evening thinking about it. What were the key elements of the day? Were there any keynote speakers who had an impact on you? Did you learn anything new? If not, why not? Write this down – perhaps using the framework in Box 70.2. Record at least one thing that you learned that you can bring into practice.

It is important to appreciate that the portfolio is a tool, so that it is used constructively to develop personally and professionally.

FUTURE DEVELOPMENTS: DEGREES, MASTERS AND PhDS/APEL/APL

There is a plethora of choice for midwives wishing to develop their knowledge and skills. A decade ago, diplomas were the highest qualification available for the majority of practitioners; now most have access to honours degrees. 12 years ago, a midwife wanting a Masters degree would normally have to settle for a Masters in Social Science, Psychology, Nursing or Education – now most universities offer Masters in Midwifery Studies or Science.

A growing number of midwives are undertaking doctoral studies (PhD), and there are a growing number of clinical doctorates. Figure 70.2 illustrated the

> **Box 70.2 Recording continuing education/development**
>
> You need to include:
>
> **Date, time and place**
>
> **Where learning took place**
> Conference centre/ward or community area/library
>
> **A review of your current role**
>
> **The learning activity:**
> - Why did you choose the particular topic/activity?
> - How did you plan this activity?
> - How many hours did you study/work?
> - Briefly describe the learning activity (i.e. reading a relevant clinical article; attending a course; observing practice)
> - Were there any disappointments or difficulties you had to face?
> - What was the best part of the learning for you?
>
> **Learning outcomes:**
> - What were the key aspects of the learning for you?
> - How will you put this into practice?
> - What sort of learning plans do you have for the future?

hierarchy, with the Master in Philosophy (MPhil) and PhD considered the pinnacle of study, requiring the practitioner to learn the knowledge and skills of research, and then apply them to a research project. As the number of midwives holding these higher degrees grows, it is likely that the status of and internal belief in midwifery will increase, though it will be important to ensure that at the heart of what is studied is knowledge pertinent and applicable to midwives, midwifery and above all to women and their babies.

Work-based Learning (WBL) may include elements of *accreditation of prior learning* (APL) or *accreditation of prior experiential learning* (APEL). This may involve guided study within the clinical area, practical sessions or activity. Some programmes include work-based learning to denote the practical part of the course, either self-assessed or under the supervision of the course tutor, or suitably qualified colleagues. Students are provided with a workbook or logbook, and this forms part of the reflection and recording necessary for demonstrating their progress.

WBL is sometimes viewed as a way of providing practitioners with learning experience, without 'losing them' while they go elsewhere for study. The National Health Service University (NHSU) has expressed its commitment to developing WBL so that all levels of workers within the health service can have good opportunities to learn and develop, in essence turning the Health Service into a learning organization (NHSU, 2003). This is a useful development, as the principle of a learning organization is positive (ENB, 1995). A learning organization is a dynamic one that can adapt and change as required, and which enables its workers to participate at all levels in the organization (ENB, 1995; Jarvis, 1992; Marsick, 1987). This requires a cultural and psychological shift in ensuring that there are appropriate opportunities for utilizing the principles of experiential learning, and providing adequate opportunities for review and reflection.

APEL and APL present some exciting possibilities for midwives, and are increasingly being used as a means by which the practitioner can validate and add value to clinical practice. It is necessary to enrol in a university or further education college, and formally apply to have academic credit applied to clinical practice and learning in that practice. This is no easy option. Time must be spent in preparing a professional portfolio documenting clinical activities, including evidence of critical reflection and a 'claim' for the academic credits appropriate to the clinical learning and development achieved.

> **Reflective Activity 70.3**
>
> Think about your clinical experience over the last year. What have you learned from your actual practice during this time? How would you describe this learning? Think about how this could be translated into a professional portfolio.

Computers, e-learning and the Net

The development of computer-assisted learning and the growth of the Internet have revolutionized learning and information retrieval, and shortened the 5-year 'sell-by date' of knowledge. It is crucial that midwives become comfortable using computers, and retrieving information through varied databases (see Ch. 4). Courses and programmes such as the European Computer Driving License (ECDL) are a way of learning a variety of computer skills including word processing and spreadsheet utilization (Jacob, 1999).

Increasingly, modules and programmes of learning are available in electronic form (Jordan, 1999) and *WebCT* (web course tools) are being developed to support different facets of learning, offering notice boards, chat rooms and a range of guided learning facilities. Research suggests that students like the variety this offers, but that development of electronic packages is time hungry (Wilson, 1998).

The NHS has gone some way to providing information and resources to practitioners within the workplace. The National Knowledge Service (NHS, 2003), a partnership between NHS Direct Online, National Electronic Library for Health, NHS.uk, Department of Health, Electronic Library for Social Care and the Modernisation Agency, provides a website offering portals into several databases and sources of evidence-based practice, with the aim of improving knowledge and information for practitioners and patients to 'base their decisions on best current knowledge' (NHS, 2003). Other NHS initiatives such as the NHSU information line will provide information for NHS employees regarding career planning, CV development and course access.

New approaches in education

Midwifery education is increasingly linking with other professions towards interprofessional education. An example of this is the Advanced Life Support in Obstetrics (ALSO) course and the Neonatal Life Support (NLS) course, but also more pre-registration courses are including significant interprofessional components in an effort to improve learning and working. Problem- and inquiry-based learning also provides an approach which is congruent with adult learning philosophy and enables students to develop higher-level problem-solving and critical skills (McCourt and Thomas, 2001; McNiven *et al.*, 2002).

LEARNING AND DEVELOPMENT

By the time students and qualified midwives have begun studying again, they have gone through a range of educational activities – some positive and some negative. These include experiences of rote learning, tests and examinations, and inevitably some failures. Often early negative experiences can colour people's approach to learning and to their own self-image.

Reflective Activity 70.4

Think about the words: *study, learning* and *assessments* and what thoughts they conjure up in your mind. Were your school days your happiest days?

Think about a positive and a negative image from your own history, and think about what made it positive and what made it negative.

There are many different models and theories around learning styles, and several questionnaires and quizzes which can be used to identify a person's learning style. One is that proposed by Honey and Mumford (1992), based on work by Kolb, which suggested that people fit into one of four main groups:

- *Pragmatist* – practical and keen to try out new ideas
- *Reflector* – prefers to observe, think and gather information before making a judgement
- *Theorist* – likes to tease out and think through information in a systematic way
- *Activist* – likes to be active, and moves straight into experimentation on learning something new.

Reflective Activity 70.5

Get a copy of the Honey and Mumford learning styles questionnaire (either from their book or web-page: http://www.ieg-net.co.uk/contents/resources/learning_styles.htm). Plot out the answers – being brutally honest – and look at which group you fit into. Surprised? Does your learning style fit into any learning activities that you have accessed?

Another model emerged from a case study investigating teachers and students going through a 'Project 2000' programme. The study primarily focused on learning and reflection, and found that styles of teaching reflection included a model which incorporated surface, impersonal to deep personal, then surface personal and deep personal approaches (Miller *et al.*, 1994).

LEARNING

The complex nature of learning has been explored by many (Bloom, 1956; Boud, 1988; Bruner, 1977; Freire, 1972; Jarvis, 1983; Mezirow, 1981). The sheer breadth and depth of previous work within this area precludes more than an overview within this chapter.

There are many approaches: behaviourist, humanistic, the cultural environs, cognitive, through the spectrum to radical and emancipatory learning and education. Most of the earlier experiments and research into learning in humans was based on experiments with animals – even birds. Only during the development of 'progressive' education did research into human learning begin to be carried out. When looking at education broadly, including children's and adult education, there is evidence of a complex interplay of many of these different theories and approaches, and indeed in most situations, experience and how learning is approached are similarly complex.

Conditioning was demonstrated by Pavlov in a series of famous experiments with dogs, who salivated in expectation of a meal heralded by a bell ringing. Once this response was learned, the dog would salivate even if no meal appeared after the bell. If food was withheld repeatedly, the dog would 'learn' that the bell did not necessarily mean food delivery, and would lose that conditioned response. This theory of learning applies in many situations – for example in how individuals learn fear and develop phobias, as in Box 70.3, and how these might be diminished.

This example illustrates that it is possible to develop fear and anxiety from one or two negative experiences, and this may lead to anxiety and panic at the thought of the examination, or even the sight of the midwife preparing the pack. This was reinforced by work by Grantley Dick-Read (1986), who advocated that those supporting women in childbirth needed to address the fear–tension–pain cycle, and this knowledge should inform the midwife's support and education approach. This means providing a safe environment for the woman, sensitively identifying her previous experiences, fears and anxieties, and then planning how best to aid understanding and learning.

Behaviourism indicated the pleasure and pain principle of learning through research using rats, pigeons and apes. Skills are learned through a process of being taught; feedback reinforces what is to be learned, and deletes what should not be. The early experiments involved animals being provided with rewards (food pellets) or punishment (no food pellets/or small electric shocks). Generally the creature swiftly learned the task with both negative and positive feedback, though learning was more effective when rewarded rather than punished. This filtered through to school activities, though food pellets and electric shocks were swapped for positive or negative reactions from the teacher. This translates to providing feedback to the person learning – which might be yourself, the student you are working with or the woman and family. Praise and criticism are substituted for food or electric shocks, remembering that positive rewards are more effective than negative reactions (see Fig. 70.6).

Positive feedback is provided first: 'You did x really well …'; followed by the negative criticism: 'This needed to be done differently … because …'; and the feedback is completed with another positive comment: 'This was really an excellent approach'. The person is then left with a clear idea of what needs to be improved, but is not swamped by thinking that nothing that was done was right or good.

Trial and error learning was proposed by Thorndike, following research with cats in puzzle boxes (Gross, 1987). Initially the cats were extremely keen to escape from the box to a food reward, and sought the escape route haphazardly. Once the cat had escaped, it was put back in the box, and was able to escape progressively more quickly, the speed of escape improving from 5 minutes to about 5 seconds. This illustrated the three 'laws' of the learning process:

- Readiness: relating to the learner's state of mind as he or she approaches the learning episode

---

Box 70.3 Learning fear – applied to midwifery

Vaginal examination (VE) during labour – woman anxious, midwife perhaps does not realize the woman's anxiety:

VE acutely painful (unconditioned stimulus) → pain/fear (unconditioned response)
Suggestion that VE is required (conditioned stimulus) + VE painful (unconditioned stimulus) → pain/fear (unconditioned response)
Suggestion that VE is required (conditioned stimulus) → fear (conditioned response)

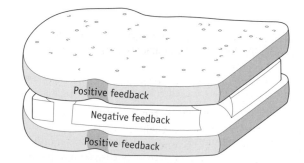

Figure 70.6   The Skinner 'sandwich'.

- Exercise: a process of reinforcement as the individual practices the successful task
- Effect: the strengthening or breaking of the relationship between the action and its consequence.

Applying this to human learning, the individual may try out different approaches to solve a problem, and then use that solution when faced with the same or a similar problem in the future.

Cognitive gestalt theory. Gestalt means pattern, shape or form, and describes the individual's need to make sense of what is being seen and learned and put this into a 'whole'. This problem-solving aptitude helps the individual gain insight into learning – the 'Aha' experience. Gestalt includes concepts such as insightful learning, the nature versus nurture debate and field theory. Gestalt theory highlighted four basic laws of organization in terms of context of perception and problem-solving (see Box 70.4).

The individual's natural tendency to seek understanding needs to be supported, and some gaps in knowledge may be useful as an impetus for learning. In teaching, this can be used to help make sense of what is being learned – perhaps planning a learning activity in which some information is provided and some not, so that the learner is encouraged to develop *closure* in composing the whole problem, and gets the experience of elements of discovery learning. Gestalt provided the tools for discovery learning and for the spiral curriculum, in which new learning is linked with existing information.

Gagne proposed the existence of phases of learning, taking the learner from simple to complex skills and understanding and bringing together the ideas of other theorists into a whole, illustrating progression to higher levels of problem-solving skills. This has echoes of Bloom's *taxonomy of learning*, which included three

domains or categories of educational activities: cognitive (mental skill), affective (growth in feelings), and psychomotor (practical and physical skills). These domains are still used to set learning objectives, and in assessment (see Table 70.2).

This framework did not include the psychomotor domain; Bloom stated that their experience of working with practical skills had been limited (Bloom, 1956). This echoes the difficulty experienced in the healthcare setting of appropriately identifying and measuring practical skills and abilities.

Bruner presented the spiral curriculum, a way of increasing depth of learning, and highlighted the importance of structure; readiness for learning; intuition as a productive but neglected area; and the importance of climate and teacher. Certainly his words: 'teaching is a superb way of learning' (Bruner, 1977: 88), which were echoed in more recent work as: '[the] teacher is not only a communicator but a model' (Eraut, 1994: 90), are useful things for midwives to think in their day-to-day life, in their own learning, and in teaching women and students.

Carl Rogers and Malcolm Knowles are probably the most influential adult education theorists in relation to midwifery. Both were American theorists who were part of the *humanist movement* within adult education.

Rogers proposed that students needed to be provided with intellectual freedom, allowing them to direct their own studies, and described some fascinating case studies recording the effects of independence on student learning and development (Rogers, 1969, 1983). The influence of this on midwifery education was manifest in the inclusion of self-directed sessions and negotiated programmes. The freedom concept cannot be wholly subscribed to, given the limited training time in which to achieve certain competencies and the need to be assessed as having learned certain knowledge in order to be deemed safe to practice (EEC, 1980; UKCC, 2000).

Knowles was very much influenced by Lindeman's early work, which suggested that the education of adults required a different approach to that of children, stressing that 'experience is the adult learner's living textbook' (Lindeman, 1926, reprinted 1961: 7). Knowles challenged educational thinking further (Knowles, 1973, 1980), by suggesting that *pedagogy* – the science of teaching – was no longer appropriate. He analysed the concept of pedagogy – which he initially viewed as only appropriate for children – and presented a new word – *andragogy – the art and science of helping adults learn* (see Table 70.3).

Box 70.4 The gestalt four basic laws of organization

- *Simplicity* – items will be organized into simple figures according to symmetry, regularity, and smoothness
- *Similarity* – items similar in some respect tend to be grouped together
- *Proximity* – phenomena tend to be grouped together according to their nearness
- *Closure* – items are grouped together if they tend to complete some entity

Table 70.2 Taxonomy of the educational objectives within the cognitive domain (after Bloom, 1956; Bloom *et al.*, 1964)

Competence	Skills	Descriptive terms used and example of application
Knowledge: • of specifics • of terminology • of specific facts • of theories and structure	Observation and recall of information – facts or theories Knowledge of dates, events, places Knowledge of major ideas Mastery of subject matter	List, define, tell, describe, identify, show, label, collect, examine, tabulate, quote, name, who, when, where, etc. *Example*: The student will list the major landmarks of the pelvis and fetal skull
Comprehension: • understanding (lowest level) • translation • interpretation • extrapolation	Understanding information Grasping meaning Translating knowledge into new context Interpreting facts, comparing, contrasting Ordering, grouping, inferring causes Predicting consequences	Summarize, describe, interpret, contrast, predict, associate, distinguish, estimate, differentiate, discuss, extend *Example*: The student will describe the significance of the major landmarks of the pelvis and fetal skull
Application	Using information Using methods, concepts, theories in new situations Solving problems using required skills or knowledge Ability to predict possible effects of a change	Apply, demonstrate, calculate, complete, illustrate, show, solve, examine, modify, relate, change, classify, experiment, discover *Example*: The student will demonstrate the mechanism of labour, describing the interaction of the fetal skull with the pelvis, and be able to teach students and women the basic principles
Analysis: • of elements • of relationships • of organizational principles	Seeing patterns Organization of parts Recognition of hidden meanings Identification of components	Analyse, separate, order, explain, connect, classify, arrange, divide, compare, select, infer *Example*: The student will be able to discuss the greater significance of different variations in shapes and sizes of pelves, and the effect on the mechanism of labour and outcomes. The student may question the sources of this knowledge
Synthesis Production of: • a unique communication • a plan or proposed set of operations • a set of abstract relations	Using old ideas to create new ones Generalizing from given facts Relating knowledge from several areas Predicting, drawing conclusions	Combine, integrate, modify, rearrange, substitute, plan, create, design, invent, what if?, compose, formulate, prepare, generalize, rewrite *Example*: The student will be able to assess pelvic capacity and identify women who may have assisted labour difficulties. The student may consider the effect of posture and mobilization, and link research to this aspect of midwifery
Evaluation Making judgements using internal and external evidence and criteria	Comparing and discriminating between ideas Assessing value of theories, presentations Making choices based on reasoned argument Verifying value of evidence, recognizing subjectivity	Assess, decide, rank, grade, test, measure, recommend, convince, select, judge, explain, discriminate, support, conclude, compare, summarize *Example*: The student is able to merge knowledge of anatomy and physiology with the research from major studies, and also the evidence of her or his own practice to provide the woman with unbiased choices, and aid the student's own process of problem-solving and decision-making

Table 70.3 Pedagogy and andragogy

	Pedagogy	Andragogy
Definition	Educating children in a didactic fashion ... to lead	The art and science of helping adults learn
The learner	Dependent	Deep need to be self-directing Occasionally dependent
Learner's previous experience	Limited Of little worth	Rich reservoir of experience – resource for learning
Learner's readiness to learn	When society says	When the individual feels ready – 'need to know'
Learner's orientation to learning	Subject-orientated	Problem-solving Developing full potential
Teacher	Holds the knowledge In control of what and how learning takes place	Is a co-learner Facilitator of learning experiences rather than teacher
Practical implications	Fixed set of knowledge to be learned, though with time and societal changes this alters	Need self-directed opportunities Problem-based enquiry Need to review previous experience (may prevent further learning) Need to explicitly value previous experience

Initially, Knowles defined *andragogy* as a completely opposite concept to *pedagogy*, and it was presumed that it was a mistake to use one method with the wrong group of students, i.e. pedagogy would be inappropriate for a group of adult learners (Knowles, 1973). Later, however, he suggested that *andragogy* and *pedagogy* could be viewed as two 'extremes on a spectrum', used according to the needs of the student group of the time (Knowles, 1980). This theory has been criticized for its assumption that adults are more self-directing than children (Tennant, 1986), the assumption that adults differ from children in their 'reservoir' of experience (Jarvis, 1983) and the different motivation and readiness to learn of the two groups (Tennant, 1986).

Andragogy has been adopted almost completely by midwifery as well as nursing and other streams of education involving adults, though some aspects do conflict with the current directive to be cost-effective, reduce teacher–student contact time, and increase the student–teacher ratio. Andragogical approaches require different classroom settings – desks and chairs arranged in semicircles or circles; more experiential learning; negotiated sessions where students set the agenda; and an increase in self-directed provision.

Teachers (or facilitators) used Knowles' assumptions and processes in the delivery of sessions, and in designing programmes of learning which incorporated a process model (as in Fig. 70.7), in which the starting point is an environment which is conducive to learning, and the end

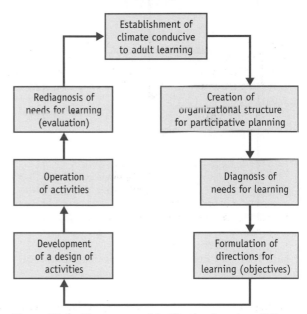

Figure 70.7 The process of facilitating learning. (After Knowles, 1973.)

point is an evaluation of the learning that has taken place, and identification of the next step required.

From andragogy to reflection

Kolb explored the work of Dewey, Piaget, Lewin and Tough, (Dewey, 1933; Kolb, 1984; Tough, 1979) to

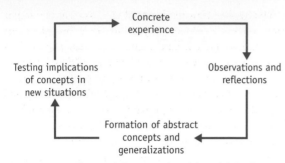

Figure 70.8 The Lewinian Experiential Model (Kolb, 1984: 21).

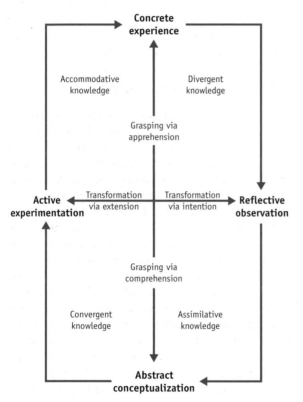

Figure 70.9 Structural diagram illustrating experiential learning and basic knowledge forms (Kolb, 1984: 42).

develop a theory of experiential learning, incorporating reflection as a crucial link between experience and learning (Fig. 70.8). His research suggested that people fit somewhere into four main groups, two on each bipolar continuum, and that this may be assessed by means of a learning styles inventory (LSI).

This has been incorporated into midwifery education – through increased use of experiential learning (Fig. 70.9) and reflection – and reflective practice has become an important part of the midwife's daily work (Box 70.5).

Box 70.5 Practical illustration of reflective cycle

Normally the cycle starts with the experience (at a concrete level) as something tangible to the senses of the individual. This might be the experience of a practical event such as witnessing a normal delivery. It might be that this delivery is a student's first experience of witnessing a birth, and the woman in labour may react as some labouring women do, by being quite noisy, but as she enters transition becomes centred on herself. The baby is delivered, and it is a huge emotional experience. The student notes that the baby looks pink, but has blue extremities. She observes and reflects as she is part of this experience. The result is a sorting out in her own mind of the practical experience and her previous knowledge plus her 'classroom knowledge', and she begins to add to her personal knowledge bank. Each component of the experience may be processed separately according to her knowledge. If we look at one aspect, say the colour of the baby, she may make sense of it by thinking that this is the way babies are, and initially this simple acceptance might serve as a temporary working knowledge. Taking this to the next step of the cycle, she will then perhaps be expecting a pink baby with blue extremities at the next birth.

However, as she becomes more experienced and, hopefully, begins to learn more about neonatal physiology, she will appreciate that this is a visual illustration of the transitional effects of birth. She will also begin to understand the individuality of the experience, for the mother, midwife and indeed the baby.

This LSI has been widely tested with different age and occupation groups and some generalizations made. The four main styles are:

- *The convergent learning style:* associated with the abstract conceptualization part of the cycle. People in this group are better able to focus on technical rather than interpersonal and social tasks.
- *The divergent learning style* (opposite to convergent): emphasizes the reflective and concrete experience aspects. Those who are divergent tend to be imaginative and 'feeling orientated' and are generally interested in people.
- *The assimilation learning style:* associated with the abstract conceptualization and reflective observation

part of the cycle. Assimilators are less interested in people, and are focused on ideas and abstract concepts.

- *The accommodative learning style*: associated with the concrete experience and active experimentation part of the cycle. Those in this group are more practically focused and use trial and error.

These learning styles link in closely with the experiential learning cycle.

People may develop the learning style congruent with their personalities, educational preparation, chosen career, or role function of the time (Kolb, 1984). In one study, individuals from the nursing profession scored heavily within the converger sector (suggesting task-orientation and a difficulty or reluctance to deal with people), and in another they fell into the accommodator/diverger group (Kolb, 1984).

Experiential learning, and thus reflection, were in keeping with the times, as a complex interaction between Dewey's pragmatic philosophy (Dewey, 1933) and Piaget's belief that all learning was linked to experience, Lewin's findings (cited by Kolb, 1984) of the need for tension and dialogue after experience, and by Tough's research findings on the extent and nature of adult learning activity (Tough, 1979).

Kolb viewed learning as a dynamic and fluid process, in which the experience and outcome are different for each person, and emphasized that, rather than being an empty vessel to be filled, the student comes to learning with a range of learning and experience, and needs to 'relearn' rather than learn 'from scratch'. The educationalist therefore assists individuals to modify or dispose of old ideas and change their belief system.

Experiential learning is an important tool in developing learning, in which more effective interaction with the concepts being taught is achieved, as the person is encouraged in a lesser or greater degree to actually feel what the concept would feel like. An example in midwifery would be students learning how to give 'bad news' to women and their families. This could be achieved by practising in a classroom setting what it feels like from the perspective of both the mother and midwife, and what words, body language or strategies are most caring and effective. A crucial part of this exercise is the debriefing and reflective phase which follows, during which all participants can present their perspective, and the group can explore events and strategies together, expanding the learning potential by the number of the participants in the group.

This type of learning is not always as easy as it might appear. To tell individuals just 'to act it out' does not provide enough guidance, and may result in limited learning or, in the worst case scenario, entering territory which may be uncharted and unsupported. An example could be a bereavement workshop, where participants may relive their own experiences of loss, during which they may need specialist support and guidance.

If the midwife uses role play, either with student midwives, or with women (i.e. during antenatal education), it is important to have clear aims and objectives; role play cards, and time for reflection and review afterwards. People may remain 'in role' after the workshop, and therefore it is useful to remind participants that the role play is at an end, and provide a 'cooling/winding down' exercise, such as a game or manual task.

Reflection and reflective practice

Around the same time as Kolb presented his work in experiential learning, Schon published *The Reflective Practitioner* (Schon, 1983), which described the crisis of the professions, and popularized reflection. Though reflection had been discussed previously, as early as the time of Aristotle, and in the early part of the 20th century (Dewey, 1933), Schon brought it to the attention of professions such as nursing, midwifery and social work. This book valued intuition and a more qualitative approach to problem-solving in practice, providing a means of understanding how practitioners make sense of and add to their repertoire of knowledge. Becoming a reflective practitioner has since become an ideal to which many practitioners aspire (Brockbank and McGill, 1998; Driscoll, 1994). Schon's work included a comparison of the practitioner who chooses to utilize a technical rationality model and work logically to address the problems of the 'high, hard ground where practitioners can make effective use of research-based theory and technique', or alternatively take a more intuitive path through the now famous 'swampy lowland where situations are confused "messes" incapable of technical solutions' (Schon, 1983: 42). Schon suggested that clients were more likely to have the sort of problems which required the more creative and holistic approach and, in a period of time when nursing and midwifery in common with other emerging professions wished to develop their professional standing, this supported the more feminine, tacit nature of clinical practice.

Certainly, clients often present with a combination of risk factors, clinical and psychosocial problems which would present a profile more akin to the swampy lowlands than those high hard grounds, and therefore this viewpoint is seductive. Though Schon described several 'exemplars' of teachers working with students to develop reflective practice, there was not really a clear tool available to assist a practitioner in developing the skills. Since that time, however, several other writers have published tools and frameworks to guide reflection.

Reflective Activity 70.6

Develop your personal philosophy of midwifery: This could be the first part of your portfolio. What does it mean for *you* to be a midwife? What is important to you? Is it evidence-based practice? Being kind and supportive? Facilitating the woman's autonomy?

Try this out with a colleague. Don't be afraid of using the word 'I'. This is *your* philosophy.

It is often helpful to try out some reflective tools to explore whether they can assist in making sense of experiences, and develop learning. There is an example of one in Box 70.6, but there are a number of different models providing trigger questions that can assist in thinking about an experience or an area of practice, and develop it into learning (Atkins and Murphy, 1993; Benner, 1984; Driscoll, 1994; Johns, 1995). This includes *critical incident analysis*, a term for an incident during which something went wrong, a crisis or a situation recorded for risk-management purposes, and also used in research and increasingly in the field of reflective practice to denote a variety of situations:

- where something went unusually well (or not)
- when things did not go as planned
- a very demanding incident
- a review of an everyday and routine situation
- one which 'captures the quintessence of what nursing is all about' (Benner, 1984).

Reflective Activity 70.7

Use the tool in Box 70.6 to reflect on an aspect of your practice – perhaps how you conduct a 'booking interview'. You may wish to do this with a peer, or write it down as a reflective piece for your professional portfolio. Do not be surprised if writing about it takes several pages.

If truly subscribed to, reflective practice can be a potent model for the practitioner to audit day-to-day practice, and continue learning and development from the complex digestion and assimilation of theory and practice. It is not without problems and does require significant investment of time and energy, plus support (Macdonald, 2002). It is seldom highlighted that reflection can be difficult, which means that many people will avoid thinking beyond the most obvious. It may also be uncomfortable as areas of practice are revisited – some long forgotten and some more enduring. Reflection needs therefore to carry something of a health warning, and an understanding that it is not always possible to reflect on all areas of practice all of the time.

One phenomenological study explored the 'dark side' of reflection. Students described feelings of 'lost innocence' and 'cultural suicide' when they returned to their workplace, utilizing their new perspectives from reflection (Brookfield, 1994). The students were at a point of challenging workmates, and this was the *cultural suicide* element. Another difficulty was that though many students expressed their excitement and commitment to reflection, they also described feelings of finding out more about themselves as practitioners, increasing self-uncertainty, even feeling like an *impostor* (i.e. 'they will find out I don't know anything').

An earlier activity provided an opportunity to explore a personal philosophy for midwifery, and there is some evidence that just thinking about the individual's philosophy, generates some reflection (Kottkamp, 1990). It is also a really useful means of articulating what is personally believed in as a midwife, and sharing this with colleagues. It is important to acknowledge at this point that reflection is an individual activity, and it is not possible to reflect for another person.

Reflection for you ... and others

In reviewing reflective models in the context of the experiential cycle, it becomes clear that others in the maternity service will be learners, who will need to be assisted through the cycle, in order to make sense of their experiences. Student midwives usually have a clinical record of some kind, and a clinical assessment tool. Increasingly, students are being required to illustrate some critical reflection on their practice, and will therefore value working with midwives who are familiar with the terminology, and will also find it helpful to have a chance to reflect on different experiences and issues in practice. Sharing reflective incident analysis

Box 70.6 A reflective model

Prior to the event/experience

How did you prepare for the incident/experience? Were you prepared?

Is this an issue that you have considered/thought about recently? Why?

What was in your mind prior to the event?

Did you have any worries/concerns about it? How did you address them?

The incident/experience

Describe what happened (no analysis at this stage):

- Who said/did what?
- Record the where's and how's
- Were your feelings:
  - discomfort?
  - troubled?
  - very positive?
- What other aspects affected your handling of the situation, i.e. busyness of ward/community, other stressors?
- What knowledge did you use (was this from textbook/research or from colleagues/routine practice)?

Analysis stage

What were you trying to achieve?

Why did you respond to the situation/event in the way you did?

What was the outcome for:

- you?
- the woman and baby?
- your colleagues?
- your student?

How did others feel about what happened:

- the woman and baby?
- your colleagues?
- your student?

And how do you know:

- from assessing body language/posture?
- from what was said to you?

Was this similar to previous responses from other similar situations/events?

What were the main thoughts/concerns in your mind at the time?

Thinking about the knowledge you were using, was it based on:

- training/text book?
- research?

- evidence?
- your assumptions?

Were there any tensions or difficulties which arose from the knowledge you were using?

Was this knowledge appropriate to the situation, and were you conscious of any gaps in your knowledge?

The 'what if' stage – alternatives and choices

How could you have dealt with this differently?

Would this have changed what happened – and how?

Were you in a position to actually influence this?

Would you do the same things if this situation happened again?

- If so, why?
- If not, why not?

Plan of action

What did you learn from this – good and bad? Don't forget your personal Skinner sandwich.

What element of practice, or what you did, did you feel was special and needs to be celebrated?

Will you use this in your future practice?

How will you share this with colleagues?

If you do not want to share with your colleagues, why not? What does that tell you, and how do you deal with it?

What do you need to update yourself or find out next:

- theory?
- practical skills?
- research?

What is your personal calendar for this – tonight, tomorrow or next week?

If you are not sure of what you have to learn, who do you use to help you find out? And why?

- Supervisor of Midwives?
- Link teacher?
- Consultant midwife?
- Doctor?
- Colleague?

Evaluation

When will you review this reflection?

With whom will you share this (supervisor/mentor or colleague)?

Perspective – suspended judgement

At this point, what are your views on this event/experience?

How have you incorporated this into your personal knowledge store?

Box 70.7 Trigger questions for assisting the woman to reflect

- You booked to have your baby with us ... how did you feel when you first met your midwives ... do you feel that account was taken of your individual needs? (antenatal)
- What did you think your antenatal care was going to be like? (antenatal)
- Did you feel you had sufficient information about becoming a parent antenatally? (postnatal)

Box 70.8 The student learns ...

Midwife X sees Mrs Brown, who is 32 weeks' pregnant, with student midwife A. On examining Mrs Brown, the midwife feels that the fetus is not growing perhaps as fast as she would expect. She asks Mrs Brown about her nutrition patterns, and whether she smokes, drinks alcohol, etc. She provides the appropriate advice, but decides to ask Mrs Brown to attend antenatal clinic the following week. She therefore makes the appointment and records this in the notes.

Student A works in the clinic a couple of weeks later, and is encouraged by midwife Y to undertake the examination and the 'talking' under her supervision. Mrs Clarke is 32 weeks' pregnant, and her observations are all within normal parameters – her fetus is growing well. Student midwife A makes an appointment for the following week.

Midwife Y is completely confused ... surely this is not what they teach in the university these days! She challenges the student, and is actually a little sharp with her.

can be an interesting exercise which can bring another perspective, and will also serve as an illustration to the student of how practitioners utilize reflection in day-to-day practice.

Perhaps most fundamentally, women themselves need to reflect. It is clearly not practical to ask women to complete pages of reflective accounts of their experiences, though some women may find this beneficial. It is good practice to review aspects of the woman's experience with her, at a point where she has had time to consider events, and has begun to question what happened and why. Many midwives focus on the labour and delivery, and will provide an opportunity for reflection on these. However, women may have had concerns and troubling experiences during the antenatal and postnatal period, and will value a chance to discuss issues with a suitable person. In reflecting with the woman, it is important to remember that, as in all reflections, she has to reflect on her own experience. Some trigger questions (Box 70.7), and a focus on her as the key player can be helpful, just providing information and clarification when asked to do so. Counselling skills (i.e. learning not to be quick to give a neatly packaged answer) are really helpful at this stage.

Issues around debriefing may need more skilled support, and it is not unusual during the 'routine' reflections to identify a woman who may require additional counselling support.

Mentorship and the midwife as a role model

An important part of developing learning and practice is through interaction with others, and possibly the most powerful way in which humans learn physical, communication and caring skills is through the medium of role modelling. This allows absorption of the culture of the service (Hindley, 1999), which may be negative as well as positive learning (Kirkham, 1999).

As a practitioner, it is important to be aware that actions, attitudes and demeanour may be perceived in different ways by students, other practitioners, women and their families and friends. Students especially are observant of their mentors, and may emulate their attitudes, though they will tend to prefer the woman-centred and flexible rather than prescriptive approach (Bluff, 2002).

It is important to share the way decisions and judgements are made with junior colleagues – demonstrating how the very complex process that takes place during the woman's care in the context of the service can be learned (see Box 70.8).

Not to share this process robs the student and practitioner of a valuable learning experience. This process of talking through what is being done and why – almost reflecting 'on your feet' which Loughran describes – is a wonderful example of both helping students understand the thought processes an experienced practitioner has, and also illustrates the complexities of those processes (Loughran, 1996, 2000).

Though students learn theory (and some practice) in the university setting, the real world practice is learned from their mentors in practice. This is a heavy responsibility to be borne, but also exciting to be part of such an intense learning experience. Whether you are the mentor or student, take advantage of the support mechanisms that exist. Ensure that the university provides copies of the documents that are needed, such as the student handbook or course document, the clinical assessment guidelines, and an outline of the programme. Midwifery educationalists are an important resource, and will often provide sessions on assessment processes either in small groups or on an individual basis.

Be positive. The first few days of working together can be hard, as a lot of guidance and support is required. If the midwife and student work as partners in learning, the student can assist the workload at the same time as learning, the midwife can teach real practice, and research and information can be shared.

Use reflection and assessment well. Students can be assisted to reflect by midwives demonstrating their own reflective processes; being encouraged to seek feedback from the woman; and being open to self-assessment.

Budgets, money and tax

Once the practitioner is earning enough to be taxed, there are various entitlements and increased allowances for professional body subscriptions (e.g. to the Royal College of Midwives (RCM) or Royal College of Nursing (RCN)); subscription to publications such as *MIDIRS Midwifery Digest* and some journals and, if the employer has not paid for study days, tax relief can be claimed on this. There are a variety of sources of information, including the RCM or RCN, who will assist their members in making such a claim – which can be made for the previous 6 years.

Funding study days and courses is often part of a contract between the local university and maternity service/hospital trust, especially if it is a work-related programme of study. Many trusts also provide local training. Contracts usually run for the financial year, though the academic year usually begins in September. It is therefore vital that midwives engage with their director of midwifery, supervisors and educationalists to identify what is required in terms of education and

development locally, which can then be fed into the Workforce Development Confederations. The NHS-supported yearly appraisals assist in providing one channel of communication, but it is important that midwives work with their multidisciplinary colleagues to identify and access what education and development are needed to improve practice.

CONCLUSION

In considering aspects of learning and education, midwives must be aware of their own learning patterns, and be willing to review their own learning history. This will assist in planning education and development activities, but perhaps more importantly, will assist them in analysing the learning and development needs of the women with whom they are working, and the students for whom they are responsible. The good teacher should be able to plan and assess learning, and this includes an analysis – even unlearning – of things that have been learned before; or unpicking and addressing assumptions that others may have about learning, or about the whole experience of pregnancy, childbirth and motherhood.

An important part of practice is to have a framework and tools which can assist in critically reflecting and assessing the effects of that practice. However, this requires the skills described many years ago of open-mindedness, wholeheartedness and responsibility (Dewey, 1933). This does carry a health warning, in that truly reflecting on practice brings new challenges and perspectives which may not always be comfortable.

This chapter has reviewed the multifaceted nature of learning, education and development. As midwifery faces new challenges and different ways of working, it is paramount that midwives continue to learn and develop. To do so well will certainly benefit the profession and the individual midwife both professionally and personally. Most importantly of all it will benefit the care provided to women, their babies and families, and thus society as a whole.

KEY POINTS

- An understanding of the structure of general education and professional education pathways is useful in viewing the opportunities which are available to those in the healthcare setting.

- Midwives should be aware of the impact of learning on themselves, their colleagues, students and the women with whom they work.

- An understanding of learning theory assists midwives in their professional and personal development and enables them to facilitate the learning of others.

- There are a wide variety of educational and development opportunities available to practitioners, often accessible locally.

REFERENCES

Atkins, S. & Murphy M. (1993) Reflection: a review of the literature. *Journal of Advanced Nursing* 18: 1188–1192.

Bartlett, H.P., Simonite, V., Westcott, E. *et al.* (2000) A comparison of the nursing competence of graduates and diplomates from UK nursing programmes. *Journal of Clinical Nursing* 9(3): 369–379.

Benner, P. (1984) *From Novice to Expert: Excellence and Power in Clinical Nursing Practice*. California: Addison-Wesley Publishing.

Bircumshaw, D. & Chapman, C.M. (1988) A follow-up of the graduates of the 3-year post-registration Bachelor of Nursing degree course in the University of Wales. *Journal of Advanced Nursing* 13(4): 520–524.

Bloom, B.S. (ed) (1956) *A Taxonomy of Educational Objectives. Handbook Part I Cognitive Domain*. New York: David McKay.

Bloom, B.S., Engelhart, M.D., Furst, E.J. *et al.* (eds) (1964) *A Taxonomy of Educational Objectives. Handbook Part I Cognitive Domain*. New York: David McKay.

Bluff, R. (2002) The midwife as role model. *International Confederation of Midwives. Midwives and Women Working Together for the Family of the World*. ICM proceedings, Vienna. The Hague: International Confederation of Midwives.

Boud, D., Keough, R. *et al.* (eds) (1988) *Reflection: Turning Experience into Learning*. London: Kogan Page.

Bower, H. (2002) Educating the midwife. In: Mander, R.F. & Fleming, V. (eds) *Failure to Progress: The Contraction of the Midwifery Profession*. London: Routledge, Taylor and Francis Books.

Brockbank, A. & McGill, I. (1998) *Facilitating Reflective Learning in Higher Education*. Buckingham: Society for Research into Higher Education and Open University Press.

Brookfield, S. (1994) Tales from the dark side: a phenomenology of adult critical reflection. *International Journal of Lifelong Education* 13(3): 206–216.

Bruner, J. (1977) *The Process of Education*. Cambridge, Massachusetts: Harvard University Press.

Department of Health (DoH) (1998) *A First Class Service*. London: HMSO.

Department of Health and Social Security (DHSS) (1972). *Report of the Committee on Nursing*. (Chair: Professor Asa Briggs) (Cmnd. 5115) London: HMSO.

Dewey, J. (1933, reprinted 1960) *How We Think*. London: DC Heath.

Dick-Read, G. (1986) *Childbirth Without Fear: The Original Approach to Natural Childbirth*. New York: Harper & Row.

Dolphin, N. (1983) Why do nurses come into continuing education programs? *Journal of Continuing Education in Nursing* 14(4): 8–16.

Donnison, J. (1988) *Midwives and Medical Men*. London, Heinemann.

Driscoll, J. (1994) Reflective practice for practise. *Senior Nurse* 13(7): 47–50.

English National Board for Nursing, Midwifery and Health Visiting (ENB) (1995) *Creating Lifelong Learners: Partnerships for Care*. London: ENB.

English National Board for Nursing, Midwifery and Health Visiting (ENB) (1988) *Refresher Courses for Practising Midwives*. London: ENB.

Eraut, M. (1994) *Developing Professional Knowledge and Competence*. London: Falmer Press.

Eraut, M.A., Alderton, J., Boylan, A. *et al.* (1995) *Learning the Use of Scientific Knowledge in Nursing and Midwifery Education*. London: ENB.

European Economic Community (1980) *European Community Directive 80/155/EEC*, Article 4. Brussels: European Economic Community.

Finlayson, L.R. & Nazroo, J.Y. (1998) *Gender Inequalities in Nursing Careers: Research Summary*. London: Policy Studies Institute.

Freire, P. (1972) *Pedagogy of the Oppressed*. Penguin: Harmondsworth.

Gross, R. (1987) *Psychology: The Science of Mind and Behaviour*. London: Hodder and Stoughton.

Hindley, C. (1999) An assessment of clinical competency on an undergraduate midwifery programme: midwives' and students' experiences. *Journal of Clinical Excellence* 1(3): 157–162.

Honey, P. & Mumford, A. (1992) *The Manual of Learning Styles*. Maidenhead: Honey.

Jacob, S. (1999) Union learning fund supporting information technology training. *RCM Midwives Journal* 2(8): 254.

Jarvis, P. (1983) *Adult and Continuing Education: Theory and Practice*. London: Croom Helm.

Jarvis, P. (1992) Quality in practice: the role of education. *Nurse Education Today* 12(3): 3–10.

Johns, C. (1995) Framing learning through reflection within Carpers's fundamental ways of knowing in nursing. *Journal of Advanced Nursing* 22: 226–234.

Jordan, G. (1999) The use of communications and information technologies (C&ITS) as a tool for continuing professional development (CPD): a case study. *CTI Nursing and Midwifery Newsletter* **4**(3): 5–6.

Kirkham, M. (1999) The culture of midwifery in the National Health Service in England. *Journal of Advanced Nursing* **30**(3): 732–739.

Knowles, M.S. (1973) *The Adult Learner: A Neglected Species.* Houston: Gulf Publishing.

Knowles, M.S. (1980) *The Modern Practice of Adult Education: From Pedagogy to Andragogy,* revised edn. Chicago: Association Press.

Kolb, D.A. (1984) *Experiential Learning: Experience as the Source of Learning and Development.* New Jersey: Prentice Hall.

Kottkamp, R.B. (1990) Means for facilitating reflection. *Education and Urban Society* **22**(2): 182–203.

Leap, N. & Hunter, B. (1993) *The Midwife's Tale.* London: Scarlet Press.

Lindeman, E.C. (1926, reprinted 1961) *The Meaning of Adult Education.* Oklahoma: Oklahoma Research Center for Continuing Professional and Higher Education.

Loughran, J. (1996) *Developing Reflective Practice: Learning about Teaching and Learning through Modelling.* London: Falmer Press.

Loughran, J. (2000) Effective reflective practice. *Making a Difference through Reflective Practice: Values and Actions.* Conference on Reflective Practice. University College Worcester, July 2000, pp. 38–44.

McCourt, C. & Thomas, B.G. (2001) Evaluation of a problem-based curriculum in midwifery. *Midwifery* **17**(4): 323–331.

Macdonald, S.E. (2002) *Reflecting on Reflection....* ICM 26th Triennial Congress Vienna, April 2002, pp. 1–19.

McKenna, H. (1991) The developments and trends in relation to men practising midwifery: a review of the literature. *Journal of Advanced Nursing* **16**(4): 480–489.

McNiven, P., Kaufman, K. & McDonald, H. (2002) A problem-based learning approach to midwifery. *British Journal of Midwifery* **10**(12): 751–755.

Marsick, V.J. (ed) (1987) *Learning in the Workplace.* London: Croom Helm.

Mezirow, J. (1981) A critical theory of adult learning and education. *Adult Education* **32**(1): 3–24.

Miller, C., Tomlinson, A. & Jones, M. (1994) *Learning Styles and Facilitating Reflection.* London: ENB.

National Academic Recognition Information Centre for the United Kingdom (UK NARIC) (2003) *The UK Educational System.* Online. Available: http://www.naric.org.uk/home.htm.

National Health Service (NHS) (2003) *The National Knowledge Service.* Online. Available: http://www.nks.nhs.uk.

National Health Service University (NHSU) (2003) Online. Available: http://www.nhsu.nhs.uk/media/press_news/nhsu_moving_forward.htm.

Nursing and Midwifery Council (NMC) (2002) *Statistical Analysis of the Register 1 April 2001 to 31 March 2002.* London: NMC.

Radford, N. & Thompson, A. (1988) *Direct Entry – A Preparation for Midwifery Practice.* Guildford: University of Surrey.

Rogers, C.R. (1969) *Freedom to Learn: A View of What Education Might Become.* Columbus, Ohio: Charles E Merrill Publishing.

Rogers, C.R. (1983) *Freedom to Learn for the 1980s.* Westerville, Ohio: Charles E Merrill.

Royal College of Midwives (RCM) (2003) *Valuing Practice: A Springboard for Midwifery Education.* London: RCM.

Schon, D.A. (1983) *The Reflective Practitioner: How Professionals Think in Action.* USA: Basic Books.

Sex Discrimination Act 1975 London: HMSO.

Tennant, M. (1986) An evaluation of Knowles' Theory of Adult Education. *International Journal of Lifelong Education* **5**(2): 113–122.

Tough, A. (1979) *The Adult's Learning Projects.* Austin, Texas: Learning Concepts.

Tuckett, A. (1997) *Lifelong Learning in England and Wales.* Leicester: National Institute of Adult Continuing Education.

United Kingdom Central Council for Nursing, Midwifery and Health Visiting (UKCC) (1986) *Project 2000: A New Preparation for Practice.* London: UKCC.

United Kingdom Central Council for Nursing, Midwifery and Health Visiting (UKCC) (1990) *The Report of the Post-Registration and Practice Project (PREPP).* London: UKCC.

United Kingdom Central Council for Nursing, Midwifery and Health Visiting (UKCC) (1997) *PREP and You.* London: UKCC.

United Kingdom Central Council for Nursing, Midwifery and Health Visiting (UKCC) (2000) *UKCC Midwifery Competencies: Requirements For Midwifery Registration Programmes.* London: UKCC.

United Kingdom Central Council for Nursing, Midwifery and Health Visiting (UKCC) (2001) *The PREP Handbook.* London: UKCC.

UKCC Commission for Education (1999) *Fitness for Practice.* London: UKCC.

While, A.E.F., Fitzpatrick, J. M. & Roberts, J.D. (1998) An exploratory study of similarities and differences between senior students from different pre-registration nurse education courses. *Nurse Education Today* **18**(3): 190–198.

Wilson, T.M. & Mires, G. (1998) Teacher versus the computer for instruction: a study. *British Journal of Midwifery* **6**(10): 655–658.

ADDITIONAL RESOURCES

http://www.refworks.com/
This enables users to create their own personal database by importing references from online databases, and to use these in writing papers, providing an automatic formatting facility.

http://www.endnote.com/
This is one of the most mature bibliographic software resources, providing subject bibliographies, flexible image handling and connectivity to explore and mobilize reference collections.

http://www.lifelonglearning.co.uk/
Lifelong Learning website.

http://www.learningandteaching.info/learning/gestalt.htm
National Grid for Learning website.

http://www.nhsu.nhs.uk/learn/learn
National Health Service University website.

71

Drugs and the Midwife

Catherine Siney

LEARNING OUTCOMES

After reading this chapter, you will be able to:

- have a clear understanding of the drugs which may be used during pregnancy and childbirth
- be familiar with the actions, interactions and contraindications for the drugs common in midwifery, and be able to access information on

drugs that are less common, but which may be prescribed for mothers and babies in your care
- be aware of the main sources of information regarding drugs and medications
- be conversant with the legislation regarding drugs and medications.

INTRODUCTION

This chapter provides an overview of the drugs commonly used in and around childbirth. It also includes information about homeopathy and drugs which may be misused, both prescribed and illicit, although if more depth is required, the annotated bibliography and appropriate references provide further information.

It must also not be forgotten that women may be on long-term or short-term prescribed medication, e.g. immunosuppressants, antidepressants, antibiotics or anticonvulsants. These drugs may interact with drugs used in pregnancy and childbirth and their effects may be increased or diminished.

It is essential that midwives are aware of their statutory obligations around drug administration, and are conversant with the legislation governing drugs and medications. In administering medications, midwives must also ensure that they are proficient in the use, dosage, effect and methods of administration of any drug used. This includes consideration that any equipment used is correct and properly maintained. Should the midwife be required to administer new drugs, or use new equipment to administer medications, this must be under the direction of a medical practitioner (UKCC, 1998).

The midwife should also use every opportunity to emphasize health and well-being through advising

about healthy diet and exercise, as this may reduce the need for medications such as iron and some vitamins and minerals.

Midwives have a long history of using substances both to ameliorate the discomforts of pregnancy, and for use during labour. Before the 1902 Midwives Act, these were as varied as the midwives' practice itself, and could include herbs, as well as more overtly powerful substances, such as laudanum (which contained opium) (Donnison, 1988).

In 1956 midwives were authorized to give chloral hydrate, syrup of chloral, potassium bromide, pethidine, tincture of opium, pil opii and Dover's powder. Chloral hydrate and potassium bromide were generally given together for their hypnotic and sedative action. These mixtures had a nauseous taste, so were usually diluted with 4 ounces (120 ml) of water to which glucose and fresh lemon juice were added. It was sipped slowly so that vomiting was less likely to occur. Tincture of opium (laudanum) was occasionally used alone but usually combined with the other sedatives, and Dover's powder (containing opium) was used in combination with aspirin for backache in early labour. Midwives were authorized to give 200 milligrams of pethidine to a patient but not more than 100 milligrams at one time. (Myles, 1956)

Midwives' practice in relation to medications is governed by the *Midwives Rules and Code of Practice*

(UKCC, 1998) and *Guidelines for the Administration of Medicines* (UKCC, 2000). The United Kingdom Central Council for Nursing, Midwifery and Health Visiting (UKCC) is now replaced by the Nursing and Midwifery Council (NMC). Midwives may carry anti-septics, sedatives, analgesics, local anaesthetics, oxytocic preparations and medications approved for use in maternal and neonatal resuscitation (UKCC, 1998). These are determined by local guidelines and 'standing orders', which should be agreed by the multidisciplinary team (including senior midwives, supervisors of midwives, obstetricians, paediatricians, and the pharmacist), and should be recorded in writing and available in a central point in the maternity unit.

Reflective Activity 71.1

What drugs and medications are included in your local standing orders. Where are the standing orders kept? Is this document signed and up to date?

SOURCES AND RESOURCES

There are a variety of sources of information for the midwife regarding drugs and medications. In the clin-ical setting, the midwife's first source would be the *British National Formulary* (BNF), which includes clear guidance on drug interactions, and the effect on pregnancy and lactation. This may also be available electronically, should there be computer facilities in the clinical area. Should an up-to-date version not be available, or the information be considered inadequate for the particular client situation, the midwife should consult the pharmacist. Other resources are UK drug information centres, or the National Teratology Information Service which can provide information over the telephone.

The midwife can also access textbooks and literature from the hospital or university library, though she needs to ensure that the editions used are as up to date as possible. The advantage in using textbooks is that this usually provides more detailed information regarding the physiological effects of drugs.

PHYSIOLOGICAL ISSUES

Any drug taken that crosses the placenta may affect development, growth or function of the fetus, and is therefore only prescribed in pregnancy (and labour) if the benefits to the woman outweigh the risks to the baby. Also, the physiological changes of pregnancy can affect blood concentrations of certain drugs. Because the total blood volume increases so markedly in pregnancy, drugs are diluted in a larger volume of fluid and so may be less effective than in non-pregnant women (Hytten and Leitch, 1971; Pirani *et al.*, 1973).

Another factor which affects some drugs in pregnancy is the increased rate of liver metabolism – drugs which rely on the activity of liver enzymes are eliminated more quickly than usual, for example phenytoin (O'Hare *et al.*, 1984). There is no change in the rate of elimination of drugs which rely on blood flow in the liver. There is a change, however, in the rate of drug elimination in pregnancy owing to increased blood flow in the kidney. This results in some drugs being excreted more quickly, mainly those which are eliminated unchanged by the kidney (Rubin, 2000).

DRUG INTERACTIONS

Two or more drugs given at the same time may exert their effects independently or may interact. The interaction may be potentiation or antagonism of one drug by another, or occasionally, some other effect.

Pharmacodynamic interactions are interactions between drugs which have similar or antagonistic pharmacological effects or side-effects. They may be due to competition at receptor sites, or occur between drugs acting on the same physiological system. They are usually predictable from a knowledge of the pharmacology of the interacting drugs; in general, those demonstrated with one drug are likely to occur with related drugs. They occur to a greater or lesser extent in most patients who receive the interacting drugs.

Pharmacokinetic interactions occur when one drug alters the absorption distribution, metabolism or excretion of another, thus increasing or reducing the amount of drug available to produce its pharmacological effects. They are not easily predicted and many of them affect only a small proportion of patients taking the combination of drugs. Pharmacokinetic interactions occurring with one drug cannot be assumed to occur with related drugs unless their pharmacokinetic properties are known to be similar. Pharmacokinetic interactions are of several types: affecting absorption, due to changes in protein binding, affecting metabolism and affecting renal excretion (BMA, 2003).

Rule 41 of the *Midwives Rules and Code of Practice* (UKCC, 1998) is concerned with the administration of medicines and other forms of pain relief:

A practising midwife shall only administer those medicines, including analgesics, in which she has been trained as to use, dosage and methods of administration.

A practising midwife shall only administer medicines including inhalational analgesics by means of apparatus if she is satisfied that the apparatus has been properly maintained and:

(a) it has a CE marking or, if it does not have such a marking,
(b) it is of a type for the time being approved by the UKCC as suitable for use by a midwife and in this paragraph, CE marking has the meaning assigned to it in the Medical Devices Regulations 1994, SI 1994 No 3017.

In a situation in which clinical trials involving new medicines including inhalation analgesics, or new apparatus, are taking place, a practising midwife may only participate under the direction of a registered medical practitioner.

LAW GOVERNING DRUG ADMINISTRATION

The Medicines Act 1968

This act classifies medicines into the following categories:

Prescription-only medicines (POMs)   These are medicines which may only be supplied or administered to a patient on the instruction of an appropriate practitioner (a doctor or dentist) and from an approved list for a nurse prescriber. The pharmacist is the expert on all aspects of medicine legislation and should be consulted.

Pharmacy-only medicines   These can be purchased from a registered primary care pharmacy, provided that the sale is supervised by the pharmacist.

General sale list medicines (GSLs)   These need neither a prescription nor the supervision of a pharmacist and can be obtained from retail outlets. Generally, no medication should be administered without a prescription. However, local policies or *patient group directions* should be developed to allow the limited administration of medicines in this group to meet the needs of patients (UKCC, 2000).

Supply, possession and use of controlled drugs

The possession and administration of controlled drugs by midwives is covered by the Misuse of Drugs Regulations 1985, SI 1985 No. 2066; the Misuse of Drugs (Northern Ireland) Regulations 1986, SR 1986 No. 52 and the Medicines Act 1968. The Misuse of Drugs Regulations provide for the supply of pethidine to midwives (and any other controlled drug listed in Schedule 5 Part III of The Prescription Only Medicines (Human Use) Order 1997, SI 1997 No. 1830) using the supply order procedure. Supply order forms can be obtained from the supervisor of midwives.

The administration of controlled drugs by midwives working in a hospital or institution should be in accordance with locally agreed policies and procedures. It may be decided locally that midwives practising in hospitals or institutions can follow the same practice as midwives working in the community.

> ### Reflective Activity 71.2
>
> In preparing for providing pain relief for a woman planning a home birth who would like to use pethidine, how would you access, store and administer this drug?

Controlled drug schedules

There are five controlled drug schedules:

- *Schedule 1*: Drugs which are often used illegally such as hallucinogens.
- *Schedule 2*: Addictive drugs including diamorphine, pethidine and morphine.
- *Schedule 3*: Some of the barbiturates, including pentazocine (Fortral) which may be used by midwives.
- *Schedule 4*: This includes 33 benzodiazepine tranquillizers, some of which may be used in obstetric practice, e.g. diazepam (Valium), nitrazepam (Mogadon) and temazepam (Euhypnos).
- *Schedule 5*: This contains medicines which include only a limited amount of a controlled drug, e.g. some analgesics and cough mixtures.

Drugs in schedules 3, 4 and 5 do not have to be kept in a controlled drug cupboard, nor do they have to be entered in a controlled drug register.

Destruction and surrender of controlled drugs

Regulation 26 of the Misuse of Drugs Regulations contains a procedure for witnessing the destruction of pethidine (or other controlled drugs approved in accordance with the Medicines Act 1968) which have been supplied to the midwife, but which are no longer required. The destruction is done by the midwife but only in the presence of an authorized person who may be one of the following:

- a supervisor of midwives in England, Scotland, Wales or Northern Ireland
- a regional pharmaceutical officer in England
- a pharmaceutical officer of the Welsh Office
- a chief administrative pharmaceutical officer of health boards in Scotland
- in Northern Ireland, an inspector appointed by the Department of Health and Social Services under the Misuse of Drugs Act 1971
- medical officers in England, Scotland or Wales
- an inspector of the Royal Pharmaceutical Society of Great Britain
- a police officer
- an inspector of the Home Office drugs branch.

There is a provision within the Misuse of Drugs Regulations for midwives to surrender stocks of unwanted controlled drugs to the pharmacist from whom they were obtained or to an appropriate medical officer, but not a supervisor of midwives.

Controlled drugs and home births

In the case of controlled drugs supplied directly to the mother on prescription from a family practitioner, the woman (to whom in law they belong) is responsible for destroying any which are unused. The woman should be advised to destroy the drugs, preferably in the midwife's presence.

Alternatively, the woman can be advised to return the unused drugs to the pharmacist from whom they were obtained. This must be done by the woman, but the midwife should record in the woman's notes the advice given and any action taken, together with details of the nature and amounts of drugs involved.

Supply of prescription-only medicines to midwives

In accordance with Part III of the Medicines Act 1968 the midwife may be supplied with certain medicines which are normally available only on prescription issued by a doctor. These medicines may be obtained from a retail or hospital pharmacist by a midwife who has notified her intention to practise. They may only be used in her professional practice.

Preparations for use by midwives are listed below. These are included in Schedule 3 (Parts I and III) of the Medicines (Products other than Veterinary Drugs) (Prescription Only) Order 1983 SI No. 1212 and any subsequent orders:

Part I

- Ergometrine maleate (tablets).
- Chloral hydrate derivatives – but Welldorm (formerly dichloralphenazone) is no longer recommended for use in pregnancy because the chemical composition has been changed.

Part III (for parenteral use)

- Pentazocine lactate
- Pethidine hydrochloride

} These drugs have to kept locked in a controlled drug cupboard and be entered in a Controlled Drug register.

- Promazine hydrochloride (Sparine).
- Lidocaine (lignocaine) hydrochloride.
- Phytomenadione (vitamin K).
- Naloxone hydrochloride (Narcan).
- Oxytocin.
- Ergometrine maleate.

The law is different in Scotland because a midwife can only administer oxytocic drugs such as ergometrine and Syntometrine, and naloxone and lidocaine (lignocaine) without a doctor's prescription.

ADMINISTRATION OF MEDICATIONS AND DRUGS

Safe and effective use of medications begins with the initial assessment of the need for the particular drug, followed by a careful consideration of the following:

- Is there actually a need for a medication?
- What are the normal dosage, route, possible interactions, contraindications and side-effects of the drug chosen?
- Do the needs of the problem outweigh the potential side-effects?
- Does the woman have any known allergies?
- Has sufficient information been given to the woman?
- Has the woman given informed consent?
- Is the prescription clear, legible and indelible, and signed by the appropriate practitioner?
- Is the generic or brand name of the drug included, and the method of administration, dosage, frequency, drug commencement and completion dates?

- Has the weight of the patient been recorded, and does this inform the dosage?
- Does administration ensure that therapeutic blood levels are maintained (i.e. is it once, twice, three or four times a day)?
- If the drug is to be added to solution, is the solution correct?

Prior to actually administering the drug, ask:

- Is this the right:
  - patient/client – are there any other patients with the same name?
  - date?
  - time?
  - drug?
  - dosage?
  - route?
- Is she allergic to this drug?

And following administration:

- Accurately record the administration.
- Sign and date that the drug has been given.
- Inform medical colleague or prescriber should any side-effects or adverse reactions occur.

In some units or contexts the midwife may be asked to prescribe and administer drugs on her own responsibility. It is considered good practice to seek another person's assistance to check the drug, especially should the drug concerned be an intravenous solution or a drug requiring complicated calculation (UKCC, 2000). It could be argued that using this strategy may prevent a number of drug errors, and the practitioner may choose to always follow this practice, using a student or qualified colleague, or in the home setting, the woman's partner.

HOMEOPATHIC AND HERBAL SUBSTANCES

Homeopathic and herbal medicines are subject to the licensing provisions of the Medicines Act 1968, although those on the market when the Act became operative, (which applies to most of those substances now available) received product licences without any evaluation of their efficacy, safety or quality.

When a woman wishes to use homeopathic or herbal substances and the midwife believes that the substances might either be an inappropriate response to the presenting symptoms or could negate or enhance the effect of prescribed medicines, she must discuss this fully with the woman. Acting in the interests of the woman and with her full knowledge, the midwife should consider contacting the relevant expert practitioner to seek advice, but must also be mindful of the need not to override the woman's rights (UKCC, 1998).

COMPLEMENTARY AND ALTERNATIVE THERAPIES

This may involve the use of substances such as essential oils or specific equipment. It is vital that practice in these respects is based upon sound principles and that the midwife practitioner is suitably qualified. Midwives should not therefore give advice or prescribe such substances unless they have received appropriate education and training in their use (UKCC, 1998).

DRUGS USED IN PREGNANCY AND DELIVERY

There now follows some basic information about the main drugs associated with pregnancy and delivery. More specific application may be found in the relevant chapters, e.g. Chapter 27.

Aperients/laxatives

Aperients are given to augment the normal rhythm of the bowel. In pregnancy, progesterone reduces the activity of plain muscle, and constipation may occur. The midwife should advise the woman regarding drinking adequate fluids, eating a high-fibre diet, and ensuring exercise such as walking and swimming. However, some women may still require aperients. Generally this might be a 'one-off' dosage, and the midwife should advise the woman against using aperients as a regular addition to her diet.

Lactulose

Indications Constipation.

Action A sugar that is broken down by gut bacteria to produce acids which result in peristalsis.

Dose 15 ml up to twice a day.

Route Oral.

Contraindications No adverse effects reported in normal pregnancy.

Side-effects Abdominal bloating.

Isogel

Indications   Constipation.

Action   Bulking agent.

Dose   Two 5 ml teaspoonfuls in water once or twice daily with meals.

Route   Oral.

Contraindications   None in normal pregnancy.

Side-effects   None.
Bulking agents for the treatment of constipation are preferable to irritants because the latter may cause high levels of abdominal discomfort (Hay-Smith, 1994).

Liquid paraffin
This softens and lubricates stools to aid defecation, but is rarely used as it can cause seepage and soiling of clothing. Long-term use may interfere with absorption of fat-soluble vitamins A, D and K.

Bisacodyl BP (Dulcolax)
Bisacodyl is a 'contact' aperient, which softens faecal mass. It is effective and safe in pregnancy and the puerperium as it is not absorbed. Bisacodyl may also be given in the form of suppositories.

Dose
- 5–10 mg orally
- 10 mg per rectum.

Haematinic substances

Iron is an essential component of haemoglobin and is necessary not only for the woman but also for the growing fetus. Women who have a good and mixed diet should not normally develop anaemia in pregnancy. If anaemia is diagnosed, however, the woman may require iron supplements. Prophylactic iron has previously been used antenatally, and present evidence suggests that there may be a case for supplementation for certain groups with iron deficiency (Mohamed, 1999). Iron often causes nausea and it is therefore wiser to begin its administration in the second trimester when the symptoms of morning sickness have passed. Digestive side-effects are also reduced when iron preparations are taken with meals.

Where the haemoglobin is very low or the date of delivery imminent, intramuscular or intravenous preparations may be used.

Ferrous sulphate compound tablets BPC (*Fersolate*)

Indications   Iron-deficiency anaemia.

Action   An iron salt which increases haemoglobin regeneration.

Dose   200 mg up to three times a day.

Route   Oral.

Contraindications   Antacids and tetracycline reduce absorption.

Side-effects   Nausea; gastrointestinal irritation; diarrhoea, and, with continued administration, constipation, black-coloured stools. (The black stools are usually due to the excess iron being excreted via the bowel.)

Folic acid BP
Folic acid is a member of the vitamin B group and is necessary for maturation of red blood cells. It is used pre- and periconceptually to prevent neural-tube defects and other congenital malformations (COMA, 2000; Czeizel, 1995, 2000).

Indications   Folate deficiency, prevention of neural tube defects.

Action   Necessary for maturation of red cells.

Dose   5 mg daily over a 4-month period for prevention of recurrence of neural tube defect, and 400 μg daily to prevent first occurrence of neural tube defect: both doses till the 12th week of pregnancy (COMA, 2000; MRC Vitamin Study Group, 1991).

Route   Oral.

Contraindications   Caution in epilepsy – folic acid occasionally reduces plasma phenytoin concentration.

Side-effects   None in short-term use. Some studies suggest that there is an increased incidence of multiple pregnancy (Czeizel et al., 1994), and that there may be a slightly increased risk of miscarriage (Hook and Czeizel, 1997).

Antihypertensive drugs

These drugs are used to control or modify blood pressure, either to manage an acute problem with hypertension or as a long-term measure for essential hypertension.

Hydralazine hydrochloride
This vasodilator hypertensive may be given in combination with a beta-blocker to reduce the side-effect of tachycardia.

Indications   Moderate–severe hypertension, hypertensive crisis.

Action   Vasodilator antihypertensive.

Dose
- Oral: 5–50 mg, twice daily
- Slow IV: 5–10 mg over 20 min repeated after 20–30 min
- IV infusion: 200–300 mg/min initially to a maintenance dose of 50–150 mg/min.

Contraindications   Idiopathic systemic lupus erythematosus, severe tachycardia, high output heart failure, myocardial insufficiency due to mechanical obstruction, cor pulmonale, dissecting aortic aneurysm, porphyria.

Side-effects   Tachycardia, fluid retention, nausea and vomiting, systemic lupus erythematosus-like syndrome after long-term high dose therapy. May also lead to a rapid hypotension.

Labetalol hydrochloride

Labetalol combines alpha- and beta-adrenoceptor blocking activity. Alpha-blocking activity in peripheral arteries lowers peripheral resistance and helps to reduce the blood pressure.

Indications   Hypertension, hypertensive crisis.

Action   Alpha- and beta-receptor blocking activity.

Dose   50–800 mg depending on route:

- Oral: 100 mg twice daily to maximum 2.4 g daily
- IV: 50 mg over 1 min – maximum 200 mg
- Phaeochromocytoma: may need higher dosage
- Pregnancy dose: IV infusion 20 mg/hour which can be doubled every 30 min to a maximum of 160 mg/hour.

If used intravenously, the upright position should be avoided after administration. Abrupt withdrawal is to be avoided.

Route   Oral, IV.

Contraindications   Asthma or history of obstructive airways disease; heart failure; second- or third-degree heart block; cardiogenic shock; after prolonged fasting, metabolic acidosis.

Side-effects   Postural hypotension, tiredness, weakness, headache, rashes, scalp-tingling, difficulty in micturition, epigastric pain, nausea, vomiting. May be a risk of intrauterine growth restriction (IUGR).

Magnesium sulphate

Magnesium sulphate is now considered the drug of choice to treat pre-eclampsia and eclampsia (Neilson, 1995). The findings from the Eclampsia Trial Collaborative Group (1995) indicate that women who develop eclampsia and are treated with magnesium sulphate are less likely to suffer recurrent fits and to die.

Indications   Eclampsia.

Action   Anticonvulsant – muscle relaxant.

Dose   Regimes may vary between hospitals and units and the following is one example:

- 5 g magnesium sulphate over a period of 20 min via infusion, by adding 8 ml of 50% magnesium sulphate solution to 200 ml normal saline
- Continue to infuse 2 g magnesium sulphate in normal saline per hour for 24 hours
- Monitor magnesium levels after 1 hour and then 4-hourly, maintaining the therapeutic range at 2–3 mmol/l.

Route   IV.

Contraindications   Renal failure.

Side-effects   Magnesium is mainly excreted by the kidneys, and is therefore retained in renal failure. There is a risk of toxicity, which can be identified by clinical signs such as loss of patellar reflexes, weakness, nausea, sensation of warmth, flushing, drowsiness, double vision and slurred speech. Toxicity may be reversed by treating with calcium gluconate.

Methyldopa BP (Aldomet)

Though vasodilators and beta-adrenoceptor drugs are now preferred for the treatment of hypertension, Methyldopa is still occasionally used.

Indications   Hypertension, hypertensive crisis.

Action   Centrally acting, antihypertensive drug.

Dose   500–3000 mg depending on route:

- Oral: 250 mg two to three times daily, maximum daily dose of 3 g
- IV: 250–500 mg infusion repeated after 6 hours if required.

Route   Oral, IV.

Contraindications   History of depression, active liver disease, phaeochromocytoma, porphyria.

Side-effects   There are a large number of side-effects – drowsiness, gastrointestinal disturbances, bradycardia, postural hypotension, oedema, arthralgia, paraesthesia, sedation, headache, dizziness, mild psychosis, depression, impaired mental acuity, parkinsonism, Bell's palsy, abnormal liver function tests, leucopenia, thrombocytopenia, hepatitis, jaundice, hypersensitivity reactions, rashes, hyperprolactinaemia.

Myometrial relaxants

Beta-adrenoceptor stimulants relax uterine muscle and may be used in selected cases in an attempt to inhibit uncomplicated preterm labour between 24–33 weeks. They are usually used over a period of 48 hours. This provides time to administer steroid therapy to increase the chances of neonatal well-being, and to reduce the risks of these drugs to the woman, which increase after 48 hours. The effect is brought about mainly by their influence on the receptors stimulated by the sympathetic nervous system. Large doses cause a rise in heart rate and a fall in blood pressure and therefore the pulse and blood pressure should be checked frequently, especially during intravenous administration. In the event of a marked fall in blood pressure it is recommended that the woman be turned into a lateral position.

Treatment is usually commenced by slow intravenous infusion followed, as contractions cease, by intermittent intramuscular doses and finally oral administration. The drug most commonly used now is ritodrine hydrochloride.

Ritodrine hydrochloride (Yutopar)

Indications   Uncomplicated preterm labour, fetal asphyxia due to hypertonic uterine action.

Action   Beta$_2$-adrenoceptor stimulant.

Dose   10–120 mg depending on route:

- IV: initial 50 mg/min increased to usual dose 150–350 mg/min
- IM: 10 mg every 3–8 hours
- Oral: 10 mg 30 min prior to the termination of IV therapy
- Oral maintenance: first 24 hours 10 mg every 2 hours; thereafter 10–20 mg every 4–6 hours; maximum 120 mg daily.

Route   Oral, IM, IV.

Contraindications   Haemorrhage, hypertension, pre-eclampsia or eclampsia, cord compression, intrauterine infection, antepartum haemorrhage which demands immediate delivery, placenta praevia, maternal cardiac disease.

Side-effects   Nausea, vomiting, flushing, sweating, tremor; and, with high doses, hypokalaemia, tachycardia and hypotension, chest pain or tightness, arrhythmias.

Atosiban

This is a newly licensed drug which may be useful when a beta$_2$-adrenoceptor stimulant is not appropriate, i.e. when the woman has a cardiac condition. *It is important to monitor blood loss after delivery.*

Indications   Uncomplicated preterm labour between 24–33 weeks.

Action   Oxytocin-receptor antagonist.

Dose   IV injection, initially 6.75 mg over 1 min, then by IV infusion 18 mg/hour for 3 hours, then 6 mg/hour for up to 45 hours; maximum duration of treatment 48 hours.

Route   IV.

Contraindications   Eclampsia and severe pre-eclampsia, intrauterine infection, intrauterine fetal death, antepartum haemorrhage (requiring immediate delivery), placenta praevia, abruptio placentae, IUGR with abnormal fetal heart rate, premature rupture of membranes after 30 weeks' gestation, hepatic and renal impairment.

Side-effects   Nausea, vomiting, tachycardia, hypotension, headache, dizziness, hot flushes, hyperglycaemia, injection site reaction; less commonly pruritus, rash, fever, insomnia.

Analgesics

These drugs are used to relieve pain but maintain consciousness. Some of these drugs may cause respiratory depression and withdrawal symptoms in the neonate.

Meptazinol (Meptid)

This synthetic narcotic analgesic drug is used for the short-term relief of moderate to severe pain, including labour and postoperative pain. Unlike many other narcotic drugs, it rarely causes euphoria and is therefore less likely to produce dependence than other drugs of this class. Unless by overdosage, it does not cause respiratory depression. Meptazinol is likely to increase the sedative effect on the central nervous system of drugs such as hypnotics, antidepressants and antihistamines. Monoamine oxidase inhibitors (MAOIs) may produce a dangerous rise in blood pressure when taken with meptazinol.

Indications   Moderate to severe pain, obstetric analgesia.

Action   Synthetic narcotic analgesic.

Dose

- Oral: 200 mg every 3–6 hours as required
- Obstetric analgesia: IM: 100–150 mg according to patient's weight (2 mg/kg) (normal adult dose 75–100 mg every 2–4 hours if necessary).

Route   IM, oral.

Contraindications   Long-term liver or kidney problems; lung disorders such as asthma or emphysema.

Side-effects   Nausea, vomiting, dizziness and drowsiness. Overdosage may cause respiratory depression, and naloxone may be used to reverse the effect.

Pethidine hydrochloride

Pethidine is a powerful analgesic and antispasmodic; it is the most widely used analgesic in the obstetric field, relieving the pain of labour without diminishing the force of uterine contraction. It is used during the first stage of labour to produce analgesia and relaxation and, when given intramuscularly, takes effect in 10–15 minutes.

Pethidine crosses the placenta and may depress the fetal respiratory centre; thus if given within 2–3 hours of delivery it may cause birth asphyxia. In most normal deliveries a total of 200 mg (usually in separate doses of 100 mg) provides adequate pain relief and therefore many health authorities and trusts will require the involvement of a medical practitioner should more than this amount be required.

In some cases pethidine may be given intravenously for rapid action and effective pain relief in labour. Pethidine should not be given to women being treated with monoamine oxidase inhibitors (MAOIs) as these drugs potentiate the action of pethidine about 10 times; thus the combination is highly dangerous.

Indications   Moderate to severe pain, obstetric analgesia.

Action   Opioid analgesic (used in labour because it is associated with less respiratory depression than are other opioids).

Dose

- SC or IM injection: 50–100 mg repeated 1–3 hours later if necessary
- Oral: 50–150 mg every 4 hours.
- IV injection: 25–50 mg (given slowly) repeated after 4 hours.

Route   SC, IM, IV, oral.

Contraindications   Severe renal impairment, raised intracranial pressure, head injury, treatment with MAOIs.

Side-effects   Nausea and vomiting, constipation, drowsiness, hypotension, respiratory depression in woman and neonate.

Overdosage or neonatal respiratory depression may be counteracted by treating with naloxone (Narcan); however, caution should be exercised should there be any suspicion that the woman has been using drugs such as morphine or heroin as this may cause acute neonatal withdrawal problems.

Diamorphine hydrochloride (heroin)

Drugs such as diamorphine and morphine are derived from opium, which in turn is prepared from the unripe seed capsules of the opium poppy. Diamorphine resembles morphine in its actions and uses, but produces better pain relief with less severe side-effects when given intravenously. Diamorphine is an extremely effective analgesic that also reduces anxiety and stress, which makes it a useful drug for pain from injury, surgery, heart attack or chronic diseases such as cancer. The effects of diamorphine wear off quickly, and when used over a short, acute period, it is unlikely to result in dependence. However, people who use this drug regularly for its euphoric effects are highly likely to become addicted.

Diamorphine may be used intramuscularly, and may have significant benefits over pethidine, in terms of improved pain relief, less nausea and less neonatal respiratory depression (Fairlie *et al.*, 1999). It is also increasingly being used for labour via epidural, subarachnoid and intrathecal single dose and infusion (Bloor *et al.*, 1999; Sneyd and Meyer-Whitting, 1992) and elective caesarean section (Barkshire *et al.*, 2001), and post-caesarean section pain relief. Results from several studies would suggest that it is an effective means of analgesia with reduced side-effect of nausea (Bloor *et al.*, 1999; Daniel and McGrady, 1995), though in one study, administration of subarachnoid diamorphine resulted in a higher incidence of pruritus (Bloor *et al.*, 2000), and another indicated that a continuous epidural infusion was preferable in terms of pain relief and reduction in side-effects (Daniel and McGrady, 1995).

Indications   Moderate and severe pain, obstetric analgesia.

Action   Opioid analgesic.

Dose   Dependent on route.

Route   May be used IM, IV and via the epidural, intrathecal and subarachnoid routes.

Contraindications   Long-term kidney or liver problems, heart/circulatory problems, asthma, bronchitis, thyroid disease. Combination with other drugs such as sedatives, alcohol, antidepressants, antipsychotics, sleeping drugs and antihistamines; monoamine oxidase inhibitors may produce a severe rise in blood pressure when taken with diamorphine.

Side-effects   Nausea, vomiting and constipation are common, especially with high doses; slow or irregular breathing, severe drowsiness or loss of consciousness.

Other analgesics that might be used   Dihydrocodeine 30 mg tablets (every 4–6 hours); diclofenac sodium 50 mg tablets/100 mg suppositories; paracetamol 500 mg (two tablets every 4–6 hours). Aspirin should be used with caution, and avoided whilst breastfeeding because of the risk of Reye's syndrome.

Antacids

These drugs are given to reduce gastric acidity and relieve heartburn; e.g. alginic acid (Gaviscon) given orally.

Ranitidine

Indications   To reduce gastric acid secretion prior to emergency caesarean section.

Action   A histamine H_2-receptor antagonist.

Dose
- Oral: 150 mg 6-hourly during labour prophylactically
- IM: 50 mg 6-hourly
- IV: 50 mg diluted to 20 ml given over 2 min.

Route   Oral, IM or slow IV.

Contraindications   Avoid in porphyria.

Side-effects   Tachycardia, agitation, visual disturbances, erythema multiforme, alopecia, hepatic impairment, renal impairment, pregnancy, and during breastfeeding.

Tranquillizers

Tranquillizers are sometimes given during pregnancy, labour or postpartum. They are antiemetic, potentiate the analgesic (if given), relieve anxiety and apprehension and help the overanxious woman to rest. These may also be used for women with mental health problems who may suffer an acute episode of anxiety.

Promazine BP (S.4B) (Sparine)

Indications   Short-term adjunctive management of psychomotor agitation.

Action   Antipsychotic.

Dose
- Oral: 100–200 mg four times daily
- IM: 50 mg for short-term adjunctive management.

Route   Oral or IM.

Contraindications   Coma caused by CNS depressants, bone marrow depression, phaeochromocytoma, cardiovascular and cerebrovascular disease.

Side-effects   Drowsiness, apathy, pallor, hypothermia, nightmares, insomnia, depression.

Diazepam (Valium)

Diazepam is a tranquillizer and an anticonvulsant and may be administered by intravenous infusion in cases of severe pre-eclampsia and eclampsia. In recent years, there has been an increased understanding of the dependence effect of diazepam. The midwife should also be aware that a woman may have been taking this drug prior to pregnancy.

Indications   Anxiety, insomnia, anticonvulsant, may be used for treatment of severe pre-eclampsia and eclampsia.

Action   Anxiolytic (sedative), anticonvulsant.

Dose
- 2 mg – depending on need and route – for pre-eclampsia and eclampsia
- IM or by IV infusion: 5–10 mg (40 mg/500 ml) to a maximum of 3 mg/kg over 24 hours.

Route   Oral, IM, IV, rectal.

Contraindications   Respiratory depression, acute pulmonary insufficiency, porphyria, sleep apnoea syndrome, severe hepatic impairment, myasthenia gravis; not for chronic psychosis, phobic or obsessional states, and should not be used alone in depression or in anxiety with depression.

Side-effects   Drowsiness and light-headedness the next day, confusion and ataxia, amnesia, dependence.

NB: Some, neonates exposed to diazepam or other benzodiazepines during the third trimester or during labour may exhibit either the 'floppy infant' syndrome, or marked neonatal withdrawal symptoms (Iqbal, et al., 2002; Peinnemann and Daldrup, 2001). Symptoms vary from mild sedation, hypotonia, and reluctance to suck, to apnoeic spells, cyanosis, and impaired metabolic responses to cold stress. These symptoms have been reported to persist for periods from hours to months after birth (McElhatton, 1994).

Hypnotics

Chloral hydrate
This is not as popular a drug as formerly, but may be used for short-term insomnia.

Indications   Insomnia (short-term use).

Action   Hypnotic.

Dose   0.5–1 g (maximum 2 g) at bedtime with plenty of water.

Route   Oral.

Contraindications   Severe cardiac disease, gastritis, marked renal or hepatic impairment, respiratory disease, porphyria; should be avoided in women with a history of personality disorder or drug or alcohol abuse.

Side-effects   Gastric irritation (nausea and vomiting reported), abdominal distension, flatulence; also vertigo, ataxia, staggering gait, rashes, headache, lightheadedness, malaise, ketonuria, excitement, nightmares, eosinophilia, reduction in white cell count; dependence (may be associated with gastritis and renal damage) on prolonged use.

Anaesthetics

Local anaesthetic drugs act by causing a temporary block to conduction along nerve fibres. Toxic effects associated with local anaesthetics may occur as a result of very high blood levels or too rapid an injection. Signs of toxicity include excitability of the central nervous system, which is characterized by nausea and convulsions, followed by depression.

The cardiovascular system may also be depressed, requiring urgent resuscitative measures. The anaesthetics most commonly used in obstetrics are as follows.

Lidocaine (lignocaine) hydrochloride

Indications   Anaesthesia, nerve blocks, epidural and caudal block.

Action   Local anaesthetic; reversible block to conduction along nerve fibres.

Dose   Adjusted according to site and response:

- For infiltration of the perineum prior to episiotomy, up to 10 ml of 0.5% solution
- Epidural and caudal block with adrenaline (epinephrine) 1 in 200 000% to a maximum of 50 ml.

Route   Topical, SC or epidural.

Contraindications   Inflamed or infected tissues (may cause a systemic rather than a local reaction), hypovolaemia, complete heart block.

Side-effects   Hypotension, bradycardia, cardiac arrest, agitation, euphoria, respiratory depression, convulsions; hypersensitivity may be present.

Bupivacaine (Marcain)
Bupivacaine is widely used for continuous epidural analgesia in labour. It takes up to 30 minutes to take full effect but then lasts for 2–3 hours.

Indications   Epidural and spinal anaesthesia.

Action   Local anaesthetic.

Dose   According to the site of operation and response of the patient.

Route   Into epidural space, e.g. in labour:

- Lumbar: 0.25–0.5% maximum 12 ml
- Caudal:
  - 0.25% maximum 30 ml
  - 0.5% maximum 20 ml.

NB: 0.75% solution is contraindicated for epidural use in pregnancy.

Contraindications   Hypovolaemia; complete heart block; avoid in porphyria; caution in intravenous regional anaesthesia, and epilepsy.

Side-effects   Hypotension; bradycardia; cardiac arrest; CNS effects include agitation; euphoria; respiratory depression; convulsions; anaesthesia.

Oxytocic drugs

Ergometrine maleate BP (S.4B)
Ergometrine was introduced to obstetric practice in the 1930s by Chassar Moir. Since then it has proved to be of immense value in the prevention and treatment of postpartum haemorrhage. It has a powerful action

on the uterus especially immediately after labour, when it produces rhythmic contractions. Its action is less rapid but more prolonged than that of oxytocin. Ergometrine is given to prevent and control haemorrhage during childbirth, especially if an anaesthetic has been used and hence uterine action is poor. It is most usually injected intramuscularly with the crowning of the head or the birth of the anterior shoulder, or intravenously when there is increased risk such as antepartum haemorrhage, postpartum haemorrhage or poor muscle tone which occurs with such conditions as grand multiparity and multiple pregnancy. It may be injected into the uterine wall by the surgeon during caesarean section. Ergometrine may be given orally postpartum to ensure good contraction of the uterus.

There are complications associated with the use of ergometrine, particularly if given intravenously (Dumoulin, 1981). Hypertension has been reported by many researchers, including Hendricks and Brenner (1970), Johnstone (1972) and Moir and Amoa (1979). Cases of pulmonary oedema in cardiac patients, cardiac arrest and cerebral haemorrhage have also been reported (DHSS, 1986). It has been shown to cause a reduction in serum prolactin levels and may reduce the production of breast milk. Finally there is a high incidence of vomiting, especially following the administration of intravenous ergometrine (Moodie and Moir, 1976). Midwives should therefore avoid giving ergometrine to women with hypertensive disorders (DoH, 1994) and those suffering from cardiac and respiratory conditions, unless the drug is prescribed by a doctor.

Indications   Prevention and treatment of haemorrhage.

Action   Oxytocic, i.e. stimulates uterine contractions.

Dose
- Third stage labour: 500 mg IM, usually with oxytocin 5 units
- Prevention in high-risk cases: 125–250 mg IV
- Secondary postpartum haemorrhage: 500 mg orally three times daily for 3 days.

Route   IM, IV, oral.

Contraindications   First and second stages of labour (only with crowning of head or birth of anterior shoulder in second stage), vascular disease, hepatic and renal impairment, severe hypertension, sepsis. Caution with multiple pregnancy, pre-eclampsia, eclampsia.

Side-effects   Nausea, vomiting, transient hypertension, vasoconstriction, stroke.

Oxytocin

Oxytocin was synthesized in 1954 by Du Vigneaud. Oxytocin may be given diluted in an intravenous infusion to induce or augment labour. The uterine contractions and fetal heart are continuously monitored, as hyperstimulation can cause fetal distress leading to intrauterine fetal death. In the presence of malpresentation or cephalopelvic disproportion such contractions can cause rupture of the uterus. Intravenous oxytocin can cause a transient but marked fall in blood pressure (Hendricks and Brenner, 1970) with tachycardia and an increased stroke volume which increases the cardiac output. It also has an antidiuretic action.

Syntocinon

Indications   For prevention or treatment of haemorrhage during the third stage of labour. For induction and augmentation of labour.

Action   Stimulates uterine contractions.

Dose
- For induction and augmentation of labour: 1–3 mU/min, adjusted according to response by slow IV infusion
- For missed abortion: as a solution containing 10–20 units/500 ml given at a rate of 10–30 drops/minute, increased in strength by 10–20 units/500 ml every hour to a maximum strength of 100 units/ 500 ml
- For postpartum haemorrhage: 20–40 units per 500 ml Hartmann's solution.

Route   IM, slow IV infusion.

Contraindications   Hypertonic uterine action, mechanical obstruction to delivery, failed trial labour, severe hypertension, fetal distress, placenta praevia.

Side-effects   High doses cause violent uterine contractions which may lead to rupture and fetal asphyxiation, arrhythmias, maternal hypertension and subarachnoid haemorrhage, and pulmonary oedema.
NB: Prolonged intravenous administration at high doses with large volume may cause water intoxication with hyponatraemia. This can be prevented by using an electrolyte-containing diluent (i.e. not glucose), using a higher concentration of oxytocin, and careful monitoring of fluid and electrolytes.

Oxytocin and ergometrine (Syntometrine (S.4B))

In 1961 Embrey combined ergometrine maleate with oxytocin to form *Syntometrine*, which is now widely used for active management of the third stage. This proprietary preparation of oxytocin 5 units and ergometrine 500 mcg in 1 ml is said to combine the best of two constituents: it acts quickly because of the oxytocin and the action is prolonged by the ergometrine. Its use is confined to the prevention and treatment of postpartum haemorrhage. Intramuscular Syntometrine takes effect in 2–3 minutes. Syntometrine 1 ml is usually injected intramuscularly with the crowning of the head or the birth of the anterior shoulder, though some agencies favour administration after delivery of the neonate, especially should there be suspicion of an undiagnosed twin. It causes a powerful contraction of the uterus which aids placental separation and the control of bleeding. Several studies have suggested that routine Syntometrine may dramatically reduce the risk of postpartum haemorrhage (Prendiville *et al.*, 1988, 2000; Rogers *et al.*, 1998) (see Ch. 30).

Indications   As for ergometrine maleate. Used for active management of the third stage of labour or routine prevention or treatment of postpartum haemorrhage.

Action   As for ergometrine maleate.

Dose   1 ml IM; 0.5–1 ml IV.

Route   IM, IV.

Contraindications   As for ergometrine maleate.

Side-effects   As for ergometrine maleate.

Prostaglandins

Prostaglandins are substances found in extracts and secretions of human prostate and seminal vesicles and in many other parts of the body. There are several preparations similar in action but slightly different in their chemical structure. Certain prostaglandins cause contraction of uterine muscle and are used in therapeutic abortion and to induce labour.

Prostaglandins are contraindicated in the same situations as oxytocin and should be used with caution in patients with raised intraocular pressure or a history of asthma. They may cause nausea, vomiting and diarrhoea.

Prostaglandin E_2 (PGE_2) may be administered vaginally, extra-amniotically or orally to ripen the cervix, when necessary, or to induce labour. Vaginal PGE_2 may be given in a gel, or as tablets or lipid-based pessaries. A PGE_2 polymer vaginal pessary (3 mg) is now available. Extra-amniotic instillation can be either intermittent or by continuous infusion through a transcervical catheter. Prostaglandin $F_{2\alpha}$ may also be administered vaginally to ripen the cervix, although some studies have shown it to be less effective for ripening the unfavourable cervix than PGE_2. Oral preparations of prostaglandins for routine induction of labour are satisfactory, provided the cervix is favourable and particularly in multiparous women. Prolonged treatment, however, such as may be required to ripen the cervix may cause side-effects. Prostaglandins are not administered intravenously because of their unpleasant side-effects, which include nausea, vomiting, diarrhoea, local tissue reaction and erythema.

Examples   *Dinoprostone* is given orally or via the vagina. *Gemprost* is given via the vagina.

Coagulants

Phytomenadione (vitamin K)

Indications   May be given prophylactically to all neonates, or selectively to those who are preterm or have had a traumatic delivery (i.e. ventouse, breech and LSCS).

Action   Production of blood clotting factors and proteins necessary for normal calcification of bone.

Dose   See Chapter 31, for more information. Refer to your locally agreed policy for neonatal use, e.g. prophylactic dose 0.5 mg orally or by injection.

If the mother is breastfeeding, the dose may be repeated on the 7th and 28th day of life.

Route   Oral, IM or IV.

Contraindications   None reported.

Side-effects   These are associated with the development of haemolytic anaemia; hyperbilirubinaemia and kernicterus have been reported. Some debate was raised regarding an increased risk of childhood leukaemia (Golding *et al.*, 1990, 1992) with routine IM vitamin K, though this has not been supported by other studies (Ekelund *et al.*, 1993; Passmore *et al.*, 1998).

Anticoagulants

Anticoagulants are widely used in the prevention and treatment of deep vein thrombosis. There should be some laboratory monitoring, and the midwife should discuss with the woman the purpose and action of the drug.

Heparin

Heparin is given to start anticoagulation and is rapidly effective although its effects are of short duration. It is therefore best given by continuous infusion. If given intermittently, the interval should not exceed 6 hours. Oral anticoagulants are started at the same time as heparin, and heparin is discontinued after 3 days.

Dose 5000 units initially, followed by continuous infusion of 40 000 units over 24 hours or 10 000 units by intravenous injection every 6 hours.

Warfarin sodium

Oral anticoagulants take 36–48 hours to take effect. The dose of oral anticoagulants is adjusted to prolong the prothrombin time. Oral anticoagulants are teratogenic and therefore should not be given in early pregnancy. They cross the placenta and thus are not given in the last few weeks of pregnancy.

Protamine sulphate

Protamine sulphate is used to counteract an overdose of heparin. It is given by slow intravenous injection, the maximum dose being 50 mg. An overdose of protamine sulphate has an anticoagulant effect.

Respiratory drugs

Respiratory stimulants which are antidotes to pethidine and other narcotics may be used if the baby shows signs of respiratory depression at birth.

Naloxone hydrochloride (Narcan Neonatal)

Naloxone hydrochloride is a narcotic antagonist which is given intramuscularly or intravenously to a baby suffering from respiratory depression at birth. It may also be used (though rarely) for a woman with respiratory depression after opioids. It has replaced earlier antidotes such as nalorphine and levallorphan because they are also partial agonists and can thus cause respiratory depression themselves.

Indications Reversal of opioid-induced respiratory depression.

Action Binds competitively to opioid receptors.

Dose

- Neonate: 10 µg/kg by SC, IM, or IV route, repeated every 2–3 min, or 200 µg (60 mg/kg) IM as a single dose at birth (onset of action slower)
- Adult: IV 100–200 µg (1.5 µg/kg). If response is inadequate, increments of 100 µg every 2 min. Further doses by IM injection after 1–2 hours if required.

Route SC, IM or IV.

Contraindications Acute opioid withdrawal may be precipitated in opioid-dependent patients.

Side-effects Not a problem at therapeutic doses.

Special note When administered to the neonate, it should be noted that this is *not* an emergency drug, and should not be given to babies who are apnoeic or without an adequate heart rate. Because of Narcan's short half-life, the midwife should also continue observing the neonate's respiratory and response rates until it is certain that the respiratory depression effect of the opioids received during labour has passed.

Reflective Activity 71.3

Get access to a computer, either at home or at your maternity unit or library.

Go to the BNF site – http://www.bnf.org/webnf/lform1/bnf/index.html – and look up Syntometrine.

After you have looked at the information on the site, consider the following:

- Was any of the information there new to you?
- Was the site easily accessible?
- How would you use this site in the future?

DRUGS AND BREASTFEEDING

Breastfeeding is regarded as one of the most important measures to improve child health in all societies. The most important question to ask is whether a breastfeeding mother needs medication. If so, then a drug regimen should be chosen which will have minimal impact on the nursing infant. With careful selection, it is seldom necessary to deny the infant the known benefits of breastfeeding. Only in a few instances is a temporary cessation of breastfeeding (expressing and discarding the milk) advisable, e.g. after use of a radio-diagnostic agent. In a small number of cases where a mother is on long-term medication with agents known to have potentially serious side-effects, e.g. psychotropic agents, timing of breastfeeding to avoid peak interval levels in milk (perhaps 1–2 hours after oral medication) will minimize exposure to the drug via breast milk.

Infant factors

The age of the infant is important in calculating the potential risk of adverse reactions. In premature or newborn infants, renal and hepatic functions are not fully developed and there is a risk of drug accumulation. Usually, renal and hepatic functions mature within 2–4 weeks after birth. Older infants will ingest decreasing amounts of drugs as they are weaned from breast milk on to solid foods.

Drug exposure depends not only on the volume of milk ingested, but also on the extent of absorption from the gastrointestinal tract. Some drugs normally given by injection are destroyed in the gut, e.g. insulin and heparin. Since the infant receives these by the oral route, they do not pass into the systemic circulation and thus pose no hazard.

The infants' tissue receptor sensitivity may also influence the risk of adverse drug reactions. A few drugs may cause idiosyncratic or allergic reactions unrelated to the amount ingested.

Drugs with an adverse effect on lactation

Only a few drugs are known to affect lactation adversely. Oestrogens, particularly in high dose, may decrease milk production and the Family Planning Association recommends that oestrogen-containing oral contraceptives should be avoided. The progestogen-only oral contraceptive does not adversely influence milk production (Grant and Golightly, 2000). Some other drugs do not actually affect the milk supply, but may have an effect on the taste of the milk for the neonate, such as the antibiotic metronidazole (Flagyl), which makes the breast milk bitter.

EFFECTS OF DRUGS OF MISUSE AND DEPENDENCE ON PREGNANCY AND THE NEONATE

It is generally accepted that drugs should be prescribed in pregnancy only if the benefit to the mother outweighs the risk to the fetus. During the first trimester, drugs may produce congenital malformations, that is they may be teratogenic, and during the second and third trimesters, they may affect growth and functional development. Women may not be in contact with any agency which can tell them about the possible risks to their baby if they take drugs, including tobacco and alcohol, during pregnancy. It is also important to remember that many of the obstetric problems commonly associated with illicit drug use are also associated with social deprivation and poor health and nutrition. Intravenous injection of drugs may also present the risk of both local and systemic infection.

There is a difference between drug misuse and drug dependence. Drug misuse, which is broadly equivalent to 'drug abuse' and 'problem drug taking', denotes drug taking which is hazardous or harmful and is unsanctioned by professional or cultural standards. Drug dependence is a term used to describe the altered physical and psychological state which results in disturbed physical and mental functioning when the drug is abruptly discontinued. It is broadly equivalent to 'drug addiction'. However, not all drug misusers are drug dependent. Generally, a drug on which a woman is dependent is likely to cause problems for the baby when it is withdrawn from the source, usually after birth. Symptoms of withdrawal vary in strength and effect, depending probably on the condition of the baby after birth. This explains the wide variation in symptoms seen even when women have taken similar amounts of illicit drugs (Siney, 1999).

It is vital therefore, that the midwife identify women who may have used drugs, or may be regular drug users as early as possible in the pregnancy. The 'booking interview' is a key opportunity to make this assessment, but it is important that at this first interview, the purpose of ascertaining this information is made explicit to the woman. This must include a discussion about issues of confidentiality, i.e. that if the woman reveals that she is using drugs which may affect the fetus or neonate, then other practitioners such as paediatricians would need to be involved. Generally the woman is more likely to be open about this information if she understands the implications for her baby, and if the pattern of care provides her with a feeling of security. In some services the woman could be referred to a midwife and/or multidisciplinary team specializing in supporting women with drug problems. Continuity of care for this woman is also an important means of support, and is more likely to assist her in firstly revealing that she has a problem, and in being able to consider strategies for withdrawal. Some women may become aware of the dangers to their baby, and attempt to withdraw without proper support and advice, and this may cause more harm to the fetus.

NURSE PRESCRIBING

District nurses and health visitors were able to become nurse prescribers under the Medicinal

Products: Prescription by Nurses Act 1992. In May 2002, ministers announced their intention to extend nurse prescribing to allow nurses working in appropriate settings to prescribe a range of medicines for certain medical conditions. This included minor injuries such as burns, cuts and sprains; ailments such as hay fever or ear infections; health promotion, i.e. vitamins for women considering pregnancy, and palliative care.

Those nurses who undertake this role normally undertake a degree-level preparation programme, which should include 25 taught days, and 12 work-based learning days under supervision, gaining the knowledge and skills in prescribing medications (DoH, 2002). Nurses put forward for the training would normally be those who wish to extend their role into prescribing, and for whom this forms a normal part of their role. This might include nurses who are working in palliative care, such as Macmillan nurses, or those who work in community settings.

Patient Group Directives (or group protocols) allow nurses to *supply* and prescribe prescription-only medicines to patients, and are developed to provide more flexibility both for the nurses and for clients and patients. These directives are specific written instructions for supply and administration of a named medicine or vaccine in a particular clinical situation. They are prepared and agreed by a multidisciplinary group, including senior doctors, and pharmacists.

This new development does not affect the midwife's ability to prescribe and administer medications; however, a number of midwives may wish to undertake the training, and extend their area of prescribing, for example midwives undertaking preconceptual care, or midwives working in transitional care.

CONCLUSION

Midwives must be knowledgeable about the range of drugs and medications that women and babies may require, but should also be aware of other less commonly used drugs.

They should be conversant with the legislation and with safe practice in storing, administering and recording drugs, and this should be clearly reflected in their day-to-day practice. Midwives should also be aware of the sources of information regarding drugs, which include local pharmacists, hospital pharmacists, and literature such as the *British National Formulary* and the *Nurse Prescribers' Formulary*. Practitioners may also wish to access more up-to-date information which is available electronically, from the BNF on-line, or the Nurse Prescribing site (see Additional resources at the end of the chapter). Midwives can also gather information from their clients regarding the effects of medications and their feelings about them. This is crucial in terms of identifying serious side-effects, but is also an important source of information for future clients. An example might be iron preparations, which might cause constipation: the midwife who is aware of this can provide information and advice to counteract that effect in women taking iron preparations. Midwives should also be vigilant about drugs and medications being discussed in the media, as this might trigger questions from women and their families. An example of this would be the links between vitamin K and childhood leukaemia, and a recent debate about the measles, mumps and rubella (MMR) vaccination.

Being up to date and knowledgeable therefore provides a higher standard of care to the mother and her baby, and more confidence to the practitioner.

KEY POINTS

- All drugs taken during pregnancy and lactation will have an effect.
- Some drugs may interact with other drugs to either lessen or increase effect.
- It is essential that the midwife follow the guidelines available for safe prescription, administration and storage of drugs and medications.
- It is important that the midwife has a strategy for accessing up-to-date and sufficiently detailed information concerning drugs and medications.

- The pharmacist or drugs information department in the trust is an excellent resource for up-to-date and appropriate drug information.
- The midwife must ensure that the woman is educated in the potential effects of different drugs on herself, her fetus and the neonate.
- Women who are drug users have particular problems, and should be supported by a multidisciplinary care team to ensure minimal harm to mother and baby.

REFERENCES

Barkshire, K., Russell, R. & Burry, J. (2001) A comparison of bupivicaine-fentanyl-morphine with bupivicaine-fentanyl-diamorphine for caesarean section under spinal anaesthesia. *International Journal of Obstetric Anaesthesia* 10(1): 4–10.

Bloor, G.K., Sinden, M. & McGregor, R. (1999) An audit of single dose epidural diamorphine during elective caesarean section at a district general hospital. *International Journal of Obstetric Anaesthesia* 8(1): 11–16.

Bloor, G.K., Thompson, M. & Chung, N.A. (2000) A randomised double blind comparison of subarachnoid and epidural diamorphine for elective caesarean section using a combined spinal–epidural technique. *International Journal of Obstetric Anaesthesia* 9(4): 233–237.

British Medical Association (BMA) and Royal Pharmaceutical Society of Great Britain (RPSGB) (2003) *British National Formulary,* 46th edn. London: BMA and RPSGB.

Committee on Medical Aspects of Food and Nutrition Policy (COMA) (2000) *Folic Acid and the Prevention of Disease: Report on Health and Social Subjects* (Chair: Sir J.G. Evans). London: Department of Health.

Czeizel, A.E. (1995) Folic acid in the prevention of neural tube defects. *Journal of Pediatric Gastroenterology and Nutrition* 20(1): 4–16.

Czeizel, A.E. (2000) Primary prevention of neural-tube defects and some other major congenital abnormalities: recommendations for the appropriate use of folic acid during pregnancy. *Paediatric Drugs* 2(6): 437–449.

Czeizel, A.E., Metneki, J. & Dudas, I. (1994) Higher rate of multiple births after periconceptional vitamin supplementation. *New England Journal of Medicine* 330(23): 1687–1688.

Daniel, M. & McGrady, E.M. (1995) Epidural diamorphine: a comparison of bolus and infusion administration in labour. *Anaesthesia* 50(1): 14–16.

Department of Health (DoH) (1994) *Report on Confidential Enquiries into Maternal Deaths in the United Kingdom 1988–1990.* London: HMSO.

Department of Health (DoH) (2002) Extension of independent nurse prescribing. Online. Available: http:// www.doh.gov.uk/nurse prescribing/index.htm March 2002.

Department of Health and Social Security (DHSS) (1986) *Report on Confidential Enquiries into Maternal Deaths in England and Wales 1979–1981.* London: HMSO.

Dumoulin, J.G. (1981) A reappraisal of the use of ergometrine. *Journal of Obstetrics and Gynaecology* 1: 178–181.

Donnison, J. (1988) *Midwives and Medical Men.* London: Heinemann.

Eclampsia Trial Collaborative Group (ETCG) (1995) Which anticonvulsant for women with eclampsia? Evidence from the Collaborative Eclampsia Trial. *Lancet* 345(8963): 1455–1463.

Ekelund, H., Finnstrom, O., Gunnarskog, J. *et al.* (1993) Administration of vitamin K to newborn infants and childhood cancer. *British Medical Journal* 307(6896): 89–91.

Fairlie, F.M., Marshall, L., Walkers, J.J. *et al.* (1999) Intramuscular opioids for maternal pain relief in labour: a randomised controlled trial comparing pethidine with diamorphine. *British Journal of Obstetrics and Gynaecology* 106(11): 1181–1187.

Golding, J., Paterson, M. & Kinlen, L.J. (1990) Factors associated with childhood cancer in a national cohort study. *British Journal of Cancer* 62(2): 304–308.

Golding, J., Greenwood, R., Birmingham, K. *et al.* (1992) Childhood cancer: intramuscular vitamin K and pethidine given in a national cohort study. *British Medical Journal* 305(6849): 341–346.

Grant, E. & Golightly, P. (2000) Principles of prescribing in lactation. In: Lee, A., Inch, S. & Finnigan, D. (eds) *Therapeutics in Pregnancy and Lactation,* pp. 14, 16–17, 19. Oxford: Radcliffe Medical Press.

Hay-Smith, J. (1994) Postpartum laxatives. In: Enkin, M.W., Keirse, M.J.N.C., Renfrew, M.J. *et al.* (eds) *Pregnancy and Childbirth Module. Cochrane Database of Systematic Reviews:* Review No. 03663. Cochrane Updates on Disk, Issue 1. Oxford: Update Software.

Hendricks, C.H. & Brenner, W.E. (1970) Cardiovascular effects of oxytocic drugs used postpartum. *American Journal of Obstetrics and Gynaecology* 108(5): 751–760.

Hook, E.B. & Czeizel, A.E. (1997) Can terathanasia explain the protective effect of folic-acid supplementation on birth defects? *Lancet* 350(9076): 513–515.

Hytten, F.E. & Leitch, I. (1971) *The Physiology of Pregnancy.* Oxford: Blackwell Science.

Iqbal, M.M., Sobhan, T. & Ryals, T. (2002) Effects of commonly used benzodiazepines on the fetus the neonate and the nursing infant. *Psychiatric Services* 53(1): 39–49.

Johnstone, M. (1972) The cardiovascular effects of oxytocic drugs. *British Journal of Anaesthesia* 44(8): 826–834.

McElhatton, P.R. (1994) The effects of benzodiazepine during pregnancy and lactation. *Reproductive Toxicology* 8(6): 461–475.

Medical Research Council (MRC) Vitamin Study Group (1991) Prevention of neural tube defects: Results of the Medical Research Council Vitamin Study. *Lancet* 238(8760): 131–137.

Mohamed, K. (1999) Iron supplementation in pregnancy. *The Cochrane Library,* Issue 3. Oxford: Update Software.

Moir, D.D. & Amoa, A.B. (1979) Ergometrine or oxytocin? Blood loss and side-effects at spontaneous vertex delivery. *British Journal of Anaesthesia* 51(2): 113–117.

Moody, J.E. & Moir, D.D. (1976) Ergometrine, oxytocin or extradural analgesia. *British Journal of Anaesthesia* 48: 57.

Myles, M. (1956) *A Textbook for Midwives*. London: Livingstone.

Neilson, J.P. (1995) Magnesium sulphate: the drug of choice in eclampsia. *British Medical Journal* **311**(7007): 702–703.

O'Hare, M.F., Kinney, C.D., Murnaghan, J.A. *et al.* (1984) Pharmacokinetics of phenytoin during pregnancy. *European Journal of Clinical Pharmacology* **27**(5): 583–587.

Passmore, S.J., Draper, G., Brownbill, P. *et al.* (1998) Ecological studies of relation between hospital policies on neonatal vitamin K administration and subsequent occurrence of childhood cancer. *British Medical Journal* **316**(7126): 184–189.

Peinnemann, F. & Daldrup, T. (2001) Severe and prolonged sedation in five neonates due to persistence of active diazepam metabolites. *European Journal of Pediatrics* **160**(6): 378–381.

Pirani, B.B.K., Campbell, D.M. & McGillivary, I. (1973) Plasma volume in normal first pregnancy. *Journal of Obstetrics and Gynaecology. British Commonwealth* **80**(10): 884–887.

Prendiville, W.J., Harding, J.E., Elbourne, D.R. *et al.* (1988) The Bristol Third Stage Trial: active versus physiological management of the third stage of labour. *British Medical Journal* **297**(6659): 1295–1300.

Prendiville, W.J., Elbourne, D. & McDonald, S. (2000) Active versus expectant management of the third stage of labour. *The Cochrane Library*, Issue 3. Oxford: Update Software.

Rogers, J., Wood, J., McCandlish, R. *et al.* (1998) Active versus expectant management of the third stage of labour: the Hinchingbrooke randomised controlled trial. *Lancet* **351**(9104): 693–699.

Rubin, P.C. (ed) (2000) *Prescribing in Pregnancy*, 3rd edn. London: BMJ.

Siney, C. (1999) An overview. In: Siney, C. (ed) *Pregnancy and Drugs Misuse*, pp. 11–12. Hale: Books for Midwives Press.

Sneyd, J.R, & Meyer-Whitting, M. (1992) Intrathecal diamorphine (heroin) for obstetric analgesia. *International Journal of Obstetric Anaesthesia* **1**(3): 153–155.

United Kingdom Central Council for Nursing, Midwifery and Health Visiting (UKCC) (1998) *Midwives Rules and Code of Practice*. London: UKCC.

United Kingdom Central Council for Nursing, Midwifery and Health Visiting (UKCC) (2000) *Guidelines for the Administration of Medicines*. London: UKCC.

STATUTES

Medical Devices Regulations 1994 SI No. 3017. London: HMSO.

Medicinal Products: Prescription by Nurses Act 1992 London: HMSO.

Medicines Act 1968 London: HMSO.

Medicines (Products other than Veterinary Drugs) (Prescription Only) Order 1983 SI No. 1212. London: HMSO.

Misuse of Drugs Act 1971 London: HMSO.

Misuse of Drugs (Northern Ireland) Regulations 1986 SR No. 52. London: HMSO.

Misuse of Drugs Regulations 1985 SI No. 2066. London: HMSO.

Prescription Only Medicines (Human Use) Order 1997 SI No. 1830. London: HMSO.

FURTHER READING

Banister, C. (1997) *The Midwife's Pharmacopoeia*. Hale: Books for Midwives Press.
This book is an easy-to-use reference guide. It is well referenced with a good index.

British Medical Association (BMA) and Royal Pharmaceutical Society of Great Britain (RPSGB) (2003) *British National Formulary*, 46th edn. London: BMA and RPSGB.
This publication provides information on drugs, their uses, dosages and interactions, and is a useful reference point. The appendices include a useful table on drugs present in breast milk.

Lee, A., Inch, S. & Finnigan, D. (2000) *Therapeutics in Pregnancy and Lactation*. Oxford: Radcliffe Medical Press.
This book summarizes the known effects of many commonly used drugs. It gives guidance on drug therapy during pregnancy and lactation, based on available evidence.

Mehta, D.K. (ed) (2001) *Nurse Prescribers' Formulary: 2002–2004*. London: BMA and RPSGB in association with Community Practitioners' and Health Visitors' Association and the Royal College of Nursing.
Primarily designed for nurses and midwives trained in prescribing, this publication contains much of the BNF information.

Siney, C. (ed) (1999) *Pregnancy and Drug Misuse*. Hale: Books for Midwives Press.
This book is written from a multidisciplinary perspective which allows the reader to look more effectively at the wider picture.

ADDITIONAL RESOURCES

http://www.npc.co.uk/
Website of the Nurses prescribing Centre, based in
Liverpool. This is a source of support and information for
practitioners, and includes different medications, news and
developments within nurse prescribing.

http://www.bnf.org/webnf/lform1/bnf/index.html
This is the British National Formulary on-line, which
provides a search facility for drugs and medications, effects,
interactions and dosages.

http://www.doh.gov.uk/nurseprescribing/index.htm
This Department of Health site provides information
regarding nurse prescribing, which includes background,
press releases, and guidelines for practitioners,
educationalists and managers.

Index

Page numbers followed by a 'f' indicate figures, page numbers followed by a 't' indicate tables, page numbers followed by a 'b' indicate boxes.
Page numbers in **bold** refer to chapter references.

A

abdomen, enlarged 240
abdominal aortic compression 991–992
abdominal changes, descent/separation of placenta 512, 516
abdominal examination
 attitude 259–260, 260
 breech presentation 896–897
 brow presentation 913
 denominator 260
 engagement 262–263, 262f
 face presentation 909
 findings throughout pregnancy 266
 hydatidiform mole 765
 instrumental vaginal deliveries 973
 labour, first stage 259–266, 439
 lie 259, 260f
 methods 263–266
  normal findings 263t
  observation 263
  palpation 263–266
  see also palpation
 neonate 552–554, 552b
  midline defects 552b
  palpation 553
 occipitoposterior position 889, 889f
 pelvic assessment 73
 position 260–261, 261f
 presentation 260, 261f
 shoulder presentation 914
abdominal exercises
 curl-ups 391
 knee rolling 391f
 musculoskeletal system 387
 postnatal exercises 390–391
  curl-ups 391, 391f
  diastasis recti postpartum 391f
  knee rolling 391
 preparation for childbirth 387
  pelvic tilting exercises 387
  transversus exercises 387

abdominal muscles
 anatomy 384
 physical preparation 384f
abdominal pain see pain
abdominal pregnancy 768
 secondary 768
abdominal preparation for childbirth 387
abnormalities see congenital anomalies
ABO blood group system 313, 687
 incompatibility 687
abortion 758–765
 classification 759f
 complete 760
 criminal 764
 delayed 761
 grief, parental 34–35
 history taking 248
 hyperemesis gravidarum 754
 incidence 114
 incomplete 760
 induced 762–764
 inevitable 760–761
 legislation 762
 mental health issues following 922
 missed see missed abortion
 psychological effects 762
 recurrent see recurrent abortion
 septic 764–765
 silent 761
 spontaneous see spontaneous abortion
 therapeutic 762–763
  see also therapeutic abortion
 threatened 643, 760
 tubal 767, 767f
 vomiting 752
Abortion Act 1967 366, 762, 1156, 1157b
 pregnancy law 1156, 1157b
abruptio placentae 772–773, 772f
 bleeding
  concealed 772–773
  partially revealed 773
  revealed 772
 causes 772

management 773
 mild 773
 moderate 773
 placenta praevia comparison 774t
 postpartum haemorrhage 988
 severe 773
 types 772–773, 772f
abscess, breast 610–611
abused child see child abuse
acanthosis nigricans 131
acardiac twins 844
acceptance, in bereavement 30
accreditation of prior experimental learning (APEL) 1194
accreditation of prior learning (APL) 1194
acetabulum 66
Acheson report 360
achondroplasia 677, 677f
 clinical features 677
aciclovir 824
acid aspiration syndrome see Mendelson's syndrome
Acidophilus tablets 272
acidosis 658
 buffering systems 658
 fetal blood sampling 658
 metabolic 537, 658
 prolonged labour 877
 respiratory 537, 658
acquired immune deficiency syndrome (AIDS) see HIV infection
ACTH see adrenocorticotrophic hormone (ACTH)
Action on Pre-eclampsia (APEC) 782, 789
action plan, in-utero transfer 568
active childbirth movement 1089
active management of labour
 expectant management vs 514
 first stage 442
 history 513
 indications 513–514
 placenta praevia 771
 postpartum haemorrhage 513
 prevention 514

active management of labour (*contd*)
  principles 515–516
  prolonged labour 878, 880–881
    second stage 880
    third stage 880–881
  technology overuse 5
  variation in practice 514
Acts, of Parliament
  Abortion Act 1967 *see* Abortion Act
    1967
  Action on Pre-eclampsia (APEC)
    782, 789
  Adoption and Children's Act 1059
  Children Act 1989 *see* Children Act
    1989
  Congenital Disabilities (civil liability)
    Act 1976 1161
  Data Protection Act, consent 1057
  Disability Discrimination Act 1995
    268, 270
  Health Act 1999 1118
  Health Service Reorganisation Act
    1973 401
  Human Fertilisation and Embryology
    Act *see* Human Fertilisation and
    Embryology Act 1990
  Human Rights Act, Children Act
    1053–1054
  Law Reform Act 1945 1149
  Maternal and Child Welfare Act of
    1918 242
  Medicinal Products: Prescription by
    Nurses Act 1992 1223–1224
  Medicines Act 1968 1211–1212
  Mental Health Act 1983 1154
  Midwives Act 1902 *see* Midwives
    Act 1902
  Midwives Act 1936 401
  Nurses, Midwives and Health
    Visitors Act (1979) 1089–1090
  Nurses, Midwives and Health
    Visitors Act (1997) 1144
  Registration of Births and Deaths Act
    1034
  Unfair Contract Terms Act 1977
    1149b
  Vaccine Damage Payments Act 1979
    1160
  see also legal issues
acupressure 342
  morning sickness treatment 752
acupuncture 342
  birth inducer 867–868
  labour pain relief 349
  morning sickness treatment 752
acute respiratory distress syndrome
    (ARDS) 980
acyanotic lesions, congenital heart
    disease 664–665
addiction *see* drug abuse/addiction
A delta fibres 462

adenine (A), genetics 174
adenohypophysis, menstrual cycle 94
adherent placenta 995
adhesions, pelvic 131, 132
adipose tissue, brown *see* brown
    adipose tissue (BAT)
adoption 1059
Adoption and Childrens Act 1059
adrenal cortex, fetal 214
adrenal glands, development 214
adrenaline (epinephrine)
  fetal 215
  fetal response to labour 418, 419f
  neonatal resuscitation 657
  oxytocin inhibition 418, 433
adrenal medulla, development 215
α-adrenergic receptors, uterine
    responses to pregnancy 305
adrenocorticotrophic hormone (ACTH)
  adenohypophysis 94
  DHEAS synthesis 214
  fetal life 214–215
  mammogenesis 601–602
  maternal/fetal significance 302
  physiological responses to pregnancy
    302
adrenoplacental hormonal regulation,
    cortisol 297–298
adult respiratory distress syndrome
    (ARDS) 980
Advanced Life Support in Obstetrics
    (ALSO), shoulder dystocia 950
advice
  antenatal *see* antenatal care
  bereavement 849
  contraception, post-termination 764
  genetic *see* genetics
  negligent 1161
  parental, fetal skull 232–233, 233b
  preconception care 148t, 149t
AFP *see* alpha-fetoprotein (AFP)
age
  fetal *see* gestational age
  maternal
    Down's syndrome 678
    shoulder dystocia 940
    spontaneous abortion 760
agnus-castus, postnatal depression 350
AIDS *see* HIV infection
aids, disability 278–279
AIMS *see* Association for
    Improvements in Maternity
    Services (AIMS)
airway management *see* resuscitation,
    neonate
ala 67
alcohol
  abuse, mental health issues 921
  antenatal care 250–251
  antenatal screening 363–364
  dependence in pregnancy 251

fetal syndrome and effects 250
  intake in pregnancy 363–364
  perinatal death 1038
  preconception care 152t
  spontaneous abortion 760
Alcopar (bephenium
    hydroxynaphthoate) 798
Aldomet (methyldopa) 785,
    1215–1216
aldosterone, physiological response in
    pregnancy 292–293
Alexander technique 343–344
alkali-denaturation (Apt) test, vasa
    praevia 776
alleles, genetic history 173
all-fours position
  shoulder dystocia 943
  Wood's manoeuvre 944
Allis sign 555
alopecia, instrumental deliveries 971
α-adrenergic receptors, uterine
    responses to pregnancy 305
alpha-fetoprotein (AFP)
  genetics screening (risk indicators)
    184–185
  level in anencephaly 317
  level in spina bifida 317
ALSO (UK), breech presentation
    training 895
alternative therapies, preconception
    care 152t
aluminium, preconception care 153t
alveolus
  breast structure 601
  lung, development 209–211, 529
ambiguous genitalia 675
  congenital adrenal hyperplasia 676,
    700
  neonatal examination 555
Ambu bag 653
ambulation, labour 447–448
amelia 677
amenorrhoea
  pregnancy 236
  primary/secondary 131b
  secondary 240
American College of Obstetricians and
    Gynecologists, exercise guidelines
    360
amino acids
  excretion, physiological response in
    pregnancy 295
  maternal nutrition 330
Amnihook 866
amniocentesis 324
  early 324
  genetics diagnostic tests 186
  multiple pregnancy 842
  psychological aspects 20
amnion 198, 519
  hormonal interactions in labour 413

amniotic band syndrome *see* congenital constriction band (amniotic band) syndrome
amniotic compartment, development 197–198
amniotic fluid
  analysis, respiratory distress syndrome 660
  increases 198
  measurement
    post-term pregnancy 870
    ultrasound scan 322–323
  meconium staining 503
  oxytocin 435
  prolactin 201f
  volume regulation 199–201
amniotic fluid embolism 1000–1001
  long-term consequences 1000
  maternal death 1045
amniotomy 865–867
  active management of labour 442
  caesarean section 979
  complications 867
  equipment 866
  instrumental vaginal deliveries 972
  oxytocic drugs 867
  prolonged labour 878–879
amoxycillin 824
ampicillin, renal disease 802
ampulla 80b, 162
ampullae 601
anaemia 793–798
  antepartum haemorrhage 776
  causes 798
  definition 793
  effects on pregnancy 794
  ethnic minority groups 268
  fetal 322
  folic acid deficiency 795
  haemolytic 796
  iron deficiency *see* iron deficiency anaemia
  late 687
  megaloblastic 795
  milk production 609
  multiple pregnancy 843
  nutritional therapy 335–336
  postpartum fatigue 743–744
  postpartum haemorrhage 988
  preconception care 146t
  preterm baby 640
  sickle cell *see* sickle cell anaemia
  signs symptoms 794
  types 794
    see also individual types
anaesthesia 1219
  caesarean section 980–981, 981
  epidural *see* epidural anaesthesia
  episiotomy, shoulder dystocia 944

Mendelson's syndrome (acid aspiration syndrome) 980
  see also Mendelson's syndrome (acid aspiration syndrome)
  postpartum haemorrhage 989
  spinal (subarachnoid) 981
  suturing the perineal 485
  toxicity 1219
anal fissure, postpartum 739
analgesia/analgesics 1216–1218
  epidural *see* epidural anaesthesia
  opioid 468
    see also pethidine
  oxytocin as 415
  preterm birth 859
  systemic 468–469
  see also pain relief
anal sphincter 478
  childbirth-associated structural damage 740
  injury 488, 488f
anal wink, neonatal examination 555
anaphylactic shock 998
anatomy
  abdominal muscles 384
  brain 225–227, 228f, 229f
  for epidural anaesthesia 470, 470f
  female 65–90
    see also female anatomy
  male 83–86
  reproductive *see* reproductive anatomy
android pelvis, occipitoposterior position 885
anencephaly 671–672
  alpha-fetoprotein (AFP) level 317
  clinical features 671–672
  face presentation 908
  incidence 672
  screening 671
angiogenin 99
  endometrium implantation preparation 190
angiotensin II, physiological response in pregnancy 292
angiotensinogen 291–292
angles and planes, pelvis 70–71
ankle
  circling, circulatory exercises 386
  examination 556
  oedema 259
ankyloglossia, breastfeeding problems 611
anomie 927
anorexia nervosa, pregnancy 754–755
anovulation 130, 131b
antacids 1218
  antenatal care 272
  Mendelson's syndrome 980
antenatal care 240–245
  aims 242

alternative schemes/models of care 244–245
  birth/care plans 267
  cardiac failure 799
  care during pregnancy 242–243
  corticosteroids *see* corticosteroids, antenatal
  development 241–242
  examinations 258–266
  first visit 245–254
  frequency of visits 255–256
  health promotion 360–367
  helping cope with changes 271–279
    gastrointestinal tract 271–272
  history 240–241
  history taking 246–253
    alcohol 250–251
    diet 251
    domestic abuse 253
    drugs/medication 249
    family history 252–253
    HIV screening 253
    medical/surgical 249
    personal details 246
    present pregnancy 247–248
    previous pregnancies 248–249
    smoking 250
  infant feeding 254–255
  investigations *see* antenatal investigations
  maternal heart disease 799
  medical examination 256–257
  mental health issues 919–924
  musculoskeletal system 273–274
  obstructive labour prevention 964
  pain education 459–460
  patterns of care 242
  perineal trauma 480
  physiology of pain education 460
  provision 242
  records 266–267
  risk factors assessment 258
  screening *see* antenatal screening
  skin changes 273
  symphysis pubis pain 277–278
  where to give birth? 243
  women with special needs 267–271
antenatal day assessment units 245
antenatal exercises, musculoskeletal system 386
antenatal investigations 312–326
  fetal well-being assessment 317–318
    see also fetal well-being assessment
  invasive tests 323–324
  MRI 323
  radiological techniques 323
  screening and diagnosis 312–313, 313t
    see also antenatal screening
  ultrasound 318–323

Antenatal Results and Choice 764
antenatal screening
  anencephaly 671
  blood tests *see* blood tests
  Down's syndrome 679
  multiple pregnancy 842
  sociological perspective 4–5
antepartum haemorrhage **769–776,**
  988
  abruptio placentae *see* abruptio
    placentae
  complications 775–776
    blood coagulation disorders
      775–776
    infection 776
    postpartum haemorrhage 776
    psychological
      disturbances/psychoses 776
    renal failure 776
    Sheehan's syndrome 776
  fetal well-being tests 775
  guidelines 777b
  management 773–775
    hospital 774–775
  monitoring 774, 775
  multiple pregnancy 844
  placenta praevia *see* placenta praevia
  small-for-gestational-age baby 643
anterior fontanelle *see* fontanelles,
  anterior
anterior pituitary necrosis 776
anteversion of uterus (pendulous
  abdomen) 832, 832f
antibiotics
  children born to HIV-infected
    mothers 818
  cystic fibrosis 700
  gonorrhoea 709
  neonatal use guidelines 712
  preterm labour prevention 855
  toxoplasmosis 706
  urinary tract infections 711
antibodies, blood testing 313–314
anticoagulants 1221–1222
anticonvulsants
  eclampsia 787
  pregnancy 811, 812
antidepressant drugs
  breastfeeding 931
  postnatal depression 927
anti-D immunoglobulin 313–314, 687
  inevitable abortion 760–761
antiembolic stockings, caesarean
  section 982
antihistamines, obstetric cholestasis 812
antihypertensive drugs 785–786,
  1214–1216
  risks 785
anti-inflammatory activities,
  implantation/development of
  placenta 192

antiretroviral therapy
  children born to HIV-infected
    mothers 818
  combination therapy
    mitochondrial dysfunction 819
    pregnancy 818
anus
  dermatitis 567
  fissure, postpartum 739
  imperforate *see* imperforate anus
  neonatal examination 555
anxiety/fear
  adrenaline/noradrenaline release 433
  complementary therapies 347
  cortisol/catecholamines rise 418
  HIV screening 819
  instrumental deliveries 971
  labour 434
  midwives, shoulder dystocia 940
  pain increase 458, 459
  predictor of painful labour 460
  pregnancy 17–18, 923
  prolonged labour 879
aorta
  coarctation *see* coarctation of the
    aorta
  fetal 649
aortic valve stenosis 665
aperients 1213–1214
Apgar scores 536–537, 536t
  neonatal resuscitation 656–657
apnoea
  preterm 634
  primary 652
  resuscitation 652, 718
  secondary (terminal) 652
apnoea alarms, sudden infant death
  syndrome 717–718
apparent life-threatening events (ALTEs),
  sudden infant death syndrome 718
appearance
  mother, at antenatal visit 256
  neonate 543–544, 544t
  in relation to communication 15–16
appetite, during labour 435
aquanatal exercise 360–361
  teaching physical skills, physical
    preparation 394
arachnoid mater 229f
arbor vitae 80b
Area Child Protection Committee
  (ACPC) 1061
areola 601
arginine vasopressin (AVP) 214
arms
  breech presentation 907–908
  newborn examination 551
  posterior delivery, shoulder dystocia
    945, 945f
arnica tablets 342
  perineal problems 351

aromatherapy 342–343
arthritis 711
  gonococcal 823
artificial feeding 613–620
  advantages 618
  bottlefeeding 616, 616f
  disadvantages 617–618
  discomfort 533
  disorder/infection risk 617b
  ecology 617
  methods 616–618
  midwife's role 618
  reasons for use 613–615
  stools 533
  see also feeding; milk formulae
artificial rupture of membranes,
  umbilical cord
  presentation/prolapse 955
asphyxia 651–652
  causes 651
  phases 652
  primary apnoea 652
  secondary (terminal) apnoea 652
  shoulder dystocia 948
aspirin, hypertension 785–786
assault, law consent trespass (to
  person) 1151
assisted conception
  costs 141
  cryopreservation 139
  donor insemination 134
  egg donation 139
  gamete intrafallopian tube transfer
    (GIFT) 135
  intrauterine insemination (IUI)
    134–135
  in vitro fertilization (IVF) *see* in vitro
    fertilization (IVF)
  micromanipulation 133
  outcome from 139–140
  ovulation induction 134
  surrogacy 139
Association for Improvements in
  Maternity Services (AIMS) 405
  active childbirth movement 1089
Association for Postnatal Illness 927
Association of Radical Midwives
  (ARM) 402
  foundation 1089
asthma 810–811
  factors effecting attacks 810
asylum seekers, pregnancy 359
asymmetrical pelvis (Naegele's type) 74t
asymptomatic bacteriuria 257, 801
asynclitism (posterior) 75f
atosiban (Tractocile) 857, 1216
atresia
  choanal 672
  duodenal 674
  oesophageal *see* oesophageal atresia
    (OA)

atrial natriuretic peptide
  amniotic fluid volume regulation
    201
  physiological response in pregnancy
    293
atrial septal defect (ASD) 664
  complex 664
  simple 664
atrial ventricular septal defect (AVSD)
  664
auscultation
  abdominal 265–266, 265f
  cardiac disorders 663
  cardiovascular system 547–548
  multiple pregnancy diagnosis 842
  neonatal examination 547–548
autonomic nervous system 534
  neonatal assessment 560
autonomy, ethics principles 1138–1139
autosomal characteristics/diseases,
  genetics inheritance modes 178–180
autosomal polycystic kidney disease
  (APKD) 675
  dominant (ADPKD) 675
  recessive (ARPKD) 675
autosomes, human genome 175
Avanti condom 116
axillary temperature measurement 583

B

Babinski reflex 560
baby see neonate
Baby Friendly Initiative 1110, 1110b
Baby Hippy manikin 557
baby to breast attachment 604, 605f,
  606f
Bach flower remedies 342
  labour pain relief 350
  panic attacks 347
bacille Calmette–Guérin vaccine (BCG)
  810
backache
  complementary therapies 346
  postnatal complications 393
  postpartum 729, 741–742
  see also back pain
back care
  musculoskeletal system 385–386
  postnatal 392
  posture 385f
back injuries, labour 448
back pain
  epidural analgesia 471
  low, pregnancy 274
  see also backache
'Back to Sleep' campaign,
  recommendations 564, 715–716
bacteraemia 712

bacterial shock 999–1000
  management 999–1000
  signs 999
Ballard score 628, 630f
Bandl's retraction 964
Barlow test 557–558, 557f
barrier creams, dermatitis 567
Bartholin's glands 77b
Bart's test 316–317
basal metabolic rate (BMR), neonatal
  heat production 577
bathing 566
  ambient temperature 581
  hypothermia risk 580–581
battery, law consent trespass
  (to person) 1151
battledore insertion of umbilical cord
  520
bean bags, in labour 448
bearing-down urge 498–499
bed bath, caesarean section 982
'bed birth myth' 448
bed/cot spacing, infection prevention
  704
bedding, sudden infant death syndrome
  716
bedrest, pre-eclampsia 785
bed sharing
  breastfeeding 608
  sudden infant death syndrome 716
behavioral change approach, health
  promotion 359t
benzathine penicillin G 706
bephenium hydroxynaphthoate
  (Alcopar) 798
bereavement 27–47
  miscarriage 34
  mourning, tasks of 28b, 30
  multiple birth 849
  parental responses 32–33
  parental support 33
  reality acceptance 30
  scan diagnosis 34
  support 29–30
  termination due to anomaly 34–35
  see also grief
bereavement room 36
bereavement skills training 29–30
beta-adrenergic agonists 857, 1216
  side effects 857
betamethasone, preterm labour 856,
  858
bicornuate uterus 830
bifidus factor, breast milk 596t
bilaminar disc 205, 206f
bile 685
bilibed 690, 692f
biliblanket 690, 691f
bilirubin 684
  conjugated 684–685
  light 686

  measurement 685–686, 685b, 686
  unconjugated 684–685
bilirubin diglucuronide 684–685
biliverdin 684
bimanual compression, postpartum
  haemorrhage 994
  external 991
  internal 991, 991f
binge drinking, perinatal death 1038
binovular twins see dizygotic twins
biochemical/serum screening, genetics
  screening (risk indicators)
  184–185
biophysical profile (BPP) scoring
  post-term pregnancy 870
  ultrasound scan 322
biparietal diameter (BPD) 248
bipartite placenta 519
birth (childbirth) 420–423
  asphyxia see hypoxic ischaemic
    encephalopathy
  care following 517–518
  criminal law 1157
  environment see birth environment
  experience, mental preparation 926
  future of 1096–1097
  home see home birth
  hospitals see hospitalization of birth
  legal issues 1156–1159
  maternal choice in 1090–1092
  morbidity following **736–747**
    extent 736–737
    implications for midwives 744
    medical consultation 737
  notification 1034
  physical preparation **383–396**
    see also physical preparation
  place of **401–409**, 1086–1087
  preparations 535–536
    at risk pregnancy 535, 536b
  records 518
  registration 1034–1035
  skilled attendance 1106–1107
  studies of nature and culture 504
  temperature control 579
  trauma, breech presentation
    898–899
birth attendance, legal issues 1157
birth balls 448
birth canal, axis in upright position 71f
birth centres 245
birth environment 435–438, 497
  continuity of career 437–438
  decisions 436–437
  home 435–436
  integrated birthing suits 437
  midwifery-led care in birth units
    436–437
birthing pool, pain relief 464
birthing position see positioning/
  posture

birthing units, midwifery-led care
436–437
birth partners 434
role of 434
birth plans 439
birth rate 1035–1036, 1035f
birthweight 630–632
extremely low (ELBW) 630, 853
incredibly low (ILBW) 853
low see low birthweight (LBW)
maternal, shoulder dystocia 940
perinatal death 1037
sudden infant death syndrome 717
very low (VLBW) 630, 853
WHO definition 630–632
bisacodyl BP (Dulcolax) 1214
Bishop's scoring system 864, 864t
bitemporal diameter 225f
Black Report 9, 356
bladder
anatomical changes in pregnancy
294
catheterization of see catheterization
of bladder
filling, umbilical cord
presentation/prolapse 957
labour
care during 447
second stage 497
retroversion of uterus 831–832
blastocyst 166–167
implantation 191, 195
bleeding
abruptio placentae 772–773
cephalhaematoma 231
cerebral, external signs 232f
implantation 758
labour third stage 510–511
vaginal see vaginal bleeding
vitamin K deficiency see vitamin K
deficiency bleeding (VKDB)
see also haemorrhage
blindness
antenatal care 269
diabetes mellitus 806
gonorrhoea 823
blisters 678
blood coagulation disorders
antepartum haemorrhage 775–776
testing 776
blood count 258, 314
blood cross-matching
antenatal care 258
massive obstetric haemorrhage 992
postpartum haemorrhage 990
blood glucose levels
assessment 808
labour 808
blood loss see bleeding; haemorrhage
blood pressure
eclampsia 766

measurement 259
antenatal care 243
caesarean section 982
hormonal contraceptives
122–123
labour, second stage 503
pregnancy 258
pre-eclampsia 782–783
shock 998
see also hypertensive disorders
blood tests
antenatal care 258
cross-matching see blood cross-
matching
fetal, acidosis 658
maternal 313–317
ABO blood grouping 313
antibodies 313–314
fetal assessment 316–317
full blood count 314
haemoglobin 314
haemoglobinopathies 315
infection screening 315–316
mean corpuscular volume 314
phenylketonuria 315
platelets 314
rhesus blood grouping 313
well-being assessment 313–314,
314t
white cell count 314
neonatal, bilirubin measurement
685–686, 685b
blood transfusions
exchange transfusion 692–693
see also exchange transfusion
haemoglobinopathies 797
iron deficiency anaemia 795
massive obstetric haemorrhage 992
postpartum haemorrhage 990, 993
refusal, legal issues 1153b
thalassaemia 797
uterine rupture 967
blood volume
maternal changes 290, 291f
physiological responses to pregnancy
290, 291f
pregnancy 423
blue cohosh, labour onset remedy
348
B-lynch suture (brace), massive
obstetric haemorrhage 992–993,
993f
body image
changes 357
pregnancy/childbirth 21, 109–110
body language 15
body mass index (BMI)
calculation 257
preconception 145
Bolam Test, law negligence breach of
duty 1146–1147

bone
growth, physiological responses to
pregnancy 306
see also individual bones
bottlefeeding 616, 616f
see also milk formulae
bowel problems, postpartum 739–740
brace suture (B-lynch), massive
obstetric haemorrhage 992–993,
993f
brachial palsy, congenital 948–949
brachial plexus injury
degrees of injury 949
fundal pressure 947
shoulder dystocia 948–949
treatment 949
brachial pulse, neonatal examination
547
bradycardia, fetal heart rate 317
brain
anatomy 225–227, 228f, 229f
bleeding, external signs 232f
development 205–206
meninges 227, 228f, 229f
trauma, instrumental deliveries 971
Braxton Hicks contractions 238
cervical effacement/dilatation 430
pain physiology 461
breach of duty, negligence 1146–1147
breast(s) 600
abscess 610–611
blood supply 601
changes
epithelial mitosis 100f
pregnancy 236
premenstrual 288
contractile tissue 601
embryology 600
examination, antenatal care 256
glandular tissue 601
growth 601–602
lymphatic drainage 601
nerve supply 601
secretion, inevitable abortion 760
stimulation, birth induction 867
see also nipple stimulation
structure 601
surgery, milk production 609
see also mammary gland
breast engorgement
complementary therapies 351
milk 609
reduction 609
symptoms 728
treatment 729
venous 609
breastfeeding 254–255, 591–613
advantages 596–598
after delivery 517
anticonvulsants 812
assistance 603–608

attachment/latching on 604, 605f
caesarean section 981, 983
contraception 125
contraindications 598–599
diabetic woman 809
drugs 599, 1212–1223
early initiation 603–604
exclusive 597
    HIV transmission 599
feeding position 604, 605f, 728
hepatitis B virus 821
HIV transmission 598–599, 707,
    817, 820
incidence 254
infection prevention 705
midwife's role 599–600
mother-baby relationship 603–604
multiple birth 843, 847–848
neonate requirements 593–594
physiological jaundice 685
postoperative care 681
preterm baby 598, 611–612, 635,
    859
problems 608–613, 728–729
    maternal 608–611
    neonatal 611–612
progestagen-only pill 121
psychological aspect 23
psychotropic drugs 931
public health issues 592–593, 608
returning to work 613
seven-point plan 600b
sexuality/sexual difficulties 110
smoking 608
stools 533
sudden infant death syndrome 717
support groups 613
thermoregulation 580
twins 613
see also breast milk; feeding;
    lactation
breastfeeding jaundice 688
Breastfriends Doncaster 613
breast milk
calorific value 593
comparison with milk formula
    614–615t
constituents 594–596
defence agents 596–597t
drugs 599
expressing 604–608
    see also expressed breast milk
        (EBM)
immunoglobulins 703
inadequate supply 608–609
breastmilk, insufficiency 608–609, 729
breast milk
lymphocytes 703
mature 595
milk formulae vs 614–615t
necrotizing enterocolitis 641

pollutants 599
preterm 598, 612
solid:fluid ratio 594
storage 607–608
transitional 594–595
volume produced 602
see also breastfeeding; lactation
breathing techniques
labour coping strategies 389–390
pain relief 459
breath sounds 547, 547f
breech presentation 894–908
associated risks 897–899
birthing position 903, 904, 905
care/management during pregnancy
    899
causes 885, 895, 896t
complementary therapies 347
congenital anomalies 895, 896t
delivery
    assisted 905–907
    complications 907–908
    mechanisms 900–902
diagnosis 896–897
fetal positions 900–902, 900f
incidence 885
labour
    first stage 903–904
    management 902–904
    second stage 904–905
lower extremities 555
meconium staining 503
types 894–895, 894f
ultrasound scan 897, 903
umbilical cord presentation/prolapse
    955
vaginal examination 897
bregma 224f
position 222f
Britain, teenage pregnancy incidence 270
British Epilepsy Association, parent
    guidance 812
broad ligaments 81
bromocriptine
inevitable abortion 760
lactation suppresser 39
bronchopulmonary dysplasia (BPD)
    see lung disease, chronic
bronzed baby syndrome 694
brow 222f
brown adipose tissue (BAT)
distribution 578
heat production 577–578
preterm baby 634
brow presentation 913–914, 914f
causes 886
diagnosis 913
incidence 886
management 913–914
skull moulding 230f, 230t
vaginal examination 913

Brushfield's spots 678
bulbocavernosus muscles 478
bulbourethral glands 84b
bulbus cordis 208
bulimia nervosa, pregnancy 755
bullae 678
bupivacaine (Marcain) 1219
epidural analgesia 470
Burns–Marshall manoeuvre 906–907,
    906f
buttocks, dermatitis 567
buzz groups 375

C

cabbage leaves, breast engorgement
    346, 351
cadmium, preconception care 153t
caesarean section (CS)
anaesthesia 980–981
breech presentation 897–898
classic upper segment 977
costs 979
elective
    HIV transmission 817–818
    physiological birth vs 503
elective lower section, lung fluid 529
epidural anaesthesia 981
facilitating mother-baby relationship
    981
fetal risks 978–979
genital tract abnormalities 831
herpes simplex virus 709, 824
HIV infection 819
implications 979
increasing rates 442, 978
indications 978t, 979
lower segment (LSCS) 977
management to reduce rates 442
maternal-infant attachment 981–982
maternal request 1092–1093
midwives' role 979–980
obstructive labour 964
physical preparation 392
placenta praevia 771
postoperative care 981–982,
    982–983
records 982
scar rupture 965
spinal (subarachnoid) anaesthesia
    981
stress incontinence 738
transient tachypnoea of the newborn
    659
trial of scar 983
umbilical cord presentation/prolapse
    957–958
uterine rupture 967
vasa praevia 776

caffeine
  miscarriage risk 328–329
  preconception care 146t
calamine lotion 273
calcification, placenta 519, 879
calcium
  deficiency, preconception care 146t
  hypocalcaemia treatment 699
  maternal nutrition 333–334
  supplementation, pre-eclampsia 334,
    782
  see also hypocalcaemia
calcium channel blockers
  hypertension 785
  preterm labour 858
calcium gluconate 787, 857–858, 1215
callus formation, bony injury 949
cancer, preconception care 150t
Candida albicans 272, 709, 824
  dermatitis 567
candidiasis (thrush) 709–710
  antenatal care 272
  CNS infection 709
  disseminated 709
  nipple pain 610
  nutritional therapy 336
  oral infection 709
  prevention 824
  transmission 824
  treatment 709
capillary filling time, neonatal
    examination 547
capillary haemangiomas 546, 678
caput succedaneum 229–231, 231f
  characteristics 229–231
carbimazole, thyrotoxicosis 800
carbohydrates
  breast milk 595
  fetal metabolism 216–217
  maternal nutrition 331
  neonatal digestion 594
carbon dioxide, arterial pressure
    (PCO$_2$), physiological responses to
    pregnancy 296
cardiac catheterization 663–664
cardiac disease, maternal 798–800
  antenatal care 799
  classification 798b
  congenital 798–799
  fetal effects 799
  labour 799
  postnatal care 799
  signs 798
cardiac disorders, fetal 649–670
  causes 663
  congenital see congenital heart
    disease
  examination 663
    auscultation 663
    feeding pattern 663
  follow-up/support 666

investigation 663–664
  prenatal diagnosis 663
  symptoms 663
cardiac failure 799
cardiac massage, neonatal resuscitation
    655–656
  breath:compression ratio 655
  cardiac compression 655–656
    monitoring 656
    recommend methods 655, 656f
  technique 655b
cardiac output
  fetal response to labour 420
  maternal changes 289–290, 291f
Cardiff ' count to ten kick chart' 317
cardiogenic shock 998
cardiopulmonary resuscitation,
    amniotic fluid embolism 1000
cardiotocograph (CTG)
  post-term pregnancy 869–870
  pre-eclampsia 784
  sociology 5
cardiovascular adaptations 289–290
cardiovascular system (CVS) 531–532
  anomalies see cardiac disorders
  development 206–209
  fetal response to labour 420
  neonatal examination 546–548
    auscultation 547–548
    chest cavity 546–547
    observation 546
    palpation 547
  postnatal changes 531, 724
    blood 531–532
  see also fetal circulation; heart
care of property, legal issues 1160
'Care of the Next Infant' (CONI)
    programme 718–719, 1041
carpal tunnel syndrome, pregnancy
    274
casein dominant formula 615, 616t
caseload/group practice midwifery
    244–245
cassette method, pregnancy diagnosis
    239–240, 239f
castor oil, birth induction 867
casuistry, deontology 1136
catecholamines
  decrease, caesarean section 978
  lung fluid absorption 591, 651
  lung maturity 652
catheterization of bladder
  caesarean section 982
  postpartum haemorrhage treatment
    991
  retroversion of uterus 831–832
caulophyllum, labour onset remedy
    348
causation, negligence 1147
cell division 175–176
  DNA replication 176

meiosis 176, 176f
  mitosis 175–176, 176f
Central Midwives Board 1083–1084
central nervous system (CNS)
  anomalies 671–672
  consciousness states 534, 535b
  development 205–206, 534, 535
  neonate 534–535
central venous pressure (CVP)
    monitoring
  postpartum haemorrhage 993
  shock 999
cephalhaematoma 231, 231f
  characteristics 231
  instrumental deliveries 971
  treatment 231
cephalic presentation 261
  meconium staining 503
  umbilical cord presentation/prolapse
    955
cephalopelvic disproportion 960–963
  dangers 961
  definition 960
  diagnosis 960–961
  immigrant women 329
  induction contraindication 864
  management 961
  trial of labour 961–963
    see also labour, trial of
  X-ray pelvimetry 961
Cerazette 121
cerclage, cervical see cervical cerclage
cerebellum 227f
cerebral bleeding, external signs 232f
cerebrum 227, 227f
Certified Midwife 1084–1085
cervical canal 80b
cervical cap 119
cervical carcinoma 768–769
  examination 769
  treatment 769
cervical cerclage 759, 762, 983f
  causes 983–984
  contraindications/complications 984
  diagnosis 984
  preterm labour prevention 855
  techniques 984
cervical dilatation/effacement
    430–431, 431f
  examination 444
  failure 881–882
  inevitable abortion 760
  monitoring 442
  movement of tissue planes 412f
  pain physiology 461
cervical dystocia 881–882
cervical endometrium 80b
cervical erosion 768
cervical incompetence 983, 984
  spontaneous abortion 759
  ultrasound scan 319

cervical intraepithelial neoplasia (CIN) 768–769
cervical ligaments 81, 477
cervical polyp 768
cervical ripening
  complications 865
  labour induction 864–865
  nipple stimulation 348
cervical secretion, use in family planning 117
cervical tears 480–481
  uterine rupture 966
cervix 80b, 82
  changes in preparation for labour 411–412
  cyclical changes 163
  damage, shoulder dystocia 947
  examination 444
  laceration 993–994
  length, preterm labour indicator 855
  menstrual cycle changes 100
  oxytocin 435
  physiological responses to pregnancy 306
  vaginal examination 444
C fibres 462
chafing 565
chamomile tea 342
  nausea/vomiting 344–345
Changing Childbirth 21, 402, 1091–1092
  future developments 1029–1030
changing stool 533
chemical thermogenesis 577
chest cavity, neonatal examination 546–547
chest X-ray
  cardiac abnormalities 663
  respiratory distress syndrome (RDS) 659
  timing during pregnancy 323
  transposition of the great arteries 665
  tuberculosis 712
chicken pox (varicella zoster) 149t, 707
chignon 232, 232f
child abuse
  categories 1061b
  Children Act 1989 1158
  disabled child 1060
  domestic violence 1060
  emotional 1062
  investigation 1055
  physical 1061–1062
  stress 1062
Child Assessment Order 1063
Child Bereavement Trust (CBT) 44
childbirth see birth
Child Growth Foundation chart 630, 631–632f

child minding 1058
Child Protection Conference 1063
Child Protection Plan 1064
Child Protection Register 1064, 1064b
  Children Act 1989 1158–1159, 1159b
children
  female circumcision 835
  legal definition 1051b
  protection 1060–1064
  support for 1054–1055
  understanding of death 41–43
  welfare 1052
Children Act 1989 249, 527, 1050–1068, 1157–1158, 1158b
  Area Child Protection Committee (ACPC) 1158, 1159b
  background 1050–1051
  child abuse 1158
  child assessment framework 1055–1057, 1056f
  child protection 1060–1064
  child protection register 1158–1159, 1159b
  children away from home 1058
  content 1052–1053
  disabled child 1059–1060
  family support 1054–1055
  Human Rights Act 1053–1054
  interagency cooperation 1158
  key features 1051–1052
  non-intervention 1052
  parental responsibility 1052–1053
  pre-birth assessment 1062–1063
  significant harm 1061–1062
  structure 1052–1053
  teenage mothers 1058–1059
  welfare promoting strategies 1053
children's laws 1156–1159
  Area Child Protection Committee (ACPC) 1158, 1159b
  see also Children Act 1989
chin examination 550, 550b
chiropractic 341
chlamydia 131, 709, 824
chlamydial conjunctivitis 709
Chlamydia psittaci, preconception care advice 149t
Chlamydia trachomatis 709, 824
chloral hydrate 1219
chloramphenicol eyedrops, gonorrhoea 709
chlorhexidine 704
choanal atresia 672
  diagnosis 672
  symptoms 672
cholestasis 273
  intrahepatic of pregnancy (obstetric cholestasis) 812
chondrocranium 220
chordee 675

choriocarcinoma 766
  spread 766
  treatment 766
chorion 198, 519
  hormonal interactions in labour 413, 414
chorion frondosum 208
chorionicity, twins 841
chorionic villi
  circulation 194f, 197
  implantation 193
chorionic villus sampling (CVS) 323–324
  complications 324
  genetics diagnostic test 185–186
  multiple pregnancy 842
chorion laeve 198
chromaffin cells 215
chromosome analysis 177–178
  karyotyping 177, 177f
chromosome anomalies 177–178, 678–679
  anovulation 131
  deletion 178
  monosomy 178
  reciprocal translocation 178
  social construction 5
  translocation 178
  trisomy 178
  X chromosome 178
    see also X chromosomes
  Y chromosome 178
    see also Y chromosome
chromosomes 174–175, 671
  genetics history 173
  X chromosome 174f
chronic lung disease see lung disease, chronic (CLD)
Church, history of midwifery 1074
ciliary movements 163
circulation maintenance, shock 998–999
circulatory exercises
  musculoskeletal system 386–387
  postnatal exercises 390
  prenatal
    ankle circling 386
    leg tightening 386
circulatory system see cardiovascular system (CVS); fetal circulation
circumcision, female 835
  see also female genital mutilation (FGM)
circumvallate placenta 519, 519f
civil law 1163–1164
  conditional fees 1164
  current developments 1163–1164
claims (England), clinical negligence 1145b
CLASP study 785–786

clavicle
  deliberate fracture 947
  examination 551
  fractures, shoulder dystocia 949
cleft lip 673
  feeding problems 611, 673
  surgery 673
cleft palate 673
  family history 673
  feeding problems 611
  incidence 673
  surgery 673
cleidotomy
  obstructive labour 964
  shoulder dystocia 947
client-centred approach, health
    promotion 359t
clinical audit 1022–1024
  change implementation 1024, 1025b
  data assessment 1023–1024
  methods 1023t
  records 1023
Clinical Audit 1021–1022
clinical beachmarks 1025
clinical governance, midwifery quality
    1024–1027
clinical indicators 1026
clinical negligence
  claims (England) 1145b
  legal issues 1145
Clinical Negligence Scheme for Trusts
  legal issues 1161–1162
  NHS Litigation Authority (NHSLA)
    1162
clinical networks 1014
clitoris 77b
clomiphene 130
clomiphene citrate 134
Clostridium welchii, shock 999
clothing
  neonatal thermoregulation 584
  during pregnancy 579
clotting factors *see* coagulation factors
coagulants 1221
coagulation factors
  placenta separation 423
  pregnancy 422
coagulation tests, pre-eclampsia 784
coarctation of the aorta 664
  associated lesions 664
  symptoms 664
cobalamin (vitamin B$_{12}$) *see* vitamin B$_{12}$
    (cobalamin)
coccydynia, postnatal complications 393
coccyx 66
Cochrane Database 55
Cochrane Library 58
Code of Professional Conduct (UKCC
    1992) 1126, 1144
  deontology 1136
  moral dilemma 1135
coitus interruptus 115

cold stress *see* hypothermia
Collaborative Low-dose Aspirin Studies
    in Pregnancy 785–786
collagen
  changes in preparation for labour
    411
  degrading enzymes 414
colostrum 237, 594
  gastrointestinal tract maturation 594
  protective constituents 594
colour, neonate 545, 546
combined contraceptive pill (COC)
    121, 768
  older mothers 125–126
comfort measures, labour, second stage
    497–498
Commission for Health Improvement
    (CHI) 1010, 1026, 1162
common law 1143
  consent 1155–1156
communication 14–17
  bad news 33, 564
  ethnic minority groups 267
  language use 16
  listening skills 16
  mother-baby relationship 562
  non-English speaking women 16
  non-verbal 14–15
  personal space 15
  physical appearance 15–16
  questioning techniques 16
  skills 245
  therapeutic counselling 16–17
  touch 15, 33
  verbal processes 14–15
  written 15–16
community, health promotion
    358–360
community midwives 402–405
  antenatal education 404
  antenatal support groups 404
  postnatal care 404–405, 731
compensation, legal issues 1150–1151
complaints, legal issues 1160
complement 704
  breast milk 596t
complementary feeds 617
complementary therapies 15, **338–354,**
    1213
  antenatal clinic integration 347–348
  commonly used types 340–344
  holistic approach 338
  implementation 339–340, 340b
    policies and protocols 340
    professional indemnity insurance
    340
  labour 348–350
    onset 348
    pain/discomfort 348–350
  morning sickness treatment 752
  postnatal period 350–351
  pregnancy 344–348

professional accountability
    338–339
  stress 347
complete breech 894–895
compound presentation 915
conception, assisted *see* assisted
    conception
conceptus maldevelopment,
    spontaneous abortion 759
conditional fees, civil law 1164
condom (sheath) 115–116
  effectiveness 116
  female 119
conduction, neonatal heat loss 576
Confidential Enquiry into Maternal
    and Child Health (CEMACH)
    931, 1036–1037
Confidential Enquiry into Maternal
    Deaths (CEMD) 919, 931–932,
    1036
  recommendations 932
Confidential Enquiry into Stillbirths
    and Deaths in Infancy (CESDI)
    1036–1037
  shoulder dystocia recommendations
    950
Confidential Enquiry into Suicides and
    Homicides (CISH) 931
confidentiality, HIV screening 821
congenital adrenal hyperplasia (CAH)
    700, 700f
  ambiguous genitalia 676
  dexamethasone 700
congenital anomalies **670–683**
  aetiology 670–671
    genetic factors 670–671
    iatrogenic factors 671
    teratogenic factors 671
  asphyxia causes 651
  breech presentation 895, 896t
  central nervous system 671–672
  chromosomal 678–679
  deformation 670
  epilepsy 811
  gastrointestinal system 673–675
  genitourinary system 675–676
  heart disease 664–666
  incidence 670
  induction indicator 864
  limb abnormalities 676–677
  malformation 670
  post-term pregnancy 868
  respiratory system 672
  skin abnormalities 677–678
  see also individual anomalies
congenital bilateral absence of vas
    deferens (CBAVD) 132
congenital brachial palsy (CBP)
    948–949
congenital constriction band (amniotic
    band) syndrome 671
  limb reduction deformities 677

Congenital Disabilities (civil liability)
  Act 1976, legal issues 1161
congenital dislocation of hip (CDH) *see*
  developmental dysplasia of hip
congenital heart disease 664–666
  acyanotic lesions 664–665
  cyanotic lesions 665–666
  genetics advice 183
congenital hypertrophic pyloric stenosis
  674
  projectile vomiting 674
congenital varicella syndrome 707
conjoined twins 844
consciousness level assessment 534, 535b
consent 1057, 1151–1156, 1152b
  blood transfusion refusal 1153b
  capacity 1153
  common law power 1155–1156
  court application 1155b
  forms 1156
  HIV screening 820
  informed 1153
  instrumental vaginal deliveries 973
  legal issues 1151–1156, 1152–1153b
  negligence 1151–1153
  neonate examination 527–528
  refusal 1154–1155
    Mental Health Act 1983 1154
  self-discharge 1156
  trespass (to person) 1151
    assault 1151
    battery 1151
    defence 1151
  vaginal examination 444
  voluntarily 1153
consent forms, legal issues 1156
constipation 739–740
  antenatal care 272
  complementary therapies 345
  neonate 555
  nutritional therapy 335, 345, 728
  postnatal 727–728, 739
continuity of care 466–467
  labour 437–438
continuous positive airways pressure
  (CPAP) 662
  complications 662
contraception **114–128**
  advice, post termination 764
  caesarean section 983
  diabetic woman 809
  factors to consider 124t
  female 116–123
    barrier methods 118–119
    care when receiving hormonal
      contraceptives 122–123
    emergency 123
    hormonal 121–123
    implants 122
    injectable contraceptives 122
    intrauterine contraceptive devices
      (IUCDs) 119–121

physiological methods *see*
  physiological methods of
  contraception
  see also individual types
male 115–116
  future developments 116
  medical disorders 126
  methods 115
  postnatal period 124–126
    see also postnatal period
  role of midwife 126
  sterilization 123–124
contraceptive pill *see* oral contraception
contractions
  Braxton Hicks *see* Braxton Hicks
    contractions
  uterine *see* uterine contractions
contributory negligence, legal issues
  1149
controlled drugs *see* drugs, controlled
convection, neonatal heat loss 576
convulsions
  eclamptic *see* eclamptic convulsion
  instrumental deliveries 971
  neonatal 562, 698
    signs 698
  pregnancy 811
  see also epilepsy
coordination of contractions *see* uterine
  contractions
coping strategies
  labour *see* labour
  pain 459, 463
cordocentesis 324
  genetics diagnostic tests 186
cornu 80b
corpus cavernosum 84b
corpus luteum
  autocrine–paracrine–endocrine
    functions 167
  demise 91
  development 167–168
  menstrual cycle 90
  position, vomiting 751
corpus spongiosum 84b
cortical reactions
  fertilization 164f, 165
  venous network 168
corticosteroid-binding globulin (CBG),
  responses to pregnancy 298–299
corticosteroids
  antenatal
    complications 650, 660
    dosage 650
    respiratory distress syndrome
      659–660
    surfactant production 650
  labour induction 868t
  preterm labour 858
  surfactant production 856
corticotrophin-like intermediate lobe
  peptide (CLIP) 215

corticotrophin-releasing hormone
  (CRH) 214, 296
  actions 300
  maternal/fetal significance 302
  physiological responses to pregnancy
    300, 301f, 302
corticotrophin-releasing hormone
  (CRH) binding protein 300, 302
  maternal/fetal significance 302
cortisol 300f
  cardiovascular system development
    206–207, 209
  competitive binding with
    progesterone 299
  fetal adrenoplacental regulation
    297–298
  hypothalamic–pituitary–adrenal–
    placental axis 298
  lung maturation 212–213
  maternal 298
  profiles in pregnancy 299f
  progesterone relation 301f
cortisone, oxidation to cortisol 297
Cot Death Research Association 1041
cot deaths 715
cotyledons 516
Council for Regulation of Healthcare
  1010
counselling
  genetic 182–183
  grief 44
  infertility 140–141
  mental health issues 922
  therapeutic 16–17
  therapeutic abortion 763
  uterine rupture 967
counselling approach 16–17
court application, consent 1155b
courts 1142
Couvelaire uterus 772–773
  postpartum haemorrhage 988, 988f
cracked nipples *see* nipple(s), cracked/
  sore
cramp, pregnancy 274
cranberry juice 801
Cranbrook Report 401
cranial nerves 560, 560t
cranial osteopathy 341
craniosacral therapy 341
craniotomy, obstructive labour 964
Creutzfeldt–Jakob disease (CJD) 149t
cricoid pressure (Sellick's manoeuvre)
  980, 981f
Cri du chat syndrome 679
Crigler–Najjar syndrome 689
criminal abortion 764
criminal law, birth 1157
Critical Appraisal Skills Programme
  (CASP) 56
crown-rump length (CRL) 248
crutches, elbow, symphysis pubis pain 278
crying, interpretation 559

cryopreservation 138
cultural aspects
  female genital mutilation 835
  health problems 267–268
  pain 463–464
cultural/religious beliefs
  childbirth 5
  communication 5
  malpresentation/malposition 884
  sudden infant death syndrome 718
  weight in pregnancy 329
cumulus cells mass 161
  oocyte maturation 95
  ovulation 96
cup-feeding
  formulae 616
  origins 564
  preterm baby 612, 612f
curl-ups, abdominal exercises 391, 391f
curriculum vitae 1191–1192b
curve of Carus 70
cyanosis 530
Cyclofem 122
cypress oil, haemorrhoid treatment 345
cyst(s), ovarian 833
cystic fibrosis (CF) 699–700
  antibiotics 700
  genetic engineering 187
  genetics inheritance modes 179
  investigation 567, 699
  periventricular haemorrhage 639
  preconception care 151t
  presentation 699
  treatment 700
cystic fibrosis transmembrane
    conductance regulator (CFTR),
    genetic engineering 187
cystine
  breast milk 595
  menstrual cycle 95
cystitis 801
cytomegalovirus (CMV) 708
  maternal screening 316
  preconception care advice 149t
  symptoms 708
  transmission rate 708
cytosine (C), genetics 174
cytotrophoblast shell 199
  development 192–193, 194f

D

daily activities, physical preparation
    392
damages
  compensation 1151
  general 1151
Danazol 131
Dancer hold 611

Darwin, Charles 172
  genetics history 172
databases
  Boolean logic 55
  searching 54–55
Data Protection Act, consent 1057
death registration 43–44, 1034–1035
decidua
  hormonal interactions in labour
      413, 414
  implantation 192
  organogenesis/placenta formation
      195
decidualization 100
  implantation 191
deciduochorial placenta formation
    193–194, 194f
deep transverse arrest (DTA) 890f, 892
deep vein thrombosis (DVT)
    1221–1222
  symphysis pubis pain 278
defences (legal) 1149–1151
  compensation 1150–1151
    general damages 1151
    special damages 1151
  contributory negligence 1149
    Law Reform Act 1945 1149
  dispute allegations 1149
  exemption from liability 1149
    Unfair Contract Terms Act 1977
      1149b
  law consent trespass (to person)
      1151
  negligence elements 1149
  time limitation 1150, 1150b
  voluntary assumption of risk 1150
    Volente non fit injuria 1150
dehydroepiandrosterone (DHAS) 292
dehydroepiandrosterone sulphate
    (DHEAS) 214
delayed abortion 761
delegation, negligence 1148
deletion, chromosome anomalies 178
Delfen foam 126
delivery
  amniotic fluid embolism 1000
  breech presentation *see* breech
      presentation
  'face-to-pubes' 890–892, 891f
  forceps *see* forceps delivery
  membranes *see* membranes
  mental health issues 924
  paternal presence 109
  placental *see* placenta delivery
  preterm baby 633
  small-for-gestational-age baby
      643–644
  therapeutic drugs 1213–1222
  vaginal *see* vaginal delivery
  ventouse *see* ventouse delivery
delivery equipment, temperature 579

delivery room temperature 579
  preterm baby 633
density gradient, intrauterine
    insemination 134–135
dental care 271
  antenatal care 256
deontology
  casuistry 1136
  code of professional conduct
      (UKCC 1992) 1136
  ethics dilemmas 1136–1137
  intuitionistic pluralism 1136
  prima facie duties 1136
  rational monism 1136
  traditional 1136
deoxycorticosterone (DOC)
  menstrual cycle 288, 288f
  renal handling of sodium 293
deoxyribonucleic acid (DNA), genetics
    history 173
Depo-Provera (DMPA) 122
depression, postnatal *see* postnatal
    depression
dermatitis, groin/buttock/anus 567
dermatocranium 220
developmental dysplasia of hip
    (congenital dislocation of hip)
    556–558
  Barlow test 557–558, 557f
  diagnosis 677
  early detection 557, 677
  examination 557
  Ortolani test 557–558, 557f
  risk factors 557
developmental problems, herpes
    simplex virus 709
dexamethasone
  chronic lung disease 660
  congenital adrenal hyperplasia
      700
  preterm labour 856, 858
Dexon (polyglycolic acid) 484
dextrose, labour 808
diabetes mellitus, maternal 804–809
  baby of diabetic woman 809
  blood glucose assessment 808
  cardiac abnormalities 663
  care during
    labour 808–809
    pregnancy 807–808
  diagnosis/classification 804–805
  diet 807–808
  fetal complications 806–807, 807b
  gestational 805
  glycosylated haemoglobin assessment
      808
  induction 862
  insulin 808
  intrauterine contraceptive devices
      (IUCDs) 809
  labour 808–809

maternal complications 806–807, 807b
oral hypoglycaemic drugs 808
postnatal care 809
preconception care 150t, 807
pregnancy 805–806
preterm labour 858
shoulder dystocia 941
type I insulin-dependent (IDD) 804
type II non-insulin-dependent (NIDD) 804–805
Diabetes UK 807
diabetic cherub 809
diabetic nephropathy 806
diagnostic tests 313t
genetics 185–186
diamorphine hydrochloride (heroin) 1217–1218
diaphragm (Dutch cap) 118–119
positioning 118f
size 119
diaphragm, second stage of labour 493
diaphragmatic hernia 661, 672
ex-utero intrapartum treatment 680
identification 672
incidence 672
intubation 661
in-utero tracheal occlusion 680
left-sided anomaly 672
right-sided anomaly 661, 672
surgery 661, 672
diastasis 277–278
incidence 275
diastasis recti 552, 724
postpartum, abdominal exercises 391f
diazepam 1218–1219
eclampsia 787
diclofenac suppositories, perineal pain relief 727
diet see nutrition/diet
dietary deficiencies, pelvis 73
diethylstilboestrol (DES) 829f
digoxin 799
dilatation see cervical dilatation/effacement
dilation and evacuation, therapeutic abortion 763
dilemmas (solving), ethics 1135–1137
direct Coombs' test 687b
direct latex agglutination tests, pregnancy diagnosis 238–239
disability
aids, symphysis pubis pain 278–279
breech presentation 897
multiple birth 850
postnatal care 269–270
preconception care 154t
Disability Discrimination Act 1995 268, 270
disabled child, legal rights 1059–1060

disabled women, antenatal care 268–270
DISCERN instrument 57
disordered uterine action see prolonged labour; uterine contractions
dispute allegations, legal issues 1149
disseminated candidiasis 709
disseminated intravascular coagulation (DIC)
antepartum haemorrhage 775–776
postpartum haemorrhage 989
diuresis, postnatal 724–725
dizygotic twins 840
causes 840
physical features 841
placentae 841
dizygous twins see dizygotic twins
DNA 174–175, 174f
adenine (A) 174
cytosine (C) 174
genetics 174–175, 174f
guanine (G) 174
history 173
replication, cell division 176
thymine (T) 174
transcription 175
translation 175
DNA probe, genetics diagnostic tests 185
DNA testing, zygosity determination 841
Döderlein's bacilli (lactobacilli) 78
domestic abuse/violence 253, 364–366
child abuse 1060
guidelines 365b
maternal/fetal risks 364–365
mental health issues 921
midwives' role 365–366
preconception care 152t
prevalence 364
signs 366b
dominant allele, genetics history 173
DOMINO scheme (domiciliary in and out scheme) 244, 1088
donor insemination (DI) 134
Doppler ultrasound 322
post-term pregnancy 870
double pumping 604–607
double test 316–317
Down's syndrome (trisomy 21) 678–679
antenatal screening tests 679
associated anomalies 679
clinical features 678–679
feeding problems 611
forms 678–679
incidence 678
infertility 133
mosaicism 678
'drop in clinics,' contraception for young patients 114

drug abuse/addiction
perinatal death 1038
pregnancy 249
see also substance abuse
drugs
controlled 1209–1212
destruction/surrender 1211–1212
home birth 1212
possession/supply/use 1211
schedules 1211
dependence 1223
history taking 249–250
misuse 1223
preconception care 152t
pregnancy 364
therapeutic 1209–1217
administration 1212–1213
breastfeeding 599, 1212–1223
controlled see above drugs, controlled
delivery 1213–1222
information 1210
interactions 1210–1211
legal issues 1160
legislation 1211–1212
neonatal resuscitation 657–658
nurse prescribing 1223–1224
physiological issues 1210
pregnancy 1213–1222
preterm labour 857–859
respiratory 1222
thermoregulation 578
see also individual drug types
Dubowitz scale/scoring 543, 628, 629f
Duchenne muscular dystrophy, genetics advice 183
ductus arteriosus 209, 649
closure 650, 651
patent see patent ductus arteriosus (PDA)
transposition of the great arteries 665
ductus venosus 649
Dulcolax (bisacodyl BP) 1214
dummies
breastfeeding 604
sudden infant death syndrome 717
duodenal atresia 674
dural puncture, accidental, postpartum headache 742
dural tap, epidural analgesia 471
dura mater 229f
dust, infection risk 565
Dutch cap (diaphragm) see diaphragm (Dutch cap)
duty of beneficence, ethics duty of care 1137–1138
duty of care
ethics 1136–1137, 1137–1138
negligence 1145–1146
duty of fidelity, ethics duty of care 1137

duty of justice, ethics duty of care 1138
duty of non-maleficence, ethics duty of care 1138
dwarfism 677
dyspareunia, postpartum 740–741
  complications 393
  risk factors 741
DZ twins see dizygotic twins

E

ear(s)
  development 206
  examination 549, 549b
eating disorders
  preconception care 146t
  pregnancy 754–755
eccentric insertion of umbilical cord 520
echocardiography, cardiac abnormalities 663
eclampsia 786–788
  dangers 787
  labour 789
  management 787–788
    post delivery 788
  observations 788
  seizures see eclamptic convulsion
  see also hypertensive disorders; pre-eclampsia
Eclampsia Collaborative Trial Group (ECTC) 1215
eclamptic convulsion 786–787
  clonic stage 787
  comatose stage 787
  management 787
  premonitory stage 786
  tonic stage 786–787
ectoderm, primary 195, 205
ectopic pregnancy 766–768
  chlamydia 824
  heterotopic 768
  secondary abdominal 768
  tubal 766–768, 767f
    abortion 767, 767f
    damage 132
    diagnosis 767
    management 767–768
    non-surgical management 768
    risk factors 766–767
    rupture 767, 767f
    symptoms 767
  ultrasound scan 319, 767
ectromelia 677
Edinburgh Postnatal Depression Scale (EPDS) 922, 927, 928f, 929f
educational approach, health promotion 359t

education and training
  bereavement skills 29–30
  computers 1194–1195
  degrees 1188–1189
  diplomas 1188–1189
  e-learning 1194–1195
  financial constraints 1205
  fitness for practice 1123
  funding 1013
  higher education 1186–1189, 1193–1195
  history of 1185–1186, 1187t
  internet 1194–1195
  learning approaches 1195–1199, 1198t, 1199t
  learning styles 1199–1201
  lifelong learning 1185–1208
  mentorship 1204–1205
  new approaches 1195
  note taking 1192–1193, 1193b
  parenthood see parent education
  portfolio 1191–1192
  postgraduate studies 1193–1194
  post-registration 1124–1125
  pre-registration midwifery 1122–1123
  profile 1189
  questioning skills 1204b
  reflective learning 1201–1204, 1203b
  scholarships 1188–1189
  standard setting 1122–1125
  supervisors 1128
  work-based learning 1194
  see also teaching physical skills
Edward syndrome (trisomy 18) 679
  clinical features 679
egg donation 139
Ehlers–Danlos syndrome 479
Eisenmenger's syndrome 798–799
elbow crutches, symphysis pubis pain 278
elbow examination 551
electrocardiography (ECG)
  cardiac abnormalities 663
  shock 999
  trial of labour 962
electronic fetal monitoring 452
electrophoresis, iron deficiency anaemia 794
embolism
  amniotic fluid see amniotic fluid embolism
  pulmonary, maternal death 1044
  see also thromboembolism
embryo(s)
  assessment, genetics 181–182
  freezing 138–139
  grading, IVF 138t
  rhythmic secretion 163
  transfer, IVF 137–138, 138f

embryonic compartment, formation 195–196, 196f
embryonic development 165–167, 166f, 205–219
emergency card 537
emergency contraception 123
emergency drills/protocols
  postpartum haemorrhage 987
  shoulder dystocia 950, 951
Emergency Protection Order 1063
emotional care
  amniotic fluid embolism 1000–1001
  in labour 433–434
  shoulder dystocia 947
  umbilical cord presentation/prolapse 958
  uterine rupture 967
employment issues
  history taking 247
  preconception care 151t
  pregnancy and health 367
  pregnant women 1054
endocrine assessment, male factor infertility 132
endocrine disorders 696–702
  screening 696
endoderm, primary 195, 205
endogenous opioids
  maternal pain threshold 303
  oxytocin and 303
  physiological responses to pregnancy 302–303
endometrial stromal differentiation 168
endometriomas 131
endometriosis 131
endometrium 79
  arterial supply 99f
  changes in epithelial mitosis 100f
  cyclic development 97–99
  implantation preparation 190
  menstrual cycle changes 97, 98f
  response to implantation/formation of placenta 191
  trophoblast interactions 191
endoparasite (fetus-in-fetu) 844
β-endorphin, physiological responses to pregnancy 302–303, 303f
endorphins 462
endothelins 97
endotracheal intubation, neonatal resuscitation 654, 655f
  larynx damage 654
endotracheal tube (ETT) 654
energy requirements
  changes in menstrual cycle 89
  labour 972
engagement, fetal head 266
  abdominal examination 262–263, 262f
England, NHS restructuring 1015

enkephalins 462
enteral feeding, hyperemesis
        gravidarum 753–754
Entonox 467–468, 468f
    minimize bearing-down urge 498
Epanutin (phenytoin sodium) 811
epiblast 195
epidemiology, fertility/childbearing
        1034–1049
epidermolysis bullosa 678
epididymis 84b, 85b
epidural anaesthesia 469–471
    breech presentation 904
    caesarean section (CS) 981
    disadvantages 470–471
    induction/anatomy 470, 470f
    long-term problems 471
    maternal heart disease 799
    mobile 471
    multiple pregnancy 845
    physiological effects 470
    postpartum backache 742
    preterm labour 858–859
    pushing techniques 499
    suturing the perineal 485
epilepsy
    maternal 811–812
    preconception care 150t
Epilim (sodium valproate) 811
epinephrine hydrochloride (adrenaline)
    see adrenaline (epinephrine)
episiotomy (surgical incision)
        481–484, 481f
    active management of labour 442
    complications 482
    controversy 483
    female genital mutilation 834–835,
        835f
    indications 482, 500
    labour, second stage 499–500
    mediolateral/posterolateral 481,
        484
    midline 481, 484
    postpartum perineal trauma 741
    procedure 482, 483t
    rates 482
    risks 482
    shoulder dystocia 944
    timing 482
        shoulder dystocia 944
epispadias 675
    surgical correction 675
epithelial cells, implantation 191
Epstein's pearls 549
equipment, instrumental vaginal
        deliveries 973
ERa (oestrogen receptor subtype) 410
ERb (oestrogen receptor subtype) 410
Erb's palsy 948, 948f
ergometrine 513
    active management of labour 515

postpartum haemorrhage 990
    prolonged labour 995
ergometrine maleate 1219–1220
    complications 1220
    with oxytocin 1220–1221
erythema infectiosum (slapped cheek
        disease), preconception care advice
        148t
erythema toxicum 546
erythropoiesis, physiological response
        in pregnancy 290–292
erythropoietin, maternal changes
        290–292
Escherichia coli
    renal conditions 801
    shock 999
    urinary tract infections 711
essential oils
    labour pain relief 349
    perineal problems 351
    postnatal depression 350
estimated date of delivery (EDD) 247
    calculation 247t
ethical issues, small-for-gestational-age
        baby (SGA) 646
ethical theory, ethics definition 1133
ethics **1133–1141**
    assisted reproduction techniques
        139–140
    definition 1133–1134
        ethical theory 1133
        meta-ethics 1133
        moral rights 1134
        practical ethics 1133
    dilemmas (solving) 1135–1137
        deontology 1136–1137
            see also deontology
        in vitro fertilization (IVF) 1136
        utilitarianism 1135–1136
    duty of care 1137–1138
        duty of beneficence 1138
        duty of fidelity 1138
        duty of justice 1138
        duty of non-maleficence 1138
    importance 1134–1135
        code of professional conduct
            (UKCC 1992) 1135
        moral conflict 1134–1135
        moral dilemma 1135
        principles 1137
    preterm baby 646
    principles 1138–1139
        autonomy 1138–1139
ethnic minority groups
    antenatal care 267–268
    health promotion 359
    mental health issues 920
    social needs 7–8
European Community Committees 1111
European Union Committee on training
        midwives 1111

European Union round table 1111
evacuation of retained products of
        conception (ERPC), inevitable
        abortion 760
evaporation, neonatal heat loss 576
evidence-based healthcare (EBHC)
        48–62
    definition 48
    expert knowledge 49
    grey literature 50
    hierarchy 51, 51f
    implementation 56–58
        evaluation 58
    meta-analysis 50–51
    midwife's involvement 58
    personal knowledge 49
    process 52–58
        critical appraisal 55–56
        database searching 54–55
        question framing 52–53, 53b
        searching 54–55, 55f
        searching skill development 54
    research knowledge 49–51
    search stimulation 51
    systematic review 50
evidence-driven audit cycle 58
exaggerated Sims' position, umbilical cord
        presentation/prolapse 955, 956f
Examination of the Newborn Tool 540
exchange transfusion 691–693
    complications 693
    indications 692
    phototherapy 693
    procedure 692
    single site method 692
    two site method 692
exercise
    active sports avoidance 361
    pelvic floor see pelvic floor exercises
    postnatal see postnatal exercises
    preconception care 151t
    during pregnancy 360–361
        guidelines 361b
    see also physical preparation for
        childbirth
exercise-to-music, teaching physical
        skills, physical preparation 395
exocrine disorders 699–700
exomphalos 674–675
    incidence 674
    management 675
expectant management
    active management of labour vs 514
    missed abortion 761
    third stage of labour see labour, third
        stage
expiratory grunting 530
expressed breast milk (EBM)
    double pumping 604–607
    production 604–607
    storage 607–608

external cephalic version (ECV), breech presentation 899, 903
external gradient 576
extra-amniotic prostaglandins, therapeutic abortion 763
extracorporeal membrane oxygenation (ECMO) 662
 complications 662
 rescue treatment 662
extraembryonic mesoderm 197
extrauterine gestation *see* ectopic pregnancy
extremely low birthweight (ELBW) 630, 853
extubation, caesarean section 981
ex-utero intrapartum treatment (EXIT) 680
eye(s)
 development 206
 examination 549, 549b, 559
 infection 710
 see also specific ocular conditions
eye protection
 labour 502
 phototherapy 692, 692f
eye-to-eye contact 15
Ez condom 116

F

face, newborn 222f
face presentation
 causes 886
 complications 909t
 delivery 909–911
 diagnosis 909
 fetal positions 910–911
 incidence 886
 management 912–913
 manual rotation 912–913
 obstructed labour 911, 913f
 primary 908
 secondary 908
 skull moulding 230f, 230t
 spontaneous delivery 911
 vaginal examination 909
'face-to-pubes' delivery 890–892, 891f
facial expression 14–15
facial palsy 971
factual causation, negligence 1147–1148
faecal incontinence 487
 instrumental deliveries 971
 perineal trauma 480
 postpartum 728, 739–740
 risk factors 740
faecal specimens, iron deficiency anaemia 794

fallopian tubes 80b
 cyclical changes 163
 damage, infertility 131–132
 fertilization 161–162, 162f
 interstitial portion 162
 non-pregnant 79f
Fallot's tetralogy 798
falx cerebri 228f
family history 252–253, 542b
family pedigree 252f
 preconception care 147
family support services 1057–1058
 access 1057–1058
fasting, labour 450, 972
father, legal rights 1053
fatherhood
 'new' 10
 traditional role 10
fatigue, postpartum 743–744
 risk factors 743–744
fat storage, diabetes in pregnancy 805
fatty acids
 breast milk 595
 maternal nutrition 330
 neonatal digestion 594, 595
fear *see* anxiety/fear
feeding 254–255, **591–627**
 artificial *see* artificial feeding
 breast 591–613
  see also breastfeeding
 equipment sterilization 620f
 HIV transmission 817
 methods 616–618, 635–636
 preterm baby 635–637
 small-for-gestational-age baby 645
 sudden infant death syndrome 717
 thermoregulation 578, 580
feet
 congenital anomalies 676
 newborn examination 555–556
 temperature measurement 583
female anatomy **65–90**
 implications for midwifery 83, 85–86
 pelvis 65–73, 66f
 reproductive 75–82
female genitalia, newborn examination 554–555
female genital mutilation (FGM) 833–835, 1063
 mortality/morbidity 834
 pregnancy/childbirth 108
 WHO classification 834, 834f
FemCap 119
Femidom 119
femoral pulse, newborn examination 547
fentanyl 471
Ferguson reflex, prolonged labour 880
Ferguson reflex 493
ferrous gluconate 795
ferrous sulphate 794

ferrous sulphate compound tablets BPC (Fersolate) 1214
Fersolate 1214
fertility
 control *see* contraception
 epilepsy 811
 problems *see* infertility
 rates 1035
 resuming relations after childbirth 115
fertilization **161–171**
 blastocyst 166–167
 corpus luteum development 167–168
 fallopian tubes 161–162, 162f
 human chorionic gonadotrophin (hCG) 167
 in vitro 136–137, 136f
 luteal phase 169
 luteinization 168
 morula 166
 oocyte/spermatozoon fusion 164–165, 164f
 relaxin 168–169
 sperm capacitation 163–164
 sperm transport 163
 vaginal/cervical tissue changes 163
 zygote 165–166, 165f
fetal adrenoplacental hormonal regulation, of cortisol 297–298
fetal alcohol effects (FAE) 250
fetal alcohol syndrome (FAS) 250
fetal assessment, magnetic resonance imaging 323
fetal axis pressure 493
fetal circulation 207–209, 210f, 531
 development 208, 208f
 differences from adult 207–208
 transition to neonatal life 531, 650–651
 see also cardiovascular system; heart
fetal development **205–219**
 skull 220–222, 221f
 testes 83
fetal distress, trial of labour 963
fetal fibronectin 855
fetal fibronectin tests
 false positive results 855
 preterm labour indicator 855
fetal growth
 abnormalities, induction 863
 assessment 320–321
 hypothalamic–pituitary–adrenal (HPA) axis 302
fetal haemoglobin 531, 685
fetal heart monitoring 238, 451–452
 acceleration patterns 451, 452f
 baseline variability 451, 452f
 electronic 452
 healthy patterns 451–452
 trial of labour 962

fetal heart rate (FHR) 317
  abnormalities, cervical ripening 865
  post-term pregnancy 869
  response to labour 420
fetal heart sounds
  breech presentation 897
  face presentation 909
fetal hypoxia
  amniotic fluid embolism 1000
  meconium staining 503
fetal macrosomia 806
  induction indicator 863
  postpartum haemorrhage 988
  post-term pregnancy 869
  ultrasound to predict 941
fetal malformations, diabetic woman 807
fetal monitoring 451–452
  caesarean section 979
  diabetic woman 808, 809
  electronic 452
  trial of labour 962
  water birth 501
  see also fetal heart monitoring
fetal mortality/morbidity
  caesarean section 978–979
  diabetes mellitus 806
  domestic violence 364–365
  fetal surgery 680
  induction 863
  obstetric cholestasis 812
  perinatal 1037–1040
    predisposing factors 1037–1038
  reduction 1036
  stillbirths 1037
  teenage pregnancy 366
  umbilical cord presentation/prolapse 956
  uterine rupture 967
  Zavanelli manoeuvre 946
fetal movements 238, 317–318
  differential diagnosis 240
  kick charts 317–318
  signs of pregnancy 237
fetal part palpation, placenta praevia 770
fetal position
  assessing 445–446, 445f, 446t
  thermoregulation 577
fetal prolactin 201f
fetal response to labour/birth 418–420
  fetoplacental blood flow 420
  heart rate 420
  pulmonary 418–420
fetal size
  cephalic disproportion 961
  shoulder dystocia 941
fetal skull **220–234**
  bones 223, 224f
  development 220–222, 221f

diameters 225
  biparietal 225f
  bitemporal 225f
  mentovertical 226f
  occipitofrontal 226f
  relative to maternal pelvis 226f
  submentobregmatic 226f
  submentovertical 226f
  suboccipitobregmatic 226f
  suboccipitofrontal 226f
injuries 229–232
  preterm birth 859
internal structures 225–227, 229f
measurement 223–225
moulding during labour 227–229, 229f, 230f, 230t
parental advice 232–233, 233b
structure 223–225, 224f, 225f
ultrasound scan 220, 221f
fetal temperature 575
fetal thermoregulation 575
fetal weight estimation, ultrasound scan 322–323
fetal well-being assessment
  nuchal translucency 320
  pre-eclampsia 784
fetocide see selective fetal reduction
fetoplacental blood flow, fetal response to labour 420
fetoscopy, genetics diagnostic tests 186
fetus
  adaptations to mother's pelvis in labour 494
  adrenal cortex 214
  age see gestational age
  anaemia treatment 322
  anomalies identification, ultrasound scan 320
  assessment, genetics 181–182
  behaviour, post-term pregnancy 869
  blood supply, umbilical cord presentation/prolapse 956
  breathing movements 211–212, 652
    preterm labour indicator 855
  Child Protection Register 1063
  circulation see fetal circulation
  head engagement see engagement, fetal head
  heartbeat monitoring 265
  hypothalamic–pituitary–adrenal (HPA) axis 302
  malpositions 884–917
  malpresentations 884–917
  maternal conditions, effects on
    diabetes mellitus 806–807, 807b
    heart disease 799
    renal 802
    thyrotoxicosis 800
  membranes 519
  oxygen supply, umbilical cord presentation/prolapse 956

pethidine effects 469
positioning in labour, second stage 500
skull see fetal skull
therapy, ultrasound scan 322
water birth 501
see also entries beginning fetal
fetus-in-fetu (endoparasite) 844
fetus papyraceous 761, 761f
fibroids (fibromyomata) 832–833, 833f
  postpartum haemorrhage 989
  umbilical cord presentation/prolapse 955
fibronectin, fetal 855
fibronectin tests, fetal 855
fimbriae 80b
finger nails examination 551
first stage of labour see labour, first stage
first-time parenthood, psychological aspect 18
Fitness for Practice report 1123
flatus incontinence, postpartum 740
flexed breech 894–895
floppy infant syndrome 1219
flucloxacillin, pemphigus neonatorum 711
fluconazole, Candida 709–710
fluid(s)
  administration
    caesarean section 982
    shock 998
  intravenous, moderate vomiting in pregnancy 753
  labour 450
fluid balance
  postpartum haemorrhage 993
  pre-eclampsia 785
folic acid 1214
  birth defect reduction 328, 1027–1028
  deficiency, preconception care 146t
  dietary sources 795
  maternal nutrition 332–333
  preterm baby 328
  supplements 251
    folic acid deficiency anaemia 795
    haemoglobinopathies 797
folic acid deficiency anaemia 795
follicles
  aspiration 136
  dominant 90–91
    selection of 91–92
  preovulatory 93f, 94–95
  secondary 90
follicle-stimulating hormone (FSH)
  dominant follicle selection 91
  in vitro fertilization 132
  male infertility 132
  mid-cycle surge 92

follicle-stimulating hormone (FSH)
  (*contd*)
  oocyte maturation 95
  ovulation 96
  physiological response to pregnancy
    298
  postnatal 724
folliculogenesis 90–91
follow-on milks 430
follow-up care after birth 517–518
fomites, infection risk 565
fontanelles 223
  anterior 224f, 225f
    position 222f
  anterolateral 224f
  mastoid 224f
  posterior 224f, 225f
fontanelles, newborn examination
  548–549
food avoidance 251
football hold 848, 848f
footling breech presentation 895
foramen ovale 208–209, 649
  closure 531, 650
forceps, history 973
forceps delivery 971, 973–974, 974f
  adjustment/articulation 974, 975f
  application 974, 975f
  first usage 1076–1077
  obstructive labour 964
  stress incontinence 738
  traction 974
  umbilical cord presentation/prolapse
    957–958
  ventouse *vs* 973
forearm, newborn examination
  551
foreign clients 245
  advocacy 435
Foresight organization 360
forewaters, labour, first stage 432–433,
  433f
fossa ovalis 650
foster carers 1058
fostering 1058
Foundation for the Study of Infant
  Deaths (FSID) 715, 1041
  'Back to Sleep' campaign 715–716
  'Care of the Next Infant' programme
    718–719
fourchette 77b
Framework for Maternity Services in
  Scotland 1015
frank breech presentation 895
fraternal twins *see* dizygotic twins
frenulum 77b
frontal bones 224f, 225f
  development 220
  at term 222
frontal suture 225f
fundal dominance 432

fundal fiddling, active management of
  labour 516
fundal palpation 264
fundal pressure, shoulder dystocia 947
funerals, sibling attendance 42

G

galactopoiesis 602–603
galactosaemia 697
  clinical features 697
galactose-1-phosphate uridyltransferase
  deficiency 697
gamete intrafallopian tube transfer
  (GIFT) 135
gap junctions, changes in preparation
  for labour 411–412
garlic
  heartburn/indigestion remedy 335
  thrush remedy 336
gastric contents, aspiration of, in
  labour 450
gastroenteritis 710
  causative organisms 710
  monitoring 710
  preventative measures 710
gastrointestinal system 532–533
  38 weeks gestation baby 532–533
  abnormalities 673–675
    see also specific abnormalities
  development 215–217, 216f
  maturation 216, 532, 594
  meconium 533
  postnatal changes 724
  stools 533
gastrointestinal tract
  neonatal maturation 594
  pregnancy changes 271–272
gastroschisis 674–675
  incidence 674
  management 675
gate theory of pain *see* pain
gel pads 535
gender 9–11
  childrearing arrangements 10
  labour divisions 10
  leadership 1179
  stereotypes 10
general practitioner (GP), postnatal role
  725
general sale list medicines (GSLs)
  1211
genes 174–175
  dominant/recessive 671
  expression 175f
gene therapy 187
genetically modified foods,
    preconception care 146t
genetic counselling 182–183

genetic disorders *see* chromosome
  anomalies
genetic engineering 186–188
  cystic fibrosis (CF) 187
  cystic fibrosis transmembrane
    conductance regulator (CFTR)
    187
  gene therapy 187
genetics **172–189**
  advice 182–183
    congenital heat disease 183
    Duchenne muscular dystrophy 183
  chromosome analysis 177–178
    karyotyping 177, 177f
  chromosome anomalies 177–178
    see also chromosome anomalies
  counselling 182–183
  diagnostic tests 185–186
    amniocentesis 186
    chorionic villus sampling (CVS)
      185–186
    cordocentesis 186
    DNA probe 185
    fetoscopy 186
    preimplantation genetic diagnosis
      (PGD) 185
  diseases, origin 181
    sickle-cell anaemia 181
  embryo assessment 181–182
  fetus assessment 181–182
  history 172–174
  inheritance pattern 179f
  preconception care 147, 151t
genetic screening 183–185
  assisted conception 140
  biochemical/serum screening 184–185
    alpha-fetoprotein (AFP) 184–185
  history-taking 184
  preconception care 147
  serum/biochemical screening
    184–185
  serum screening, alpha-fetoprotein
    (AFP) 184
  ultrasound scanning (USS) 184
genital herpes 823–824
genital tract abnormalities **829–837**
  developmental anomalies 829–831,
    829f
  female genital mutilation 833–835
    see also female genital mutilation
    (FGM)
  fibromyomata (fibroids) 832–833
  implications for midwife 836
  ovarian cysts 833
  uterus displacements 831–832
    see also uterus displacements
genital tract infection, preterm labour
  854
genital tract injuries
  instrumental deliveries 971
  postpartum haemorrhage 993–994

genital tract sepsis, maternal death 1045
genitourinary system
  abnormalities 675–676
    see also ambiguous genitalia
  development 213–215
  newborn examination 554–556, 554b
genome, human 175
  see also Human Genome Project
German measles (rubella virus) see rubella (German measles)
gestational age
  assessment 543–544, 628, 629f, 630f
    post-term pregnancy 868
    ultrasound scan 320
  ultrasound parameters 318–319
gestational diabetes 805
gestational trophoblastic disease 765–766
gestures 15
Gilbert syndrome 688
Gillick criteria 125
ginger, morning sickness treatment 752
gingival oedema 271
gingivitis 271
girth, abdominal examination 263
glans penis 84b
globin 796
glomerular filtration rate (GFR), physiological response in pregnancy 289, 295
glucose
  blood levels 808
  co-transfer 805–806
  excretion, in pregnancy 295
  metabolism 533–534
    fetal 533–534
    neonatal 534
  in pregnancy 805–806
  reabsorption 806
glucose-6-phosphate dehydrogenase (G6PD) deficiency 697, 798
  triggers 688, 697
glucose tolerance, impaired 805
glucose tolerance test (GTT) 805
glyceryl trinitrate (GTN), preterm labour 858
glycodelin A, implantation 192
glycogen, hepatic 216–217
glycoproteins, organogenesis/placenta formation 195
glycosuria 257
  in pregnancy 295
glycosylated haemoglobin (HbA$_1$) 806
  assessment 808
GnRH agonist, in vitro fertilization 135–136
gonadotrophin 134
  ovarian cycle 91

gonadotrophin-releasing hormone (GnRH)
  menstrual cycle 92–94
  neurochemical reactions controlling 93
  physiological response in pregnancy 298
gonococcal arthritis 823
gonorrhoea 709, 822–823
  treatment 709
Government initiatives 371, 373–374
grandparents, grief 43
grasp reflex 559
Graves' disease (hyperthyroidism, thyrotoxicosis) 800–801
  neonatal thyrotoxicosis 701
gravidin 413
great vein of Galen 228f
grief 27–47
  abortion 762
  death registration 43–44
  dual process model 32, 32f
  friends and family 43
  labour when baby has died 35–36, 967
  mourning, tasks of 28b, 30
  pain 30–31
  parental response 32–33
  post-mortem examination 39–40
  postnatal period 39
  respectful disposal of the body 44
  respecting parents 41
  siblings 41–43
  spiritual needs 41
  support agencies 44, 47
  taking a baby home 43
  understanding of 30–32
  unexpected death 36–38
  see also bereavement; neonatal mortality/death
groin
  dermatitis 567
  newborn examination 554
group B streptococcus (GBS) 709
growth
  fetal see fetal growth
  mammary 601–602
  uterus 304–305
growth hormone, fetal overproduction 806
guanine (G), genetics 174
Guedel airway insertion, neonatal resuscitation 654
Guidelines for Records and Record Keeping 1126
Guidelines for the Administration of Medicines 1126, 1210
Guidelines for the Management of Massive Obstetric Haemorrhage 777b

Guthrie test 566, 696
  cystic fibrosis 699
  haemorrhagic disease 696
GyneFix 120

H

H2 receptor antagonist, Mendelson's syndrome 980
haem 684, 795
haematinic substances 1214
haemoglobin (Hb)
  adult 531–532
  blood tests 314
  combinations, sickle cell disease 796t
  fetal 531, 685
  glycosylated see glycosylated haemoglobin (HbA$_1$)
haemoglobinopathies 315, 795–796
haemolysis elevated liver enzymes low platelets (HELLP) syndrome 782, 784
haemolytic anaemia 796
haemolytic disease of the newborn 686–687
  ABO incompatibility 687
  anti-D treatment 687
  hydrops fetalis 687
  immunization 686, 686f
  investigations 687b
  rhesus factor 686–687
haemorrhage
  antepartum 769–776
    see also antepartum haemorrhage
  difficulties in defining 514
  estimations 987–988
  labour 423
    third stage 509
  massive obstetric 992–993
  maternal death 1044–1045
  measuring 517
  periventricular see periventricular haemorrhage (PVH)
  postpartum see postpartum haemorrhage (PPH)
  pulmonary 645
  retinal, instrumental deliveries 971
  shock 998
  subaponeurotic, vacuum extraction cup 232
  subgaleal, instrumental deliveries 971
  uterine rupture 967
  warning 771
haemorrhagic disease of the newborn (HDN) see haemolytic disease of the newborn; vitamin K deficiency bleeding

haemorrhoidal arteries 78
haemorrhoids
  complementary therapies 345–346
  postnatal 727–728, 739
hair examination 548b, 549
hand(s)
  congenital anomalies 676–677
  newborn examination 551
hand expression 606b, 606f
handling, during labour 448
handpumps 606, 607f
handwashing, infection prevention
  565, 638, 704
harm, negligence 1148
hats, neonatal thermoregulation 584
hazardous substances, preconception
  care 152t
head
  breech presentation 908
  circumference measurement
    544–545
    mentovertical 222f
    occipitofrontal 222f
    suboccipitobregmatic 222f
  deflexion 890
  engagement see engagement, fetal
    head
  entrapment 908, 908f
  extension 892
  flexion 890, 890f
  newborn examination 548, 548b,
    559
  nodding 15
  temperature loss 580
  see also fetal skull
headache
  complementary therapies 346–347
  postpartum 742
    without backache 742
health
  definition 355
  models 355–356
  reducing inequalities in health
    356
  top-down commitment bottom-up
    approach 356
Health Act 1999 1118
Health Action Zone 359
health and safety, legal issues 1159
health authorities, child protection
  1061
Health Belief Model 356
healthcare premises, adaptations
  269–270
healthcare team, mental health issues
  923
Health Divide, The, health inequalities
  9
Health Locus of Control 356
Health of a Nation Report, teenage
  pregnancy rates 366

Health of the Nation, health
  inequalities 9
health promotion **355–370**
  antenatal period 360–367
  approaches 358
  definition 356
  evaluation 367–368
  midwife's role 358–360
    community action 358–360
  models 358, 358f
  in practice 359t
  preconception care 360
  what is it? 356–368
health screening, preconception care
  143, 145
Health Service Reorganisation Act
  1973 401
health visitor, postnatal role 725
hearing
  disability, antenatal care 268–269
  loss, unconjugated
    hyperbilirubinaemia 693
  newborn examination 549
  testing 567
heart
  development 207
  disorders see cardiac disease,
    maternal; cardiac disorders
  examination 256
  failure 799
  fetal 208–209, 649
  monitoring, fetal see fetal heart
    monitoring
  murmurs 548
  newborn examination 547–548
    gallop sounds 548
    murmurs 548
  see also entries beginning cardiac
heartburn
  antenatal care 271–272
  complementary therapies 345
  nutritional therapy 335, 345
heart rate
  fetal response to labour 420
    see also fetal heart rate (FHR)
  maternal changes 290
  monitoring, shock 999
heat clamp 575
heated mattress
  gel filled 588
  water filled 588
heat loss
  mechanisms 576–577
  newborn 575–577
heat production, newborn 577–578
heat shields 588
heat stress see hyperthermia
heel-prick test, pain relief 681
Hegar's sign 238
height
  antenatal care 256

maternal, cephalic disproportion
  predictor 960–961
Helicobacter pylori infection
  diagnosis 753
  hyperemesis gravidarum 753
  treatment 753
HELLP syndrome 782, 784
HELPERR mnemonic 950
hemabate, massive obstetric
  haemorrhage 992
heparin 1222
hepatitis 708
  maternal screening 315–316
  transplacental infection 708
hepatitis B (HBV) 708
  breastfeeding 821
  maternal screening 315–316
  preconception care advice 149t
  pregnancy 821
  transmission, water birth 501
hepatitis C (HCV) 708
  breastfeeding 599
  maternal screening 316
hermaphroditism 676
hernia, diaphragmatic see
  diaphragmatic hernia
heroin (diamorphine hydrochloride)
  1217–1218
herpes simplex virus (HSV) 709,
  823–824
  developmental problems 709
heterotopic pregnancy 768
heterozygous, genetics history 173
high-frequency oscillatory ventilation
  (HFOV) 662
highly active antiretroviral therapy
  (HAART), pregnancy 818
HighScope study 373
hindwaters, labour, first stage
  432–433, 433f
hip
  development, supine sleeping 716
  developmental dysplasia see
    developmental dysplasia of hip
    (congenital dislocation of hip)
  newborn examination 556–558,
    556b
Hirschsprung's disease 674
  diagnosis and repair 674
histamine-2 receptor antagonist,
  Mendelson's syndrome 980
history-taking
  antenatal care see antenatal care
  genetics screening (risk indicators)
    184
HIV infection 706–707
  acute primary infection 816
  antibody-positive phase 816
  breastfeeding 598–599, 707, 817,
    820
  clinical features 707

disease progression 816–817
late symptomatic disease 816–817
legal issues 1150
maternal screening 316
midwives' rules and code of practice (UKCC 1998) 821
neonatal 818
preconception care advice 148t
pregnancy 108
prevalence in pregnancy 816, 816f
remission 817
screening see HIV screening
symptomatic disease 816–817
syphilis treatment failure 822
terminal phase 817
transmission
   risk 706, 707
   water birth 501
vertical transmission 706
   reduced rates 817–818
   risk 819
HIV screening 815–821
antenatal care 253
autonomy 820–821
beneficence 817–819
   baby 818
   family 818–819
   mother 818
confidentiality 821
ethical principles 816
harmful effects 819
information 820
informed consent 820
non-maleficence 819–820
home
antepartum haemorrhage management 773–774
children living away from 1058
postnatal care 404–405, 731
pre-eclampsia care 786
symphysis pubis pain 278–279
home birth 243–244, 405–407, 435–436
controlled drugs 1212
experience 406–407
facilitation 405–406
obstructive labour 964
pain perception 463–464
preparation 406
resuscitation, neonate 581
retained placenta 996
safety issues 405
homeopathy 341–342, 1213
heartburn 345
labour induction 867–868
nausea/vomiting 345
regulation 341
home ovulation predictor tests 236
home pregnancy tests 240
homozygous, genetics history 173
hookworm infestation 798

hormonal regulation
cardiovascular system 297
cervical effacement 430
renal haemodynamic changes 289
respiratory system 297
hormones, fertilization 167
Horner's syndrome (ipsilateral ptosis) 949
hospital, postnatal care 730–731
hospitalization of birth
bias 435
pain perception 463–464
safety aspects 435
see also National Health Service (NHS)
hot water bottles 584
human chorionic gonadotrophin (hCG)
DHEAS synthesis 214
ectopic pregnancies 132
effects in early pregnancy 167
fertilization 167
implantation 191
in vitro fertilization 132
levels, vomiting 751
luteotrophic 167
mammogenesis 601
nausea and vomiting 751
pregnancy diagnosis 238, 240
Human Fertilisation and Embryology Act 1990 and 1992 130, 1157
pregnancy law 1157
Human Fertilisation and Embryology Act 1991, gestation limits for termination 762–763
Human Fertilisation and Embryology Authority (HFEA) 130
human genome 175
autosomes 175
genetics 175
X chromosome 175
Y chromosome 175
Human Genome Project 172–189
genetics 172–189
human milk fortifiers 636
human placental lactogen (hPL)
mammary gland regulation 304
mammary growth 601–602
Human Rights Act, Children Act 1053–1054
humerus
damage, shoulder dystocia 949
newborn examination 551
hurdle concept 18
hyaline membrane disease 659
hyaluronic acid 411
hyaluronidase, labour induction 868t
hydantoin syndrome 811
hydatidiform mole 240, 765–766
abdominal examination 765
appearance 765, 765f
continued growth 766

incidence 765
karyotype 765
signs/symptoms 765
treatment 765–766
ultrasound scan 319, 765
hydralazine hydrochloride 785, 1214–1215
hydrocele 554
hydrocephalus 672
diagnosis 672
head circumference 672
periventricular haemorrhage 639
postnatal surgery 672
hydrops, twin-to-twin transfusion syndrome 843
hydrops fetalis 687
β-hydroxysteroid dehydrogenase (11βHSD) 297–298
hygiene
labour, second stage 497–498
newborn 565
hymen 77b
newborn examination 554–555
hyperbilirubinaemia
conjugated 693–694
   causes 693
   complications 694
   investigation 694
   management 694
unconjugated see unconjugated hyperbilirubinaemia
hyperemesis gravidarum 753–754
care and management 753–754
   intravenous infusion 753
causes 753
complications 753
fetal effects 753
Helicobacter pylori infection 753
investigation 753–754
Mallory–Weiss syndrome 753
medication 754
patient records 754
pregnancy termination 754
psychological support 754
ptyalism 753
symptoms 753
Wernicke's encephalopathy 753
hyperglycaemia 698, 806
hypernatraemia 699
milk powder 699
signs 699
treatment 699
hypertension, preconception care 150t
hypertensive disorders **780–792**
chronic 790
classification 780–781
drugs 785–786
essential 790
induction 862
maternal death 1044
postpartum haemorrhage 988

hypertensive disorders (*contd*)
  psychological care 789–792
  terminology 780–781
  see also eclampsia; pre-eclampsia
hyperthermia 576, 587
  causes 587
  effect 587
  heat stress reversal 587
  labour risk factors 579
  signs 587
hyperthyroidism (thyrotoxicosis,
    Graves' disease) 800–801
  neonatal 701
hyperventilation, luteal phase 288
hypnotherapy 343
  labour pain relief 349, 464
hypnotics 1219
hypo-birthing 464
hypoblast 195
hypocalcaemia 638, 698–699
  calcium treatment 699
  pre-eclampsia 782
  signs 699
  symptoms 699
  transient 698–699
hypogastric arteries 209, 649
hypoglycaemia 697–698
  causes 698
  hypothermia 586
  management 698
  maternal nausea 335
  neonatal brain damage 697
  preterm baby 634, 698
  prevention 698
    blood sugar monitoring 698
  risk factors 698
  signs 698
  small-for-gestational-age baby 644
  symptoms 698
  vomiting 335
hypoglycaemic drugs, pregnancy 808
hypomagnesaemia 699
  congenital (primary) 699
hyponatraemia 699
hypoplastic left heart syndrome
    665–666, 667f
hypospadias 675
  newborn examination 554
  surgical correction 675
hypotension, epidural analgesia 471
hypothalamic–pituitary–adrenal (HPA)
    axis 298
  fetal significance 302
  maternal significance 302
hypothalamic–pituitary–adrenal–
    placental axis 298–303
hypothalamus, development 206
hypothermia 585–587
  complications 586, 587
  definition 585
  hypoglycaemia 586

labour risk factors 579
  management 586–587
  parental education 584, 585b
  physiology 586, 586f
  rewarming 586–587
  risk minimization 584
  signs/symptoms 585–586
  small-for-gestational-age baby 644
hypothyroidism 801
  testing 567
hypothyroidism, congenital 700–701
  clinical signs 701
  hormonal dysfunction 701
  symptoms 701
  thyroid dysgenesis 700
  treatment 701
  unconjugated hyperbilirubinaemia
    688–689
hypovolaemic shock 998
  postpartum haemorrhage 993
hypoxia
  fetal
    amniotic fluid embolism 1000
    meconium staining 503
  inspiration stimulant 651
hypoxic ischaemic encephalopathy
    (HIE) 638–639
  clinical presentation 638–639
  investigation 639
  small-for-gestational-age baby 644
  treatment 639
hysterotomy, therapeutic abortion
    763–764

I

ice packs, perineal pain 727
identical twins *see* monozygotic twins
identification
  baby 538–539
  twins 845, 846
iliac arteries 78
  ligation 993
iliac crest 66
iliac spines 66, 67
iliococcygeus muscles 478
ilium 66
immunization
  hepatitis B virus 821
  sudden infant death syndrome 717
  see also vaccine
immunoglobulin 703
  breast milk 596t
  unconjugated hyperbilirubinaemia
    693
immunoglobulin A (IgA) 594, 703
immunoglobulin D (IgD) 703
immunoglobulin G (IgG) 703
immunoglobulin M (IgM) 703

immunoreactive trypsinogen (IRT) test,
    cystic fibrosis 567, 699
immunosuppression, implantation/
    development of placenta 192
Immunosuppressive drugs, pregnancy
    803
imperforate anus 674
  meconium 674
  surgery 674
Implanon 122
implantation *see* placental
    implantation/development
implantation bleeding 758
inadequate lactation, complementary
    therapies 350–351
incompetent cervix *see* cervical
    incompetence
incontinence, postpartum
  faecal 728, 739–740
  flatus 740
  stress 737–738
  see also faecal incontinence; urinary
    incontinence
incredibly low birthweight (ILBW)
    853
incubators, thermoregulation 587
indigestion, nutritional therapy 335
indometacin
  fetal effects 858
  patent ductus arteriosus 664
  preterm labour 858
induced abortion 762–764
induced labour **862–875**
  breech presentation 903
  contraindications 864
  fetal indications 863–864
  maternal indications 862–863
  maternal request 863
  maternal views 871
  methods 864–868
    medical 864–867, 868t
    non-medical 867–868
  place 871–872
  planning 871
  postpartum haemorrhage 989
  post-term pregnancy 870
  prolonged labour 995
  RCOG national guidelines 871–872
  timing 864
inevitable abortion 760–761
infant(s), physiological/biological
    outcomes, elective CS *vs*
    physiological birth 503
infant feeding *see* feeding
infant formulae *see* milk formulae
infant mortality 1040–1041
  causes 1040
  reduction 1036
  social factors 1041
infant mortality rate 1040, 1040f
  reduction 1041

infant therapy, ultrasound scan 322
infarction, placenta 516, 519
infection 703–714
  abortion 759, 762
  antepartum haemorrhage 776
  antibiotics 712
  cervical ripening 865
  delivery acquired 709–710
  maternal see maternal infection
  maternal screening 315–316
  neonatal defences 535, 703–704
  perinatal 708–710
    ascending infections 708–709
    invasive prenatal procedures 708
  postnatal 710–712
  postpartum haemorrhage 989
  preconception care 147
  prenatal 705–708
    presentation 705–706
    TORCH 705
  preterm baby 638
  prevention 704–705
    breastfeeding 705
    carer illness 565, 705
    cross-infection 565–566
    environment 704
    equipment 565, 704
    handwashing 565, 638, 704
    invasive procedures 704–705
    isolation procedures 704
    labour 448, 450
    preconceptual and antenatal care
      704
  recognition 705
    dramatic presentation 705
    management 705
    subtle presentation 705
  suturing of perineum 484
  transient tachypnoea of the newborn
    659
  water births 501
  see also individual infections
inferior vena cava, fetal 649
infertility 129–142
  assisted conception see assisted
    conception
  causes 130–133, 131t
    anovulation 130–131
    endometriosis 131
    male factor 132–133
    tubal factors 131–132
  chlamydia 824
  counselling 140–141
  male see male infertility
  poor nutrition 328
  stress 140–141
infibulation 834–836, 834f, 835f
inflammation, preparation for labour
  412
informed consent 1153
infundibulum 162, 206

inguinal glands 76
inhaled nitric oxide 662
inheritance
  genetics history 173
  history 173
inheritance modes 178–181
  autosomal characteristics/diseases
    178–180
    cystic fibrosis 179
  genetics 178–181
  multifactorial characteristics 181
  polygenic characteristics 181
  sex-linked characteristics/diseases
    180–181
    X-linked dominant inheritance
      180–181
    X-linked recessive inheritance
      180, 180f
    Y-linked 180
inheritance pattern, genetics 179f
Innocenti Declaration 591, 592b,
  613–620
instrumental vaginal deliveries
  970–977
  amniotomy 972
  cervical tears 481
  contraindications 972
  diet/fasting/nutrition 972
  history 970
  indications 972
  maternal complications 971
  midwifery aspects 971–972
  neonatal complications 971
  pain relief 972
  physical preparation 392
  policies 972
  position 972
  postnatal care 977
  procedure 972–973
  supportive presence 972
  syntocinon 972
  ventouse vs forceps 973
insulin
  fetal anabolic hormone 216, 533–534
  labour 808
  lung maturity 652
  pregnancy 808
interagency cooperation, Children Act
  1989 1158
interferons 703
intermittent positive-pressure
  ventilation (IPPV) 661
  complications 661
internal gradient 576
internal iliac veins, fetal 649
International Confederation of
  Midwives (ICM) 1110–1111,
  1110b
international organizations 1107–1111
International Year of the Family 373
intertrigo 566

intervillous space 193
intracranial trauma, instrumental
  deliveries 971
intracytoplasmic sperm injections
  (ICSI) 133, 133f
  outcome of 140
intrahepatic cholestasis of pregnancy
  (obstetric cholestasis) 812
intrapartum death, reduction measures
  1039
intrauterine contraceptive devices
  (IUCDs) 119–121, 120f
  contraindications 120
  diabetic woman 809
  emergency 123
  mode of action 120
  older mothers 125–126
  preconception care 153t
intrauterine growth restriction
  320–321, 321f
intrauterine insemination (IUI)
  134–135
intravenous feeding 636
intravenous fluid
  hyperemesis gravidarum 753
  moderate vomiting in pregnancy 753
intravenous line, caesarean section 982
intubation of pregnant women 980
intuitionistic pluralism, deontology
  1136
in-utero tracheal occlusion 680
in-utero transfer 568
investigation procedure, sudden infant
  death syndrome 718
in vitro fertilization (IVF) 129,
  136–137, 136f
  blastocyst transfer 138, 139f
  chlamydia 824
  costs 140
  drug management 135–136, 135f
  embryo grading 137, 138t
  embryo transfer 137–138, 138f
  ethics dilemmas 1135–1136
  fertilization 136–137, 136f
  fragmentation 137, 138f
  GnRH agonists 135, 136
  sperm preparation 136
  stress 140
involution of uterus 723–724
  progress assessment 726
iodine deficiency 800
iron
  deficiency, blood tests 314
  malabsorption 794
  maternal nutrition 334–335
  serum levels 794
  supplementation 794–795
    in pregnancy 793
    preterm baby 636–637
    side effects 795
  uptake, breast milk 595–596

iron-binding capacity 794
iron deficiency anaemia 794–795
    following postpartum haemorrhage
        994
iron–dextran complex (Imferon)
        795
ischial spine 67, 476
ischial tuberosity 66
ischiocavernosus muscles 478
ischiococcygeus muscles 478
ischiorectal fossa 478–479
ischium 66
isogel 1214
isolation procedures 704
isthmus 80b, 162

J

Jacquemier's sign 238
jaundice **684–695**
    causes 684
    conjugated hyperbilirubinaemia
        693–694
    instrumental deliveries 971
    newborn 545–546
    physiological 685
    physiology 684–685
    unconjugated hyperbilirubinaemia
        686–693
jaw thrust, resuscitation, neonate
        653–654, 654f
Jectofer 795
Jehovah's witness, refusal of blood
        1139
jitteriness 561–562
joint mobility, physiological responses
        to pregnancy 306
Journal of the American Medical
        Association, User guides to
        medical literature 56

K

Kallmann's syndrome 132
Kangaroo care 583
karyotyping
    chromosome analysis 177, 177f
    hydatidiform mole 765
kell cell antibodies 542–543
kernicterus 684, 689
    acute symptoms 689, 689t
    complications 689
    MRI 689
    risk factors 689
ketoacidosis, labour 972
ketones 257
kick charts 317–318

kidney(s)
    maternal changes 289, 293–294
    see also entries beginning renal
Kielland's forceps 971
Klebsiella, shock 999
Kleihauer test 687b
Klinefelter's syndrome 133
Klumpke's paralysis 949
knee presentation 895
knee rolling, abdominal exercises 391,
        391f
Kramer tool 687, 688f

L

labetolol hydrochloride 785, 1215
labial lacerations 487
labium majora 77b
labium minora 77b
laboratory diagnosis, pregnancy
        confirmation 238–240
labour
    active, definition 877
    active management see active
        management of labour
    anatomic issues 85
    characteristics 430
    complementary therapy use
        348–350
        see also complementary therapies,
            labour
    concept of care 466
    continuity of care 437–438
    continuum of 429–430
    coping strategies 389–390
        breathing 389–390
        relaxation 389
    environment 435–438
        see also birth environment
    female genital mutilation 834–835
    fetal response see fetal response to
        labour/birth
    fibroids (fibromyomata) 833
    first stage see labour, first stage
        (below)
    haemoglobinopathies 797
    heart disease in 799
    hypothermia 579
    induced see induced labour
    maternal preparation see maternal
        preparation for labour
    mental health issues 924
    multiple pregnancy see multiple
        pregnancy, labour
    obstructed 963–964
        causes 963
        face presentation 911, 913f
        management 964
        mortality/morbidity 964

    prevention 964
    signs/symptoms 963–964
    uterine rupture 966
occipitoposterior position 889–892
physiological/biological outcomes,
        elective CS vs physiological birth
        503
physiological changes in **410–427**
postpartum haemorrhage prevention
        989–990
precipitate 881
pre-eclampsia 789
preterm see preterm labour
previous traumatic, mental health
        issues 922, 924
prolonged see prolonged labour
relaxin 168–169
renal transplant 803
second stage see labour, second stage
        (below)
sexuality and 107
small-for-gestational-age baby
        643–644
stages 430
    time taken 430t
    see also individual stages (below)
symphysis pubis pain 277–278
temperature control 579
third stage see labour, third stage
        (below)
thyrotoxicosis 801
trial of
    conditions necessary 962
    management 962–963
    safety issues 962
    variety 428–429
    see also birth; delivery
labour, first stage 430
    active phase 442–443
        active management 442
    care in **433–435**
        advocacy 434–435
        emotional/psychological care
            433–434
        partnership in care 433
        role of birth supporter 434
    fetal condition 451–452
        electronic fetal monitoring 452
        healthy heart patterns 451–452
        see also fetal monitoring
    historically 1073
    latent phase 441–442
    midwifery care during 441–450
        assessment of progress 441–443
        bladder care 447
        infection prevention 448, 450
        loss per vaginam 447
        membrane rupture 447
            see also membranes
        mobility/ambulation 447–448
        moving/handling 448

positioning 449f
    see also positioning/posture
psychological examination
    446–447
upright posture 448
uterine activity 447
vaginal examination 443–446
new research 452
nutrition in 450–451
observations 439–441
    abdominal examination 439
    general examination 439
    records 440–441, 440f, 441f
    vaginal examination 439–440,
        443–446
    see also vaginal examination
onset 438–439
    contact of midwife 439
    mucoid/bloody show 438
    rupture of membranes 438–439
    uterine contractions 438
physiological changes 430b
    cervical effacement/dilatation
        430–431, 431f
    forewaters/hindwaters 432–433,
        433f
    mucoid/bloody show 433, 438
    rupture of membranes 433, 438–439
    uterine contractions 430–431
    see also uterine contractions
labour, second stage 430, **492–506**
bearing-down urge
    delayed 499
    early 498
definition 492
duration 496–497
episiotomy, assessing need 500
expulsive phase 493
    support during 498–500
future developments 503–504
historically 1073
mechanisms 494–496
    after birth 496
    crowning 494, 495f
    descent 494, 494f
    extension 495
    flexion 494
    internal rotation 494, 494f, 495f
    lateral flexion 495
    restitution 495
    shoulders, internal rotation 495,
        495f, 496f
midwifery care 497–500
    activities during birth 502–503
    expulsion support 498–500
    hygiene/comfort measures
        497–498
    transition support 498
observations/records 503
optimal fetal positioning 500
perineal practices 499

physiology 493–496
positions 497
preparation for birth 501–502
prolonged 880
pushing techniques 435, 499
signs of progression 492–493
transition 492–493
    support during 498
labour, third stage 430, **507–523**
active management 493, 513–516
    see also active management of
        labour
choices 508
complications **987–1002**, 1000
    see also individual complications
definition 507
expectant management 507–508,
    511–513
    active management *vs* 514
    lack of skill in midwives
        513–514
management 511–517
midwives' role 508
mismanagement
    acute inversion of uterus 996
    postpartum haemorrhage 989
physiology 508–511
    factors affecting 511
prolonged *see* prolonged labour
risks 507
lacerations
    cervix 993–994
    fetal skull 232
    labial 487
lactation
    drug suppression 729, 1223
    following postpartum haemorrhage
        994
    initiation 602, 724
    maintenance 602–603
    natural suppression 729
    physiology 601–603
        puberty to pregnancy 601–602
    preparation 303–304
    see also breastfeeding; breast milk
lactational amenorrhoea method
    (LAM) 117
lactic acid 78
lactiferous ducts
    embryology 600
    structure 601
lactobacilli (Döderlein's bacilli) 78
Lactobacillus bifidus, breast milk
    703
lactoferrin, breast milk 596t, 703
lactogenesis 602
lactose, breast milk 595
lactulose 272, 1213
La Leche League's (LLL) Peer
    Counsellor programme 613
Lamaze preparation 464

language
    problems
        antenatal care 267
        mental health issues 920
    social construction 5
    value 5
lanugo 633
laparotomy, uterine rupture 967
large-for-gestational-age baby (LGA),
    hypoglycaemia 698
large luteal cells (LLC) 168
laryngeal mask airway (LMA) 654–655
    meconium 654
last menstrual period (LMP) 247
    post-term pregnancy dating 868
'late' anaemia 687
    symptoms 687
law and midwives *see* legal issues
Law Reform Act 1945, law defences
    contributory negligence 1149
laxatives 272, 1213–1214
lead, preconception care 153t
leaders
    career development 1180–1182
    definition 1171–1172
    distinguishing features 1175t, 1178t
leadership
    gender/race 1179
    midwives **1167–1184**
    styles 1179–1180, 1180t
    theories 1174–1177
Lea's shield 119
lecithin (L), lung maturation marker
    660
left mentoanterior position (LMA), face
    presentation 910f, 911
    delivery 911, 911f, 912f
left mentolateral position (LML), face
    presentation 910, 910f
left mentoposterior position (LMP),
    face presentation 910, 910f
left sacroanterior position (LSA),
    breech presentation 900, 900f
left sacrolateral position (LSL), breech
    presentation 900, 900f
left sacroposterior position (LSP),
    breech presentation 900, 900f
legal issues **1142–1166**
    abortion 762
    Acts *see* Acts, of Parliament
    birth 1156–1159
        attendance 1157
        criminal law 1157
    care of property 1160
    children 1156–1159
        see also Children Act 1989
    civil law 1163–1164
        see also civil law
    classification 1142–1143
        private law 1143
        public law 1143

legal issues (*contd*)
clinical negligence 1145
claims (England) 1145b
Clinical Negligence Scheme for
Trusts 1161–1162
NHS Litigation Authority
(NHSLA) 1162
Commission for Health
Improvement, The (CHI) 1162
complaints 1160
Congenital Disabilities (civil liability)
Act 1976 1161
consent 1151–1156, 1152b
health and safety 1159
litigation 1145
medicines 1160
National Institute of Clinical
Excellence, The (NICE) 1162
national service framework (NSF)
1162–1163
negligence 1145–1149
see also negligence
perineal trauma 488
pregnancy 1156–1159
record keeping 1159–1160
sources 1143–1145
code of professional conduct 1144
common law 1143
Human Rights Act, The 1998
1143–1144
legislation 1143
midwife rules 1144, 1144b
Nurses, Midwives and Health
Visitors Act (1997) 1144
ratio decidendi 1143
supervision 1145
stillbirth, registration 1156
vaccine damage 1160–1161
legislation *see* midwifery legislation
legs
cramp
labour 497
pregnancy 274
examination 555
tightening, circulatory exercises 386
see also limb
length, newborn 544, 545f
leptin
fertilization 165
menstrual cycle 95
lesbians, pregnancy/childbirth 108
let-down reflex 602
leucocytes, breast milk 597t
levator ani 477
Levonelle 2 123
levothyroxine sodium (thyroxine
sodium), congenital
hypothyroidism 701
liability exemption 1149
lidocaine (lignocaine) hydrochloride
500, 1219

lie
abdominal examination 259, 260f
induction 863
transverse/oblique *see* shoulder
presentation
see also malpresentations
'Life will never be the same' report 374
ligamentum teres 650
ligamentum venosum 650
lightening 238
lignocaine (lidocaine) hydrochloride
500, 1219
limb
abnormalities 676–677
see also arms; legs
limb reduction deformities 677
causes 677
linea nigra 263
lip reading, health care setting
268–269
liquid paraffin 272, 1214
Listeria monocytogenes 251, 707
preconception care advice 148t
listeriosis 707
intrauterine infection 707
maternal presentation 707
maternal screening 316
neonatal symptoms 707
preconception care advice 148t
lithium, breastfeeding 931
lithotomy pole (leg restraints), suturing
perineal trauma 485
lithotomy position
acute inversion of uterus 997
instrumental vaginal deliveries 973
Wood's manoeuvre 944
litigation, legal issues 1145
liver
development 216–217
fetal carbohydrate metabolism 216
newborn examination 553
liver function tests, pre-eclampsia 784
local anaesthesia
bupivacaine 470, 1219
see also epidural anaesthesia
local authority
child minding regulations 1058
children living away from home
1058
Local Supervising Authority (LSA)
1128
function 1128
proposed standards 1127–1128
responsible midwifery officers 1128
Local Supervising Authority Midwife
1128
lochia 724
alba 724
duration 726
rubra 724
serosa 724

locked twins 844
long-chain polyunsaturated fatty acids
(LCPUFA), breast milk 595
lover/mother syndrome 110
Lövset's manoeuvre 907–908, 907f
low back pain, pregnancy 274
low birthweight (LBW) 630
milk formulae 635b
lower segment caesarean section
(LSCS), fetal lung fluid 651
lumbar vertebra (5th) 66
lumbosacral joint 68
lung(s)
development 209–211, 210f
examination, antenatal care 256
fetal 649
volume, alterations in pregnancy
296f
see also entries beginning pulmonary
lung buds 650
lung disease, chronic (CLD) 637–638,
660
risk factors 660
survival 638
treatment 660
lung fluid 529, 651
fetal 650
absorption in caesarean section
978
displacement 651
function 529
luteal phase, fertilization 169
luteinization 168
luteinizing hormone (LH)
dominant follicle selection 91
fertilization 167
luteinization 168
male infertility 132
mid-cycle surge 92
natural family planning 117
oestrogen 117
oocyte maturation 95
physiological response in pregnancy
298
luteotrophic human chorionic
gonadotrophin (hCG) 167
lying-in hospitals 1078
lymphatic drainage
breasts 601
uterus 82
vagina 78
lymphocytes 703
lysozyme, breast milk 596t, 703

M

macrosomia *see* fetal macrosomia
magnesium sulphate 1215
eclampsia 787

preterm labour 857–858
toxicity 787
magnesium supplementation,
hypomagnesaemia 699
magnetic resonance imaging (MRI)
cardiac abnormalities 663
fetal assessment 323
kernicterus 689
maternal assessment 323
neonatal assessment 323
placental assessment 323
malaria 712
male genitalia
anatomy 20b, 21b, 83–86
newborn examination 554
male infertility
luteinizing hormone 132
poor nutrition 328
male midwives 1075–1076, 1186
male pill 116
Mallory–Weiss syndrome, hyperemesis
gravidarum 753
malpositions **884–917**
clinical assessment 886
identification 884–885
incidence 885–886
labour
prolonged 496
second stage 500
occiput see occipitoposterior position
ultrasound scan 321
umbilical cord presentation/prolapse
955
malpresentations **884–917**
clinical assessment 886
identification 884–885
incidence 885–886
multiple pregnancy 844
placenta praevia 770
ultrasound scan 321–322
see also breech presentation; brow
presentation; face presentation;
shoulder presentation
mammary gland 303–304
hormonal regulation 304
menstrual cycle changes 100–101
pre-lactational adaptations 303–304
see also breast(s)
mammogenesis 601–602
management, midwives **1167–1184**
management styles 1179–1180, 1180t
management theories 1174–1177
manager
distinguishing features 1175t
role 1172–1173
mandible 224f
man-midwife 1075–1076, 1077f
manual rotation, occipitoposterior
position 892
Marcain (bupivacaine) 1219
epidural analgesia 470

Marfan's syndrome 798–799
marital status, history taking 246–247
mask of pregnancy 236
massage 15, 343
constipation 345, 345f
oedema 15, 346, 346f
pain relief 464–465
massive obstetric haemorrhage
992–993
mastitis 610–611, 729
diagnosis 611
infective 611
non-infective 610–611
Maternal and Child Welfare Act of
1918 241
maternal assessment, magnetic
resonance imaging 323
maternal dehydration, prolonged
labour 877
maternal examination
abdominal see abdominal
examination
cephalic disproportion 960
vaginal examination 439–440
see also vaginal examination
maternal history 542, 542b
maternal hypothalamic–pituitary–
placental axis 298
maternal-infant attachment 423
caesarean section 981–982
sensory contact 421, 421f
see also mother-baby relationship
maternal infection
screening 315–316
shoulder dystocia 947
spontaneous abortion 759
maternal instinct 563
maternal monitoring, water birth 501
maternal mortality/morbidity 1103
acute inversion of uterus 997
amniotic fluid embolism 1000
caesarean section (CS) 978
causes 1043t, 1101–1102, 1102f
confidential enquiries 1043
definition 1041–1043
domestic violence 364–365
eclampsia 786, 787
epidemiological factors 1104, 1104b
epilepsy 811–812
fetal surgery 680
historical issues 1076, 1085,
1104–1106, 1106t
indirect causes 1045–1046
instrumental vaginal deliveries 971
modernity 1104, 1105f
obstructive labour 964
postpartum haemorrhage 987, 994
prolonged labour 877–878
reduction 1027, 1027b
recommendations 1044, 1045
Registrar-General's Office 1109

risk 1102–1103, 1102t
Royal Maternity Charity 1110
skilled attendance requirement
1104–1105
symphysiotomy 946–947
Zavanelli manoeuvre 946
see also birth, morbidity following
maternal mortality rate 1041, 1042f,
1100–1101, 1101t
maternal mortality ratio (MMR)
1100–1101
maternal nutrition **327–337**
breastfeeding 608
essential nutrients 330–335
labour 450–451, 972
necessity 327–328
periconceptional 328–329
perinatal death 1038
pre-eclampsia 782
therapeutic intervention 335–336
weight in pregnancy 329
maternal preparation for labour
410–418
cervical changes 411–412
contractions/spontaneous pushing
417
expulsive phase 418
inflammation 412
myometrial changes 411–412
oestrogens and oxytocin receptors
411
oxytocin 414–418
placental steroids 410–411
progesterone 412
prostaglandins 413–414
spontaneous breathing 418
tissue changes 412
uterine changes 411
maternal prolactin 201f
see also prolactin
maternal serum screening for Down's
syndrome (MSSDS) 316–317
Maternity Alliance (1994) 268
mental health issues 924
maternity services
nurse training 1186
perinatal death 1039–1040
reduction measures 1039
planning 20
Matthew Duncan presentation 510
Mauriceau–Smellie–Veit manoeuvre
905–906, 906f
maxilla 224f
McDonald suture 984
McRoberts' manoeuvre 908, 941–942,
943f
mean corpuscular haemoglobin
(MCH), iron deficiency anaemia
794
mean corpuscular volume (MCV), iron
deficiency anaemia 794

meconium 533
  breech presentation 897
  imperforate anus 674
  neonatal resuscitation 656–657
  passage 533
    breast milk 594
    preterm baby 634–635
  staining 503
meconium aspiration syndrome 503, 658–659
  causes 658
  post-term pregnancy 869
  shoulder dystocia 948
  small-for-gestational-age baby 644
meconium ileus, cystic fibrosis 699
median nerve compression 274
medical approach, health promotion 359t
Medical Certificate of Stillbirth 44, 1037
medical examination, antenatal care 256–257
medical herbalism 342
medical history 249
Medical Subject Headings (MeSH) 55
Medicinal Products: Prescription by Nurses Act 1992 1223–1224
medicines
  legal issues 1160
  see also drugs
Medicines Act 1968 1211–1212
Medline 55
medulla oblongata 227f
megaloblastic anaemia 795
meiosis
  cell division 176, 176f
  zygote 165
melanocyte-stimulating hormone (MSH) 215
membranes
  artificial rupture of, umbilical cord presentation/prolase 955
  delivery 512–513
    active management of labour 516
    examination after 516–517, 517f
  examination 444–445
    multiple pregnancy 846
  intact, prostaglandins 413–414
  preterm prelabour rupture see preterm prelabour rupture of the membranes (PPROM)
  rupture of 433, 438–439
    assessment 447
    prostaglandins 414
    umbilical cord presentation/ prolapse 955
  stripping the 865
  sweeping 865
men see entries beginning male
Mendel, Gregor 172–173
  genetics history 172–173

Mendelson's syndrome (acid aspiration syndrome) 450
  caesarean section 980
meningitis 712
menopause, sexuality 110–111
menstrual cycle 89–97, 89f
  adenohypophysis 94
  changes during 163
  folliculogenesis 90–91
  menses 90
  mid-cycle LH/FSH surge 92
  oocyte maturation 95
  ovarian cycle 91
  ovarian regulation 91–94, 92f
  ovulation 96–97, 96f
  physiological changes 116f
  preovulatory follicle 94–95
  proliferative phase 89–90
  secretary phase 90
menstrual history 247
mental health
  history 924, 926
  preconception care 154t
  problems see mental health problems
Mental Health Act 1983, consent refusal 1154
mental health care, midwives' role
  antenatal period 919–924
  confidential enquiries into maternal deaths (CEMD) 931–932
  labour/delivery 924
  postnatal 926–927
  puerperal psychosis 930–931
mental health problems **918–935**
  at risk patients 919
  confidential enquiries into maternal deaths (CEMD) 931–932
  drugs/breastfeeding 931
  history taking 249
  incidence 919
  labour/delivery 924
  maternal mortality 919
  midwife's role in antenatal period 919–924
  see also mental health care
  postnatal 924–931, 925t
mental health promotion 357
mentovertical circumference, newborn skull 222f
meptazinol (Meptid) 469, 1216–1217
Meptid (meptazinol) 469, 1216–1217
mercury, preconception care 153t
messenger RNA (mRNA) 175
metabolic acidosis 537, 658
metabolic changes, nausea 751
metabolic disorders **696–702**
  acquired 697–699
  inborn 697
  screening 696
metabolism, neonatal see neonatal metabolism

meta-ethics, ethics definition 1133
methyldopa (Aldomet) 785, 1215–1216
methylprednisolone, hyperemesis gravidarum 754
metoclopramide, Mendelson's syndrome 980
metronidazole 824
microcephaly 672
  causes 672
  types 672
micturition
  frequency of, pregnancy 236
  labour 497
  postnatal 727
midwifery care
  birth units 436–437
  history 241
  TENS usage 466
Midwifery Leadership Competency Model 1169, 1169f
midwifery legislation 1116–1119, 1143
  current 1118–1119
  history 1116–1117
  licensing 1075
  recent changes 1117–1118
  registration 1082, 1084–1085
  statutory bodies 1116–1117, 1116f
  supervision 1127–1130
midwifery practice audits
  audit of practice 904
  standing breech birth 904
midwifery standards 1022
midwife ventouse practitioners (MVP) 977
midwives
  advocacy 434–435
  breastfeeding knowledge 599–600
  care during labour 441–450
    first stage see labour, first stage, midwifery care during
    second stage see labour, second stage, midwifery care
  career development 1180–1182
  child protection 1060–1061, 1060b
  children in need assessment 598
  competence lack 1125
  contact of, labour onset 439
  continuity of career 437–438
  cultural context 3–13
  development of **1071–1099**
  education see education and training
  future of 1095–1097
  history of 6, **1071–1099**
    church and law 1074
    governing 1074–1075
    under threat 1076–1078
  international perspectives **1100–1115**
  leadership **1167–1184**

lifelong learning **1185–1208**
male 1075–1076, 1077f, 1186
management **1167–1184**
mental health care *see* mental health care
minimum educational standard 1189
models of working 402–404
NHS reform 1015–1016, 1086
office of 1071–1073
partnership in care 433
postnatal role 725
psychological context 14–26
public health role 358–360
quality **1021–1033**
recruitment/retention problems 1094–1095
self-development 1180–1182
sociology 4
state control 1085–1086
statutory requirements **1116–1132**
supervision *see* supervision
working overseas 1111–1112
Zavanelli manoeuvre 946
Midwives Act 1902 241–243, 401, 1209
history and development 1082–1085
Midwives Act 1936 401
Midwives' Institute 1082
Midwives Liaison Committee 1111
The Midwives Rules 266
midwives' rules and code of practice (UKCC 1998) 1125–1126
HIV infection 821
law sources 1144, 1144b
medication 1127, 1209–1210, 1211
midwifery practice 1126–1127
perineal trauma 488
pre-registration education 1123–1124
supervision 1127
water births 500
mifepristone 763
labour inducer 868t
licensing 763
milk duct, blockage 729
milk formulae
breast milk *vs* 614–615t
casein dominant 615, 616t
hypernatraemia 699
low birth weight 635b
preparation 618, 619f, 620f
ready-to-feed 616
regulations 615
types available 616
whey dominant 615, 616t
see also artificial feeding
milk insufficiency 608–609, 729
milk powder *see* milk formulae
MIND 918
minerals

breast milk 595–596
supplements, preterm baby 636–637
Mirena intrauterine system (IUS) 120–121
miscarriage
cervical cerclage 984
history taking 248
parental grief 34
ultrasound scan 319
misconduct 1121, 1125
Nursing and Midwifery Council (NMC) 1121f, 1125
misoprostol
active management of labour 515
labour inducer 866t, 868t
missed abortion 761
expectant management 761
fetus papyraceous 761
medical inducement 761
ultrasound scan 319
misshapen head, supine sleeping 716
Misuse of Drugs Regulations 1211–1212
mitochondrial dysfunction, antiretroviral combination therapy 819
mitosis, cell division 175–176, 176f
mobility, labour 447–448
Modernisation Agency 1010
Mongolian spots 545
monoamine oxidase inhibitors (MAOIs), contraindications 1216, 1217
monoamniotic twins 844
monoclonal antibody tests/indirect agglutination, pregnancy diagnosis 239
monosomy, chromosome anomalies 178
monozygotic (monozygous) twins 840
cause 840
fetal abnormalities 844
incidence 840
placentae 841
zygosity determination 840–841
mons veneris 77b
moral conflict, ethics importance 1134–1135
moral dilemma
code of professional conduct (UKCC 1992) 1135
ethics importance 1135
principles 1137
moral rights, ethics definition 1134
morning sickness 752
see also vomiting
Moro reflex (startle reflex) 559, 949
morphine 468, 1217
mortality
perinatal *see* perinatal mortality/ morbidity

see fetal mortality/morbidity; maternal mortality/morbidity; neonatal mortality/death
morula 166
mother
advantages of breastfeeding 598
heat source 583
hypothalamic–pituitary–adrenal (HPA) axis 302
pethidine effects 468–469
see also entries beginning maternal
mother and baby homes 1058
mother-baby relationship 10, 562–563
breastfeeding 603–604
communication 562–563
delayed 24
identity 563
initial reactions 538
multiple births 848–849
preterm baby 637
psychological aspect 23–24
stages 563
symphysis pubis pain 278
motherhood
early days 24
ideology 10
social construction 6
moulding of skull 227–229, 229f, 230f, 230t
sugar loaf 887
mourning
tasks of 28b, 30
see also grief
mouth
newborn examination 549, 550b
pregnancy changes 271
mouth-to-mouth resuscitation 652–653
movements, fetal *see* fetal movements
moving, during labour 448
moxibustion, breech presentation 347, 899
mRNA (messenger RNA) 175
MUC-1, implantation 192
mucoid/bloody show 433, 438
assessment 447
Müllerian duct anomalies 794, 829
multidisciplinary practice, NHS 1014
multifactorial characteristics, genetics inheritance modes 181
multifetal pregnancy reduction 850
multigravida women
antenatal visits 255
labour, second stage 501–502
multiparity
placenta praevia 769
umbilical cord presentation/prolapse 955
see also multiple pregnancy
Multiple Births Foundation (MBF) 842
bereavement advice 849

multiple pregnancy **839–852**
  antenatal
    preparation 842–843
    screening 842
  assisted contraception 129
  breastfeeding 843, 847–848
  complications 843–844
  diagnosis 841–842
    auscultation 842
    inspection 842
    palpation 842
  following assisted conception 140
  incidence 839–840, 839f, 839t
  labour
    anesthesia 845
    complications 844–845
    first stage 845
    intrapartum care 844–847
    onset 845
    preterm 844, 845
    prolonged 844
    second stage 845–846
    third stage 846
  malpresentation 844, 846
  mortality rates 849, 849f
  mother-baby relationship 848–849
  parental education 842–843
  parental support 848
  placenta/membrane examination 846
  placenta praevia 769, 844
  postnatal care 847–850
  postpartum haemorrhage 988
  pre-eclampsia 843
  ultrasound scan 319, 841–842
  umbilical cord presentation/prolapse 955
  see also dizygotic twins; monozygotic twins; triplets; twins
multiple sclerosis, preconception care 150t
Munchausen syndrome by proxy 1062
mural granulosa cells 91
  proliferation 92
murmurs, heart in newborn 548
muscles, myometrium responses to pregnancy 305, 305f
musculoskeletal system
  antenatal care 273–274
  newborn 534
  newborn examination 550–551
    lower extremities 555–556, 555b
    spine 556
    upper extremities 551, 551b
  physical preparation for childbirth
    abdominal exercises 387
    antenatal exercises 386
    back care 385–386, 385f
    circulatory exercises 386–387
    pelvic floor exercises 387
    physiological effects 385
    posture 385f

postnatal changes 724
  relaxin 385
musculoskeletal systems, adaptations to pregnancy 306
myelomeningocele reconstruction 680
myomectomy, fibroids (fibromyomata) 833
myometrial relaxants 1216
myometrium 79
  changes in preparation for labour 411–412
  following birth 420
  implantation 191
  oxytocin 414, 435
  physiological responses to pregnancy 304–305
  rupture 966
MZ twins *see* monozygotic twins

N

Naegele's rule 247, 248
Naegele's type (asymmetrical pelvis) 74t
naevus flammeus (port-wine stain) 546, 678
naevus simplex 678
naloxone hydrochloride (Narcan) 469, 1222
  neonatal resuscitation 657
nappy, changing 533
nappy rash 567
Narcan (naloxone hydrochloride) 1222
  neonatal resuscitation 657
narcotic antagonists, neonatal resuscitation 657
nasal flaring 530
naso/orogastric feeding 636f
naso/orojejunal feeding 636, 636f
nasopharyngeal suction 503
National Birth Centre Study 437
National Childbirth Trust (NCT) 927
  active childbirth movement 1089
  birth partners 434
  mental health issues 924
National Clinical Assessment Authority 1010
National Gamete Donation Trust 139
National Health Service (NHS) **1005–1020**
  caesarean section costs 979
  clinical governance 1009–1010
  contraception 114
  cultural change 1018
  current problems 1007–1009
  future of 1016–1018
  health inequalities 1011–1012
  history of 1006

multidisciplinary practice 1014
  organization structure 1167–1170
  partnership development 1014–1015
  patient involvement 1012
  performance improvement 1009–1010
  plan 358
  primary care 1010–1011
  public health promotion 1011–1012
  quality issues **1021–1033**
  reform 1009–1016, 1086
  restructuring 1015
  social care 1014
  staff development 1012–1013
  staff shortage 1013, 1017
  staff support 1012–1013
  targets 1009
National Health Service University (NHSU) 1194
National Institute for Clinical Excellence (NICE) 57, 1010
  breech presentation guidelines 904
  confidential enquiries 1036
  legal issues 1162
National Patient Safety Agency 1010
National Sentinel Caesarean Section Audit 977–978
National Service Framework (NSF) 1009, 1025
  legal issues 1162–1163
nausea 240, **751–757**
  antenatal care 236, 271
  causes 751–752
  complementary therapy 344–345
  diagnostic tests 751–752
  history 248
  nutritional therapy 344–345, 751–757
  see also vomiting
neck, newborn examination 550, 550b
necrobiosis (red degeneration) 833
necrotizing enterocolitis (NEC) 641, 710
  breast milk 641
  predisposing factors 641
  radiography 641, 642f
negligence
  breach of duty 1146–1147
    Bolam Test 1146–1147
  causation 1147
  consent 1151–1153
  delegation 1148
  duty of care 1145–1146
  factual causation 1147–1148
  harm 1148
  intervening causes 1148
  legal issues 1145–1149
  personal liability 1148
  reasonably foreseeable harm 1148
  student liability 1148
  supervision 1148

unqualified assistant liability 1148
vicarious liability 1148
negligence elements 1149
negligent advice 1161
legal issues 1161
Neisseria gonorrhoeae 709, 822
neonatal convulsions 562, 698
signs 698
neonatal herpes 823
neonatal intensive care unit (NICU),
environment 641–642
neonatal metabolism 594
carbohydrate digestion 594
fat digestion 594, 595
protein digestion 594
neonatal mortality/death 36–38, 1040
complications 35–36
instrumental vaginal deliveries 971
parental grief 35–36
parental memories 37
photographs 38
time with the baby 37–38
washing/dressing the baby after
death 38
neonatal mortality rate 1040, 1040f
neonatal pain 681–682
causes 561
relief *see* pain relief
responses 681
signs 561
neonatal problems
diabetic woman 809
renal transplant 803
neonatal respiration 530–531
abnormal signs 530
assessment 547
breathing movements 530
chest moving symmetrically 530
diaphragm moving symmetrically
530
breathing rate 530, 545
control 530–531
rib cage and respiratory musculature
530
neonatal skin 532
abdominal 552
assessment 545–546, 545b, 559
colour 545
neonatal skull, external structures
222–223, 222f
circumferences 222f
layers 223
neonatal surgery 680–681
postoperative care 681
preoperative care 680
thermoregulation 584
neonatal tetany *see* hypocalcaemia
neonatal thyrotoxicosis 701
neonatal transport 568–570
incubator 569
midwife skills required 568–569

parental support 569–570
record-keeping 570
status monitoring 569
thermoregulation 582
neonatal varicella zoster
immunoglobulin 707
neonatal ventilators 661
neonatal withdrawal syndrome 1219
neonate
antibiotics use guidelines 712
assessment, magnetic resonance
imaging 323
bathing 565–566
behaviour 563–564
breastfeeding problems 611–612
consciousness level 534, 535b
diabetic woman 809
examination **539–541**, 518
abdominal examination *see*
abdominal examination,
neonate
bony injury 949
equipment 540f, 541, 541b
instrumental deliveries 977
musculoskeletal system *see*
musculoskeletal system,
newborn examination
neurological *see* neurological
function, newborn examination
preparation 540–541
testes 554
thermoregulation 536
feeding 591–627
follow-up 565
gastrointestinal tract maturation 594
general appearance 543–545, 544t
HIV infection 818
hygiene 565
identification 538–539
immediate care 518
jaundice *see* jaundice
legal rights of 527–528
maternal thyrotoxicosis 800
nutrition
full-term requirements 593–594
preterm 608, 635–637
physical assessment 541–564
physiological/biological outcomes,
elective CS *vs* physiological birth
503
positioning after birth 512
active management of labour 515
postnatal care 564–567
record keeping 567–568
resuscitation *see* resuscitation, neonate
saliva 597
screening tests 566–567
skin *see* neonatal skin
temperature control *see*
thermoregulation
see also entries beginning neonatal

nephropathy, diabetic 806
nerve transmission, pain physiology
461–462
neural folds 206
neural plate 206
neural tube 206
neural tube defects
folic acid supplements 332–333
maternal blood tests 316–317
neurocranium 220
neuroendocrine reflex, oxytocin
synthesis and secretion 416f
neurogenic shock 998
neurohormonal reflex 602
neurological damage, extracorporeal
membrane oxygenation 662
neurological function, newborn
examination 558–562, 558b
consciousness level 534, 535b
mental status 559
physical 558–559
reflexes 559–560
newborn *see* neonate
New Man 10
NHS *see* National Health Service
(NHS)
NHS Executive (1999), evidence-based
practice 52
NHS Litigation Authority (NHSLA),
Clinical Negligence Scheme for
Trusts 1162
niacin (vitamin B_3), maternal nutrition
332
nifedipine 785, 858
nipple(s)
antenatal preparation 254–255
care 254
cracked/sore 609–610, 728
cracked /sore 609–610
damage assessment 610
moist healing 610
inverted 254
pain, Raynaud's phenomenon 610
shields
cracked/sore nipples 610
milk production 609
structure 601
nipple stimulation
active management of labour 515
cervical ripening 348
labour 107
nitric oxide, respiratory support 662
nitrous oxide 467–468
absorption though placenta 468f
non-identical twins *see* dizygotic twins
nonoxynol 9 119
non-shivering thermogenesis 577
noradrenaline (norepinephrine)
fetal response to labour 419f
oxytocin inhibition 433
shock 998–999

Noristerat 122
'normal' birth 1093–1094
normal saline, neonatal resuscitation 658
normogram 876, 877f
norpethidine 469
Northern Ireland, NHS restructuring 1015
North Staffordshire Changing Childbirth Research Team (NSCCRT), shared care scheme 244
nose, newborn examination 549–550, 550b
nose to nipple feeding position 604, 605f
nuchal translucency thickness measurement 320
    cardiac abnormalities 663
    multiple pregnancy 842
nurse cells 161
Nurses, Midwives and Health Visitors Act (1979) 1089–1090
Nurses, Midwives and Health Visitors Act (1997), law sources 1144
Nursing and Midwifery Council (NMC)
    complaints procedure 1121f
    conduct standards 1125
    consultation document 1118
    establishment 1118, 1119
    functions 1119–1120, 1122–1130
    legal assessors 1121
    medical assessors 1121
    medication guidelines 1210
    membership 1120
    misconduct 1121f, 1125
    Register 1122
    registrant assessors 1121
    statutory committees 1120–1121
        conduct and competence 1120, 1125
        health 1120
        investigating 1120
        midwifery 1120
        orders 1120–1121
    striking off 1121
    structure 1119, 1119f
    visitors 1122
nutritional therapy 335–336, 344
nutrition/diet
    changes in menstrual cycle 89
    diabetic woman 251, 807–808
    ethnic minority groups 267
    labour 450–451, 972
    maternal 327–337
        see also maternal nutrition
    neonate 593–594
    preconception care 145, 146t
    pregnancy 251
    preterm baby 608, 635–637
    supplements
        constipation 272
        preconceptual care 146t

O

obesity
    maternal, shoulder dystocia 940
    polycystic ovary syndrome 131
    preconception care 146t
    pregnancy 256–257
obliques (external), abdominal muscles 384
obliques (internal), abdominal muscles 384
obliterated hypogastric arteries 650
obstetric care
    diabetic woman 808
    information 379
obstetric cholestasis (intrahepatic cholestasis of pregnancy) 812
obstetric history, preconception care 154t
obstetrician 1071
    trial of labour 962
obstetric manipulations, umbilical cord presentation/prolapse 955
obstetrics, procedures in 970–986
    caesarean section 977–983
    cervical cerclage 983–984, 983f
    instrumental vaginal deliveries 970–977
    see also individual procedures
obstructed labour see labour, obstructed
obturator foramen 66
occipital bone 224f, 225f
    development 220
occipital protuberance 224f
occipitofrontal circumference, newborn skull 222f
occipitoposterior position 886–893
    care in labour 893
    causes 885
    complications 893t
    diagnosis 889
    fetal head
        deflexion 890f
        extension 892
        flexion 890, 890f
    fetal position 886–887, 887f, 888f
    incidence 885
    labour 889–892
    manual rotation 892
    persistent 890–892, 891f
    umbilical cord presentation/prolapse 955
    vaginal examination 889
occiput 222f
occlusive caps 118–119, 118f
    spermicide with 119
occult sphincter damage 740
occupation see employment issues

oedema 259
    ankle 259
    complementary therapies 346
    gingival 271
    massage 15, 346, 346f
    pre-eclampsia 783, 785
    pulmonary see pulmonary oedema
oesophageal atresia (OA) 673–674
    at birth 673
    complications 674
    nursing 674
    surgery 674
    survival rates 674
oestradiol 100
    fertilization 168
oestrogen
    FSH/LH inhibition 298
    hypersensitivity 812
    mammary gland regulation 304
    menstrual cycle 288, 288f
    musculoskeletal system physiological effect 385
    myometrium responses to pregnancy 305
    oral contraceptives 121
    oxytocin receptors and 411
    prolactin, effects on 298
    receptors, subtypes 410
    renal haemodynamic changes 289
oligohydramnios
    associated conditions 322
    post-term pregnancy 869
oliguria, pre-eclampsia 785
omphalitis 710
oocytes
    collection 136
    freezing 139
    fusion with spermatozoon 164–165
    maturation 95
    ovarian cycle 91
    rhythmic secretion 163
    transport 162
operative procedures see obstetrics, procedures in
ophthalmia neonatorum 710
    causative organisms 710
    presentation 710
opioid analgesia 468
    see also endogenous opioids
oral contraception 121
    breastfeeding 602, 1223
    care of woman 122–123
    diabetic woman 809
    emergency 123
    hydatidiform mole 766
    nutrient deficiency 328
    postpartum 114, 125
    preconception care 153t
Order for Burial, stillbirth 1037
Orem's self-care model 246
organ donation 40

organogenesis 144, 194, 205–217
Origin of the Species 172
Ortolani test 557–558, 557f
Osiander's sign 238
ossification
    intramembranous 220
    physiological responses to pregnancy 306
    skull bones 220–222, 221f
osteitis 711
osteochondrodysplasias 677
osteomalacic pelvis 74t
osteopathy 341
    regulation 341
otitis media 711
outcome measurement 1026
out-door charities 1078
ovarian arteries 82
ovarian cycle 91
ovarian cysts 833
ovarian failure 131
ovarian hyperstimulation syndrome (OHSS) 134
ovarian ligaments 80b
ovarian veins 82
ovaries 80b
    non-pregnant 79f
overheating, sudden infant death syndrome 716–717
overseas, working 1111–1112
ovulation 96–97
    mediators participating 96f
    postnatal period 724
ovulation induction 134
oxygen consumption, changes in pregnancy 295–296, 296f
oxygen tension, organogenesis/placenta formation 195
oxygen therapy 661
    complications 661
    preterm baby 634
    shock 999
    thermoregulation 581–582, 588
    umbilical cord presentation/prolapse 957
oxytocic drugs 1219–1221
    active management of labour 513
    amniotomy 867
    bleeding control 511
    labour, second stage 502
    massive obstetric haemorrhage 992–993
    maternal heart disease 799
    postpartum haemorrhage treatment 990, 991
    trial of labour 962, 963
    uterine rupture 965–966
    see also active management of labour
oxytocin 1220
    active management of labour 515
    after birth 421

daytime plasma levels 415f
endogenous opioids and 303
with ergometrine 1220–1221
inhibition 415, 433
intrauterine 416–417
labour inducer 866t, 867
lactogenesis 602, 1210
late pregnancy to birth 414
levels during labour 415f
mammogenesis 601
menstrual cycle 94
nocturnal release 414
pattern of systemic 415–416
pregnancy to labour 414–415
prolonged labour 879–880, 995
receptors, oestrogen 411
synthesis and secretion 416f
trial of labour 963
uterine responses to pregnancy 305
    see also oxytocic drugs
oxytocinase 414

P

pacifiers see dummies
packed cell volume (PCV), iron deficiency anaemia 794
pain **458–472**
    coping strategies 459, 463
    cultural aspects 463–464
    definition 458–459
    education, antenatal care 459–460
    endogenous opioids role in 303
    gate theory 462–463
        TENS 465
    maternal threshold, endogenous opioids 303
    neonates see neonatal pain
    nipples 609–610, 728
    origins of labour pain 460–463
    pathways 462f
    physiological effects 460
    preparation for childbirth 459–460
    psychology of 459
    symphysis pubis 277–278
pain relief
    acupuncture 349
    asthma 811
    caesarean section 982
    concept of support 466–467
    first use 1081–1082
    instrumental vaginal deliveries 972
    lumbar epidural 469–471
    newborn
        environmental 681
        interventional techniques 681
        management 560–561
        pharmacological 681
        sucrose 561, 681

perineal 727
pharmacological 467–471
    nitrous oxide 467–468
    systemic analgesia 468–469
    positions/massage 464–465
    postnatal period 729–730
    prolonged labour 496
    self-hypnosis 464
    shock 999
    transcutaneous electrical nerve stimulation (TENS) 465–466
        see also transcutaneous electrical nerve stimulation (TENS)
    water as 464
    see also analgesia/analgesics
palpation
    abdominal examination 263–266, 265f
        deep pelvic 264
        fundal palpation 264
        lateral 264
    neonatal examination 547
pancreas, fetal 534
panic, complementary therapies 347
paracetamol, perineal pain 727
paraesthesias, postpartum 744
paralysed hemidiaphragm 948–949
paralytic ileus 982
parental responsibility 1052–1053
    birth registration 1035
parental support, multiple pregnancy 848
parent-baby relationship, preterm baby 637
parentcraft 372
parentcraft classes, multiple pregnancy 842
parent education **371–382**
    activities 378f
    affective, skills and knowledge (ASK) 378
    content of programmes 378–379
    group process 377–378
        integration phase 378
        warm-up phase 377
        work phase 377–378
    group work 374–379, 375f
        buzz groups 375
        games 376–377
        problem solving 376
        quizzes 375
        snowballing 376
        stories/scenarios 375–376
    hypothermia 584, 585b
    multiple pregnancy 842–843
    what is it? 372
    see also parent education classes
parent education classes 269
    ethnic minority groups 268
    group size 377
    'icebreakers' 377

parent education classes (*contd*)
  mental health issues 926
  structures of sessions 379, 380f
  teenagers 271
Parenting Education and Support
  Forum 373
parents, prospective, information for
  145
Parents in Partnership – Parent Infant
  Network (PIPPIN) Programme
  374
parietal bones 224f, 225f
  development 220
parietal eminence 224f, 225f
paronychia 711
partial liquid ventilation (PVL) 662
Partners for Safe Motherhood 1104
  priorities 1104b
partogram 440, 440f, 876, 877f
  obstructive labour 964
  trial of labour 962
Patau's syndrome (trisomy 13) 679
patent ductus arteriosus (PDA) 650,
  664
  clinical features 664
  closure 531
  preterm baby 650
  treatment 664
paternity leave 1055
paternity rights 1053
patient advice and liaison service
  (PALS) 1012
patient satisfaction 1028–1029,
  1029b
Patient's Charter, The 1028
Pawlik's grip 264
Peel Report 401, 463
pelvic adhesions 131, 132
pelvic brim 72t
  angles and planes 70
  dorsal position 943f
  McRoberts' manoeuvre 943f
  measurements 68–69, 69f
  shapes 71f
pelvic cavity, measurements 69
pelvic conjugates 70, 70f
pelvic examination, preterm labour
  indicator 855
pelvic fascia 477
pelvic floor **476–491**
  blood, lymph, nerve supply 478
  displacement, second stage of labour
  493
  injuries *see* perineal trauma
  innervation damage, stress
  incontinence 686, 727
  muscles 477f
    function 385
    postnatal changes 724
  structure 476–479
    deep muscle layer 477–478

pelvic fascia 477
pelvic peritoneum 476–477
  superficial perineal muscles
    477–479
surgery, history taking 249
pelvic floor exercises 361, 479
  antenatal 480
  musculoskeletal system 387
  postnatal exercises 391–392
  stress incontinence 686–687
pelvic infection, tubal damage 132
pelvic inflammatory disease (PID),
  gonorrhoea 823
pelvic injury, history taking 249
pelvic outlet 72t
  angles and planes 70
  measurements 69
pelvic peritoneum 476–477
  rupture 966
pelvic support, symphysis pubis pain 277
pelvic tilting exercises 387
pelvic vasocongestion 106
pelvimetry, breech presentation 903
pelvis (female) 65–73, 66f
  abnormalities, shoulder dystocia 941
  angles and planes 70–71
  assessment 73
    labour 446
  bony 65, 67
  characteristics 72t
  injury/disease 73
  joints/ligaments 67, 68f
    pregnancy 67
  measurements 68–69, 69t
  organs 78f
  physiological responses to pregnancy
    306
  true 67–68
    axis 68f
  unusual types 74t
  variations 71, 73
pemphigus neonatorum 711
pendulous abdomen (anteversion of
  uterus) 832, 832f
penicillin
  gonorrhoea 709
  syphilis 822
penicillinase-producing *Neisseria
  gonorrhoeae* (PPNG) 823
penis 84b
periconceptional nutrition 328–329
perimetrium 79
  protection during labour 499
perinatal mortality/morbidity
  ethnic minority groups 267
  reduction 1027–1028, 1028b
  smoking 1038
  social class 1037–1038
perinatal mortality rate 1037
  reduction 1038–1039
  standards indicator 1039

perineal body 479
perineal care 109
  labour, second stage 499
perineal massage 480, 499
perineal muscles 478
  superficial 477–479
perineal pain
  instrumental deliveries 971
  postnatal 726–727, 740
perineal trauma 479–488
  aetiology 479–480
  antenatal preparation 480
  complementary therapies 351
  definition 479
  first degree 480
  fourth degree 480–481
  legal issues 488
  midwives' rules and code of practice
    (UKCC 1998) 488
  non-suturing 485, 487
  postpartum 740–741
    trauma 741
  prevalence 479
  risk factors 480
  second degree 480
  short/long term effects 480
  spontaneous 480–481
  suturing 484–485, 487
    materials 484
    procedure 485, 485f, 486t, 487
    techniques 484
  third degree 480
  third/fourth degree tears 487–488
    repair 488
  water births 500–501
  see also episiotomy
perineum 77b
peripheral arterial vasodilatation
  hormonal regulation 297
  maternal changes 290
peristaltic movement, newborn
  examination 553
peritoneum 476–477
periventricular cystic leucomalacia
  (PVL) 639
periventricular haemorrhage (PVH)
  639–640
  causes 639
  complications 639
  management 639
  ultrasound 639, 639f
persistent occipitoposterior position of
  the vertex (POP) 890–892, 891f
  skull moulding 230f, 230t
persistent pulmonary hypertension of
  the newborn (PPHN), inhaled
  nitric oxide 662
Persona 117–118
personal details, history taking 246
personality disorder, pregnancy 923
personal liability, negligence 1148

personal space 15
petechiae 545
pethidine 468–469
  antagonists 469
  fetal effects 469
  maternal effects 468–469
  prolonged labour 496
  thermoregulation 578
pethidine hydrochloride 1217
  multiple pregnancy 845
  overdose 1217
pets, preconception care 152t
PGFM plasma levels 423f
pH, vaginal, preterm labour indicator
  855
pharmacodynamic interactions 1210
pharmacokinetic interactions 1210
pharmacy-only medicines 1211
Phenergan see promethazine
  hydrochloride
phenothiazines, breastfeeding 931
phenylalanine hydroxylase deficiency
  697
phenylketonuria (PKU) 697
  features 697
  Guthrie test 566, 696
  maternal blood tests 315
  preconception care 150t
phenytoin sodium (Epanutin) 811
phocomelia 677
phosphatidylglycerol (PG), lung
  maturation marker 660
phototherapy 690–691
  assessment 691
  conjugated hyperbilirubinaemia 694
  double 690–691
  effectiveness 690
  equipment 690, 691f, 692f
  eye protection 691, 692f
  guidelines 690t
  light spectrum 690
  other care implications 691
  thermoregulation 588
  triple 691
phrenic nerve palsy 948–949
physical examination
  abdominal see abdominal
    examination
  antenatal 256–257
  neonate see neonate, examination
  vaginal see vaginal examination
physical preparation for childbirth
  383–396
  abdominal muscles 384f
    anatomy 384
    function 384
  back care 392
  caesarean delivery 392
  childbirth 383–396
  daily activities 392
  instrumental delivery 392

labour see labour, coping strategies
musculoskeletal system see
  musculoskeletal system
  Randall 384
  relaxation 388
    exercises 389b
  stress 388
physical signs, mental health issues
  920
physiological jaundice 685
physiological methods of contraception
  116–118
  2 day method 117
  changes within reproductive system
    117f
  lactational amenorrhoea method
    (LAM) 117
  persona 117–118
  standard days method (SDM) 117
physiological response to pregnancy
  288–310, 357
  anatomical renal adaptations
    293–294
  cardiovascular adaptations 289–290
  fetal adrenoplacental hormonal
    regulation of cortisol 297–298
  hypothalamic–pituitary–placental
    axis 298–303
  mammary gland 303–304
  maternal hypothalamic–pituitary–
    placental axis 298
  musculoskeletal adaptations 306
  renal haemodynamic changes 289
  uterine adaptations 304–306
  ventilation 295–297
physiotherapist, symphysis pubis pain
  277
physiotherapy (women's health)
  383–384
  physical preparation 383–384
phytomenadione (vitamin K) 1221
  maternal epilepsy 811
  obstetric cholestasis 812
  oral use 539
  preterm birth 859
  prophylaxis 539, 640
  treatment refusal 527–528
  see also vitamin K deficiency
    bleeding (VKDB)
pia mater 229f
Pierre Robin syndrome 673
  nursing 673
pigmented naevi 678
pituitary gland
  development 206
  hormones 298–303
  neurovascular pathways 94f
  pregnancy adaptations 298
placenta 200f
  abnormalities 518–519, 769–770
    see also individual abnormalities

absorption of pharmacological
  agents 468
arterial supply 199f
assessment, MRI 323
bipartite 519
calcification 519, 869
circumvallate 519, 519f
cortisol regulation 297
examination
  after delivery 516–517, 517f
  multiple pregnancy 846
fetal surface 518
fetal thermoregulation 575
hypothalamic–pituitary–adrenal
  (HPA) axis 302
hypothalamic–pituitary regulation
  214–215
infarction 516, 519
location, ultrasound scan 320
maternal surface 518
nutrient/gaseous exchange 420
physiological responses to pregnancy
  298
presentation at vulva 510
retained 994–995
  postpartum haemorrhage 989
  reflexology 350
steroids 298–300
  uterine responses to pregnancy
    305–306
succenturiate lobe 518–519, 519f
at term 518, 518f
weighing 517
placenta accreta 519, 772
  prolonged labour 995
placenta delivery 421–423, 422f,
  512–513
  active management 515–516
  descent/separation 508–509,
    509–510
    control of bleeding 510
    detection of 512, 515–516
    mechanisms 510f
    signs 516
  detachment 509
  examination 991
  expulsion 509, 510f
    control of bleeding 510–511
  latent phase 509
  manual 990–991, 997
    acute inversion of uterus 996
    hydrostatic methods 997
    prolonged labour 995–996,
      996f
  phases 509f
  postpartum haemorrhage 990–991
placenta diffusa 769–770
placenta increta, prolonged labour
  995
placental hormones, diabetes in
  pregnancy 805

placental implantation/development **190–204**, 198f
  cytotrophoblast shell development 192–193, 193f
  deciduochorial placenta formation 193–194, 194f
  definitive placenta formation 199
  endometrial preparation 190
  endometrial responses 191–192
  immunosuppression/anti-inflammatory activities 192
  optimal environment 194
  organogenesis 194
  pre-decidualization 191
  trophoblast-endometrial interactions 191
placental separation, breech presentation 899
placental steroids 298–300, 410–411
placenta membranacea 769
placenta percreta, prolonged labour 995
placenta praevia 769–772
  associated conditions 769
  causes 769
  classification 769t, 770f
  differential diagnosis 774t
  induction contraindication 864
  multiple pregnancy 769, 844
  outcome 771
    active treatment 771
    conservative treatment 771
    delivery 771
    third stage of labour 771
  postpartum haemorrhage 988
  shoulder presentation 914
  signs/symptoms 770–771
  smoking 769
  umbilical cord presentation/prolase 955
  vaginal examination 771, 772
  warning haemorrhages 771
plagiocephaly, supine sleeping 716
plasma substitute solutions, neonatal resuscitation 658
plasma volume 291f
  maternal changes 290
Plasmodium falciparum 712
platelet-activating factor (PAF) 211
plexus of Lee–Frankenhäuser 78
Pneumocystis carinii pneumonia (PCP), HIV-infected children 818
pneumocyte 528
  type 1 211, 529
  type 2 211, 529
pneumonia, neonatal 710–711
  causative organisms 710
pneumothorax 660
  diagnosis and treatment 660
pollutants, breastfeeding 599

polycystic ovary syndrome (PCO) 130–131, 131f
  tubal damage 131–132
polycythaemia, small-for-gestational-age baby 644–645
polydactyly 676–677, 676f
polygenic characteristics, genetics inheritance modes 181
polyglactin 910 (Vicryl) 484
polyglycolic acid (Dexon) 484
polyhydramnios
  acute, multiple pregnancy 843
  associated conditions 322
  postpartum haemorrhage 988
  umbilical cord presentation/prolapse 955
pons varolii 227f
port-wine stain (naevus flammeus) 546, 678
positioning/posture
  breech presentation 903, 904, 905
  labour 448, 449f
    active management of 515
    fetus 500
    second stage 497
    third stage 512
    minimize bearing-down urge 498
    pain relief 464–465
    prone *see* prone position
    sleeping *see* sleeping position
possets 553–554
posterior fontanelle 224f, 225f
post-maturity syndrome 869
post-mortem examination 39–40
  necessity 40
  organ donation 40
  procedural information 40
postnatal back care 392
postnatal blues 730, 925
  see also postnatal depression
postnatal care **723–735**
  aims 723
  complementary therapies 350–351
  debriefing 730
  effectiveness 731–732
  examinations 725b
  maternal heart disease 800
  midwifery implications 732–733
  multiple pregnancy 847–850
  observations 725b
  organization 730–731
  physical health 726–730
  psychological health 730
  psychosocial support 730
  trials 732
postnatal complications 392–393, 1027
  backache 393
  coccydynia 393
  dyspareunia 393
  physical preparation 392–393

separated symphysis 393
  urinary problems 393
postnatal depression 278, 730, 742–743, 925–929
  aetiology 926
  complementary therapies 350
  detection 927
  history of 922, 923
  incidence 925
  midwife's role 926–927
  multiple pregnancy 849
  risk factors 743
  signs/symptoms 927b
  symptoms 730
  treatment 927, 929
postnatal exercises 390–392
  abdominal 390–391
    curl-ups 391f
    knee rolling 391f
    see also abdominal exercises, postnatal
  circulatory 390
  pelvic floor exercises 391–392
  physical preparation 390–392
postnatal period
  anatomic issues 85
  contraception
    factors considered 124
    older mothers 125–126
    oral 121
    special groups 125–126
    teenagers 125
    timing of starting 124–125
  health professional's role 725
  physiological health changes 723–725
  symphysis pubis pain 278–279
postnatal support groups 927
postnatal weight gain, sudden infant death syndrome 717
postpartum *see* postnatal period
postpartum blues 730, 977
postpartum haemorrhage (PPH) 776, 987–994
  active management of labour 513
  caesarean section 982
  causes 988
  cervical tears 481
  definition 987
  estimating blood loss 987–988
  following 994
  massive obstetric haemorrhage 992–993
    observations 993
  pregnancy following 994
  prevention 989
  primary 987
  primary from placenta site 988–993
    after placenta delivery 991
    before placenta delivery 990–991
    predication/risk factors 988–989

prophylaxis 989–990
treatment 990–991
secondary 987
shoulder dystocia 947
subsequent pregnancies 994
traumatic 993–994
post-registration education and practice
(PREP) 1124, 1189
portfolio 1191–1192
post-term pregnancy **868–871**
classification 868
dating 868
economics 870–871
features 869
incidence 868
induction from 41 weeks 870
management 869–870
surveillance 869–870
post-traumatic stress syndrome 24
hypertensive disorders 789
instrumental deliveries 971, 977
shoulder dystocia 947
post-traumatic stress syndrome,
symphysis pubis pain 278
posture
back care 385f
in labour 448
see also positioning/posture
Potter's syndrome 679
poverty 1054–1055
PR-A (repressor of progesterone genes)
410
PR-B (activator of progesterone genes)
410
precipitate labour 881
preconception care **143–157**
aim 144
assessment 144–145
diabetic woman 807
disability 149–150
environment/lifestyle 147, 149,
151–153t
genetics 147, 151t
health promotion 360
hepatitis B (HBV) 149t
history taking 144
infection 147, 148–149t
information for prospective parents
145
medical conditions 147, 150t
midwifery and 150, 154
nutrition 145, 146t
objectives 144
renal transplant 803
reproductive sexual health 149, 153t
screening tests 145
sexually transmitted disease 147
stress 151t
prednisone
asthma 811
pregnancy 803

pre-eclampsia 781–786
aetiology 781–782
calcium supplementation 334, 782
care at home/community 786
delivery mode 788–789
diabetic woman 807
diagnosis 782–783
hydatidiform mole 765
investigation 783, 784
labour 789
management 785–786
post delivery 789
multiple pregnancy 843
pathophysiology 781
postpartum haemorrhage 988
psychological care 789–790
ranitidine 980
recurrent 789
severe 784–786
symptoms 783, 786
see also eclampsia; hypertensive
disorders
pregnancy
abdominal 768
anatomic issues 85–86
bleeding during see vaginal bleeding,
during pregnancy
care of women 240–279
combined 768
complementary therapies 344–348
confirmation **236–240**
differential diagnosis 240
home ovulation predictor tests
236
laboratory diagnosis 238–240
positive signs 238
signs and symptoms 236–238, 237t
ultrasound scan 319
vaginal examination 238
drugs 1213–1222
eating disorders 754–755
ectopic see ectopic pregnancy
employment rights 1054
female genital mutilation 834
hCG effects 167
heterotopic 768
legal issues 1156–1159
maternal changes see physiological
response to pregnancy
medical disorders of **793–814**
see also individual disease
multiple see multiple pregnancy
optimal fetal positioning 500
pelvis joints/ligaments 67, 68f
physiological response, fetal/maternal
see physiological response to
pregnancy
planning 143
see also preconception care
postpartum haemorrhage see
postpartum haemorrhage (PPH)

post-term see post-term pregnancy
previous 248–249
psychological factors see
psychological factors, pregnancy
risk of mental health illness 918
sex during 106
sexuality 357
smoking 361–363
see also smoking, in pregnancy
stress 22
teenage see teenage pregnancy
temperature control 578–579
pregnancy law
Abortion Act 1967 1156, 1157b
Human Fertilisation and Embryology
Act 1990 and 1992 1157
preimplantation genetic diagnosis
(PGD), genetics diagnostic test
185
prelabour rupture at term (PROM) 863
induction 863
premenstrual syndrome, poor nutrient
328
prepuce 77b, 84b
prescription-only medicines (POMs)
1211
supply to midwives 1212
preterm baby **628–648**, 633
asphyxia causes 651
breastfeeding 598, 611–612, 635,
859
causes 632–633
characteristics 633, 633f
complications 633–635, 637–641
delivery 633
ethical issues 646
feeding 635–637
follow-up 645–646
gestational age estimation 628, 629f,
630f
hypoglycaemia 634, 698
infection prevention 638
labour 633
management 633
mother-baby relationship 637
nutrition 608, 635–637
prognosis 645–646
thermoregulation 634
see also preterm labour
preterm delivery
gonorrhoea 823
prolonged labour 995
preterm fetus, umbilical cord
presentation/prolapse 955
preterm labour **853–861**
aetiology 853–854
definition 853
delivery 858–859
diabetic woman 807
incidence 853
management 856–859

preterm labour (*contd*)
  monitoring 858
  multiple pregnancy 844, 854
  parental reaction 859
  prediction 854–856
  preterm prelabour rupture of the
      membranes 856
  prevention 854–856
  risk factors 853–854
  signs 856
  see also preterm baby
preterm prelabour rupture of the
    membranes (PPROM) 856
  causes 856
  induction 863
  monitoring 856
prima facie duties, deontology 1136
primary care trusts (PCTs) 1010
primary ectoderm 195, 205
primary endoderm 195, 205
primigravida women
  antenatal visits 255
  breech presentation 897
  labour, second stage 501–502
primitive bronchioles 650
primitive streak 205
prisoners 9
private law, classification 1143
problem solving, parent education 376
professional indemnity insurance,
    complementary therapies 340
progestagen-only pill (POP) 121
progesterone
  competitive binding with cortisol
      299
  cortisol relation 301f
  endometrium implantation
      preparation 190
  implantation 191
  milk secretion prevention 601
  ovulation 96
  preparation for labour 412
  pulmonary changes 297
  receptor subtypes 410
  renal haemodynamic changes 289
  renal handling of sodium 293
progestogen
  erythropoiesis 292
  mammary gland regulation 304
  myometrium responses to pregnancy
      305
  oral contraceptives 121
Project 2000, midwifery education
    1187–1188
prolactin 201f
  adenohypophysis 94
  amniotic fluid volume regulation
      200
  breast development 601
  DHEAS synthesis 214
  elevated levels 130

lactogenesis 602, 724
lung maturation 212–213, 215
lung maturity 652
maternal 201f
physiological response in pregnancy
    298
suckling 602
prolactin-inhibiting factor (PIF) 601
  build-up 602
  function 602
prolactin-releasing factor 602
prolonged labour **876–883**, 994–996
  active management 878
      see also active management of
          labour, prolonged
  causes 878, 995
  definition 876–877
  epidural analgesia 471
  fetal dangers 877–878
  inefficient uterine action 878
  management 995–996
  maternal dangers 877–878
  midwife's role 879–881
  multiple pregnancy 844, 878
  oxytocin use 879–880, 995
  placental morbid adherence 995
  postpartum haemorrhage 988
promazine (Sparine) 1218
promethazine hydrochloride
    (Phenergan)
  moderate vomiting in pregnancy 753
  obstetric cholestasis 812
prone position
  play 564
  sudden infant death syndrome 716
property, care of, legal issues 1160
propylthiouracil (PTU), thyrotoxicosis
    800
prostaglandin dehydrogenase (PGDH)
  immunosuppression/anti-
      inflammatory activities 192
  preparation for labour 412
prostaglandin E,
  immunosuppression/anti-
      inflammatory activities 192
prostaglandin E_2 (PGE_2) 865, 866t,
    1221
  amniotic fluid volume regulation
      200–201
  decidual cells 413
  fetal response to labour 418
  immunosuppression/anti-
      inflammatory activities 192
  labour 413, 414
  ovulation 96
prostaglandin $F_2\alpha$ 866t, 1221
  decidual cells 413
  labour 413
  massive obstetric haemorrhage 992
prostaglandins 1221
  active management of labour 515

complications 865
corticotrophin-releasing hormone 302
ductus arteriosus patency 649
extra-amniotic, therapeutic abortion
    763
labour inducer 865, 866t
pain physiology 461, 461b
preparation for labour 413–414
therapeutic abortion 763
uterine rupture 965–966
prostate gland 84b
protamine sulphate 1222
proteins
  breast milk 595
  digestion, neonatal 594
  maternal nutrition 330
proteolytic enzymes 97
  oocyte/spermatozoon fusion
      164–165, 164f
pruritus gravidarum 273
pseudocyesis 240
pseudohermaphroditism 676
psychiatric unit, postnatal depression
    929
psychological care
  caesarean section 983
  pre-eclampsia 789–790
psychological examination, care during
    labour 446–447
psychological factors
  caesarean section 978
  labour 428
  in labour 433–434
  pain/pain relief 467
  perception of pain 459
  pregnancy **17–24**
    adaptation 18–19
    birth experiences 22–23
    early days of motherhood 24
    information needs 19–20, 19cs
    involvement 19–20, 19cs
    maternal reaction 20–21
    post delivery 23
    relationships 18
    transition adjustment 21–22
  symphysis pubis pain 278
  umbilical cord presentation/prolapse
      956
  vomiting 751
  see also mental health problems
psychological support
  postnatal care 730
  during pregnancy 20–21
psychological trauma, prolonged
    labour 877, 881
psychoprophylaxis, preparation for
    childbirth 459
psychosis, puerperal *see* puerperal
    psychosis
psychosocial support, postnatal care
    730

psychotropic drugs, breastfeeding 931
puberty 105–106
pubic arch 66
pubic ramus 67
pubis 66
public law, classification 1143
public-private partnerships (PPP)
    1014–1015
pubocervical ligaments 81, 477
pubococcygeus muscles 477–478
pudendal arteries 76
puerperal psychosis 730, 929–931
    aetiology 929–930
    incidence 929
    midwives' role 930–931
    signs/symptoms 930b
puerperal sepsis, following postpartum
    haemorrhage 994
puerperium, definition 723
pulmonary embolism, maternal death
    1044
pulmonary haemorrhage, small-for-
    gestational-age baby 645
pulmonary oedema
    pre-eclampsia 785
    symptoms 857
pulmonary system
    fetal response to labour/birth
        418–420
    pregnancy 296t
    see also respiratory system
pulmonary valve stenosis 665
pulsatilla
    haemorrhoid treatment 345–346
    heartburn treatment 345
pulse rate, shock 998
pulse taking
    caesarean section 982
    labour, second stage 503
    neonatal examination 547
pushing techniques 435, 499
pyelonephritis 711, 801–802
pyloric stenosis, congenital
    hypertrophic 674
pyoderma 711
pyridoxine (vitamin B₆) see vitamin B₆
    (pyridoxine)

Q

Qi Gong 344
qualitative research 50
quality, midwifery **1021–1033**
Quality Assurance Agency, midwifery
    benchmarks 1123
quality cycle 1022, 1022f
quality of life, morbidity following
    childbirth 737
quality spiral 1022

quantitative studies 49–50
questionnaires, history taking 246
quickening 237
quizzes 375

R

rachitic pelvis 74t
racial issues
    history taking 247
    leadership 1179
    sociology 9–11
radiation
    neonatal heat loss 576
    preconception care 153t
radiography
    necrotizing enterocolitis 710
    pregnancy diagnosis 238
Ramadan, weight in pregnancy 329
randomized controlled trials 5
ranitidine 1218
    antenatal care 272
    Mendelson's syndrome 980
raspberry leaf tea
    labour pain relief 350
    onset of labour remedy 348
ratio decidendi, common law 1143
rational monism, deontology 1136
Raynaud's phenomenon, nipple pain
    610
ready-to feed formulae 616
reasonably foreseeable harm,
    negligence 1148
rebound retinal hypoxia 641
recessive allele, genetic history 173
reciprocal translocation, chromosome
    anomalies 178
record keeping 16
    audit 1023
    birth 518, 1034–1035
    caesarean section 982
    guidelines 1126
    labour
        first stage 440–441, 440f, 441f
        second stage 503
    legal issues 1159–1160
    newborn 567–568
    rules 1127
    shoulder dystocia 950
    supervision 1130
    see also registration
records
    antenatal care 266–267
    'shared notes' 266–267
rectal examination 487, 488
rectovaginal fistula, obstructive labour
    964
rectum
    examination 487, 488

newborn 555
    temperature measurement 583
recurrent abortion 761–762
    antiphospholipid antibodies 762
    causes 761–762
    cervical cerclage 762
    infection 762
    poor nutrition 328
red blood cells (RBC), volume,
    maternal changes 290, 291f
red degeneration (necrobiosis) 833
reflex assessment 559–560
reflexology 343
    heartburn 345
    milk shortage 350–351, 351f
    nausea/vomiting 345
    retained placenta 350
refugees
    mothers 7–8
        special health/social needs 8
    pregnancy 359
refusal, consent 1154–1155
Register of nurses and midwives 1122
registration
    birth 518, 1034–1035
    death 43–44
    stillbirth 44, 762, 1034–1035, 1037,
        1156
Registration of Births and Deaths Act
    1034
relaxation 388
    exercises 389b
        physical preparation 389b
    labour coping strategies 389
    physical preparation 388
    techniques
        pain relief 459
        parent classes 372
    therapies 344
relaxin 168–169
    functions 168
    labour inducer 868t
    musculoskeletal system physiological
        effect 385
    pelvic muscles 479
    renal haemodynamic changes 289
religious issues, history taking 247
renal agenesis 675
renal anatomical adaptations 293–294
renal disease, pregnancy 801–804
    causative agents 801
    chronic disease 802–803
    diagnosis 802
    fetal effects 802
    management 802
    signs/symptoms 802
renal failure, acute in pregnancy
    803–804
    causes 803–804, 804
    management 804
renal function tests, pre-eclampsia 784

renal haemodynamic changes 289
renal system 213–214, 213f
  development 213–214, 213f
    problems 675
  fetal 533
  neonatal 533
renal transplant 803
renal tubules, physiological response in
  pregnancy 295
renin, physiological responses to
  pregnancy 292
renin–angiotensin system, physiological
  responses to pregnancy 292
reproductive anatomy 75–82
  external genitalia 75–76, 76f
  fetal development 75
  internal genitalia 76–79, 80b, 81–82
  male 20b, 21b, 83
    fetal development 83, 83f
  see also testes
Reproductive Health for Refugees
  Consortium 359
reproductive history, preterm labour
  854
reproductive physiology (female)
  89–104
  cyclical changes in organs 97–101
  see also menstrual cycle
reproductive sexual health
  genital tract abnormalities 829–830
  preconception care 149
reproductive system, postnatal changes
  724
Requirements for Pre-registration
  Midwifery Programmes 1122–1123
Rescue Remedy 342
  labour pain relief 349
  panic attack remedy 347
respiration, neonates see neonatal
  respiration
respiration changes, shock 998
respiration establishment 651
respiratory acidosis 537, 658
respiratory arrest, epidural analgesia
  471
respiratory depression
  amniotic fluid embolism 1000
  pethidine 469
respiratory distress, fetal, caesarean
  section 978
respiratory distress syndrome (RDS)
  637, 659–660
  airway collapse 661
  diagnosis 659
  investigation 660
  occurrence 659
  post-mortem 659
  prevention 659–660
  surfactant 650, 659
    prophylactic 660
  symptoms 659

respiratory drugs 1222
respiratory support 661–662
  continuous positive airways pressure
    662
  extracorporeal membrane
    oxygenation 662
  high-frequency oscillatory ventilation
    662
  intermittent positive-pressure
    ventilation, complications 661
  nitric oxide 662
  oxygen therapy 661
  parental 661
  partial liquid ventilation 662
  synchronous intermittent mandatory
    ventilation 662
respiratory system 528–531, 650
  abnormalities 672
  development 209–213, 528–529,
    650
    hormonal regulation 212–213
    stages 528–529
  disorders 649–670
  lung buds 650
  lung fluid see lung fluid
  lung maturity factors 530
  newborn examination 546–548
  physiological response in pregnancy
    295–297, 296
    hormonal regulation 296
  postnatal changes 724
  problems, maternal 809–811
  surfactant 529, 650
  transition to neonatal life 650–651
  ultrasound scan 650
  see also pulmonary system
'rest and thankful' phase 493
resuscitaires, radiant heater 581
resuscitation, neonate 652–653,
  652–658, 656–657, 981
  airway management 653–655
    airway opening 653, 653f
    bag and mask ventilation 653
    endotracheal intubation 654,
      655f
    Guedel airway insertion 654
    jaw thrust 653–654, 654f
    laryngeal mask airway 654–655
    suction under direct vision 654
  drugs and fluids 657–658
  equipment 652b
  home environment 581
  initial treatment 652–653
  meconium 656–657
  mouth–nose breathing 652–653
  preparation 537–538
  procedure 657b
  sudden death syndrome 718
  thermoregulation 581–582
retained placenta see placenta, retained
rete testis 85b

retinal haemorrhages, instrumental
  deliveries 971
retinal hypoxia, rebound 641
retinopathy of prematurity (ROP) 641
  preventative care 641
retrograde ejaculation 133
retroplacental blood clot 509–510
rhesus factor 686–687
  antenatal care 258
  inheritance 687f
  testing 313
rhesus isoimmunization, induction
  indicator 863
rheumatic heart disease 798
rhomboid of Michaelis 493
ribcage, changes in pregnancy 295f
riboflavin (vitamin B_2), maternal
  nutrition 331–332
ribonucleic acid (RNA) 175
ribosomal RNA (rRNA) 175
right mentoanterior position (RMA),
  face presentation 910f, 911
right mentolateral position (RML), face
  presentation 910, 910f
right mentoposterior position (RMP),
  face presentation 910, 910f
right sacroanterior position (RSA),
  breech presentation 900, 900f
  vaginal birth mechanism 901–902,
    901f, 902f
right sacrolateral position (RSL),
  breech presentation 900, 900f
right sacroposterior position (RSP),
  breech presentation 900–901,
    900f
Ringer's lactate solution, neonatal
  resuscitation 658
The Rising Caesarean Section Rate: A
  Public Health Issue 978–979
risk indicators (screening) 183–185
  see also genetic screening
risk management 1025–1026
risk measurement 1093–1094
risk-scoring systems, preterm labour
  854
ritodrine hydrochloride (Yutopar) 857,
  1216
Robert's pelvis 74t
rooting reflex 559, 604
round ligaments 81, 477
Royal College of Midwives 1082
  education strategy 1188
Royal College of Obstetricians and
  Gynaecologists (RCOG)
  Clinical Green Top guidelines
    897–898
  induction guidelines 862, 871–872
  sweeping the membranes guidelines
    862
  vaginal examination guidelines 444
Royal Maternity Charity 1110

rubella (German measles) 707–708
  cross-infection risk 708
  maternal screening 315
  preconception care advice 148
  vaccination 707
  viraemia 707
Rubin manoeuvre, shoulder dystocia
  944f, 945

S

sacral angle 70
sacral foramina 67
sacral promontory 66
sacrococcygeal joint 68
sacroiliac joint pain, complementary
  therapies 346
sacroiliac joints 68
sacroiliac ligaments 68
sacrospinous ligaments 68
sacrotuberous ligaments 68
sacrum 66, 72t
Safe Motherhood Initiative 1043,
  1103–1104, 1103b
  co-sponsors 1104b
  specific countries 1104t
Safe Motherhood Midwifery Modules
  1109
safe period, contraception 116
safety, teaching physical skills 394–395
salbutamol, preterm labour 857
salmonella 251
sauna use, congenital abnormality risk
  579
Saving Lives: Our Healthier Nation,
  health inequalities 9
scalp 222f
Schultze presentation 510
sciatica, complementary therapies 346
sciatic notch, greater 67, 72t
sclerema, hypothermia 585
Scotland
  drug legislation 1212
  midwifery history 1078
  NHS restructuring 1015
screening
  antenatal see antenatal screening
  definition 312
  genetics 183–185
    see also genetic screening
  health, preconceptual 143, 145
  HIV see HIV screening
  preconception care 145
scrotum 84b
  newborn examination 554
secondary abdominal pregnancy 768
second-stage of labour see labour,
  second stage
sedation, puerperal psychosis 930

seizures see convulsions
selective fetal reduction 322, 763
  anesthesia 764
  first trimester 764
  multiple pregnancy 849
  second trimester 764
self-discharge, consent 1156
self-harm, pregnancy 923
self-hypnosis, pain relief 464
Sellick's manoeuvre (cricoid pressure)
  980, 981f
seminal vesicle 84b
seminiferous tubules 85b
senna preparations 272
Sentinel study, caesarean section 978
separated symphysis, postnatal
  complications 393
septic abortion 764–765
  causative organisms 764–765
  examination 764
  post surgical risks 764
septicaemia 712
  causative organisms 712
  complications 712
  treatment 712
septic shock 999
  see also bacterial shock
Serratia, shock 999
serum/biochemical screening, genetics
  184–185
sex see sexual intercourse
sex education 106, 270
sex-linked characteristics/diseases,
  genetics inheritance modes
  180–181
sexual abuse victims
  mental health issues 921, 924
  pregnancy/childbirth 108
  vaginal examination 443
sexual health
  preconception care 149, 153t
  promotion 357–358
sexual intercourse
  after childbirth 109, 115
  milk ejection during 110
  pregnancy 21, 106–107, 357–358
  problems 740–741
sexuality 105–113
  breastfeeding 110
  definition 105
  labour and 107
  menopause 110–111
  paternal presence at delivery 109
  perineal care 109
  pregnancy 357
  puberty 105–106
  sex after childbirth 109, 740
  sex during pregnancy 106–107
  teenage pregnancy 105–106
  women requiring special care
  107–108

sexually transmitted disease (STDs)
  108, **815–828**
  chlamydia 709, 824
  gonorrhoea 709, 822–823
  hepatitis B virus 821
  herpes simplex virus (HSV) 709,
  823–824
  HIV screening 815–821
    see also HIV infection; HIV
    screening
  neonate
    delivery acquired 709–710
    prenatal infection 706–707
  preconception care 147
  syphilis 822
    see also syphilis
  Trichomonas 824–825
sexual problems, postpartum 740–741
shaken baby syndrome 1041
sheath see condom (sheath)
Sheehan's syndrome 776
  following postpartum haemorrhage
  994
  milk production 609
shiatsu 342
  constipation remedy 345, 346f
  heartburn remedy 345, 345f
  labour pain relief 349, 349f
Shirodkar suture 984
shock 997–1000
  acute inversion of uterus 997
  bacterial 999–1000
    see also bacterial shock
  shoulder dystocia 947
  signs of deterioration 998
  treatment 998
short bowel malabsorption syndrome
  641
Short Report 401
shoulder dystocia **939–953**, 940f
  birth injury 948–950, 949b
  bony injury 949
  calling for help 948
  cleidotomy 947
  definition 939
  degrees of seriousness 939
  education/training/development 950
  fetal outcomes 948–950, 951
  fundal pressure 947
  incidence 940
  management 941–946
    all-fours position 943
    episiotomy 944
    McRoberts' manoeuvre 941–942,
    943f
    posterior arm delivery 945, 945f
    Rubin manoeuvre 944f, 945
    suprapubic pressure 944, 944f
    Woods' manoeuvre 944–945, 944f
    Zavanelli manoeuvre 946, 946f
  maternal outcome 947

shoulder dystocia (*contd*)
  mechanism 939–940
  notes/record keeping 950
  postpartum haemorrhage (PPH) 947
  predicting 941
  risk 940
  risk factors 940–941
    diabetes 941
    fetal size 941
    maternal age 940
    maternal birthweight 940
    maternal obesity 940
    pelvic abnormality 941
    previous shoulder dystocia 941
  symphysiotomy 946–947
  ultrasound to predict macrosomic fetus 941
shoulder presentation 914–915, 914f
  causes 885–886, 914
  diagnosis 914
  incidence 885–886
  induction contraindication 864
  management 914–915
  twins 915
  umbilical cord presentation/prolapse 955
  undiagnosed 915
  vaginal examination 915
show, mucoid/bloody 433, 438, 447
sickle cell anaemia
  ethnic minority groups 268
  genetics diseases origin 181
  preconception care 151t
sickle cell disease
  blood tests 315
  haemoglobin combinations 796t
  management 797
  patterns of inheritance 796t
  pregnancy effect 797
sickle cell trait 796–797
sign language interpreter 269
silent abortion 761
silver swaddler 584
Simmonds' disease 776
sinciput 222f
sinus 223
  confluence of 228f
  lateral 228f
  sagittal 228f
  straight 228f
skin
  abnormalities 677–678
  changes
    bacterial shock 999
    pregnancy 236, 273
    shock 998
  layers 532
  pigmentation 273
  preterm baby 634
  temperature measurement 583

skull
  base of 223, 224f
  fetal *see* fetal skull
  fractures, instrumental deliveries 971
  neonatal *see* neonatal skull
slapped cheek disease (erythema infectiosum), preconception care advice 148t
sleep
  disturbances, mental health issues 926
  fetal breathing 211
  increased desire, physiological changes of pregnancy 289
  during labour 435
sleeping position 564, 564f
  developmental problems 716
  sudden infant death syndrome 716
SLEEP mnemonic 950
small-for-gestational-age baby (SGA) **642–645**
  causes 642–643
  characteristics 643
    asymmetrical growth restriction 643
    symmetrical growth restriction 643
  complications 644–645
  delivery 643–644
  ethical issues 646
  follow-up 645–646
  hypoglycaemia 698
  hypothermia 644
  incidence 661
  labour 643–644
  management 643
  prognosis 645–646
  substance abuse 645
small luteal cells (SLC) 168
smell, heightened sense 289
SmokeScreen 1030b
smoking
  antenatal care 250
  breastfeeding 608
  perinatal death 1038
  placenta praevia 769
  preconception care 152t
  in pregnancy 361–363
    cessation, midwives' role 362–363
    damage limitation 363
    model of behaviour changes 362
  reduction programmes 1029
  spontaneous abortion 759
  sudden infant death syndrome 717
smooth muscle formation, myometrium responses to pregnancy 305, 305f
snowballing, parent education 376
social class *see* socioeconomic status
social differentiation 7–11
  gender 9–11

race 7–8
  social class 8–9
Social Exclusion Unit (SEU) 366
social services
  child protection 1061
  National Health Service 1014
  referrals 1056
  symphysis pubis pain 278
social support, mental health issues 922
societal change approach, health promotion 359t
socioeconomic status 8–9
  classification 9t
  communication 16
  female stereotypes 9
  health inequalities 9
  history taking 247
  mental health issues 920
  perinatal death 1037–1038
  prisoners 9
sociological perspective 4–6
sociology **3–13**
  historical development 3–4
  and midwives 4
  scientific knowledge 4–6
sodium bicarbonate, neonatal resuscitation 658
sodium citrate, Mendelson's syndrome 980
sodium supplementation, hyponatraemia 699
sodium valproate (Epilim) 811
'soft markers,' ultrasound scan 320
soft tissue damage, shoulder dystocia 947
solvents, preconception care 153t
sore nipples 609–610
soya milk formulae 616
Sparine (promazine) 1218
sperm
  capacitation 163–164
  freezing 139
  transport 163
spermatic cord 84b
spermatogenesis, genes responsible 132
spermatozoa
  fertilization 161
  fusion with oocyte 164–165
  transport 163
  zona pellucida binding 164
sperm count, WHO criteria for normal 133t
spermicide
  caps 119
  condoms 116
sperm preparation, in vitro fertilization (IVF) 136
spherical primordial sex cells 197
spherocytosis 697
sphincters 478

sphingomyelin (S), lung maturation marker 660
spina bifida 671
  alpha-fetoprotein (AFP) level 317
  clinical features 671
  cystica 671
  fetal surgery 671
  occulta 671
spinal anaesthesia (subarachnoid), caesarean section 981
spinal injury, history taking 249
spine
  deformity 556
  newborn examination 556, 556b
spiral arterioles, pre-eclampsia 781
splanchnic mesoderm 196
spleen, newborn examination 553
spondylolisthetic pelvis 74t
spontaneous abortion 758–762
  amniocentesis 324
  causes 759–760
  chorionic villus sampling 324
  genital tract abnormalities 831
  smoking 759
  vomiting 752
spontaneous breech presentation 899
Sprengel's deformity 556
squamocolumnar junction 82
squaw vine, postnatal depression 350
standard days method (SDM) 117
staphylococcal scalded skin syndrome 711
staphylococci, shock 999
Staphylococcus aureus
  paronychia 711
  sudden infant death syndrome 717
startle reflex (Moro reflex) 559, 949
STAT3 protein, fertilization 165
status epilepticus 812
stepping reflex 560
stercobilinogen 685
sterilization 123–124
steroids, asthma 811
sticky eye 710
stillbirth
  bereaved mothers 28
  definition 1037
  registration 44, 762, 1034–1035, 1037
  legal issues 1156
Stillbirth and Neonatal Death Society (SANDS), teardrop sticker 31–32
stools
  artificially-fed baby 533
  breast-fed baby 533
  changing 533
  newborn assessment 555
stork bite 678
strawberry naevi 678
streptococci

group B (GBS), preconception care advice 149t
  preterm labour infection 854
  shock 999
stress 388
  child abuse 1062
  complementary therapies 347
  infertility 140–141
  physical preparation 388
  preconception care 151t
  reduction 22
stress incontinence
  pelvic floor innervation damage 686, 727
  postpartum 727, 737–738
    delivery method 686
stretch marks (striae gravidarum) 263, 273
  zinc deficiency 334
stridor 530
striking off, Nursing and Midwifery Council (NMC) 1121
stripping the membranes 865
stroke volume, maternal changes 290
stromal cells 99
  decidualization 191
stromal fibroblasts 98
student liability, negligence 1148
subaponeurotic haemorrhage, vacuum extraction cup 232
subarachnoid anaesthesia (spinal), caesarean section 981
subarachnoid space 229f
subdural space 229f
subepithelial capillary plexus 99
  endometrium implantation preparation 190
subfertility, poor nutrition 328
subgaleal haemorrhage, instrumental deliveries 971
suboccipitobregmatic circumference, newborn skull 222f
subpubic angle 71
subpubic arch 72t
subseptate uterus 830
substance abuse
  mental health issues 921
  small-for-gestational-age baby 645
  see also drug abuse/addiction
substance P 462, 463
succenturiate placenta 518–519, 518f
sucking, nutritive/non-nutritive 533, 564
sucking reflex 559
suckling
  ineffective 604
  prolactin release 602
  saliva production 597
suction curettage, hydatidiform mole 766
suction evacuation 763, 763f

sudden infant death syndrome (SIDS) 715–720
  apnoea alarms 717–718
  apparent life-threatening events 718
  diagnosis 715
  epidemiological features 717
  family care 718–719
  follow-up 718
  illness 717
  incidence/trends 715–716, 715f
  investigation procedure 718
  reduction 1041
  risk factors 716–717
  smoking effects 363
  subsequent pregnancies 718–719
  thermoregulation 716–717
sudden unexpected death in epilepsy (SUDEP) 812
sudden unexpected death in infancy (SUDI) 715
  immunization 717
suicide
  attempt, pregnancy 923
  postnatal depression 929
superficial perineal muscles 477–479
superior vena cava, fetal 649
supervision 1127–1130
  benefits 1129
  clinical governance 1129–1130
  history 1128
  management comparison 1129, 1130t
  Midwives Rules and Code of Practice 1127
  negligence 1148
  proposed standards 1127–1128
  quality 1026
  supervisors 1128–1129
Supervisor of Midwives 1128–1129
supine hypotensive syndrome 980
supine sleeping, developmental problems 716
supplementary feeds 617
supplementer tubes 617f
  preterm feeding 612
supplement nursing system (SNS) 616–618, 617f
supplements
  constipation 272
  preconception care 146t
  see also nutrition/diet
support agencies/groups
  breastfeeding 613
  grief 44, 47
  symphysis pubis pain 279
'Supporting Families,' Government's consultative document 373
Supporting Families initiatives 358
suprapubic pressure, shoulder dystocia 944, 944f

Sure Start initiatives 373, 404, 613, 1039, 1055
Sure Start programmes 359
surfactant 211
    antenatal corticosteroids 650, 856
    functions 591, 650
    inspiration aid 651
    phospholipid concentrations 211
    production 529, 650
    respiratory distress syndrome 650, 659, 660
    types 650
surgery
    acute inversion of uterus 997
    fetal 679–680
        associated problems 680
        diaphragmatic hernia 661, 672
        spina bifida 671
        wound healing physiology 680
    massive obstetric haemorrhage 992–993
surgical history 249
surrogacy 139
suture lines, newborn examination 548
sutures (skull) 223
    coronal 224f, 225f
    frontal 225f
    lambdoidal 224f, 225f
    sagittal 225f
swaddling 573–574, 584
sweeping the membranes 865
swim up procedure, intrauterine insemination 134
symphysiotomy
    shoulder dystocia 946–947
    spontaneous, McRoberts' manoeuvre 943
    trial of labour 963
symphysis pubis 66, 68, 84b
    diastasis, complementary therapies 346
    joint 276f
    pain 274–279
        antenatal 277–278
        incidence 275
        labour 277–278
        management 277–279, 278
        physiology 275–277
        postnatal period 278
        recovery 279
        risk factors 279
        symptoms 275–276
        transfer home 278–279
symphysis pubis dysfunction (S-PD) 729
synchronous intermittent mandatory ventilation (SIMV) 662
syncytium 192
syndactyly 676–677, 676f
syntocinon 502, 1220
    active management of labour 442, 515

contractions 1087
    history of 1087
    instrumental vaginal deliveries 972
    maternal heart disease 799
    missed abortion 761
    postpartum haemorrhage 990, 992
    trial of labour 962
    umbilical cord presentation/prolapse 957
syntometrine 502, 513, 1220–1221
    active management of labour 514–515
    postpartum haemorrhage 990
    prolonged labour 995–996
syphilis 706, 822
    neonatal symptoms 706
    screening 316, 706
    treatment 706
syringe feeding 616
systemic lupus erythematosus (SLE), preconception care 150t

T

T-ACE questionnaire 364
tachycardia, fetal heart rate 317
tachypnoea, neonatal see transient tachypnoea of newborn (TTN)
Tai Chi 344
talipes 676
talipes calcaneovalgus 676, 676f
talipes equinovarus 676, 676f
talipes metatarsus varus 676
taurine, breast milk 595
Tay–Sachs disease, preconception care 151t
teaching physical skills 393–395
    preparation before childbirth 393–395
        aquanatal sessions 394
        contraindications 395
        exercise to music 395
        points to consider 393
        safety precautions 394–395
        when to begin 393–395
    see also education and training
team midwifery 244
technology 5
    sociology 5–6
teenage mothers 1058–1059
    legal issues 1058–1059
    see also teenage pregnancy
The Teenage Parenthood Network 271
teenage pregnancy 105–106, 366–367
    actions to reduce 366
    antenatal care 270–271
    midwives' role 367
    postpartum contraception 125
    rates 366
    risks associated 366–367

temperature
    control see thermoregulation
    fetal 575
    measurement 583
        caesarean section 982
        shock 998
temporal bones 224f
    development 220
Ten Steps to Successful Breastfeeding 591, 592b, 1110b
tentorial tear 232
    signs 232
tentorium cerebelli 228f
    tear 232
terbutaline 857
    side effects 857
Term Breech Trial 895, 898
terminal air sac, development 529
termination see abortion
testes 84b
    blood/nerve supply 85b
    efferent ductule 85b
    fetal development 83
    lobules 85b
    newborn examination 554
    structure 85f
    undescended see undescended testes (UDT)
test-tube baby 129
tetanic uterine action 881
tetanus, preconception care advice 149t
tetralogy of Fallot 665, 666f
thalamus, development 206
thalassaemia 797–798
    blood tests 315
    ethnic minority groups 268
    preconception care 151t
thalidomide 149t
    limb reduction deformities 677
theca cells 91
theory of child development 4
therapeutic abortion 762–764
    counselling 763
    first trimester 763
        mifepristone 763
        suction evacuation 763
    follow-up care 763
    legal requirements 762–763
    pre-procedure tests 763
    second trimester 763–764
        dilation and evacuation 763
        extra-amniotic prostaglandins 763
        hysterotomy 763–764
        oral prostaglandins 763
        placental expulsion 763
        selective fetal reduction 763
therapeutic counselling 16–17
therapeutic distance 17
thermoregulation 532, 573–590
    bathing 580–581

birth 579
feeding 578, 580
fetal 575
heat loss 576–577
heat production 577–578
historical background 573–574
labour 579
maintenance 583
midwife's role 578–582
monitoring 582–583
normal function 575
phototherapy 588
physiology 574–578
preterm baby 634
resuscitation, neonate 581–582
sudden infant death syndrome 716–717
surgery 584
Thermospot 583
thiamin (vitamin B₁), maternal nutrition 331
Thinking Sociologically 4
third stage of labour *see* labour, third stage
Thorn manoeuvre 912–913, 913f
threatened abortion 760
small-for-gestational-age baby 643
thromboembolism
maternal death 1044
venous, oral contraceptives 121
thrombosis
deep vein *see* deep vein thrombosis (DVT)
maternal death 1044
thrush *see* candidiasis (thrush)
thymine (T), genetics 174
thyroid activity, hyperemesis gravidarum 753
thyroid-binding globulin (tBG) 800
thyroid conditions 800–801
preconception care 150t
thyroid hormone, lung maturation 212–213
thyrotoxicosis (hyperthyroidism, Graves' disease) 800–801
hydatidiform mole 765
thyroxine 800, 801
lung maturity 652
thyroxine sodium (levothyroxine sodium), congenital hypothyroidism 701
tidal volume, changes in pregnancy 295
tissue changes, preparation for labour 412
tocolytic drugs 857–858
postpartum haemorrhage 989
tongue, newborn examination 549, 550b
tongue tie, breastfeeding problems 611
tonic uterine action 881

TORCH, prenatal infection 705
total fertility rate (TFR) 1035
total parenteral nutrition (TPN)
hyperemesis gravidarum 753–754
thiamine 754
total quality management (TQM) 1022
toxic shock 998
Toxoplasma gondii 706
transmission 316
toxoplasmosis 251–252, 706
maternal screening 316, 706
preconception care advice 148t
prenatal antibiotics 706
transmission risk 706
Toxoplasmosis Trust 252
tracheo-oesophageal fistula (TOF) 673–674, 673f
at birth 673
nursing 674
surgery 674
traction reflex 559
Tractocile (atosiban) 857, 1216
tranquillizers 1218–1219
transcription, DNA 175
transcutaneous electrical nerve stimulation (TENS) 465–466
advantages 465
electrode positioning 465f
transfer home, symphysis pubis pain 278–279
transfer RNA (tRNA) 175
transient tachypnoea of newborn (TTN) 634, 659
caesarean section 659
characteristics 634
infectious cause 659
temperature maintenance 659
translation, DNA 175
translocation, chromosome anomalies 178
transport incubator, thermoregulation 588
transposition of the great arteries 665, 665f
transversus abdominis 384
function 384
transversus exercises, abdominal exercises 387
travel advice, pregnancy 367
Trendelenburg position, bladder filling 957
Treponema pallidum 706, 822
Treponema pallidum haemagglutination assay (TPHA) 706
trespass (to person), consent 1151
Trichomonas 824–825
tricyclic antidepressants, breastfeeding 931
trilaminar disc 205, 207f

triple test 243, 316–317
triplets
breastfeeding 613
delivery 846–847
incidence 840, 840f
see also multiple pregnancy
trisomy, chromosome anomalies 178
trisomy 13 (Patau's syndrome) 679
trisomy 18 (Edward syndrome), clinical features 679
trisomy 21 *see* Down's syndrome
trofolastin 273
trophoblast, infiltration 194f
secondary phase 198–199
trophoblast-endometrial interactions 191
trophoblastic barrier 194f
trophoblasts, implantation 191
tuberculosis (TB) 712, 809–810
diagnosis 809
drug treatment 810t
immunization 712
preconception care advice 148t
pregnancy care 809–810
treatment 712
tubigrip, symphysis pubis pain 277
tubulus rectus 85b
tumours, ultrasound scan 321
tunica albuginea 85b
tunica vaginalis 85b
Turner's syndrome 131, 679
X chromosome 679
turtle sign 939
twin clinics 843
twin reversed arterial perfusion (TRAP) 844
twins
acardiac 844
birth complications 844–845
breastfeeding 613
causes 840
chorionicity 841
conjoined 844
death of 849
deferred delivery 845
identification 845, 846
locked 844
monoamniotic 844
prolonged labour 878
shoulder presentation 915
undiagnosed 846
zygosity determination 840–841
see also dizygotic twins; monozygotic twins; multiple pregnancy
Twins and Multiple Births Association (TAMBA) 842
twin-to-twin transfusion syndrome (TTTS), multiple pregnancy 843–844
management 844
tympanic temperature measurement 583

U

UDP-glucuronyl transferase 685
  deficiency 688
UK Amniotic Fluid Embolism Register
  1000
UK Baby Friendly Initiative 591
UK Central Council for Nursing,
  Midwifery and Health Visiting
  (UKCC), complementary therapy
  guidelines 339
UK Council of Health Regulators
  1118–1119
ultrasound scanning (USS)
  antenatal investigations 318–323
  cephalic disproportion 961
  Doppler 322
  fetal breathing movements 650
  fetal skull 221f
  first 10 weeks' pregnancy 193
  first trimester scan indications
    318–320
  genetics screening (risk indicators)
    184
  genital tract abnormalities 831
  grief/bereavement 34
  macrosomic fetus prediction 941
  method 318
  multiple pregnancy 319, 841–842
  perineal pain relief 727
  post-term pregnancy dating 868
  pregnancy diagnosis 238
  psychological aspects 20
  second trimester scan indications
    320
  third trimester scan indications
    320–321
  umbilical cord presentation/prolapse
    955
    management 956
    prelabour/first stage 956–957
    second stage 957–958
umbilical arteries 209, 649
umbilical cord 520f
  abnormalities 520
  after delivery 421, 519–520
    care 518
  clamping 509–510
    respiration establishment 651
  cleaning 553
  compression, preterm labour 858
  cutting 503
    active management of labour
      515
    when to cut 512
  examination
    after birth 519–520
    second stage of labour 502
  function 520
  insertion abnormalities 520, 520f

length
  descent/separation of placenta
    512, 516
  presentation/prolapse 955
  newborn examination 552–553
  sepsis 710
  thickness 553
  traction, active management of
    labour 516, 516f
  water birth 501
umbilical cord presentation/prolapse
  954–959, 954f
  bladder filling 957
  causes 954–955
  dangers 956
  definitions 954
  diagnosis 955
  management 956–958
  manual replacement 957
  multiple pregnancy 844
  occult cord presentation 954
  shoulder presentation 885
  ultrasound scan see ultrasound
    scanning (USS), umbilical cord
    presentation/prolapse
umbilical vein 209, 649
unconjugated hyperbilirubinaemia
  686–693
  complications 689
    kernicterus 689
  conjugation failure 688–689
    genetic causes 688–689
  enterohepatic circulation increase
    689
  evaluation 685–686
    bilirubin measurement 685–686,
      685b
    bilirubin records 686
    clinical 687
  follow-up 693
    blood tests 693
  genetic causes 687
  increased red cell breakdown
    686–688
    haemolytic disease of the newborn
      686–687
  management 690–693
    exchange transfusion 691–693
    immunoglobulin 693
    initial assessment 690
    phototherapy see phototherapy
    post-discharge risk 690b
    supportive measures 690
  oxytocin 867
undescended testes (UDT) 675
  newborn examination 554
Unfair Contract Terms Act 1977,
  exemption from liability 1149b
unicornuate uterus 830
uniovular twins see monozygotic
  twins

United Kingdom Central Council for
  Nursing, Midwifery and Health
  Visiting (UKCC) see Nursing and
  Midwifery Council
United Nations Children's Fund
  (UNICEF) 1109–1111
unqualified assistant liability,
  negligence 1148
upright position, axis in birth canal 72f
upright position/posture
  descent/separation of placenta 512
  labour
    first stage 448
    second stage 497
ureters 84b
  changes in pregnancy 294
  obstruction 294, 294f
  physiological changes 801
urethra 84b
urethral meatus 13b
urethral sphincter 478
urethral valves 675
  fetal surgery 680
urinalysis 257
  pre-eclampsia 783
urinary catheter, caesarean section 982
urinary incontinence
  perineal trauma 480
  stress see stress incontinence
urinary output 533
  newborn examination 555
urinary problems
  postnatal complications 393
  postpartum 737–738
urinary retention, postpartum 739
urinary system
  development 213–215
  postnatal changes 724–725
urinary tract infections 711
  Escherichia coli 711
  postpartum 739
  retroversion of uterus 832
  sample collection 711
  treatment 711
urinary voiding difficulties, postpartum
  739
urine dipstick testing, bilirubin levels
  686
urine, fetal 214
urine samples 257, 259, 711
  iron deficiency anaemia 794
urobilinogen 685
uterine abnormalities, spontaneous
  abortion 759
uterine action
  disordered see prolonged labour
  inefficient 878
  overefficient 881
  preterm labour indicator 854
  tetanic 881
  tonic 881

uterine arteries 82
 embolization, massive obstetric
  haemorrhage 992
 pulsation 238
uterine blood flow 194f
 physiological responses to pregnancy
  304
uterine contractions 431
 assessment 447
 coordination 431–432
  intensity/amplitude 432
  polarity 432
  resting tone 432
  retraction 432, 432f
 inadequate 995
 labour onset 438
 oxytocin 435
 second stage of labour 493
 uterine rupture 966
uterine exhaustion 964
uterine hyperstimulation
 oxytocin 867, 879
 trial of labour 963
uterine ligaments 81, 81f
uterine muscles 81f
uterine obliquity, face presentation
 908
uterine retroversion, spontaneous
 abortion 759
uterine rupture 965–967
 aftercare 967
 causes 965
 management 967
 scar rupture 965, 966
 shoulder dystocia 947
 signs/symptoms 966–967
 silent 966
 spontaneous 966
 traumatic rupture 965–966
 unscarred rupture 966
uterine temperature, teratogenic
 abnormalities 575
uterine veins 82
uteroplacental circulation 193, 194f,
 195
uteroplacental insufficiency, post-term
 pregnancy 869
uterosacral ligaments 81, 477
uterotonic drugs, active management of
 labour 513
 see also oxytocic drugs
uterus 78–79, 79, 81–82
 abdominal examination 263
 abnormalities 995
 acute inversion 996–997
  causes 996
  dangers 997
  diagnosis 997
  management 997
  postpartum haemorrhage 989
  spontaneous 996

anteversion (pendulous abdomen)
 832, 832f
blood supply 81, 81f, 82f
body/corpus 80b
contractions see uterine
 contractions
description 78
double (uterus didelphys) 830
enlargement, pregnancy 236
fibroids 832–833, 833f
first trimester pregnancy 193f
functions 79
fundus 80b
growth 304–305
guarding of, active management of
 labour 516
infection 999
involution see involution of uterus
lymphatic drainage 82
malformations 793f, 829–831
 see also uterus displacements
massage, postpartum haemorrhage
 treatment 990, 990f, 991
menstrual cycle changes 97
 pre-decidualization 99–100
nerve supply 82
 pain physiology 461
non-pregnant 79f
physiological responses to pregnancy
 304–306
preparation for labour 411
rupture see uterine rupture
structure 79
subseptate/bicornuate 830
unicornuate 830
uterus didelphys (double uterus) 830
uterus displacements 831–832
 anteversion (pendulous abdomen)
  832, 832f
 incarceration 831f
 prolapse 832
 retroversion 831–832
  dangers 832
  diagnosis 831
  treatment 831–832
utilitarianism, ethics dilemmas (solving)
 1135–1136

vaccine
 legal issues 1160–1161
 Vaccine Damage Payments Act 1979
  1160
 see also immunization
Vaccine Damage Payments Act 1979,
 vaccine damage 1160
vacuum extraction see ventouse
 delivery

vagina 77–78
 anatomic relations 78t
 angle 77
 blood supply 78
 cyclical changes 163
 damage, shoulder dystocia 947
 dryness, breastfeeding 110
 function 78
 lymphatic drainage 78
 menstrual cycle changes 100
 structure 78
vaginal birth after caesarean (VBAC)
 965–966, 983
vaginal bleeding
 caesarean section 982
 postnatal 724, 726
 during pregnancy 758–779
  before 24th week 758–769
  after 24th week 769–776
 ultrasound scan 319
vaginal delivery
 elective CS vs 503
 gonorrhoea 823
 herpes simplex virus 824
 instrumental see instrumental vaginal
  deliveries
 symphysis pubis pain 277–278
 see also birth; delivery; labour
vaginal examination 439–440,
 443–446
 antenatal care 256
 breech presentation 897
 brow presentation 913
 cervix 444
 contraindications 443
 face presentation 909
 fetal position 445–446, 445f, 446t
 flexion and station of head 446,
  446f
 indications 444
 informed consent 444
 instrumental vaginal deliveries 973
 membranes 444–445
 methods 444
 occipitoposterior position 889
 pelvic assessment 73, 446
 placenta praevia 771, 772
 pregnancy confirmation 238
 presentation 445
 risks 443–444
 shoulder presentation 915
 signs in pregnancy 238
 transition 493
 umbilical cord presentation/prolapse
  955
vaginal loss
 during labour 447
 mucoid/bloody show 433, 438
  assessment 447
  labour, first stage 447
 see also vaginal bleeding

V

vaginal orifice/introitus 77b
vaginal pH, preterm labour indicator 855
vaginal secretions 78
vaginal septum 830–831, 830f
Valium *see* diazepam
valve stenosis, cardiac catheterization 664
vanishing twin syndrome 319, 840
varicella zoster 707
varicose veins 259, 273
vasa praevia 776
vascular endothelial growth factor (VEGF) 97, 99
   endometrium implantation preparation 190
vascular naevi 546
vas deferens 85b
   congenital bilateral absence 132
   ligation 123, 124f
vasectomy 123–124
vasopressor agents, shock 998–999
vasovagal shock, acute inversion of uterus 997
vault caps 119
vault of skull 223, 224f
velamentous insertion of umbilical cord 520
Venereal Disease Research Laboratory (VDRL) test, syphilis 706
venous thromboembolism (VTE), oral contraceptives 121
ventilators, neonatal 661
ventouse delivery 971, 975–976
   chignon 232
   contraindications 975
   equipment/procedure 976, 976f
   forceps *vs* 973
   midwife ventouse practitioners 977
   obstructive labour 964
   subaponeurotic haemorrhage 232
ventricular septal defect (VSD) 664
vernix caseosa 532, 566
vertex, newborn skull 222f
vertex presentation, skull moulding 230f, 230t
very low birthweight (VLBW) 630, 853
vesicovaginal fistula, obstructive labour 964
vestibule 77b
vicarious liability, negligence 1148
Vicryl (polyglactin 910) 484
Vicryl Rapide 484
vimule 119
violence *see* domestic abuse/violence
viscerocranium 220
visually impaired women, antenatal care 269
vital signs, assessment 544–545
vitamin A, maternal nutrition 331

vitamin B$_1$ (thiamin), maternal nutrition 331
vitamin B$_2$ (riboflavin), maternal nutrition 331–332
vitamin B$_3$ (niacin), maternal nutrition 332
vitamin B$_6$ (pyridoxine) 271
   maternal nutrition 332
   morning sickness treatment 752
vitamin B$_{12}$ (cobalamin)
   deficiency, folic acid deficiency anaemia 795
   deficiency tests 314
   maternal nutrition 332
vitamin C
   maternal nutrition 333
   preterm baby 636
   supplementation 795
vitamin D
   maternal nutrition 333
   postpartum deficiency 744
vitamin E, maternal nutrition 333
vitamin K *see* phytomenadione
vitamin K deficiency bleeding (VKDB) 532, 640, 701
   signs/symptoms 539
vitamins
   breast milk 595
   deficiency, preconception care 146t
   see also individual vitamins
Volente non fit injuria, law defences voluntary assumption of risk 1150
volume expanders, neonatal resuscitation 657–658
voluntary consent, legal issues 1153
voluntary assumption of risk 1150
voluntary organization, family support 1057
vomiting **751–757**
   antenatal care 271
   brain stimulation 751
   causes 751–752
   complementary therapies 344–345
   congenital hypertrophic pyloric stenosis 674
   diagnostic tests 751–752
   eating disorders 754–755
   hyperemesis gravidarum *see* hyperemesis gravidarum
   hypoglycaemia 335
   mild 752
   moderate 752–753
     intravenous fluid 753
     medication 753
   morning sickness 752
   newborn 553
   placental development enhancement 751
   spontaneous abortion risk 752
   symptoms 752–753
   therapeutic nutrition 335, 344–345

vulval haematoma 994
vulval hygiene, inevitable abortion 760
vulval toilet, caesarean section 982

W

Wales, NHS restructuring 1015
walking reflex 560
warfarin 799, 1222
warning haemorrhages, placenta praevia 771
water, pain relief 464
waterbirth 500–501
   cleaning protocols 704
   embolism from 501
   midwives' rules and code of practice (UKCC 1998) 500
   prolonged labour 879
   temperature 501
   time of entry 501
   water temperature 579
water embolism 501
water loss, neonatal heat loss 576–577
webbed digits 676–677
weighing 259
   pregnancy 256–257
   scales, thermoregulation 587
weight
   gain
     pregnancy 256–257
     sudden infant death syndrome 717
   newborn 544
   sudden infant death syndrome 717
Welldorm 1212
Wernicke's encephalopathy
   hyperemesis gravidarum 753
   symptoms 753
whey dominant formula 615, 616t
white coat hypertension 258
White Ribbon Alliance on Safe Motherhood 1111
Who's Fit to be a Parent 6
wick method, pregnancy diagnosis 239–240, 239f
Winterton Report 402, 405
withdrawal, during labour 435
women, in medicine 6
Woods' manoeuvre, shoulder dystocia 944–945, 944f
work-based learning (WBL) 1194
Working for Patients, quality in healthcare 1021
working overseas 1111–1112
Working Together to Safeguard Children, social services referral 1056
World Alliance for Breastfeeding (WABA) 1110

World Breastfeeding Week 1110, 1110b
World Health Organization (WHO) 1108–1109
  birthweight definition 630–632
  female genital mutation classification 834, 834f
  function 1108
  health definition 355
  health promotion definition 356
  structure 1108, 1109f
wound care
  caesarean section 982–983
  fetal surgery 680
wrapping, newborn 573–574, 584
wrist examination 551

X

X chromosomes 174f
  anomalies 178
  congenital abnormalities 679
  human genome 175
  hydatidiform mole 765
X-linked dominant inheritance, sex-linked characteristics/diseases 180–181

X-linked recessive inheritance
  genetics inheritance modes 180f
  sex-linked characteristics/diseases 180
X-ray, antenatal investigations 323
X-ray pelvimetry 323
  cephalic disproportion 961

Y

Y chromosome
  anomalies 178
  human genome 175
Y-linked, sex-linked characteristics/diseases 180
yoga 343
yolk sac
  first trimester pregnancy 193f
  primary 195
  secondary
    composition 197
    energy metabolism/digestion 197
    formation/degeneration 195–197, 197f
    layers 197

Yutopar (ritodrine hydrochloride) 857, 1216

Z

Zavanelli manoeuvre, shoulder dystocia 946, 946f
zidovudine
  HIV transmission 817
  neonatal effects 819
  pregnancy 817
zinc
  cadmium neutralizer 334
  maternal nutrition 334
  preconception care 153t
zona pellucida, differentiation 166
zygosity determination 840–841
  DNA testing 841
  physical features 841
  placentation 840–841
zygote
  division 165, 165f
  fertilization 165–166, 165f